Medical Toxicology

A SYNOPSIS AND STUDY GUIDE

Medical Toxicology

A SYNOPSIS AND STUDY GUIDE

Seth Schonwald, MD, FACEP, ACMT

DIRECTOR OF TOXICOLOGY
DEPARTMENT OF EMERGENCY MEDICINE
DEACONESS-NASHOBA HOSPITAL
AYER, MASSACHUSETTS

Based on the Works of
Matthew J. Ellenhorn, MD

LIPPINCOTT WILLIAMS & WILKINS
A **Wolters Kluwer** Company
Philadelphia • Baltimore • New York • London
Buenos Aires • Hong Kong • Sydney • Tokyo

Acquisitions Editor: Anne M. Sydor
Developmental Editor: Jenny Kim
Production Editor: Toni Ann Scaramuzzo
Manufacturing Manager: Colin Warnock
Cover Designer: QT Design
Compositor: Techbooks Inc.
Printer: R. R. Donnelley-Willard, Ohio

530 Walnut Street
Philadelphia, PA 19106 USA
LWW.com

Printed in the USA

Library of Congress Cataloging-in-Publication Data

Schonwald, Seth.
Medical toxicology : a synopsis and study guide / Seth Schonwald.
p. ; cm.
Includes bibliographical references and index.
ISBN 0-7817-2613-1
1. Toxicology—Examinations, questions, etc. 2. Toxicology—Outlines, syllabi, etc. I. Title.
[DNLM: 1. Poisoning—Examination Questions. 2. Poisoning—Handbooks. 3. Emergencies—Examination Questions. 4. Emergencies—Handbooks. 5. Poisons—toxicity—Examination Questions. 6. Poisons—toxicity—Handbooks. 7. Toxicology—methods—Examination Questions. 8. Toxicology—methods—Handbooks. QV 607 S371m 2001]
RA1216 .S347 2001
615.9′0076—dc21

00-052018

---

10 9 8 7 6 5 4 3 2 1

For my father . . .

Contents

PART IV
Chemical Products

PART V
Natural Toxins

Preface

My foremost goals in this project have been to organize, clarify, summarize, edit, and update *Ellenhorn's Medical Toxicology: Diagnosis and Treatment of Human Poisoning, Second Edition.* I have included material from the first edition to better define or clarify the text. Since the publication of *Ellenhorn's Medical Toxicology, Second Edition,* numerous new pharmaceutical and industrial products have been introduced, and numerous important contributions to the field of medical toxicology have been made. Many of these agents and observations have been incorporated into this synopsis. Some products mentioned in this work have been discontinued in the United States or are rarely involved in current reviews of poisoning. I have included some for their historical importance, some for their ongoing worldwide availability, and some for their illustrative profiles. In general, I have eliminated products only available outside the United States. I have maintained a clinical focus throughout the book and have eliminated references to animal research unless conventional thought emphasizes relevant extrapolation to human presentations.

Controversies in toxicology exist. While general approaches to management and identification of toxic presentations are identified in this book, many disagreements persist. I have listed selected readings at the conclusion of each chapter of this synopsis, and identified where controversies remain. Hundreds of additional references and supporting literature are also available in the first and second editions of *Ellenhorn's Medical Toxicology.*

Some generic products are produced by more than one company, and are known by more than one trade name. Trade names mentioned in the text, in no way indicate a preference or incentive of any sort. I have listed them in certain contexts so that readers may better identify a variety of agents quickly. I hope that the trade names I have mentioned will be familiar to the interested reader.

I have included hundreds of questions in this synopsis. They are meant as study aids, and to emphasize highlights of the sections to which they are appended. Depending on one's level of toxicologic sophistication, some individuals may consider them too easy, too hard, too broad, or too limited. They are meant as a cross-section of medical toxicology and will hopefully be helpful to students and practitioners in the field.

Thoughts, corrections, and comments are appreciated.

Seth Schonwald, MD, FACEP, ACMT

Acknowledgments

I initially met Dr. Matthew Ellenhorn in Los Angeles in 1989 during my years as an Emergency Medicine resident at UCLA. In 1990, in Tucson, Arizona, I humbly thanked him for guiding me through my boards in toxicology and a long friendship began.

Dr. Ellenhorn died on February 2, 1996. During my exegesis and summary of his works, *Medical Toxicology: Diagnosis and Treatment of Human Poisoning*, the first (co-authored with Dr. Donald Barceloux) and second Editions, I have realized more and more how important his contribution to the field of toxicology has been. Through this work, I have come to appreciate how much the toxicology world misses him. My heartfelt thanks go to Dr. Ellenhorn, and to Mrs. Syma Ellenhorn for her unwavering support and encouragement during this project.

I would like to thank those teachers who introduced me to, and nurtured my interests in Medicine and Toxicology during my training and tenure as an Internal Medicine and Emergency Medicine physician. These include Jerome Hoffman, MD at UCLA in Los Angeles, Charles Hatem, MD, John Patrick, MD and Gary Setnik, MD at Mount Auburn Hospital in Cambridge, Massachusetts, and Alan Woolf, MD and Michael Shannon, MD at the Massachusetts Poison Control System in Boston.

I would also like to express my sincere thanks and tremendous appreciation to those colleagues who contributed thoughts, questions and encouragement to this project. These include Steven Balser, MD, George Bosse, MD, David Huckins, MD, Chris Keyes, MD, Ira Leviton, MD, Michael Leviton, MD, Richard Levy, MD, Blake L. Powell, MD, JD, Harry Stanger, MD, George Stedman, MD, Ann Marie Testarmata, MD and Jonathan Weinstock, MD. My special thanks to Alison Deutsch, MD who contributed a great deal of support and questions throughout this work. Additional thanks to Dina Kacandes, PT, Jennifer Schonwald, MS and Liesa Lessard, MEd for their typing assistance and organization.

Medical Toxicology

A SYNOPSIS AND STUDY GUIDE

PART I

Principles of Medical Toxicology

CHAPTER 1

Introduction to Medical Toxicology

GENERAL EPIDEMIOLOGY

It has been estimated that there are 4–5 million cases of poisoning per year in the United States. About 2.3 million of these were reported to the American Association of Poison Control Centers (AAPCC) Toxic Exposure Surveillance System (TESS) by 66 poison centers in 1997. Most of these (86.2%) were unintentional, and the vast majority (74.9%) was managed in a non-health care facility (usually in the patient's home). Of those cases managed in a health care facility, 58% were treated without admission.

Many cases of recognized poisoning go unreported, and many cases of poisoning are never reported. Occupational and medical examiner data are often unreported. Much of the accumulated knowledge of medical toxicology is based on case reports involving single overdoses, chronic overexposures, epidemiologic studies, and animal experiments. Case reports demonstrate a temporal but not necessarily a causative relationship between exposure and health effects. This information is often confounded by the inability to exclude other causes of illness.

Over time, approaches to poison management change and experience with toxins, and groups of toxins, changes. In 1983, ipecac was administered in 13.4% of recorded poisoning exposures, and activated charcoal was used in 4%. By 1997, use of ipecac declined to 1.5% and activated charcoal use increased to 7.1%. The four most frequent substances used in poisonings reported to the AAPCC in 1997 were cleaning substances (10.4%), analgesics (10.3%), cosmetics and personal care products (9.0%), and plants (5.6%). In children under 6 years old, the substances most frequently involved are cosmetics and personal care products (12.7%), followed by cleaning substances (11.2%).

The average child presents to a health care facility about 1.5 hours after exposure. The average adult presents to a health care facility about 3.5 hours after exposure. Ingestion accounts for about 74.0% of exposure routes, followed in frequency by dermal exposure, inhalation, ocular exposure, bites and stings, parenteral exposure, and aspiration exposure. The overwhelming majority of human exposures are acute.

Questions—Introduction to General Epidemiology

1. **It has been estimated that there are ____ cases of poisoning per year in the U.S.**
   A. 100,000
   B. 1 million
   C. 2.3 million
   D. 4–5 million
   E. More than 10 million

2. **Of poisonings reported to the American Association of Poison Control Centers (AAPCC) Toxic Exposure Surveillance System (TESS) in 1997**
   A. Most were unintentional
   B. Most were managed in a non-health care facility
   C. Most cases managed in a health care facility were treated and released without admission
   D. All of the above
   E. A and B

3. **Many cases of recognized poisoning go unreported or are never reported**
   A. True
   B. False

FATALITIES

In 1997, 786 deaths (0.036% of reported cases) were reported to the AAPCC. Four hundred eighteen (53.2%) of these were suicides. The categories with the largest number of deaths changed between 1988 and 1997. In 1988, the most frequent cause of drug deaths was antidepressants, followed by analgesics, stimulants and street drugs, and sedative/hypnotics/antipsychotics. By 1997, analgesics led the list, followed by antidepressants, sedative/hypnotics/antipsychotics, and stimulants and street drugs.

Children less than 17 years of age account for most poisoning exposures, but account for only about 10% of fatalities. Fatalities in children under the age of 6 are uncommon, representing about 3.2% of fatalities. Common toxins lethal to children include gases, fumes and vapors such as carbon monoxide, toxic alcohols, analgesics, iron, antidepressants, cleaning substances and cardiovascular toxins. In adults, carbon monoxide also leads the list, followed by antidepressants, drugs of abuse, cardiovascular toxins, and analgesics.

In children, poisoning is usually accidental and is generally associated with low morbidity and mortality. In adults, self-poisoning is more common and is associated with a higher morbidity and mortality rate. Data suggest that a few drugs (e.g., camphor, chloroquine, tricyclic antidepressants, phenothiazines, quinine, methyl salicylate, and theophylline) are fatal to toddlers 2 years of age or younger after ingestion of one commercially available dose unit.

Factors that tend to increase the lethality of an overdose include greater age (over 60 years), suicidal intent, previous attempts, psychosocial stress factors such as a recent loss, chronic or serious illnesses, drug abuse, organic or drug-induced psychosis, depression or sense of helplessness, and lack of a supportive family system.

Questions—Fatalities

1. **The number of deaths from poisoning in 1997 reported to the AAPCC was**
   A. Less than 100
   B. Less than 1000
   C. 6,000
   D. 10,000
   E. 15,000

2. **Most reported deaths from poisoning are suicide attempts.**
   A. True
   B. False

3. **In the U.S., the category with the largest number of deaths in 1997 was**
   A. Stimulants and street drugs
   B. Sedative/hypnotics/antipsychotics

Answers to questions in shaded boxes appear at the end of the chapter.

C. Alcohol
D. Antidepressants
E. Analgesics

4. A few drugs may be fatal to toddlers 2 years of age or younger after ingestion of one commercially available dose unit. These include all of the following, except
A. Camphor
B. Chloroquine
C. Acetaminophen
D. Methyl salicylate
E. Quinine

PEDIATRIC POISONING

The American Association of Poison Control Centers (AAPCC) Data Collection System collects data and reports on pediatric poisoning exposures. In 1988, infants younger than 12 months accounted for 15% of all cases of poisoning less than 6 years of age reported to the AAPCC. Poisoning peaked at 10 months and between 2 and 4 years. Most cases (80%) occurred in the home; 61% occurred in the kitchen, 24% in the bedroom, 10% in the living room, and 8% in the bathroom. In 1977, 52.5% of all poison exposure cases reported to the AAPCC occurred in children younger than 6 years of age.

Limitations of the AAPCC data include (1) underreporting of chronic pediatric poisonings; (2) important poisonings requiring hospitalization in which clinicians feel they are competent and do not require the assistance of a poison center; (3) deaths occurring in the community in which a poison center is not notified; and (4) applicability of a national data set to local policy levels.

A major portion (30%) of pediatric ingestions reported to poison centers in the United States involve children with a history of at least one prior poisoning episode. Children tend to repeat with the same type of substance. The mother is the caretaker in 70% of these cases. The caretaker (43%) often placed the infant near the substance. The infant was usually playing alone (66%) and the substance was within easy reach (78% on the floor or edge of tub or changing table).

Childhood poisoning from prescription drugs has dropped since a federal regulation requiring child-resistant packaging was passed in 1974. Still, the Consumer Products Safety Commission has found that many drugs involved in childhood poisoning are in no container at all, and are found loose. Almost one-third of all medicines that were in a prescription container at the time of the accident was not in child-resistant packaging.

Woolf and Lovejoy, at Children's Hospital in Boston, have suggested that impaired impulse suppression, hyperactivity, inability to discriminate safe from unsafe activities, living in a hazardous environment, and inadequate parental vigilance are all possible behavioral and developmental determinants of childhood overdose. Family stress also creates supervisory lapses conducive to childhood poisoning.

Questions—Pediatric Poisoning

1. Most cases of pediatric poisoning occur
A. At the mall
B. At a grandparent's home
C. In the home
D. In the presence of a baby-sitter
E. In a bathroom

MEDICATION ERRORS AND ADVERSE REACTIONS

There are inherent risks, both known and unknown, associated with the therapeutic use of prescription and nonprescription drugs and with other pharmaceutical agents. The incidents or hazards that result from such risks have been defined as drug misadventures and include adverse drug events (ADEs) and medication errors. Despite increasing awareness of these problems, and the institution of incident reporting systems to detect adverse drug events, ADEs continue to appear.

Medication errors in and out of the hospital may result in unintentional poisoning. Such errors may be committed by experienced and inexperienced staff, including nurses, pharmacists, physicians, and supportive personnel including technicians, students, clerical staff, administrators, pharmaceutical manufacturers, patients and their caregivers.

Medication errors may follow inappropriate prescribing, patient noncompliance, dispensing errors, and medication administration problems. Errors resulting in preventable ADEs may also include ordering errors, transcription errors, drug interactions, and dispensing errors. Many of these errors, such as those arising during the prescribing phase, may yield potentially "severe" or "serious" outcomes.

Some look-alike or sound-alike medication pairs have been implicated in a number of ADEs. Many adult and elderly patients are potential poisoning victims because of their inability to read and comprehend label instructions. Many errors result from "misplacing" the decimal point on prescriptions or medication orders. In one nursing study, 25% of potential ADEs were attributed to an error that would have resulted in an administration of an amount that was 10 times higher or lower than the dose ordered. Numerous institutional solutions to these problems have been proposed.

Questions—Medication Errors and Adverse Reactions

1. Medication errors may follow
A. Inappropriate prescribing
B. Patient noncompliance
C. Transcription errors
D. Decimal point errors
E. All of the above

POISON CENTERS

Since 1978, the American Association of Poison Control Centers (AAPCC) has maintained standards for staffing, staff qualifications, data resources, and service provisions required to achieve designation as an AAPCC Regional Poison Control Center. Regional centers surpass non-regional centers in population served, call volume, call volume per capita, center staffing, medical direction, and follow-up protocols.

In 1997, 66 poison centers reported exposure data to the AAPCC. It has been estimated that 250.1 million Americans are served by participating centers in 41 entire states, portions of 4 states and the District of Columbia. Poison center peak call volumes are noted between 4 p.m. and 10 p.m.

The AAPCC Data Collection System collects data regarding all reported poisoning exposures. Periodically, these data are published and distributed. Data collected include route of exposure, intent (accidental or intentional), demographic information such as age and sex, specific poisons involved, quantity, outcomes, and circumstances surrounding exposures. Various poisoning severity scores have also been devised.

Questions—Poison Control Centers

1. **In 1997, ____ poison centers reported exposure data to the AAPCC**
   A. 16
   B. 66
   C. 206
   D. 506
   E. 806
2. **Most calls to poison centers occur**
   A. Between 8 a.m. and noon
   B. Between 10 p.m. and 2 a.m.
   C. At lunch, between 11 a.m. and 2 p.m.
   D. Between 4 p.m. and 10 p.m.
   E. Between 4 a.m. and 10 a.m.

IDENTIFICATION OF TOXIC SYNDROMES

Various drugs and toxins are associated with syndromes, or constellations of symptoms, which result from specific pharmacologic principles. Drugs may interact with certain receptors or neurotransmitters (e.g., by promoting their release or blocking their reuptake), and lead to stimulation (i.e., sympathomimetic, or parasympathomimetic action) or inhibition (i.e., sympatholytic, or parasympatholytic action) of nerves and their actions.

In addition to the following "Toxidromes," numerous other constellations have been identified. A "serotonin syndrome" is now recognized, as well as a "narcotic syndrome," a "hallucinogenic syndrome" and a "solvent syndrome." Please see specific chapters for better elucidation of these other "toxidromes."

Cholinergic Toxidrome

Acetylcholine is the ubiquitous neurotransmitter responsible for the parasympathetic nervous system. Sites of innervation include the peripheral nervous system at the somatic neuromuscular junction, autonomic ganglia, the adrenal medulla, the central nervous system (brain and spinal cord), and postganglionic parasympathetic fibers. Cholinergic receptors are divided into muscarinic and nicotinic receptors.

Muscarinic receptors are present in postganglionic parasympathetic fibers, at autonomic ganglia, and at cortical and subcortical neurons. Muscarine-like drugs, therefore, affect both peripheral and central nervous systems. Muscarinic symptoms include miosis, vasodilation, bradycardia, depressed myocardial contractility, depressed myocardial conduction, bronchorrhea, increased gut motility, micturition, and sweating. The mnemonic "DUMBBELS" describes the peripheral effects of muscarinic poisoning: **D**iarrhea, **U**rination, **M**iosis, **B**radycardia, **B**ronchorrhea, **E**mesis, **L**acrimation, **S**weating.

Activation of cholinergic agonists initially stimulates autonomic ganglia and neuromuscular junctions and then, in high doses, produces blockade. Nicotinic actions primarily affect the neuromuscular junction and may produce fasciculations, weakness, and paralysis. D-Tubocurarine blocks both the nicotinic effects in the neuromuscular junction and the muscarinic effects on the autonomic ganglia. Drug examples include organophosphates, carbamates, and pilocarpine. Atropine inhibits muscarinic effects.

Anticholinergic Toxidrome

Parasympatholytic agents such as atropine, and the belladonna alkaloids, block cholinergic effects. In general, clinical presentations resemble sympathomimetic actions (e.g., elevated blood pressure and temperature, erythema, delirium, and mydriasis) except that parasympatholytic agents produce silent bowel sounds and dry skin. A popular mnemonic for anticholinergic overdose is as follows: Hot as Hades, Blind as a bat, Red as a beet, Dry as a bone, Mad as a hatter. Drug examples include antihistamines, jimsonweed, benztropine, tricyclic antidepressants, baclofen, and the phenothiazines. Physostigmine inhibits anticholinergic effects.

Sympathomimetic Toxidrome

Catecholamines are the neurotransmitters of the sympathetic nervous system. These neurotransmitters include epinephrine (certain central nervous system neurons and the adrenal medulla), dopamine (extrapyramidal tracts of the thalamus), and norepinephrine (peripheral sympathetic fibers that innervate the skin, eyes, heart, lungs, gastrointestinal tract, and exocrine glands). Adrenergic receptors are divided into alpha and beta types, depending on their response to catecholamines and adrenoreceptor blocking agents.

Beta-adrenoreceptors are sub-classified as beta-1 (primarily responsible for cardiovascular effects) and beta-2 (responsible for smooth muscle dilation, insulin release, lipolysis, and gluconeogenesis). Most beta-adrenergic drugs have both properties in varying degrees.

Alpha-adrenoreceptors are excitatory in the eye, gastrointestinal tract, and vascular smooth muscle. Although classification is incomplete, alpha receptors are sub-classified as alpha-1 (these receptors are primarily postjunctional and initiate postsynaptic excitatory smooth muscle and exocrine gland events) and alpha-2 (these receptors are primarily presynaptic inhibitors that mediate negative feedback of norepinephrine release and oppose alpha-1 stimulation).

Most synthetic sympathomimetics bear structural resemblance to natural catecholamines. Signs of sympathomimetic syndrome include restlessness, euphoria, mydriasis, hypertension, tachycardia, hyperpyrexia, diaphoresis, increased motor activity, tremor and insomnia. Drug examples include amphetamines, caffeine, ephedrine, cocaine, PCP and methylphenidate. Benzodiazepines inhibit many of these effects.

Questions—Identification of Toxic Syndromes

1. **Signs of cholinergic poisoning include all of the following except**
   A. Urinary incontinence
   B. Mydriasis
   C. Bradycardia
   D. Diaphoresis
   E. Vomiting
2. **Signs of anticholinergic poisoning include all of the following except**
   A. Dry skin
   B. Ileus
   C. Delirium
   D. Hypertension
   E. Hypothermia

3. In general, anticholinergic presentations resemble sympathomimetic actions except that parasympatholytic agents produce silent bowel sounds and dry skin.
A. True
B. False

4. Signs of sympathomimetic syndrome include
A. Restlessness
B. Euphoria
C. Mydriasis
D. All of the above
E. A and B

CLINICAL SIGNS OF SPECIFIC TOXINS

Numerous signs and symptoms have been associated with various drugs, chemicals, toxins, or classes of drugs. The following list represents some of these commonly encountered signs and symptoms, and some of the agents and conditions associated with them. This list is by no means complete, nor is the potential spectrum of clinical effects from drugs completely represented here.

Acute Renal Failure

Numerous nephrotoxins may cause acute renal failure. These include boric acid, cadmium, carbon tetrachloride, chromium, diethylene glycol, dichloropropane, diesel fuel, dioxane, dynamite, ethylene dibromide, gasoline, methylchloride gas, bromide gas, methylene chloride, phenol, polyethylene glycol, iodine, tetrachloroethylene, toluene and trichloroethylene.

Acute Respiratory Distress Syndrome (ARDS)

See Noncardiogenic Pulmonary Edema.

Acute Tubular Necrosis

Associated indirect precipitants include arsine gas, aniline, chlorate, copper, cresol, naphthalene, bromates, propylene glycol, fava beans (hemoglobin deposition), carbon monoxide, PCP, amphetamines, copper, lindane, mercuric chloride, zinc phosphide, and licorice (myoglobin deposition). Numerous direct nephrotoxins include arsenic, barium chloride, carbon tetrachloride, chlordane, chloroform, 2,4-D, chromium, diquat, paraquat, ethylene dichloride, ethylene dibromide, mercury salts, methylene chloride, thallium, tetrachloroethylene, turpentine, Djenkol beans, colchicine, amanita phalloides and Cortinarius mushrooms, and yellow phosphorous. See Nephrotoxins.

Aggression

Drugs that may induce or aggravate aggression include alcohol, amitriptyline, amphetamines, barbiturates, benzodiazepines, hallucinogens, opiates, phencyclidine, and propranolol. Violence is behavior characterized by an aggressive assault or combativeness. It may be precipitated by a mental disease, situational frustration, or organic disease. Drugs inducing violent reactions include ethanol (intoxication, intolerance, and withdrawal), amphetamines, anticholinergics, aromatic hydrocarbons, cocaine, corticosteroids, LSD (lysergic acid diethylamide), phencyclidine, and sedative-hypnotics (intoxication or withdrawal). Factors contributing to violent behavior may include anemia, dementia, electrolytic abnormalities, endocrinopathies, head trauma, hypoglycemia, hypoxia, postictal states, and vitamin deficiencies. See Psychosis, Mania.

Agranulocytosis

Agranulocytosis has followed exposure to analgesic antiinflammatory drugs, antiarrhythmics, anticonvulsants, antidepressants, antihypertensive agents, antimicrobial agents, antipsychotic drugs, antithyroid drugs, diuretics, and numerous other drugs. Certain drugs such as chloramphenicol may be associated with aplastic anemia. Drugs, foods and vitamins may cause abnormal platelet function.

Akathisias

Cyclic antidepressants, monoamine oxidase inhibitors, fluoxetine, lithium, buspirone, and levodopa are the principal causes of akathisias.

Alopecia

Anticoagulants, retinol and its derivatives, interferons, and antihyperlipidemic drugs can cause hair loss. Such loss is usually reversible on the interruption of treatment.

Anaphylaxis

Numerous agents have been responsible for acute anaphylactic reactions. These include insect and snake venoms, antibiotics such as the penicillins, cephalosporins and sulfonamides, anesthetics such as lidocaine, preservatives such as metabisulfites and benzoates, foods such as peanuts, milk, eggs and seafood, as well as steroids, ethylene oxide, pollens, latex, radiocontrast media, opiates, aspirin, and numerous other agents.

Anemia

Reduced hemoglobin levels result from drugs that cause upper gastrointestinal tract bleeding (e.g., heavy metals such as iron, alcohols, anticoagulants, phenylbutazone, indomethacin, nonsteroidal antiinflammatory drugs, hydralazine, adrenocortical steroids, and reserpine) as well as drugs that produce hemolysis or hepatic failure. See Hemolytic Anemia.

Anion Gap Acidosis

Causes of a high anion gap acidosis include metabolic acidosis, dehydration, infusions of salts of organic acids (e.g., lactate, acetate, citrate), reduced unmeasured cations (e.g., potassium, calcium, magnesium), alkalemia, lab error, and underestimation of serum chloride. A suggested mnemonic for the causes of an anion gap acidosis is "I Love Chocolate Raspberry Truffle MUDPIES." (**I**ron, isoniazid, ibuprofen, **L**ithium, lactate, **C**arbon monoxide, cyanide, caffeine, **R**espiratory dysfunction, **T**oluene, **M**ethanol, **U**remia, **D**iabetic ketoacidosis (DKA), **P**araldehyde, phenformin, **I**ron, INH, idiopathic, **E**thylene glycol, ethanol, **S**alicylates, strychnine, seizures, hydrogen sulfide, starvation, and sympathomimetics).

ARDS (Acute Respiratory Distress Syndrome)

See Noncardiogenic Pulmonary Edema.

Arrhythmias

Arrhythmias may occur in conjunction with antiarrhythmic drugs, as well as tricyclic antidepressants, phenothiazines, sedative-hypnotics such as chloral hydrate, stimulants, halogenated hydrocarbons, phosphorus, carbon monoxide, scorpion and spider stings. Other precipitants include theophylline, beta-blockers, digoxin, organophosphates, carbamates, antimony, lithium, arsine and arsenic. See Torsade de Pointes and Complete Heart Block.

Asthma

Nonsteroidal antiinflammatory drugs account for more than two- thirds of drug-induced asthmatic reactions, with aspirin accounting for more than half of these. Beta-blockers, cholinergic agonists, chemotherapeutic agents, antibiotics, radiographic contrast agents, muscle relaxants, and intravenous anesthetic agents have also caused bronchospasm associated with systemic reactions. See Chapter 45, Airborne Toxins.

Atherosclerosis

Atherosclerosis is definitely caused by carbon disulfide and possibly by carbon monoxide, combustion products and arsenic.

Benign Intracranial Hypertension

Drugs most often associated with pseudotumor cerebri (benign intracranial hypertension) include tetracycline, minocycline, nifedipine, nalidixic acid, vitamin A and retinoid analogs, cotrimoxazole, cimetidine, atenolol, and glyceryl trinitrate.

Bezoars

See Concretions.

Bradycardia

Cholinergics, digitalis, clonidine, ethchlorvynol, narcotics, calcium channel blockers, beta-blockers, and other anti-arrhythmic drugs may cause bradycardia.

Bronchiolitis Obliterans

Bronchiolitis obliterans has been associated with ammonia, chlorine, nitrogen dioxide, ozone, phosgene, sulfur dioxide, and beryllium.

Bronchitis

Ammonia, chlorine, ozone, sulfur, mercury, osmium tetroxide, nitrogen dioxide, carbon disulfide, formaldehyde, hydrogen chloride, cadmium, vanadium pentoxide, acrolein, hydrogen fluoride, chromates, acetaldehyde, and formic acid may produce acute tracheobronchitis characterized by cough, sore throat, chest pain, and lightheadedness. See Chapter 45, Airborne Toxins.

Bullae

Bullous lesions may suggest barbiturates, carbon monoxide, sedative hypnotics, narcotics, and prolonged coma. See Pemphigus below.

Cerebrovascular Accident (CVA)

See Stroke.

Cholestasis

Indirect hepatotoxins cause hepatic damage by interfering with essential metabolic pathways, which leads to cytotoxic (necrosis or steatosis) and/or cholestatic (biliary stasis) injury patterns. Agents associated with cholestasis include icterogenin (Lippia rhemani alkaloid), anabolic and contraceptive steroids, novobiocin, rifamycin, gallbladder dyes, methylenediamine (Epping jaundice), and paraquat. See Hepatotoxins and Hepatic Necrosis.

Chorea

Chorea is commonly associated with the anticonvulsant drugs, especially phenytoin. Chorea has also been observed with anabolic steroids, amphetamines, methylphenidate, pemoline, cimetidine, levodopa and dopamine, as well as ethanol, toluene, manganese, and cocaine. See Tremor.

Coagulopathy

Prolonged prothrombin times can occur with substances that cause hepatotoxicity (e.g., acetaminophen, carbon tetrachloride, and Amanita phalloides toxin), and anticoagulant agents (e.g., coumarin and difenacoum). See Disseminated Intravascular Coagulation.

Cognitive Impairment

Impairment of consciousness is associated with the use of amphetamines, barbiturates, benzodiazepines, insulin, opiates, alcohols, phenothiazines, tricyclic antidepressants, and numerous other agents. All agents capable of producing psychosis (see Psychosis), coma (see Coma), and/or seizures (see Seizures) may also impair consciousness. Conditions predisposing to drug-induced cognitive impairment include age, brain disease, and addiction to alcohol and/or other drugs. The elderly are at particular risk because of multiple diseases, multiple drug use, and age-associated alterations in metabolism. See Dementia.

Colonic Effects

Colonic ischemia is associated with cocaine, ergotamine, estrogen, amphetamines, digitalis, methysergide and vasopressin. Colonic pseudoobstruction is associated with narcotics, phenothiazines, vincristine, atropine, anticholinergics, tricyclic antidepressants and ganglionic blocking agents. Infectious or necrotizing enterocolitis is associated with antibiotics and pseudomembranous colitis. Allergic colitis has been associated with gold, NSAIDs, methyldopa, flucytosine, methotrexate, salicylates and sulfa drugs.

Coma

The presence of coma is a nonspecific sign. The occurrence of coma necessitates a careful physical examination to distinguish between structural and toxic-metabolic causes. Rapid onset of coma due to toxic causes includes cyanide, hydrogen sulfide, carbon monoxide, nicotinic acid, rapidly acting narcotics, or barbiturates. Alternating levels of consciousness suggest phencyclidine (PCP) or glutethimide. Central nervous system depression occurs with aliphatic alcohols (ethanol, isopropanol, methanol), anxiolytic drugs (sedative-hypnotics, benzodiazepines), anticholinergic drugs, anticonvulsants (phenytoin, valproic acid), antidepressants (monoamine oxidase inhibitors, cyclic antidepressants), antihistamines, barbiturates, bromides, opiates, and tranquilizers. Hypoglycemic agents, envenomations, drugs that cause seizures, and drugs that cause acidosis must also be considered.

Complete Heart Block

Class I antiarrhythmic agents (procainamide, quinidine), calcium channel blockers, beta-blockers, digitalis, organophosphates, cocaine, clonidine, phenytoin, neuroleptic agents, and cyclic antidepressants may cause complete heart block. See Arrhythmias.

Concretions

Concretions represent medications that form a gastric mass. Medications reported to cause bezoars or concretions include aluminum hydroxide, aspirin, bromide, calcium phosphate, carbamazepine, cholestyramine, cyanocobalamin (vitamin B12), iron, meprobamate, nifedipine, sodium polystyrene sulfonate, sucralfate, theophylline (sustained-release), and vitamin C. Of these, aluminum hydroxide, aspirins (coated / buffered), calcium combinations, cyanocobalamin (vitamin B12), iron, sucralfate and some vitamins have been reported to be radiopaque. Those reported not to be radiopaque include meprobamate, nifedipine, theophylline in all its forms, bromide, cholestyramine and sodium polystyrene sulfonate.

Contact Dermatitis

Numerous agents have been associated with contact dermatitis. These include germicides such as formaldehyde and parabens, foods such as grains and spices, metals such as chromium, cobalt and nickel, organic dyes, plastic resins, rubber products, fragrances, perfumes and the classic rhus plants (poison ivy, oak and sumac).

Crystalluria

Crystalluria may follow poisoning with sulfonamides, carbon tetrachloride, primidone, and ampicillin. Crystalluria is commonly associated with the ingestion of oxalates or ethylene glycol.

Cyanosis

Cyanosis indicates hypoxia, methemoglobinemia (the characteristic chocolate-brown color of the methemoglobin pigment produces cyanosis out of proportion to observed clinical response), or ergotamine ingestion. See Methemoglobinemia.

Deafness

See Ototoxicity.

Delirium

See Dementia.

Dementia

Numerous drugs and chemicals have been associated with dementia (chronic cognitive deficits) and delirium (temporary cognitive deficits). Among others, these include major tranquilizers, antidepressants, sedative hypnotics, narcotics, anticholinergic agents, antihypertensive agents, anticonvulsants, digoxin, antiparkinsonian agents such as levodopa, amantadine, and bromocriptine, high-dose penicillin or chloramphenicol, gastrointestinal agents such as cimetidine, antineoplastic agents, lead, arsenic, solvents and insecticides. See Cognitive Impairment.

Dental Discoloration

Agents known to effect tooth color include fluorides, tetracycline, chlorhexidine, and liquid iron preparations.

Depression

Among the numerous drugs that cause depression include beta-blockers, corticosteroids, fenfluramine, interferon, levodopa, methyldopa, methylphenidate, oral contraceptives, pemoline, and phenylpropanolamine. Additional anecdotes suggest an association with benzodiazepines, cimetidine, diltiazem, metoclopramide, nifedipine, ranitidine, and verapamil.

Diaphoresis

Diaphoresis and increased salivation occur with organophosphates, cholinergics, mercury, sympathomimetics, salicylates, and arsenic.

Disseminated Intravascular Coagulation (DIC)

Disseminated intravascular coagulation can result from shock, rattlesnake bite, phencyclidine, monoamine oxidase inhibitors, mushroom poisoning, and iron.

Dry Mouth

See Xerostomia.

Dyspnea

Dyspnea may result from pulmonary parenchymal damage (caused by respiratory irritants), bronchospasm (caused by isocyanates or asthma), physical asphyxiants (carbon monoxide, cyanide, acrylonitrile, hydrogen sulfide), or methemoglobinemia (caused by aniline, nitrites, dapsone, nitrobenzene, sodium chlorates). See Chapter 45, Airborne Toxins.

Dystonic Reactions

Dystonias are associated principally with phenothiazines, butyrophenones, metoclopramide, and tricyclic antidepressants. They may be associated with phenytoin, carbamazepine, and propranolol in high doses, and with antiemetics, cocaine, chloroquine, phencyclidine, mercury, lead, arsenic, lithium, and hydroxychloroquine. See Tremor.

Erythema

Diffuse erythema is frequently seen with anticholinergic poisoning and rarely with carbon monoxide and cyanide. Erythema may also be associated with rifampin, niacin, vancomycin, and borates.

Erythema Multiforme

Erythema multiforme has been associated with penicillins, tetracyclines, clindamycin, sulfonamides, and certain anticonvulsants.

Esophageal Injury

Pill-induced esophageal injury may follow use of tetracycline, doxycycline, ipratropium bromide, slow-release potassium chloride, acetylsalicylic acid, nonsteroidal antiinflammatory drugs, and quinidine. Symptoms of sudden onset of dysphagia, often accompanied by substernal chest pain and odynophagia, typically occur 4 to 12 hours after ingestion.

Fasciculations

Fasciculations may be associated with organophosphates, nicotine, lithium, and glyceryl trinitrate.

Gastrointestinal Obstruction

Numerous agents may be associated with drug-induced gastrointestinal obstruction. Agents, which may cause obstruction in a lumen without a predisposing lesion, include barium sulfate, cholestyramine, potassium supplements, bulk laxatives, and aluminum hydroxide.

Gingival Hyperplasia

Agents known to induce gingival hyperplasia include phenytoin, sodium valproate, phenobarbital, cyclosporine, nifedipine, diltiazem, and verapamil.

Glossitis

See Tongue Effects.

Headache

Numerous agents have been associated with headache during drug use. These include amyl nitrate, atenolol, captopril, cimetidine, cocaine, diclofenac, dipyridamole, griseofulvin, indomethacin, isosorbide dinitrate, isotretinoin, metoprolol, nalidixic acid, nifedipine, nitroglycerin, piroxicam, ranitidine, and trimethoprim-sulfamethoxazole. Analgesics, caffeine, ergotamine, and methysergide have been associated with headaches during a withdrawal period.

Hemolytic Anemia

Hemolysis may accompany arsine, stibine and dichloroethane poisoning. It is also caused by direct erythrocyte binding (penicillin, cephalothin, streptomycin), binding to plasma protein (quinine, quinidine, sulfonylurea derivatives), and undetermined mechanisms (methyldopa, levodopa, mefenamic acid). Some drugs and chemicals can induce a hemolytic anemia in persons with glucose-6-phosphate dehydrogenase deficiency. These include doxorubicin, methylene blue, nalidixic acid, nitrofurantoin, primaquine and sulfamethoxazole.

Hemolytic Uremic Syndrome

Drugs that have been associated with a hemolytic uremic syndrome include cyclosporine, anticancer drugs (e.g., mitomycin), ticlopidine, and quinine.

Hemoptysis

Hemoptysis may follow exposure to irritant respiratory gases and anticoagulants.

Hepatic Necrosis

Direct hepatotoxins produce direct cellular injury characterized by necrosis and / or steatosis. Cytotoxic agents include aflatoxin, ochratoxin, cycasin, pyrrolizine alkaloids, Amanita phalloides, tannic acid, safrole, hypoglycin A, ethionine, puromycin, tetracycline, L-asparaginase, methotrexate, mithramycin, bromobenzene, 6-mercaptopurine, urethane, ethanol, vinyl chloride, galactosamine, dimethylnitrosamine and other nitrosamines. Other examples include carbon tetrachloride, chloroform, other chlorinated hydrocarbons, acetaminophen, iron, copper, paraquat, DDT, phosphorus, arsenic, thallium, and borates.

Hepatotoxins

Symptoms of hepatic disease include malaise, lethargy, nausea, vomiting, pruritus, right upper quadrant pain, and anorexia. Signs of hepatic disease include scleral icterus, hepatic enlargement and tenderness, dark urine, light-colored stools, and loose stools. Numerous classification schemes have been proposed to identify hepatotoxins. Intrinsic hepatotoxins are predictable and idiosyncratic hepatotoxins are unpredictable. At times, the pattern of necrosis (centrilobular, midzonal, peripheral) helps identify offending agents. Indirect hepatotoxins cause hepatic damage by interfering with essential metabolic pathways, which leads to cytotoxic (necrosis or steatosis) and / or cholestatic (biliary stasis) injury patterns. A variety of potential chemical and natural hepatotoxins found in natural or synthesized chemical products remain unclassified. See Hepatic Necrosis and Cholestasis.

Drug-induced hepatitis is characterized by (1) clinical and laboratory evidence of hepatocellular injury; (2) onset of symptoms related in time to drug therapy; (3) lack of serologic evidence for current infection with hepatitis A, B or C, cytomegalovirus, or Epstein-Barr virus; (4) absence of an acute hepatic insult such as septic shock; (5) lack of evidence of chronic liver disease; and (6) absence of other concomitantly administered drugs, especially any known hepatotoxins. The presence of fever, rash, eosinophilias, or lymphadenopathy is supportive but not essential.

Hirsutism

Hirsutism may follow the use of testosterone, danazol, corticotropin, metyrapone, anabolic steroids, and glucocorticoids. Hypertrichosis has been observed after use of cyclosporine, minoxidil, and diazoxide.

Hypercalcemia

Hypercalcemia may be induced by calcium-containing antacids, other exogenous forms of calcium (e.g., vitamin supplements), and vitamin D.

Hyperkalemia

Drug-induced hyperkalemia may follow inhibition of potassium entry into cells via inhibition of Na / K ATPase activity. This has been seen with digitalis, beta-2 adrenoceptor antagonists, and drugs that cause acidosis. Reduced potassium excretion is observed with potassium-sparing diuretics, angiotensin-converting enzyme inhibitors, nonsteroidal antiinflammatory drugs, and agents that impair renal tubular function. Hyperkalemia also follows renal Na channel blockade with amiloride. Hyperkalemia may be associated with abdominal pain, diarrhea, muscle pain, weakness, electrocardiographic changes (tall peaked T waves, ST-segment depression, prolonged PR interval, QRS prolongation), and cardiac arrhythmias (ventricular tachycardia, ventricular fibrillation).

Hypernatremia

Drug-induced hypernatremia follows excessive intake of sodium, salt emetics, enemas, and intravenous saline solutions. Drugs causing diabetes insipidus, including lithium, phenytoin, and alcohol, may also cause hypernatremia.

Hyperpnea

Hyperpnea is a nonspecific sign resulting from drugs that cause elevated temperature, hypoxia, or metabolic acidosis.

Hyperprolactinemia

Hyperprolactinemia may be associated with neuroleptic agents such as phenothiazines, thioxanthenes and butyrophenones, monoamine oxidase inhibitors, tricyclic antidepressants, reserpine, methyldopa, metoclopramide, amoxapine, verapamil, and cocaine.

Hypersensitivity

Virtually any drug may yield hypersensitivity in a susceptible subject. Certain agents, such as aromatic antiepileptic agents like phenytoin, carbamazepine, and phenobarbital, and sulfonamides are frequent causes of hypersensitivity reactions. Other drugs, especially allopurinol, gold salts, and dapsone, are also associated with a hypersensitivity syndrome. The syndrome typically develops 2 to 6 weeks after a drug is first used, later than most other serious skin reactions. With antiepileptic drugs, fever and rash are the most frequent presenting symptoms. Lymphadenopathy is frequent and usually due to benign lymphoid hyperplasia. Hepatitis, interstitial nephritis, and hematologic abnormalities, especially eosinophilia and atypical lymphocytosis, are also common.

Hypertension

Hypertension may be caused by sympathomimetics such as cocaine, amphetamines, and phenylpropanolamine, oxymetazoline, anticholinergics, phencyclidine, ergotamine, organophosphates, ethanol, scorpion venoms, and spider venoms. Other causes include glucocorticoids, mineralocorticoids (e.g., certain types of black licorice, carbenoxolone, fluoroprednisolone, fluorocortisol, ketoconazole), estrogen, progesterone, androgens, danazol, ketamine, fentanyl, and scopolamine.

Hyperthermia

Numerous mechanisms may be responsible for an elevated temperature after exposure to drugs or toxins. Complications from high temperatures include coagulopathy, rhabdomyolysis with secondary renal failure, electrolyte disturbances, cardiorespiratory depression, hepatic dysfunction, and convulsions. Certain drugs cause "drug fevers" that are difficult to distinguish from those of infectious etiology. Drug fevers usually begin 7–10 days after initial drug exposure, however reexposure can produce elevated temperatures within hours. Examples of common drugs that cause drug fever include antibiotics (penicillins, sulfa compounds, tetracycline, streptomycin), antiarrhythmics (procaine, quinidine), isoniazid, nonsteroidal anti-inflammatory drugs (ibuprofen, sulindac), phenytoin, allopurinol, and clofibrate.

Some drugs increase temperature by interfering with oxidative metabolism. Examples include salicylates, dinitrophenol, pentachlorophenol, thyroid hormones, and chlorophenoxy compounds like 2,4-D. Heat illness may be exacerbated by drugs which prevent or block sweating, a natural cooling mechanism. These include anticholinergic agents (antihistamines, tricyclic antidepressants, phenothiazines) and sympathomimetics (cocaine, ephedrine, amphetamines).

Malignant hyperthermia is a rare, autosomal dominant condition, associated with a variety of anesthetic agents such as halothane, and succinylcholine. Increased muscle rigidity may yield hyperpyrexia after strychnine, water hemlock, or phencyclidine use. Increased activity has been associated with a variety of agents that may also yield hyperpyrexia. Examples include amphetamines, lysergic acid diethylamide (LSD), cocaine, phencyclidine (PCP), mescaline, monoamine oxidase inhibitors, methaqualone, glutethimide, and tricyclic antidepressants. Also, see Neuroleptic Malignant Syndrome.

Hypocalcemia

Among other causes, drugs associated with hypocalcemia include citrate loads from blood products, and aggressive phosphate replacement. Hypocalcemia may be observed after poisoning with hydrogen fluoride, oxalates, ethylene glycol, and organic tin compounds and is often observed in critically ill patients in association with cardiovascular or neuromuscular insufficiency.

Hypoglycemia

Hypoglycemia may be induced by ethanol, isopropanol (inhibits gluconeogenesis), barbiturates, beta-blockers (inhibit glycogenolysis), oral hypoglycemics, insulin, ethacrynic acid, and salicylates. Agents which destroy beta islet cells include Vacor, streptozotocin, alloxan and pentamidine. Agents capable of producing hepatic necrosis may inhibit gluconeogenesis and indirectly cause hypoglycemia as well.

Hypokalemia

Drug-induced hypokalemia via increased Na/K ATPase activity and enhanced cellular potassium entry may occur with beta-2 agonists, theophylline, and insulin. Hypokalemia may also be induced by competitive blockade of potassium channels (chloroquine, barium), gastrointestinal losses, and drug-induced metabolic alkalosis. Hypokalemia can result in generalized muscle weakness, paralytic ileus, electrocardiogram changes (flat or inverted T waves, prominent U waves, ST-segment depression), and cardiac arrhythmias (atrial tachycardia heart block, atrioventricular dissociation, ventricular tachycardia, and/or ventricular fibrillation). Drugs that may cause a hypokalemic myopathy include the thiazide diuretics, amphotericin, carbenoxolone, emetine, and alcohol.

Hypomagnesemia

Decreased serum magnesium may be associated with cisplatin therapy, cyclosporine and diuretic use. Torsade de Pointes may be associated with hypomagnesemia. See Torsade de Pointes.

Hyponatremia

Drug-induced hyponatremia may follow excessive water intake and impaired water excretion by the kidney due to increased activity of antidiuretic hormone. Drugs associated with this phenomenon include carbamazepine, chlorpropamide, and nonsteroidal antiinflammatory drugs.

Hypophosphatemia

Decreased serum phosphate may be associated with aluminum-containing antacids, corticosteroids, high serum insulin, and aggressive calcium replacement.

Hypopigmentation

Agents associated with hypopigmentation include benzylchlorophenol, butylphenol, cresol, hydroquinone, phenylphenol, pyrocatechol, and tertiary butylcatechol.

Hypotension

Agents associated with decreased preload include heavy metals, colchicine, and food poisoning agents. Agents associated with decreased afterload include alpha-blockers and phenothiazines. Agents associated with decreased contractility include clonidine, barbiturates, sedative-hypnotics, narcotics and tricyclic antidepressants. Agents associated with dysrhythmias or conduction disturbances include fluorocarbons, solvents, phenol, fluoroacetate, dinitrophenol, arsenic, phosphorous, organophosphates, carbamates, lithium, carbon monoxide, cyanide, methemoglobin-formers, hydrogen sulfide, chloral hydrate, tricyclic antidepressants, phenothiazines, succinylcholine, cocaine, digitalis, beta-blockers, quinidine, quinine, chloroquine, theophylline, hydantoins and calcium channel blockers.

Hypothermia

Hypothermia is diagnosed as a core temperature below 35° C (95° F). In urban settings, ethanolism is the most common cause, followed by drugs of abuse and psychiatric disorders. Occult infections are frequent and are the most serious causes of hypothermia. Besides ethanol, substances involved in hypothermia include narcotics, sedative-hypnotics (especially barbiturates, chloral hydrate, and glutethimide), phenothiazines, tricyclic antidepressants, general anesthetics, carbon monoxide, and insulin. Other etiologies include acute intracranial lesions, gastrointestinal bleeding, diabetic ketoacidosis, and pancreatitis. The J or Osborne wave on the electrocardiogram is pathognomonic for hypothermia but may not be present in mild hypothermia (32–35° C).

Incontinence

Medications that have the potential to cause incontinence include sedatives such as benzodiazepine and alcohol. Diuretics such as furosemide may predispose to incontinence as well. Drugs with the potential to weaken bladder contraction include anticholinergics. Drugs which affect sympathetic nerves such as phenylpropanolamine, pseudoephedrine, and central sympathetic antagonists (Aldomet®, Catapres®, and Minipress®), may also predispose to incontinence.

Interstitial Fibrosis

Interstitial fibrosis has been associated with aluminum, asbestos, beryllium, coal dust, cobalt, copper, bleomycin, nitrofurantoin, mercury, paraquat, silica and talc.

Interstitial Nephritis

Nephrotoxins which cause interstitial nephritis, include mineral spirits, cadmium, fluoride (Vichy water), lead, and Worcestershire sauce.

Mania

Drug-induced mania may be associated with steroids, levodopa and other dopaminergic agents, iproniazid, sympathomimetic amines, triazolobenzodiazepines, and hallucinogens. See Psychosis.

Metabolic Acidosis

See Anion Gap Acidosis.

Methemoglobinemia

Some agents associated with methemoglobinemia include aniline dyes, arsine, benzocaine, bismuth subnitrate, chlorates, chlorobenzene, dapsone, dinitrobenzenes, dinitrophenol, dinitrotoluene, hydroquinone, lidocaine, menthol, methylene blue, naphthalene, nitrates, nitrites, nitrogen oxide, nitroglycerin, nitrophenol, phenacetin, phenols, phenazopyridine, primaquine, quinones, sulfonamides, toluenediamine, toluidine and trinitrotoluene.

Miosis

Miosis (small pupils) is associated with narcotics (except meperidine), propoxyphene, phenothiazines in light stages of coma; barbiturates, ethanol, and benzodiazepines in deep coma; organophosphates, pontine hemorrhage, and bromides.

Motor Neuron Disease

Excitatory amino acid neurotransmitters such as glutamate have been implicated in the pathogenesis of certain neurodegenerative disorders. Glutamate analogs such as methylaminoalanine, oxalylaminoalanine, and domoic acid are neurotoxic and have been linked to neurologic disorders in humans. Lathyrism (i.e., using chick peas as a food staple) is associated with weakness and spasticity associated with corticospinal tract dysfunction.

Movement Disorders

Drug-induced movement disorders occur during the early phase of neuroleptic administration. Drug-induced parkinsonism is clinically indistinguishable from idiopathic Parkinson's disease. Drugs and toxins that induce parkinsonism include clebopride, 1-methyl-4-phenyl-1, 2,3,6-tetrahydropyridine (MPTP) (a designer drug), disulfiram, lithium, manganese, carbon disulfide, organophosphates, metoclopramide, amoxapine, carbon monoxide, phenylpropanolamine, and antihistamines. The most frequent causes are the phenothiazine or butyrophenone groups, and the major tranquilizers. See Tremor.

Myasthenia Gravis

Drug-induced myasthenic crisis may be associated with the aminoglycosides, polymyxin, penicillamine, tetracycline, quinidine, lidocaine, quinine, morphine, meperidine, curare, succinylcholine, and procainamide. Recovery may occur within a few weeks of withdrawal of the toxic offender.

Mydriasis

Many causes exist for mydriasis (enlarged pupils), including hypoxic encephalopathy from any source. This sign is not specific, but may indicate the presence of sympathomimetics (amphetamine, cocaine, LSD), anticholinergic drugs (atropine, tricyclic antidepressants), drug withdrawal, glutethimide, and antihistamines.

Myocardial Injury

Organic nitrates cause nonatheromatous ischemic heart disease. See Atherosclerosis. Carbon monoxide, cyanide and hydrogen sulfide are myocardial asphyxiants. Direct myocardial injury has been associated with cobalt, arsenic, arsine, lead, antimony and organic solvents. See Arrhythmias, and Hypertension.

Myoclonus

Phencyclidine, cadmium, Cicuta species (water hemlock), bismuth, methyl bromide, tetraethyl lead, chloralose, and toxic cooking oil syndrome have been associated with myoclonus.

Myopathy

Drug-induced myopathy can result from a direct local effect, when drug is injected into muscle. Diffuse myopathy may result after systematic use. Myopathies may also be associated with electrolyte disturbances, muscle compression, ischemia, and immunologic reactions. Repeated injections of antibiotics or drugs of addiction can lead to severe muscle fibrosis and contractures. Clofibrate and e-aminocaproic acid cause an acute or subacute painful necrotizing myopathy with myoglobinuria and acute renal failure. Other drugs that induce toxic myopathies are the lipid-lowering agents, succinylcholine, halothane, corticosteroids, and chloroquine. Inflammatory myopathies have followed use of d-penicillamine, procainamide, hydralazine, phenytoin, and penicillin. Environmental agents associated with myositis include foods (adulterated rapeseed oil, l-tryptophan), occupational exposures (silica), and medical devices (collagen and silicone implants).

Nail Effects

A variety of drugs, chemicals, and other natural agents affect nail color when applied locally. Asymptomatic pigmentary abnormalities are the most common change and may suggest general disease or a specific diagnosis. Antibiotics such as tetracycline, chloramphenicol, and minocycline may produce photosensitivity with onycholysis. Cancer chemotherapeutic agents can cause hyperpigmentation of the nails, particularly among black patients. Antimalarial drugs also produce pigmentary changes.

Nephrotoxins

Nephrotoxins include drugs, chemicals, foods, plants, and animal venoms. Attempts to classify nephrotoxins by histopathology or mechanism of action have been confusing and unsatisfactory. Manifestations of renal damage are not specific and include some or all of the common syndromes of nephrotoxicity including nephrogenic diabetes insipidus, renal tubular acidosis, Fanconi syndrome, acute or chronic renal failure, and nephrotic syndrome. Clinical signs of nephrotoxicity are variable, often involving nonspecific symptoms (nausea, vomiting, decreased mental activity, pruritus, hiccups, muscle twitching, fatigue, anorexia, malaise, weakness) and / or secondary complications (hypertension, edema, peripheral neuropathy, congestive heart failure, electrolyte imbalance, oliguria, gastric ulcers, malnutrition, acidosis, proteinuria, hematuria, hyperuricemia, and decreased drug clearance). See Acute Renal Failure, and Interstitial Nephritis.

Neuroleptic Malignant Syndrome

Neuroleptic malignant syndrome (NMS) is a rare and frequently fatal complication of therapy with neuroleptic drugs (phenothiazines, lithium, butyrophenones, thioxanthenes, and loxapine) and of levodopa withdrawal characterized by hyperpyrexia, hypertonicity of skeletal muscles, autonomic instability, and fluctuating consciousness.

Neuropathy

Peripheral nerve damage produces changes in deep (position, vibration), superficial (pain, temperature, touch), and cortical (stereognosis, graphesthesia) sensitization, as well as reduced reflexes and motor function. The most common identified sources include trauma, drugs, toxins, vitamin deficiencies, metabolic and storage diseases, infections, immune diseases, malignancies, vasculitis, leprosy, alcoholism, diabetes mellitus, and thyroid disorders. Often the cause is not identified.

Neuropathy may be subdivided into pathologic sites of injury. Axonopathy manifests as axon degeneration, myelin degeneration, partial recovery, and "dying-back" neuropathy. Examples of agents that may be involved are acrylamide (sensory motor), hexacarbons such as n-hexane, and methyl-n-butyl ketone (stocking and glove sensory motor and autonomic neuropathy), carbon disulfide (sensory motor), tri-o-cresyl phosphate (motor paralysis), metals such as thallium, arsenic, mercury, and platinum (motor), and colchicine, podophyllum, vincristine, Taxol, ethanol, Vacor, disulfiram, isoniazid, nitrous oxide, metronidazole, and dapsone.

In myelinopathies, the axon is spared, and myelin is selectively destroyed. Proprioception, touch, and vibration are impaired (large fibers). Pain, temperature, and autonomic responses are intact, there is areflexia, and healing is rapid. Responsible agents include lead (motor neuropathy, wrist drop), buckthorn (ascending paralysis), diphtheria toxin, hexachlorophene, amiodarone, and trichloroethylene. Neuronopathy may be caused by doxorubicin (dorsal root ganglia, and autonomic ganglia) and pyridoxine (sensory loss, ataxia).

Toxins affecting nerve function without nerve injury include botulism, tetanus, strychnine, elapid venom, and black widow spider venom. Methanol, disulfiram, carbon monoxide, and 1-methyl-4-phenyl-1, 2,3,6-tetrahydropyridine (MPTP) (a designer drug) cause necrosis of the basal ganglia. Cranial neuropathy may be associated with botulism, carbon disulfide, trichloroethylene and ethylene glycol.

Noncardiogenic Pulmonary Edema

Many drugs have been associated with noncardiogenic pulmonary edema (NCPE), a common cause of acute respiratory distress syndrome (ARDS). NCPE is characterized by the simultaneous presence of severe hypoxemia, bilateral infiltrates on chest roentgenogram, and a normal pulmonary capillary wedge pressure with exclusion of other risk factors. Agents known to cause ARDS include amiodarone, heroin and opiates, antidepressants, bleomycin, calcium channel blockers, cocaine, sedative-hypnotics, salicylates, lidocaine, vinca alkaloids, haloperidol, paraquat, phenothiazines, irritant gases such as phosgene and nitrogen dioxide, and smoke inhalation.

Nystagmus

Horizontal nystagmus suggests alcohol, sedative-hypnotics, primidone, carbamazepine, phencyclidine, or phenytoin. Combined vertical and horizontal nystagmus most commonly involves phencyclidine intoxication, but is also seen in Wernicke's syndrome, phenytoin intoxication, and deep sedative-hypnotic overdose. Downbeat nystagmus has been associated with lithium, alcohol, toluene, and felbamate.

Odors

Physicians rarely use the sense of smell to diagnose, in part because of the difficulty in describing smells objectively. A variety of diseases and drugs have been identified with odors. Classic examples include the sweet smell of ketones associated with diabetic and alcoholic ketoacidosis, a garlic odor associated with arsenic and organophosphate poisoning, the roasted almond smell of cyanide, the rotten eggs smell of sulfur dioxide, the wintergreen smell of methyl salicylate, the pear-like aroma of chloral hydrate, and the solvent smell of xylene, kerosene and other hydrocarbons.

Ophthalmoplegia

Ophthalmoplegia has been associated with sedative-hypnotics, Wernicke's encephalopathy, and botulism.

Optic Neuritis

Methanol, organic arsenic, chloramphenicol, ethambutol, ethchlorvynol, isoniazid, lead, and sulfonamides have been associated with optic neuritis.

Osmolal Gap

The osmolal gap represents the difference between measured osmolality (measured by freezing point depression) and calculated osmolality. Elevated osmolal gaps result from decreased serum water (e.g., hyperlipidemia and hyperprothrombinemia) or high concentrations of low-molecular-weight substances. For toxicologic purposes, if the serum does not appear lipemic, an osmolal gap indicates the presence of low-molecular-weight toxin(s). A gap greater than 10 mosm is abnormal. A suggested mnemonic for the causes of an osmolal gap is "ME DIE" (**M**ethanol, **E**thanol, **D**iuretics (e.g., mannitol, sorbitol, and glycerol), **I**sopropanol, **E**thylene glycol).

Other causes include glycerin, diatrizoate sodium, isoniazid, acetone, ether, trichloroethane, paraldehyde, and chloroform. The presence of toxic levels of many low-molecular-weight substances including ethylene glycol is not easily detected by the serum osmolality. A normal gap does not exclude toxic levels of methanol or ethylene glycol.

Ototoxicity

Diuretics and antiinflammatory agents (e.g., salicylates) are associated with acute and transient impairment of hearing or tinnitus. Some antineoplastic agents and aminoglycoside antibiotics are associated with delayed and often irreversible loss of hearing. Erythromycin, aspirin, gentamicin, cisplatin, metronidazole, and naproxen may precipitate drug-associated tinnitus and deafness. Deafness alone is occasionally observed after erythromycin, gentamicin, cisplatin, furosemide, metronidazole, and azithromycin. Tinnitus is more common with aspirin, quinine, indomethacin, sulindac, metoprolol, naproxen, and procaine penicillin.

Oxalosis

Oxalosis has been associated with diethylene glycol, ethylene glycol, ethylene glycol butyl ether, and rhubarb ingestion.

Pancreatitis

Drugs can cause acute pancreatitis, but with the exception of ethanol, drugs rarely cause chronic pancreatitis. Reports of acute pancreatitis are generally anecdotal. Pancreatitis has definitely been associated with asparaginase, azathioprine, didanosine, estrogens, furosemide, mercaptopurine, pentamidine, sulfonamides, sulindac, tetracyclines, thiazides and valproic acid.

Paralysis

Paralysis is associated with botulism, organophosphates, carbamates, Conium maculatum (poison hemlock), and, of course, paralytic drugs such as succinylcholine and curare.

Parkinsonism

See Movement Disorders.

Parotitis

Parotitis has been associated with bretylium, methyldopa, clonidine, guanethidine, phenylbutazone, oxyphenbutazone, and thioridazine.

Pemphigus

Pemphigus may be secondary to penicillamine, captopril, penicillin, rifampin, pyrazolone compounds, beta-blockers, progesterone, heroin, piroxicam, levodopa, lysine acetyl salicylate, gold, phenobarbital, cephalexin, enalapril, pentachlorophenol, phosphatide, hydantoins, and barbiturates. Most of these drugs induce pemphigus rarely, considering their widespread use.

Peripheral Neuropathy

See Neuropathy.

Pleural Effusion

Agents associated with pleural effusion include chemotherapeutic agents, nitrofurantoin, bromocriptine, dantrolene, methysergide, l-tryptophan, drugs that induce systemic lupus erythematosus, tocolytics, amiodarone, esophageal variceal sclerotherapy agents, and interleukin-2.

Pneumonitis

Chromates, zinc, vanadium, mercury, or hydrocarbons may cause toxic pneumonitis. See Chapter 46, Hydrocarbons and Chapter 45, Airborne Toxins.

Primary Biliary Cirrhosis

Primary biliary cirrhosis has been associated with acetaminophen, chlorpromazine, phenylbutazone, tolbutamide, thiabendazole, benoxaprofen, and a compound containing glycyrrhizin, cysteine, and glycine.

Psychogenic Illness

Headache, nausea, vomiting, myalgias, nonspecific neurological symptoms, and / or dyspnea may characterize acute illnesses of psychogenic origin ("hysteria"). Numerous features have been identified that help differentiate mass hysteria from toxic exposures. The preponderance of psychogenic illness occurs in adolescents or preadolescents, specifically in girls or women. There may be transmission by sight, sound, or smell and there is typically a rapid onset and resolution. There may be evidence of unusual physical or emotional stress, absence of laboratory or physical evidence identifying a specific cause, and relapse of illness in the setting of the original outbreak.

Psychosis

Numerous agents may cause psychosis. Among others, these include phencyclidine (PCP), lysergic acid diethylamide (LSD), cocaine, amphetamines, caffeine, theophylline, anticholinergics, chronic heavy metals, bromide, digitalis, carbon monoxide, drug withdrawal, cimetidine, solvent abuse, acyclovir, albuterol, amantadine, aminocaproic acid, high-dose phenytoin, tricyclic antidepressants, antihistamines, bromocriptine, corticosteroids, disopyramide, ketamine, levodopa, morphine, procaine, quinacrine, and vincristine. See Mania.

Pulmonary Edema

Drug-induced pulmonary edema has been associated with heroin, salicylates, chlorine, phosgene, paraquat, nitrogen dioxide, hydrogen chloride, phenothiazines, organophosphates, cadmium, glutethimide, and ethchlorvynol. See also Noncardiogenic Pulmonary Edema.

Raynaud's Disease

Drugs associated with Raynaud's Disease include beta-blockers, ergot alkaloids and bleomycin.

Retinal Hemorrhage

Retinal hemorrhage may be seen after carbon monoxide, methaqualone, warfarin, heparin, and super-warfarin exposures.

Rhabdomyolysis

Rhabdomyolysis is a clinical syndrome characterized by sufficient skeletal muscle injury to permit the escape of intracellular contents into the plasma. Creatine phosphokinase is the most sensitive laboratory marker of rhabdomyolysis. A fivefold elevation of this muscle enzyme in the absence of cardiac or brain injury indicates rhabdomyolysis. Red urine in the absence of red blood cells on microscopic exam may indicate rhabdomyolysis. Myoglobinuria may be absent on initial examination in up to 20% of rhabdomyolysis cases, and myoglobinuria does not correlate with the extent of myoglobinemia.

Ethanol, muscle compression, seizures, and trauma are the most common etiologies. Drugs involved include heroin, methadone, phencyclidine (PCP), phenylpropanolamine, amphetamines, lysergic acid diethylamide (LSD), glutethimide, salicylates, succinylcholine, clofibrate, and e-aminocaproic acid. Toxins associated with rhabdomyolysis include ethanol, p-phenylenediamine, isopropanol, carbon monoxide, ethylene glycol, toluene, Cicuta (water hemlock) ingestion, strychnine, and envenomations (rattlesnake, brown recluse spider, hornet, and wasp). Complications of rhabdomyolysis include hyperkalemia, hyperphosphatemia, hypocalcemia, hyperuricemia, and acute renal failure.

Rigidity

Drugs which induce neuroleptic malignant syndrome (see above) and / or dystonic reactions (see above) may cause rigidity. Paralytics, phencyclidine (PCP), strychnine, monoamine oxidase inhibitors (MAOIs) and haloperidol may cause rigidity. Black widow spider bite is also associated with rigidity.

Scleroderma

Scleroderma may follow use of carbidopa, hydroxytryptophan, diethylpropion, pentazocine, local anesthetics, bromocriptine, phytonadione, cocaine, and appetite suppressants.

Seizures

Toxin-induced seizures are usually grand mal convulsions rather than absence or complex partial seizures. Common drug-related causes of seizures are penicillin, hypoglycemic agents, lidocaine and other local anesthetics, methylxanthines, and neuroleptic drugs. Other drugs and conditions which may cause seizures include phencyclidine (PCP), propoxyphene, cyclic antidepressants, isoniazid, strychnine, camphor, cicutoxin, cocaine, organophosphates, carbon monoxide, lithium, lead, chlorinated hydrocarbons, barbiturate withdrawal, phenol, drug-induced hypoxia, propranolol, 2,4-D, lindane, antihistamines, disulfiram, alcohol withdrawal and other sedative-hypnotic withdrawal. Isoniazid, bronchodilators, lidocaine, and insulin may cause multiple seizures or status epilepticus. Noncompliance with prescribed anticonvulsant therapy by epileptic patients is a frequent cause of seizures.

Initial diagnostic evaluation of seizures may include determination of antiepileptic drug levels, serum chemistry studies including glucose, sodium, calcium, magnesium and blood urea nitrogen determination. Urine and blood samples may be obtained for toxicologic screening. Oxygenation should be confirmed by oximetry or arterial blood gas determination. Lumbar puncture may be performed unless contraindicated by intracranial hypertension, suspected cerebral mass lesion, or obstructed cerebrospinal fluid flow (e.g., hydrocephalus). Brain imaging by CT scan or magnetic resonance imaging scan is usually performed before a lumbar puncture in adults.

Serum Sickness

Agents associated with serum sickness include serum preparations and vaccines. Beta-blockers, streptokinase, and beta-lactam antibiotics may yield reactions resembling serum sickness.

Sexual Dysfunction

It may be difficult to distinguish drug-induced sexual dysfunction from the effects of depression or disease. Drug-induced sexual dysfunction is reversed when drug use is stopped.

Frequent offenders include antihypertensive agents, antipsychotic drugs, and antidepressants.

Sialadenitis

Sialadenitis has been associated with phenylbutazone, isoproterenol, nitrofurantoin and iodine.

Sialorrhea

Pilocarpine, neostigmine, iodides, and cholinergic agents such as the organophosphates may cause sialorrhea.

Skin Necrosis

Intravenous drugs known to cause skin necrosis include chemotherapeutic agents such as bleomycin, dacarbazine, vinca alkaloids, doxorubicin, daunorubicin, dactinomycin, mitomycin, fluorouracil, streptozocin, chlorozotocin and nitrogen mustard. Other agents which may cause skin necrosis after i.v. administration include dextrose (10%), mannitol, sodium bicarbonate, calcium and potassium salts, nafcillin, norepinephrine, dopamine, radiologic dyes and methylene blue.

Stomatitis

Agents associated with stomatitis include nitrogen mustard, methotrexate, fluorouracil, mercaptopurine, chlorambucil, doxorubicin, daunorubicin, bleomycin, penicillamine, gold salts, topical chloral hydrate, and Gentian violet.

Stroke

Sympathomimetic drugs such as oxymetazoline, phenazoline, amphetamine, ephedrine, phenylpropanolamine, methamphetamine, pseudoephedrine and cocaine can cause stroke.

Systemic Lupus Erythematosus

As many as 10% of cases of systemic lupus erythematosus (SLE) are drug related. Procainamide and hydralazine are the drugs most commonly implicated. A definite association has also been shown for isoniazid, methyldopa, quinidine, and chlorpromazine. Drugs less frequently implicated include certain anticonvulsants, beta-blockers, sulfasalazine, penicillamine, lithium, and antithyroid drugs. Drug-induced SLE usually occurs after long-term (6–12 months) high-dose therapy with the suspected agent. Clinical manifestations may include arthralgias, arthritis, fever, skin rash, adenopathy, myalgias, pericarditis, pleuritis, pleural effusion, hepatosplenomegaly, and renal and central nervous system involvement. The antinuclear antibody (ANA) test is positive and may remain positive up to 2 years. Rapid remission typically follows discontinuation of the drug.

Tachycardia

Drugs which cause hyperthermia (see Hyperthermia), seizures (see Seizures), and hypoglycemia (see Hypoglycemia) may cause tachycardia. Among others, cocaine, amphetamines, phencyclidine, antihistamines, anticholinergics, cyclic antidepressants, phenothiazines, theophylline, ethanol or sedative-hypnotic withdrawal, and carbon monoxide may cause tachycardia.

Tardive Dyskinesia

Phenothiazines constitute the principal group of drugs associated with this disorder. Metoclopramide has also been suspect.

Taste and Smell Disorders

Chemosensory dysfunction may be divided into numerous categories. These include ageusia (absence of taste), hypogeusia (diminished taste sensitivity), dysgeusia (taste distortion), anosmia (absence of smell), hyposmia (diminished smelling capacity), and dysosmia (distorted smell). A variety of nervous, nutritional, endocrine, infectious, and localized nasal diseases produce disorders affecting taste and smell. Medications associated with a metallic or bitter taste include penicillamine, levodopa, methimazole, propylthiouracil, phenylbutazone, amphotericin B, griseofulvin, azathioprine, salicylazosulfapyridine (Azulfidine®), sodium lauryl sulfate, chlormezanone, carbamazepine, baclofen, phenformin, ethambutol, vitamin D, sodium thiosulfate, clarithromycin and allopurinol.

Tinnitus

See Ototoxicity.

Tongue Effects

"Glossitis" and tongue ulceration has followed use of trimethoprim-sulfamethoxazole, diclofenac, naproxen, metronidazole, sulindac, amoxicillin, erythromycin, captopril, and piroxicam. Ketamine may cause tongue protrusion as may the agents associated with tardive dyskinesia.

Torsade de Pointes

Antiarrhythmic agents which increase the QT interval (e.g., quinidine, disopyramide, procainamide, lidocaine, and amiodarone), psychotropics (e.g., phenothiazines, tricyclic antidepressants, tetracyclic antidepressants, and maprotiline), and organophosphates have been associated with Torsade de Pointes. See Arrhythmias.

Toxic Epidermal Necrolysis

Toxic epidermal necrolysis has been associated with certain viruses, butazones, hydantoins, sulfonamides, barbiturates, and antibiotics.

Tremor

Resting tremor is most pronounced at rest and decreases with activity. See causes of toxin-induced parkinsonism in Movement Disorders. Postural tremor is most pronounced with an outstretched hand and is associated with beta agonists, phenytoin, valproic acid, cyclic antidepressants, monosodium glutamate, lithium, arsenic, and alcohol withdrawal. Kinetic tremor is most pronounced with motion and is associated with alcoholic cerebellar degeneration, mercury, lithium, and sedative-hypnotic intoxication.

Chorea tremor consists of repetitive dance-like movements and is associated with anticonvulsants (e.g., phenytoin, carbamazepine), anticholinergics, dopamine agonists (e.g., amantadine, bromocriptine), ethanol, toluene, manganese, and sympathomimetics (e.g., amphetamine, cocaine). See Chorea. Dystonic tremor consists of muscle group spasms (e.g., oculogyric crises, torticollis, tortipelvis, and opisthotonus) and is associated with neuroleptics, antiemetics, cocaine, chloroquine, and hydroxychloroquine. See Dystonic Reactions.

Vasculitis

Drugs associated with vasculitis include allopurinol, penicillin, sulfonamides, thiazides, pyrazolone, hydantoins, and propylthiouracil.

Xerostomia

Agents associated with xerostomia include centrally acting hypertensive agents, diuretics, antipsychotics, tricyclic antidepressants, antihistamines, anticholinergics, anticonvulsants, laxatives, muscle relaxants, narcotics and hypnotics.

Questions—Clinical Signs of Specific Toxins

1. **Which of the following associations is incorrect?**
   A. Vasculitis-Sulfonamides
   B. Tremor-Carbamazepine
   C. Torsade de Pointes-Digitoxin
   D. Tardive Dyskinesia-Phenothiazines
   E. Miosis-Organophosphates
2. **Which of the following is not associated with methemoglobinemia?**
   A. Aniline dyes
   B. Methyl salicylate
   C. Dinitrotoluene
   D. Dapsone
   E. Phenazopyridine
3. **Which of the following is not associated with hypothermia?**
   A. Ethanol
   B. Narcotics
   C. Jimsonweed
   D. Phenothiazines
   E. Carbon monoxide
4. **Which of the following associations is incorrect?**
   A. Drug-induced pulmonary edema-Heroin
   B. Raynaud's Disease-Ergot alkaloids
   C. Rhabdomyolysis-Rattlesnake envenomation
   D. Scleroderma-Cocaine
   E. Seizures-Camphor
5. **Which of the following is not associated with drug-induced seizures?**
   A. Cocaine
   B. Lindane
   C. Propranolol
   D. Cicutoxin
   E. Succinylcholine

Answers

Introduction to General Epidemiology

1. D 2. D 3. A

Fatalities

1. B 2. A 3. E 4. C

Pediatric Poisoning

1. C

Medication Errors and Adverse Reactions

1. E

Poison Centers

1. B 2. D

Identification of Toxic Syndromes

1. B 2. E 3. A 4. D

Clinical Signs of Specific Toxins

1. C 2. B 3. C 4. D 5. E

CHAPTER 2

Basic Approach to the Poisoned Patient

INTRODUCTION

The initial approach to all poisoned patients is identical to the initial approach to all patients. All patients must be stabilized by a preestablished systematic approach based on the ABCDs of resuscitation. The initial patient survey is directed toward correcting immediate life-threatening problems of Airway, Breathing, Circulation, and Depression of the central nervous system.

STABILIZATION

The basic approach to the poisoned patient includes

STABILIZATION
- This includes a brief screening examination directed toward identifying measures necessary in the first several minutes to prevent further deterioration of the patient.
- Attention is directed toward the ABCDs of resuscitation.

DECONTAMINATION
- After a patient is stabilized, attention is directed toward decontaminating the patient and those in his environment.
- Specific methods include eye decontamination, skin decontamination, and gut decontamination.

PATIENT EVALUATION
- Once a patient has been stabilized, he or she is evaluated by history, physical examination, and laboratory tests.
- A complete survey directed toward identifying and quantifying toxin(s), evaluating the severity of clinical effects, and searching for associated complications and trauma, is undertaken.
- Laboratory work complements the history and physical examination.

ELIMINATION ENHANCEMENT

- In certain cases, there may be appropriate measures to improve elimination of toxin.
- These include urine pH alteration, diuresis, hemodialysis, hemoperfusion, peritoneal dialysis, and activated charcoal.

ANTIDOTES

- Some toxins may respond to specific antidotes.
- Specific antidotes are effective in less than 5% of poisonings, but naloxone and glucose may be administered to all patients exhibiting central nervous system depression.

CONTINUING CARE

- After diagnosis and initial treatment, an adequate observation period should be established.
- Poison prevention education or psychiatric counseling may be appropriate, and a referral source should be identified for follow-up treatment.

EVALUATION OF (A) AIRWAY

Airway obstruction may result from mucosal swelling, secretions, posterior displacement of the tongue, foreign bodies, and/or trauma. Symptoms include dyspnea, dysphonia, air hunger, and/or hoarseness. Signs include stridor, intercostal and/or substernal retractions, cyanosis, diaphoresis, drooling, and tachypnea.

- If a cervical fracture is suspected (all unconscious patients should be assumed to have a cervical fracture until proven otherwise), a chin lift or jaw thrust should be applied until radiographs of the cervical spine exclude a fracture.
- Clear the airway of secretions with suction and remove any foreign body.
- Nasopharyngeal or oropharyngeal airways may be used in obtunded patients to prevent pharyngeal obstruction caused by collapse of the posterior base of the tongue.
- Comatose patients without a gag reflex require intubation to prevent aspiration.
- An emergency cricothyroidotomy or, if time permits, a tracheostomy may be necessary in acute upper airway obstruction if an endotracheal tube cannot be passed from above the vocal cords.
- Cricothyroidotomies are difficult procedures in young children because of excessive tracheal mobility and therefore are not recommended in children under 12 years of age.

Questions—Evaluation of (A) Airway

1. Airway obstruction may result from

A. Vomitus
B. The tongue
C. Mucosal swelling
D. Foreign bodies
E. All of the above

EVALUATION OF (B) BREATHING, VENTILATION, AND OXYGENATION

Respiratory depression leading to hypoventilation is by far the most common drug-induced pulmonary complication. Other etiologies of pulmonary dysfunction, including those associated with drug abuse, include aspiration pneumonia, noncardiogenic and cardiogenic pulmonary edema, pneumonitis, lung abscess, septic pulmonary emboli, atelectasis, pneumothorax, pulmonary fibrosis, chronic obstructive pulmonary disease from smoking, bronchospasm from numerous environmental and occupational sources, and, rarely, tetanus-induced respiratory failure.

Ventilation

The partial pressure of arterial carbon dioxide ($PaCO_2$) measures the ability of the lungs to remove carbon dioxide, and is an accurate estimate of alveolar ventilation. Normal arterial carbon dioxide levels are 37–43 mm Hg. During each breath, most air reaches the alveoli where gas exchange occurs (alveolar ventilation, VA), and some air remains in the conducting airways (dead-space ventilation, VD), where no exchange occurs. Minute ventilation (VE) is the amount of air exhaled in 1 minute and reflects the 1-minute sum of dead-space and alveolar ventilation.

When alveolar ventilation decreases, arterial $PaCO_2$ levels rise. The mechanism is either decreased minute ventilation (e.g., respiratory depression) or increased anatomic and/or physiologic dead-space (e.g., emphysema). Since alveolar oxygen tension (PaO_2) depends on arterial $PaCO_2$, the PaO_2 decreases with increasing alveolar carbon dioxide levels. For calculation purposes, alveolar and arterial carbon dioxide levels are considered equivalent as carbon dioxide exchange occurs easily across the alveolar membrane.

Portable flow meters can measure individual tidal volumes. Minute ventilation is the product of tidal volume and respiratory rate over 60 seconds. In general, minute ventilation below 4–6 L/min, vital capacity below 10 mL/kg, and tidal volumes below 4–5 mL/kg suggest the need for assisted ventilation. The dynamic state of the patient must always be considered in interpreting those measurements, since they are not steady-state measurements.

Oxygenation

Arterial oxygen tension (PaO_2) and arterial oxygen saturation (O_2 sat) are the two dependent parameters that measure the degree of arterial oxygenation. The sigmoidal oxyhemoglobin dissociation curve expresses their relationship, so that knowledge of one allows determination of the other. In most clinical situations, the PaO_2 is measured. The O_2 sat may be calculated and misreported as normal when carboxyhemoglobinemia or methemoglobinemia occurs.

Above a PaO_2 of 60 mm Hg, the dissociation curve is relatively flat with an O_2 sat over 90%. Since small decreases in PaO_2 below 60 mm Hg produce large decrements in oxygen saturation, PaO_2 changes at this level are therapeutically significant. Changes above 60 mm Hg are important for diagnostic purposes and may reflect trends towards or away from hypoxemia.

Signs of inadequate oxygenation include cyanosis, tachypnea, hypoventilation, diaphoresis, suprasternal and/or intercostal retractions, and altered mental status. Any clinical suspicion of inadequate ventilation or oxygenation should be evaluated with arterial blood gas measurements, chest x-ray, and, if appropriate, tidal volume measurements.

A normal PaO_2 does not guarantee adequate tissue oxygenation, since cellular respiration depends on both oxygen delivery and tissue utilization. Certain toxins may adversely affect both these parameters. Normal oxygen delivery requires adequate hemoglobin oxygen saturation (carbon monoxide reduces arterial oxygen saturation but not PaO_2), adequate hemoglobin levels (anemia reduces oxygen-carrying capacity), normal oxygen-unloading mechanisms (hypothermia, alkalosis, and decreased

2,3-diphosphoglycerate levels reduce oxygen release, as revealed by a leftward shift of the oxyhemoglobin dissociation curve), and an adequate cardiac output.

Metabolic acidosis in the presence of a normal PaO_2 suggests a toxin that either decreases oxygen-carrying capacity (e.g., carbon monoxide, or methemoglobinemia) or reduces tissue oxygen utilization (e.g., cyanide, or hydrogen sulfide). In such cases, the appropriate antidote must be given to maintain cellular respiration.

Hypoxemia

The arterial oxygen tension (PaO_2) depends on the inspired oxygen tension (FiO_2), the alveolar ventilation, and the distribution of ventilation and perfusion in the lungs. Reduced arterial oxygen levels may result from a number of abnormalities that can be diagnosed via arterial blood gas interpretation. These include:

ALVEOLAR HYPOVENTILATION

- Elevated arterial carbon dioxide ($PaCO_2$) levels reflect alveolar hypoventilation.
- Central nervous system depressants classically produce respiratory depression in serious overdose, leading to $PaCO_2$ levels above 45 mm Hg.
- Increased minute ventilation corrects this defect.

VENTILATION-PERFUSION (V/Q) MISMATCH

- Bronchoconstriction and aspiration pneumonia are examples of pulmonary abnormalities in which the alveoli are underperfused and overventilated or overperfused and underventilated.
- The resultant mismatch causes a reduced arterial oxygen tension, which can generally be corrected with oxygen.

SHUNT

- Perfusing areas of the lung that receive no ventilation, or ventilating areas with no perfusion, cause a reduced PaO_2 level that does not normalize with 100% oxygen.
- Such patients receiving 100% oxygen have decreased PaO_2 levels and abnormal alveolar-arterial oxygen gradients.
- Atelectasis and pulmonary emboli are examples of parenchymal defects that produce shunting.

DIFFUSION DEFECTS

- Rarely, fibrosis of the alveolar membrane impairs the diffusion of gas between the alveolar sac and the pulmonary vasculature.
- The carbon monoxide diffusing capacity distinguishes this abnormality from ventilation-perfusion mismatch.

DECREASED INSPIRED OXYGEN CONCENTRATION

- Reduction of inhaled oxygen concentration (e.g., by high altitude, by respiratory asphyxiants such as methane and carbon dioxide) causes decreased alveolar oxygen and therefore reduced PaO_2.
- In normal patients, acute hypoxemia first compromises brain function. When the PaO_2 falls below 55 mm Hg, euphoria, impaired judgment, and loss of short-term memory occur. Progressive loss of cognition and motor function results from worsening hypoxemia until loss of consciousness occurs at 30 mm Hg. Increasing hypoxemia produces myocardial dysfunction and dysrhythmias, depending on underlying cardiovascular disease.

Alveolar-Arterial Oxygen Gradient

Calculating the alveolar-arterial oxygen difference (A-a gradient) can assess the presence of pulmonary parenchymal defects. A normal A-a gradient indicates normal lung function and an extrapulmonary cause of hypoxemia. An abnormal A-a gradient implies intrinsic lung dysfunction such as ventilation-perfusion mismatch, shunt, or diffusion defect.

Early in the course of toxic pulmonary conditions (e.g., aspiration pneumonia, pulmonary edema, or chemical pneumonitis) arterial PaO_2 levels may be normal. Estimating the alveolar-arterial oxygen gradient (PaO_2-PaO_2) yields a more sensitive indicator of pulmonary disease than the PaO_2 alone. The average alveolar-arterial oxygen tension is obtained from the following formula:

$$PaO_2 = (PB - 47) \times (FiO_2) - \frac{PaCO_2}{0.8} \text{ where}$$

$$PB = \text{barometric pressure (760 mm Hg at sea level) and}$$

$$FiO_2 = \text{inspired oxygen tension (21\% at room air or 0.21) and}$$

$$PaCO_2 = \text{alveolar carbon dioxide level (measured by arterial blood gas)}$$

For room air at sea level, the alveolar-arterial oxygen difference (A-a gradient) is:

$$\begin{aligned} \text{A-a gradient} &= PaO_2 - PaO_2 \\ &= (760 - 47) \times (0.21) - \frac{PaCO_2}{0.8} - PaO_2 \\ &= 150 - 1.2\,(PaCO_2) - PaO_2 \end{aligned}$$

The $PaCO_2$ and PaO_2 are both measured by arterial blood gas. In healthy young adults, the normal A-a gradient is approximately 10–15 mm Hg. The gradient increases with age. Normal elderly patients often have gradients over 30 mm Hg.

Supplemental Oxygen

Oxygen should be given to all poisoned patients with depressed mentation or hypoxemia. In the absence of hypercarbia ($PaCO_2$ levels over 45 mm Hg), the risk of worsening alveolar ventilation by oxygen administration is virtually nonexistent. Even in patients with severe chronic obstructive lung disease, supplemental oxygen aimed at providing a PaO_2 level of at least 60-mm Hg is associated with minimal risk of increasing hypercarbia.

Supplemental oxygen does not correct hypoventilation (identified by hypercarbia). Hypoventilation requires assisted ventilation and supplemental oxygen delivered by nasal catheters and cannulae (for FiO_2 ranging from 24–50% with flow rates up to 6 L), oxygen masks (for FiO_2 ranging from 35–50% at rates of 5 L or greater), or masks with reservoir bags (disposable nonrebreathing and partial-rebreathing masks which provide FiO_2 levels over 50% depending on minute ventilation and inspiratory flow rate).

Complications of oxygen therapy result from physical hazards (e.g., drying of mucous membranes, fires, or trauma associated with tubes, catheters, or masks), physiological effects (e.g., atelectasis, hypercarbia), and direct cytotoxicity. Increased formation of free radicals (e.g., superoxide anions, hydrogen peroxide, and hydroxyl radicals) probably interacts with cellular enzymes and membranes to produce toxic effects.

A number of drugs and toxins, including paraquat, bleomycin, Adriamycin, disulfiram, diethyldithiocarbamate, daunorubicin, and certain antibiotics generate free radicals and potentially enhance oxygen toxicity. Ozone and nitrogen dioxide are also capable of damaging the lungs through free radical formation. The only effective treatment for oxygen poisoning is prevention. In general, pure oxygen can be safely administered for brief periods involved in cardiopulmonary resuscitation or the transport of critically ill patients.

Intubation

Intubation is the definitive procedure to control both the airway and ventilation. Indications include inadequate oxygenation and ventilation despite supplemental oxygen, as measured by arterial blood gases or the inability to protect the airway from aspiration (e.g., coma with loss of gag reflex). The decision to intubate also requires clinical judgment of the anticipated clinical course and the extent of cellular hypoxia. The gag reflex alone is not a reliable indicator of the need for intubation, since alert patients may have depressed gag reflexes.

Nasotracheal intubation is usually preferred in the spontaneously breathing patient, whereas orotracheal intubation is preferred in the comatose patient whose muscle relaxation allows direct visualization of the epiglottis. Pharmacologic aids to intubation must be administered cautiously in the presence of overdose. Succinylcholine is the muscle relaxant of choice for intubation (1–2 mg/kg intravenously), producing a rapid onset (1 min) and short duration (5–10 min) of action. Relaxation of esophageal sphincters may cause regurgitation of stomach contents. Pressure on the cricoid cartilage helps prevent aspiration during the procedure.

Succinylcholine can exacerbate the cholinergic side effects of certain drugs, leading to worsening bradycardia, salivation, and bronchorrhea in cholinergic overdoses. Since plasma cholinesterase hydrolyzes succinylcholine, substances such as organophosphates or cocaine, which reduce this enzyme, would be expected to prolong the effects of succinylcholine.

Following passage of the tube, proper tube placement should be confirmed by auscultation of the midepigastric region, axilla, and lower lateral chest. Alignment of the 23-cm mark on the endotracheal tube with the teeth in the average male adult (21 cm in the average female) generally places the tube in the proper position, 2 cm above the carina. Required postintubation laboratory tests include chest x-ray and arterial blood gas measurements.

Questions—Evaluation of (B) Breathing, Ventilation, and Oxygenation

1. The ____ is an accurate estimate of alveolar ventilation.
A. $PaCO_2$
B. PaO_2
C. FiO_2
D. PaO_2

2. Minute ventilation
A. Is the total amount of air inspired over 1 minute
B. Reflects the 1-minute difference between dead-space and alveolar ventilation
C. Is the product of tidal volume and respiratory rate over 60 seconds
D. None of the above
E. A and C

3. The sigmoidal oxyhemoglobin dissociation curve expresses the relationship between arterial oxygen tension (PaO_2) and arterial oxygen saturation (O_2 sat) so that knowledge of one allows determination of the other.
A. True
B. False

4. The following moves the oxyhemoglobin dissociation curve to the left
A. Hyperthermia
B. Acidosis
C. Decreased 2,3-diphosphoglycerate levels
D. None of the above
E. A and B

5. Reduced arterial oxygen levels may result from all of the following, except
A. Alveolar hypoventilation
B. Ventilation-perfusion (V/Q) mismatch
C. Shunt
D. Decreased inspired carbon dioxide concentration
E. Diffusion defects

6. Calculating the alveolar-arterial oxygen difference (A-a gradient) can assess the presence of pulmonary parenchymal defects. A normal A-a gradient indicates normal lung function and an extrapulmonary cause of hypoxemia. An abnormal A-a gradient implies intrinsic lung dysfunction such as ventilation-perfusion mismatch, shunt, or diffusion defect.
A. True
B. False

7. Drugs and toxins which generate free radicals and enhance oxygen toxicity include all except
A. Paraquat
B. Bleomycin
C. Triamcinolone
D. Adriamycin
E. Disulfiram

EVALUATION OF (C) CIRCULATION

This portion of the initial patient examination determines whether the tissues are receiving adequate amounts of blood. Shock is the clinical picture in which the patient demonstrates signs and symptoms of inadequate tissue perfusion. Although hypotension and decreased cardiac output usually occur together, these two clinical measurements are not synonymous with shock.

Patients may have blood pressures within the normal range and still show clinical evidence of tissue hypoperfusion. Conversely, patients with blood pressures below the normal range may not demonstrate evidence of shock. Occasionally, patients with elevated cardiac output may show evidence of tissue hypoperfusion. The diagnosis of inadequate tissue perfusion is a clinical diagnosis characterized by depressed consciousness, decreased blood pressure, peripheral vasoconstriction, metabolic acidosis, and/or oliguria.

Mechanisms of Poor Perfusion

Cardiac output, the main determinant of tissue perfusion, is the product of heart rate and stroke volume. The amount of blood volume pumped depends on preload, afterload, and contractility. Drugs and chemicals can affect each of the four parameters determining the cardiac output (i.e., preload, afterload, contractility, and heart rate) but relative hypovolemia manifested by reduced preload is the most common cause of reduced blood pressure and/or cardiac output. The introduction of a Swan-Ganz catheter into the pulmonary artery allows the quantitation of these parameters in order to optimize treatment.

PRELOAD

Physiologically, preload is the amount of stretch on ventricular muscle fibers resulting from the left ventricular volume at the end of diastole. Pulmonary artery wedge pressures measured by Swan-Ganz catheter, below 10-mm Hg, suggest inadequate preload or filling pressures in the presence of hypotension.

AFTERLOAD

The amount of resistance the heart pushes against during its emptying phase is afterload. The best measurement of afterload is the systemic vascular resistance, which normally ranges from 900 to 1,400 dyne.sec.cm-5.

CONTRACTILITY

The intrinsic strength of ventricular muscle is called contractility. Contractility is difficult to measure directly, but a rough correlation is the left ventricular stroke work index (LVSWI). Depression of myocardial contractility can result from overdoses with many agents including sedative-hypnotics and tricyclic antidepressants.

HEART RATE

Cardiac rates below 60 beats per minute and above 150 beats per minute often reduce cardiac output and blood pressure. Numerous toxins produce dysrhythmias and/or conduction disturbances, which can appreciably alter heart rate.

Shock

Signs and symptoms of shock reflect end organ failure, sympathomimetic excess, and compensatory mechanisms. Responses to inadequate tissue perfusion include tachycardia, narrowing of the pulse pressure (difference between systolic and diastolic pressure), decreased urinary output (adult volumes below 25 mL/h), hypotension (usually less than 90 mm Hg systolic), and decreased capillary blanching. Symptoms of shock may appear when the blood pressure is above 90 mm Hg, especially in older patients whose usual blood pressures are elevated. Early signs of shock, such as anxiety and agitation, reflect sympathomimetic excess. Late signs include delirium, stupor and coma.

Signs of dehydration in children include tenting of the skin, dry mucous membranes, a depressed anterior fontanelle, decreased tearing, and dry diapers. Volume loss in adults results in thirst, lightheadedness, near-syncope, postural hypotension, increased urine specific gravity, and decreased urine sodium (less than 10 mEq/L). Prolonged capillary blanching occurs in the presence of inadequate tissue perfusion. Testing for capillary refill involves depressing the patient's hypothenar eminence or fingernail and watching for the red blush to return. Normally the color returns in about 2 seconds.

Treatment

- Hypotension is treated with fluids, position change and pressors as needed. A large-bore peripheral intravenous line (16 gauge or larger) is inserted and crystalloid solution is administered. A second line is used in severe cases to administer more fluids and drugs.
- Initially, a fluid challenge of 200 mL is given (10–20 mL/kg in a child) and improvement in blood pressure is monitored over 10 minutes. The patient is also placed in the Trendelenburg position. If blood pressure fails to normalize, a re-bolus is given and signs of fluid overload are carefully watched for. Hemodynamic monitoring should be considered in those adult patients who do not respond to 2-L infusion and short-term, low-dose vasopressors.
- All patients with hypotension or exposure to arrhythmogenic toxins (e.g., cardiac glycosides, beta-blocking agents, quinidine, quinine, etc.) are placed on a cardiac monitor. An electrocardiogram is also obtained. Careful attention to rate, rhythm, dysrhythmias, and conduction delay is given.
- In patients who do not respond to initial fluid challenges, central venous pressures and hourly urinary output are monitored. Patients with existing cardiac disease or severe hypotension often need more sophisticated hemodynamic monitoring such as a pulmonary artery catheter and/or intra-arterial pressure monitoring.

VASOPRESSORS

- If adequate fluid challenges do not raise the systolic blood pressure above 80–90 mm Hg, and signs of shock persist after several liters of fluid, a vasopressor should be used and hemodynamic monitoring considered.
- Dopamine is the usual vasopressor of choice. At low doses dopaminergic stimulation dominates, resulting in renal and mesenteric dilation. Medium range doses cause beta-1 stimulation, increasing contractility, and mildly increasing pulse rate. High doses cause primarily alpha stimulation, producing systemic vasoconstriction including the renal vessels.
- Norepinephrine is the vasopressor of choice for drugs that cause alpha-blockade (e.g., phenothiazines, tricyclic antidepressants) and that inhibit dopamine beta-hydroxylase (e.g., disulfiram). It is a naturally occurring catecholamine with potent alpha and beta-1 properties, which causes both peripheral vascular constriction and increased cardiac contractility. High doses cause intense vasoconstriction, which increases blood pressure but decreases tissue perfusion. Low doses may be added to medium-range dopamine doses for refractory hypotension, but close hemodynamic monitoring is advised to assess efficacy accurately.
- Hypovolemia should be corrected before norepinephrine is administered. Constant cardiac monitoring must be initiated and the blood pressure monitored every 5 minutes until a clear trend is established. An intraarterial monitor may be necessary to monitor blood pressure accurately because of intense vasoconstriction. Excessive blood pressure elevation may result from therapeutic overshoot.

Questions—Evaluation of (C) Circulation

1. Which of the following is false?

A. Shock is the clinical picture in which the patient demonstrates signs and symptoms of inadequate tissue perfusion
B. Hypotension and decreased cardiac output are synonymous with shock.
C. Patients with elevated cardiac outputs may show evidence of tissue hypoperfusion.
D. Inadequate tissue perfusion is characterized by depressed consciousness, metabolic acidosis, and/or oliguria.
E. Cardiac output is the product of heart rate and stroke volume.

2. Relative hypovolemia manifested by reduced preload is the most common cause of reduced blood pressure and/or cardiac output.

A. True
B. False

3. Which of the following associations is incorrect?
A. Preload-the amount of stretch on ventricular muscle fibers resulting from the left ventricular volume at the end of diastole
B. Afterload-the amount of resistance the heart pushes against during the emptying phase
C. Contractility-the ability of the cardiac valves to contract and distend in a concerted manner
D. None of the above
E. B and C

4. Responses to inadequate tissue perfusion include all of the following, except
A. Tachycardia
B. Widening of the pulse pressure
C. Decreased urinary output
D. Decreased capillary blanching
E. Anxiety and agitation

5. ____ is the vasopressor of choice for drugs that cause alpha-blockade
A. Epinephrine
B. Norepinephrine
C. Neo-synephrine
D. Dopamine
E. Dobutamine

EVALUATION OF (D) DEPRESSION OF THE CENTRAL NERVOUS SYSTEM

Numerous drugs and clinical entities are capable of depressing the central nervous system. Many aspects of assessment and treatment remain constant despite specific etiologies. The Glasgow Coma Scale may be used to assess and follow the depth of coma or unresponsiveness. The predictive value of this and other scales in overdose remains to be determined.

Pupillary size and responsiveness is assessed quickly and easily. The maximum miotic response to sympathetic paralysis or parasympathetic excess is 1.5–2 mm, whereas the maximal mydriatic response to sympathetic excess or parasympathetic paralysis is 8–9 mm. Good prognostic indicators of recovery from hypoxic/ischemic coma include initial presence of the pupillary light reflex, motor responses to pain, and/or spontaneous eye movements. The applicability of these indicators to overdose-induced coma is variable.

Because pupillary pathways are relatively resistant to toxic-metabolic insults, the presence or absence of the light reflex is the single most important physical sign differentiating toxic-metabolic from structural coma. In coma from metabolic causes, with the exception of anticholinergic drugs and glutethimide, pupillary reactivity is usually preserved. Unilateral pupillary dilation strongly suggests a structural cause of coma (e.g., subdural hematoma). Rarely, the use of mydriatic or miotic eye drops obscures a diagnosis based on pupillary response.

The Coma Cocktail

Many (but not all) clinicians have advocated that a "coma cocktail" or group of antidotes be administered to all individuals who present with depressed mental status. These antidotes include glucose, thiamine and naloxone. Oxygen is also routinely administered. Glucose 0.5–1.0 gram/kg is given as 50% dextrose in water in adults, 25% dextrose in water in children, and 10% dextrose in water in neonates. A blood glucose level is drawn before the dextrose is administered. If hypoglycemia is not suspected a Dextrostix determination may be made before glucose infusion.

Thiamine, 100 mg intramuscularly or intravenously, is given as treatment and prevention of Wernicke's encephalopathy. Glucose administration may theoretically deplete thiamine stores and precipitate or worsen Wernicke's encephalopathy. It is generally advised, therefore, that thiamine is given before dextrose is administered. Eye movement paralysis, ataxia, and mental status changes characterize Wernicke's encephalopathy, occasionally seen in alcoholics and other individuals with poor nutritional status. Korsakoff's psychosis is characterized by retrograde and anterograde amnesia with confabulation.

Naloxone (Narcan®) is also given to comatose patients or those with depressed neurologic signs. The dose is 2 mg (at least) in adults and 0.03 mg/kg in children. Naloxone is a specific opiate antagonist with minimal side effects. Agitation and withdrawal signs may develop in opiate-dependent patients. Additional naloxone doses may be required in overdoses involving diphenoxylate-atropine (Lomotil®), propoxyphene (Darvon®), pentazocine (Talwin®), or codeine overdoses. Naloxone may be given via an endotracheal tube if necessary

All patients with depressed mental status should also have supplemental oxygen. Many agents or conditions alter hemoglobin-carrying capacity (such as carbon monoxide, or methemoglobinemia) or alter tissue utilization of oxygen (such as cyanide, hydrogen sulfide). Additional antidotal and other therapies may be required according to individual toxins.

Seizures

Generalized seizures secondary to toxins are usually brief and self-limited. Attention should always be directed toward maintaining adequate oxygenation with suction and supplemental oxygen. Seizures are treated with diazepam (Valium®) or other benzodiazepines such as lorazepam (Ativan®). Phenytoin (Dilantin®) is also utilized if seizure activity is refractory to benzodiazepines, or if there is a clinical expectation that seizures will persist.

Phenobarbital is a third-line drug, which may also be used to treat seizures. Coadministration of phenobarbital and diazepam causes synergistic respiratory depression and should be avoided unless the patient is intubated. Paraldehyde has been used as an alternative. General anesthesia is the method of last resort when status epilepticus persists despite these measures. Intubation and muscle paralysis may be necessary in cases where hyperthermia complicates persistent seizures. Intravenous pyridoxine effectively stops seizures secondary to isoniazid (INH) overdose.

Seizures unresponsive to diazepam may result from altered body homeostasis and trauma (e.g., acidosis, hypocalcemia, electrolyte imbalance, hypoxia, hypoglycemia, meningitis, intracranial hematoma, and subarachnoid hemorrhage). The presence of seizures may also indicate a serious toxic condition that requires methods to enhance elimination (e.g., hemoperfusion or hemodialysis use in seizures induced by theophylline, lithium, and salicylates).

Questions—Evaluation of (D) Depression of the Central Nervous System

1. The maximum miotic response to sympathetic paralysis or parasympathetic excess is
A. 0.5–1.0 mm
B. 1.5–2.0 mm

C. 2.5–3.0 mm
D. 3.5–4.0 mm
E. 4.5–5.0 mm

2. Elements of the typical "coma cocktail" include all of the following, except
A. Thiamine
B. Oxygen
C. Naloxone
D. Saline
E. Dextrose

3. Which of the following regarding seizures secondary to toxins is false?
A. They are usually brief and self-limited.
B. They may require benzodiazepines to control them.
C. They generally indicate a poor prognosis.
D. They may be unresponsive to diazepam in the setting of acidosis.
E. All of the above.

DECONTAMINATION

Once a patient has been stabilized and potential poison(s) have been identified, methods to decontaminate are instituted to prevent further toxicity, and to protect those in the immediate environment from additional exposure. See Chapter 4, Gut Decontamination regarding the various gastrointestinal methods utilized to decrease drug toxicity.

Eye contamination is treated with immediate irrigation. Eyes are flushed copiously for at least 15–20 minutes with normal saline or water. Acid or alkaline irrigating solutions are avoided. Alkaline corneal burns are ophthalmologic emergencies requiring ophthalmologic consultation.

Skin contamination is a common occurrence. It has been estimated that one in four industrial substances represent an appreciable hazard for skin absorption. Cutaneous absorption depends on several factors such as lipid solubility, skin condition, location, caustic effect, physical conditions, and the presence of certain chemical vehicles. Serious toxicity has resulted from cutaneous absorption, and health personnel should be cautious when decontaminating their patients.

Toxic substances such as organophosphates, organic metal compounds (e.g., lead), aniline, phenol, hydrocyanic acid, and ethylene dibromide may penetrate intact skin and must be handled with proper protective equipment. All contaminated clothes must be quickly and carefully removed. Skin contaminated by corrosives is treated with copious water or saline irrigation as soon as possible and continuous irrigation for at least 15 minutes. Neutralizing substances are not advised. Exposed persons should be rinsed with cold water and washed thoroughly (including skin folds, nail beds, and hair) with a nongermicidal soap. Green soap is highly effective but often not available.

Some chemical exposures require special treatment. Lime (calcium oxide) and cement exposures are treated like alkali burns. In burns by flammable metals (e.g., lithium, sodium), large particles are removed, and the exposed surface is covered with mineral oil. Application of polyethylene decreases tissue penetration in burns caused by phenols (cresols). Copper sulfate solution improves debridement and reduces the toxicity of white phosphorus burns. For hydrofluoric acid burns, use of intradermal or intraarterial calcium gluconate decreases tissue necrosis.

Specially trained hazardous materials (HAZMAT) teams handle chemical spills when available. In contrast to human skin decontamination, water is not always used to neutralize and wash away a spill. Priorities of cleanup include containment, absorption, and dilution with agents specific for individual toxins.

Questions—Decontamination

1. Certain toxic substances may penetrate intact skin and must be handled with proper protective equipment. These include
A. Chlorhexidine
B. Organophosphates
C. Phenol
D. All of the above
E. B and C

2. Neutralizing substances may be helpful in decontaminating skin contaminated by corrosives.
A. True
B. False

3. Which of the following associations is incorrect?
A. Polyethylene-phenols
B. Copper sulfate-white phosphorus burns
C. Hydrofluoric acid burns-calcium gluconate
D. Flammable metals-mineral oil
E. Hydrochloride gel-lye

THE VIOLENT PATIENT

Violence may be associated with numerous toxins, such as phencyclidine, alcohol, heroin, amphetamines, and LSD, as well as head trauma, cerebral edema, stroke, meningoencephalitis, central nervous system bleeds, and metabolic abnormalities capable of altering consciousness (e.g., hypoglycemia or hyponatremia). An initial approach should focus on establishing rapport with the patient, ideally by talking. An attempt should be made to address the patient's immediate needs. An offer of food or water may calm the patient and avoid physical confrontation. If these methods fail, medication may be required.

A combination of an antipsychotic medication (e.g., haloperidol or droperidol) with a benzodiazepine (e.g., lorazepam or diazepam) is generally more effective than an antipsychotic alone in treating a violent patient. Many adult patients respond to haloperidol 5 mg and lorazepam 2 mg intramuscularly in the same syringe. In the elderly, only 1–2 mg of haloperidol is used. Side effects of rapid tranquilization with haloperidol include extrapyramidal symptoms in about 10% of patients. These usually develop within 24 hours and may include dystonia, torticollis, opisthotonus, oculogyric crises, laryngospasm, and/or akathisia. Extrapyramidal symptoms may be treated with diphenhydramine 25–50 mg (intravenously or intramuscularly) or benztropine 2 mg i.m. or i.v. repeated every 5 minutes up to three doses or until resolution of symptoms. Relief usually occurs within 1–3 minutes after an intravenous injection.

The blood sugar concentration should be established quickly in any individual who presents violently. If the patient is hypoglycemic, 50% dextrose in water is administered. Benzodiazepines such as lorazepam or diazepam may be quite helpful in sedating aggressive individuals, however overuse can result in hypotension, shallow respirations, and/or apnea. For this reason, medicated violent patients must be carefully monitored in a controlled setting. As the differential diagnosis of altered mental status and/or violent behavior is large, a broad, general laboratory and/or radiographic approach is often warranted.

It is generally advised that a buffer of at least two armlengths between staff and the violent patient be maintained. The presence of security personnel or police officers is vital. Hard restraints should be used quickly but carefully in the seriously violent individual. Rhabdomyolysis has been associated with violent individuals struggling against their restraints and should be checked for in appropriate settings. Haloperidol and droperidol should be avoided in patients suffering from anticholinergic toxic psychosis or who are hot to the touch, especially those who are combative and phencyclidine or cocaine intoxicated. These agents can induce a neuroleptic malignant syndrome.

Questions—The Violent Patient

1. Which of the following regarding the violent patient is false?

A. Metabolic abnormalities may cause violence.
B. Rhabdomyolysis has been associated with violent individuals struggling against their restraints.
C. A combination of an antipsychotic medication with a benzodiazepine is generally more effective than an antipsychotic alone in treating a violent patient.
D. Hard restraints are rarely required to manage the seriously violent patient.
E. Haloperidol and droperidol should be avoided in patients suffering from anticholinergic toxic psychosis.

THE SUICIDAL PATIENT

Most persons who attempt suicide either do not want to kill themselves or are ambivalent about the consequences. The suicide act represents a maladaptive, destructive coping response usually to the emotional turmoil of an acute crisis. The suicidal crisis tends to be episodic and often involves a loved one. Only rarely are patients unequivocal in their desire to die. Health care professionals must thoroughly evaluate the suicide risk of each attempt to identify those patients who represent a continuing risk and who require hospitalization. Risk remains high when the patient feels the attempt has accomplished nothing. Low-risk patients should have a therapeutic treatment plan and psychiatric follow-up should be established before discharge.

The interview should be conducted in an unhurried, quiet environment and should include the interview of family members and / or significant others if possible. The classic successful suicide patient is the middle-aged, single, unemployed male with a recent loss. Three times as many men as women commit suicide, but women make more gestures. The peak age for suicide attempts is between 24 and 44, whereas completed suicides occur more often between 55 and 64. Suicide rates have been highest among divorced persons followed by widows and singles; married persons (except teenagers) have the lowest rates.

Patients who have attempted suicide account for an estimated 0.3–1.0% of all emergency department visits, but this figure may be as high as 12% in the adolescent age group. Up to 80% of patients who successfully complete suicide were seen by a physician within the 6 months immediately before their death, and 50% of them within 1 month. Suicide is the ninth leading cause of death in the United States and accounts for thousands of fatalities annually. It is the second most common cause of death in young adults. Demographic factors only identify potential suicide patients and should not be used alone to determine suicide risk.

Most suicidal patients do not deal effectively with loss. Frequently, the precipitating event for the suicide act will be some real or perceived loss and the patient should be questioned closely about temporal events. Common contributing factors include divorce, death or anniversary of the death of a loved one, and / or rejection by a significant other. Economic stressors may include the loss of a job or home, or other financial reversals. Physical stressors may include medical illness, particularly when terminal, in either the patient or a close family member.

Risk Factors

Two-thirds or more of persons who complete suicides have communicated their intent to others. In at least one study, three-fourths of patients had signs of depressive illness. The degree of lethality in a suicide plan appears to correlate better with a degree of hopelessness than with the presence of depressive illness. The clinician should question the patient for evidence of cognitive, emotional, and biological dysfunction suggestive of depression. Any person who believes that his or her situation will not improve is a high-risk suicide candidate. The degree of hopelessness should be thoroughly explored. The intensity of distress and melancholia correlates with suicide risk.

Acute panic states in schizophrenics unpredictably aggravate a tendency toward suicide by loosening impulse control and distorting reality. Such patients may respond to hallucinogenic commands by violent means including suicide attempts. The delirium caused by ethanol and mind-altering drugs can mobilize suicidal impulses and release normal inhibitions. It has been estimated that 15–25% of people who commit suicide have alcohol addiction problems and about 5% of chronic alcoholics end their lives by suicide. Patients who have previously overcome the taboo of suicide are more likely to try again. Each unsuccessful attempt increases the statistical probability of a completed suicide. Suicide attempts by important role models increase the risk of similar actions by the patient who may harbor reunion fantasies with the dead loved one.

Treatment

- After medical stabilization, the most important aspects of emergency department management of a suicidal patient are determination of the suicide risk and arrangement for appropriate disposition. Potential dispositions include sending the patient home, general medical admission, voluntary psychiatric unit admission, or involuntary psychiatric hospitalization.
- Psychiatric consultation should be obtained for any patient who the physician believes is suicidal. Immediate psychiatric evaluation is necessary for high-risk patients, and all patients who intentionally expose themselves to toxic substances should receive a psychiatric referral. For patients who have passed their suicidal crisis and have regained hope, a discharge plan may be formulated provided the patient has a supportive living environment and will follow a treatment plan. Elements of such plans include establishing contact with a therapist, formulating an agreement or "pact" requiring the patient to re-establish contact if they feel unsafe, and arranging with the family to remove high-risk items and to provide observation.
- Actively suicidal patients should be hospitalized in a secure psychiatric unit with close observation. When medical care is necessary, one-to-one staffing and frequent checks should be provided. All potentially harmful objects including glass, belts, shoelaces, and mirrors are removed. Depending on local

law, appointed psychiatrists, health care teams, or physicians may institute a temporary involuntary commitment. Those patients who constitute a danger to themselves, a danger to others, or who are incapable of caring for themselves will generally be candidates for involuntary commitment if necessary.

Questions—The Suicidal Patient

1. Which of the following is false?

A. Most persons who attempt suicide either do not want to kill themselves or are ambivalent about the consequences.
B. The suicidal crisis tends to be episodic and often involves a loved one.
C. Three times as many men as women commit suicide, but men make only twice as many gestures.
D. Suicide rates have been highest among divorced persons followed by widows and singles.
E. Up to 80% of patients who successfully complete suicide were seen by a physician within the 6 months immediately before their death, and 50% of them within 1 month.

Answers

Evaluation of (A) Airway

1. E

Evaluation of (B) Breathing, Ventilation, and Oxygenation

1. A 2. C 3. A 4. C 5. D 6. A 7. C

Evaluation of (C) Circulation

1. B 2. A 3. C 4. B 5. B

Evaluation of (D) Depression of the Central Nervous System

1. B 2. D 3. C

Decontamination

1. E 2. B 3. E

The Violent Patient

1. D

The Suicidal Patient

1. C

CHAPTER 3

The Diagnosis of Poisoning

INTRODUCTION

The management of patients who overdose on drugs and chemicals is often independent of the specific agent(s) that are implicated in that overdose. Fundamental concepts of management in medical toxicology, such as aggressive support of ventilatory, cardiovascular, metabolic, and neurologic functions, are often performed with partial or absent information regarding offending agents. While knowledge of specific agents is helpful, particularly where antidotal intervention may be applicable, it may be impossible to ascertain in depressed, pediatric, obtunded, or evasive patients.

Discrepancies between clinical impressions and certain laboratory results may be multifactorial. Patients and friends may give unreliable histories. Finding an empty medicine container, for example, does not necessarily imply ingestion of that agent. Threshold concentrations required by laboratories to detect individual agents might influence the performance of the laboratory. Errors in toxicology have been documented in both false-positive and false-negative directions. The laboratory is not always the absolute "gold standard."

Potentially important unsuspected drugs are found in only a small minority of patients. Clinical characteristics of patients with unsuspected drug identifications are not significantly different from those of other patients and unexpected laboratory results rarely lead to changes in patient management and probably never affect outcome. Laboratory discovery of an unsuspected drug often does not appear as a marker for severity of illness and does not, in itself, identify patients requiring closer observation or having a poorer prognosis. While objective data may identify agents and confirm historical elements, clinical management is unlikely to be affected.

The ultimate value of identifying poisons or toxins must be weighed against the economic impact of performance of such tests in many patients who do not require them. The health care professional should ascertain whether the local hospital laboratory is capable of performing tests in a timely manner for those drugs whose identification or concentration exhibit a useful correlation with the clinical status of the patient.

Questions—Introduction to the Diagnosis of Poisoning

1. Which of the following statements is false?

A. Finding an empty medicine container does not necessarily imply ingestion.
B. Clinical characteristics of patients with unsuspected drug identifications are not significantly different from those of other patients and unexpected laboratory results rarely lead to changes in patient management and probably never affect outcome.
C. Fundamental concepts of management in medical toxicology, such as aggressive support of ventilatory, cardiovascular, metabolic, and neurologic functions, are often performed with partial or absent information regarding offending agents.

Answers to questions in shaded boxes appear at the end of the chapter.

D. Errors in toxicology have been both false-positive and false-negative.
E. The laboratory is always the "gold standard."

THE TOXIC SCREEN

Drug screening is one tool used to evaluate patients with altered mental status, unexplained symptoms, or coma of unclear etiology. In known overdose cases, comprehensive toxicology screening contributes little when patients are responsive to verbal stimuli and stable during hours of observation. It may be reasonable to obtain general toxicology screens in seriously ill patients in whom antidotes, dialysis, or hemoperfusion may be beneficial.

Clinical judgment must ultimately guide decisions regarding the use of toxic screens and the laboratory. A drug screen may be indicated when the history is unreliable, in multiple-drug ingestions, in delirious or comatose patients, after head trauma, in a seizing patient with unclear etiology, for the identification of specific drugs, as a medico-legal adjunct, to indicate when antagonists may be used, and to aid in the estimation of prognosis. A toxic screen is not necessary in stable individuals who give reliable histories, in patients who have been observed by reliable individuals, in stable psychiatric patients, and as a matter of course in all patients who present with unexplained symptoms.

Limitations

Toxicology laboratories use several methods to screen for toxins, because there is no single, accurate, inexpensive method to detect them all. Each method differs in cost, accuracy, complexity, speed, and specificity. Individual test reliability depends on analyst expertise, equipment, method, and the number of requests processed. Problems arise from changes that occur in the storage of biologic fluids, the transfer of drugs from tube to tube, and the standards used to test drugs. Familiarity with specific laboratory requirements, processes, and limitations is critical to the proper utilization of the laboratory.

The use of toxicology testing as a broad screen without an understanding of its limitations is hazardous. Many drugs are often not detected by toxicology screen. While specifics may vary between institutions, agents commonly not found in toxic screens include hemoglobins, metals, diuretics, halogens, solvents, pesticides, radioactive compounds, antibiotics, vitamins, many nonsteroidal antiinflammatory compounds, calcium channel blockers and beta blockers. Laboratories may group similar classes of drugs into classes or panels (e.g., drugs of abuse, anticonvulsants, alcohols, etc.). Ordering the "wrong" panel can yield false-negative results if the clinician's initial impression is wrong or misguided.

Again, few potentially important unsuspected drugs are found in most poisoned patients and discovery of a clinically unsuspected drug does not serve as a marker of the severity of illness. While the toxicology screen may change management based on clinical history in overdose with certain agents (e.g., acetaminophen, salicylates, lithium, theophylline, methanol, ethylene glycol, and digoxin) it is not universally required to manage overdoses with most agents. Furthermore, a positive urine toxic screen (in the workplace or elsewhere) for drugs of abuse does not indicate that an individual was clinically affected when the specimen was collected, or predict the frequency of use, the pattern of use, or addiction.

Questions—The Toxic Screen

1. A qualitative drug screen may be indicated in each of the following, except
A. When the history is unreliable
B. In multiple-drug ingestions
C. In delirious or comatose patients
D. As a medico-legal adjunct
E. To determine eligibility for intensive care

2. Which of the following is false?
A. Few potentially important unsuspected drugs are found in most poisoned patients and discovery of a clinically unsuspected drug often serves as a marker of toxic severity.
B. While the toxicology screen may change management based on clinical history in overdose with certain agents, it is not universally required to manage overdoses with most agents.
C. A positive urine toxic screen for drugs of abuse does not indicate that an individual was clinically affected when the specimen was collected.
D. Toxicology laboratories use several methods to screen for toxins.
E. Problems arise from changes that occur in the storage of biologic fluids, the transfer of drugs from tube to tube, and the standards used to test drugs.

THE LABORATORY APPROACH

Of the thousands of agents available for poisoning, non-research laboratories are able to detect only about 100, and quantitate far fewer, in body fluids. Expectations of the clinical toxicology laboratory often exceed reality, especially in the present environment of cost containment. Because of the limitations of time, expense, and number of drugs commonly encountered, toxicology screens do not include all toxic possibilities.

In general, the laboratory remains a selective adjunct to the clinical evaluation of the patient. Good clinical communication, proper specimens, knowledge of specific laboratory procedures, and the proper use of each test are required to maximize the effectiveness of a clinical laboratory. Laboratories may not reliably identify drugs in the serum of overdosed patients, partly because of technical limitations, partly because of laboratory error, and possibly because of inadequate specimens. Drugs judged responsible for an overdose are not always identified, depending on the standards and capabilities of individual laboratories.

General Methods

Since about 15—20 drugs account for almost 90% of pharmaceutical poisonings, most laboratories limit drug screens to those substances commonly involved in poisonings. Initially the samples are separated into bases and acids. Weak acids (e.g., barbiturates) are un-ionized in acid pH and easily extracted from an acidified sample. Weak bases (e.g., phenothiazines and opiates) are extracted under alkaline conditions.

Simple, rapid screening methods (1.5-hour turnaround time) can detect 94–98% of all substances eventually found by sophisticated chromatographic methods, by combining spot tests, immunoassay, and thin-layer chromatography (TLC). Urine spot tests (i.e., rudimentary tests generally involving the addition of a reagent to a urine specimen) are available for salicylates, acetaminophen, phenothiazines, glucose, ketone bodies, opiates, barbiturates, benzodiazepines, benzoylecgonine, phencyclidine, and tetrahydrocannabinol. Many such tests have not been subject to clinically controlled studies.

Although screens vary between laboratories, gas-liquid chromatography (GLC) generally screens for volatiles (i.e., alcohols) and enzyme-mediated immunoassay technique (EMIT) screens for drugs of abuse such as benzodiazepines, opiates, cocaine metabolites, phencyclidine, methaqualone, barbiturates, and propoxyphene. TLC screens both the urine and serum. Positive results are generally confirmed by another method, generally TLC or EMIT. If questions persist, gas-liquid chromatography is generally used.

Urine and Blood Samples

Urine samples are preferred when blood concentrations of known or suspected compounds are too low for detection by conventional means. Such drugs usually have either rapid elimination or large volumes of distribution. Examples are phenothiazines, barbiturates, benzodiazepines, sedative-hypnotics, tricyclic antidepressants and antihistamines.

Blood samples are preferred when detectable levels occur in blood, because these concentrations are more representative of the concentrations at receptor sites. Blood levels are quantitative, whereas urine levels are qualitative. Not all blood levels correlate with clinical effects. Basic drugs have large volumes of distribution and often are better detected in the urine, whereas acid and neutral drugs are more easily detected in blood screens.

Hair Samples

Reports on the detection of drugs of abuse in human hair have appeared for opiates, cocaine, benzoylecgonine, morphine, phencyclidine, methadone, methamphetamine, caffeine, nicotine, phenobarbital, haloperidol, digoxin, antidepressants, chloroquine, and desethylchloroquine. The presence of a dose-response relationship between administered dose and hair drug level, and the time course of drug appearance in hair has not yet been demonstrated. The clinical usefulness of hair screening techniques is yet to be defined or rejected by clinical studies.

Hair analyses have been performed by radioimmunoassay with confirmation by standard gas chromatography-mass spectrometry (GC-MS) techniques. Sampling of hair is subject to contamination by passive means, cross-reaction, or leaching by toiletries. Once incorporated into hair, drugs remain there indefinitely and can be detected as long as the hair is available. It may be possible, depending on hair length, to trace the drug intake of an addict over periods longer than 6 months.

Drug concentrations differ in head hair, axillary hair, and pubic hair. Secretion of drugs in perspiration affects this mechanism of deposition and remains a confounding factor. Laboratory analysis of hair is laborious and tedious. Diffusion of drugs within hair may cause difficulties in interpretation of positive and negative results. No protocols have addressed the stability of drugs in hair, particularly in hair that has been bleached, dyed, or treated with sprays, rinses, or other preparations available to beauticians and to the public.

Meconium Samples

Meconium drug analysis is useful for drug testing in the newborn period and may be highly specific and sensitive. Meconium analysis can be performed with common laboratory techniques for screening purposes and confirmed by GC-MS. Collection of meconium is easy and noninvasive, and analysis of serial meconium samples can reflect the type, chronology, and amount of in utero drug exposure by the infant. Drugs in meconium are present up to 3 days after birth.

Meconium represents the entire intestinal contents of the fetus before birth and is composed of desquamated epithelial cells, bile, pancreatic and intestinal secretions, and the residue of swallowed amniotic fluid. Serial analysis of meconium may be a useful tool to determine the pattern of drug use by the mother throughout gestation. Meconium is available during the first day of life. Its passage may occur in the first hour of life but usually occurs by the tenth hour.

Studies have suggested that cocaine, benzoylecgonine, and morphine in meconium can correlate with the amounts of drugs used by the mother during pregnancy. Nicotine metabolites in meconium may provide a quantifiable measure of fetal exposure to nicotine by active and passive maternal smoking. Cocaethylene, a metabolite of cocaine and ethanol appears in the meconium. Its presence may corroborate neurobehavioral abnormalities seen in the cocaine baby syndrome.

Saliva Samples

Marijuana, cocaine, phencyclidine, opiates, barbiturates, amphetamines, and benzodiazepines have all been detected in saliva by various analytic methods including immunoassay, GC-MS, and TLC. Initial studies with cocaine and phencyclidine suggest a correlation between saliva and plasma concentrations of these drugs, indicating a dynamic equilibrium between saliva and blood.

Concentrations of drug are usually lower in saliva than in urine; however, assay methods now available can detect the quantities present. Saliva may eliminate privacy issues and possible adulterations during sample collection. Drug concentrations in saliva provide an estimate of the actual circulating amount, and the results may be used to determine intoxication.

Sweat Samples

Drugs that have been detected after use of a "sweat patch" include cocaine, heroin, methamphetamine, phencyclidine, and Δ^9-tetrahydrocannabinol. Further studies are needed to delineate the clinical importance of sweat sample analysis.

Qualitative Tests

Qualitative tests confirm the presence of chemicals above certain minimum concentrations. Their primary use is confirmation of clinical diagnosis as no direct correlation exists between qualitative screens and clinical effects. Qualitative drug screens require blood samples (5–10 mL of both clotted and anticoagulated blood), urine samples (50 mL), and/or gastric samples (25–50 mL).

Pills, capsules, and other contraband may help the laboratory by providing high concentrations of the drug that may be present in the screen. Gastric aspirates provide high concentrations of unmetabolized drug, and the first 25–50 mL should be saved and refrigerated. Urine samples are required, because many basic drugs do not achieve high blood levels.

Quantitative Tests

The usefulness of quantitative levels in the management of poisoned patients depends on the correlation of drug level to clinical effects. Clinical responses to the few drugs that do correlate with identifiable serum concentrations may be modified by a variety of patient and drug factors. These include individual variations in pharmacokinetics, individual variations in metabolism including tolerance, underlying medical diseases, formation of toxic metabolites, and the presence of other drugs. Quantitative blood tests should be limited to those drugs for which blood levels predict subsequent toxicity or guide specific therapy, such as hemodialysis, hemoperfusion, or administration of antidotes.

Quantitative drug screens require blood samples. Since toxicity usually correlates with peak receptor levels, samples should ideally be taken after complete absorption. The duration of effect depends on pharmacokinetic parameters that are influenced by both patient and drug variables. As these factors may delay toxicity, serial drug levels (2–4 hours apart) should be taken in cases in which blood levels influence management, until a clear trend is established.

Agents for which blood levels may help management include acetaminophen (e.g., the Rumack-Matthew nomogram may be used to determine the need for n-acetylcysteine), salicylates (e.g., the Done nomogram may help estimate toxicity and concentrations may guide the need for dialysis), carboxyhemoglobin (there may be a rough correlation with clinical picture), methemoglobin (concentration may suggest the need for methylene blue), methanol and ethylene glycol (concentration may suggest the need for dialysis, ethanol or 4-methylpyrazole), lithium (concentration may guide the need for dialysis), and iron (concentration may suggest the need for deferoxamine).

Other agents for which blood levels may help management include paraquat (the concentration may predict outcome and guide the use of hemoperfusion), digoxin (concentration may suggest the need for fab fragments), theophylline (concentration may suggest the need for dialysis or hemoperfusion), organophosphates (the RBC cholinesterase level may predict outcome or guide the use of oxime therapy), ethanol (concentration may confirm diagnosis and predict length of intoxication), phenytoin (there may be a rough correlation with clinical picture), and metals such as lead, cadmium, mercury and arsenic (concentration may suggest the need for chelation therapy).

Questions—The Laboratory Approach

1. Non-research labs are able to detect
- A. Thousands of poisons.
- B. About 100 agents.
- C. Only 2 or 3 drugs reliably.
- D. No drugs. All testing must be sent to research labs for reliability.
- E. None of the above.

2. Which of the following is true?
- A. About 15–20 drugs account for almost 90% of pharmaceutical poisonings.
- B. About 2–5 drugs account for almost 90% of pharmaceutical poisonings.
- C. Weak acids (e.g., barbiturates) are ionized in acid pH.
- D. Weak bases (e.g., phenothiazines) are best extracted under acidic conditions.
- E. None of the above.

3. Which of the following is false?
- A. Although screens vary between laboratories, gas-liquid chromatography (GLC) generally screens for volatiles (e.g., alcohols).
- B. Enzyme-mediated immunoassay technique (EMIT) screens for drugs of abuse such as benzodiazepines, opiates, cocaine metabolites, phencyclidine, methaqualone, barbiturates, and propoxyphene.
- C. Thin-layer chromatography (TLC) can only screen urine.
- D. Positive results are generally confirmed by another method.
- E. None of the above.

4. All of the following are true except
- A. Urine samples are preferred when blood concentrations of known or suspected compounds are too low for detection by conventional means.
- B. Blood samples are preferred when detectable levels occur in blood, because these concentrations are more representative of the concentrations at receptor sites.
- C. Blood levels are quantitative, whereas urine levels are qualitative.
- D. Blood levels, rather than urine levels, typically correlate with clinical effects.
- E. Basic drugs have large volumes of distribution and often are better detected in the urine, whereas acid and neutral drugs are more easily detected in blood screens.

5. Which of the following is false?
- A. Drug concentrations differ in head hair, axillary hair, and pubic hair.
- B. Meconium drug analysis is useful for drug testing in the newborn period and may be highly specific and sensitive.
- C. Meconium analysis requires rarely used laboratory techniques for screening
- D. Collection of meconium is easy and noninvasive, and analysis of serial meconium samples can reflect the type, chronology, and amount of in utero drug exposure by the infant.
- E. Drugs in meconium are present up to 3 days after birth.

6. Drugs which have been identified in meconium include
- A. Cocaine
- B. Morphine
- C. Cocaethylene
- D. All of the above
- E. A and C

7. Which of the following is true?
- A. Marijuana, cocaine, phencyclidine, opiates, barbiturates, amphetamines, and benzodiazepines have all been detected in saliva by various analytic methods.
- B. Initial studies with cocaine and phencyclidine suggest no correlation between saliva and plasma concentrations of these drugs.
- C. Concentrations of drugs are usually higher in saliva than in urine.
- D. Drug concentrations in saliva provide an estimate of inhaled amount, and the results may be used to determine intoxication.
- E. None of the above.

ANALYTIC METHODS

Chromatography, the most frequently used analytic technique, involves a separation method based on the flow of a mobile liquid or gas over a solid or stationary phase containing the unknown. Immunoassays such as enzyme multiple immunoassay technique (EMIT) or radioimmunoassay are sensitive techniques which are less specific than chromatographic or mass spectrometry methods.

Atomic Absorption Spectrophotometry

Atomic absorption spectrophotometry is the usual method for detecting inorganic agents such as lead, mercury, thallium, and cadmium but is not suitable as a screening technique. Most toxicology screens do not detect heavy metals. Inductively coupled plasma atomic emission spectroscopy allows simultaneous multi-element analysis and is useful in the industrial workplace. This method quantitatively measures 17 elements from a single sample.

Enzyme-Mediated Immunoassay Technique

The enzyme-mediated immunoassay technique (EMIT) is a fast, expensive, and simple method with intermediate accuracy and specificity. This system works on the principle that the amount of drug present in a specimen is proportional to the inhibition of an enzyme-substrate reaction. A known quantity of drug is labeled by chemical attachment to an enzyme. Drug-specific antibodies added to the specimen bind the drug-enzyme complex, thereby reducing enzyme activity. Free drug in the specimen competes with enzyme-labeled drug and limits the antibody-induced enzyme inactivation. Enzyme activity correlates with drug concentration in the specimen. This is measured by absorbance changes resulting from the enzyme's catalytic action on a substrate.

EMIT is preferred over other radioimmunoassay methods in emergent situations because of its simplicity and speed in providing information on toxic drug concentrations. EMIT eliminates the complex separation phase necessary in radioimmunoassays. Two systems available are EMIT-ST (single test), consisting of a compact spectrophotometer for small laboratories, and EMIT-dau (drugs of abuse) for larger hospitals. Negative tests do not exclude the ingestion of a drug that may be present in undetectable quantities.

The most common cause of false-positive results from EMIT is antibody cross-reactivity with substances which bear structural similarities to the drug being tested. Examples include poppy seeds, which may contain opium congeners, resulting in a drug screen that is positive for opiates. Dextromethorphan, chlorpromazine, and diphenoxylate can also yield false-positive opiate results. Nasal decongestants such as ephedrine and phenylpropanolamine can produce a false-positive urine drug screen for amphetamines. Phenylephrine, pseudoephedrine, n-acetylprocainamide, chloroquine, and procainamide can also yield false-positive amphetamine results. False-positive detection of phencyclidine may occur with dextromethorphan, diphenhydramine, chlorpromazine, doxylamine and thioridazine.

False-negative screens may result from technological shortcomings, if the drug screen does not seek the drug in question, structural dissimilarity of drug from drug-class prototype (e.g., fentanyl), poor quality assurance, toxicokinetic characteristics, large volumes of distribution, and short elimination half-lives. False-negatives may also result from intentional specimen alteration or adulteration (e.g., use of a colleague's "clean" urine, use of a fluid other than urine, drinking excessive fluids, use of a diuretic, and/or addition of bleach, caustics, golden seal tea, lemon juice, salt, soap, or vinegar to urine).

Gas Chromatography-Mass Spectrometry

Gas chromatography-mass spectrometry (GC-MS) combines substance retention times seen in gas chromatography with characteristic fragmentation patterns seen with mass spectroscopy. Libraries of fragmentation patterns may be used to screen for a large variety of agents simultaneously. Although gas chromatography-mass spectroscopy is probably the best, almost "foolproof" technique to determine the presence of chemicals or drugs, it is also quite costly. The high capital equipment expense and operating costs limit its use to reference centers.

Gas-Liquid Chromatography

Gas-liquid chromatography (GLC) is a sophisticated but somewhat slow method that is highly accurate and specific. Liquid or dissolved solid specimens are injected into the column and vaporized by heat. Inert gases carry the specimen out of the column where chemical detectors record the emergence of the specimen as a function of time. The comparison of retention times and peak areas with known standards allows identification and quantitation. This method is effective for quantitation of blood levels of volatile liquids such as methanol, ethanol, and ethylene glycol.

High-Pressure Liquid Chromatography

High-pressure liquid chromatography (HPLC) is similar in speed, specificity, and expense to GLC, but is not restricted to volatiles. Complex compounds, including conjugated metabolites, are well separated by facilitating the movement of specimens with high pressures (1,000–6,000 psi).

Radioimmunoassay

Radioimmunoassay is a slow, expensive method, but has good accuracy. Mixing known quantities of drug-specific antibody and amounts of radioactive labeled drug allows analysis of a resulting precipitate with a gamma counter. The amount of emittance inversely correlates with the presence of assayed drug. This test is excellent for detection of drugs in extremely low blood concentrations such as cannabinoids (marijuana), LSD, digoxin, and paraquat.

Thin-Layer Chromatography

Thin-layer chromatography (TLC) is a simple, inexpensive technique that is effective for qualitative screening, but not for quantitative measurements. Separation of substances results from absorption or partition as mobile solvent moves across a stationary sorbent phase (usually silicic acid or aluminum oxide). A characteristic amount of migration occurs for a specific test substance after the test specimen is applied to the base of the liquid solvent system. These tests take about 2 hours and must be interpreted carefully by experienced technicians.

There are commercially available thin-layer chromatographic systems with less performance expertise required (than for standard TLC) that chromatographically screen for drugs.

Ultraviolet Spectrophotometry

Ultraviolet spectrophotometry (UVS) is an easy, economical, and quantitative test that can detect toxic blood acetaminophen and salicylate levels as well as elevated urine phenothiazine levels. However, interference by multi-drug ingestions seriously impairs its accuracy and restricts its use.

Questions—Analytic Methods

1. **Which of the following is false?**
   A. Atomic absorption spectrophotometry is the usual method for detecting inorganic agents such as lead, mercury, thallium, and cadmium but is not suitable as a screening technique.
   B. Most toxicology screens detect heavy metals.
   C. Inductively coupled plasma atomic emission spectroscopy allows simultaneous multi-element analysis and is useful in the industrial workplace.
   D. The enzyme-mediated immunoassay technique (EMIT) is a fast, expensive, and simple method with intermediate accuracy and specificity.
   E. EMIT is preferred over other radioimmunoassay methods in emergent situations because of its simplicity and speed in providing information on toxic drug concentrations.

2. **Which of the following is false?**
   A. EMIT eliminates the complex separation phase necessary in radioimmunoassays.
   B. The most common cause of false-positive results from EMIT is antibody cross-reactivity with substances which bear structural similarities to the drug being tested.
   C. Poppy seeds can produce a false-positive urine drug screen for amphetamines.
   D. Phenylephrine, pseudoephedrine, n-acetylprocainamide, chloroquine, and procainamide can also yield false-positive amphetamine results.
   E. False-positive detection of phencyclidine may occur with dextromethorphan, diphenhydramine, chlorpromazine, doxylamine and thioridazine.

3. **False-negative screens may result**
   A. From technological shortcomings
   B. If the drug screen does not seek the drug in question
   C. From poor quality assurance
   D. From long elimination half-lives
   E. A, B and C

4. **Which of the following is false?**
   A. Gas chromatography-mass spectrometry (GC-MS) combines substance retention times seen in gas chromatography, with characteristic fragmentation patterns seen with mass spectroscopy.
   B. Gas chromatography-mass spectroscopy is probably the best, almost "foolproof" technique to determine the presence of chemicals or drugs.
   C. GC-MS is an excellent screening tool because it detects many drugs.
   D. Gas-liquid chromatography (GLC) is a sophisticated but somewhat slow method that is highly accurate and specific.
   E. GLC is effective for quantitation of blood levels of volatile liquids such as methanol, ethanol, and ethylene glycol.

5. **High-pressure liquid chromatography (HPLC)**
   A. Is similar in speed, specificity, and expense to GLC, but is restricted to volatiles.
   B. Can separate complex compounds, including conjugated metabolites, by facilitating the movement of specimens with high pressures.
   C. Is rarely used as GC-MS has replaced its usefulness.
   D. A and B
   E. All of the above.

6. **Which of the following is false?**
   A. Radioimmunoassay is a slow, expensive method, but has good accuracy.
   B. Mixing known quantities of drug-specific antibody and amounts of radioactive labeled drug allows analysis of a resulting precipitate with a gamma counter in radioimmunoassay.
   C. The amount of emittance directly correlates with the presence of assayed drug.
   D. Radioimmunoassay is excellent for detection of drugs in extremely low blood concentrations such as cannabinoids (marijuana), lysergic acid diethylamide (LSD), digoxin, and paraquat.
   E. None of the above.

7. **Thin-layer chromatography (TLC)**
   A. Is a complex, expensive technique that is effective for qualitative screening, but not for quantitative measurements.
   B. Involves separation of substances from absorption or partition as mobile solvent moves across a stationary sorbent phase (usually silicic acid or aluminum oxide).
   C. Must be interpreted carefully by experienced technicians.
   D. A and C
   E. B and C

ANION GAP

The anion gap is calculated from serum electrolytes as Anion Gap (AG) = [Sodium] − ([Bicarbonate] + [Chloride]) where the normal AG is about 12–14 mEq/L. The normal gap represents the difference between unmeasured anions (e.g., proteins, organic acids, phosphates, and sulfates) and unmeasured cations (e.g., potassium, calcium, and magnesium).

Metabolic acidosis results from ingestion, increased production, or decreased excretion of nonvolatile acids, or from the loss of body alkali. The serum anion gap (AG) distinguishes between two types of metabolic acidosis: increased anion gap acidosis or normal anion gap acidosis. Some toxins produce an increased anion gap acidosis characterized by the accumulation of organic acids.

Causes of a high anion gap acidosis include metabolic acidosis, dehydration, infusions of salts of organic acids (e.g., lactate, acetate, and citrate), reduced unmeasured cations (e.g., potassium, calcium, and magnesium), alkalemia, lab error, and underestimation of serum chloride. A number of agents have been associated with a decreased anion gap. A suggested mnemonic for this list is "BLIND" (**B**romide, **L**ithium, **I**odide, **N**itrate, and **D**iatrizoate sodium).

A suggested mnemonic for causes of a high anion gap acidosis is "I Love Chocolate Raspberry Truffle MUDPIES." (**I**ron, isoniazid (INH), idiopathic, **L**actate, **C**arbon monoxide, cyanide, **R**espiratory dysfunction, **T**oluene, **M**ethanol, **U**remia, **D**iabetic ketoacidosis (DKA), **P**araldehyde, phenformin, **I**ron, isoniazid (INH), idiopathic, **E**thylene glycol, ethanol, **S**alicylates, strychnine, seizures, hydrogen sulfide, starvation, sympathomimetics).

Normal or non-anion gap acidosis results from loss of bicarbonate (e.g., diarrhea, and/or renal tubular acidosis) or from the addition of chloride-containing acids (e.g., ammonium chloride or calcium chloride). Drugs associated with a non-anion gap metabolic acidosis include acetazolamide, amphotericin B, amiloride, spironolactone, and toluene. The anion gap may be normal in the early stages of methanol and ethylene glycol poisoning when ethanol coingestion prevents formation of their metabolites.

The anion gap calculation may not signal the presence of all cases of clinically important lactic acidosis. Increased blood lactate is a reflection of ineffective tissue oxygenation and carries a poor prognosis in critically ill patients. Lactic acidosis may be defined as a pH less than 7.4 and a blood lactate greater than 2.5 mmol/L. Lactate elevations are considered high (usually 100% mortality) when levels are more than 10 mmol/L, moderate (usually 75% mortality) between 5 and 9.9 mmol/L, and mild (approximately 35% mortality) between 2.5–4.9 mmol/L.

When the lactate level is very high, the anion gap will be at the upper limits of normal or elevated. However, the anion gap may not be elevated in 50% of patients with a moderate lactate elevation and in up to 80% of those with mild elevation. Therefore, elevated serum lactate should be included in the differential diagnosis of non-anion gap acidosis.

Questions—Anion Gap

Case Study (Questions 1 and 2)

A 23-year-old homeless man presents to the emergency room after drinking 8 ounces of ethylene glycol. On arrival, he is obtunded. His laboratory results include: Sodium 143, Potassium 5.0, Chloride 92, Bicarbonate 20.

1. **His anion gap is**
   A. Cannot be calculated from these lab tests alone
   B. 36
   C. 25
   D. 51
   E. 31
2. **His anion gap**
   A. Is normal.
   B. Reflects lactic acidosis.
   C. Reflects metabolic acidosis.
   D. Reflects metabolic alkalosis.
   E. Cannot be calculated.
3. **Causes of a high anion gap include all of the following except**
   A. Iron
   B. LSD
   C. Carbon monoxide
   D. Diabetic ketoacidosis
   E. Ethylene glycol
4. **Drugs associated with a non-anion gap metabolic acidosis include**
   A. Acetazolamide
   B. Amphotericin B
   C. Spironolactone
   D. A and C
   E. All of the above.
5. **Agents associated with a decreased anion gap include all of the following except**
   A. Bromide
   B. Lactate
   C. Iodide
   D. Nitrate
   E. Diatrizoate sodium

OSMOLAL GAP

Osmolality is the concentration of osmotically active particles in a solution. The degree to which any chemical substance contributes to the osmolality of a solution is simply based on the number of molecules present. One millimole of substance will contribute 1 mOsm to the measured osmolality. One ethanol molecule (molecular weight 46), for example, has the same osmotic activity as one molecule of albumin (molecular weight 66,500).

The osmolal gap represents the difference between measured osmolality (measured by freezing point depression) and calculated osmolality. Osmolality may be calculated from the major osmotically active substances in the serum. These substances include sodium, glucose, and blood urea nitrogen (BUN).

$$\text{Osmolal Gap} = \text{Osmolality (measured)} - \text{Osmolality (calculated)}$$

$$\text{Calculated Osmolality} = 2(\text{Na}) + \frac{\text{glucose}}{18} + \frac{\text{BUN}}{2.8}$$

Elevated osmolal gaps result from decreased serum water (e.g., hyperlipidemia and hyperprothrombinemia) or high concentrations of low-molecular-weight substances. For toxicologic purposes, if the serum does not appear lipemic, an osmolal gap indicates the presence of low-molecular- weight toxin(s). A gap greater than 10 mosm is abnormal.

A suggested mnemonic for the causes of an osmolal gap is "ME DIE." (**M**ethanol, **E**thanol, **D**iuretics (e.g., mannitol, sorbitol, and glycerol), **I**sopropanol, and **E**thylene glycol). Other causes include glycerin, diatrizoate sodium, isoniazid, acetone, ether, trichloroethane, paraldehyde, and chloroform. The presence of toxic levels of many low-molecular-weight substances including ethylene glycol is not easily detected by the serum osmolality. A normal gap does not exclude toxic levels of methanol or ethylene glycol.

The osmolal gap can provide a rough estimation of serum ethanol levels by the formula:

$$\text{Estimated Ethanol (mg/dL)} = \frac{\text{Osmolal Gap}}{10} \times 46$$

Serum osmolality should be used as a screening measure for the presence of selected solvents rather than as an estimation of blood ethanol levels. In the absence of an increased osmolal gap, ethanol is an unlikely cause of coma and other causes should be considered (e.g., subdural hematoma, stroke, another drug). The finding of both an osmolal and an anion gap, in the absence of detectable ethanol, is considered strong evidence for poisoning by methanol or ethylene glycol or for alcoholic ketoacidosis (AKA).

Dehydration and rehydration may affect the accuracy of formulas used to calculate the osmolal gap. Most formulas are based on the assumption that serum is about 93% water. However, this numeric "constant" may change as the hydration state changes. A dehydrated patient may have a fraction as low as 0.89 or as high as 0.94 when rehydrated. Pathologic processes associated with alcoholism may contribute to the osmolal gap.

Alcoholic ketoacidosis, for example, with an unexplained osmolal gap and a large anion gap could mimic ethylene glycol or methanol poisoning.

Questions—Osmolal Gap

1. One ethanol molecule (molecular weight 46) has the same osmotic activity as one molecule of albumin (molecular weight 66,500).
A. True
B. False

2. Causes of an osmolal gap include all of the following except
A. Methanol
B. Ethanol
C. Certain Diuretics
D. Isopropanol
E. Iron

Case Study (Questions 3, 4 and 5)
A 23-year-old homeless man presents to the emergency room after drinking 8 ounces of ethanol. His laboratory results include: Sodium 143, Potassium 5.0, Chloride 92, Bicarbonate 20, Glucose 180, BUN 56, Creatinine 1.7, Osmolality 346.

3. His calculated osmolality is
A. 316
B. It cannot be calculated
C. 326
D. 31.6
E. 379

4. His osmolal gap is
A. 10
B. 20
C. 30
D. 40
E. 316

5. His estimated ethanol (in mg/dL) calculated from his osmolal gap is
A. It cannot be calculated
B. 13.8
C. <10
D. 138
E. 154

RADIOLOGIC TECHNIQUES

Some pills and substances may be detected by radiologic techniques. While certain substances are radiopaque in ideal, *in vitro* circumstances, their detection in patients may be difficult. The radiopacity of a pill or toxin depends on the radiodensity of surrounding tissues and may be affected by the position of the patient, previous substances in the gastrointestinal tract, and its physical form (e.g., liquid, solid, pill matrix, etc).

In general, the number of poisons that are consistently detected by simple radiograph is quite limited. While detection may confirm the presence of certain toxins, plain films rarely affect management issues. The use of an abdominal x-ray to screen obtunded patients with possible overdoses is generally not helpful.

Abdominal X-Ray

In certain cases, identification of toxins by radiography may be helpful. These include substances that have been shown to be radiodense with *in vitro* models, and by experience in actual human poisonings. Iron tablet ingestion may demonstrate pills or pill fragments by x-ray. Serial x-rays may be helpful in following the progress of decontamination techniques such as whole bowel lavage and in roughly quantifying the amount of iron ingested. Heavy metals and certain mothballs may be seen. Foreign objects such as button batteries, coins, pica (e.g., clay and paint chips) and radiopaque packets containing illicit drugs (i.e., with body "packers" and "stuffers") may also be identified and followed.

The well-known mnemonic "CHIPE" has been used to describe radiodense substances potentially detectable on the abdominal flat plate or KUB. (**C**hloral hydrate, carbon tetrachloride, **H**eavy metals, **I**odine, **P**henothiazines, and **E**nteric coated tablets). This mnemonic is limited in that it does not refer to all radiodense pills, and does not reflect the physical conditions of the toxins it suggest (e.g., not all chloral hydrate will be seen on KUB). The presence of tablets following ingestion, and the absence of opacities after decontamination measures, may aid diagnostic or therapeutic decisions but by themselves do not dictate management.

The abdominal flat plate may also yield a variety of clues not associated with the radiodensity of a toxin. Perforation and subdiaphragmatic air may follow caustic ingestions. Pneumoperitoneum may be seen after forceful vomiting associated with ipecac or after insertion of a gastric lavage tube. An ileus may be associated with numerous anticholinergic toxins and opiates. Mechanical obstruction may be due to concretion formation or bezoars. Intestinal infarction has been seen with cocaine, ergots, contraceptives and hypotensive agents.

Bone X-Ray

Numerous bony abnormalities have been associated with certain toxins. The appearance of lead lines and metaphyseal changes may corroborate chronic lead exposure. Chronic steroid use may yield osteoporosis and osteonecrosis. Hypervitaminosis D may also yield osteoporosis. Hypervitaminosis A may be associated with cortical hyperostosis and subperiosteal bone formation. Acro-osteolysis has been associated with vinyl chloride. Chronic fluoride exposure may be associated with osteosclerosis and ligamentous calcifications.

Chest X-Ray

An x-ray of the chest should be taken in all patients with tachypnea, coma, or obtundation to search for potential causes of hypoxemia. These might include toxic pneumonitis (e.g., from respiratory irritants such as nitrogen oxides, phosgene, and metals), aspiration pneumonitis (e.g., from hydrocarbon ingestions or gastric contents after seizures), cardiogenic or noncardiogenic shock (e.g., from opiate or salicylate toxicity), pulmonary edema, and atelectasis. Pneumomediastinum may be seen after crack use. Diaphragmatic and pleural plaques may be seen after chronic asbestos exposure, and other pneumoconioses (e.g., silicosis, and beryllium) may yield abnormal interstitial patterns.

Head CT Scan and MRI

Computed tomography of the head (CT or CAT scan) and/or other methods of central nervous system visualization, such as magnetic resonance imaging (MRI), can yield numerous diagnostic clues. An emergency CT scan in an obtunded or comatose patient may yield numerous toxic and non-toxic possibilities. Findings include intracerebral bleeds, tumors, subdural and epidural hematomas, subarachnoid hemorrhage, and strokes.

Cocaine, amphetamines, phencyclidine, and sympathomimetics have been associated with intraparenchymal bleeds. Trauma related to alcohol and drugs of abuse may yield brain contusions and hematomas. Focal necrosis of certain brain regions, such as the basal ganglia, may be associated with carbon monoxide, cyanide, hydrogen sulfide, and methanol. Vasospastic cerebrovascular accident or stroke has been associated with cocaine and the ergots. Cerebellar atrophy may be seen with alcoholism or toluene exposures.

Ultrasound

Diphenhydramine, theophylline, propoxyphene, and phenobarbital (substances poorly visualized on plain radiography) may be detected by ultrasound. Ferrous sulfate, enteric-coated aspirin, and chloral hydrate may also be detected by this method. While more studies are needed, ultrasound may be useful in confirming ingestions of certain non-radiopaque substances, determining success of attempts at gastric decontamination of such substances, assessing the number of pills ingested, and assessing toxic ingestions in situations where radiography may be contraindicated (e.g., pregnant women).

Questions—Radiologic Techniques

1. Which of the following is false?
- A. While certain substances are radiopaque in ideal, *in vitro* circumstances, their detection in patients may be difficult.
- B. The radiopacity of a pill or toxin depends on the radiodensity of surrounding tissues and may be affected by the position of the patient, previous substances in the gastrointestinal tract, and its physical form (e.g., liquid, solid, pill matrix, etc).
- C. Numerous poisons may be consistently detected by simple radiograph.
- D. While detection may confirm the presence of certain toxins, plain films rarely affect management issues.
- E. The use of an abdominal x-ray to screen obtunded patients with possible overdoses is generally not helpful.

2. All of the following may be seen on abdominal x-ray, except
- A. Iron tablets
- B. Certain mothballs
- C. Button batteries
- D. Certain packets of cocaine
- E. Diphenhydramine

3. Which of the following statements is false?
- A. Lead lines and metaphyseal changes may corroborate chronic lead exposure.
- B. Chronic steroid use may yield osteoporosis and osteonecrosis.
- C. Hypervitaminosis D may yield osteoporosis.
- D. Acro-osteolysis has been associated with vinyl chloride.
- E. None of the above.

4. Which of the following concerning chest x-ray is true?
- A. An x-ray of the chest should be taken in all patients with tachypnea, coma, or obtundation to search for potential causes of hypoxemia.
- B. Pneumomediastinum may be seen after crack use.
- C. Classic diaphragmatic and pleural plaques may be seen after chronic asbestos exposure and other pneumoconioses (e.g., silicosis, coal dust and beryllium) may yield abnormal interstitial patterns.
- D. A and C
- E. All of the above.

5. Which of the following statements is false?
- A. Cocaine, amphetamines, phencyclidine, and sympathomimetics have been associated with intraparenchymal bleeds.
- B. Trauma related to alcohol and drugs of abuse may yield brain contusions and hematomas.
- C. Focal necrosis of certain brain regions, such as the basal ganglia, may be associated with carbon monoxide, carbon tetrachloride, cyanide, hydrogen sulfide, and methanol.
- D. Vasospastic cerebrovascular accident or stroke has been associated with cocaine and ergots.
- E. Cerebellar atrophy may be seen with alcoholism or toluene exposures.

Answers

Introduction to the Diagnosis of Poisoning

1. E

The Toxic Screen

1. E 2. A

The Laboratory Approach

1. B 2. A 3. C 4. D 5. C 6. D 7. A

Analytic Methods

1. B 2. C 3. E 4. C 5. B 6. C 7. E

Anion Gap

1. E 2. C 3. B 4. E 5. B

Osmolal Gap

1. A 2. E 3. A 4. C 5. D

Radiologic Techniques

1. C 2. E 3. E 4. E 5. C

SELECTED READINGS

The Diagnosis of Poisoning

1. Gabow PA, Kachney WD, Fennessey PV, et al. Diagnostic importance of an increased serum anion gap. N Engl J Med 1980;303:854–858.
2. Goldfrank, LR, Flomenbaum, NE, Lewin, NA, et al. Goldfrank's toxicologic emergencies, 6th Edition. Appleton & Lange, Stamford, Connecticut. 1998; 77–103.

3. Hepler BR, Sutheimer CA, Sunshine I. The role of the toxicology laboratory in emergency medicine. J Toxicol Clin Toxicol 1982;19:353–365.
4. Hoffman RS, Smilkstein MJ, Howland MA, Goldfrank LR. Osmolal gaps revisited: Normal values and limitations. Clin Toxicol 1993;31:81–93.

CHAPTER 4
Gut Decontamination

INTRODUCTION

A foundation of toxicology, albeit persistently controversial, concerns gastrointestinal methods used to reduce absorption and enhance expulsion after overdose. These include emesis with ipecac syrup, gastric lavage, activated charcoal, cathartics, and whole bowel irrigation. Although certain *in vitro* studies have confirmed the effectiveness of these measures in decreasing drug absorption within the first hour, well-controlled clinical trials that unequivocally determine the optimal combination of emesis, lavage, charcoal, and cathartics are not available. Consequently, increasing concern over the efficacy of traditional methods of gut decontamination has been expressed in the medical literature.

In 1993, the American Academy of Clinical Toxicology (AACT) and the European Association of Poison Centres and Clinical Toxicologists (EAPCCT) agreed to collaborate and formulate position statements on the primary methods of gut decontamination. Each statement reviewed animal and human studies, rationale, indications, contraindications, complications and dosing regimens. Essential elements of these statements are noted below.

EMESIS

Ipecac is the dried root of the indigenous Brazilian and Central American shrubs Cephaelis ipecacuanha and Cephaelis acuminata. Commercially, ipecac is available as the syrup (syrup of ipecac USP). The active ingredients are two ether-soluble alkaloids, emetine (contains methoxylated groups) and cephaeline (contains a free phenol group), which together constitute 90% of the total alkaloid content. Emetine is methyl cephaeline. Syrup of ipecac is sold over-the-counter in 15 and 30-mL containers. The effectiveness of expired ipecac remains controversial, although the use of expired products was equally effective as controls in several studies.

Indications

Many studies have indicated that ipecac is highly effective at inducing emesis. Use of ipecac is non-invasive and simple, yet its use remains controversial. There are still insufficient data to support or exclude its use after poison ingestion. Its use should only be contemplated in individuals who are alert, who have ingested potentially toxic amounts and types of poisons, and who are not likely to seize or become obtunded. It is widely used to treat pediatric ingestions of household products and plants.

It should be considered only if it can be given within 60 minutes of toxin ingestion as its effect diminishes with time. The use of emesis to reduce absorption usually is not effective more than 4–6 hours after ingestion, unless the toxin itself delays absorption. Additional factors that may delay absorption include food in the stomach, other drugs (anticholinergics, narcotics, ganglionic blockers, aluminum hydroxide), and associated alterations in clinical status (e.g., pain, ulcer, ileus, acute abdomen, trauma, and myocardial infarction).

Dosage Regimens

Ipecac is generally not considered safe in children up to 6 months of age. In children 6–12 months, 5–10 mL of ipecac is ingested with 120–240 mL of water. In children 1–12 years, 15 mL of ipecac is ingested with 120–240 mL of water. In adults, 15–30 mL of ipecac is given with 240 mL of water. The dose may be repeated in all groups if emesis has not occurred in 30 minutes.

Contraindications

Ipecac should never be given to individuals with compromised airways (as in comatose or seizing patients), or with absent or impaired gag reflexes. If an individual has ingested a toxin which may potentially compromise airway reflexes, due to seizure activity for example, ipecac is absolutely contraindicated. Certain toxins, such as hydrocarbons with high aspiration potential and corrosives such as strong acids and bases should not be used with ipecac. Other contraindications include children less than 6 months of age, and coingestion of sharp solid objects.

Complications

The most common complications of ipecac use are diarrhea, lethargy, drowsiness and prolonged vomiting. All complications, while well documented, are rare. The use of ipecac may delay the use of charcoal by 1–2 hours. Other complications, including Mallory-Weiss tears, pneumomediastinum, aspiration pneumonia, hyperactivity, fever, diaphragmatic hernia, intracranial bleed, and gastric rupture are all rare.

Chronic Abuse

Chronic use of syrup of ipecac several times daily over several months has resulted in cardiomyopathy, ventricular fibrillation, and death. Chronic ipecac consumption complicating anorexia nervosa has resulted in reversible myopathies, with nerve conduction abnormalities that are indistinguishable from experimental emetine neuropathy. Emetine is a direct myotoxin that inhibits protein synthesis, disrupts mitochondrial oxidative phosphorylation, and produces both skeletal and cardiac myopathies. As a cumulative poison, emetine causes a cardiomyopathy in doses exceeding 1 gram over several weeks. Chronic abuse of syrup of ipecac caused at least several deaths from biventricular congestive heart failure.

Questions—Emesis

1. Ipecac use should be considered in patients who
A. Are comatose
B. Have seizure disorders
C. Have ingested potentially toxic amounts of poisons and who are unlikely to become obtunded
D. Have ingested insoluble substances
E. Have ingested any toxin within 30 minutes

2. The effectiveness of expired Ipecac is uncontested.
A. True
B. False

Answers to questions in shaded boxes appear at the end of the chapter.

3. **The use of emesis to reduce adsorption usually is not effective 4–6 hours after ingestion unless the toxin itself delays absorption.**
   A. True
   B. False
4. **All of the following are complications of ipecac use except**
   A. Aspiration pneumonia
   B. Intracranial bleed
   C. Gastric rupture
   D. Hypothermia
   E. Hyperactivity
5. **The organ most significantly involved in chronic ipecac use is the**
   A. Heart
   B. Liver
   C. Kidney
   D. Brain
   E. Lung

LAVAGE

Gastric lavage involves the introduction of a nasogastric or an orogastric tube into the stomach and the removal of stomach contents by suction or syringe. Numerous substances, including water, or saline, or charcoal have been instilled into the stomach before its contents, and presumably toxin remnants, are removed. One prospective controlled study of acutely self-poisoned patients indicated that little clinical deterioration occurs in asymptomatic patients treated without gastric emptying.

Gastric emptying procedures in symptomatic patients did not significantly alter the length of stay in the emergency department, mean length of time intubated, or mean length of stay in the intensive care unit. In fact, gastric lavage was associated with a higher prevalence of medical intensive care unit admissions and aspiration pneumonia. Other studies in volunteers have indicated that gastric lavage is more effective than syrup of ipecac when performed immediately after exposure, but no statistical difference between lavage and emesis exists in the reduction of drug absorption when markers are administered 1 hour postingestion.

Indications

As clinical studies have not confirmed the benefit of gastric lavage alone, gastric lavage should generally not be considered unless a life-threatening amount of poison has been ingested within 60 minutes of presentation. Involvement of drugs that delay absorption, ingestion of large quantities of toxic drugs, and absence of bowel sounds on physical examination may lead to increased drug recovery at later times postingestion. Even then, clinical benefit has not been confirmed. Lavage does not benefit the patient who has ingested a nontoxic agent or a nontoxic amount of a toxic agent. Lavage is not useful as a deterrent to subsequent ingestions. In conclusion, gastric emptying procedures in the emergency department are usually ineffective, may result in increased morbidity, and appear to offer no clinical advantage over charcoal alone.

Technique

If possible, the technique should be explained to the patient. A reliable suction device must be readied in case of aspiration. Intubation must precede this technique in any individual with a compromised mental status or airway. Patients should be placed in the left lateral, head down position. A 36–40 French orogastric tube should be used in adults and a 24–28 French tube should be used in children. After lubricating the firm, yet rounded end, the tube is inserted via the mouth or nose, gently. Force should not be used. Aliquots of water or saline should be used. In a child, 10 mL/kg of warm saline is recommended. In adults, 200–300 mL is used. Lavage is done until particulate toxic material is no longer noted in the return. There is some evidence that certain toxins may still be present in lavage fluid even after this visual test is satisfied.

Contraindications

Contraindications include ingestion of strong corrosives, coingestion of sharp objects, and, most importantly, in individuals with an unprotected airway who exhibit a depressed level of consciousness. Patients who are at increased risk of bleeding, such as those with varices or bleeding dyscrasias, should not undergo this technique.

Complications

Complications are well-documented; however, serious problems arise rarely. These may include pulmonary aspiration during tube insertion, esophageal perforation, tension pneumothorax, and empyema. Hypothermia may occur in young children given large volumes of cold fluid. Epistaxis, especially when large tubes are inserted nasally, may occur. Electrolyte imbalance, particularly when lavage solutions other than saline (e.g., Fleet's Phospho-Soda) are used in young children, has been reported. Laryngospasm, hypoxia, hypercapnia, and mechanical injury to the throat, esophagus and stomach have been reported.

Questions—Lavage

1. **Gastric lavage should generally not be considered unless a life-threatening amount of poison has been ingested within 60 minutes of presentation.**
   A. True
   B. False
2. **Lavage is not useful to**
   A. A patient who ingested a nontoxic agent
   B. A patient who ingested a nontoxic amount of a toxic agent
   C. Deter subsequent ingestions
   D. All of the above
   E. None of the above
3. **The following steps are taken when lavage is performed except**
   A. The patient is placed in a left lateral head down position
   B. A 36-40 French orogastric tube is chosen for all adults and children
   C. The firm round end is lubricated
   D. The tube is inserted gently into the mouth or nose
   E. Warm saline is instilled
4. **Contraindications to lavage include**
   A. Ingestion of antidepressants by patients with psychiatric histories
   B. Ingestion of several cardiac and diuretic medications

C. Ingestion of strong corrosives
D. Patients with previous abdominal surgeries
E. All of the above

5. Complications of gastric lavage include all the following except
A. Hyperthermia
B. Epistaxis
C. Electrolyte imbalance
D. Hypoxia
E. Hypercapnia

ACTIVATED CHARCOAL

Activated charcoal is produced by heating wood pulp to 900° C, washing, and then activating the substance with steam or strong acids. The subsequent network of tiny pores is capable of trapping toxins ranging in molecular weight from 100–1,000 daltons. One gram of charcoal contains approximately 1,000 m^2 of surface area. Presently, several activated charcoal-70% sorbitol mixtures are marketed, possibly because of the improved palatability and catharsis of sorbitol. A mixture of 30 grams activated charcoal and 120 mL 70% sorbitol produced a mean transit time of 90 minutes in healthy adult volunteers. Such doses cause no significant change in serum osmolality, electrolytes, magnesium, hepatic enzymes, or complete blood count.

Activated charcoal effectively binds a variety of drugs and chemicals and is effective in preventing absorption of many ingested substances when given within 1 hour of exposure. Thereafter, its efficacy diminishes significantly and depends on several factors (e.g., delayed absorption, the charcoal to drug ratio, pH, stomach contents, drug dose, and time since ingestion). Activated charcoal does not bind well to elemental metals (lead, lithium, boron), boric acid, some pesticides (malathion, DDT, methyl carbamate), ferrous sulfate, cyanide, strong acids and alkali, ethanol, and petroleum distillates.

Charcoal therapy involves the oral administration or instillation via nasogastric or orogastric tube of activated charcoal to adsorb poisons in the GI tract. Activated charcoal is emerging as a sole decontamination measure in view of the relative lack of efficacy of both syrup of ipecac and gastric lavage demonstrated in recent controlled clinical trials. The effectiveness of several combined decontamination measures (e.g., charcoal-lavage-charcoal, charcoal 5 minutes after 60-mL syrup of ipecac) has not been clinically evaluated in large controlled studies. Serial activated charcoal can significantly reduce certain drug half-lives. See also Chapter 5, Antidotes.

Indications

When given within 1 hour, activated charcoal may be more effective than either lavage or emesis. Charcoal should be considered in individuals who have ingested a potentially toxic amount of poison within one hour of presentation. Charcoal may be considered more than 1 hour after ingestion; however, studies to document clinical efficacy are lacking.

The use of repeated doses of activated charcoal, as compared with other modalities of gut decontamination, has not been subjected to controlled clinical trials and has generally not been shown to reduce morbidity and mortality. Enhanced elimination may occur via nonrenal mechanisms, such as interruption of enterohepatic or enteroenteric circulation. Serial charcoal resulted in reductions in the half-lives of both theophylline and phenobarbital after intravenous administration. Studies suggest that serial activated charcoal may produce a gastrointestinal dialysis whereby certain drugs back diffuse from high serum levels, through intestinal villi into lower intraluminal concentrations.

Pharmacokinetic characteristics of compounds favoring enhanced serial activated charcoal elimination include significant enterohepatic or enteroenteric circulation, limited protein binding, and small volume of distribution. The intoxication from drugs producing chronic toxic effects through long terminal elimination half-lives potentially may be ameliorated by serial activated charcoal. Examples of such compounds are dioxins, organochlorine pesticides, polychlorinated biphenyls, chlordecone, methylmercury, penicillamine, isotretinoin (13-cis-retinoic acid), and amiodarone. The clinical efficacy of this modality in reducing the toxicity of these compounds remains to be proven.

At present, multiple-dose activated charcoal is probably of value in the treatment of theophylline overdose, but is not likely to be very important in the presence of most other intoxications. It can be considered if a life-threatening amount of phenobarbital, carbamazepine, quinine, dapsone, or aspirin is ingested. Its value in the treatment of digoxin, digitoxin, phenytoin, sodium valproate, meprobamate, dapsone, carbamazepine, and cyclosporine intoxications has yet to be established by controlled studies. It does not hasten the elimination of cyclic antidepressants.

Dosage Regimens

An optimal dosage scheme is unknown; however, 1 gram/kg is generally recommended in children up to one year. Twenty-five to 50 grams is recommended in the 1–12 year age group, and adults are given 25–100 grams. The charcoal slurry must be mixed thoroughly to prevent the formation of charcoal plugs. A minimum of 8 ounces of fluid is recommended if the powder form is used. Palatability may be improved by the addition of saccharin at a concentration of 1:20 or the use of an opaque container. Premixed activated charcoal offers some practical advantages: improved palatability, good shelf life, and reduced preparation times. Cherry syrup, chocolate, and saccharin do not reduce the efficacy of activated charcoal.

Contraindications

An unprotected airway is the primary contraindication to charcoal therapy, as aspiration may develop. Evidence of gastrointestinal perforation and overdose from non-toxic or poorly bound toxins also preclude the use of charcoal. Corrosive ingestions contraindicate the use of activated charcoal because of the lack of efficacy and obscuration of endoscopy. The administration of activated charcoal following acetaminophen overdose may be a relative contraindication to charcoal use because activated charcoal binds the antidote N-acetylcysteine (NAC) *in vitro*. Whether or not activated charcoal reduces the efficacy of NAC remains to be determined. Patients with concomitant ingestion of other serious toxins who present within 4 hours may benefit from activated charcoal.

Complications

Complications are well described, but rare. Constipation may occur. The use of multiple doses of activated charcoal has been associated with several cases of intestinal obstruction, particularly in the cecum, both with and without the concomitant use of cathartics. A poorly mixed charcoal slurry produced atelectasis corrected by bronchoscopy in an 8-month-old child. Fortunately, an aspiration pneumonitis did not develop. A charcoal-containing empyema has been described 4 weeks after gastric lavage that probably was complicated by an esophageal perforation.

Questions—Activated Charcoal

1. **One gram of charcoal contains a surface area of approximately**
   A. 1,000 square meters
   B. 100 square meters
   C. 10 square meters
   D. 1 square meter
   E. 1 square centimeter
2. **The efficacy of charcoal partially depends on**
   A. Serum pH
   B. Stomach contents
   C. Urine pH
   D. All of the above
   E. None of the above
3. **Repeated doses of activated charcoal**
   A. Have been studied with controlled clinical trials
   B. Have been shown to reduce morbidity and mortality
   C. Have resulted in reduced half-life of theophylline after i.v. administration
   D. Have resulted in reduced half-life of carbamazepine after i.v. administration
   E. Should always be offered in polypharmacy ingestions
4. **All of the following are contraindications to activated charcoal use except**
   A. Loss of the gag reflex
   B. History of acetaminophen use
   C. Gastrointestinal perforation
   D. Overdose of corrosive ingestions
   E. Overdose of poorly bound toxins
5. **Complications of activated charcoal are rare.**
   A. True
   B. False

CATHARTICS

The use of cathartics may reduce the transit time of drugs in the gut and decrease the constipating effects of multiple doses of charcoal, but they have never been shown to improve morbidity and mortality or to decrease hospital stay. Although cathartics are routinely used in overdoses, there are no unequivocal experimental data demonstrating that cathartics reduce the gastrointestinal absorption of drugs or poisons.

Commonly used cathartics are classified as saline (magnesium citrate) and saccharide (sorbitol). Saline cathartics act by altering the physical - chemical forces within the intestinal lumen. The osmotic retention of fluid within the gastrointestinal tract activates motility reflexes and enhances expulsion. The latency period between administration and catharsis depends on a number of factors that affect gastric mobility, including stress, physical activity, and the toxin's effect on bowel motility. See Chapter 39, Over the Counter Products.

Indications

There are no definite indications for cathartics in the management of the poisoned patient.

Dosage Regimens

Magnesium citrate is the most palatable of saline cathartics; it contains 16 mEq of magnesium per gram of salt. The adult dose is 8 ounces or 250 mL. The pediatric dose is 4 mL/kg. Commercial sorbitol suspension is marketed as 20% (weight per volume) activated charcoal in 70% sorbitol. Dilution of this solution is recommended for ambulatory adults and children. The recommended dose is 70% sorbitol 1–2 mL/kg in adults and 35% sorbitol 4.3 mL/kg in children

Contraindications

Magnesium cathartics should be avoided in patients with preexisting renal failure or in those patients likely to develop renal dysfunction (e.g., in patients with myoglobinuria, or prolonged seizures). Avoid sodium in severe hypertension, renal failure, or heart failure. Avoid cathartic use in corrosive ingestion, severe diarrhea, adynamic ileus, electrolyte problems, and recent bowel surgery. Use cathartics with caution in the absence of bowel sounds.

Complications

Patients, especially children, should be carefully monitored for evidence of impaired fluid and electrolyte balance during administration of multiple doses of activated charcoal and sorbitol. Severe dehydration and hypernatremia may develop. If volume depletion develops, cathartics should be withheld. Hypermagnesemia may follow excessive intake, impaired excretion, or parenteral administration of magnesium. Patients treated for overdose of drugs with frequent oral dosage of magnesium-containing cathartics may develop signs and symptoms of hypermagnesemia. Fatal hypermagnesemia has followed rectal administration of magnesium preparations in cases of megacolon and bowel obstruction. Common undesirable effects of cathartic use include abdominal cramps, excessive diarrhea, and abdominal distension.

Questions—Cathartics

1. **All of the following affect the latency period between administration of cathartic and resulting catharsis except**
   A. Stress
   B. Physical activity
   C. The toxin's effect on bowel motility
   D. The molecular weight of the toxin
   E. Gastric motility
2. **There are clearly documented indications for the use of cathartic in the poisoned patient.**
   A. True
   B. False
3. **Contraindications to cathartic use include**
   A. Preexisting renal failure
   B. Active bowel sounds
   C. Constipation
   D. Oncologic history
   E. All of the above

WHOLE GUT LAVAGE

The previously used instillation of large volumes of isotonic saline as a means of preparing the bowel for diagnostic procedures or for gastrointestinal tract surgery was associated with electrolyte and fluid imbalance, and concern about these complications has limited the use of whole bowel irrigation in treatment of overdoses. The recent development of isotonic solutions that use polyethylene glycol and sodium sulfate instead of sodium chloride has resulted in a procedure more suitable for clinical trials. Examples of isotonic solutions are GoLYTELY® and Colyte®. The use of polyethylene glycol (PEG) solution in whole gut lavage produces no significant changes in serum electrolytes, serum osmolality, body weight, or hematocrit.

Whole-bowel irrigation (WBI) is probably a useful and rapid method to empty the gut in 4–6 hours. It is messy and labor intensive for patients who present to a hospital many hours after an overdose. WBI produces a more thorough cleansing of the intestinal tract than cathartics.

Indications

There are no established indications for the use of whole bowel irrigation. Potential uses for WBI as a decontamination measure include ingestion of massive amounts of highly toxic drugs and ingestion of large amounts of drugs in patients presenting late (4 hours postexposure). An additional possible use may be in ingestion of toxic substances that can be detected by radiography (e.g., arsenic, carbon tetrachloride, mercury, and thallium).

Whole-bowel irrigation is a safe and effective decontamination procedure for potentially lethal iron ingestions, especially if the iron tablets have passed the pylorus. Activated charcoal does not adsorb iron or other metal compounds (e.g., lithium, potassium). Whole-bowel irrigation effectively removes miniature disk batteries from the gut and may be of theoretical benefit in removing cocaine-filled packets in body packers and body stuffers. Lead, lithium, sustained-release verapamil and theophylline may be cleared from the gastrointestinal tract by this method, but there is little evidence to indicate a lessening of morbidity or mortality from this procedure.

Dosage Regimens

The technique for WBI involves the insertion of a nasogastric tube into the stomach and the instillation of PEG-ELS solution while the patient sits on a commode. Alternatively, the solution can be ingested orally. Activated charcoal may be administered before WBI. The use of intravenous metoclopramide (10 mg adults, 0.1–0.3 mg/kg) may reduce the incidence of nausea and vomiting. The usual rate of fluid administration is 2 L/hour in adults and 0.5 L/hour (25–40 mL/kg) in children under 12 years of age. PEG-ELS solution should be given at room temperature to prevent hypothermia. The endpoint occurs when the rectal effluent is similar in appearance to the infusate. The usual infusion lasts 2–6 hours. This does not ensure that the toxin or foreign body is eliminated.

Contraindications

Contraindications to the use of WBI include gastrointestinal pathology or dysfunction (obstruction, ileus, hemorrhage, perforation) and inadequate airway protection.

Complications

Few complications occur following the use of WBI for preparation of the bowel for radiographic examination or for surgery in either adults or children, even in the presence of cardiac, renal, or pulmonary disease. Complaints usually are minor and include nausea, vomiting, abdominal distension, cramps, sleep loss, and anal irritation. Propylene glycol electrolyte lavage solution may occupy activated charcoal binding sites. It may also displace toxin from activated charcoal, possibly leading to an increase in toxin bioavailability.

Questions—Whole Gut Lavage

1. **There are no established indications for the use of whole-bowel irrigation.**
   A. True
   B. False
2. **Potential and possible uses of whole-bowel irrigation include**
   A. Ingestion of massive amounts of highly toxic drugs
   B. Ingestions of large amounts of drugs in patients presenting late
   C. Ingestions of toxic substances that can be detected by radiography
   D. All of the above
   E. None of the above
3. **Whole-bowel irrigation may be beneficial in all of the following except**
   A. Potentially lethal ingestions
   B. Lessening morbidity of theophylline in the gastrointestinal tract
   C. Removal of miniature disc batteries
   D. Clearing the gastrointestinal tract of lead and lithium
   E. Serious iron ingestions
4. **Contraindications to whole-bowel irrigation include**
   A. Intact, protected airway
   B. History of whole-bowel irrigation for the same patient
   C. Pregnancy
   D. Gastrointestinal dysfunction
   E. History of seizure disorder

Answers

Emesis

1. C 2. B 3. D 4. D 5. A

Lavage

1. A 2. D 3. B 4. C 5. A

Activated Charcoal

1. A 2. B 3. C 4. B 5. A

Cathartics

1. D 2. B 3. A

Whole Gut Lavage

1. A 2. D 3. B 4. D

SELECTED READINGS

Gut Decontamination

1. Kulig K. Initial management of ingestions of toxic substances. N Engl J Med 1992;326:1677–1681.
2. Lovejoy FH Jr, Shannon M, Woolf AD. Recent advances in clinical toxicology. Curr Problems Pediatr 1992(Mar.):119–129.
3. Olson KR. Is gut emptying all washed up? Am J Emerg Med 1990; 8:560–561. Editorial.
4. Perrone J, Hoffman RS, Goldfrank LR. Special considerations in gastrointestinal decontamination. Emerg Med Clin North Am 1994;12:285–289.
5. Position Statements: Gut Decontamination. Clin Tox 1997;35(7):695–762.

ACKNOWLEDGMENT

Thanks to Alison Deutsch, MD for contributing the questions in this chapter.

CHAPTER 5
Antidotes

INTRODUCTION

While relatively few antidotes exist, some may be lifesaving. Some antidotes (e.g., naloxone, flumazenil) exhibit rapid and dramatic clinical effects. Some do not affect all the toxic effects of a particular poison (e.g., chelating agents), and a few are useful adjuncts to treatment without specific antidotal effects (e.g., diazepam in the treatment of organophosphate poisoning). Controlled clinical studies have generally been limited by ethical concerns. Many uses are experimental or anecdotal and have not been thoroughly studied.

The purpose of antidotal therapy is to reduce toxicity by inhibiting the translocation of the toxin to an effector site, by reducing toxin concentration, or by reducing toxin action at effector sites. Antidotes should generally not be administered indiscriminately. Although an effective antidote may be available, its use should depend on an evaluation of the patient's clinical state, appropriate laboratory values, and the expected pharmacologic action of the toxin.

Antidotes are drugs and may themselves precipitate undesirable reactions. Consequently, both the risk and benefit of antidotal therapy must be carefully evaluated in every case before an antidote is given. After the antidote is administered, the patient must be observed until the effects of the toxin have subsided in the absence of the antidote. The therapeutic half-life of some antidotes (e.g., naloxone) is shorter than that of the toxins (e.g., methadone), and initial improvement seen with antidotal therapy may be followed by a disastrous deterioration unless the patient is closely observed.

Antidotes may reflect national practices (e.g., 4-dimethylaminophenol for cyanide intoxication in Germany, hydroxocobalamin for cyanide poisoning in France, silibinin for amanitin poisoning in Austria and Germany), but most antidotes, thanks to widely publicized information are widely used. The American Academy of Clinical Toxicology (AACT) has proposed facility assessment guidelines for Regional Poison Treatment Centers, which include recommendations for a pharmacy stock of common antidotes in amounts adequate to meet regional needs.

ANTIDOTES

Activated Charcoal

See Chapter 4, Gut Decontamination.

Aminophylline

USES

- Many reported uses have not been subject to controlled clinical trials. Reports are often anecdotal. May be useful in antagonizing the effects of flurazepam, midazolam, and lorazepam. See also Flumazenil (Romazicon®).
- Aminophylline improves ventilation in lorazepam-induced neonatal apnea.
- May antagonize morphine and fentanyl induced respiratory depression.
- May reduce the depth and duration of sedation by thiopental.

MECHANISM OF ACTION

Aminophylline antagonizes diazepam-induced somnolence and reverses sedation associated with lorazepam by enhancing the level of extracellular adenosine in the central nervous system. This apparently occurs by blocking adenosine reuptake into neuronal and glial cells and antagonizing the depressant action of adenosine by competitively binding to adenosine receptors. Aminophylline is rarely used for benzodiazepine-induced sedation since the advent of flumazenil. See Flumazenil (Romazicon®).

CAUTIONS

Aminophylline may cause tachycardia, seizures, arrhythmias, hypokalemia, and vomiting.

DOSE

Aminophylline has been administered in doses of 1–2 mg/kg intravenously to reverse sedation induced by diazepam, flunitrazepam, lorazepam, and midazolam.

4-Aminopyridine (4-AP)

USES

- Pancuronium overdose.
- Potentiates neostigmine and Pyridostigmine Bromide (Mestinon®) reversal. See Pyridostigmine Bromide (Mestinon®).
- Possibly effective in verapamil intoxication and in human botulism (improves peripheral but not respiratory paralysis).
- Of possible use, orally, in disorders of neuromuscular transmission (Eaton-Lambert syndrome, congenital myasthenia, myasthenia gravis and multiple sclerosis).

MECHANISM OF ACTION

4-Aminopyridine (4-AP) is used as an antagonist of nondepolarizing neuromuscular blocking agents. This agent enhances transmembrane calcium influx, which results in facilitation of synaptic transmission. Aminopyridine also increases the release of acetylcholine at the neuromuscular junction by selectively blocking potassium channels. The rate of efflux of potassium determines the duration of the action potential. Blocking of potassium channels prolongs the action potential and allows more calcium to move into the cell. The intracellular uptake of calcium is essential for the release of acetylcholine. Increased influx of calcium following treatment with aminopyridine may result in an increased release of acetylcholine. 4-Aminopyridine is not commercially available in the United States.

CAUTIONS

4-Aminopyridine may induce central nervous system stimulant effects, including seizures. Treat overdose with 4-aminopyridine with supportive therapy, prevention of absorption, treatment of seizures with diazepam, and the possible use of pancuronium.

DOSE

Administer 10 mg i.v. slowly, or 0.35 to 0.5 mg/kg with neostigmine or pyridostigmine.

Antihistamines

USES

- Antihistamine drugs, such as benztropine and diphenhydramine effectively relieve drug-related dystonias associated with neuroleptic drugs (e.g., haloperidol, phenothiazines, thioxanthenes) and metoclopramide.

MECHANISM OF ACTION

Benztropine and diphenhydramine reverse drug-induced dystonias through competitive inhibition of muscarinic receptors and blockade of dopamine reuptake.

CAUTIONS

The adverse effects of benztropine and other antihistamines result from their anticholinergic side effects. Diphenhydramine is the preferable agent in patients expected to tolerate anticholinergic drugs poorly (e.g., with angle-closure glaucoma).

DOSE

Benztropine should be given to adults either intramuscularly or intravenously at doses of 1–2 mg for dystonic reactions. Diphenhydramine (1–2 mg/kg up to 50 mg given intramuscularly or slowly intravenously) rapidly reverses dystonias. All patients with drug-induced dystonias should be placed on oral medication for 2–3 days to prevent recurrence (benztropine, 1–2 mg twice daily, or diphenhydramine, 25–50 mg three times daily).

Antivenin, Black Widow Spider (Latrodectus Mactans)

USES

- The antivenin is effective against all American black widow spiders (Latrodectus species).
- Use in patients with seizures, respiratory failure, pain and muscle spasms due to Latrodectus bites not entirely controlled with calcium gluconate, benzodiazepines and opiates. See Calcium Gluconate and Calcium Chloride.

MECHANISM OF ACTION

Like crotalid antivenin, this product is derived by immunizing healthy horses against the black widow spider (Latrodectus mactans) and collecting venom-neutralizing serum globulins.

CAUTIONS

All patients should be skin tested for serum sensitivity before antivenin administration. Desensitization should be considered only in the rare circumstance where the patient's life is clearly threatened. Serum sickness may occur. Children less than 5 years old and adults greater than 60 are at increased risk of toxicity.

DOSAGE

Except in young children and the elderly, Latrodectus envenomation often is treated effectively with supportive care alone. One to two vials in 50–100 cc of normal saline infused intravenously over 1 hour is the average dose.

Antivenin, Crotalidae Polyvalent

USES

- In mild, moderate or severe envenomations by rattlesnakes (Crotalus, Sistrurus), copperheads, cottonmouths and cantil (Agkistrodon), fer-de-lance (Bothrops species), and bushmaster (Lachesis mutus).
- Whether or not antivenin should be administered after snake bites depends on a careful assessment of the degree of envenomation and the clinical response of the patient. Mild symptoms include local swelling, and pain with obvious fang marks. Moderate symptoms may include profound swelling, ecchymosis, some systemic signs and laboratory abnormalities. Severe signs include blisters, profound edema, necrosis, systemic involvement and seriously altered lab values.

MECHANISM OF ACTION

The lyophilized polyvalent serum is a direct preparation of venom-neutralizing globulin derived from the serum of horses gradually immunized against certain crotalid snakes (Crotalidae). It is reconstituted with bacteriostatic water for intravenous use and contains antibodies for all American members of the Crotalidae family.

CAUTIONS

Sensitivity to anti-venin may be profound. In all patients where time allows and the use of antivenin is contemplated, sensitivity testing should be performed. For patients with a history of horse serum allergy, 1:100 or greater test dilutions should be administered. The use of antivenin in skin test-positive patients requires careful evaluation of potential risks and benefits. In certain grave situations (i.e., severe rattlesnake bites), antivenin has been given to sensitive patients, following consultation with appropriate specialists. The use of antivenin requires an intensive care setting and the immediate availability of epinephrine and diphenhydramine.

Serum sickness (malaise, fever, myalgias, urticaria, arthralgias, nausea, vomiting, lymphadenopathy, edema, muscle weakness, and peripheral neuritis, usually in the upper extremity) often occurs within 1–3 weeks of antivenin administration, particularly when large doses are given. Great care should be undertaken in those with a history of asthma, urticaria, or prior allergic reactions to horses or horse products.

DOSAGE

Mild envenomations are treated with 5–10 vials in 250–500 cc of normal saline. Moderate indications are treated with 10–20 vials of antivenin in 500 cc of normal saline. Severe bites are treated with 20 or more vials in 500–1000 cc of normal saline. Each infusion is run over 4–6 hours. Additional antivenin may be required based on the severity of poisoning. Maximal effectiveness results from i.v. dosing within 4 hours of envenomation. The effectiveness of antivenin beyond 12–24 hours postenvenomation is questionable, except perhaps for the reversal of coagulopathy.

Antivenin, North American Coral Snake

USES

- The antivenin is effective for the Texas or Eastern coral snake (Micrurus fulvius) but not for the Arizona or Sonoran coral snake (Micrurus euryoxanthus).

MECHANISM OF ACTION

This commercial product contains venom-neutralizing globulins derived from serum of immunized horses.

CAUTIONS

All patients should be skin-tested for sensitivity. Desensitization procedures require the presence of life-threatening signs.

DOSAGE

Following negative skin tests, three to five reconstituted vials are given intravenously to all patients with confirmed envenomation. The appearance of neurologic symptoms indicates the need for an additional three to five vials.

Antivenins, Other

A variety of antivenins are available from noncommercial and research sources. Most of these products do not have Food and Drug Administration approval, because too few data exist on their efficacy or indications for use.

EXOTIC SNAKE SPECIES

Many large zoos stock exotic antivenin. Your local poison control center would be the best source of referral for locally available exotic antivenin sources.

SCORPION ANTIVENIN

The Departments of Botany and Microbiology have developed a goat serum product at Arizona State University in Tempe that appears to be effective in severe envenomations by Centruroides scorpions. The antivenin has not been adequately tested and is not approved by the Food and Drug Administration.

SEA SNAKE ANTIVENIN, (HYDROPHIIDAE)

The Commonwealth Serum Laboratory in Australia distributes an equine antivenin.

SEA WASP ANTIVENIN, (CHIRONEX FLECKERI)

A sheep antivenin is available in Melbourne, Australia.

Atropine

USES

- Anticholinesterase pesticides (organophosphates, carbamates). Atropine reverses the muscarinic but not nicotinic (muscle weakness, muscle fasciculations, respiratory depression) side effects of these toxic agents.
- Physostigmine excess. See Physostigmine Salicylate (Antilirium®).
- Antimyasthenic agents (e.g., pyridostigmine). See Pyridostigmine Bromide (Mestinon®).
- Nerve gas agents (e.g., Sarin, Soman, and Tabun).
- Synthetic choline esters (e.g., Urecholine) and cholinergic agonists (e.g., bethanechol).
- Clitocybe and Inocybe mushrooms only when clear muscarinic symptoms are present.
- As an adjunct in treating bradyarrhythmias induced by numerous cardiac medications (e.g., beta-blockers, calcium channel blockers, digitalis glycosides, clonidine and guanabenz).

MECHANISM OF ACTION

Atropine is a racemic mixture of hyoscyamine of which l-hyoscyamine is almost totally responsible for its antimuscarinic properties. At pharmacologic doses, atropine antagonizes cholinergic stimuli at muscarinic receptors while exhibiting little or no effect at the nicotinic receptors of the autonomic ganglia or neuromuscular junction.

CAUTIONS

All patients should be closely observed for signs of atropine excess (dilated pupils, flushed facies, tachycardia, fever, ileus, disorientation, delirium, dry mouth, urinary retention, drying of secretions). Adequate oxygenation is vital as atropine may cause ventricular fibrillation in the presence of hypoxia. Atropine should be used cautiously in the presence of glaucoma (relatively contraindicated for angle-closure glaucoma), hypertension, hyperthermia, and hypothyroidism. Physostigmine may be used to reverse atropine effects only if no cholinergic symptoms are present.

DOSAGE

The initial dose for symptomatic patients ranges from 0.015–0.05 mg/kg to a maximum of 1–4 mg in adults, with careful monitoring for clinical improvement or signs of atropinization. It is repeated every 15–30 minutes until the desired therapeutic response (i.e., drying of excessive secretions) is achieved. Pupillary dilation is not a reliable therapeutic end-point. In severe pesticide poisonings, atropine doses as high as 1–2 g/day have been required to control muscarinic symptoms.

BAL in Oil

See Dimercaprol.

Benztropine (Cogentin®)

See Antihistamines.

Calcium Disodium EDTA (Versenate®)

USES

- Acute lead poisoning. See D-Penicillamine (Cuprimine®) and Succimer, DMSA (Chemet®).
- Acute cadmium, copper, and zinc poisoning.
- Ocular exposures to calcium oxide, lime, and cement.

MECHANISM OF ACTION

Divalent and trivalent heavy metals displace the calcium in calcium disodium ethylenediaminetetraacetate ($CaNa_2EDTA$), forming a stable complex that is excreted renally. $CaNa_2EDTA$ chelates lead, zinc, and, to a lesser extent, iron, copper, manganese, and cadmium. $CaNa_2EDTA$ is preferred to NaEDTA, because the latter sequesters calcium, leading to hypocalcemia.

CAUTIONS

Adequate fluids should be given and the urine volume monitored, since reversible acute tubular necrosis can occur with $CaNa_2EDTA$ therapy. Prolonged chelation may cause zinc and vitamin B6 deficiency. $CaNa_2EDTA$ can be nephrotoxic and hemodialysis may be required in patients with inadequate urine flow despite the use of fluids and diuretics. Rapid intravenous infusions may cause intracranial hypertension. Adverse effects may also include chills, thirst, malaise, anemia, hypotension, increased prothrombin time and inverted T waves. $CaNa_2EDTA$ should not be given orally for lead poisoning.

DOSAGE

Administer 50–75 mg/kg per day in three divided doses for up to 5 days either intravenously or intramuscularly up to a maximum dose of 1 g/15 kg per day. $CaNa_2EDTA$ intravenous solutions should be diluted to a concentration of 2–4 mg/mL and infused over 1–2 hours. For intramuscular use, add 1 ml of 1% procaine per mL of $CaNa_2EDTA$. A 2-day rest period and evaluation of the effectiveness of chelation (blood, urine lead and erythrocyte protoporphyrin levels) should precede further courses. The concurrent use of dimercaprol (BAL in Oil) may enhance lead excretion in cases of acute lead encephalopathy. In ocular exposures, irrigate eyes for at least 15 minutes with 0.01–0.05 M disodium EDTA (Disotate®), Endrate®).

Calcium Gluconate and Calcium Chloride

USES

- Hydrofluoric acid burns of the skin and ingestion of fluoride salts.
- Calcium channel blocker overdose.
- Possible use in beta-blocker overdose and in sodium fluoroacetate exposures.
- Used to treat hyperkalemia, and hypermagnesemia (one of several treatments).
- Symptomatic relief of muscle spasm following Latrodectus (e.g., Black Widow spider) envenomation.

MECHANISM OF ACTION

In concentrated hydrofluoric acid skin burns, calcium binds to the fluoride ion, preventing further skin penetration. Calcium may reverse the neuromuscular paralysis associated with hyperkalemia and hypermagnesemia as well as the muscle spasms occurring after widow spider envenomation. Calcium may reverse the effects of calcium channel blockers in overdose.

CAUTIONS

Intravenous calcium gluconate should be given slowly through a patent line. The heart rate and blood pressure should be monitored during administration. Calcium salts are locally irritating, with the gluconate salt better tolerated than chloride. Administration of calcium to patients with chronic renal failure may result in hypercalcemia, although calcium administration in healthy patients rarely leads to elevated calcium levels. Intravenous calcium should be avoided, if possible, in patients receiving cardiac glycosides. Sodium bicarbonate and calcium should not be administered through the same intravenous line.

DOSAGE

Hydrofluoric Acid Burns

- In less than 20% concentration hydrofluoric acid burns, massage 2.5% gel (may not be commercially available-contact local poison center or pharmacy for instructions on preparation), into exposed area for 15 minutes, repeating as necessary for pain.
- In cases of greater than 20% concentration or failure to respond to calcium gluconate gel, one may infiltrate each square centimeter of exposed area with 0.5 mL of 10% calcium gluconate subcutaneously using a 30-gauge needle.
- Intradermal injections of calcium gluconate should not be used in digits. Intra-arterial injections in these cases may be used.

Fluoride Salts or Serious Systemic Toxicity from Dermal or Oral Hydrofluoric Acid Exposure

- Intravenous calcium gluconate (10% solution) should be given slowly at 0.1–0.2 mL/kg up to 10 mL in adults. A repeat dose may be administered in 15–20 minutes, but subsequent doses require monitoring of serum calcium levels.

Calcium Channel Blocker Overdoses

- Children: 0.1–0.3 mL/kg of 10% calcium chloride (10–30 mg/kg) over 5 minutes, then repeat as necessary.
- Adults: 10 mL of 10% calcium chloride (1 g) or 30 mL of 10% calcium gluconate (3 grams) over 5 minutes, then repeat every 10–20 minutes for 3–4 doses as necessary.

Chelators

See Calcium Disodium EDTA (Versenate®) for acute lead poisoning, cadmium poisoning, copper poisoning, and zinc poisoning.

See Deferoxamine Mesylate (Desferal®) for iron and aluminum poisoning.

See Diethylenetriaminepenta-acetic Acid (DPTA) for plutonium poisoning, and exposure to transuranium metals, berkelium, californium, americium, and curium. It may also be useful for chelation of some rare earth metals (cerium, yttrium, lanthanum, promethium, and scandium) and some transitional metals (zirconium and niobium).

See Dimercaprol (BAL in oil) for arsenic, but not arsine gas, poisoning, adjunctive therapy for acute lead encephalopathy but not other forms of lead toxicity, gold poisoning, and inorganic mercury poisoning. Dimercaprol may possibly be useful in antimony, bismuth, chromium, nickel, copper, zinc, and tungsten poisoning. See D-Penicillamine (Cuprimine®) for the possible treatment of copper, lead, mercury, arsenic, and bismuth poisoning.

See Sodium Diethyldithiocarbamate (Dithiocarb) for the treatment of nickel dermatitis and nickel carbonyl poisoning. It is an investigational drug in the United States and is classified as an orphan drug.

Cyanide Antidotes (Amylnitrite, Sodium Nitrite, and Sodium Thiosulfate)

USES

- Symptomatic cyanide poisoning.
- Nitroprusside.
- Acetonitrile and acrylonitrile.
- Plants containing cyanogenic glycosides, such as apricot pits, peach pits and Laetrile.
- Smoke inhalation that results in the formation of cyanogenic gases from synthetic materials.
- Hydrogen sulfide.
- Sodium thiosulfate alone may be useful in bromate and chlorate poisoning.
- Alternate cyanide antidotes have been developed in other countries. See Dicobalt Edetate, 4-Dimethyl-para-aminophenol Hydrochloride (4-DMAP), and Hydroxocobalamin.

MECHANISM OF ACTION

Cyanide binds to ferric ion, interferes with cytochrome oxidase, and reduces cellular respiration. Nitrites, exogenously given in cases of cyanide poisoning, induce methemoglobin formation, which in turn attracts cyanide off cytochrome oxidase. Thiosulfate enhances renal elimination of cyanide by forming thiocyanate when combined with cyanomethemoglobin.

Reaction 1: Hemoglobin-$Fe2^+$ + sodium nitrite → methemoglobin-$Fe3^+$

Reaction 2: Methemoglobin-$Fe3^+$ + cyanide/cytochrome oxidase complex → cyanide-methemoglobin-$Fe3^+$ + cytochrome oxidase (free)

Reaction 3: Cyanide-methemoglobin-$Fe3^+$ + thiosulfate → hemoglobin-$Fe2^+$ + thiocyanate (less toxic, easily eliminated renally).

Although included in a Cyanide Antidote Kit (produced by Eli Lilly), amyl nitrite ampules are questionably effective, as they produce very low methemoglobin levels. Intravenous sodium nitrite, also in the kit, produces a methemoglobin level of 25%, which must be reduced in the presence of anemia. In Europe, Dicobalt edetate (see Dicobalt Edetate) and hydroxocobalamin (see Hydroxocobalamin) are considered safer antidotes than the sodium nitrite and sodium thiosulfate combination. In Germany, 4-DMAP is also used in cyanide poisoning. See 4-Dimethyl-para-aminophenol Hydrochloride (4-DMAP).

In hydrogen sulfide poisoning, the methemoglobin resulting from intravenous sodium nitrite produces metsulfhemoglobin, which is nontoxic and easily excreted by the body. Therefore, the administration of sodium thiosulfate is unnecessary.

CAUTIONS

As nitrites may produce or aggravate hypotension, blood pressure should be monitored closely. Dosages must be adjusted for weight and hemoglobin level in children, because fatal methemoglobinemias result from excessive sodium nitrite doses. Oxygen saturation and methemoglobin levels must be monitored closely. Pure oxygen should be administered concurrently. Check methemoglobin level 30 minutes after sodium nitrite. The therapeutic goal is 20-30% methemoglobinemia. Consider exchange transfusion if methemoglobinemia is excessive.

DOSAGE

Begin treatment at the first sign of known exposure or if exposure is strongly suspected. Amyl nitrite ampules are first crushed in gauze and given to patients to inhale for 15 seconds. Use a fresh ampule every 3 minutes. Children under 25 kg require reduced doses based on hemoglobin. Contact your local poison center for specifics. In adults, sodium nitrite (10 mL of 3% solution) is given intravenously over 2–5 minutes. Subsequently, 25% sodium thiosulfate (1.65 mL/kg up to 50 mL) is administered intravenously over 10 minutes. Use 1.65 mL/kg in children. Nitrite therapy, and not thiosulfate, may be indicated in hydrogen sulfide poisoning.

Dantrolene

USES

- Dantrolene appears to diminish hyperthermic states and muscle rigidity associated with amphetamine overdose, carbon monoxide poisoning, monoamine oxidase overdose, organophosphate poisoning, and in neuroleptic malignant syndrome (NMS). Confirmation of its usefulness for these indications requires further controlled study.
- Dantrolene may be useful in controlling the hypermetabolic state associated with rhabdomyolysis secondary to theophylline poisoning.

MECHANISM OF ACTION

Dantrolene sodium acts in the treatment of hypercatabolic syndromes such as malignant hyperthermia or neuroleptic malignant syndrome by affecting calcium flux across the sarcoplasmic reticulum of skeletal muscle cells, resulting in rapid resolution of hyperthermia, dysrhythmias, muscle rigidity, tachycardia, hypercapnia, and metabolic acidosis.

CAUTIONS

Use of oral dantrolene as a prophylactic drug in patients supposedly susceptible to malignant hyperthermia induced nausea, vomiting, dizziness, and diarrhea. Watch for lightheadedness, drowsiness, phlebitis, muscle weakness, and respiratory failure. Acute pulmonary edema and severe cardiac insufficiency have been reported with dantrolene use. Animal studies demonstrate an increase in lethality with a concomitant decrease in seizures when dantrolene is added to theophylline. Complete heart block and hyperkalemia developed in animals pretreated with verapamil who were then given dantrolene in one study.

DOSAGE

Oral dantrolene is not recommended for prophylaxis or treatment due to variability in plasma levels attained, especially in children, delay in achieving therapeutic levels, and hepatotoxicity after oral use. In malignant hyperthermia, intravenous dose is 1 mg/kg. Dose may be repeated up to a cumulative dose of 10 mg/kg as needed.

Deferoxamine Mesylate (Desferal®)

USES

- Specific iron chelator that does not enhance the excretion of electrolytes or trace metals. Use if peak serum iron approximately 4–6 hours post-ingestion is greater than 350 ug/dL. In addition, deferoxamine is used in symptomatic individuals or if serum iron determination is unavailable. Symptoms of iron poisoning include gastrointestinal distress, acidosis, hypotension, bloody vomitus, or coma. Multiple radiopacities may be seen on X-ray.
- Aluminum toxicity (experimental).

MECHANISM OF ACTION

Deferoxamine is a siderochrome produced by the bacteria Streptomyces pilosus that specifically chelates iron to form ferrioxamine. This complex is water soluble and readily excreted by the kidney. The urine characteristically turns a pink to vin rose color, although one case report documented a lack of urine discoloration in the presence of elevated serum iron levels. Complex formation is more rapid in acid pH, but renal excretion is more rapid in alkaline urine.

CAUTIONS

Although the use of 2 grams of deferoxamine as a lavage solution has been proposed for treatment of acute iron poisoning, and several studies demonstrate decreased iron absorption after such lavage, no studies have compared deferoxamine with other oral complexing agents. In view of the fact that oral deferoxamine may increase the total body burden of iron (the ferrioxamine complex is readily absorbed), oral deferoxamine is not currently recommended as a lavage solution in iron poisoning.

Rapid intravenous administration may cause flushing, erythema, urticaria, hypotension, and shock. Blood pressure should be monitored during infusions. Cataract formation has been reported in patients undergoing prolonged deferoxamine therapy but not in patients treated for acute iron intoxication. Long-term use of deferoxamine has been associated with hearing loss, night blindness, visual field defects, retinal pigmentary degeneration, optic neuropathy, and visual loss.

DOSAGE

The goal of deferoxamine therapy is elimination of free iron and enhancement of the renal excretion of iron. The usual dose for moderate to severe toxicity is 15 mg/kg/h intravenously up to 90 mg/kg over 8 hours. The maximum recommended dose is 6 grams over 24 hours. An alternative regimen is 90 mg/kg intramuscularly every 8 hours for 24 hours, but this route should not be used in hypotensive patients because of erratic drug absorption. One case in which 30 mg of deferoxamine per kilogram per hour was required to achieve chelant excess suggests that the traditional therapeutic ceiling (15 mg/kg/h) may not apply to massive iron overdoses.

Dextrose and Octreotide

USES

- Dextrose may be used to treat hypoglycemia induced by insulin or oral hypoglycemic agents.
- Dextrose may also be used to treat hypoglycemia induced by ethanol overdose, or by other toxins such as salicylates, beta blockers, MAO inhibitors, and Akee Fruit poisoning.
- Octreotide is potentially useful for the hyperinsulinemia induced by sulfonylurea overdose.

MECHANISM OF ACTION

Dextrose replenishes a lack of blood glucose in its pure form. Octreotide is a synthetic, somatostatin analog peptide, which suppresses plasma insulin, and C-peptide levels.

CAUTIONS

Some evidence suggests that dextrose solutions be avoided or used sparingly in patients at risk for cerebral ischemia, impending cardiac arrest, severe hypotension, or those receiving cardiopulmonary resuscitation.

DOSAGE

A 50 mL i.v. bolus of 50% glucose is given to adults after blood is withdrawn for analysis. The pediatric dose is 4 mL/kg of 25% glucose. Bedside determination of normoglycemia will determine use. Octreotide 50 μg every 12 hours subcutaneously may be useful in sulfonylurea overdose.

Dicobalt Edetate

USES

- Dicobalt edetate is used in Europe in the treatment of cyanide poisoning.
- See Cyanide Antidotes (Amyl Nitrite, Sodium Nitrite, and Sodium Thiosulfate).

MECHANISM OF ACTION

Cobalt salts may form a relatively nontoxic stable ion complex with cyanide. Dicobalt edetate is currently used in the United Kingdom and is not approved for use in the United States.

CAUTIONS

If cyanide toxicity has not been diagnosed, free cobalt ions, which are usually present in solutions of Dicobalt edetate, may lead to serious cobalt toxicity. Glucose may protect against cobalt toxicity and should be given at the same time as Dicobalt edetate. Vomiting, urticaria, facial, laryngeal and neck edema, anaphylactic shock, chest pain, hypotension, and ventricular arrhythmias have been reported with the use of Dicobalt edetate. Fully conscious patients are unlikely to require Dicobalt edetate. There is little experience in pregnancy.

DOSAGE

A suggested dose is 300 mg of Dicobalt edetate administered by intravenous injection over 1 minute. If there is no response, a further dose of 300 mg may be given 5 minutes later. Each injection of Dicobalt edetate should be followed immediately by 50 mL of 50% glucose intravenously.

Diethylenetriaminepenta-acetic Acid (DTPA)

USES

- The U.S. Food and Drug Administration has approved the use of zinc trisodium diethylenetriaminepenta-acetic acid (DTPA) as an investigational drug for the decorporation of plutonium, berkelium, californium, americium, and curium.
- It may also be useful for chelation of some rare earth (e.g., cerium, yttrium, lanthanum, promethium and scandium) and some transitional metals (e.g., zirconium and niobium).

MECHANISM OF ACTION

DTPA enhances the elimination of radionuclides and metals from the body by a process involving the exchange of organic compounds for inorganic ions to form a relatively stable, non-ionized ring complex which is readily excreted by the kidney. The FDA approval of DTPA covers only its use for the transuranium metals.

CAUTIONS

A urinalysis should be performed before each treatment. Potential contraindications to the drug are leukopenia, thrombocytopenia, and serious kidney dysfunction.

DOSAGE

Adults are given 1 gram in 250 mL normal saline or 5% glucose in water, infused over 1 hour. Infusions may be repeated on 5 successive days per week. Adults may also be given 1 gram in a 4-mL vial placed in a nebulizer. The entire volume is usually inhaled in 15–30 minutes. Inhalation administration can be repeated daily or, if indicated, 2–3 times per week.

Digoxin-specific Antibody (Fab) Fragments

USES

- The antibody fragments are used in life-threatening digitalis and digitalis glycoside poisoning. Indications include life-threatening arrhythmias, a serum digoxin level greater than 10 ng/mL in an acute ingestion, a potassium level greater than 5 mEq/L in the setting of digitalis ingestion, and the ingestion of greater than 10 mg in adults or 4 mg in children.
- Possibly effective for cardiac glycoside containing plants include oleander and foxglove.

MECHANISM OF ACTION

Antibodies to digoxin are derived from sheep immunized with a digoxin-serum albumin conjugate, and are split by papain digestion into fragments (Digibind®). The Fab fragments retain the antigen-binding properties, but are less immunogenic, are more easily excreted, and diffuse more rapidly than the whole antibody. Sheep Fab fragments have been used successfully to neutralize severe human digoxin poisoning with minimal adverse reactions. Serum digoxin levels rise dramatically after Fab fragment therapy, reflecting large amounts of inactive, antibody-bound digoxin, whereas free digoxin drops to undetectable levels. Fab fragments have a small volume of distribution and are eliminated through renal filtration.

CAUTIONS

Rapid withdrawal of positive inotropic effects in patients with poor cardiac reserves, and hypersensitivity reactions, remain potential problems. As Fab fragments are themselves immunogenic, patients treated more than once may experience an acute IgE-mediated hypersensitivity reaction. Monitor potassium levels and electrocardiogram for signs of recurrent congestive heart failure and hypokalemia. Delayed digoxin toxicity may occur in individuals with renal insufficiency due to impaired elimination of digoxin-Fab complexes.

DOSAGE

Equimolar doses are recommended for neutralization of digoxin although lower doses may be equally effective. The Fab fragment has a molecular weight of about 50,000 daltons and digoxin, 780 daltons. Therefore, about 65 mg Fab fragments is the molar equivalent necessary to bind and neutralize 1 mg of digoxin. The dose in number of vials = the steady state digoxin level in ng/mL, × kg of body weight ÷ (100). Four to six vials will generally be sufficient, except in extremely large overdoses. Administer i.v. over 30 minutes through a filter. A bolus injection may be used in cases of impending cardiac arrest.

Dimercaprol (BAL in Oil)

USES

- Arsenic, but not arsine gas, poisoning.
- Adjunctive therapy for acute lead encephalopathy.
- Gold poisoning and inorganic mercury poisoning. Dimercaprol has increased the central nervous system uptake of organic mercury in experimental animals compared with controls.
- Possibly useful in antimony, bismuth, chromium, nickel, copper, zinc, and tungsten poisoning.

MECHANISM OF ACTION

Heavy metals inhibit sulfhydryl-containing enzymes, which are essential factors for chemical processes throughout the body, including cell respiration. Like most chelating agents, dimercaprol (British Anti-Lewisite or BAL in Oil) contains ligands that bind heavy metals in preference to the body's sulfhydryl groups. The resulting chelated mercaptide product is less toxic and more easily excreted from the body than the heavy metals. The dimercaprol-metal complex can disassociate and release the bound metal, particularly at low pH or low dimercaprol concentrations. Further data are required to substantiate the clinical importance of this postulate.

CAUTIONS

Blood pressure should be monitored, and dimercaprol must be given cautiously in hypertensive patients. Dimercaprol must be administered by deep intramuscular injection because of its propensity to produce pain and sterile abscesses at the injection site. It must never be given intravenously. Fever occurs commonly in children following the second or third dose and frequently persists until dimercaprol is withdrawn.

Dimercaprol is potentially nephrotoxic. The drug must be used with caution in patients with renal dysfunction and oliguria. Alkalinization of the urine may produce disassociation of the dimercaprol-metal complex and may prevent renal toxicity. Dimercaprol elimination requires hepatic metabolism and therefore must be used cautiously, if at all, in patients with hepatic dysfunction. Dimercaprol is contraindicated in methylmercury poisoning due to exacerbation of central nervous system symptoms. Dimercaprol may cause hemolysis in G6PD deficiency.

DOSAGE

A typical dosage schedule for arsenic toxicity is 3–5 mg/kg intramuscularly (i.m.) every 4 hours for 2 days, 3 mg/kg i.m. every 6 hours for 1 day, and then 3 mg/kg i.m. every 12 hours for 7 days until symptoms clear or the urine arsenic level drops below 50 ug/24 hours. When doses exceed 5 mg/kg, most patients will experience vomiting, seizures or coma, within 1-6 hours.

Dimercaptosuccinic Acid (DMSA)

See Succimer.

4-Dimethyl-para-aminophenol Hydrochoride (4-DMAP)

USES

- 4-DMAP has been the drug of choice in Germany for cyanide poisoning. Its use is generally restricted to cyanide-poisoned patients in deep coma, with dilated nonreactive pupils and deteriorating cardiorespiratory function. See Cyanide Antidotes (Amyl Nitrite, Sodium Nitrite, and Sodium Thiosulfate).
- It may be useful in cyanide poisoning following prolonged use of sodium nitroprusside.
- It may possibly be of use in severe hydrogen sulfide poisoning.

MECHANISM OF ACTION

4-Dimethyl-para-aminophenol hydrochloride (4-DMAP) rapidly induces methemoglobin formation. Methemoglobin, in turn, combines with cyanide. Cyanomethemoglobin, a less toxic compound, is then excreted after combination with exogenous thiosulfate.

CAUTIONS

Even at recommended doses, 4-DMAP may produce an excessive methemoglobinemia ranging up to 70%. Excess methemoglobinemia may be corrected with methylene blue; however, this may release cyanide. Exchange transfusion may be useful in severe cases. Hemolysis has been seen on the second day after administration of a therapeutic dose. Treatment with 4-DMAP is contraindicated in patients with glucose-6-phosphatase dehydrogenase (G6 PD) deficiency. In contact with air, 4-DMAP is readily oxidized and the solution changes color. Headache, dizziness, hyperventilation, cyanosis, and green/brown discoloration of the urine may be seen.

DOSAGE

A dose of 3.25 mg/kg body weight is given intravenously immediately. This is followed by sodium thiosulfate, 150–200 mg/kg, intravenously. Artificial respiration is implemented as required.

Diphenhydramine (Benadryl®)

See Antihistamines.

DMSA

See Succimer.

Ethanol

USES

- Pending confirmation of toxic levels, the administration of ethanol is recommended whenever the history or physical examination suggests significant ingestion of methanol or ethylene glycol.
- Acidosis or peak plasma levels of methanol or ethylene glycol exceeding 20 mg/dL indicate the need for ethanol therapy.

Ethanol is also indicated if blood concentration is not readily available or if ingestion of these toxins is suspected.
- 4-Methylpyrazole (4-MP) is an alternative antidote in these settings. See 4-Methylpyrazole.

MECHANISM OF ACTION
Ethanol reduces the formation of toxic metabolites produced after methanol and ethylene glycol ingestion. Specifically, ethanol delays the formation of formic acid in methanol poisoning, and both glycolic and glyoxylic acid in ethylene glycol poisoning. Ethanol acts by competitively inhibiting alcohol dehydrogenase.

CAUTIONS
Serum glucose, serum ethanol levels, and arterial pH must be monitored during ethanol infusion. Ethanol administration is not a substitute for hemodialysis in serious intoxications. Maintenance ethanol infusions should be increased during dialysis. Solutions of 10% ethanol in D5W (5% dextrose in water) should be used for intravenous infusions, because absolute alcohol is highly irritating to veins.

DOSAGE
The therapeutic objective is maintenance of a plasma ethanol level of 100 mg/dL. The intravenous loading dose is 7.6–10 mL/kg of 10% ethanol in D5W over 30 minutes. Maintenance dose is 1.4 mL/kg/hour of 10% ethanol in D5W. Maintenance doses are based on the fact that the average patient metabolizes about 125 mg/kg body weight per hour. Alcoholic patients and patients undergoing dialysis require higher maintenance levels. An oral alternative loading dose is 800 mg/kg and a maintenance dose of 125–150 mg/kg every hour diluted in juice.

Flumazenil (Romazicon®)

USES
- Flumazenil is indicated primarily in the treatment of symptoms of benzodiazepine overdose.
- Flumazenil is also effective in treating zolpidem (Ambien®) overdose, and may be helpful in Zopiclone overdose.
- Flumazenil is possibly effective in improving consciousness in ethanol intoxication, where it may aid in improving blood gas analyses and permitting extubation.

MECHANISM OF ACTION
Flumazenil antagonizes the actions of benzodiazepines by competitively inhibiting benzodiazepine activity at the GABA-benzodiazepine receptor complex. Flumazenil has little or no agonist activity in humans.

CAUTIONS
Ventricular tachycardia, complete heart block, and death may follow flumazenil use. Seizures and acute anxiety states may be provoked in patients dependent on benzodiazepines. Acute withdrawal symptoms may be seen in the benzodiazepine-dependent patient given flumazenil in an emergency facility. Seizures are more common if the patient has taken a tricyclic antidepressant, isoniazid, cocaine, or propoxyphene in addition to the benzodiazepine. In these cases flumazenil antagonizes the anticonvulsant properties of the benzodiazepines, leaving drugs that may be epileptogenic. Repeat doses may be required because of the short duration of action of flumazenil (1 hour).

DOSAGE
As a diagnostic tool in the evaluation of comatose drug overdose, flumazenil should be given as a 0.2-mg bolus intravenously, with an additional 0.1 mg/min until the patient is awake. Most patients respond to 3 mg or less. A continuous infusion of flumazenil has not been shown superior to a repeat bolus technique, often preferred for routine clinical use. An intravenous dose of 5 mg may improve consciousness in alcohol intoxication but does not improve psychomotor function.

Folinic Acid (Leucovorin®) and Folic Acid

USES
- Leucovorin "rescue" is used in folic acid antagonist overdose. These overdoses are manifested by bone marrow depression. Folic acid antagonists include methotrexate, trimethoprim, and pyrimethamine.
- Folic acid possibly is effective as adjunctive therapy for methanol intoxication.

MECHANISM OF ACTION
Folic acid is a B-complex vitamin that is required for nucleoprotein synthesis and normal erythropoiesis. Folic acid is not the metabolically active form, but it is the precursor of the active tetrahydrofolic acid. Folic acid antagonists (e.g., methotrexate) inhibit folic acid reductase and prevent the formation of tetrahydrofolic acid. Therefore, overdoses of folic acid antagonists require leucovorin, which is a derivative of tetrahydrofolic acid rather than folic acid. Folic acid probably accelerates the detoxification of the toxic metabolite, formic acid, in methanol intoxication.

CAUTIONS
Allergic reactions may occur following oral or parenteral administration of folic acid or leucovorin. Folate and sodium bicarbonate may precipitate if given together.

DOSAGE
Leucovorin should be given within the first hour of a methotrexate, trimethoprim or pyrimethamine overdose. The initial route should be intravenous using a dose equal to the amount of folic acid antagonist consumed. Usually, 10–100 mg/m^2 is given i.v. or i.m. every 3–6 hours for 72 hours. Folate doses for methanol toxicity are 1 mg/kg up to 50 mg i.v. every 4–6 hours for 2 days.

Glucagon

USES
- Glucagon is used in symptomatic beta-adrenergic blocker overdose.
- Preliminary reports indicate a potential usefulness for glucagon in the management of hemodynamic instability associated with calcium channel blocker poisoning.
- Treatment of hypoglycemia or hypoglycemic agent overdoses. See Dextrose and Octreotide.
- Anecdotal reports suggest a use for glucagon 0.5 mg intravenously over 30 seconds to facilitate passage of foreign bodies from the distal esophagus into the stomach.

MECHANISM OF ACTION
Glucagon stimulates the production of cyclic AMP (cAMP). By increasing myocardial cAMP, glucagon increases the chronotropic and inotropic activity of the heart, and reverses the overdose effects of beta-blockers and calcium-channel blockers. Glucagon also stimulates the release of glucose from liver stores, and the release of catecholamines. It may be used as a treatment for hypoglycemic states.

CAUTIONS

Nausea, vomiting, hypersensitivity reactions, and elevated blood glucose levels may result from glucagon administration. Hypokalemia may result from glucagon-induced insulin secretion with intracellular transfer of glucose and potassium. Glucagon should be given cautiously to hypertensive patients, because of catecholamine induction in all patients and particularly in those with pheochromocytoma. Monitor serum glucose levels carefully if glucagon is administered to patients suspected of having an insulinoma. Significant hypoglycemia may occur. Glucagon is classified as pregnancy category B.

Other adverse reactions may include erythema multiforme, Stevens-Johnson syndrome, hypersensitivity reactions, and thrombophlebitis. These may be lessened by diluting the drug before use in large doses or by continuous infusion. Failure of glucagon therapy in calcium channel blocker overdose may be associated with both hypo- and hypercalcemic states. Careful monitoring of the total serum calcium and, preferably, total serum ionized calcium, as well as supplemental infusion of calcium chloride, may be required.

DOSAGE

Calcium channel blocker overdoses may require glucagon doses higher than those used to reverse the myocardial depression associated with beta-blocker overdoses. If an initial bolus of 2–10 mg i.v. over 1 minute is unsuccessful at increasing blood pressure, it is probably reasonable to double that dose. If glucagon improves the hemodynamic status of the patient, a glucagon infusion should be started at a rate of 2 to 5 mg/h. Isoproterenol and dobutamine often are necessary to augment contractility in beta-blocker overdose. Severe beta-blocker overdoses may require higher-than-usual vasopressor doses. In hypoglycemic states, give an initial bolus of 0.5–1 mg over 1 minute, then 0.5–1 mg every 20 minutes as needed.

Hydroxocobalamin

USES

- Treatment of cyanide poisoning, especially that resulting from excessive sodium nitroprusside infusions. Hydroxocobalamin is an investigational orphan drug in the U.S. It is not available commercially in the U.S.
- Possibly in cyanide-intoxicated smoke inhalation victims.
- As therapeutic treatment after exposure to acetonitrile, propionitrile, and potassium and sodium cyanide by oral, inhalational, or dermal routes.
- For treatment of diseases caused by chronic, low-level cyanide exposure (tobacco amblyopia, Leber's hereditary optic atrophy). See Cyanide Antidotes.

MECHANISM OF ACTION

Hydroxocobalamin binds to cyanide to form cyanocobalamin (Vitamin B12). It does not interfere with tissue oxygenation. Cyanocobalamin is excreted unchanged in urine.

CAUTIONS

Anaphylactoid reactions and acne have been observed. Hepatotoxicity, myocardial, and renal changes have been observed in animals. Hydroxocobalamin causes muscle twitching, spasm and hypertension with reflex bradycardia. A transient reddish discoloration of skin, mucous membranes, and urine may be observed. This discoloration may last 12 hours. In prolonged infusions, the solution must be protected from light. The presence of hydroxocobalamin in serum interferes with a number of laboratory tests (bilirubin rises, creatinine falls, and serum iron cannot be measured).

DOSAGE

In France, a formulation is available which contains 4 grams of hydroxocobalamin powder. This is diluted in more than 220 mL of 5% dextrose solution. Give 50 times the estimated cyanide dose. For an approximate fatal dose of 200 mg of cyanide, this would represent a hydroxocobalamin dose of 10 g. If the amount of cyanide ingested is not known, give 50 mg/kg. A 5-gram dose binds 100 mg of cyanide. Five grams of hydroxocobalamin in combination with 12.5 grams of sodium thiosulfate appears to be a safe and effective treatment for cyanide poisoning patients.

Serum thiocyanate levels should be measured in patients who receive nitroprusside infusions at rates higher than 10 mg/kg/min for longer than 48 hours or who have renal insufficiency. The suggested dose of hydroxocobalamin for preventing nitroprusside-induced cyanide toxicity is 25 mg/h for 10 hours at the end of a nitroprusside infusion.

Hyperbaric Oxygen (HBO)

USES

- Carbon monoxide poisoning in symptomatic patients, or if carboxyhemoglobin level is > 40%, or > 15% in a pregnant patient.
- Carbon monoxide poisoning in patients who have had any period of unconsciousness or who develop cardiac ischemia or arrhythmias.
- Carbon monoxide poisoning in children or in patients with preexisting cardiovascular disease who have a carboxyhemoglobin level > 20%.
- Possibly helpful in methylene chloride poisoning.
- May be helpful in cyanide and hydrogen sulfide poisoning and in severe cases of methemoglobinemia.
- Possibly useful in carbon tetrachloride poisoning.
- Suggested for treatment of severe brown recluse spider envenomation (Loxosceles reclusa bites).

MECHANISM OF ACTION

Oxygen displaces carbon monoxide from hemoglobin, myoglobin and cytochrome oxidase enzymes. The half-life of carboxyhemoglobin may be reduced to 23 minutes at 3 atmospheres with 100% oxygen. Hyperbaric oxygen may decrease cerebral edema and delayed neuropsychiatric sequelae, however more research is needed. Carbon monoxide may decrease hepatotoxicity in carbon tetrachloride toxicity.

CAUTIONS

Patients may be denied necessary intensive care, especially in monoplace chambers. Traumatic rupture of the tympanic membrane, acute sinusitis and optic neuritis have all been described. Refractive errors, particularly in elderly patients treated for prolonged periods, may occur. Pneumothorax may occur in those with pre-existing pulmonary blebs. The use of hyperbaric oxygen therapy is also complicated by potential safety hazards such as explosion and fire, oxygen toxicity, and seizures.

DOSAGE

Two to three atmospheres of 100% oxygen are administered in chambers. Treatment protocols and indications are controversial.

Methionine

USES

- In Europe, oral methionine is approved as an agent to prevent hepatotoxicity after large acetaminophen ingestions.

- N-Acetyl-L-cysteine remains the preferred antidote for acetaminophen overdose in the United States and Canada. See N-Acetylcysteine (NAC), (Mucomyst®).

MECHANISM OF ACTION
Restores depleted glutathione stores in hepatotoxic acetaminophen ingestions.

CAUTIONS
Is not generally available in the U.S., as N-acetylcysteine has proven so efficacious.

DOSAGE
Ten grams, orally, is given over 12 hours.

Methylene Blue

USES

- Methylene blue is administered to symptomatic patients who have been exposed to methemoglobin-forming compounds and whose methemoglobin levels exceed 20–30%. Blood may appear chocolate brown if methemoglobin concentration exceeds 15%.
- Methemoglobin inducers include aniline dyes, nitrites, nitrates, local anesthetics such as benzocaine, phenazopyridine, dapsone, naphthalene, nitrobenzene and dinitrophenol.

MECHANISM OF ACTION
Methylene blue acts as an electron carrier for the hexose monophosphate pathway, which reduces methemoglobin to hemoglobin. In patients with methemoglobinemia, the erythrocyte methemoglobin reductase reduces methylene blue to leukomethylene blue (colorless form), which in turn reduces methemoglobin to hemoglobin.

CAUTIONS
Large intravenous doses (more than 7 mg/kg) produce nausea, vomiting, abdominal pain, chest pain, dizziness, diaphoresis, confusion, and cyanosis because of methemoglobin formation. Arterial blood gases should follow oxygen saturation and methemoglobin levels. Pulse oximetry overestimates oxygen saturation and can not be used to rule out methemoglobinemia. Methylene blue causes hemolysis in glucose-6-phosphate dehydrogenase (G6PD)-deficient patients and exchange transfusion should be seriously considered as an alternative to methylene blue therapy. Since methylene blue is eliminated mostly by renal excretion, the drug should be used cautiously in the presence of renal dysfunction. This drug is contraindicated as an agent to reverse methemoglobinemia after the use of sodium nitrite as an antidote for cyanide poisoning.

DOSAGE
A dose of 0.2 mL/kg of a 1% (10 mg/mL) solution, or 1–2 mg/kg, should be administered over several minutes. The dose may be repeated in 60 minutes and every 4 hours up to 15 mg/kg. The treatment goal is a methemoglobin level less than 20%.

4-Methylpyrazole (4-MP), (Antizol®)

USES

- 4-Methylpyrazole (4-MP) is used in ethylene glycol poisoning and possibly in methanol poisoning. See Ethanol.

MECHANISM OF ACTION
4-Methylpyrazole is an inhibitor of alcohol dehydrogenase, the enzyme responsible for metabolizing methanol and ethylene glycol to their toxic metabolites. 4-Methylpyrazole administered by the oral or intravenous route appears to lead to the rapid excretion of free ethylene glycol in the urine, an increase in plasma ethylene glycol half-life, and return to normal levels of plasma and urinary oxalate in 2 days. It also leads to the correction of metabolic acidosis within hours, and prevents the development of renal failure. Few serious side effects have been observed at doses of 10–20 mg/kg/d. 4-MP is useful for patients with normal renal function admitted less than 3 hours after ingestion. If renal function is impaired, dialysis may be necessary.

CAUTIONS
Patients must be treated soon after ingestion (ideally within 3 hours). Patients may experience nausea, dizziness, rashes, and vertigo. Multiple doses may induce a slight rise in blood pressure and hepatic aminotransferase levels. Diarrhea and headache may also be observed. Treatment with 4-MP is more effective for patients with normal renal function. If renal function is impaired, dialysis may be required. Intravenous bolus dosing may induce a phlebosclerosis with local pain during injection.

DOSAGE
4-Methylpyrazole is administered by the oral or intravenous route at a dose of 10–20 mg/kg/d, perhaps for 3–5 days.

N-Acetylcysteine (NAC), (Mucomyst®)

USES

- N-Acetylcysteine (NAC) is used for the treatment of acetaminophen overdoses. Survival improves in patients with acetaminophen-induced fulminant hepatic failure given acetylcysteine soon after acetaminophen ingestion. Improvement may also be observed after encephalopathy and other signs of severe liver damage, including coagulopathy, have developed. Toxicity may be predicted by the Matthew-Rumack nomogram. Serum acetaminophen does not peak until 4 hours post-ingestion.
- Only the oral form of NAC has been approved by the FDA. The intravenous form is available in the U.S. only through an investigational protocol. Intravenous NAC is available in the United Kingdom and Canada.
- Numerous anecdotal reports indicate potential uses of acetylcysteine in addition to acetaminophen poisoning. These include toxicity secondary to halogenated hydrocarbons which may deplete glutathione (chloroform-phosgene metabolite, carbon tetrachloride, bromobenzene), paraquat, acrylonitrile, naphthalene (epoxide metabolite conjugates with glutathione), sulfur mustard, cytotoxic agents (ifosfamide, bleomycin), and prevention of delayed neuropsychiatric complications in carbon monoxide poisoning.
- Other proposed uses include improvement of macrophage function in the bronchioalveolar lavage fluid of smokers, treatment of inflammatory joint disease, prevention of HIV expression (AIDS), use in the adult respiratory distress syndrome (free radical scavenger), potentiation of the cardiovascular effects of nitroglycerin, treatment of dichromate intoxication, amanitin poisoning, and reduction of lipoprotein. No clear conclusions have emerged from these studies to provide definitive guidelines for clinical usefulness. Controlled clinical studies are required to place most of these observations in perspective.

MECHANISM OF ACTION
N-Acetyl-L-cysteine (NAC) acts as a glutathione substitute that prevents the formation of toxic intermediary metabolites after

acetaminophen overdose. It is the N-acetyl derivative of the naturally occurring amino acid cysteine. N-Acetylcysteine may increase oxygen consumption and improve microcirculatory blood flow.

CAUTIONS

NAC is most effective if given within 16 hours of ingestion of acetaminophen and preferably within 8–12 hours postingestion. New evidence indicates that some deleterious effects of acetaminophen poisoning may be curtailed if NAC is even given up to 24 hours post-ingestion. When the results of the acetaminophen level will not be available before 8 hours postingestion, and the ingested dose is suspected to be toxic, a loading dose of NAC should be given pending laboratory results. Activated charcoal absorbs NAC *in vitro* and possibly *in vivo.* They may be co-administered, however, particularly if multiple drugs are suspected.

NAC has a wide margin of safety, and the loading dose may be repeated if vomiting occurs within the first hour. It is quite foul tasting and may be administered with carbonated beverages or juices. Adverse reactions (nausea, vomiting, rhinitis, fever, chills) to oral NAC may occur. Hypersensitivity-like reactions occur more frequently with intravenous administration and are manifested as urticaria, flushing, diaphoresis, pruritus, and rarely, transient hypotension, tachycardia, and bronchospasm. Such reactions usually respond to antihistamines and slowing of the infusion.

DOSAGE

The oral NAC course approved in the U.S. is a loading dose of 140 mg/kg (diluted in soda pop or juice to 5% solution), then 70 mg/kg every 4 hours for 17 additional doses. Antiemetics such as metoclopramide, ondansetron or droperidol may be helpful. The intravenous route is preferred in Europe for its shorter duration, ease of administration in nauseated patients, and ability to administer activated charcoal concurrently. The intravenous loading dose is 150 mg/kg in 200 mL 5% dextrose over 15–60 minutes, followed by 50 mg/kg in 500 mL 5% dextrose over 4 hours, and 100 mg/kg in 1 L 5% dextrose over the next 15 hours (total dose, 300 mg/kg over 20 hours).

Naloxone (Narcan®) and Nalmefene (Revex®)

USES

- Natural and synthetic opiate overdoses (e.g., codeine, fentanyl, heroin, meperidine, and morphine).
- Opiate partial agonist overdose (e.g., butorphanol, propoxyphene, pentazocine, and tramadol).
- Diphenoxylate overdose.
- Dextromethorphan overdose.
- Possible reversal or partial reversal of ethanol-induced coma.
- Possibly effective against alpha-2 agonists such as clonidine, guanabenz and guanfacine.
- Possibly effective against imidazoline nasal sprays such as tetrahydrozoline and oxymetazoline.

MECHANISM OF ACTION

Naloxone is a semisynthetic, pure opiate antagonist derived from thebaine and structurally similar to oxymorphone. Its presumed mechanism of action is competitive antagonism at mu, kappa, and sigma opiate receptors in the central nervous system. Mu receptors have the highest affinity for naloxone. Unlike levallorphan and nalorphine, naloxone has minimal agonist activity at clinical doses. Nalmefene is a derivative of naltrexone, which also exhibits opioid antagonist effects without producing opiate agonist effects.

CAUTIONS

Naloxone is a pure opiate antagonist with few adverse reactions at clinical doses. Hypertension as well as atrial and ventricular dysrhythmias have been associated with the postoperative use of naloxone, mostly in patients with organic heart disease or abstinence syndrome. Postoperative sudden death has been reported in healthy young adults following intravenous naloxone. Naloxone and nalmefene can produce opioid withdrawal in dependent patients.

Slow intravenous titration of naloxone to reverse the respiratory and central nervous sytem depression of opioid use avoids serious withdrawal symptoms. The naloxone therapeutic half-life for reversal of respiratory depression is 30–60 minutes, shorter than the drug half-life for most opiates. Naloxone may be readministered when opiate symptoms reappear until the patient is symptom-free for 2–4 hours after the last naloxone dose. Methadone overdoses require longer periods of observation. Nalmefene may last many hours and may particularly be advantageous in cases involving long-acting opiates.

DOSAGE

Naloxone: For children, use 0.03–0.1 mg/kg intravenously. For adults, start with 0.4–2.0 mg boluses. If there is no response, give several 2.0 mg boluses up to 10 mg. i.v. drip: Maintain drip at 2/3 dose necessary to achieve initial response. Add 10 times this amount to 1 liter of D5W and infuse at 100 mL/hour. Naloxone (0.4 mg) may be administered via endotracheal tube if intravenous access is unavailable. The subcutaneous and intramuscular routes are alternative routes of administration as well. Certain opioid drugs (e.g., propoxyphene, pentazocine, Lomotil® and codeine) may require large naloxone doses to reverse opiate effects. At least 5 mg (0.1 mg/kg in children) should be administered in these overdoses and more should be given if a partial response is noted.

Nalmefene: 0.5–1.0 mg i.v. every 2 minutes as needed to a total of 2 mg.

Octreotide

See Dextrose and Octreotide.

D-Penicillamine (Cuprimine®)

USES

- D-Penicillamine may be useful for the treatment of copper, lead, mercury, arsenic, and bismuth poisoning.
- It may be used following dimercaprol therapy in arsenic exposures, and in the presence of toxic blood or urine levels in arsenic, mercury and copper poisoning.

MECHANISM OF ACTION

The D-isomer of penicillamine is an oral chelating agent that is a non-bacteriocidal degradation product of all penicillins.

CAUTIONS

D-penicillamine is contraindicated in penicillin-allergic patients. Food, antacids, and iron salts reduce penicillamine absorption. Adverse reactions include fever, proteinuria, rash, bone marrow depression, gastrointestinal distress, renal and hepatic dysfunction, taste disorders, and autoimmune diseases such as Goodpasture's syndrome, myasthenia gravis, polymyositis, and systemic lupus erythematosus (SLE). Pyridoxine, 10–25 mg/d, should be administered concomitantly because penicillamine inhibits pyridoxal-dependent enzymes.

DOSAGE

For mercury and copper exposures in adults, 15–40 mg/kg/d up to 1–2 grams, divided into four doses, should be administered for 5 days. In arsenic exposures, 100 mg/kg/day to a maximum of 1 gram/day may be required. Penicillamine should be given on an empty stomach. Urine heavy metal levels should be monitored to determine the continued effectiveness of penicillamine.

Phentolamine Mesylate (Regitine®)

USES

- Cocaine-induced myocardial ischemia, vasospasm, and hypertension.
- Is used to treat vasopressor (e.g., norepinephrine, dopamine, epinephrine) extravasation (e.g., as might occur by inadvertently injecting lidocaine with epinephrine into a digit).
- Possibly useful in naloxone-induced pulmonary edema.
- Management of hypertensive crises secondary to overdose with sympathomimetic agents, including monoamine oxidase inhibitors.

MECHANISM OF ACTION

Phentolamine mesylate is an alpha-adrenergic blocking agent that causes peripheral vasodilation by direct relaxation of smooth muscle and by competitively blocking $\alpha 1$ and $\alpha 2$ receptor sites. Phentolamine also acts as a weak antagonist of 5-hydroxytryptamine and releases histamine from mast cells.

CAUTIONS

Do not use in hypotensive patients or with other hypotensive agents. Epinephrine should not be used in a phentolamine overdose, as it may result in hypotension and increase the tachycardia due to its unopposed beta-2 action.

DOSAGE

For Vasoconstriction

Remove venous access device and inject in a circle around the area where extravasation has occurred, using a new 24-gauge needle for each injection. The recommended dose with this method is a total of 5–10 mg (in normal saline) depending on the size of the extravasated area. Phentolamine, 7.5 mL of a solution containing 5 mg of phentolamine in 10 mL of normal saline, slowly infiltrated into ischemic subcutaneous tissue has been used for dopamine infiltration.

For Cocaine-Induced Myocardial Ischemia

Phentolamine may be used as an intravenous infusion in 5% dextrose or saline at a rate of 0.2–2.0 mg/min, titrating the dose to a desired blood pressure response. As much as 5–20 mg may be required in hypertensive crisis. Blood pressure and pulse should be monitored. A cardiac monitor must be available for continuous use.

Physostigmine Salicylate (Antilirium®)

USES

- May be useful in atropine and anticholinergic poisoning in rare, severe cases. Life-threatening complications include severe hypertension, refractory hallucinations, seizures, and arrhythmias.
- Plants containing anticholinergic alkaloids include jimson weed and deadly nightshade.
- Controversial role in baclofen and tricyclic antidepressant overdose, where it is almost never indicated except as a drug of last resort.
- Second-line agent for envenomation by certain Asian snakes or intoxication with tetradotoxin if edrophonium supplies are depleted.

MECHANISM OF ACTION

Physostigmine reversibly inactivates cholinesterases by carbamylation, leading to cholinergic actions lasting several hours. There is a high incidence of serious, possibly fatal side effects, so the risks of administration usually outweigh the benefits.

CAUTIONS

Physostigmine is generally contraindicated in patients with cardiovascular disease (especially conduction disturbances), gastrointestinal obstruction, and asthma. Seizures, bradycardia, or asystole may result from physostigmine administration, particularly with rapid infusion. The maximum intravenous rates are 0.5 mg/min in children and 1 mg/min in adults. Physostigmine should be used extremely cautiously, if at all, to reverse excessive atropinization in organophosphate toxicity. Signs of cholinergic crisis, such as bradycardia, hypersalivation and bronchospasm may accompany physostigmine use. Physostigmine excess may be treated with atropine. See Atropine. Serious consideration should be given to poison control center consultation before physostigmine use.

DOSAGE

The initial intravenous dose is 0.5 mg (0.02 mg/kg) repeated every 5 minutes up to 2 mg or until the desired effect in an adult. The minimal effective dose should be used; additional doses may be necessary every 30–60 minutes because of rapid physostigmine elimination.

Phytonadione (Aqua Mephyton®, Mephyton®)

See Vitamin K1.

Pralidoxime, 2-PAM (Protopam®)

USES

- Pralidoxime is used to reverse nicotinic cholinergic effects associated with organophosphate exposures. Pralidoxime effectively reverses nicotinic cholinergic effects (e.g., fasciculations, muscle twitches, weakness, pallor, tachycardia, and hypertension) but not the muscarinic reactions (e.g., bronchospasm, dyspnea, excessive secretions, miosis, hypotension, bradycardia, incontinence, vomiting and diarrhea). Atropine (see Atropine) is used to combat the muscarinic effects in organophosphate exposures.
- May be used to treat poisoning by antimyasthenic agents such as pyridostigmine (see Pyridostigmine Bromide), tacrine, and nerve gas agents (e.g., Sarin, Soman, and Tabun).

MECHANISM OF ACTION

Pralidoxime is an effective reactivator of cholinesterases recently inactivated by exposure to organophosphates. By removing a phosphoryl group from an inhibited enzyme, an oxime complex is formed and active cholinesterase is regenerated by pralidoxime. Pralidoxime also detoxifies certain organophosphates and may actually protect cholinesterases from inhibition by directly reacting with them. The efficacy varies with the organophosphate involved and decreases with increasing age of inactivation.

CAUTIONS
Pralidoxime is most effective when given within 24 hours postexposure and probably has no value more than 36–48 hours postexposure. Approximately 80–90% of pralidoxime is excreted unchanged in the urine. Dosages should be reduced in the presence of renal dysfunction. Succinylcholine, theophylline, and respiratory depressants must be used cautiously in patients with organophosphate exposures. Rapid i.v. administration may cause tachycardia, rigidity, hypertension, neuromuscular blockade, and laryngospasm, which apparently are dose and rate related.

Pralidoxime must be used cautiously in patients with myasthenia gravis because it may precipitate a myasthenic crisis in those patients who require anticholinesterase drugs. Carbamate poisoning usually causes transient signs of cholinergic excess that respond to atropine. The use of pralidoxime in the setting of carbamate insecticide poisoning is controversial and may enhance carbaryl toxicity.

DOSAGE
A dose of 25–50 mg/kg, up to 1–2 grams in adults, should be administered intravenously over 5 minutes. Repeat dosing may be required every 6 hours for several days. Atropine must be administered concurrently to reverse muscarinic cholinergic effects. See Atropine.

Protamine Sulfate (Prosulf®)

USES
- Protamine is used in heparin, dalteparin and enoxaparin overdoses that result in bleeding.

MECHANISM OF ACTION
Protamine is a protein derived from fish sperm that complexes with heparin to form a stable salt. The protamine-heparin complex has no anticoagulant properties. Protamine sulfate has weak anticoagulant actions itself, resulting from mild inhibition of thromboplastin generation and activity, and subsequent decreased conversion of prothrombin to thrombin.

CAUTIONS
Rapid intravenous administration may cause anaphylactoid reactions (hypotension, dyspnea, flushing, and bradycardia). The dose should not exceed 100 mg because of protamine's anticoagulant properties. Partial thromboplastin times (PTT) should be monitored 15 minutes after administration to assess the effectiveness of therapy. Pregnancy risk factor C.

DOSAGE
One mg of protamine neutralizes 90–115 units of heparin. The appropriate dose should be calculated up to a 50-mg maximum and infused intravenously over 5 minutes at 10 mg/mL.

Prussian Blue

USES
- Prussian blue is possibly effective in thallium toxicity.
- Prussian blue salts have been used as an antidote after radiocesium and thallium contamination

MECHANISM OF ACTION
Thallium is exchanged for potassium in the molecular lattice and subsequently the complex is excreted in the feces.

CAUTIONS
Prussian blue is not commercially available or FDA-approved for use.

A decomposition product in Prussian blue salts may be cyanide.

DOSAGE
Use 250 mg/kg/d in four divided doses orally or through a nasogastric tube.

Pyridostigmine Bromide (Mestinon®)

USES
- Widespread use as a nerve agent pretreatment under wartime conditions. See Atropine and Pralidoxime, 2-PAM (Protopam®).
- Used by anesthesiologists to antagonize nondepolarizing neuromuscular blockade.
- Used in the treatment of myasthenia gravis.

MECHANISM OF ACTION
Pyridostigmine is an anticholinesterase agent that inhibits the hydrolysis of acetylcholine by competing with acetylcholine for attachment to acetylcholinesterase.

CAUTIONS
Patients may experience flatus, diarrhea, abdominal cramps, urinary urgency, nausea, headache, daydreams, rhinorrhea, tingling of the extremities, muscle weakness, cramps, and twitching. Patients with a history of asthma may experience bronchospasm. Acute hypertension is rare.

DOSAGE
For prevention of the effects of anticholinesterase chemical warfare agents, 30 mg is given orally every 8 hours. For myasthenia gravis, adults are given 60 mg orally three times daily with a maintenance daily dose of 60 mg to 1.5 grams. Children may be started on 7 mg/kg or 200 mg/m^2 daily, divided into five or six doses.

Pyridoxine Hydrochloride (Vitamin B6)

USES
- May prevent or control isoniazid-induced seizures and subsequent lactic acidosis. Should be given to any symptomatic patient with isoniazid poisoning or any asymptomatic patient suspected of ingesting 80 mg/kg of isoniazid or more.
- May reduce the central nervous system symptoms that result from the monomethylhydrazine block of pyridoxine metabolism in hydrazine-containing false morel (Gyromitra) mushroom poisoning. Should be given to anyone with a known or suspected ingestion of these mushrooms. Probably does not reduce the hepatic and renal consequences of these mushrooms.
- May combat optic neuritis due to chloramphenicol.
- Possibly effective in cycloserine and acrylamide toxicity.
- Is a cofactor in the metabolism of toxic intermediaries of ethylene glycol and may enhance the elimination of these toxic products. Should be given to anyone with a known or suspected ingestion of ethylene glycol.

MECHANISM OF ACTION

Pyridoxine is a water-soluble B-complex vitamin involved in the transamination of amino acids and conversion of tryptophan to niacin. This vitamin appears to be essential in the synthesis of gamma-aminobutyric acid (GABA) within the central nervous system. Isoniazid-induced seizures are thought to result from decreased GABA levels because of isoniazid inhibition of brain pyridoxal-5-phosphate activity.

CAUTIONS

Pyridoxine usually is nontoxic even in large doses. Several years of daily doses ranging from 500 mg to 2 grams has led to a progressive sensory neuropathy that improved after discontinuation of the vitamin. Nausea and allergic reactions have been reported.

DOSAGE

For isoniazid toxicity, a single intravenous (i.v.) infusion over 30–60 minutes of a gram-for-gram equivalent dose, or 5 grams, is used. For monomethylhydrazine toxicity, the dose is 25 mg/kg i.v.. If the initial dose is effective, additional doses may be administered as symptoms reappear up to 300 mg/kg/d. In ethylene glycol cases, 100 mg administered i.v. may be given daily. See Ethanol and 4-Methylpyrazole (4-MP), (Antizol®).

Sodium Bicarbonate

USES

- Tricyclic antidepressant poisoning.
- May be useful in poisoning by phenothiazines, propoxyphene, carbamazepine, amantadine, cocaine, quinidine, chloroquine, amoxapine, diethylene glycol, ethylene glycol, formaldehyde, maprotiline, methanol, propylene glycol, and strychnine.
- Useful in treating weakly acidic toxins such as barbiturates (e.g., phenobarbital), salicylates, chlorpropamide, and chlorophenoxy herbicides.
- May reverse respiratory symptoms induced by chlorine gas.
- Used to treat hyperkalemia and hypercalcemia.

MECHANISM OF ACTION

Dissociates to produce bicarbonate, which neutralizes hydrogen ions and raises pH. Sodium bicarbonate can reverse QRS prolongation in antidepressant and propoxyphene overdose. It reverses cardiac conduction defects caused by quinidine-like effects of cardiotoxic drugs and increases protein binding of tricyclic antidepressants. Neutralizes respiratory injury induced by chlorine gas.

CAUTIONS

Sodium bicarbonate may cause cerebral edema, metabolic alkalosis, hypokalemia, and hypocalcemia. Extravasation may cause local tissue necrosis. Sodium load may exacerbate congestive heart failure.

DOSAGE

In tricyclic overdose with QRS widening greater than 10 milliseconds, goal of therapy is an arterial pH of 7.45–7.55. One to two mEq/kg may be pushed intravenously and repeated as necessary in severe cases. To enhance urinary elimination by weakly acidic toxins such as salicylates and barbiturates, the therapeutic goal is a urine pH of 7.5–8.0. This may be achieved by adding 2–3 amps (equals 88 to 132 mEq) of sodium bicarbonate to 1 liter of D5W, and infusing the solution at 2–3 mL/kg/hour. Attempts at alkalinization may be dangerous in patients with renal dysfunction or congestive heart failure. In chlorine gas exposures, a nebulized 3.75–5% solution may be used. In adult hyperkalemia, 50 mEq over 5 minutes may be administered intravenously. In children, dose is 1–2 mEq/kg every 2–4 hours.

Sodium Diethyldithiocarbamate (Dithiocarb)

USES

- Dithiocarb has been used to treat nickel dermatitis and nickel carbonyl poisoning. It is an investigational drug in the U.S. and is classified as an orphan drug.
- Previously, Dithiocarb was recommended as a chelator for thallium poisoning.
- Where Dithiocarb has not been available, disulfiram (Antabuse) has been administered because it is metabolized to two molecules of Dithiocarb and is hypothetically of value. The absence of clinical studies and the toxicity of disulfiram do not make it a proven alternative to Dithiocarb.

MECHANISM OF ACTION

Dithiocarb is a chelating agent that increases the excretion of nickel in the urine and feces. It is metabolized to disulfiram, an agent used in the treatment of chronic ethanolism.

CAUTIONS

Patients are advised not to drink alcohol for 12 hours before and 48 hours after treatment because of the potential disulfiram effect. Patients have reported a metallic taste and abdominal discomfort (gastric complaints, flatulence, diarrhea) following the use of Dithiocarb.

DOSAGE

In mild cases, give 2 grams of Dithiocarb orally in divided doses every 4 hours. In moderate or severe poisoning, give 2 grams at first, then 1 gram in 4 hours, 0.6 grams in 8 hours and 0.4 grams in 16 hours. On subsequent days, give 0.4 grams every 8 hours.

Succimer, DMSA (Chemet®)

USES

- An oral medication, DMSA, was approved in 1991 by the FDA for the treatment of severe lead poisoning in children whose blood level is greater than 45 $\mu g/dL$. See also Calcium Disodium EDTA (Versenate®) and D-Penicillamine (Cuprimine®). The therapeutic goal is weekly lead levels less than 15 mcg/dL.
- It may be used in cases of lead encephalopathy with contraindications to Dimercaprol.
- DMSA is specific for arsenic, lead, mercury, methylmercury, and silver but does not bind iron, calcium, or magnesium. DMSA may be of benefit in severe thallium intoxication.
- DMSA may increase mercury excretion and decrease blood mercury concentrations in mercury vapor poisoning.

MECHANISM OF ACTION

Dimercaptosuccinic acid (DMSA) provides two sulfhydryl groups that can chelate metals.

CAUTIONS

Rashes, nausea, vomiting, and an elevation in alanine aminotransferase concentration may be seen following DMSA. All patients should be adequately hydrated before treatment. Use of DMSA in the presence of diminished renal function must proceed with great caution. In cases of lead poisoning, measure blood lead level before therapy and on day 3, day 7, and weekly for evidence of rebound. Monitor complete blood count and platelets, ferritin, bilirubin, alkaline phosphatase, aminotransferases, blood urea nitrogen, creatinine, uric acid, calcium, phosphorus, glucose, total protein, albumin, urinalysis, and urine lead.

The efficacy of DMSA compared with $CaNa_2EDTA$ for lead poisoning has been questioned. Unlike $CaNa_2EDTA$, DMSA does not increase elimination of essential minerals like calcium, magnesium, copper and zinc. Unlike D-penicillamine, DMSA does not increase the gastrointestinal absorption of lead. Identification and removal of the source of lead exposure should accompany therapy, because the drug cannot prevent lead poisoning in a lead-containing environment.

DOSAGE

The dose is 10 mg/kg or 350 mg/m^2 every 8 hours for 5 days. Reduce to 10 mg/kg or 350 mg/m^2 every 12 hours (two-thirds initial dose) for an additional 2 weeks of therapy. A course of therapy lasts 19 days. A minimum of 2 weeks is recommended between courses. In young children who cannot swallow the capsule, open the capsule, and sprinkle the medicated beads on a small amount of soft food or place the beads in a spoon and follow with a soft drink. In children 1–5 years old, oral DMSA has been given in doses of 30 mg/kg/d for 5 days, then 20 mg/kg/d for 14 days.

Vitamin B6

See Pyridoxine Hydrochloride.

Vitamin K1 (Phytonadione), (Aqua Mephyton®)

USES

- Phytonadione is used to treat moderate to severe hemorrhages caused by coumarin or indandione overdoses. It will not reverse heparin-induced hemorrhage.
- Used in long-acting rodenticide poisoning by brodifacoum, bromadiolone, chlorphacinone and diphacinone.

MECHANISM OF ACTION

Phytonadione is a fat-soluble naphthoquinone derivative required for the synthesis of blood coagulation factors II (prothrombin), VII (proconvertin), IX (Christmas), and X (Stuart-Prower) in the liver. In adequate doses, vitamin K1 reverses the inhibitory action of coumarin and indandione compounds on these factors.

CAUTIONS

Although phytonadione is relatively nontoxic, hypersensitivity reactions or anaphylactoid reactions may follow intravenous administration. Slow infusions may ameliorate but not always eliminate these reactions. Phytonadione is relatively contraindicated in patients requiring Coumadin for heart valves.

DOSAGE

Use 1.5–10 mg intramuscularly or subcutaneously every 4–8 hours based on serial prothrombin times. Intravenous infusions should not exceed 1.0 mg/min, and should be attempted only in severe cases. The oral dose in adults is 2.5–10 mg every 12–48 hours.

Questions—Antidotes

1. Which of the following antidotes is incorrectly matched with the toxin(s) it counteracts?
A. 4-Aminopyridine (4-AP)- Pancuronium
B. Polyvalent Crotalidae Antivenin-Rattlesnakes, Fer-de-lance (Bothrops species), and Bushmaster (Lachesis mutus)
C. North American Coral Snake Antivenin-Sonoran Coral Snake
D. Atropine-Nerve Gases
E. Calcium Disodium EDTA-Lead, Copper, Zinc

2. Which of the following antidotes is incorrectly matched with the toxin(s) it counteracts?
A. Calcium Gluconate-Latrodectus Envenomation
B. Sodium Nitrite-Acetonitrile
C. Deferoxamine-Iron, Aluminum
D. Octreotide-Sulfonylureas
E. Dicobalt Edetate-Sodium Thiosulfate

3. Which of the following antidotes is correctly matched with the toxin(s) it counteracts?
A. Diethylenetriaminepenta-acetic acid (DTPA)-Methylene Chloride
B. Digoxin-Specific Antibody (Fab) Fragments-Jimsonweed
C. Dimercaprol-Arsenic
D. 4-Dimethyl-para-aminophenol hydrochloride (4-DMAP)-Californium
E. Ethanol-Isopropyl Alcohol

4. Which of the following antidotes is correctly matched with the toxin(s) it counteracts?
A. Folic Acid-Methanol
B. Glucagon-Azathioprine
C. Hydroxocobalamin-Methemoglobinemia
D. Hyperbaric Oxygen-Sulfur Dioxide
E. 4-Methylpyrazole (4-MP)-Ethanol

5. Which mechanism of action is incorrect?
A. 4-Methylpyrazole (4-MP) is an inhibitor of alcohol dehydrogenase.
B. N-Acetyl-L-cysteine (NAC) acts as a glutathione substitute.
C. Naloxone is a non-competitive antagonist at mu, kappa, and sigma opiate receptors in the central and peripheral nervous systems.
D. Phentolamine mesylate is an alpha-adrenergic blocking agent.
E. Physostigmine reversibly inactivates cholinesterases by carbamylation.

6. Which of the following is false?
A. Pralidoxime is most effective when given within 24 hours postexposure of organophosphates and probably has no value more than 36–48 hours postexposure.
B. Rapid intravenous administration of protamine may cause anaphylactoid reactions.
C. Pyridostigmine is an anticholinesterase agent that inhibits the hydrolysis of acetylcholine by competing with acetylcholine for attachment to acetylcholinesterase.
D. Isoniazid-induced seizures are thought to result from increased GABA levels as a consequence of isoniazid stimulation of brain pyridoxal-5-phosphate activity.
E. Dithiocarb is a chelating agent that is metabolized to disulfiram.

Answers to questions in shaded boxes appear at the end of the chapter.

7. Which of the following is false?
A. Dimercaptosuccinic acid (DMSA) provides two sulfhydryl groups that can chelate metals.
B. DMSA is approved for the treatment of lead poisoning in children whose level is > 45 ug/dL.
C. Phytonadione is a fat-soluble naphthoquinone derivative required for the synthesis of blood coagulation factors II, VII, IX and X in the liver.
D. Benztropine and diphenhydramine reverse drug-induced dystonias through non-competitive stimulation of nicotinic receptors and blockade of norepinephrine reuptake.
E. At pharmacologic doses, atropine antagonizes cholinergic stimuli at muscarinic receptors while exhibiting little or no effect at the nicotinic receptors of the autonomic ganglia.

8. Possible indications for hyperbaric oxygen include
A. Carbon monoxide poisoning
B. Methylene chloride poisoning
C. Latrodectus mactans envenomations
D. Hydrogen sulfide poisoning
E. A, B and D

9. Complications of hyperbaric oxygen therapy include all of the following except
A. Rupture of the tympanic membrane
B. Acute sinusitis
C. Pneumocephaly
D. Refractive errors
E. Pneumothorax

Answers

Antidotes

1. C 2. E 3. C 4. A 5. C 6. D 7. D
8. E 9. C

CHAPTER 6
Elimination Enhancement

INTRODUCTION

With supportive treatment alone, spontaneous recovery after toxicologic exposure occurs in 98% of intensive care unit admissions. However, in certain instances, various extracorporeal techniques are useful in the treatment of poisoning. Extracorporeal techniques may be useful in salicylate, methanol, ethylene glycol, lithium, and theophylline overdose, and are of limited use in sedative-hypnotic, industrial, and household poisonings.

An American Association of Poison Control Centers (AAPCC) survey found that hemodialysis in 1986 was used predominantly for ethylene glycol, lithium, methanol, and aspirin poisoning. Hemoperfusion was used mostly in theophylline, cyclic antidepressant, and barbiturate overdose. By 1992, hemodialysis was used mainly for lithium, theophylline, ethylene glycol, aspirin, methanol, and ethanol poisoning, in that order of frequency. Hemoperfusion was used mainly for theophylline, long-acting barbiturates, benzodiazepines, and carbamazepine, in order of frequency.

All the extracorporeal techniques (hemodialysis, hemoperfusion, and hemofiltration) have not been subject to controlled clinical trials in poisoned patients. Their clinical benefit remains to be firmly established in most instances.

Questions—Introduction to Elimination Enhancement

1. With supportive treatment alone, spontaneous recovery after toxicologic exposure occurs in 98% of intensive care unit admissions.
A. True
B. False

HEMODIALYSIS

Although hemodialysis has been recommended for a variety of toxins, only relatively few severely poisoned patients actually benefit from dialysis. To be effective, dialysis should improve the removal of a toxin at least 30% compared with unaided clearance. The physical characteristics of the toxin are the major factors that limit the efficacy of dialysis. The drug or toxin must be able to pass easily across the dialysis membrane (e.g., molecular weights below 500 daltons, high water solubility, and low protein binding).

Either rapid equilibration with tissue stores or a high plasma concentration (i.e., small volume of distribution) is necessary to ensure that adequate amounts of drug are available for clearance by dialysis. Plasma drug levels should correlate with clinical effects so that serum measurements can confirm the effect of hemodialysis on the duration of toxic effects. Available objective data on renal drug clearance do not permit a consensus on which drug overdose patients benefit from hemodialysis. Specific agents for which hemodialysis should be considered even before blood levels are analyzed are methanol and ethylene glycol. The use of dialysis for salicylates, phenobarbital, isopropanol, lithium, and theophylline depends on both serum levels and clinical condition.

Indications

The decision to initiate hemodialysis depends on clinical evaluation of both patient-related and drug-related parameters, in addition to the knowledge that hemodialysis will significantly improve drug clearance. The following factors favor dialysis:

- Severe clinical intoxication with vital sign abnormalities such as hypotension, apnea, or hyperthermia that do not respond to supportive care.
- Impairment of normal excretion routes or the presence of disease states that reduce drug clearance (e.g., ethchlorvynol overdose in a severely cirrhotic patient).
- Progressive clinical deterioration or the development of complications such as aspiration pneumonia despite maximum supportive care.
- Prolonged coma that may produce complications such as aspiration pneumonia, sepsis, or peripheral neuropathy secondary to pressure ischemia.
- Presence of an underlying disease, such as chronic obstructive pulmonary disease (COPD), that may progress during coma.
- Ingestion and probable absorption of a potentially lethal dose determined despite gut decontamination.
- Documentation of a potentially lethal drug level.
- Presence of a significant quantity of a toxin that is metabolized to a toxic metabolite (e.g., methanol, ethylene glycol).

Answers to questions in shaded boxes appear at the end of the chapter.

Adverse Reactions

Acute adverse reactions from hemodialysis include hypotension, electrolyte and osmolar imbalance (muscle cramps, dysequilibrium syndrome characterized by confusion, coma, or convulsions), hypoxemia, spontaneous bleeding (retroperitoneal or subdural hematoma), and mechanical complications (air embolism, ruptured arteriovenous fistula, blood leak). Sudden death during dialysis has resulted from machine malfunction or fistula rupture, electrocution, cardiac dysrhythmias, complete heart block secondary to triglyceride emulsion, coagulopathy, or hyperkalemia from overheated solutions.

Complications

Contraindications include the concomitant presence of antidotes (e.g., naloxone in opiate overdose, or n-acetylcysteine in acetaminophen overdose), coagulopathy, or cardiogenic shock. Bleeding may occur secondary to anticoagulation.

Questions—Hemodialysis

1. **Hemodialysis may be helpful in each of the following overdoses, except**
   A. Lithium
   B. Methanol
   C. Salicylates
   D. Tricyclic antidepressant
   E. Theophylline
2. **Physical conditions that favor hemodialysis include**
   A. Molecular weights below 500 daltons
   B. High water solubility
   C. High protein binding
   D. All of the above
   E. A and B
3. **Adverse reactions from hemodialysis include**
   A. Hypertension
   B. Electrolyte and osmolar imbalance
   C. Bleeding
   D. Mechanical complications
   E. All of the above

HEMOPERFUSION

In 1965, Yatzid first introduced hemoperfusion as a method for removing toxic material in which the blood is pumped through a cartridge of absorbent material. After heparinization, hemodialysis pumps push blood from vascular catheters through the absorbent cartridges and back into the circulation. Although it shows some of the same pharmacokinetic and patient-related limitations as hemodialysis, high molecular weight, protein binding or poor water solubility does not limit hemoperfusion. Because it is a relatively new technique, large comparative studies are not available to guide treatment. However, clinical studies to date indicate a role for hemoperfusion in the clearance of nonbarbiturate sedative-hypnotics, disopyramide, and theophylline.

Charcoal and resin are the two distinct cartridge types and have different drug affinities. Charcoal-coated absorbent material removes both polar (e.g., salicylates, methotrexate) and nonpolar drugs as well as metabolites. Amberlite XAD-4 resin effectively clears nonpolar, lipid-soluble drugs (e.g., ethchlorvynol) better than charcoal-coated cartridges.

Problems that limit the usefulness of hemoperfusion include late initiation of treatment, presence of compounds with a large volume of distribution or with a rapid distribution, poisonings that are more easily treated with hemodialysis, and usefulness of symptomatic therapy during the critical phase. There is little benefit to hemoperfusion over hemodialysis. Clearance of some drugs may be higher with hemoperfusion than with hemodialysis, but this probably is not significant.

General Indications

- An established intoxication causing a severe disturbance of one or more vital functions with a drug having a small distribution volume and displaying a clear relationship between blood levels and toxic effects.
- Deterioration of the clinical state of an intoxicated patient with initially less severe symptoms, despite optimal conservative treatment.
- Intoxication with a drug known to be metabolized to a more toxic one.
- Intoxication with a drug known to produce delayed toxicity.
- Severe intoxication with midbrain dysfunction.
- Development of complications of coma.
- Impairment of normal drug excretory function.
- Intoxication with an extractable drug that can be removed at a rate greater than that of endogenous elimination.

POSSIBLE INDICATIONS FOR HEMOPERFUSION

- Short-acting barbiturates and nonbarbiturate sedative-hypnotics (i.e., ethchlorvynol, glutethimide, meprobamate, and methaqualone) where supportive care is inadequate and blood levels suggest a lethal ingestion. Clearance by hemoperfusion usually exceeds hemodialysis clearance. The patient-related criteria for hemoperfusion are the same as those for hemodialysis.
- Drugs with delayed toxicity. Hemoperfusion for Amanita phalloides, paraquat, diquat, and methotrexate toxicity is theoretically useful, but the efficacy of the procedure in these intoxications remains to be determined.
- Theophylline. When seizures or dysrhythmias cannot be controlled, hemoperfusion produces greater clearance than hemodialysis.
- Disopyramide. Clearance by hemoperfusion exceeds that by hemodialysis.
- Salicylates. Although hemoperfusion produces good clearance, the electrolyte and acid-base imbalance is better controlled by hemodialysis.
- Phenytoin. Patients with severe phenytoin overdose may benefit from hemoperfusion, which is less limited by protein binding than hemodialysis.
- Chloramphenicol. An anecdotal case demonstrates the successful clinical use of charcoal hemoperfusion in the gray baby syndrome.

Adverse Reactions

Numerous adverse reactions may occur during hemoperfusion. These include thrombocytopenia (often a 30% reduction) and loss of clotting factors. As heparinization is required, hemorrhage may occur during use. Leukopenia (often a 10% reduction) may occur, but infection is rare. Fever and chills may occur without the presence of sepsis. Air embolism has been reported. Glucose, calcium, and urate levels may be reduced. Occasional "rebound" elevation of drug levels may occur as a result of redistribution of the compound from deep compartments. Hypotension (usually mild) and hypothermia (rare except in infants) may occur.

Complications

Situations in which hemoperfusion should not be used are similar to hemodialysis. These include adequacy of supportive care alone in maintaining the patient, cardiogenic shock, and coagulopathy or contraindication to heparinization (e.g., gastric ulcer).

Questions—Hemoperfusion

1. **Which of the following regarding hemoperfusion is false?**
   A. In hemoperfusion, blood is pumped through a cartridge of absorbent material.
   B. Unlike hemodialysis, high molecular weight, protein binding, or poor water solubility does not limit hemoperfusion.
   C. There may be a role for hemoperfusion in the clearance of nonbarbiturate sedative-hypnotics, disopyramide, and theophylline.
   D. Charcoal and cholestyramine are two distinct cartridge types and have different drug affinities.
   E. Substances with a large volume of distribution are not amenable to hemoperfusion.
2. **Complications of hemoperfusion include all of the following, except**
   A. Thrombocytopenia
   B. Loss of clotting factors
   C. Leukocytosis
   D. Air embolism
   E. Glucose, calcium, and urate levels may be reduced

HEMOFILTRATION

During hemofiltration, an arteriovenous pressure difference induces a convective transport of solutes through a hollow fiber or flat sheet membrane. This permits a substantial flow of plasma water and a high permeability to compounds with a relative molecular weight less than or equal to 40,000. Hemofiltration is performed similar to hemodialysis except that the blood is pumped through a hemofilter. It can be performed intermittently or continuously. The advantage of hemofiltration over hemodialysis and hemoperfusion is its ability to remove compounds with large (4,500 to 40,000) molecular weights. Such compounds include the aminoglycoside antibiotics and metal chelate complexes such as aluminum or iron deferoxamine.

Indications

The indications to remove toxic compounds by hemofiltration are limited. Clinical studies suggest that continuous arteriovenous hemofiltration (CAVH) does not appear to substitute for hemodialysis or hemoperfusion. If a compound is amenable to removal by hemodialysis, its clearance will be greater than that achieved by hemofiltration. Hemofiltration and plasmapheresis remain potentially hazardous forms of treatment. CAVH, compared with hemodialysis, may be useful for eliminating agents like lithium, methanol, ethanol, ethylene glycol, vancomycin, aminoglycosides, and N-acetylprocainamide, however confirmatory studies are largely lacking.

Adverse Reactions

Complications of hemofiltration include clotting of the filter and mild bleeding.

Questions—Hemofiltration

1. **Hemofiltration is performed similar to hemodialysis except that the blood is pumped through a hemofilter.**
   A. True
   B. False
2. **The advantage of hemofiltration over hemodialysis and hemoperfusion is its ability to remove compounds with large (4,500 to 40,000) molecular weights.**
   A. True
   B. False
3. **Numerous indications for hemofiltration have been identified.**
   A. True
   B. False

FORCED DIURESIS AND pH ALTERATION

Many drugs are weak acids or bases and in solution become ionized when they gain or lose a hydrogen ion. At physiologic pH, most drugs are partially ionized. The extent of ionization depends on the dissociation constant (K) and the pH of the medium. The pKA of a drug is the pH at which equal amounts of drug are in the ionized (polar) form and the un-ionized (nonpolar) form. Weak acids have a pKA between 3.0 and 7.5, whereas the pKA of weak bases ranges from 7.5 to 10.5. The goal of forced diuresis with urine pH alteration is to enhance renal excretion by increasing the amount of the ionized (polar) form in the urine. Conceptually, altering urine pH produces an ion trap within the renal tubules. Cell membranes are more permeable to nonpolar drug forms, which easily diffuse across the tubular membrane and are reabsorbed. Peak excretion rates then require maximal ionization, because the ionized form is "trapped" in the renal tubule and excreted. Maximal excretion of drugs with an acid pKA (e.g., weak acids such as salicylate, phenobarbital, phenoxyacetate herbicides) occurs in the alkaline pH range, whereas enhancement of renal excretion of drugs with an alkaline pKA (e.g., amphetamines, quinidine, phencyclidine) occurs in the acid pH range.

The reverse is true for absorption from the stomach. In acidic solutions, weak acids such as salicylates are less ionized and more easily absorbed. Weak bases are better absorbed in alkaline media (e.g., duodenum) and are more trapped in an acidic environment (e.g., stomach). Generally, weak acids are better candidates for enhanced excretion because they tend to remain in plasma (i.e., have smaller volumes of distribution). Plasma has a relatively higher pH (approximately 7.4) than intracellular fluid pH (approximately 7.0). Weak bases are less ideal candidates for enhanced excretion because they easily enter cells where they are trapped in a more acidic intracellular environment. Hence, weak bases are less available to the kidney for renal excretion.

General Indications

Because of potential complications and unique drug characteristics required to enhance renal excretion effectively, indications for forced diuresis with pH alteration are few. Drugs considered for this method must have low protein binding, limited metabolism, high renal clearance, and primarily extracellular fluid distribution (i.e., a small volume of distribution). Furthermore, the pKA of the drug must be in a range that maximal renal excretion can be achieved by realistic alterations in urine pH.

Alkaline Diuresis (Weak Acids)

INDICATIONS

The use of alkaline diuresis is an effective and safe method to enhance salicylate excretion particularly in mild to moderate intoxications. The potential complications of cerebral and pulmonary edema in severe, acute, and chronic ingestions make hemodialysis a safer method than alkaline diuresis in severe overdose cases. The importance of forced diuresis (urinary flow rate of 2 to 6 mL/kg/h) is controversial, because urinary alkalinization alone will significantly increase excretion. Alkaline diuresis also is effective in phenobarbital overdose, but usually is not necessary. Supportive care often suffices in mild and moderate overdoses. In more severe overdoses, hemodialysis is safer because excessive fluid loads may precipitate pulmonary edema. Severe cases of 2,4-dichlorophenoxyacetic acid (2,4-D) poisoning may benefit from alkaline diuresis.

METHODS

One to 2 mEq/kg of sodium bicarbonate (in 15 mL/kg 5% dextrose) is added to 0.45% saline and run over 3 to 4 hours. Urine pH in 1 hour should be at least 7.5 and preferably 8.0. Additional intravenous boluses of sodium bicarbonate (0.5 mEq/kg) may be needed to alkalinize the urine, but the arterial pH must be monitored. Fluid deficits, hypokalemia, and acidosis must be corrected. Baseline laboratory values should include serum creatinine, electrolytes, glucose, arterial blood gases, plasma drug concentrations, and urine pH. Renal dysfunction contraindicates the use of alkaline diuresis. Urine volumes for adults should be kept above 3 mL/min. The use of large fluid volumes (9 to 12 mL/min) is controversial and may not significantly increase renal excretion. When large volumes and diuretics are given, careful supervision in an intensive care setting is required, along with monitoring of fluid balance (central venous pressure, hourly urine output), serum electrolytes, and acid-base balance (urine and plasma).

COMPLICATIONS

Complications may include pulmonary edema, cerebral edema, and electrolyte and acid-base disturbances (e.g., hypomagnesemia, hypokalemia, hypernatremia, alkalosis, and/or hypocalcemia).

Acid Diuresis (Weak Bases)

INDICATIONS

The current indications for acid diuresis are essentially nil. Adverse reactions are common and the process is technically difficult. Initial enthusiasm for enhancing phencyclidine (PCP) elimination is waning because its large volume of distribution (VD) limits the amount of drug available for renal excretion. Furthermore, acid diuresis is dangerous if myoglobinuria is present, because of the precipitation of myoglobin in the renal tubules and the subsequent development of acute tubular necrosis.

The urinary excretion of quinidine does not appear to be significantly increased by acid diuresis because quinidine is about 80% metabolized. In view of the fact that renal elimination is small and cardiac complications are difficult to manage in quinidine overdoses, the use of acid diuresis is not recommended, at least until more clinical data are available. In strychnine overdose, there is a theoretical advantage to acid diuresis, but the rapid onset of symptoms limits its use.

METHODS

Ammonium chloride, 75 mg/kg/24 hours, is divided into 4 to 6 oral doses or given intravenously as a 2% solution. Intensive care unit monitoring is required to follow electrolyte and acid-base status. An alternative method is the administration of 0.2 mEq/kg/hour of a 0.1-molar hydrochloric acid solution through a central venous line. The endpoint of acidification is a urine pH of 5.5 to 6.0.

COMPLICATIONS

Contraindications to urinary acidification include hepatic insufficiency, renal dysfunction, and myoglobinuria. Ammonia encephalopathy has resulted from the use of ammonium chloride.

Questions—Forced Diuresis and pH Alteration

1. **The pKA of a drug**
   A. Is the pH at which equal amounts of drug are in the ionized (polar) form and the un-ionized (nonpolar) form
   B. Represents the dissociation constant of a particular drug at a given pH
   C. Determines whether hemodialysis will be helpful
   D. Depends on relative protein binding
   E. Is the Michaelis-Menton constant
2. **The goal of forced diuresis with urine pH alteration is to enhance renal excretion by increasing the amount of the unionized form in the urine.**
   A. True
   B. False
3. **Maximal excretion of weakly acidic drugs occurs in the acidic pH range.**
   A. True
   B. False
4. **Drugs with an alkaline pKA include**
   A. Amphetamines
   B. Quinidine
   C. Phencyclidine
   D. All of the above
   E. None of the above
5. **The current indications for acid diuresis are essentially nil because adverse reactions are common and the process is technically difficult.**
   A. True
   B. False

PERITONEAL DIALYSIS

Peritoneal dialysis is almost never used in the management of drug overdoses or poisoning, and is generally not an acceptable substitute for hemodialysis. Peritoneal dialysis operates on principles similar to those of hemodialysis, with diffusion of toxins from mesenteric capillaries across the peritoneal membrane into dialysate dwelling in the peritoneal cavity. The blood flow rate depends on intrinsic mesenteric circulation and cannot be adjusted as in hemodialysis.

As the clearance of small, dialyzable substances depends on blood and dialysate of low rates, clearance of toxins is consistently higher with hemodialysis than with peritoneal dialysis. Addition of albumin, lipids, or furosemide to the peritoneal dialysate enhances clearance but not to the levels achieved with hemodialysis. The role of peritoneal dialysis is limited to the rare patient who is a candidate for hemodialysis, for whom hemodialysis is unavailable or contraindicated.

Indications

Acute peritoneal dialysis is used principally to treat patients with acute renal failure, especially in patients with bleeding disorders or venous access problems or in centers without access to hemodialysis. The slow rate of drug removal by this technique is offset by the ability of peritoneal dialysis to be carried out for 24 hours versus the typical 2- to 4-hour cycles of hemodialysis or hemoperfusion. It does not require anticoagulation and uses minimal equipment.

Methods

Acute peritoneal dialysis involves either placing a stylet catheter at the bedside under local anesthesia or surgically inserting a Tenckhoff catheter in the abdomen. Dialysate fluid is instilled, and 1 to 2 L is exchanged each hour.

Complications

Multiple complications have been reported with peritoneal dialysis. These include pain, hemorrhage from vascular laceration, perforated viscus, peritonitis, volume overload or depletion, electrolyte imbalance, skin infection, and leakage.

Questions—Peritoneal Dialysis

1. **Peritoneal dialysis is almost never used in the management of drug overdoses or poisoning, and is generally not an acceptable substitute for hemodialysis.**
   A. True
   B. False

PLASMAPHERESIS AND PLASMA EXCHANGE

Plasmapheresis separates cellular blood components from plasma. The cells may be resuspended in colloid, albumin, or fresh-frozen plasma, and then are reinfused. In plasmapheresis, removed plasma is replaced with crystalloid solution. In plasma exchange, a protein-containing solution substitutes for the missing plasma. These methods eliminate toxic substances but sacrifice part of a patient's own plasma proteins.

Indications

A practical role for these methods has not been firmly established in medical toxicology. Case reports on the use of plasmapheresis have been described in overdoses with vincristine, paraquat, inorganic mercury, thyroxine, orellanus, amanita, theophylline, antithymocyte globulin, digoxin antibody complexes, phenytoin, dapsone, propoxyphene, hemlock, and carbamazepine. Plasmapheresis theoretically may be applicable in overdoses of toxic compounds that are highly protein bound and not eliminated effectively by hemoperfusion or hemodialysis.

Methods

This automated process removes a volume of blood from the patient and returns all of the blood elements. Variable therapeutic responses to this process have been reported in a number of diseases, including myasthenia gravis, Guillain-Barré syndrome, systemic lupus erythematosus, and rheumatoid arthritis. The rationale for use in drug overdose is that agents soluble in plasma or bound to plasma proteins would be removed by plasma exchange.

Complications

Complications may include disseminated intravascular coagulation (DIC), thrombocytopenia, nausea, hypovolemia, hypertension, hypercoagulability, infection, anaphylaxis, vascular perforation, seizures, and arrhythmias.

Questions—Plasmapheresis and Plasma Exchange

1. **A practical role for plasmapheresis and plasma exchange has not been firmly established in medical toxicology.**
   A. True
   B. False

EXCHANGE TRANSFUSION

This infrequently used method involves the removal of the patient's blood and replacement with fresh whole blood. A double-exchange transfusion implies that an amount of blood equivalent to twice the patient's total blood volume has been exchanged.

Indications

There are anecdotal case reports on the use of exchange transfusion in iron, quinine, ethchlorvynol, meperidine, glutethimide, chloral hydrate, diphenhydramine, and neonatal chloramphenicol overdoses. In these cases, the efficacy of exchange transfusion was not documented with pharmacokinetic data. Potentially, the most effective application of exchange transfusion is in severe methemoglobinemia in patients who do not respond to or cannot tolerate appropriate doses of the antidote, methylene blue.

Nitro and amino derivatives of aromatic hydrocarbons (e.g., aniline), nitrates, nitrites, and chlorates will produce methemoglobinemia. Anecdotal case reports demonstrate the successful use of exchange transfusion in methemoglobinemia, but do not document reduced methemoglobin elimination half-lives compared with methylene blue therapy.

Methods

Various regimens involve phlebotomy followed by transfusion with whole blood.

Complications

As with any transfusion, potential complications may include mismatches, chills, hypotension, infection, and bleeding.

Questions—Exchange Transfusion

1. **Exchange transfusion has been used to treat all of the following overdoses, except**
   A. Iron
   B. Ibuprofen
   C. Quinine
   D. Chloral hydrate
   E. Diphenhydramine

Answers

Introduction to Elimination Enhancement

1. A

Hemodialysis

1. D 2. E 3. E

Hemoperfusion

1. D 2. C

Hemofiltration

1. A 2. A 3. B

Forced Diuresis and pH Alteration

1. A 2. B 3. B 4. D 5. A

Peritoneal Dialysis

1. A

Plasmapheresis and Plasma Exchange

1. E

Exchange Transfusion

1. B

SELECTED READINGS

Elimination Enhancement

1. Litovitz T, Veltri JC. The role of hemoperfusion and hemodialysis in toxicology. Am J Emerg Med 1988;6:80.
2. Pond SM. Extracorporeal techniques in the management of poisoned patients. Med J Aust 1991;154:617–622.
3. Shannon M. Extracorporeal drug removal. II. Other methods. Clin Toxicol Rev 1990;12(9):1–2.

CHAPTER 7
Pharmacokinetics

INTRODUCTION

Pharmacokinetics is the mathematical study of drugs, which describes dynamic changes in body drug concentrations with respect to absorption, distribution, metabolism, and excretion. The duration and intensity of drug effects depend on factors that influence drug movement within the body. Drug effects generally depend on active drug concentration at receptor sites. Anatomically, the sites or compartments that typically are sampled to assess drug concentration (i.e., blood, urine) may not reflect the concentration of drug at its receptors. Consequently, drug effect does not always correlate with plasma concentration.

Mathematically, a two-compartment model predicts the changes in plasma concentration for most drugs with predominant renal elimination. The central compartment represents the plasma and organs of high perfusion (e.g., heart, brain, and kidney), whereas tissue stores and poorly perfused organs account for the peripheral compartment. For calculation purposes, drugs are eliminated from and absorbed into the central compartment. The resulting plasma concentration (Cp), when plotted against time shows three phases: absorption, distribution, and elimination. Distribution half-life describes the rate of distribution into the peripheral compartment, and elimination half-life describes the rate of drug elimination from the central compartment.

Drug Interactions

Drug interactions may delay or enhance excretion, alter binding to serum proteins or receptor sites, change metabolism, and/or reduce the volume of distribution. Although drugs that interact may be administered concurrently, cognizance of frequently encountered drug interactions is important, and dosages should be adjusted accordingly. Some interactions may occur only at high dosage. See individual toxins for specific, relevant drug interactions.

Patients particularly susceptible to drug interactions include elderly patients and other patients receiving many drugs, patients who have acute illness (e.g., severe anemia, left ventricular failure, status asthmaticus, and pneumonia), patients who have unstable diseases (e.g., epilepsy, diabetes mellitus, cardiac arrhythmia, and dementia), patients dependent on drug treatment (e.g., transplant recipients, patients with connective tissue disorders, and patients with Addison's disease), patients who have considerable renal or hepatic impairment (e.g., cirrhosis, congestive cardiac failure, and uremia), and patients who have more than one presribing doctor.

Questions—Introduction to Pharmacokinetics

1. **Which of the following is false?**
   A. Pharmacokinetics is the mathematical study of drugs, which describes dynamic changes in body drug concentrations with respect to absorption, distribution, metabolism, and excretion.
   B. Drug effects generally depend on active drug concentration at receptor sites.
   C. Mathematically, a two-compartment model predicts the changes in plasma concentration for most drugs with predominant renal elimination.
   D. Distribution half-life describes the rate of distribution into the central compartment.
   E. Drug interactions may delay or enhance excretion, alter binding to serum proteins or receptor sites, change metabolism, and/or reduce the volume of distribution.
2. **Patients particularly susceptible to drug interactions include all of the following, except**
   A. Elderly patients and other patients receiving many drugs

B. Patients who have acute illness
C. Patients who have considerable renal or hepatic impairment
D Patients allergic to antibiotics
E. Patients who have more than one prescribing doctor.

DEFINITIONS

Absolute Bioavailability

For a drug in a dosage form administered by an extravascular route, the fraction of the administered dose that reaches the systemic circulation when the reference is the same dose of drug administered intravenously.

Accumulation

Increase in drug concentration in whole blood (plasma or serum) or tissue, or the amount of drug in the body, until steady state is reached.

Area Under The Curve

Concentration of drug in blood (plasma or serum) integrated over time [from zero to time (t) or to infinity] after a single dose or during a dosage interval at steady state.

Bioavailability

Bioavailability is the relative amount of drug that enters the systemic circulation from an administered dosage form and the rate at which the drug appears in the systemic circulation.

Bioequivalence

Bioequivalence of a drug product is achieved if its extent and rate of absorption (bioavailability) are not substantially different from those of the standard when administered at the same molar dose.

Biophase

Immediate environment surrounding the site of action of a drug in the body.

Central Compartment

Sum of all body regions (organs, tissues, and fluids) in which the drug concentration approaches immediate equilibrium with that in blood or serum. See multicompartment model.

Clearance

Ratio of the overall elimination rate of a drug to its concentration in the reference fluid (e.g., plasma). Under steady-state conditions, clearance relates systematically available dose rate (i.e., maintenance dose per dosage interval) to the average steady-state concentration of drug in a specified biological fluid. It must be defined according to site of measurement (e.g., blood, plasma, and plasma water).

Compartment

Mathematical entity that can be described by a volume (not necessarily physiologic) and its drug concentration.

Concentration

Measured amount of drug or metabolite per unit volume of any biological fluid. Also called a "level." Free drug plus protein-bound drug equals total drug concentration. The plasma concentration (Cp) = the total amount of active drug in the body (A) divided by the volume of distribution (Vd).

Creatinine Clearance

Ratio of the excretion rate of creatinine in urine to the concentration of creatinine in plasma or serum. It is used as a measure of renal function (glomerular filtration rate).

Disposition

All the processes and factors that are involved from the time the drug reaches the circulation to the time when it, or one or more of its metabolites, leaves the body in the urine, feces, bile, expired air, or sweat.

Distribution Half-Life

Describes the rate of distribution into the peripheral compartment.

Distribution Phase

Portion of the plasma concentration-time curve during which the drug distributes primarily into the peripheral compartment. Drugs that follow a one-compartment model do not have an identifiable distribution phase.

Dosage Regimen

Dose and dosage interval required to produce clinical effectiveness or to maintain a therapeutic concentration in the body. Also called dose rate.

Dose

Amount of drug administered.

Dose-Response Curve

Graphic presentation of the pharmacologic or clinical effectiveness or toxicity (i.e., response) versus dose.

Dosing Interval

Time between doses.

Drug

Substance of synthetic, semisynthetic, natural, or biological origin that prevents, cures, or reduces disease or distress in humans or animals.

Drug Product

Final pharmaceutical form containing the active ingredient(s) and vehicle substances necessary in formulating a desired dosage, desired volume, and desired application form, ready for administration. Also called dosage form.

Drug Release

Delivery of the active ingredient from a dosage product into solution. The dissolution medium is either a biological fluid (e.g., gastric contents) or an artificial test fluid. The speed (dissolution rate constant) and amount of drug in solution characterize drug release.

Elimination Half-Life

Elimination half-life describes the rate of drug elimination from the central compartment. It is the time necessary to decrease the drug concentration (Cp) in the blood (plasma or serum) by one half during the elimination phase. It is determined by the volume of distribution and total body clearance. It may or may not agree with therapeutic or response half-life. It is also called the biological half-life or β T 1/2. See Half-Life.

Elimination Phase

Portion of the plasma concentration-time curve during which the drug is eliminated primarily from the central compartment.

Enterohepatic Recirculation

Phenomenon in which drugs emptied via bile into the small intestine can be reabsorbed from the intestinal lumen into systemic circulation.

Enzyme Induction

Increase in enzyme content (activity or amount) that may result in faster metabolism of a compound.

Enzyme Inhibition

Decrease in rate of metabolism of a compound (usually by competition) by enzymes.

Excretion

Final elimination of drug from the body's systemic circulation into urine, feces, sweat, air, and milk.

Extraction Ratio

Ratio of organ clearance (i.e., hepatic, renal) to blood or plasma flow through the organ.

Extravascular Administration

All routes of administration except those where the drug is directly introduced into the bloodstream. Examples of extravascular routes are intramuscular (IM), subcutaneous (SC), peroral (PO), oral, rectal (PR), intraperitoneal (IP), and topical.

First-Order Kinetics

Process of elimination in which the rate of drug disappearance is directly proportional to plasma concentration.

First-Pass Effect

Phenomenon whereby drugs may be metabolized (not chemically degraded) following absorption but before reaching systemic circulation. Hepatic first-pass effect may occur following peroral and rectal administration. It may be avoided by using sublingual and buccal routes of drug administration. Pulmonary first-pass effect cannot be avoided by intravenous, buccal, or sublingual routes.

Generic Product

Drug product marketed under the nonproprietary or common name of the drug(s).

Half-Life (T 1/2)

Time required to reduce the peak drug concentration by half. The term "half-life" should apply to both a specific phase and a specific fluid (e.g., "plasma elimination half-life") because drug concentrations vary in the plasma, urine, and cerebrospinal fluid. Excretion of the drug from the body is almost complete after five to six elimination half-lives. Overdoses may prolong half-life based on therapeutic doses. Published elimination rate tables are useful for drugs for which the half-life remains constant during overdose (i.e., first-order kinetics) but less so for drugs (e.g., salicylates) that convert to zero-order kinetics or Michaelis-Menten kinetics after overdose.

Hepatic Clearance

Rate of total body clearance accounted for by the liver. The magnitude depends on intrinsic hepatic clearance, fraction of unbound drug in blood, and liver blood flow.

Intravascular Administration

All routes of administration where the drug is directly introduced into the bloodstream. These include intravenous (IV), intraarterial, and intracardiac. Bioavailability is 100%.

Intrinsic Clearance

Theoretical unrestricted maximum clearance of unbound drug by an eliminating organ.

Intravenous Bolus

In common usage, rapid intravenous administration (i.e., intravenous injection).

Lag Time

Interval between drug administration and drug concentration measurable in blood. Lag times may occur after oral administration and result from slow disintegration and dissolution of tablets or capsules or delayed gastric emptying.

Lean Body Weight

Body weight minus fat mass.

Level

See concentration.

Loading Dose

Dose used in initiating therapy. This dose is usually larger than the maintenance dose and is used to provide rapid therapeutic concentrations. The need for a loading dose depends on elimination half-life, dosage interval, and therapeutic concentration to be achieved. The amount of biologically active drug absorbed into the body (A) required to rapidly reach therapeutic levels = volume of distribution (Vd) × the desired concentration. Also called the priming dose.

Maintenance Dose

Dose required to maintain clinical effectiveness or a therapeutic concentration. It is determined by drug clearance, distribution volume, elimination rate, desired steady-state concentration, and desired therapeutic effectiveness of the drug.

Michaelis-Menten Kinetics

Mathematical description of certain zero-order processes that usually involve saturable enzymatic reactions.

Multicompartment Model

A mathematical model whereby a drug equilibrates with more than one compartment (different tissues) in the body. In a two-compartment model, there is a central compartment composed of plasma and highly perfused tissues (e.g., brain, heart, liver, kidneys and gastrointestinal tract) and a peripheral compartment composed of everything else in the body.

Multiple-Dose Administration

Use of repeated single doses. It may result in accumulation when a drug is given repeatedly at intervals shorter than those required to eliminate the previously given dose.

Nonlinear Kinetics

The rate of the process is not directly proportional to the concentration, as it is in first-order kinetics. These processes may be described by Michaelis-Menten kinetics, Langmuir equation, and so on. See zero-order kinetics.

Oral Administration

Strictly speaking, includes buccal, sublingual, and perlingual administration routes where the drug is adsorbed from the mouth cavity (no first-pass effect). Not to be confused with peroral (PO).

Peripheral Compartment

Sum of all body regions (i.e., organs, tissues, or parts of them) to which a drug eventually distributes, but is not in immediate equilibrium with central compartment. The peripheral compartment is sometimes further subdivided into shallow and deep compartments. See multicompartment model.

Peroral Administration (PO)

Indicates that the dosage form is swallowed and the drug is absorbed from the gastrointestinal tract (first-pass effect possible). Not all drugs are absorbed such as charcoal, kaolin, and some antacids. Not to be confused with oral administration.

PKA

Is the pH at which a substance exists half in an ionized form and half in an un-ionized form. Knowing the pKA helps predict whether altering serum and urine pH may enhance a substance's elimination.

Plasma Concentration

See concentration.

Priming Dose

See loading dose.

Protein Binding

Phenomenon that occurs when a drug combines with plasma or tissue protein. The unbound drug is in equilibrium with the biophase.

Rate-Limiting Step

Process with the slowest rate constant in a system of sequential kinetic processes. If rate constants are nearly identical, then identification of the rate-limiting step may be difficult.

Relative Bioavailability

Term used to indicate both the relative amounts of a drug that reach the general circulation unchanged and the relative rates of appearance of a drug administered to the same subjects in two or more different dosage forms by the same or two different extravascular routes.

Relative Dosage Interval

For a specified dosage regimen, the variable period between closely spaced multiple doses given at irregular intervals.

Renal Clearance

Rate of total body clearance accounted for by the kidney. The net effects of glomerular filtration, tubular secretion and reabsorption, blood flow, and protein binding determine its magnitude.

Saturation Kinetics

Nonlinear or zero-order kinetics generally involving hepatic enzymes. See Zero-Order Kinetics.

Single-Compartment Model

A mathematical model whereby a drug equilibrates with all tissues in the body.

Steady State

Strictly speaking, this is achieved only during constant rate infusion when input and output are equal. The steady-state drug concentrations during multiple-dose administration fluctuate between a maximum (peak) and a minimum (trough) steady-state concentration within each dosage interval.

Therapeutic Drug Range

The concentration of a drug at which the majority of a given population can expect to receive therapeutic benefit.

Total Clearance

The sum of individual clearances of eliminating organs.

Toxic Blood Range

The concentration of a drug at which the majority of a given population can expect to exhibit toxic manifestations.

Toxicokinetics

Deals mathematically with the changes in drug and / or metabolite concentration in the human or animal body in an overdosed situation.

VMAX

Vmax is defined as the maximum rate of metabolism (mg / h) of drugs following zero-order or saturation kinetics.

Volume of Distribution

Not a "real" volume, but a hypothetical volume of body fluid that would be required to dissolve the total amount of drug at the same concentration as that found in the blood or plasma. It is a proportionality constant relating the amount of drug in the body to the measured concentration in biological fluid.

Xenobiotics

Chemicals including drugs, environmental substances, industrial agents, and pesticides. Xenobiotics may be natural or manufactured.

Zero-Order Kinetics

Also called saturation or nonlinear kinetics. Is the process of elimination in which the rate of drug elimination is not proportional to concentration, and hence small increases in active drug may cause large increases in drug concentration.

INTERPRETATION OF PHARMACOKINETIC DATA

Pharmacokinetic principles must be applied cautiously because they are only an aid in management. Supportive care remains the mainstay of therapy. Pharmacokinetic data often change in the overdose state, and data based on therapeutic doses may be misleading (e.g., salicylates change from first-order to zero-order kinetics near upper therapeutic limits). Adults also may ingest multiple drugs that may interact to change pharmacokinetics. Alterations in body hemostatic mechanisms (e.g., blood flow) or preexisting disease states (e.g., cirrhosis, alcoholism, and renal failure) change drug absorption, distribution, and elimination.

Pharmacokinetic data help estimate duration and severity of symptoms given an amount ingested. The volume of distribution (Vd) suggests when measures to enhance elimination are useful and helps verify the quantity ingested. Dialysis usually is not helpful when the Vd exceeds 1 L / kg. The plasma concentration confirms ingestion and can help guide therapy and management of overdose in certain instances. The pKA helps predict which drugs benefit from the manipulation of urinary pH in order to enhance ion trapping and increase excretion. Such applications are limited to very few drugs.

The rate of absorption suggests how long emesis or lavage may be effective. Knowing when peak plasma levels occur helps predict the appropriate time to sample plasma levels. Pharmacokinetic data also help determine the potential for delayed or prolonged toxicity in overdose (e.g., delayed gastric emptying, slowed intestinal mobility). Drugs that follow first-order kinetics (primarily renal elimination) have predictable half-lives that allow estimation of the duration of toxicity. However, drugs that rely on hepatic metabolism usually follow nonlinear kinetics and are less predictable.

Drug Concentrations

The patient's clinical assessment, and not his drug concentrations, guides treatment in the majority of circumstances. Plasma drug concentrations may be useful in monitoring compliance, individualizing therapy, diagnosing wider treatment, avoiding toxicity, diagnosing toxicity, monitoring and detecting drug interactions, and guiding withdrawal of therapy.

Some drug levels are commonly obtained in clinical practice and routinely help guide patient management. Free drug level methods may not easily be available to the local community hospital laboratory. There is a considerable lack of data establishing correlations between therapeutic or toxic response and free drug concentrations. Knowing certain drug concentrations, such as acetaminophen and salicylates, are useful in overdose.

Routine drug concentrations include digoxin, certain antiarrhythmics (disopyramide, lidocaine, procainamide and its main metabolite, n-acetylprocainamide, quinidine), anticonvulsants (carbamazepine, ethosuximide, phenobarbital, phenytoin, primidone, valproic acid), antibiotics (amikacin, chloramphenicol, gentamicin, tobramycin, vancomycin), theophylline, psychoactive agents (lithium, tricyclic antidepressants), and other agents such as cyclosporine and methotrexate.

Questions—Interpretation of Pharmacokinetic Data

1. **Drug levels which routinely help guide patient management include all except**
   A. Digoxin
   B. Carbamazepine
   C. Diazepam
   D. Theophylline
   E. Cyclosporine
2. **The volume of distribution suggests when measures to enhance elimination are useful and helps verify the quantity ingested. Dialysis usually is not helpful when the Vd exceeds ____ L/kg.**
   A. 0.01
   B. 0.10
   C. 1
   D. 10
   E. 100

PHARMACOKINETIC FORMULAS AND EXAMPLES

Knowledge of the volume of distribution (Vd) allows prediction of the plasma concentration (Cp) when the amount of drug administered (A) is known:

$$\text{Cp (mg/L)} = \frac{\text{A(mg/kg)}}{\text{Vd(L/kg)}}$$

$$\text{Vd (L/kg)} = \frac{\text{A(mg/kg)}}{\text{Cp(mg/L)}}$$

Loading dose (Ld), or the amount of drug initially administered, may be calculated as:

$$\text{A (mg/kg)} = \text{Cp (mg/L)} \times \text{Vd(L/kg)}$$

The Cp is measured in milligrams per liter, which often is not a practical value for computation. Useful conversion factors exist for Cp:

$$\begin{aligned}\text{Cp (mg/L)} &= 10\text{(mg/dl), also known as mg\%}\\ &= \mu\text{g/mL} = \text{mg/L}\\ &= \frac{\text{ng/mL}}{1{,}000}\end{aligned}$$

Assuming a process of elimination in which the rate of drug disappearance is directly proportional to plasma concentration (first-order kinetics) the half-life of a substance is defined as:

$$\text{T 1/2(h)} = \frac{0.693}{\text{Ke (elimination rate constant)}}$$

Clearance (CL), or elimination of drug(s) following first order kinetics may be defined as:

$$\text{CL(L/kg/h)} = \frac{0.693 \times \text{Vd(L/kg)}}{\text{T 1/2(h)}}$$

For drugs following first-order kinetics, the maximum rate of metabolism (Vmax) and the elimination rate are constant. The elimination rate (ER) may be defined as:

$$\text{ER(mg/kg/h)} = \frac{0.693 \times \text{Cp(mg/L)}}{\text{T 1/2(h)}}$$

The following defines the relationship between elimination rate(ER) and clearance(CL):

$$\text{ER(mg/kg/h)} = \text{CL(L/kg/h)} \times \text{Cp(mg/L)}$$

Maintenance dose (M), or the amount of drug to be administered over time, depends on a drug's half-life (elimination rate constant) and may be calculated as:

$$\text{M(mg/kg/h)} = \frac{0.693 \times \text{Cp(mg/L)} \times \text{Vd(L/kg)}}{\text{T 1/2(h)}}$$

Example 1

What plasma concentration is achieved from 0.2-mg digoxin, given a Vd of 7 L/kg, and a patient weight of 70 kg?

$$\begin{aligned}\text{Cp(mg/L)} &= \frac{\text{A(mg/kg)}}{\text{Vd(L/kg)}} = \frac{0.2/70}{7} = \frac{0.2}{490}\\ &= 0.0004\ \text{mg/L}\\ &= 0.4\ \text{ng/mL (therapeutic is 0.5–2 ng/mL)}\end{aligned}$$

Example 2

Calculate the plasma ethanol concentration of a 9-kg, 10-month-old whose sibling gave him 2 tbsp (30 mL) of whiskey. Assume that whiskey = 80 proof = 40% ethanol = 40 mL absolute ethanol per 100 mL. The Vd of ethanol in children = 0.7 L/kg and specific gravity = 0.8 g/mL.

$$\begin{aligned}\text{Dose(A)} &= 30\ \text{mL} \times \frac{40\ \text{mL absolute ethanol}}{100\ \text{mL whiskey}}\\ &= 12\ \text{mL of absolute ethanol}\end{aligned}$$

To convert the volume to milligrams, use the specific gravity of alcohol, 0.8.

$$\begin{aligned}\text{A} &= 12\ \text{mL} \times (0.8\ \text{g/mL})\\ &= 9.6\ \text{g} = 9{,}600\ \text{mg}\\ \text{Cp} &= \frac{\text{A(mg/kg)}}{\text{Vd(L/kg)} \times \text{body weight(kg)}}\\ &= \frac{9{,}600\ \text{mg}}{0.7\text{(L/kg)} \times 9\ \text{kg}}\\ &= 1{,}524\ \text{mg/L} = 152.4\ \text{mg/dL}\end{aligned}$$

Example 3

A 30-kg child ingests fifteen 100-mg phenytoin tablets. The Vd of phenytoin = 0.7 L/kg. Calculate the peak plasma phenytoin concentration, assuming rapid, complete absorption.

$$\begin{aligned}\text{Cp} &= \frac{\text{A(mg/kg)}}{\text{Vd(L/kg)} \times \text{body weight(kg)}}\\ &= \frac{1500\ \text{mg}}{0.7\text{(L/kg)} \times 30\ \text{kg}}\\ &= 71\ \mu\text{g/mL}\end{aligned}$$

Example 4

How many 30-mL drinks of 80-proof whiskey (40% ethanol) are required to reach a plasma ethanol concentration of 100 mg/dL in a 70-kg man? Assume that the drinks are consumed within 1 hour and no metabolism occurs. Vd of ethanol in adults = 0.6 L/kg and specific gravity = 0.8 g/mL.

$$\text{Cp} = \frac{\text{A(mg/kg)}}{\text{Vd(L/kg)} \times \text{body weight(kg)}}$$

$$\text{Cp} = 100\ \text{mg/dL} = 1{,}000\ \text{mg/L}$$

therefore

$$\begin{aligned}\text{A(mg/kg)} &= \text{Cp} \times \text{Vd(L/kg)} \times \text{body weight(kg)}\\ &= 1{,}000\ \text{mg/L} \times 0.6\ \text{L/kg} \times 70\ \text{kg}\\ &= 42{,}000\ \text{mg} = 42\ \text{grams}\end{aligned}$$

If one drink contains 30 mL of 80-proof ethanol, then

$$\begin{aligned}\text{ethanol(g)} &= 30 \times 0.4 \times 0.8\\ &= 9.6\ \text{grams}\end{aligned}$$

(where the factor 0.8 represents the specific gravity of ethanol that converts milliliters to milligrams)

Therefore, the number of 30-mL drinks required would be

$$= 42/9.6, \text{ or 4 drinks.}$$

Example 5

A drug is ordered in a dose of 0.8 mg/kg intravenously. The patient weighs 64 kg. In 2 hours, toxic symptoms develop. If the Vd is 0.8 L/kg and the peak serum level in 2 hours is 8 (μg/mL, was the appropriate dose administered?

$$\text{Cp} = 8\ \mu\text{g/mL} = 8\ \text{mg/L}$$

and

$$\begin{aligned}\text{Vd} &= 0.8\ \text{L/kg} \times 64\ \text{kg}\\ &= 51.2\ \text{L.}\end{aligned}$$

$$A(mg/kg) = Cp \times Vd(L/kg) \times body\ weight(kg)$$
$$= 8\ mg/L \times 51.2\ L$$
$$= 409.6\ mg$$

The ordered dose was 0.8 mg/kg, however the administered dose was 409.6 mg or

$$= 409.6\ mg/64\ kg = 6.4\ mg/kg.$$

Therefore, the appropriate dose was NOT administered.

Example 6

You want to achieve a serum level of 10 μg/mL of theophylline in a 70-kg patient. Theophylline follows first-order kinetics. Calculate the loading dose (Ld) and maintenance dose (M) required if the T 1/2 = 5 hours, and the Vd = 0.45 L/kg.

$$Cp = 10\ \mu g/mL = 10\ mg/L$$

and $$Vd = 0.45\ L/kg \times 70\ kg$$
$$= 31.5\ L$$

therefore $$Ld = Vd(L/kg) \times Cp(mg/L)$$
$$= 31.5\ L \times 10\ mg/L$$
$$= 315\ mg\ theophylline$$

and $$M = \frac{0.693 \times Cp(mg/L) \times Vd(L/kg)}{T\,1/2(h)}$$
$$= \frac{0.693 \times 10\ (mg/L) \times 0.45\ L/kg}{5\ (h)}$$
$$= 0.6\ mg/kg/h$$

Example 7

A 5-year-old, 15-kg girl ingests an unknown amount of Pepto Bismol containing salicylate. The plasma salicylate level is 1,080 mg/L, 4 hours after ingestion. How much salicylate did the child ingest? The Vd of salicylate = 0.3 L/kg.

$$Vd = 15\ kg \times 0.3\ L/kg = 4.5\ L$$
$$Cp(mg/L) = \frac{A(mg/kg)}{Vd(L/kg)}$$
$$Vd(L/kg) = \frac{A(mg/kg)}{Cp(mg/L)}$$
$$A(mg/kg) = Cp(mg/L) \times Vd(L/kg)$$
$$A = 1{,}080\ (mg/L) \times 4.5\ L$$
$$A = 4{,}824\ mg = 4.8\ grams, a toxic amount.$$

Questions—Pharmacokinetic Formulas and Examples

1. **What plasma concentration is achieved from 0.2-mg digoxin, given a Vd of 7 L/kg, and a patient weight of 70 kg?**
   A. 0.4 ng/mL
   B. 4.0 ng/mL
   C. 4.4 ng/mL
   D. 0.2 ng/mL
   E. 0.4 ng/L
2. **What is the dose of absolute ethanol in 100 mL of 100-proof whiskey?**
   A. 0.5 mL of absolute ethanol
   B. 5.0 mL of absolute ethanol
   C. 50 mL of absolute ethanol
   D. 100 mL of absolute ethanol
   E. 500 mL of absolute ethanol
3. **A 50-kg child ingests twenty 100-mg phenytoin tablets. Calculate the peak plasma phenytoin concentration, assuming rapid, complete absorption. The Vd of phenytoin = 0.7 L/kg.**
   A. 5.7 μg/mL
   B. 57 μg/mL
   C. 570 μg/mL
   D. 0.57 μg/mL
   E. 0.057 μg/mL
4. **Knowledge of the volume of distribution (Vd) allows prediction of the plasma concentration (Cp) when the amount of drug administered (A) is unknown.**
   A. True
   B. False

ABSORPTION

The small intestine absorbs most drugs, and reduction of small bowel surface area (e.g., by malabsorption) limits absorption. Decreased gastric emptying delays both absorption and toxicity. Numerous factors such as the fat content or state (e.g., liquid or solid) of food in the stomach affect gastric emptying. Gastric acids limit the absorption of certain drugs (e.g., benzyl penicillin), whereas metabolizing enzymes in the brush border impair the absorption of certain drugs (e.g., levodopa and isoprenaline). Common drugs that delay gastric emptying include aspirin, iron, anticholinergics, alcohol, and barbiturates. Delayed absorption means that early blood levels (i.e., within the first 4 hours) may be misleading (e.g., phenytoin, salicylates, and tricyclic antidepressants).

Peak absorption in overdose may be difficult to predict because of chronic drug dosing, product formulation (e.g., sustained-release tablets), and delayed absorption from numerous causes. Peak level calculations are sometimes useful in estimating toxic effects because certain signs of toxicity from certain drugs develop at specific concentrations. For example, nystagmus frequently occurs at phenytoin levels between 20 and 50 μg/mL.

Sustained-release formulations cause marked delays in toxicity (e.g., theophylline, aspirin, and cold preparations). For some drugs (e.g., aspirin and digoxin), tablet dissolution may be the rate-limiting step for absorption. Certain drugs (e.g., aspirin, iron, carbamazepine, meprobamate, glutethimide, and ethchlorvynol) form concretions (e.g., bezoars) that delay absorption. Slowed intestinal motility (potentially caused by opiates, anticholinergics, phenytoin, and Lomotil) alters absorption and delays peak clinical effects. High-molecular-weight substances (e.g., cholestyramine) are poorly absorbed.

Questions—Absorption

1. **Drugs that delay absorption include all of the following, except**
   A. Griseofulvin
   B. Diphenhydramine
   C. Iron
   D. Barbiturates
   E. Aspirin

2. Drugs known to form concretions include all of the following, except
A. Ampicillin
B. Carbamazepine
C. Iron
D. Aspirin
E. Meprobamate

DISTRIBUTION

Most drugs distribute easily through the extracellular space, whereas lipoprotein membranes inhibit transport of polar compounds across cell walls. Lipophilic or nonpolar compounds freely cross the lipoprotein membranes of the brain, cerebrospinal fluid, and cells, distributing widely into tissue stores. Tight junctions between endothelial cells form a blood-brain barrier that limits drug penetration into brain cells. Ionized or polar drugs are less able to penetrate lipoproteins than nonpolar compounds and display a relatively smaller volume of distribution.

Only free, unbound drug possesses pharmacologic effects. The free drug concentration, therefore, most closely represents the amount of active drug. The free drug fraction is the ratio of free drug to total plasma drug concentration. Although the free drug fraction may increase dramatically, drug concentration depends on whether the newly freed drug is cleared from the plasma. Numerous factors influence the relative amount of free drug in plasma.

Drug-Binding Proteins

Albumin is the most important plasma drug protein and binds most acidic and some basic drugs. Alpha-1 acid glycoprotein binds most basic drugs and some hormones. Stress, inflammation, malignancy, and blood diseases elevate the plasma protein level, whereas liver disease, nephrotic syndrome, and malnutrition reduce the plasma concentration. Other drug-binding proteins include lipoproteins and gammaglobulins.

Binding Site Saturation

Albumins usually have more drug sites than drug available and hence saturation is unusual. Disopyramide and valproic acid have a narrow therapeutic index and display concentration-dependent binding. Because active drug increases without a change in the total drug concentration after saturation of binding sites, these plasma drug levels do not correlate well with clinical effects.

Binding Site Affinity

When salicylates, for example, bind to albumin, acetylation modifies the protein structure. Acetyl albumin demonstrates decreased affinity for other drugs and enhances their clinical effects.

Displacement

An increase in the free fraction of one drug, resulting from displacement by another drug, represents a common drug interaction. For example, high levels of salicylate displace phenytoin. The increased free phenytoin fraction reduces the total steady-state phenytoin concentration because of increased elimination.

Protein Concentrations

Hypoalbuminemia increases the free fraction because it decreases the amount of bound drug. Total drug concentration decreases because the rate of metabolism is proportional to free drug concentration. Diseases causing hypoalbuminemia include cirrhosis and the nephrotic syndrome. Hepatic dysfunction increases the free drug concentration because it decreases metabolism, although the total concentration remains the same.

Volume of Distribution

The volume of distribution (Vd) is not a "real" volume, but is a hypothetical volume of body fluid that would be required to dissolve the total amount of drug at the same concentration as that found in the blood or plasma. A proportionality constant relates the amount of drug in the body to its measured concentration in biological fluids. A "large" Vd exceeds 1 L/kg. The plasma concentrations (Cp) of drugs with large volumes of distribution usually are measured in ng/mL.

Artificial elimination procedures (e.g., hemodialysis, hemoperfusion) do not effectively enhance the excretion of drugs with large volumes of distribution. For drugs with a small Vd (i.e., less than 1 L/kg), the plasma concentration of drug (Cp) generally is measured in micrograms per milliliter. Dialysis effectively enhances the elimination of these drugs if they possess good water solubility and poor protein binding.

The volume of distribution of drugs during acute overdosage is often different from that during chronic drug overdose. Overdoses with theophylline, salicylate, and lithium for example, may be associated with seizures, arrhythmias and other life-threatening events at serum drug concentrations that usually are therapeutic or mildly toxic.

pH Effects

Drugs are weak acids or bases and, in solution, they become ionized when they lose or gain a hydrogen ion. These drugs become trapped in the compartment in which they are more ionized, because ionized (polar) compounds do not cross cell membranes easily. If the urine pH favors the ionized form of the drug, trapping will occur in the renal tubular space, resulting in increased excretion. Weak acids (e.g., aspirin) are better absorbed in acid media and better excreted in alkaline media. Weak bases (e.g., quinidine) are better absorbed in alkaline environments and better excreted in acid urine.

Manipulation of the urine pH can increase the excretion of certain acidic (quinidine, phencyclidine, and amphetamines) and basic (phenobarbital, aspirin, and 2,4-D) drugs. Specific pharmacokinetic parameters (e.g., large volume of distribution, heavy protein binding, rapid hepatic clearance, and low renal clearance) limit the applicability of pH manipulation to very few drugs.

Intracellular fluid is more acidic than extracellular fluid at physiologic pH; therefore, bases cross the cell membrane and are trapped in the intracellular compartment. The consequences of this relative partition are that bases have a higher volume of distribution (more widely disseminated) and a longer half-life that translates to prolonged intoxication and metabolism. These compounds are relatively harder to eliminate by artificial means than acidic drugs. They are better excreted in acidic urine. If a single therapeutic dose is less than 75 mg, or the volume of distribution exceeds 1 L/kg, the drug usually is a weak base.

Acids exist more frequently in the ionized or polar form at physiologic pH. Compared with basic drugs, these drugs have higher Cp, larger therapeutic doses, and smaller volumes of distribution because of their reduced ability to penetrate cells. Acidic drugs are eliminated more rapidly because of their relatively greater concentration in plasma. Hence, ion trapping is more useful for acidic than basic drugs. These compounds are better excreted in alkaline urine and better absorbed in acid media.

Receptor Effects

A receptor is a specific tissue protein (membrane-bound or intracellular) capable of binding the members of a specific group of drugs or endogenous substances. The interaction of a drug with its receptor leads to pharmacologic effect through a series of incompletely understood mechanisms. Different types of receptors may be defined by their most potent endogenous agonist (e.g., histamine receptors). See Part E, Receptor Toxicology.

A ligand is a drug or endogenous substance that binds to a receptor (e.g., histamine is a ligand at histamine receptors). An agonist is a ligand that produces an appropriate response when it binds to its receptor (e.g., histamine is an agonist at histamine receptors). An antagonist is a ligand that prevents the effects of an agonist. Pure antagonists do not cause any effects by binding to receptors (e.g., cimetidine is an antagonist of the actions of histamine at one subtype of histamine receptor, H2). A partial agonist is a ligand that has both agonist and antagonist properties.

Receptors may be divided into subtypes on the basis of the selectivity of a range of agonists or antagonists (e.g., histamine receptors can be divided into two subtypes: that for which conventional antihistamines have a high antagonist selectivity, H1, and that for which drugs such as cimetidine and ranitidine have high antagonist selectivity, H2). Downregulation and upregulation are loose terms used to indicate a decrease or increase, respectively, in the number of receptor sites in a tissue. Changes of this kind often occur in response to long-term administration of a drug or in disease.

Questions—Distribution

1. **Numerous factors influence the amount of free drug in plasma. These include all except**
   A. Drug-binding proteins
   B. Binding site saturation
   C. Binding site affinity
   D. Displacement by other agents
   E. Rh type
2. **The volume of distribution (Vd)**
   A. Is not a "real" volume, but is a hypothetical volume of body fluid that would be required to dissolve the total amount of drug at the same concentration as that found in the blood or plasma
   B. Is considered large if it exceeds 1 L/kg
   C. Remains constant in acute drug overdoses and in chronic situations
   D. All of the above
   E. A and B
3. **Drugs are weak acids or bases and, in solution, they become ionized when they lose or gain a hydrogen ion.**
   A. True
   B. False
4. **Drugs become trapped in the compartment in which they are less ionized.**
   A. True
   B. False
5. **Weak acids are better absorbed in alkaline media and better excreted in acidic media.**
   A. True
   B. False
6. **Manipulation of the urine pH can increase the excretion of certain acidic (quinidine, phencyclidine, and amphetamines) and basic (phenobarbital, aspirin, and 2,4-D) drugs.**
   A. True
   B. False
7. **Intracellular fluid is more alkaline than extracellular fluid at physiologic pH; therefore, bases cross the cell membrane and are trapped in the intracellular compartment.**
   A. True
   B. False

METABOLISM

Most metabolism occurs in the liver and is an important route of elimination for lipid-soluble drugs that the kidneys do not easily excrete. Examples include β-blockers, acetaminophen, tricyclic antidepressants, and tranquilizers. Metabolites tend to be water-soluble and can be excreted in the bile and/or urine. Other metabolic products usually, but not always, possess reduced pharmacologic activity. In overdose, enzyme pathways may saturate, leading to prolonged half-lives and extended clinical effects.

Certain drugs and chemicals are metabolized to active compounds. Procainamide, for example, is metabolized to n-acetylprocainamide (NAPA) and concentrations of both are generally utilized in guiding therapy. Some active metabolites may be toxic. Acetonitrile, for example, is converted to cyanide. Meperidine is metabolized to normeperidine, a central nervous system stimulant. Acetaminophen is partly metabolized to the toxic intermediate n-acetyl-p-benzoquinoneimine (NAPQI). Methanol is metabolized to toxic formaldehyde and formic acid, and ethylene glycol is metabolized to the toxic glycolic acid.

"Prodrugs" are compounds that are inactive in their parent forms but which, after administration, are transformed chemically to the active derivative. The most common prodrug linkage is an ester bond, and phosphate salts form most of the rest. Activation of most prodrugs is by an enzymatic process that cleaves off the active moiety. Examples include glucocorticoids, which are transformed into methylprednisolone and hydrocortisone, and aminophylline, which is transformed into theophylline.

Numerous factors influence drug metabolism. These include age (metabolizing enzymes decrease with age), sex (the plasma half-life for some drugs may be longer in men), pharmacogenetic factors (e.g., certain groups are rapid acetylators), body size and weight, pregnancy, nutritional status (albumin level), and disease status (e.g., the reduced hepatic blood flow seen in congestive heart failure decreases the metabolism of drugs with large first-pass effects). Hepatitis slows elimination of drugs that are metabolized by the cytochrome P450 microsomal enzyme system and prolongs their half-lives. Other factors include drug interactions (e.g., enzyme inhibitors), individual variation, toxic doses (e.g., change in pharmacokinetics), and biochemical status.

First-Pass Effect

The liver biotransforms some drugs during their initial pass through the portal circulation after oral administration. Hence, a large portion of drug fails to reach the systemic circulation in the original form. This is called the "first-pass effect." The first-pass effect accounts for the difference in peak plasma levels between oral and intravenous doses. Parenteral, sublingual, and buccal administration of drugs avoids the first-pass effect. Drugs with large first-pass effects (e.g., propranolol) display wide discrepancies between oral and intravenous doses. Variations in hepatic blood flow in diseases such as congestive heart failure significantly alter metabolism of drugs with large hepatic clearance and may cause toxicity at usual pharmacologic doses.

Biotransformation

There are two phases of biotransformation of drugs in humans. These include phase I, or preconjugation reactions, and phase II, or conjugation reactions. Some drugs require only phase I for inactivation and phase II reactions may occur without phase I oxidation, reduction, or hydrolysis. Some drugs must pass through both phases to be inactivated.

PHASE I REACTIONS

These chemical processes unveil suitable chemical groups within the drug (e.g., OH, NH_2, and COOH) after oxidation (hydroxylation), reduction, and hydrolysis reactions. The common hydroxylating enzymes are included in the cytochrome P450 pathway that is affected by microsomal enzyme inducers (e.g., barbiturates).

PHASE II REACTIONS

Chemical groups revealed by phase I reactions are coupled to endogenous compounds such as glucuronic acid and sulfates during this phase. Reaction speed varies and, for some metabolic enzymes, depends on genetic factors. About 50% of whites, for example, are fast acetylators, whereas 90% of Eskimos are slow acetylators.

Drug-Metabolizing Enzymes

The vast majority of phase I metabolism is catalyzed by enzymes located in the liver termed the cytochrome P450 mixed-function oxidase system. This term derives from the fact that these enzymes initially were believed to be similar to mitochondrial cytochromes and they maximally absorb light at 450-nm wavelength under certain conditions. More than 20 different P450s have been identified in humans. P450s also are found in the intestines and kidney. The majority of P450s involved in drug metabolism appear to belong to three distinct gene families. Many drugs may be dependent on single forms of P450 for their metabolism in the liver because each P450 has a unique substrate-binding site that determines the affinity with which it binds to and metabolizes a drug.

Certain medications inhibit cytochrome P450 drug metabolism and may influence dosing regimens and clinical effects. These include acute ethanol ingestion, allopurinol, amiodarone, chloramphenicol, cimetidine, ciprofloxacin, danazol (androgens), diltiazem, disulfiram, enoxacin, erythromycin (macrolides), fluconazole, fluoxetine, imipramine, ketoconazole, metoprolol, metronidazole, nortriptyline, omeprazole, oral contraceptives, primaquine, propoxyphene, propranolol, quinidine, ranitidine, trimethoprim-sulfamethoxazole, valproic acid, and verapamil.

Certain medications increase cytochrome P450 drug metabolism and may influence dosing regimens and clinical effects as well. These include barbiturates, carbamazepine, chronic alcohol use, cigarette smoking, glutethimide, griseofulvin, haloperidol, meprobamate, omeprazole, phenytoin, polycyclic aromatic hydrocarbons, primidone, and rifampin. Major effects of microsomal enzyme induction involve enhanced drug metabolism, enhanced carcinogen metabolism, enhanced steroid hydroxylation, enhanced bilirubin metabolism, and increased agranular endoplasmic reticulum.

First-Order Kinetics

For more than 90% of drugs, most renal excretion follows first-order (linear) kinetics, where the elimination half-life is independent of concentration, in contrast to the saturation kinetics of hepatic metabolism. Because the drug elimination rate (ER) is defined as:

$$\mathrm{ER(mg/kg/h)} = \frac{0.693 \times \mathrm{Cp(mg/L)}}{\mathrm{T\,1/2(h)}}$$

if plasma concentration (Cp) doubles, the rate of elimination doubles. If T 1/2 doubles, the elimination rate is halved. The elimination rate does not change with concentration, but the amount excreted does. No accumulation occurs at dosing intervals longer than the plasma half-life.

Plasma clearance (CL) is the volume of plasma from which all drug is removed in a specific time period. The term "clearance" is in units of volume per weight per time, whereas the elimination rate represents the amount of drug removed per weight per time. The following defines the relationship between elimination rate (ER) and clearance (CL):

$$\mathrm{ER\ (mg/kg/h)} = \mathrm{CL\ (L/kg/h)} \times \mathrm{Cp\ (mg/L)}$$

Zero-Order Kinetics

Most drugs detoxified by hepatic metabolism follow zero-order (saturation) or nonlinear kinetics. The rate of this process is independent of drug concentration. A fixed amount of drug is eliminated over a period of time. Drug elimination is limited by the capacity of enzymes involved, which ultimately become saturated near the upper limits of a therapeutic range. Small increments in dose may produce large increases in plasma concentration.

There is no predictable half-life decline as there is in first-order kinetics. The T 1/2 will change with concentration of hepatically metabolized drugs at therapeutic concentrations. Vmax is defined as the maximum rate of metabolism (mg/h), and the elimination rate is constant. The metabolic rate becomes more complex than a simple, fixed maximum rate. Michaelis-Menten kinetics describes this situation with the following equation:

$$\mathrm{ER\ (mg/kg/h)} = \frac{\mathrm{Vmax\ (mg/kg/h)} \times \mathrm{Cp\ (mg/L)}}{\mathrm{Km} + \mathrm{Cp\ (mg/L)}}$$

where Vmax = maximum rate of metabolism (mg/kg/h)
Cp = plasma concentration (mg/mL)
Km = specific Michaelis constant for enzyme process

For zero-order kinetics, the serum levels will continue to rise disproportionately to dose when the rate of administration exceeds the Vmax (maximum rate of metabolism). Phenytoin is an example of a drug that follows zero-order kinetics.

Questions—Metabolism

1. Most metabolism occurs in the liver and is an important route of elimination for lipid-soluble drugs that the kidneys do not easily excrete. Examples include all of the following, except
A. Phenazopyridine
B. β-Blockers
C. Acetaminophen
D. Tricyclic antidepressants
E. Many tranquilizers

2. Certain drugs and chemicals are metabolized to active compounds. Which is false?
A. Procainamide-n-acetylprocainamide (NAPA)
B. Acetonitrile-cyanide
C. Meperidine-normeperidine
D. Methanol-ethanol
E. Ethylene glycol-glycolic acid

3. Theophylline is an example of a "prodrug" because it is derived from another active compound, aminophylline.
A. True
B. False

4. Numerous factors influence drug metabolism. These include all of the following, except
A. Age
B. Sex
C. Body size and weight
D. Pregnancy
E. All of the above

5. Most drugs detoxified by hepatic metabolism follow zero-order (saturation) or nonlinear kinetics. The rate of this process is dependent on drug concentration.
A. True
B. False

6. For more than 90% of drugs, most renal excretion follows first-order (linear) kinetics, where the elimination half-life is independent of concentration.
A. True
B. False

ELIMINATION

Artificial Elimination

Dialysis, hemoperfusion, exchange transfusion, and hyperbaric oxygen can increase the elimination of certain toxins and are the methods most frequently used to enhance elimination. The effectiveness of methods that enhance drug elimination (e.g., hemodialysis) depends on both the plasma clearance and the plasma concentration. Although such methods may significantly increase plasma clearance of a specific drug, they may not effectively remove a large amount of drug if the volume of distribution is large. See Chapter 6, Elimination Enhancement.

Biliary Elimination

Drugs with molecular weight greater than 500 daltons and specific chemical structures enhance biliary excretion. Carrier-mediated active transport is important in concentrating compounds in bile. For many drugs, there exists an enterohepatic circulation whereby drugs are excreted in the bile and absorbed into the intestine. Data on the clinical significance of enterohepatic circulation is limited in humans. Substances with varying amounts of enterohepatic circulation include chloral hydrate, colchicine, digitalis, glutethimide, halogenated hydrocarbons, isoniazid, methaqualone, nonsteroidal antiinflammatory drugs, phencyclidine, phenothiazines, phenytoin, salicylates and tricyclic antidepressants. Drugs excreted in the bile theoretically may be bound in the gut by activated charcoal or cholestyramine.

Pulmonary Elimination

The body excretes volatile anesthetics primarily by the lungs. Paraldehyde is partially eliminated by the lungs. Factors affecting rate of excretion include tidal volume, minute ventilation, drug solubility, and the ventilation-perfusion relationship.

Renal Elimination

Numerous compounds are excreted renally to some degree. The amount of drug eliminated by glomerular filtration is determined by cardiac output and is related to plasma volume. Renal disease and old age reduce the amount filtered. Drugs eliminated by the proximal tubule include penicillin, cephalosporins, and probenecid. Lipid-soluble compounds are eliminated by passive reabsorption in the distal convoluted tubule. Excretion is pH dependent. Alkaline urine traps weakly acidic drugs (e.g., phenobarbital, aspirin) and acidic urine traps weakly alkaline drugs (e.g., phencyclidine, amphetamines). Forced diuresis increases the excretion of a few drugs but usually does not increase renal clearance.

Questions—Elimination

1. Substances with varying amounts of enterohepatic circulation include
A. Phenytoin
B. Methotrexate
C. Halogenated hydrocarbons
D. All of the above
E. A and C

2. Drugs excreted in the bile theoretically may be bound in the gut by activated charcoal or cholestyramine.
A. True
B. False

GERIATRIC PHARMACOKINETICS

It has been estimated that drug reactions account for up to 10% to 15% of geriatric admissions. The elderly are at increased risk of developing drug side effects because of many different factors. These include age-related drug sensitivity, altered pharmacokinetics, multiple medications and potential drug interactions, greater use of drugs compared with other segments of the population, and greater use of more potent drugs compared with other segments of the population. Failure to take drugs as prescribed is often because of failure to understand the importance of therapy, failure to understand the directions for use, high dosing frequency, cost of medication, and failure to get prescriptions filled. The majority of poisonings that occur in persons 60 years and older are unintentional and may be amenable to poison prevention education.

Symptoms caused by drug-induced poisonings may be interpreted as normal signs of aging and include disorientation, tremors, lethargy, depression, forgetfulness, loss of appetite, and constipation. Poor eyesight, failure to read instructions, eating or swallowing an improperly stored product, taking medicines in the dark, stopping a drug suddenly without physician direction, transferring a drug from its original container to another, and failure to use proper protection when using a dangerous product add to the probability of undesirable drug effects in the elderly.

Clinical drug effects also depend on pharmacokinetic and host factors. Sedation is more likely in the elderly. Lean muscle mass decreases in the elderly, whereas body fat increases 35%. Total body water decreases 17%, extracellular water 40%, and plasma volume 8%. Plasma protein concentration, especially of serum albumin, also decreases. Organ blood flow decreases as does cardiac index, which specifically affects the hepatic first-pass effect. Renal plasma flow and glomerular filtration may affect elimination, which typically decrease 50% between the ages 40 years and 80 years. Effect is not predicted by creatinine alone, because both production and clearance are reduced. Mixed function oxidase activity (P450s) decreases with age, leading to reduced enzyme induction.

Increasing drug interactions in the elderly may follow an increase in the number of drugs ingested daily, alterations in pharmacokinetics, long-term drug use, alteration in gut surface area, decrease in gastric motility, decreased gastric acid secretion, use of antacids, drugs competing for binding sites on serum albumin, increase in the proportion of fat to body mass, decreased body water, reduced liver size with diminished ability to metabolize drugs, less efficient renal clearance of drugs, and heightened drug receptor sensitivity, especially to cardiovascular and psychotropic drugs.

Questions—Geriatric Pharmacokinetics

1. It has been estimated that drug reactions account for ____ geriatric admissions.
A. 2%
B. 10%
C. 50%
D. Most
E. Rare

2. The elderly are at increased risk of developing drug side effects because of many different factors. These include all of the following, except
A. Age-related drug sensitivity
B. Tendency to live in warmer climates
C. Altered pharmacokinetics
D. Multiple medications and potential drug interactions
E. Greater use of more potent drugs compared with other segments of the population

3. Body fat ____ in the elderly.
A. Increases
B. Decreases

Answers

Introduction to Pharmacokinetics

1. D 2. D

Interpretation of Pharmacokinetic Data

1. C 2. C

Pharmacokinetic Formulas and Examples

1. A 2. C 3. B 4. B

Absorption

1. A 2. A

Distribution

1. E 2. D 3. A 4. B 5. B 6. A 7. B

Metabolism

1. A 2. D 3. B 4. E 5. B 6. A

Elimination

1. E 2. A

Geriatric Pharmacokinetics

1. B 2. B 3. A

SELECTED READINGS

Introduction to Pharmacokinetics

1. Done AK. Everything you've always wanted to know about pharmacokinetics but were afraid to ask. Emerg Med 1978;10(6):67–69, 75–76,81.
2. Greenblatt DJ, Koch-Weser J. Clinical pharmacokinetics. Part I. N Engl J Med 1975;293:702-705; Part II. N Engl J Med 1975;293:963–969.
3. Sue Y-J, Shannon M. Pharmacokinetics of drugs in overdose. Clin Pharmacokinet 1992;23:93–105.

Definitions of Pharmacokinetics

1. Done AK: Everything you've always wanted to know about pharmacokinetics but were afraid to ask. Emerg Med 1978;10:(6):67–69,75–76,81.
2. Gibaldi M, Levy G: Pharmacokinetics in clinical practice: I. Concepts. JAMA
3. Greenblatt DJ, Koch-Weser J: Clinical pharmacokinetics, Part I. N Engl J Med 1975;293:702–705; Part II. N Engl J Med 1975; 293:963–969.

Distribution

1. Gibaldi M, Nagashima R, Levy G: Relationship between drug concentration in plasma or serum and amount of drug in the body. J Pharm Sci 1969;58:193–197.
2. Koch-Weser J: Bioavailability of drugs. N Engl J Med (First of two parts) 1974;291:233–236; (Second of two parts) 1974;291:503–508.

Metabolism

1. Adverse Drug Interaction Program. New Rochelle, NY: The Medical Letter, 1993.
2. Gillette JR: Factors affecting drug metabolism. Ann NY Acad Sci 1971;179:43–66.
3. Wrighton SA, Stevens JC. The human hepatic cytochromes P450 involved in drug metabolism. Crit Rev Toxicol 1992;22:1–21.

Elimination

1. Viccellio, P: *Handbook of Medical Toxicology.* Little, Brown and Company, Boston. 1993:12–27.

Geriatric Pharmacokinetics

1. Kroner BA, Scott RB, Waring ER, Zanga JR. Poisoning in the elderly: Characterization of exposures reported to a poison center. J Am Geriatr Soc 1993; 41:842–846.
2. Woolf A, Fish S, Azzara C, Dean D. Serious poisonings among older adults: A study of hospitalization and mortality rates in Massachusetts 1983–1985. Am J Pub Health 1990;8:867–869.

CHAPTER 8

The Pregnant Patient

INTRODUCTION

The pregnant female ingests prescribed or over-the-counter drugs at all stages of pregnancy. These chemical substances enter the altered pharmacokinetics of the pregnant mother and may induce changes in the physiology and development of the embryo and the fetus. The pregnant mother may be exposed to an intentional overdose of a drug, therapeutic agent, or occupational chemical. The resultant damage, if any, to the unborn child (embryo, fetus, neonate, and infant) often depends on the period (first, second, or third trimester) during which toxic exposure has occurred.

Most studies correlating toxic exposure with pregnancy outcome have examined structural malformations (teratogenesis) that develop during first trimester organogenesis. Other adverse effects on reproduction, such as chromosomal and biochemical factors, may be equally important in toxin-exposed pregnant patients. Most available reports of adverse outcomes deal with anecdotal cases of overdose or therapeutic exposure of potentially toxic agents during pregnancy. Information on poisoning of the mother and, inferentially, of her embryo or fetus, is severely limited. Systematic prospective clinical studies focusing on specific drugs, drug dose, type of exposure, period of fetal development, and clinical outcomes on pregnancy, labor, and neonates, are generally lacking.

Considerable teratogenic literature has been published, but most of these observations concern therapeutic dosages of a suspect drug. Although an overdose probably produces teratogenic changes at least equal to those following therapeutic dose and causes profound alterations in the pharmacokinetics of both mother and fetus, such conclusions are not yet supported by adequate clinical studies.

Questions—Introduction to the Pregnant Patient

1. Knowledge about toxic exposures during pregnancy

A. Is mostly based on large, case-controlled studies
B. Mostly concerns the deleterious effects of therapeutic doses
C. Centers around chromosomal more than structural abnormalities
D. Does not rely on anecdotal cases for any doses of drugs
E. None of the above

DRUG USE DURING PREGNANCY

The thalidomide disaster emphasized to both the public and the medical profession that drugs ingested by a mother could harm her developing baby. Despite this, pregnant mothers continue to use prescription and over-the-counter drugs extensively. Reviews indicate that up to 90% or more of all pregnant women continue to take one or more drugs, including dietary supplements, during pregnancy. Despite extensive dissemination of information and ubiquitous warning labels in our society, women continue to smoke, drink alcohol, and take illicit drugs during pregnancy.

Pregnancy Risk Factors

The Food and Drug Administration has proposed risk factors to help health care workers quickly ascertain the danger that drugs pose to the developing fetus. Newly approved drugs are required to contain this information in the "Precautions" section of package inserts. These categories tend to simplify a complex topic and must be viewed as only part of a decision process when prescribing drugs during pregnancy.

These risk factors do not distinguish use of drugs by trimester or length of use. Some older drugs have not been assigned categories, and manufacturers may assign a risk category that differs from perceptions in the medical community. Nonetheless, they are a starting point to consider when drug therapy during pregnancy is proposed. They do not apply to breastfeeding.

Category A

Controlled studies show no risk. Adequate, well-controlled studies in pregnant women have failed to demonstrate a risk to the fetus in any trimester of pregnancy.

Category B

No evidence of risk in humans. Adequate, well-controlled studies in pregnant women have not shown increased risk of fetal abnormalities despite adverse findings in animals.

Category C

Risk cannot be ruled out. Adequate, well-controlled human studies are lacking, and animal studies have shown a risk to the fetus or are lacking as well. There is a chance of fetal harm if the drug is administered during pregnancy, but the potential benefit may outweigh the potential risk.

Category D

Positive evidence of risk. Studies in humans, or investigational or post-marketing data have demonstrated fetal risk. Nonetheless, potential benefits from the use of the drug may outweigh the potential risk. For example, the drug may be acceptable if needed in a life-threatening situation or serious disease for which safer drugs cannot be used or are ineffective.

Category X

Contraindicated in pregnancy. Studies in animals or humans, or investigational or post marketing reports have demonstrated positive evidence of fetal abnormalities or risk that clearly outweighs any possible benefit to the patient.

Questions—Drug Use During Pregnancy

1. A drug that has been found to adversely affect an animal fetus when used in a pregnant mother is classified as

A. Category A
B. Category B
C. Category C
D. Category D
E. Category X

Answers to questions in shaded boxes appear at the end of the chapter.

2. A drug that has failed to demonstrate risk to a fetus in the first trimester in controlled studies is classified as
   A. Category A
   B. Category B
   C. Category C
   D. Category D
   E. Category X

3. A drug shown to have risk clearly outweighing any possible benefit is classified as
   A. Category A
   B. Category B
   C. Category C
   D. Category D
   E. Category X

4. A drug that has been shown to have an adverse effect in animal reproduction, which was not confirmed in controlled studies of women in their first trimester, is classified as
   A. Category A
   B. Category B
   C. Category C
   D. Category D
   E. Category X

5. A drug that has been shown to have human fetal risk but may have benefits acceptable despite the risk is classified as
   A. Category A
   B. Category B
   C. Category C
   D. Category D
   E. Category X

PHARMACOKINETICS OF PREGNANCY

A number of significant physiologic alterations occur during pregnancy that may profoundly affect the pharmacokinetics of drugs administered during this period, both therapeutically and in overdose.

Absorption

The rate of gastric emptying is reduced in pregnancy, especially after a high-osmolality meal. This change is most pronounced at the time of labor when drugs administered orally may be absorbed very slowly. Gastric emptying procedures following an overdose during pregnancy may be effective for longer intervals after ingestion than would be the case in the nonpregnant patient. An increase in small intestine transit time may lead to slower but more complete drug absorption. An overdose early in pregnancy may coincide with first trimester nausea and vomiting, and serious drug effects may be considerably mitigated.

Distribution

During pregnancy, the apparent volume of distribution of drugs may be altered by an expansion in the mean plasma volume (2.6 L in the nonpregnant state, increasing by 20% at midgestation and by 50% at term). This expansion is greater than the increase in red cell mass, which explains the usual drop in hematocrit seen in pregnant patients.

An increase in the development of organs associated with pregnancy (uterus, breasts, products of conception, plus an increase in extravascular water) leads to an increase in total body water. For relatively polar drugs with a normally small apparent volume of distribution, the effect is more marked than for lipophilic drugs with a large volume of distribution.

The pregnant woman gains an average of 12 kg, of which 3 to 4 kg consists of fat. Body fat may act as a depot or reservoir for fat-soluble drugs. An increase in the apparent volume of distribution of many drugs not only reduces the plasma concentration of such drugs, but may also prolong their half-lives. Because clearance is independent of the volume of distribution, it may take longer for eliminating organs to clear drugs.

Pregnancy is one of the few situations in which monitoring of the free drug level may be clinically useful, especially after an overdose. Free fractions of drugs such as propranolol and lidocaine that bind to alpha-acid glycoprotein also are increased in pregnancy. With therapeutic doses, any increase in free drug usually is well cleared by the body, because processes of elimination are not normally saturated.

Plasma albumin concentration decreases in normal pregnancy, and the protein-binding capacity of plasma decreases. This change increases the volume of distribution of a drug as freer drug passes into tissues. Highly protein-bound drugs include anticoagulants, anticonvulsants, and benzodiazepines. Changes in protein binding during pregnancy may not be clinically important after therapeutic doses. In an overdose setting, such elimination processes may be overwhelmed and lead to deleterious clinical effects because of free drug accumulation.

Metabolism

Hepatic alterations that may affect drug or chemical metabolism in the overdosed pregnant woman include hepatic blood flow, bile excretion, and enzyme induction. There is little clinical evidence to support any significant effect resulting from changes in hepatic blood flow or biliary excretion. Decarboxylase reactions are depressed because of a relative deficiency during pregnancy of the decarboxylase coenzyme precursors, thiamine, and pyridoxine.

Folic acid deficiency also reduces many microsomal enzyme systems. Such deficiency may be enhanced when chronic anticonvulsant therapy, which is known to cross the placenta, is administered during pregnancy. Folic acid supplementation before and during pregnancy may prevent congenital deformities that may develop after the first trimester use of antiepileptic drugs.

At term, the human fetal liver has a relatively well-developed ability to metabolize drugs. However, during pregnancy, its contribution to overall metabolism is small. Toxic metabolites may be generated in the fetus itself during the first part of gestation.

Excretion

During pregnancy, renal plasma flow almost doubles. Drugs such as lithium, cephalexin, and gentamicin, the elimination of which depends almost entirely on renal clearance, show an increase in overall clearance. Digoxin and ampicillin both are metabolized and excreted unchanged into the urine. Their half-lives also are altered by pregnancy. Drugs such as anticonvulsants and tricyclic antidepressants, which usually are dependent on metabolism for their elimination, are not affected significantly by the alterations in renal function that occur in pregnancy.

The glomerular filtration rate during pregnancy behaves similarly to the renal plasma flow. This increase also tends to increase elimination of free drug present in the plasma. Consequently, an increase in elimination of lithium, digoxin, and antibiotics (e.g., ampicillin, cephalosporins, and aminoglycosides) may be considerable during pregnancy. In preeclampsia, proteinuria may result in reduced plasma albumin levels, reduced drug binding, an increase in free drug distribution to tissues, and a substantial loss of bound and unbound drug in the urine.

Questions—Pharmacokinetics of Pregnancy

1. **The rate of gastric emptying in pregnancy**
   A. Is reduced when compared to women who are not pregnant
   B. Is most reduced at the time of labor
   C. Allows gastric lavage to be more effective for longer intervals after ingestion than for a nonpregnant patient
   D. Is particularly reduced after a high osmolality meal
   E. All of the above
2. **Which of the following is false regarding pregnant patients?**
   A. Pregnancy is one of the few situations in which monitoring of the free drug level may be clinically useful, especially after an overdose.
   B. With therapeutic doses, any increase in free drug usually is poorly cleared by the body because processes of elimination are not normally saturated.
   C. Plasma albumin concentration decreases in normal pregnancy, and the protein-binding capacity of plasma decreases.
   D. During pregnancy, renal plasma flow almost doubles
   E. Changes in protein binding during pregnancy may not be clinically important after therapeutic doses. In an overdose setting, such elimination processes may be overwhelmed and lead to deleterious clinical effects because of free drug accumulation.
3. **The pregnant woman's**
   A. Relative deficiency of thiamine and pyridoxine depresses decarboxylase reactions
   B. Folic acid deficiency counteracts the effects of anticonvulsants
   C. Increased hepatic blood flow enhances effects of anticonvulsants
   D. Exposure to toxic metabolites reflects her own metabolism and not that of the fetus
   E. None of the above
4. **All of the following have altered elimination in the pregnant woman except**
   A. Tricyclic antidepressants
   B. Lithium
   C. Cephalexin
   D. Digoxin
   E. Ampicillin

THE PLACENTA

The placenta transfers oxygen and nutrients from the mother to the fetus and conveys carbon dioxide and other metabolic products from the fetus to the mother. A number of variables determine the effectiveness of the human placenta as an organ of transfer. These include the concentration of specific drug under consideration (and, in some instances, the extent to which it is bound to another compound), the rate of maternal blood flow through the intervillous space, and the area available for exchange across the villous epithelium.

Other variables include the physical properties of the tissue barrier interposed between blood in the intervillous space and blood in the fetal capillaries (in case the substance is transferred by diffusion), the capacity of the biochemical machinery of the placenta to effect active transfer (in case the substance is transferred actively), the amount of substance metabolized by the placenta during transfer, the area for exchange across the fetal capillaries in the placenta, the concentration in the fetal blood of the substance (exclusive of any that is bound), and the rate of fetal blood flow through villous capillaries.

Most drugs present in the maternal blood reach the fetal circulation in some concentration. The placenta, which contains enzymes capable of altering drugs during their passage through the membrane, can metabolize compounds to form active metabolites. Drugs also may change the normal patterns of circulation and the activity of the placenta itself. The fetus, with immature kidney and liver functions and inadequate enzyme systems, is less able to eliminate drugs than an adult.

Most drugs ingested in therapeutic quantities by the mother produce no ill effects on the fetus. However, different doses of the same drug may exert widely varied actions on the fetus. Many women are not aware that over-the-counter products are drugs that possibly could have an effect on their babies. In addition, the period of greatest fetal susceptibility occurs early in pregnancy when both the woman and her physician may be unaware of her pregnancy.

Simple diffusion appears to be the mechanism for transfer of oxygen, carbon dioxide, water, most electrolytes, and anesthetic gases. Most substances with a molecular weight below 500 to 1,000 daltons readily diffuse through the placental tissue interposed between the maternal and fetal circulation. Uncharged materials such as urea pass through the placenta easily, and compounds with high lipid solubility often pass unmetabolized into the fetal circulation.

Questions—The Placenta

1. **Most drugs ingested in therapeutic quantities produce no ill effects on a fetus.**
   A. True
   B. False
2. **Most substances with a molecular weight below 5,000 daltons readily diffuse through the placental tissue interposed between the maternal and fetal circulation.**
   A. True
   B. False
3. **The placenta, which contains enzymes capable of altering drugs during their passage through the membrane, can metabolize compounds to form active metabolites.**
   A. True
   B. False

REPRODUCTIVE TOXICOLOGY

The Parents: Preconception

A drug overdose or chemical exposure may, by its interaction with a gamete (sperm or ova), either impair fertilization or cause such severe alterations in the resulting zygote that an early unrecognized abortion occurs. Either paternal or maternal exposure to mutagenic agents at this stage may result in the inhibition of fertilization, impaired placental implantation, spontaneous abortion, or production of an abnormal embryo.

Diminished fertility in both men and women may result from the toxic effects of chemicals. For example, up to 15% of men exposed to dibromochloropropane (DBCP) may be azoospermic and another 21%, oligospermic. Screening procedures for known and potential reproductive hazards currently are under development. Various factors may render individual case reports unreliable in establishing a causal connection between a potential offending agent and a destructive reproductive response. These may include problems in semen collection, difficulties in obtaining an accurate reproductive history, other possible associations with male reproductive hazards (e.g., loss of libido, impotence, sterility, anatomic lesions), drugs (e.g., antifertility drugs, antimetabolites), radiation, endocrine abnormalities, and problems in interpreting endocrine laboratory tests.

The Parents: Postconception

The pregnant woman may be subject to unusual or unpredictable reactions to drug overdose during gestation as a result of alterations in pharmacokinetics, drug detoxification mechanisms, and / or changes in hepatic, renal, or pulmonary function. These changes may seriously affect absorption, distribution, metabolism, and excretion of drug, resulting in production of unusual metabolites, deviations from protein binding, and changes in first-pass effect, half-life, and excretion.

It has been estimated that 42% of pregnancies occur in working women. Chemical teratogenicity may follow maternal exposures to lead, mercury, carbon monoxide, and some pesticides. Many of these data are based on animal studies and statistically significant corroborating evidence after human exposure has been lacking. An increase in central nervous system toxicity (neural tube defects) and oral clefts has been observed after exposure to organic solvents during pregnancy. More studies are needed to better assess this enormous topic.

The Embryo

THE FIRST WEEK (PREIMPLANTATION)

During the first week after fertilization and before placental implantation, quantities of an absorbed drug or its metabolites may reach the zygote, morula, or blastocyst in sufficient concentrations to alter normal development. Few studies of drug pharmacokinetics have been performed at this stage of embryo development following therapeutic or toxic drug administration. During this period, some therapeutic substances administered in normal doses and some drugs ingested in overdose probably are embryocidal, leading to defective implantation, or inducing spontaneous abortion.

EIGHTH DAY TO TWENTY-FIRST DAY

Between the first and third weeks, when implantation has occurred, similar effects on the embryo may result after a toxic exposure. An "all-or-none" effect, or death or normal development, has been described. In animals, some chemical insults cause malformations during this predifferentiation stage (before the end of the third week). No data on humans are available to corroborate this all-or-none concept.

TWENTY-FIRST DAY TO END OF EIGHTH WEEK

During the period of active organ differentiation, drugs, chemicals, or physical agents can induce profound teratogenic changes in the embryo. The central nervous system, heart, gut, skeletal system, and muscle all begin to differentiate in the somite stage, although at different rates. Teratogenic drugs acting in this period may affect any of these systems.

Adverse effects on embryo and fetal development depend on the time of exposure, the dose of the chemical agent, the efficiency with which the mother metabolizes the agent, placental transfer, vulnerability of fetal tissues (e.g., limb buds were especially vulnerable to thalidomide), ability of the embryo or fetus to metabolize the agent, and pharmacogenetic differences. After the 8th to the 12th weeks of intrauterine life, the embryo is fully differentiated and drugs usually are no longer teratogens, though they may still affect the fetus in other ways.

During much of the critical period for malformation, the mother may not know she is pregnant. The embryo may be more susceptible to toxic exposure than the mother because of its rapid cell turnover, inadequate detoxification and excretion mechanisms, immature biologic barriers, poor immunosurveillance, and exposure to multiple drugs or chemicals.

EIGHTH WEEK TO BIRTH(FETUS)

During fetal development, there is further differentiation of the embryonic primordium into definitive organs, general growth (i.e., cell proliferation, increase in cell size), storage of energy substrates, and increase in cellular protein content. Environmental threats to the fetus may be biological (e.g., viruses), physical (e.g., radiation), or chemical (e.g., drugs). Threats may occur through the general environment (e.g., rubella virus), occupation (e.g., exposure to anesthetic gases), therapeutic intervention (e.g., diethylstilbestrol, thalidomide), or substance abuse (e.g., cigarettes, alcohol).

Precise mechanisms of harm on the germinal, embryonic, or fetal cells are not known but may involve mutation, chromosomal changes, interference with mitosis or nucleic acid function, lack of precursor substrates for developing cell chemical processes, altered energy sources, changed membrane characteristics, osmotic disturbances, and enzyme inhibitions. Fetotoxicity may be manifested by infertility, fetal or neonatal death, growth retardation, malformations or structural defects, and later genetic, carcinogenic, behavioral, and reproductive effects.

Perinatal Period (Infant)

Physical growth, maturation of the central nervous system, and development of certain endocrine glands is not completed until months after birth. The newborn may be exposed via airborne contamination to chemicals, resulting from either paternal or maternal carriage on clothes, following occupational exposure. The presence of chemicals in the milk of lactating mothers may subject the newborn to unwanted toxic effects.

Questions—Reproductive Toxicology

1. Paternal or maternal exposure to mutagenic agents before fertilization can

A. Inhibit fertilization
B. Impair placental implantation
C. Cause spontaneous abortion
D. Produce an abnormal embryo
E. All of the above

2. Exposure to organic solvents during pregnancy

A. Is associated with neural tube defects
B. Is associated with oral clefts
C. Has not been associated with specific fetal abnormalities
D. A and B
E. None of the above

3. During the first three weeks of gestation
A. Numerous studies on drug pharmacokinetics have definitively shown the effects of drugs on embryo development
B. Only overdoses of drugs are embryocidal
C. Human data has proven that toxins cause death but not malformations compatible with life.
D. Some chemical insults in animal studies have been shown to cause malformations.
E. None of the above

4. During the last 2 trimesters of gestation,
A. Viruses are never a threat
B. Therapeutic interventions have never been harmful
C. Precise mechanisms of harm may include mutation, chromosomal changes, or changed membrane characteristics.
D. The heart begins to differentiate
E. None of the above

SPECIFIC TOXIN CONSIDERATIONS DURING PREGNANCY

Excellent reviews and books have summarized the effects of drugs (usually after therapeutic doses), toxins, and chemicals during pregnancy. Certain drugs are known to adversely affect the fetus during the first trimester, later in pregnancy, and during the perinatal period. It has been estimated that approximately half of the drugs used by pregnant patients are over-the-counter, self-administered medications. Specific topics relating to drugs and their effects on the pregnant patient are listed below. This list is by no means exhaustive. Specific details regarding pregnancy and lactation may be found within individual chapters.

Acetaminophen

In 1982, the first case of an acetaminophen overdose (22.5 g) in the third trimester of pregnancy (36 weeks gestation) was reported. An oral N-acetylcysteine (Mucomyst®) protocol was instituted and 6 weeks later, a healthy normal infant was delivered. The early fetus, on the other hand, is at risk from acetaminophen, because its ability to conjugate toxic metabolites with glutathione may only be a fraction of an adult's capacity. It is recommended that treatment with oral N-acetylcysteine is given to appropriate, pregnant, acetaminophen-overdose patients, and that delivery not be induced. Activated charcoal also may be useful. No studies have been published indicating fetal malformations after acetaminophen overdose and N-acetylcysteine has not been reported to produce teratogenic effects.

Amanita Phalloides

An *Amanita phalloides* mushroom ingestion has been reported in a 21-year-old pregnant woman and confirmed by measurement of α-amanitin levels. She developed nausea, vomiting, abdominal pain, and diarrhea within 10 hours of ingestion. No amatoxins were detected in the amniotic fluid by high-performance liquid chromatography or immunoassay methods. She later gave birth to a healthy baby with no biochemical evidence of hepatocellular danger, suggesting that α-amanitin does not cross the placental barrier during the acute phase of intoxication.

Angiotensin-Converting Enzyme Inhibitors

Fetal anuria, renal tubular dysgenesis, fetal renal malfunction, and acute renal failure have been reported in babies whose mothers have been treated with angiotensin-converting enzyme inhibitors during pregnancy.

Antithrombotic Agents

Heparin probably is safe for the fetus during pregnancy, but oral anticoagulants may not be, especially in the first trimester. Warfarin may be associated with congenital abnormalities. Heparin may cause a persistent anticoagulant effect at the time of delivery, increasing the risk of maternal bleeding and should be stopped 24 hours before elective induction of labor. Heparin can be given safely to mothers who are breastfeeding. It is not secreted in breast milk. Warfarin also does not appear to induce an anticoagulant effect in the breast-fed infant. Low-dose aspirin (150 mg/dL) (see Salicylates, below) during the second and third trimesters appears to be safe, but the safety of aspirin in higher doses or when taken in the first trimester is still questionable.

β-Agonists

Betamimetic tocolytic therapy is inadvisable for patients with inherent cardiac disease. Maternal effects may include hypotension with reflex tachycardia, increase in stroke volume, increased cardiac output, and increased systolic blood pressure. The most common arrhythmia reported is supraventricular tachycardia, although atrial fibrillation, atrial premature contractions, and ventricular ectopy also have been observed. Continuous electrocardiogram monitoring of a patient receiving intravenous betamimetic therapy should be performed.

Chest pain is relatively uncommon. Transient ST-segment depression is common and appears to be dose related. About 5% of maternal patients receiving intravenous betamimetic therapy develop pulmonary edema. Use of betamimetics may lead to an acute rise in plasma glucose concentration and an increase in insulin release. Neonates delivered after recent exposure to maternal betamimetic therapy should be monitored for hypoglycemia. See Ritodrine, below.

β-Blockers

β-Blockers, frequently cardioselective, have been widely used for the treatment of pregnancy-induced hypertension. Adverse reactions are believed to be rare and the effects on the fetus or infant are thought to be minimal. However, propranolol after long-term use may produce intrauterine growth retardation, neonatal hypoglycemia, and neonatal bradycardia.

Caffeine

Caffeine readily crosses the placenta. The enzyme or enzymes necessary to metabolize caffeine is absent until several days after birth. Fetal arrhythmias may follow excessive intake of caffeine by the mother during pregnancy. The weight of evidence suggests that ingesting more than 300 mg per day of caffeine during pregnancy may cause intrauterine growth retardation, decreased birthweight, and possibly spontaneous abortion. Few adverse pregnancy outcomes have been reported in women who consume less than 300 mg/day of caffeine during pregnancy. No solid conclusions have been made regarding the safety of caffeine at lower levels.

Infants exposed to high maternal levels of caffeine for the majority of the pregnancy may develop irritability, jitteriness, and vomiting in the immediate newborn period. Caffeine is excreted in breast milk and is found in umbilical cord blood. The half-life of caffeine is prolonged in pregnancy. In 1980, the FDA advised pregnant women to avoid or limit use of caffeine-containing foods and drugs.

Calcium Channel Blockers

Nifedipine, nicardipine, and verapamil are capable of inhibiting uterine contractions. There may be a profound reduction in uteroplacental blood flow. Nifedipine can be used orally or parenterally. After oral use, maximum plasma concentrations are achieved in 15 to 90 minutes with a plasma half-life of 2 to 3 hours.

Carbon Monoxide

Although teratogenetic effects following maternal exposure to carbon monoxide have not been described, fetotoxic effects following toxic maternal exposure do occur. During acute carbon monoxide intoxication, maternal carboxyhemoglobin (HbCOM) concentration increases rapidly, then reaches a plateau in 7 to 8 hours. Fetal carboxyhemoglobin (HbCOF) levels show little change during the first hours of maternal intoxication, then increase slowly over 24 hours and may exceed the maternal carboxyhemoglobin levels.

With normobaric oxygen, HbCOM and HbCOF half-lives are respectively 90 minutes and 3 to 4 hours. HbCOF half-life with pure hyperbaric oxygen is not accurately known. Because fetal accumulation of carbon monoxide is higher and its elimination is slower than in the maternal circulation, hyperbaric oxygen may decrease fetal hypoxia and improve outcome. Consideration should be given to the use of hyperbaric oxygen in pregnant women with acute carbon monoxide intoxication, irrespective of their HbCOM or presenting clinical features, although controlled clinical trials to support this treatment are not available.

Ciguatera Poisoning

A 20-year-old mother who developed ciguatera poisoning during the second trimester experienced increased fetal movements for a few hours. She endured multisystemic symptoms typical of ciguatera for 8 weeks. The newborn, at term, was normal with adequate respiratory and neurologic reflexes and developed normally during the first 10 months. It is unknown whether ciguatoxin can cross the placenta. It may appear in breast milk.

Cocaine

Many women use cocaine while pregnant. Cocaine-using women have a significantly higher rate of spontaneous abortion. Infants of cocaine-using women may have depression of interactive behavior with poor organizational response to environmental stimuli. Cocaine-using women may feel contractions and increased fetal activity within minutes of using cocaine and experience early onset of labor. There are some indications that infants of cocaine-using women are at increased risk for the development of congenital malformations and for perinatal mortality. Women who use cocaine during pregnancy are at risk for premature deliveries, abruptio placentae and maternal death.

Diazepam

Sodium benzoate, a solubilizing agent in injectable diazepam, competes with bilirubin and, in an overdose, displaces it from its protein-binding site. The benzoate freely crosses to the fetus and competes for protein-binding sites, resulting in hyperbilirubinemia in the neonate.

Digitalis

Few data are available on intrauterine digitalis toxicity. Digitalis compounds pass through the placenta. Data on the transplacental passage of Fab antibody fragments are not available. The pregnant patient with an acute digitalis overdose should be treated similarly to a nonpregnant patient when indicated. The antidigoxin antibody fragment should be given to the mother when required, although its safety and efficacy for the fetus are unknown. Fetal cardiac rhythm should be monitored. A viable fetus can be delivered as an emergency and the antidote administered to the neonate as indicated by blood levels if necessary.

Drug Abuse And Withdrawal

A large number of neonates who have been exposed to drugs in utero, particularly those whose mothers denied the use of drugs, appear normal at birth. Noting the maternal profile (e.g., single, multigravida, no previous maternal care, preoccupation with daily procurement of drugs, prostitution) and drug screening of the newborn can enhance detection of the newborn at risk by meconium analysis (radioimmunoassay for metabolites of cocaine, morphine, and cannabinoids).

The onset of neonatal withdrawal syndrome may occur within 1 to 4 days of birth for most drugs except phenobarbital, for which symptoms appear 10 to 14 days after birth, and chlordiazepoxide, for which symptoms may appear 24 days after birth. Drugs with longer elimination half-lives tend to result in withdrawal manifestations later than those with short elimination half-lives. Neonatal withdrawal syndrome usually does not develop in neonates of mothers who have been drug free for a week or more prior to delivery.

Ethanol

Ethanol may act as a tocolytic and inhibits the secretion of the neurohypophyseal hormones, antidiuretic hormone, and oxytocin. Ethanol appears to suppress uterine activity through inhibition of oxytocin release, reduction of myometrial oxytocin receptors, and noncompetitive antagonism at the uterine level. In controlled studies, ethanol is a less-effective tocolytic than isoxsuprine, ritodrine, terbutaline, or magnesium sulfate. Children exposed in utero to alcohol as a tocolytic only have shown no abnormalities.

Consumption of at least one to two alcoholic drinks daily has been associated with a significant decrease in birth weight. A safe level of ethanol use during pregnancy has not been established. One to two drinks per day taken by the mother during the first trimester may not be associated with more teratogenicity than that associated with nondrinkers. Neonatal withdrawal and acute ethanol intoxication are potential risks in children born to alcoholic mothers.

Studies on the human placenta suggest that the placenta oxidizes ethanol to acetaldehyde and releases acetaldehyde to the fetus. This may be a factor in the fetal alcohol syndrome. The fetal alcohol syndrome defines specific facial characteristics seen in children born to alcoholic mothers. Numerous birth abnormalities have been reported. Long-term follow-up studies of these children indicate severe growth deficiencies and intellectual handicaps that correlate with a degree of craniofacial abnormalities. Dental malocclusions, malalignments, and eustachian tube dysfunction occurs as a result of facial hypoplasia.

Iron

Acute iron intoxication in pregnancy poses a dilemma to the clinician. Toxic levels of iron often are associated with severe complications and can be fatal. The effective iron chelator, deferoxamine, has possible teratogenic potential. If delivery occurs, the infant should be evaluated for iron overload or iron deficiency secondary to maternal deferoxamine therapy. The fetus seems to fare better than the mother does after maternal iron overdose. Although the maternal serum iron level is high, little iron appears to pass to the fetus. The risk to the fetus is not from the iron itself, but is secondary to the induced pathophysiologic derangements (i.e., acidosis) in the mother. Emergency delivery of a viable fetus should be reserved only for documented maternal or fetal distress.

Lead

Lead crosses the placenta. It is unlikely that the chelator, calcium disodium edetate, passes through the placenta. Few studies have been performed during pregnancy following the use of dimercaprol (BAL in Oil) or dimercaptosuccinic acid (DMSA). During pregnancy, maternal and not fetal indications must guide the administration of lead chelators.

Lindane

An anecdotal case report suggests that lindane crosses the placenta, is excreted in human breast milk, and may be fetotoxic.

Lithium

One prospective study of 148 women who had used lithium during their first trimester and who had consulted teratogen information centers suggests that lithium is not an important human teratogen. Based on this study, it has been suggested that women with major affective disorders who wish to have children may, after consultation with their health provider, continue lithium therapy, provided that adequate screening tests are done, including ultrasound and fetal echocardiography.

Magnesium

Magnesium is an effective tocolytic. Serum magnesium concentrations of 4 to 8 mEq/L appear to inhibit uterine activity. Magnesium is eliminated by renal excretion. Serum magnesium level should be monitored, especially in the presence of depressed renal function. Loss of deep tendon reflexes occurs at serum levels of 4 to 8 mEq/L. Respiratory depression may be seen at 12 to 15 mEq/L. Above this level, cardiac conduction defects and cardiac arrest may occur. Side effects include transient hypotension and flushing. Transplacental transfer of magnesium to the fetus occurs. Neonatal hypotonia and drowsiness have been observed. Treatment includes cessation of administration, mannitol, and calcium.

Methyl Isocyanate

The Bhopal gas disaster on December 2, 1984, in which a large amount of methyl isocyanate was liberated, was one of the most damaging industrial accidents in history. A study of pregnant women exposed to this toxic gas indicated a high incidence of spontaneous abortion compared with those not exposed. Rates of stillbirths and congenital malformations were not found to be different. Perinatal and neonatal mortality was increased in the affected area.

Methylene Blue

In addition to its use as an antidote to methemoglobinemia, methylene blue may be used during diagnostic laparoscopy to examine the patency of the fallopian tubes, and during pregnancy to provide a marker in amniocentesis for multiple pregnancies and to verify premature rupture of the membranes. Undesirable effects have included hyperbilirubinemia and secondary hemolysis in the newborn, Heinz body formation, methemoglobinemia, and a strikingly deep blue baby in which assessment of hypoxia is difficult. It appears that methylene blue may be especially hazardous during the second trimester.

Nutmeg

Ingestion of nutmeg by a 29-year-old primigravida at the 30th week of gestation led to palpitations, agitation, blurred vision, apprehension, chest tightening, and dry mouth. Anticholinergic hyperstimulation caused by nutmeg ingestion is treated with supportive and symptomatic care.

Opiates

Pregnant women addicted to opiates have an increased incidence of antepartum hemorrhage, premature labor, and intrauterine death, which often occurs during withdrawal. From the infant's point of view, heroin may be preferable to methadone because the abstinence syndrome is less prolonged and severe.

Organophosphates

There are few data on the human transplacental passage of many organophosphate pesticides. In addition, little is known regarding cholinesterase development during fetal development. Relative transplacental passage and possibly differing fetal and maternal sensitivities may be important. Atropine, a principal antidote, has agonist properties and therefore a potential atropine dose may be either subtherapeutic or toxic for the fetus.

The pregnant patient should be treated like the nonpregnant patient however, using life support, gastrointestinal decontamination, aggressive respiratory care, atropine, and pralidoxime as required. The fetus should be monitored closely. If the mother is doing well, but the potentially viable fetus exhibits distress, consideration should be given to immediate delivery and appropriate therapy of the newborn.

Phenytoin

There is an increased incidence of congenital malformations in children born to epileptic women who have taken anticonvulsants during pregnancy. If a mother has epilepsy and is taking anticonvulsant drugs, her chance of having a child with a major congenital abnormality may be as high as 6%. Several studies suggest that abnormalities are more likely if more than one anticonvulsant is used or if particularly large doses are taken.

Teratogenic effects with phenytoin use, the so-called "fetal hydantoin syndrome" has been observed for over 20 years. Beause the risk of congenital malformations among infants exposed in utero to antiepileptic drugs is estimated to be two to three times greater than in the general population, folic acid has been recommended as an addition to the regimen of an epileptic woman who wishes to become pregnant. Vitamin K is administered to the newborn.

Prostaglandins

Prostaglandins are natural products that act as initiators and regulators of labor. When administered at any stage of gestation they cause uterine contractions and expulsion of the conceptus. Certain prostaglandins are effective in inducing abortion and labor. Intramyometrial injection of prostaglandins has been advocated to control postpartum hemorrhage secondary to placenta accreta and uterine hypotonia. Prostaglandins exert their effect on the smooth muscle of blood vessels, the bronchi, and the uterus. The prostaglandins may have vasodilator effects leading to a decrease in blood pressure with increase in heart rate and cardiac output. Prostaglandins have both inotropic and chronotropic effects on the myocardium. In the bronchi, they may cause bronchoconstriction or dilation of the smooth muscle of the bronchioles.

Prostaglandins have resulted in life-threatening profound hypotension, myocardial infarction, bronchospasm, seizures in epileptic patients, uterine rupture in midtrimester abortion, amniotic fluid embolism, third-trimester intrauterine deaths, ventricular tachycardia, gastric outlet obstruction in neonates, respiratory distress in a neonate, uterine hyperstimulation, and hypokalemia. Cardiac arrest has followed intramyometrial injection of prostaglandin E2.

Prostaglandin Synthetase Inhibitors

Indomethacin, a prostaglandin synthetase inhibitor, inhibits preterm labor. Following oral use, peak plasma concentrations are reached in 1 to 2 hours. Indomethacin is readily transferred across the placental unit to the fetus within 15 minutes. Maternal side effects generally are minimal and include nausea and heartburn. Potential fetal and neonatal complications associated with prostaglandin synthetase inhibitors include premature closure of the ductus arteriosus and neonatal primary pulmonary hypertension. One study suggested that using indomethacin for preterm labor appears to increase the risk of serious neonatal complications such as necrotizing enterocolitis and intracranial hemorrhage, in infants born at or before 30 weeks gestation.

Radiation

The possibility of pregnancy should be considered in deciding whether to examine a woman of reproductive age with x-rays. In the first 10 days after menstruation, it is unlikely that there is a conceptus and x-radiation is unlikely to be an additional risk. During the rest of the first month, any risk is likely to be so small that no special limitation on diagnostic exposures is required. During the second month of gestation, malformation of specific organs has occurred in experimental animals exposed to radiation. Between 8 and 15 weeks after conception, irradiation of the forebrain may result in mental retardation, but no evidence of this has been shown in the first 8 weeks.

Practical guidelines for the use of x-rays assume that a woman in her reproductive years is pregnant unless proved otherwise. Generally acceptable proofs that she is not pregnant include onset of menses in the last 10 days, oral contraceptive use, intrauterine device use, surgical sterilization, or a negative pregnancy test. If a woman may be in the first trimester of pregnancy, avoid inclusion of the pelvis in the primary x-ray beam if possible. Where feasible, always shield the pelvis and abdomen of women when performing diagnostic roentgenographic studies.

If there is a valid medical indication to perform a diagnostic study using radiation on a pregnant woman, this will generally outweigh the remote possibility of harm to the patient or her fetus. If a woman receives a relatively large amount of radiation (5 to 15 rads) to the pelvis in the first trimester of pregnancy, the increased risk of a congenital anomaly of the fetus is from 1% to 3%.

Retinoids

The association between vitamin A and human teratogenicity is unclear. Women in their reproductive years should be informed that excessive use of vitamin A shortly before and during pregnancy can be harmful to their babies and that a bioaccumulation of vitamin A from continuous high doses is a concern. Women of childbearing potential should consult with their physicians concerning birth control before consuming these products. Doses lower than 10,000 IU probably are not teratogenic.

Reports of birth defects and spontaneous abortions have followed exposure to isotretinoin during the first trimester of pregnancy. Teratogenicity has been associated with both isotretinoin (oral, cream) and etretinate. Defects have included external ear malformations, cleft palate, micrognathia, heart defects, ventricular septal defects, aortic arch malformations, and some brain malformations. Fetal malformation has followed 4 months to 1 year after the last dose of etretinate. Limb reduction defects have followed maternal use of isotretinoin in the first trimester of pregnancy. Both isotretinoin and etretinate carry category X labeling.

Women should not use isotretinoin and etretinate who are pregnant or who may become pregnant while taking the drug. Pregnancy should be ruled out before treatment begins. This precaution may be accomplished best by obtaining a negative pregnancy test no more than 2 weeks prior to the beginning of therapy and starting therapy on the second or third day of the patient's next menstrual period. An effective form of contraception should be used for at least 1 month before therapy begins. Women who have received isotretinoin should continue using an effective form of contraception for 1 month after discontinuing treatment.

The period during which pregnancy must be avoided after treatment is discontinued has not been determined for women who have received etretinate. Since isotretinoin has a half-life of only 1-day, after 1 month off therapy and the completion of one full menstrual cycle, women may safely become pregnant. This must still be confirmed by controlled clinical studies. Female patients should be counseled on the risk of major birth defects associated with first-trimester exposure to isotretinoin or etretinate. Should a pregnancy occur during treatment (or after treatment, in the case of etretinate), the woman should consult her physician about the management of her pregnancy.

Ribavirin

Animal studies have shown that the antiviral agent ribavirin is teratogenic, causing severe malformations in offspring of exposed females. Exposure of health care workers who tend patients receiving ribavirin aerosol via oxygen tent or mist mask may exceed the recommended safety levels to protect against reproductive harm. Surgical masks and similar respiratory protection are not likely to reduce exposure to the aerosol sufficiently. Hospitals are advised to consider alternative job assignments for health care workers who are at risk and to develop policies to minimize occupational exposure to the drug.

Ritodrine

Ritodrine is a tocolytic β-adrenergic agonist with predominant effects on β-2 receptors. Intravenous ritodrine usually is given until uterine contractions have ceased, unacceptable side effects have developed, or a maximum dosage of 350 mg/min has been achieved. An initial-phase half-life of 6 to 9 minutes is followed by biphasic elimination with a half-life of about 21.3 hours. There is rapid transplacental transfer of intravenous ritodrine. Maternal pulmonary edema, myocardial ischemia with ST-T wave changes, agranulocytosis, salivary gland enlargement, increases in plasma glucose, increases in plasma insulin, and maternal deaths have been associated with ritodrine. Overdose with ritodrine leads to flushing, tremulousness, tachycardia, hypotension, and hypokalemia. Treatment is symptomatic and supportive.

Salicylates

Unlike acetaminophen, the parent compound, and not the metabolites, produce the toxicity of salicylate overdose. This places the fetus at risk. Salicylate traverses the placenta and is found in higher concentrations in the fetus. Treatment of the mother with salicylate poisoning requires intensive supportive care. Fetal factors such as higher serum concentrations, larger proportion of salicylate in the brain, lower buffering capacity, and decreased salicylate metabolism mitigate against the positive effects of maternal gastrointestinal decontamination and extracorporeal removal. When the fetus is potentially viable outside of the uterus, consideration should be given to prompt delivery.

Salicylates cross the placenta. A possible teratogenic effect and an increase in stillbirths occur after therapeutic ingestion, but the effects are not firmly established. Fetal death may occur in utero after the mother ingests significant salicylate. Salicylates delay the onset of labor by inhibiting prostaglandin synthesis, increasing postmaturity, and increasing the duration of spontaneous delivery. The FDA recommends no aspirin administration in the last trimester of pregnancy. Ingestion of aspirin late in gestation may result in infants born with abnormalities in hemostasis, acid-base balance, tachypnea, and glucose metabolism. A prospective study of premature infants indicated that aspirin was associated with an increase in intracranial hemorrhage in this group.

Daily small doses (100 mg) of aspirin administered during the third trimester of pregnancy have been shown to reduce the incidence of pregnancy-induced hypertension and preeclampsia in women at high risk for these disorders. Aspirin is not curative for mild pregnancy-induced hypertension but may be a preventive treatment. There is insufficient evidence to justify the administration of low-dose aspirin to all primigravid women. The evidence appears sufficiently strong to justify its use in pregnant women judged to be at increased risk of developing toxemia.

Snake Bites

Few detailed studies of snakebites in pregnant women are available. Death from supine hypotensive syndrome of pregnancy has followed mild snake envenomation. A 32-week pregnant woman was bitten by *Bothrops jararaca* in Brazil and developed abruptio placentae, evidence of disseminated intravascular coagulation, and acute renal failure. Labor was induced and the infant was stillborn. In Sri Lanka, two patients were bitten by cobras and two others by vipers. Slowing of fetal movements in all four patients occurred before evidence of systemic poisoning. Antivenin may be indicated if there is slowing of fetal movements even if the mother has no evidence of systemic poisoning.

Spermicides

The active ingredient in spermicides is nonoxynol-9. Such contraceptive agents are marketed over-the-counter as creams, jellies, suppositories, and foam in aerosol containers as well as sponges. These preparations work by providing a physical barrier to sperm penetration as well as a chemical spermicidal action. Maternal use of spermicides is not associated with adverse fetal outcome.

Terbutaline

Terbutaline inhibits uterine contractions and is effective in treating premature labor. A maternal infusion of terbutaline has a half-life of about 4 hours. There is a rapid transplacental transfer within 1 hour. After subcutaneous administration, the absorptive half-life is 7 minutes. Doses of 0.25 mg subcutaneously are used every 20 to 60 minutes until contractions have subsided. Maternal side effects such as tachycardia, hypotension, chest pain, arrhythmias, and hypokalemia, have occurred with both terbutaline and ritodrine. Sudden maternal death has followed terbutaline.

Tobacco

The term "fetal tobacco syndrome" has been proposed when the mother smoked five or more cigarettes a day throughout the pregnancy, the mother had no evidence of hypertension during pregnancy (specifically no preeclampsia and documentation of normal blood pressure at least once after the first trimester), and the newborn has symmetric growth retardation at term defined as a birth weight less than 2,500 grams and a ponderal index (weight in grams/length in centimeters) greater than 2.32. There also must be no other obvious cause of intrauterine growth retardation such as congenital infection or anomaly.

Other relationships between maternal cigarette smoking and adverse pregnancy outcomes have included abruptio placentae, bleeding during pregnancy, premature rupture of membranes, fetal death, neonatal mortality, sudden infant death syndrome, deficits in growth, intellectual, behavioral, and emotional development. Mothers aged 35 years and older who smoke may have a higher risk of delivering infants with minor malformations.

Tocolytic Agents

Pharmacologic inhibition of uterine contractions is the mainstay of treatment for preterm labor. Tocolytic agents include aminophylline, ethanol, isoxsuprine, β-adrenergic agents, calcium channel blockers, magnesium sulfate, prostaglandin synthetase inhibitors, terbutaline, and ritodrine. See specific agents within this section. Betamimetics and magnesium sulfate are common therapeutic agents of choice in the United States today. Prostaglandin synthetase inhibitors, calcium channel blockers, and phosphodiesterase inhibitors currently are undergoing clinical evaluation.

Toluene

Women workers exposed to high air concentrations of toluene appear to have a higher incidence of spontaneous abortion than a similar group of women with no occupational exposure to toluene. Further studies are required to validate this finding. Animal studies indicate that toluene readily crosses the placenta. Maternal spray paint or glue sniffing leads to maternal complications including renal tubular acidosis, hypokalemia, hypocalcemia, cardiac arrhythmias, rhabdomyolysis, and premature labor. Premature toluene exposure leads to a characteristic pattern of anomalies similar to findings in infants exposed to alcohol in utero consisting of an increased incidence of malformations, poor growth, and developmental delays.

Questions—Specific Toxin Considerations During Pregnancy

1. The pregnant patient with an acetaminophen overdose
   A. Should receive oral N-acetylcysteine and activated charcoal
   B. Should be induced
   C. Should only receive oral N-acetylcysteine after the first trimester
   D. Should be warned of likely teratogenic effects of N-acetylcysteine
   E. Should be warned of likely fetal malformations as a result of acetaminophen

2. Which of the following antithrombotic agents is likely to be safest in the first trimester?
   A. Warfarin
   B. Heparin
   C. Low-dose aspirin
   D. High-dose aspirin
   E. All are equally safe

3. Long-term use of propranolol may produce
   A. Intrauterine growth retardation
   B. Neonatal hypoglycemia
   C. Neonatal bradycardia
   D. All of the above
   E. None of the above

4. Caffeine ingestion during pregnancy
   A. Has few reported adverse outcomes at less than 300 mg/day
   B. Has no clinical manifestations in the newborn period
   C. Is not transferred through the umbilical cord
   D. Causes macrosomia
   E. None of the above

5. Neonatal withdrawal
   A. Occurs earlier after phenobarbital exposure than most other drugs
   B. Lasts longer when resulting from drugs with long elimination half-lives
   C. Rarely occurs in neonates whose mothers have been drug free for more than 24 hours before delivery
   D. Can be predicted by drug screening the newborn but not by identifying maternal risk
   E. None of the above

6. Magnesium effects include all of the following except
   A. Neonatal drowsiness
   B. Neonatal hypertonia
   C. Maternal loss of deep tendon reflexes
   D. Maternal respiratory depression
   E. Maternal flushing

7. Methylene blue
   A. Is used to treat methemoglobinemia
   B. Is used to examine the patency of fallopian tubes
   C. Is used to verify rupture of membranes
   D. Can cause hyperbilirubinemia
   E. All of the above

8. Prostaglandins
   A. Cause uterine contractions
   B. Cause hypertension
   C. Cause bronchospasm
   D. Only induce labor in the third trimester
   E. None of the above

9. Maternal cigarette smoking is associated with
   A. Deficits in behavioral and emotional development of the child
   B. Placenta accreta
   C. Postdated delivery
   D. Head sparing growth retardation
   E. All of the above

BREAST MILK

Most substances found in breast milk are accounted for by passive transfer. The efficiency of passive transfer usually is represented by the ratio of the concentration of a substance in milk to the concentration of the substance in plasma. Agent-specific factors and maternal factors affect passive transfer.

Blood Flow

The rate of milk formation is 0.8 L/day. With a blood flow of 300 to 400 L/day, even relatively low maternal blood levels of a substance have the potential to produce high levels in milk.

Chemical Properties

Agents chemically similar to milk constituents or transported like milk constituents may be actively excreted in milk.

Ionization Constant

Only the un-ionized, lipid-soluble portion of an organic compound diffuses readily into milk. Weak acids tend to give milk/plasma ratios less than one, whereas weak bases tend to give ratios greater than one.

Lipid Solubility

Lipid-soluble compounds are found at higher levels in milk than blood. Those substances that are highly lipid soluble are stored in fat and slowly eliminated from the body.

Metabolism

Metabolism of drugs usually produces less lipid-soluble, less toxic compounds than the parent drug. Chemicals that are rapidly metabolized and eliminated from blood have less time to partition into milk and do not reach significant levels. Agents eliminated or metabolized slowly are more available for transmission into milk.

Molecular Weight

Agents with molecular weights less than 200 daltons tend to partition more effectively into milk.

Protein Binding

Highly protein-bound substances tend to partition to a lesser extent into milk than non-protein-bound substances.

Specific Drugs and Breastfeeding

The American Academy of Pediatrics and independent researchers have studied numerous drugs, chemicals, foods, and environmental agents and their relationship to breastfeeding. Drugs contraindicated during lactation include cimetidine (inhibits drug metabolism, suppresses gastric acidity, causes central nervous system stimulation, and is concentrated in breast milk), cytotoxic agents such as cyclophosphamide, methotrexate, and doxorubicin (possible immune suppression), ergotamine (vomiting, diarrhea, convulsions), thiouracil, methimazole (interferes with thyroid function), phenindione (hemorrhage), bromocriptine (suppresses lactation), gold salts, lithium, cyclosporine (possible immune suppression), cocaine, phencyclidine (PCP), and clemastine. Drugs that require temporary cessation during lactation are metronidazole (allow 24 hours for excretion) and certain radiopharmaceuticals.

Drugs that have caused significant effects on some nursing infants and should be given to nursing mothers with caution include salicylates (have caused dose-related metabolic acidosis, may affect platelet function and have caused rash), clemastine (has caused drowsiness, irritability, refusal to feed, high-pitched cry, and neck stiffness), phenobarbital (has been associated with sedation, infantile spasms and methemoglobinemia), primidone (has caused sedation and feeding problems) and sulfasalazine (has caused bloody diarrhea in one infant).

Questions—Breast Milk

1. **Drugs contraindicated during pregnancy include all of the following, except**
   A. Cimetidine
   B. Cyclophosphamide
   C. Methotrexate
   D. Codeine
   E. Bromocriptine
2. **Drugs found in breast milk are**
   A. Lipid soluble
   B. Rapidly metabolized and eliminated from blood
   C. Those with molecular weights greater than 200 daltons
   D. Likely to be highly protein-bound
   E. All of the above

TREATMENT GUIDELINES DURING PREGNANCY

Certain drugs should be avoided or used with caution in pregnancy. In addition to the descriptions regarding some of these agents above, see individual chapters for more comments regarding the risks of specific agents during pregnancy. In general, no drug should be considered 100% safe to the developing fetus, including topical preparations. A true indication must be present for the administration of any drug and the potential benefits should always be weighed against the possible hazards of the drug to the mother and the fetus. It must be remembered that the effect of a drug on the fetus may not necessarily be the same as the intended pharmacological effect on the mother. Certain drugs may have delayed effects on the fetus. Symptoms and signs may not develop until later in life.

Treatment

- Active measures required to stabilize a pregnant patient exposed to a toxic substance are similar to those applied to the nonpregnant overdosed patient.
- These may include gut decontamination by charcoal or lavage, methods of elimination including hemodialysis, and antidotal therapy.
- Drugs that are life saving must be employed when it is determined that an imminent danger of death or significant morbidity exists for both the mother and the fetus. Conservative measures without drug use can be employed when a serious danger to maternal or fetal life does not exist and where insufficient data have been accumulated to provide for safe use of a specific pharmacologic agent.
- Supportive measures that may specifically be applied to the pregnant individual include monitoring of the fetal heart rate, ultrasonography, obstetric and neonatal consultation, and use of cesarean sections as required late in pregnancy.
- As drug metabolism during pregnancy may be slower than in the nonpregnant state, due consideration must be given to the dosage of drug and the route of administration.
- No known dysmorphogenic drug should be administered to any woman of childbearing age unless she is using a reliable form of contraception. Even then, errors may occur and an unfortunate outcome may be precipitated.
- In general, women should be strongly discouraged from self-medication during pregnancy.

Questions—Treatment Guidelines During Pregnancy

1. **When a pregnant patient is exposed to a toxic substance,**
   A. Fetal monitoring should be considered
   B. Antidotes are never used
   C. Cesarean section anytime in pregnancy is preferable to vaginal delivery.
   D. Gut decontamination is a particularly dangerous intervention.
   E. All of the above

Answers

Introduction to the Pregnant Patient

1. B

Drug Use During Pregnancy

1. C 2. A 3. E 4. B 5. D

Pharmacokinetics of Pregnancy

1. E 2. B 3. A 4. A

The Placenta

1. A 2. B 3. A

Reproductive Toxicology

1. E 2. D 3. D 4. C

Specific Toxin Considerations During Pregnancy

1. A 2. B 3. D 4. A 5. B 6. B 7. E
8. C 9. A

Breast Milk

1. D 2. A

Treatment Guidelines During Pregnancy

1. A

SELECTED READINGS

The Pregnant Patient

1. Tenenbein M. Poisoning in pregnancy. In: Koren G, ed. Maternal-Fetal Toxicology: A Clinician's Guide. New York: Marcel Dekker, 1990:89–114.
2. Teratology Society Public Affairs Committee: FDA classification of drugs for teratogenic risk. Teratology 1994;49:446–447.

ACKNOWLEDGMENT

Thanks to Alison Deutsch, MD for contributing the questions in this chapter.

PART

II

Drugs

SECTION

A

Analgesics

CHAPTER 9

Acetaminophen

INTRODUCTION

Acetaminophen (Paracetamol, Tylenol®) was discovered at Johns Hopkins University in 1877. In 1950, it was marketed in the United States as an analgesic to replace its nephrotoxic analogue, phenacetin. Acetaminophen is a synthetic, nonopiate derivative of p-aminophenol. It has analgesic and antipyretic properties, but lacks antiinflammatory properties. In 1966, Davidson and Eastham reported the first case of hepatic necrosis following massive acetaminophen overdose.

In 1993, about 60,000 inquiries involving acetaminophen were reported by the Toxic Exposure Surveillance System of the American Association of Poison Control Centers. Only a small minority of patients is at risk of severe liver damage. Recovery from even severe damage usually is rapid and complete, and the overall mortality rate is low. Synonyms include APAP, paracetamol, and n-acetyl-p-aminophenol.

Pathophysiology

Acetaminophen shares analgesic and antipyretic properties with its analogues, phenacetin and acetanilid. It acts by inhibiting prostaglandin synthesis. Advantages over salicylates include relative lack of sensitization, absence of gastrointestinal irritation, lack of effect on coagulation, and absence of association with Reye's disease. Risk factors that enhance the development of liver toxicity after an overdose of acetaminophen include chronic ingestion of agents that induce hepatic microsomal enzymes (e.g., isoniazid, anticonvulsants). Starvation depletes glutathione stores and is a risk factor. Patients who consume excessive quantities of acetaminophen in multiple doses may present with acetaminophen levels in the toxic range.

Pharmacokinetics

ABSORPTION

- Usually rapid and complete and occurs at a rate that depends on gastric emptying.
- Peak therapeutic concentration occurs within 1 hour.

DISTRIBUTION

- Plasma protein binding is 25% to 50% and volume of distribution is 0.75 to 1.0 L/kg.
- The half-life is about 2 to 3 hours, and in overdose the elimination half-life increases.

ELIMINATION

- The liver biotransforms 90% of acetaminophen by conversion to sulfate or glucuronide.
- The sulfate pathway predominates in children under 12, whereas adults primarily use the glucuronide pathway (60%). Unchanged renal excretion accounts for less than 5% of elimination.
- A small portion of the therapeutic dose is metabolized by the P450 mixed-function oxidase pathway to a reactive, toxic intermediary [N-acetyl-p-benzoquinoneimine (NAPQI)].

Clinical Presentations

When first seen, the severity of intoxication with acetaminophen cannot be determined on clinical grounds alone. Consciousness generally is not depressed, even in the presence of high serum levels of acetaminophen, unless other drugs have also been taken.

HEPATIC EFFECTS

Nausea and vomiting usually develop within a few hours of ingestion of a hepatotoxic dose of acetaminophen. At this stage, liver function tests may be normal. From about 18 to 72 hours after ingestion, there may be hepatic tenderness and abdominal pain. Unless hepatic failure develops, there usually is rapid improvement after the third day with eventual complete recovery. The maximum abnormality of liver function tests usually is delayed until the third day.

Most hepatotoxicity probably results from a toxic intermediary (NAPQI) that binds covalently to hepatocytes and causes a centrilobular hepatic necrosis. The liver metabolizes most therapeutic doses of acetaminophen by glucuronide and sulfate conjugation. Only small amounts of acetaminophen are converted to NAPQI by the cytochrome P450 mixed-function oxidase system. Glutathione rapidly detoxifies this intermediate. When glutathione stores are depleted below a critical value (about 30% of normal stores) NAPQI binds with hepatic cell macromolecules, producing tissue necrosis.

There is significant individual susceptibility to the toxic effects of acetaminophen, as 20% or more of patients with toxic acetaminophen plasma levels do not develop hepatotoxicity. Severe liver damage develops in about 8% of all acetaminophen overdose patients who do not receive antidotal therapy, despite the fact that about 15% may display plasma acetaminophen levels in the toxic range. Fatal hepatic failure occurs in about 1% to 2% of these patients who have received no specific therapy. Age, diet, nutritional status, metabolic state, and concomitant drug ingestion affect individual changes in cytochrome P450 mixed-function oxidase activity and susceptibility to hepatotoxicity.

Fulminant hepatic failure may develop in severely poisoned patients from the third to the sixth day. It is characterized by jaundice, encephalopathy, increased intracranial pressure, disseminated intravascular coagulation (DIC), hemorrhage, hyperventilation, acidosis, hypoglycemia, and renal failure. Fulminant hepatic failure after acetaminophen overdose has a mortality of 50%. The survival rate for hepatic failure following acetaminophen overdose depends on age, use of N-acetylcysteine (NAC), and degree of encephalopathy on presentation. Delay in performing liver transplantation adversely affects the chances of survival by increasing the risk of cerebral edema, hemorrhage, hypotension, and renal failure. Candidates for liver transplantation should be identified early.

RENAL EFFECTS

Renal impairment has been reported in about 1% of patients who have ingested an acetaminophen overdose. The kidney also metabolizes acetaminophen to a toxic intermediate, which binds to renal macromolecules, leading to cell death. Oliguric renal failure may become apparent within 24 to 48 hours of acetaminophen overdose, and it usually is associated with back pain, microscopic hematuria, and proteinuria. Acetaminophen may cause analgesic nephropathy and end-stage renal disease. Renal papillary necrosis has been reported following consumption of acetaminophen.

CARDIOVASCULAR EFFECTS

Myocardial changes may include fatty degeneration of myocytes, focal myocardial muscle necrosis, left ventricular dilation, subendocardial necrosis, and focal infiltration of neutrophils into the myocardium. Cardiomyopathy and myocarditis have been reported. Acetaminophen-induced cardiotoxicity rarely is clinically significant. Dysrhythmias and other electrocardiographic abnormalities occur frequently in patients with acetaminophen-induced hepatic coma, but ST-T wave changes develop rarely in nonencephalopathic patients.

PANCREATIC EFFECTS

Doses of acetaminophen as low as 9.75 grams have been associated with pancreatitis. Hyperamylasemia may be observed in significant overdoses.

HYPERSENSITIVITY EFFECTS

Allergic reactions to acetaminophen are rare, often occurring during the first hour of treatment, and usually involve the skin. Reported dermatological presentations include bullae, eczema, urticaria, and exfoliative dermatitis. Bronchospasm and urticaria have been reported in adults and children. Dose-dependent anaphylactoid reactions (characterized by vomiting, diarrhea, pruritus, urticaria, angioedema, dyspnea, and hypotension) also have been reported.

HEMATOLOGIC EFFECTS

In addition to disseminated intravascular coagulation often associated with hepatic necrosis, thrombocytopenia associated with therapeutic acetaminophen use appears in the medical literature.

ALCOHOLIC PATIENTS

The alcoholic patient may be more susceptible to the hepatic effects of an overdose of acetaminophen. In chronic alcoholics, glutathione depletion is probably a more important risk factor for hepatotoxicity than increased metabolic activation of acetaminophen. Liver toxicity and acute renal tubular necrosis in alcoholics have been associated with daily doses of only 4 to 6 g of acetaminophen for 3 to 4 days. However, definitive proof linking alcoholism with an increased risk of hepatotoxicity at therapeutic doses has not been clearly established. Most reports of acetaminophen-induced hepatotoxicity in alcoholics involve excessive doses of acetaminophen.

CHRONIC EFFECTS

Chronic acetaminophen poisoning in adults is uncommon but often results in an encephalopathy together with other clinical and laboratory manifestations of hepatic failure. Chronic excessive use by adults who seek pain relief and fever control may lead to a toxic hepatitis.

Toxic Dosage/Death

In adults, the single acute threshold dose for severe liver damage is 150 to 250 mg/kg. Children younger than 10 years old appear to be more resistant than adults.

Pregnancy/Lactation

Both the mother and the fetus are at risk for hepatotoxicity following an overdose of acetaminophen because acetaminophen, but not the conjugated metabolites, freely diffuses across the placenta. There is no clear evidence, however, that either acetaminophen or NAC (the antidote for acetaminophen toxicity) is teratogenic. Treatment of pregnant patients should follow standard protocols. Acetaminophen is classified as pregnancy risk factor B.

Neonates whose mothers have taken an overdose of acetaminophen experience a relatively lower degree of hepatic damage than adults and older children. However, the fetus remains at risk if a large dose of acetaminophen crosses the placental barrier, because the fetal liver forms a toxic metabolite through oxidation.

Laboratory

ANALYTIC METHODS

Acetaminophen is measured by immunoassay.

BLOOD LEVELS

Therapeutic concentration ranges from 5 to 20 μg/mL. Some feel that a serum acetaminophen level in all cases of drug overdose can be cost-effective. Acetaminophen is widely available, is usually an initially silent overdose, is a drug that has the potential for significant morbidity or mortality, and effective treatment is available if the diagnosis is confirmed. A standard approach to toxicity based on quantitative levels, and the Rumack nomogram, has been widely accepted (Fig. 1).

Treatment

GUT DECONTAMINATION

Activated charcoal should be given within the first several hours of ingestion of acetaminophen. Activated charcoal may reduce the serum level of acetaminophen even after absorption is complete. Activated charcoal adsorbs some of the antidote NAC *in vitro;* however, there is no clinical evidence that the administration of activated charcoal inhibits the efficacy of oral NAC. There also is little evidence to support the practice of increasing the dose of oral NAC therapy after the administration of activated

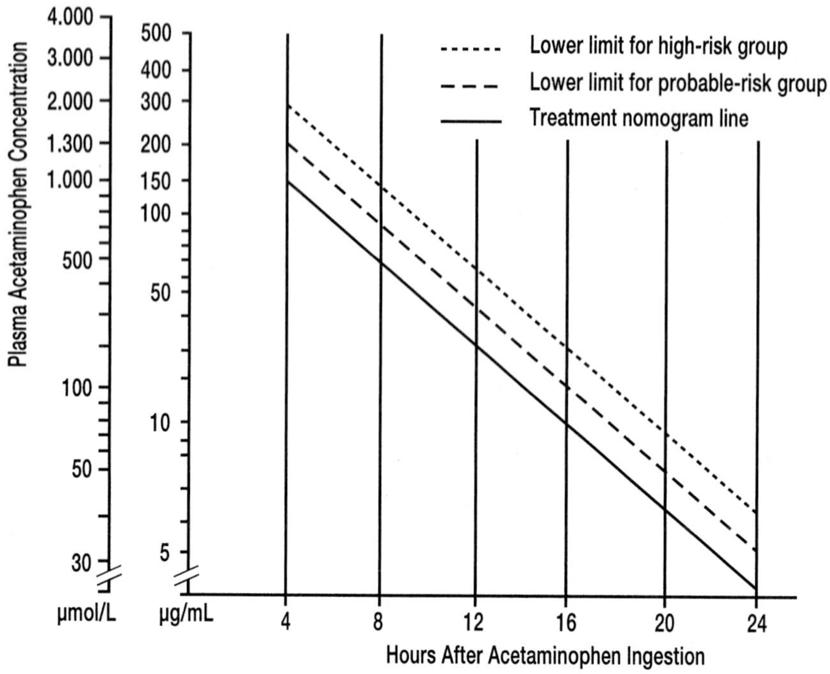

Figure 1. Nomogram lines used to define risk groups, according to initial plasma acetaminophen concentration. (From Smilkstein MJ, Bronstein AC, Linden C, et al. Acetaminophen overdose: A 48-hour intravenous N-acetylcysteine treatment protocol. Ann Emerg Med 1991;20:1058–1063)

charcoal. There is no contraindication to the administration of activated charcoal and intravenous NAC. NAC dosing is not based on acetaminophen blood levels. The optimal dose of activated charcoal has not been determined. An acceptable standard dose for adults is 1 gram/kg.

If a patient presents within 1 to 2 hours of an acetaminophen overdose, emesis or activated charcoal therapy may reduce the availability of acetaminophen and result in lower blood levels. For the patient who presents more than 1 to 2 hours after a pure acetaminophen overdose, it is unlikely that gastrointestinal decontamination will be useful. It seems reasonable to give activated charcoal and to wait for a 4-hour acetaminophen level, as NAC is most effective when it is started within 8 hours of ingestion. If the level is in a potentially toxic range according to the nomogram, NAC therapy should be initiated. In significant acetaminophen overdoses, which present 8 hours after ingestion, NAC is still recommended, however its efficacy may be less pronounced. Gastric emptying procedures and activated charcoal administration are of limited value, if any, in chronic cases.

ELIMINATION ENHANCEMENT

Exchange transfusion has been used in neonates following acetaminophen ingestion by the mother shortly before birth. Arteriovenous hemofiltration has been employed for treatment of the associated hepatic encephalopathy, but there is little evidence that this procedure removes significant amounts of acetaminophen. The primary use of hemodialysis in overdoses of acetaminophen is for the treatment of renal failure. There is little clinical evidence at present that supports the effectiveness of early hemodialysis for overdose therapy. Peritoneal dialysis is ineffective. Hemoperfusion does not have a well-defined role in the treatment of acetaminophen overdose.

SUPPORTIVE MEASURES

- Baseline blood tests for hospitalized patients should include complete blood count, liver function tests, glucose, electrolytes, and creatinine. Repeat liver function tests daily for 3 days, then as indicated by the appearance of hepatic encephalopathy. No further tests are necessary for those patients whose acetaminophen levels fall below the "toxic line" on the Rumack nomogram.
- Hepatotoxicity is characterized by elevated serum levels of alanine and aspartate transaminase, lactic dehydrogenase, and total bilirubin levels; long prothrombin and partial thromboplastin times; hypoalbuminemia; hypoglycemia; and elevated serum ammonia levels. Early signs of hepatotoxicity include hypoglycemia and metabolic acidosis. The severity of the liver function abnormality is not a reliable predictor of outcome.
- The prothrombin time is the best laboratory guide to the severity of hepatic encephalopathy. The development of an encephalopathy is likely when the prothrombin time exceeds 25 seconds at 48 hours postingestion, or 40 seconds at 72 hours. A peak prothrombin time exceeding 100 seconds or a prothrombin time that continues to increase 4 days after an overdose indicates a poor prognosis (8% chance of survival) and suggests the need for a liver transplant.
- Administer vitamin K1 for elevated prothrombin time (1.5x normal). Fresh frozen plasma should be used for severe prolongation (3x normal). Follow serial hemoglobin and stool guaiac tests for evidence of gastrointestinal bleeding.
- Elevated amylase and lipase may occur in pancreatitis and DIC may yield consumption of fibrinogen. Hyperlactatemia may occur in severely poisoned patients. Thrombocytopenia may occur as well. A moderate reduction in the platelet count may occur during acute liver failure, but severe thrombocytopenia with a nadir in the platelet count 2 days postingestion may occur in the absence of hepatic encephalopathy.
- Repeat acetaminophen levels are unnecessary once serial levels indicate that peak levels have occurred and the last level is below the toxic line.
- Maintain normal hydration and electrolyte balance and avoid forced diuresis.
- Regular lactulose and enemas assist the elimination of nitrogenous substances and endotoxins from the bowel in encephalopathic patients.

- Cerebral edema is a major cause of death following the development of hepatic encephalopathy and may be treated with mannitol and fluid restriction.

Antidotes

N-ACETYLCYSTEINE

A nomogram developed by Rumack and Matthew in 1975 relates plasma levels of acetaminophen, at specific times postingestion, to potential hepatotoxicity. Acetaminophen levels "above the lower line" have about a 60% chance of developing severe liver abnormalities (as defined by elevation of alanine and aspartate transaminase activities above 1,000 IU/L). Levels above a second, higher line increase this probability to 90%. Patients with values above either line often do not develop liver damage, whereas severe liver damage may rarely occur in patients with relatively low acetaminophen concentrations.

NAC is the N-acetyl derivative of L-cysteine, a naturally occurring amino acid. It helps replenish diminished glutathione stores in acetaminophen overdoses. In the United States, oral NAC is suggested in patients whose acetaminophen level (at given times) exceeds the lower lines on the Rumack-Matthew nomogram. It should be noted that treatment lines initially were developed from observations of untreated patients. The usefulness of the nomogram lines in young children, and after 15 hours postingestion, has never been validated. They do not, in themselves, predict life or death.

Oral NAC is the only antidote currently approved for general use in acetaminophen poisoning in the United States, but intravenous NAC is available under a restricted investigational drug protocol. NAC provides maximum protection against hepatotoxicity when administered within 8 to 12 hours of an acetaminophen overdose. The efficacy of NAC decreases after this period, but few deaths in treated cases occur when NAC is administered by 16 hours postingestion. The effectiveness of NAC beyond 14 to 36 hours is controversial. Late therapy with NAC is not associated with an increased incidence of adverse effects. NAC administration would appear justified in the presence of hepatotoxicity caused by acetaminophen, no matter what the time course or interval since the last dose.

Once NAC therapy begins, a full course of NAC should be administered regardless of the location of subsequent levels of acetaminophen on this nomogram. Subsequent plasma levels of acetaminophen that fall below the treatment line are not an indication to stop NAC therapy. A 5% solution of NAC should be given as an oral loading dose of 140 mg/kg. The available commercial preparations of NAC are 10% and 20% solutions and need to be diluted. This can be done using water or a commercial carbonated or flavored drink. Seventeen further doses of 70 mg/kg NAC should be given as a 5% solution in diluent every 4 hours. The total dose given is 1,330 mg/kg over 72 hours.

NAC has no hepatotoxic effects. Drinking NAC through a straw minimizes its unpleasant odor. Alternatives in patients unable to retain oral NAC include placement of a nasogastric or duodenal tube and intravenous administration of metoclopramide to reduce nausea. Ondansetron, another antiemetic, improves tolerance to oral NAC in intravenous doses of 0.15 mg/kg repeated every 8 hours for three doses.

The acetaminophen nomogram has not been validated for chronic prolonged ingestions. Hepatic damage may occur despite acetaminophen concentrations in the "nontoxic" range on the nomogram if the time when ingestion was completed rather than the time ingestion commenced is used to plot the results. Chronic, excessive, continuous, or prolonged ingestions do not provide easy predictors, unlike overdose at a single point. An initial nontoxic acetaminophen blood level at 4 hours after ingestion may be followed by a delayed toxic concentration.

METHIONINE

Methionine is an oral antidote used in Great Britain. Experience in the United States has not been sufficient for adequate evaluation of its safety or efficacy. Methionine acts as a glutathione precursor and protects against acetaminophen-induced hepatic and renal toxicity if it is administered within 8 to 10 hours of overdose.

CIMETIDINE

Cimetidine reduces acetaminophen-induced liver toxicity in animal models, but the amount of cimetidine required to inhibit the formation of toxic metabolites substantially following an overdose of acetaminophen probably is beyond a clinically acceptable dose. The role of cimetidine as adjunctive therapy to NAC is unproved.

4-METHYLPYRAZOLE

Animal studies suggest inhibition of acetaminophen-induced hepatotoxicity when 4-methylpyrazole (4-MP) is administered within 4 hours of a toxic acetaminophen dose. 4-MP is an inhibitor of the main cytochrome P450 enzyme involved in acetaminophen activation in humans. Clinical studies are required to validate this observation.

Questions—Acetaminophen

1. **Clinical and biochemical signs of acetaminophen hepatotoxicity usually develop**
   A. Within 1 to 4 hours of ingestion
   B. Within 4 to 8 hours of ingestion
   C. Within 8 to 18 hours of ingestion
   D. Within 18 to 72 hours of ingestion
   E. 72 hours after ingestion
2. **Fulminant hepatic failure caused by severe acetaminophen poisoning is characterized by**
   A. Encephalopathy
   B. Hemorrhage
   C. Hypoglycemia
   D. Renal failure
   E. All of the above
3. **The minimal toxic dose of acetaminophen in adults is**
   A. 50 to 150 mg/kg
   B. 150 to 250 mg/kg
   C. More than 250 mg/kg
   D. 2,000 mg
   E. More than 2,500 mg
4. **Which does not enhance the development of liver toxicity after an acetaminophen overdose?**
   A. Salicylate use
   B. Glutathione depletion
   C. Isoniazid use
   D. Starvation
   E. Anticonvulsant use
5. **Which serum test is the best laboratory guide to the severity of hepatic encephalopathy?**
   A. Alanine transaminase
   B. Prothrombin time
   C. Ammonia
   D. Lactate
   E. Glucose

Answers to questions in shaded boxes appear at the end of the chapter.

6. **Acetaminophen plasma levels above the higher line on the Rumack nomogram indicate what risk of developing severe liver abnormalities?**
   A. 60%
   B. 75%
   C. 90%
   D. 100%
   E. The nomogram cannot be used to answer this question
7. **The following are true regarding oral NAC used for acetaminophen overdose except**
   A. The course of NAC should not be stopped if subsequent acetaminophen levels are nontoxic
   B. The loading dose is 140 mg/kg of oral NAC
   C. 17 doses of 70 mg/kg of NAC should follow the loading dose
   D. Oral NAC should not be given with activated charcoal as clinical evidence suggests that charcoal inhibits the efficacy of NAC
   E. Metoclopramide or ondansetron may be used to maximize NAC tolerability
8. **The following toxicities are reported consequences of acetaminophen overdose except**
   A. Gastritis and esophagitis
   B. Cardiomyopathy and myocarditis
   C. Pancreatitis and hyperamylasemia
   D. Bronchospasm and urticaria
   E. Thrombocytopenia
9. **The Rumack nomogram is limited in that**
   A. It can be applied only to small children
   B. Its usefulness has not been validated for levels drawn more than 15 hours after ingestion
   C. It can predict only mortality, not morbidity
   D. It is best applied to chronic prolonged ingestions
   E. B and C
10. **NAC provides maximum protection against hepatotoxicity when administered**
   A. Intravenously rather than enterally
   B. At a higher dose if given concurrently with charcoal
   C. Within 8 to 12 hours of acetaminophen overdose
   D. In cases of chronic overdose
   E. All of the above

CASE STUDY (QUESTIONS 11 AND 12)
A 22-year-old female is brought in by paramedics after ingesting a bottle of Tylenol following a fight with her boyfriend. She arrives with stable vital signs, is tearful and alert.

11. **All of the following would be useful in determining intervention and prognosis except**
   A. The estimated time of ingestion
   B. The estimated amount she ingested
   C. An immediate Tylenol level, regardless of the time of ingestion
   D. What medications she used on a regular basis prior to this event
   E. Her history of alcohol abuse
12. **You find that her ingestion occurred 5 hours before her presentation, and she has a 5-hour acetaminophen level of 250 μg/mL. Appropriate intervention at this time includes**
   A. Activated charcoal, taken orally or via nasogastric tube
   B. Loading dose of NAC, taken intravenously or enterally
   C. Placement of a large catheter in case hemofiltration is needed
   D. Informing the nearest transplant team that a liver transplant may be needed
   E. A and B
13. **The toxic intermediary involved in acetaminophen poisoning is called**
   A. N-Acetyl-p-benzoquinoneimine or "NAPQI"
   B. Glutathione
   C. N-Acetylsulfone
   D. Benzoylecgonine
   E. Hydroxyapatite

Answers

Acetaminophen

1. D	2. E	3. B	4. A	5. B	6. A	7. D
8. A	9. B	10. C	11. C	12. B	13. A	

SELECTED READINGS

Acetaminophen

1. Davidson DGD, Eastham WN: Acute liver necrosis following overdose of paracetamol. Br Med J 1966;2:497–499.
2. Prescott LF: Paracetamol overdosage. Pharmacological considerations and clinical management. Drugs 1983;25:290–314.
3. Rumack BH, Peterson RC, Koch GG, et al.: Acetaminophen overdose. 662 cases with evaluation of oral acetylcysteine treatment. Arch Intern Med 1981;414:380–385.
4. Smilkstein MJ, Knapp GL, Kulig KW, et al.: Efficacy of oral N-acetylcysteine in the treatment of acetaminophen overdose. Analysis of the national multicenter study (1976 to 1985). N Engl J Med, 1988,319(24):1557–1562.

ACKNOWLEDGMENT

Thanks to Alison Deutsch, MD for contributing the questions in this chapter.

CHAPTER 10

Nonsteroidal Antiinflammatory Drugs

INTRODUCTION

Nonsteroidal antiinflammatory drugs (NSAIDs) constitute a rapidly expanding group of drugs that are useful for a great variety of medical conditions. Their increasing use and availability have led to increased reports of overdose. Most overdose cases are benign. Chronic exposure to NSAIDS may lead to acute and chronic renal failure, gastroduodenal damage, colitis, infrequent liver injury, occasional neutropenia, hypertension, and antagonism to antihypertensive medications.

In 1989, the Food and Drug Administration required all manufacturers of NSAIDs to add special warnings regarding the risk of gastrointestinal ulceration, bleeding, and perforation with NSAID therapy. Structurally, NSAIDs have been classified as either carboxylic acids or enolic acids. Enolic acid NSAID overdoses (e.g., phenylbutazone, piroxicam) appear to be more serious than carboxylic acid NSAID overdoses. NSAIDs are used for the treatment of multiple musculoskeletal conditions, dental pain, dysmenorrhea, renal colic, and postpartum pain. Phenylbutazone is used as an antiinflammatory drug in veterinary medicine.

Pathophysiology

NSAIDs act by inhibiting prostaglandin synthesis. As prostaglandins maintain the gastric mucosal barrier, inhibition of prostaglandin synthesis by NSAIDs may be the cause of gastritis, peptic ulcers, and gastrointestinal bleeding observed with these drugs. NSAIDs also uncouple mitochondrial oxidative phosphorylation. During absorption, enterocytes become ATP deficient, setting off a cascade of events detrimental to the cell. The combined effect of uncoupled oxidative phosphorylation and decreased prostaglandin production is damaging to cells.

Pharmacokinetics

ABSORPTION

- After therapeutic doses, absorption is rapid. Maximum blood concentrations appear in 1 to 2 hours.

DISTRIBUTION

- NSAIDs are 95% bound to plasma protein, especially albumin.
- With extensive protein binding, there is a small volume of distribution (0.10 to 0.17 L/kg).

ELIMINATION

- NSAIDs are mostly conjugated with glucuronic acid, although some may undergo oxidation or hydroxylation before conjugation. Indomethacin and sulindac undergo enterohepatic recirculation.
- The kidney excretes only 1% to 5% of the absorbed dose as unchanged drug.
- About 50% of a 25-mg IV dose of indomethacin are excreted in bile as unchanged drug.
- Renal clearance and elimination half-lives vary among NSAIDs (2 to 125 mL/min), producing a wide range of serum half-lives, from 1 to 1.5 hours (tolmetin) to 50 to 100 hours (phenylbutazone).
- Other half-lives of NSAIDs after therapeutic doses include fenoprofen (3 hours), ibuprofen (2 hours), naproxen (13 hours), diflunisal (8 to 12 hours), meclofenamate (2 hours), mefenamic acid (3 hours), and piroxicam (50 hours).

Clinical Presentations

Ibuprofen overdose usually is benign with a low risk of life-threatening complications, but large ingestions can present with coma, metabolic acidosis, bradycardia, hypotension, seizures, or apnea. Fatalities from ibuprofen have been reported, mostly in children. Acute reversible renal failure can occur. There is a poor correlation between ibuprofen serum concentrations and clinical findings.

GASTROINTESTINAL EFFECTS

NSAID toxicity may involve the stomach and duodenal bulb as well as the small and large intestine. Virtually all classes of NSAIDs have been implicated in the development of enteropathy with erosions, strictures, ulcerations, perforations, blood loss, diarrhea and villous atrophy. Symptoms do not reflect extent of mucosal damage and may occur without demonstrating mucosal injury. Such lesions heal quickly when drugs are withdrawn, and healing can take place while therapy continues.

Risk factors for serious gastrointestinal bleeding include age greater than 60 years, history of peptic ulcer disease, dyspepsia with NSAID use, cigarette and alcohol use, high dose and prolonged NSAID use, concomitant use of steroids, and serious concomitant disease.

NEUROLOGIC EFFECTS

Disorientation, hallucinations, and loss of consciousness have been described. Convulsions, coma, and brainstem signs have been associated with mefenamic acid and phenylbutazone.

RESPIRATORY EFFECTS

Most NSAIDs have induced an eosinophilic pneumonia characterized by cough, low-grade fever, dyspnea, malaise, and, less commonly, lymphadenopathy, pleuritic chest pain, pleural effusion, noncardiogenic edema, and diffuse myalgias. Bilateral infiltrates are visible on chest roentgenogram. Patients recover on withdrawal of the offending drug.

CARDIOVASCULAR EFFECTS

Atrial fibrillation has been reported following an ibuprofen overdose. A hypertensive effect occasionally has followed the use of NSAIDs in both normotensive and hypertensive patients. NSAID overdose patients, however, infrequently exhibit a significant increase in blood pressure.

RENAL EFFECTS

NSAID nephrotoxicity appears in at least three distinct forms: Acute renal insufficiency resulting from a reduction in renal blood flow, acute tubular necrosis, and papillary necrosis have been reported. Risk factors for acute renal insufficiency include age greater than 60 years, vascular disease, renal or functional volume depletion, preexisting renal insufficiency, and systemic lupus erythematosus. Acute renal failure has followed a simple 60-mg intramuscular dose of ketoralac.

HEPATIC EFFECTS

Risk factors for hepatotoxicity following an overdose with a NSAID include advanced age, renal insufficiency, multiple-drug use, alcohol use, and higher NSAID drug dose.

HEMATOLOGIC EFFECTS

Like aspirin, NSAIDs may increase the bleeding time of a normal person from less than 1 day for flurbiprofen, ibuprofen, indomethacin, and sulindac, to 2 weeks for piroxicam. Case reports indicate a low risk of neutropenia following use of NSAIDs. Phenylbutazone and piroxicam may cause aplastic anemia.

Toxic Dosage/Death

Death from ingestion of NSAIDs is very rare but may occur from excessively large doses or coingestion of drugs such as salicylates or antidepressants. Phenylbutazone-associated fatalities have occurred after the appearance of gastrointestinal distress, convulsions, coma, metabolic acidosis, hepatic necrosis, and renal failure. A 2-gram ingestion of phenylbutazone in a 1-year-old resulted in death. Death following an ibuprofen overdose was associated with a blood ibuprofen (heart blood, postmortem) level of 518 mg/mL.

Drug Interactions

There is a considerable potential for interactions between NSAIDs and other drugs. Other gastric irritants such as salicylates may exacerbate NSAID gastropathy. There is increased bleeding potential when NSAIDs are used simultaneously with warfarin.

Pregnancy/Lactation

Ibuprofen is classified as pregnancy risk factor B, or D if used in the third trimester. Indomethacin, a prostaglandin synthetase inhibitor, can inhibit preterm labor. It also is classified as pregnancy risk factor B. Maternal side effects are generally minimal and include nausea and heartburn.

Potential fetal and neonatal complications associated with prostaglandin synthetase inhibitors include premature closure of the ductus arteriosus and neonatal primary pulmonary hypertension. One study suggested that using indomethacin for preterm labor appears to increase the risk of serious neonatal complications such as necrotizing enterocolitis, and intracranial hemorrhage, in infants born at or before 30 weeks gestation.

Laboratory

ANALYTIC METHODS

High-performance liquid chromatography assays have been described for most NSAID drugs in human plasma.

BLOOD LEVELS

The lack of a specific antidote or definitive treatment and the poor predictive value of an ibuprofen nomogram suggest that routine serum concentration determinations are not considered useful in management of an overdose.

Treatment

GUT DECONTAMINATION

Patients with a history of NSAID ingestion who present with no symptomatology should be given a dose of activated charcoal and observed in the emergency department for 6 hours. The efficacy of cathartics in NSAID treatment has not been validated. Ipecac should never be administered to patients who have ingested an overdose of mefenamic acid or phenylbutazone, as seizures may occur after ingestion. Emesis following ipecac use may induce a gastric mucosal tear, and could delay the use of activated charcoal.

Decontamination measures should be instituted in cases involving mefenamic acid or phenylbutazone that present within 2 to 4 hours postingestion. Gastric lavage with tracheal protection followed by immediate instillation of activated charcoal would appear to be a reasonable approach. Clinical judgment dictates that the necessity of decontamination in other NSAID cases should be based on dosage, weight, time since ingestion, and concomitant drugs.

ELIMINATION ENHANCEMENT

The effectiveness of hemodialysis, hemoperfusion, or peritoneal dialysis appears to be limited because of high protein binding. Hemoperfusion, however, was found to reduce the serum half-life and to increase the clearance of phenylbutazone after an overdose. As the kidney excretes only a small proportion of absorbed NSAIDs in the urine, forced diuresis or alkalinization of the urine would not be expected to increase clearance of NSAIDs. Although its role has not been established, cholestyramine use in some severely symptomatic patients may be of benefit.

SUPPORTIVE MEASURES

- A possibility of seizures, metabolic acidosis, and other complications exists in serious, large NSAID overdoses. Patients who have any significant symptomatology should be admitted to a hospital for 24 hours, placed on seizure precautions, and evaluated for impaired hepatic function and acid/base balance.
- For refractory hypotension, institute a central line, employ positioning, and administer fluids and dopamine as required. Seizures may be treated with diazepam. For respiratory depression, employ assisted ventilation.
- Monitor renal and hepatic function. In renal failure, consider hemodialysis or hemofiltration.
- Watch for gastrointentinal bleeding by monitoring stool guaiacs. Consider an H2-receptor antagonist.
- Screening tests in severe overdoses include complete blood counts, electrolytes, creatinine, liver function tests, arterial blood gases (re: the possibility of metabolic acidosis), and coagulation studies. Metabolic acidosis occurs rarely and is most frequent in mefenamic acid and phenylbutazone overdoses. Hyperkalemia has been described after indomethacin, ibuprofen, and piroxicam therapy.
- Hypoprothrombinemia without hepatocellular toxicity has been reported with overdoses of aspirin, etodolac, mefenamic acid, indomethacin, naproxen, and ibuprofen.

Questions—Nonsteroidal Antiinflammatory Drugs

1. NSAIDs have a wide range of serum half-lives because

A. The absorption of different preparations is so varied.
B. The renal clearance and elimination half-lives are so varied.
C. The percent of plasma protein-bound drug varies so much.
D. The volume of distribution of different NSAIDs is so varied.
E. They actually have a narrow range of serum half-lives.

2. The following are true statements regarding gastrointestinal effects of NSAID toxicity except

A. The stomach, duodenal bulb, small and large intestine may be involved.
B. Symptoms do not reflect the extent of mucosal damage.
C. Lesions heal quickly when drugs are withdrawn.
D. Only a few classes of NSAIDs have been implicated in the development of enteropathy.
E. GI effects include erosions, ulcerations, perforations, blood loss, and villous atrophy.

3. Risk factors for gastrointestinal bleeding in the setting of NSAID overdose include all except

A. Age greater than 60
B. Cigarette and alcohol use
C. Vascular disease
D. Concomitant steroid use
E. History of peptic ulcer disease or other serious disease

Answers to questions in shaded boxes appear at the end of the chapter.

4. **Death from NSAID ingestion**
   A. Is very rare
   B. May occur from an excessively large dose
   C. May occur from coingestion of drugs such as salicylates and antidepressants
   D. A and B
   E. A, B and C
5. **NSAID serum concentration determinations are not useful in overdose management because**
   A. The ibuprofen nomogram has poor predictive value
   B. There is no specific antidote or treatment
   C. Unpredictable absorption makes levels unreliable
   D. A and B
   E. A, B and C
6. **Emesis should never be induced after ingestion of phenylbutazone**
   A. True
   B. False

CASE STUDY (QUESTIONS 7 AND 8)

A 45-year-old female with systemic lupus erythematosus ingested 30 tablets of Naprosyn® in a suicide attempt 2 hours before presentation. On arrival, she is alert with a temperature of 104° F, RR 40, HR 95, and BP 120/70. A nasogastric tube is placed and she is given activated charcoal.

7. **A chest x-ray is ordered because of the concern for**
   A. Dilated cardiomyopathy caused by NSAID toxicity
   B. Bacterial pneumonia caused by NSAID-induced immunosuppression
   C. Eosinophilic pneumonia caused by NSAID toxicity
   D. Appropriate nasogastric tube placement
   E. Pneumothorax as a complication of nasogastric tube placement
8. **This patient is at high risk for acute renal failure because of**
   A. Age greater than 40
   B. Concomitant lung disease
   C. History of systemic lupus erythematosus
   D. Intermittent NSAID use with previously normal renal function
   E. All of the above
9. **Fatalities resulting from ibuprofen overdose have been reported mostly**
   A. In children
   B. In adolescents
   C. In the elderly
   D. A and B
   E. A and C
10. **Treatment of patients with isolated NSAID overdoses may include all of the following except**
    A. Gut decontamination
    B. Monitoring of renal function
    C. Hemoperfusion
    D. Hydration
    E. N-Acetylcysteine (NAC)

Answers

Nonsteroidal Antiinflammatory Drugs

1\. B 2. D 3. C 4. E 5. D 6. A 7. C
8\. C 9. A 10. E

SELECTED READINGS

Nonsteroidal Antiinflammatory Drugs

1. McElwee NE, Veltri JC, Bradford DC, Rollins DE. A prospective population-based study of acute ibuprofen overdose: Complications are rare and routine serum levels are not warranted. Ann Emerg Med 1990;19:657–662.
2. Smolinske SC, Hall AH, Vandenberg SA, et al. Toxic effects of nonsteroidal anti-inflammatory drugs in overdose: An overview of recent evidence on clinical effects and dose-response relationships. Drug Saf 1990;5:252–274.
3. Verbeeck RK. Pharmacokinetic drug interactions with nonsteroidal anti-inflammatory drugs. Clin Pharmacokinet 1990;19:44–68.

ACKNOWLEDGMENT

Thanks to Alison Deutsch, MD for contributing the questions in this chapter.

CHAPTER 11
Salicylates

INTRODUCTION

More than 200 products contain salicylates (e.g., aspirin, acetylsalicylic acid or ASA) and 20 billion tablets are consumed annually in the United States. The general accessibility of aspirin has increased with its potential uses as a preventive medication for cerebrovascular ischemic events, colon cancer, angina pectoris, migraine, and recurrent myocardial infarction.

Deaths of young children following acute ingestion has declined notably because of strict packaging laws and reduced consumption. Acetaminophen now causes more toxic exposures in children. Chronic salicylate toxicity occurs in all age groups because of the saturation of metabolizing enzymes, and the incidence of toxicity from multiple doses apparently has increased. Serious sequelae may result from misuse. Chronic salicylate poisoning in children causes more hyperventilation, dehydration, acidosis, and central nervous system symptoms than acute poisoning.

Bismuth subsalicylate (Pepto-Bismol®, etc.) has been suggested to minimize salicylate-induced gastric irritation. The salicylate in bismuth subsalicylates is almost entirely available. Unfortunately, a recommended dose (15 mL up to eight times per 24 hours) when added to an antiinflammatory dose regimen of aspirin, may yield serious salicylate intoxication. Elderly patients who ingest large amounts of Pepto-Bismol® daily may develop agitation, confusion, lethargy, disorientation, slurred speech, and acute pulmonary edema. Barium-like contrast densities may be seen on an abdominal plain film. Available preparations include:

Acetylsalicylic Acid

Most salicylate poisonings involve aspirin ingestion. Children's flavored tablets contain 80 mg ($1\frac{1}{4}$ grain) of acetylsalicylic acid, whereas adult aspirin is either regular strength (5 grains = 325 mg) or extra strength (500 mg). Enteric coated tablets may delay peak concentrations many hours after ingestion.

Bismuth Subsalicylate

Each milliliter of Pepto-Bismol® contains the equivalent of 8.77 mg of salicylic acid. A dose of 60 mL produces a peak plasma salicylate level of 4 mg/dL, similar to the usual analgesic dose of aspirin. The 240-mL dose recommended for traveler's diarrhea is equivalent to 8 regular-strength (325 mg) adult aspirin tablets. This dose should be administered cautiously, if at all, to patients with bleeding disorders and aspirin sensitivity and to those receiving antiplatelet drugs or probenecid.

Methyl Salicylate

Salicylates such as Oil of Wintergreen or Ben Gay® are an infrequent but dangerous cause of salicylate poisoning. One teaspoon contains 7,000 mg of salicylate (equivalent to 21 aspirin tablets) and childhood fatalities after ingestion of as little as 4 mL of Oil of Wintergreen has been reported. A 1-oz tube of external liniment (20% methyl salicylate) is equivalent to the above fatal dose of Oil of Wintergreen. When applied to large areas of skin, topical salicylic acid may cause sufficient dermal absorption to produce toxic serum salicylate levels.

Pathophysiology

Salicylates inhibit prostaglandin synthesis, prevent the formation of thromboxane, a platelet aggregating substance, and inhibit various clotting factors. Salicylates uncouple oxidative phosphorylation leading to an increased metabolic rate. Important compensatory mechanisms include increased oxygen consumption. This results in an increased pulse rate, increased CO_2 formation (hyperventilation), increased heat production (elevated temperature), and increased glucose utilization (reduced tissue glucose levels).

Salicylates also interfere with the Krebs cycle and block both lipid and carbohydrate metabolism. Metabolic acidosis resulting from the formation of organic acids occurs. Because children are less able than adults to maintain a compensatory respiratory alkalosis, systemic metabolic acidosis appears earlier in children.

Pharmacokinetics

ABSORPTION

- Acetylsalicylic acid is a weak acid with a pKA of 3. The low pKA means that about 50% of the salicylate appears in the un-ionized form in the stomach and hence is rapidly absorbed.
- The stomach and blood hydrolyze acetylsalicylic acid to salicylic acid and acetic acid. The rate-limiting factor for absorption is tablet dissolution. Since ASA is poorly soluble in the acid media of the stomach, precipitates may coalesce to form concretions in large overdoses.
- Concretions may delay absorption, and thus toxicity, 8 to 24 hours.
- The large surface area of the small bowel also absorbs salicylate despite the higher pH.

DISTRIBUTION

- Albumin binds approximately 50% to 80% of salicylate, whereas the rest appears in plasma in the active, ionized state. Within the usual therapeutic plasma levels, protein binding is concentration dependent and contributes to nonlinear kinetics.
- Saturation of binding sites increases tissue distribution of drug and decreased binding sites (e.g., associated with cirrhosis, hypoalbuminemia, competitive drugs) lead to more free salicylate and increased toxicity. Serum protein binding of salicylates decreases with age.
- The volume of distribution is 0.1 to 0.2 L/kg, but acidosis increases the volume of distribution because of enhancement of tissue penetration by salicylates.
- For therapeutic doses, the plasma salicylate half-life is approximately 2 to 4.5 hours, but untreated overdose prolongs it as long as 18 to 36 hours. Peak therapeutic levels occur within 2 hours.
- The antiinflammatory and toxic effects result from salicylic acid, whereas the antiplatelet effect results only from acetylsalicylic acid.

ELIMINATION

- For small doses 80% of the hepatic metabolism results from conjugation with glycine to form salicyluric acid and with glucuronic acid to form salicyl acyl and phenolic glucuronide. The two parallel pathways (glycine, glucuronide conjugation) have limited capacity and saturate easily above therapeutic doses.
- Renal elimination becomes more important with large or multiple doses. Renal elimination depends on pH. This is the most important factor because increasing urine pH causes a major increase in renal excretion. Drugs that affect urinary pH will alter plasma salicylate levels.
- Renal elimination also depends on potassium level and renal function. An adequate serum potassium level, especially in children, is necessary to maintain an alkaline pH. Increased potassium excretion as well as systemic acidosis in salicylate overdose leads to hypokalemia and reduces salicylate excretion from the kidney.
- Saturation of hepatic enzymes causes the excretion of larger amounts of unchanged salicylic acid in the urine. Only small portions of single, therapeutic doses (5%) appear in the urine as unchanged drug. A substantial first-pass effect occurs at therapeutic doses.
- With large salicylate doses the time needed to eliminate the salicylate increases with increasing dose, and salicylate kinetics switch from first order to zero order (Michaelis-Menten kinetics). Blood levels then increase significantly with small increases in dose.

Clinical Presentations

METABOLIC EFFECTS

Most patients poisoned with aspirin have either a simple respiratory alkalosis secondary to direct stimulation of the respiratory center and subsequent hyperventilation, or a mixed respiratory alkalosis and metabolic acidosis. Acidemia frequently is associated with neurologic features, pulmonary edema, and a fatal outcome. Respiratory alkalosis may not be present or may be transient in infants. Hyperglycemia occurs more commonly than hypoglycemia in salicylate overdoses. Children appear more susceptible to hypoglycemia. The mechanisms of reduced blood sugar levels probably include a combination of increased peripheral glucose demand, increased rate of tissue glycolysis, and impaired rate of glucose synthesis from noncarbohydrate substrate.

HEMATOLOGIC EFFECTS

Hemostatic defects rarely cause clinical manifestations unless there is a preexisting bleeding disorder (e.g., ulcer, hemophilia). Decreased factor VII, hypoprothrombinemia, decreased platelet adhesiveness, and decreased blood platelet levels may occur after salicylate overdose. A single 650-mg dose of aspirin may increase the bleeding time of a normal person for 4 to 7 days, probably because of decreased formation of the platelet aggregation stimulator thromboxane A2. Impaired coagulation may compromise surgical results, particularly grafts, flaps, or microsurgical procedures.

CARDIOVASCULAR EFFECTS

Acute salicylate intoxication may induce cardiac depression and asystole. The exact mechanism has not been defined. Hypokalemia can produce dysrhythmias. Rhabdomyolysis may be associated with a salicylate-induced hyperthermia. The creatine kinase serum levels are elevated and diffuse myalgias are observed. Salicylate overdose has also been linked with shock.

GASTROINTESTINAL EFFECTS

Endoscopic studies have shown that all human control subjects who ingest ASA have benign gastric erosions; 60% have duodenal erosions after use of ASA for only 1 day. More prolonged use of ASA can lead to more severe lesions. Surreptitious use of ASA should be considered in the differential diagnosis of patients with recurrent peptic ulcers. Nausea and vomiting usually occur early along with epigastric pain in acute overdose. Hematemesis may develop from gastric irritation but only several cases of gastric perforation have been associated with acute salicylate overdose. Hepatotoxicity can develop when salicylate levels exceed 20 mg/dL and usually are mild, dose dependent, and reversible.

OTOLOGIC EFFECTS

Hearing loss and tinnitus usually are reversible and increase progressively with increasing aspirin dosage. Unbound plasma salicylate concentration may be a better predictor of salicylate-induced ototoxicity than plasma salicylate concentration.

PSEUDOSEPSIS SYNDROME

Patients with chronic salicylate intoxication may present with a syndrome resembling occult sepsis including fever, leukocytosis, a leftward shift in the differential cell count, hypotension, reduced systemic vascular resistance, and multiple-organ system failure (adult respiratory distress syndrome, acute renal failure, coagulopathy, disseminated intravascular coagulation, and/or encephalopathy). A source of infection is not documented.

NEUROLOGIC EFFECTS

Neurologic effects may include tinnitus and lethargy in even mild intoxications. Patients may become irritable or disoriented. Asterixis, hallucinations, seizures, or coma may characterize serious overdose. The presence of seizures indicates a serious prognosis after acute overdose. Convulsions may reflect an electrolyte and/or metabolic disorder in addition to direct salicylate-induced toxicity. Confusion, bizarre behavior, stupor, movement disorders, papilledema, and cerebral edema can develop after multiple therapeutic doses of salicylates.

PULMONARY EFFECTS

Noncardiogenic pulmonary edema develops in a small percentage of acute and chronic overdose cases. Proposed mechanisms include CNS mediation through stimulation of the hypothalamus leading to excessive adrenergic discharge, inhibition of prostaglandins resulting in increased pulmonary lymphatic flow, and/or a direct toxic effect of salicylates on pulmonary endothelium producing extravasation of fluid. Risk factors include age over 30, cigarette smoking, chronic salicylate ingestion, metabolic acidosis, and neurologic symptoms. Salicylate levels usually exceed 40 mg/dL in these cases.

Aspirin may precipitate bronchial asthma up to 3 hours after administration through an alteration in the immune mechanism or pharmacological reaction in some patients. Susceptible patients generally are in the 20 to 50 age group and may have a history of nasal polyps, asthma, and chronic urticaria. Acute airway obstruction secondary to angioedema may develop in sensitized patients and 5% of aspirin-sensitive patients have a cross-reaction to acetaminophen.

RENAL EFFECTS

Analgesic-associated nephropathy is the leading cause of renal papillary necrosis and cortical interstitial nephritis. Analgesics probably produce renal damage through toxic metabolites, ischemia, or some combination of these two factors. Salicylates in combination with phenacetin or acetaminophen are much more likely to cause nephropathy than either agent alone. Salicylates have been associated with Fanconi syndrome involving the proximal renal tubule and the syndrome of inappropriate antidiuretic hormone (SIADH).

REYE'S SYNDROME

Reye's Syndrome is a rare, biphasic illness characterized by encephalopathy and fatty infiltration of viscera. This clinical entity probably develops from a virus-host reaction in susceptible patients. Although an association exists between ASA consumption and Reye's syndrome, the presence of a direct causal effect remains controversial.

The disease usually occurs in children under 16 years of age, however it may occur in adults. It typically begins with a prodromal viral syndrome (especially varicella and influenza). After recovery from the viral illness, vomiting starts and symptoms of encephalopathy develop within 48 hours. Lethargy and muscle tenderness may progress to delirium, coma, pupillary dilation, and death. The mortality rate is 10% to 40% and permanent neurologic sequelae may occur. The Surgeon General now recommends not giving salicylates to children with influenza and chicken pox. The incidence of Reye's syndrome fell in the United States from a peak of 0.88 per 100,000 children less than 18 years of age in 1980 to 0.09 per 100,000 in 1989.

The clinical picture of Reye's syndrome in adults is similar to that seen in children. Vomiting and encephalopathy develop a few days after influenza, gastroenteritis, or an upper respiratory infection. The association with salicylates seems less strong in adults than in children. About one third of adults die, a mortality rate similar to that seen in children. In adults, the diagnosis is best confirmed by percutaneous liver biopsy (microvesicular fatty change within the hepatocytes with little or no inflammatory infiltrate or narcosis). The differential diagnosis includes causes of fulminant hepatic failure in adults (e.g., viral hepatitis, isopropanol, amanitin, or carbon tetrachloride poisoning, acetaminophen overdose, and halothane anesthesia).

Toxic Dosage/Death

Mortality is less than 2% after acute salicylate overdoses but may reach 25% after severe, chronic salicylate intoxication. Death following salicylate overdose appears to be increased in patients over 70 years of age. Delayed presentation, coma, hyperpyrexia, pulmonary edema, and acidemia are more common in fatal cases. The mean plasma salicylate concentration in fatal cases is often between 70 and 90 mg/dL. The prognosis of acute salicylate poisoning cannot be determined from the plasma concentration of the blood alone. Ingestion of 66 Pepto-Bismol tablets by a 36-kg patient (a salicylate dose of 187 mg/kg) was fatal.

Drug Interactions

Drug interactions related to the ulcerogenic and irritating potential of aspirin include caffeine, phenylbutazone, indomethacin and alcohol. Factors that reduce aspirin absorption include food, chelation with iron, and complexation with caffeine and indomethacin. ASA is largely protein bound. As such, it competes for protein binding sites and the free drug fraction of other drugs seeking the same sites may be increased. Examples include displacement of bishydroxycoumarin and displacement of certain antimicrobial agents.

ASA potentiates penicillins and sulfonamides and displaces oral hypoglycemia agents. ASA antagonizes the uricosuric effect of probenecid, sulfinpyrazone, and phenylbutazone. It also diminishes the effects of spironolactone diuretics.

Pregnancy/Lactation

Salicylates cross the placental barrier. A possible teratogenic effect and an increase in stillbirths occur after therapeutic ingestion, but the effects are not firmly established. Fetal death may occur in utero after the mother ingests significant salicylate. Salicylates delay the onset of labor by inhibiting prostaglandin synthesis, increasing postmaturity, and increasing the duration of spontaneous delivery.

Ingestion of aspirin late in gestation may result in infants born with abnormalities in hemostasis, acid-base balance, tachypnea, and glucose metabolism. A prospective study of premature infants indicated that aspirin was associated with an increase in intracranial hemorrhage in this group.

However, daily small doses (100 mg) of aspirin administered during the third trimester of pregnancy have been shown to reduce the incidence of pregnancy-induced hypertension and preeclampsia in women at high risk for these disorders. Aspirin is not curative for mild pregnancy-induced hypertension but may be a preventive treatment. There is insufficient evidence to justify the administration of low-dose aspirin to all primigravid women. The evidence appears sufficiently strong to justify its use in pregnant women judged to be at increased risk of developing toxemia.

Laboratory

ANALYTIC METHODS

The Trinder method (Ferric Chloride Test) is a quick, bedside colorimetric test used to determine the presence of salicylic acid. In the Trinder spot test, 1 mL of urine and 1 mL of Trinder reagent are mixed in a test tube. A color change occurs immediately if salicylate is present. If the color change has a discernible violet or purple color, the result is considered positive. Another quick, bedside colorimetric test involves Phenistix. The presence of urinary salicylates produces an immediate brownish-purple color on the Phenistix test, similar to phenothiazines.

Gas chromatography with extraction procedures and high-performance liquid chromatography can distinguish aspirin (acetylsalicylic acid) from salicylic acid in contrast to colorimetric procedures.

BLOOD LEVELS

Toxic salicylate blood levels appear over 25 mg/dL. Serious symptoms may develop at lower levels because of dehydration, fever, renal dysfunction, or delayed salicylate metabolism. In overdose, the formation of concretions, enteric coated tablets, and delayed gastric emptying may delay toxic reactions and cause salicylate levels to rise over the first 12 to 24 hours.

The Done nomogram (Fig. 1) applies to a single ingestion of non-enteric-coated salicylate at a known time. It displays good predictive value at 6 hours after a single, acute ingestion, but not after chronic ingestions. The nomogram starts at 6 hours to ensure that levels will not be interpreted before they have reached their peak. It can be used earlier if more than one level is obtained to establish that the salicylate level is declining. Acidosis, dehydration, fever, and renal failure complicate its use. Concretions, delayed gastric emptying, and enteric coatings can prolong absorption. The nomogram tends to overpredict the severity of intoxication in moderate and severe intoxications and the nomogram has a higher predictive index when used for concentrations drawn 6 to 12 hours after ingestion.

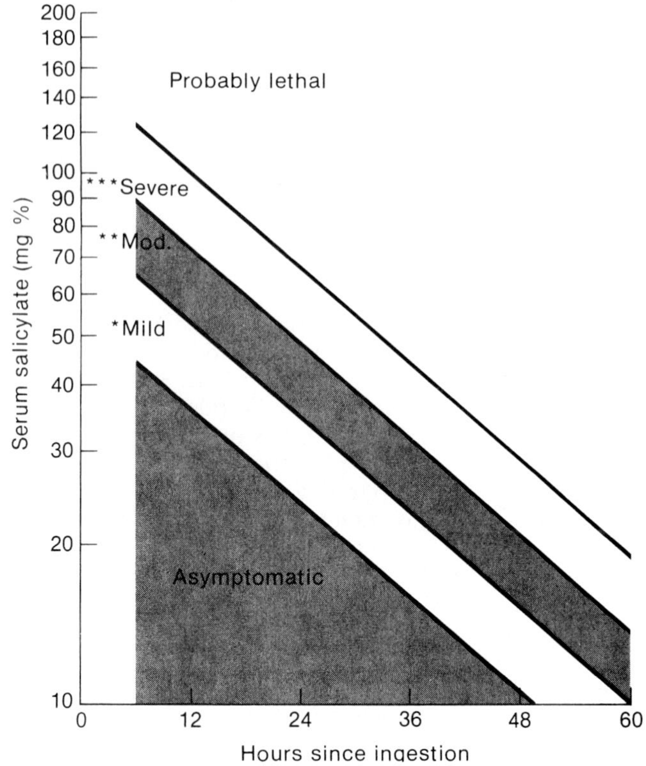

Figure 1. Nomogram relating serum salicylate level to severity of intoxication at varying intervals after acute ingestion of single doses of aspirin. Nomogram starts at 6 hours to ensure that levels will not be interpreted before they have reached their peak; it can be used earlier if more than one level is obtained to establish that the salicylate level is declining. (Adapted from Done AK. Aspirin overdose: incidence, diagnosis and management. Pediatrics 1978;62(suppl.):895.Reproduced by permission.)
*Mild toxicity: mild to moderate hyperpnea without acidosis, lethargy, and vomiting; slight fever may be present.
**Moderate toxicity: severe hyperpnea with acidosis, marked lethargy or excitability but no coma or convulsions, and marked gastrointestinal distress.
***Severe toxicity: severe hyperpnea, severe neurologic impairment that may include coma or convulsions, and marked metabolic acidosis.

Treatment

GUT DECONTAMINATION

Toxic doses of salicylates may cause pylorospasm and decrease the rate of gastric emptying. If enteric-coated or sustained-release preparations are ingested, peak plasma levels may not occur until 12 to 24 hours or more. Gastric lavage may remove pill fragments up to 12 hours after ingestion, however a significant effect on clinical outcome with this intervention has not been proved.

Confirmation of the usefulness of activated charcoal in actual salicylate poisoning cases is still required. Nonetheless, there may be some benefit to charcoal, and it is still recommended

(1 gram / kg by mouth in adults) in significant overdoses. Multiple dose charcoal or whole bowel irrigation has not been shown to enhance the excretion of previously absorbed salicylate in poisoned patients. Multiple human aspirin studies have not shown any benefit from the addition of cathartics to charcoal and hypermagnesemia has been reported with repeated doses of cathartic.

ELIMINATION ENHANCEMENT

Hemodialysis effectively increases clearance and improves fluid and electrolyte balance in severely poisoned patients. Indications include the presence of cardiac or renal failure, intractable acidosis, and severe fluid imbalance. Serum salicylate levels greater than 100 to 120 mg / dL in single acute ingestions serve as a rough guide for the need for hemodialysis. Seizures indicate a poor prognosis and may indicate the necessity to dialyze at lower levels. Chronic salicylate intoxications may be dialyzed at lower levels such as 60 to 80 mg / dL. Charcoal hemoperfusion produces better salicylate clearance than hemodialysis but does not correct fluid and electrolyte balance like hemodialysis. Peritoneal dialysis clearly is inferior to hemodialysis and hemoperfusion, but does improve salicylate clearance.

SUPPORTIVE MEASURES

- Patients with clinically significant symptoms usually are dehydrated. These patients should receive generous fluid replacement with hypotonic glucose solutions (0.25 to 0.5 N saline) using urinary output (3 mL / kg / hour or 100 to 200 mL / hour in adults) as a measure of adequate hydration.
- Relative vitamin K deficiency may be treated with 2.5 to 5 mg vitamin K daily.
- If a rectal temperature is higher than 40°C, a cooling blanket or ice in the axilla and groin may be used. The temperature should be followed closely with a rectal probe and the cooling measures discontinued when rectal temperature falls below 38.5°C.
- Helpful laboratory tests in mild, acute intoxications include complete blood count, electrolytes, BUN, creatinine, glucose, arterial blood gases, and urinalysis. For moderate to severe intoxications a platelet count, prothrombin time, calcium and liver function tests may be helpful.
- A widening arterial-alveolar oxygen gradient is a sensitive early detection test for the development of noncardiogenic pulmonary edema. Because salicylate-induced pulmonary edema is noncardiogenic, digoxin, and diuretics are not useful. If a significant arterial-alveolar (A-a) oxygen gradient is present, fluids must be administered cautiously and alternate methods of enhancing elimination should be considered (e.g., hemodialysis). The mainstay of therapy is oxygen, intubation, and positive end expiratory pressure (PEEP) ventilation. Pulmonary catheters may be necessary to maintain adequate filling pressures.
- Proton pump inhibitors may prevent morphologic lesions induced by aspirin. Antacids, misoprostol, prostaglandins, H2 blockers and sucralfate, may effectively protect the gastric mucosa from lesions induced by aspirin as visualized by gastroscopy.
- Salicylism should be considered in any elderly patient with unexpected delirium or dementia. Symptoms of chronic salicylism are difficult to diagnose in this age group. These symptoms may include fever, dehydration, confusion, hearing loss, falling, agitation, hallucinations, an acute mental status change, lethargy, memory impairment, an inability to care for self, and poor hygiene. Consider a bedside Ferric Chloride Test or salicylate level in all of these patients.

URINARY ALKALINIZATION

- Acidosis is treated aggressively because decreased serum pH increases tissue penetration of salicylates, especially into the central nervous system. Urinary salicylate excretion increases when the urinary pH is greater than 7.5 and is optimal between 8.0 and 8.5. Urinary alkalinization, therefore, is an effective method to treat and increase the excretion of salicylates. For mild toxicity, 1 mEq / kg sodium bicarbonate is added to a liter of 5% dextrose.
- If alkalinization is not achieved within several hours, the dose may be repeated. Moderate to severe intoxications requires bolus therapy (50 to 100 mEq / kg sodium bicarbonate) over 1 to 2 hours plus close monitoring of blood or urinary pH. Alkalinization may be stopped when repeat salicylate levels decline below 35 to 40 mg / dL.

METABOLIC SUPPORT

- Electrolyte status must be followed closely. Patients often are hypokalemic and should be given potassium supplements based on serum potassium and creatinine levels. Acidosis may mask hypokalemia. The rate of potassium replacement should be limited to 10 mEq / h in an adult unless severely hypokalemic. Hypokalemia must be corrected by a separate intravenous line as bicarbonate salts may precipitate. Hypokalemia must also be corrected to alkalinize the urine.
- All patients who present with central nervous system depression and / or serum hypoglycemia should receive intravenous glucose (50 mL of 50% dextrose or 1 mL / kg of D50). Central nervous system hypoglycemia may occur even with normal serum glucose levels. Blood glucose levels must be measured on admission and whenever central nervous system symptoms develop.
- Signs of hypocalcemia and the development of pulmonary edema with hydration must be closely monitored. As ionized calcium may be decreased, intravenous calcium gluconate, 5 to 10 mL in an adult, may be used. Forced alkaline diuresis may worsen hypocalcemia-induced symptoms.

SEIZURES

- Convulsions indicate a serious prognosis and suggest the need to enhance elimination by hemodialysis. Seizures are treated with diazepam intravenously, 0.1 to 0.2 mg / kg per dose in children or 5 mg in adults.
- Metabolic abnormalities such as hypernatremia, hypoglycemia, and hypocalcemia, and cerebral edema (manifested by papilledema) should be considered. The use of glucose and calcium should be considered if seizures do not resolve immediately.

REYE'S SYNDROME

- Management of Reye's syndrome is directed towards encephalopathy and, in particular, towards lowering raised intracranial pressure. Patients should be admitted to an intensive care unit where the head of the bed is raised to minimize the effect of increased jugular venous pressure on intracranial pressure. Mannitol may be infused (in a dose of 0.2 to 1.0 gram / kg) in severe cases.
- Acute hyperventilation, continuous monitoring of intracranial pressure by surgically placed extradural sensors, and short-acting barbiturates may be helpful.

Antidotes

There are no antidotes for salicylate ingestions, but these patients often coingest acetaminophen, for which N-acetylcysteine (NAC) is the antidote. If the history does not exclude acetaminophen coingestion, an acetaminophen blood level should be drawn at least 4 hours postingestion.

Questions—Salicylates

1. **Which of the following carries the largest dose of salicylate if taken orally?**
   A. 240 mL (one dose) of Pepto-Bismol®
   B. One regular strength aspirin
   C. One teaspoon of Ben-Gay®
   D. B and C are equal doses
   E. A, B, and C are equal doses
2. **Which of the following is not true regarding the pharmacokinetics of salicylates?**
   A. ASA is a weak acid, resulting in rapid absorption in the stomach
   B. Alkalosis increases tissue penetration
   C. Untreated overdose can prolong the plasma half-life of salicylates by as much as 8 times that of therapeutic doses.
   D. Hypokalemia impairs renal clearance of salicylates.
   E. Renal elimination becomes more important with large or multiple doses.
3. **Most patients poisoned with aspirin have either a simple respiratory alkalosis or a mixed respiratory alkalosis and metabolic acidosis.**
   A. True
   B. False
4. **One 650-mg dose of aspirin will increase the bleeding time of a normal individual for**
   A. less than 24 hours
   B. 24 to 48 hours
   C. 48 to 72 hours
   D. 4 to 7 days
   E. Up to 1 month
5. **The following metabolic sequelae may occur as direct result of acute salicylate toxicity except**
   A. Hypokalemia
   B. Elevated creatine kinase
   C. Hyperglycemia
   D. Hypercalcemia
   E. Hyperthermia
6. **Which of the following central nervous system effects can be seen with salicylate overdose?**
   A. Seizures
   B. Coma
   C. Asterixis
   D. Papilledema
   E. All of the above
7. **Pulmonary sequelae of salicylate overdose include all of the following except**
   A. Noncardiogenic pulmonary edema
   B. Precipitation of bronchial asthma
   C. Angioedema with resulting airway obstruction
   D. Pneumothorax
   E. Hyperventilation
8. **The Done nomogram should be used with caution in the following situation(s)**
   A. Fever
   B. Renal failure
   C. Delayed gastric emptying
   D. Multiple ingestions
   E. All of the above
9. **Potentially helpful therapeutic maneuvers in the setting of acute salicylate ingestion include all of the following, except**
   A. Hemodialysis, if the serum salicylate level exceeds 100 mg/dL
   B. Urine alkalinization with sodium bicarbonate to achieve a urine pH of 8 to 8.5
   C. Potassium supplementation
   D. Hypertonic fluid replacement
   E. Ventilatory support
10. **Regarding Reye's syndrome, the following is (are) correct**
    A. Rarely occurs over the age of 7
    B. the mortality exceeds 80%
    C. Children with chickenpox or influenza should not be given salicylates.
    D. The incidence of Reye's syndrome rose through the 1980's
    E. A and C

CASE STUDY (QUESTIONS 11 AND 12)

A 68-year-old female is brought to the Emergency Department via ambulance, found to be lethargic and ill appearing, following ingestion of an unknown, but large, amount of aspirin tablets. She is barely arousable, tachypneic, and hypotensive.

11. **The following laboratory studies are helpful except**
    A. Complete blood count
    B. Arterial blood gases
    C. Urinalysis
    D. Erythrocyte sedimentation rate
    E. Creatinine
12. **The following information is obtained: Serum salicylate level = 100 mg/dL, pulmonary edema on chest X-Ray, PaO_2 on 100% oxygen = 58. Interventions may include all of the following except**
    A. Hemodialysis
    B. Administration of IV furosemide
    C. H2 blockers
    D. Ventilatory assistance
    E. Sodium bicarbonate

Answers

Salicylates

1. C 2. B 3. A 4. D 5. D 6. E 7. D
8. E 9. D 10. C 11. D 12. B

SELECTED READINGS

Salicylates

1. Bailey RB, Jones SR. Chronic salicylate intoxication: A common cause of morbidity in the elderly. J Am Geriat Soc 1989;37:556–561.

Answers to questions in shaded boxes appear at the end of the chapter.

2. Bennett WM, De Broe ME. Analgesic nephropathy: a preventable renal disease. N Engl J Med 1989;320:1269–1271.
3. Chapman BJ, Proudfoot AT. Adult salicylate poisoning: Deaths and outcome in patients with high plasma salicylate concentrations. Q J Med 1989;72:699–707.
4. Done AK. Salicylate intoxication: Significance of measurements of salicylates in blood in cases of acute ingestion. Pediatrics 1960;26:800–807.
5. Krause DS, Wolf BA, Shaw LM. Acute aspirin overdose: Mechanisms of toxicity. Ther Drug Monit 1992;14:441–451.
6. Proudfoot AT. Acute Poisoning: Diagnosis and Management. 2nd ed. Oxford: Butterworth-Heinemann, 1993:205–209.

ACKNOWLEDGMENT

Thanks to Jonathan Weinstock, MD for contributing the questions in this chapter.

CHAPTER 12
Muscle Relaxants

INTRODUCTION

Skeletal muscle relaxants are used to relieve spasticity. They include baclofen, dantrolene, chlormezanone, methocarbamol, benzodiazepines (such as diazepam), carisoprodol, cyclobenzaprine, and orphenadrine. Overdose with baclofen may be more common than heretofore presumed. Dantrolene rarely has been reported in overdose. Chlormezanone is a tranquilizer with muscle relaxant properties and has been the subject of a few reports of poisoning. Methocarbamol has been involved in a few fatalities associated with overdose. Diazepam is discussed in detail in Chapter 28, Psychotropic Drugs. Carisoprodol has skeletal muscle relaxant properties, which may be largely secondary to its related sedation.

Symptoms of overdose with antispasticity agents appear to be an exaggeration of therapeutically desired effects. Generally, there is diminished consciousness or coma, profound muscle hypotonia, absent limb reflexes, and respiratory depression. Laboratory studies are usually normal. Patients given good supportive care usually survive.

BACLOFEN, DANTROLENE, CHLORMEZANONE, AND METHOCARBAMOL

Baclofen and dantrolene are used to alleviate spasticity, clonus, spinal automatic movements, flexor spasms, and pain in patients with multiple sclerosis and spinal disorders. Baclofen probably is used most often as an antispasticity drug, because it is often effective at doses that are free of undesired side effects. Baclofen also has been effective in relieving intractable hiccups. Intrathecal baclofen is available in the United States for amelioration of spasticity caused by multiple sclerosis or spinal cord injury in patients unresponsive to oral baclofen. In particular, respiratory depression, somnolence, and coma have been observed with this route of administration.

Chlormezanone is mainly a tranquilizer that may have some muscle relaxant qualities. Methocarbamol is used for the symptomatic relief of muscle spasm.

Dantrolene has been used to treat malignant hyperthermia and neuroleptic malignant syndrome. Dantrolene appears to diminish hyperthermic states and muscle rigidity associated with amphetamine overdose, carbon monoxide poisoning, monoamine oxidase inhibitor overdose, and organophosphate poisoning. Dantrolene also may be useful in controlling the hypermetabolic state associated with rhabdomyolysis secondary to theophylline poisoning.

Pathophysiology

Baclofen (Lioresal®) is a derivative of the inhibitory neurotransmitter γ-aminobutyric acid (GABA). Dantrolene (Dantrium®) is a hydantoin derivative. Chlormezanone is a substituted metathiazonone. Methocarbamol (Robaxin®) is a carbamate derivative. All are synthetic chemicals.

Baclofen acts mainly as a mimetic of GABA in the spinal cord, blocking the excitatory effects of the sensory input from limb muscles. Baclofen is not a GABA receptor agonist, but appears to act at a novel site on the nerve terminal. Baclofen also is thought to inhibit substance P, which normally acts to stimulate monoaminergic neurons in the brainstem. Dantrolene acts peripherally on muscle by interfering with calcium release. This, in turn, prevents membrane excitation and contraction.

Pharmacokinetics

ABSORPTION

- Baclofen is almost completely absorbed from the gastrointestinal tract.
- Its bioavailability is 70% to 80% complete.
- A single oral dose of 40 mg begins to act in 30 to 45 minutes.
- Plasma levels for the unchanged drug peak within 2 hours.
- Plasma concentrations of dantrolene peak in 4 to 8 hours.

DISTRIBUTION

- The apparent volume of distribution of baclofen is about 0.8 L/kg. Animal studies indicate a wide tissue distribution (liver, kidneys) with slow release from brain and nervous tissue.
- The apparent volume of distribution of dantrolene is 0.65 L/kg.
- Dantrolene interacts with human serum albumin *in vitro* but its binding to serum proteins has not been reported.
- Baclofen is 30% bound to plasma proteins.
- Protein binding of methocarbamol ranges between 46% to 50%.

ELIMINATION

- Approximately 85% to 90% of an oral dose of baclofen is excreted unchanged in urine and 10% is excreted in feces.
- In the first 6 hours, two-thirds of baclofen is excreted. By 24 hours, 80% is excreted and by 72 hours, all is excreted.
- The elimination half-life of baclofen averages about 3.6 hours and ranges from 2 to 6 hours.
- Baclofen half-life in overdose may rise to 34 hours or longer.
- Methocarbamol exhibits a half-life of 1.14 hours in normal control subjects.
- Chlormezanone, after therapeutic dose, exhibits a mean half-life of 24 hours; this value may rise to as many as 29 hours in overdose.
- After intravenous dantrolene administration in children, the elimination half-life was approximately 10 hours.
- Approximately 15% to 25% of an orally administered dose of dantrolene is excreted renally; almost 80% appears as 5-hydroxydantrolene.

Clinical Presentations

The clinical features of baclofen overdose in both adults and children include coma, muscle flaccidity, hyporeflexia, and respiratory depression.

NEUROLOGIC EFFECTS

On admission, the severely poisoned patient may be tearful and agitated, but within 3 to 5 hours, patients may become flaccid, lose limb reflexes, develop coma, become unresponsive to painful stimuli, have no spontaneous respirations, and exhibit absence of doll's-eyes and the ice-water caloric response. Involuntary movements may be observed initially, and grand mal seizures may develop 6 hours after ingestion. Seizures have not been reported in intrathecal overdose. Muscle twitching and jerking is often noted. Behavioral disturbances and delirium also have been observed. Consciousness, muscle function, and neurologic function may not return for several days.

CARDIOVASCULAR EFFECTS

Hypotension and hypertension have been observed after baclofen overdose. Normal sinus rhythm, sinus bradycardia, and supraventricular tachyarrhythmias all have been seen.

MISCELLANEOUS EFFECTS

Hypothermia, blue and mottled extremities, and cerebral edema have been reported in baclofen overdose. Elevation of liver enzymes has been seen in chlormezanone overdose. Use of oral dantrolene as a prophylactic drug in patients suspected to be susceptible to malignant hyperthermia may induce nausea, vomiting, dizziness, and diarrhea.

CHRONIC EFFECTS

Fatigue, lassitude, giddiness, mental confusion, depression, headaches, euphoria, muscle weakness, nausea, vomiting, and diarrhea all have been observed with chronic baclofen use. After at least 2 months of therapy with dantrolene, patients may develop hepatotoxicity, which can be fatal.

WITHDRAWAL EFFECTS

Abrupt cessation of baclofen, after its use for many months, may lead to grand mal seizures, auditory and visual hallucinations, paranoid ideas, insomnia, confusion, dyskinesias, sleeplessness, agitation, belligerence, hyperactivity, and grandiose ideas within 12 to 96 hours. Symptoms may last up to 8 days. Similar symptoms are seen after withdrawal from benzodiazepines, chlormezanone, and many sedative-hypnotic drugs. Restoring baclofen in normal dosage with gradual tapering may be an effective approach to management. Therapeutic dosages of chlormezanone may be associated with a hypersensitivity type of hepatitis occurring 1 to 2 months after ingestion.

Toxic Dosage/Death

Adult patients have ingested up to 1.12 grams of baclofen and survived, although serious poisoning has occurred with doses of 150 and 300 mg. Ingestion of 1.25 to 2.5 grams by a patient led to fatality. A 30-year-old man who probably ingested between 1,000 and 1,800 mg of baclofen became comatose and died in 5 days.

Drug Interactions

As baclofen is a neuronal depressant in the central nervous system, it may potentiate other sedative drugs such as diazepam and alcohol. Animal studies demonstrate an increase in lethality with a concomitant decrease in seizures when dantrolene is added to theophylline. Ethanol and methocarbamol taken together can lead to severe central nervous system depression and death.

Pregnancy/Lactation

Insufficient data are available regarding the passage of baclofen, chlormezanone, or methocarbamol through the placenta or into breast milk. Dantrolene is known to cross the placental barrier. At least one pregnant patient reported to have taken an overdose of dantrolene has given birth to a healthy baby.

Laboratory

ANALYTIC METHODS

Accurate levels of baclofen are available with gas/liquid chromatography. A reverse-phase HPLC method can detect quantities of baclofen in plasma and urine to 5 ng. Dantrolene and its metabolites may be determined by high-performance liquid chromatography (HPLC). Plasma methocarbamol concentrations are fluorometrically determined by HPLC.

BLOOD LEVELS

Therapeutic blood levels of methocarbamol are reported to range from 16 to 41 mg/L. Plasma baclofen levels are confirmatory of a clinical diagnosis but do not function to dictate management, which must remain supportive and based on clinical evaluations. Toxic blood levels have been reported to range from 1,100 to 3,500 ng/mL.

Treatment

GUT DECONTAMINATION

Syrup of ipecac should not be used in baclofen overdoses, as absorption is rapid and obtundation and coma can develop rapidly. Gastric lavage with endotracheal intubation may be performed early after overdose. Activated charcoal can be introduced through a gastric lavage tube (1 gram/kg in adults) although its effect on clinical outcome has not been proved. Cathartics have not been evaluated in the treatment of baclofen overdose.

ELIMINATION ENHANCEMENT

Forced diuresis may be useful in view of the largely unchanged excretion of baclofen in urine, however this has not been formally proved in clinical settings. Five percent dextrose and 0.45% saline, accompanied by diuretics such as furosemide (1 mg/kg to a maximum of 40 mg in a single intravenous dose) may be administered to obtain a urine flow of 3 to 6 mL/kg/hour. Enhancement of elimination of baclofen by extracorporeal means, such as peritoneal dialysis, or hemodialysis, has not been evaluated. The low protein binding of baclofen and the urinary excretion of almost all drug may favor such measures in the treatment of overdose.

SUPPORTIVE MEASURES

- Patients who overdose on muscle relaxants may be conscious on admission but may quickly lapse into coma with profound respiratory depression and generalized flaccidity. Treatment of severe overdose should be provided in a hospital intensive care facility with respiratory assistance available. Children who have ingested more than 5 mg/kg of baclofen or adults who have ingested more than 100 mg should be admitted.

- Such care may be required for several days before the patient resumes unassisted ventilation.
- The airway should be maintained by endotracheal intubation if respiratory depression or obstruction occurs. Assisted ventilation may be required early after overdose as severe respiratory depression may supervene.
- Continuous monitoring of the electrocardiogram and vital signs is mandatory. Hypotension can be managed by placing the patient in Trendelenburg position, starting an infusion of intravenous fluids, and, if required, administering pressor amines such as dopamine or norepinephrine.
- Occasional transient elevations of lactic dehydrogenase and aspartate transaminase levels have been observed. Periodic evaluation of renal and hepatic function and encephalographic evaluation are useful during coma.
- Seizures following baclofen overdose should be managed with intravenous diazepam. If there is an inadequate response to diazepam then intravenous phenytoin may be required.
- Baclofen withdrawal hallucinations can be managed by reintroducing the drug and tapering it gradually. Withdrawal reactions occur after use of baclofen for many months and have not been reported after acute poisonings.

Antidotes

No specific antidote is available for the treatment of overdose with baclofen, chlormezanone, methocarbamol, or dantrolene. Anecdotal reports suggest a role for intravenous physostigmine in the treatment of intrathecal baclofen overdose. Respiratory depression, somnolence, coma, pinpoint pupils, and areflexia appeared to respond to a dose of 1 to 2 mg of physostigmine. Precautions and dangers associated with physostigmine use include lacrimation, miosis, salivation, bradycardia, heart block, bladder spasm, diarrhea, seizures, asystole, and bronchospasm. Physostigmine should not be administered to patients with cardiorespiratory depression.

Questions—Baclofen, Dantrolene, Chlormezanone, and Methocarbamol

1. Both baclofen and dantrolene treat the following disorders except
A. Spasticity
B. Malignant hyperthermia
C. Flexor spasms
D. Pain in patients with multiple sclerosis
E. Spinal automatic movements

2. Baclofen and dantrolene
A. Are poorly absorbed from the gastrointestinal tract
B. Have similar elimination half-lives
C. Have wide tissue distribution with slow release from brain
D. Have no renal elimination
E. All of the above

3. Clinical manifestations of baclofen overdose include all the following except
A. Hyperreflexia
B. Coma
C. Respiratory depression
D. Muscle flaccidity
E. Agitation

4. Chronic baclofen use can cause
A. Fatigue
B. Confusion
C. Depression
D. Euphoria
E. All of the above

5. The effects of baclofen
A. Have not been reported as fatal
B. May be similar to those caused by its abrupt cessation
C. Are not affected by concomitant use of other medications
D. Do not involve the fetus if ingested by a pregnant woman
E. All of the above

6. Appropriate baclofen overdose treatment may include
A. Syrup of ipecac
B. Gastric lavage, up until 12 hours after ingestion
C. Diureses with intravenous fluids and diuretics
D. Physostigmine, regardless of the severity of symptoms
E. All of the above

CARISOPRODOL

Carisoprodol is used as an adjunct to analgesics, rest, and physical therapy for the relief of pain in acute musculoskeletal conditions. Its clinical efficacy has not been convincingly established.

Carisoprodol (Soma®) is a centrally acting skeletal muscle relaxant, which is structurally and pharmacologically similar to meprobamate. Its skeletal muscle relaxant effects are minimal and probably are secondary to its sedative effect. It has weak anticholinergic, antipyretic, and analgesic properties. Overdose can be fatal and similarities to meprobamate intoxication should be noted. Overdose patients who are symptomatic should be admitted for intensive observation. Carisoprodol is a synthetic chemical.

Pathophysiology

Carisoprodol produces prolonged symptoms of central nervous system depression resulting from its metabolism to meprobamate.

Pharmacokinetics

ABSORPTION

- Carisoprodol has a pKA of 4.2.
- Peak serum levels appear in about 1 hour.

DISTRIBUTION

- Carisoprodol is rapidly distributed into the central nervous system.
- Its apparent volume of distribution and protein binding in humans are not available.

ELIMINATION

- The drug is rapidly metabolized in the liver.
- Meprobamate is the major metabolite.

Clinical Presentations

Drowsiness, lethargy, agitation, tachycardia, and nystagmus on lateral gaze may be seen in overdose. Headache, dizziness, vertigo, ataxia, and double vision may occur. Massive overdose may yield seizures, coma, and death in rare, severe cases.

Chronic adverse effects may include skin rash, drowsiness, nausea, vomiting, vertigo, facial flush, fatigue, pruritus, ataxia, tremor, headache, irritability, epigastric distress, and fixed drug eruption. Carisoprodol may, like other skeletal muscle relaxants, become a drug of abuse.

Toxic Dosage/Death

Severe toxic overdoses manifested by central nervous system stimulation, depression, and death, have followed ingestion of 9.4 grams, 8.4 grams, and as little as 3.5 grams in a pediatric case.

Drug Interactions

Central nervous system depression with carisoprodol may follow concomitant use of alcohol, other central nervous system depressants, antihistamines, or anesthetics.

Pregnancy/Lactation

Carisoprodol is excreted in human milk in a concentration two to four times that in maternal plasma. Its distribution through the placenta in humans has not been evaluated however animal data indicate placental penetration. Pregnancy risk factor C.

Laboratory

ANALYTIC METHODS

A colorimetric assay for carbamates is available, and specific gas chromatography method for carisoprodol has been devised.

BLOOD LEVELS

There appears to be some correlation of plasma levels of carisoprodol (and meprobamate) with sedation and toxic effects, however the clinical management of overdose cases should not rely on blood levels.

Treatment

GUT DECONTAMINATION

Gastric lavage with tracheal protection may be useful within the first 3 to 4 hours, however the effect on clinical outcome has not been proved. Similarly, activated charcoal and cathartics may be of assistance, but there are no studies to establish their value. There is no evidence for the formation of gastric masses (bezoars) in carisoprodol overdoses, as is occasionally seen in meprobamate overdoses.

ELIMINATION ENHANCEMENT

Intravenous fluids (5% dextrose in water or 5% dextrose in normal saline) should be administered only in sufficient quantity to maintain normal urine flow. There are no data substantiating the use of forced diuresis, hemodialysis, peritoneal dialysis, exchange transfusion, charcoal or resin hemoperfusion, plasmapheresis, or whole-bowel irrigation.

SUPPORTIVE MEASURES

- Supportive care is the mainstay of management for a carisoprodol overdose. Patients with any symptoms of overdose should be observed in a hospital care facility for at least 24 hours.
- If there are no typical clinical signs or symptoms in the first 8 hours after reported ingestion, consideration may be given to discharge from intensive observation.
- Airway, breathing, and circulatory status should be monitored until the patient is awake and breathing normally. Assisted ventilation is generally not required.

Questions—Carisoprodol

1. Effects of therapeutic doses of carisoprodol include
- A. Skeletal muscle relaxation
- B. Analgesia
- C. Antipyresis
- D. Sedation
- E. All of the above

2. Carisoprodol
- A. Is slowly distributed into the central nervous system
- B. Is metabolized in the liver
- C. Is metabolized in the kidneys
- D. Has peak serum levels in 8 to 10 hours
- E. Does not metabolize into recognizable products

3. Treatment of carisoprodol overdoses may include all of the following except
- A. Gastric lavage if within 3 to 4 hours of ingestion
- B. High suspicion and investigation for bezoar formation
- C. Intravenous fluids without diuretics
- D. 24-hour observation
- E. Careful monitoring of respiration

CYCLOBENZAPRINE

Cyclobenzaprine (Flexeril®) is a synthetic chemical used for the relief of spasm associated with acute, painful musculoskeletal conditions. Its efficacy is controversial. No fatalities from overdose have been described. Cyclobenzaprine is a tricyclic amine similar in structure and pharmacologic action to amitriptyline (a tricyclic antidepressant). Originally studied during the 1960s as an antidepressant, it was subsequently evaluated for its use in chronic tension headache and for rigidity in Parkinson's disease. There is no evidence of its effectiveness in the treatment of spasticity associated with cerebral or spinal cord disease or in children with cerebral palsy.

Pathophysiology

Cyclobenzaprine toxicity is related to its ability to produce central and peripheral antimuscarinic anticholinergic blockade. It blocks muscarinic cholinergic receptors, augments the activity of exogenous norepinephrine (by releasing endogenous catecholamines from presynaptic neurons and by reducing reuptake), and acts as an antihistamine. Cyclobenzaprine was shown to abolish certain forms of muscular rigidity in animals.

Pharmacokinetics

ABSORPTION

- Cyclobenzaprine is completely but slowly absorbed from the intestine.
- Average plasma levels increase with increasing daily dosage. Time to peak plasma level varies from 3 to 8 hours, however if given intravenously, this is reduced to 0.5 to 2 hours.

DISTRIBUTION

- Cyclobenzaprine is rapidly taken up by tissues and slowly released into the blood.
- About 93% are bound to plasma proteins.

ELIMINATION

- The drug is almost completely metabolized. First-pass hepatic metabolism may be important in cyclobenzaprine metabolism. Enterohepatic recirculation has been postulated.
- Very little unchanged drug is excreted in the urine.
- The half-life of cyclobenzaprine is approximately 1 to 3 days.

Clinical Presentations

At therapeutic doses, manifestations of both peripheral and central anticholinergic blockade are frequently observed. Prominent side effects include dry mouth, drowsiness, dizziness, nausea, and unpleasant taste sensations. Less frequent undesirable effects include rash, ataxia, weakness, headache, fatigue, and nervousness. Rare patients have reported tachycardia, disorientation, hallucinations, cardiac arrhythmias, and seizures. Although only a few patients with overdose have been reported to date, it is clear that most develop only mild symptoms similar to those reported as adverse effects to therapeutic dosages.

Serious overdose patients may present with agitation, confusion, and hallucinations. Peripheral anticholinergic findings (e.g., dry skin, dry mucous membranes, tachycardia, decreased gastrointestinal motility, and urinary retention) may be present as well. Unlike tricyclic antidepressant poisoning, reports of coma, convulsions, hypotension, arrhythmias, or impaired cardiac conduction and contractility, have not been reported. Pupils typically are midposition, equal, and reactive.

Toxic Dosage/Death

Poisoning has followed pure overdoses of cyclobenzaprine in quantities of 600 mg to approximately 1,000 mg. A 15-year-old who ingested about 800 mg of cyclobenzaprine died on the eighth day. A 45-year-old adult who ingested 900 mg became comatose, developed cardiac arrest in 4 days, and died.

Drug Interactions

Skeletal muscle relaxants are frequently used in combination with alcohol, benzodiazepines, or narcotics to prolong the effect of these co-ingested substances. They also are used to increase the efficacy of the primary drug of abuse or to achieve the same effects with a smaller amount of alcohol or narcotic.

Pregnancy/Lactation

It is not known whether cyclobenzaprine crosses the placenta or is distributed into breast milk. Pregnancy risk category B.

Laboratory

ANALYTIC METHODS

Gas-liquid chromatography methods are available for quantitative analysis of cyclobenzaprine in the plasma and urine. Toxicology urine screens also may include a qualitative test for cyclobenzaprine. Because of its structural similarity to amitriptyline, cyclobenzaprine is not easily distinguished from amitriptyline by conventional laboratory methods. This reinforces the necessity of obtaining a careful clinical history in conjunction with analytical techniques.

BLOOD LEVELS

Blood levels are not helpful in managing the clinical effects of cyclobenzaprine overdose. These procedures are not performed routinely in clinical laboratories and have not been correlated either with side effects after therapeutic dosage or with toxicity associated with overdose.

Treatment

GUT DECONTAMINATION

As anticholinergic effects may delay gastric emptying, gastric lavage may be effective for many hours after overdose, however the clinical effectiveness of this procedure has not been proved.

ELIMINATION ENHANCEMENT

The utility of extracorporeal methods of elimination has not been studied or proven in cyclobenzaprine overdose.

SUPPORTIVE MEASURES

- Treatment of cyclobenzaprine overdose should follow the steps recommended for overdose of tricyclic antidepressant drugs. See Chapter 28, Psychotropic Drugs.
- Ventricular arrhythmias, QRS widening, or intraventricular conduction defects may be treated with sodium bicarbonate (1 mEq/kg IV) sufficient to increase the arterial or urine pH to 7.5.

Antidotes

Physostigmine use for anticholinergic symptoms in cyclobenzaprine poisoning may be reserved for patients with very serious symptoms (e.g., severe agitation, delirium, hypertension, or life-threatening arrhythmias), however is only recommended in particularly serious cases.

Questions—Cyclobenzaprine

1. Cyclobenzaprine
- A. Is rarely used but commonly fatal
- B. Is structurally similar to selective serotonin reuptake inhibitors
- C. Is established as effective in relief of spasm associated with painful musculoskeletal conditions
- D. All of the above
- E. None of the above

2. Side effects of cyclobenzaprine include
- A. Increased secretions
- B. Agitation
- C. Unpleasant taste sensations
- D. Hyperactivity
- E. None of the above

3. Overdoses of cyclobenzaprine
- A. May present with agitation, confusion, and hallucinations
- B. Have been reported frequently
- C. Can be distinguished from tricyclic overdoses by conventional urine testing
- D. Have been reported to include coma, seizures, and hypotension
- E. All of the above

4. Treatment of cyclobenzaprine overdose
A. Is helped by blood levels
B. May include gastric lavage many hours after ingestion
C. Usually includes extracorporeal elimination
D. Always includes physostigmine
E. None of the above

ORPHENADRINE

Orphenadrine (Norflex®) is a synthetic chemical used to treat discomfort associated with acute, painful muscular conditions. Orphenadrine is an anticholinergic drug that has been used as a skeletal muscle relaxant and to combat the parkinsonian effects of phenothiazines. In children, it has produced severe poisoning and death after ingestion. Serious symptoms such as convulsions or cardiac arrest may lead to death within a few hours. Treatment must be aggressive. Physostigmine may be a useful antidote in certain cases.

Pathophysiology

Orphenadrine is an antimuscarinic agent closely related to the antihistamine diphenhydramine. Its difference from diphenhydramine is sufficient to reduce its antihistaminic activity, increase its anticholinergic activity, and permit it to have central effects on muscle tone.

Orphenadrine may exert a direct depressant effect on myocardial contraction and cardiac conduction, and produce a significant cardiotoxic effect in overdose. Orphenadrine works peripherally as a cholinergic blocker but also has central effects, which may explain its ability to reduce skeletal muscle spasm. It does not have direct skeletal muscle relaxant activity. It also has some antihistaminic and local anesthetic effects.

Pharmacokinetics

ABSORPTION

- Orphenadrine is rapidly and completely absorbed from the stomach and intestines.
- Plasma levels peak in about 2 to 4 hours after an oral dose and in about 1 hour after an intramuscular dose. Plasma levels tend to increase in proportion to the dose administered.

DISTRIBUTION

- High concentrations are found in the liver and lungs.
- Orphenadrine may undergo an enterohepatic cycle in its path from the intestine to the liver and then into the bile. Orphenadrine has a pKA of 8.4 and is about 20% protein bound.

ELIMINATION

- Orphenadrine is almost completely metabolized by a first-order kinetic process to at least eight metabolites. The clinical activity of the metabolites has not been clinically evaluated.
- The major metabolite appears to compete for biotransformation with orphenadrine and may be active. The elimination half-life of orphenadrine is about 15 hours.
- Approximately 50% to 60% are excreted in the urine as metabolites; about 8% are excreted unchanged. Large amounts are excreted in the bile and feces.

Clinical Presentations

Convulsions, coma, mydriasis, and tachycardia may occur within two hours of orphenadrine overdose. These effects are similar to those following tricyclic antidepressant overdoses. Athetoid movements, cardiac arrest, shock, and hypothermia all have been described. Hypoglycemia, elevated transaminase levels, a fall in the prothrombin time, disseminated intravascular coagulation (DIC), hepatomegaly, pulmonary hemorrhage, and hypokalemia all have been seen. Pathologic changes may include brain edema, hemorrhagic pulmonary edema, hepatic necrosis, and renal congestion.

Anticholinergic effects are most evident following long-term use of higher-than-therapeutic doses. Dry mouth, urinary retention, tachycardia, blurred vision, pupillary dilation, nausea, vomiting, headache, dizziness, agitation, drowsiness, tremors, and mental confusion may be observed. Rare cases of aplastic anemia, urticaria, and anaphylactic reaction have been reported. Reduction in dosage eliminates undesirable side effects.

Toxic Dosage/Death

A dose of 650 to 700 mg resulted in severe toxicity and death in a 2-year-old child. Another 2-year-old ingested 1.4 grams and recovered. In adults, an overdose of 2 to 3 grams has been associated with death, however a 19-year-old woman recovered after reportedly ingesting 7.5 grams. In severe cases, death is rapid and occurs within 2 to 5 hours. Death is often a result of cardiac or respiratory arrest and may follow status epilepticus.

Drug Interactions

Orphenadrine may be additive with other anticholinergic agents such as the phenothiazines, antiparkinsonian drugs, atropine, antihistamines, and tricyclic antidepressants. Additive effects with propoxyphene may result in mental confusion, anxiety, and tremors. All the skeletal muscle relaxants possess sedative properties and may be abused for this effect. Skeletal muscle relaxants are frequently used in combination with other depressants, such as alcohol, benzodiazepines, or narcotics, to prolong the effect of these co-ingestants.

Pregnancy/Lactation

Orphenadrine may appear in breast milk and is classified as pregnancy risk category C.

Laboratory

ANALYTIC METHODS

A gas chromatographic procedure has been described for orphenadrine and its major metabolite. A high-performance liquid chromatography method also can be employed.

BLOOD LEVELS

Toxicity appears to begin at a blood level of about 2 mg/mL. Concentrations of 4 to 8 mg/mL may be fatal. Use of laboratory studies is not available in many community hospitals. When used, they can confirm the presence of orphenadrine. Treatment, which frequently must be immediate and aggressive, should be guided by clinical evaluations and should not be delayed while laboratory studies of blood levels are being obtained.

Treatment

GUT DECONTAMINATION

Orphenadrine may be retained in the stomach for several hours because of its anticholinergic properties. Emesis induction should be avoided because of the rapid onset of symptoms, such as seizures, in the first hours after ingestion. Gastric lavage with tracheal protection may be instituted within 4 hours of ingestion. Activated charcoal (adults, 1 gram/kg and children, 15 to 50 grams) can be given orally or introduced through a gastric lavage tube. As slurry, 240 mL of diluent is given per 30 grams of charcoal. Cathartics have not been evaluated in the treatment of orphenadrine overdose but may be useful in preventing additional absorption.

ELIMINATION ENHANCEMENT

No reports are available on the use of forced diuresis or extracorporeal methods of drug removal such as hemodialysis, peritoneal dialysis, or hemoperfusion.

SUPPORTIVE MEASURES

- Electrocardiographic monitoring should be instituted on arrival. Continuous monitoring of vital signs in an intensive area is mandatory in significant overdoses. Equipment for cardiac resuscitation should be immediately available.
- The orphenadrine-depressed heart is responsive to the positive inotropic and chronotropic actions of catecholamines.
- Seizures may begin within 20 minutes of ingestion or en route to the hospital. Intravenous diazepam may be effective in controlling seizures. Avoid barbiturates or other central nervous system depressants if possible.
- Institute endotracheal intubation with assisted ventilation in hypoxic patients.
- Follow hepatic transaminases, prothrombin time, blood sugar, acid/base balance, and electrolytes. Hypokalemia may require potassium replacement under careful electrocardiographic monitoring.

Antidotes

PHYSOSTIGMINE

Physostigmine may be useful in the treatment of hallucinations, arrhythmias, hypertension, coma, myoclonic seizures, and life-threatening tachycardia when anticholinergic signs and symptoms are present. The dose is 0.5 mg intravenously, slowly. The patient must be observed carefully for evidence of cholinergic effects. If there is no improvement, the dose is repeated at 5-minute intervals to a maximum of 2 mg. A continuous drip should not be used. Ventilatory therapy and gastric lavage should be instituted with careful cardiovascular evaluation before physostigmine is used.

Questions—Orphenadrine

1. Orphenadrine
- A. Is used to treat parkinsonian effects of phenothiazines
- B. Has produced seizures and cardiac arrest within a few hours of ingestion
- C. Has less antihistaminic effect than diphenhydramine
- D. May directly depress myocardial contraction
- E. All of the above

2. After ingestion of orphenadrine,
- A. Absorption from the stomach and intestines is rapid
- B. Peak levels are in 1 hour
- C. Elimination half-life is about 5 hours
- D. All excretion is in the urine
- E. The liver is not usually involved in metabolism

3. Overdose of orphenadrine
- A. Is similar to MAO inhibitors
- B. Usually becomes symptomatic 24 hours after ingestion
- C. May include disseminated intravascular coagulation
- D. Has not been reported in children
- E. All of the above

Answers

Baclofen, Dantrolene, Chlormezanone, and Methocarbamol

1. B 2. C 3. A 4. E 5. B 6. C

Carisoprodol

1. E 2. B 3. B

Cyclobenzaprine

1. E 2. C 3. A 4. B

Orphenadrine

1. E 2. A 3. C

SELECTED READINGS

Baclofen, Dantrolene, Chlormezanone, and Methocarbamol

1. Bismuth C, de Rohan-Chabot P, Goulon M, et al. Dantroline: A new therapeutic approach to the neuroleptic malignant syndrome. Acta Neurol Scand 1984;70(suppl. 100):193–198.
2. Fraser AD, MacNeil W, Isner AF. Toxicological analysis of a fatal baclofen (Lioresal®) ingestion. J Forens Sci 1991;36:1596–1602.
3. May CR. Baclofen overdose. Ann Emerg Med 1983;12:171–173.

Carisoprodol

1. Goldberg D. Carisoprodol toxicity. Milit Med 1969;134:597–601.
2. McEvoy GK, ed. AHFS Drug Information 86. Bethesda, MD: American Society of Hospital Pharmacists, 1986:617–618.
3. Reynolds JEF, ed. Martindale: The Extra Pharmacopoeia. 30th ed. London: Pharmaceutical Press, 1993:1202.

Cyclobenzaprine

1. Linden CH, Mitchiner JC, Lindzon RD, et al. Cyclobenzaprine overdosage. J Toxicol Clin Toxicol 1983;20:281–288.
2. Tasset JJ, Schroeder TJ, Pesce AJ. Cyclobenzaprine overdose: The importance of a clinical history in analytical toxicology. J Anal Toxicol 1985;10:258.

Orphenadrine

1. Bennet MB, Kohn J. Orphenadrine overdose: Cerebral manifestations treated with physostigmine. Anaesth Intens Care 1976;4:67. Case Report.
2. Blomquist M, Bonnichsen R, Schubert B. Lethal orphenadrine intoxications: A report of five cases. Z Rechtsmed 1971;68:111.
3. Robinson AE, Holder AT, McDowall RD, et al. Forensic toxicology of some orphenadrine-related deaths. Forens Sci 1977;9:53–62.
4. Snyder BD, Kane M, Plocher D. Orphenadrine overdose treatment with physostigmine. N Engl J Med 1976;295:1435.

ACKNOWLEDGMENT

Thanks to Alison Deutsch, MD for contributing the questions in this chapter.

SECTION

B

Antiinfective Drugs

CHAPTER 13

Antibiotics and Antituberculosis Drugs

INTRODUCTION

Antibiotics are ubiquitous. While an attempt is made here to summarize the major classes of antibiotics currently used in the United States, one must be cognizant of the fact that many new products, not to mention entirely new classes of antiinfective agents, are being introduced yearly. Among many relevant side issues, pseudomembranous colitis deserves special mention as it is seen commonly by general practitioners.

Pseudomembranous Colitis

Antibiotic-associated pseudomembranous colitis (PC) can arise with almost any antimicrobial agent. A patient who receives antibiotic therapy that is not active against Clostridium difficile is at increased risk of developing pseudomembranous colitis. PC is caused by the production of a cytotoxic toxin by Clostridium difficile during intestinal overgrowth. The relative risk of developing pseudomembranous colitis after exposure to clindamycin is substantially higher than for third-generation cephalosporins, broad-spectrum penicillins, or any other antibiotic.

Clostridium difficile may be acquired by patients in a hospital setting, and the risk of nosocomial acquisition is probably greater than that in the community, where the carriage rate in healthy adults has been estimated to be about 5%. The incubation period for Clostridium difficile colitis ranges from several days up to 6 weeks following antibiotic treatment, so the disease may develop in some patients after discharge from the hospital. Clostridium difficile colitis can be distinguished from a benign or nonspecific diarrhea that occurs in some patients given antibiotics in that the latter is not accompanied by fever or leukocytosis and usually disappears promptly on stopping therapy with the offending agent.

Stool smears are positive for fecal leukocytes in about 50% of patients with Clostridium difficile colitis. Pseudomembranes may be observed on sigmoidoscopy or colonoscopy; however, this finding does not establish the etiology. Stools should be cultured for enteric pathogens because they are occasionally acquired nosocomially. The finding of Clostridium difficile on culture is insufficient to make a definitive diagnosis of Clostridium difficile colitis. Establishing the presence of Clostridium difficile toxin in the stool using an *in vitro* enzyme-linked immunosorbent assay or a cytotoxic assay makes the definitive etiologic diagnosis. Besides stopping the responsible antibiotic, management is directed toward eradicating toxin-producing Clostridium difficile with oral vancomycin or metronidazole.

Abdominal pain, low-grade fever, hypoalbuminemia, and leukocytosis are frequently present. Complications secondary to diarrhea or high fever occur more often in debilitated patients and those at age extremes. They include a protein-losing enteropathy, colonic perforation, toxic megacolon, and death. The colon may be involved proximally, distally, or universally.

Questions—Introduction to Antibiotics and Antituberculosis Drugs

1. Which of the following concerning pseudomembranous colitis is false?
A. Stool smears are positive for fecal leukocytes in about 50% of patients with Clostridium difficile colitis.
B. Pseudomembranes may be observed on sigmoidoscopy or colonoscopy; however, this finding does not establish the etiology.
C. The finding of Clostridium difficile on culture is insufficient to make a definitive diagnosis of Clostridium difficile colitis.
D. Clostridium difficile colitis can be distinguished from a benign or nonspecific diarrhea that occurs in some patients given antibiotics in that the latter is not accompanied by fever or leukocytosis and usually disappears promptly on stopping therapy with the offending agent.
E. The relative risk of developing pseudomembranous colitis after exposure to third-generation cephalosporins is substantially higher than for clindamycin.

AMINOGLYCOSIDES

Aminoglycosides are antibiotics and semisynthetic antibiotic derivatives derived from cultures of Streptomyces species or Micromonospora species. They are active against a number of Gram-negative organisms and are routinely used to combat urosepsis, pseudomonal infections, and diabetic problems. The drugs contain one or two amino sugars glycosidically linked to an aminocyclitol nucleus. Examples include amikacin, gentamicin, neomycin, kanamycin, netilmicin, streptomycin, and tobra-

Answers to questions in shaded boxes appear at the end of the chapter.

mycin. Wide interpatient variation may occur, necessitating variable dose schedules dependent on renal function and other pharmacokinetic factors. Serial monitoring of blood levels may be indicated.

Pathophysiology

Aminoglycosides are bactericides. They appear to inhibit protein synthesis in susceptible bacteria by binding to 30S ribosomal subunits. Auditory toxicity appears to be related to the selective destruction of the outer hair cells of the organ of Corti. Retrograde degeneration of the auditory nerve occurs later. Vestibular system damage occurs, mostly to type I hair cells of the summit of the ampulla cristae. Cochlear or ampullar cell damage appears to be related to concentrations of aminoglycosides in the perilymph and endolymph. Hearing loss is usually bilateral and the degree of loss is dose related.

Aminoglycosides may produce proximal tubular cell damage with an accumulation of structures within lysosomes called myeloid bodies. Aminoglycoside-induced neuromuscular paralysis appears to result from both an inhibition of presynaptic acetylcholine release and a blockade of postsynaptic acetylcholine receptor sites. Calcium ion concentration at the myoneural junction is depressed. The paralysis is associated with very high concentrations of drug at the neuromuscular junctions.

Pharmacokinetics

ABSORPTION

- Less than 1% of gentamicin is absorbed orally.

DISTRIBUTION

- Volume of distribution of gentamicin is 0.2–0.3 L / kg in adults.
- Protein binding of gentamicin is less than 30%.

ELIMINATION

- The half-life of gentamicin in adults is 1.5–3.0 hours, and the half-life of amikacin is 1.6 hours.
- Clearance of gentamicin is directly related to renal function and occurs via glomerular filtration.
- From 94 to 98% of amikacin is excreted unchanged via glomerular filtration.

Clinical Presentations

Ototoxicity and nephrotoxicity are the most serious adverse effects of aminoglycoside administration. They are most likely to occur in the elderly, in dehydrated patients, in patients with renal impairment, in those who have been receiving high doses of the drug, in those who have been receiving the drug for long periods, or in those receiving other ototoxic and / or nephrotoxic drugs. Pharmacokinetic monitoring (serum antibiotic levels, creatinine levels) must be individually adjusted to attain effective, yet nontoxic, delivery of antibiotics.

OTOTOXIC EFFECTS

The initial symptom of cochlear damage is often tinnitus, which is usually high-pitched and continuous. By the time hearing loss is reported, significant high-frequency loss has probably already occurred, along with a 25- to 30-dB loss in the lower speech frequencies. Serial audiometric testing may be used to pick up early asymptomatic loss of high frequency hearing loss for patients on a long-term course of aminoglycosides (e.g., >1 month).

Patients may develop dysequilibrium if they are ambulatory, with an ataxic gait, stumbling, and loss of balance on turning. Most clinically observed ototoxicity is chronic and is generally accepted to be largely irreversible.

Vestibular symptoms may be observed with dizziness, nystagmus, vertigo, and ataxia. Risk factors include older age, prolonged duration of therapy, bacteremia, poor physical condition, fever, liver and renal impairment, and the combination of an aminoglycoside with another ototoxic agent.

NEUROMUSCULAR EFFECTS

All the aminoglycosides are capable, in rare circumstances, of causing neuromuscular blockade and paralysis. The mechanism appears to involve blockade of calcium uptake, which results in both inhibition of presynaptic acetylcholine release and blockade of postsynaptic acetylcholine receptors. Factors known to enhance neuromuscular blockade in association with the use of aminoglycosides include the concurrent use of curare-like drugs, succinylcholine, and the simultaneous presence of botulinum toxin.

RENAL EFFECTS

Most patients with nephrotoxicity develop a nonoliguric azotemia. Renal toxicity may be reversible although death resulting from uremia has occurred. Laboratory evidence of nephrotoxicity includes increases in the blood urea nitrogen and serum creatinine, decreases in urine specific gravity and creatinine clearance, proteinuria, or cells or casts in the urine. The various aminoglycosides have different potentials to cause nephrotoxicity.

Risk factors for aminoglycoside nephrotoxicity include the choice of aminoglycoside, prolonged duration of therapy, greater total aminoglycoside dose, hypotension, volume depletion, high peak or trough serum aminoglycoside concentrations, and concurrent liver disease. Other risk factors include metabolic acidosis, potassium depletion, hypomagnesemia, increased parathyroid hormone activity, and obesity.

HYPERSENSITIVITY EFFECTS

Rash, urticaria, stomatitis, pruritus, fever, and eosinophilia have been recorded. Cross-allergenicity has been demonstrated among the aminoglycosides. Topical use of neomycin may result in rashes and skin sensitization.

Toxic Dosage/Death

Gentamicin and amikacin nephrotoxicity have been correlated with peak serum levels over 10 μg / mL and 38.5 μg / mL respectively, and trough levels of 1 μg / mL and 10 respectively.

Drug Interactions

Agents that may have additive nephrotoxicity with the aminoglycosides include amphotericin B, vancomycin, piperacillin, clindamycin, cisplatin, calcium channel blockers, nonsteroidal antiinflammatory drugs, and radiocontrast agents. Additive ototoxic and / or nephrotoxic effects may be observed with ethacrynic acid, urea, and mannitol. Furosemide use is not considered a major risk factor for the development of aminoglycoside-induced nephrotoxicity or auditory toxicity. Dimenhydrinate and other antiemetics may mask symptoms of vestibular ototoxicity.

Succinylcholine, tubocurarine, decamethonium, pancuronium, polymyxins, myasthenia gravis, and Clostridium botulinum toxin potentiate neuromuscular blockade and may cause respiratory paralysis. Oral neomycin potentiates the effect of oral anticoagulants and decreases absorption of digoxin, methotrexate, and spironolactone. Oral neomycin may potentiate the effects of oral anticoagulants by interfering with gastrointestinal absorption or synthesis of vitamin K.

Pregnancy/Lactation

Gentamicin and amikacin are classified as pregnancy risk category C.

Laboratory

ANALYTIC METHODS

Aminoglycosides may be measured by high-pressure liquid chromatography.

BLOOD LEVELS

Serum aminoglycoside concentrations should be monitored serially. The risks of ototoxicity and nephrotoxicity are both increased when relatively moderate elevations of peak (more than 12 μg/mL for gentamicin or tobramycin) or trough (more than 2 μg/mL) concentrations persist.

Treatment

GUT DECONTAMINATION

Activated charcoal and cathartics may be effective after oral overdose; however, no systematic clinical studies of their efficacy are available.

ELIMINATION ENHANCEMENT

Peritoneal dialysis, hemodialysis, hemoperfusion, and exchange transfusion are rarely required and are of little value after aminoglycoside overdose except in the presence of renal failure, where such procedures have had limited success. Furosemide has not been shown to increase the rate of clearance of aminoglycosides.

SUPPORTIVE MEASURES

- For most aminoglycoside overdosages, supportive symptomatic therapy, maintenance of life support measures and administration of sufficient fluids to maintain a urine flow of 3–6 mL/kg per hour are adequate.
- Caution must be exercised to avoid fluid overload and pulmonary edema, especially when overaggressive therapy is administered to patients with renal insufficiency.
- Eighth cranial nerve function (auditory, vestibular) must be carefully monitored in the period (weeks or months) after an aminoglycoside overdosage.
- Monitor renal function (serum creatinine and blood urea nitrogen) serially.
- Rare hypomagnesemia may occur after prolonged (at least 2 days) or recurrent courses of aminoglycosides. This may lead to hypocalcemia and tetany. Serial magnesium, calcium, and potassium monitoring should be performed before, during, and after therapy in patients at risk.

Antidotes

There are no known antidotes for aminoglycoside overdosage. Calcium gluconate intravenously may be useful in treatment of the neuromuscular paralysis.

Questions—Aminoglycosides

1. The most serious adverse effects of aminoglycoside administration are
A. Ototoxicity and nephrotoxicity
B. Ototoxicity and hepatotoxicity
C. Hepatotoxicity and cardiotoxicity
D. Cardiotoxicity and nephrotoxicity
E. Nephrotoxicity and hematotoxicity

2. Most patients with nephrotoxicity develop
A. Nephrotic syndrome
B. Uremia
C. Membranoproliferative glomerulonephritis
D. Papillary necrosis
E. Nonoliguric azotemia

3. Risk factors for aminoglycoside nephrotoxicity include all of the following except
A. Metabolic acidosis
B. Duration of therapy
C. Previous ototoxicity
D. Hypotension
E. High total aminoglycoside dose

4. All the aminoglycosides are capable, in rare circumstances, of causing neuromuscular blockade and paralysis.
A. True
B. False

5. Treatment of aminoglycoside toxicity/overdose usually includes which of the following?
A. Hemodialysis
B. Intravenous hydration with 3% sodium chloride.
C. Intravenous furosemide
D. Intravenous calcium gluconate
E. None of the above

β-LACTAMS

β-lactam antibiotics in use are the penicillins, the cephalosporins, and the carbapenems (imipenem). Monobactams include aztreonam and do not contain a β-lactam ring.

Penicillins

Toxicity associated with penicillin use is common; however, poisonings are relatively rare. Large ingestions of oral penicillin-type drugs are usually nontoxic. Serious neurotoxic overdosages with penicillin have largely occurred during periods of hospitalization for treatment of serious infections. Immediate and delayed hypersensitivity responses to penicillin may follow either therapeutic use or overdosage and are often seen in an emergency facility.

All penicillins contain a 6-aminopenicillanic acid nucleus. This is composed of a β-lactam ring fused to a five-member thiazolidine ring. Different side chains are attached resulting in different penicillin derivatives with unique spectra of activity, stability against hydrolysis by β-lactamases, acid stability, gastrointestinal absorption, and protein binding. Penicillins are used against susceptible Gram-positive aerobic cocci, Gram-negative aerobic cocci, Gram-positive aerobic bacilli, Gram-positive anaerobic bacteria, and certain spirochetes.

PATHOPHYSIOLOGY

Penicillins are bactericidal. The antibacterial activity results from inhibition of glycopeptide synthesis in bacterial cell walls. Penicillins reversibly bind to enzymes in the bacterial cytoplasmic membrane. Penicillins may have a direct seizure-provoking effect when placed in contact with cortical cells of the brain.

PHARMACOKINETICS

Absorption

- Most available penicillins (except penicillin G, methicillin, and carbenicillin) are relatively resistant to destruction by gastric acid.
- Only about 30–50% of an orally administered dose reaches the systemic circulation.
- Food delays absorption (except for phenoxymethyl penicillin, ampicillin and amoxicillin).
- Peak serum concentrations are attained 30–60 minutes after oral administration and 15–30 minutes after parenteral injection.

Distribution

- The penicillins are well distributed in muscle, lung, interstitial fluid, skin abscesses, and synovium.
- Sites that are difficult to access are the central nervous system, eye, and prostate.
- The volume of distribution of most penicillins ranges from 0.13–0.70 L/kg.

Elimination

- Penicillins are largely eliminated by excretion in unchanged form in the urine.
- The metabolic products of penicillin rather than penicillin itself form allergenic haptenic moieties. The penicilloyl moiety, the major metabolic product, is the major determinant, and is most often responsible for accelerated urticarial reactions but not for anaphylaxis.
- About 5% of penicillin is metabolized to approximately 10 other antigens known as minor determinants. The minor determinant mixture is composed of crystalline penicillin, its hydrolysis product, sodium penicillate, and other penicillin products.
- Biotransformation of penicillin V and oxacillin is considerable (49–56%), especially when orally administered.
- The half-life of most penicillins is about 1 hour or less. However, in renal failure, the half-life is prolonged to 12 hours (penicillin G) and 20 hours (carbenicillin).

CLINICAL PRESENTATIONS

Penicillin, worldwide, is probably one of the most commonly prescribed drugs, and untoward reactions constitute a significant health problem often seen first by emergency room personnel. Hypersensitivity reactions are the most frequent and life-threatening.

Hypersensitivity Effects

Immediate hypersensitivity reactions occur in approximately 1–10% of patients treated with penicillin. Anaphylactic shock occurs in 1–5 per 10,000 patient courses of treatment and is the most common cause of anaphylaxis. Penicillin may be responsible for as many as 75% of anaphylactic deaths in the U.S. and may cause 400–800 deaths per year. Reactions occur more often when penicillin is injected but may occur after oral use. Anaphylactic reaction occurs most commonly between the ages of 20 and 49 years, but may rarely occur in children under 12 years of age and in the elderly. Sex, race, and histocompatibility leukocyte antigen (HLA) phenotype do not appear to affect the incidence of penicillin allergy.

Immunologic Effects

Penicillin can cause a number of immunopathologic states including anaphylaxis, urticaria, angioedema, immune hemolytic anemia, and serum sickness-like reactions. Serum sickness-like reactions (characterized by fever, rash, arthralgias, renal involvement and lymphadenopathy related to IgG, or IgM complexes) may begin 2–15 weeks after withdrawal of penicillin therapy. Most reactions are mild, resolve spontaneously in days to weeks, and respond to cessation of penicillin therapy.

IgE of minor determinant specificity is considered responsible for most episodes of penicillin anaphylaxis. Positive skin tests indicate a 41–67% chance that a clinically detectable reaction will occur, with up to 50% of reactions involving respiratory obstruction or hypotension. Patients without a history of penicillin allergy have a 7% or fewer incidence of positive skin tests. Clinical histories suggestive of IgE-mediated reactions yield a 17–46% positive skin test rate.

If penicillin is considered the drug of choice in the face of positive skin test, oral desensitization done safely and effectively may be indicated. The 6-aminopenicillanic nucleus of the penicillin molecule is antigenic and is present in all semisynthetic penicillins. Therefore, a person with a history of an allergic response to "penicillin" is assumed allergic to all penicillins.

Hematologic Effects

Hemolytic anemia rarely occurs. A positive Coombs test will develop in approximately 3% of patients receiving large doses (10–20 million units per day) of intravenous penicillin. Only a small percentage of these reactors actually develop hemolytic anemia. Penicillin therapy should not be discontinued merely because of the development of a positive direct Coombs test, since clinically significant hemolysis may not develop. Neutropenia and leukopenia are seen in 1–4% of patients using penicillin or semisynthetic penicillins. Immunologically mediated thrombocytopenia and pancytopenia have been reported.

Renal Effects

Nephritis in serum sickness-like reactions may develop into acute renal failure with anuria after a single dose of penicillin. Acute interstitial nephritis is seen in 1–2% of patients receiving methicillin, mezlocillin, carbenicillin, nafcillin sodium, ampicillin, and oxacillin.

Dermatologic Effects

Dermatologic effects represent the most frequent category of side effects from penicillins. Ampicillin therapy has been associated with a higher incidence (5–10%) of maculopapular rash compared with the other penicillins (approximately 2%). Other cutaneous states including erythema multiforme, Stevens-Johnson syndrome, exfoliative dermatitis, epidermal necrolysis, erythema nodosum, and cutaneous necrotizing angiitis have been reported. Maculopapular eruptions may occur during penicillin therapy as part of serum sickness-like reaction.

Metabolic Effects

Sodium overload and hypokalemia have followed treatment with carbenicillin. Potassium penicillin G has been associated with hyperkalemia, ventricular fibrillation, and asystole.

Gastrointestinal Effects

Elevated aspartate aminotransferase is observed in 1–4% of patients and most frequently in those receiving oxacillin, nafcillin, or carbenicillin. Diarrhea is seen in up to 25% of patients receiving ampicillin. Pseudomembranous colitis has been rarely reported with oral penicillin V.

Neurologic Effects

Central nervous system toxicity in the form of myoclonic seizures can follow massive doses of penicillin G, ampicillin, carbenicillin, or methicillin. Direct application of penicillin to the cortex will provoke seizure activity. Intrathecal penicillin or its derivatives are rarely used for meningitis in view of its history of neurotoxicity. Penicillin neurotoxicity should be suspected if a patient exhibits myoclonic jerks, hyperreflexia, a decreasing level of consciousness, lethargy, irritability, confusion, clonus, hallucinations, impaired memory, seizures, or electroencephalogram abnormalities after massive doses of penicillin.

Inadvertent intra-arterial injections intragluteally or intramuscularly in the thigh may result in occlusion, thrombosis, and severe neurovascular damage. Transverse myelopathy has been reported with permanent paralysis and gangrene requiring amputation of digits, necrosis, and sloughing at and surrounding the injection site.

TOXIC DOSAGE/DEATH

There is no correlation between penicillin reactivity and personal or familial history of allergy. Most deaths from penicillin anaphylaxis have occurred in persons with no history of allergy. Seizures are observed with cerebrospinal fluid penicillin levels over 12 U/mL. Cerebrospinal fluid levels with no risk of seizures are usually below 7.8 U/mL.

DRUG INTERACTIONS

High concentrations of carbenicillin and ticarcillin will inactivate aminoglycosides *in vitro* in the same syringe or intravenous infusion container. This may also occur *in vivo* when renal impairment permits high concentrations of drugs to accumulate. Antibacterial activity may be additive or synergistic when penicillins are used with cephalosporins. The bactericidal activity of penicillins *in vitro* may be antagonized when used concomitantly with chloramphenicol, erythromycin, or tetracycline.

Penicillin V or ampicillin may decrease the efficacy of oral contraceptives and increase the incidence of breakthrough bleeding. The serum half-life of penicillin G may be increased when used with nonsteroidal antiinflammatory drugs such as indomethacin, and salicylates. Hyperkalemia may be seen when penicillin G potassium is used with potassium-sparing drugs. Concomitant use with probenecid causes higher and prolonged serum concentrations of penicillin.

PREGNANCY/LACTATION

Penicillin passes through the placenta and is found in small quantities in breast milk. Pregnancy risk category B.

LABORATORY

Analytic Methods

Penicillin may be detected by high-pressure liquid chromatography.

Blood Levels

Blood levels are rarely indicated in managing overdoses by these agents. Penicillins may interfere with urine, cerebrospinal fluid, or serum proteins, urinary glucose, and urine specific gravity. They may increase serum uric acid falsely and cause a positive direct antiglobulin (Coombs') test.

TREATMENT

Gut Decontamination

Gut decontamination procedures are rarely required, since large ingestions of oral penicillin-type drugs are usually nontoxic. Gastric lavage and/or instillation of activated charcoal with endotracheal intubation is safe, and possibly useful, in treating the rare convulsing patient or comatose individual known to have recently ingested large quantities of penicillins.

Elimination Enhancement

Forced diuresis may increase excretion of penicillins; however, caution is required in view of potential alterations in electrolyte balance. Where severe overdosage has occurred and renal impairment exists, hemodialysis may be considered. Peritoneal dialysis is of little value in removing most penicillins.

Supportive Measures

- Supportive measures generally suffice, as most overdoses are inconsequential and nontoxic.
- Seizures may be managed with intravenous diazepam (adults, 5–10 mg, repeated every 15 minutes as required and children, 0.25 mg/kg every 2–5 minutes to a total of 10 mg). If seizures cannot be controlled, phenytoin, phenobarbital or even general anesthesia may be required.
- Penicillin is the most common cause of drug-induced serum sickness. In these cases, discontinue penicillin immediately. Oral diphenhydramine every 4 hours may be used for generalized pruritus or urticaria. Aspirin or nonsteroidal antiinflammatory drugs may be used for pain or fever. Corticosteroids, such as 60 mg of prednisone or equivalent, may be given orally for fever with arthralgias or proteinuria.
- Anaphylaxis may be lethal. Immediate attention to an adequate airway is vital. Anaphylaxis, manifested by angioedema, respiratory failure, and/or hypotension may require intravenous saline and aqueous epinephrine 1:1,000 (adult and child, 0.01 mL/kg per dose subcutaneously to a maximum dose of 0.5 mL. Repeat as needed every 10-20 minutes for three to four doses or begin continuous drip). If vascular collapse has occurred, 5 mL of a 1:10,000 solution of epinephrine can be administered intravenously. Pressor amines such as dopamine or norepinephrine may be required.
- Allergic phenomena such as angioedema, hoarseness, or dysphagia suggestive of laryngeal edema may require 0.3–0.5 mL of aqueous epinephrine 1:1,000 subcutaneously together with diphenhydramine 50 mg i.v. The dose of epinephrine may be repeated every 15 minutes in view of its short half-life, and may be given as a drip in severe cases.
- Management of acute interstitial nephritis includes immediate cessation of penicillin. Hemodialysis and steroids may be required in severe cases. The prognosis is generally good.
- Monitor electrolytes, electrocardiogram, urinalysis, serum creatinine, blood urea nitrogen, and complete blood count. Observe for cardiac effects of hyperkalemia.

Questions—Penicillins

1. Which of the following is false?
A. Large ingestions of oral penicillin-type drugs are usually nontoxic.
B. All penicillins contain a 6-aminopenicillanic acid nucleus that is composed of a β-lactam ring fused to a five-member thiazolidine ring.
C. Penicillins are bacteriostatic.
D. Penicillin can cause a number of immunopathologic states including anaphylaxis, urticaria, angioedema and immune hemolytic anemia.
E. Serum sickness-like reactions may begin 2–15 weeks after withdrawal of penicillin therapy.

2. Which of the following is false?
A. Immediate hypersensitivity reactions occur in about 1–10% of patients treated with penicillin.
B. Anaphylactic shock from penicillin is the most common cause of anaphylaxis.
C. Anaphylactic reactions occur more often when penicillin is ingested but may occur after i.v. or i.m. use.
D. Sex, race, and histocompatibility leukocyte antigen (HLA) phenotype do not appear to affect the incidence of penicillin allergy.
E. Acute interstitial nephritis may be seen after penicillin use.

3. Central nervous system toxicity due to penicillin in the form of myoclonic seizures
A. Can follow any dose of intravenous penicillin
B. Can follow massive doses of penicillin G
C. Is not associated with penicillin use
D. Occurs more frequently when penicillins are used with aminoglycosides.
E. None of the above

4. Which of the following is the most common category of side effects caused by penicillins?
A. Jaundice
B. Thrombocytopenia or hemolytic anemia
C. Rash
D. Anaphylaxis
E. Serum sickness

Cephalosporins

Cephalosporins are semisynthetic antibiotics derived from cephalosporin C, a natural antibiotic produced by the mold Cephalosporium acremonium. The active nucleus is 7-aminocephalosporanic acid, which is closely related to the penicillin nucleus, 6-aminopenicillanic acid. Cross-reactivity between the cephalosporins and the penicillins has been reported. It has been estimated that 1–5% of patients who have had an adverse response to penicillins will have one from cephalosporins. Patients known to have had an anaphylactic reaction to penicillin should avoid cephalosporins. Those who have had a delayed-type reaction (e.g., rash, fever, and eosinophilia) to penicillin should use cephalosporins with caution. Overdoses with cephalosporin are rare.

PATHOPHYSIOLOGY

Cephalosporins are bactericidal and act by inhibiting synthesis of the bacterial cell wall. Compounds with an N-methylthiotetrazole (NMTT) side chain (such as moxalactam, cefotetan, cefoperazone, cefmetazole or cefamandole) have been associated with a higher incidence of bleeding. Free NMTT inhibits vitamin K epoxide reductase, thus interfering with the carboxylation of several factors in the coagulation cascade.

PHARMACOKINETICS

Absorption

- The peak serum concentration is generally achieved 0.5–1.5 hours with these agents.
- They are generally well absorbed from the gastrointestinal tract.

Distribution

- The volume of distribution of cephalosporins generally ranges from 0.1–0.4 L/kg.

Elimination

- Cefadroxil, cefazolin, cephalexin, cephradine, cefaclor, cefuroxime, and ceftizoxime are not metabolized.
- Cephalothin and cefotaxime are partially metabolized in the liver and kidneys to desacetyl metabolites that also have antibacterial activity.

CLINICAL PRESENTATIONS

Large doses of cephalosporins do not appear to induce severe toxicity. Experience with therapeutic use of cephalosporins indicates that adverse effects may occur in the course of use.

Gastrointestinal Effects

Nausea, vomiting, and diarrhea are the most frequent reactions to oral cephalosporins. Abdominal pain, tenesmus, dyspepsia, glossitis, and heartburn may be seen. Intramuscular or intravenous cephalosporins may also cause adverse gastrointestinal effects.

Renal Effects

Nephrotoxicity is rarely observed with cephalosporins, but may occur in those with diminished renal function, those over age 50, and those taking other nephrotoxic drugs.

Hematologic Effects

Cephalosporins may have several adverse effects, including hemolytic anemia, neutropenia, thrombocytopenia, and coagulation defects. Coagulopathies have been associated with the use of moxalactam, cefazolin, cefoperazone, cefmetazole, cefamandole, and cefmenoxime. Neutropenia, probably immune-mediated, has been associated with cephalothin, cefotaxime, cephradine, and cefonicid. Occasionally, transient thrombocytosis and eosinophilia may occur.

Hypersensitivity Effects

Reactions have occurred in some patients receiving cephalosporins including urticaria, pruritus, rash, fever, chills, reactions resembling serum sickness, joint pain, angioedema, exfoliative dermatitis, and, rarely, anaphylaxis.

Neurologic Effects

Drowsiness, coma, convulsions, reversible confusional states, hallucinations, and delirium have been reported after large doses of cephalosporins, especially in those with renal failure. Intrathecal administration of large doses has resulted in hallucinations, nystagmus, and seizures.

DRUG INTERACTIONS

Disulfiram-like reactions may occur when alcohol is ingested within 48–72 hours in patients taking cephalosporins containing a methyltetrazolethiol side chain such as cefamandole, cefoperazone, and moxalactam. Nausea, vomiting, flushing, headache, and hypotension manifest the reaction. Simultaneous administration of oral probenecid competitively inhibits tubular secretion, resulting in higher and more prolonged serum concentrations of cephalosporins.

Concurrent use of nephrotoxic agents such as aminoglycosides, colistin, polymyxin B or vancomycin may increase the risk of nephrotoxicity associated with many cephalosporins. Similar nephrotoxic changes may be potentiated by concurrent use of rapid-acting diuretics, such as furosemide and ethacrynic acid. High-dose heparin, oral anticoagulants, and other drugs that affect hemostasis (such as aspirin) may increase the risk of hemorrhage with moxalactam.

PREGNANCY/LACTATION
Cephalosporins cross the placenta and are found in low concentrations in breast milk.

LABORATORY

Analytic Methods
These agents may be detected with high-pressure liquid chromatography.

Blood Levels
Plasma levels of cephalosporins are confirmatory of their presence but not otherwise useful.

TREATMENT

Gut Decontamination
Gastric lavage with tracheal protection may be indicated after oral overdose; however, there is no evidence that activated charcoal or cathartics are effective in cephalosporin overdose.

Elimination Enhancement
Peritoneal dialysis or hemodialysis may be effective (low apparent volume of distribution), but insufficient evidence to support their use has been documented.

Supportive Measures
- Coagulopathies can be treated with vitamin K. For patients with hypoprothrombinemia but without apparent bleeding, a single 10-mg dose of vitamin K administered subcutaneously will cause the prothrombin time to return to baseline rapidly (usually within several hours).
- If the drugs have a methylthiotetrazole substitution, the defect may continue for 24–36 hours after administration of vitamin K. Active bleeding may require fresh frozen plasma.
- Hypersensitivity reactions are managed with attention to airway, epinephrine, antihistamines, and pressor agents, if indicated (see Penicillins section above). Since many cephalosporins are excreted into the urine, the patient should be well hydrated.
- Laboratory studies in a suspected overdose should include liver function tests, blood urea nitrogen, serum creatinine, urinalysis, prothrombin time, platelet count, partial thromboplastin time, fibrinogen levels, fibrin split products, bleeding time, platelet aggregation tests, and complete blood count.
- Positive direct and indirect antiglobulin (Coombs) tests have been reported in some patients receiving cephalosporins. This may interfere with hematologic studies or transfusion cross-matching procedures.

Questions—Cephalosporins

1. Cephalosporins are derived from
A. Bacteria
B. Mold
C. Amoebae
D. Penicillin
E. Stem cells

2. Cephalosporins
A. Interfere with bacterial DNA replication
B. Interfere with protein synthesis
C. Destroy endoplasmic reticulum
D. Inhibit synthesis of the bacterial cell wall
E. Bind to protoplasmic glycoproteins

3. Cephalosporins may yield several adverse hematologic effects including
A. Hemolytic anemia
B. Neutropenia
C. Thrombocytopenia
D. Coagulation defects
E. All of the above

4. Disulfiram-like reactions have been associated with the concomitant use of certain cephalosporins and alcohol.
A. True
B. False

5. It has been estimated that _____ % of patients who have had an adverse response to penicillins will have one from cephalosporins.
A. 0
B. 1–5
C. 10
D. 15
E. 20

Imipenem

Imipenem (Primaxin®) is the first of the carbapenems, a newer class of β-lactam antibiotics. Imipenem is an antibiotic produced by Streptomyces cattelya. It is marketed in combination with cilastatin, a nonantibiotic enzyme inhibitor that prevents the breakdown of imipenem to nephrotoxic metabolites. The combination is available only for intravenous use.

PATHOPHYSIOLOGY
Imipenem inhibits bacterial wall synthesis by binding to penicillin binding proteins.

PHARMACOKINETICS

Absorption
- Bioavailability is less than 5%.
- Peak plasma level is 14–80 mg / mL after 250 mg to 1 gram i.v.

Distribution
- Volume of distribution is 0.22 L / kg (0.33 L / kg in children).

Elimination
- The elimination half-life is 0.8–1.2 hours.
- Five to 40% is excreted unchanged.

CLINICAL PRESENTATIONS
Imipenem should be administered with caution to patients known to be hypersensitive to other β-lactam antibiotics because

of the possibility of cross-reactivity. The most common adverse effects are phlebitis or pain at the site of infusion, nausea, and vomiting. Seizures have been reported in up to 5% of patients. Seizures generally begin about 7 days after the onset of therapy. As with other β-lactam antibiotics, central nervous system lesions are strong risk factors for seizures. In addition, more than recommended doses, particularly in patients with renal insufficiency, are associated with an increased risk of seizures.

TOXIC DOSAGE/DEATH
A toxic or lethal dose has not been established.

DRUG INTERACTIONS
There is increased efficacy and/or toxicity when used with probenecid. Use of theophylline and/or ganciclovir may potentiate seizures.

PREGNANCY/LACTATION
Pregnancy risk category C.

LABORATORY

Analytic Methods
Imipenem may be detected by high-pressure liquid chromatography.

Blood Levels
Following imipenem levels in overdose has not been demonstrated to help guide therapy.

TREATMENT

Gut Decontamination
Reduction of potentially elevated serum levels may be afforded by prompt gastric emptying. Charcoal may be a useful adjunct in significant overdose; however, its use has not been studied.

Elimination Enhancement
Use of dialysis has not been tested in imipenem overdose.

Supportive Measures
- Cautions must be taken for the potential of seizures in overdose.

Questions—Imipenem

1. Which of the following is false?

A. Imipenem is an antibiotic produced by Streptomyces cattelya.

B. Imipenem is marketed in combination with cilastatin, a nonantibiotic enzyme inhibitor that prevents the breakdown of imipenem to nephrotoxic metabolites.

C. Imipenem inhibits bacterial wall synthesis by binding to penicillin binding proteins.

D. Imipenem should be administered with caution to patients known to be hypersensitive to other β-lactam antibiotics because of the possibility of cross-reactivity.

E. Unlike penicillins, seizures have not been associated with the use of imipenem.

Aztreonam

Aztreonam (Azactam®) is the first synthetic monobactam to be marketed in the U.S. Aztreonam differs from penicillins and cephalosporins in having a monocyclic rather than a bicyclic nucleus.

PATHOPHYSIOLOGY
The mode of action of aztreonam is similar to that of the β-lactams. It has a high affinity for a penicillin-binding protein found in Gram-negative bacteria and interferes with synthesis of the bacterial cell wall.

PHARMACOKINETICS

Absorption
- The bioavailability of aztreonam is about 100% after i.m. injection, and only 1% after oral use.
- Time to peak plasma level is 1 hour.

Distribution
- Volume of distribution is 0.21 L/kg.
- Plasma protein binding is 56%.

Elimination
- Elimination half-life is 1.6 hours.
- 1-7% is excreted unchanged.

CLINICAL PRESENTATIONS
The most frequently reported undesired effects after intravenous or intramuscular use have been local reactions to injections, skin rash or pruritus, nausea, vomiting, and diarrhea. Aztreonam has little cross-allergenicity with penicillins and cephalosporins. Clostridium difficile pseudomembranous colitis may develop. Bone marrow suppression has been observed and seizures may be associated with very high doses and in patients with diminished renal function.

TOXIC DOSAGE/DEATH
A toxic or lethal dose of aztreonam has not been established.

PREGNANCY/LACTATION
Pregnancy risk category B.

LABORATORY

Analytic Methods
Aztreonam levels are not routinely obtained in hospital labs. They may be determined by high-pressure liquid chromatography.

Blood Levels
Following aztreonam levels in overdose is not helpful in guiding therapy.

TREATMENT

Gut Decontamination
Gastric lavage, activated charcoal, and cathartics have not yet been evaluated in aztreonam overdose. As there may be a clinical concern about possible seizure development, in certain cases syrup of ipecac is not advisable.

Elimination Enhancement
In view of the moderate degree of protein binding (56%) and the low volume of distribution (0.21 L/kg), it would appear useful to initiate hemodialysis or hemoperfusion to accelerate elimination of aztreonam from the serum if clinically indicated.

Supportive Measures

- Cautions must be taken for the potential of seizures in overdose.

Questions—Aztreonam

1. **Which of the following about aztreonam is false?**
   A. Cross-reactivity with penicillins is common.
   B. A lethal dose has not been established.
   C. Myelosuppression and pseudomembranous colitis have been associated with its use.
   D. It interferes with synthesis of the bacterial cell wall.
   E. Following aztreonam levels in overdose is not helpful in guiding therapy.

MACROLIDES

Erythromycin

Poisoning with erythromycin is rare. Adverse effects are infrequent, and significant toxicity with acute overdoses is unusual. Although erythromycin is considered one of the safest antibiotics known, hepatotoxicity and ototoxicity have been reported. Erythromycin is produced from Streptomyces erythraeus. The erythromycin base is poorly soluble in water, is rapidly inactivated by gastric acid, and is inconsistently absorbed after oral administration. Erythromycin consists of a macrocyclic lactone ring or macrolide attached to two sugar moieties.

A number of preparations of erythromycin have been developed to diminish destruction by gastric acid and to promote better absorption. At least six preparations for oral use are available. These include enteric-coated tablets, enteric-coated pellets and "film"-coated tablets of the base; stearate salts; ethylsuccinate ester and lauryl sulfate salts of the propionyl ester (the estolate). There are two preparations for intravenous use, lactobionate and gluceptate. Intramuscular administration is avoided because of severe pain. Erythromycin is also available as an ophthalmic ointment and in topical preparations.

PATHOPHYSIOLOGY

Erythromycin interferes with bacterial protein synthesis by reversibly binding to the 50S ribosomal subunit in bacterial RNA, resulting in blockage of transpeptidation reactions.

PHARMACOKINETICS

Absorption

- Erythromycin base is absorbed intact. Erythromycin stearate is absorbed as the base.
- The esters and ester salts of erythromycin are relatively acid stable, form a stable suspension in water, and are tasteless. They are absorbed more completely in the fasting state.
- Erythromycin ethylsuccinate is absorbed as the intact ester and free base after intestinal hydrolysis.
- Absorption of oral erythromycin occurs mostly in the duodenum.
- Its bioavailability depends on the specific erythromycin derivative, the formulation, the acid stability, the presence of food in the gastrointestinal tract, and the gastric emptying time.

Distribution

- Erythromycin is distributed throughout the total body water to all tissues. All tissues except the brain, middle ear, prostate, and eye have higher erythromycin concentrations than the serum.
- Erythromycin is concentrated in the liver and bile.
- The apparent volume of distribution is 0.72 L/kg.
- Protein binding approximates 75%.

Elimination

- Erythromycin is partly metabolized by demethylation in the liver.
- Up to 4.5% of an oral dose and 15% of an intravenous dose are recoverable in the urine, but elimination is mainly by biliary excretion of the intact drug.
- The serum half-life in normal subjects is 2 hours and in anuric subjects is 4–6 hours.
- Dosage reduction in patients with renal failure is usually not necessary.

CLINICAL PRESENTATIONS

Erythromycin is among the safest antibiotics in use, and life-threatening effects are rare. Overdosage and poisoning have rarely been reported in the medical literature.

Gastrointestinal Effects

Abdominal pain, cramps, nausea, vomiting, diarrhea, and flatulence are most frequently associated with both oral and intravenous erythromycin use and are dose related, especially with doses in excess of 4 grams per day. Cholestatic hepatitis has occurred after use of the estolate preparation and is characterized by nausea, vomiting, abdominal pain, jaundice, fever, abnormal liver function tests with or without rash, leukocytosis, and eosinophilia. This syndrome clears in a few days to weeks after the drug is stopped. The hepatitis appears to be a hypersensitivity reaction. Pancreatitis has been described. Pseudomembranous colitis is rare. Superinfection of the gastrointestinal tract or vagina with Candida species or Gram-negative bacilli may occur.

Cardiovascular Effects

QT prolongation and Torsade de Pointes may occur with intravenous administration of erythromycin. Susceptibility seems to be related to electrolyte alterations such as hypokalemia, hypocalcemia, and hypomagnesemia, myocardial ischemia, left ventricular dysfunction, hepatic dysfunction or immaturity, and concomitant use of certain drugs. See Drug Interactions below. Hypotension may be observed after both intravenous and oral administration. Thrombophlebitis has been reported with intravenous use.

Ototoxic Effects

Ototoxicity is rarely associated with large oral or intravenous doses of erythromycin, more commonly in elderly patients with renal failure, and is apparently related to high serum concentrations of the drug. Ototoxicity is temporary and goes away after the antibiotic is stopped because actual nerve damage does not occur.

Hypersensitivity Effects

Skin rash, Stevens-Johnson syndrome, fixed drug eruptions, and eosinophilia have occasionally been described.

TOXIC DOSAGE/DEATH

A lethal dose of erythromycin has not been established. Toxic blood levels in overdosage have not been defined.

DRUG INTERACTIONS

Erythromycin can interact with many other drugs through the cytochrome P450 enzyme system. It can increase blood levels of fentanyl, carbamazepine, clozapine, colchicine, cyclosporine, digoxin, ergotamine, midazolam, nadolol, theophylline, triazolam, valproic acid, vinblastine, and warfarin. Concomitant use of erythromycin with astemizole (Hismanal®) or terfenadine (Seldane®) was associated with serious ventricular arrhythmias, Torsade de Pointes, and rash. Their manufacturers have discontinued both of these products.

Erythromycin may itself cause action potential prolongation by altering sodium channel function, similar to class IA and III antiarrhythmic agents. Erythromycin increases the effect of theophylline, oral anticoagulants, digoxin, and carbamazepine. It is known to decrease the effect of clindamycin, lincomycin, and penicillin.

PREGNANCY/LACTATION

Erythromycin crosses the placental barrier. It is found in breast milk in concentrations as high as 50% of those seen in plasma. Pregnancy risk factor B.

LABORATORY

Analytic Methods

Blood levels are not generally available and have not been used to establish a correlation with therapeutic or toxic response.

Blood Levels

Therapeutic blood levels are about 1.0–2.0 μg/mL. Peak blood levels of 0.1–1.9 μg/mL are obtained 3–4 hours after a single oral therapeutic dose, and levels of 3–10 μg/mL follow 1 hour after a single intravenous dose.

TREATMENT

Gut Decontamination

Gastric lavage and cathartics may be useful, but their efficacy has not been established. Activated charcoal probably is useful in reducing the amount of drug absorbed after an oral overdose, but its role in altering outcome is unknown.

Elimination Enhancement

Hemodialysis or peritoneal dialysis does not significantly remove the drug. Hemoperfusion (charcoal or resin) is not indicated. The value of exchange transfusion has not been established.

Supportive Measures

- General measures include monitoring of cardiovascular status and monitoring labs such as electrolytes, liver function tests, and kidney function tests. If liver toxicity is evident by clinical exam or laboratory tests (alanine aminotransferase, aspartate aminotransferase, bilirubin, and alkaline phosphatase), withdrawal of the drug should be sufficient to ameliorate hepatotoxic effects with no permanent sequelae.
- Audiograms may help assess rare instances of hearing loss. This occurs after erythromycin lactobionate is administered parenterally and is usually reversible on withdrawal of the drug.
- Intravenous erythromycin should be infused over at least 60 minutes, with cardiovascular monitoring in premature newborns and patients with cardiovascular disease. If QT prolongation or any form of ventricular arrhythmias is detected, the infusion should be promptly discontinued. Patients may experience QT prolongation, ventricular arrhythmias or hypotension.
- Lidocaine (1.0–1.5 mg/kg intravenous bolus) may be used to treat erythromycin-induced ventricular tachycardia or fibrillation.
- In the group of patients with Torsade de Pointes, magnesium sulfate is the drug of choice. The adult dose is 2.0 grams as an intravenous bolus in unstable patients.
- Erythromycin may cause false elevations in concentrations or urinary catecholamines, 17-hydroxycorticosteroids, and 17-ketosteroids and may interfere with colorimetric assays for alanine and aspartate aminotransferase concentrations.

Questions—Erythromycin

1. Which of the following is true regarding erythromycins (macrolides)?
- A. Their most common side effect is deafness, which is rare.
- B. They freely cross the blood-brain barrier.
- C. The stearate form of erythromycin is more toxic than the ethylsuccinate form because it is absorbed better.
- D. The most common side effect is superinfection by Gram-negative rods or fungi.
- E. Most of an administered dose is metabolized in tissues or the liver before renal excretion.

2. Which of the following is a side effect of erythromycins?
- A. Prolongation of the QT interval.
- B. Hemolytic uremic syndrome.
- C. Seizures.
- D. Myonecrosis.
- E. Renal failure.

3. How does erythromycin increase levels of most other medications with which it interacts?
- A. Competition with enzymes in the hepatic cytochrome P450 system.
- B. Induction of the cytochrome P450 system, leading to higher levels of toxic metabolites.
- C. Competition for binding sites on albumin.
- D. Competition for renal excretion mechanisms.
- E. Induction of acid production by the stomach, allowing for better absorption.

Azithromycin and Clarithromycin

Azithromycin (Zithromax®), clarithromycin (Biaxin®) and dirithromycin (Dynabac®) are antimicrobial macrolides similar to erythromycin. Azithromycin is a 15-membered macrolide compound referred to as an azalide, and clarithromycin is a 14-membered macrolide similar to erythromycin. Both azithromycin and clarithromycin are used as antimicrobial agents useful against atypical mycobacteria, toxoplasmosis and, possibly, Haemophilus influenzae. The spectrum of activity of dirithromycin is the same as the older erythromycin preparations, but its half-life is long enough to allow for once-a-day dosing.

PATHOPHYSIOLOGY

Like other macrolides, these agents inhibit protein synthesis by binding to a component of the 50S subunit of the bacterial ribosome.

PHARMACOKINETICS

Absorption

- The oral bioavailability of azithromycin is 37%, and that of clarithromycin is 55-68%.

Distribution

- Azithromycin and clarithromycin distribute well into the lungs, sputum and tonsils, but poorly into the cerebrospinal fluid.

Elimination

- The elimination half-life of azithromycin is 11–14 hours, and that of clarithromycin is 4.9 hours.
- The biliary excretion of unchanged drug is the primary route of elimination of azithromycin.
- Twenty to 30% of clarithromycin is excreted unchanged in the urine.

CLINICAL PRESENTATIONS

Few reports of overdose with these compounds appear in the medical literature. Macrolide antibiotics can be associated with reversible hearing loss. Gastrointestinal side effects including diarrhea, nausea, abdominal pain, dyspepsia, vomiting or gastritis have been reported in 10–20% of clarithromycin-treated patients and 10% of azithromycin-treated patients (compared with 20–35% of patients treated with erythromycin).

TOXIC DOSAGE/DEATH

Toxic doses have not been established for these agents and deaths have not been reported.

DRUG INTERACTIONS

Magnesium or aluminum antacids decrease peak serum levels without affecting the extent of absorption of these agents. Clarithromycin may be associated with increased plasma levels of theophylline and carbamazepine.

PREGANCY/LACTATION

Azithromycin is pregnancy risk category B and clarithromycin is pregnancy risk category C.

LABORATORY

Analytic Methods

Blood levels are not generally available and have not been used to establish a correlation with therapeutic or toxic response.

Blood Levels

Following blood concentrations in overdose is not expected to be helpful.

TREATMENT

Gut Decontamination

Lavage and/or charcoal may be helpful; however, definitive studies demonstrating decreased morbidity with these agents have not been undertaken.

Elimination Enhancement

There is no experience with these methods in azithromycin or clarithromycin overdose.

Supportive Measures

- Treatment of an overdose is largely supportive and symptomatic.

Questions—Azithromycin and Clarithromycin

1. Like other macrolides, azithromycin and clarithromycin inhibit protein synthesis by binding to a component of the ____ subunit of the bacterial ribosome.
A. 30S
B. 40S
C. 50S
D. 60S
E. 80S

QUINOLONES AND FLUOROQUINOLONES

Nalidixic acid, the first quinolone antibacterial agent, was introduced in 1963. Because of its narrow antibacterial spectrum, frequent development of resistance, poor absorption from the gastrointestinal tract, and relatively high incidence of side effects, the use of nalidixic acid has been limited to lower urinary tract infection caused by a few susceptible bacteria. Vomiting, seizures, hyperglycemia, benign intracranial hypertension, behavioral disturbances, and metabolic acidosis characterize acute toxicity resulting from overdose.

Fluoroquinolones are broad-spectrum antiinfective agents active against a wide range of aerobic Gram-positive and Gram-negative organisms. Levofloxacin (Levaquin®), norfloxacin (Norflox®), ciprofloxacin (Cipro®), and ofloxacin are a few of the fluoroquinolones currently approved for use in the U.S. Another quinolone, trovafloxacin (Trovan®), was removed after reports of hepatic injury.

These agents have been effective in treating upper and lower respiratory tract infections, and infections of the urinary tract, gastrointestinal tract, skin, soft tissues and bone. The quinolones and fluoroquinolones may induce undesirable effects relating to the gastrointestinal tract and central nervous system. Infrequent allergic reactions and cartilage erosions in weight-bearing joints have been reported.

PATHOPHYSIOLOGY

Quinolones inhibit DNA-gyrase in susceptible organisms. All fluoroquinolones are gamma-aminobutyric acid (GABA) inhibitors and may cause seizures.

PHARMACOKINETICS

Absorption

- Nalidixic acid is absorbed almost entirely from the gastrointestinal tract, with peak plasma concentrations of 20–50 mg/mL reported 2 hours after 1 gram has been ingested.
- The absorption of norfloxacin is 35–70%; that of ciprofloxacin is 75–85%, and that of ofloxacin is 70–80%.

Distribution

- The protein binding of nalidixic acid is 90%, that of norfloxacin is 15%, that of ciprofloxacin is 20–40%, and that of ofloxacin is 10–20%.
- The volume of distribution of ciprofloxacin is 2.1–3.5 L/kg.

Elimination

- Nalidixic acid has an elimination half-life of 1 to 2 hours, and is excreted as both the parent compound (5%) and the active metabolite hydroxynalidixic acid (95%). Nearly all of a dose is excreted within 24 hours.

Toxic Dosage/Death

A patient who ingested 8 grams of trimethoprim survived. There is no known lethal dose of trimethoprim or TMP-SMX. Deaths following TMP-SMX ingestion have been due to drug-induced hemolytic anemia, toxic epidermal necrolysis, and anaphylaxis.

Drug Interactions

Trimethoprim appears to inhibit the hepatic metabolism of phenytoin. It also decreases the renal clearance of procainamide. TMP-SMX should be used with caution with methotrexate, as sulfonamides can displace methotrexate from plasma protein binding sites.

Pregancy/Lactation

Trimethoprim readily crosses the placenta and is found in breast milk. Sulfamethoxazole also crosses the placenta and appears in breast milk. Trimethoprim is pregnancy risk category C and sulfonamides are pregnancy risk category B.

Laboratory

ANALYTIC METHODS

Trimethoprim may be quantitated in the serum by a high-performance liquid chromatographic (HPLC) method. Simultaneous measurement of trimethoprim and sulfamethoxazole is available by HPLC as well.

BLOOD LEVELS

A peak serum concentration of about 1 μg/mL is reached 1–4 hours after an oral dose. A single dose of trimethoprim 160 mg and sulfamethoxazole 800 mg produces peak serum concentrations of 1-2 μg/mL trimethoprim and 36-40 μg/mL sulfamethoxazole in 1–4 hours. The serum trimethoprim concentration after ingestion of 8 grams was 19.6 μg/mL. A suicide following trimethoprim overdose had a blood level of 133 μg/mL postmortem. It is unclear what dose of trimethoprim was ingested.

Treatment

GUT DECONTAMINATION

Gastric emptying, if performed within a few hours of ingestion, may aid in removing some of these drugs and prevent rapid induction of toxic serum levels. Activated charcoal has been used, but its efficacy, as well as that of cathartics, has not been studied.

ELIMINATION ENHANCEMENT

Acidification of the urine may enhance the elimination of trimethoprim but is generally not recommended. Hemodialysis may remove only moderate amounts of trimethoprim in view of its protein binding and large volume of distribution.

SUPPORTIVE MEASURES

- For most patients with trimethoprim or TMP-SMX overdose, symptomatic and supportive treatment is indicated. If patients are asymptomatic and able to eat without difficulty, they can be discharged to be followed as outpatients. Patients should be hospitalized in severe cases where cardiac monitoring, intravenous fluids, and oxygen, if required, are available.
- Anaphylaxis and allergic reactions may require epinephrine, fluids, and steroids based on clinical presentation.
- Patients should be followed for any evidence of hematologic depression both in hospital and as outpatients in the following weeks. Hematologic evaluation may require bone marrow in certain cases according to clinical judgment.
- Seizures can be treated with diazepam.
- Electrolytes should be determined and adjusted together with adequate fluid replacement.
- Serum transaminase levels may be elevated after overdose with trimethoprim.

Questions—Trimethoprim and Trimethoprim Sulfamethoxazole

1. The most common side effect of sulfonamides is
   A. Seizures
   B. Renal failure
   C. Hepatic failure
   D. Rash
   E. Anaphylaxis

2. Which of the following statements about trimethoprim-sulfamethoxazole is true?
   A. Side effects are usually not seen with oral dosing because absorption is poor.
   B. Both components are mostly metabolized before renal excretion.
   C. Both components are mostly metabolized before hepatic excretion.
   D. The half-life can be tripled by the concurrent administration of probenecid.
   E. The cross-allergenicity with β-lactams is 5–10%.

3. In anaphylaxis due to trimethoprim or sulfonamides, which of the following may be given?
   A. Sodium bicarbonate, to alkalinize urine
   B. 0.1N hydrochloric acid, to acidify urine
   C. Phenytoin, to induce hepatic cytochrome P450 enzymes
   D. Leucovorin, to block further damage to alveolar cells
   E. Epinephrine, fluids, and (if necessary) steroids

VANCOMYCIN

Vancomycin (Vancocin®) is a bactericidal antibiotic that may induce acute renal failure in overdose. It has been associated with sensorineural hearing loss. Intravenous vancomycin is used in the treatment of potentially life-threatening Gram positive infections and to treat antibiotic-associated pseudomembranous colitis produced by Clostridium difficile.

Pathophysiology

Vancomycin inhibits bacterial cell wall synthesis by blocking the attachment of D-alanine-D-alanine in the transpeptidation step.

Pharmacokinetics

ABSORPTION

- Minimal absorption of vancomycin follows oral administration.

DISTRIBUTION

- The apparent volume of distribution is 0.39–0.92 L/kg.
- Protein binding has been reported to be 10–82%.

ELIMINATION

- Intravenous vancomycin is excreted 80–100% unchanged in the urine in the first 24 hours.
- The elimination half-life is 3–10 hours.
- Its serum half-life is directly proportional to the serum creatinine level.

Clinical Presentations

Vancomycin use commonly results in a "red man syndrome" or "red neck syndrome" associated with pruritus and an erythematous rash or flushing over the face, neck, upper chest, and arms. Hypotension may also occur. "Red man syndrome" may involve histamine release. Its severity may be related to the dose of vancomycin, rate of injection, or amount of endogenous histamine released. It may be prevented by pretreatment with antihistamines and by running an intravenous infusion slowly, over at least 60 minutes. "Red man syndrome" has also been reported following intravenous infusions of erythromycin, and rifampin.

Vancomycin in overdose may cause oliguria and acute renal failure. Rapid intravenous administration has been associated with cardiopulmonary arrest. Nephrotoxicity, a sensorineural hearing loss, toxic epidermal necrolysis, Clostridium difficile colitis, and hematologic depression characterized by leukopenia, neutropenia, and / or thrombocytopenia have followed vancomycin use.

Toxic Dosage/Death

An adult who received a total of 56 grams over 10 days developed acute renal failure and survived. A premature infant received three 12-mg doses of intravenous vancomycin and six 240-mg doses, and survived. A lethal dose has not been established.

Drug Interactions

Patients receiving concurrent vancomycin and aminoglycoside antibiotics are at substantial risk for nephrotoxicity. Other antibiotics such as amphotericin B, bacitracin, cisplatin, colistin, and polymyxin B, given systemically or topically, may add to renal toxicity as well. Intravenous vancomycin enhances the neuromuscular blockade of vecuronium.

Pregnancy/Lactation

Vancomycin has not been extensively studied in pregnant women or lactating mothers. One study of 10 pregnant women suggests that vancomycin use during the second and third trimesters of pregnancy does not produce sensorineural hearing loss or nephrotoxicity in the infant.

Laboratory

ANALYTIC METHODS

A high-performance liquid chromatography method is available that is sensitive to 1 mg / mL.

BLOOD LEVELS

The serum concentration following an intravenous dose reaches a peak of 15 mg / mL in 2 hours. Following serum concentrations is not helpful in overdose. In-hospital monitoring may be helpful in preventing ototoxicity or nephrotoxicity. Serum levels of 25–100 mg / mL have been associated with ototoxicity.

Treatment

GUT DECONTAMINATION

In the rare case of oral vancomycin misuse or overdose, gastric emptying within the first 2 hours may lessen the absorption of vancomycin. Multidose activated charcoal may reduce the absorption of an overdose of vancomycin when ingested or administered intravenously. There are no data on the use of cathartics or whole-bowel irrigation after an overdose of vancomycin.

ELIMINATION ENHANCEMENT

Continuous arteriovenous hemofiltration may aid in reducing elevated serum levels of vancomycin; however, routine use has not been justified by clinical studies. The drug is not appreciably removed by hemodialysis.

SUPPORTIVE MEASURES

- In significant overdoses, patients should be hospitalized where they can be monitored for fluid balance, electrolytes, renal function, hearing function, and hematologic status, especially white blood cells and platelets.
- Serial serum creatinine levels should be monitored, and urinalysis performed.
- Furosemide and dopamine may be used to increase urine flow.
- Hydroxyzine, 50 mg administered 2 hours before a vancomycin infusion, may be of value in mitigating the severity of symptoms in "red man syndrome." Pretreatment with an H1 blocker may be helpful as well. An infusion must be stopped if there is a clinically significant drop in blood pressure or if there is an onset of chest or muscle pain.
- Total white blood cell count, neutrophils, and platelets should be followed both in hospital and for several weeks after discharge.
- Contributing factors leading to ototoxicity are renal insufficiency, simultaneous use of other antibiotics, and a history of previous hearing loss. Patients should be followed with serial audiograms in significant overdoses.

Questions—Vancomycin

1. A common side effect of vancomycin is
   A. Clostridium difficile (pseudomembranous) colitis
   B. Leukopenia
   C. "Red man" or "red neck" syndrome
   D. Renal failure
   E. Seizures

2. Which of the following statements about vancomycin is true?
   A. Its most serious side effect is respiratory depression.
   B. Its serum half-life is directly proportional to the serum creatinine level.
   C. Serious side effects usually occur due to interactions with other medications.
   D. Overdoses or serious toxicity should be treated with steroids.
   E. Overdoses or serious toxicity should be treated with hemodialysis.

3. Which of the following about "red man" or "red neck" syndrome is true?
   A. It may be prevented by pretreatment with antihistamines.
   B. It is due to the induction of endogenous pyrogen (interleukin-1) production.

C. It is due to IgE antibodies that are already circulating in the bloodstream.
D. It is more common in patients with a history of atopy.
E. It is more common in patients with renal failure.

LEPROSTATIC DRUGS

Clofazimine

Clofazimine (Lamprene®) is a substituted iminophenazine dye that has been used since 1962 as an anti-leprosy drug. After prolonged use it may lead to abdominal pain, anorexia, vomiting, diarrhea, and weight loss. Death has followed development of serious gastrointestinal symptoms. Few overdoses have been reported. Treatment is symptomatic and supportive. Clofazimine is effective in the prevention and treatment of erythema nodosum leprosum reactions and is useful in the treatment of dapsone-resistant leprosy cases.

PATHOPHYSIOLOGY

Clofazimine may bind to mycobacterial DNA; however, the precise mechanism is unclear. It likely chelates intracellular iron with the simultaneous production of oxygen radicals.

PHARMACOKINETICS

Absorption

- Bioavailability is about 20%.
- Peak plasma level is 0.5–1.0 mg/mL.

Distribution

- Time to peak plasma level is 8-12 hours.

Elimination

- Elimination half-life is 70 days.
- 0.1% is excreted unchanged.

CLINICAL PRESENTATIONS

In general, clofazimine is well tolerated and virtually nontoxic. A reversible dose-related pink to brownish skin discoloration is the most commonly observed side effect of clofazimine. Discoloration of the sweat, hair, sputum, urine, and feces may occur. A bull's-eye retinopathy has been described. Conjunctival pigmentation has been described, and generalized retinal degeneration has been observed in a patient with AIDS. Clofazimine crystals may be found within the cytoplasm of alveolar macrophages.

Gastrointestinal Effects

A late syndrome, commencing in months or years in individuals on high dosage, may present with persistent diarrhea, loss of weight, abdominal pain, and may lead to death. This syndrome is often associated with the deposition of clofazimine crystals in the submucosa of the small intestine and in the mesenteric lymph nodes. Eosinophilic enteritis has also been described.

TOXIC DOSAGE/DEATH

An acute toxic or lethal dose has not been described.

DRUG INTERACTIONS

Clofazimine reduces rifampin absorption. Plasma levels of vitamin A appear to decrease with increased duration of treatment with clofazimine.

PREGNANCY/LACTATION

Clofazimine crosses the placenta and is present in breast milk. Infants may be pigmented at birth or from ingesting the drug in maternal milk. Three neonatal deaths have been reported in three pregnancies in which clofazimine was used. The cause of death was not determined. Pregnancy risk category C.

LABORATORY

Analytic Methods

A thin-layer chromatography method has a limit of detection of 5 ng/g.

Blood Levels

Blood levels of clofazimine are generally not available in community hospital settings. Blood levels may confirm the presence of clofazimine but are probably not useful in treating overdoses.

TREATMENT

Gut Decontamination

Gastric lavage and/or charcoal may be useful within the first 6–8 hours of ingestion.

Elimination Enhancement

There are no studies relating to enhancement of elimination of clofazimine.

Supportive Measures

- In prolonged clofazimine administration, liver function tests, kidney function tests, serum albumin, and fasting blood sugar levels should be determined at 3-month intervals.
- Funduscopic examination is advised every 4 months while a patient receives clofazimine.
- Radiologic abnormalities of the small bowel, particularly the ileum, may consist of alternating segments of constriction and dilation, cogency of the mucosal folds, and circumscribed "polypoid" areas with chronic use.

Questions—Clofazimine

1. Which of the following side effects have been observed with clofazimine?
A. Adrenal failure
B. Strongyloides stercoralis hyperinfection syndrome
C. Colonic polyposis
D. Reversible discoloration of the skin
E. Renal failure

Dapsone

Dapsone, a sulfone similar in structure to the sulfonamides, has been associated with a number of overdoses in children and adults in the United States and overseas. Dapsone poisoning may be associated with methemoglobinemia and sulfhemoglobinemia. Deep cyanosis, impairment of oxygen transport and oxygen delivery by red blood cells, and central nervous system dysfunction may occur. Treatment depends largely, but not consistently, on the use of repeated doses of activated charcoal and good supportive care. Methylene blue, possibly ascorbic acid, and the use of extracorporeal methods to rid the body of excess dapsone and its metabolites are measures that have yet to prove themselves unequivocally useful. Fatalities have been reported in spite of aggressive management.

Dapsone is the drug of choice for all forms of leprosy. It is usually used alone or in combination with rifampin plus clofazimine depending on the type of leprosy under treatment. It is also used to treat dermatitis herpetiformis. In conjunction with pyrimethamine, it may be useful for the suppression or prophylaxis of malaria caused by chloroquine-resistant Plasmodium falciparum when pyrimethamine-sulfadoxine cannot be used. Other indications for its use have included pyoderma gangrenosum, pustular psoriasis, and acne vulgaris.

PATHOPHYSIOLOGY

Dapsone interacts with hemoglobin to produce several pigmented compounds, among them methemoglobin, and sulfhemoglobin, and this leads to clinical cyanosis. Dapsone also interacts with the red cell stroma to produce lysis of red cells. All of the above effects are dose-dependent and may occur after large doses of dapsone in glucose-6-phosphate dehydrogenase normal individuals, or after smaller doses in those with severe glucose-6-phosphate dehydrogenase deficiency. Effects on hemoglobin and red cells decrease the oxygen-carrying capacity of the blood, and lead to alterations in brain metabolism. Ordinarily, such effects are mild and reversible (at blood levels under 20 μg/mL), but in overdose (over 400 mg), may be life-threatening.

Methemoglobinemia

In an overdose of an oxidant such as dapsone is introduced, excess methemoglobin is formed. Methemoglobinemia is caused by the oxidation of the ferrous iron (Fe^{2+}) in heme to ferric iron (Fe^{3+}). Ferric iron cannot carry oxygen or carbon dioxide. At least 90 products are known to produce methemoglobinemia.

Nicotinamide adenine dinucleotide (NADH)-dependent methemoglobin reductase catalyzes the reduction of methemoglobin back to hemoglobin. Nicotinamide adenine dinucleotide phosphate (NADPH)-dependent methemoglobin reductase, usually inactive, becomes active when methemoglobin rises over 1–2%. NADH methemoglobin reductase remains of paramount importance for the reconversion of methemoglobin to hemoglobin.

The red cell relies on glycolysis and the hexose monophosphate shunt for its energy supply. In the hexose monophosphate shunt, NADPH is produced which reduces oxidants that cause hemolytic anemias and Heinz body formation. Normally, this system results in a daily turnover of 1–2% of total red blood cell hemoglobin to methemoglobin. Methylene blue (see Antidotes below) accelerates the NADPH-dependent methemoglobin reductase reaction.

Sulfhemoglobinemia

Sulfhemoglobinemia develops after a sulfur atom displaces one of the nitrogen atoms in the pyrrole ring of the hemoglobin molecule. It is present normally in very small amounts (0.5% of total blood volume). Unlike methemoglobin, there is no mechanism for its reconversion to hemoglobin. It is irreversible and remains for the life of the red blood cell. Methylene blue has no effect on sulfhemoglobinemia. The hypoxia resulting is seldom life-threatening. In dapsone overdosage, sulfhemoglobin may increase on the fourth day and is associated with continued cyanosis even after methemoglobin levels have returned to nontoxic levels.

PHARMACOKINETICS

Absorption

- Dapsone is well-absorbed from the gastrointestinal tract.
- Peak blood levels are reached about 2–6 hours after ingestion.

Distribution

- The volume of distribution is 1–2 L/kg, indicating diffusion through the total body water.
- At physiologic pH, the drug is highly lipid soluble, and this favors transport across membranes.
- It is about 73% bound to plasma proteins and its main metabolite, monoacetyldapsone, is nearly 100% protein bound.
- Dapsone may be detected in tissues up to 3 weeks after treatment has been terminated.

Elimination

- Dapsone undergoes acetylation in the liver to a monoacetyl derivative, its major metabolite, and a diacetyl derivative.
- The acetylation of dapsone is subject to genetic polymorphism. Approximately 72% of individuals are rapid acetylators.
- The half-life of diaminodiphenylsulfone (DDS) after therapeutic dosage varies widely between 9–45 hours with a mean of 30 hours. In toxic overdose, the half-life may rise to 2–4 days.
- Dapsone is eliminated largely in the urine as unchanged dapsone (15%) and as water-soluble metabolites (70–85%).
- Slow gut absorption, enterohepatic recycling, or saturation of metabolic pathways may cause the correlation of a prolonged toxic course with slow elimination.
- Enterohepatic recycling may be of considerable importance since repeated doses of activated charcoal appear to decrease the half-lives of both dapsone and its major metabolite.

CLINICAL PRESENTATIONS

Varying clinical pictures such as restlessness, dyspnea, extensive hemolysis, anemia, and/or serious central nervous system dysfunction may reflect dapsone toxicity. Tachycardia and elevated systolic and diastolic blood pressure may be seen. Nausea and vomiting, often brownish tinged, have been reported. Nephrotic syndrome and renal papillary necrosis are occasionally observed. In addition to the cyanosis noted above, minor rashes, morbilliform eruptions, erythema nodosum, and toxic epidermal necrolysis have been observed.

Hematologic Effects

Patients who overdose on dapsone may have a normal blood picture including reticulocytes, hemoglobin, hematocrit, haptoglobin, red blood cells, and red blood cell fragility. Methemoglobinemia, chocolate brown venous blood, agranulocytosis, or hemolytic anemia may begin early or after a lag of several days. Anemia, hemolytic anemia, and Heinz body formation appear to be dose related. Bone marrow suppression appears to be an idiosyncratic reaction, as are leukopenia and agranulocytosis. A rare megaloblastic anemia may be observed.

Dapsone may produce hemolysis at low therapeutic doses, with an increase in reticulocyte levels and diminished red blood cell life, but the hemoglobin level remains normal because of compensatory marrow hyperplasia. Hemolytic anemia has begun as late as 9 days after ingestion and may result from a direct toxic effect of dapsone on the phospholipids of the red blood cell membrane. Signs may include an increase in reticulocytes, and lactic dehydrogenase, and a fall in plasma haptoglobin. Hemolysis may be especially severe in patients with G6PD deficiency, methemoglobin reductase deficiency, or hemoglobin M.

Methemoglobinemia and Sulfhemoglobinemia

Methemoglobinemia may not be dose related. Methemoglobin levels may be elevated or nondetectable. Methemoglobin levels of 10–25% are usually associated with cyanosis. Cyanosis of the lips, nails, buccal and palatal mucosa, and extremities may be present in an otherwise alert individual. The patient may have a bluish-gray color. The cyanosis may remain for 3–10 days and does not respond to oxygen. Exertional dyspnea, headache, tachycardia, dizziness, and fatigue accompany levels of 35–40%. At 60%, stupor is observed and at levels >70%, death may supervene.

Although cyanosis, dyspnea, headache, and nausea may be correlated with methemoglobin levels, cyanosis may persist after return of levels to normal. Sulfhemoglobinemia may be delayed and associated with prolonged cyanosis. Cyanosis has disappeared when the sulfhemoglobin level decreases below 5%.

Neurologic Effects

Restlessness and diminished consciousness are often observed. In children, early agitation and hyperexcitability may be seen. Later, torpor, depression, incoordination and tonic-clonic seizures may occur. Behavior may be aggressive. Adults may become euphoric, confused, and may hallucinate. Protrusions of the tongue, grinding of teeth, truncal ataxia, and choreiform movements have been observed. Headache, lethargy, delirium, motor weakness, and decreased deep tendon reflexes may be apparent. Peripheral motor neuropathy and psychosis are rarely seen. Less than 50% of patients have a mild sensory impairment. Optic atrophy or blurred vision after several weeks of normal vision has been observed. No eye damage has been reported with therapeutic doses.

"DDS" Syndrome

Diaminodiphenylsulfone (DDS) syndrome has been observed in about 5% of patients on long-term dapsone therapy after the fifth or sixth week of treatment, although it may begin as early as 2 weeks after treatment is begun. This syndrome is manifested by a sudden papular or exfoliative rash, fever, malaise, and weakness followed, after a few days, by an enlarged tender liver, jaundice, epigastric or hypogastric pain, lymphadenopathy and monocytosis.

TOXIC DOSAGE/DEATH

A dose of 1,450 mg has been lethal in a 16-year-old boy, whereas 1,200 mg was not fatal in another boy. Recovery has followed ingestions of 7.5 and 10 grams in adults. A 5-gram ingestion in a 22-month-old resulted in death. A lethal serum concentration has not been established. At post mortem, dapsone is found in the blood, urine, liver, and brain.

DRUG INTERACTIONS

Dapsone may add to the effects of any drug that can induce hemolysis in patients with glucose-6-phosphate dehydrogenase (G6PD) deficiency. Among others, these include aniline, nitrites, phenylhydrazine, naphthalene, nitrofurantoin, and primaquine.

PREGNANCY/LACTATION

Dapsone appears to pass into the fetal circulation, and both dapsone and monoacetyl dapsone have been found in breast milk in quantities sufficient to produce a mild hemolytic anemia in an infant. Dapsone is a weak base favoring its entrapment in milk, which is relatively acidic compared to plasma. Pregnancy risk category C.

LABORATORY

Analytic Methods

Dapsone and monoacetyl dapsone blood and urine levels may be determined by fluorometry, by high-performance liquid chromatography, or by high-performance thin-layer chromatography.

Blood Levels

There is no close correlation between blood levels of dapsone and clinical course as manifested by cyanosis, methemoglobinemia, and/or hemolytic anemia. Serum dapsone levels over 1–2 μg/mL have been associated with toxicity.

TREATMENT

Gut Decontamination

Patients are frequently conscious and alert despite profound cyanosis. Activated charcoal appears to be effective in ridding the body of excess dapsone and metabolites by interfering with its enterohepatic metabolism. When given orally in a dose of 20 grams, four times daily, it lowered the half-life of dapsone from 88 to 13.5 hours and that of monoacetyl dapsone, from 67 to 14 hours in one study. Activated charcoal should be administered for at least 3 days. There is no clinical evidence that cathartics increase the elimination of dapsone from the gut.

Elimination Enhancement

Dapsone and monoacetyl dapsone are very slowly eliminated from the body through the renal route. In view of the high volume of distribution, a high degree of protein binding, minimal excretion of unchanged drug, and problems related to extracorporeal procedures, the usefulness of charcoal hemoperfusion, hemodialysis, peritoneal dialysis, exchange transfusion, and plasma exchange to enhance dapsone removal has not been established. Administration of sufficient fluids, orally or intravenously, should be provided to maintain a normal urine flow, prevent hemoconcentration, and maintain normal parameters of renal function.

Supportive Measures

- Patients may present with cyanosis without any other disturbing symptoms.
- Methemoglobinemia may be present, and there may be signs of hemolysis including an increased reticulocyte count, decreased hemoglobin, and Heinz body formation. Such patients should be hospitalized in an intensive care unit for careful clinical monitoring and treatment. Airway, breathing, and circulatory status should be immediately evaluated.
- Hemolysis may develop 3–9 days after dapsone ingestion and may continue long after both methemoglobin and sulfhemoglobin levels have returned to normal. Patients must therefore be kept under close observation for a prolonged period.
- Blood should routinely be drawn for arterial blood gases, blood methemoglobin levels, reticulocyte count, plasma hemoglobin, serum haptoglobin, lactic acid dehydrogenase, and complete blood count. Examination of the color of the venous blood should be made visually while waiting for laboratory results. A G6PD evaluation should be made on the blood sample.
- Packed red blood cell transfusions may be required for symptomatic treatment of hemolytic anemia. Intravenous hydrocortisone has not been useful in treating hemolysis.
- Blurred vision may occur after an initial period of normal vision. This may be evaluated by assessing macular function, using fluorescein angiography.

- Oxygen inhalation therapy is not useful in dapsone overdosage. Chest x-ray is usually within normal limits.
- Ascorbic acid has not been determined to be clinically useful in dapsone overdose.
- Seizures should be treated with diazepam (adults, 5 to 10 mg i.v. slowly and children, 0.1–0.3 mg/kg slowly). If unresponsive, use phenytoin, 15 mg/kg i.v. at 0.5 mg/kg/min with electrocardiographic monitoring. Intramuscular phenobarbital and intramuscular paraldehyde have had no ameliorative effect on decreasing the restlessness observed after dapsone overdose.
- On admission, most patients have normal liver function and kidney function tests, serum electrolytes, electroencephalograms, and electrocardiograms. A mild leukocytosis and an increase in blood urea nitrogen may be observed.

ANTIDOTES

Methylene Blue

Methylene blue is a specific treatment for cyanosis resulting from excessive methemoglobinemia such as that induced by dapsone. An effective dose initially is 1–2 mg/kg given intravenously over a 5–10 minute period. Cyanosis may be lessened temporarily and methemoglobin blood levels decreased, but rebound methemoglobinemia may require multiple injections of methylene blue over several days, as dapsone is continually absorbed and slowly eliminated.

Use of methylene blue must be dictated by clinical evaluation of the patient to determine whether the deep, often dramatic, cyanosis is accompanied by other adverse effects of methemoglobinemia sufficient to warrant the use of this product. If methylene blue is used, methemoglobin levels must be monitored frequently. The cyanosis itself is not a good guide to therapy, as methylene blue may induce a grayish discoloration of the skin. Further, severe anemia may disguise cyanosis even in the presence of elevated methemoglobin levels.

Methylene blue is ineffective against toxic methemoglobinemia resulting from either a congenital deficiency in methemoglobin reductase or a G6PD deficiency where the generation of NADP via the hexose monophosphate shunt may be impaired. In excessive dose, methylene blue itself may cause hemolysis in otherwise normal individuals or in those with G6PD deficiency and may also produce paradoxical methemoglobin formation.

Questions—Dapsone

1. **When possible, before initiating treatment with dapsone, which test may be helpful?**
   A. Measurement of a glucose-6-phosphate dehydrogenase (G6PD) level
   B. Hemoglobin electrophoresis
   C. Resting arterial oxygen pressure (PaO_2) or saturation (O_2 sat)
   D. Nicotinamide adenine dinucleotide or nicotinamide adenine dinucleotide phosphate levels
   E. Hexose monophosphate level
2. **Which of the following is part of the treatment for some cases of methemoglobinemia that are caused by dapsone?**
   A. Exchange transfusion
   B. Hemodialysis
   C. Hemofiltration
   D. Steroids
   E. Methylene blue

ANTITUBERCULOSIS DRUGS

Ethambutol

Ethambutol (Myambutol®) is used in combination with other drugs to treat tuberculosis. It is not used alone, either in the initial treatment or in re-treatment of tuberculosis. When used, it is given as a single oral dose every 24 hours.

PATHOPHYSIOLOGY

Ethambutol is a tuberculostatic agent acting as an antimetabolite affecting RNA synthesis.

PHARMACOKINETICS

Absorption

- Ethambutol is 75–80% absorbed.

Distribution

- Volume of distribution is 1.6 L/kg.
- Protein binding is 10–30%.

Elimination

- About 80% of the drug and its inactive metabolites are excreted in the urine.

CLINICAL PRESENTATIONS

Therapeutic toxic effects are restricted largely to the nervous system. Retrobulbar neuritis, manifested by impaired visual acuity and color vision, is reported with dosages of 50 mg/kg/d. There may be constriction of visual fields. Blindness in the elderly has occurred with 15 mg/kg/d. Rarely, allergic reactions, gastrointestinal disturbance, and cholestatic jaundice may occur. Acute overdose symptoms include nausea, abdominal pain, fever, mental confusion, visual hallucinations, and optic neuropathy (retrobulbar neuritis).

TOXIC DOSAGE/DEATH

Death from ethambutol overdose has not been reported.

DRUG INTERACTIONS

Aluminum may decrease intestinal absorption.

PREGNANCY/LACTATION

Pregnancy risk category B.

LABORATORY

Analytic Methods

Ethambutol levels are not routinely available from hospital labs.

Blood Levels

A peak plasma level of 5 mg/mL after a dose of 25 mg/kg has been reported. Following blood levels in overdose does not guide clinical management.

TREATMENT

Gut Decontamination

Charcoal and/or gastric lavage may be helpful in overdose although formal studies to confirm their use are lacking.

Elimination Enhancement

Ethambutol may be slightly dialyzable and theoretically helpful in serious ingestions.

Supportive Measures

- Management is primarily supportive.

Questions—Ethambutol

1. Which is the chief side effect of chronic ethambutol ingestion?

A. Cholestatic hepatitis due to direct hepatotoxicity
B. Impaired visual acuity or color vision due to optic neuritis
C. Renal failure due to deposition of ethambutol crystals in glomeruli
D. Pulmonary edema due to cardiac failure
E. Constipation due to impairment of the parasympathetic nervous system.

Isoniazid

Isoniazid (isonicotinic hydrazine or INH) is the cornerstone of treatment for active tuberculosis and is the drug of choice for prophylactic therapy of individuals who demonstrate a positive tuberculosis skin test reaction. In overdose, INH produces serious morbidity and mortality. The diagnosis of INH overdose should be considered in any patient that exhibits otherwise unexplained metabolic acidosis and seizure activity.

The drug of choice in the treatment of INH overdose is pyridoxine (vitamin B6). Though rarely used, hemodialysis, peritoneal dialysis, hemoperfusion, and exchange transfusion have been effective in INH removal. INH overdosages have been reported in the American Indian population, where tuberculosis is common and suicide is prevalent.

PATHOPHYSIOLOGY

INH causes pyridoxine deficiency. INH, a hydrazone, competitively inhibits pyridoxine kinase, the enzyme that converts pyridoxine to the physiologically active pyridoxal phosphate. INH also inactivates pyridoxal phosphate directly. Reduction in pyridoxine, and the resultant reduction in pyridoxal phosphate, has an adverse effect on both the formation and the catabolism of the inhibitory neurotransmitter, gamma aminobutyric acid (GABA).

INH also blocks the conversion of lactate to pyruvate by interfering with NAD, the enzyme that catalyzes this reaction. This mechanism may also contribute to the lactate acidosis produced by INH-induced seizures.

PHARMACOKINETICS

Absorption

- Isoniazid is absorbed from the gastrointestinal tract and from intramuscular sites.
- Peak plasma levels of 1–7 mg/mL are reached in 1 to 2 hours.
- Plasma concentrations of rapid INH inactivators are 20 to 50% those of slow inactivators.

Distribution

- Protein binding is 10%.
- Isoniazid is distributed into all body fluids and tissues.
- Its apparent volume of distribution is 0.6 L/kg.

Elimination

- Seventy-five to 95% is excreted in the saliva, feces and urine.
- Excretion is completed in 24 hours. Less than 10% is excreted in the bile.
- The plasma half-life is 1–4 hours in normal subjects.
- INH is inactivated in the liver.

CLINICAL PRESENTATIONS

The clinical triad of acute INH overdose consists of repetitive seizures refractory to usual anticonvulsants, metabolic acidosis often refractory to sodium bicarbonate, and coma. Patients who ingest higher than therapeutic doses of INH over a prolonged period may develop signs and symptoms of chronic INH poisoning. Nausea and vomiting may be an early warning sign, but seizures may occur without signs of acute INH toxicity such as coma, status epilepticus, severe metabolic acidosis, and hyperglycemia.

Hepatitis occurs in 0.46% of patients receiving INH as preventive therapy. Its incidence is greater with increasing age, is more frequent in those who regularly use ethanol, and may occur more often in patients also receiving phenobarbital or rifampin treatment. A prodrome of vague gastrointestinal complaints with anorexia, nausea, vomiting, and abdominal distress may be its early manifestation. However, patients may be asymptomatic in the presence of seriously elevated aminotransferase levels. The patient may ultimately develop fever, chills, rash, urticaria, dark urine, clay-colored stools, diarrhea, malaise, fatigue, and joint and muscle pains.

Serum alanine and aspartate aminotransferases are usually elevated from slight to 50 times normal. They may normalize even when INH is continued. Hyperbilirubinemia, increased alkaline phosphatase, and lengthened prothrombin time may be observed with eosinophilia. The liver may exhibit patchy or massive hepatic necrosis similar to viral hepatitis. Bridging or multilobular necrosis or both may be present.

TOXIC DOSAGE/DEATH

As little as 1.5 grams of INH can induce toxicity in an adult. A 2–3 gram ingestion is generally toxic. The acute ingestion of 6–10 grams can cause severe toxicity and death, and 10–15 grams are often fatal if not treated. Put another way, 35–40 mg/kg produces seizures in some patients, and 80–150 mg/kg induces seizures and high mortality. Three mg/kg has produced fatal status epilepticus in a patient with a prior history of epilepsy.

DRUG INTERACTIONS

Additive dizziness and drowsiness may occur with cycloserine and ethionamide. Bacille Calmette-Guerin (BCG) vaccine may not be effective if administered during therapy with INH. INH inhibits the hepatic metabolism of phenytoin, resulting in increased plasma phenytoin levels, especially in slow acetylators. INH hepatotoxicity is enhanced by carbamazepine. INH hepatitis risk is increased with alcohol, and hepatic necrosis is increased by phenobarbital. Rifampin increases transformation to more toxic metabolites and may increase the incidence of INH hepatitis. INH and disulfiram concurrently lead to coordination difficulties, ataxia, and psychotic episodes.

INH, closely related to monoamine oxidase inhibitors, has induced a typical "tyramine syndrome" consisting of palpitations, flushing, conjunctival injection, headache, dyspnea, tightness of the chest, tachypnea, and sweating when taken with tyramine containing substances (e.g., parmesan cheese, burgundy wine).

PREGNANCY/LACTATION

INH appears in fetal blood if administered during pregnancy. It is found in the breast milk of nursing mothers. Milk concentration may be equal to maternal plasma concentration. Pregnancy risk factor C.

LABORATORY

Analytic Methods

A qualitative urine test for INH and its metabolites can be performed with commercially available reagent-impregnated paper strips.

Blood Levels

INH quantitative serum levels are performed by few clinical laboratories and, in an acute situation, are usually not available. Treatment should not await the results of these tests.

TREATMENT

Gut Decontamination

As seizures may occur spontaneously, induction of emesis is not advised. Asymptomatic patients who have ingested a potentially toxic amount of INH should be observed for at least 4 hours after activated charcoal has been administered, since there is often a latent period before toxicity develops. If it can be established unequivocally that toxicity has not occurred when more than 4 hours have elapsed since the ingestion of INH in amounts less than 20 mg/kg (1.5 g in an adult), only careful observation may be indicated.

If the patient has had seizures and is postictal, the airway has been protected (endotracheal intubation), and pyridoxine has been administered, the stomach may be emptied by gastric lavage and the lavage returns sent for toxicology evaluation. After the stomach has been emptied, activated charcoal and cathartics should be administered.

Elimination Enhancement

With very little protein binding and a low volume of distribution, INH is a good candidate for dialysis, but in view of its short half-life and efficient antidote, such procedures are often unnecessary. If peritoneal dialysis is used, pyridoxine may be added to each liter of fluid used in the dialysis. Hemoperfusion may be useful in reducing the half-life and serum concentration of INH. Exchange transfusion has successfully been used in children.

Supportive Measures

- Establish an airway that is dependable and easily managed. Endotracheal intubation is indicated if status epilepticus is present, and in obtunded or unconscious patients.
- In the unresponsive patient in whom an airway has been established, dependent positioning of the head, left lateral position of the body, and gastric suction together with assisted respiration should be instituted. Mechanical assisted ventilation may be required for respiratory depression.
- Adequately hydrate overdosed individuals with saline.
- Diazepam acts synergistically with pyridoxine to attenuate seizures (5–10 mg of i.v. diazepam is the starting dose). If convulsions persist, the same dose of diazepam may be repeated in 10–20 minutes.
- If acidosis is not responsive to specific therapy (pyridoxine, diazepam, fluids), sodium bicarbonate may be given by i.v. bolus. Do not mix sodium bicarbonate with pyridoxine solution. Monitor acidotic patients with ECG and watch for hypokalemia or hyperkalemia.
- Periodic serum transaminase levels should be obtained in all INH patients, especially in those who are ethanol users, in those with a history of liver disease, and in those receiving other potentially hepatotoxic agents. Stop INH if the transaminase is two to three times its normal concentration.
- On admission, blood should be obtained for estimation of glucose, electrolytes, bicarbonate, arterial blood gases, liver function tests, serum blood urea nitrogen, creatinine, lactic acid, and complete blood count.

ANTIDOTES

Pyridoxine

If in doubt whether INH overdosage is the cause of convulsions or coma, consider an early therapeutic trial of pyridoxine intravenously, because of its relative safety and potential benefits. Give pyridoxine in alleged or definite cases of INH overdosage even if seizures have not occurred. The optimal pyridoxine dose should be at least equal to the maximum amount of INH allegedly ingested. Mix pyridoxine as a 5% or 10% solution with water and administer intravenously over a 5-minute period (i.e., 5 grams/5 minutes in a 50-mL volume). Repeat in 5–20-minute intervals as needed in a comatose or convulsing patient. Pyridoxine is available commercially in vials of 1 gram/10 mL.

If the ingested dose of INH is unknown, start with 5.0 grams of pyridoxine and follow in 30 minutes with an additional 5.0 grams until seizures cease or consciousness is regained. Do not mix pyridoxine with sodium bicarbonate in an intravenous bottle. When convulsions are controlled, seizure-induced lactic acidosis will resolve and sodium bicarbonate may not be required.

Tachypnea, postural reflex abnormalities, paralysis, and convulsions may follow excessive pyridoxine dosage, however up to 52 grams intravenously has been tolerated by INH overdose patients without adverse effects. No adverse effects were observed with pyridoxine in one study at doses from 70–357 mg/kg.

Questions—Isoniazid

1. Treatment for INH overdose includes which of the following?
A. Methylene blue
B. Steroids
C. Epinephrine
D. Salicylates
E. Pyridoxine (vitamin B6)

2. The clinical triad of acute INH overdose consists of
A. Methemoglobinemia, acidosis, skin discoloration
B. Nausea, seizures, myelopathy
C. Repetitive seizures, metabolic acidosis, and coma.
D. Seizures, mydriasis, hypothermia
E. Hematuria, chest pain, seizures

3. INH, a hydrazone, competitively inhibits pyridoxine kinase, the enzyme that converts pyridoxine to the physiologically active pyridoxal phosphate.
A. True
B. False

Thiacetazone

Thiacetazone is one of the mainstays of antituberculosis treatment in the developing world. It is not available in the United States, but is widely used in China, Ethiopia, and India, mainly in combination with isoniazid. Thiacetazone was introduced and continues to be used because of its low cost. This drug is especially toxic to patients with HIV. Cutaneous, gastrointestinal and central nervous system toxicity are the predominant toxic responses to thiacetazone. Death has followed its use.

Thiacetazone is a third-line drug (as are ethionamide, cycloserine, kanamycin, capreomycin, and viomycin) for the treatment of tuberculosis. Its main role is in the prevention of emergence of resistance to other drugs, especially isoniazid.

PATHOPHYSIOLOGY

Either thiacetazone or a reactive metabolite appears to be responsible for cutaneous hypersensitivity reactions in patients treated with tuberculosis, regardless of HIV status.

PHARMACOKINETICS

Absorption

- Peak plasma concentrations during treatment are reached in 4-5 hours and average 1.8 mg/mL.

Distribution

- A concentration of 0.4 mg/mL completely inhibits 75–100% of some strains of Mycobacterium tuberculosis.

Elimination

- The major route of metabolism is probably ring hydroxylation followed by conjugation with glucuronic acid.
- About 20–35% of thiacetazone is excreted unchanged in the urine.
- The elimination half-life is about 12–14 hours.

CLINICAL PRESENTATIONS

Nausea, vomiting, and anorexia occur in about 10% of patients taking 200 mg daily and are more common at higher doses. Conjunctivitis is common but not severe. Giddiness, seizures, choreiform movements, and cerebral edema have been observed.

Dermatologic Reactions

Skin eruptions have been classified as mild (uncomplicated pruritus, acneiform eruptions, morbilliform erythema), moderate (extensive maculoerythematous eruptions, urticaria, purpura), and severe (erythroderma, Stevens-Johnson syndrome, and Lyell's disease). The risk of severe cutaneous hypersensitivity reactions and death is increased in HIV-positive patients.

TOXIC DOSAGE/DEATH

Toxicity and death may follow use of therapeutic doses.

DRUG INTERACTIONS

Thiacetazone potentiates streptomycin ototoxicity in some patients. Giddiness develops after about 6 weeks of treatment in patients receiving concomitant streptomycin therapy.

LABORATORY

Analytic Methods

The preferred analytical method is high-performance liquid chromatography using a reversed-phase column packing with ultraviolet detection.

Blood Levels

Toxic effects have not been correlated with blood levels.

TREATMENT

Gut Decontamination

Charcoal may bind available thiacetazone in the gastrointestinal tract; however, its clinical efficacy has not been studied.

Elimination Enhancement

These methods have not been studied in the context of thiacetazone overdose.

Supportive Measures

- Treatment is generally supportive. Seizures are treated with benzodiazepines.
- If hepatotoxicity is involved, serum transaminase concentrations may be increased.

Questions—Thiacetazone

1. Which of the following is seen with chronic thiacetazone ingestions?

A. Renal failure
B. Hallucinations
C. Rash
D. Pulmonary edema
E. Renal failure

Cycloserine

Cycloserine is a synthetic broad-spectrum antibiotic produced by a strain of Streptomyces orchidaceus. It is considered a second-line drug in the treatment of tuberculosis and in retreatment regimens. Cycloserine poisoning is uncommon.

PATHOPHYSIOLOGY

Cycloserine acts by inhibiting cell wall synthesis in susceptible strains of Gram-positive and Gram-negative bacteria, and in Mycobacterium tuberculosis.

PHARMACOKINETICS

Absorption

- About 70–90% of an oral dose of cycloserine is readily absorbed.
- Peak serum levels (therapeutic) of 15–25 μg/mL are reached in 3–4 hours.

Distribution

- Protein binding is 0.5%.
- The volume of distribution is 0.6 L/kg.
- The normal serum half-life is 10 hours.

Elimination

- Thirty to 35% of cycloserine is metabolized in the liver and 60% is excreted in the urine unchanged.

CLINICAL PRESENTATIONS

Behavioral disturbances, hallucinations, extrapyramidal signs, dizziness, headache, difficulty in sleeping, seizures, coma, and death have been reported. Other signs include increased tendon reflexes, patellar clonus, Babinski sign, and paresthesias.

TOXIC DOSAGE/DEATH

Death has been reported in overdose and a toxic dose has not been established.

DRUG INTERACTIONS

Drug interactions include increased convulsions with chronic alcohol abuse, and dizziness, and drowsiness with isoniazid.

PREGNANCY/LACTATION
Pregnancy risk factor C.

LABORATORY

Analytic Methods
Methods to detect cycloserine are not routinely available in hospital labs.

Blood Levels
Following cycloserine levels in overdose has not been shown to be helpful in guiding therapy.

TREATMENT

Gut Decontamination
Charcoal may bind available cycloserine in the gastrointestinal tract; however, its clinical efficacy has not been studied.

Elimination Enhancement
These methods have not been studied in the context of cycloserine overdose. However, peritoneal dialysis and hemodialysis may be useful.

Supportive Measures
- Treatment is generally supportive. Discontinue the drug.

Questions—Cycloserine

1. Which of the following is true about the main side effects of cycloserine?
   A. They result from effects on the central nervous system.
   B. Patients are at increased risk if they are on concurrent nephrotoxic agents.
   C. Since the molecule is small and dialyzable, treatment should include hemodialysis.
   D. Alkalinization of urine with sodium bicarbonate should be attempted to speed excretion by renal mechanisms.
   E. Liver biopsy results may be identical to those seen in acute hepatitis B.

Rifampin

Rifamycins are macrocyclic antibiotics produced by Streptomyces mediterranei. Rifampin (Rifadin®) is used in the treatment of clinical tuberculosis and other mycobacterial diseases when given together with isoniazid. It is also used for the treatment of asymptomatic meningococcus carriers, in the prophylaxis of Haemophilus influenzae type b infections, and in tuberculoid leprosy, with dapsone.

PATHOPHYSIOLOGY
The rifamycins exert a bactericidal effect by inhibition of DNA-dependent RNA polymerase, preventing chain initiation but not elongation. Continuous use of rifampin generally does not lead to significant toxicity. Intermittent use, however, leads to a number of toxic reactions that are considered to result from antibody production causing hypersensitivity reactions in a variety of organ systems (blood, liver, kidney).

PHARMACOKINETICS

Absorption
- Rifampin is well absorbed orally (90%), reaching a peak plasma concentration in 2–4 hours.

Distribution
- Protein binding is 75%.
- Rifampin is well distributed throughout the body and is present in effective concentrations in many body fluids, including the cerebrospinal fluid.
- Its apparent volume of distribution is 1.6 L/kg.

Elimination
- The serum half-life of rifampin is 1.5–5 hours.
- Rifampin is deacetylated in the liver to desacetylrifampicin. The deacetylated rifampin is excreted in the feces.
- Both the parent drug and the metabolite are excreted in the bile.
- Rifampin undergoes some enterohepatic recirculation.
- About 6–30% of an oral dose is excreted in the urine.

CLINICAL PRESENTATIONS
Many adverse reactions are observed after intermittent, but not continuous, rifampin use. Gastrointestinal disturbances may include nausea, vomiting, anorexia, constipation, mild abdominal pain, and diarrhea. Cutaneous reactions include rashes, pruritus, and facial flushing, and are mild and transient. Other reactions may include hepatitis, acute renal failure, influenzalike syndrome, thrombocytopenia, hemolytic anemia, leukopenia, eosinophilia, and pseudomembranous colitis.

Other symptoms associated with intermittent use may include petechiae, purpura, nasal and tongue bleeding, prolonged bleeding time, fever, chills, arthralgias, menstrual irregularities, obtundation, lethargy, organic brain syndrome, ataxia, dizziness, blurred vision, and transient hearing loss. Obtundation and lethargy may be seen. Fatalities may occur. Suspicion of rifampin drug poisoning should be considered in a patient with unexplained orange, orange-red, or red discoloration of the skin susceptible to mechanical removal, hyperemesis, and pruritus, in a previously healthy afebrile patient.

Gastrointestinal Effects
Nausea, vomiting, and abdominal pain may be seen. Hepatic reactions in patients with previously normal liver function are usually mild and nonspecific and regress with symptomatic care within a few days. In a small number of cases, a raised aspartate aminotransferase may be associated with a slow acetylator phenotype. Serum concentrations of rifampin are higher in cirrhotic patients than in those with normal livers. Effective blood concentrations can be achieved with smaller doses in cases of previous hepatocellular insufficiency. A hepatorenal syndrome has been described after resumption of intermittent rifampin therapy.

Renal Effects
Intermittent therapy may result in the production of antibodies sufficient to induce hypersensitivity reactions. Acute renal failure has been attributed to this and is associated, in some patients, with eosinophilia, skin rash, and tubulo-interstitial nephritis on renal biopsy. Acute renal failure may accompany hepatic dysfunction. Rifampin hypersensitivity reactions in the kidney

may also be manifested by a light-chain proteinuria, especially in dehydrated patients.

Dermatologic Effects

A "red man syndrome," characterized by an orange-red color in the skin, mucous membranes, urine, feces, sweat, tears has been reported. Washing or scrubbing can remove the skin color. Flushing, generalized pruritus, angioedema of the face, and sweating may be observed. Scleral discoloration may be absent initially or present but, in any case, appears within 6–10 hours.

TOXIC DOSAGE/DEATH

All patients suspected of ingesting over 6–9 grams (adults) or over 600–1,000 mg (children) should be evaluated in an emergency facility. Death from rifampin overdosage has been associated with alcohol ingestion at the time of death or a history of chronic alcoholism. Death is more likely to occur if there is underlying liver disease, frequent use or abuse of alcohol, and lack of previous rifampin therapy. Death may also occur with therapeutic doses in patients taking the drug at irregular intervals.

DRUG INTERACTIONS

Rifampin is a strong hepatic microsomal enzyme inducer. When rifampin is used in combination with isoniazid, especially in those with a previous history of liver damage, a considerable number of patients may develop jaundice, serious liver damage and hepatitis.

PREGNANCY/LACTATIONS

Rifampin crosses the placenta and is found in breast milk. Pregnancy risk category C.

LABORATORY

Analytic Methods

Serum rifampin levels are not easily available at most clinical laboratories and are not usually useful in management of an overdose patient.

Blood Levels

Peak plasma levels after a 600-mg dose are 7–12 μg/mL.

TREATMENT

Gut Decontamination

If the patient is not comatose, obtunded, vomiting, or convulsing or has not lost the gag reflex, gastric lavage with endotracheal intubation may be employed, followed by activated charcoal. Since rifampin undergoes an enterohepatic recirculation, repeated (every 2–6 hours) doses of activated charcoal orally may result in additional total clearance of rifampin. However, there is no reported proof that "pulsed" charcoal in rifampin overdoses is helpful.

Elimination Enhancement

Use of fluids orally and parenterally may encourage some urinary elimination of rifampin. In view of its extensive volume of distribution and high protein binding, rifampin does not lend itself well to hemodialysis, hemoperfusion, peritoneal dialysis, or exchange transfusions.

Supportive Measures

- Most patients without a history of excess alcohol intake, hepatocellular damage, or intermittent rifampin therapy will respond well to symptomatic, supportive therapy.
- Cutaneous reactions are usually mild and transient. If a reaction is persistent and the rash has subsided, desensitization after appropriate challenge doses may be carried out under careful supervision. Gastrointestinal reactions are rarely serious and can be treated symptomatically.
- Presence of clinical jaundice, and/or hepatomegaly, should be investigated. Patients usually recover completely from rifampin hepatitis and can begin taking the drug once liver function has returned to normal. If treatment is resumed, liver function tests must be periodically repeated and the drug discontinued if they become abnormal or there is clinical evidence of recurrent hepatic involvement. Blood alcohol levels indicating the presence of excess alcohol may suggest the possibility of subsequent hepatotoxicity.
- Monitor platelets carefully in rare cases of thrombocytopenic purpura. Stop rifampin use and do not resume its use. The platelet count should return to normal in a few days. In cases of hemolytic anemia, stop drug use. Admit patient to hospital and monitor renal function.
- Monitor complete blood counts, platelet counts, liver function tests (aspartate aminotransferase, bilirubin, alkaline phosphatase), kidney function tests (urinalysis, serum creatinine, blood urea nitrogen), electrolytes, skin and scleral color, and fluid intake and output in all overdose cases.

Questions—Rifampin

1. Which of the following is true about rifampin?

A. It often causes an asymptomatic elevation of arterial ammonia levels.
B. After administration, it can be found in all body cavities and fluids.
C. Most of an administered dose is excreted in urine.
D. Most of an administered dose is not absorbed.
E. It is stored in fat, resulting in a half-life of more than 48 hours.

2. A "red man syndrome," characterized by an orange-red color in the skin, mucous membranes, urine, feces, sweat, tears has been reported after rifampin use.

A. True
B. False

NITROFURANTOIN

Nitrofurantoin was introduced 40 years ago for the treatment of urinary tract infections. It is rapidly absorbed from the gastrointestinal tract, well concentrated in the urine, and active against a variety of common urinary tract pathogens. Few reports of nitrofurantoin overdose are available despite its extensive use.

Pathophysiology

Nitrofurantoin inhibits bacterial acetyl coenzyme A and cell wall synthesis.

Pharmacokinetics

ABSORPTION

- Bioavailability is 90%.
- Time to peak plasma level is 2 hours.

DISTRIBUTION
- Volume of distribution is 0.6 L/kg.
- Plasma protein binding is 90%.

ELIMINATION
- Excreted unchanged in 30 minutes
- Active metabolites 33%
- Half life is 20–60 minutes.

Clinical Presentations

Excessive doses of nitrofurantoin may be expected to induce nausea and vomiting. Acute pulmonary reactions, such as interstitial fibrosis, interstitial pneumonitis, dyspnea, cough, and chest pain, are more common in the elderly and rare in children. Hepatotoxicity is infrequently observed. Leukopenia and agranulocytosis have rarely been reported in overdose. Methemoglobinemia is also described. Hematologic reactions may be seen in patients with glucose-6-phosphate dehydrogenase (G6PD) deficiency.

Peripheral neuropathy may occur within 6 weeks of starting treatment. Total or partial recovery is common. Hypersensitivity reactions occur in 1 to 5% of patients and may rapidly subside after cessation of therapy. A rust or brown colored urine may be seen with use.

Toxic Dosage/Death

The most frequent adverse reactions to nitrofurantoin are anorexia, nausea, and vomiting, occurring more often with doses greater than 7 mg/kg daily.

Drug Interactions

The effect of nitrofurantoin is decreased with concomitant use of antacids, quinolones and nalidixic acid. Probenecid increases its effect.

Pregnancy/Lactation

Nitrofurantoin may cause hemolytic anemia in the newborn and its use is therefore contraindicated in the latter stages of pregnancy. Pregnancy risk factor B. Nitrofurantoin crosses the placenta and is found in breast milk.

Laboratory

ANALYTIC METHODS
Nitrofurantoin levels are generally not available in hospital settings.

BLOOD LEVELS
Urinary nitrofurantoin levels range from 50–100 mg/mL after a 100 mg dose. Blood levels, however, are not useful in monitoring overdose.

Treatment

Gut Decontamination
Charcoal and/or lavage may decrease bioavailability after excessive overdose.

ELIMINATION ENHANCEMENT
Hemodialysis has not been effectively used to treat nitrofurantoin overdose.

SUPPORTIVE MEASURES
- A high fluid intake should be provided to promote urinary excretion of the drug.
- Rare methemoglobinemia is treated with methylene blue.

Questions—Nitrofurantoin

1. Which of the following is a side effect of nitrofurantoin?
A. Pulmonary edema
B. Pulmonary fibrosis
C. Pneumothorax
D. Respiratory distress syndrome
E. Pulmonary hypertension

CHLORAMPHENICOL

Chloramphenicol, the first broad-spectrum antibiotic to be discovered, is produced synthetically as a derivative of dichloroacetic acid. It has a nitrobenzene moiety, a chemical group that may be responsible for aplastic anemia associated with the drug. Major toxic effects of overdosage relate to the hematopoietic system. A "gray baby syndrome" has been described with neonatal use.

Pathophysiology

Chloramphenicol appears to inhibit protein synthesis in susceptible organisms by binding to 50S ribosomal subunits. It causes inhibition of peptide bond formation similar to that seen with erythromycin, clindamycin, lincomycin, oleandomycin, and troleandomycin.

Pharmacokinetics

ABSORPTION
- Bioavailability after oral administration is 55–92%.

DISTRIBUTION
- Chloramphenicol is widely distributed to all tissues, cerebrospinal fluid, saliva, ascites fluid, pleural fluid, synovial fluid, and aqueous and vitreous humor.
- Highest concentrations are found in the liver and kidneys.
- The apparent volume of distribution is approximately 0.92–1.4 L/kg.
- Protein binding is 50–60%.

ELIMINATION
- The plasma half-life in adults with normal renal and hepatic function is a short 1.6–3.3 hours.
- Chloramphenicol is inactivated primarily in the liver by glucuronyl transferase.
- In children with normal renal and hepatic function, 6–80% is excreted unchanged, whereas in the adult 5–30% is excreted unchanged.
- The remainder is excreted as inactive metabolites, mostly the glucuronide.

Clinical Presentations

Occasional undesirable toxic side effects associated with chloramphenicol include blood dyscrasias, gray baby syndrome, and gastrointestinal disturbances. Rare occurrences of fatal aplastic anemia, allergic or febrile reactions, peripheral and optic neuritis, and pseudomembranous colitis have been reported. Leukemia after prolonged aplastic anemia continues to be a controversial finding. Nausea, vomiting, diarrhea, glossitis, pruritus ani, and enterocolitis have been infrequently reported. Rashes, drug fevers, and anaphylaxis are rare. Herxheimer-like responses have occurred in patients receiving chloramphenicol for the treatment of syphilis, brucellosis, and typhoid fever.

HEMATOLOGIC EFFECTS

Bone marrow toxicity is the most important toxic effect of chloramphenicol. Reversible and irreversible constellations of signs have been described. Reticulocytopenia, anemia, leukopenia, thrombocytopenia, or any combination of these findings manifests reversible bone marrow depression, resulting from a direct pharmacologic effect of chloramphenicol. This type of depression is relatively common, occurs during the course of therapy, is dose related (over 4 grams or more per day), is found where serum levels are above 25 μg/mL, and is reversible on discontinuance of the antibiotic.

A fatal "idiosyncratic" aplastic anemia occurs once in 25,000–40,000 patients receiving the antibiotic, a risk 13 times that for aplastic anemia in the general population. It is not necessarily dose related and occurs weeks to months after cessation of oral, parenteral, or eye drop therapy, although 22% of cases occur concurrently. Its cause has not been established but it may be associated with the nitrobenzene moiety. There is no test for predicting this reaction. Chloramphenicol may also induce a hemolytic anemia in patients with G6PD deficiency.

GRAY BABY SYNDROME

Gray baby syndrome is the other major fatal form of chloramphenicol toxicity. It has been described in neonates receiving the drug in the first few days of life in a dose of more than 15–50 mg/kg, and is associated with toxic blood levels (over 25 μg/mL). The classic picture begins a few days after the initiation of therapy, with vomiting, abdominal distension, anorexia, and respiratory distress. Hypotension, hypothermia, acidosis, a characteristic gray color, greenish diarrhea, and progressive shock soon follow this. Within a few days, almost half of these infants die. The syndrome has also been reported in older infants and adults.

NEUROLOGIC EFFECTS

Optic neuritis, which may result in blindness, has been described in patients receiving prolonged high-dose chloramphenicol therapy. Symptoms may be reversible. Other neurologic sequelae such as peripheral neuritis, headache, depression, ophthalmoplegia, and mental confusion have also been described.

Toxic Dosage/Death

A toxic or fatal dose has not been established.

Drug Interactions

Disulfiram-like symptoms may be experienced with chloramphenicol use after alcohol ingestion. Chloramphenicol inhibits hepatic microsomal enzymes and interferes with the biotransformation of dicumarol (increased anticoagulant effects), chlorpropamide (increased incidence of hypoglycemia), and phenytoin (toxic serum levels). Phenobarbital and phenytoin taken concurrently may cause a decrease in chloramphenicol concentrations. Acetaminophen may induce increased toxicity with chloramphenicol. Chloramphenicol may delay the response of anemic patients receiving iron, folic acid, and vitamin B12 and may increase the effect of other myelosuppressive agents.

Pregnancy/Lactation

Chloramphenicol should not be used by the mother near term. It crosses the placenta and is found in breast milk. Pregnancy risk category C.

Laboratory

ANALYTIC METHODS

Chloramphenicol may be detected by high-pressure liquid chromatography.

BLOOD LEVELS

Since overdoses with chloramphenicol are frequently associated with elevated chloramphenicol plasma levels, monitoring baseline and periodic blood levels, especially in infants and children, enhances its safe use. An oral dose of 1 gram reaches a peak serum level of 10–13 μg/mL in 1–3 hours. After 1 gram i.v., a peak serum level of 4.9–12 μg/mL is reached in 1 hour.

Treatment

GUT DECONTAMINATION

Activated charcoal (50–100 grams in adults and 15–30 grams in children) may be helpful if administered shortly after significant ingestions.

ELIMINATION ENHANCEMENT

Peritoneal dialysis and hemodialysis are ineffective. In view of the short half-life, these procedures are not fast enough to be useful and chloramphenicol is minimally removed. Charcoal hemoperfusion has been useful in the presence of severe hepatic dysfunction and signs of acute chloramphenicol toxicity. If no hepatic dysfunction is present, charcoal hemoperfusion may result in rapid improvement of cardiovascular collapse. If charcoal hemoperfusion is not available, exchange transfusion has been used but there is no evidence that it is more effective than supportive therapy.

SUPPORTIVE MEASURES

- Immediate attention, as always, should be directed towards airway, breathing and hemodynamic stability. Discontinue medication, establish an airway, and check adequacy and rate of respirations. Endotracheal intubation with mechanical assisted ventilation may be required. Support circulation with an intravenous line, use of fluids, and pressor agents as required. Monitor cardiac function, respiratory function, arterial blood gases, and vital signs.
- Baseline blood studies should include a complete blood count, chloramphenicol blood levels (although not helpful in managing an acute overdose), liver and kidney function studies, arterial blood gases, electrolytes, and hematologic parameters such as bleeding time, clotting time, prothrombin time, partial thromboplastin time, and platelet count.
- Rare anaphylaxis may be treated with epinephrine, pressors, fluids, and/or steroids.
- Dose-related reversible bone marrow depression may be treated with blood products and followed with hematologic monitoring. Aplastic anemia may be amenable to bone marrow transplants, steroids, and blood products.
- Infants with markedly elevated serum concentrations of chloramphenicol but with no clinical or laboratory abnormalities

can be safely observed after discontinuation of chloramphenicol.

- If reticulocytopenia, leukopenia, thrombocytopenia, or anemia is observed, the drug should be discontinued immediately. Unfortunately, this does not exclude the possibility after some weeks, of the irreversible type of bone marrow depression described above. Bone marrow studies should be performed as indicated in all individuals with declining blood counts.
- Infants with gray baby syndrome should receive general supportive care. Use intravenous fluids, pressors, and sodium bicarbonate as required. Treat shock with pressors and fluids, apnea with mechanical support guided by blood gases, metabolic acidosis, hypothermia, and hypoglycemia. Decontamination of the gut may proceed with life support measures when feasible and with constant airway protection.

Questions—Chloramphenicol

1. **What is the mechanism of action of chloramphenicol?**
   A. Inhibition of bacterial respiration
   B. Formation of oxygen radicals, which are toxic to bacteria
   C. Inhibition of bacterial DNA replication
   D. Inhibition of bacterial cell wall synthesis
   E. Inhibition of bacterial protein synthesis
2. **The principal side effect of chloramphenicol that may occur after treatment is finished is?**
   A. Gallstones
   B. Pulmonary hypertension
   C. Aplastic anemia
   D. Pseudomembranous (Clostridium difficile) colitis
   E. Hepatic failure
3. **Gray baby syndrome**
   A. Is a fatal form of chloramphenicol toxicity
   B. Has been described in neonates receiving the drug in the first few days of life
   C. Is characterized by methemoglobinemia and shock
   D. All of the above
   E. A and B

METRONIDAZOLE

Metronidazole (Flagyl®) is a synthetic chemical drug used in the treatment of trichomoniasis, amebiasis, giardiasis, anaerobic bacterial infections, acne rosacea, and Gardnerella infections. It is also used in the treatment of dracunculiasis, pseudomembranous colitis, and in active inflammatory bowel diseases such as Crohn's disease. When used as an antimicrobial drug, it is usually used for a short time, whereas its use in inflammatory bowel disease may involve prolonged periods of therapy, frequently longer than 12 months. With long-term therapy, the incidence of side effects, manifested as peripheral neuropathy, increases.

Acute overdoses with metronidazole (Flagyl®) are uncommon. When they do occur, few serious manifestations of toxicity appear. Most cases are treated with supportive therapy alone. A disulfiram-like reaction may occur with concomitant ingestion of alcohol. Chronic accumulation of substantial doses of metronidazole may be associated with central and peripheral nervous system dysfunction. Central effects are generally ameliorated with the discontinuation of medication, however peripheral neuropathies may linger for long periods.

Pathophysiology

Metronidazole is bactericidal, amebicidal, and trichomonacidal. The drug acts by entering the bacterial cell and is chemically reduced to a product that causes disruption of DNA and nucleic acid synthesis. Inactive end products are then released. Metronidazole is equally effective against dividing and nondividing cells.

Pharmacokinetics

ABSORPTION

- Eighty to 98.9% of an oral dose is absorbed from the gastrointestinal tract.
- Peak plasma concentrations are reached in 3 hours.

DISTRIBUTION

- Metronidazole is widely distributed into most body tissue and fluids, including bone, saliva, pleural fluid, peritoneal fluid, vaginal secretions, seminal fluid, cerebrospinal fluid, and cerebral and hepatic abscesses.
- Distribution is similar by oral or intravenous administration.
- The apparent volume of distribution is 0.6–0.8 L/kg. After 400 mg i.v., it is 1.05 L/kg.
- Protein binding is less than 20%.

ELIMINATION

- The elimination half-life is 6–12 hours.
- Metronidazole is metabolized by the liver and excreted through the kidneys.
- Metronidazole and its metabolites are eliminated primarily in the urine (60–80% of the dose). Urinary excretion of unchanged metronidazole is less than 10% of a dose.
- The urine may be dark or reddish brown after oral or intravenous use of metronidazole.

Clinical Presentations

There are few reports of acute metronidazole overdose reported in the medical literature. High cumulative metronidazole dosage has been associated with toxicity to the nervous system. Total dose appears to be important in the pathogenesis of central nervous system toxicity.

Clinical effects include nausea and vomiting, anorexia, malaise, seizures, mental status changes and coma. Central nervous system effects do not appear related to renal or hepatic function or to the level of metronidazole in cerebrospinal fluid. Chronic manifestations of toxicity may include nausea, headache, dry mouth, metallic taste, vomiting, diarrhea, insomnia, weakness, stomatitis, vertigo, rash, and gynecomastia. Infrequently observed are pseudomembranous colitis and leukopenia. Stocking-glove loss of sensation, depressed vibration sense, and distal sensory axonal neuropathy have been described with chronic use.

Toxic Dosage/Death

Single oral overdoses of metronidazole up to 15 grams have been used in suicide attempts, and have resulted in nausea, vomiting, and ataxia. Doses from 3.6–19.5 grams have not resulted in death or prolonged morbidity. Hepatotoxicity has developed after a 12.5 gram exposure.

Drug Interactions

With alcohol, metronidazole may cause a disulfiram-like reaction consisting of flushing, headache, nausea, vomiting, abdominal cramps, and sweating. Metronidazole inhibits alcohol dehydrogenase. With disulfiram, it may produce confusion and psychotic behavior. With warfarin, it increases the anticoagulant effect. A decrease in metronidazole effect is observed when it is used together with phenobarbital, phenytoin, or oxytetracycline. With cimetidine, the half-life of metronidazole is increased, and its renal clearance is decreased. Metronidazole has no effect on the oxidative drug metabolism of diazepam or phenytoin, at therapeutic concentrations.

Pregnancy/Lactation

Metronidazole crosses the placenta. It is distributed into milk in concentrations equal to concurrent plasma concentrations. The highest concentrations in breast milk occur 2–4 hours after administration. There is minimal risk to the fetus, however facial abnormalities have been noted in newborns of mothers who used metronidazole in their first trimester. Pregnancy risk category B.

Laboratory

ANALYTIC METHODS

There is a lack of specificity of bioassays for the measurement of metronidazole because of the antibiotic activity of the metabolite hydroxymetronidazole. A specific high-performance liquid chromatography assay can measure metronidazole and its major metabolites in plasma and urine.

BLOOD LEVELS

In overdose or in the presence of hepatic disease, close monitoring of metronidazole levels and the neurologic status of patients may be indicated. As levels may take quite a while to come back, they are generally not helpful in guiding acute management of overdose. A therapeutic dose results in peak and trough steady-state plasma levels averaging 25 and 18 $\mu g/mL$. There does not seem to be a relationship between serum metronidazole levels and neurotoxicity.

Treatment

GUT DECONTAMINATION

Seizures may occur in extreme overdoses, and emesis induction with syrup of ipecac is generally contraindicated. If the patient is comatose, obtunded, convulsing, or has lost the gag reflex, gastric lavage with prior tracheal protection may be helpful. Activated charcoal and cathartics may follow lavage, but there is no clinical evidence of efficacy.

ELIMINATION ENHANCEMENT

Forced diuresis may not be effective in accelerating metronidazole excretion in view of the small amount of unchanged drug excreted in the urine and its limited renal clearance. Hemodialysis has not been used in overdose patients. Its wide volume of distribution potentially limits hemodialysis. There are inadequate data to support the use of peritoneal dialysis, hemoperfusion, or exchange transfusion.

SUPPORTIVE MEASURES

- Metronidazole overdoses are infrequent and rarely fatal, and usually do not lead to prolonged periods of morbidity. Basic life support (airway, breathing, and circulation) must be maintained and stabilized. Vital signs should be monitored.
- Baseline complete blood counts and renal and hepatic function tests should be obtained during treatment of overdose.
- In the chronic high-dose patient, seizure precautions must be maintained.
- Neurologic monitoring of chronically toxic metronidazole patients is required, especially concerning the peripheral nervous system. Head CT, EEG, motor nerve conduction velocity, and sensory nerve action studies should be performed periodically as indicated.
- Diazepam is the drug of choice in metronidazole-induced seizures. An intravenous bolus (adult, 5–10 mg repeated every 15 minutes up to 20 mg and children, 0.25 mg / kg up to 5–10 mg) will usually control seizures. If seizures are not controlled with diazepam, phenytoin, phenobarbital, or general anesthesia may be required.

Antidotes

There is no specific antidote. Metronidazole bears close structural resemblance to a precursor of thiamine. To overcome the possible conversion of metronidazole by gut flora to an antagonist of vitamin B1, the use of prophylactic thiamine with metronidazole therapy, or therapeutically for the treatment of neurotoxic manifestations of overdose, may be considered. There are no firm data to support this hypothesis.

Questions—Metronidazole

1. **The major side effects of metronidazole are usually due to its effects on which organ/system?**
   A. Eyes
   B. Skeletal muscle
   C. Liver
   D. Nervous system
   E. Kidneys
2. **The treatment of acute and/or chronic overdoses of metronidazole includes?**
   A. Hemodialysis or hemoperfusion
   B. Alkalinization of urine with sodium bicarbonate
   C. Exchange transfusions
   D. Methylene blue
   E. None of the above
3. **Because metronidazole inhibits alcohol dehydrogenase, a disulfiram-like reaction may occur with concomitant ingestion of alcohol and metronidazole.**
   A. True
   B. False

TETRACYCLINES

Tetracyclines were discovered as a result of screening soil samples for antibiotic activity. The first tetracycline, chlortetracycline (Aureomycin ®, no longer in use), was obtained from Streptomyces aureofaciens. Antibiotics in this group that are currently used include oxytetracycline (Terramycin®), tetracycline (Achromycin®), doxycycline (Vibramycin® and Monodox®), minocycline (Minocin®, Vectrin®, and Dynacin®), and demeclocycline (Declomycin®). They all have the same fundamental structure of four joined rings, with the side chains on the rings determining their pharmacologic and antibiotic properties.

Pathophysiology

All tetracyclines are bacteriostatic antibiotics that inhibit protein synthesis by reversibly binding to the 30S subunit of the bacterial ribosome. They obstruct the access of aminoacyl tRNA molecules to the mRNA-ribosome-peptide complex, thereby preventing the addition of amino acids to the peptide chain.

Pharmacokinetics

ABSORPTION

- Following oral administration, short-acting tetracyclines are incompletely absorbed by the stomach.
- The most important factor determining absorption is the absence of divalent and trivalent cations. Ca^{+2}, Mg^{+2}, Al^{+3}, and Fe^{+3} all chelate tetracyclines and prevent their absorption. These substances are contained in a variety of substances, including dairy products, antacids, vitamins, and iron pills.

DISTRIBUTION

- After absorption, tetracyclines are widely distributed to all tissues, including the central nervous system, bone, synovial fluid, and human milk.
- Their volume of distribution is 1–3 L/kg, depending on the tetracycline studied.

ELIMINATION

- The short-acting tetracyclines (tetracycline and oxytetracycline) have half-lives in the range of 8-9 hours. That of intermediate-acting (demeclocycline) is 12 hours, and long-acting tetracyclines (doxycycline and minocycline) 16–18 hours.
- The urinary recovery is as high as 70% for oxytetracycline and as little as 6% for minocycline.
- The degree of hepatic metabolism, as well as the types of metabolic degradation products, is determined by the side chains on the rings.

Clinical Presentations

GASTROINTESTINAL EFFECTS

Gastrointestinal effects are relatively mild and reversible, and include nausea, vomiting, abdominal pain, diarrhea, enterocolitis, and pancreatitis. The nausea may limit dosing. Additionally, esophageal ulceration has been observed, frequently in patients who took a tablet shortly before going to bed and with little water.

DERMATOLOGIC EFFECTS

Morbilliform rashes occasionally occur, but are not serious. Anaphylaxis and urticaria occur rarely. Phototoxicity occurs relatively commonly, especially with demeclocycline.

TEETH AND BONES

Staining of teeth during their calcification (from a fetal age of about five months to about age 8–12 years in children) is related to the total dose of tetracycline ingested, and probably results from its chelation by calcium. For this reason, tetracyclines should be used very sparingly in young children, and only if no alternative antibiotic is available.

HEPATOTOXICITY

Fatty necrosis of the liver occurs in pregnant women, in patients who are treated with at least 2000 mg per day of tetracycline, and in patients who develop excessively high serum levels due to renal insufficiency. This complication is often fatal.

NEUROLOGIC EFFECTS

The tetracyclines have been associated with pseudotumor cerebri (benign intracranial hypertension) in adults. Minocycline causes reversible lightheadedness, vertigo, and tinnitus as early as the second day of treatment.

RENAL EFFECTS

By inhibiting protein synthesis, the tetracyclines may worsen pre-existing azotemia. Demeclocycline causes nephrogenic diabetes insipidus, which has caused it to be exploited more as a treatment for the syndrome of inappropriate antidiuretic syndrome (SIADH) than as an antibiotic.

Toxic Dosage/Death

Death due to fatty necrosis of the liver has occurred with as little as 2 g/day of tetracycline.

Drug Interactions

Since tetracyclines decrease prothrombin activity, patients on oral anticoagulation require careful monitoring of their coagulation times. Oral contraceptives may be less effective if taken with a tetracycline. Food or medication that contains divalent or trivalent cations (as noted earlier) significantly decreases absorption and effectiveness of tetracyclines.

Pregnancy/Lactation

Because of fatty necrosis of the liver and the staining effect on teeth, tetracyclines should be used in pregnancy only if no alternatives are available. Tetracyclines are excreted in human milk. Pregnancy risk category D.

Laboratory

ANALYTIC METHODS

Tetracycline may be measured by high-performance liquid chromatography or by bioassay.

BLOOD LEVELS

These are not routinely available in hospital laboratories, and are not monitored in patients. A 500 mg oral dose of tetracycline gives a peak serum level of 4 μg/mL; an equivalent intravenous dose results in a serum level of 8 μg/mL. A 200 mg oral dose of doxycycline or minocycline yields a peak level of 2.5 μg/mL, with a peak level of 4 μg/mL obtained following the same intravenous dose.

Treatment

GUT DECONTAMINATION

Charcoal and cathartics may be effective. However, systematic studies have not been done.

ELIMINATION ENHANCEMENT

Dialysis does not alter the serum half-life and is not expected to be beneficial.

SUPPORTIVE MEASURES

- Adequate hydration should be given to maintain urine flow.
- Liver enzymes should be monitored serially.

Questions—Tetracyclines

1. **Which of the following classes of medications interact with the tetracyclines?**
   A. Narcotics
   B. Inhalation anesthetics
   C. Oral anticoagulants
   D. H2 blockers
   E. β-blockers
2. **Which of the following side effects of tetracyclines may occur in pregnant women?**
   A. Fatty necrosis of the liver
   B. Renal failure
   C. Hemorrhagic colitis
   D. Respiratory distress syndrome
   F. Spontaneous rupture of membranes

Answers

Introduction to Antibiotics and Antituberculosis Drugs

1. E

Aminoglycosides

1. A 2. E 3. C 4. A 5. E

Penicillins

1. C 2. C 3. B 4. C

Cephalosporins

1. B 2. D 3. E 4. A 5. B

Imipenem

1. E

Aztreonam

1. A

Erythromycin

1. E 2. A 3. A

Azithromycin and Clarithromycin

1. C

Quinolones and Fluoroquinolones

1. E 2. C 3. A 4. B

Trimethoprim and Trimethoprim-Sulfamethoxazole

1. D 2. B 3. E

Vancomycin

1. C 2. B 3. A

Clofazimine

1. D

Dapsone

1. A 2. E

Ethambutol

1. B

Isoniazid

1. E 2. C 3. A

Thiacetazone

1. C

Cycloserine

1. A

Rifampin

1. B 2. A

Nitrofurantoin

1. B

Chloramphenicol

1. E 2. C 3. E

Metronidazole

1. D 2. E 3. A

Tetracyclines

1. C 2. A

SELECTED READINGS

Introduction to Antibiotics and Antituberculosis Drugs

1. Fekety R, Shah AB. Diagnosis and treatment of Clostridium colitis. JAMA 1993;269:71–75.

Aminoglycosides

1. Barclay ML, Begg EJ. Aminoglycoside toxicity and relation to dose regimen. Adverse Drug React Toxicol Rev 1994;13:207–234.
2. Little PJ: Accidental gentamicin overdosage. NZ Med J 1973;78:301–302.
3. Silverblatt F: Pathogenesis of nephrotoxicity of cephalosporins and aminoglycosides: A review of current concepts. Rev Infect Dis 1982;4(suppl):S360–S365.
4. Taketomo RT, McGhan WF, Fushiki MR: Gentamicin nephrotoxicity: Application of multivariate analysis. Clin Pharm 1982;1:544–548.

Penicillins

1. Brunner EH, Haddad ZH: Penicillin induced anaphylaxis. West J Med 1984;141:508–509.
2. Erffmeyer JE: Adverse reactions to penicillin. Ann Allergy 1981;47:288–293 (part I); 294–300 (part II).
3. Saxon A, Beall GN, Rohr AS, Adelman DC. Immediate hypersensitivity reactions to beta-lactam antibiotics. Ann Intern Med 1987;107:204–215.

Cephalosporins

1. Bailey RR: Bleeding tendency in patients on cephalosporins. Lancet 1983;1:822.
2. Cephalosporins, in McEvoy GK (Ed): Drug Information 85: American Hospital Formulary Service. Bethesda, Md, American Society of Hospital Pharmacists. 1985, 71–111.

Imipenem

1. Imipenem/cilastatin: A new type of antibiotic. Drug Ther Bull 1991;29(11):43.
2. Job ML, Dretler RH. Seizure activity with imipenem therapy: Incidence and risk factors. DICP Ann Pharmacother 1990;24:467–469.

Aztreonam

1. Westley-Horton E, Koestner JA. Aztreonam: A review of first monobactam. Am J Med Sci 1991;302:46–49.

Erythromycin

1. Brandress MW, Richardson WS, Barold SS. Erythromycin induced QT prolongation and polymorphic ventricular tachycardia (Torsade de pointes): Case report and review. Clin Infect Dis 1994;18:995–999.
2. Mondolfi AA. Erythromycin. Clin Toxicol Rev 1995;17(9):1–2.

Azithromycin and Clarithromycin

1. Kanatani MS, Guglielmo BJ. The new macrolides. Azithromycin and clarithromycin. West J Med 1994;160:31–37.

Quinolones and Fluoroquinolones

1. Ball P. Ciprofloxacin, an overview of adverse experiences. J Antimicrob Chemother 1986;18(suppl. D):187–193.
2. Hooper D. Fluoroquinolone antimicrobial agents. N Engl J Med 1991; 324:384–94.
3. Walker RC, Wright AJ. The fluoroquinolones. Mayo Clin Proc 1991;66:1249–1259.
4. Walker RC, Wright AJ. The quinolones. Mayo Clin Proc 1987;62:1007–1012.

Trimethoprim and Trimethoprim Sulfamethoxazole

1. Cockerill F III, Edson RS. Trimethoprim-sulfamethoxazole. Mayo Clin Proc 1987;62:921–929.
2. Hoppu K, Partanen S, Koskela E. Trimethoprim poisoning. Lancet 1980;1:778.
3. Stevens RC, Laizare SC, Stein DS, Holden CL. Pharmacokinetics and toxicity of co-trimexazole following pneumocystis-dosing in healthy subjects. Clin Pharmacol Ther 1991;49:199.

Vancomycin

1. Bailie GR, Neal D. Vancomycin in ototoxicity and nephrotoxicity: A review. Med Toxicol 1988;3:376–386.
2. Wallace MR, Mascola JR, Oldfield EC III. Red man syndrome: Incidence, etiology, prophylaxis. J Infect Dis 1991;164:1180–1185.

Clofazimine

1. Cunningham CA, Friedberg DN, Carr RE. Clofazimine-induced generalized retinal degeneration. Retina 1990;10:131–134.
2. Holdiness MR. Clinical pharmacokinetics of clofazimine: A review. Clin Pharmacokinet 1989;16:74–85.
3. Yawalker SJ, Vischer W. Lamprene (clofazimine) in leprosy. Lepr Rev 1979;50:135–144.

Dapsone

1. Adverse reactions to dapsone. (Editorial) Lancet 1981;2:184-185.
2. Berlin G, Brodin B, Hilden J-O, et al: Acute dapsone intoxication. A case treatment with continuous infusion of methylene blue, forced diuresis and plasma exchange. Clin Toxicol 1984/1985;22(6):537–548.
3. Curry S: Methemoglobinemia. Ann Emerg Med 1982;11:214–221.
4. Kromann N, Vilhelmsen R, Stahl D: The dapsone syndrome. Arch Dermatol 1982;118:531–532.

Ethambutol

1. Ethambutol hydrochloride. In: Physicians' Desk Reference. Montvale, NJ: Medical Economics, 1995:1271.
2. Holdiness MR. Clinical pharamcokinetics of the antituberculosis drugs. Clin Pharmacokinet 1984;9:511–544.

Isoniazid

1. Ducobu J, DuPont P, Laurent M, et al. Acute isoniazid/ethambutol, rifampicin overdosage. Lancet 1982;1:632.
2. Kingston RL, Saxena K. Management of acute isoniazid overdosages. Clin Toxicol Consult 1980;2:37–44.
3. Manoguerra AS. Acute isoniazid toxicity. Clin Toxicol 1980;16:407–408.
4. Sievers M, Herrier R, Chin L, et al. Treatment of isoniazid overdose. JAMA 1982;247:583–84.

Thiacetazone

1. Nunn P, Porter J, Winstanley P. Thiacetazone: Avoid like poison or use with care? Trans R Soc Trop Med Hyg 1993;87:578–582.

Cycloserine

1. Handbook of Antimicrobial Therapy, rev ed. Medical Letter on Drugs and Therapeutics. New Rochelle, NY, The Medical Letter, Inc, 1984.
2. Miyakawa T, Suzuki T, Nakamura K, et al: An autopsy case of cycloserine poisoning. Folia Psychol Neurol Japon 1977;31(2):235–241.

Rifampin

1. Ducobu J, DuPont P, Laurent M, et al: Acute isoniazid / ethambutol / rifampicin overdosage. Lancet 1982;1:632.
2. Farr B, Mandell GL: Rifampin. Med Clin North Am 1982; 66:157–168.
3. Girling DJ, Hitze KL: Adverse reactions to rifampicin. Bull WHO 1979;57:47–49.
4. Meisel S, Brower R: Rifampin: A suicidal dose. Ann Intern Med 1980;92:262–263.

Nitrofurantoin

1. Chudnofsky DR, Otten EJ. Acute pulmonary toxicity to nitrofurantoin. J Emerg Med 1989;7:15–19.
2. Shah RR, Wade G. Reappraisal of the risk/benefit of nitrofurantoin: Review of toxicity and efficacy. Adverse Drug React Acute Poison Rev 1989;8:183–201.

Chloramphenicol

1. Chloramphenicol toxicity. Lancet 1969;2:476.
2. Chloramphenicol, in McEvoy GK (Ed): Drug Information 86: American Hospital Formulary Service. Bethesda, Md, American Society of Hospital Pharmacists, 1986:147–150, 1325–1326, 1735.
3. Powell DA, Nahata MC: Chloramphenicol: New perspectives on an old drug. Drug Intell Clin Pharmacol 1982;16:295–300.
4. Thompson WL, Anderson SE, Lipsky JJ, et al: Overdoses of chloramphenicol. JAMA 1975;234:149–150.

Metronidazole

1. Alston TA: Neurotoxicity of metronidazole. Ann Intern Med 1985;103:161.
2. Neu HC: The pharmacology and toxicology of antimicrobial agents, in Braude AI, Davis CE, Fierer J (Eds): Microbiology. Philadelphia, WB Saunders, 1982:275.

Tetracyclines

1. Frost P, Weinstein GD, Gomez EC. Phototoxic potential of minocycline and doxycycline. Arch Derm 1972;105:681.
2. Schultz JC, Adamson JS Jr, Workman WW, et al. Fatal liver disease after intravenous administration of tetracycline in high doses. N Eng J Med. 1963;269:999.

ACKNOWLEDGMENT

Thanks to Ira Leviton, MD for contributing the questions in this chapter and for contributing the entire "Tetracyclines" section.

CHAPTER 14
Antifungal Drugs

INTRODUCTION

Systemic fungal infections are largely treated by amphotericin B, flucytosine, miconazole, fluconazole, and ketoconazole. The incidence of systemic fungal infections has been increasing because of AIDS, immunocompromised patients who are living longer, addiction to intravenous drugs, and greater use of invasive procedures and broad-spectrum antibiotics. There are four major groups of antifungal drugs.

Polyene Group

The polyene group includes amphotericin B, natamycin, and nystatin. Though all are used topically for treating superficial candidiasis, only amphotericin B is used intravenously and is an important agent for therapy of systemic fungal infections. Overdoses with amphotericin B may be fatal but amphotericin B is now available in several new preparations that allow the delivery of doses up to five times as much as was previously possible. A new formulation of nystatin for intravenous administration is in the late stages of clinical development.

Flucytosine

Flucytosine is a synthetic nucleotide analog, and is the only member of the second group of antifungal drugs. There have been no reports of overdosage with flucytosine.

Griseofulvin

Griseofulvin has also been used in the treatment of dermatophyte infections as well as in a number of nonfungal disease states.

Imidazoles

Imidazoles are the third major group of antifungal drugs. Most, such as clotrimazole, miconazole, econazole, isoconazole, and tioconazole, are used topically. Ketoconazole and itraconazole are active systemically after oral administration. Miconazole must be administered parenterally. Fluconazole is also helpful in the treatment of systemic candidal infections.

Questions—Introduction to Antifungal Drugs

1. Which of the following is false?
- A. The polyene group includes amphotericin B, natamycin, and nystatin.
- B. Flucytosine is a synthetic nucleotide analog.
- C. Griseofulvin has also been used in the treatment of dermatophyte infections as well as in a number of nonfungal disease states.
- D. Imidazoles are only effective after oral administration.
- E. Overdoses with amphotericin B may be fatal.

AMPHOTERICIN B

Amphotericin B deoxycholate (Fungizone®) is considered the "gold standard" of antifungal therapy, especially for systemic mycoses. Amphotericin A and B are produced together during the fermentation of Streptomyces nodosus, but only amphotericin B is used clinically. Its drawbacks include the need for intravenous administration, and intolerance by many patients because of side effects such as fever, chills, headache, myalgias, and poor penetration into the cerebrospinal fluid. Although renal dysfunction and bone marrow suppression frequently follow chronic use, overdosed infants, children and adults have developed life-threatening arrhythmias and death.

The high incidence of serious toxicity due to amphotericin B deoxycholate, in combination with new technology, has led to three new formulations: amphotericin B colloidal dispersion (ABCD, formerly known as Amphocil®, now Amphotec®), amphotericin B lipid complex (ABLC, Abelcet®), and liposomal amphotericin B (AmBisome®). The amphotericin component of all these is dosed several times higher than that of the deoxycholate preparation.

Pathophysiology

Amphotericin B exerts its antifungal activity by binding to sterols in the fungal cell membrane. The membrane ceases to function as a selective barrier, and potassium and other cell constituents are lost.

Pharmacokinetics

ABSORPTION

- Only about 10% is absorbed with oral forms.

DISTRIBUTION

- Volume of distribution is 3 L/Kg.
- Protein binding is around 90%.

ELIMINATION

- Amphotericin has a biphasic half-life. Its initial peak is around 15–48 hours with a terminal half-life of about 1–2 weeks.
- The method of elimination is unknown. Most of an administered dose is not recovered in ether urine or stool, and is assumed to be very slowly metabolized in the body.

Clinical Presentations

In many patients amphotericin B causes fever, chills, hypotension, and tachypnea, often beginning 1–3 hours after starting an infusion and lasting 1 or more hours. The incidence of fever and chills due to the newer preparations of amphotericin B is the same as that seen with the deoxycholate preparation. Abdominal distention, hepatotoxicity and bloody diarrhea have been reported with the deoxycholate preparation. Respiratory depression, delirium, seizures, and hemiparesis have also been observed in acute overdose.

CARDIOVASCULAR EFFECTS

The most commonly reported cardiovascular effects of amphotericin B are tachycardia and changes in blood pressure, including both hypertension and hypotension. Sinus bradycardia is uncommon. Ventricular fibrillation has been reported after rapid infusions of the drug, especially in patients with renal insufficiency.

RENAL EFFECTS

Amphotericin B deoxycholate almost invariably causes a decrease in renal function, including a decline in glomerular filtration rate, renal tubular acidosis, decreased serum potassium, and diminished renal concentrating ability. A mild to moderate permanent reduction in glomerular filtration rate should be expected following a long course of amphotericin B deoxycholate. The advantage of the newer preparations of amphotericin B over the deoxycholate formulation is that the former are much less nephrotoxic.

HEMATOLOGIC EFFECTS

A normochromic normocytic anemia accompanied by a depression of erythropoietin production usually occurs in patients on

Answers to questions in shaded boxes appear at the end of the chapter.

prolonged amphotericin treatment. Thrombocytopenia may be seen. No permanent renal or bone marrow function abnormalities have been reported following amphotericin overdose.

Toxic Dosage/Death

Up to 14 mg in infants and 200 mg in adults have been ingested with only moderate sequelae. Cardiac arrest and death have followed 5 mg intravenously. Four infants and children developed cardiac arrest and died after up to 10–50 times the recommended dose was inadvertently administered.

Drug Interactions

Amphotericin B with gentamicin may induce a synergic nephrotoxicity. Similarly, other drugs with a nephrotoxic potential may be additive to the nephrotoxic effects of amphotericin. As amphotericin B may cause hypokalemia, this effect may be potentiated by corticosteroids. The hypokalemia may potentiate digoxin toxicity, may be associated with rhabdomyolysis, and may enhance the effect of nondepolarizing (curariform) drugs.

Pregnancy/Lactation

The U.S. FDA has placed amphotericin B in pregnancy risk category B. Controlled clinical studies have not been conducted with amphotericin in pregnant women.

Laboratory

ANALYTIC METHODS

Bioassay or high-pressure liquid chromatography measures amphotericin B in fluids.

BLOOD LEVELS

Blood levels do not aid in the management of amphotericin overdose.

Treatment

GUT DECONTAMINATION

There is no indication for gastrointestinal contamination, as amphotericin B is generally administered by the intravenous route. Emesis, lavage, and activated charcoal or cathartics may be useful if large amounts of ointment, creams, or lozenges are orally ingested. However, there are no clinically controlled data to support the use of gastric or intestinal emptying procedures.

ELIMINATION ENHANCEMENT

Amphotericin B is poorly dialyzable. There are no clinical data to support the use of forced diuresis or of other extracorporeal methods.

SUPPORTIVE MEASURES

- Patients with amphotericin B overdose should be hospitalized for symptomatic and supportive treatment. Rare hepatotoxicity and arrhythmias represent the greatest immediate threats to life.
- Chest x-ray and arterial blood gases should be obtained where there is evidence of respiratory depression or distress. Baseline renal and liver function tests should be drawn and followed during therapy.
- Agents that appear to aid in preventing amphotericin B-induced chills include ibuprofen, hydrocortisone, and meperidine.
- Amiloride twice daily may reduce potassium wasting.
- Normal saline must be administered to patients receiving amphotericin to reduce nephrotoxicity.
- Periodic neurologic evaluation should be performed to rule out impending neurologic deficits.

Questions—Amphotericin B

1. Which of the following is false?

A. Amphotericin B is considered the "gold standard" of antifungal therapy, especially for systemic mycoses.
B. Amphotericin A and B are produced together during the fermentation of Streptomyces pneumoniae, but only amphotericin B is used clinically.
C. The drawbacks of amphotericin B deoxycholate use include the need for intravenous administration, and intolerance by many patients because of side effects.
D. Renal dysfunction and bone marrow suppression frequently follow chronic use of amphotericin B.
E. Amphotericin B with gentamicin may induce a synergic nephrotoxicity.

2. Symptoms of Amphotericin B toxicity include all of the following except

A. Fever, chills, hypotension, and tachypnea.
B. Abdominal distention, hepatotoxicity and bloody diarrhea have been reported.
C. Respiratory depression, delirium, seizures, and hemiparesis
D. The most commonly reported cardiovascular effect of amphotericin B is bradycardia.
E. Ventricular fibrillation has been reported after rapid infusions of the drug, especially in patients with renal insufficiency.

3. Regarding the renal toxicity of Amphotericin B,

A. Amphotericin B almost invariably causes a decrease in renal function.
B. Effects include a decline in glomerular filtration rate.
C. Effects may include renal tubular acidosis, decreased serum potassium, and diminished renal concentrating ability.
D. A and B
E. A, B, and C

FLUCYTOSINE

Flucytosine is associated with bone marrow suppression, hepatic dysfunction, and diarrhea. Rapid development of fungal resistance has limited its use. Acute or chronic toxicity may be manifested by severe bone marrow suppression or gastrointestinal disorders.

Pathophysiology

Flucytosine is deaminated to 5-fluorouracil and then converted to 5-fluorodeoxyuridylic acid monophosphate, a substance that interferes with DNA synthesis.

Clinical Presentations

Flucytosine toxicity is especially manifest in rapidly proliferating tissues, such as the bone marrow and the lining of the gastrointestinal tract. The risk of bone marrow toxicity appears to be increased with prolonged high concentrations. Adverse gastrointestinal effects may include nausea, vomiting, anorexia, abdominal bloating, diarrhea, and hemorrhagic colitis prior to bowel perforation. Elevations of serum hepatic enzyme levels appear to be dose-related and reversible.

In the presence of azotemia or concomitant amphotericin B use, leukopenia, thrombocytopenia, and enterocolitis have been reported and may be fatal. Anaphylactic reactions have also been reported.

Toxic Dosage/Death

A fatal dose of flucytosine has not been determined.

Laboratory

ANALYTIC METHODS

Bioassay and gas chromatographic methods are available.

BLOOD LEVELS

Monitoring blood levels in acute overdose is not helpful; however, blood levels should be monitored in patients being treated with flucytosine.

Treatment

GUT DECONTAMINATION

As absorption is slow but relatively complete, and toxic effects following flucytosine ingestion may be dose-related, gastric emptying should be considered if the patient is conscious, and has a gag reflex. The usefulness of activated charcoal, cathartics, syrup of ipecac, and gastric lavage has not been clinically confirmed.

ELIMINATION ENHANCEMENT

Flucytosine may be removed more quickly with the use of extracorporeal methods such as hemodialysis and peritoneal dialysis, but clinical confirmation of these methods is unproved.

SUPPORTIVE MEASURES

- Blood studies should include a complete blood count, differential, platelet count, hepatic function tests, and an evaluation of renal function. Crystalluria may occasionally be seen.
- All patients should be hospitalized until evidence of bone marrow suppression, serious gastrointestinal disturbance, and hepatic or renal dysfunction has been fully evaluated.
- Follow-up hematology studies should be arranged.

Questions—Flucytosine

1. **Which of the following is false?**
   A. Flucytosine is associated with bone marrow suppression, hepatic dysfunction, and diarrhea.
   B. Rapid development of fungal resistance has limited its use.
   C. Acute or chronic toxicity may be manifested by severe bone marrow suppression or gastrointestinal disorders.
   D. Flucytosine is deaminated to 5-fluorouracil.
   E. The risk of bone marrow toxicity can be associated with minimal exposures.
2. **Symptoms of flucytosine toxicity may include all of the following except**
   A. Nausea, vomiting
   B. Unilateral headache, pruritus and myoclonic jerking
   C. Anorexia, abdominal bloating, and diarrhea
   D. Elevations of serum hepatic enzyme levels
   E. Anaphylaxis

FLUCONAZOLE

Fluconazole (Diflucan®) is one of the more recent members of the azole family to be licensed for the treatment of systemic fungal infections. Fluconazole differs from other azoles with respect to its toxicokinetic and toxicity profiles.

Pathophysiology

The azole antifungal agents interrupt the conversion of lanosterol to ergosterol, the main sterol of yeast and fungal cell membranes. Fluconazole acts by binding to fungal cytochrome P450, thus inhibiting the demethylase enzyme involved in the synthesis of ergosterol.

Pharmacokinetics

ABSORPTION

- Fluconazole may be administered orally or parenterally.

DISTRIBUTION

- Fluconazole is water-soluble, has a long serum half-life, low protein binding (approximately 10%), and penetrates well into the cerebrospinal fluid.

ELIMINATION

- Fluconazole is eliminated by the kidney. As the glomerular filtration rate diminishes, the half-life (normally approximately 30 hours) becomes prolonged. Dosage should be reduced accordingly.

Clinical Presentations

Fluconazole has been associated with abdominal discomfort, nausea and, less commonly, signs of liver damage. In rare instances, it has been linked to severe skin rashes and fatal hepatic necrosis. Dizziness, headache, somnolence, delirium/coma, psychiatric disturbances, malaise, fatigue, and seizures have been reported. There are rare reports of fever, edema, pleural effusion, oliguria, and arthralgias. Alopecia is commonly associated with higher doses given for 2 months or longer.

Toxic Dosage/Death

There are no published reports of overdose in humans; however, fatal hepatic necrosis has followed its use.

Drug Interactions

Fluconazole may increase phenytoin concentration and inhibit coumarin.

Pregnancy/Lactation

There are no adequate and controlled studies in pregnant women. Fluconazole attains concentrations in breast milk that may be harmful to the nursing infant. Pregnancy risk category C.

Laboratory

ANALYTIC METHODS
Fluconazole is analyzed by a high-performance liquid chromatography assay.

BLOOD LEVELS
Monitoring blood levels is not helpful in managing acute overdose.

Treatment

GUT DECONTAMINATION
Activated charcoal and cathartics may be of value, but no confirmatory studies are available. There is no evidence to support the use of gastric lavage.

ELIMINATION ENHANCEMENT
As most of fluconazole is excreted unchanged by the kidney, consideration should be given to hemodialysis for serious overdoses. There are no data to substantiate the use of forced diuresis, peritoneal dialysis, exchange transfusion, charcoal or resin hemoperfusion, plasmapheresis, or whole-bowel irrigation after a fluconazole overdose.

SUPPORTIVE MEASURES
- As always, airway, breathing, and circulatory status should be monitored until it becomes evident that the patient is awake, breathing normally, and otherwise stable.
- If clinical judgment indicates the presence of symptoms of overdose, the patient should be carefully observed in a hospital facility for at least 24 hours.
- The patient should be observed for clinical or laboratory signs of hepatic or renal damage.
- Potential eosinophilia, anemia, leukopenia, neutropenia, and thrombocytopenia should be monitored. Hypokalemia may require replacement potassium therapy.

Questions—Fluconazole

1. **Which of the following about fluconazole is false?**
   A. Fluconazole has been associated with abdominal discomfort, nausea and liver damage.
   B. In rare instances, it has been linked to severe skin rashes and fatal hepatic necrosis.
   C. Dizziness, headache, somnolence, delirium/coma, psychiatric disturbances, malaise, fatigue, and seizures have been reported.
   D. There are rare reports of fever, edema, pleural effusion, oliguria, and arthralgias.
   E. Irreversible alopecia is commonly associated with short-term use.
2. **Which of the following about fluconazole is true?**
   A. Limited information is available on the acute toxicity of fluconazole in humans. If acute overdosage occurs, supportive and symptomatic treatment should be initiated.
   B. Fluconazole may be administered orally only.
   C. Fluconazole acts by binding to fungal cytochrome P450.
   D. A and B
   E. A and C

KETOCONAZOLE

Ketoconazole (Nizoral®) is a synthetic substituted imidazole derivative structurally related to clotrimazole, miconazole, tioconazole, and econazole. It was the first broad-spectrum oral antifungal drug synthesized and has been used in the United States for more than a decade.

Pathophysiology

Ketoconazole exerts its antifungal effects by inhibiting the biosynthesis of ergosterol, the main sterol in the membranes of fungi. In addition, ketoconazole may inhibit the synthesis of cholesterol in mammalian cells, and it appears to interfere with cytochrome P450 enzyme systems in several organs.

Pharmacokinetics

ABSORPTION
- Rapid oral absorption.

DISTRIBUTION
- Volume of distribution is 0.36 L/kg. Ketoconazole is highly protein bound.

ELIMINATION
- Initial half-life is 2 hours and terminal half-life is 8 hours.
- Peak serum concentration generally is in 1–4 hours.

Clinical Presentations

Chronic use of ketoconazole may lead to anorexia, nausea or vomiting, pruritus, rash, and dizziness. Anaphylaxis rarely occurs after the first dose. As ketoconazole appears to interfere with gonadal function, it may suppress testosterone concentrations and can lead to gynecomastia, decreased libido, loss of potency in men, and menstrual irregularities in women. Adrenal crisis has followed as ketoconazole may lower cortisol concentration.

Hemolytic anemia, hypertension, and hypoglycemia have been observed. Hallucinations have been infrequently associated with ketoconazole and may reflect its penetration into the central nervous system. Serious hepatic toxicity is rare. Hepatitis associated with ketoconazole is usually reversible when treatment is stopped.

Toxic Dosage/Death

Ketoconazole has rarely been associated with overdose, although fatal hepatotoxicity has been reported.

Drug Interactions

Concomitant use with terfenadine (Seldane®, no longer available) has yielded Torsades de Pointes. Ketoconazole requires gastric acidity for absorption. Cimetidine (Tagamet®), ranitidine (Zantac®), famotidine (Pepcid®), and nizatidine (Axid®) decrease its absorption. Concurrent use of rifampin and ketoconazole markedly decreases the effects of both drugs. Ketoconazole may increase the effect of oral anticoagulants, the toxicity of cyclosporine, and the toxicity of corticosteroids. When ketoconazole is used with phenytoin, the serum concentrations of both drugs may be altered. A disulfiram-like reaction has been reported with alcohol.

Pregnancy/Lactation

Ketoconazole is embryotoxic in rats when administered in the first trimester of pregnancy. To date there are no adequate and controlled studies on the use of ketoconazole by pregnant women. Ketoconazole is probably distributed into human milk, suggesting that lactating women receiving the drug should not breast-feed until definitive studies reflect its safety. Pregnancy risk category C.

Laboratory

ANALYTIC METHODS

Serum and plasma levels of ketoconazole have been determined by bioassay and by more sensitive high-performance liquid chromatography methods.

BLOOD LEVELS

Blood levels are not helpful in guiding therapy.

Treatment

GUT DECONTAMINATION

There is no clinical evidence to support the efficacy of emesis or gastric lavage.

ELIMINATION ENHANCEMENT

As most of the parent drug ketoconazole is metabolized and little unchanged drug is found in the urine, extracorporeal methods to enhance elimination should not be expected to be useful.

SUPPORTIVE MEASURES

- For most patients with ketoconazole overdose, supportive symptomatic therapy, maintenance of life support measures (airway, respiration, and circulation), and administration of fluids to maintain sufficient urine flow would appear to be adequate.
- If hepatic and renal function tests are normal, and there is no evidence of adrenal or gonadal dysfunction, hypoglycemia, hemolytic anemia, hypertension, or central nervous system abnormalities, the patient can be discharged after being monitored for 24 hours (cardiovascular function, fluids, electrolytes).

Questions—Ketoconazole

1. Which of the following about ketoconazole is false?
- A. Concomitant use with terfenadine has yielded Torsades de Pointes.
- B. Ketoconazole requires gastric acidity for absorption.
- C. Cimetidine (Tagamet®), ranitidine (Zantac®), famotidine (Pepcid®), and nizatidine (Axid®) increase its absorption.
- D. Ketoconazole may increase the effect of oral anticoagulants, the toxicity of cyclosporine, and the toxicity of corticosteroids.
- E. When ketoconazole is used with phenytoin, concentrations of both drugs may be altered.

2. Clinical effects of ketoconazole use may include
- A. Anorexia, nausea or vomiting, pruritus, rash, and dizziness
- B. Anaphylaxis
- C. Gynecomastia, decreased libido, and menstrual irregularities in women
- D. All of the above
- E. None of the above

3. Other effects from ketoconazole include
- A. Hyperlipidemia
- B. Hemolytic anemia
- C. Hyperglycemia
- D. Avascular necrosis
- E. Sheehan's Syndrome

ITRACONAZOLE

Itraconazole (Sporanox®) is used in the treatment of blastomycosis, aspergillosis, and histoplasmosis. It can be used orally, is well absorbed, and undergoes extensive hepatic metabolism. It does not penetrate the brain or cerebrospinal fluid in therapeutic concentrations, is highly specific for fungal cytochrome P450, has no effect on mammalian steroid biosynthesis or hepatic drug metabolism, and does not appear to alter pituitary, testicular, or adrenal function. It is not recommended for pregnant or lactating mothers. An intravenous preparation is in late stages of clinical testing.

Serious toxicity has not been experienced with itraconazole except for mild gastrointestinal intolerance. Other reactions observed include hypokalemia, hypertriglyceridemia, and hepatic enzyme elevations. No fatal reactions have been noted. Gynecomastia and rashes are infrequent occurrences. Hypokalemia and hypertension have been observed. Further studies are required to evaluate the possible relationship of dose to toxicity.

Questions—Itraconazole

1. Which of the following is false?
- A. Itraconazole (Sporanox®) is used in the treatment of blastomycosis, aspergillosis, and histoplasmosis.
- B. It can be used orally, is well absorbed, and undergoes extensive hepatic metabolism.
- C. It penetrates the blood-brain barrier and may cause seizures.
- D. It is highly specific for fungal cytochrome P450, has no effect on mammalian steroid biosynthesis or hepatic drug metabolism, and does not appear to alter pituitary, or adrenal function.
- E. It is not recommended for pregnant or lactating mothers.

MICONAZOLE

Miconazole (Lotrimin®) is a synthetic imidazole derivative available for parenteral use and as miconazole nitrate for topical and vaginal use.

Pathophysiology

Miconazole, similar to other imidazoles, exerts its antifungal action by altering fungal cell membranes and interfering with intracellular enzymes. Overdosage with the intravenous form of miconazole may lead to arrhythmias, hyponatremia, lethargy, and seizures.

Pharmacokinetics

ABSORPTION

- Only 25–30% is absorbed orally.
- Dermal absorption is 0.1–0.3%.

DISTRIBUTION

- Protein binding is 90–93%.

ELIMINATION

- Approximately 50% is excreted in the feces after hepatic metabolism.
- Initial half-life is 40 minutes and secondary half-life is 2 hours.

Clinical Presentations

Adverse effects following intravenous miconazole have included nausea, vomiting, thrombophlebitis, anemia, and hyponatremia. Cardiac arrest and anaphylaxis may occur if given too fast intravenously. Cardiac monitoring in an overdose may disclose bradycardia, prolonged intraventricular conduction, and premature atrial beats.

Critical adverse reactions have been attributed to its vehicle (Cremophor EL). Seizures have also been reported. Because the commercial miconazole injection contains methylparaben and propylparaben as bactericidal agents, lactic acid as a buffering agent, and castor oil, it is not possible to exclude one or more of these agents as a cause of seizure activity.

Toxic Dosage/Death

A lethal dose has not been reported.

Drug Interactions

Miconazole may prolong prothrombin time in patients on warfarin or other coumarin anticoagulants. Drug interactions with cyclosporine, phenytoin, and rifampin may occur based on the structural similarity of miconazole to ketoconazole. There appears to be an antagonism between miconazole and amphotericin B.

Pregnancy/Lactation

Safe use of miconazole in pregnant women or nursing mothers has not been established. Pregnancy risk category C.

Treatment

GUT DECONTAMINATION

Gastrointestinal decontamination procedures have not been evaluated in imidazole overdoses.

ELIMINATION ENHANCEMENT

In view of its substantial apparent volume of distribution, high protein binding, extensive metabolism, and minimal renal excretion of unchanged drug, hemodialysis is probably ineffective after an overdose.

SUPPORTIVE MEASURES

- Severely intoxicated patients should receive an intravenous line, cardiac monitoring, electrocardiogram, and oxygen. Mechanical ventilation may be required.
- If acute shortness of breath, choking, hypotension, cyanosis, or laryngeal edema is observed, immediate treatment with epinephrine, oxygen, and an adequate airway may be indicated.
- Laboratory examination in an overdose should include complete blood count including platelet count, serum electrolytes, blood lipid profile, chest x-ray, electrocardiogram, cardiac monitoring, and appropriate diagnostic neurologic examinations.
- Seizures appear to respond to diazepam.

Questions—Miconazole

1. The vehicle in miconazole that has been associated with adverse reactions is

A. Cremophor EL
B. Polyethylene glycol
C. Benzoic acid
D. Hydroflourous acid
E. Gentian violet

2. Which of the following is false?

A. Miconazole, similar to other imidazoles, exerts its antifungal action by altering fungal cell membranes and interfering with intracellular enzymes.
B. Overdosage with the intravenous form of miconazole may lead to arrhythmias, hyponatremia, lethargy, and seizures.
C. Miconazole may shorten prothrombin time in patients on warfarin or other coumarin anticoagulants.
D. Drug interactions with cyclosporine, phenytoin, and rifampin may occur based on the structural similarity of miconazole to ketoconazole.
E. Adverse effects following intravenous miconazole have included nausea, vomiting, thrombophlebitis, anemia, and hyponatremia.

GRISEOFULVIN

Griseofulvin (Fulvicin®) is an oral fungistatic antibiotic produced by Penicillium griseofulvin that is effective in the treatment of dermatophytoses. It has been available for several decades. The incidence of adverse reactions to therapeutic doses is very low. Interest in griseofulvin, which may have waned with the appearance of the newer imidazoles, has increasingly focused on its use in a number of nonfungal diseases such as Raynaud's phenomenon, progressive systemic sclerosis, lichen planus, mycosis fungoides, herpes zoster, eosinophilic fasciitis, and molluscum contagiosum.

Pathophysiology

Although the precise mechanism of action of griseofulvin is still unknown, it is presumed to disrupt the fungal mitotic spindle structure and arrest fungal growth in the M phase of the life cycle.

Pharmacokinetics

ABSORPTION

- Absorption is enhanced by a fatty meal.
- Absorption of the "ultra-micro" size variety of griseofulvin is excellent.

DISTRIBUTION

- Half-life is 9–22 hours.

ELIMINATION

- Griseofulvin is metabolized extensively in the liver.

Clinical Presentations

Therapeutic use can lead to headaches, nausea, vomiting, anorexia, abdominal cramps, flatulence, and diarrhea. Hypersensitivity reactions to griseofulvin that may be life-threatening include urticaria, erythema multiforme, angioedema, and a reaction resembling serum sickness. Disabling neurologic phenomena such as vertigo, blurry vision, mental depression, lethargy, and insomnia have been observed. Rarely, life-threatening hepatotoxicity has been reported. Renal and hematopoietic toxicity following griseofulvin use is extremely rare.

Toxic Dosage/Death

A toxic or lethal dose in humans has not been established.

Drug Interactions

Concomitant use of griseofulvin with alcohol may cause tachycardia and flushing. Blood griseofulvin concentrations decrease when used with phenobarbital. There is a decrease in warfarin effectiveness. Concomitant use with oral contraceptives may enhance metabolism of the estrogenic component of the oral contraceptive and lead to amenorrhea, increased breakthrough bleeding, and decreased contraceptive efficacy.

Pregnancy/Lactation

Griseofulvin may be fetotoxic in pregnant patients. Its use in human pregnancy has been limited. Pregnancy risk category C.

Laboratory

ANALYTIC METHODS

Griseofulvin assay is not generally available in a hospital setting.

BLOOD LEVELS

Serum levels have not been correlated with toxic effects.

Treatment

GUT DECONTAMINATION

Gastric emptying with airway protection may be useful, although it has not been proved. There is no evidence to support the use of activated charcoal, or cathartics.

ELIMINATION ENHANCEMENT

There is no evidence to support the use of extracorporeal aids to elimination.

SUPPORTIVE MEASURES

- There are no specific data suggesting specific therapeutic measures for treatment of a griseofulvin overdose. Supportive and symptomatic therapy are indicated.
- After prompt evaluation of the airway, breathing, and circulatory status, attention must focus on any life-threatening complication such as a hypersensitivity reaction (angioedema, serum sickness) or a serious hepatotoxic reaction.
- Treatment of a hypersensitivity response may require intravenous fluids, central monitoring in patients with underlying cardiovascular disease, electrocardiographic monitoring, epinephrine, diphenhydramine, or β-adrenergic agonists for bronchospasm.
- Patients with serious renal, hepatotoxic, hemapoietic, or hypersensitivity reactions should be admitted to the hospital and, if required, followed in an intensive care facility with careful respiratory and cardiovascular monitoring. Patients may be discharged after renal, hepatic, and hematopoietic functions have been stabilized, the patient has no neurologic deficit, vital signs are normal, and there is no imminent threat of a recurrent hypersensitivity reaction.

Questions—Griseofulvin

1. Which of the following is false?

A. Therapeutic use of griseofulvin can lead to headaches, nausea, vomiting, anorexia, abdominal cramps, flatulence, and diarrhea.
B. Hypersensitivity reactions to griseofulvin that may be life-threatening include urticaria, erythema multiforme, angioedema, and a reaction resembling serum sickness.
C. Disabling neurologic phenomena such as vertigo, blurry vision, mental depression, lethargy, and insomnia have been observed with griseofulvin use.
D. Renal and hematopoietic toxicity following griseofulvin use is common.
E. A toxic or lethal dose has not been established.

2. Which of the following is true?

A. Griseofulvin (Fulvicin®) is an oral fungistatic antibiotic produced by Penicillium griseofulvin that is effective in the treatment of dermatophytoses.
B. The incidence of adverse reactions to therapeutic doses of griseofulvin is very low.
C. Interest in griseofulvin, which may have waned with the appearance of newer imidazoles, has increasingly focused on its use in a number of nonfungal diseases such as Raynaud's phenomenon, progressive systemic sclerosis, lichen planus, mycosis fungoides, herpes zoster, eosinophilic fasciitis, and molluscum contagiosum.
D. A and C
E. All of the above.

Answers

Introduction to Antifungal Drugs

1. D

Amphotericin B

1. B 2. D 3. E

Flucytosine

1. E 2. B

Fluconazole

1. E 2. E

Ketoconazole

1. C 2. D 3. B

Itraconazole

1. C

Miconazole

1. A 2. C

Griseofulvin

1. D 2. E

SELECTED READINGS

Antifungal Drugs

1. Araujo DE, Flowers FP, King MM. Griseofulvin: A new look at an old drug. DICP Ann Pharmacother 1990;24:851–854.
2. Drugs for treatment of fungal infections. Med Lett Drugs Ther 1990; 32(82a):58–60.
3. Fluconazole. Med Lett Drugs Ther 1990;32 (818):50–52.
4. Graybill JR, Carven PC. Antifungal agents used in systemic mycoses: Activity and therapeutic use. Drugs 1983;25:41–62.
5. Jacobs PH, Nael N. The action and safety of ketoconazole: A brief literature review. Cutis 1988;42:276–282.
6. Maddux MS, Barrier SL. A review of complications of amphotericin B therapy: Recommendations for prevention and management. Drug Intell Clin Pharm 1980;14:177–181.
7. Sabra R, Branch RA. Amphotericin B nephrotoxicity. Drug Saf 1990;5:94–108.
8. Van Tyle JH. Ketoconazole. Mechanism of action, spectrum of activity, pharmacokinetics, drug interactions, adverse reactions and therapeutic use. Pharmacotherapy 1984;4:343–373.

ACKNOWLEDGMENT

Thanks to Ira Leviton, MD for his help in developing this chapter.

CHAPTER 15

Antiparasitic and Antimalarial Drugs

INTRODUCTION

Numerous antiparasitic and antimalarial drugs have been identified. Major groups include alcohols such as mefloquine and halofantrine, 4-aminoquinolines such as chloroquine, hydroxychloroquine, and amodiaquine, and 8-aminoquinolines such as primaquine. Certain antibiotics such as tetracycline and erythromycin are also effective against various parasites. Other groups include the cinchona alkaloids of which quinine is a prime example and dihydrofolate reductase inhibitors such as proguanil and pyrimethamine.

Dihydrofolate reductase inhibitors are often combined with antibiotics, e.g., pyrimethamine plus sulfadoxine (Fansidar®) and pyrimethamine plus dapsone (Malparim®). This list is by no means exhaustive. Numerous agents, too many to review, have been tested against the hundreds of parasitic and helminthic illnesses around the world. Overdose reports are sporadic.

CHLOROQUINE AND AMINOQUINOLINES

Chloroquine (Aralen®), a synthetic 4-aminoquinoline derivative, is a primary drug for the treatment of malaria and is available in tablet form as chloroquine hydrochloride. 4-Aminoquinolines are related to hydroxychloroquine (Plaquenil®) and primaquine, an 8-aminoquinoline derivative.

Chloroquine causes severe poisoning in overdosage that may be rapidly fatal without therapeutic intervention. Chloroquine is currently used for prophylaxis and treatment of malaria, in extraintestinal amebiasis, for babesiosis, in rheumatoid arthritis, for lupus erythematosus as an adjunct to steroids in both the discoid and systemic forms, in porphyria cutanea tarda, and as an abortifacient.

Hydroxychloroquine, a synthetic 4-aminoquinoline derivative, is used for the suppression or chemoprophylaxis of malaria and for treatment of rheumatoid arthritis and lupus erythematosus. Overdoses and suicide attempts with hydroxychloroquine are rare. Few published data are available on the toxicokinetics of this compound after an overdose. Amodiaquine is another 4-aminoquinoline antimalarial agent. Reports of agranulocytosis and hepatitis have dampened enthusiasm for use of amodiaquine and it is no longer recommended for malaria prophylaxis.

Pathophysiology

4-Aminoquinoline derivatives appear to bind to nucleoproteins and inhibit DNA and RNA polymerase. High drug concentrations are found in the parasites' digestive vacuoles. Chloroquine has some antiinflammatory activity. In vitro, it has antihistaminic, antiserotonin, and prostaglandin inhibitory activity. 4-Aminoquinolines depress cardiac muscle, impair cardiac conductivity, and produce vasodilatation with resultant hypotension; they depress respiration and cause diplopia, dizziness, and nausea.

Pharmacokinetics

ABSORPTION

- Chloroquine is rapidly and almost completely absorbed (90%) from the gastrointestinal tract after oral administration. Bioavailability is greater with food.

DISTRIBUTION

- Chloroquine is widely distributed into liver, spleen, kidney, lungs, brain, and spinal cord. It binds to melanin-containing cells in the eyes and skin. In the blood, chloroquine concentrates in the erythrocytes and binds to platelets and leukocytes.
- Protein binding is 55%. Its volume of distribution is 93.6 L/kg, but values as high as 1,000 L/kg have been reported.

ELIMINATION

- The terminal half-life after a single 250-mg oral dose is 3.1 hours; after a single 500-mg oral dose, 42.9 hours; and after a single 1-gram oral dose, 312 hours.
- 10–20% is excreted unchanged in urine, 25% as the metabolite desethyl chloroquine.
- Small amounts are found in urine for months to years after the last known ingestion of the drug.

Clinical Presentations

CHLOROQUINE

The clinical features of an acute chloroquine poisoning episode may develop within 30 minutes of ingestion and rapidly lead to death if treatment is not rapidly instituted. Gastrointestinal effects include nausea and vomiting. Rapid superficial breathing, Cheyne-Stokes breathing, sudden apnea, respiratory failure, or, terminally, respiratory arrest may be observed.

Neurologic Effects

Drowsiness and lethargy are seen early. Later the patient may become excitable and uncooperative. Headache, photophobia, and seizures appear either as presenting signs or terminally. Signs and symptoms may include difficulty in swallowing, a constricting feeling in the throat, paresthesias, analgesia in the face and neck area, tremors, difficulty speaking, absence of deep tendon reflexes, athetoid movements and coma. Diplopia, abnormal eye movements, wandering gaze, opacities in the cornea, and retinal injury may be seen after chronic administration.

Cardiovascular Effects

The cardiovascular system is the most profoundly affected site of action of chloroquine. Chloroquine is a powerful cardiotoxin, reducing the excitability and conductivity of cardiac muscles similar to that observed with quinidine. Sudden hypotension may occur, with absence of peripheral pulses, vasodilatation, cyanosis of the lips and face, arrhythmias, and cardiac arrest may be seen early. The electrocardiogram may show bradycardia, atrial standstill, a widened QRS, prolonged intraventricular conduction, inverted or flattened T waves, S-T segment depression, ventricular tachycardia, nodal rhythm, prolongation of QT, complete heart block, or ventricular fibrillation.

HYDROXYCHLOROQUINE

Hydroxychloroquine is rarely associated with cardiotoxicity. Abuse of hydroxychloroquine may impair conductivity and decrease excitability. Other signs of hydroxychloroquine overdose may include seizures, vomiting, arrhythmias, cardiac arrest, death, acute necrotizing eosinophilic myocarditis, myopathy, ventricular arrhythmias, and hepatic failure.

AMODIAQUINE

Amodiaquine overdose has been associated with syncope, spasticity, speech problems, seizures, involuntary movements, agranulocytosis, and hepatitis.

Toxic Dosage/Death

Myocardial toxicity and arrhythmias are probably the cause of death in chloroquine poisoning. Toxic blood levels range from 3–99 μg/mL. Possible predictors of death from chloroquine poisoning include a systolic blood pressure less than 85 mm Hg, dose ingested greater than 5 grams, QRS prolongation of at least 0.12 second, and a blood chloroquine concentration greater than 25 mmol/L (8 mg/mL).

Pregnancy/Lactation

Chloroquine crosses the placenta. Chloroquine, 250 mg daily, was administered to one mother during two pregnancies from 6 weeks after conception until term. Both offspring exhibited severe deafness and vestibular damage. An insignificant amount is found in breast milk. Chloroquine and hydroxychloroquine are classified as pregnancy risk category C.

Laboratory

ANALYTIC METHODS

High-performance liquid chromatography (HPLC) can be used to detect chloroquine and its main metabolite desethylchloroquine. HPLC may also be used to analyze amodiaquine and hydroxychloroquine.

BLOOD LEVELS

Peak plasma concentrations are reached in 1–2 hours. Orally, 500 mg results in a peak serum concentration of 0.12 μg/mL. A single 1-gram oral dose results in a peak serum level of 0.34 μg/mL. Chloroquine and chloroquine metabolite blood levels are not of practical assistance in the management of a chloroquine poisoning.

Treatment

GUT DECONTAMINATION

Emesis should be avoided because of rapid onset of symptoms. If gastric emptying is preferred, it should be performed with prior endotracheal intubation. The drug is rapidly absorbed however, and if symptoms are already present, gastric emptying may not be effective. Gastric lavage may precipitate cardiac manifestations. Activated charcoal can prevent absorption of more than 95% of an ingested chloroquine dose still in the stomach and should be administered as soon as possible after oral ingestion of chloroquine. Activated charcoal (adults, 60–100 grams and children, 30–60 grams) may be placed into the gastric lavage tube after lavage.

ELIMINATION ENHANCEMENT

Forced diuresis and/or urinary acidification may increase the excretion of unchanged chloroquine, but neither procedure is recommended. Charcoal hemoperfusion may be effective if begun very early after ingestion in a severely toxic patient, however, clinical studies have not adequately proven its usefulness. Peritoneal dialysis and hemodialysis are not effective. The high volume of distribution of chloroquine in tissue limits dialysis and hemoperfusion techniques. Exchange transfusion may prove to be useful, as chloroquine concentrations are high in red blood cells, whole blood cells, and platelets. However no studies are available to validate this concept.

SUPPORTIVE MEASURES

- Death may result in the first hour after ingestion, especially in children. Treatment is largely supportive. As cardiac and respiratory arrest may quickly supervene, preparations should be made for tracheal airway protection (endotracheal intubation) and mechanical ventilation. Defibrillators and cardiac pacemakers may be required.
- Treat seizures with diazepam (up to 10 mg i.v. slowly in adults and 0.1–0.3 mg/kg i.v. slowly in children). If unresponsive: phenytoin, 15 mg/kg i.v. at up to 0.5 mg/kg/min, and ECG monitoring may be given. Studies in rats and one clinical report show that diazepam may have a protective effect in chloroquine intoxication.
- Treat hypotension with intravenous fluids and Trendelenburg's position initially. Epinephrine has been used to treat chloroquine-induced hypotension. An initial dose of 0.25 mg/kg per minute is followed by increments of 0.25 mg/kg per minute until an adequate systolic arterial pressure (about 100 mm Hg) is obtained. Dopamine and norepinephrine may also be used.
- Hemolytic anemia may be seen in patients with glucose-6-phosphate dehydrogenase (G6PD) deficiency. Methemoglobinemia, anemia, leukopenia, and thrombocytopenia have been observed. Monitor methemoglobin in cyanotic patients. For methemoglobinemia greater than 30%, methylene blue is administered. For hemolysis, transfusion, alkalinization, and diuresis are employed. Monitor liver and renal function.

- Acute chloroquine intoxication is associated with a hypokalemia that is correlated with the severity of the intoxication. Plasma potassium levels should be followed closely, particularly in patients receiving catecholamine infusions. The physician should avoid repleting with too much potassium and thereby inducing hyperkalemia.
- Arrhythmias may require lidocaine. Avoid class IA antiarrhythmics (quinidine, disopyramide, and procainamide). Intraventricular block may be treated with isoproterenol and/or pacemaker.

Antidotes

There are no antidotes. Diazepam may have a protective effect in diminishing chloroquine toxicity but this has not been established. Anecdotal reports note that the combination of diazepam and epinephrine may be effective in reversing large (i.e., > 5 gram) overdoses.

Questions—Chloroquine and Aminoquinolines

1. Which of the following is false?
A. High-performance liquid chromatography can be used to detect chloroquine and its main metabolite desethylchloroquine.
B. Forced diuresis and/or urinary alkalinization may increase excretion of unchanged chloroquine but neither procedure is recommended.
C. Acute chloroquine intoxication is associated with a hypokalemia that is correlated with the severity of the intoxication.
D. Chloroquine crosses the placenta.
E. Chloroquine causes severe poisoning in overdosage that may be rapidly fatal without therapeutic intervention.

2. Chloroquine has each of the following, except
A. Some anti-inflammatory activity
B. Antihistaminic activity
C. Anti-serotonergic activity
D. Prostaglandin inhibitory activity
E. Antidopaminergic activity

3. Which of the following regarding the cardiotoxicity of chloroquine is true?
A. The cardiovascular system is rarely affected by chloroquine.
B. Chloroquine is a powerful cardiotoxin, reducing the excitability and conductivity of cardiac muscles similar to that observed with quinidine.
C. Sudden hypertension may occur, with absence of peripheral pulses, vasodilatation, cyanosis of the lips and face, arrhythmias, and cardiac arrest often seen early.
D. The electrocardiogram may reveal QRS narrowing.
E. Ventricular fibrillation has not been associated with chloroquine use.

4. Which of the following is false?
A. Amodiaquine overdose has been associated with syncope, spasticity, speech problems, seizures, involuntary movements, agranulocytosis, and hepatitis.
B. Hydroxychloroquine, like chloroquine, is frequently associated with cardiotoxicity.
C. Hemolytic anemia may be seen in patients with glucose-6-phosphate dehydrogenase (G6PD) deficiency after chloroquine exposures.
D. Activated charcoal can prevent absorption of more than 95% of the fraction of an ingested chloroquine dose still in the stomach and should be administered as soon as possible after oral ingestion of chloroquine.
E. Signs of hydroxychloroquine overdose may include seizures, vomiting, arrhythmias, cardiac arrest, death, acute necrotizing myocarditis, myopathy, ventricular arrhythmias, and hepatic failure.

QUININE

Quinine (Quinamm®) poisoning has been increasingly reported during the past 10–20 years. Quinine overdoses primarily occur because of abortion attempts, suicide attempts, and accidental ingestions. Death generally follows renal failure, acute hemolytic anemia, and respiratory arrest. The major causes of morbidity in nonfatal cases of quinine overdose include reversible renal failure, cinchonism, prolonged hearing deficits, and blindness.

Heroin addicts who inject heroin diluted with quinine intravenously may develop convulsions, coma, or death. Although quinine is not used as often for adulteration of heroin as previously, narcotic addicts who present with atrioventricular conduction defects should have their urine examined for quinine. Drug screening for employment has frequently included urine testing for quinine as an indirect indication of heroin or other drug abuse. As an 8-oz bottle of tonic mixer contains approximately 2.2 mg of quinine per fluid ounce, an individual who has recently had a gin and tonic may be suspected of heroin usage.

Quinine is used to treat chloroquine-resistant malaria. It is also used for nocturnal cramps, in patients with myotonia, and occasionally as an illicit abortifacient. When an initial dosage fails to produce an abortion, the dosage may be repeated until toxic levels are inadvertently reached. Quinine, like quinidine, is an alkaloid obtained from the bark of the cinchona tree. It is the levorotatory isomer of quinidine, and is available commercially as the sulfate salt.

Pathophysiology

Quinine appears to interfere with the function of plasmodial DNA. It is a local irritant, has a local anesthetic action, and acts on all muscle groups. Subcutaneously or intramuscularly, it is very painful. It acts similarly to quinidine on cardiac muscle when given intravenously, and may cause severe hypotension. It may be oxytocic to the pregnant uterus. On skeletal muscle, it decreases tetanic response, excitability of the motor end plate, and calcium distribution. When ingested orally, it produces gastric pain, nausea, and vomiting. When administered intravenously quinine may cause venous thrombosis. In the kidney, it may induce tubular damage. Quinine may cause inappropriate insulin release, leading to symptomatic hypoglycemia.

Pharmacokinetics

ABSORPTION

- Over 90% of quinine is absorbed orally, mainly from the small intestine.
- Peak plasma levels are reached in 1–3 hours.

DISTRIBUTION

- Protein binding is 70%. The apparent volume of distribution is 1.2–1.7 L/kg.
- Quinine is widely distributed to body tissues including cerebrospinal fluid.

Answers to questions in shaded boxes appear at the end of the chapter.

ELIMINATION

- Quinine is metabolized in the liver by hydroxylation. Quinine is eliminated mainly in urine as metabolic products. Less than 5% is normally excreted unchanged in the urine, whereas in overdose, less than 25% is excreted unchanged.
- Its half-life in plasma is 5 hours; however in overdose patients, its elimination half-life is 25 hours.
- There is some evidence that quinine is excreted more rapidly in acidic urine. However, there is considerable doubt that forced acid diuresis is useful in quinine overdose.

Clinical Presentations

OPHTHALMOLOGIC EFFECTS

Eye changes may appear the next day or after the patient awakens from a heavy sleep or coma. Eye changes may also begin as early as an hour after overdose and partial or complete blindness may be sudden. Resolution of blindness may take hours to weeks and patients may remain permanently blind. The pupils are fixed and dilated in most cases of quinine poisoning. Constriction in the visual fields is probably the most constant sign. As amaurosis or amblyopia passes, the patient may be hampered by loss of his peripheral vision even when central vision returns to normal. Improvement may take place over months or years.

Some enlargement of pupils may remain permanently, which do not react to accommodation. In the acute stages of vision loss, the electroretinogram may remain almost normal. It becomes abnormal during the phase of visual improvement and parallels the changes in visual acuity on the second or third day. Visual evoked potential, dark adaptation, and color testing measurements are often abnormal. Ophthalmoscopic changes include pallor of the optic disks, extreme contraction of the arteries and veins of the retina, cherry spot at the macula, and retinal edema.

OTOTOXIC EFFECTS

Deafness is an early sign. It usually passes quickly and completely. Deafness may also be accompanied by tinnitus, a feeling of fullness in the head, headache, giddiness, and dizziness. The patient may also present with mutism.

CARDIAC EFFECTS

The cardiotoxicity of quinine is similar to that of class IA antiarrhythmic drugs. Cardiotoxicity is usually the cause of death from overdose. Quinine has a negative inotropic action. It slows the rate of depolarization and conduction and increases action potential duration and effective refractory period of the myocardium. Sinus tachycardia, high-degree atrioventricular block, prolongation of the PR interval, sinoatrial block and arrest, AV dissociation, ventricular fibrillation, Torsade de Pointes, and prominent U waves may be seen. Quinine also has α-adrenergic blocking effects. Hypotension may follow vasodilation, myocardial depression, or dysrhythmia.

CINCHONISM

Tinnitus, dizziness, rash, cardiovascular effects, headache, fever, intestinal cramping, diarrhea, vomiting, apprehension, confusion, and seizures compose the constellation of symptoms associated with cinchonism. The patient feels fine the next day if quinine is discontinued. With small doses, a hypersensitivity response may occur, consisting of flushing, pruritus, rashes, fever, gastric distress, dyspnea, tinnitus, or visual impairment. Angioedema has also been described.

MISCELLANEOUS EFFECTS

Symptoms usually disappear except for residual optic nerve or auditory damage. Hypoglycemia may be present. Rarely anuria, uremia, tubular necrosis, acute hemolytic anemia, hemoglobinuria, hypoprothrombinemia, purpura, agranulocytosis, abortion, asthma, peripheral neuropathy and sensory loss may be observed.

Toxic Dosage/Death

After overdose, the fatal oral dose in adults is approximately 8 grams in sensitive individuals. However, doses of less than 1 gram have proven fatal. Fatalities have occurred with a 900-mg dose in children under 2 years. Untoward effects are typically observed in the 2.5–4.0 gram range. Plasma levels associated with toxic effects average 10 μg/mL. Fatal plasma quinine levels taken before death averaged 9.1–16.0 μg/mL in one study.

Drug Interactions

Alcohol intake may exacerbate quinine toxicity. Increased serum digoxin, and decreased renal clearance of digoxin may occur with quinine use. Delayed or decreased absorption of oral quinine may occur with aluminum-containing antacids. Concomitant use with neuromuscular blocking agents such as pancuronium, succinylcholine, and tubocurarine may potentiate their effects. The effect of oral anticoagulants with quinine use is enhanced.

Pregnancy/Lactation

Quinine passes through the placenta and into breast milk. Use of quinine as an abortifacient can produce poisoning in the fetus and result in infant deafness. Other suspected teratogenic effects of quinine are blindness and physical malformations. Pregnancy risk category D.

Laboratory

ANALYTIC METHODS

Plasma quinine levels can be performed with a modification of the test used to measure quinidine levels using high-performance liquid chromatography.

BLOOD LEVELS

When plasma quinine determinations can be quickly performed (within a few hours after ingestion) in a patient who has not yet developed eye signs or symptoms, they may be a predictor of visual change. A dose of 10 mg/kg produces peak levels of 7–17 μg/mL. Ocular toxic effects are most likely to occur in patients with plasma quinine levels over 15 μg/mL less than 10 hours after ingestion and over 10 μg/mL 10 hours postingestion. Plasma concentrations over 16 μg/mL may be associated with cardiac arrhythmias. Tinnitus is usually associated with plasma levels of 9–10 μg/mL, but levels as low as 2–3 μg/mL have been reported with this symptom.

Treatment

GUT DECONTAMINATION

Early emesis induction is relatively contraindicated due to the rapidity of absorption. Gastric lavage and/or repeated administration of activated charcoal may be preferable for patients in whom rapid clinical deterioration is suspected. Repeated activated charcoal reduces the plasma half-life of quinine and should be administered early in quinine overdosage. It may be the only effective way to lessen the potentially disastrous consequences of permanent blindness and fatal cardiotoxicity.

ELIMINATION ENHANCEMENT

Measures to enhance the elimination of quinine have been generally ineffective. Hemodialysis combined with resin hemoperfusion may be effective in the treatment of quinine blindness refractory to usual therapy. Exchange transfusion has not been successful. The extensive protein binding and volume of distribution of the drug limit the efficacy of these procedures. Forced acid diuresis is unlikely to produce a sufficiently rapid reduction in plasma concentration or to have a substantial effect on visual disturbance.

SUPPORTIVE MEASURES

- Supportive care remains the mainstay of treatment for quinine toxicity. On admission, blood is drawn for a complete blood count, blood sugar, prothrombin time, renal function tests, urinalysis, and electrolytes. Blood for evaluation of plasma quinine level should be drawn even if visual symptoms are absent as they may be of prognostic value.
- The overdose patient should be hospitalized in an intensive care facility. Immediate attention to vital signs with careful monitoring of electrocardiograms and ventilation should be instituted. Preparations must be made for assisted ventilation as necessary.
- Treatment includes careful eye examinations (visual fields, electroretinography, electrooculogram, visual evoked potentials, dark adaptations, color testing) and ear evaluations.
- Class I, II, and III antiarrhythmic agents should be avoided. Direct-current cardioversion is used to treat ventricular tachycardia or ventricular fibrillation. Overdrive pacing or isoproterenol may be useful for Torsade de Pointes. Transvenous pacing can be useful for complete heart block or marked prolongation of the QRS complex.
- Stellate ganglion block has been advocated by some for the treatment of quinine amblyopia, but is considered by others to have no rational basis and to be ineffective. It may also result in death or serious complications such as aphasia or hemiparesis.
- For angioedema, epinephrine and diphenhydramine may be useful.
- Fluid and electrolyte monitoring and repeated evaluations of renal function should be performed. Acidosis, electrolyte imbalance, and hypoxia must be treated aggressively to halt the progression of cardiotoxicity.
- Hyperbaric oxygen has been suggested by some, but remains controversial.
- Unfortunately, there is no evidence that any treatment affects visual prognosis.

Questions—Quinine

1. **Which of the following is false?**
   A. Quinine poisoning has been increasingly reported during the past 20 years.
   B. Quinine overdoses primarily occur because of abortion attempts, suicide attempts, and accidental ingestions.
   C. Death generally follows renal failure, acute hemolytic anemia, and respiratory arrest.
   D. The major causes of morbidity in nonfatal cases of quinine overdose include reversible renal failure, cinchonism, prolonged hearing deficits, and blindness.
   E. Contrary to popular belief, tonic water can not give a false positive result on toxic screen.
2. **Which of the following is true?**
   A. Heroin addicts who inject heroin diluted with quinine intravenously may develop convulsions, coma, or death.
   B. Quinine is no longer used to adulterate heroin.
   C. Drug screening for employment does not detect quinine.
   D. Measures to enhance the elimination of quinine have been generally effective.
   E. Exchange transfusion has been successful in quinine overdose.
3. **Signs of cinchonism include all of the following except**
   A. Tinnitus
   B. Dizziness
   C. Impotence
   D. Cardiovascular effects
4. **Which of the following concerning the cardiotoxicity of quinine is false?**
   A. The cardiotoxicity of quinine is similar to that of class IA antiarrhythmics.
   B. Cardiotoxicity is rarely the cause of death from overdose.
   C. Quinine has a negative inotropic action.
   D. Quinine slows the rate of depolarization and conduction and increases action potential duration and effective refractory period of the myocardium.
   E. Sinus tachycardia, high-degree atrioventricular heart block, prolongation of the PR interval, sinoatrial block and arrest, complete dissociation, ventricular fibrillation, Torsade de Pointes, and prominent U waves may be seen in quinine overdose.
5. **The ototoxic effects of quinine include**
   A. Deafness
   B. Tinnitus
   C. Dizziness
   D. All of the above
   E. None of the above

PROGUANIL AND PYRIMETHAMINE

Proguanil hydrochloride is a synthetic antimalarial agent that may, after long-term use, lead to renal failure and megaloblastic anemia. Overdoses are generally followed by complete recovery, although deaths have been reported. Treatment is symptomatic and supportive.

Pyrimethamine (Daraprim®) is a folic acid antagonist. It is the best known of the many 2,4-diaminopyrimidines synthesized for antimicrobial activity and is the most active against plasmodia. It is structurally related to trimethoprim. Pyrimethamine-sulfadoxine is currently the drug of choice for the prophylaxis of malaria caused by chloroquine-resistant Plasmodium falciparum. Pyrimethamine can be used with dapsone as an alternative. Pyrimethamine is of little value in treating acute malaria alone with the exception of its use with quinine in Plasmodium falciparum-resistant malaria when pyrimethamine-sulfadoxine cannot be used.

In conjunction with a sulfonamide, pyrimethamine is used for the treatment of toxoplasmosis. Some pyrimethamine intoxications are due to overdosages in infants treated for congenital toxoplasmosis. Trials of pyrimethamine-sulfadoxine (Fansidar®) have evaluated its prophylactic role in the prevention of Pneumocystis pneumonia seen in AIDS.

Pathophysiology

Proguanil and pyrimethamine are dihydrofolate reductase inhibitors. Pyrimethamine is a folic acid antagonist. It binds to and reversibly inhibits dihydrofolate reductase in parasites, preventing the reduction of dihydrofolic acid to tetrahydrofolic acid (folinic acid).

Pharmacokinetics

ABSORPTION

- Pyrimethamine is well absorbed from the GI tract and reaches a peak serum level in 2 hours.

DISTRIBUTION

- The apparent volume of distribution of pyrimethamine is 2.8–2.9 L/kg.
- Pyrimethamine is distributed to the kidneys, lungs, liver, and spleen.

ELIMINATION

- The half-life of pyrimethamine is 4–6 days.
- About 20–30% of a dose is excreted in the urine. Metabolites are excreted in the urine for weeks.

Clinical Presentations

PROGUANIL

Proguanil may cause mouth ulcers, diarrhea, vomiting, abdominal pain, chronic renal failure, megaloblastic anemia, and pancytopenia.

PYRIMETHAMINE

Anorexia, nausea, vomiting, abdominal cramps, atrophic glossitis, and gastritis may be seen. Dyspnea, apnea, bilateral rales, and respiratory failure have been reported. Stevens-Johnson syndrome and cyanosis may be seen.

Hematologic Effects

High doses may lead to folic acid deficiency, which may yield reversible bone marrow depression, megaloblastic anemia, leukopenia, thrombocytopenia, agranulocytosis, and pancytopenia. Hemolysis may occur in patients with glucose-6-phosphate dehydrogenase (G6PD) deficiency when used in combination with sulfadoxine.

Neurologic Effects

Ataxia, tremors, refractory seizures, malaise, fatigue, irritability, photosensitivity, and blindness have occurred with pyrimethamine. Pupils may be dilated. The electroencephalogram shows slow amplitude. There may be motor weakness and hyperactive deep tendon reflexes.

Toxic Dosage/Death

Poisonings with pyrimethamine have been observed in areas indigenous to its use and are frequently fatal. Toxic blood levels of proguanil are >100 ng/mL.

Pregnancy/Lactation

Pyrimethamine is distributed into breast milk. Six hours after 50–75 mg is taken orally, levels of 3.1–3.3 μg/mL are found in milk and are still detectable at 48 hours. Pregnancy risk category C.

Laboratory

ANALYTIC METHODS

High performance liquid chromatography may be used to analyze these agents.

BLOOD LEVELS

Blood levels of pyrimethamine are not clinically useful in the treatment of overdosage. Peak plasma levels of pyrimethamine (after 25 mg orally) are 0.13–0.4 μg/mL. Peak sulfadoxine plasma levels (after 500 mg orally) are 51–76 μg/mL, reached in 2.5–6 hours.

Treatment

GUT DECONTAMINATION

Since convulsions may start soon after significant ingestions, endotracheal intubation should be performed before gastric lavage and charcoal administration.

ELIMINATION ENHANCEMENT

There are no reports of dialysis being used to treat these agents.

SUPPORTIVE MEASURES

- Treat hematologic consequences by discontinuing pyrimethamine. Folate deficiency is treated with calcium leucovorin injection, 3–9 mg/d i.m. for 3 days, or more, and oral folic acid, 10 mg/d.
- For gastrointestinal toxicity, reduce dosage and try to administer medication with meals.
- In case of seizures, ascertain airway patency. Give diazepam or phenytoin intravenously. Severe convulsions may ultimately require general anesthesia.
- Respiratory failure is treated with mechanical ventilation, positive pressure breathing, endotracheal intubation, and oxygen as required.
- Labs should include complete blood counts including platelets and reticulocyte counts. Renal and hematopoietic systems should be monitored for at least 1 month after overdosage with pyrimethamine alone or in combination with sulfadoxine.

Antidotes

There are no known antidotes for all adverse effects. However, folate and leucovorin may reverse hematologic consequences induced by folate depletion.

Questions—Proguanil and Pyrimethamine

1. Which of the following is false?

A. Proguanil hydrochloride is a synthetic antimalarial agent that may, after long-term use, lead to renal failure and megaloblastic anemia.
B. Pyrimethamine (Daraprim®) is a folic acid antagonist.
C. Pyrimethamine is structurally related to dapsone.
D. Pyrimethamine-sulfadoxine is currently the drug of choice for the prophylaxis of malaria caused by chloroquine-resistant P. falciparum.
E. In conjunction with a sulfonamide, pyrimethamine is used to treat toxoplasmosis.

2. **Which of the following is true?**
   A. Some pyrimethamine intoxications are due to overdoses in infants treated for congenital toxoplasmosis.
   B. Pyrimethamine may cause mouth ulcers, diarrhea, vomiting, abdominal pain, chronic renal failure, megaloblastic anemia, and pancytopenia.
   C. Blood levels of pyrimethamine are clinically useful in the treatment of overdose.
   D. Ataxia, tremors, refractory seizures, malaise, fatigue, irritability, photosensitivity, and blindness have occurred with proguanil.
   E. Poisonings with pyrimethamine have been observed in areas indigenous to its use and are rarely fatal.

MEFLOQUINE AND HALOFANTRINE

Mefloquine (Lariam®), a 4-quinoline methanol derivative, is an antimalarial drug chemically related to quinine. It is available for the prevention and treatment of Plasmodium falciparum and Plasmodium vivax malaria. Halofantrine, an amino alcohol, together with mefloquine and artemisinine derivatives, is used in the treatment of chloroquine-resistant malaria. Halofantrine is not available in the United States.

Clinical Presentations

MEFLOQUINE

Adverse effects from mefloquine include seizures, vertigo, nausea, dizziness, fatigue, and acute psychosis. An "acute brain syndrome," consisting of encephalopathy with disorientation and mental dysfunction, sometimes complicated by status epilepticus and coma, has been described. A psychiatric syndrome consisting of acute psychosis, memory loss, confusion, hallucinations, and behavioral abnormalities (such as aggression, agitation, hyperactivity or hypoactivity) has been noted with mefloquine use. Depression can be severe, with suicide attempts, and may persist as long as 9 months. Other psychiatric symptoms generally do not last more than 10 days. Toxic blood levels of mefloquine are >1000 ng/mL.

HALOFANTRINE

Acute adverse effects include abdominal pain, diarrhea, intravascular hemolysis, increases in liver enzyme levels, and pruritus. Prolongation of the QT interval has also been reported.

Laboratory

ANALYTIC METHODS

High performance liquid chromatography is used to analyze mefloquine and halofantrine.

BLOOD LEVELS

As these levels are not readily available, their use in overdose is not generally warranted.

Treatment

GUT DECONTAMINATION

Since convulsions may start soon after significant ingestions, endotracheal intubation should be performed before gastric lavage and charcoal administration.

ELIMINATION ENHANCEMENT

There are no reports of dialysis being used to treat these agents.

SUPPORTIVE MEASURES

- Seizures are treated with diazepam. Treatment is symptomatic and supportive.

Questions—Mefloquine and Halofantrine

1. **Signs of mefloquine toxicity include**
   A. Seizures, vertigo, nausea, dizziness, fatigue, and acute psychosis.
   B. An "acute brain syndrome," consisting of encephalopathy with disorientation and mental dysfunction, sometimes complicated by status epilepticus and coma.
   C. A psychiatric syndrome consisting of acute psychosis, memory loss, confusion, hallucinations, and behavioral abnormalities.
   D. Depression.
   E. All of the above.

Answers

Chloroquine and Aminoquinolines

1. B 2. E 3. B 4. B

Quinine

1. E 2. A 3. C 4. B 5. D

Proguanil and Pyrimethamine

1. C 2. A

Mefloquine and Halofantrine

1. E

SELECTED READINGS

Chloroquine and Aminoquinolines

1. Chloroquine and other antimalarials. In: Reynolds JEF, ed.Martindale: The Extra Pharmacopoeia. 30th ed. London: Pharmaceutical Press, 1993: 393–411.
2. Mofenson H, Caraccio TR. Treatment of severe chloroquine poisoning. N Engl J Med 1988;319:50.
3. Wang R. Hydroxychloroquine cardiotoxicity. Clin Toxicol 1995;33:475–486. Abstract 164.
4. Wilkinson R, Mahatane J, Wade P, Parvol G. Chloroquine poisoning. Br Med J 1993;307:504.

Quinine

1. Bateman DN, Blain PG, Woodhouse KW, et al. Pharmacokinetics and clinical toxicity of quinine overdosage: Lack of efficacy of techniques intended to enhance elimination. Q J Med N Ser 1985;54:125–131.
2. Boland ME, Roper S, Henry JA. Complications of quinine poisoning. Lancet 1985;1:384–5.
3. Schonwald S, Shannon M. Unsuspected quinine intoxication presenting as acute deafness and mutism. Am J Emerg Med 1991;9:318–320.
4. Wolf LR, Otten EJ, Spadafora MP. Cinchonism: Two case reports and review of acute quinine toxicity and treatment. J Emerg Med 1992;10:295–301.

Proguanil and Pyrimethamine

1. Helsby NA, Ward SA, Edwards G, et al. The pharmacokinetics and activations of proguanil in man: Consequences of variability in drug metabolism. Br J Clin Pharmacol 1990;30:593–598.
2. Pyrimethamine. In: McEvoy GK, ed. AHFS Drug Information 94. Bethesda, MD: American Society of Hospital Pharmacists, 1994:460–464.

Mefloquine and Halofantrine

1. Halofantrine in the treatment of malaria. Lancet 1989;2:537–538. Editorial.
2. Hennequin C, Bouree P, Bazin N, et al. Severe psychiatric side effects observed during prophylaxis and treatment with mefloquine. Arch Intern Med 1994;154:2360–2362.
3. Patchen LC, Campbell CC, Williams SB. Neurologic reactions after a therapeutic dose of mefloquine. N Engl J Med 1989;321:1415–1416.

CHAPTER 16

Antiviral and AIDS Drugs

INTRODUCTION

Multiple drugs are currently in use for the treatment of viral infections in the United States. These include a multitude of ever changing AIDS drugs: acyclovir (Zovirax®), valacyclovir (Valtrex®), famciclovir (Famvir®), ganciclovir (Cytovene®), cidofovir (Vistide®), amantadine (Symmetrel®), rimantadine (Flumadine®), ribavirin (Virazole®), interferon (Intron® or Roferon®) and foscarnet (Foscavir®).

Acyclovir is used for genital herpes, herpes encephalitis, neonatal herpes, herpes zoster (shingles), and mucocutaneous disease due to herpes simplex in the immunocompromised host. Ganciclovir is used for the treatment of cytomegalovirus. Amantadine is used to treat influenza A virus. Overdose with fatalities has been reported following acyclovir and amantadine. Treatment is largely symptomatic and supportive.

ACYCLOVIR AND GANCICLOVIR

Acyclovir (Zovirax®) is a synthetic purine nucleoside derived from guanine. Its active form is acyclovir triphosphate, which accumulates in infected cells as a result of transformation by viral thymidine kinase. It is used for the treatment of genital and other herpes simplex virus infections. Related products, valacyclovir, and famciclovir are also used to combat herpes simplex virus (HSV).

Ganciclovir (Cytovene®) is used to treat cytomegalovirus (CMV) retinitis, colitis and esophagitis-complications notably present in the HIV positive population. Ganciclovir is also active against all the viruses that are treated by acyclovir. Ganciclovir resembles acyclovir except for the addition of a hydroxy-methyl group, a change that may enable the compound to be incorporated into both viral and host DNA. A related product, cidofovir (Vistide®), is also used to treat CMV.

Pathophysiology

Acyclovir is an antiviral agent only after it is phosphorylated in infected cells by a virus-induced enzyme. After phosphorylation, it becomes an inhibitor of viral DNA polymerase. Once acyclovir is incorporated into the growing viral DNA chain, further DNA elongation cannot occur and the virus cannot replicate. It is the first antiviral drug to require a viral enzyme for activation. Ganciclovir is also phosphorylated to a substrate, which ultimately inhibits viral DNA synthesis.

Pharmacokinetics

ACYCLOVIR

Absorption

- Bioavailability is 25–30%, and time to peak plasma level is 2 hours.

Distribution

- Volume of distribution is 0.8 L/kg. Plasma protein binding is 15–20%.

Elimination

- Elimination half-life is 3 hours and 90–92% is excreted unchanged.

GANCICLOVIR

Absorption

- Ganciclovir is well absorbed.

Distribution

- Plasma protein binding is 1–2%.

Elimination

- Elimination half-life is 2–6 hours, and 94–99% is excreted unchanged.

Clinical Presentations

ACYCLOVIR

Topical use of acyclovir may yield occasional burning or stinging on application, with mild erythema on drying. Short-term oral use of acyclovir has been associated with nausea and vomiting. Long-term oral use is generally well tolerated, with nausea, vomiting, diarrhea, abdominal pain, rash, and headache occurring in less than 5% of patients. The adverse reactions most frequently reported with intravenous acyclovir are inflammation and phlebitis at the injection site.

Neurologic and psychiatric effects may include lethargy, tremors, confusion, hallucinations, and seizures. Susceptibility to neurotoxic manifestations is increased with end-stage renal disease. Acyclovir crystals may precipitate in renal tubules when it is given at high doses, resulting in renal dysfunction, renal failure, or anuria. Acute nonoliguric renal failure may follow the intravenous use of acyclovir. Unlike ganciclovir, acyclovir has no dose-related effect on bone marrow.

GANCICLOVIR

The occurrence of significant neutropenia averages 30% with normal ganciclovir use and appears to be the most important dose-limiting effect. The neutropenia is both dose-related and idiosyncratic and appears to be reversible. Thrombocytopenia and anemia may also occur. A number of overdoses have been reported. Adverse effects include reversible neutropenia, renal failure, abdominal pain, nausea, vomiting and lethargy. Hematopoietic parameters should be followed periodically for at least 1 month following an overdose.

Toxic Dosage/Death

ACYCLOVIR

High oral doses of 800–4800 mg/day appear to be generally well tolerated. Several patients have ingested up to 100 capsules of oral acyclovir without adverse effects. One adult ingested 4800 mg with no apparent sequelae. Renal failure has followed the administration of high dose bolus injections in patients whose fluid and electrolyte balance were not properly monitored. Some patients for up to 2 weeks have tolerated parenteral doses up to 84 mg/kg.

GANCICLOVIR

Patients who have received 5–7 grams of ganciclovir have developed acute renal failure and survived. No fatalities have been reported from ganciclovir overdose. In animal studies, ganciclovir has been shown to be mutagenic, carcinogenic, and teratogenic. The manufacturer states that the drug should be handled and disposed of in accordance with guidelines issued for cytotoxic drugs, including the use of protective gloves and eyewear.

Drug Interactions

Profound drowsiness and lethargy have been reported when zidovudine and acyclovir are used together. Ganciclovir with zidovudine may be additive or synergistic in producing myelosuppression. This results in increased half-life, and decreased excretion of these drugs. Amphotericin B and ketoconazole may potentiate the antiviral effects of acyclovir.

Pregnancy/Lactation

ACYCLOVIR

Acyclovir crosses the placenta. It is distributed into breast milk at concentrations higher than maternal plasma concentrations. The Centers for Disease Control and Prevention state that systemic acyclovir treatment should not be used in pregnant women without life-threatening disease. Acyclovir has been successfully used in a pregnant patient with herpes simplex virus encephalitis. All formulations of acyclovir are assigned to pregnancy risk category C, which indicates that safety in human pregnancy has not been determined.

GANCICLOVIR

Ganciclovir is teratogenic and carcinogenic and causes aspermatogenesis in animals. Ganciclovir crosses the placenta. It may carry a high risk of damage to fetuses. Ganciclovir should not be given to pregnant women. It is not known whether ganciclovir is excreted in breast milk.

Laboratory

ANALYTIC METHODS

Serum levels of acyclovir can be measured with accuracy using radioimmunoassay, high-performance liquid chromatography, or bioassay. Reverse-phase high-performance liquid chromatography is the most commonly used method of quantifying ganciclovir concentrations. Radioimmunoassay and enzyme-linked immunosorbent assay systems are also available.

BLOOD LEVELS

Specific blood levels of these agents are not helpful in guiding management in overdose.

Treatment

GUT DECONTAMINATION

Gut decontamination after oral overdose with acyclovir may decrease the development of neurotoxic and renal changes, especially in the patient with prior evidence of neurotoxicity and diminished renal function. Gastric lavage within 2 hours of ingestion may be helpful but has not been proved. There is no evidence to support the usefulness of activated charcoal. Following intravenous overdose, there is no evidence that gut decontamination procedures are of value.

ELIMINATION ENHANCEMENT

Removal of acyclovir is accelerated during hemodialysis. If severe overdose has occurred or renal impairment exists, hemodialysis should be considered. There have been no controlled clinical studies, however, to substantiate its usefulness in acyclovir overdose. Exchange transfusions and peritoneal dialysis do not remove the drug. Hemodialysis appears to effectively reduce ganciclovir plasma concentrations and may be useful in the treatment of renal failure in critically ill patients.

SUPPORTIVE MEASURES

Acyclovir

- Patients who take a significant acyclovir overdose should be hospitalized for observation, neurologic and renal evaluation. Patients may require long-term monitoring and symptomatic treatment for neurotoxic and renal sequelae.
- With normal renal function and no evidence of cardiovascular instability, simply increasing fluid flow via intravenous saline may be sufficient to preclude renal problems. Dehydration, preexisting renal insufficiency, and high-dose bolus infusion may result in crystallization of acyclovir within the kidney causing a reversible crystalline nephropathy.
- Symptomatic treatment with neuroleptic agents may assist in controlling unusual behavior.
- Extravasation phlebitis is treated by discontinuing infusion and by applying warm compresses.
- Adverse hemodynamic effects generally have not been observed.

Ganciclovir

- Patients with a history of ganciclovir overdose should be hospitalized and monitored for evidence of bone marrow suppression, renal, hepatic and gastrointestinal dysfunction.
- Daily labwork should include complete blood counts, platelet counts, renal function, and electrolytes. Neutrophil counts should be followed during the first month after ingestion.
- Gastric lavage with adequate airway protection may be useful within the first 4 hours of significant ingestion, however ipecac, gastric lavage, activated charcoal, cathartics, and whole-bowel irrigation have not been systematically studied in patients with ganciclovir overdose.
- Hepatocellular enzyme studies, blood glucose determinations, and renal function tests should be obtained periodically in the ganciclovir overdose patient.

Questions—Acyclovir and Ganciclovir

1. Which is the dose-limiting side effect of ganciclovir?
A. Neutropenia
B. Anemia
C. Thrombocytopenia

Answers to questions in shaded boxes appear at the end of the chapter.

D. Aplastic anemia
E. The volume of the intravenous infusion or the number of pills required

2. When acyclovir is given at high doses, which of the following often occurs?
A. Seizures, confusion, hallucinations, and obtundation
B. Asymptomatic production of anti-acyclovir antibodies
C. Deposition of acyclovir in fat
D. Precipitation of acyclovir crystals in urine
E. Deposition of acyclovir in peripheral nerves

3. Which of the following is true?
A. Ganciclovir is less toxic than acyclovir.
B. Ganciclovir is active against a broader array of viruses than is acyclovir.
C. Most of a dose of both ganciclovir and acyclovir are metabolized in the liver.
D. Ganciclovir and acyclovir act by inhibiting reverse transcriptase of herpes viruses.
E. None of the above.

AMANTADINE

Amantadine (Symmetrel®) poisoning has been reported infrequently; however when it occurs, it may be deadly. There is no specific treatment and management is essentially supportive. Amantadine is a synthetic, water-soluble, primary amine with a uniquely structured tricyclic ring. Amantadine is used for the prophylaxis and symptomatic treatment of respiratory infections caused by influenza A. It does not inhibit strains of influenza B.

Amantadine has been used to treat all forms of Parkinson's disease and for the relief of parkinsonian signs and symptoms in carbon monoxide poisoning and antipsychotic-induced extrapyramidal effects. A related product, rimantadine (Flumadine®) is also used for the prophylaxis and treatment of influenza A.

Pathophysiology

Amantadine prevents penetration of absorbed virus into host cells. It blocks dopamine reuptake into presynaptic neurons, and alters the accumulation, release, and uptake of catecholamines in the central and peripheral nervous systems. These dopamine-enhancing properties probably account for its beneficial effect in patients with parkinsonian symptoms. Both amantadine and rimantadine inhibit viral RNA and protein synthesis.

Pharmacokinetics

ABSORPTION

- The bioavailability of amantadine is > 80%.
- Time to peak plasma level is 1–4 hours.

DISTRIBUTION

- Volume of distribution is 4–10 L / kg. Plasma protein binding is 65%.

ELIMINATION

- Elimination half-life is 12 hours.
- Fifty-six percent is excreted unchanged.

Clinical Presentations

Chronic use of therapeutic doses in the patient with diminished renal function may lead to signs and symptoms of neurotoxicity such as hallucinations, delirium, disorientation, weakness, fatigue, and falling in elderly patients. Rarely, ocular toxicity with blurred vision, vision loss, oculogyric crisis, and mydriasis have been reported following therapeutic amantadine use. Long-term use of amantadine has been associated with livedo reticularis, peripheral edema, congestive heart failure, and urinary retention. Amantadine may increase seizure activity in patients with a preexisting seizure disorder.

In acute overdose, anticholinergic signs such as dry mouth, pupillary dilation, toxic psychosis, and urinary retention may be observed. Cardiopulmonary arrest, ventricular fibrillation, prolonged QT interval, Torsade de Pointes, ventricular tachyarrhythmias, and death may occur. Cardiac abnormalities may begin up to 36 hours after an overdose. Central nervous system manifestations include agitation, psychosis, increased motor activity, tremors, disorientation, hallucinations, and seizures. Adult respiratory distress syndrome (ARDS), pulmonary hemorrhage and pulmonary edema have also been observed.

Toxic Dosage/Death

Amantadine administered or ingested in doses of more than 2 grams is potentially lethal, although survival has occurred after the ingestion of 2.8 grams. Death may not occur for several days, and does not necessarily follow a predictable course of decline.

Drug Interactions

Renal clearance may be reduced in patients simultaneously taking hydrochlorothiazide with triamterene. Toxic delirium may occur in patients concurrently taking amantadine and trimethoprim-sulfamethoxazole. Co-ingesting anticholinergic drugs may potentiate the anticholinergic effects.

Pregnancy/Lactation

Teratogenic effects have been described in animal studies. Treatment with amantadine in women of childbearing age is not justified except perhaps in life-threatening influenza pneumonia. Pregnancy risk category C.

Laboratory

ANALYTIC METHODS

Amantadine is analyzed by gas chromatography / mass spectrometry.

BLOOD LEVELS

Blood levels generally correlate with dose ingested.

Treatment

GUT DECONTAMINATION

Although there have been no controlled studies on the efficacy of syrup of ipecac or gastric lavage in amantadine-poisoned patients, the clinician must exercise judgment in deciding which procedure is indicated for a specific patient, recognizing that fatalities do occur, that the history is often inaccurate, that seizures may occur, that blood levels rise quickly after amantadine ingestion, and that renal insufficiency may not be apparent on first emergency evaluation.

Following an overdose, especially in elderly patients with diminished renal function, in patients who have ingested more than one drug, in patients with preexisting cardiovascular disease, or in those with evidence of disturbed mental status, gastric lavage and/or charcoal may be useful within the first 4 hours.

ELIMINATION ENHANCEMENT

Elimination of unabsorbed amantadine may be enhanced by single or multiple-dose activated charcoal. The large volume of distribution of amantadine indicates that active elimination methods such as dialysis would be unhelpful. Hemoperfusion has not been evaluated.

SUPPORTIVE MEASURES

- Treatment of most patients with amantadine toxicity is expectant and supportive. Usually simple observation and occasional sedation may be all that is required. Patients with significant overdoses should be admitted to an intensive care facility where cardiac monitoring and immediate attention to airway, breathing, and circulation are available.
- As ventricular arrhythmias may appear up to 36 hours following amantadine overdose, continuous cardiac monitoring is indicated for at least 36 to 48 hours.
- In the overdose patient with agitated behavior, sedation should be considered after the patient has been admitted, is on a cardiac monitor, and is under intensive care.
- Symptoms of toxicity in the elderly, particularly hallucinations and disorientation, can appear with therapeutic doses.
- Acidification of urine may increase the rate of excretion of amantadine; however, this method is generally not advised.
- Care must be taken when using adrenergic agents concurrently, as these agents, in combination with amantadine, further dispose the patient to serious ventricular tachyarrhythmias.
- Lidocaine may be the drug of choice to stop ventricular arrhythmias in the overdose patient, as Class I antiarrhythmics may exacerbate prolonged QT intervals.

Antidotes

Physostigmine (0.5 mg intravenously given initially) may ameliorate anticholinergic symptoms such as agitation, tremors, and hallucinations but must be used with great caution. Seizures, bronchospasm, bradycardia, and asystole have all been observed with physostigmine use.

Questions—Amantadine

1. **Besides being used for both treatment and prophylaxis of influenza, amantadine is also indicated for the treatment of which of the following disorders?**
   A. Rotavirus
   B. Varicella (chicken pox)
   C. Zoster (shingles)
   D. Parkinson's disease
   E. Trigeminal neuralgia
2. **Life-threatening side effects of amantadine are usually due to which condition?**
   A. Fulminant hepatic necrosis
   B. Cardiac arrhythmias
   C. Cerebral edema
   D. Malignant hypertension
   E. Respiratory arrest
3. **Which may be helpful in treating a patient with an amantadine overdose?**
   A. Alkalinization of urine with sodium bicarbonate
   B. Intravenous mannitol
   C. Mucomyst inhalation
   D. Control of blood pressure with pseudoephedrine
   E. Treatment of arrhythmias with intravenous lidocaine

FOSCARNET

Foscarnet sodium (phosphonoformic acid or Foscavir®) is used to treat cytomegalovirus (CMV), and acyclovir resistant-herpes simplex virus and varicella zoster infections. Its most serious adverse effect is impairment of renal function. It is predominantly used to treat AIDS patients and transplant patients with CMV infections. There have been no published reports of overdose.

Pathophysiology

Foscarnet is a virostatic, noncompetitive inhibitor of viral enzymes. It acts by resembling phosphate and taking the place of the terminal phosphate on deoxyribonucleotide triphosphate molecules. When these defective nucleotides are incorporated into viral DNA, the DNA chain can no longer be elongated.

Pharmacokinetics

ABSORPTION

- Oral bioavailability is poor, thus i.v. therapy is required.

DISTRIBUTION

- Volume of distribution is 0.3–0.6 L/kg. Plasma protein binding is 14–17%.

ELIMINATION

- Elimination half-life is 3 hours.
- Twenty-eight percent is excreted unchanged in the urine.

Clinical Presentations

Overdose may result in seizures, renal function impairment, paresthesias and electrolyte disturbances involving primarily calcium and phosphate. Foscarnet should not be administered by rapid or bolus intravenous injection as toxicity may be increased as a result of excessive plasma levels. Care with an infusion pump should be taken to avoid unintentional overdose by carefully controlling the rate of infusion.

Toxic Dosage/Death

Malaise, nausea, vomiting, fatigue, and headache may be associated with plasma concentrations above 350 mmol/L (about 100 mg/mL). A lethal dose for foscarnet has not been reported.

Laboratory

ANALYTIC METHODS

Phosphonoformic acid is determined in ultrafiltrate by reversed-phase liquid chromatography by electrochemical detection.

BLOOD LEVELS

Blood levels are generally not available in the acute setting and have not been shown to be helpful in managing overdose.

Treatment

GUT DECONTAMINATION

Gastric lavage and charcoal may lessen the probability of high serum levels of foscarnet. However, clinical trials have not been performed to gauge the clinical efficacy of these interventions.

ELIMINATION ENHANCEMENT

Hemodialysis and hydration may be of benefit in reducing drug plasma levels in patients who receive an overdose of foscarnet, but these have not been evaluated in a clinical trial setting.

SUPPORTIVE MEASURES

- Patients who have overdosed should be ensured an adequate airway and efficient respiratory and circulatory status. Preparation should be made for possible seizure onset. Seizures are treated with benzodiazepines.
- Blood should be drawn for renal function tests and electrolyte levels (calcium and phosphorus).
- Fluid balance should be maintained for at least 24 hours. Follow-up of renal function for several weeks may be indicated.

Questions—Foscarnet

1. Which of the following is associated with foscarnet?
A. Thrombocytopenia
B. Respiratory arrest
C. Electrolyte disturbances
D. Hyperosmolar coma
E. Neutropenia

AIDS DRUGS

Introduction

Since the discovery of the human immunodeficiency virus (HIV), numerous drugs have been developed. A large number of new antiretroviral drugs have made their way to the market in the past several years. In addition to the medications discussed in this section, these include the nucleoside analogues lamivudine (3TC, Epivir®) and abacavir (ABC, Ziagen®); the protease inhibitors saquinavir (formerly Invirase®, now Fortovase®), ritonavir (Norvir®), indinavir (Crixivan®), nelfinavir (Viracept®), and amprenavir (Agenerase®); and the non-nucleoside reverse transcriptase inhibitors (NNRTI's) delavirdine (Rescriptor®), nevirapine (Viramune®), and efavirenz (Sustiva®).

Overdoses have rarely been reported. Little toxicologic information is available about many of these at this time. The protease inhibitors are known to interact with a large number of other medications, including rifampin, cisapride, astemizole (Hismanal®, no longer marketed), terfenadine (Seldane®, no longer marketed), amiodarone, and benzodiazepines. The "other" medication and not the protease inhibitor usually causes the side effects. More anti-retrovirals are in the late stages of clinical testing and may be marketed by the time this synopsis is published.

Patients with AIDS who receive multiple medications appear to be at increased risk of developing Stevens-Johnson syndrome, toxic epidermal necrolysis, scalded skin syndrome, and a generalized morbilliform exanthem. The HIV-positive patient is subject to polypharmacy, iatrogenic toxicity, unusual drug reactions and interactions, and, possibly, increased drug allergies. AIDS represents a significant risk factor for suicide. Self-poisoning with drugs represents the most common method of committing suicide among AIDS victims. Several drugs used to treat AIDS-related infections (including pentamidine, trimethoprim-sulfamethoxazole, and amphotericin B) have been associated with psychosis and delirium, conditions that increase suicide risk.

Zidovudine

Zidovudine (3′, 5′ azidothymidine, AZT or Retrovir®) was the first drug approved in the United States for use in the management of HIV infections. Zidovudine therapy delays progression to AIDS and late stages of HIV disease, increases CD4 cell counts, and suppresses viral replication in patients with asymptomatic or mildly symptomatic HIV infection. Overdoses of zidovudine alone are relatively asymptomatic. There have been no fatalities following zidovudine overdoses. Zidovudine is a synthetic chemical available in oral and parenteral forms.

PATHOPHYSIOLOGY

AZT is a reverse transcriptase inhibitor of HIV-1.

PHARMACOKINETICS

Absorption

- Rapid and nearly complete absorption from the gastrointestinal tract follows oral administration.

Distribution

- The systemic bioavailability of zidovudine capsules and solution is about 63% and reflects a substantive first-pass effect.

Elimination

- Zidovudine is glucuronidated in the liver.

CLINICAL PRESENTATIONS

Patients may develop nystagmus, lethargy, and ataxia at doses of 5000–7500 mg when sedative-hypnotic agents, benzodiazepines, and marijuana are also ingested. Long-term administration of zidovudine is associated with myopathy, manifested by myalgia, proximal muscle wasting, and an increase in serum creatine kinase concentration. Macrocytosis, anemia, and mild neutropenia have also been associated with long-term use. Anemia is an expected side effect of zidovudine, even when it is used at proper doses.

TOXIC DOSAGE/DEATH

Doses up to 450 mg/kg have been ingested with few, if any, abnormal symptoms or signs. No lethal dose for zidovudine has been reported.

DRUG INTERACTIONS

Acetaminophen administered with zidovudine may increase the rate of bone marrow suppression. Acetaminophen hepatotoxicity is probably augmented by zidovudine through its competition for glucuronidation metabolic pathways. Drugs, which are subject to glucuronidation, may alter the glucuronidation of zidovudine.

PREGNANCY/LACTATION

Zidovudine and its glucuronide metabolite cross the placenta, and are found in all body fluids of the infant. Use of zidovudine throughout pregnancy in a known HIV-infected mother is now considered standard medical care, since studies have shown that it can reduce the rate of transmission to the fetus from approximately 25% to 8%. In several large studies, no pattern of intrauterine growth retardation, asphyxia, or serious hematologic toxicity has been observed.

LABORATORY

Analytic Methods

A radioimmunoassay procedure is available to determine the presence of zidovudine and its metabolite zidovudine glucuronide. A high-performance liquid chromatography method also analyzes both the drug and its metabolite simultaneously.

Blood Levels

Blood may be drawn to confirm the presence of zidovudine. However, the delay in obtaining results makes this generally unimportant clinically. Following blood levels in overdose has not been shown to help guide management.

TREATMENT

Gut Decontamination

Seizures may occur after ingestion of high doses of zidovudine, and therefore use of syrup of ipecac is not advisable. If gastric lavage is contemplated, adequate tracheal protection should be provided. Activated charcoal may be beneficial if other drugs, particularly sedative-hypnotics, have been ingested. There is no clinical evidence that gastric lavage, activated charcoal or cathartics are useful in zidovudine overdose treatment.

Elimination Enhancement

With the high volume of distribution and relatively benign course following supportive therapy, hemodialysis and hemoperfusion are not likely to be helpful. Whole-bowel irrigation has not been used, but may possibly be beneficial in high-volume ingestions.

Supportive Measures

- Patients who have ingested an overdose of solely zidovudine are usually alert and have normal vital signs. They should be treated symptomatically and supportively in hospital, where they should be observed for at least 24 hours.
- On admission to an emergency facility, blood should be drawn for complete blood count, liver function tests, and renal function studies. A urine toxic screen is generally recommended.
- Seizures may be treated with diazepam. Electroencephalography and computed brain scans may be indicated to search for other causes of seizures.
- Follow-up blood counts, including neutrophil and platelet counts, should be performed during the first few weeks. Liver abnormalities may occur.
- Multiple doses of acetaminophen should be avoided in zidovudine-treated patients.

Questions—Zidovudine

1. Which of the following is an expected side effect of zidovudine, even at proper doses?
A. Anemia
B. Thrombocytopenia
C. Mild renal insufficiency
D. Peripheral neuropathy
E. Leukocytosis

2. How does the human body handle zidovudine?
A. Slow deamination inside T-helper (CD4) cells
B. Glucuronidation by hepatocytes
C. Deacetylation by hepatocytes
D. Renal excretion without metabolism
E. None of the above.

3. Use of zidovudine throughout pregnancy in a known HIV-infected mother is now considered standard medical care, since studies have shown that it can reduce the rate of transmission to the fetus from approximately 25% to 8%.
A. True
B. False

Pentamidine

Pentamidine (Pentam-300®) is an antiparasitic drug structurally similar to procainamide and to "potassium-sparing" diuretics such as amiloride and trimethoprim. Pentamidine has been used for many years in the treatment of African trypanosomiasis and leishmaniasis. For many years it has also been effective therapy, along with trimethoprim-sulfa, for the treatment of Pneumocystis carinii pneumonia, a common infection associated with HIV.

Pentamidine has been administered prophylactically by inhalation to prevent Pneumocystis carinii pneumonia in high risk, HIV-infected patients. Parenteral administration of pentamidine is associated with a high risk of toxicity. Inhaled pentamidine produces high concentrations of the drug on bronchoalveolar surfaces with minimal systemic absorption. There have been only anecdotal reports of overdose with pentamidine.

PATHOPHYSIOLOGY

The mechanism of action of pentamidine is unknown. It may be a folic acid antagonist and may bind to DNA, but the exact mechanism has not yet been determined.

PHARMACOKINETICS

Absorption

- Peak plasma level is 0.2–1.0 mg/mL.

Distribution

- Volume of distribution is 3 L/kg.

Elimination

- Elimination half-life is 9 hours (i.m.) and 6 hours (i.v.). Thirty to 60% is excreted unchanged.
- Concentrations in the bronchoalveolar sediment 18–24 hours after administration are greater following comparable doses of aerosolized pentamidine than with intravenous doses.

CLINICAL PRESENTATIONS

Intramuscular pentamidine may induce mild azotemia, hypoglycemia, injection site reactions, leukopenia, and rash. Reactions immediately following its use may include hypotension, tachycardia, nausea, vomiting, metallic taste, hallucinations, and syncope. Hypoglycemia may be fatal. Nephrotoxicity, thrombocytopenia, hallucinations, hypotension, and ventricular tachycardia have all been observed after intravenous use. Torsade de Pointes, QTc interval prolongation, and ventricular fibrillation may develop.

Pancreatitis, which may be fatal, may follow parenteral pentamidine therapy. Hypomagnesemia, hypokalemia, hyperkalemia and hypocalcemia may occur. Inhalation of pentamidine may yield pancreatitis, acute renal failure, maculopapular rash, hypoglycemia, pneumothorax, atypical Pneumocystis carinii infection, and extrapulmonary pneumocystosis. Cough and bronchospasm are frequently observed. Torsade de pointes has followed inhalation.

TOXIC DOSAGE/DEATH

As of 1985, only 5 pentamidine-associated deaths were reported. Since then, additional deaths have followed acute pancreatitis or hypoglycemia. No lethal dose has been established.

PREGNANCY/LACTATION

Few pregnancy studies have been done in large human populations. Pentamidine has been placed in pregnancy risk category C. Pentamidine should not be given to a pregnant woman or nursing mother unless the potential benefits are judged to outweigh the unknown risks. Pregnant health care workers should avoid pentamidine exposure.

LABORATORY

Analytic Methods

A high-performance liquid chromatography method is available for quantitation of pentamidine in whole blood, plasma, and urine. A reverse-phase chromatographic system with fluorescence detection is used. A bioassay is also available that appears sensitive and specific.

Blood Levels

There has been no evidence correlating the clinical picture with blood levels.

TREATMENT

Gut Decontamination

These methods have not been proved effective in pentamidine overdose.

Elimination Enhancement

In view of the high apparent volume of distribution of pentamidine, it is unlikely that hemodialysis, hemoperfusion, or other extracorporeal methods would aid in its rapid elimination.

Supportive Measures

- Patients with an overdose of intravenous or inhaled pentamidine are usually in a health care facility. The patient with significant pentamidine overdose should always be transferred to an intensive care area. An intravenous line, oxygen, and cardiac monitoring should be available.
- Ventricular arrhythmias may be life threatening. Patients who develop polymorphic (Torsade de Pointes) or monomorphic ventricular tachycardia during pentamidine therapy may benefit from bolus magnesium sulfate injection. If the arrhythmia persists, overdrive pacing or isoproterenol infusion may be useful. Lidocaine therapy may be useful as well.
- Hypomagnesemia and hypokalemia may predispose to the development of Torsade de Pointes. Therefore, potassium and magnesium should be closely followed and aggressively replaced.
- Frequent electrocardiograms should be obtained. Medications that may potentiate the development of arrhythmias (e.g., procainamide) should be avoided.
- Severe hypoglycemia may occur during pentamidine therapy or even days after the last dose. Patients must be closely monitored for hypoglycemia during treatment and for several weeks thereafter. Diabetes mellitus may be induced and is likely to be dose dependent, time dependent, and irreversible.

Questions—Pentamidine

1. Which of the following may occur after treatment with pentamidine is finished?
   A. Non-Hodgkin's lymphoma
   B. Pericarditis
   C. Hypoglycemia
   D. Respiratory distress syndrome due to destruction of pulmonary surfactant
   E. Aplastic anemia

Other Anti-HIV Medications

DIDANOSINE (DDI, DIDEOXYINOSINE)

Didanosine (DDI, Dideoxyinosine, Videx®), a purine nucleoside analog, is a potent inhibitor of the replication of HIV in culture systems, and appears to have promise as a therapeutic agent against HIV in humans. Didanosine is a treatment option for adults and children with severe HIV infection who are unable to tolerate, or whose condition has deteriorated on, zidovudine. Overdoses have not been reported. Mild phlebitis, maculopapular rash, palpitations, and a mild headache have been observed with intravenous use.

Major toxic effects after oral use include pancreatitis and peripheral neuropathy. Peripheral neuropathy (pain, burning, aching in the soles of the feet) is the primary dose-limiting toxicity seen in patients. Ocular effects such as amblyopia, diplopia, optic atrophy, and blindness have been reported. Conduction abnormalities, congestive heart failure, and cardiac arrest have been observed. Treatment of an overdose is symptomatic and supportive as it is with other synthetic nucleoside antiviral agents such as acyclovir, ganciclovir, and zidovudine.

STAVUDINE (D4T)

Stavudine, (Zerit®, formerly known as D4T), is a nucleoside analog of thymidine approved in the U.S. in 1994. It is used to treat adults with advanced HIV infection who are intolerant of other therapies with proven clinical benefit, or who have experienced significant clinical or immunologic deterioration while receiving these therapies. Reversible, peripheral neuropathy is the most serious adverse event. Chills, fever, nausea, vomiting, insomnia, depression, anorexia, and dyspepsia have all been reported. Chronic features of overdose generally include peripheral neuropathy and hepatotoxicity. Treatment is mainly symptomatic and supportive. Gastric evacuation may be useful if the patient is seen within 1–2 hours of ingestion. No data are available on the use of extracorporeal methods to hasten elimination. Patients may be discharged in 6 hours if liver function tests are stable.

ZALCITABINE (DDC, DIDEOXYCYTIDINE)

Zalcitabine (DDC, dideoxycytidine, Hivid®), is a reverse transcriptase inhibitor of HIV-1, similar to zidovudine (AZT). Zalcitabine may induce adverse effects such rash, fever, and aphthous stomatitis during the first month of treatment. The major clinical toxic effects are a painful sensorimotor peripheral neuropathy involving predominantly the lower extremities and, less frequently, pancreatitis. Symptoms of peripheral neuropathy typically resolve over several weeks. Overdose with zalcitabine has not been reported.

Questions—Anti-HIV Medications

1. Which one of the following is a side effect of both zalcitabine and dideoxyinosine?
A. Serum sickness
B. Peripheral neuropathy
C. Hepatitis
D. Renal failure
E. Hypoglycemia

Answers

Acyclovir and Ganciclovir

1. A 2. D 3. B

Amantadine

1. D 2. B 3. E

Foscarnet

1. C

Zidovudine

1. A 2. B 3. A

Pentamidine

1. B

Anti-HIV Medications

1. B

SELECTED READINGS

Acyclovir and Ganciclovir

1. Drugs for non-HIV viral infections. Med Lett Drugs Ther 1994;36(919):27–31.
2. Keeney RE, Kirk LE, Bridgen D. Acyclovir tolerance in humans. Am J Med 1982;73(1A):176–181.
3. Nightingale SC. Ganciclovir approved. Lancet 1989;2:281.

Amantidine

1. Amantadine. In: McEvoy GK, ed. AHFS Drug Information 94. Bethesda, MD: American Society of Hospital Pharmacists, 1994:392–395, 2426-2428.
2. Douglas RG. Prophylaxis and treatment of influenza. N Engl J Med 1990;322:443–450.
3. Tominack RL, Hayden FG. Rimantadine hydrochloride and amantadine hydrochloride use in influenza A virus infections. Infect Dis Clin North Am 1987;1:459–478.

Foscarnet

1. Chrisp P, Clissold SP. Foscarnet: A review of its antiviral activity, pharmacokinetic properties and therapeutic use in immunocompromised patients with cytomegalovirus retinitis. Drugs 1991;41:104–129.
2. Safrin S, Berger TG, Gilson I, et al. Foscarnet therapy in five patients with AIDS and acyclovir-resistant Varicella-zoster virus infection. Ann Intern Med 1991;115:19–21.

Introduction to AIDS Drugs

1. AIDS drugs being studied. FDA Consumer 1992;26(3):8–9.
2. Drugs for AIDS and associated infections. Med Lett Drugs Ther 1993;35:79–81.
3. Lee BL, Safrin S. AIDS commentary: Interactions and toxicities of drugs used in patients with AIDS. Clin Infect Dis 1992;14:773–779.
4. Peters BS, Carlin E, Weston RJ, et al. Adverse effects of drugs used in the management of opportunistic infections associated with HIV infection. Drug Saf 1994;10439–454.

Zidovudine

1. Casals A, Ribelles N, Clotet B, Fox M. Zidovudine overdose. Med Clin 1989;5:199.
2. Heard JM, Slovis CM. Zidovudine (AZT) (Retrovir®) overdose. Vet Hum Toxicol 1988;30:365–366.
3. Pickus OB. Overdose of zidovudine. N Engl J Med 1988;318:1206.
4. Zidovudine. Med Letter Drugs Ther 1990;32:78.

Pentamidine

1. Collins RJ, Pien FD, Houk JH. Case report: Insulin dependent diabetes mellitus associated with pentamidine. Am J Med Sci 1989;297:174–175.
2. Engrav MB, Coodley G, Magnusson AR. Torsade de pointes after inhaled pentamidine. Ann Emerg Med 1992;21:1403–1405.
3. Wispelwey B, Pearson R. Pentamidine: A risk-benefit analysis. Drug Saf 1990;5:212–219.

Anti-HIV Medications

1. Broder S, Yarchoan R. Dideoxycytidine: Current clinical experience and future prospects. Am J Med 1990;88(suppl. 5B):5B-31S–5B-33S.
2. Lai KK, Gang DL, Zawacki JK, Cooley TP. Fulminant hepatic failure associated with 2′,3′-dideoxyinosine (ddI). Ann Intern Med 1991;115:283–284.
3. Schindzielorz A, Pike I, Daniels M, et al. Rates and risk factors for adverse events associated with didanosine in the expanded access program. Clin Infect Dis 1994;19:1076–1083.
4. U.S. Food and Drug Administration. Stavudine approved for certain patients with advanced HIV.

ACKNOWLEDGMENT

Thanks to Ira Leviton, MD for contributing the questions in this chapter.

SECTION

C

Alcohols and Drugs of Abuse

CHAPTER 17

Alcohols, Glycols, and Disulfiram

INTRODUCTION

Ethyl alcohol is a serious and ubiquitous fact of life. Alcohol determination is the most frequently performed medicolegal test and remains the most common single drug taken by patients visiting emergency departments. In one study, positive blood-alcohol levels were found in over one-third of male victims involved in fatal single automobile accidents. Alcohol misuse is the leading killer of persons aged 15 to 45 years and is associated with 67% of drownings, 70% of fire deaths, 67% of murders, 35% of suicides, and the vast majority of deaths from hepatic failure. An increase in blood alcohol also has been associated with fatal aircraft accidents and fatal pedestrian deaths.

Nationally, between 40% and 55% of all drivers involved in fatal crashes have blood ethanol concentrations greater than or equal to 100 mg/dL (100 mg/dL = 0.10%). In 1983, there were 37,971 reported fatal motor vehicle accidents in the United States resulting in 42,584 fatalities. Alcohol was an important contributing factor in 17,847 (42%) of these deaths. More than 200,000 Americans die annually from alcohol-related disorders, and alcohol dependency afflicts 5% to 10% of the American population. For untreated alcoholics, normal life expectancy decreases 12 to 15 years compared with population norms.

ETHANOL

Ethanol is a central nervous system (CNS) depressant. Neurologic impairment depends on a number of variables, including genetic factors, amount ingested, prior alcohol use, rate and direction of blood ethanol elevation, coingestion of other drugs and alcohol products, trauma, nutritional status, and complications of chronic ethanolism. In nontolerant individuals, decrements in cognitive ability, motor coordination, and sensory perception may begin at ethanol concentrations as low as 50 mg/dL.

Alcoholism is a chronic disease with genetic, psychosocial, and environmental factors influencing its development and manifestations. The disease is often progressive and fatal. It is characterized by impaired control over drinking, preoccupation with alcohol, use of alcohol despite adverse consequences, and distortions in thinking, most notably denial. Each of these symptoms may be continuous or periodic.

While late in the course of illness, its medical and social consequences become obvious; early detection may be less apparent and generally requires a careful medical and psychosocial evaluation. The "Brief Michigan Alcoholism Screening Test" and "CAGE Questionnaire" (CAGE indicates a mnemonic for questions about **C**utting down on drinking, **A**nnoyance at others' concern about drinking, feeling **G**uilty about drinking, and using alcohol as an **E**ye-opener in the morning) are useful, well known, screening measures to detect occult alcoholics in hospitalized populations, but are much less sensitive in the general community.

Alcoholism tends to appear in families, and studies in twins indicate that genetic factors partly control normal alcohol use. Recent research on alcoholism has focused on metabolic factors, individual CNS responses to alcohol, and a possible genetic association with depression and personality disorders. Alcohol sensitivity may be related to an atypical isoenzyme of hepatic alcohol dehydrogenase that causes rapid formation of acetaldehyde after ethanol use.

Ethyl alcohol is a clear, colorless, aliphatic hydrocarbon. Ethanol is a "universal diluent" that is mildly polar and easily crosses cell membranes. Commercial products containing ethyl alcohol include beverages; solvents for perfumes, aftershaves, and colognes; medicinal liquids (e.g., cold preparations may contain up to 20% ethanol); mouthwashes; liniments; and some rubbing alcohols. Distilled spirits typically contain ethanol volumes of 40% to 50% (80 to 100 proof), that reliably are displayed on labels.

Wines vary more widely in ethanol content, ranging from 10% to 20% (20 to 40 proof) and average 12% ethanol by volume. The greatest variation occurs in beers, which contain from 2% to 6% ethanol (4 to 12 proof); with regular domestic American beers averaging 4% to 5% ethanol by volume. Mouthwashes may contain up to 75% ethanol, and colognes, up to 40% to 60% ethanol. More than 700 American medicinal preparations contain ethanol, ostensibly as an inert diluent or solvent, in concentrations ranging from 0.3% to 68%.

Pathophysiology

Ethanol is a CNS depressant that selectively depresses the reticular activating system (RAS). The mechanism of action probably involves interference with ion transport (i.e., sodium flux) at the cell membrane rather than at synapses, similar to the action of anesthetic agents. The frontal lobes are sensitive to a low concentration, resulting in alteration of thought and mood before changes in vision (occipital lobe) and coordination (cerebellum). Preferential suppression of inhibitory neurons probably causes the excitation seen at low ethanol concentrations.

CHRONIC EFFECTS

Chronic ethanolism leads to multiple metabolic changes caused, at least in part, by alterations in a cellular redox, which results from a decreased oxidized to reduced nicotinamide adenine dinucleotide (NAD^+/NADH) ratio. Among other biochemical effects, there is a shift from pyruvate to lactate that results in acidosis, and an elevation of serum uric acid which results from reduced clearance. Lipid metabolism is altered with accumulation of fat in the liver, and there is a possible increase of collagen disposition and depressed protein synthesis.

HYPOGLYCEMIA

Alcohol impairs hepatic gluconeogenesis in the presence of significant hepatic glycogen store depletion, generally secondary to starvation or fasting. It probably does this by reducing the intracellular NAD^+/NADH ratio. Hypoglycemia occurs more commonly in children in whom small amounts of ethanol may cause hypoglycemic seizures or even death. The majority of these children are under 5 years of age. Children may drink large amounts in relation to their body weight and quickly produce high blood-alcohol concentrations. In a child under 5 years, hepatic alcohol dehydrogenase activity is not mature and the ability to metabolize any alcohol load is limited. The hypoglycemia appears to be related primarily to the inhibition of hepatic gluconeogenesis.

ALCOHOLIC KETOACIDOSIS

Alcoholic ketoacidosis (AKA) follows withdrawal from alcohol. It tends to develop in chronic alcoholics who have recently been binging. Typically, these patients become volume depleted and have abruptly stopped or decreased their alcohol intake 1 to 3 days before presentation. These patients often have no measurable blood alcohol levels when first seen in a health care facility. Signs and related symptoms may include nausea, vomiting, abdominal pain, anorexia, hepatitis, pancreatitis, or aspiration pneumonia. The patient may be confused, drowsy, or even comatose. Tachypnea and tachycardia are common signs, and the patient may present with Kussmaul respirations. Most patients will respond to glucose-containing intravenous fluids without insulin.

Moderate to severe ketoacidosis is a result of the formation of β-hydroxybutyrate and acetoacetate. β-Hydroxybutyrate usually predominates and testing with Ketostix® or Acetest® (which are most sensitive to acetoacetate, less so to acetone, and not at all to β-hydroxybutyrate) may show only a weakly positive reaction. The finding of ketonuria without glycosuria suggests the diagnosis and serum ketones are elevated markedly. Electrolyte, glucose, and arterial blood-gas measurements are essential in making a diagnosis. Patients with AKA will have an elevated anion-gap metabolic acidosis. Hypokalemia and hypochloremia often are seen because of prolonged vomiting. Respiratory alkalosis may be seen as a compensatory response to metabolic acidosis or a result of alcohol withdrawal.

Pharmacokinetics

ABSORPTION

- Both gastrointestinal and respiratory tracts are effective routes of toxicity. The small intestine extracts about 80% of an oral ethanol dose; the stomach absorbs the remainder.
- Factors that delay gastric emptying may decrease absorption of alcohol.
- The rate of increase in blood ethanol depends on the type of beverage and ethanol concentration (beer slows absorption), gastric contents (high protein and high volumes decrease absorption), and gastrointestinal motility (trauma, prior gastric surgery, and drug-induced ileus all reduce motility). Such factors may delay peak blood-ethanol levels several hours after consumption.
- In healthy adults, 80% to 90% of absorption occurs within 30 to 60 minutes, but food may delay complete absorption for 4 to 6 hours.

DISTRIBUTION

- Because it is both water and lipid soluble, ethanol distributes into total body water and easily penetrates the blood-brain barrier and placenta.
- The approximate volume of distribution is 0.6 L/kg in adults and 0.7 L/kg in children.
- Women have a slightly smaller volume of distribution than men do because women have relatively less water and more fat.
- Acetaldehyde, produced by all known oxidative pathways of ethanol metabolism, is converted to acetate by aldehyde dehydrogenase. Asians often harbor an inactive aldehyde dehydrogenase variant that causes them to experience high blood-acetaldehyde levels when they drink, with subsequent development of ethanol intolerance and flushing.

ELIMINATION

- The hepatic metabolism of ethanol is characterized by zero-order kinetics (i.e., the elimination rate is concentration independent) except at very low or very high concentrations. Some authors believe ethanol metabolism follows Michaelis-Menten kinetics.
- Blood ethanol decreases more rapidly at concentrations over 300 mg/dL, perhaps because of oxidation by the microsomal ethanol-oxidizing system. The kidney and lungs excrete only 5% to 10% of an absorbed dose unchanged.
- The maximum rate of metabolism is 100 to 125 mg/kg/hour, although, by enzymatic induction, tolerant individuals can increase their metabolic rates to 175 mg/kg/hour.
- The average adult metabolizes 7 to 10 g/h and reduces the ethanol level 15 to 20 mg/dL/h. Chronic alcoholics, in contrast, may have metabolic rates as high as 30 to 40 mg/dL/h. Children have higher metabolic rates than adults do, ranging up to 28 mg/dL/h.
- Hepatocytes contain three main ethanol metabolic pathways. The alcohol dehydrogenase pathway (in the cytosol) is the major pathway of ethanol oxidation in the body. Conversion of ethanol to acetaldehyde by alcohol dehydrogenase is the rate-limiting step. Both alcohol and aldehyde dehydrogenase require NAD, which reduces the hepatic NAD/NADH ratio. The shift in this ratio causes profound metabolic abnormalities in chronic alcoholics.
- A microsomal ethanol-oxidizing system (MEOS), represents the second major metabolic pathway and is located in the endoplasmic reticulum. The MEOS is separate from the cytochrome P450 system. This pathway becomes more important as ethanol concentration rises.
- A peroxidase-catalase system is a minor pathway located in peroxisomes.

Clinical Presentations

Ethanol is a selective central nervous system depressant in low doses and a generalized depressant in high doses. Comparison of cognitive and psychomotor skills at blood-ethanol levels of 90 and 135 mg/dL indicates that attention, concentration, motor coordination, and reaction time are significantly more affected at the higher level. Initially, ethanol produces exhilaration, which progresses to loss of restraint, behavioral abnormalities, loquaciousness, slurred speech, ataxia, gait disturbances, irritability, drowsiness, stupor, and coma.

A flushed face, dilated pupils, excessive sweating, and gastrointestinal distress (manifested as pancreatitis, gastritis, esophagitis, and/or alcoholic hepatitis) may accompany CNS symptoms. Ethanol can produce dysrhythmias (e.g., atrial fibrillation) in nontolerant binge drinkers, as well as in chronic alcoholics. Ethanol is a venodilator that produces decreased preload, afterload, and systemic vascular resistance in healthy adults after ingestion. Ingestion of ethanol also has a myocardial depressant effect. Tolerance lessens acute ethanol effects, but may exacerbate chronic metabolic effects.

Chronic Effects

NEUROLOGIC EFFECTS

Diminished fine motor skills, diminished cognition, peripheral motor/sensory neuropathy, and Wernicke-Korsakoff syndrome have been observed. Movement disorders may occur. Heavy consumption (over 400 grams per week) of alcohol appears to predispose to both hemorrhagic and nonhemorrhagic strokes.

GASTROINTESTINAL EFFECTS

Acute and chronic pancreatitis may occur. Alcoholic cirrhosis with or without alcoholic hepatitis occurs in about half of proven chronic alcoholics. There is still controversy relating to the reversibility of cirrhosis and to whether abstinence from alcohol improves survival. Other gastrointentinal (GI) effects include esophageal varices secondary to increased portal hypertension from cirrhosis, dysphagias, Mallory-Weiss syndrome, ulcers, small intestinal malabsorption, motility problems, and fatty liver.

MUSCULOSKELETAL EFFECTS

Patients may develop proximal-muscle weakness with elevated serum creatine kinase levels and myoglobinuria. Myopathy generally appears in middle-aged alcoholics after many years of drinking. Hip fractures, osteopenia, and fractures are associated with osteoporosis. Short-term alcohol administration causes a decline in the secretion of parathyroid hormone and this may account at least in part for the transient hypocalcemia, hypercalciuria, and hypermagnesemia that follow alcohol ingestion.

HEMATOLOGIC EFFECTS

Hematologic abnormalities include bone marrow suppression, megaloblastic hematopoiesis with increased mean corpuscular volume, interference with iron utilization, and thrombocytopenia.

CARDIOVASCULAR EFFECTS

"Holiday Heart syndrome" reflects supraventricular arrhythmias induced by drinking binges. Atrial fibrillation is the most common arrhythmia, but atrial flutter, atrial tachycardia, junction tachycardia, and multiple atrial premature beats have been observed. Cardiac decompensation, cardiomyopathy, and right and left sided failure may become apparent after many years of heavy alcohol use. Electrocardiographic changes include left ventricular hypertrophy with abnormal T-waves and nonspecific ST-T wave changes.

Primary ventricular arrhythmias culminating in fibrillation may partially explain why alcoholics may die suddenly and unexpectedly. Most episodes of cardiac arrhythmias terminate within 24 to 48 hours either spontaneously or after treatment with β-blockers, sedation, rehydration, and treatment of electrolyte depletion. Acutely, alcohol causes a modest fall in blood pressure. Chronic, significant consumption results in a dose-dependent rise in blood pressure.

NUTRITIONAL EFFECTS

Vitamin deficiencies of B1, B6, B12, zinc, and magnesium occur with nutritional neglect. Alcoholism probably is the most important cause of magnesium deficiency. Alcoholics ingest low levels of magnesium in their diet and excrete more in their urine. Hypomagnesemia may be present, but serum levels of magnesium do not predict body deficits accurately. Magnesium deficiency interferes with thiamine action. Thiamine should be administered with magnesium to prevent Wernicke-Korsakoff syndrome.

RENAL EFFECTS

Patients with chronic alcoholism may have a variety of renal tubular abnormalities. These abnormalities can be reversible, disappearing after 4 weeks of abstinence despite many years of alcohol abuse.

ENDOCRINE EFFECTS

Increased secretion of cortisol, aldosterone, and insulin may occur, in addition to decreased release of oxytocin and testosterone.

PEDIATRIC ISSUES

Alcohol abuse may occur in very young children. Percutaneous alcohol intoxication has been described in young children after use of alcohol-soaked gauze pads. In juvenile alcohol intoxication, metabolic acidosis may be correlated with blood-alcohol concentration and loss of consciousness. Hypoglycemia is the most common reported symptom in children under 5 years of age. The hypoglycemic effects of ethanol are not dose dependent. The fasting state may predispose a child to ethanol-induced hypoglycemia. Hypokalemia is an important concomitant finding.

Withdrawal Syndromes

The withdrawal of ethanol may lead to unopposed compensatory mechanisms, which are clinically manifested as autonomic hyperexcitability. The exact mechanism of withdrawal is not known. Hypomagnesemia and hypokalemia may contribute to withdrawal effects. Sharply decreased consumption of alcohol or intercurrent illness may cause a hyperadrenergic state ranging from minor tremor and anxiety to hallucinations and convulsions. Withdrawal syndromes develop more often in regular heavy drinkers than in binge drinkers. The severity of the syndrome depends more on intensity than duration and may develop in extremely heavy drinkers over months rather than years. Appreciable individual differences in response to the abrupt cessation of alcohol consumption do occur among chronic alcoholic patients.

COMMON ABSTINENCE SYNDROME

Symptoms typically develop 6 to 8 hours after cessation of drinking. Although most patients are asymptomatic at 72 hours, some symptoms may continue for over 1 week. Symptoms may include tremor, agitation, sleep disturbance, hyperexcitability, and preoccupation with personal misery. Nausea, vomiting, weakness, headache, insomnia, flushed face, conjunctival injection, and diaphoresis also may occur. Prognosis is excellent with appropriate management. Although barbiturates, phenothiazines, antihistamines, and paraldehyde all have been used successfully, benzodiazepines are safe and most effective in this setting. Studies with clonidine suggest that it may be effective in reducing some of the adrenergic manifestations of alcohol withdrawal.

ALCOHOLIC HALLUCINOSIS

Symptoms develop 24 to 36 hours after cessation of alcohol intake. This disorder of perception ranges from delusions to visual and auditory hallucinations. The patient often remains fully oriented. This syndrome is managed effectively with benzodiazepines, Haldol® when necessary, and by protecting individuals from harm in a supportive environment.

ALCOHOLIC SEIZURES

Grand mal seizures, so-called "rum fits," may occur 8 to 48 hours after cessation of drinking, with a peak incidence at 24 hours. Loss of consciousness may not occur during tonic-clonic activity. Only 3% of these patients develop status epilepticus and more than 50% have only one seizure. Seizures rarely develop after hallucinations, but one-third of withdrawal seizures progress to delirium tremens (DTs). Most seizures are brief and self-limited, so that no therapy other than protection from harm and support of the airway is needed. Any patient arriving at an emergency department with seizures should be questioned about alcohol intake. It is involved in up to 40% of adults with seizures admitted to a hospital and in about 15% of patients with status epilepticus. Intravenous benzodiazepines are the anticonvulsants of choice, and prophylactic or long-term phenytoin therapy generally is not helpful.

DELIRIUM TREMENS

Symptoms usually develop 3 to 5 days after cessation of ethanol consumption but may occur up to 14 days later and persist for several months. Seizures occur in approximately one-third of patients with DTs and usually precede the development of DTs. Classic effects include profound confusion, delusions, vivid hallucinations, autonomic hyperactivity, agitation, and disorientation. Fever, sweating, tachycardia, dilated pupils, hypertension, and piloerection may be dramatic. Delirium tremens is a true medical emergency with a 9% to 15% mortality rate. Always consider concurrent illness (e.g., infection, metabolic disease, and/or trauma) in the differential diagnosis.

WERNICKE-KORSAKOFF SYNDROME

Thiamine deficiency produces Wernicke's encephalopathy, the most common neuropathological cause of cognitive impairment in chronic alcoholics. Ocular abnormalities, ataxia, vestibular paresis, seizures, hypotension, hypothermia, and coma may characterize its presentation. Ocular changes include diplopia, blurred vision, bidirectional nystagmus, and lateral gaze palsy. Ataxia results from polyneuropathy manifested by decreased deep tendon reflexes and sensation. Tremor is often present.

Change in mental status occurs in over 90% of patients and is poorly responsive to treatment. Eighty percent of patients with Wernicke's encephalopathy develop Korsakoff's psychosis characterized by retrograde (inability to recall information) and anterograde (inability to assimilate new information) amnesia. Confabulation and decreased initiative may occur, but impairment of sensorium is minimal. About one-quarter of Korsakoff patients require long-term institutional care.

Toxic Dosage/Death

Death may occur from respiratory depression at ethanol levels exceeding 500 mg/dL. However, chronic alcoholics may exhibit few clinical signs of intoxication at blood levels between 300 and 450 mg/dL and may survive levels exceeding 500 mg/dL. One patient survived acute alcohol intoxication with a blood ethanol level of 1,500 mg/dL. Although the reported lethal ethanol dose is 5 to 8 grams/kg for adults and 3 grams/kg for children, variation in toxicity occurs as a result of the concurrent presence of hypoglycemia and drug interactions. The American Academy of Pediatrics has established a blood level of 25 mg/dL as the maximum concentration of ethanol a single dose of alcohol-containing medication should be able to produce in a child.

Drug Interactions

Certain drugs produce a disulfiram-like reaction when taken with alcohol, possibly by inhibiting the enzyme aldehyde dehydrogenase. These include metronidazole, sulfonamides, hypoglycemia agents, the mushroom *C. atramentarius*, and industrial chemicals like amides, oximes, carbamates, dithiocarbamates, and thiuram derivatives. Common direct interactions involve either central nervous system depression, when there is a concomitant ingestion of sedative-hypnotics, or prolonged bleeding times, when normal subjects ingest at least five drinks and a single aspirin tablet. In ordinary doses, neither amphetamines nor caffeine significantly improves ethanol-impaired performance. The interaction of central nervous system stimulants and ethanol is unpredictable.

Pregnancy/Lactation

Ethanol may act as a tocolytic and inhibits the secretion of the neurohypophyseal hormones, antidiuretic hormone, and oxytocin. Ethanol appears to suppress uterine activity through inhibition of oxytocin release, reduction of myometrial oxytocin receptors, and noncompetitive antagonism at the uterine level. In controlled studies, ethanol is a less effective tocolytic than isoxsuprine, ritodrine, terbutaline, or magnesium sulfate. Children exposed in utero to alcohol as a tocolytic have shown no abnormalities.

Consumption of at least one to two alcoholic drinks daily has been associated with a significant decrease in birth weight. A safe level of ethanol use during pregnancy has not been established. One to two drinks per day taken by the mother during the first trimester may not be associated with more teratogenicity than that associated with nondrinkers. Neonatal withdrawal and acute ethanol intoxication are potential risks in children born to alcoholic mothers.

Studies on the human placenta suggest that the placenta oxidizes ethanol to acetaldehyde and releases acetaldehyde to the fetus. This may be a factor in production of the fetal alcohol syndrome. The fetal alcohol syndrome defines specific facial characteristics seen in children born to alcoholic mothers. Numerous birth abnormalities have been reported. Long-term, follow-up studies of these children indicate severe growth deficiencies and intellectual handicaps that correlate with the degree of craniofacial abnormalities. Dental malocclusions, malalignments, and eustachian tube dysfunction, occurs as a result of facial hypoplasia.

Following ingestion of ethanol by the lactating mother, breast milk samples will contain alcohol that can be perceived by odor. Alcohol in breast milk leads to reduced consumption of milk by infants.

Laboratory

ANALYTIC METHODS

Gas chromatography is the method of choice. This procedure is highly specific for ethanol. Rapid quantitative determination of blood alcohol concentration (BAC) also may be determined by an electrochemical method. A saliva test limited by cross-reactivity with congeners such as methanol, mouthwash, phenol-containing lozenges, tobacco products, and patient cooperation also exists. Vomitus containing alcohol may produce a falsely elevated test result.

Within 24 hours of death, little ethanol is formed by decomposition, even at room temperature. No blood specimen from bodies refrigerated within 4 hours of death and stored up to 28 hours contained more than 10 mg ethanol per deciliter. Blood ethanol produced by postmortem decomposition rarely exceeds 50 mg/dL. Fluoride ion, mercuric ion, and cold storage inhibit the tissue formation of ethanol by microorganisms. Femoral and jugular veins are the best postmortem blood sampling sites.

With knowledge of the body weight, concentration of alcohol, and amount ingested, the peak blood ethanol level can be estimated using the general pharmacokinetic formula:

$$\text{Plasma concentration (Cp)} = \frac{\text{dose (A)}}{\text{volume of distribution } (V_D)}$$

$$\text{Ethanol blood level (Cp in mg/dL)} = \frac{\text{dose (mg ethanol consumed)}}{\text{VD (L/kg)} \times \text{weight (kg)} \times 10}$$

(Where V_D = 0.6 L/kg for adults and 0.7 L/kg for children. The factor 10 in the denominator changes the blood ethanol level from mg/L to the more commonly used units, mg/dL).

Ethanol dose (mg) = ethanol ingested (mL) × ethanol concentration (%) × 800

(Where 800 = an approximation using the specific gravity of ethanol to convert mL to mg).

EXAMPLE

A 15-kg, 3-year-old boy, ingesting four swallows of cologne (50% ethanol), would achieve what ethanol-blood level? Assume that one swallow is equal to 5 mL.

$$\text{Blood ethanol level} = \text{Cp (mg/dL)} = \frac{\text{dose (mg)}}{V_D \times \text{body weight (kg)} \times 10}$$

$$\text{Ingested ethanol dose (mg)} = (4)(5\text{ mL})(0.5)(800\text{ mg/mL})$$

$$\text{therefore, Cp} = \frac{(4)(5)(0.5)(800)}{(0.7)(15)(10)} = 76\text{ mg/dL}$$

BLOOD LEVELS

Ethanol blood levels roughly correlate with clinical signs. One must treat the patient however, and not the blood level, because tolerance, trauma, hypoglycemia, drug interactions, and disease factors may complicate the clinical picture. The clinical presentation of a tolerant patient at a given blood-ethanol level is less predictable for example, as clinical evidence of intoxication may be minimal in chronic alcoholics at significantly elevated blood ethanol levels. Most states accept a BAC of 0.08% to 0.10% (i.e., 80 to 100 mg/dL) as evidence of impairment.

The American Medical Association's Council on Scientific Affairs believes that deterioration of driving skills begins at a BAC of 0.05% and progresses to more serious impairment as levels rise. Psychomotor testing indicates early impairment in processing and acquisition of information, performance on divided-attention tasks, and judgment; however, biological differences between individuals cause substantial differences in ethanol effects.

Caution should be exercised when correlating blood ethanol levels to presumed dose. One glass of wine, one shot of whiskey, or one can of beer generally raises the blood ethanol level about 25 mg/dL. The average elimination rate in nontolerant individuals is 15 to 20 mg/dL/h. Pitfalls in correlating blood-ethanol levels with consumption include exact time of consumption, peak ethanol time, accuracy of test method, appropriate marking of sample, time between incident and withdrawal of sample, time between sample withdrawal and analysis, storage methods, collection methods, variability in volume of distribution, and sampling site. Proper collection technique involves the use of nonalcoholic skin antiseptics, although at least one study found no significant difference between alcoholic and nonalcoholic preps in measurement of the blood ethanol level. Another study also showed that performing venipuncture through a pool of 100% ethanol on skin does not affect ethanol results.

BREATH SAMPLES

Portable breath detection devices have been developed as rapid, simple, and noninvasive methods to estimate ethanol levels. Variables altering accuracy include recent use of alcohol or alcohol-containing products (within 15 to 30 minutes), recent belching or vomiting, inadequate end expiratory specimen from poor cooperation, obstructive pulmonary disease, and poor technique.

SERUM OSMOLALITY

Ethanol is one of several solvents that achieve sufficient toxic concentrations to be detected by an osmolal gap as measured by freezing-point depression. Measurement of osmolality by vapor pressure changes is not accurate. The normal osmolal gap is less than 10 mosm/kg H_2O. Other solvents that cause an osmolal gap include ethyl ether, isopropanol, methanol, acetone, and ethylene glycol. Serum osmolality should be used as a screening measure for the presence of selected solvents rather than as an estimation of blood ethanol levels. In the absence of an increased osmolal gap, ethanol is an unlikely cause of coma and other causes should be considered (e.g., subdural hematoma, stroke, another drug).

$$\text{Calculated Osmolality} = 2(\text{Na}) + \frac{\text{glucose}}{18} + \frac{\text{BUN}}{2.8}$$

$$\text{Osmolal Gap} = \text{Osmolality (measured)} - \text{Osmolality (calculated)}$$

Serum ethanol levels can be estimated roughly by the following equation:

$$\text{Estimated Ethanol (mg/dL)} = \frac{\text{Osmolal Gap} \times 46}{10}$$

Treatment

GUT DECONTAMINATION

Rapid absorption of alcohol makes decontamination unhelpful more than a few minutes after ingestion. Even the administration of charcoal before ethanol consumption does not produce different peak concentrations or time-to-peak concentrations in human volunteers. Cathartics are probably not helpful as well.

ELIMINATION ENHANCEMENT

Fructose may accelerate metabolism by 25%, but the modest reduction in alcohol levels is outweighed by the serious side effects of fructose, including vomiting, abdominal pain, pruritus, lactic acidosis, and shock. Hemodialysis increases ethanol clearance by three to four times, but supportive care usually suffices. Comatose, unstable patients with ethanol levels exceeding 500 mg/dL may indicate the need for dialysis if supportive care fails.

SUPPORTIVE MEASURES

- In all acutely inebriated patients, search for concurrent trauma, underlying disease, and coingestion of drugs and toxic alcohol substitutes (i.e., methanol, ethylene glycol).
- Evidence of trauma in the alcoholic patient indicates the need for cervical immobilization, cervical x-rays, and a careful search for cervical and cerebral injury.
- Acute ingestions in nontolerant patients usually respond to supportive care with special attention to prevention of aspiration and replacement of fluid and electrolytes.
- Comatose patients should be treated with initial attention to airway, breathing, circulation, and a "coma cocktail" to potentially correct easily reversible conditions (i.e., 1 amp of D50 for hypoglycemia, 2.0 mg of naloxone for possibly opiate intoxication, and 100 mg of thiamine for potential Wernicke-Korsakoff syndrome).
- Replace nutritional deficiencies in the chronic alcoholic (2 grams of magnesium sulfate, 100 mg of thiamine, 5 mg of folate, 1 ampule of multivitamins).
- Watch for development of withdrawal syndromes.
- Asymptomatic children who ingest ethanol and remain symptom free for 2 hours can safely be managed at home.

DELIRIUM TREMENS

- Correct fluid and electrolyte imbalances with crystalloid solutions. This may require many (i.e., greater than 5 L) within 24 hours. Adjust electrolytes, such as magnesium, as required by serum levels. Replace thiamine, pyridoxine, and folate as well.
- Monitor for dysrhythmias in an intensive care setting.
- Search for concurrent illness (e.g., hypoglycemia, pancreatitis, thiamine deficiency, alcoholic ketoacidosis, gastrointestinal bleeding, cerebral trauma, or other diseases of chronic alcoholism).
- Intravenous diazepam is effective in a 10-mg intravenous loading dose followed by 5 mg every 5 to 10 minutes until the patient is calm. Large doses of diazepam have been used safely. Oxazepam also may be used. Severe agitation or hallucinations also may respond to haloperidol, 2 to 5 mg intramuscularly.
- Watch for oversedation and hepatic encephalopathy.
- Restraints may be required in severely uncontrollable patients.
- Obtain skull films, computer tomography of head, and/or lumbar puncture as indicated for refractory cases.
- Studies with carbamazepine suggest that it may be effective in treating alcohol withdrawal, including delirium tremens.

ALCOHOLIC KETOACIDOSIS

- Management of these patients requires correction of volume depletion and administration of glucose. The volume depletion is usually amenable to an infusion of normal saline with dextrose.
- Intravenous therapy is continued until the serum bicarbonate level reaches 18 to 20 mEq/L, signs of orthostasis have resolved, and oral fluids are well tolerated.
- Patients typically will respond to replacement therapy within 12 hours.
- Close monitoring (every 4 to 6 hours) and supplementation of serum potassium and phosphorus levels during treatment is vital as hypokalemia and hypophosphatemia may ensue quickly.
- Sodium bicarbonate administration has not been shown to be particularly beneficial.
- Insulin therapy is not required.

Antidotes

The efficacy of naloxone in ethanol-induced coma is questionable. There are some case studies which describe the reversal of ethanol-induced coma by naloxone, however, no substantive series or well-controlled study confirms the usefulness of naloxone. A study on alcohol intoxication failed to show the effectiveness of naloxone in reversing ethanol-induced central nervous system depression. Flumazenil may aid in reversing the respiratory depression associated with ethanol ingestion, but this observation has not been clinically validated. Analeptic agents should not be used.

Questions—Ethanol

1. Ethanol is no longer a diluent or a solvent in American medicinal preparations.
A. True
B. False

2. In children who ingest small amounts of ethanol then have seizures, the cause may be
A. Hyponatremia
B. Coingestion of cocaine
C. Hypoglycemia
D. Genetic predisposition to epilepsy
E. None of the above

3. Alcoholic ketoacidosis usually develops
A. In adolescents drinking for the first time
B. In children ingesting a small amount of ethanol
C. In chronic drinkers who ingest more than their usual amount of alcohol
D. In chronic drinkers who recently binged then withdraw from alcohol
E. C and D

4. Absorption of alcohol is increased by
A. Factors that delay gastric emptying
B. High protein gastric contents
C. High volume of gastric contents
D. All of the above
E. None of the above

5. Heavy chronic consumption of alcohol appears to predispose patients to
A. Hemorrhagic strokes
B. Ischemic strokes
C. Thrombocytosis
D. A and B
E. A and C

6. Ethanol withdrawal
A. May lead to autonomic hyperexcitability
B. Is more often symptomatic in binge drinkers than in regular heavy drinkers
C. Has symptoms dependent more on duration than intensity of drinking
D. Is not affected by hypomagnesemia or hypokalemia
E. None of the above

7. Alcoholic seizures, or "rum fits," occurring after cessation of alcohol ingestion
A. Have a peak incidence at 48 hours after cessation
B. Usually continue into status epilepticus
C. Are best treated with intravenous benzodiazepines

Answers to questions in shaded boxes appear at the end of the chapter.

D. Very rarely precede the development of delirium tremens
E. All of the above

8. **Which does not** produce a disulfiram-like reaction when taken with alcohol?
A. Oxytocin
B. Metronidazole
C. Sulfonamides
D. Hypoglycemic agents
E. Oximes

9. **A safe level of ethanol use in pregnancy is**
A. One glass of red wine each day
B. One glass of red wine each week
C. One beer each week
D. One shot of liquor each week
E. Has not been established

10. **Ethanol blood levels roughly correlate with clinical signs.**
A. True
B. False

ISOPROPYL ALCOHOL

Isopropyl alcohol or isopropanol is a common solvent, disinfectant, "rubbing alcohol" and glass cleaner that shares central nervous system depressant properties with ethanol. At room temperature, isopropanol is a clear, volatile liquid with a burning, bitter taste and an aromatic odor. The principal metabolite of isopropanol, acetone, does not cause the renal, cardiac, retinal, or metabolic toxicity that results from ethylene glycol or methanol metabolites.

Isopropanol is second to ethanol as the most commonly ingested alcohol and remains a common cause of drug overdose. In 1996, the Annual Report of the American Association of Poison Control Centers reported 28,072 cases. Toxicity results from ingestion, and from inhalation as may occur when young children are given isopropanol sponge baths in a poorly ventilated area.

Pathophysiology

Isopropanol is a potent central nervous system depressant and causes cardiovascular depression in large doses. The metabolite, acetone, may potentiate and lengthen the duration of central nervous system symptoms. Mild acidosis may develop by conversion of acetone to acetic acid and formic acid. The shift in the NAD/NADH ratio brought about by the action of alcohol dehydrogenase may cause decreased gluconeogenesis and hypoglycemia similar to ethanol.

Pharmacokinetics

ABSORPTION

- Intestinal uptake of isopropanol is rapid.
- 80% of an oral dose is absorbed within 30 minutes. Complete absorption occurs within 2 hours, although large overdose may delay absorption.
- Skin absorption is relatively small but contributes to toxicity with prolonged contact. Toxicity may occur after isopropanol sponge baths from inhalation and dermal absorption.

DISTRIBUTION

- Isopropanol distributes in body water with an apparent volume of distribution of 0.6 to 0.7 L/kg.
- Two hours are required for complete tissue distribution.

ELIMINATION

- The kidney excretes 20% to 50% of an absorbed dose unchanged.
- Hepatic alcohol dehydrogenase metabolizes approximately 80% of isopropanol to acetone, which the lung or kidney slowly eliminates.
- Urine tests positive for acetone are measurable by 3 hours postingestion. A positive urine test for acetone still may be present at 24 hours postingestion.
- Serum acetone is measurable within 30 minutes postingestion. If no acetone is quantified by 30 minutes postexposure, exposure to isopropyl alcohol is unlikely.
- Acetone is further metabolized to acetate, formate, and carbon dioxide. The kinetics of isopropanol most closely follows concentration-dependent (first-order) kinetics.
- The half-life of isopropanol is about 2.5 to 3.2 hours.
- The elimination half-life of its active metabolite, acetone, is more prolonged.

Clinical Presentations

Isopropanol intoxication has a rapid onset of action (30 to 60 minutes), with peak effects within several hours. The clinical picture is similar to that of ethanol intoxication, except that the early elation phase usually is absent, the duration of action is longer because of acetone formation, and the odor of acetone is more prominent.

NEUROLOGIC EFFECTS

Dizziness, poor coordination, headache, and confusion progress to stupor, ataxia, coma, and loss of deep tendon reflexes in serious cases. Serious nervous system depression may persist for 24 hours. The early elation phase seen in ethanol intoxication is not present. Pupils often are miotic, and nystagmus may be present.

GASTROINTESTINAL EFFECTS

Gastric irritation appears early, with abdominal pain and vomiting often prominent. Hematemesis may occur.

CARDIOVASCULAR EFFECTS

Hypotension associated with large overdoses probably results from peripheral vasodilation. Serious arrhythmias have not been reported. Tachycardia is common.

MISCELLANEOUS EFFECTS

Acute tubular necrosis, hepatic dysfunction, hemolytic anemia, and myoglobinuria have been reported. Mild hypothermia may occur as a result of central nervous system depression and peripheral vasodilation.

Toxic Dosage/Death

Isopropanol is considered twice as potent a central nervous system depressant as ethanol. The toxic dose is about 1 mL/kg of a 70% isopropanol solution (as commonly seen in rubbing alcohol), but as little as 0.5 mL/kg may cause symptoms. The lethal dose is roughly 150 to 240 mL (2 to 4 mL/kg), although adults have survived 1-L ingestions. Isopropanol levels of 128 to 200 mg/dL have been associated with coma and death. More than three swallows of 70% isopropanol usually result in symptoms in children, and such ingestion requires medical observation.

Drug Interactions

Isopropanol potentiates the hepatic and renal toxicity produced by haloalkenes such as carbon tetrachloride.

Laboratory

ANALYTIC METHODS

Gas chromatographic methods similar to those used for ethanol detection constitute the method of choice. High acetone levels may interfere with creatinine determinations.

BLOOD LEVELS

A given isopropanol blood level is roughly twice as toxic as the same blood ethanol level. Blood isopropanol levels of 50 mg/dL are associated with mild intoxication in the nontolerant individual. Endogenous isopropanol may be found in insulin-dependent diabetes mellitus patients not exposed to isopropyl alcohol who are hyperglycemic and acidotic, indicating that acetone may be converted to isopropanol in physiologic conditions in which reduced NAD is elevated.

OSMOLAL GAP

Isopropanol is an alcohol that produces an osmolal gap. A 50-mg/dL toxic blood level typically produces an 8 to 9 mosm increase in the osmolal gap. Elevations of endogenous glycerol, acetone, and acetone metabolite levels also may be causes for an increased osmolal gap in the alcoholic patient. Any contribution of ethyl alcohol to the increased osmolal and anion gap can be evaluated from an initial serum ethyl alcohol level.

Treatment

GUT DECONTAMINATION

Rapid absorption of isopropanol precludes the usefulness of emesis or lavage unless coingested drugs or coma delay absorption. Activated charcoal and cathartics are not useful clinically. Children who ingest more than 0.5 mL of 70% isopropanol per kilogram may be given syrup of ipecac within 30 minutes postingestion unless contraindicated.

ELIMINATION ENHANCEMENT

Severe isopropanol overdoses have been managed successfully with both peritoneal dialysis and hemodialysis. Indications for dialysis include hypotension not easily corrected with fluids, deteriorating vital signs, coma and predicted peak blood isopropanol levels higher than 400 mg/dL.

SUPPORTIVE MEASURES

- Rapid-onset respiratory depression and hypotension indicate serious ingestions that require careful cardiac and respiratory monitoring together with immediate intravenous access.
- Consider coingestion of other toxic alcohols when osmolal gap and clinical picture do not correlate with blood isopropanol level.
- Ice-water lavage and serial hemoglobin levels are indicated for those patients with evidence of GI bleeding. Treat hypotension with fluids and vasopressors such as dopamine, if necessary.
- Ingestion of more than three swallows (15 mL) of 70% isopropanol by a 10-kg child (i.e., 1.5 mL/kg) is an indication for several hours of medical observation. Asymptomatic or minimally symptomatic children may be discharged at the end of the observation period.
- Consider dialysis if hypotension is not corrected easily with fluids. Also, consider dialysis in the setting of deteriorating vital signs, coma, and predicted peak blood isopropanol levels higher than 400 mg/dL.
- Screening for electrolytes, blood urea nitrogen, creatinine, glucose, complete blood count, arterial blood gases, serum acetone, and hepatic aminotransferases is indicated in severe isopropanol ingestion with depressed mental status. Hypoglycemia may occur, especially in children.
- High serum ketones with minimal acidosis are characteristic of isopropanol ingestion.

Questions—Isopropyl Alcohol

1. **The principal metabolite of isopropanol, acetone, causes the renal, cardiac, retinal, and metabolic toxicities that result from ethylene glycol and methanol metabolites.**
   A. True
   B. False
2. **A positive urine test for acetone**
   A. Is measurable by 3 minutes postingestion
   B. Is measurable by 3 hours postingestion
   C. May still be positive 24 hours postingestion
   D. A and C
   E. B and C
3. **If no serum acetone is quantified by 30 minutes postexposure,**
   A. Exposure to isopropyl alcohol is unlikely
   B. Exposure to isopropyl alcohol was likely combined with ethanol
   C. Exposure to isopropyl alcohol was likely combined with vinegar
   D. Exposure to isopropyl alcohol cannot be commented upon
   E. None of the above
4. **Compared to ethanol,**
   A. Isopropyl alcohol has a more prominent early elation phase.
   B. Isopropyl alcohol has a longer duration of efficacy.
   C. Isopropyl alcohol has a less notable odor.
   D. A and B
   E. A and C
5. **A lethal dose of isopropanol is roughly**
   A. 20 to 50 mL
   B. 50 to 100 mL
   C. 100 to 150 mL
   D. 150 to 250 mL
   E. None of the above
6. **Effective treatment of isolated isopropanol overdose may include**
   A. Lavage
   B. Activated charcoal
   C. Cathartics
   D. Hemodialysis
   E. Forced diuresis

METHANOL

Methanol, methyl alcohol, or "wood alcohol" is produced from the destructive distillation of wood. Methanol toxicity may result from methanol-contaminated whiskey, or more commonly, from the ingestion of antifreeze, windshield wiper fluids, deicing solutions, paints, and paint thinners. In 1996, a report of the American Association of Poison Control Centers reported 2,589 exposures.

Elimination of methanol depends on the folate pool, a variable among species. Methanol is a colorless, volatile liquid with the structural formula CH_3OH. Methanol has a distinctive odor that may be masked by impurities added during the production process. Methanol is widely available as a solvent and antifreeze. Formulations include antifreeze (95% concentration), windshield washer fluid (35% to 95%), Sterno canned heat (4%), shellacs, various paints, paint removers, varnishes, duplicating fluids, gasoline additives, ethanol denaturants, and rarely, nail polish removers.

Pathophysiology

Methanol toxicity results from the accumulation of two metabolites, formaldehyde and formic acid. Marked species variation in toxicity occurs as a result of differential rates of formate metabolism. Formaldehyde is rapidly metabolized to formic acid. The accumulation of formic acid accounts for most of the metabolic acidosis that follows methanol ingestion and probably correlates better with clinical toxicity than serum methanol levels.

Lactate may appear late in the course of severe methanol poisoning as a result of both formate-induced inhibition of mitochondrial respiration and of tissue hypoxia. Serum lactate can increase after methanol intoxication despite normal ventilation and perfusion and accounts for a significant bicarbonate deficit in severe poisoning. Methanol has inherent central nervous system depressant effects similar to those of ethanol.

Pharmacokinetics

ABSORPTION

- Methanol is well absorbed from the gastrointestinal tract, with peak levels reached within 30 to 90 minutes.
- Skin and lung absorption may be significant enough to cause methanol toxicity in the home environment and in the industrial setting (e.g., a painter may develop blindness after working in methanol-soaked clothes).

DISTRIBUTION

- Methanol is distributed like ethanol, with an apparent volume of distribution of 0.6 to 0.7 L/kg.
- The highest concentrations are found in the kidney, liver, and gastrointestinal tract, with smaller concentrations in the brain, muscle, and adipose tissue. Concentrations in the vitreous humor and optic nerve are high.

ELIMINATION

- Hepatic metabolism in humans accounts for most elimination (90% to 95%).
- Unchanged renal excretion accounts for 2% to 5% of methanol elimination.
- Pulmonary excretion accounts for small amounts of methanol elimination in human oral ingestions.
- Elimination in overdose follows saturation (zero-order) kinetics.
- Alcohol dehydrogenase oxidizes methanol to formaldehyde, which is converted rapidly to formic acid by aldehyde dehydrogenase.
- The folate-dependent pathway oxidizes formic acid to carbon dioxide, and a rate constant determines variation in toxicity among species.
- Methanol is oxidized 10 times more slowly than ethanol and has a longer elimination half-life.
- Ethanol has a 10 to 20 times greater affinity for alcohol dehydrogenase than methanol. Therefore, ethanol is metabolized preferentially by alcohol dehydrogenase.
- The serum half-life of methanol after mild toxicity is 14 to 20 hours and, after severe toxicity, 24 to 30 hours.
- Concurrent administration of ethanol increases the serum half-life to 30 to 35 hours.

Clinical Presentations

The onset of symptoms varies between 40 minutes and 72 hours. Coingestion of alcohol delays symptoms and the absence of symptoms on initial presentation does not exclude serious toxicity. The usual latent period is 12 to 24 hours. Symptoms and signs usually are limited to the central nervous system, eyes, and gastrointestinal tract. Inhalation may result in conjunctival and respiratory tract irritation. Severe metabolic acidosis may produce dyspnea and shock. Coma, seizure, and severe metabolic acidosis are serious prognostic signs. Death generally is from respiratory arrest.

NEUROLOGIC EFFECTS

Headache, vertigo, lethargy, and confusion occur commonly in mild to moderate intoxications. Coma and seizures may occur in severe cases, probably as a result of cerebral edema. Methanol produces little euphoria compared with ethanol.

OPHTHALMOLOGIC EFFECTS

Blurred vision, decreased visual acuity, photophobia, and "feeling of being in a snowfield" are common complaints. Signs include constricted visual fields, fixed and dilated pupils, retinal edema, and hyperemia of the optic disk. Prompt initiation of therapy is necessary to reverse symptoms, but even when treated appropriately, visual defects may persist in 25% of severe cases.

GASTROINTESTINAL EFFECTS

Methanol is a mucosal irritant and produces nausea, vomiting, and abdominal pain in many cases. Pancreatitis may occur. Absence of gastrointestinal symptoms does not rule out toxicity.

RENAL EFFECTS

Acute, reversible, renal failure in association with myoglobinuria has been described after methanol exposure.

HEMATOLOGIC EFFECTS

Mean corpuscular volume (MCV) is elevated in severe methanol poisoning. Leukocytosis and anemia also may occur.

Toxic Dosage/Death

Generally, 1 mL/kg is considered lethal. Fatalities have been reported after ingestion of 15 mL of a 40% solution, although 30 mL generally is considered a minimal lethal dose. Adults have survived ingestions of 500 to 600 mL with aggressive medical care. Consumption of as little as 0.1 mL/kg, or 6 to 10 mL, may cause blindness, but wide individual variation exists.

Laboratory

ANALYTIC METHODS

A modified gas chromatographic method may be used to analyze blood formate levels.

BLOOD LEVELS

Reports correlating blood methanol to clinical effects show variation of toxicity because of differences in sample timing, individual variation, concentration of toxic metabolites, and coingestion of ethanol. Peak methanol levels below 20 mg/dL usually are associated with asymptomatic individuals. Generally, central nervous system symptoms appear above 20 mg/dL, ocular symptoms appear above 100 mg/dL (however, ocular toxicity may correlate better with formate concentration than with methanol concentration), and fatalities in untreated patients occur at 150 to 200 mg/dL. Peak methanol levels guide treatment, but levels must be correlated to the presence of symptoms, since time of ingestion often is unknown. Coingestion of ethanol reduces methanol toxicity.

METABOLIC ACIDOSIS

A profound metabolic acidosis occurs in severe methanol poisoning. Most patients with a serum bicarbonate level under 18 mEq/L have a methanol level over 50 mg/dL. All symptomatic patients should have an arterial pH measured. Mortality correlates best with severity of acidosis rather than with blood methanol levels. Formate accounts for over 50% of the bicarbonate deficit. When formate levels exceed 20 mg/dL, ocular injury and metabolic acidosis are likely.

OSMOLAL GAP

Methanol causes a significant osmolal gap. For each milligram of methanol per deciliter, the osmolal gap rises by about 0.34 mosm. A methanol level of 50 mg/dL raises the osmolal gap by 17 mosm/kg H_2O. Other osmotically active alcohols include isopropanol, ethylene glycol, and ethanol.

Treatment

GUT DECONTAMINATION

Lavage is recommended for patients presenting within 2 hours of ingestion and may be useful up to 4 hours after ingestion if coma or coingested drugs reduce gastrointestinal motility. Charcoal does not adsorb methanol well and probably is not efficacious. There is no scientific evidence to substantiate the usefulness of cathartics in methanol poisoning.

ELIMINATION ENHANCEMENT

Forced diuresis is not effective, but hemodialysis effectively removes methanol as well as formaldehyde and formic acid. Hemodialysis is about eight times more effective than peritoneal dialysis. Dialysis does reduce the intensive care time required for ethanol therapy at methanol levels above 50 mg/dL. Dialysis may be stopped when the methanol level falls below 25 mg/dL. Ethanol also is dialyzed and maintenance levels must be increased during dialysis. Hemoperfusion is ineffective.

Indications for dialysis are somewhat controversial. A peak methanol level over 50 mg/dL is recommended in the medical literature, but the exact level is debatable. Similarly, formate levels over 20 mg/dL have been recommended as a cut-off. Refractory metabolic acidosis, any visual impairment, and renal failure are other indications for dialysis.

SUPPORTIVE CARE

- Frequent assessment of vital signs is mandatory. Watch for variations in blood pressure, hypothermia, tachycardia, arrhythmias, cyanosis, and dyspnea.
- Evaluate airway, breathing, and circulation in all patients. Give naloxone, glucose, and thiamine to all obtunded patients. Because methanol causes central nervous system depression and sudden apnea, carefully monitor respiratory status. For all patients with significant methanol ingestions, immediately draw blood for arterial blood gases to screen for metabolic acidosis and hypoxemia.
- Bicarbonate therapy, guided by arterial blood gases when the arterial pH falls below 7.2, may be a helpful adjunct.
- Plasma bicarbonate levels correlate poorly with the time after ingestion.
- Routine laboratory tests after a serious methanol ingestion should include methanol and ethanol levels, electrolytes with calculation of anion and osmolal gaps, calcium, complete blood count, blood urea nitrogen, creatinine, urinalysis, serum osmolality, hepatic aminotransferase enzymes, amylase, and creatine kinase.
- Phenytoin may be preferable to diazepam for controlling seizures because phenytoin does not synergistically depress consciousness.

Antidotes

ETHANOL

Administration of ethanol blocks the formation of formaldehyde and formic acid because of the preferential affinity of ethanol for alcohol dehydrogenase. Ethanol levels should be maintained between 100 and 150 mg/dL to completely inhibit toxic metabolite formation. Intravenous administration is more reliable than oral administration, but ethyl alcohol is irritating to veins. Blood must be drawn frequently before, during, and after dialysis until a steady-state ethanol level is confirmed. Continue ethanol infusion until the methanol level falls below 20 to 25 mg/dL. As ethanol prolongs the elimination half-life of methanol to 24 to 30 hours, several days may be required to reduce the methanol level below 25 mg/dL when hemodialysis is not used.

Indications for ethanol include peak methanol levels over 20 mg/dL. Ethanol should be considered in any patient with a history of ingestion of 0.4 mL/kg of methanol. Any symptomatic patient should receive ethanol pending confirmatory blood methanol levels. Patients who are being considered for hemodialysis and all patients with metabolic acidosis due to methanol poisoning should be considered for ethanol therapy.

FOLATE

Administration of folate provides increased cofactor for the oxidation of formic acid to carbon dioxide. Folic acid, 50 mg intravenously every 4 hours for several days, has been recommended as a large but safe dose. The use of folate is especially important in alcoholics, who may be folate depleted. Folate efficacy in humans has not been proven. Leucovorin is the active form of folate and may be substituted for folic acid.

4-METHYLPYRAZOLE

4-Methylpyrazole (4-MP) or fomepizole decreases methanol toxicity by inhibiting alcohol dehydrogenase. In most cases, administration of 20 mg/kg 4-MP adequately inhibits formate formation for 24 hours. Fomepizole may be preferential to ethanol therapy as ethanol treatment requires frequent monitoring, results in CNS depression, and may induce hypoglycemia.

Questions—Methanol

1. **Methanol toxicity results from the accumulation of its toxic metabolites**
   A. Formic acid and acetone
   B. Acetone and formaldehyde
   C. Formic acid and formaldehyde
   D. Formaldehyde and propylene glycol
   E. None of the above
2. **Peak levels of methanol occur how long after ingestion?**
   A. 10 to 20 minutes
   B. 30 to 90 minutes
   C. 3 to 4 hours
   D. 6 to 8 hours
   E. None of the above
3. **Skin and lung absorption of methanol may be significant enough to cause toxicity in the home environment and in the industrial setting.**
   A. True
   B. False
4. **Symptoms of methanol toxicity may include all of the following except**
   A. Blurred vision
   B. Vomiting
   C. Pinpoint pupils
   D. Abdominal pain
   E. Vertigo
5. **Severe methanol poisoning primarily causes**
   A. Respiratory alkalosis
   B. Respiratory acidosis
   C. Metabolic alkalosis
   D. Metabolic acidosis
   E. None of the above
6. **Treatment of methanol poisoning may include**
   A. Lavage
   B. Charcoal
   C. Cathartics
   D. Forced diuresis
   E. All of the above
7. **Indications for consideration of the use of ethanol to treat methanol poisoning includes**
   A. Peak methanol level over 20 mg/dL
   B. History of ingestion of 0.4 mL/kg
   C. Any symptoms of methanol toxicity
   D. Metabolic acidosis
   E. All of the above
8. **4-MP or fomepizole**
   A. Requires closer monitoring than ethanol treatment
   B. Results in less central nervous system depression than ethanol
   C. Can cause hypoglycemia, just like ethanol
   D. All of the above
   E. None of the above

ETHYLENE, PROPYLENE, AND DIETHYLENE GLYCOL

Ethylene glycol is a colorless, odorless, sweet-tasting compound that is used as an antifreeze, coolant, hydraulic brake fluid, glass cleaner, preservative, and glycerine substitute. Ethylene glycol has intoxicating properties similar to those of ethanol. Its metabolites yield central nervous system, cardiopulmonary, and renal dysfunction, as well as severe metabolic acidosis. TESS documented 5,548 reported exposures were documented by the Toxic Exposure Surveillance System (TESS) compiled by the American Association of Poison Control Centers in 1996.

Propylene glycol has been used as nontoxic antifreeze in dairies and breweries and as a component of automotive brake fluids. It has been used in the production of varnishes and synthetic resins, as a flavoring agent in baking and candy production, and as an emulsifier and nontoxic preservative in the foods industry. It can be found in several oral antibiotics, and it is a major ingredient in the formulation of several parenteral preparations, including diazepam (Valium®) and phenytoin (Dilantin®) in which its concentration may be as high as 40%.

Diethylene glycol is used in industrial solvents and antifreeze. Poisoning from this agent is rare but often fatal. The Elixir Sulfanilamide disaster of 1937 was one of the most consequential mass poisonings of the 20th century. This tragedy occurred shortly after the introduction of sulfanilamide, the first sulfa antimicrobial drug, when diethylene glycol was used as the diluent in its liquid formulation. A total of 105 patients died from its use.

Pathophysiology

Ethylene glycol produces roughly the same central nervous system depression as ethanol, but ethylene glycol produces toxic metabolites, which may prove deadly. The metabolic acidosis and anion gap seen with ethylene glycol ingestion result from glycolic (primarily) and lactic acid formation. The citric acid cycle is inhibited as a result of a reduced NAD/NADH ratio. This results in some oxalic acid formation, which contributes to the metabolic acidosis. Oxalate formation produces myocardial depression and acute tubular necrosis. Glycoaldehydes, glycolic acid, and glyoxylic acid may contribute to central nervous system depression and may contribute to renal toxicity by producing renal edema.

Liver metabolism of propylene glycol produces lactic acid, which enters the glycolytic pathway and, after large exposures, causes an anion gap and metabolic acidosis.

Pharmacokinetics

ABSORPTION

- Ethylene glycol is rapidly absorbed orally, but not by lung or dermal routes.
- Peak levels occur 1 to 4 hours after ingestion.
- Absorption of propylene glycol through intact skin is minimal, but the application of propylene glycol-containing compounds to infants with large areas of desquamation (e.g., silver sulfadiazine therapy in toxic epidermal necrolysis) has resulted in cardiorespiratory arrest.

DISTRIBUTION

- Because ethylene glycol is highly water soluble, it distributes evenly throughout body tissue.
- The volume of distribution of ethylene glycol is 0.83 L/kg.
- Propylene glycol has a half-life of 1.8 to 3.3 hours, and a volume of distribution of 0.51 to 0.88 L/kg.

ELIMINATION

- Approximately 20% of a 1-mg/kg dose of ethylene glycol are excreted unchanged. Less than 1% of ethylene glycol is metabolized to oxalic acid at this dose.
- The liver oxidizes ethylene glycol primarily to glycoaldehyde, glycolate, and then glyoxylate.
- The metabolism of glyoxylate follows several pathways that depend on the cofactors thiamine and pyridoxine.
- The oxidation of ethylene glycol to glyoxylate and subsequently to oxalate requires the conversion of NAD to NADH. The altered NAD/NADH ratio shifts pyruvate to lactate and thereby helps produce lactic acidosis.
- The acidic metabolites are more toxic than the parent compound. The order of toxicity appears to be glyoxylate > glycoaldehyde > ethylene glycol.
- The plasma half-life of ethylene glycol is approximately 3 to 5 hours.
- At ethanol levels of 100 to 200 mg/dL, the half-life of ethylene glycol is prolonged to 17 hours because of the 100-times-greater affinity of ethanol for alcohol dehydrogenase.
- The kidney excretes 45% of an absorbed dose of propylene glycol unchanged, and the remainder is metabolized by hepatic alcohol dehydrogenase to lactate, acetate, and pyruvate.
- The elimination half-life of propylene glycol averages about 19 hours.

Clinical Presentations

ETHYLENE GLYCOL

Ethylene glycol toxicity may be assumed with an ethanol-like intoxication with no odor, a large anion-gap acidosis, coma, osmolal gap, calcium oxalate crystals, and mental status changes. The presentation of ethylene glycol poisoning is classically divided into three stages, and depends on the severity of ingestion.

Stage 1

This "Central Nervous System (CNS) Depression" stage occurs 1 to 12 hours postingestion. Transient exhilaration occurs without the odor of ethanol. Gastrointestinal complaints include nausea and vomiting. Acidosis, coma, convulsions, and myoclonic jerks may be present. The optic fundus usually is normal, although the occasional presence of papilledema may confuse the clinical presentation with that of methanol. Nystagmus and ophthalmoplegia may occur. Cerebral edema secondary to cytotoxic damage and calcium oxalate deposition synergistically depresses central nervous system activity in severe poisoning.

Stage 2

Cardiopulmonary symptoms occur 12 to 24 hours after ingestion. Tachycardia, tachypnea, and mild hypertension often occur. Congestive heart failure and circulatory collapse are seen in severe ingestions.

Stage 3

This renal stage occurs 24 to 72 hours postingestion. This stage is characterized by oliguria, flank pain, acute tubular necrosis, and renal failure. Renal damage may be transient or permanent.

PROPYLENE GLYCOL

Propylene glycol primarily is a central nervous system depressant in large doses, and may cause hypoglycemia, lactic acidosis, and seizures in susceptible patients. In experimental animals, propylene glycol possesses one-third the central nervous system depressant properties of ethanol. The Food and Drug Administration considers propylene glycol safe in small doses for pharmaceutical preparations. Propylene glycol also may cause hemolysis, deafness, a high anion-gap acidosis from elevated lactate levels, cardiac arrhythmias, asystole, hepatic damage, renal damage, and serum hyperosmolarity with a marked osmolar gap.

DIETHYLENE GLYCOL

Symptoms of oral diethylene glycol poisoning occur within 24 hours of ingestion and include nausea, anorexia, vomiting, abdominal pain, and diarrhea. Neurologic effects include headache, dizziness, and narcosis. Polyuria and oliguria may occur. Jaundice and ascites may indicate liver pathology. In severe cases, the patient may exhibit seizures, coma, anuria, edema, fluid and electrolyte imbalance, and acidosis. At autopsy, renal tubular damage and centrilobular liver necrosis are observed.

Toxic Dosage/Death

A minimum lethal dose of ethylene glycol in humans is approximately 1.0 to 1.5 mL/kg or 100 mL in an average adult, however doses as little as 30 mL may be fatal. Levels greater than 85 mg/dL generally are fatal. Patients have survived 1- and 2-L ingestions that were treated within 1 hour of their suicide attempts. A single fatal oral dose of diethylene glycol in humans is about 1.2 mL/kg.

Laboratory

ANALYTIC METHODS

Glycol levels require gas chromatography and are not included routinely on toxicology screens.

BLOOD LEVELS

Serum propylene glycol levels up to 1,000 mg/dL do not correlate well with clinical status. Patients have been conscious with serum levels of 760 mg/dL.

URINE

Although oxalate normally is a minor metabolic product of ethylene glycol metabolism, urinary oxalate crystals are a common, but not invariable, feature of ethylene glycol intoxication. Two forms of calcium oxalate crystal are noted in urine: a tent-shaped form or dihydrate crystal, and a prism or dumbell-shaped monohydrate form. The dihydrate form appears only during high urinary calcium and oxalate concentrations, as seen in ethylene glycol poisoning. Some commercial ethylene glycol antifreeze products contain fluorescein as a colorant to aid in the detection of automobile cooling system leaks. The urine of a patient suspected of antifreeze ingestion may disclose visually detectable fluorescein under a Wood's lamp in the first several hours after ingestion.

Treatment

GUT DECONTAMINATION

Lavage may be effective only for a few hours, unless coingested drugs or coma delay the generally rapid absorption of ethylene glycol. Reducing absorption is important in massive, recent overdose. Charcoal and cathartics probably are not effective.

ELIMINATION ENHANCEMENT

Deteriorating vital signs, significant metabolic acidosis not amenable to correction with hydration and sodium bicarbonate, crystalluria, and serum ethylene glycol levels over 50 mg/dL are indications for early dialysis. The endpoint for dialysis is a serum ethylene glycol level of 10 mg/dL. During hemodialysis, there is no need for ethanol administration intravenously or in the dialysate because glycolate is effectively eliminated. For clearance of ethylene glycol and its metabolites, hemodialysis is superior to peritoneal dialysis. Continuous arteriovenous hemofiltration dialysis may be an alternative when hemodialysis and fomepizole therapy is not available.

SUPPORTIVE CARE

- Correct acidosis, fluid and electrolyte imbalance, and respiratory depression aggressively. Renal clearance of ethylene glycol is inversely related to water absorption. Maintenance of good urine output is necessary to enhance urinary elimination.
- Anion gap metabolic acidosis indicates the production of organic acids. Systemic acidosis below 7.2 may be treated with sodium bicarbonate. The serum bicarbonate concentration also may be increased when bicarbonate dialysate is used during hemodialysis.
- Toxicity may occur without significant elevation of the osmolal gap. Serious ethylene glycol toxicity (50 mg/dL) produces an approximate rise in the osmolal gap of 10 mosm.
- Propylene glycol is osmotically active and produces a concentration-dependent increase in serum osmolality.
- Osmolal and anion gaps may remain elevated despite low ethylene glycol levels because of the accumulation of glycolate.
- Check the urine each hour for at least 5 hours after presumed ethylene glycol ingestion before significant intoxication is ruled out. If urine oxalate crystals are seen and confirmed by a second urine specimen in 1 hour, begin intravenous (IV) alcohol or fomepizole, and hemodialyze.
- Check urine under Wood's lamp. If antifreeze has been ingested, the urine may fluoresce from fluorescein dye included in the product. If urine fluoresces, begin IV alcohol or fomepizole, and hemodialyze.
- Hypocalcemia secondary to calcium oxalate deposition may occur, and may be manifested by QT prolongation on electrocardiogram. Replace as indicated with 10% calcium gluconate intravenously.
- Tetany, myalgias, elevated creatinine levels, and increased creatine phosphokinase (CPK) levels may be seen in ethylene glycol poisoning and should all be monitored.
- In diethylene glycol poisoning, decontamination is recommended within 1 to 2 hours of an acute oral ingestion. Syrup of ipecac is not advised because of the potential for early seizures. Ethanol therapy has not been subjected to controlled clinical studies. Seizures are treated with standard anticonvulsants. Hemodialysis is indicated in unstable and acidotic patients.

Antidotes

4-METHYLPYRAZOLE

4-MP or fomepizole is a competitive inhibitor of alcohol dehydrogenase and effectively blocks the formation of toxic metabolites from ethylene glycol. A 15-mg/kg IV loading dose is followed by 10 mg/kg IV every 12 hours for 4 doses, then 15 mg/kg IV every 12 hours until the ethylene glycol level falls below 20 mg/dL. In all suspected cases, do not wait for symptoms to appear or for a serum level to return before treatment. Fomepizole is dialyzable and must be given every 4 hours during dialysis.

ETHANOL

Alcohol competitively inhibits alcohol dehydrogenase and blocks the metabolism of ethylene glycol. Ethanol therapy prolongs the half-life of ethylene glycol and reduces the formation of toxic metabolites. In severe ethylene glycol intoxication, acidemia, glycolic acid production, and serum ethylene glycol levels may persist despite ethanol infusions.

Indications for ethanol therapy include a strong suspicion of significant ethylene glycol ingestion pending determination of serum levels, peak serum ethylene glycol levels over 20 mg/dL (with or without symptoms), and acidemia, regardless of ethylene glycol levels. The ethanol must be administered as soon as possible as the elimination half-life of ethylene glycol is 3 hours at low concentrations. The dosage is the same as that for methanol poisoning and may be given intravenously or orally.

After termination of hemodialysis, ethanol may be administered in IV boluses of 500 mL 5% glucose with 10% ethanol over 20 to 30 minutes, followed by a continuous infusion of 70 to 100 mL/hour. Serum ethanol level is monitored every hour until a constant level of 90 to 130 mg/dL is maintained. For severe adult poisoning in which medical care may be delayed, four 1-oz "shots" of whiskey before or during transport may be used.

COFACTORS

Pyridoxine (50 mg IM per dose) and thiamine (100 mg IM per dose) are cofactors in the metabolism of ethylene glycol and should be given four times each day for two days. Magnesium also is a cofactor and should be replenished aggressively, guided by serum magnesium levels, particularly in alcoholic patients.

Questions—Ethylene, Propylene, and Diethylene Glycol

1. Ethylene glycol is absorbed rapidly when exposure is
   A. Oral
   B. Inhalational
   C. Dermal
   D. A and B
   E. A and C

2. Stage one of the presentation of ethylene glycol poisoning
   A. Occurs 12 to 24 hours after ingestion
   B. Primarily has renal involvement
   C. May include transient exhilaration followed by central nervous system depression
   D. Usually involves tachycardia, tachypnea, and hypertension
   E. None of the above

3. Ethylene glycol ingestion is always associated with a positive Wood's lamp test of urine.
   A. True
   B. False

4. Which of the following statements is true?
   A. Quantitative ethylene levels are included routinely on toxicology screens.
   B. Some commercial ethylene glycol antifreeze products contain fluorescein as a colorant to aid in the detection of automobile cooling system leaks.
   C. Urinary oxalate crystals invariably are a feature of ethylene glycol intoxication.
   D. No patient has survived ingestion of 1 to 2 L of ethylene glycol.
   E. None of the above

5. Indications for early dialysis in ethylene glycol poisoning include
A. Crystalluria
B. Serum ethylene glycol level over 50 mg/dL
C. Deteriorating vital signs
D. All of the above
E. None of the above

6. 4-Methylpyrazole is dialyzable and must be given every 4 hours during dialysis.
A. True
B. False

BENZYL ALCOHOL

Benzyl alcohol is an aromatic alcohol used as a bacteriostatic preservative. Parenteral medications formulated with benzyl alcohol include atropine, glycopyrrolate, physostigmine, pyridostigmine, heparin, crystalloid solutions, succinylcholine, atracurium, pancuronium, tubocurarine, and metoclopramide. One milliliter or 5 mg of diazepam contains 15.7 mg of benzyl alcohol.

Pharmacokinetics

Benzyl alcohol is oxidized to benzoic acid, conjugated with glycine, and excreted as hippuric acid. Conjugation may be limited by an immature liver in neonates, leading to toxicity.

Clinical Presentations

Several deaths have occurred in premature neonates weighing less than 2,500 grams after the intravenous injection of benzyl alcohol-containing solutions. Metabolic acidosis, bradycardia, skin breakdown, respiratory depression, gasping respirations, hypotonia, hepatorenal failure, hypotension, and cardiovascular collapse characterize the clinical picture. All patients received intravenous flushes with bacteriostatic saline containing an average of 130 to 405 mg of benzyl alcohol per kilogram per day. High urine benzoate and hippurate levels and elevated serum benzoic acid levels were found.

The term "gasping baby syndrome" describes the progressive neurologic deterioration of premature infants suffering from benzyl alcohol poisoning. Retrospective studies of neonates revealed a substantial decline in mortality and intraventricular hemorrhage among infants weighing less than 1 kg after the use of benzyl alcohol-containing solutions was discontinued.

Toxic Dosage/Death

Acute toxicity is minimal. Adult humans safely tolerate 30 mL by rapid infusion. With dosages of benzyl alcohol ranging from 99 to 234 mg/kg/day, hypotension, severe metabolic acidosis with an increased anion gap secondary to increased blood concentrations of benzoic acid, changes in consciousness, leukopenia, thrombocytopenia, hyperammonemia, and respiratory gasping are observed with high mortality rates.

Treatment

GUT DECONTAMINATION

Management primarily is supportive. Charcoal and other gut decontamination methods have not been proven effective in the treatment of benzyl alcohol poisoning.

ELIMINATION ENHANCEMENT

Benzyl alcohol elimination would probably be enhanced by dialysis, but no case studies document its effectiveness.

SUPPORTIVE MEASURES

- Do not use bacteriostatic saline with benzyl alcohol with premature neonates.
- When a continuous intravenous diazepam infusion is administered for status epilepticus, no dosage of more than 1 mg/kg/hour should be used. When using dosages between 0.5 and 1 mg/kg/hour, frequent cardiovascular and respiratory monitoring is required.
- Serum electrolytes, blood gases, and anion gap should be measured at least every 6 to 12 hours.
- Serum and urine benzoic acid concentrations may be determined every 24 hours in severe cases.

Questions—Benzyl Alcohol

1. The clinical picture of benzyl alcohol toxicity includes all of the following except
A. Metabolic acidosis
B. Hypotonia
C. Hypertension
D. Hepatorenal failure
E. Respiratory depression

2. Treatment of benzyl alcohol poisoning includes
A. Charcoal
B. Gastric lavage
C. Induced emesis
D. Serum and urine benzoic acid concentrations
E. None of the above

DISULFIRAM

During the 1930s, disulfiram was introduced into medicine as a scabicide. In 1948, Hald and Jacobsen drank ethyl alcohol after they had ingested disulfiram and noted a highly disagreeable reaction. Based on this experience, disulfiram was proposed for the prophylactic treatment of chronic alcoholism. Disulfiram is now widely used all over the world as an alcohol deterrent. In the United States, as many as 200,000 persons have been under treatment with disulfiram.

In spite of the large number of individuals maintained on disulfiram and the common occurrence of disulfiram (Antabuse®) reactions, reports of overdose are relatively uncommon. Disulfiram use in the ambulatory and supportive care of the chronic alcoholism patient nevertheless has been associated with serious and sometimes fatal toxic effects.

Disulfiram is used as an alcohol deterrent together with supportive psychotherapy in the management of alcohol dependence in highly motivated patients. Its efficacy has not been established. Subjects must abstain from alcohol at least 12 hours before use. The patient must specifically be made aware that disulfiram is being ingested and warned regarding ingestion of alcohol in any form.

Disulfiram also is used as a fungicide, a rubber accelerator, a seed disinfectant, and a vulcanizer. It has been used in the treatment of chronic nickel dermatitis based on the chelating action of diethyldithiocarbamate, a metabolite of disulfiram. Disulfiram is a thiuram derivative (tetraethylthiuram disulfide). It is closely related to other thiurams used in industry.

Pathophysiology

Disulfiram inhibits the enzymatic oxidation of acetaldehyde to acetate, which occurs in the liver during normal alcohol catabolism by competing with NAD for aldehyde dehydrogenase. When alcohol is ingested after disulfiram ingestion, acetaldehyde concentration in blood may increase 5 to 10 times the concentration observed after the metabolism of alcohol alone. Elevated acetaldehyde may produce the unpleasant symptoms of the disulfiram-alcohol reaction.

Others feel that the carbon disulfide metabolite of disulfiram produces many of the disagreeable symptoms. Carbon disulfide may react with pyridoxal 5-phosphate to inhibit monoamine oxidase. In turn, this may deplete pyridoxine, an important cofactor. Decreased pyridoxine can lead to a decrease in brain gamma-aminobutyric acid (GABA) and yield an increase in seizure production.

Disulfiram also inhibits erythrocyte aldehyde dehydrogenase (ALDH) for 36 to 120 hours. Erythrocyte ALDH activity can be monitored to measure patient compliance. Inhibited erythrocyte ALDH activity is not regenerated until new erythrocytes are made. Significant extrahepatic acetaldehyde metabolic capacity remains inhibited for long periods after disulfiram is discontinued.

Pharmacokinetics

ABSORPTION

- Disulfiram is slowly and incompletely absorbed (70% to 90%) from the gastrointestinal tract.
- Up to 20% of an ingested dose may be found in the feces.
- An interval of approximately 3 to 12 hours after disulfiram ingestion may be required before the disulfiram-alcohol reaction occurs.
- Peak plasma levels of disulfiram occur approximately 8 to 10 hours after oral ingestion.
- Diethyldithiocarbamate (DDC) and diethylamine metabolites in plasma also peak at 6 to 8 hours after dosing.
- Very little disulfiram is found in the plasma after 24 hours and none of the drug or its metabolites is found after 36 hours.

DISTRIBUTION

- Protein binding has been reported as 50%.
- Disulfiram and its metabolites have been found in the thyroid, adrenals, pancreas, stomach, small and large intestine, muscle, liver, testes, kidney, lung, spleen, and heart.
- Disulfiram has high lipid solubility and accumulates in various fat deposits.

ELIMINATION

- Metabolism occurs in the erythrocytes and the liver. Disulfiram is metabolized in the liver to carbon disulfide. The erythrocyte glutathione reductase system reduces disulfiram to DDC.
- DDC is metabolized in the liver by glucuronidation, nonenzymatic degradation, methylation and oxidation. Approximately 5% to 20% is excreted in the feces and 50% to 70% in the urine as free and esterified sulfate and conjugated DDC.
- The lungs excrete 10% to 60% as carbon disulfide.
- Approximately 90% of an ingested dose is out of the body in 3 days.

Clinical Presentations

Symptoms of disulfiram toxicity in the adult are similar to those associated with carbon disulfide poisoning. Symptoms induced by carbon disulfide include parkinsonism and peripheral neuropathies. Other symptoms include ataxia, paraesthesias, dementia, seizures, vomiting, lethargy, dehydration, garlic or rotten-egg breath, and flushing. Acute disulfiram-induced hepatitis is rare, perhaps unlikely to occur in more than one out of 25,000 patients treated. Fatalities have been reported. Nickel hypersensitivity dermatitis may be initiated by contact with nickel on the skin as disulfiram metabolizes to dithiocarbamate, an effective nickel chelator.

Chronic disulfiram use has been associated with numerous undesirable effects, however alcohol use prior to and intermittently during disulfiram maintenance therapy may have contributed to some of these reported experiences. Basal ganglia lesions that develop after disulfiram toxicity may be because of carbon disulfide, one of the disulfiram metabolites. Disulfiram-induced parkinsonism and catatonia is well documented. Following long-term disulfiram use (weeks to years) and occasionally in the acute setting, patients have developed tremor, dysphagia, dysarthria, staggering gait, myoclonic jerks, and signs of polyneuropathy. Marked behavioral and personality disorders have been observed.

DISULFIRAM-ETHANOL REACTION

Patients who ingest disulfiram 3 to 12 hours before ethanol are subject to an uncomfortable reaction that begins 5 to 15 minutes after the alcohol is ingested. There is no correlation between the amount of ethanol ingested and the severity of the disulfiram-ethanol reaction. Skin flushing, malaise, headache, nausea, palpitations, dyspnea, hyperventilation, tachycardia, fever, chest pain, weakness, and vomiting may occur within 20 to 30 minutes and generally resolve within 2 to 4 hours.

Severe reactions may include respiratory distress, chest pain, electrocardiographic changes consistent with myocardial ischemia, hypotension, seizures, ventricular and atrial dysrhythmias, and even death from cardiovascular collapse. A disulfiram-ethanol reaction may occur even weeks after the last dose of disulfiram and may be precipitated by any prescription or over-the-counter medication containing alcohol.

Toxic Dosage/Death

DISULFIRAM

Toxicity in children may occur with an ingested dose of 2.5 grams of disulfiram. Single doses of disulfiram up to 6 grams have been reported without ill effects.

DISULFIRAM-ETHANOL REACTION

Mild symptoms of a disulfiram-ethanol reaction have been observed with as little as 7 mL of alcohol. In some patients, ingestion of as much as 1.5 grams per day of disulfiram is required for a significant, reversible, and only mildly symptomatic alcohol challenge response. Death, a rare occurrence with disulfiram, has followed a "test drink" of 1 ounce of whiskey (15 mL of alcohol).

Drug Interactions

Disulfiram-drug interactions without alcohol may inhibit hepatic metabolism and may prolong half-life, therapeutic, and toxic effects. Drugs implicated include antidiabetic agents, barbiturates, caffeine, chlordiazepoxide, Coumadin®, ethylene dibromide, paraldehyde, phenytoin, rifampin, and sedative-hypnotics.

Isoniazid use with disulfiram may cause behavioral changes and incoordination. Concurrent metronidazole use may cause acute psychosis and confusion. Disulfiram use with anesthetics has been associated with hypotension; with Digoxin® has been associated with hypokalemia; with tricyclic antidepressants has potentiated the severity of disulfiram-ethanol reactions.

Pregnancy/Lactation

Adequate information is not available relating to passage of disulfiram or its metabolites through the placenta or the presence of disulfiram or its metabolites in the fetus or in breast milk. Disulfiram is classified as pregnancy risk category C.

Laboratory

ANALYTIC METHODS

A high-performance liquid chromatographic method is available for the determination of disulfiram, DDC, carbon disulfide, and other metabolites from a single sample of plasma or urine.

BLOOD LEVEL

The usual "toxic screen" does not detect disulfiram or its metabolites. To confirm an overdose, levels must be obtained specifically for disulfiram or its metabolites. Levels for these chemical products may not be available at most community hospitals. Disulfiram is quickly metabolized and levels are generally not of any value by the time a patient arrives at a hospital facility. Furthermore, elevated blood levels have not yet been established to correlate with severity of clinical symptoms.

Treatment

GUT DECONTAMINATION

Because gastrointestinal absorption is very slow, gut decontamination theoretically may be advantageous up to 10 hours or more after ingestion. Activated charcoal (1 gram/kg) may be used and repeated every 4 hours, although there are no data to substantiate its usefulness. This may be sufficient to encourage further fecal excretion of DDC glucuronide during its enterohepatic circulation. Syrup of ipecac contains ethanol and may precipitate a disulfiram-ethanol reaction. Cathartic use has not been studied in disulfiram overdose.

ELIMINATION ENHANCEMENT

The lipophilic properties of disulfiram, with its conversion to metabolites that are partially excreted through the respiratory tract, render extracorporeal procedures such as hemodialysis, hemoperfusion, and forced diuresis, probably ineffective.

SUPPORTIVE MEASURES

- If the clinical course is, as is usually the case, mild and self-limited and all clinical, electrocardiographic, and other laboratory evidence of a disulfiram reaction indicate no abnormalities, the patient can, after a period of at least 8 to 12 hours, be discharged.
- Because symptoms may not appear for 3 to 12 hours after ingestion, active measures can be instituted to eliminate tablets already ingested.
- On admission to the hospital, blood should be drawn for a complete blood count, glucose, blood urea nitrogen, creatinine, electrolytes, and liver function studies. Careful observation must be made for evidence of decreased serum potassium, leukocytosis, or eosinophilia.
- Airway protection (endotracheal intubation) and assisted ventilation may be required in the comatose patient. Seizures may be treated with diazepam or phenytoin.
- Pyridoxine, 1 gram IV, may be useful in the treatment of patients with evidence of neurologic toxicity.
- Serum ethanol levels should be determined in any patient who is suspected to have taken an overdose of disulfiram. This may aid in the evaluation and confirm that symptoms are related to a disulfiram-alcohol interaction.
- Hypotension may be controlled with Trendelenburg position, intravenous fluids, and/or pressor amines such as norepinephrine.
- Exposure to any form of alcohol should be prevented for at least 2 weeks after a disulfiram poisoning.
- Computed tomography (CT) scans performed within 1 week to a few months after the onset of neurologic symptoms may show symmetric, bilateral, low-density lesions of the basal ganglia. Such lesions may be seen within a few days after the onset of symptoms.
- Motor nerve conduction velocity studies and electromyography should be done if peripheral neuropathy is evident.

DISULFIRAM-ETHANOL REACTION

- Treatment is mainly supportive. Patients with any evidence of coronary ischemia should be admitted to an intensive care unit and placed under continuous cardiac monitoring. Myocardial ischemia, infarction and arrhythmias, both atrial and ventricular, may occur.
- Respiratory tract patency must be established and maintained. Assisted ventilation may be required. Supplemental oxygen should be administered to all patients.
- Seizures can be managed with endotracheal intubation, respiratory protection, and diazepam (up to 10 mg IV in an adult and 0.1 to 0.3 mg/kg IV slowly in a child). Phenytoin also may be used.
- Hypokalemia can be treated with oral or intravenous potassium supplements.
- Do not use phenothiazines as their α-blocking potential may induce or further exacerbate hypotension.

Antidotes

There is no antidote. Ferrous chloride and ascorbic acid were, at one time, proposed as antidotes for the treatment of a severe disulfiram-ethanol reaction, however they have not been proven to be clinically helpful.

Questions—Disulfiram

1. The unpleasant symptoms of the disulfiram-alcohol reaction may be a result of

A. Elevated blood acetate concentration
B. Elevated blood acetaldehyde concentration
C. Carbon disulfide
D. A and B
E. B and C

2. Peak plasma levels of disulfiram occur at

A. 2 to 4 hours after ingestion
B. 4 to 6 hours after ingestion
C. 6 to 8 hours after ingestion
D. 8 to 10 hours after ingestion
E. None of the above

3. Chronic disulfiram use has been associated with

A. Alzheimer's
B. Parkinsonism
C. Huntington's

D. A and B
E. B and C

4. **The disulfiram-alcohol reaction**
A. May include skin flushing, headache and chest pain
B. Has severity which correlates with the amount of alcohol ingested
C. Usually begins 2 to 4 hours after ingestion
D. Usually resolves 6 to 8 hours after ingestion
E. All of the above

5. **One should avoid use of all of the following drugs with disulfiram except**
A. Isoniazid
B. Metronidazole
C. Penicillin
D. Digoxin
E. Tricyclic antidepressants

Answers

Ethanol

1. B 2. C 3. D 4. E 5. D 6. A,
7. C 8. A 9. E 10. A

Isopropyl Alcohol

1. B 2. E 3. A 4. B 5. D 6. D

Methanol

1. C 2. B 3. A 4. C 5. D 6. A,
7. E 8. B

Ethylene, Propylene, And Diethylene Glycol

1. A 2. C 3. B 4. B 5. D 6. A

Benzyl Alcohol

1. C 2. D

Disulfiram

1. E 2. D 3. B 4. A 5. C

SELECTED READINGS

Ethanol

1. Criteria Committee, National Council on Alcoholism. Criteria for the diagnosis of alcoholism. Am J Psychiatry 1972;129:129.
2. Duffens K, Marx JA. Alcoholic ketoacidosis-a review. J Emerg Med 1987;5:399–406.
3. Ellenhorn MJ. The alcohols. In: Hall JB, Schmidt GA, Wood LDH eds. Principles of critical care. New York: McGraw-Hill, 1992, 2080–2093.
4. Gibson PJ, Cant AJ, Mant TG. Ethanol poisoning. Acta Paediatr Scand 1985;74:977–978.
5. Guppy A. At whole blood concentration should drunk-driving be illegal? Something lower than 17.4 mmol/L (0.8 g/L). Br Med J 1994;308:1055–1056.
6. Kaplan NM. Alcohol and hypertension. Lancet 1995;345:1588–1589.
7. Milas AA, Tavassoli M. Laboratory markers of ethanol intake and abuse: a critical appraisal. Am J Med Sci 1992;303:425–428.
8. MMWR. Update. Alcohol-related traffic fatalities-United States 1982–1993. JAMA 1994;272:1892.
9. Morse RM, Flavin DK. Joint Committee of the National Council on Alcoholism. JAMA 1992;268:1012–1014.
10. Redetzki HM. Ethanol (Management Treatment Protocol): Poisindex Information System. Rumack BH, ed. Colorado: Micromedex, Inc. Edition expires 8/30/92.
11. Schenker S, Speeg KV. The risk of alcohol intake in men and women. All may not be equal. N Engl J Med 1990;322:127–129.
12. Wax PM, Hoffman RS, Goldfrank LR. Rapid quantitative determination of blood alcohol concentration in the emergency department using an electrochemical method. Ann Emerg Med 1992;21:254–259.

Isopropyl Alcohol

1. Braden GL, Strayhorn CH, Germain MJ, Mulhern JG, Skutcher CL. Increased osmolal gap in alcoholic acidosis. Arch Intern Med 1993;153:2377–2380.
2. Kelner M, Beuley DN. Isopropanol ingestion: interpretation of blood concentrations and clinical findings. J Toxicol Clin Toxicol 1983;20:497–507.
3. Rich J, Scheife RT, Katz N, Caplan LR. Isopropyl alcohol intoxication. Arch Neurol 1970;417:322–324.
4. Stead AN, Moffat AC. A collection of therapeutic, toxic and fatal blood drug concentrations in man. Hum Toxicol 1983;3:437–464.

Methanol

1. Bennett JL, Cary FH, Mitchell GL, et al. Acute methyl alcohol poisoning: a review based on experiences in an outbreak of 323 cases. Medicine 1953;32:431–463.
2. Martensson E, Olofsson U, Heath A. Clinical and metabolic features of ethanol-methanol poisoning in chronic alcoholics. Lancet 1988;1:327–328.
3. McCoy HG, Cipolle RJ, Ehlers SM et al. Severe methanol poisoning: application of a pharmacokinetic model for ethanol therapy and hemodialysis. Am J Med 1979;67:804–807.
4. McGuigan MA. Analysis of the temporal development of acidosis in uncomplicated methanol poisoning. Ann Emerg Med 1995;26:725.
5. Palatnick W, Redman LW, Sitar DS, Tenenbein M. Methanol half-life during ethanol administration: implications for management of ethanol poisoning. Ann Emerg Med 1995;26:202–207.

Ethylene, Propylene, And Diethylene Glycol

1. Baud FJ, Galliott M, Astier A, et al. Treatment of ethylene glycol poisoning with intravenous 4-methylpyrazole. N Engl J Med 1988;319:97–100.
2. Brown CG, Trumbull D, Klein-Schwartz W et al. Ethylene glycol poisoning. Ann Emerg Med 1983;12:501–506.
3. Cate JC, Hendricks R. Propylene glycol intoxication and lactic acidosis. N Engl J Med 1980;303:1237.
4. Goodkin DA. Ethylene glycol poisoning. Am J Med 1990;88:201.
5. Scully R, Galdabini J, McNealy B. Case records of the Massachusetts General Hospital. Discussion of Levinsky NG. Case 38:1979. N Engl J Med 1979;301:650–657.
6. Winter ML, Ellis MD, Snodgrass WR. Urine fluorescence using a Wood's lamp to detect the antifreeze additive sodium fluorescein: a qualitative adjunctive test in suspected ethylene glycol ingestion. Ann Emerg Med 1990;19:663–667.
7. Woolf AD. Diethylene glycol. Clin Toxicol Rev 1994;17(3):1–2.

Benzyl Alcohol

1. Gershanik J, Boecler B, Ensley H, et al. The gasping syndrome and benzyl alcohol poisoning. N Engl J Med 1982;307:1384–1388.
2. Hiller JL, Benda GI, Rahatzad M, et al. Benzyl alcohol toxicity: impact on mortality and intraventricular hemorrhage among very low birth weight infants. Pediatrics 1986;77:500–506.
3. Lopez-Herce J, Bonet C, Meana A, Albajara L. Benzyl alcohol poisoning following diazepam intravenous infusion. Ann Pharmacother 1995;29:632.
4. Weissman DB, Jackson SH, Heicher DA, Rockoff MA. Benzyl alcohol administration in neonates. Anesth Analg 1990;70:673.

Disulfiram

1. Manoguerra AS, Kerney TE. Acute disulfiram toxicity. Vet Hum Toxicol 1982;24(4):282.
2. Raing JM. Disulfiram toxicity and carbon disulfide poisoning. Am J Psychiatry 1977;134:371–378.
3. Wright C, Moore R, Grodin DM, Spyker DA. Disulfiram hepatotoxicity: incidence of enzyme elevation and predictors of fatal outcome. Vet Hum Toxicol 1991;33:38.

ACKNOWLEDGMENT

Thanks to Alison Deutsch, MD for contributing the questions in this chapter.

CHAPTER 18
Amphetamines

INTRODUCTION

Amphetamine was first synthesized in 1887, but its pharmacological effects were not investigated until the late 1920s when a substitute for ephedrine was sought. Amphetamine was used in the 1930s in over-the-counter nasal decongestants called "Benzedrine inhalers." Around that time, the stimulant and appetite-suppressant properties of amphetamines, as well as their clinical usefulness for narcolepsy and hyperactivity in children, were discovered. In 1937, amphetamines became available only by prescription because of their abuse potential. Both the Germans and the allies used amphetamines to counter battle fatigue and maintain alertness in their military troops during World War II. The Japanese distributed amphetamine compounds extensively to their civilian workers, in addition to their military troops, to increase productivity. After the war, the availability of large stockpiles of over-the-counter amphetamines contributed to widespread abuse in Japan.

Amphetamines have strong central nervous system effects, which last longer than those of cocaine do. Because they increase physical and mental alertness, amphetamines are popular among college students, athletes, and truck drivers who require prolonged vigilance or short periods of high energy. Long-term use may lead to psychological dependence and tolerance, although physical withdrawal symptoms are mild compared with those of opiates and barbiturates. Depression may follow chronic use or binges and may result in continued use.

Legitimate uses of amphetamines and methylphenidate include treatment of properly documented narcolepsy in adults and attention deficit disorder in children. Occasionally, both these drugs may be indicated when attention deficit disorder extends into adulthood. The use of amphetamines for short-term (8 to 12 weeks) suppression of appetite remains a legal indication, although this use is highly controversial. Long-term benefit of amphetamines for appetite suppression is clinically insignificant because of tolerance and is potentially harmful because of the common complication of abuse. These drugs cannot be legally prescribed for the treatment of drug dependence, fatigue, anxiety reactions, or chronic anxiety or to generate a sense of well being.

Habitual use or massive doses may result in a toxic psychosis characterized by paranoia, delusions, hallucinations, or bizarre violent behavior. The amphetamine user may present as a restless, tremulous individual who is garrulous, suspicious, and anxious. Some individuals become hostile and aggressive. Although memory, orientation, and insight usually are preserved, high or prolonged amphetamine doses may cause the individual to act upon his or her delusions, leading to suicidal or homicidal actions. Perhaps because of the rapid development of tolerance, fatalities occur uncommonly and usually in newer, less experienced amphetamine users. In a series of amphetamine-induced deaths, trauma-related deaths accounted for two-thirds of the victims. Medical causes of death include cerebrovascular hemorrhage, acute cardiac failure, hyperthermia, cerebral edema with brain stem compression, and seizures.

Clandestine laboratories produce many amphetamine analogues (see Chapter 24, Designer Drugs). Some synthetic amphetamine compounds have gained popularity as hallucinogenic "love" drugs with relatively mild toxicity. Such a reputation is not deserved as certain analogues are equipotent to amphetamines and may produce hyperthermia, seizures, rhabdomyolysis, coma, or death. The psychoactive amphetamine derivative, 3,4-methylenedioxymethamphetamine (MDMA), may yield an amphetamine-like reaction, which includes anxiety, dysphoria, tachycardia, hypertension, hypertonicity, and seizures. The illicit hallucinogen p-methoxyamphetamine (PMA) and the methylene-dioxyamphetamine compounds (MDA, MMDA, MDEA, and MDMA) have no legal indications.

Pathophysiology

Amphetamine is the prototype of a class of noncatecholamine compounds that produce strong central nervous system stimulation. Technically, the name amphetamine refers specifically to phenylisopropylamine, however commonly this name refers to a number of structurally related compounds including methamphetamine, fenfluramine, phentermine, and synthetic amphetamine analogues that share similar pharmacological and toxic effects. Amphetamine (Benzedrine) is racemic β-phenylisopropylamine and the dextrorotatory isomer of amphetamine is available as dextroamphetamine (Dexedrine®). Methamphetamine is closely related chemically to both amphetamine and ephedrine but has more prominent central than peripheral effects at low dose. See Chapter 24, Designer Drugs.

Both long- and short-term amphetamine administration produce large concentration changes in norepinephrine, dopamine, and dopamine metabolites. Amphetamine or one of its metabolites also may produce a direct effect by acting as a false neurotransmitter. Some experimental evidence suggests that large doses of methamphetamine enhance synaptic catecholamine levels by inhibiting monoamine oxidase, which is the enzyme responsible for the oxidation of norepinephrine and serotonin. Some amphetamine derivatives, including MDMA, may cause an acute release of serotonin and lead to long-term depletion of serotonin that correlates with morphologic damage to serotonergic nerve endings.

Because of the close structural resemblance of amphetamines to the neurotransmitters dopamine and norepinephrine, most investigators believe that alterations of these chemicals mediate at least some of the behavioral effects of amphetamines. Amphetamines block reuptake of dopamine in therapeutic doses, but in overdose may act as dopamine receptor blockers, resulting in movement disorders that usually resolve in the acute setting without any specific intervention. Increasing the synaptic concentration of these neurotransmitters either by direct release from storage vesicles or by inhibition of reuptake is the most likely mechanism of action.

Amphetamines and amphetamine analogues have variable peripheral and central α- and β-adrenergic effects that cause anorexia and sympathomimetic effects. Amphetamine contains a basic β-phenylamine moiety, which possesses strong stimulant, cardiovascular, and anorectic activity. Addition of an α-methyl group, substitution of a terminal amine or an α-phenyl group, and cyclization of the side chain reduce stimulant and cardiovascular effects, but maintain the anorectic properties. Modification of the side chain into a heterocyclic structure attenuates the anorectic and cardiovascular effects, but maintains the stimulant activity. The illicit production of p-methoxyamphetamine (p-methoxy group addition) and methylenedioxyamphetamine results in hallucinogenic street drugs that are equipotent in α-adrenergic properties to amphetamine.

Pharmacokinetics

ABSORPTION

- Single pharmacological doses of amphetamines (i.e., 10 to 25 mg) given to human volunteers produce peak plasma levels in 1 to 2 hours and are rapidly absorbed from the gastrointestinal tract.
- Amphetamine absorption usually is complete by 4 to 6 hours.
- Phentermine absorption is slightly slower (i.e., peak levels at 4 hours in therapeutic doses); other amphetamine analogues and methamphetamine have absorption characteristics similar to those of amphetamines.
- At pharmacological doses, methylphenidate and fenfluramine produce peak plasma levels about 3 hours postingestion and are absorbed almost completely from the gastrointestinal tract.
- Sustained-release preparations are available as resin-bound rather than soluble salts. These compounds display reduced peak blood levels compared with standard amphetamine preparations, but total bioavailability and time to peak levels remain similar.

DISTRIBUTION

- Amphetamines concentrate in the kidney, lungs, and brain.
- The extent of protein binding and the volume of distribution are not well understood for many amphetamine compounds and analogues. Reported variations in protein binding range from 15% (methylphenidate) and 16% (amphetamine) to 34% (fenfluramine).
- The volume of distribution of amphetamine and phentermine in therapeutic doses is 3 to 5 L/kg.
- Fenfluramine (12 to 16 L/kg) and methylphenidate (11 to 33 L/kg) have exceedingly large volumes of distribution.

ELIMINATION

- The major metabolic pathway for amphetamine involves deamination to phenylacetone. This latter compound subsequently is oxidized to benzoic acid and excreted as glucuronide or glycine conjugates. Smaller amounts of amphetamine are converted to norephedrine by oxidation.
- β-Hydroxylation produces the active metabolite O-hydroxynorephedrine, which acts as a false neurotransmitter and may account for some drug effect especially in chronic users.
- Normally, about 30% of a therapeutic amphetamine dose are excreted unchanged in the urine by 24 hours, but the actual amount of urinary excretion and metabolism is highly pH dependent. When the urinary pH is acidic (pH 5.5 to 6.0), amphetamine is excreted primarily unchanged by the kidney, whereas under alkaline conditions (urinary pH 7.5 to 8.0) metabolism by deamination is the major route of elimination.
- Within the first 48 hours, about 60% of an amphetamine dose is excreted by the kidney unchanged in acid urine, whereas only 3% to 7% is excreted during that period in alkaline urine.
- The elimination half-life is also urine-pH dependent. The normal half-life is approximately 12 hours, but ranges from 8.0 to 10.5 hours in acid urine and from 16 to 31 hours in alkaline urine.
- Demethylation of methamphetamine produces the active metabolite, amphetamine.
- Methamphetamine has a pKA of 9.9. Therefore, metabolism and renal excretion are urine-pH dependent and similar to those for amphetamine.
- Phentermine is less susceptible to metabolism than amphetamine. The kidney excretes up to 80% of a therapeutic dose within 24 hours. Elimination half-life is approximately 7 to 8 hours in acid urine (pH 5), compared with 19 to 24 hours under normal conditions.
- Rapid deesterification of methylphenidate to ritalinic acid produces an inactive metabolite that is excreted in the urine unchanged or as oxoritalinic acid.
- Urinary acidification increases 48-hour urinary excretion of unchanged fenfluramine and norfenfluramine from 7% to 23% and 19%, respectively. Deamination of fenfluramine to benzoic acid and glycine conjugation accounts for the major metabolites.
- Demethylation converts phendimetrazine to the active metabolite, phenmetrazine, which is metabolized further by p-hydroxylation and conjugation. Urinary acidification increases unchanged 24-hour renal elimination of phenmetrazine from 19% to at least 46%.

Clinical Presentations

ABUSE

Intermittent Low-Dose Misuse

Many individuals occasionally take 5 to 20 mg of oral amphetamines to allay fatigue, elevate mood, or prolong wakefulness. Students studying for exams, military personnel on extended exercises, athletes wanting to excel, and truck drivers on prolonged trips commonly use amphetamines. Professional football players have consumed these drugs to induce analgesia and rage, improve speed, and reduce weight. These drugs do seem to improve the performance of tired individuals on repetitive tasks, unless jitteriness or impaired judgment adversely affects the outcome. Most sporadic users do not develop a habitual craving for amphetamines. Rarely, hallucinations and sudden death occur during strenuous exercise in warm environments. In addition, these drugs may push the user to greater expenditures of energy, resulting in excessive fatigue.

Sustained Oral Misuse

Some people who have been using amphetamines either illicitly or through legitimate prescriptions continue to ingest them in regular daily doses of 20 to 40 mg. Attempts to reduce the dose may result in depression and lethargy. Unfortunately, such patients may become incapable of accurately evaluating the physical or psychological effects of amphetamine use on their mind or performance. Individuals who enjoy the euphoric effects are particularly vulnerable to excessive doses. Tolerance may develop and consumption of daily doses ranging from 50 to 150 mg is not unusual. An additional risk is polydrug abuse, because alcohol or sedative-hypnotics may be administered to combat the insomnia associated with habitual amphetamine misuse.

High-Dose Intravenous Abuse

Individuals who relish the euphoria discover that intravenous injections produce a more intense feeling of pleasure. The "rush" has been compared to sexual orgasm. Other attractive feelings apparent between injections include a sense of power, hyperactivity, hyperexcitability, euphoria, and heightened sexual awareness. Although the abuse pattern involves fewer individuals than those who orally abuse amphetamines, violent and bizarre behavior, emaciated appearance, and major medical complications have focused public and professional attention on this abuse pattern.

"Speed" is the term given to methamphetamine. A "speed freak" is a compulsive user. Stereotyped behavior, which includes skin picking, bead stringing, pacing, and interminable chattering, may be apparent. During the action phase, the "speed freak" may not sleep or eat. Orgasm and ejaculation are difficult or impossible to achieve, leading to marathon sexual activity in some users. High methamphetamine doses may result in suspiciousness or paranoid psychosis, which, along with hyperactivity and poor impulse control, may produce unpredictable violent behavior. This person continues to perpetuate the "high" by repeated intravenous injections until fatigue, paranoia, confusion, or lack of drug stops use.

During the reaction phase, exhaustion develops and the user may sleep for 24 to 48 hours and subsequently eat ravenously. Once the hunger is satisfied, severe depression may ensue. To relieve the depression, the amphetamine addict starts intravenous use again, thus beginning another cycle or "speed binge." Certain individuals feel too anxious on amphetamines and turn to polydrug combinations such as intravenous barbiturate-amphetamine or heroin-amphetamine. If an intravenous dosage is increased too rapidly, an individual may develop a peculiar condition called "overamped," in which he or she is conscious but unable to speak or move. Elevated blood pressure, temperature, and pulse, as well as chest distress, may occur in this setting. Death from overdose is infrequent in tolerant individuals.

Inhalant Abuse

One Benzedrine inhaler contains the equivalent of 250 mg of racemic amphetamine. An abuser would chew and swallow the enclosed paper strip, preferably with chewing gum to reduce irritation. The strips were occasionally soaked in beverages or swallowed whole. A 1959 Food and Drug Administration ban on over-the-counter amphetamine inhalers led to the introduction of the Benzedrex inhaler, which contained 250 mg of propylhexedrine, 12.5 grams of methanol, and various aromatics. By the mid-1970s, both the oral and intravenous abuse of these inhalers had been reported in the medical literature. Most methamphetamine and amphetamine analogues have been removed from inhalants.

Overdose

Acute overdoses of amphetamine, amphetamine analogues, and cocaine produce a similar clinical syndrome manifested primarily as an accentuation of their pharmacological effects on the cardiovascular system and central nervous system (CNS). For acute oral amphetamine overdoses, CNS symptoms and signs begin within 30 to 60 minutes and persist for 4 to 6 hours. Large overdoses, amphetamine analogues, sustained-release preparations, and alkalinization of the urine prolong the effects. The clinical picture of amphetamine overdose may be categorized by severity.

MILD

Restlessness, talkativeness, irritability, insomnia, tremor, hyperreflexia, mydriasis, flushing, diaphoresis, combativeness, dry mucous membranes, nausea, vomiting, pallor.

MODERATE

Hyperactivity, confusion, hypertension, tachypnea, tachycardia, premature ventricular contractions, chest discomfort, vomiting, abdominal pain, profuse diaphoresis, mild temperature elevation, impulsivity, repetitive behavior, hallucinations, panic reaction.

SERIOUS

Delirium, marked hypertension or tachycardia, hyperpyrexia (over 40°C), convulsions, focal neurologic signs, hypotension, coma, hemodynamically significant cardiac dysrhythmias.

CARDIAC EFFECTS

Amphetamines raise both systolic and diastolic blood pressure and initially slow heart rate. High doses cause tachycardia, palpitations, and dysrhythmias. L-Amphetamine is a slightly stronger cardiovascular stimulant than d-amphetamine. Methamphetamine produces cardiovascular effects only in large doses, but it displays more prominent CNS effects at low doses. The amphetamine analogues cause cardiovascular effects in healthy patients only at very large doses. Premature ventricular contractions are well documented in overdose. Ventricular dysrhythmias have been suspected as the cause of sudden death in propylhexedrine abusers. An acute cardiomyopathy has been associated with intravenous amphetamine use. Pulmonary edema, hypotension, myocardial infarction, and pericardial effusion have been associated with propylhexedrine contained within a Benzedrex inhaler. Chronic oral abuse of dextroamphetamines has led to a chronic cardiomyopathy.

VASCULAR EFFECTS

Diffuse vascular spasm and progressive paresthesias, coldness, and pain has followed the ingestion of certain amphetamines. Perivascular infiltration of amphetamines can produce local necrosis, cellulitis, granulomas, and abscess formation. Intraarterial injection causes intense vasospasm with distal cyanosis, ecchymosis, petechiae, edema, paresthesias, pain, weakness, necrosis, and decreased capillary filling. Immediate intense vasospasm is obvious after intraarterial injections.

HEMATOLOGIC EFFECTS

Leukocytosis frequently occurs after amphetamine use. Microangiopathic hemolytic anemia has occurred in intravenous polydrug users who abuse amphetamines as well as barbiturates and heroin. Disseminated intravascular coagulation (i.e., thrombocytopenia, hypofibrinogenemia, hypoprothrombinemia, reduced partial thromboplastin levels, and elevated fibrin split products) can occur after intravenous or oral amphetamine use, especially in association with rhabdomyolysis or hyperpyrexia.

NEUROLOGIC EFFECTS

Amphetamines are stimulants that induce alertness, euphoria, increased confidence, gregariousness, enhanced mental and physical activity, and improved self-esteem. As dose or tolerance increases, anxiety, dysphoria, confusion, depression, nausea, vomiting, headache, sweating, apprehension, tremulousness, confusion, and fatigue supervene. Amphetamines increase wakefulness and delay the onset and duration of rapid eye movement (REM) sleep. Withdrawal from chronic use produces the opposite pattern, which may require several months to return to normal. Analgesic effects are minimal and therapeutically insignificant.

The etiology of intracerebral and subarachnoid hemorrhage associated with amphetamine use appears multifactorial. Virtually all patients present with the onset of severe headache with or without nausea. Most patients remain conscious but may be confused or disoriented. Unilateral motor or sensory deficits may develop. The admission blood pressure is normal in the majority of cases, although some patients present with marked hypertension.

Hypertension seen in amphetamine use may lead to vessel rupture and hemorrhage. Seizures often are not part of the initial presentation but may complicate convalescence. Intracerebral hematomas may progress to brain stem herniation and death. The average mortality is approximately 30%, and most survivors develop mild residual deficits. Central nervous system vasculitis has occurred in the setting of oral acute dextroamphetamine overdose, amphetamine withdrawal, and therapeutic use as an anorectic drug.

Gilles de la Tourette's disorder, characterized by chronic, fluctuating somatic and vocal tics (e.g., eye blinking, jaw jerks, hip turning, humming, panting, muscle jerks) either has been precipitated or exacerbated by the use of amphetamine or methylphenidate. A dopaminergic mechanism has been suggested, because haloperidol treatment helps alleviate symptoms.

ANORECTIC EFFECTS

Weight loss from therapeutic doses results almost entirely from reduced food consumption. Increased physical activity contributes somewhat to initial weight reduction, but tolerance after several months abolishes anorectic properties at the usual doses. Patients often regain lost weight after tolerance develops or drug administration ceases.

RENAL EFFECTS

Acute renal failure may develop secondary to acute tubular necrosis (because of hypotension), rhabdomyolysis, intravascular coagulation, hypovolemia, or hyperpyrexia. Dialysis may be required to correct electrolyte abnormalities.

HEPATIC EFFECTS

Markedly elevated hepatic aminotransferases have been noted after intravenous abuse of amphetamine and amphetamine analogues, but differentiation between direct hepatotoxicity and viral hepatitis has not been reported. Therapeutic doses of methylphenidate have been associated with hepatotoxicity.

PSYCHIATRIC EFFECTS

Paranoid delusions, hallucinations, and bizarre behavior seen in amphetamine users usually occur in the setting of chronic abuse. Hallucinations and stereotyped compulsive behavior can occur during therapeutic use even without excessive medication, especially in children and patients with borderline personalities. Hallucinations usually disappear within several days, but delusions may remain for days to months. Typically, amphetamine psychotics are volatile, suspicious, hyperactive, aggressive, hostile, and anxious. Hallucinations occur often and usually are visual. Tactile hallucinations are distinctive features of amphetamine and cocaine abusers. These alterations of thinking may lead to delusions of parasitosis and destructive excoriation of the skin.

At low doses, MDMA produces disinhibition of emotions and relaxation, but at high doses, an amphetamine-like reaction predominates that may include emotional lability, dysphoria, grandiose thoughts, anxiety, paranoia, and rarely hallucinations. Cocaine and amphetamine psychoses closely resemble one another and usually are indistinguishable on the basis of signs and symptoms.

PULMONARY EFFECTS

Pulmonary granulomas are a well-known complication of intravenous drug use. Pulmonary fibrosis, right ventricular hypertrophy, and pulmonary hypertension are frequent findings at postmortem examinations, particularly in propylhexedrine addicts. Hypoxemia may result from respiratory paralysis secondary to seizures, noncardiac pulmonary edema, or acute cardiac failure. Pulmonary hypertension occurs in intravenous (IV) drug users, especially those who abuse propylhexedrine.

MUSCULOSKELETAL EFFECTS

Rhabdomyolysis with myoglobinuria, hyperpyrexia (up to 42.8°C), leukemoid reaction, disseminated intravascular coagulation, and azotemia have been reported after large, acute amphetamine ingestions and intravenous administration of phenmetrazine and methamphetamine. Headache, myalgias, lightheadedness, paresthesias, weakness, and delirium characterize the syndrome, which may progress several days before the patient seeks medical attention.

Laboratory changes may include elevated serum muscle enzymes (creatine kinase and aldolase), myoglobinuria, hyperbilirubinemia, hyperuricemia, hypocalcemia, hyperkalemia, azotemia, hyperphosphatemia, and hypokalemia. Associated coagulopathies, which produce intramuscular hemorrhage and elevated compartment pressures, increase rhabdomyolysis.

TOLERANCE

Marked tolerance may develop after both oral and intravenous use and often leads to rapid escalation of dose. Large oral doses in habitual amphetamine users range from 50 to 150 mg daily. As much as 1 gram may be injected every 2 to 3 hours by a "speed freak" during a binge. Daily doses exceeding 5 to 8 grams for several days can be administered parenterally by these addicts until exhaustion, psychosis, or drug unavailability ends the "speed run." A methylphenidate user may use intravenous doses of 20 to 2,000 mg / day. Although tolerance develops to the pharmacological effects of amphetamines, narcolepsy has been treated for years without an increase in dose. Children usually do not experience the mood elevation or euphoria seen in adults with methylphenidate use, even upon initiation of therapy.

WITHDRAWAL EFFECTS

Abrupt discontinuance of amphetamines produces neither seizures nor life-threatening symptoms, even in those patients who habitually consume large quantities. Apathy, depression, lethargy, anxiety, and sleep disturbances characterize the abstinence syndrome associated with chronic use of amphetamine, methylphenidate, and fenfluramine. Myalgias, abdominal pain, voracious appetite, and a profound depression with suicidal tendencies may complicate the immediate post-withdrawal period and peak in 2 to 3 days.

Toxic Dosage/Death

Fatalities from amphetamine and amphetamine analogues are infrequent. Deaths have been associated with cardiovascular (e.g., acute left ventricular failure, ventricular fibrillation), cerebrovascular (e.g., subarachnoid hemorrhage, intracerebral hematoma, cerebral edema with brain stem compression), and hyperthermic (e.g., seizures, rhabdomyolysis, cardiovascular collapse) causes. Intravenous propylhexedrine abusers appear susceptible to sudden death secondary to dysrhythmias and pulmonary edema during periods of physical and emotional stress. Patients who die of cardiovascular causes often have predisposing factors such as coadministration of stimulants or dysrhythmogenic drugs, hypokalemia, or preexisting cardiovascular disease. In one series, two-thirds of fatalities resulted from violence, including accidents, suicide, and, less often, homicide.

The minimal lethal amphetamine dose varies with age and animal species. Children appear more susceptible than adults do. Methamphetamine is twice as toxic in animal models. In humans, death has been reported with as little as 1.5 mg methamphetamine per kilogram, whereas survival occurred after an ingestion of 28 mg amphetamine per kilogram. An adult fenfluramine death resulted after an oral dose of 1.6 grams. Predicting toxicity in chronic users is difficult. Because of tolerance, amphetamine addicts can inject 1 to 5 grams of amphetamine intravenously.

Drug Interactions

There is an increased stimulatory effect when amphetamines are used concomitantly with monoamine oxidase inhibitors.

Pregnancy/Lactation

Methylphenidate (Ritalin®) is pregnancy risk category C.

Laboratory

ANALYTIC METHODS

Urine samples may be analyzed for amphetamine, methamphetamine, and MDMA by gas chromatography-mass spectrometry. The detection limit for amphetamine, methamphetamine, and MDMA with this procedure is 50 ng/mL. Gas chromatography is the procedure of choice for analyzing amphetamine levels. Gas-liquid chromatography can detect concentrations of 100 ng/mL, which are present in the blood after large, single therapeutic doses (e.g., 30-mg amphetamine base). Thin-layer chromatography (TLC) is an accurate urine screening procedure at levels of 100 ng/mL when equivocal results are confirmed by more sensitive methods. Positive TLC urine tests for synthetic amphetamine compounds (MDA, MMDA, MDMA, and MDEA) must be confirmed by gas chromatography-mass spectrometry because of frequent false positive results.

Most compounds, except methamphetamine, do not produce cross-reactivity during thin-layer chromatography. Immunological methods are sensitive, relatively specific, and semiquantitative. Their greatest defect is a lack of specificity, so that all positive results should be confirmed by more sensitive methods (e.g., gas chromatography) if specificity is important. Slight cross-reactivity occurs with phenylpropanolamine (PPA).

BLOOD LEVELS

Toxicological analyses of blood and urine confirm amphetamine ingestion but do not guide clinical management. Amphetamine doses of 10 mg produce a peak plasma level of about 35 ng/mL at 2 hours in nontolerant individuals. The euphoriant effect appears to correlate with peak plasma levels after intravenous administration. Peripheral sympathomimetic effects (i.e., elevated heart rate and blood pressure) begin at a plasma level of 20 ng/mL. Tolerant individuals who daily consume over 1 gram of amphetamines maintain steady-state plasma levels of 2,000 to 3,000 ng/mL.

Postmortem amphetamine blood levels ranged from 0.5 to 41 μg/mL with an average of 8.6 μg/mL. Similar blood levels of methamphetamine and fenfluramine have been present in fatalities, whereas phenmetrazine, propylhexedrine, and phentermine have been associated with death at lower concentrations (i.e., 0.1 to 5 μg/mL). Therapeutic plasma concentrations of fenfluramine usually are in the range 0.05 to 0.15 μg/mL. Toxic effects appear at concentrations greater than 0.5 μg/mL and death has occurred at concentrations greater than 6.0 μg/mL.

Treatment

GUT DECONTAMINATION

Ingestion of more than 1 to 2 mg/kg within an hour of presentation may warrant lavage or activated charcoal. Although amphetamines do delay gastric emptying as much as 40% and decrease motility, attempts to remove the drug from the stomach more than 4 hours postingestion probably are not efficacious. Activated charcoal may be effective up to 12 hours when sustained-release or resin-complexed capsules have been ingested.

ELIMINATION ENHANCEMENT

Because amphetamine is a weak base, urinary acidification increases the excretion of unmetabolized drug and causes a decrease of the plasma half-life. The efficacy of this therapeutic maneuver on clinical outcome remains controversial, however, because cardiovascular complications of forced diuresis and plasma acidification may develop. Hemodialysis and hemoperfusion have not been studied in amphetamine overdose. Rhabdomyolisis is treated with urinary alkalinization.

SUPPORTIVE MEASURES

- Severely intoxicated patients should receive an intravenous line, cardiac monitoring, electrocardiogram (ECG), and oxygen. Respiratory depression is uncommon in pure amphetamine intoxication, but either cardiogenic pulmonary edema or the adult respiratory distress syndrome may develop.
- Most patients tolerate sinus tachycardia well, but propranolol may be used to slow tachydysrhythmias in symptomatic patients.
- Hypotension may respond to fluid challenges, but a vasopressor may be needed. Shock is a poor prognostic sign and indicates the need for right heart catheterization to measure right-sided filling pressures and cardiac output. Mannitol diuresis may enhance myoglobin clearance and prevent acute renal failure in cases of rhabdomyolysis.
- Seizures should be treated with airway management, ventilatory support, and intravenous diazepam. Seizures refractory to diazepam may be controlled with phenytoin.
- Laboratory work-up may include complete blood count, electrolytes, calcium, phosphorus, uric acid, muscle enzymes, hepatic aminotransferases, creatinine, glucose, blood urea nitrogen, coagulation profile, urinalysis (including myoglobin), arterial blood gases, chest x-ray, ECG, and cardiac monitoring.
- Appropriate diagnostic neurologic examinations (e.g., computerized axial tomography) to rule out other causes of agitation also may be required.

AGITATION

- Agitation may be treated with diazepam (intravenous doses of 5 to 10 mg in adults or 0.1 to 0.3 mg/kg in children). Chlorpromazine (1 mg/kg to 25 to 50 mg in adults) has been recommended for moderate to severe agitation, but the added risk of seizures, hypotension, and anticholinergic excess (especially from adulterants of street amphetamines) theoretically complicates its use.
- Haloperidol probably is safer. The haloperidol dose for adults is 2 to 5 mg intramuscularly. Droperidol also has been used successfully in amphetamine intoxications. The usual dose is 0.1 mg/kg. Slow administration of droperidol (2.5 mg/min maximum) to poisoned adults has resulted in the alleviation of agitation within 15 minutes of a 13-mg dose. Hypotension, respiratory depression, and dystonic reactions are potential complications. A calm environment and familiar faces also help alleviate agitation.
- Psychosis in chronic amphetamine abusers requires hospitalization to provide a protective environment, especially since suicidal ideation may be prominent during withdrawal. Chlorpromazine can be instituted at dosages of 50 mg orally or intramuscularly every 4 hours. Depending on adverse effects (sedation, orthostatic hypotension) and clinical response, the total daily dose varies up to 200 to 800 mg divided in four to six doses. Haloperidol in doses of 2 to 5 mg orally or intramuscularly every 6 hours is an alternative. Long-term

management of the habitual amphetamine user is difficult because of frequent relapses.

HYPERTENSION

- α-Adrenergic blocking agents (e.g., phentolamine) have been recommended for hypertension, but they have not been proven clinically superior to intravenous sodium nitroprusside (0.5 to 8 μg/kg/min).
- Oral nifedipine (10 mg) is untested clinically but has a rapid onset of action (5 to 10 minutes sublingually, 20 minutes ingested) and potentially may be useful when elevated blood pressures require treatment acutely.

HYPERTHERMIA

- Severe temperature elevation (i.e., over 42°C) is a poor prognostic sign. Elevated body temperature as measured by rectal probes should be treated aggressively, especially when temperatures exceed 39° to 40°C. Cooling measures include hypothermic blankets, ice baths, and sedation.
- Dantrolene infusions may rapidly correct hyperpyrexia and the hypermetabolic state seen in MDMA overdose. If dantrolene is ineffective in controlling the fever, the patient should be paralyzed and mechanically ventilated. Chlorpromazine may reduce shivering as well as physical activity. Vital signs should be followed closely (i.e., every 15 to 20 minutes) and cooling measures continued until rectal temperatures are below 38.5°C.

Questions—Amphetamines

1. Abrupt withdrawal of amphetamines may produce
A. Abdominal pain
B. Seizures
C. Lethargy
D. A and B
E. A and C

2. Massive doses of amphetamines may cause
A. Paranoia
B. Delusions
C. Hallucinations
D. Bizarre violent behavior
E. All of the above

3. After amphetamine ingestion
A. Peak plasma levels occur in 6 to 8 hours
B. Complete absorption usually is by 4 to 6 hours.
C. Peak plasma levels are earlier if preparation is the sustained-released form
D. Amphetamines concentrate in the liver
E. Urinary alkalinization increases 48-hour urinary excretion

4. High-dose intravenous abuse of amphetamines
A. Includes constant hyperactivity and no depression
B. Is mostly characterized by depression without euphoria
C. May make orgasm and ejaculation difficult to reach
D. Frequently causes death in tolerant individuals
E. None of the above

5. Cardiac effects of oral amphetamine overdose include
A. Premature ventricular contractions
B. Acute cardiomyopathy
C. Atrial standstill
D. A and B
E. A, B and C

6. Intraarterial injection of amphetamines causes
A. Intense vasospasm
B. Petechiae
C. Paresthesias
D. All of the above
E. None of the above

7. The admission blood pressure of most patients with intracerebral hemorrhage associated with amphetamine use is markedly elevated.
A. True
B. False

8. Overdoses of methylphenidate have been associated with hepatotoxicity, while therapeutic doses have not.
A. True
B. False

Case Study (Questions 9 and 10)

A 20-year-old female presents after ingesting one-half a bottle of her brother's sustained-release Ritalin® in a suicidal gesture. She also takes MAO inhibitors for depression. She presents euphoric, febrile to 41.5°C, and weak, with decreased urine output.

9. The most likely cause of her brown urine is
A. Hepatitis
B. A flu syndrome which predisposed her to her overdose
C. Rhabdomyolysis
D. Meningococcemia
E. Drug reaction

10. Treatment should include
A. Activated charcoal if within 1 hour of ingestion
B. Urinary alkalinization
C. Hypothermic blankets, ice bath, sedation
D. All of the above
E. None of the above

Answers

Amphetamines

1. E	2. E	3. B	4. C	5. A	6. D
7. B	8. B	9. C	10. D		

SELECTED READINGS

Amphetamines

1. Barrett PJ. "Ecstasy" misuse: Overdose or normal dose? Anaesthesia 1993;48:83.
2. Council on Scientific Affairs. Clinical aspects of amphetamine abuse. JAMA 1978;240:2317–2319.
3. Gorard DA, Davier SE, Clark ML. Misuse of Ecstasy. Br Med J 1992;305:309.
4. Henry JA. Ecstasy and the dance of death: Severe reactions are unpredictable. Br Med J 1992;305:566.
5. Kalant H, Kalant O. Death in amphetamine users: Causes and rates. CMA J 1975;112:299–304.
6. Nichol AM. The nontherapeutic use of psychoactive drugs: A modern epidemic. N Engl J Med 1983;308:925–933.
7. Ong BH. Dextroamphetamine poisoning. N Engl J Med 1962; 266:1321–1322.
8. Rittoo DB, Rittoo D. Complications of "Ecstasy" misuse. Lancet 1992;340:725–727.

Answers to questions in shaded boxes appear at the end of the chapter.

9. Skeers VM. Illegal methamphetamine drug laboratories: A new challenge for environmental health personnel. J Environ Health 1992;55:6–10.
10. Watson CJE, Thomson HJ, Johnston PS. Body-packing with amphetamines: An indication for surgery. J R Soc Med 1991;84:311–312.
11. Zalis EG, Parmley LF. Fatal amphetamine poisoning. Arch Intern Med 1963;101:822–826.

ACKNOWLEDGMENTS

Thanks to Alison Deutsch, MD for contributing the questions in this chapter.

CHAPTER 19
Cocaine

INTRODUCTION

Cocaine is the most potent naturally occurring central nervous system stimulant. Cocaine shares many pharmacological and adverse effects with stimulants such as the amphetamines, and accordingly has a long history of use and abuse. Archaeological findings in Ecuador indicate that pre-Inca inhabitants discovered the mind-altering properties of the shrub Erythroxylon coca. The Incas felt the plant was a divine gift created to alleviate hunger and thirst. Coca cultivation was tightly controlled so that primarily the ruling class chewed the leaves on special occasions. Less frequently, the working class was rewarded for special deeds by a gift of coca leaves.

History

Amerigo Vespucci mentioned the Indian practice of chewing coca with alkaline ash, which later was proven to increase cocaine absorption. Spanish entrepreneurs used coca leaves to attract Indians to hard labor. Although Pizarro probably brought coca leaves to the 16th-century Spanish court, Europeans did not adopt the custom of coca chewing, in part because these leaves do not retain their potency after long periods of travel. Recreational use awaited the development of chemical methods to extract the active ingredient.

The alkaloid cocaine was first characterized in 1859 by Albert Niemann, who also recognized cocaine's anesthetic properties. Sigmund Freud wrote reports in 1884 about the ability of cocaine to relieve depression and cure morphine addiction. In that same year, Carl Koller recognized the importance of the ability of cocaine to anesthetize the cornea in ophthalmologic surgery. The American surgeon Halstead demonstrated the peripheral nerve-blocking properties of cocaine injections. Unfortunately, Halstead became one of the first victims of cocaine dependency when he tried to cure his morphine addiction with cocaine.

Robert Louis Stevenson wrote the first draft of Dr. Jekyll and Mr. Hyde while being treated with cocaine for tuberculosis. Sir Arthur Conan Doyle's character Sherlock Holmes used artificial stimulants until he became tired, wasted, and paranoid. Later, he reappeared in good health, with his pipe replacing the cocaine habit. John Stith Pemberton marketed a cocaine-caffeine mixture called Coca-Cola® in 1886. By 1891, the serious adverse effects of cocaine were recognized and there had been 200 reports of systemic cocaine intoxication, including 13 deaths. Freud had been accused of unleashing the third great scourge of humanity (after alcohol and opiates), and he subsequently removed all reference to cocaine abuse from his autobiography.

The United States tried to control cocaine use through the Pure Food and Drug Act of 1906, and subsequently, the Coca-Cola Company decocainized their coca leaves before making their drink. The 1914 Harrison Narcotic Act labeled cocaine as a narcotic with the same restrictions and penalties as heroin. In 1970, the Comprehensive Drug Abuse Prevention and Control action classified cocaine as a schedule II drug (i.e., high abuse potential with limited medical application), which again allowed its legal use. The major clinical indication for the use of cocaine is as a topical anesthetic and vasoconstrictor for ear, nose, and throat surgery.

In the 1960s, cocaine emerged as a substance commonly used with heroin (called a "speedball") by intravenous polydrug users, but by the 1970s its reputation changed to that of an expensive, high-status drug that was insufflated (sniffed) or smoked rather than injected. The attraction of cocaine to successful and independent members of the middle and upper class includes exhilaration, ecstasy, enhanced self-confidence, and heightened physical prowess. In addition, it has a reputation as an aphrodisiac, although long-term use has been associated with sexual dysfunction. Concern over the illicit use of cocaine has increased because of its accelerated use among all social classes and the prevalence of more hazardous forms of abuse (e.g., freebasing).

Sources

Cocaine is one of at least 14 alkaloids extracted from the leaves of two coca shrubs indigenous to South America. The Erythroxylon coca bush requires a moist, tropical climate found in Peru, Ecuador, Bolivia, Mexico, the West Indies, and Java. The bush grows to 8 ft. in height over 40 years. This plant is the main source of illicit cocaine trade. The leaves are soaked in gasoline drums containing alkali, sulfuric acid, kerosene, and other solvents. The fluid and leaves are discarded, leaving a thick brown coca paste that is sold to clandestine laboratories. There the paste is refined into white crystalline powder containing cocaine hydrochloride. The coca plant should not be confused with the cocoa plant, which contains caffeine rather than cocaine.

The Erythroxylon novogranatense plant grows in the drier mountainous region of Colombia, the Caribbean coast of South America, and the north coast of Peru. The leaves of the Trujillo variety are grown legally in Peru and are exported to the Stepan Chemical Company in Maywood, NJ. This facility is the only legally recognized manufacturer of cocaine for pharmaceutical purposes in the United States.

Structure

Cocaine is an ester type of local anesthetic and belongs to the tropane family of natural alkaloids. Other members of the family include scopolamine and atropine. Structurally, cocaine is benzoylmethylecgonine. As an ester of benzoic acid and the nitrogen-containing base methylecgonine, cocaine hydrolyzes to benzoylecgonine, ecgonine methyl ester, and ecgonine. Cocaine hydrochloride is a white crystalline powder, which is the formulation of legal and most illicit cocaine. The hydrochloride salt is poorly volatile. Conversion to the freebase with sulfate and ether produces a salt that resists heat decomposition and allows inhalation of the active compound (freebasing).

Although an increased supply of cocaine has improved the purity of street cocaine, invariably the street drug still contains a variety of adulterants. Cocaine content in street samples may range from 15% to 90%. The presence of impurities should always be considered in adverse reactions that complicate cocaine use. A proliferation of cocaine look-alikes such as ephedrine, caffeine, phenylpropanolamine, and local anesthetics are widely available as cocaine substitutes. Use of these substitutes has been associated with hypertension, nausea, vomiting, sneezing, insomnia, anxiety, palpitations, tremor, abdominal cramps, and diarrhea.

Synonyms

Street names for cocaine include coke, snow, cadillac, champagne of drugs, flake, gold dust, green gold, blow, speedball (heroin and cocaine), liquid lady (alcohol and cocaine), dama blanca, happy trails, pimp's drug, rock, Bernice, jam, star-spangled powder, toot, C, lady, white girl or lady, nose candy, her, and she. Snort, hit, line, and dose represent the street nomenclature for individual measures of cocaine that range up to 200 mg per measure depending on purity. Large quantities of cocaine are sold in grams or spoons (i.e., one-half or a whole gram). Crack is alkaloidal cocaine. The name is derived from the popping sound that occurs during heating. Rock is a synonym for this form of cocaine because of its appearance. Both these names apply to the free-base form of cocaine, which is suitable for smoking, in contrast to the hydrochloride salt, which decomposes with heat.

Pathophysiology

The only well-accepted medical uses of cocaine are mucous membrane anesthesia and vasoconstriction. The dual pharmacological vasoconstriction and local anesthetic actions of cocaine are unequaled among clinical drugs. Doses as low as 20 to 50 mg provide satisfactory vasoconstriction for ear, nose, and throat surgery within 2 to 4 minutes. The maximum safe cocaine dose is 1 to 3 mg/kg, and solutions should not exceed cocaine concentrations of 10%. Four milliliters of a 5% cocaine solution contains the absolute maximum allowable adult dose (i.e., 200 mg). Although cocaine was administered first as a topical anesthetic of the cornea, newer agents (e.g., cyclopentolate) have replaced cocaine, primarily because repeated cocaine application causes corneal opacification and delayed epithelization.

CENTRAL NERVOUS SYSTEM EFFECTS

Cocaine is a powerful central nervous system stimulant and sympathomimetic agent that produces these effects through the potentiation of neurotransmitters, principally norepinephrine and epinephrine. Cocaine in increasing doses causes rostral-caudal stimulation beginning with the cortex. Initially, euphoria, hyperactivity, restlessness, and garrulity occur. Progressive activation of the lower brain centers results in tremor, hyperreflexia, and convulsions. In high doses, after the excitatory phase, a period of depression develops. Coma, hyporeflexia, and respiratory or cardiovascular depression may characterize this period.

About 10% to 30% of strokes in young adults are associated with drug use, rising to 90% of patients in the third and fourth decade. Drugs most often implicated in stroke are sympathomimetic agents such as the amphetamines, phencyclidine, phenylpropanolamine, methylphenidate, cocaine, and opiates such as heroin. Neurologic symptoms develop immediately or within 3 to 6 hours of use of cocaine in most cases of cocaine-related strokes. Cocaine-associated strokes occur in both first-time users and long-time users and are independent of the route of administration.

The alkaloid form of cocaine has been associated with both occlusive and hemorrhagic strokes. The hydrochloride form has been related mainly to hemorrhagic strokes. Cocaine blocks serotonin reuptake and acutely increases serotonin levels. Serotonin is a strong vasoconstrictor and may contribute to decreasing blood flow to the brain. Cerebral vasculitis also may induce a cerebrovascular accident.

Both subarachnoid and intracerebral hemorrhages have been associated with cocaine use. Patients with sudden onset of a severe headache several minutes to hours after cocaine use, especially if it is associated with nausea, vomiting, neck stiffness, or loss of consciousness, should be admitted for evaluation of a possible subarachnoid hemorrhage. Preexisting lesions (cerebral aneurysm or arteriovenous malformation) form the substrate for this complication. Patients may present either hypertensive or normotensive. In about 80%, an aneurysm or arteriovenous malformation has been detected. Cerebral angiographic examination is recommended in cases of cocaine-related intracerebral hemorrhage, especially if the hemorrhage is lobar or intraventricular.

Between approximately 2% and 10% of patients presenting to an emergency department with cocaine toxicity have seizures. Cocaine-related grand mal seizures have been reported as long as 12 hours after cocaine use. Those with no history of prior seizures usually experience single generalized convulsions occurring after intravenous or crack cocaine use. Cranial computed tomography (CT) scans and electroencephalograms usually are normal and these patients usually recover without neurologic deficits. Focal seizures are associated with cerebral infarction, subarachnoid hemorrhage, or intraparenchymal hemorrhage.

Status epilepticus usually is observed in cocaine users with no prior seizure history who have used large amounts of cocaine (2 to 8 grams). Patients with a history of non-cocaine-related seizures will, after using cocaine, usually experience focal motor seizures, which are usually multiple. These frequently occur after intranasal use. If they have a single generalized seizure, they usually have a normal cranial CT scan, electroencephalogram, and neurologic outcome.

Numerous other neurologic complications after cocaine use have been described. Cocaine may trigger migraine headaches. Withdrawal from cocaine also may trigger headaches. Headache also may be related to trauma after a seizure or to trauma to the head from problems related to a drug deal. Subdural or epidural hematoma or skull fracture must be considered. If the drug is used intravenously, headache also can be caused by central nervous system infections.

Chronic intranasal use of cocaine may lead to vasospasm, chronic inflammatory changes, and damage to the cribriform plate. Surgical repair may be necessary. Intravenous cocaine users may experience fungal cerebritis. Cocaine abuse has been associated with stereotyped movements, such as picking and stroking, tics, Tourette's syndrome, chorea, and dystonic reactions. Cocaine snorting has been associated with frontal sinusitis and may subsequently yield a brain abscess. Chronic cocaine abusers with no discrete evidence of cerebral infarction or history of significant head trauma, HIV infection, or other neurologic disease may have CT evidence of diffuse frontotemporal cerebral atrophy.

CARDIOVASCULAR EFFECTS

Although 5 million Americans are thought to use cocaine regularly, only 100 to 200 cases of cocaine-related acute myocardial infarction have been reported in the North American literature. Because of this, many patients with cocaine-related chest pain are admitted to the hospital with a diagnosis of possible myocardial infarction. Cocaine-related myocardial infarction is associated with a high prevalence of coronary thrombi and anterior wall involvement in otherwise normal coronary arteries. Cocaine-induced myocardial infarction may follow cocaine abuse by the intranasal, intravenous, and inhalation routes. About one-half of patients who experience a myocardial infarction have had previous chest pain. Nine of ten have been cigarette smokers and two-thirds have had their myocardial infarcts within 3 hours of cocaine usage. Most patients presenting to an emergency department with cocaine-induced chest pain do not have a myocardial infarction.

Proposed mechanisms for cocaine-induced myocardial infarction include coronary artery spasm, *in situ* thrombus formation and platelet aggregation, direct myocardial injury, accelerated atherosclerosis, nonatherosclerotic intimal proliferation, and increased myocardial oxygen demand. Cocaine-induced myocardial infarction in patients with normal coronary arteries probably involves adrenergically mediated increases in myocardial oxygen consumption, vasoconstriction of large epicardial arteries or small coronary resistance vessels, and coronary thrombosis. Accelerated atherosclerosis and impairment of endothelium vasodilation may occur after chronic cocaine use.

Intranasal cocaine induces recurrent coronary vasoconstriction. The initial vasoconstriction is noted 30 minutes after drug administration, and is temporally related to the peak blood concentration of cocaine. As the blood concentration of cocaine declines, this vasoconstriction is alleviated. At 90 minutes after drug administration, coronary vasoconstriction recurs and is temporally related to increased concentrations of the principal metabolites of cocaine, benzoylecgonine and ethyl methyl ecgonine. Angina and myocardial infarction occurring hours after cocaine inhalation may be a result of the coronary vasoconstrictive influence of such metabolites.

Cocaine increases thromboxane production and platelet aggregation, which may exacerbate ischemia by increasing vasoconstriction activity. Abnormal coronary resistance vessels (small epicardial vessels on endomyocardial biopsy) indicate that when a chronic change in coronary blood vessels reaches a critical stage, presumably chest pain can be induced by plugging of the small vessels by platelet thrombi activated by further cocaine abuse. Release of thromboxane A2 from stimulated platelets could also exacerbate ischemia by increasing vasoconstrictor activity.

Chest pain of presumed cardiac origin in a cocaine-abusing individual should be considered an ischemic event. Patients may require admission to the coronary care unit. Chest pain is the most frequent cocaine-associated complaint, occurring in as many as 40% of such patients presenting to the emergency department. Chest pain may often be seen in emergency departments following insufflation, inhalation, or intravenous use of cocaine. Such pain in the cocaine user may be a result of pneumomediastinum and pneumothorax (inhalation use), foreign particle or septic emboli (intravenous use), associated trauma, and myocardial ischemia and infarction (any route). All patients presenting to the emergency room with chest pain should be questioned about cocaine.

The electrocardiogram (ECG) is less sensitive in identifying myocardial infarction in patients with cocaine-induced chest pain than in other patients presenting with chest pain. Recurrent myocardial infarction may occur in patients with normal coronary angiograms who use cocaine.

RESPIRATORY EFFECTS

Initially, central neurogenic stimulation causes increased ventilation manifested by tachypnea and an elevated tidal volume. Increasing doses may cause respiratory depression, cyanosis, and hypoxemia. Death may result from respiratory depression, often in association with seizures, from ventricular fibrillation, or from cardiovascular collapse.

OPHTHALMOLOGIC EFFECTS

Cocaine causes mydriasis by both local and central α-adrenergic effects on the radial muscles of the iris. Partial cycloplegia also occurs. As with other mucous membranes, cocaine produces anesthesia and vasoconstriction locally.

GASTROINTESTINAL EFFECTS

Cocaine can produce nausea and vomiting via central stimulation of vomiting centers. Diarrhea and abdominal cramps may result from sympathomimetic effects on the intestinal wall. In animal models, hepatotoxicity reminiscent of acetaminophen toxicity has been seen, however, hepatotoxicity is not a well-recognized complication of human intoxication.

HYPERSENSITIVITY EFFECTS

True anaphylactic reaction to pure cocaine is extremely rare, although street samples may contain known allergenic drugs, such as quinine. Immediate reactions to cocaine use more likely result from massive overdose or rapid intravenous injection.

Pharmacokinetics

ABSORPTION

- Cocaine is rapidly and well absorbed from the nasal, oral, and pulmonary routes at levels commonly associated with therapeutic use.
- Plasma cocaine concentration rapidly increases for the first 20 to 30 minutes after insufflation, reaching a peak between 15 and 60 minutes.
- Absorption by the nasal route at therapeutic doses is 98% complete after 4 hours.
- A 25-mg intravenous cocaine dose produces subjective and physiological effects similar to those of a 100-mg intranasal dose. Oral administration produced detectable plasma cocaine at 30 minutes, with peak levels reached between 50 and 90 minutes.
- Free-base cocaine is rapidly and completely absorbed into the pulmonary circulation. Inhalation of 15 mg free-base cocaine produces as much psychological and physiological effect as intravenous administration of 20 mg cocaine hydrochloride.
- Most free-base cocaine is delivered to the lungs within the first four puffs. Subjective euphoria occurs within 6 to 11 minutes. As much as two-thirds of the drug may be lost before reaching alveoli.
- Intravenous injection produces kinetics similar to those of free-base smoking, with physiological and psychological effects appearing several minutes earlier.

DISTRIBUTION

- The volume of distribution of cocaine is 1.2 to 1.9 L/kg.
- At autopsy, the highest cocaine concentrations are found in the urine and kidney, followed by brain, blood, liver, and bile.
- The apparent plasma half-life of cocaine is about 0.9 hour after therapeutic oral doses, compared with 1.3 hours for insufflation, which may reflect continuing nasal absorption.
- Cocaine plasma levels remain detectable for 4 to 6 hours. In chronic cocaine users, the plasma cocaine half-life averages 48 minutes after a 32-mg intravenous injection.
- Cocaine easily diffuses across the blood-brain barrier. In contrast to cocaine, the metabolite benzoylecgonine passes poorly into brain tissue.

COCAETHYLENE

- Cocaethylene, the ethyl homolog of cocaine (ethylbenzoylecgonine), is a pharmacologically active metabolite of cocaine, and is found in cocaine users who have simultaneously consumed cocaine and ethanol.

- Cocaethylene is formed in the liver from cocaine and ethanol by transesterification.
- Its concentration in blood may approach or surpass that of cocaine (highest found in one study, 1,600 mg/mL).
- The longer half-life (2 hours) compared with cocaine (38 minutes) may explain why some individuals whose cocaine blood levels are low experience cocaine-related strokes or myocardial infarction.
- Cocaethylene penetrates the blood-brain barrier. Cocaethylene may explain why so many cocaine users use alcohol. They apparently get a higher and longer high.
- Cocaethylene is found in the blood and brain when cocaine and ethanol are present.
- Cocaethylene may be active at cocaine binding sites in the central nervous system (dopamine, norepinephrine, serotonin, opioid sigma, and muscarinic cholinergic receptors) and may be active at the sodium channel.
- The presence and concentration of cocaethylene cannot be accurately deduced from simultaneous serum levels of cocaine or ethanol.

ELIMINATION

- Cocaine is rapidly and extensively metabolized. Less than 10% is excreted unchanged in the urine.
- Plasma and liver cholinesterases hydrolyze cocaine to the major inactive metabolite ecgonine methyl ester, which accounts for 32% to 49% of urine metabolites.
- The other major metabolite is benzoylecgonine, which accounts for 29% to 45% of urinary metabolites. This metabolite may be hydrolyzed nonenzymatically.
- Conversion of cocaine to norcocaine by N-methylation accounts for only 2.6% to 6.2% of cocaine metabolism. Although norcocaine is active, its contribution to the effect of cocaine is questionable.
- Cocaine elimination half-life by the intranasal route is 75 minutes, 48 minutes for oral, and 54 minutes for intravenous administration. Half-life varies significantly between individuals, perhaps because of differences in cholinesterase levels.
- Elimination half-lives of the two main metabolites, benzoylecgonine and ecgonine methyl ester (5 to 7 and 4 to 5 hours, respectively), exceed those of urinary cocaine (about 1.5 hours). Consequently, cocaine detection methods rely on the urinary excretion of metabolites rather than unchanged cocaine.
- Cocaine generally can be detected for 8 hours in urine after intranasal doses of 1.5 mg/kg.
- Benzoylecgonine remains detectable in urine by chromatographic techniques or immunoassay (EMIT) for 48 to 72 hours, whereas radioimmunoassay identifies metabolites for 90 to 144 hours.

Clinical Presentations

The clinical effects of cocaine in acute overdose develop rapidly. Delayed diagnosis seldom is a problem. Smugglers who ingest bags filled with cocaine (body packers) are an exception because they may develop an acute toxic condition if these bags (often containing 3 to 11 grams of cocaine each) rupture during intestinal transit.

Cocaine toxicity can be divided sequentially into three phases: early stimulation, late stimulation, and depression. In severe overdose cases, progression through this sequential pattern is accelerated. Terminal convulsions, ventricular dysrhythmias, or respiratory arrest usually develops within the first 30 minutes. Resolution of major symptoms occurs within 1 to 3 hours, unless secondary damage (e.g., hypoxic encephalopathy) or complications of hyperthermia supervene. Recognition of the early stimulation phase (e.g., anxiety, talkativeness, agitation, and muscle hyperactivity) is vital when treating the cocaine body packer whose ingested bags rupture.

RESPIRATORY EFFECTS

Severe overdoses can cause hypoxemia and hypercarbia because of respiratory depression and/or protracted seizures. Drug-induced pulmonary edema may develop after intravenous administration of free-base cocaine and, in rare cases, contributes to hypoxemia. Insufflation may cause reactive hyperemia of nasal mucosa and persistent rhinitis. Erosions and, less often, nasal perforation complicate chronic use. Deep inhalation may deposit adulterants leading to sinusitis. Pulmonary granulomas, dyspnea on exertion, pulmonary opacities, and cerebrospinal fluid rhinorrhea have been reported after administration via the nasal route. Chronic cough and bronchitis productive of black or blood-tinged sputum may result from habitual free-base smoking. Pneumomediastinum and pneumothoraces have been reported after prolonged Valsalva maneuvers associated with freebasing.

CARDIOVASCULAR EFFECTS

Sinus tachycardia is the most frequent ECG finding. Illicit use of cocaine can cause elevations in pulse and blood pressure as well as ventricular dysrhythmias, particularly in patients with underlying cardiovascular disease. Chest pain and elevated cardiac enzymes may be seen in individuals with structurally normal coronary arteries. Multiple case histories suggest that cocaine may adversely affect coronary artery tone or thrombogenesis even in the absence of underlying disease. Ventricular bigeminy and multifocal premature ventricular contractions have complicated high-dose topical anesthesia during laryngoscopy and may be seen in overdoses by any route. In addition to respiratory depression, hypotension resulting from cocaine-induced reduction in myocardial contractility and, perhaps, ventricular fibrillation contribute to mortality.

NEUROLOGIC EFFECTS

Seizures, agitation, tremor, and mental status change have all been reported. Patients may present with a confused toxic psychosis that includes disorientation, short-term memory impairment, and organic brain dysfunction. See Pathophysiology section regarding additional presentations.

PSYCHIATRIC EFFECTS

Depending on dose, chronicity, personality, genetic predisposition, and expectations, cocaine produces a continuum of psychiatric syndromes ranging from euphoria and dysphoria to a schizophreniform psychosis similar to amphetamine-induced psychosis. Acute overdose or habitual use may lead to mood changes characterized by paranoid thinking, agitation, irritability, restlessness, and impulsivity. Chronic users may become depressed, suspicious, irritable, and impotent, which reinforces continual cocaine use.

Distorted thought processes can cause aggressive suicidal and homicidal behavior and impaired judgment and attentional deficits increase the chance of accidental trauma. Tactile hallucinations (i.e., "coke bugs," formication) are the most frequent type in psychotic individuals and have been given the eponym "Magnan's sign." Visual misperceptions may involve flashing lights in the peripheral vision called "snow lights." Persistence of psychiatric symptoms beyond 5 to 7 days suggests an underlying psychiatric disorder.

Abuse Patterns

Cocaine does not produce the classical addiction pattern seen with opiates and sedative-hypnotics, despite the fact that heavy users develop acute tolerance to the euphoric effects of cocaine as well as physical withdrawal symptoms (e.g., depression, insomnia, headaches, fatigue, irritability, gastrointestinal distress). Major physiological changes and strong tolerance do not characterize medical or casual cocaine use.

INSUFFLATION (SNIFFING OR SNORTING)

Most recreational cocaine users favor this route. The cocaine crystals are chopped into a fine powder and placed in lines on a hard smooth surface such as a mirror. Each line typically represents between 10 and 35 mg of cocaine depending on purity, but drug effect is not always predictable because of the presence of adulterants. The user draws the powder into the nostril (snorting) with a rolled paper. The euphoric effects begin within minutes and last approximately 20 to 45 minutes. After the elation subsides, restlessness, irritability, and depression may appear, which reinforce continual cocaine use. Binges or runs may last several days until either physical, financial, or drug resources are exhausted. Often, sedative-hypnotics, alcohol, and even heroin are administered to counteract the rebound dysphoria ("crash") associated with cocaine use.

FREEBASING

The free alkali base of cocaine is an intermediate compound in the extraction of the hydrochloride salt from coca leaves. Commercial paraphernalia shops sell simple extraction kits, which dissolve the hydrochloride salt in an alkaline solution, separate it with a volatile solvent (ether), and dry the product as the benzoylmethylecgonine amino alcohol base. The remaining product is volatile and may be smoked in a cigarette or water pipe. "Crack" is the popular term for the tiny crystalline pieces or "rocks" of free-base cocaine that are smoked in a pipe. Ether is highly flammable and explosions can result during the extraction or drying process.

The cocaine base is rapidly absorbed by the lungs and produces an immediate feeling of euphoria and general stimulation. The intensely pleasurable feeling may be more exhilarating than that elicited by intravenous injection. This pattern has a high potential for dependency and overdose, since the period of euphoria is quickly followed by a powerful dysphoric mood swing that leads to further drug use. Unlike intranasal users, smokers do not appear to titrate or adjust the dose. Generally, larger quantities of cocaine are used than via the intranasal route, and correspondingly more concomitant drug use occurs (e.g., alcohol, sedative-hypnotics, heroin).

INTRAVENOUS USE

Many intravenous polydrug users try cocaine when it is available but return to their customary mind-altering substance when supplies are exhausted. Cocaine produces too much hyperactivity and excitement for some addicts who prefer to combine it with a narcotic such as heroin. Intravenous drug-combination use appears to be increasing, perhaps because of the increased availability of cocaine. Intravenous cocaine habits are expensive and produce reactions and adverse effects similar to those produced by free-base cocaine habits.

COCA PASTE SMOKING

Coca paste is the first product of the cocaine extraction process and contains up to 80% cocaine sulfate as well as other impurities. The white semisolid product is sprinkled on tobacco or marijuana cigarettes. Smoking causes an immediate euphoria similar to that of free-base smoking, however coca paste is relatively inexpensive compared with cocaine hydrochloride or freebase. This practice started in South America and is seen sporadically in the United States.

TOLERANCE

Although tolerance does not appear with therapeutic cocaine doses, most chronic drug users develop tolerance to the euphoric and physiological effects after habitual consumption of high doses. Some chronic users, particularly free-base cocaine smokers, anecdotally have developed tolerance to quantities exceeding suspected human lethal doses of 1 gram.

Toxic Dosage/Death

The maximum safe adult dose of intranasal cocaine is 80 to 200 mg (4 mL of 5% cocaine solution). Twenty-five milligrams of intranasal cocaine may produce a slight elevation in systolic blood pressure and a subjective feeling of euphoria. A 16-mg intravenous dose simulates the effects of the average dose that subjects self-inject on the street. Both intravenous and intranasal doses produce significant physiological and psychological changes. Fatalities can occur via nasal, oral, intravenous, and pulmonary routes. The oral route of administration is associated with death when associated with massive ingestions by cocaine smugglers (e.g., body packers). Dysphoric reactions may occur with intranasal cocaine doses as low as 20 to 30 mg, and the typical adult fatal range is considered to be 1 to 1.2 grams. Toxic reactions are difficult to predict, because of variations in street impurities, adulterants, cocaine content, and individual tolerance.

Postmortem cocaine blood levels are highly variable, ranging from 0.1 to 2.11 μg/mL in several reviews. Mean blood cocaine levels are similar for various routes of administration and average about 6 μg/mL in overdose deaths. Sudden death may occur at lower cocaine concentrations (mean, 0.6 mg/L) when associated with agitational psychosis. When evaluating blood cocaine levels, a number of variables must be considered. These include tolerance, previous history of cocaine use, individual susceptibility (e.g., cardiovascular disease, pseudocholinesterase deficiencies), concomitant drug use (illicit or licit), role of adulterants, storage techniques, and time between administration and death.

Most cocaine fatalities result from accidental overdoses, although suicides, homicides, and accidental trauma contribute significantly to mortalities. Terminal symptoms of cocaine overdose involve tonic-clonic seizures followed by respiratory arrest. Status epilepticus, hyperthermia, respiratory arrest, and ventricular dysrhythmias represent the greatest risk in cocaine overdose. Frequently, the association with cocaine is missed, since routine drug screens may be negative for cocaine because of its rapid clearance. Cocaine can precipitate myocardial infarction and dysrhythmias and may cause sudden death in patients with undiagnosed cardiovascular disease. Up to 30% of cocaine-related deaths in one study involved the simultaneous use of heroin.

Drug Interactions

Hereditary pseudocholinesterase deficiency, reserpine, dopamine, tricyclic antidepressants, α-methyldopa, guanethidine, and monoamine oxidase inhibitors potentiate the adverse effects of cocaine. The use of cocaine "mud" (dry cocaine powder moistened with epinephrine solution for nasal surgery) causes dangerous drug interactions and has resulted in successful litigation. Although vasoconstrictors such as adrenaline intensify shrinkage of mucous membranes, they do not retard cocaine absorption or the onset of action.

Pregnancy/Lactation

Studies on the teratogenicity of cocaine in animals are conflicting. Spontaneous abortion rates and the incidence of abruptio placentae (especially after intravenous cocaine injection) is increased in pregnant cocaine addicts, perhaps because of placental constriction and increased uterine contractility that occur after cocaine use. Neonates exposed to cocaine from this group of mothers may display significant depression of interactive behavior and poor organizational response to external stimuli.

In at least one study, reduced birth weights, increased malformation rates, and higher incidences of abruptio placentae and stillbirths were detected. Cocaine is excreted in breast milk and can induce cocaine intoxication in the breast-fed infant. Apnea and seizures have been induced in an infant from the direct ingestion of cocaine used as a topical anesthetic for nipple soreness. Cessation of cocaine exposure early in pregnancy by social cocaine users does not appear to be associated with any subsequent adverse pregnancy outcomes.

Laboratory

ANALYTIC METHODS

Screening procedures for detecting cocaine use usually involve thin-layer chromatographic analysis of urine specimens for the principal cocaine metabolite, benzoylecgonine. This method identifies unchanged cocaine and other drugs of abuse, as well as benzoylecgonine concentrations as low as 2 μg/mL. A special thin-layer chromatography solvent system is necessary to separate cocaine from the ethyl homologue cocaethylene formed in the presence of ethanol. Gas chromatography-ion trap mass spectrometry and gas chromatography with electron-capture detection may perform quantification of cocaethylene and cocaine in blood and urine.

Gas-liquid chromatographic techniques are more sensitive for benzoylecgonine and efficiently detect low cocaine levels found in blood and plasma. High-performance liquid chromatography can identify low cocaine concentrations, but lidocaine and droperidol interfere with cocaine determinations and meperidine invalidates tetracaine as an internal standard. Both radioimmunoassay, which cross-reacts with cocaine, and enzyme immunoassay are sensitive quantitative detectors of urinary benzoylecgonine.

Illicit samples commonly contain impurities (e.g., ecgonine, methylecgonine, and benzoylecgonine), several resulting from the incomplete esterification of the ecgonine base during crude leaf extract, purification, or cocaine decomposition. High-performance liquid chromatography and infrared spectroscopy can separate cocaine from commonly encountered adulterants such as lidocaine, procaine, tetracaine, benzocaine, and lactose. The degradation of cocaine to benzoylecgonine continues postmortem under alkaline and warm conditions.

BLOOD LEVELS

Measurements of blood cocaine levels do not guide clinical management. Higher urinary drug concentrations (particularly cocaine metabolites that are excreted for longer periods) make urine screens for cocaine metabolites more effective than blood sampling. Nasal application of cocaine doses of 2 mg/kg produced an average peak plasma concentration of 0.161 μg/mL at 1 hour. Equivalent oral doses cause higher peak plasma levels at 1 hour (0.21 μg/mL). Because euphoric effects occur before peak plasma concentrations are reached, the rate of change may be more important than the absolute plasma concentration.

Treatment

GUT DECONTAMINATION

Because most cocaine users inhale or inject, drug decontamination procedures frequently are not warranted. The exception is the person who ingests cocaine packets or "rock" cocaine. Depending on the type of bag (i.e., propensity for breakage), the location, and the presence of symptoms, the patient may be managed conservatively. All ingestions should receive activated charcoal, 1 gram/kg. Symptomatic patients are operative candidates. Asymptomatic patients can be treated expectantly on the basis of abdominal radiographic evaluation of the ingested packets. Attempts at endoscopic removal of gastric bags have resulted in breakage and toxicity. Similarly, vaginal or rectal bags must be handled with caution. The prevalence of better-wrapped packets has reduced the risk of internal deterioration. The development of intestinal obstruction or toxicity is an indication for emergency surgery.

ELIMINATION ENHANCEMENT

The short biological half-life, small urinary excretion of unchanged cocaine, and relatively large volume of distribution make elimination enhancement measures impractical. Asymptomatic cocaine body packers may be aided by the use of whole-bowel irrigation with polyethylene glycol electrolyte lavage solution, followed by contrast radiography to confirm the adequacy of removal. This technique has not been shown safe and effective with early presentations, with poorly wrapped substances, or for symptomatic cocaine body packers.

SUPPORTIVE MEASURES

- For most patients with mild cocaine-induced stimulation, central nervous system sedation with a benzodiazepine (e.g., diazepam) generally is effective.
- Intractable seizures, respiratory arrest, hyperthermia, and dysrhythmias represent the greatest immediate risk to life. The first priority is to assess ventilation and establish an airway.
- Immediate intravenous access should be established along with cardiac monitoring for all patients with serious vital sign abnormalities.
- Nasotracheal intubation and use of paralyzing agents (succinylcholine, 1 mg/kg, with or without thiopental, 1 to 3 mg/kg) are useful alternative methods to endotracheal intubation when seizures limit oral access.
- With the exception of delayed intestinal rupture of cocaine bags, major symptoms usually present within the first hour of exposure.
- The ingestion of cocaine base ("rock") may delay serious symptoms for several hours.
- A chest x-ray and arterial blood gas should be obtained when the patient's clinical condition indicates respiratory depression or distress.
- The presence of pulmonary edema requires the placement of a Swann-Ganz catheter to maximize hemodynamic variables.
- The importance of naloxone (2 mg intravenously) in lethargic or comatose patients should not be ignored, since many intravenous users simultaneously inject heroin.

SEIZURES

- Diazepam (0.1 to 0.3 mg/kg up to an adult dose of 10 mg) is the drug of choice in treating seizures. If diazepam is not effective, then phenytoin loading should be tried. If phenytoin is not effective, phenobarbital loading and general anesthesia may be tried.

- After seizures are controlled, an investigation of the patient should rule out other causes of seizures, stroke, subarachnoid hemorrhage, and infection. A CT scan, lumbar puncture, and electroencephalogram may be of value if indicated.
- Cocaine-associated status epilepticus is a relatively rare complication of cocaine abuse. It may follow all methods of cocaine use. Frequently it follows an unusually large dose of cocaine and often concurrent use of other drugs such as heroin, amphetamines, or marijuana.
- Cocaine-associated status epilepticus may be resistant to medical treatment.
- Endotracheal intubation, assisted ventilation, and neuromuscular blockers are required for persistent seizures and subsequent acidosis.
- Persistent seizures, especially in the presence of hyperthermia, indicate the need for early neuromuscular paralysis (i.e., pancuronium).

HYPERTHERMIA AND RHABDOMYOLYSIS

- The most life-threatening presentation of acute cocaine intoxication is severe hyperthermia, occasionally presenting with temperatures of 41°–45°C.
- Hyperthermia can prevent gluconeogenesis causing hypoglycemia. If glucose is low, 50 to 100 mL of 50% dextrose, and 100 mg of thiamine intravenously, are indicated.
- Core temperatures, as measured by rectal thermocouple, exceeding 40.5°C (105°F) require immersion in an ice bath and monitoring of vital signs every 10 to 15 minutes after airway, breathing, and circulation have been stabilized.
- Packing in ice and use of hypothermic blankets are alternative measures when an ice bath is not available. The patient should be removed when the core rectal temperature drops to 39°C.
- Patients who do not respond to diazepam and vigorous cooling measures have been treated with dantrolene 1 mg/kg every 6 hours or bromocriptine orally via a nasogastric tube. The efficacy of dantrolene in the treatment of cocaine-induced hyperthermia has not been established. It can lead to cardiac insufficiency and pulmonary edema.
- Hyperthermia may induce rhabdomyolysis. Monitor these patients with serial serum creatine kinase and urine myoglobin studies. Attempt to differentiate rhabdomyolysis-induced enzyme increases from those resulting from myocardial infarction. Use alkalinization, diuretics (e.g., mannitol, furosemide), and fluids to diminish the precipitation of myoglobin in the urine and lessen the possibility of renal failure.
- Perhaps one-third of patients with rhabdomyolysis develop renal failure following myoglobin-induced tubular injury. Hemodialysis aids in reversing the renal failure. Dopamine and furosemide may reduce renal vascular resistance and assist in reducing the number of hemodialyses required to reverse oliguria.
- Less severe temperature elevations (38° to 40°C) can be treated by placement in a cool room, removal of clothes, minimization of physical activity, and tepid sponging.

HYPERTENSION AND CARDIAC ISCHEMIA

- The stimulant phase of cocaine usually is short, so that treatment of hypertension and tachycardia often is not necessary.
- Labetalol 10 to 20 mg intravenously repeated at 10-minute intervals up to a total of 300 mg may be helpful in life-threatening hypertension and tachycardia.
- Propranolol by slow titration (1 mg intravenously every 2 to 3 minutes up to 6 to 8 mg) previously has been used, however the use of intravenous propranolol (or any β-blocker) may cause unopposed α stimulation in this setting.
- Criteria for admitting cocaine abusers with chest pain to rule out myocardial infarction should include sustained or persistent chest pain, chest pain with known risk factors for coronary artery disease, or chest pain with electrocardiographic changes suggestive of ischemia.
- Some of the routine pharmaceutical interventions for the treatment of acute myocardial infarction may be harmful in a patient with cocaine-induced ischemia. β-Adrenergic blockade in cocaine-induced coronary vasoconstriction may induce a further decrease in coronary artery diameter, but the effect of β-blockers on mortality has not been studied in patients with cocaine-associated infarction.
- As a period of myocardial ischemia may persist up to 2 weeks following cessation of cocaine abuse, it seems prudent to avoid β-blockers in patients with suspected cocaine-induced myocardial ischemia for as long as 2 weeks following withdrawal of the toxin.
- In patients with cocaine-induced hypertension with chest pain, institute a nitroglycerin drip. Use benzodiazepines to reduce excess production of catecholamines by the central nervous system. Administer oxygen by nasal cannula at 5 L/min. Monitor cardiac status and initiate an intravenous line. If pain is refractory to nitroglycerin, use morphine.
- Early therapy of cocaine-induced myocardial infarction should be similar to that of the typical patient with myocardial ischemia. If pain does not resolve with nitroglycerin, administer nifedipine 10 mg orally or phentolamine 1 to 5 mg intravenously, followed by a drip of 10 mg in 1,000 mL of 5% dextrose in water at 10 mL/min while monitoring the blood pressure. Treat with aspirin per myocardial infarction protocol.
- Administer thrombolytic agents if required. Do not use thrombolysis in a hypertensive patient or in a cocaine-using patient with seizures until a head CT scan is proven normal. As cocaine users are at increased risk for subarachnoid hemorrhage and aortic dissection, these possibilities must be ruled out (clinically or otherwise) before thrombolytics are instituted.
- The success of thrombolysis is not universal. Approximately 20% of infarct-related arteries fail to open with thrombolytic regimens, and approximately 15% of reperfused arteries reclose in subsequent hours and days.
- Calcium-channel blockers may alleviate coronary spasm and, as noted above, β-blockers may potentiate cocaine-induced coronary vasoconstriction. In general, acute myocardial infarction after cocaine use should be treated as myocardial infarction in noncocaine users except for the use of β-blockers.
- If hyperacute anterolateral myocardial infarction with seizures is present, do a CT scan to rule out an intracerebral bleed before instituting thrombolytic therapy.
- Hypertensive crises with or without propranolol use in cocaine intoxication may be treated with sodium nitroprusside drip (0.5 μg/kg/min initial dose titrated in slow increments to effect, with careful monitoring of blood pressure).
- Esmolol, another β-blocker with an extremely short half life, may be titrated as a drip. Unopposed α stimulation also may occur with its use.

DYSRHYTHMIAS

- Cardioversion should be considered for all unstable dysrhythmias. Correcting ischemia, administering calcium-channel blockers and α- or β-adrenergic blockers, or cardioversion may treat unstable supraventricular dysrhythmias.
- Lidocaine, procainamide, quinidine, and cyclic antidepressants are sodium-channel blockers and can enhance arrhyth-

mias and seizures. Sodium bicarbonate may be considered for wide-complex arrhythmias resulting from cocaine overdoses. Although acidosis may depress myocardial function and potentiate ventricular dysrhythmias, the use of bicarbonate remains controversial.

- Avoid lidocaine and procainamide in the treatment of ventricular ectopy in the first 1 to 2 hours after acute use of cocaine if possible. Lidocaine is effective, but commonly lidocaine is an adulterant of cocaine, and patients may already have toxic lidocaine levels. Lidocaine and procaine share pharmacologic characteristics with cocaine and the possibility exists that they may enhance cocaine toxicity.
- Ventricular ectopy occurring more than 2 hours after an acute cocaine exposure may be an indication for use of lidocaine and procainamide.
- Propranolol has been used successfully to treat ventricular bigeminy and multifocal premature ventricular contractions that developed during therapeutic use of cocaine, but whether or not these dysrhythmias deteriorate into more malignant rhythms in the setting of cocaine overdose is unclear.
- Accelerated ventricular rhythms usually require no treatment.
- Ventricular tachycardia, fibrillation, and asystole are treated per Advanced Cardiac Life Support (ACLS) criteria of the American Heart Association.

HYPOTENSION

- Often, fluids do not reverse the hypotension seen in the late depressive phase of cocaine overdose. Frequently, dopamine or norepinephrine is needed.

THE COMBATIVE PATIENT

- It may be impossible to insert an intravenous line into a very combative patient. In such cases, give diazepam 10 mg or lorazepam 2 mg IM acutely and repeat if needed with continuous cardiorespiratory monitoring until the effects of both the cocaine and the sedative cease.
- Much larger doses of diazepam, up to 100 to 150 mg, have been suggested and used to control the extremely combative patient however experience with these doses is limited.
- Use hard restraints as required.
- Sedatives with butyrophenones (such as haloperidol and droperidol) or phenothiazines (such as chlorpromazine) are not recommended. These agents are anticholinergic and can precipitate malignant hyperthermia. These drugs also lower the seizure threshold by blocking inhibitory central nervous system dopaminergic receptors.
- Acceptance, reduction of stimuli (i.e., rest, quiet, cool environment), and sincere reassurance are generally effective therapeutic interventions.
- When psychosis clears, each patient should be evaluated for suicidal and homicidal ideation. Besides potential self-harm, reasons for psychiatric hospitalization include chronic freebasing or intravenous injection, concurrent dependence, severe psychiatric or medical problems, severe psychosocial impairment, lack of social or family support, repeated outpatient failure, and poor motivation.

Antidotes

Butyrocholinesterase is present in the blood at low levels and metabolizes cocaine to inactive compounds. A method for isolating butyrocholinesterase from human plasma has been developed, but is unavailable commercially. Increasing the amount of butyrocholinesterase in the blood may be a possible approach to enhancing more rapid inactivation of cocaine.

Questions—Cocaine

1. Cocaine content of street samples
A. Is usually less than 5%
B. Is usually 15%
C. Is usually 90%
D. Varies widely
E. None of the above

2. "Rock" is a synonym for
A. Cocaine mixed with amphetamine
B. Caffeine substituted for cocaine
C. Alkaloidal cocaine, also called "crack"
D. Cocaine sold illegally
E. None of the above

3. Cocaine is well accepted for medical use in
A. Mucous membrane anesthesia
B. Mucous membrane vasoconstriction
C. Esophageal anesthesia
D. A and B
E. A and C

4. What proportion of patients presenting to emergency rooms with cocaine toxicity have seizures?
A. Up to 10%
B. 25 %
C. 50%
D. 75%
E. Almost 100%

5. Status epilepticus usually is observed in
A. Cocaine users with seizure disorders using large amounts of cocaine
B. Cocaine users without seizure disorders using large amounts of cocaine
C. Cocaine users without seizure disorders using small amounts of cocaine
D. Heavy cocaine users using small amounts of cocaine from a new supplier
E. None of the above

6. Cocaine-induced myocardial infarction may follow cocaine abuse via
A. Intranasal use
B. Intravenous use
C. Inhalation use
D. All of the above
E. None of the above

7. The most frequent cocaine-associated complaint is
A. Chest pain
B. Nausea and vomiting
C. Tachypnea
D. Allergic reactions
E. Migraine

8. Cocaethylene
A. Is formed in the liver by transesterification
B. Is found in cocaine users who consume cocaine and ethanol simultaneously
C. Has a shorter half-life than cocaine
D. A and B
E. A and C

9. Cocaine's elimination half-life is the same with intranasal, oral and intravenous use.
A. True
B. False

Answers to questions in shaded boxes appear at the end of the chapter.

10. The most frequent electrocardiogram abnormality in cocaine overdose is
A. Ventricular bigeminy
B. Premature ventricular contractions
C. Sinus tachycardia
D. Ventricular fibrillation
E. None of the above

11. "Magnan's Sign" refers to
A. Chest pain with elevated cardiac enzymes in patients without cardiac histories
B. Tactile hallucinations which occur in cocaine-using psychotic patients
C. Pneumomediastinum or pneumothorax resulting from prolonged Valsalva maneuvers associated with freebasing
D. Pulmonary edema induced by intravenous freebase cocaine
E. None of the above

12. One line of snorted cocaine typically represents how much cocaine?
A. Less than 5 mg
B. 10 to 35 mg
C. 50 to 100 mg
D. 100 to 200 mg
E. Over 200 mg

13. Tolerance does not appear to develop with therapeutic cocaine doses
A. True
B. False

14. Most cocaine fatalities result from
A. Suicide
B. Homicide
C. Accidental overdose
D. Accidental trauma
E. None of the above

15. Pregnant cocaine addicts have an increased incidence of
A. Placental abruption
B. Placenta previa
C. Large for gestational age infants
D. Hypoglycemic infants
E. None of the above

16. Serum cocaine levels
A. Guide clinical management of cocaine overdoses
B. Peak before euphoric effects occur
C. Have higher peaks when taken orally than when taken via inhalation
D. A and B
E. A and C

17. Treatment of patients with mild cocaine-induced stimulation often responds well to sedation with benzodiazepines
A. True
B. False

Answers

1. D	2. C	3. D	4. A	5. B	6. D
7. A	8. D	9. B	10. C	11. B	12. B
13. A	14. C	15. A	16. C	17. A	

SELECTED READINGS

Cocaine

1. Brody SL, Slovis CM, Wrenn KD. Cocaine-related medical problems: Consecutive series of 233 patients. Am J Med 1990;88:325–331.
2. Garvin FH, Ellinwood EH Jr. Cocaine and other stimulants. Actions, abuse and treatment. N Engl J Med 1988;318:1173–1182.
3. Goldfrank L, Lewin N, Weisman RS. Cocaine. Hosp Physician 1981;17(5): 26–44.
4. Hoffman B, Derlet R. Cocaine intoxication considerations, complications and strategies: Point and counterpoint. Emerg Med 1992;1:1–6.
5. Hoffman RS, Smilkstein MJ, Goldfrank LR. Whole bowel irrigation and the cocaine body-packer: A new approach to a common problem. Am J Emerg Med 1990;8:523–527.
6. Hollander JE, Hoffman RS, Gennis P, et al. Cocaine associated chest pain: One year follow-up. Acad Emerg Med 1995;2:179–184.
7. Hollander JE, Hoffman RS, Gennis P, et al. Prospective multicenter evaluation of cocaine-associated chest pain. Acad Emerg Med 1994;1:330–339.
8. Lovejoy FH Jr, Shannon M, Woolf AD. Recent advances in clinical toxicology. Curr Prob Pediatr 1992;22:119–129.
9. Miller NS, Summers GL, Gold MS. Cocaine dependence: Alcohol and other drug dependence and withdrawal characteristics. J Addict Dis 1993;12:25–35.
10. Mule SJ. The pharmacodynamics of cocaine abuse. Psychiatr Ann 1984; 14:724–727.
11. Pirwitz MJ, Willard JE, Landau C, et al. Influence of cocaine, ethanol or their combination on epicardial coronary arterial dimensions in humans. Arch Intern Med 1995;155:1186–1191.
12. Tokarski GF, Paganussi P, Urbanski R, et al. An evaluation of cocaine-induced chest pain. Ann Emerg Med 1990;19:1088–1092.
13. Wasserberger J, Ellenhorn MJ, Landers S, et al. The emergency management of acute cocaine toxicity. Top Emerg Med 1993;15:27–40.
14. Welti CV, Mittleman RE. The "body packer syndrome"-toxicity following ingestion of illicit drugs packaged for transportation. J Forensic Sci 1981; 26:492–500.
15. Zimmerman JL, Dellinger RP, Majid PA. Cocaine-associated chest pain. Ann Emerg Med 1991;20:611–615.

ACKNOWLEDGMENTS

Thanks to Alison Deutsch, MD for contributing the questions in this chapter.

CHAPTER 20
Hallucinogenic Drugs

INTRODUCTION

A number of compounds are abused for their ability to produce visual illusions, perceptual distortion, and synesthesia (i.e., the overflow of sensory input so that colors are heard and music becomes palpable). Most of these agents are derived from plant sources. Lysergic acid diethylamide (LSD) is the most potent on a weight basis. The term "hallucinogen" commonly is applied to this drug group. Classically, the term actually refers to drugs that alter the perception of reality to the extent that the subject believes that his altered perceptions are real. Most persons who use these drugs retain their insight and recognize that what they see or hear is drug induced.

Each hallucinogen produces behavioral effects related to its serotonergic, dopaminergic, or adrenergic activity. A flashback is a recurrence of imagery associated with hallucinogen use that occurs after the acute effects of the drug have worn off. Flashbacks have been described with LSD, mescaline, phencyclidine, and marijuana use and may occur months to years after cessation of use. Hallucinogens generally exhibit agonist or partial agonist effects at numerous serotonin receptors. Levels of growth hormone, prolactin, β-endorphin, corticotropin, and cortisol are increased with hallucinogen use presumably related to the serotonergic properties of these drugs.

Of the estimated 400,000 to 800,000 plant species in the world, only about 60 plants have been used as hallucinogens. To date, only about 20 of these species are considered clinically important. Natural hallucinogens include nutmeg (*Myristica frangans*), the ergot fungus (*Claviceps purpurea*), morning glory seeds (*Ipomoea violacea*), peyote (*Lophophora williamsii*), Mimosa species, psilocybin-containing mushrooms (e.g., Psilocybe or Panaeolus), ibotenic acid-containing mushrooms (e.g., *Amanita muscaria*), and marijuana (Cannabis species).

Ergot alkaloids have a long psychopharmacological history. The parasitic fungus *C. purpurea*, which infects grain, is believed to be the primary cause of the visionary Eleusinian rite of classical times as well as the epidemic ergotism (St. Anthony's fire) of the Middle Ages. The actual ingredient in both these biological sources was lysergic acid, from which the diethylamide derivative (LSD) is formed.

Questions—Introduction to Hallucinogenic Drugs

1. **Flashbacks have been described with each of the following substances except**
   A. Mescaline
   B. LSD
   C. *Claviceps purpurea*
   D. Phencyclidine
   E. Marijuana

2. **Which of the following statements is false?**
   A. Most hallucinogens are plant derived.
   B. Thousands of plant species are hallucinogenic.
   C. Ergot alkaloids are known to have caused hallucinations in the Middle Ages.
   D. Certain mushrooms may cause hallucinations.
   E. Nutmeg can be hallucinogenic.

LYSERGIC ACID DIETHYLAMIDE

Hofmann discovered the powerful psychotropic properties of LSD in 1943 when he inadvertently ingested it. Subsequent research confirmed that D-lysergic acid diethylamide is the only one of four isomers derived from lysergic acid that has powerful mind-altering properties. Physiological effects are primarily sympathomimetic and include mydriasis, tachycardia, hyperglycemia, leukocytosis, piloerection, and elevated body temperature. Salivation, lacrimation, tremor, paresthesias, hyperreflexia, ataxia, hyperactivity, nausea, and vomiting occur after ingestion of large doses.

The main psychological experience involves visual illusions, alterations in sound and in intensity of colors, subjective slowing of time, euphoria, loss of physical boundaries, and crossover of sensory modalities. Medical uses in the 1950s included the treatment of alcoholism, psychoneurosis, sexual abnormalities, autism in children, sociopathy, and analgesia in terminal patients. Double-blind controlled studies failed to substantiate the advantage of LSD over psychotherapy alone for these indications. Complications associated with inadvertent or intentional ingestion are seizures, anxiety and depressive states, acute panic or paranoid reactions, and hallucinations.

Illicit use of LSD reached its peak popularity in the mid-1960s and subsequently declined in the 1970s. Presently, its popularity is regional but may be increasing in some localities within the United States. D-lysergic acid diethylamide is synthesized from lysergic acid and diethylamine. The precursor lysergic acid occurs naturally as an ergot alkaloid in grain parasitized by the fungus *C. purpurea* and in members of the morning glory family (e.g., *I. violacea*, *Rivea corymbosa*). Frequently, LSD is manufactured abroad and smuggled into the United States. The Federal Controlled Substances Act classifies LSD as a schedule I drug (high abuse potential, no medical uses in the United States).

Of all illicit drugs, LSD probably is the least adulterated. LSD appears illicitly as tablets, capsules, powder, solution, or impregnated on a variety of substances (e.g., gelatin, sugar cubes, blotting paper). Most LSD derivatives have fewer psychotomimetic properties than the parent drug. The ergot alkaloid D-lysergic acid amide contained in morning glory seeds has about one-tenth the hallucinogenic activity of LSD. LSD is colorless, tasteless, odorless, and water-soluble.

Because of its high potency, it is effective in dosages as low as 35 μg and is 3,000 to 5,000 times more powerful on a weight basis than mescaline. LSD is commonly called acid. It also is referred to as blue, pink, or yellow drops; window panes; orange or purple wedges; sunshine; California sunshine; blotter acid; microdots; paper acid; purple haze; yellow, blue, brown, or green caps; white lightning; the ghost, hawk, or beast.

Pathophysiology

LSD is a potent agonist at certain serotonin (5-HT1A) receptors, whereas mescaline and other phenylethylamines have little affinity for 5-HT1A receptors. Phenethylamine hallucinogens (e.g., mescaline) have an affinity for postsynaptic 5-HT2 receptors in the locus ceruleus and the cerebral cortex. Most 5-HT2 receptors in the brain are located in the cerebral cortex, where hallucinogens exert an effect on perceptual and cognitive functions. LSD binds to areas of the hippocampus, corpus striatum, cerebral cortex, and, to a much lesser extent, cerebellum. LSD- and serotonin-binding sites closely resemble each other, and serotonin has a high affinity for both sites.

LSD usually is administered orally and the intravenous, pulmonary, and nasal routes are used rarely. Use tends to be intermittent rather than intense and sustained (i.e., binge), reflecting the rapid tolerance that develops with continued use. Physical withdrawal symptoms do not occur, but the LSD drug experience may become the focal point of the user's life (e.g., cult). Drug use among LSD users often is multiple (e.g., alcohol, marijuana, amphetamines), but self-administration of sedative-hypnotics and opiates occurs infrequently.

Pharmacokinetics

ABSORPTION

- LSD is well absorbed from the gastrointestinal tract.
- Clinical toxicity after insufflation indicates that absorption also occurs from the nasal mucosa.
- The usual adult oral dose is 100 μg. Onset occurs 40 to 90 minutes postingestion and the duration is 8 to 12 hours. Peak effect develops between 3 to 5 hours.

DISTRIBUTION

- Peak LSD levels after an oral dose of 2 μg/kg appear 30 to 60 minutes after ingestion, with food apparently reducing and slightly delaying the peak levels.
- Intravenous doses of 2 μg/kg produce peak LSD levels at 30 minutes and 1-hour plasma levels ranging from 4 to 6 ng/mL. After an intravenous (IV) dose of 2 μg/kg, the volume of distribution is 0.27 L/kg.

Answers to questions in shaded boxes appear at the end of the chapter.

ELIMINATION

- Human LSD elimination is not well studied. Studies on animals suggest that the major metabolic route is hydroxylation of the benzene ring to form phenols, with the subsequent conjugated glucuronide salts excreted in the bile.
- The urine may be positive for LSD 34 to 120 hours after ingestion.
- The serum elimination half-life of LSD in man is about 3 hours, and there is marked variation among animals. Only small amounts of LSD are excreted unchanged in the urine.

Clinical Presentations

At doses of 1 to 2 μg/kg, effects develop 40 to 90 minutes postingestion, although some individuals experience symptoms as early as 15 minutes. Recovery from peak effects begins by about 4 hours and usually is completed by 8 hours. Intoxication seldom lasts beyond 12 hours. Pupillary dilation is the most frequent and consistent sign of LSD use. Heart rate, body temperature, and respirations are slightly increased but blood pressure remains normal. Peripheral signs include piloerection, uterine contraction, and, at high doses, bronchiolar constriction. Parasympathomimetic effects may be present, including salivation, lacrimation, nausea, and vomiting.

PSYCHOTOMIMETIC EFFECTS

Misrepresentation of sensory cues is the most notable and consistent alteration after the administration of LSD. Afterimages become prolonged, with flat surfaces assuming depth and fixed objects undulating. Illusions are common at therapeutic doses, but visual hallucinations are not, because the individual's insight into reality usually is preserved. Hyperacusis and amplification of background noise occur. Auditory hallucinations suggest an underlying psychosis rather than drug-induced perceptual distortions. The overflow of sensory modalities simulates a state in which colors are heard and music is palpable (synesthesias). Subjectively, time appears slowed. Loosening of associations, alteration of body image and concrete thinking, and depersonalization occur. Orientation is preserved, but judgment may be poor because of paranoia or ideas of persecution.

BEHAVIORAL EFFECTS

Behavioral patterns are difficult to predict because they depend on setting, expectation, personality, and emotional stress in addition to dose. Subjects tend to be quiet, passive, self-centered, and withdrawn, but hostility may develop as a result of the lessening of impulse control. The use of straitjackets to control LSD violence has been associated with rhabdomyolysis and renal failure. Sociability is reduced, and drives, including sexual ones, ordinarily are diminished. Mood may be labile, ranging from euphoria to depression. Rarely, catatonia, paranoid rages, or acute panic attacks occur. No single factor guarantees a pleasurable LSD experience.

Neither historical elements nor current clinical features separate patients hospitalized for adverse LSD reactions from control groups. Individuals who have previously used LSD many times without difficulty may experience an untoward reaction on a subsequent dose. Acute panic attack is the most common side effect of LSD therapy and frequently accompanies incidental consumption. Both amphetamines and LSD can produce toxic psychoses, although the amphetamine psychosis more closely resembles schizophrenia. Depressive reactions culminating in suicide, paranoid or delusional behavior leading to accidental trauma, and antisocial, impulsive behavior all have been associated with LSD use.

FLASHBACKS

Visual alterations, time distortions, and image changes may recur in LSD users after a period of abstinence. Prolonged flashbacks, defined by episodes extending beyond 6 months, occur more commonly in schizoid and obsessive personalities. Both physiological (e.g., fatigue, driving, sepsis, electrolyte disorders) and emotional stress can precipitate flashbacks. The afterimages, trailing, and induction of geometric pseudohallucinations interpreted as flashbacks may result from chronic visual disturbances. Chronic LSD users may develop impaired color perception lasting as long as 2 years postingestion.

NEUROLOGIC EFFECTS

Neuromuscular effects are weakness, tremor, hyperreflexia, and ataxia. Convulsions can complicate either experimental or street use of LSD, particularly in polydrug users and epileptic patients. Status epilepticus has been reported but is extremely rare. Focal cerebral deficits have developed after LSD use, which suggests that LSD may produce central vasospasm and vascular insufficiency similar to those produced by the structurally related compound methysergide. Generalized headache, nausea, vomiting, and hemiparesis have been described. Individuals have become comatose after insufflating large quantities of LSD.

SYMPATHOMIMETIC EFFECTS

Dilated pupils, tachycardia, hypertension, diaphoresis, flushing, and gastrointestinal (e.g., diarrhea, vomiting) signs may be prominent. Temperature elevations after LSD ingestion usually are mild. Neuroleptic malignant syndrome may be observed following LSD use. Muscle biopsy in these cases may show myoedema, focal necrosis, glycogen and lipid depletion. Dantrolene may reduce the high temperature and rigidity and can lead to an improved level of consciousness.

TOLERANCE

Tolerance develops rapidly among patients given LSD. Complete tolerance depends on both dosage and frequency and typically develops after three to four daily doses. This tolerance disappears 4 to 5 days after drug withdrawal. Cross-tolerance develops among LSD, psilocybin, and mescaline but not amphetamine.

Toxic Dosage/Death

There have been no well-documented deaths resulting from the medical consequences of LSD intoxication. More often, LSD-related fatalities result from either suicide or accidental trauma. LSD-related homicides occur infrequently. The minimal, clinically perceptible adult oral dose is 25 μg, with optimal psychedelic doses ranging from 100 to 1,000 μg. The usual street dose varies between 50 to 300 μg and averages 100 to 150 μg. Death and coma have not been associated with specific amounts of LSD. The lethal adult dose of LSD has been predicted to be 14 mg (0.2 mg/kg).

Drug Interactions

Patients taking fluoxetine and lithium in therapeutic doses may develop seizures after adding LSD for recreational use. Patients with a history of LSD use may experience flashbacks if they use selective serotonin reuptake inhibitor drugs such as sertraline, and paroxetine.

Pregnancy/Lactation

Elevated chromosomal abnormalities have been detected in the leukocytes of LSD users, but these changes are not correlated to drug dose, frequency of use, or total dosage. Rare congenital abnormalities such as anophthalmia (absence of ocular tissue), true limb aplasia (absence of entire limb bud), and multiple cerebral and cerebellar malformations have been associated with illicit maternal use of LSD.

Uncontrolled studies of women using LSD during pregnancy show elevated incidences of spontaneous abortions and major congenital abnormalities compared with national averages. However, the ingestion of other illicit drugs, the presence of infectious diseases, and poor maternal nutrition preclude a definite correlation between LSD and human birth defects.

Laboratory

ANALYTIC METHODS

Gas chromatography-mass spectrometry is useful in confirming positive LSD urine levels. An instrumental high-performance thin-layer chromatographic technique and radioimmunoassay for determination of LSD also is available.

BLOOD LEVELS

LSD concentrations in isolated serum or urine specimens are of limited value except to confirm the presence of LSD. Between 1 to 2 hours after intravenous administration of 2 μg/kg, plasma LSD concentrations range from 4 to 6 ng/mL and appear to correlate with performance scores.

Treatment

GUT DECONTAMINATION

The usual methods of decontamination usually are unnecessary, as LSD is rapidly absorbed, and their use intensifies behavioral abnormalities.

ELIMINATION ENHANCEMENT

Because of the short half-life and few serious medical reactions, hemoperfusion, hemodialysis, and peritoneal dialysis have not been used for LSD intoxication.

SUPPORTIVE MEASURES

- Monitor vital signs and ensure airway and circulatory status.
- Life-threatening medical reactions to LSD intoxication are extremely rare, but do occur. All patients with depressed mental status should be observed for respiratory depression, especially since aspiration is a definite hazard. Vital signs should be followed in all patients. Changes usually are mild and transient, except perhaps in patients with underlying cardiovascular disease.
- Avoid restraints if possible as these may yield rhabdomyolysis in severe cases. All patients who require the continued use of restraints should have the first-voided urine specimen sent for myoglobin and urinalysis. A positive dipstick test for hematuria in the absence of microscopic evidence of red blood cells suggests myoglobinuria.
- Sedate the patient with quiet reassurance and diazepam. Diazepam (5 to 10 mg intravenously in an adult) is the drug of choice for sedation and seizures. Avoid phenothiazines as these may diminish seizure threshold.
- In cases of acute panic attack, supportive care, reassurance, and the reduction of sensory stimuli are the most important aspects of management. The patient should be placed in a safe, quiet environment, preferably with a familiar person who can provide constant reassurance (i.e., "talk the patient down").
- Haloperidol may be administered as a second-line drug if the above measures fail to calm the patient and continued agitation represents an increased medical risk.
- In the setting of acute psychotic reactions, neuroleptic drugs should be administered cautiously. Phenothiazine use has been associated with hypotension, sedation, and potentiation of anticholinergic effects, decreased seizure threshold, and extrapyramidal reactions.
- Frequently, the actual psychedelic drug involved is not known, and phenothiazines can potentiate drugs with anticholinergic effects. When antipsychotic drugs are necessary, haloperidol probably is the safest neuroleptic agent.
- Psychotherapy, antianxiety agents, and neuroleptic drugs are used to treat flashbacks.
- LSD produces laboratory evidence of a nonspecific stress reaction (i.e., leukocytosis). In acutely psychotic patients hospitalized after LSD use, a mild temporary rise in serum creatine kinase occurs. Marked elevation of serum muscle enzymes and uric acid may be noted in restrained psychiatric patients who became agitated and psychotic after LSD ingestion.

Questions—Lysergic Acid Diethylamide

1. The usual oral dose of LSD is
- A. 100 μg
- B. 100 mg
- C. 100 grams
- D. 100 ng
- E. 100 kg

2. Tolerance from LSD use
- A. Develops rapidly
- B. Has not been described
- C. Is associated with increased flashbacks
- D. Manifests in amphetamine users
- E. Usually develops after daily use for a month

3. Sympathomimetic effects from LSD use may include
- A. Dilated pupils
- B. Tachycardia
- C. Hypertension
- D. Diaphoresis
- E. All of the above

4. Restraints should be avoided when treating the LSD-intoxicated individual because
- A. This creates added heat which exacerbates toxicity
- B. Suicide rates among LSD users has been associated with this maneuver.
- C. Studies have shown that LSD users tend to use more drugs after restraints.
- D. Rhabdomyolysis has been described after their use.
- E. Restraints may be used as a weapon by the LSD-intoxicated individual.

5. Which of the following is false?
- A. Auditory hallucinations are common with LSD use.
- B. Neuromuscular effects may include weakness, tremor, hyperreflexia, and ataxia.
- C. Individuals who have previously used LSD many times without difficulty may experience an untoward reaction on a subsequent dose.
- D. LSD usually is taken orally and the intravenous, pulmonary, and nasal routes are used rarely.
- E. Recovery from peak effects begins by about 4 hours and usually is completed by 8 hours.

N, N-DIMETHYLTRYPTAMINE

N, N-Dimethyltryptamine (DMT) is an endogenous mammalian hallucinogen and drug of abuse. Effects are felt almost instantaneously, peak within 2 minutes, and resolve within 20 to 30 minutes and include visual hallucinatory phenomena, bodily dissociation, extreme shifts in mood, and auditory effects in about 50% of subjects. N, N-Dimethyltryptamine is obtained from the seeds and leaves of *Piptadenia pergyina* (Mimosaceae) and other South American plants.

Pathophysiology

Hallucinogens are agonists or partial agonists at serotonin (5-HT) receptors, specifically at 5-HT2, 5-HT1A, and 5-HT1C subtypes. The 5-HT2 subtype probably mediates the hyperthermic effects of DMT.

Pharmacokinetics

ABSORPTION

- Dimethyltryptamine fumarate, 0.2 to 0.4 mg/kg elicits nearly instantaneous onset of visual hallucinatory phenomena, bodily dissociation and extreme shifts in mood.

DISTRIBUTION

- Lower doses between 0.05 to 0.1 mg/kg are not hallucinogenic. Emotional and somesthetic effects predominate. The threshold dose for hallucinogenic effects is 0.2 mg/kg.
- At doses of 0.4 mg/kg, visual imagery predominates. Auditory effects are observed in about half of individuals using DMT. There is an almost complete loss of control.

ELIMINATION

- Effects peak within 2 minutes after injection and resolve quickly within 20 to 30 minutes.

Clinical Presentations

DMT, like other classic hallucinogens, induces pupillary dilation, which may be 5-HT2 mediated. Diastolic blood pressure may rise transiently. Temperature may increase and heart rate and mean arterial blood pressure are elevated. Behavioral and psychotomimetic effects resemble the clinical profile of LSD (see above). Seizures have been reported in severe overdoses.

Laboratory

ANALYTIC METHODS

Blood levels of DMT (freebase) are assayed by a gas chromatography-mass spectrometry technique whose limit of detectability is 1 ng/mL.

BLOOD LEVELS

The time course of blood DMT levels matches the development of subjective effects, peaking at 2 minutes after completion of an injection. Peak values range from 32 to 200 ng/mL after a 0.4 mg/kg injection. Plasma levels of DMT are correlated with the psychological effects. A 0.4 mg/kg injection leads to peak plasma levels of 32 to 300 ng/mL. A dose of 0.2 mg/kg is a threshold dose for hallucinogenic effects.

Treatment

GUT DECONTAMINATION

The usual methods of decontamination usually are unnecessary, as DMT is rapidly absorbed, and their use intensifies behavior abnormalities.

ELIMINATION ENHANCEMENT

Because of the short half-life and few serious medical reactions, hemoperfusion, hemodialysis, and peritoneal dialysis have not been used for DMT intoxication.

SUPPORTIVE MEASURES

- Supportive measures are similar to those utilized for LSD.

Questions—N, N-Dimethyltryptamine

1. Which of the following is false?

A. N, N-Dimethyltryptamine (DMT) is a mammalian hallucinogen and drug of abuse.
B. Because of the short half-life and few serious medical reactions, hemoperfusion, hemodialysis, and peritoneal dialysis have not been used for DMT intoxication.
C. Hypothermia is a unique feature in overdose.
D. DMT, like other hallucinogens, induces pupillary dilation, which may be 5-HT2 mediated.
E. N, N-Dimethyltryptamine is obtained from the seeds and leaves of *Piptadenia pergyina* (Mimosaceae) and other South American plants.

2. Which of the following is true?

A. DMT is manifested at β-adrenergic sites in the mesolimbic system.
B. DMT generally is measured by EMIT.
C. DMT induces hallucinogenic symptoms 1 to 2 hours after use.
D. DMT has been isolated in mammalian species.
E. The usual methods of decontamination usually are unnecessary, as DMT is rapidly absorbed, and their use intensifies behavior abnormalities.

COLORADO RIVER TOAD

The dried venom of the *Bufo alvarius* or Colorado River toad contains 5-methoxy-N, N-dimethyltryptamine (Meo-DMT), a hallucinogen related to DMT. "Smoking toad" induces hallucinations lasting about 5 minutes. A clinical picture of profound drooling, seizure activity, arrhythmias, and cyanosis may follow the oral application of a toad to an individual's tongue. Such activity is called "toad kissing."

Questions—Colorado River Toad

1. Which of the following is false?

A. Tasting *Bufo alvarius* skin can cause hallucinations.
B. Toads actually can be smoked.
C. Bufo toads contain a hallucinogen related to N, N-dimethyltryptamine.
D. Anticholinergic symptoms following *B. alvarius* exposures are common.
E. Seizures have been described after large exposures to the Colorado River toad.

PEYOTE

In the United States, the hallucinogenic peyote cactus grows almost exclusively in "peyote gardens," a narrow strip of the South Texas chaparral country east of Laredo. In its natural form the cactus, whose scientific name is *Lophophora williamsii*, is a squat ground-hugging plant about one inch tall and 2 to 3 inches across, with a tapering, turnip-shaped root. Dealers known as "peyoteros" clip off the above-ground portion of the plant and dry it.

The dried plant, or button, generally is chewed, although it is sometimes used to brew a hallucinogenic tea. Peyote buttons are round, fleshy tops from the cactus that are sliced and dried for prolonged storage. The plant is called peyote, mescal button, or mescal. The toxin, mescaline, is the major hallucinogenic agent among at least 16 alkaloids derived from this plant.

Clinical Presentations

Mescaline is rapidly absorbed and produces a phase of mild gastrointestinal distress (nausea, vomiting, and rarely diarrhea) within 30 to 60 minutes followed by a phase of sympathomimetic effects (mydriasis, tachycardia, hypertension, diaphoresis, and tremor). Nystagmus, ataxia, and hyperreflexia also may occur. The sensory phase begins after the nausea and vomiting subsides and peaks between 4 to 6 hours after ingestion. The phase is similar to LSD intoxication and is characterized by vivid visual hallucinations. Although the sensorium remains clear, emotional lability, anxiety, and panic reactions predispose such patients to self-inflicted or accidental trauma. Symptoms usually resolve about 12 hours after ingestion.

Toxic Dosage/Death

An average mescaline dose of 5 mg / kg produces psychic effects and visual hallucinations. Each button contains the equivalent of 45 mg of mescaline. Mescaline doses over 20 mg / kg can be associated with hypertension, bradycardia, and respiratory depression, but death from the drug is less common than traumatic fatalities resulting from altered perception.

Treatment

- A quiet dark environment and calm reassurance provide the best setting.
- Diazepam is the sedative of choice (orally or intravenously) if a reassuring environment does not calm the patient.

Questions—Peyote

1. Which of the following regarding the peyote cactus is false?
   A. Peyote can be ingested via tea.
   B. Peyote is produced frequently in clandestine labs.
   C. Mescaline is the major hallucinogenic agent derived from this plant.
   D. Scientific name is *Lophophora williamsii*.
   E. B and D

2. A peyote "button"
   A. Is part of a plant chewed for its hallucinogenic effect.
   B. Is a shell found near the roots of the plant.
   C. Contains about 1 gram of mescaline.
   D. Is a type of rash associated with peyote use.
   E. Is a rare type of peyote.

MORNING-GLORY FAMILY

The seeds of certain members of the morning glory family contain psychotomimetic indole compounds that are structurally related to LSD. *Ipomoea violacea* and *Turbina corymbosa* (popularly known as ololiuqui) have been used in religious rites since Aztec times in Mexico. In the 1960s, the publication of the hallucinogenic properties of these seeds in the popular press led to an upsurge of morning glory seed consumption among experimenting teenagers and young adults.

Other members of the Convolvulaceae (e.g., Argyreia and Strictocardia) also contain large amounts of these mind-altering indole compounds. The black seeds of *Argyreia nervosa* (wood rose) have been used by poorer Hawaiians as an inexpensive hallucinogen, but adverse side effects (e.g., constipation, lethargy, nausea, and blurred vision) limit its use.

Pathophysiology

The mind-altering compounds of the morning glory family are identical to the ergot alkaloids found in the ergot fungus (*C. purpurea*), which probably was responsible for the epidemic outbreaks of St. Anthony's Fire (ergotism) during the Middle Ages. These compounds are closely related to LSD, isoergine, chanoclavine, elymoclavine, lysergol, ergonovine, and pennilavine. Ergine, which has about 10% of LSD's potency, appears to be the major alkaloid. The alkaloids chanoclavine and elymoclavine probably have no psychotomimetic effects.

Clinical Presentations

Clinical effects are dose dependent and similar to those caused by the sympathomimetic and hallucinogenic properties of LSD. Ingestion of violacea seeds may produce dilated pupils, hyperreflexia, facial erythema, a dissociative state, and emotional lability within 3 hours. Other reported adverse effects include nausea, vomiting, numbness, cool extremities, lethargy, uterine stimulation, and hypotension after intravenous injection. Like LSD, morning glory seeds can cause panic reactions, paranoia, violent behavior, and changes in perception and sensation when ingested.

Treatment

- Management involves reassurance to calm the patient and a protective environment to prevent self-harm, similar to LSD treatment. Diazepam is the sedative of choice.
- Normally, symptoms resolve within 8 hours.

Questions—Morning Glory Family

1. Which of the following is false?
   A. The mind-altering compounds of the morning glory family are identical to the ergot alkaloids found in the ergot fungus (*Claviceps purpurea*), which probably was responsible for the epidemic outbreaks of St. Anthony's Fire (ergotism) during the Middle Ages.
   B. Diazepam may be used to sedate individuals high on morning glory seeds.
   C. Like LSD, morning glory seeds can cause panic reactions, marked paranoia, violent behavior, and persistent changes in perception and sensation when ingested.

D. In the 1960s, the publication of the hallucinogenic properties of these seeds in the popular press led to an upsurge of morning glory seed consumption among young adults.
E. None of the above

2. **Signs of morning glory intoxication include**
A. Nausea, vomiting, numbness, cool extremities and lethargy
B. Hallucinations
C. Uterine atony
D. A and B
E. A, B and C

NUTMEG

Nutmeg (*Myristica fragrans*) has been widely used as a medicinal agent for such diseases as rheumatism, cholera, madness, and flatulence, and as an aphrodisiac and abortifacient. Hallucinations may occur after large ingestions. Mace toxicity is reported rarely, whereas numerous cases of nutmeg toxicity appear in the medical literature.

Nutmeg is a bushy tree, 30 to 40 feet high, with spreading branches and a yellow fleshy fruit. When the husk splits, a scarlet aril appears covering a single glossy brown seed. The tree is grown commercially on the island of Grenada. When dried, the scarlet aril is known as mace.

Pathophysiology

Nutmeg contains from 5% to 15% volatile oils, which apparently contain the active ingredient responsible for toxicity. A number of aromatic ethers have been isolated, of which myristicin is the major compound. However, pure myristicin does not completely reproduce nutmeg toxicity in either animals or humans. Part of the effects of nutmeg may be attributed to suspected metabolic products of myristicin. These include the amphetamine derivatives 3-methoxy-4, 5-methylenedioxyamphetamine (MMDA) and p-methoxyamphetamine (PMA).

Clinical Presentations

Symptoms appear within 3 to 6 hours of ingestion and generally resolve by 24 hours. Initially, nausea, vomiting, abdominal pain, chest pain, restlessness, agitation, tremor, and a feeling of doom occur. Alternating periods of lethargy and delirium may follow. Earlier case studies suggest the appearance of cold extremities, weak pulses, and shallow respirations as well as hallucinations (visual changes are more common) resulting from spacial and color distortions. Facial flushing, tachycardia, hypertension, dry mouth and delirium may simulate anticholinergic poisoning, but miosis is more common than mydriasis.

Toxic Dosage/Death

Approximately 10 to 50 grams of nutmeg is required to produce symptoms. (One nutmeg weighs about 6 grams.) Variation in toxicity may result from the loss of essential oils from the ground nutmeg. Two whole nutmegs have caused moderate toxicity while 18 grams of finely ground nutmeg powder has resulted in prolonged periods of obtundation.

Treatment

GUT DECONTAMINATION

Decontamination measures theoretically are beneficial within the first several hours, but little recent medical literature is available to guide treatment.

ELIMINATION ENHANCEMENT

These methods have not been utilized with nutmeg ingestions.

SUPPORTIVE MEASURES

- Management is supportive. Sedatives must be used with caution because alternating periods of delirium and lethargy are possible.

Questions—Nutmeg

1. **Nutmeg (*Myristica fragrans*) has not been widely used as a medicinal agent for**
A. Rheumatism
B. Cholera
C. Madness
D. Flatulence
E. Leprosy

2. **Symptoms in overdose may include**
A. Nausea, vomiting, abdominal pain, and chest pain
B. Restlessness, agitation, tremor, and a feeling of doom
C. Facial flushing, tachycardia, hypertension, hypersalivation and delirium
D. A and B
E. All of the above

KHAT

Khat (*Catha edulis*) is a euphoriant and sympathomimetic that is an integral part of the Yemen culture, where urban khat sessions are a common social gathering after lunch. Khat is a 20-foot-high, leafy bush that grows in Yemen, Ethiopia, and East Africa.

Pathophysiology

Fresh khat leaves contain cathine (phenylpropanolamine), cathinone, and norephedrine, which are similar structurally to amphetamine and possess strong stimulant properties. Cathinone is the ketone congener of cathine and probably is the principal active sympathomimetic ingredient. Urine screens for phenylpropanolamine will be positive after khat chewing, because most methods cannot distinguish between cathinone and phenylpropanolamine. In addition, phenylpropanolamine is a khat metabolite.

Clinical Presentations

Most khat is consumed in a social setting where mild euphoria and hyperactivity result. Like other sympathomimetic drugs, khat can produce mydriasis, hypertension, tachycardia, hyperthermia, anorexia, garrulousness, mood elevation, and arousal. Social and medical problems such as depression, malnutrition, insomnia, emotional lability, gastritis, and impotence have been attributed to its use. Toxic psychosis has resulted from khat chewing and is characterized by hyperactivity, pressured speech, anorexia, insomnia, and paranoid ideations.

Treatment

- Treatment is supportive. Symptoms have disappeared with thioridazine therapy and by ceasing khat use.

Questions—Khat

1. **Which of the following is false?**
   A. Toxic psychosis has resulted from khat chewing and is characterized by hyperactivity, pressured speech, anorexia, insomnia, and paranoid ideations.
   B. Fresh khat leaves contain cathine (phenylpropanolamine), cathinone, and norephedrine, which are structurally similar to amphetamine and possess strong stimulant properties.
   C. Urine screens for phenylpropanolamine generally will not be positive after khat chewing.
   D. Most khat is consumed in a social setting where mild euphoria and hyperactivity result.
   E. Khat is a 20-foot-high leafy bush that grows in Yemen, Ethiopia, and East Africa.

Answers

Introduction to Hallucinogenic Drugs

1. C 2. B

Lysergic Acid Diethylamide

1. A 2. A 3. E 4. D 5. A

N, N-Dimethyltryptamine

1. C 2. E

Colorado River Toad

1. D

Peyote

1. B 2. A

Morning Glory Family

1. E 2. D

Nutmeg

1. E 2. E

Khat

1. C

SELECTED READINGS

1. Aghajanian G. Serotonin and the action of LSD in the brain. Psychiatr Ann 1994;24:137–41.
2. Farnsworth NR. Hallucinogenic plants. Science 1968;162:1086–1092.
3. Gallagher L. Smoking toad. NY Times Mag, June 5, 1994, pp. 48–49.
4. Ingram AL. Morning glory seed reaction. JAMA 1964;190:107–108.
5. Payne RB. Nutmeg intoxication. N Engl Med J 1973;269:36.
6. Schultes RE. Hallucinogens of plant origin. Science 1969;163:245–254.
7. Wason S. LSD intoxication. Ann Emerg Med 1985;14:487.

CHAPTER 21

Marijuana and Cannabinoids

INTRODUCTION

Marijuana is the most commonly used illicit drug in the United States. Marijuana refers to the dried leaves and flowers of the Indian hemp plant, *Cannabis sativa*, which are cultivated in temperate and tropical environments for their psychological effects. Cannabis is the collective term for the bioactive substances derived, either naturally or synthetically, from this plant. Δ^9-Tetrahydrocannabinol (Δ^9-THC) is believed to be the most active ingredient. Dronabinol is an oral Δ^9-THC drug approved as a schedule II drug in the United States for the treatment of nausea and vomiting in chemotherapy patients.

Herbal use of marijuana dates back to the Chinese Emperor Shen Nung in 2737 BC. By the middle of the 19th century, medicinal use of marijuana for asthma, analgesia, seizures, sedation, muscle relaxation, and anorexia was common in Western Europe. Concern over the association of marijuana with heroin abuse, violent behavior, sexual deviation, and physical addiction led to the 1937 Marijuana Tax Act, which banned both medical and recreational use. Illicit use of marijuana spread enormously during the 1960s.

Whether or not habitual marijuana use causes chronic adverse effects remains controversial. The ambiguity surrounding the dangers of this drug as well as its cheap availability adds to its popularity. Suspected chronic effects of marijuana smoking include impairment of short-term memory and learning, reduced pulmonary function, a possibly increased risk of cancer and other lung diseases, decreased sperm count and motility, interference with ovulation and prenatal development, reduced immune response, adverse cardiovascular effects, and development of an "amotivational syndrome" in adolescents.

Marijuana may be useful in the treatment of acute glaucoma, asthma, and the severe nausea and vomiting associated with chemotherapy. Cardiovascular effects such as tachycardia, conjunctival erythema, and a slight rise in blood pressure commonly occur during therapeutic marijuana use.

Drowsiness, dry mouth, dizziness, disorientation, and inability to concentrate also are common. Patients may exhibit anxiety, paranoia, visual hallucinations, and manic psychosis. An individual's response to recreational use of marijuana depends on dose, personality, expectation of the user, and setting. Initial effects range from euphoria, perceptual alterations, and relaxation at low dose to depersonalization, pressured speech, paranoia, and manic psychosis at high dose.

Questions—Introduction to Marijuana and Cannabinoids

1. **The schedule II drug Δ^9-tetrahydrocannabinol also is known as**
   A. Droperidol
   B. Dronabinol
   C. Demerol
   D. Dexedrine
   E. None of the above

Answers to questions in shaded boxes appear at the end of the chapter.

2. Marijuana may be useful in treatment of all the following except
A. Amblyopia
B. Acute glaucoma
C. Asthma
D. Nausea and vomiting associated with chemotherapy
E. A and B

MARIJUANA AND CANNABINOIDS

The Indian hemp plant, C. *sativa*, is an annual herb that is well adapted and easily cultivated in temperate and tropical environments. All parts of both female and male plants contain the primary psychoactive substance, Δ^9-THC. Cannabinoids are monoterpenoid compounds that are extracted from C. *sativa* and their carboxylic acid metabolites, analogues, and transformation products. The Cannabis plant contains at least 61 unique cannabinoids as well as over 300 natural compounds including alcohols, steroids, sugars, fatty acids, phenols, and terpenes. During pyrolysis, little interconversion or isomerization of cannabinoids occurs.

The content of natural cannabinoids in marijuana is highly variable and depends on factors such as rainfall, sunshine, temperature, genetic composition, altitude, and soil fertility. The highest drug concentrations are found in the flowering tops (bracts), with decreasing levels in the flowers, leaves, stems, seeds, and roots. Usually, the plant is dried, cut, and formed into cigarettes. Numerous terms and definitions have arisen from drug use with these compounds.

Bhang

Dried, mature leaves and flower stems that are less potent than hashish.

Blunts

Are cheap, fat, approximately 5-inch cigars that can be filled with marijuana, crack cocaine, or other drugs. The combination can stretch the use of small quantities of cheap marijuana. The harsh stench of the cheap cigar is prized for its ability to mask the sweet smell of marijuana.

Cannabis

Collective term for psychoactive compounds derived from C. *sativa*.

Ganja

Resinous mass composed of small leaves and bracts from female plants.

Hashish

The dried resin collected from flower tops. It contains varying concentrations of Δ^9-THC up to 10%. Hashish is used commonly in the Middle East and North Africa. Hashish oil is a dark viscous alcohol or gasoline extract that can contain Δ^9-THC levels up to 20%.

Marijuana

Also spelled marihuana, this refers to any part of the plant or its extract that is used to induce psychotomimetic or therapeutic effects. Synonyms include pot, Mary Jane, MJ, weed, grass, puff, hagga, and macohna.

Sinsemilla

Seedless unpollinated female marijuana that grows widely, especially in California, and has accounted for up to 85% of domestic production. The Δ^9-THC content averages about 5%.

Pathophysiology

CARDIOVASCULAR EFFECTS

In healthy subjects smoking one marijuana cigarette, cardiac output and pulse rate increase immediately whereas stroke volume and blood pressure remain constant. Peak exercise performance is reduced. Increased cardiac output, which is related solely to elevated heart rate, appears to be mediated by mechanisms other than β-adrenergic stimulation. Nicotine produces physiological changes similar to the marijuana-induced tachycardia and elevated plasma norepinephrine levels. Tachycardia is dose related, with the usual increase averaging 20 to 50 beats per minute. In higher doses, a heart rate of 140 and mild elevation of systolic blood pressure can occur.

PULMONARY EFFECTS

The inhalation of marijuana smoke or Δ^9-THC and the ingestion of Δ^9-THC produce acute bronchodilation in both healthy and asthmatic subjects that lasts at least 1 hour. The reduction of bronchoconstriction appears mediated by mechanisms other than those of current bronchodilators, since propranolol does not block the bronchodilator response. In some individuals, cough and bronchoconstriction may develop after inhalation of marijuana smoke.

OPHTHALMOLOGIC EFFECTS

Administration of marijuana smoke to normal human volunteers causes slight pupillary constriction with preservation of light reflex, marked congestion of conjunctival vessels, reduced tearing, and a dose-related reduction of intraocular pressure. The drop in intraocular pressure lasts 4 to 5 hours, and no cumulative effect or tolerance to the pressure reduction occurs. Visual acuity is not significantly altered directly, but blepharospasm, photophobia, and decreased accommodation may reduce vision. Reddened conjunctivas are a sensitive indicator of marijuana effect and are a more reliable measure of blood levels and psychotomimetic effect than tachycardia.

NEUROLOGIC EFFECTS

The mechanism of Δ^9-THC action on the central nervous system is unclear. Psychotomimetic effects (e.g., alteration in mood, sensory perception, cognition, sensorium, motor coordination, and self-perception) begin within several minutes of smoking, maximize by 20 minutes, and seldom last more than 2 or 3 hours. Heavier doses prolong effect. Ingestion delays the onset of symptoms (30 to 120 minutes) as well as peak effects (2 to 3 hours) and duration (2 to 5 hours).

In volunteers, smoking one Δ^9-THC cigarette produces euphoria, relaxation, and sleepiness, whereas group smoking promotes social interaction, friendliness, and laughter. Lethargy is prominent at high doses, especially after several hours. Subjectively, time passes more slowly, visual imagery appears more vivid, and hearing seems keener. Decreases in balance, steadiness, and muscle strength can be noted even at low doses, although impairment of simple motor tasks and reaction times requires higher doses.

Stability of stance is a sensitive measurement of marijuana-induced impairment of psychomotor function. Individuals given doses equivalent to one to two standard marijuana cigarettes tend to show reduced performance on complex tasks such as driving and flying which involve attention, sensory input, judgment, and information processing.

GASTROINTESTINAL EFFECTS

Stimulation of appetite and dry mouth are commonly reported adverse reactions to recreational marijuana use. Nausea may occur especially in inexperienced users, but Δ^9-THC also possesses antiemetic properties, as has been reported in chemotherapy patients.

ENDOCRINE EFFECTS

Chronic Δ^9-THC exposure may cause depression of plasma testosterone levels. In addition to the suppression of testicular steroid genesis and pituitary luteinizing hormone release, Δ^9-THC may disrupt the feedback regulation of the pituitary-gonadal axis.

Pharmacokinetics

ABSORPTION

- Approximately 20% of a single inhaled Δ^9-THC dose are absorbed, whereas the bioavailability of an oral dose is significantly less.
- Gastrointestinal absorption of Δ^9-THC is high. Low oral bioavailability results from a large first-pass effect because of extensive liver metabolism.
- Peak plasma levels of Δ^9-THC occur 7 to 8 minutes after initiation of smoking or intravenous infusion and decline thereafter, despite continued smoking.
- Subjective feelings of euphoria and maximal heart rate acceleration occur about 20 minutes after peak plasma Δ^9-THC levels are reached.
- After oral administration, absorption is slow and erratic. Plasma Δ^9-THC levels reach peak levels about 45 minutes after ingestion and remain relatively constant for 4 to 6 hours.
- Clinical effects begin 30 to 60 minutes after oral consumption and peak 2 to 3 hours postingestion.
- Although not rigorously tested, approximately three times larger oral doses are required to produce the same effects as smoking.

DISTRIBUTION

- Δ^9-THC is highly lipid soluble; plasma levels decline rapidly after inhalation and a slow elimination phase follows. Δ^9-THC is almost 100% protein bound.
- The volume of distribution after intravenous administration is approximately 10 L/kg.
- The mean plasma Δ^9-THC terminal half-life after intravenous infusion in chronic users is 20 hours.
- Chronic users appear to metabolize Δ^9-THC faster than nonusers do, with a mean terminal half-life for cannabinoid metabolites of 28 hours.
- The comparable terminal half-life in nonusers is slower, ranging from 25 to 57 hours.

ELIMINATION

- Δ^9-THC is almost entirely metabolized by liver enzymes, with less than 1% excreted unchanged by the kidneys.
- Hydroxylation by hepatic microsomal enzymes converts the parent drug to metabolites.
- The active metabolite is further metabolized to the inactive, polar compound 8,11-dihydroxy-Δ^9-THC, which is excreted in the urine and feces.
- Urinary excretion of Δ^9-THC metabolites is minor, accounting for about 13% to 16% of the parent compound after 3 days, and may persist for more than 8 days.
- Biliary excretion via the feces is the major route of elimination of unconjugated cannabinoid metabolites; 30% of an intravenous dose and 50% of an oral dose are excreted after 3 days.
- Up to 15% of the metabolites appear in the enterohepatic circulation, which contributes to prolonged metabolite excretion.
- Clinical studies have reported that heavy cannabis users show positive urinary cannabinoid levels for many weeks after discontinuation from the drug. This prolonged excretion could be explained by accumulation of THC in deep tissue compartments such as fat, followed by return of THC to plasma with subsequent elimination.
- The mean terminal elimination half-life of THC in plasma (4.3 days) of frequent marijuana users is longer than previously reported (range, 2.6 to 12.6 days).

Clinical Presentations

An individual's response to marijuana depends on their personality, the existing scene, prior experience, and the amount of Δ^9-THC absorbed. High doses can produce anxiety, fear, paranoia, depression, disorientation, confusion, delusions, and hallucinations. Children and patients with underlying psychiatric disorders are particularly susceptible. Most adverse reactions respond to reassurance given by peers.

PULMONARY EFFECTS

Bronchial and pulmonary irritation secondary to marijuana smoke is well documented. Because of its relatively poor combustibility, marijuana smoke contains 50% more polyaromatic hydrocarbons than tobacco smoke, as well as increased concentrations of pulmonary irritants such as tars, sterols, and terpenes. Serious dyspnea may be seen after intravenous use with crude marijuana extract. Few reports of marijuana-associated fatalities appear in the medical literature, and cases are not well documented clinically.

PEDIATRIC EFFECTS

Ataxic gait, labile affect, vertical and horizontal nystagmus, fine tremor, stupor, tachycardia, conjunctival hyperemia, and pallor have been noted in children who ingest marijuana cookies. Symptoms begin within several hours of exposure and usually resolve by 6 hours postexposure. Although orthostatic hypotension can occur, supine blood pressure usually is normal.

Cannabis ingestion in children should be suspected if the following constellation of symptoms are noted: drowsiness, pupillary dilation, hypotonia, presence of dark particles (e.g., granules, leaves, or resin) in the mouth, lid lag, and the absence of history or symptoms indicative of trauma, central nervous system infection, or seizures. Hashish resin ingestion in children has led to rapid obtundation, occasional opisthotonic-like movements alternating with hypotonia, or meningismus. Occasional cyanosis, right bundle-branch block, tachycardia or apnea with bradycardia may be observed. Children usually recover completely 10 to 36 hours after ingestion.

PSYCHIATRIC EFFECTS

Acute toxic psychosis associated with marijuana use has been reported. Suicidal ideation, anxiety, and paranoia accompany the organic psychosis, and may last for 1 to 11 days. The development of acute psychosis after chronic use remains controversial because of questions about the contribution of premorbid personalities and multiple-drug use. Undifferentiated manic, schizophreniform, and confusional psychoses have been reported in heavy marijuana users admitted to psychiatric hospitals.

CARDIOVASCULAR EFFECTS

Elevated plasma norepinephrine levels and tachycardia represent theoretical risks to patients with cardiovascular disease. Myocardial infarction and pulmonary edema have been reported in close association with marijuana smoking. Such cases are rare, and cardiovascular risks are speculative at this time.

HYPERSENSITIVITY EFFECTS

Marijuana sensitivity occurs commonly in patients with airborne plant pollen allergies, on the basis of skin test reactivity.

CHRONIC PULMONARY EFFECTS

Lung samples taken at autopsy from heavy marijuana smokers show focal infiltrates of heavily pigmented macrophages around bronchioles, focal ulceration of columnar epithelium, and focal fibrosis. These accelerated histopathological changes seem dose related and may appear in the absence of concomitant tobacco smoking. Although paraquat may contaminate marijuana products, high combustion levels in marijuana cigarettes tend to pyrolyze the paraquat and render it biologically inactive.

The prevalence of bronchitis or emphysema among heavy marijuana users remains to be determined. Studies have shown that most illegally obtained marijuana is contaminated with Aspergillus species, most often *Aspergillus flavus* and *Aspergillus fumigatus*. In immunocompromised patients, invasive pulmonary aspergillosis may ensue.

CHRONIC PSYCHIATRIC EFFECTS

Chronic marijuana use among adolescents has been associated with an entity called "amotivational syndrome" characterized by apathy, loss of effectiveness at completing complex tasks, easy frustration, poor concentration, diminished goal-directed behavior, and overestimation of one's productivity and accomplishments. Whether or not this syndrome represents a pharmacological effect of chronic marijuana use or developmental frustration remains to be determined. The similarity of psychosocial patterns between problem drinking and habitual marijuana use, as well as the correlation of marijuana use with adolescent problem drinking, suggests that marijuana use in this setting is at least a part of the syndrome of adolescent problem behavior.

CARCINOGENIC EFFECTS

Several studies suggest an association between chronic marijuana smoking and cancer of the mouth and larynx. Marijuana smoking also may be associated with an increased risk for the development of respiratory tract malignancies. Several cases have been reported of respiratory tract malignancy in young, long-term marijuana smokers. The smoking of one marijuana cigarette leads to the deposition in the lower respiratory tract of a fourfold greater quantity of tar than smoking a filtered tobacco cigarette of comparable weight.

INTRAVENOUS EFFECTS

Severe multisystemic organ dysfunction may result from the intravenous administration of crude marijuana. Symptoms such as severe headache, blurred vision, diaphoresis, chills, dizziness, and dyspnea typically begin within 20 minutes, followed in several hours by fever, diffuse myalgias, and gastrointestinal distress. Hypotension, renal insufficiency, and rhabdomyolysis have been reported. Laboratory abnormalities include transient leukocytosis, thrombocytopenia, mild hepatic aminotransferase elevation, transient hypoalbuminemia, moderately elevated muscle enzymes, myoglobinuria, and electrolyte imbalance.

Toxic Dosage/Death

Prediction of toxic reactions is complicated by the fact that clinical effects of Δ^9-THC depend on personality, setting, mode, and dose. Marijuana plants grown in the United States contain low levels of Δ^9-THC, ranging from 1% to 3%. Hence, an average 500-mg marijuana cigarette contains between 5 and 15 mg of Δ^9-THC. More potent home-grown varieties may attain Δ^9-THC levels as high as 5% to 6%.

Exotic varieties (e.g., Acapulco Gold, Thai Stick, Buddha, and Colombian) are more potent than less expensive commercial varieties, with Δ^9-THC concentrations ranging from 6.9% to 19.1%. Most adult intoxications are benign, with the exception of multisystemic failure resulting from intravenous injection of crude marijuana extract. Children are more susceptible to toxic reactions but usually recover uneventfully.

Drug Interactions

Additive effects on psychomotor performance may follow concomitant use of marijuana and ethanol. Combinations of cocaine and marijuana appear to increase heart rates above levels seen with either drug alone. Increases plateau at about 50 beats/minute above normal. Multiple-drug abuse (alcohol, amphetamines, benzodiazepines, cocaine, and opiates) continues to be a problem with marijuana users. Cocaine-dependent individuals often appear to be dependent on marijuana. Phencyclidine may be intentionally combined with marijuana ("superweed") to obtain a more intense hallucinogenic experience.

Pregnancy/Lactation

In experimental animals, Δ^9-THC crossed the placenta but was present in lower concentrations (by a factor of 5 to 6) in fetal blood than in maternal tissue. Infants whose mothers had positive urine assays for marijuana exhibited impaired fetal growth (lower birth weight, decrease in length) in one study. The study did not demonstrate a cause-and-effect relationship, however. There does not appear to be an increased risk of spontaneous abortion, effects on birth weight or head circumference, or effects on the rate of minor or major physical anomalies because of prenatal marijuana use. Long-term development and behavioral effects remain to be determined.

Analysis of breast milk in a chronic heavy marijuana user revealed an eightfold accumulation of Δ^9-THC in breast milk compared with maternal plasma. Examination of the baby's stool showed that both Δ^9-THC and its active metabolite, Δ^9-THC, were present. The result suggests that a nursing infant can absorb Δ^9-THC from mother's milk.

Laboratory

ANALYTIC METHODS

Enzyme-multiplied immunoassay technique (EMIT) may detect urine cannabinoids for an average of 27 days (maximum, 46 days) after cessation of chronic marijuana use. An EMIT screen may test false negative if a specimen is adulterated by the acidity of bleach, detergent, salt, or vinegar or diluted in water from a tap or a toilet bowl. Passive inhalation of marijuana smoke is unlikely to result in a positive cannabinoid urine screening test, except for heavy prolonged exposure.

BLOOD LEVELS

The subjective "high" of marijuana smoking lags 20 to 30 minutes behind peak plasma levels (usually obtained 7 to 8 minutes after initiation of smoking) and then declines slowly to baseline over 4 hours. Effects are dose related, and smoking higher-potency cigarettes prolongs psychotomimetic effects. Initial peak levels sampled 15 minutes after the initiation of smoking are between 50 and 70 ng/mL. An average "high" occurs when the Δ^9-THC level is about 9 ng/mL. Conjunctival injection consistently occurred with plasma Δ^9-THC levels exceeding 5 ng/mL and was more reliable than tachycardia in predicting clinical effect. Generally, impairment of driving as judged by trained observers does not correlate well with Δ^9-THC levels.

URINE

A combination of screening by an EMIT and confirmation by gas chromatography/mass spectrometry (GC/MS) will yield almost 100% accuracy in testing for marijuana. Positive urine tests indicate only the likelihood of prior use and do not correlate with psychomotor impairment. The urine cannabinoid concentration is at best a poor guide to the amount actually taken, as a low level may result from either a large dose taken a long time previously or a small dose taken recently. Cannabinoids are detectable for an average of 1 to 2 days and as long as 7 days after a single marijuana cigarette. Smoking an additional marijuana cigarette extends the detection time 1 to 2 days.

Treatment

GUT DECONTAMINATION

Adults require only supportive care postingestion, except for obtunded patients, for whom lavage is recommended within several hours of ingestion. Syrup of ipecac has some theoretical advantages in children within 2 hours of the ingestion of a whole marijuana cigarette or cookie. Consumption of less than one cigarette causes minimal toxicity. Activated charcoal and cathartics may also be administered within the first 2 to 3 hours.

ELIMINATION ENHANCEMENT

Such methods have not been shown to impact on the treatment of marijuana intoxication.

SUPPORTIVE MEASURES

- Serious alterations of vital signs in casual users are extremely rare. Minor decreases in blood pressure often respond well to Trendelenburg's position and intravenous fluids.
- Hypovolemia from severe gastrointestinal fluid loss after administration of intravenous crude marijuana extract is common and requires large amounts of crystalloid fluids. Careful management of both fluid and electrolyte balance is necessary, because adult respiratory distress syndrome and acute renal failure may develop several days after intravenous use.
- Depressed levels of consciousness should be treated with usual measures, including glucose, naloxone, and thiamine. Most drug-induced psychoses are self-limited and resolve within 6 hours. Chronic marijuana users may display prolonged psychosis lasting up to a week.
- If possible, physical restraints and neuroleptic drugs should be avoided. However, both the patient and medical staff must be protected from aggressive behavior. Most patients do well in a normally lit room with a few familiar people. Reassurance by the physician is helpful and should not involve attempts to dissuade the patient from further use while the patient is intoxicated.
- Diazepam may be necessary to sedate the psychotic patient. Psychotic symptoms also may respond to haloperidol (5 mg IM), but dystonic reactions or seizures may complicate its use.
- Most patients who display dysphoric reactions require no laboratory studies to aid management other than those necessary to confirm the diagnosis.
- Because rare cases of intravenous crude marijuana extract produce multisystemic failure, laboratory analysis should include complete blood count, electrolytes, calcium, glucose, creatinine, blood urea nitrogen, hepatic transaminases, coagulation studies, electrocardiogram, chest x-ray, and urinalysis for myoglobin and protein.

Questions—Marijuana and Cannabinoids

1. Which of the following terms is associated with the incorrect definition?
   A. Bhang is dried, mature leaves, flowers and stems.
   B. Blunts are cheap, fat cigars filled with marijuana and other illicit drugs.
   C. Cannabis is a collective term for compounds derived from *Cannabis sativa.*
   D. Ganja is seedless, unpollinated, female marijuana that accounts for 85% of domestic production.
   E. Hashish is dried resin collected from flower tops containing up to 10% Δ^9-THC

2. Smoking marijuana causes
   A. No cardiac effects on healthy patients
   B. Dose related tachycardia
   C. Increased peak exercise performance
   D. Blood pressure increase with one cigarette smoked by a healthy patient
   E. None of the above

3. Marijuana smoke causes
   A. Bronchodilation
   B. Conjunctival congestion
   C. Reduced tearing
   D. Reduced intraocular pressure
   E. All of the above

4. Absorption of marijuana
   A. Results in peak levels 7 to 8 hours after smoking is initiated
   B. Results in peak levels 7 to 8 hours after oral ingestion
   C. Is slow and erratic after oral administration.
   D. Results in clinical effects 7 to 8 minutes after oral ingestion
   E. None of the above

5. Children who ingest cannabis or hashish
   A. May be drowsy and hypotonic
   B. May have symptoms suggestive of meningitis
   C. May have electrocardiogram abnormalities
   D. A and B
   E. A, B and C

6. Chronic cough in a chronic marijuana user may reflect
   A. Respiratory tract malignancy
   B. Aspergillosis, particularly if the patient is immunocompromised
   C. Tics, a common neurologic side effect
   D. A and B
   E. A, B and C

7. **Conjunctival injection is more reliable than tachycardia in predicting clinical effect of marijuana smoking.**
   A. True
   B. False

8. **Low urine cannabinoid levels may result from**
   A. A large dose taken a long time previously
   B. A small dose taken recently
   C. Brief passive exposure to marijuana smoke
   D. A and B
   E. A, B and C

DRONABINOL

Dronabinol (Marinol®) is Δ^9-tetrahydrocannabinol. It has been available since 1985 to treat nausea and vomiting associated with cancer chemotherapy in patients who fail to respond to conventional antiemetic therapy. It was approved by the Food and Drug Administration (FDA) in 1992 for the treatment of anorexia associated with weight loss in patients with acquired immunodeficiency syndrome (AIDS).

Dronabinol has an antiemetic effect similar to that of prochlorperazine but less than that of metoclopramide. The results of small clinical trials of THC suggest that it can reduce tremor and spasticity in some patients with multiple sclerosis. Overdose may be accompanied by disturbing psychotic symptoms such as hallucinations, delusions, and paranoid feelings. Few deaths have been reported from the use of dronabinol. Dronabinol is naturally occurring and is extracted from C. *sativa*.

Pathophysiology

Dronabinol is a centrally acting sympathomimetic drug that acts at cannabinoid receptor sites in the brain.

Pharmacokinetics

ABSORPTION

- Dronabinol is absorbed slowly from the gastrointestinal tract.
- It undergoes first-pass metabolism and its bioavailability after oral administration is 10% to 20%.

DISTRIBUTION

- Dronabinol has a large volume of distribution (about 10 L/kg).
- It is 97% to 99% bound to plasma proteins.

ELIMINATION

- Dronabinol is metabolized to 11-hydroxydronabinol, which is similar in activity to the parent compound.
- Less than 5% of an oral dose is recovered unchanged in the feces.

Clinical Presentations

Signs and symptoms following dronabinol intoxication include drowsiness, euphoria, heightened sensory awareness, altered time perception, reddened conjunctiva, dry mouth, and tachycardia. Following moderate intoxication, memory impairment, depersonalization, mood alteration, urinary retention, and reduced bowel motility may be present. Following severe intoxication, symptoms and signs may include decreased motor coordination, lethargy, slurred speech, and postural hypotension. Apprehensive patients may experience panic reactions and seizures may occur in patients with existing seizure disorders. Psychological and physiologic dependence has been noted in healthy individuals. Addiction is uncommon and may follow prolonged high-dose administration.

Toxic Dosage/Death

The estimated lethal human dose of intravenous dronabinol is 30 mg/kg. Significant central nervous system symptoms have followed oral doses of 0.4 mg/kg.

Pregnancy/Lactation

The FDA has placed dronabinol in pregnancy risk category C. Dronabinol is concentrated in and secreted in human breast milk.

Laboratory

ANALYTIC METHODS

Analysis of body fluids can be performed by either EMIT or radioimmunoassay (RIA) of metabolites in urine. Metabolites may remain for a few days or longer after a single dose and up to a month after chronic exposure.

BLOOD LEVELS

Laboratory tests do not differentiate acute from chronic intoxication and are not useful in managing acute overdoses.

Treatment

GUT DECONTAMINATION

A potentially serious oral ingestion, if recent, should be managed with gut decontamination. In unconscious patients with a secure airway, instill activated charcoal (1 gram/kg) via nasogastric tube. A saline cathartic or sorbitol may be added to the first dose of activated charcoal.

ELIMINATION ENHANCEMENT

Such methods have not been shown to impact the treatment of dronabinol intoxication.

SUPPORTIVE MEASURES

- Patients experiencing depressive, hallucinatory, or psychotic reactions should be placed in a quiet room and offered reassurance. Benzodiazepines may be used for the treatment of agitation.
- Hypotension usually responds to Trendelenburg's position and/or intravenous fluids. Pressors rarely are required.

Questions—Dronabinol

1. **Dronabinol is legally used for**
   A. Treatment of anorexia nervosa in teenagers not previously using illicit drugs
   B. Treatment of nausea and vomiting with cancer chemotherapy in patients who were unresponsive to conventional treatment
   C. Treatment of spasticity in multiple sclerosis
   D. Treatment of nausea and vomiting with motion sickness
   E. All of the above

2. **Dronabinol intoxication can cause**
   A. Dry mouth
   B. Urinary retention
   C. Postural hypotension
   D. Mood alteration
   E. All of the above

Answers

Introduction

1. B 2. A

Marijuana and Cannabinoids

1. D 2. B 3. E 4. C 5. E 6. D
7. A 8. D

Dronabinol

1. B 2. E

SELECTED READINGS

Marijuana and Cannabinoids

1. Council on Scientific Affairs: Marijuana: Its health hazards and therapeutic potentials. JAMA 1981;246:1823–1827.
2. Doblin R, Kleiman MAR. Medical use of marijuana. Ann Intern Med 1991; 114:809–810.
3. Gerostamoulos J, Drummer OH. Incidence of psychoactive cannabinoids in drivers killed in motor vehicle accidents. J Forens Sci 1993;38:649–656.
4. Miller NS, Klahr AL, Gold MS, et al. The prevalence of marijuana (cannabis) use and dependence in cocaine dependence. NY State J Med 1990;90:491–492.
5. Morland J, Bugge A, Shuterud B, et al. Cannabinoids in blood and urine after passive inhalation of cannabis smoke. J Forens Sci 1985;30:997–1002.
6. Qazi QH, Milman DH. Nontherapeutic use of psychoactive drugs. N Engl J Med 1983;309:797–798.
7. Wu T-C, Tashkin DP, Djahed B, Rose JE. Pulmonary hazards of smoking marijuana as compared with tobacco. N Engl J Med 1988;318:347–351.

Dronabinol

1. Hellinger FJ. The cost of Marinol (dronabinol). JAMA 1993;270:2810.
2. Jaffe JH. Drug addiction and drug abuse. In: Gilman AG, Rall TW, Nies AS, Taylor P, eds. Goodman and Gilman's the Pharmacological Basis of Therapeutics. 8th ed. New York: Pergamon Press, 1990:549–553.
3. Relman AS. Marijuana and health. N Engl J Med 1982; 306:603–605.

ACKNOWLEDGMENTS

Thanks to Alison Deutsch, MD for contributing the questions in this chapter.

CHAPTER 22
Phencyclidine

INTRODUCTION

Phencyclidine (PCP) was first synthesized in 1926, however its medical effects were not explored until the 1950s when chemists at Parke-Davis and Company discovered its anesthetic properties. The US Government issued a patent for phencyclidine in 1963. Adverse psychological reactions, including hallucinations, delirium, disorientation, extreme agitation, muscle rigidity and seizures were subsequently noted in humans postanesthesia. These adverse effects led to the voluntary discontinuation of marketing of the drug.

Many street names have been associated with PCP use. These include angel dust, dust, hog, KJ, mist, peace, peace pill, Shermans, snorts, T, wacky weed, and zombie dust. The most popular form of use involves the sprinkling of varying amounts of PCP (1 to 100 mg) on parsley or marijuana and smoking the substance in a "joint." Special cigarettes called "Shermans" are dipped in liquid PCP before smoking. PCP usually appears as the ready soluble hydrochloride salt, because the pure base is insoluble. When sold as "angel dust" for marijuana, PCP is incorporated into the leafy mixture. Many active, inert, and volatile substances may be found in illicit phencyclidine.

The structurally related anesthetic ketamine is a legal derivative, which is marketed as a dissociative anesthetic. Illicit uses included the "peace pill" in San Francisco and "hog" in New York City in the late 1960s. More widespread use occurred in the 1970s. PCP often is disguised or used with other drugs such as LSD, cocaine, or marijuana. The effectiveness of PCP by oral, nasal, pulmonary, and intravenous (IV) routes permits its use as an adulterant in many drugs of abuse.

By the late 1970s, synthetic PCP analogues began to appear in street samples. These include PCE (cyclohexamine), TCP (the thiophene analogue), PHP (phenylcyclohexylpyrrolidine), PCC (a synthetic intermediate containing a cyano group), and ketamine (a legal derivative). Deaths have been reported, mostly as the result of disordered thought processes or poor neurosensory control that leads to trauma or drowning. The direct effects of the drug usually are not fatal.

Pathophysiology

Although classified as a dissociative anesthetic, PCP has stimulant, depressant, hallucinogenic and analgesic properties depending on personality, dosage, route of administration and, possibly, genetic predisposition.

Pharmacokinetics

ABSORPTION

- PCP is well absorbed by oral, pulmonary, and nasal routes.
- Oral bioavailability averages 72% of 1-mg doses in human volunteers.

DISTRIBUTION

- The volume of distribution of PCP is 6.2 L/kg. The plasma protein binding of PCP is 65%.
- Half-life is 24 and 21 hours after smoking and ingestion in human volunteers, respectively.

ELIMINATION

- PCP is lipid soluble and hydroxylation occurs in the liver after slow release from adipose tissue.
- Urine samples are positive an average of 2 weeks and most samples are negative by 30 days.
- Without acidification, renal clearance of unchanged drug averages only 9%.

Clinical Presentations

Most patients present with altered behavioral and thought patterns, which may lead to poor judgment and bizarre actions that can cause serious trauma. As the dose increases, medical consequences such as coma, hyperthermia, catatonia, and rhabdomyolysis may occur. Patients may present with various combinations of central nervous system stimulation and depression, cholinergic (e.g., diaphoresis, miosis, bronchospasm, salivation) and anticholinergic effects (e.g., tachycardia, mydriasis, urinary retention), and adrenergic effects. The most common physical findings are nystagmus (horizontal, vertical, or rotatory) and hypertension. Extremely high blood pressure is unusual, as are hypertension-induced complications.

Intoxication may be graded according to clinical presentation. Minor intoxications generally recover quickly and do not require hospitalization. Such patterns include lethargy, stupor, or bizarre behavior. Mild agitation is associated with a clear sensorium and nonviolent behavior, which is associated with increased motor activity. Generally, agitation resolves within hours. Euphoria, mimicking alcohol intoxication, may be present.

Major intoxications may be associated with consciousness ranging from fully alert to comatose. Coma may occur suddenly, but often develops after a period of bizarre behavior. Coma may be short-lived or last up to a week. Mental status changes include confusion, disorientation, auditory and visual hallucinations, delusions, and psychosis identical to acute schizophrenia. Acute toxic psychosis manifested by extremely combative behavior and agitation, may require physical or chemical restraints to manage.

Medical complications of PCP may include seizures, hyperthermia, hypertension, rhabdomyolysis (possibly associated with acute renal failure), intracranial hemorrhage, catatonic posturing, apnea, aspiration pneumonia and cardiac arrest. Medical complications generally dictate need for hospitalization.

Toxic Dosage/Death

Low doses (1 to 10 mg) are associated with mild agitation, ataxia, nystagmus, confusion, euphoria, and emotional lability. Moderate doses (5 to 20 mg) may be associated with muscle rigidity, vomiting, salivation, hypertension, catatonia, toxic psychosis, and bizarre behavior. High doses (100 mg and above) may be associated with coma, seizures, rigidity, opisthotonus, alternating periods of consciousness, delirium, agitation, hallucinations, and death.

Pregnancy/Lactation

In utero exposure may yield symptoms of neonatal narcotic withdrawal, temperament problems, and sleep problems during the first year of life. Growth and development at 1 year are within normal limits.

Laboratory

ANALYTIC METHODS

PCP may be measured by gas chromatography/mass spectrometry.

BLOOD LEVELS

PCP blood levels do not correlate well with clinical findings. Depending on its pH, urine concentrates phencyclidine and represents an excellent screening fluid when available.

Treatment

GUT DECONTAMINATION

Emesis, lavage, and/or charcoal are of limited use. Most patients present hours after inhalation, insufflation, and/or ingestion, and generally are not helped after elimination by these methods. Presentation after oral ingestion within a few hours of use may benefit from charcoal.

ELIMINATION ENHANCEMENT

Urinary acidification, although theoretically advantageous, is virtually never indicated. Acidification does not effect liver metabolism, the main site of drug elimination.

SUPPORTIVE MEASURES

- Agitation and seizures may be treated with intravenous benzodiazepines. Other causes of agitated behavior, such as central nervous system infections, intracranial bleeds, etc., must be searched for and treated appropriately.
- Severe hypertension may be treated with antihypertensive therapy including nitroprusside and nitrates. Polydrug ingestions, such as those including cocaine, must be clinically ascertained to best guide the physician in choice of antihypertensive therapy.
- Aggressive cooling measures should be instituted for hyperthermic patients.
- Urine should be screened for myoglobin and patients should be hydrated liberally to prevent rhabdomyolysis.
- If myoglobinuria is demonstrated, volume depletion is corrected with mannitol and sodium bicarbonate in D5W.

Antidotes

PCP-specific antigen binding fragments (Fab) are being studied.

Questions—Phencyclidine

1. A legal derivative of phencyclidine used for anesthesia in the United States is
A. Urecholine
B. Halothane
C. Ketamine
D. Muscarinic acid
E. Benzocaine

2. Clinical signs of PCP use may include
A. Mydriasis
B. Miosis
C. Hypertension
D. A and B
E. A, B and C

3. A low dose of PCP is
A. 1.0 mg
B. 1.0 μg
C. 1.0 gram
D. 100 mg
E. 50 kg

4. The leading cause of death from phencyclidine is
A. Intracranial bleeding
B. Trauma related to bizarre behavior
C. Homicide related to angry drug dealers
D. Accidental overdoses
E. Malignant hypertension

Answers to questions in shaded boxes appear at the end of the chapter.

5. **The following toxicokinetic data are true about PCP, except**
   A. PCP is highly lipophilic
   B. PCP is a mild acid
   C. PCP is mostly metabolized in the liver
   D. Half life is less than 24 hours
   E. Serum levels do not correlate with clinical effects

Case Study (Question 6)

A 23-year-old male is brought in from a rock concert by police. He was found, disrobed, climbing up a wire fence in the parking lot. His friends say he was smoking "wacky weed." On arrival to the emergency department, he is screaming something about "Jimmy lives!" His vital signs reveal a blood pressure of 200/100, a respiratory rate of 22, temperature of 102.5°F, and pulse of 120. Physical exam reveals bilateral horizontal gaze nystagmus, 6-mm pupils, and abrasions.

6. **Treatment options may include all of the following, except**
   A. Mannitol for rhabdomyolysis
   B. Benzodiazepines
   C. Chemical or physical restraints
   D. Syrup of ipecac for the "weed" scenario
   E. Cooling blanket
7. **Pharmacologic symptoms suggestive of PCP use include all of the following, except**
   A. Signs of narcotic use, such as decreased respirations
   B. Anticholinergic signs, such as urinary retention
   C. Cholinergic signs, such as hypersalivation
   D. Adrenergic signs, such as hypertension
   E. Central nervous system depression
8. **Nystagmus seen in PCP overdose may be**
   A. Rotatory
   B. Horizontal
   C. Vertical
   D. B and C
   E. A, B and C
9. **A common street name for PCP is**
   A. Hog
   B. LJ
   C. Smack
   D. MPTP
   E. None of the above
10. **Which of the following is not** a synthetic PCP analogue
    A. TCP
    B. PCE
    C. Ketamine
    D. PHP
    E. MPTP

Answers

Phencyclidine

1. C	2. E	3. A	4. B	5. B	6. D
7. A	8. E	9. A	10. E		

SELECTED READINGS

1. Baldridge EB, Bessen HA. Phencyclidine. Emerg Med Clin North Am 1990; 8:541–550.
2. McCarron MM, Schulze BW, Thompson GA, et al. Acute phencyclidine intoxication: Incidence of clinical findings in 1,000 cases. Ann Emerg Med 1981;10: 237–242.
3. Thomas H, Schwartz E, Petrilli R. Droperidol versus haloperidol for chemical restraint of agitative and combative patients. Ann Emerg Med 1992;21:407–413.
4. Wasserberger J, Ordog GJ, Hardin E, et al. Violence in the emergency department. Top Emerg Med 1992;14:71–78.

CHAPTER 23
Opiates

INTRODUCTION

Opiates are controlled substances in the U.S. Interest in opiate toxicity derives from its multiple ramifications in the fields of clinical pharmacology, neurology, neurochemistry, sociology, criminology, clinical toxicology, and psychopathology. The knowledge of opiates reaches into every facet of clinical medicine. Opiate overdose produces constricted pupils, respiratory depression, and coma and is treated with naloxone and good supportive care.

Pathophysiology

Opiates are products derived from the juice of the opium poppy. The term is loosely applied to morphine derivatives. Opioids are compounds whose effects are stereospecifically antagonized by naloxone. Peptides with this property are called "opioid peptides." Opioid peptides form chemical messengers, including neurotransmitters, hormones, and neurohormones. In humans, opioid peptides are found in those areas of the nervous system where they act as part of an inhibitory system. These include the sensory and autonomic systems, limbic structures, and neuroendocrine systems. Opioid peptides normally are quiescent and are active only in stress states (e.g., anesthesia, surgery, pain, hypoxia, shock, neonatal states). Opioid receptors are divided into mu, kappa, sigma and delta types.

There are numerous naturally occurring opioid peptides including enkephalins, dynorphins and endorphins. Enkephalins are contained in short neurons and are found in the globus pallidus, hypothalamus, limbic system, raphe nuclei, spinal cord, adrenal medulla, sympathetic ganglia, and myenteric plexus of the gastrointestinal tract. Dynorphins are found in neurons of the posterior pituitary, hypothalamus, and submucosal plexus of the gastrointestinal tract. Endorphins are located in neurons in the anterior lobe of the pituitary and in the hypothalamus. So-called "beta" endorphins are elevated in runners who may even collapse without being sensitive to discomfort. Neurotransmission is largely subserved by shorter-length opioid peptides, enkephalins, and dynorphins. Neuronal or hormonal modulation is a function of longer-length peptides of all three families.

Opiates can influence host immunity. Opioid receptors are present on monocytes, neutrophils, lymphocytes, and mast cells. Infections such as viral hepatitis, pulmonary infections, endocarditis, bacteremia, cellulitis, and abscesses are common among opiate addicts. Lymphocytosis and hypergammaglobulinemia are frequently observed in opiate addicts. There are structural similarities among interferon, corticotropin, and endorphins.

Pharmacokinetics

The half-life, volume of distribution, presence of active metabolites, and peak plasma levels vary widely among the opiates and opioids. Short-acting opiates, such as fentanyl, have a half-life of 30 minutes. Methadone and buprenorphine, on the other hand, may have an 8-hour duration of action and longer half lives. See opiates below for individual toxicokinetic profiles.

Clinical Presentations

Opiate intoxication yields a conscious, yet sedated individual. Mood is normal to euphoric and the patient may appear to be "nodding." Pupils are generally pinpoint. Overdose is universally associated with pinpoint pupils, shallow and decreased respirations, and often, unconsciousness. Much of the chronic toxicity associated with opiate use is behavioral and includes crime, unsterile drug administration, impulsive behavior, family disruption, and unemployment. There is little evidence of mental illness produced by opiates, whereas abusers of depressants may exhibit depressive illness, and intellectual deterioration. Abusers of stimulants are frequently hospitalized for chronic psychosis.

OPIATE WITHDRAWAL

An opiate withdrawal syndrome consists of both "purposive" and "nonpurposive" symptoms. "Purposive" behaviors are goal-oriented, highly dependent on the observer and environment, and directed at getting more drugs. They include pleas, demands, manipulation, and symptom mimicking. Purposive behavior becomes prominent as withdrawal signs become increasingly evident.

"Nonpurposive" symptoms of withdrawal are not goal-oriented. They include lacrimation, rhinorrhea, yawning, and perspiration, which appear 8–12 hours after the last dose (in the case of heroin or methadone). These signs increase in intensity during the first 24 hours, and then become constant. Twelve to 14 hours after his last dose, the patient falls into a tossing, restless sleep known as the "yen," which lasts several hours, and then awakens more restless and miserable than before. Dilated pupils, anorexia, gooseflesh, restlessness, irritability, and tremor begin to appear.

At peak withdrawal, the patient may exhibit insomnia, anorexia, extreme restlessness and anxiety, violent yawning, sneezing, lacrimation, coryza, weakness, depression, nausea, vomiting, intestinal spasm, diarrhea, elevated heart rate, hypertension, and complaints of chilliness alternating with flushing and excessive sweating. The skin resembles that of a plucked turkey; thus the expression "cold turkey" to denote abrupt withdrawal without treatment. Pains and spasms are felt in the bones and muscles, associated with uncontrollable muscle twitching, and kicking movements—thus the expression "kicking the habit." With morphine and heroin, these symptoms peak at 36–48 hours, continue in intensity as long as 72 hours, and gradually subside over 5–10 days.

NEONATAL WITHDRAWAL

Signs of withdrawal in infants born to opiate-dependent mothers include irritability, rhythmic tremors, and high-pitched crying. Such infants frequently do not respond to holding, cuddling, or rocking and may have hypertonicity of muscles, marked sucking of hands, fists, or fingers, poor feeding, hyperactivity, sleeplessness, sweating, tachypnea, excoriations, sneezing, yawning, vomiting that may lead to dehydration, electrolyte imbalance, low-grade fever, diarrhea, and convulsions.

Hypoglycemia can cause jitteriness, irritability, and tachypnea. Such withdrawal is worse after methadone than after heroin use by the mother. Addicts taking huge quantities of opiates may have offspring with mild signs, and women receiving less than 20 mg of methadone per day may give birth to babies who are very symptomatic. Symptoms after heroin use are observed within 24 hours and those after methadone, within 72 hours. No infant should die of narcotic withdrawal; however, sudden infant death syndrome may occur. Growth patterns in these infants are often slower.

Pregnancy/Lactation

Many narcotic-dependent women are sterile with diminished libido and, if pregnant, frequently abort. They often have a poor self-image, are depressed, feel inadequate, and can be hostile. Anemia, hepatitis, cellulitis, venous thrombosis, subcutaneous abscesses, bacterial endocarditis, and venereal diseases are common. Obstetrical complications become severe if addiction is uncontrolled. These may include abortion, abruptio placentae, low-birth-weight infants with intrauterine growth retardation, and preterm birth.

Questions—Introduction to Opiates

1. Which of the following clinical manifestations would be unexpected in opiate overdose?
A. Constricted pupils
B. Respiratory depression
C. Coma
D. Euphoric mood
E. Piloerection

2. Neonatal opiate withdrawal would be expected to result in all of the following clinical manifestations except
A. Yawning
B. Seizures
C. Hypoglycemia
D. Miosis
E. Vomiting

3. The "yen" is
A. A characteristic tossing restless sleep pattern in opiate withdrawal
B. A unit of South Korean currency
C. A characteristic type of seizure seen with propoxyphene overdose
D. A term used to describe the social problems that occur with chronic opiate use (e.g., crime, family disruption and unemployment)
E. None of the above

OPIATE AGONISTS

Heroin

Heroin was first synthesized from morphine in 1874. In 1898, heroin, a trade name of the Bayer Company for diacetylmorphine, was commercially introduced as a cough remedy. It proved at least as addicting as morphine and became the drug of choice among American narcotic addicts. In the 1960s, the popularity of psychedelic substances such as LSD and the quick rise of marijuana use drew attention to the variety of drugs available. The number of heroin addicts rose. By the early 1980s, it was estimated that 550,000 persons in the U.S. were dependent

Answers to questions in shaded boxes appear at the end of the chapter.

on heroin, of whom 110,000 were in prison, 140,000 in treatment, and 310,000 neither in prison nor in treatment. At present, heroin is classified as a Schedule I substance in the U.S. as there is no currently accepted medical use.

There have been periodic resurgences of the use of heroin in the U.S. In 1994, for example, the product became more available and of sufficient purity to be used by snorting similar to cocaine. Heroin users inadvertently use multiple heroin additives, some toxic and some non-toxic. Nonfatal overdoses are common. Overdoses are frequent in subjects who use heroin with alcohol, benzodiazepines, cannabis, or amphetamines. Heroin is produced in subtropical countries from plants and may be susceptible to contamination by aflatoxins, which may in turn cause suppression of cell-mediated immunity. Heroin is generally "cut" with bulk diluent powders including mannitol, dextrose, lactose, talc, and baking soda. Bitter-tasting products such as quinine, strychnine, caffeine, phenacetin, procaine, lidocaine, lemon juice, antipyrine, boric acid, mercurous salts, and dog manure are also used to cut heroin.

Heroin is referred to as smack, TNT, white junk, noise, dujie, horse, stuff, junk, snow, harry, h, crap, Mexican brown, Persian, rufus, and dana. Illicit heroin varies in chemical and physical appearance among different countries or regions of origin. It originates from a number of different areas: Southeast Asia, India, Iran, Turkey, the Near East, Nigeria, and Pakistan. Laboratories that can provide heroin of varying purity also exist in Western countries. Heroin may be smoked, nasally insufflated or "snorted," used orally, sublingually, rectally, and intravenously. Heroin is often sold in aluminum foil wrappers, wax-paper envelopes, or in "bags" (rubber balloons). A heroin substitute, "Loads," was found in the New York area when two prescription drugs (glutethimide and codeine) were taken together.

BODY PACKERS AND STUFFERS

Heroin "body packers" are drug smugglers or "mules" who transport large amounts of concentrated heroin from foreign centers by swallowing wrapped packages or inserting packages into their rectum or vagina. So-called "body stuffers" are individuals who hurriedly ingest large quantities of heroin, often in flimsy or ineffective wrappers, in an effort to conceal their heroin use from authorities. Upon reaching their destination, "body-packers" use cathartics, rectal suppositories, or enemas to retrieve the packages rectally. Cocaine is also "body-packed."

The danger of death from heroin intoxication is the major concern in heroin body packing and stuffing. Larger packages may lead to obstruction, initially at the pylorus or later at the ileocecal valve. Patients may have no symptoms, or may exhibit diffuse abdominal tenderness and a distended abdomen with palpable packages. Simple manual examination, anoscopy, and rectal lavage usually disclose rectally inserted packs of drugs and often indicate smuggling for personal use. Professional smugglers are more liable to swallow narcotics, in which case the method of choice is abdominal x-ray. Heroin urine tests in these cases are usually negative. A negative urine toxicologic screen does not exclude the possibility of body packing or stuffing. A normal abdominal roentgenogram does not preclude further investigation if there is a high possibility of body packing or stuffing.

PATHOPHYSIOLOGY

See the Introduction above regarding the general pathophysiology of narcotics. Heroin is a semisynthetic morphine derivative that, in humans, is metabolized to morphine.

PHARMACOKINETICS

Absorption

- Heroin may be absorbed from multiple sites (nasal mucosa, pulmonary capillaries, subcutaneously, intramuscularly, intravenously, rectally), but is generally administered parenterally.
- Heroin has high lipid membrane solubility, leading to rapid absorption from the blood and through the blood-brain barrier. This is responsible for the "rush" experienced by users after intravenous administration.

Distribution

- The half-life of heroin in blood is less than 20 minutes.
- It is distributed widely in tissues, where it is deacetylated to 6-monoacetylmorphine (6-MAM) and morphine in the brain, kidney, liver, blood, and lungs. 6-MAM is the major opiate leaving the bloodstream after heroin overdose and exerts the major effect at receptor sites.

Elimination

- The liver converts 6-MAM to morphine. Heroin and 6-MAM have little affinity for opiate receptors in the brain. Morphine probably accounts for most of the narcotic activity of heroin.
- Heroin passes into breast milk.
- Urine yields primarily morphine in the free or conjugated form.
- After administration of heroin intravenously to normal volunteers, 45% of the dose was recovered as urinary metabolites over a 40-hour period: morphine, 4.2%; conjugated morphine, 38.3%; 6-MAM, 1.3%; unchanged heroin, 0.1%.

CLINICAL PRESENTATIONS

See Clinical Presentations in the Introduction section above for typical clinical presentations of narcotics use. Physical findings may be present, but absence does not exclude the diagnosis. Look for miosis, depressed respirations, scarred veins, heroin in the nostrils, milk in the pharynx, ice about the testicles, and needle marks.

Neurologic Effects

Multiple noninfectious neurologic complications have been described. These include coma, seizures, increased intracranial pressure, acute delirium, chronic organic brain damage, postanoxic encephalopathy, cerebral vascular accidents, involuntary movement disorders, deafness, Horner's syndrome, toxic amblyopia from concomitant quinine use, transverse myelitis, spongiform leukoencephalopathy, brachial and lumbosacral plexitis and neuropathies.

A delayed encephalopathy may develop after an overdose. Magnetic resonance imaging a few weeks later may disclose bilateral infarcts in the putamen and caudate. Infectious neurologic complications may include bacterial meningitis, mycotic aneurysm, brain, subdural or epidural abscesses, and cerebral complications of viral hepatitis and tetanus.

Musculoskeletal Effects

Acute rhabdomyolysis with myoglobinuria may be seen. Associated crush injury may yield ischemic contractures, rhabdomyolysis with increase in serum myoglobin and potassium, myoglobinuria, and acute renal failure. Myositis ossificans—from needle injury to muscles, "drug abusers' elbow," osteomyelitis, infectious spondylitis, infectious sacroiliitis, septic arthritis, and arthralgias have been reported.

Pulmonary Effects

Diluents and contamination may yield various pulmonary complications. These include pulmonary arteritis from cotton, pulmonary thrombosis and pulmonary hypertension from talc, and septic emboli, lung abscesses and right-sided endocarditis from bacteria. Bacterial pneumonia may develop from aspiration during coma or via hematogenous spread. Pulmonary edema, atelectasis, respiratory arrest, and bronchospasm may be seen with heroin overdose. Aspiration is the usual cause of pneumonitis and may share the symptoms of septic pulmonary emboli. Intravenous injection of milk in heroin overdose may produce a respiratory catastrophe, but is still believed by the drug culture to have curative properties.

Pulmonary Edema

Pulmonary edema may be a complication of heroin overdose and may be associated with anoxia and acidosis. Pulmonary hypertension with normal pulmonary capillary pressure and elevated pulmonary artery pressure may develop. Pneumonia and death may occur in three-fourths of those who present with pulmonary edema. Pulmonary edema may be obvious with pink froth in the nasopharynx and rales or wheezes on auscultation, but pulmonary edema cannot be excluded by clinical examination alone. A hypersensitivity reaction, cerebral disease, adulterant toxicity, or anoxia may cause pulmonary edema as well.

Gastrointestinal Effects

Hepatitis B from needles, associated alcoholic liver disease, hepatitis C, chronic active hepatitis, and malnutrition may be seen.

Dermatologic Effects

Cutaneous abscesses, cellulitis, lymphangitis, lymphadenitis, phlebitis, "track" hyperpigmentation, cutaneous scarring, necrotic punched rib, and cutaneous/penile ulcers from injections may occur. Pseudogynecomastia may follow "skin popping" into breast tissue.

Cardiovascular Effects

Quinine adulteration may cause bradycardia and/or tachycardia. Other cardiovascular effects may include atrial fibrillation, QT prolongation, and endocarditis. Hyperkalemic cardiac arrests from rhabdomyolysis and prolonged immobility, and mycotic aneurysms have also been reported.

Renal Effects

Nephrotic syndrome and amyloidosis have been described. Myoglobinuria with rhabdomyolysis may occur.

Ophthalmologic Effects

Crystals in the small vessels about the macula, particles in arterioles or veins, macular edema, venous engorgement, blotch hemorrhages, reduced vision, and central scotomas have been described.

Heroin Withdrawal

Symptoms of heroin withdrawal depend on the time lapsed since the last dose of heroin is taken. Symptoms include early craving for the drug and anxiety. An intermediate period of yawning, perspiration, runny nose, and lacrimation may ensue. Later, an increase in intensity of the above symptoms plus insomnia, hypertension, fever, tachypnea, tachycardia, restlessness, and nausea may predominate. In time, there may be an increase in the preceding symptoms plus flushing, vomiting, diarrhea, weight loss, spontaneous ejaculation or orgasm, hemoconcentration, leukocytosis, and hyperglycemia. Numerous drugs and modalities have been used for heroin withdrawal including heroin itself, methadone, morphine, naloxone, and numerous sedatives.

TOXIC DOSAGE/DEATH

The mechanism of death from heroin is not always known. Death may occur within a few minutes and may not necessarily be due to a pharmacological cause. Causes of death may be associated with suicidal intent, accidental narcotic overdose as in heroin "body-packing," "sudden death," violent death, anaphylactic shock or hypersensitivity to heroin or one of its adulterants, toxic reaction to quinine or other adulterants, angiothrombotic pulmonary hypertension relating to injection of particulate materials, and septic conditions.

In one District of Columbia study, persons with heroin-related deaths were 22 times as likely to have blood ethanol levels over 100 mg/dL as under 100 mg/dL. Cheaper, more plentiful, and purer heroin availability has historically caused a dramatic increase in deaths and emergency room admissions for heroin overdoses.

"Friends" of addicts may also cause complications and death. Common problems involve allowing the addict to "sleep it off" while coma and respiratory depression quickly ensue, home remedies (e.g., milk) believed to be a restorative antidote for reviving addicts who have overdosed, and placing the addict in a cold shower. This may make hypotension more severe. Injecting amphetamines or other stimulant drugs is also a "street remedy." Such a practice often confuses the clinical findings at the hospital. Placing wadded paper in the addict's mouth to prevent him from swallowing his tongue may occur. Applying vigorous artificial respiration, a practice that can cause rib fractures and lacerate the liver, has been reported.

DRUG INTERACTIONS

Heroin interacts synergistically with other opiates and central nervous system depressants.

PREGNANCY/LACTATION

Heroin crosses the placenta. Babies of heroin-dependent mothers are heroin-dependent themselves. Most pregnant addicts are young and unmarried. Seventy-five percent of pregnant heroin addicts give birth without prenatal care, unless they are in methadone maintenance programs. Although methadone may reduce maternal complications from heroin, it has the same fetal side effects as heroin: intrauterine growth retardation and neonatal withdrawal after birth. Sudden withdrawal (i.e., cold turkey detoxification) during pregnancy can lead to fetal death. Abrupt detoxification during pregnancy is therefore not recommended; rather, a switch to methadone to prevent withdrawal is advised. This requires hospitalization.

Malnutrition, infections, and anemia in the pregnant heroin user lead to premature labor, infants of low birth weight, and high perinatal mortality. Problems during labor and delivery include increased obstetrical complications, premature rupture of membranes, neonatal sepsis, pre-eclampsia, placenta previa, and abruptio placentae. After birth, withdrawal symptoms including hyperactivity, hyperirritability, coarse tremors, poor feeding, poor weight gain, and skin abrasions are present in almost all infants of heroin addicts. Sneezing, yawning, sweating, vomiting, diarrhea, and hyperthermia may also be present. Seizures occur in 5% of infants of heroin addicts and 15% of infants of methadone addicts.

LABORATORY

Analytic Methods

A gas chromatography/mass spectrometry assay method for quantitation of urinary 6-acetylmorphine (6-AM), free morphine, and total morphine is available.

Blood Levels

Plasma heroin levels are not clinically useful but may be detected for 36 hours. Following heroin administration, 6-acetylmorphine (6-AM), is excreted rapidly with a half-life of 0.6 hour. The blood level of 6-monoacetylmorphine (6-MAM) is usually very low or not detectable. The half-life of free morphine is 3.6 hours, and that of total morphine, 7.9 hours.

Urine

The presence of 6-AM in the urine indicates that heroin or 6-AM was administered within 24 hours of specimen collection and that the 6-AM in the urine is not due to morphine or codeine administration. Because it is so rapidly metabolized, the absence of detectable levels of 6-MAM does not exclude the possibility of heroin ingestion.

TREATMENT

Gut Decontamination

Gastric lavage or charcoal is ineffective in treating intravenous or insufflated heroin. Gut decontamination, however, is vital in cases involving "body packers" or "body stuffers." Syrup of ipecac or gastric lavage should not be used for patients who have ingested heroin packages because of the large size of the packages. Vomiting may cause obstruction at the proximal esophagus.

Initially a bisacodyl suppository may be inserted to empty the rectum if body packing is suspected. Attempts to remove rectal packages manually may cause them to break. Whole-bowel irrigation is not performed as polyethylene glycol in GoLYTELY can dissolve and rupture heroin-containing packages. Endoscopic removal of packages in the stomach may induce heroin intoxication if the snare used for removal causes a package to break. Activated charcoal, 60 grams in 250 or 500 mL of 3% sodium sulfate solution, is administered orally in case packages break or other substances have been co-ingested. Activated charcoal, 60 grams, can be given orally every 6 hours. Any signs of heroin toxicity should be treated with intravenous naloxone.

Elimination Enhancement

Dialysis techniques, hemoperfusion, hemodialysis, and peritoneal dialysis are not indicated.

Supportive Measures

- Establish adequacy of airway, breathing pattern and circulation. Create an artificial airway by endotracheal intubation as necessary. Tidal volume should be at least 10–15 mL/kg.
- All obtunded adult patients should be given 50 mL of 50% glucose intravenously, 100 mg of thiamine and naloxone 0.8–1.2 mg intravenously. Suspect opiate overdose if increased responsiveness and reversal of miosis are noted with naloxone. See Naloxone in Antidotes section below.

Body Packing and Stuffing

- Take a complete history of the heroin overdose, including the nature, route, and quantities of drug or drugs used, the degrees of addiction, the period of abstinence, and attempts at resuscitation. Establish an intravenous line and place the patient on a cardiac monitor.
- If body packing or stuffing is suspected, obtain an abdominal x-ray to confirm the diagnosis, to determine the location of packages in the gastrointestinal tract, and to follow the movements of the packages.
- Indications for surgical consultation are repeated bouts of heroin toxicity, radiologic evidence of retention of packages and bowel obstruction. A surgical consult should be obtained early. Patients are not to be discharged until all packages are accounted for and negative abdominal radiographs are obtained.
- Packet ingestion with subsequent rupture can usually be managed non-surgically with naloxone.

General Issues

- Be aware of other causes of obtundation (i.e., sepsis, ketosis). They may coexist or be masked by narcotics. Physical findings should be apparent, but their absence does not exclude the diagnosis. Pinpoint pupils are usually present, but pupils may be dilated where there is associated hypoxia, severe respiratory depression, or acidosis.
- Scarred veins, depressed sensorium or coma, heroin in nostrils, milk in the pharynx, single needle mark, pulmonary edema, pink froth in nasopharynx, rales or wheezes on auscultation may be present. Pulmonary edema cannot be excluded by clinical examination alone.
- On admission, blood should be drawn for complete blood count, platelets, VDRL, arterial blood gases, glucose, toxic screen, blood cultures, electrolytes, creatinine, blood urea nitrogen, liver function tests, and hepatitis serologies.
- Monitor the ECG for overdose with any contaminant (e.g., quinine).
- Multiple blood cultures should be obtained if there is evidence of septic emboli or endocarditis. Do skin cultures as necessary.
- Hypotension is treated with position change and pressor amines as needed. Continuous ECG monitoring in this setting is essential.
- Steroids may be used with an aspiration pneumonitis, but their value is questionable.
- Once stabilized, a baseline chest roentgenogram and interval blood gases may be obtained to assess pulmonary edema. Be aware of the administration of excessive fluids if there is evidence of edema on chest x-ray.
- Oxygen may be administered under intermittent positive pressure (PEEP) in severe cases. Digitalization and diuretics are probably of little value in treating heroin-induced pulmonary edema, as the problem is primarily pulmonary and not cardiac.
- Check tetanus status and skin test for tuberculosis. Check for signs of trauma and do x-ray studies or CT scans as indicated.
- A 5-day protocol using clonidine (0.1–0.3 mg) and naltrexone (1–4 mg) three times daily may have potential for the outpatient treatment of heroin withdrawal.

Treatment of Heroin Withdrawal in Infants

- Withdrawal treatment in infants includes holding and rocking the baby, using a pacifier, providing normal fluid balance, and administering paregoric, phenobarbital, and methadone. Withdrawal may take weeks or months.
- Sudden infant death syndrome occurs in 2% of infants after heroin or methadone withdrawal.
- Methadone detoxification of the mother in the prenatal period is performed slowly with decreasing amounts over a 6-day period, beginning with 10 mg four times daily, and then 5 mg/d. After the sixth day, methadone is given only as needed for withdrawal symptoms.

ANTIDOTES

Naloxone

Naloxone (Narcan®), a pure narcotic antagonist, is the drug of choice in heroin and other opiate overdoses. Naloxone may be given as a single bolus or "test dose," or by continuous infusion for longer acting opiates. The single-dose method involves administering 0.4–2.0 mg i.v. in adults and 0.03 mg/kg in children (followed by 0.1 mg/kg if no response). The dose may be repeated every few minutes until there is an increase in respiratory rate and clearing of sensorium. If no response is observed after 10 mg of naloxone is administered, consider other drugs, diagnoses, or clinical conditions. If adequate veins for intravenous naloxone are not available, intramuscular or subcutaneous routes may be used providing there is adequate perfusion, but absorption by these routes is erratic and undependable. If peripheral perfusion is inadequate, sublingual or endotracheal administration may be indicated, however the endotracheal route has not yet been approved.

If repeated doses of naloxone are required to produce respiratory and sensorium responses and continuous monitoring techniques are in place, continuous naloxone infusion may be initiated after an initial bolus. Give 0.4–0.8 mg naloxone per hour (children, 0.03 mg/kg/h). Use 2.0 mg of naloxone in 500 mL D5W infused at 100 mL/h (0.4-mg naloxone/h). Increase the rate of infusion as required. Vital signs and pulmonary status must be closely observed. Note that withdrawal symptoms may begin after the patient wakens if he or she is a chronic heroin addict.

Physostigmine

Physostigmine (Antilirium®), 0.04 mg/kg body weight intravenously, has been used in heroin-addicted patients admitted for respiratory depression and coma. Physostigmine, like naloxone, has resulted in resumption of normal spontaneous respirations and consciousness within 10 minutes without inducing opiate withdrawal. Opiates diminish brain acetylcholine content, which results in somnolence and respiratory depression. Physostigmine appears to reverse these effects by increasing CNS acetylcholine content. Unfortunately, physostigmine may induce significant bradycardia and/or asystole. As naloxone is quite effective and generally well tolerated, use of physostigmine has not been clinically justified.

Questions—Heroin

1. All of the following are true with respect to heroin overdose except
   A. Miosis is common.
   B. Pulmonary edema is very unlikely to occur.
   C. Low-dose naloxone may be appropriate in order to avoid withdrawal responses in physically dependent individuals.
   D. Rhabdomyolysis may occur.
   E. All of the above are true.

2. Heroin withdrawal would be expected to cause all of the following except
   A. Spontaneous ejaculation
   B. Lacrimation
   C. Yawning
   D. Vomiting
   E. Central nervous system depression

3. Pulmonary edema associated with heroin overdose
   A. Is never seen
   B. Is generally easy to correct quickly
   C. Is a bad prognostic sign
   D. Is best treated with digitalis
   E. Is frequently seen

4. Heroin packet ingestion with subsequent rupture can usually be managed non-surgically with naloxone administration.
   A. True
   B. False

5. The half-life of heroin is long, approximately 24 hours.
   A. True
   B. False

6. Heroin is classified as Schedule I in the U.S. (not currently accepted for medicinal purposes).
   A. True
   B. False

7. Heroin withdrawal during pregnancy can lead to fetal death.
   A. True
   B. False

8. Heroin "body stuffers" are drug smugglers or "mules" who transport large amounts of concentrated heroin from foreign centers by swallowing wrapped packages or inserting packages into their rectum or vagina.
   A. True
   B. False

Morphine

Morphine is used for pain relief in the terminally ill, in postoperative and obstetrical care, for headache, sedation, and sleep associated with pain or cough, and for dyspnea in left ventricular failure, acute pulmonary edema, and for spinal anesthesia. It is obtained from opium. Morphine, an alkaloid derivative of opium, was first described in 1803. Opium is obtained from the milky exudate of incised unripe seed capsules of the poppy plant, *Papaver somniferum*, indigenous to Asia Minor. It was an abused drug of choice for addicts until largely superseded by heroin in the post-World War II period. Morphine has been referred to as M, dreamer, Ms. Emma, cube juice, hard stuff, hocus, morph, morpho, and unkie.

PATHOPHYSIOLOGY

See the Introduction above regarding the general pathophysiology of narcotics. Morphine is metabolized in the liver to its 2- and 6-glucuronides, both of which bind to opiate receptors. The 6-glucuronide is a more potent analgesic than morphine itself, and the 3-glucuronide antagonizes the analgesic activity of 6-glucuronide in experimental animals. Patient analgesic response to morphine appears to depend on the 3-glucuronide:6-glucuronide ratio, the 6-glucuronide being responsible for the analgesic effect.

PHARMACOKINETICS

Absorption

- Morphine is well absorbed from the gastrointestinal (GI) tract, but because of rapid metabolism, plasma levels of free morphine are relatively low and levels of conjugated morphine are relatively high.
- Thirty percent of an oral dose reaches the systemic circulation if the dose is completely absorbed by the GI tract. After oral administration, the urinary excretion of free morphine is low, but total urinary excretion (free and conjugated) is similar to that after intravenous, intramuscular, or subcutaneous administration.

- Intramuscular morphine is rapidly absorbed. Time to peak concentration after intramuscular administration is 15.5 minutes.

Distribution

- The apparent volume of distribution after intravenous administration is 3.2 L/kg. In young subjects (under 30 years), the volume of distribution is double that found in older age groups (over 60 years). Protein binding is 35%.
- After therapeutic use, it is distributed in the blood, lung, liver, and bile. Very little is found in the adult brain. In addicted infants, it is present in the brain stem, thymus, spleen, cerebellum, lungs, and liver.

Elimination

- Oral morphine undergoes extensive first-pass metabolism. Most of the morphine is converted in the liver to morphine-3-glucuronide, which is excreted in the bile and feces.
- Morphine-3-glucuronide has no pharmacological activity, does not cross the blood-brain barrier, and does not react with the opiate receptors. It appears in the serum within 20 minutes and exceeds the concentration of free morphine after 2 hours.
- Morphine-6-glucuronide appears to be 10–20 times more potent than the parent drug in the central nervous system.
- The half-lives of morphine, morphine-3-glucuronide (M3G), and morphine-6-glucuronide (M6G) are 15, 11, and 13 hours, respectively.
- There is a large enterohepatic circulation of conjugated and intestinally unconjugated morphine.
- Seventy-five percent of a morphine dose is eliminated in the urine as glucuronide, and 10% is excreted as free morphine.
- Urinary codeine appears after morphine is administered, but this is due to its presence as an impurity in commercial morphine. Eighty-four percent of morphine is eliminated via urine within 8 hours.
- Intact renal function may be essential for total morphine clearance. Patients with renal impairment have increased systemic effects (prolonged respiratory depression), decreased morphine clearance, and potential toxicity after morphine. This may support a role for renal glucuronidation.

CLINICAL PRESENTATIONS

Clinical morphine poisoning is similar to heroin poisoning; however, it is infrequently seen in emergency rooms. There are few reports in the medical literature relating to morphine overdose or its clinical complications. In nontolerant adults, the triad of coma, pinpoint pupils, and depressed respiration is seen in varying degrees after toxic doses are administered. Morphine may produce profound physical dependence manifested by increasing doses needed to obtain desired pain relief.

Dependent individuals may demonstrate tolerance to high doses that would ordinarily be toxic or fatal to new users. Such individuals may rely on antisocial acts to obtain more drugs. Morphine may cause thrombocytopenia, hyperglycemia, decreased high-density lipoprotein (HDL) cholesterol, decreased ventilatory response to hypoxia and hypercapnia, and attenuated sympathetic control of cutaneous circulation. Consumption of large amounts of poppy seeds does not lead to symptoms of opiate impairment although the consumer may have positive urine results.

Withdrawal symptoms may occur with abrupt cessation of use and may be suppressed with recurrent use. Withdrawal symptoms common to opioids are also seen with morphine and include anxiety, hyperactivity, insomnia, opioid craving hypertension, tachycardia, abdominal cramps, diarrhea, mydriasis, muscular tightness, twitching, and piloerection.

TOXIC DOSAGE/DEATH

The toxic dosage in a nontolerant adult is 30 mg parenterally or 40–60 mg orally. An oral lethal dose in an adult is around 120 mg. Blood morphine concentrations higher than 100 μg/dL in addicts represent acute overdoses. In fatal cases in which morphine levels were lower than 30 μg/dL adulterants such as quinine may be present.

DRUG INTERACTIONS

Phenothiazines, monoamine oxidase inhibitors, and tricyclic antidepressants exaggerate and prolong the depressant effects of morphine. Sedative-hypnotics, ethanol, and other opiates potentiate the effects of morphine. Furosemide, when used with morphine in the treatment of pulmonary edema, may potentiate the ability of morphine to increase venous capacitance and cause further hypotension and respiratory embarrassment.

PREGNANCY/LACTATION

Maternal morphine addiction with subsequent neonatal withdrawal after illicit use is well known. Like all narcotics, morphine is transferred through the placenta very rapidly. Only trace amounts of morphine enter breast milk; its significance is unknown.

LABORATORY

Analytic Methods

A gas chromatography-mass spectrometry and radioimmunoassay method is available to differentiate conjugated from unconjugated morphine but is not useful for management of most clinical overdoses.

Blood Levels

Blood and urine levels are useful only as confirmation of the presence of morphine. The peak blood level after administration of a single 10-mg intravenous dose in adults is 60 ng/mL; after 36 hours, it is 3 ng/mL. After a single 10-mg intramuscular injection, the peak level is 70 ng/mL after 10–20 minutes and 10 ng/mL after 4 hours.

Ingestion of a number of baked goods that contain poppy seeds can lead to positive screening tests for opiates. This is due to the presence of morphine and codeine as well as other natural products on the surface of inadequately washed poppy seeds.

Urine

There is little correlation between morphine urine levels and clinical state in overdose situations. Detection of 6-MAM in urine is important for ruling out poppy seed ingestion as a cause of a "false" positive result in immunoassay screens for opiates. 6-MAM is not present in poppy seeds or in urine after the ingestion of poppy seeds.

TREATMENT

Gut Decontamination

Activated charcoal and lavage with protected airway may be useful in oral morphine ingestions. Emesis is contraindicated as stupor may predominate.

Elimination Enhancement

Dialysis procedures have not been evaluated, but a large volume of distribution would preclude the probability of their usefulness.

Supportive Measures

- Supportive measures are similar to those employed in heroin overdose. Assure adequacy of airway, breathing, and circulation.
- Management of morphine withdrawal includes symptomatic treatment of anxiety (benzodiazepines are generally used), insomnia, gastrointestinal complaints, and pain.
- Clonidine has also been used, carefully, in doses of 0.1 mg every 6–8 hours. It is titrated by 0.1-mg increments, with a daily dose not exceeding 1.2 mg.
- Obtain samples of blood, urine, and gastric contents and test for ethanol, other sedatives, tricyclic antidepressants, and phenothiazines when a morphine overdose is under investigation.

ANTIDOTES

Please see the Antidotes section under Heroin above for a complete discussion of opiate antagonists. Naloxone may be administered by repeated single injection or by continuous infusion.

Questions—Morphine

1. Which of the following about morphine overdose is false?

A. Poisoning is similar to heroin poisoning, however is infrequently seen in emergency rooms.
B. Like heroin, morphine may present with coma, pinpoint pupils, and depressed respirations.
C. May produce profound physical dependence manifested by increasing doses needed to obtain desired pain relief
D. May cause thrombocytopenia, hyperglycemia, decreased high-density lipoprotein (HDL) cholesterol, decreased ventilatory response to hypoxia and hypercapnia, and attenuated sympathetic control of cutaneous circulation
E. Toxicity may occur when large amounts of poppy seeds are ingested.

2. Each of the following may prolong the depressant effects of morphine, except

A. Aminoglycosides
B. Phenothiazines
C. Monoamine oxidase inhibitors
D. Tricyclic antidepressants
E. Ethanol

Methadone

Methadone is a synthetic diphenylpropylamine similar in structure to propoxyphene. Methadone and morphine differ chemically, but their actions and analgesic potency are similar. From 7.5 to 10 mg methadone is roughly equivalent to 10 mg of morphine. Intramuscularly, as analgesics, methadone and morphine exhibit similar durations of action. Orally, methadone retains 50% of its intramuscular potency. There is a slower development of tolerance and dependence with methadone than with morphine. Methadone is employed in detoxification and methadone maintenance programs for the management of narcotic dependence.

METHADONE MAINTENANCE

Methadone maintenance is a standard medical treatment for narcotic dependence. It provides pharmacological stability and cross-tolerance to opiate drugs and, hopefully, eliminates their necessity. Extra methadone is frequently ingested by the self-user on maintenance, irrespective of the presence of withdrawal symptoms or reduction of symptoms after dose ingestion. Strict adherence to guidelines does not necessarily prevent signs of therapeutic failure such as continued drug abuse, loitering, drug selling, and disorderly conduct.

Retention on a program for at least 1 year is critical. More than 90% of the persons who drop out or are discharged for administrative reasons after a shorter period of treatment relapse, go to jail, or die of a drug-related cause. Failure to eliminate or greatly reduce the use of heroin while the patient is receiving maintenance therapy is due, in almost all cases, to an inadequate dose of methadone.

When addiction reaches a state in which the daily administration of heroin or other morphine-like drugs is required to avoid the onset of signs of withdrawal, an individual is said to be drug-dependent. Methadone detoxification involves the administration or dispensing of methadone as a substitute narcotic drug in decreasing doses to reach a drug-free state in a period not to exceed 21 days. It is designed to allow an individual who is dependent on heroin or other morphine-like drugs to withdraw from the use of these drugs.

"Maintenance treatment" using methadone for an individual dependent on heroin involves the continued dispensing of methadone, in conjunction with the provision of appropriate social and medical services, at relatively stable dosage levels for a period in excess of 21 days as an oral substitute for heroin or other morphine-like drugs. Methadone maintenance does not stop alcoholism, nonnarcotic drug abuse, psychopathic behavior, or delinquency. Low-dose maintenance programs (30–40 mg/d, maximum of 50 mg/d) often result in a high rate of continuing illicit narcotic use by patients during treatment, have a high dropout rate (less than 50% 1-year retention), exhibit a disorderly clinic, and show poor results in rehabilitation. In one study, within 2 years after discharge from methadone maintenance, 70% of former methadone-treated addicts became re-addicted to narcotics and 52% returned for additional treatment.

PATHOPHYSIOLOGY

See the Introduction above regarding the general pathophysiology of narcotics. Among other effects, methadone lowers plasma cortisol levels in humans. Opiate receptor stimulation by exogenous opiates may, through a feedback mechanism, reduce the release and possibly the synthesis of pro-ACTH/endorphin and decrease ACTH and endogenous opiates or endorphins. Chronic methadone administration decreases the synthesis, storage, and quantity of available pro-ACTH/endorphin and endorphin/endogenous opiate reserves.

PHARMACOKINETICS

Absorption

- Methadone is well absorbed from the gastrointestinal tract, after subcutaneous administration, and from intramuscular sites.
- After oral administration, a measurable amount is present in the plasma in 30 minutes.

Distribution

- Methadone is widely distributed to the lung, liver, kidney, spleen, blood, and urine. The apparent volume of distribution is approximately 5 L/kg.
- Protein binding is 85%.
- The half-life is 10–18 hours after a therapeutic dose and up to 25 hours in methadone maintenance patients receiving 100–120 mg/d. The plasma concentration peaks 1–2 hours after high doses and 4 hours after an oral 15-mg dose.

- Blood levels decline, so that at 24 hours, the plasma levels equal 40% of peak levels (30 ng/mL).

Elimination

- Methadone is metabolized in the liver to pyrrolidine metabolites, which are excreted as glucuronides. None of these metabolites are usually found in the plasma, and none have measurable pharmacological activity.
- The kidneys become a major route of methadone excretion only at doses exceeding 50 mg/d.
- Methadone is reabsorbed in the renal tubules; the degree of such reabsorption decreases as the urinary pH decreases.
- Renal excretion can be hastened by acidifying the urine, but this is rarely necessary, since the toxic effects may be countered by naloxone.

CLINICAL PRESENTATIONS

Rhabdomyolysis, myoglobinuria, muscle necrosis, and renal failure may occur secondary to methadone intoxication and may result from muscle damage related to prolonged coma and immobilization or from a direct toxic effect of methadone. Pulmonary edema occurs rarely with methadone. All the complications seen with heroin overdose can be found with methadone overdose, especially after illicit parenteral use.

Side effects of long-term (3 years) high-dose (80–120 mg/d) maintenance treatment include increased sweating (the most common side effect), constipation (which commonly occurs during the first year even with daily laxative usage), insomnia and dozing during the day, decreased libido, and difficulty in achieving orgasm. Treatment doses of methadone ingested accidentally or purposefully by nontolerant or partially tolerant individuals can result in a potentially lethal overdose syndrome within 30 minutes to 6 hours.

Pediatric Effects

Methadone poisoning in children has been reported since the inception of methadone maintenance clinics in the late 1960s. Poisoning and fatalities in children have been attributed to lack of uniformity in the packaging of methadone supplies and inadequate parental education regarding use and storage of methadone. Methadone mothers should be encouraged to bottle feed their babies in view of its secretion in breast milk. Symptoms in children are those of classic opiate overdose with pupillary miosis; however, the pupils may be normoactive or, rarely, fixed and dilated. Infants may have drowsiness, coma, and apnea.

Withdrawal

The abrupt withdrawal of methadone, even after large doses have been ingested, produces symptoms that develop more slowly, are less intense, and are more prolonged than those seen in morphine withdrawal. Few symptoms occur until the second day or later. Symptoms may include weakness, anxiety, insomnia, abdominal discomfort, headache, sweating, and hot and cold flashes. The intensity of the symptoms often peaks on the 6th day with the onset of vomiting and diarrhea. Muscle cramps and aches are not present. Symptoms subside by the 10th day and are minimal by the 14th day, but lethargy may persist for longer periods.

TOXIC DOSAGE/DEATH

Death caused by methadone is increasing in urban areas because of its widespread availability. Most fatalities occur after oral administration. A lack of opiate tolerance is a large factor. The blood methadone concentration of victims of methadone overdose overlaps that of methadone maintenance subjects. When initial doses higher than 15–30 mg are used in an unsupervised setting, respiratory depression may ensue. Death may occur during induction of methadone maintenance when tolerance is incorrectly assessed and during maintenance when several days' doses are combined. Death can also follow accidental ingestion. Doses of 50 mg or less have been known to be lethal to nontolerant adults. The fatal dose in children is 10–20 mg.

DRUG INTERACTIONS

Chronic ingestion of methadone results in an increase in hepatic microsomal drug-metabolizing enzymes. Rifampin lowers plasma levels of methadone, increases methadone urinary excretion, and increases fecal excretion of the major pyrrolidine metabolite. Rifampin is also known to be a hepatic microsomal enzyme inducer. Diazepam taken with methadone enhances the pupillary constricting and opioid effects of methadone.

Disulfiram enhances the demethylation of methadone and increases urinary excretion of the major pyrrolidine metabolite. However, it has no effect on opiate intoxication or abstinence symptoms and, when used for the treatment of alcoholism in a patient on methadone maintenance, has no significant interaction with methadone. Central nervous system depressants (e.g., alcohol, tranquilizers, and barbiturates) may enhance the respiratory depression of methadone and may produce confusion and coma. Phenytoin may accelerate methadone metabolism.

PREGNANCY/LACTATION

Methadone crosses the placenta, causes respiratory depression in the fetus, and is secreted in breast milk in concentrations approaching plasma levels. Secretion in breast milk may prevent withdrawal symptoms in addicted infants. At least one infant death has been attributed to methadone obtained through breast milk. Methadone metabolism may be increased during pregnancy, leading to lower plasma methadone concentrations and, in some cases, symptoms of methadone withdrawal. In such cases, the methadone dose may need to be increased or to be given in divided doses. Although withdrawal symptoms in the methadone infant can be severe, the average birth weight for methadone babies is higher than that for heroin infants, but is lower than that for normal infants.

LABORATORY

Analytic Methods

A high-performance liquid chromatography method for quantitation of plasma methadone levels has a detection limit of 5 ng. A gas chromatography-mass spectrometry assay is available to determine both methadone and its metabolite EDDP in the urine.

Blood Levels

There does not appear to be any relationship between plasma levels and symptom complaints. Blood levels of methadone are not of practical value in methadone maintenance programs. A good correlation exists between plasma methadone concentrations and dose at steady-state over a wide dosage range (3–100 mg of methadone per day). Plasma methadone concentration appears to increase by 263 ng/mL for every milligram of methadone consumed per kilogram of body weight.

To stop heroin use, the amount of methadone taken per day by the patient has been correlated with a blood methadone concentration of at least 200 ng/mL. Methadone maintenance serum levels after an oral 30-mg dose display a mean trough concentration of 70–90 ng/mL.

TREATMENT

Gut Decontamination
Activated charcoal, 60 grams, can be given orally every 6 hours; however, aspiration is a significant risk in obtunded individuals and care must be undertaken to protect the airway. Any signs of methadone toxicity should be treated with opiate antagonists.

Elimination Enhancement
Dialysis procedures are inadequate because of the high tissue distribution, minute blood content, and high protein binding of methadone.

Supportive Measures
- Treatment of methadone overdose is similar to treatment of heroin overdose. Administer opiate antagonists (see Antidotes below) as needed. Successful resuscitation with a narcotic antagonist may be followed by relapse.
- As adverse effects from methadone can be delayed as long as 5 hours after ingestion, observe the patient in the hospital at least 6 hours.
- Known or suspected methadone-intoxicated children should be hospitalized, since respiratory depression may be observed for as long as 48 hours after ingestion.
- The treatment of symptomatic addicted infants is similar to the treatment of heroin-addicted infants. Paregoric USP, 3–7 drops every 4 hours, is increased as needed. Phenobarbital, 5 mg/kg body weight per day, may be added. Infants may require treatment for days to a few weeks.
- The appearance of withdrawal signs in babies born to methadone addicts later than in those born to heroin addicts is due to a difference in the pharmacokinetics of these drugs. Babies born to methadone mothers should be observed for 7 days.

ANTIDOTES

Naloxone
Please see the Antidote section under Heroin above for a complete discussion of opiate antagonists. Naloxone may be administered by repeated single injection or by continuous infusion. Naloxone intravenous infusion is specifically useful. An initial infusion rate of naloxone hydrochloride of 0.4 mg/h is used, regardless of the size and age of the patient. If an adequate response is not achieved, the infusion rate may be increased approximately every 30 minutes until an optimal clinical response is obtained.

Close monitoring for at least 2 hours after discontinuation of the infusion is required for complete recovery. In the elderly, use of methadone as an analgesic at relatively low doses (15 mg/d) may, with just a few doses, result in a clinical picture similar to that of narcotic overdose, and will respond to naloxone. Clonidine and naltrexone are effective treatments for successful withdrawal from methadone therapy as well.

Questions—Methadone

1. Regarding methadone maintenance, which of the following is false?
A. Methadone maintenance is a standard medical treatment for narcotic dependence.
B. Patients on methadone maintenance are generally self-disciplined. Extra methadone is rarely ingested by the self-user on maintenance.
C. Retention on a program for at least 1 year is critical. More than 90% of the persons who drop out or are discharged for administrative reasons after a shorter period of treatment relapse, go to jail, or die of a drug-related cause.
D. Failure to eliminate or greatly reduce the use of heroin while the patient is receiving maintenance therapy is due, in almost all cases, to an inadequate dose of methadone.
E. "Maintenance treatment" using methadone for an individual dependent on heroin involves the continued dispensing of methadone in conjunction with the provision of appropriate social and medical services, at relatively stable dosage levels for a period in excess of 21 days as an oral substitute for heroin or other morphine-like drugs.

2. Regarding methadone and pregnancy,
A. Methadone crosses the placenta, causes respiratory depression in the fetus, and is secreted in breast milk in concentrations approaching plasma levels.
B. Secretion in breast milk may prevent withdrawal symptoms in addicted infants.
C. Methadone metabolism is decreased during pregnancy, leading to higher plasma methadone concentrations.
D. All of the above.
E. A and B

3. Blood levels of methadone are not of practical value in methadone maintenance programs.
A. True
B. False

Diphenoxylate and Atropine

Diphenoxylate-atropine (Lomotil®) is an antidiarrheal agent often used to treat traveler's diarrhea. It prolongs the transit time of intestinal contents by acting on smooth muscle of the gut. Diphenoxylate and atropine poisoning represents a unique opiate-anticholinergic overdose that appears to be more serious and often more fatal in children than in adults. It may have delayed deleterious effects and, at least in children, appears to present no correlation between dose ingested and severity of toxicity. Each tablet, or 5 mL of liquid, contains 2.5 mg diphenoxylate hydrochloride and 0.025 mg (25 μg) atropine sulfate (a subtherapeutic amount of the latter is added to discourage its abuse).

PATHOPHYSIOLOGY
Diphenoxylate is a synthetic phenylpiperidine derivative closely related to meperidine (Demerol®), fentanyl (Sublimaze®), and fentanyl derivatives (e.g., China White). Both opiates and anticholinergic medications, such as atropine, decrease gut motility. Their combination synergistically decreases diarrhea by acting on smooth muscle.

PHARMACOKINETICS

Absorption
- After oral ingestion, diphenoxylate-atropine is easily absorbed through the gastrointestinal tract.
- Absorption is slowed in overdose because of a delay in gastrointestinal motility. Such delays may be as long as 30 hours.
- Diphenoxylate and its salts are largely insoluble, thus making parenteral abuse unlikely.

Distribution

- The apparent volume of distribution of diphenoxylate is 4.6 L/kg, and that of atropine, is approximately 2–4 L/kg.
- Peak plasma levels of diphenoxylate and diphenoxylic acid, an active metabolite, are reached in 2 hours.

Elimination

- The major metabolite, diphenoxylic acid, formed in the liver, is five times more active than diphenoxylate as an antidiarrheal agent.
- The half-life of diphenoxylate is 2.5 hours, and that of diphenoxylic acid, 4.4 hours, after therapeutic dosage. The half-life in overdose may be prolonged to more than 12 hours.
- Diphenoxylate is excreted in the feces (49%) and urine (14%) as conjugated products, over a 96-hour period. Enterohepatic recycling may be important in the metabolism of diphenoxylate.
- Less than 0.1% of diphenoxylate and less than 0.8% of diphenoxylic acid are excreted in the urine unchanged.

CLINICAL PRESENTATIONS

Moderate to severe diphenoxylate (opiate) symptoms appear 2–3 hours after ingestion and include slow pulse, slow depressed respirations, drowsiness, convulsions, and coma. There may be abdominal pain or pancreatitis. The pupils are constricted and cortical blindness secondary to cerebral hypoxia may occur. Cyanotic skin, hypothermia, and muscle fasciculations may be present. Respiratory depression and coma are the most prevalent and feared complications of diphenoxylate-atropine poisoning.

Adults do not appear to have the same susceptibility to opiate toxicity as children. Symptoms, especially coma and respiratory depression, may be delayed up to 30 hours because of delayed gastrointestinal motility. Opiate overdose (central nervous system and respiratory depression with miosis) may predominate or occur without signs of atropine toxicity. All patients appear to exhibit opioid effects sometime during the course of the overdose. Diphenoxylate-atropine intoxication can be considered an overdose of a long-acting opioid that may include manifestations of atropine toxicity.

There appears to be little correlation between dose ingested and severity of signs or symptoms in diphenoxylate-atropine overdose. Children may develop signs of atropinism even with a normal dose. It is not possible to predict which dose is toxic to children. Symptoms may respond to treatment and recur many hours later (24–36 hours). Because of the long elimination half-life (12–24 hours) of diphenoxylic acid in overdose, it seems likely that the recurrence of respiratory depression and opioid symptoms after apparent recovery from diphenoxylate-atropine overdose is due to the accumulation of this metabolite.

Mild atropinism effects predominate in the first 2–3 hours, but patients may present with apnea, coma, and respiratory depression. Symptoms may include tachycardia, disorientation, excitement, convulsions, hyperpyrexia, a silent bowel, mydriasis, hot, dry, and red skin, diminished muscle tone, and urinary retention. Atropine may exert its effects in children before, during, or after opioid effects. In most cases, atropine effects last from 2–12 hours. Delayed gastric emptying and gastrointestinal atony may be a factor in the occurrence of central nervous system and respiratory depression up to 15–18 hours after ingestion. Diphenoxylate abuse has rarely been reported.

TOXIC DOSAGE/DEATH

The lowest reported dose associated with signs and symptoms of poisoning was 2 tablets. Six tablets produced poisoning in another series. The lowest fatal dose reported was 1.2 mg/kg. In adults, 15–30 tablets did not produce respiratory depression or coma in one study.

DRUG INTERACTIONS

Diphenoxylate inhibits the microsomal hepatic enzyme system and has the potential to prolong the half-lives of drugs whose rate of elimination is dependent on this system.

PREGNANCY/LACTATION

These compounds are excreted in breast milk. Pregnancy risk factor C.

LABORATORY

Analytic Methods

The determination of plasma diphenoxylic acid, the major metabolite of diphenoxylate, has been performed by gas chromatography-mass spectrometry and radioimmunoassay. Plasma diphenoxylate levels are not easily obtained at most clinical laboratories.

Blood Levels

Plasma or urinary diphenoxylate levels have little clinical usefulness in the management of overdose because the rapid conversion of diphenoxylate to diphenoxylic acid generally renders diphenoxylate undetectable.

TREATMENT

Gut Decontamination

Administration of an emetic is undesirable because patients may become apneic and drowsy rapidly, increasing the possibility of aspiration. Because of the enterohepatic circulation of certain metabolites, serial activated charcoal may be of value; however, attention must be made to assuring a safe airway. Intravenous infusion of naloxone may be an alternative to oral activated charcoal when the patient has intestinal ileus or gastric atony.

Elimination Enhancement

Forced diuresis, hemodialysis, hemoperfusion, and peritoneal dialysis are not useful in removing diphenoxylate or its metabolites, in view of their high volumes of distribution.

Supportive Measures

- Airway, breathing, and circulation must be monitored and abnormalities must be addressed. Tidal volume should be maintained between 10–15 mL/kg. An artificial airway should be created by endotracheal intubation as required. If there is respiratory embarrassment, adequate oxygenation must be instituted.
- Patients with signs of atropinism or central nervous system depression should be admitted.
- For urinary retention, catheterization may be required.
- Intensive care monitoring of vital signs, fluid balance, level of consciousness, pupil size, and arterial blood gases must be continually recorded to guide patient status concerning naloxone administration and fluid infusions.
- Patients should not be discharged until the respiratory rate and state of consciousness have returned to normal and other opioid symptoms are absent. Symptomatic patients should be kept under intensive observation for at least 24 hours irrespective of whether they have already responded to the above modalities and appear asymptomatic.
- Parents should be instructed to keep such tablets out of the reach of any children in the house.

- No effect on serum electrolytes, blood urea nitrogen, hemoglobin, hematocrit, white cell count, blood glucose, or spinal fluid glucose is generally observed.

ANTIDOTES

Naloxone

Respiratory depression and coma are indications for initiating naloxone. The dosage in the adult is 0.4–2.0 mg intravenously repeated every few minutes as needed. In children, the initial dose is 0.01–0.1 mg / kg intravenously followed by an additional dose of 0.1 mg / kg as required. If there is no response, consideration must be given to exclusion of propoxyphene, or methadone as the causative agent. If there is a response, multiple doses of naloxone every 20–45 minutes may be required, as the half-life of naloxone is short and an opioid antagonist may be effective for only 45–70 minutes.

If frequent intravenous boluses are required to maintain adequate respiration and consciousness, a continuous intravenous naloxone infusion should be instituted. Naloxone, 4–8 mg, is added to each liter of 5% dextrose in water, and the solution is infused at a rate of 100 mL / h (0.4–0.8 mg naloxone per hour).

Questions—Diphenoxylate and Atropine

1. A 12-month-old child presents to the emergency room one hour after ingestion of an unknown number of Lomotil® tablets. Which of the following is true?
A. Cholinergic signs may be present.
B. Hospitalization for about 24 hours is required even if asymptomatic on initial presentation.
C. Naloxone should not be used if pupillary dilatation is present.
D. Ipecac should be used for gastrointestinal decontamination.
E. None of the above

2. Which of the following regarding the clinical effects of diphenoxylate and atropine is true?
A. Moderate to severe diphenoxylate (opiate) symptoms may appear 2–3 hours after ingestion and include slow pulse, slow depressed respirations, drowsiness, convulsions, and coma.
B. Adults do not appear to have the same susceptibility to opiate toxicity as children.
C. Symptoms, especially coma and respiratory depression, may be delayed up to 30 hours because of delayed gastrointestinal motility.
D. All of the above
E. A and B

3. In diphenoxylate and atropine overdose, opiate overdose (central nervous system and respiratory depression with miosis) may predominate or occur without signs of atropine toxicity.
A. True
B. False

4. Which of the following statements regarding the clinical effects of diphenoxylate and atropine is false?
A. All patients appear to exhibit opioid effects sometime during the course of the overdose.
B. Diphenoxylate-atropine intoxication can be considered an overdose of a long-acting opioid that may include manifestations of atropine toxicity.
C. There appears to be a significant correlation between dose ingested and severity of signs or symptoms in diphenoxylate-atropine overdose.
D. Children may develop signs of atropinism even with a normal dose.
E. Symptoms may include tachycardia, disorientation, excitement, convulsions, hyperpyrexia, a silent bowel, mydriasis, hot, dry, and red skin, diminished muscle tone, and urinary retention.

Meperidine

Meperidine (Demerol®) is used for the relief of moderate to severe pain, for preoperative medication (parenteral form), for support of anesthesia, and as an obstetrical analgesic. Meperidine is the prototype of the phenylpiperidine derivatives, which include fentanyl, and alphaprodine (Nisentil®). There are few reports of poisoning or fatalities related to meperidine in the medical literature. Myoclonic jerks or generalized convulsions may occur in overdoses. The clinical features of tolerance and physical dependence are similar to those for morphine. The analgesic potency of meperidine is one-sixth that of morphine. Meperidine, a synthetic chemical, is a Schedule II drug under the Controlled Substances Act.

PATHOPHYSIOLOGY

The chief pharmacological action of meperidine is on the central nervous system, where it produces respiratory depression. In addicts tolerant to the depressant effects of meperidine, repeated administration of large doses at short intervals may produce tremors, dilated pupils, and convulsions. Meperidine and its metabolites also have a direct effect on myoneural tissues, resulting in twitching.

PHARMACOKINETICS

Absorption

- Meperidine is absorbed from all routes of administration.
- The oral route results in lower meperidine and higher normeperidine levels compared with the parenteral route, possibly indicating extensive first-pass metabolism.
- If a toxic dose of meperidine is administered intramuscularly or intravenously, the absorption rate exceeds the rate of normeperidine formation, and central nervous system depression ensues.
- If a toxic dose of meperidine is administered orally, the rate of absorption is lower than the rate of conversion of meperidine to normeperidine by the liver. Stupor and convulsions may follow.

Distribution

- The volume of distribution is 3.84 L / kg for therapeutic doses, 5.2 L / kg in patients with cirrhosis, and 4.5 L / kg in the elderly. Meperidine distributes widely into the liver, kidney, and muscle.
- Protein binding is 65–75%.
- Peak plasma levels are obtained in 1.2 minutes after an intravenous injection, 1 hour after an intramuscular injection, and 2 hours after oral administration.
- The half-life is 2.4–4.0 hours after a therapeutic dose. No change in half-life is found in the elderly.

Elimination

- Meperidine undergoes metabolism in the liver to normeperidine, a convulsant.

- Normeperidine is not measurable after one single dose of meperidine, but accumulates with repeated doses or large quantities of meperidine. It has one-half the analgesic activity of meperidine, but appears to be two to three times more toxic.
- Normeperidine is more active as a convulsant and has a longer half-life (15–30 hours) than meperidine. Its peak plasma level is reached in 2–8 hours.
- Meperidine is excreted in the urine: 5% is excreted unchanged, 5% as normeperidine unchanged in the urine, 12% as meperidinic acid, 12% as normeperidinic acid, and the remainder as other metabolites. Enterohepatic recycling is of minor importance.

CLINICAL PRESENTATIONS

The clinical picture in overdose is similar to that after morphine overdose and may include respiratory depression and circulatory depression. Meperidine has a convulsant threshold lower than that of morphine. Prolonged use of intramuscular meperidine may result in fibrosis of tissue that may result in functional damage to muscle groups and nerves.

Neurologic Effects

High doses of meperidine produce convulsions because of its conversion to normeperidine. Myoclonus usually precedes convulsions. Plasma normeperidine levels and central nervous system irritability are significantly correlated. Predisposing factors for meperidine-induced seizures include doses greater than 100 mg every 2 hours for longer than 24 hours, renal failure, an alkaline urine, coadministration of enzyme-inducing drugs, coadministration of phenothiazines that lower seizure threshold, and a history of seizures.

Dependence

Members of the medical or allied professions are most frequently subjected to meperidine dependence. Patients who are treated with meperidine may also become dependent on it. There are some differences between meperidine- and morphine-dependent subjects. Meperidine produces tremor, twitching, confusion, hallucinations, and convulsions at large doses (3–4 grams/day). It is shorter acting and induces an abstinence syndrome that begins in 3 hours and peaks in 8–12 hours. The abstinence syndrome consists of severe muscular twitching, restlessness and fewer autonomic signs (such as lacrimation, rhinorrhea, yawning, sweating, pupillary dilatation) than morphine withdrawal.

TOXIC DOSAGE/DEATH

Daily doses of meperidine greater than 25 mg/kg may be associated with seizures due to normeperidine toxicity, especially in patients with renal failure or if taken orally.

DRUG INTERACTIONS

Administration of monoamine oxidase inhibitors with meperidine may lead to hypotension, hypertension, agitation, tremor, hyperpyrexia, convulsions, and coma. Atropine, tricyclic antidepressants, orphenadrine, benztropine, amantadine, and disopyramide may potentiate parasympathetic blockade induced by meperidine. Ethanol, hypnotics, sedatives, tranquilizers, tricyclic antidepressants, other narcotic analgesics, anticonvulsants, antihistamines, methyldopa, clonidine, and reserpine may enhance central nervous system depression induced by meperidine.

Meperidine slows gastric emptying and reduces the rate of absorption of other drugs. Phenobarbital increases formation of the toxic metabolite, normeperidine, enhancing central nervous system depressant effects. Hepatic microsomal drug-metabolizing enzyme induction may increase formation of normeperidine.

PREGNANCY/LACTATION

Meperidine crosses the placenta and is found in breast milk. Meperidine administered in excess to some mothers before birth may result in newborns with delayed respirations, decreased respiratory minute volume, decreased oxygen saturation, and a requirement for resuscitation. Feeding and ventilation problems may remain for 48 hours. Effects of meperidine on the fetus are related to maternal metabolism, placental transfer, fetal metabolism, and fetal central nervous system penetration.

Naloxone can reverse the depressant effect of narcotic analgesics when administered to the mother before delivery or when injected into the umbilical vein. Post-cesarean patient-controlled analgesia with meperidine leads to accumulation of normeperidine in breast milk. This may be associated with neonatal neurobehavioral depression in the first days of life.

LABORATORY

Analytic Methods

Meperidine may be detected by gas-liquid chromatography and confirmed by gas chromatography/mass spectrometry.

Blood Levels

Plasma normeperidine levels may correlate with clinical effects but are generally unhelpful in overdose. Shakiness is associated with levels greater than 422 ng/mL, tremors with levels greater than 463 ng/mL and seizures with levels greater than 814 ng/mL.

TREATMENT

Gut Decontamination

Gastric lavage with prior endotracheal intubation, activated charcoal through a lavage tube, and cathartics may be effective in view of the possible enterohepatic recirculation of meperidine. Attention to airway protection is vital due to the potential for seizure activity.

Elimination Enhancement

Dialysis procedures have not been evaluated. However, high protein binding and a large volume of distribution would tend to preclude an effective role.

Supportive Measures

- Establish an adequate airway, monitor breathing and circulation as necessary.
- Intravenous barbiturates may be effective in quieting the agitated state and multifocal myoclonus occasionally associated with meperidine toxicity. Treat seizures with diazepam or phenytoin, administered by slow intravenous push, if benzodiazepines are ineffective. Carbamazepine may be useful in managing hypomanic symptoms.

ANTIDOTES

Naloxone does not antagonize the tremors, twitching, or seizures caused by normeperidine. However, it does antagonize the opiate effects such as sedation, respiratory depression, hypotension, and coma.

Questions—Meperidine

1. **Which of the following about meperidine is false?**
   A. Meperidine is used for the relief of moderate to severe pain, for preoperative medication, for support of anesthesia, and as an obstetrical analgesic.
   B. There are few reports of poisoning or fatalities related to meperidine in the medical literature.
   C. Myoclonic jerks or generalized convulsions may occur in overdoses.
   D. The clinical features of tolerance and physical dependence are similar to those for morphine.
   E. The analgesic potency of meperidine is equal to that of morphine.
2. **Which active metabolite of meperidine is a proconvulsant?**
   A. Hydromeperidine
   B. Normeperidinic acid
   C. Normeperidine
   D. Fentanyl
   E. Glycomeperidine
3. **Administration of monoamine oxidase inhibitors with meperidine may lead to hypotension, hypertension, agitation, tremor, hyperpyrexia, convulsions, and coma.**
   A. True
   B. False

Propoxyphene

Propoxyphene (Darvon®) has been used in the U.S. since 1957 and continues to be a widely prescribed drug. Addiction to propoxyphene was first described in 1963 and by 1970, propoxyphene was shown to be no more effective than aspirin or codeine. In fact, propoxyphene is probably inferior to these analgesics. Unfortunately, propoxyphene is associated with many fatalities in overdose and in combination with other drugs such as tranquilizers, alcohol, and sedatives. In 1972, the patent for Darvon expired and the marketplace was subsequently flooded with brand name and generic propoxyphene.

In 1977, naloxone was used successfully in the treatment of propoxyphene overdose coingested with alcohol. By 1979, at least 500 propoxyphene-related deaths were caused by abuse and addiction each year; this number has since declined. That year, FDA warnings regarding suicide, addiction, alcohol use, and fatalities were issued. In 1980, it was recognized that although naloxone was an effective antagonist, rapidity of deterioration with sustained irreversible cerebral damage still resulted in 40% of patients before they reached resuscitation facilities.

Propoxyphene is used as a mild narcotic analgesic and has been used as an alternative to methadone to maintain and detoxify heroin-dependent individuals. It has also been used in the detoxification and maintenance of individuals addicted to methadone, pentazocine, codeine, meperidine, and oxycodone.

PATHOPHYSIOLOGY

Propoxyphene, a synthetic chemical, is structurally and pharmacologically related to methadone. Propoxyphene is a narcotic agonist and antagonist that exhibits physical and psychological dependence, tolerance, and withdrawal symptoms. Its action on opioid receptor sites is blocked by naloxone.

PHARMACOKINETICS

Absorption

- Propoxyphene is subject to pronounced first-pass biotransformation after oral administration.
- Only a small fraction of the absorbed dose enters the general circulation in unmetabolized form. Intestinal and hepatic enzymes during absorption metabolize the rest.
- Single-dose kinetics indicates complete oral absorption.

Distribution

- The volume of distribution is 10–18 L/kg. Propoxyphene is distributed in liver, lung, brain, kidney, and comparatively little in the blood.
- Protein binding is 73–80%.

Elimination

- Propoxyphene is eliminated by mono-N-demethylation via a mixed-function oxidase in the liver to form the cardiotoxic metabolite norpropoxyphene.
- Elimination half-lives are 14.6 hours for propoxyphene, 22.9 hours for norpropoxyphene (oral), and 26.7 hours for norpropoxyphene (intravenous).
- Less than 10% of the parent drug is excreted in the kidneys. Norpropoxyphene and its conjugates are excreted in the urine.
- Norpropoxyphene is cleared from the body much more slowly than propoxyphene and reaches higher plasma levels.
- Like propoxyphene, norpropoxyphene is cardiotoxic in high concentrations and may be the cause of the cardiotoxicity in propoxyphene intoxication. Narcotic antagonists do not effectively counteract the cardiotoxic effects of propoxyphene and its metabolites.

CLINICAL PRESENTATIONS

Symptoms and signs occur early, within 30 minutes after ingestion, and consist of nausea, vomiting, and drowsiness, which may progress to central nervous system depression. Within 1 hour, generalized or local seizures, respiratory depression, and cardiovascular collapse may occur. Less commonly, diabetes insipidus, pulmonary edema, and a myopathic syndrome with muscle pain, tenderness, muscle weakness, and rhabdomyolysis have been seen.

Cardiac conduction disturbances observed after propoxyphene overdose are not those usually seen with other narcotic agents. They may include transient right heart block, bigeminy, QRS prolongation, and ST-T wave abnormalities. Narcotic antagonists do not alter them. Hepatic dysfunction and papular eruption have also been described. As in other opiate ingestions, miotic pupils are seen. Propoxyphene differs from other narcotics in that abusers may have grand mal seizures in the presence of a normal EEG and brain scan when their addiction requires the use of propoxyphene in excess of 1,000 mg per day.

TOXIC DOSAGE/DEATH

Oral propoxyphene, 100–500 mg, may produce a "high" associated with nausea, vomiting, dizziness, delirium, slurred speech, and hallucinations. At doses above 500 mg, euphoria, convulsions, and coma have been reported. At 35 mg/kg, propoxyphene has produced cardiac and respiratory arrest, and at 0.9–1.3 grams, death has ensued. Smaller amounts may cause death when ingested with ethanol or other central nervous system depressants. A 1.2-gram daily dose of propoxyphene is equivalent to 20–25 mg of morphine. The cause of death from propoxyphene overdose is usually respiratory depression; however, cardiac arrhythmias may be a contributing factor. Most deaths occur before the patient reaches the hospital.

DRUG INTERACTIONS

Propoxyphene potentiates the action of alcohol, barbiturates, tricyclic antidepressants, tranquilizers, other narcotics, and anesthetics. It increases the blood levels of phenytoin, carbamazepine, phenobarbital, and doxepin. Propoxyphene effects may be potentiated by antihistamines, so called "P's and Blues." Effects include increased analgesia and mild euphoria as well as moderately severe symptoms of opiate withdrawal at therapeutic doses.

PREGNANCY/LACTATION

Withdrawal symptoms occur within 24 hours in passively addicted neonates of addicted mothers. Propoxyphene has generally not been found in breast milk, although this route may excrete it if taken in high doses. Twice as much norpropoxyphene as propoxyphene is excreted into breast milk.

LABORATORY

Analytic Methods

Propoxyphene may be detected by gas-liquid chromatography and confirmed by gas chromatography/mass spectrometry.

Blood Levels

Serum and urine levels of propoxyphene do not indicate the amount of drug ingested or the severity of the poisoning. Drug levels identify only the intoxicant and are of little value in clinical management or prognosis. Peak plasma levels of propoxyphene after an oral 65-mg dose are 84–94 ng/mL and are reached in 1.1–1.5 hours. The peak plasma level of propoxyphene after a 130-mg oral dose is 226 ng/mL and is reached in 2 hours.

Toxic levels are considered $> 20\ \mu g/100$ mL and lethal levels are generally in the 50–120 $\mu g/100$ mL range. Ethanol or other drugs are often found in propoxyphene fatalities. Overdoses of commercial formulations containing propoxyphene require analysis of salicylates or acetaminophen.

TREATMENT

Gut Decontamination

If the patient is alert, not convulsing, and has an intact gag reflex charcoal may be given, and lavage attempted, if the patient is seen within 30 minutes of ingestion. If the patient is obtunded, comatose, seizing, or rapidly developing respiratory depression, gastric lavage is only indicated with adequate protection of the trachea by endotracheal intubation. Activated charcoal binds up to 60% of the ingested drug when given within 2 hours. Cathartics, magnesium sulfate or sodium sulfate can be tried, but data substantiating their efficacy are not available.

Elimination Enhancement

Propoxyphene has a large volume of distribution, a high degree of protein binding, and a high organ concentration. Hemodialysis does not remove significant amounts of propoxyphene or norpropoxyphene from the body and is of little value in a propoxyphene overdose. As renal clearance is a small factor in removing parent compound, forced diuresis is not only of little usefulness, but may produce or exacerbate cases with pulmonary edema.

Supportive Measures

- Airway, breathing, and circulatory status must be immediately ascertained. If breathing is compromised, insert an endotracheal tube and mechanically ventilate. Monitor vital signs, consciousness, arterial blood gases, fluid intake and output, pupil size, and electrolytes.
- Serum electrolytes, liver and kidney function tests, and an electrocardiogram should be performed on admission and periodically thereafter on patients who are symptomatic or otherwise suspected of serious overdose.
- Naloxone and oxygen may initially increase seizure threshold. Intravenous diazepam (10 mg in an adult and 0.1–0.3 mg/kg in a child) should be used to treat seizures initially, however it may potentiate central nervous system depression.
- Phenytoin is the second drug of choice. However, its action may begin up to 30 minutes postinjection. Phenobarbital may be used, but it also potentiates nervous system depression.
- Clonidine may be helpful in detoxifying addicted patients.
- If propoxyphene with acetaminophen has been ingested in overdose, acetaminophen levels must be checked. If such levels are in the hepatotoxic range (see Acetaminophen chapter), appropriate N-acetyl-l-cysteine (Mucomyst®) therapy should be initiated.
- Circulatory failure may respond to dopamine infusions in patients suffering from acute propoxyphene overdose.

ANTIDOTES

Naloxone

Repeat doses of naloxone may be required to reverse signs and symptoms of respiratory depression, since symptoms may recur within 10–20 minutes of an initial naloxone dose. Continuous intravenous infusion of naloxone may be required, since the symptoms of propoxyphene ingestion often last 8–12 hours. Increased respiratory rate, dilation of pupils, rapid awakening, and improved cardiovascular status may be seen in 1–3 minutes. Continuous monitoring of pulse, respiratory rate, mental status, and pupillary size is indicated.

High doses (i.e., greater than 2.0 mg intravenously) of naloxone may be required initially. Naloxone may provoke a withdrawal reaction. Withdrawal symptoms may be blocked by clonidine, an α-2 agonist, which is known to block the release of norepinephrine associated with opiate withdrawal.

Questions—Propoxyphene

1. Which of the following regarding propoxyphene is false?

A. Addiction to propoxyphene is well described.
B. Propoxyphene is associated with many fatalities in overdose and in combination with other drugs such as tranquilizers, alcohol, and sedatives.
C. Naloxone is an effective antidote.
D. Propoxyphene, a synthetic chemical, is pharmacologically related to methadone.
E. The analgesic potency of propoxyphene approximates that of meperidine.

2. Regarding the cardiotoxic effects of propoxyphene,

A. Cardiac conduction disturbances observed after propoxyphene overdose are not those usually seen with other narcotic agents.
B. Electrocardiographic effects may include transient right heart block, bigeminy, QRS prolongation, and ST-T wave abnormalities.
C. Narcotic antagonists do not alter them.
D. All of the above
E. B and C

Codeine, Hydrocodone, and Dihydrocodeine

Codeine has been used as an analgesic and antitussive for about 150 years. Fatal intoxications resulting from codeine alone are rare. Fatalities and poisonings occur after ingestion of preparations combining codeine with other agents including aspirin, acetaminophen, antihistamines, sedatives, caffeine, or antitussive preparations such as terpin hydrate. Hydrocodone has an antitussive and analgesic potency approximately six times greater than that of codeine on a mg per mg basis.

Codeine is structurally similar to morphine. Hydrocodone and dihydrocodeine are structurally similar to codeine. Codeine is prepared commercially as the salt of the natural opium alkaloid codeine and has been referred to as schoolboy, cough syrup, and number 4s.

During the 1970s, an oral drug combination known as a "hit" or "loads" consisting of codeine (60 mg)—usually in combination with aspirin, phenacetin, or caffeine—and glutethimide (500 mg), was responsible for a large number of deaths in some U.S. cities. It is readily available, relatively inexpensive, and considered an oral substitute for heroin. A lethal comatose state is produced at unpredictable low levels of each drug when they are taken together.

PATHOPHYSIOLOGY

Codeine is a mu receptor agonist, which acts pharmacologically like other opiates.

PHARMACOKINETICS

Absorption

- Codeine is well absorbed throughout the intestinal tract.
- After a single 30-mg dose of codeine, maximum plasma concentrations are observed at about 1 hour (codeine) and 1.28 hours (codeine 6-glucuronide).
- Hydrocodone is also well absorbed.

Distribution

- The volume of distribution of codeine is 5.0 L/kg after oral administration and 2.6 L/kg after intramuscular injection.
- The volume of distribution of dihydrocodeine is 1.28 L/kg after intravenous administration.

Elimination

- Codeine is metabolized to codeine-6-glucuronide (80%), norcodeine (2%), morphine (0.5%), morphine-3-glucuronide (2%), morphine-6-glucuronide (0.8%), and normorphine (2.5%).
- Morphine-6-glucuronide has a stronger analgesic effect than morphine itself. Its plasma concentration is higher than that of morphine. Codeine-6-glucuronide probably possesses an activity similar to codeine. The plasma concentration of codeine-6-glucuronide is probably higher than that of codeine.
- The half-life of codeine is 1.5 hours, that of codeine-6-glucuronide is 2.75 hours, that of morphine-3-glucuronide is 2.75 hours, and that of morphine-3-glucuronide is 1.7 hours.
- The kidney excretes two-thirds of its alkaloid metabolites within 6 hours.
- The half-life of dihydrocodeine is 3.3–4.5 hours, and of hydrocodone, 3.8 hours. The kidney is the main site of excretion. Prolonged narcosis with dihydrocodeine overdose has been observed in renal failure.

CLINICAL PRESENTATIONS

In children, symptoms begin within the first hour and may include somnolence, rash, miosis, vomiting, itching, ataxia, and puffiness. In adults, signs may include lethargy, miosis, nausea, vomiting and weakness. Teenagers and college students have abused cough syrup containing codeine and alcohol. Terpin hydrate and codeine may contain as much as 43% ethanol (86 proof).

Fatalities may result from respiratory depression. Similar experiences have resulted from consumption of cough medicine containing hydrocodone. Few fatalities resulting solely from oral ingestion of codeine have been reported, because codeine is seldom marketed or prescribed except in combination with other drugs. When fatalities resulting solely from codeine have occurred, they have generally followed intravenous injection by narcotic addicts.

TOXIC DOSAGE/DEATH

The adult lethal dose from codeine has been reported to be 0.5–1.0 grams. Attainment of a lethal amount of codeine through commercial preparations would generally require the ingestion of 8–15 one-grain tablets or one-half to 1 pint of cough syrup. A single oral overdose of codeine (5–15 mg/kg) is often tolerated by small children, however even at 5 mg/kg, serious respiratory depression may occur in some children. In one case, two doses of a cough syrup containing 10 mg of codeine phosphate per 5 mL given to a prematurely born 3-month-old infant produced apnea, coma, and pinpoint pupils, which responded to mouth-to-mouth resuscitation and later naloxone. The lethal dose of hydrocodone is approximately 90 mg.

Peak blood levels of dihydrocodeine are reached 1.6–1.8 hours after oral (30 and 60 mg) or intravenous (30 mg) administration. Toxic blood levels of codeine have been reported to range from 1.0–8.8 μg/mL, and toxic levels of dihydrocodeine average about 1 μg/mL. Fatal blood levels of codeine range from 1.4–5.6 μg/mL, and those of dihydrocodeine, from 0.8–12 μg/mL.

PREGNANCY/LACTATION

Use of codeine during labor produces neonatal depression to the same degree as other narcotic analgesics. Neonatal codeine withdrawal may occur. Codeine passes into breast milk.

LABORATORY

Analytic Methods

Codeine, norcodeine, morphine, and normorphine with their corresponding glucuronide conjugates can be quantitated in human plasma and urine by high-performance liquid chromatography with electrochemical detection. One method for isolation and identification of dihydrocodeine uses gas chromatography and mass spectrometry. A procedure for the determination of hydrocodone in serum uses electron-capture gas chromatography.

Blood Levels

Plasma concentrations are not closely correlated with brain concentration, relief of pain, or severity of overdose symptoms. Codeine sulfate, 60 mg orally, produces peak blood levels of 150 ng/mL in 30 minutes. At 3 hours, the levels are down to 65 ng/mL, and by 12 hours, they are less than 20 ng/mL. After oral codeine use, unconjugated morphine concentrations peak at 1 hour with a level of 11 ng/mL. Codeine phosphate or unconjugated codeine produces a peak level of 200 ng/mL in 30 minutes, 120 ng/mL at 3 hours and 20 ng/mL at 12 hours.

TREATMENT

Gut Decontamination

Gastric lavage is preferable to induced emesis if there is any evidence of diminished alertness or loss of gag reflex. It is doubtful whether this procedure is useful more than 2 hours after ingestion, unless large amounts of codeine have been ingested.

Activated charcoal (in adults, 30–50 grams and in children, .5–1 g/kg) may be helpful.

Elimination Enhancement

Dialysis procedures are probably unnecessary due to excellent renal clearance and the usefulness of narcotic antagonists such as naloxone. There have been no clinical studies evaluating extracorporeal procedures.

Supportive Measures

- Respiratory depression must be urgently countered with endotracheal intubation if necessary. Arterial blood gases must be monitored carefully.

ANTIDOTES

Naloxone may be useful when administered by continuous infusion. (See guidelines in the Introduction). Therapeutic measures in dihydrocodeine overdose are similar to those used for codeine overdose. Several cases have required continuous i.v. naloxone infusions for 1–3 days.

Questions—Codeine, Hydrocodone, and Dihydrocodeine

1. Which of the following regarding codeine is false?

A. Codeine has been used as an analgesic and antitussive for about 150 years.
B. Fatal intoxications resulting from codeine alone are rare.
C. Fatalities and poisonings occur after ingestion of preparations combining codeine with other agents including aspirin, acetaminophen, antihistamines, sedatives, caffeine, or antitussive preparations such as terpin hydrate.
D. Hydrocodone has an antitussive and analgesic potency approximately six times greater than that of codeine on a milligram per milligram basis.
E. During the 1970s, an oral drug combination known as a "hit" or "loads" consisting of codeine (60 mg)—usually in combination with paregoric—and glutethimide (500 mg), was responsible for a large number of deaths in some U.S. cities.

2. Codeine is a(n) _____ receptor agonist, which acts pharmacologically like other opiates.

A. Epsilon
B. Delta
C. Mu
D. Beta
E. Alpha

Pentazocine

Pentazocine (Talwin®) is a narcotic agonist and antagonist. It has less abuse potential than morphine but may lead to physical dependence, psychological dependence, and tolerance. Naloxone can reverse the respiratory depression produced by pentazocine and induce withdrawal symptoms in patients who are also using other narcotics, including methadone. Abrupt discontinuation of pentazocine after extended use leads to withdrawal symptoms. As an agonist, it produces analgesia. It is a weak antagonist to analgesic, cardiovascular, respiratory, and behavioral depression effects induced by morphine and meperidine. The analgesic potency of pentazocine, 20–40 mg, is equivalent to 10 mg of morphine.

Ill effects, including hallucinations, have been noted since the FDA first approved the drug in 1967. At that time, drowsiness, dizziness, inability to think, vertigo, vomiting, euphoria, incoordination, extrapyramidal effects, confusion, rhinorrhea, hives, nausea, muscular tremor, and tightness of the chest were reported. By 1969, reports of physical dependence appeared. Ultimately, a high incidence of abuse was noted in the medical profession. Pentazocine abusers may suffer the same medical complications as other parenteral drug abusers. Problems after parenteral use may produce cutaneous change ("woody" fibroma) and/or glomerulonephritis. In the U.S., the oral drug form has been reformulated to include an opioid antagonist (naloxone) to reduce abuse potential.

Uses of pentazocine include treatment of moderate to severe pain, as a preoperative or preanesthetic medication, and as a supplement to surgical anesthesia. Oral Talwin NX contains pentazocine hydrochloride (50-mg base) and naloxone hydrochloride (0.5 mg). If this preparation is misused and taken intravenously, withdrawal symptoms may result. Drug abusers or addicts may experience nausea, vomiting, hypertension, hyperirritability, and sweating.

T'S AND BLUES

Pentazocine in combination with the antihistamine tripelennamine has been termed "T's and Blues." It has also been called "T's and B's," "Tops and Bottoms," and "Teddies and Betties." Tripelennamine was synthesized in 1946 and used in the late 1940s by addicts treating themselves for morphine withdrawal. Later, it was used with paregoric, heroin, or morphine in a combination known as "Blue Velvet." There is no significant metabolic interaction between pentazocine and tripelennamine.

"T's and Blues" are created by crushing two pentazocine tablets with one tripelennamine tablet, dissolving in water, straining through cotton, and injecting intravenously. The effect consists of an immediate "flash" or euphoric sensation similar to a heroin "rush" which lasts 5–10 minutes. A feeling of well-being, which slowly subsides over 4–6 hours, follows this. When dysphoria supervenes, repeated injections may be administered to ameliorate this feeling. Malaise, restlessness, irritability, and mild abdominal cramping are frequently observed.

Other abused pentazocine combinations include pentazocine and diazepam, pentazocine and diphenhydramine ("Soup"), and pentazocine and methylphenidate ("Tea and Crackers"). See also "P's and Blues" (propoxyphene and antihistamines) under Propoxyphene.

PATHOPHYSIOLOGY

Pentazocine is a benzomorphan, which is pharmacologically related to butorphanol tartrate (Stadol®). It is a white, crystalline, synthetic chemical. Pentazocine has both agonist and antagonist properties as a central nervous system depressant. It shares physiologic properties with other opiates. Pentazocine has agonist effects at the kappa and delta receptors and antagonist effects at the mu receptor.

PHARMACOKINETICS

Absorption

- Pentazocine is not as well absorbed from the gastrointestinal tract as it is from parenteral sites.
- There is a large first-pass effect.

Distribution

- High levels are found in the brain, blood, liver, bile, kidney, and urine. Because of the very high volume of distribution

(4.89 L/kg), brain concentrations (unchanged pentazocine) often exceed blood levels.
- The pKA is 9, and 60–70% is protein bound in the plasma.

Elimination

- Pentazocine is metabolized by oxidation and glucuronide conjugation in the liver.
- Its elimination half-life is 2 hours.

CLINICAL PRESENTATIONS

Signs and symptoms of overdose include those seen with pentazocine alone or in combination with acetaminophen or aspirin. Anxiety, nightmares, and hallucinations may be seen. Pentazocine occasionally produces mild to severe psychotomimetic effects in therapeutic dosage. Elevated blood pressure, tachycardia, nausea, vomiting and abdominal pain may be seen.

Respiratory Effects

As in all opiate overdoses, respiratory depression, decreased respiratory rate, decreased tidal volume, increased $PaCO_2$ levels, and apnea are possible. It can be a respiratory depressant in therapeutic dosage. Talc pulmonary granulomas, pulmonary hypertension, and pulmonary fibrosis may follow long-term use with "T's and Blues."

Neurologic Effects

Dizziness, lethargy, and paresthesias have been reported. Use of more than one or two tablets of tripelennamine in combination with pentazocine ("T's and Blues") increases the risk of toxic central nervous system stimulation and seizures.

Dermatologic Effects

Local burning sensations resulting from venous irritation has been observed in those injecting "T's and Blues." Local cellulitis and abscess formation may follow subcutaneous administration.

T'S and Blues Withdrawal

Shaking, nausea, vomiting, hallucinations, psychosis, headaches, blurred vision, loss of memory, chest pains, and palpitations have been seen in withdrawal situations.

TOXIC DOSAGE/DEATH

Any dose over the therapeutic dose can be considered toxic. Toxic oral doses of pentazocine also may involve toxic ingestions of salicylates or acetaminophen, and patients must be evaluated and treated simultaneously for these overdoses. Hypersensitivity to pentazocine, acetaminophen, or salicylate can occur with therapeutic doses. Plasma levels in pentazocine fatalities have ranged from 1–5 mg/L.

DRUG INTERACTIONS

Respiratory depression from pentazocine may be potentiated by simultaneous administration of alcohol, sedative-hypnotics, general anesthetics, monoamine oxidase inhibitors and tranquilizers including phenothiazines, other narcotic analgesics, and tricyclic antidepressants.

PREGNANCY/LACTATION

Pentazocine has not been found in breast milk. Maternal ingestion of 150–300 mg/d may result in withdrawal symptoms, including coarse tremors, irritability, vomiting, diarrhea, and hyperhidrosis, in infants within the first 24 hours after birth. Paregoric and chlorpromazine may be used to counteract these effects. Respiratory depression and apnea have occurred in newborn infants whose mothers received pentazocine during labor.

In Chicago and St. Louis, many pregnant women were reported to have used "T's and Blues" during pregnancy. This resulted in the birth of infants whose mean birth weight and head circumference were smaller than normal, who had poor neurologic development, and who went through withdrawal.

LABORATORY

Analytic Methods

A high-performance liquid chromatography method using fluorometric detection rapidly quantifies pentazocine in plasma.

Blood Levels

Blood and urine levels may confirm the qualitative presence of pentazocine, but insufficient data have been accumulated to correlate such levels with clinical course in overdose states. Peak plasma levels of pentazocine after therapeutic oral use (75 mg) are reached in 2–3 hours and average about 0.16 mg/L. After intramuscular use (45 mg), peak levels are reached in 15–60 minutes (0.14 mg/L). After an intravenous injection of 30 mg, peak values occur in 5–10 minutes and average approximately 0.2–1.0 mg/L.

TREATMENT

Gut Decontamination

Gut decontamination measures including gastric lavage, activated charcoal, and cathartics must be determined by the clinical state of the patient and the route of poisoning overdosage. If ingested within a few hours, charcoal may effectively bind pentazocine.

Elimination Enhancement

There are no adequate data to substantiate use of dialysis or hemoperfusion in pentazocine overdose. However, the large volume of distribution and high degree of protein binding would tend to lessen the effectiveness of such procedures.

Supportive Measures

- As in all opiate overdoses, attention must first focus on airway, breathing, and circulation issues. Intubate as necessary. Treatment is supportive and symptomatic.
- Pentazocine has been associated with elevated levels of serum aminotransferases and EEG epileptiform abnormalities. Renal and hepatic function tests must be monitored during treatment of pentazocine overdose.
- Electrocardiographic changes may occur, especially in the presence of hypertension or myocardial ischemia.
- Monitoring of arterial blood gases is indicated in pentazocine overdose with respiratory depression. Monitor fluids, electrolytes, baseline blood alcohol, and screen for other drugs.

ANTIDOTES

Naloxone

Naloxone, in higher than usual doses, may be required to reverse pentazocine overdose signs and symptoms. Since pentazocine has agonist effects at the kappa and delta receptors and antagonist effects at the mu receptor, naloxone, which exerts its primary effect on the mu receptor, may not effectively antagonize the agonist actions at these receptor sites. This difference may account for the observed failure of naloxone to block the effects of "T's and Blues." As naloxone is short-acting when compared with pentazocine, a continuous infusion of naloxone should be considered.

Questions—Pentazocine

1. **Because pentazocine is a narcotic agonist and antagonist, it has less abuse potential than morphine and does not lead to physical dependence, psychological dependence, and tolerance.**
   A. True
   B. False
2. **Naloxone can reverse the respiratory depression produced by pentazocine and induce withdrawal symptoms in patients who are also using other narcotics, including methadone.**
   A. True
   B. False
3. **Pentazocine in combination with the antihistamine tripelennamine has been termed "T's and Blues." There is no significant metabolic interaction between pentazocine and tripelennamine.**
   A. True
   B. False
4. **Other abused pentazocine combinations include pentazocine and diazepam, pentazocine and diphenhydramine ("Soup"), and pentazocine and methylphenidate ("Tea and Crackers").**
   A. True
   B. False

Oxycodone

Oxycodone (OxyContin®) is a semisynthetic, modified codeine narcotic agonist. It is available in a long-acting pure form, OxyContin®, and popularly with acetaminophen (Percocet®) and aspirin (Percodan®). Its analgesic potency is slightly less than that of morphine, but its duration of action is similar (4–5 hours). It is a Schedule II narcotic under the Controlled Substances Act. It has morphine-like potential for addiction and withdrawal. Like codeine and methadone, oxycodone retains about one-half of its analgesic potency orally.

PATHOPHYSIOLOGY

Oxycodone is similar to other opiate agonists. See chapters on Acetaminophen and Salicylates regarding the additive effects of these agents when taken with oxycodone.

PHARMACOKINETICS

Absorption

- Oxycodone is absorbed from the gastrointestinal tract and produces peak blood levels in 1 hour.

Distribution

- Oxycodone is found in the blood, brain, liver, bile, and gastric contents.
- Oxycodone by intravenous bolus exhibits a half-life of about 4 hours, clearance of 0.78 L/min, and volume of distribution at steady state of 2.6 L/kg.

Elimination

- Oxycodone, like hydrocodone, appears to be detoxified in the liver and excreted in the urine. Noroxycodone is an active metabolite.
- The elimination half-life is about 4 hours.

CLINICAL PRESENTATIONS

The clinical picture is similar to that of codeine and other opiate overdoses. Pulmonary edema has been described after oxycodone use.

TOXIC DOSAGE/DEATH

Blood levels of oxycodone in an addicted patient maintained on high doses (25 tablets every 4 hours) averaged 0.12 μg/mL. The blood noroxycodone level was 0.15 μg/mL 30 minutes after a dose of 25 tablets. The urine level of oxycodone was 14 μg/mL. Death has usually been associated with blood levels greater than 4 mg/L.

DRUG INTERACTIONS

Additive central nervous system depression may occur with other narcotic analgesics, general anesthetics, phenothiazines, tranquilizers, sedative-hypnotics, and central nervous system depressants such as alcohol. Special-risk patients include the elderly, debilitated patients with severe impairment of hepatic or renal function, hypothyroidism, Addison's disease, and those with sensitivity to salicylates or acetaminophen.

PREGNANCY/LACTATION

Pregnancy risk category B (D if used for prolonged periods or in high doses at term).

LABORATORY

Analytic Methods

Thin-layer chromatography can be used to detect oxycodone. Gas chromatography with electron capture may also be useful. A high-performance liquid chromatography method with electrochemical detection can detect 2 ng/mL in 2 mL of plasma.

Blood Levels

Therapeutic concentrations of oxycodone range up to 0.1 mg/L. Analysis of blood concentration does not aid in the management of oxycodone overdose. Blood should be taken for analysis of salicylate and acetaminophen, 4–6 hours respectively after any significant overdose.

TREATMENT

Gut Decontamination

Gastric lavage and charcoal may be helpful within the first few hours of overdose. As lethargy may be evident, care must be taken to protect a patient's airway above all else.

Elimination Enhancement

Hemodialysis is not helpful in the management of pure oxycodone overdoses, but may be helpful if a significant quantity of aspirin (see Salicylates chapter) is coingested.

Supportive Measures

- Airway, breathing, and circulation issues are the first concern. Mechanical ventilatory support may be necessary in cases involving profound respiratory depression.
- Fluids, oxygen, and vasopressors may be used as required.
- Symptoms and signs of salicylate overdose (Percodan®) or acetaminophen overdose (Percocet®) may require confirmation by blood salicylate or blood acetaminophen levels to institute specific therapy. Where toxic acetaminophen levels exist in blood, serious hepatotoxicity may ensue and acetylcysteine treatment must be instituted.

Questions—Oxycodone

1. **Which of the following about oxycodone is false?**
   A. Oxycodone is a narcotic agonist which is a modified hydromorphone compound.
   B. It is frequently combined with aspirin or acetaminophen in commercial preparations.
   C. It is available in a long-acting pure form.
   D. It has morphine-like potential for addiction and withdrawal.
   E. Like codeine and methadone, oxycodone retains about half of its analgesic potency orally.
2. **Pulmonary edema has been described after oxycodone use.**
   A. True
   B. False

Butorphanol

Butorphanol (Stadol®) was introduced in 1978 for the relief of moderate to severe pain. As an agonist, it is 3.5–7 times more potent than morphine by the intramuscular or subcutaneous route, 30–40 times more potent than meperidine, and 20 times more potent than pentazocine. It appears to be effective in the treatment of migraines, cancer pain, musculoskeletal pain, and post-cesarean section pain.

Butorphanol tartrate is available as a nasal spray (Stadol®) and has been approved to treat pain for which an opioid analgesic is appropriate. Little is known about abuse potential, development of tolerance, or craving. However, butorphanol may induce withdrawal in patients dependent on opiates. It also may cause respiratory depression. Adverse effects of butorphanol include sedation, nausea, dizziness, confusion, headache, and sweating. It also produces psychotomimetic reactions.

PATHOPHYSIOLOGY

Butorphanol is a potent synthetic opiate agonist and antagonist similar to pentazocine.

PHARMACOKINETICS

Absorption

- The oral, nasal, or parenteral routes absorb butorphanol.
- Peak blood levels are reached 1.0–1.5 hours after oral administration and 0.5–1 hours after intramuscular injection. Oral bioavailability is 17% because of a first-pass hepatic effect.

Distribution

- Protein binding is 80%.

Elimination

- Butorphanol is metabolized to hydroxybutorphanol (no pharmacological activity) and has an elimination half-life of 2.5–3.5 hours.
- It is excreted largely in the urine (70%) and in the biliary tract (11%).

CLINICAL PRESENTATIONS

Use of butorphanol nasal spray for migraine treatment has been associated with hallucinations, feelings of being "extremely stoned" or "stuporous," and feelings of inability to move. Sedation, dizziness, nausea, vomiting, insomnia, and nasal congestion have been observed. Miosis may be seen. Hypotension, syncope, and severe hypertension have also been reported. Overdose may induce respiratory depression and cardiovascular changes including increased pulmonary artery pressure, pulmonary wedge pressure, left ventricular end-diastolic pressure, systemic arterial pressure, and pulmonary vascular resistance.

TOXIC DOSAGE/DEATH

Death from cardiopulmonary arrest has followed use of butorphanol in surgery. The butorphanol blood level in this case was 6 mg/L.

DRUG INTERACTIONS

Butorphanol may potentiate the effects of narcotic analgesia, phenothiazines, monoamine oxidase inhibitors, sedatives and hypnotics, general anesthetics, alcohol, and tricyclic antidepressants.

PREGNANCY/LACTATION

Butorphanol passes through the placenta to the fetus, producing cord serum levels averaging 84% of maternal concentrations. It also passes into breast milk in concentrations paralleling levels in maternal serum.

LABORATORY

Analytic Methods

Butorphanol has been analyzed in biological fluids by radioimmunoassay, electron-capture gas chromatography, and gas chromatography-mass spectrometry.

Blood Levels

Blood levels have not been reported as being helpful in the management of butorphanol effects. A 1-mg intravenous injection of butorphanol is followed within 15 minutes by plasma butorphanol concentrations up to 1.3 mg/L, declining to 0.6 mg/L by 1 hour.

TREATMENT

Gut Decontamination

Gastric lavage and activated charcoal are indicated when butorphanol is taken orally.

Elimination Enhancement

These methods have not been applied to the management of butorphanol in overdose.

Supportive Measures

- Attention to airway, breathing and circulation is the foremost concern. Oxygen, intravenous fluids, and vasopressors may be required. Intubation with controlled respirations may be indicated.

ANTIDOTES

Naloxone, per aforementioned protocols for opiate overdoses, is indicated in severe cases.

Questions—Butorphanol

1. **Which of the following is true?**
   A. Use of butorphanol nasal spray for migraines has been associated with hallucinations.
   B. Paradoxical mydriasis may be seen as butorphanol is an opiate agonist and antagonist.

C. Hypotension and hypertension have been reported with butorphanol use.
D. A and B
E. A and C

Nalbuphine

Nalbuphine (Nubain®) is a synthetic opiate agonist/antagonist. It is chemically related to naloxone (a narcotic antagonist) and oxymorphone (a narcotic agonist). Nalbuphine appears useful in reversing respiratory depression that occurs after post-surgical epidural opioid administration. It may be used by intramuscular, intravenous, or subcutaneous administration. Nalbuphine is, milligram for milligram, equal to morphine and three times as potent as pentazocine. Its abuse potential is equal to that of pentazocine and probably less than that of codeine.

PATHOPHYSIOLOGY

Nalbuphine is an agonist at kappa receptors in the spinal cord and an antagonist at other opioid receptors.

PHARMACOKINETICS

Absorption

- After intravenous use, its action begins in 2–3 minutes and lasts 3–6 hours.

Distribution

- Peak plasma levels of 48 ng/mL have been reached 30 minutes after intramuscular administration.

Elimination

- It is metabolized in the liver to inactive metabolites. Metabolites are excreted in the bile and in the urine.
- The elimination half-life after intravenous administration of nalbuphine was 0.9 hour in children (after 0.2 mg/kg) and 2.3 hours in the elderly (10 mg) in one study.

CLINICAL PRESENTATIONS

Clinical effects include miosis, lethargy, hypotension, nausea, vomiting, respiratory depression, rare pulmonary edema, hallucinations, confusion, anxiety and headache. Skin rash and urticaria have also been seen.

TOXIC DOSAGE/DEATH

A single 72-mg subcutaneous injection into normal volunteers produced only sleepiness and mild dysphoria.

DRUG INTERACTIONS

Its effects may be additive when used with other central nervous system depressants such as alcohol, narcotics, general anesthetics, phenothiazines, other tranquilizers, sedatives, and hypnotics.

PREGNANCY/LACTATION

Pregnancy risk category B. It passes through the placenta and may produce respiratory depression in the neonate comparable to that induced by meperidine. Fetal plasma concentrations are about the same or higher than maternal concentrations and may be associated with respiratory and cardiac depression.

TREATMENT

Gut Decontamination

Lavage and charcoal may be helpful in the unusual case that a parenteral form is ingested.

Elimination Enhancement

No reports of treatment with these methods are available.

Supportive Measures

- Oxygen, fluids, and vasopressors may be required in individual cases.

ANTIDOTES

The manufacturer recommends the immediate intravenous administration of naloxone hydrochloride as a specific antidote.

Question—Nalbuphine

1. Which of the following about nalbuphine is false?
A. Nalbuphine is a synthetic opiate agonist and antagonist.
B. It is related to naloxone (a narcotic antagonist) and oxymorphone (a narcotic agonist).
C. Nalbuphine is less potent than morphine and three times as potent as pentazocine.
D. Its abuse potential is equal to that of pentazocine and probably less than that of codeine.
E. Nalbuphine is an agonist at kappa receptors in the spinal cord and an antagonist at other opioid receptors.

Paregoric

Paregoric (camphorated tincture of opium) is used as an antidiarrheal agent and is often mixed with other agents of unproved effectiveness. Paregoric is a mixture of powdered opium, anise oil, benzoic acid, camphor, dilute alcohol, and glycerin. In 3 ounces of paregoric, there may be 40 mg of morphine (opium contains about 10% morphine), smaller amounts of codeine, and other alkaloids. Usual oral doses do not produce euphoria or analgesia. Paregoric is considered the treatment of choice for neonatal abstinence syndrome and is more effective than diazepam in controlling seizures in neonatal abstinence periods associated with narcotic withdrawal.

Paregoric was actually sold over the counter until 1971. Since then, it has been available only by prescription. In the 1950s, some large cities had more paregoric addicts than heroin addicts. At that time, it was taken orally and intravenously.

PATHOPHYSIOLOGY

The physiology of paregoric resembles that of any other opiate. It increases smooth muscle tone throughout the gastrointestinal tract. For the pathophysiology of other ingredients, please see relevant chapters.

PHARMACOKINETICS

Absorption

- It is well absorbed after oral use.

Distribution

- Duration of action is 4–5 hours.

Elimination

- It is metabolized in the liver and excreted via the kidneys.

CLINICAL PRESENTATIONS

Prolonged use of paregoric has produced physical dependence despite its unappealing taste. Parenteral paregoric has produced local severe inflammatory reactions and scarring, especially over the jugular vein. Pulmonary hypertension, granulomas, and fibrosis have resulted from concomitant use of talc. Abscesses, cellulitis, thrombophlebitis, hepatitis, bacterial endocarditis and septicemia may occur with intravenous use. The camphor in paregoric is capable of causing seizures, and there is no therapeutic rationale for its presence in the mixture.

DRUG INTERACTIONS

Its effects may be additive when used with other central nervous system depressants such as alcohol, narcotics, general anesthetics, phenothiazines, other tranquilizers, sedatives, and hypnotics.

PREGNANCY/LACTATION

Pregnancy risk category B.

TREATMENT

Gut Decontamination

Lavage and charcoal may be helpful. As camphor may cause the rapid presentation of seizures, attention must focus on protecting the airway if these measures are utilized. Emesis is contraindicated.

Elimination Enhancement

No reports of treatment of paregoric with these methods are available.

Supportive Measures

- Oxygen, fluids, and vasopressors may be required in individual cases.
- Intravenous benzodiazepines may be vital in treating camphor-induced seizures.

ANTIDOTES

Naloxone may reverse the respiratory depression induced by paregoric.

Questions—Paregoric

1. **Prolonged use of paregoric does not produce physical dependence.**
   A. True
   B. False
2. **Pulmonary hypertension and fibrosis have resulted from use of talc with paregoric.**
   A. True
   B. False
3. **The camphor in paregoric is capable of causing seizures, and there is no therapeutic rationale for its presence in the mixture.**
   A. True
   B. False
4. **Paregoric is considered the treatment of choice for neonatal abstinence syndrome; however, it is less effective than diazepam in controlling seizures in neonatal abstinence periods associated with narcotic withdrawal.**
   A. True
   B. False

Hydromorphone

Hydromorphone (Dilaudid®) is used for the relief of severe pain and as a cough suppressant. Hydromorphone has an analgesic potency five to six times that of morphine and three times that of heroin. Hydromorphone is a hydrogenated ketone of morphine. It is a Schedule II narcotic under the Controlled Substances Act and is frequently abused through street sources.

PATHOPHYSIOLOGY

The physiology of hydromorphone resembles that of any other opiate.

PHARMACOKINETICS

Absorption

- About 60% of an oral dose is absorbed.

Distribution

- The volume of distribution of hydromorphone is approximately 1.2 L/kg.
- It is distributed to skeletal muscle, kidneys, liver, intestinal tract, lungs, spleen, and brain.

Elimination

- Hydromorphone is excreted as the glucuronidated conjugate (30%), as unchanged drug (6%), and as the 6-hydroxy metabolite (traces).
- Oral hydromorphone is metabolized to hydromorphone-3-glucuronide, which accumulates in renal failure.
- The elimination half-life after intravenous use is 2.6 hours and after oral use is 2.48 hours.

CLINICAL PRESENTATIONS

Serious overdose may lead to respiratory depression and somnolence, progressing to stupor or coma, skeletal muscle flaccidity, cold clammy skin, constricted pupils, occasional hypotension, and bradycardia. After intravenous injection, apnea, circulatory collapse, cardiac arrest, and death may occur. Hydromorphone produces psychological dependence, physical dependence, and tolerance.

TOXIC DOSAGE/DEATH

The minimally effective plasma concentration of hydromorphone in patients with chronic severe pain is about 4 ng/mL.

DRUG INTERACTIONS

Effects may be additive when it is used with other opiates or central nervous system depressants such as alcohol, anesthetics, phenothiazines, tranquilizers, sedatives, and hypnotics.

PREGNANCY/LACTATION

It crosses the placental membranes, and low levels are detected in human milk. Infants born to mothers physically dependent on hydromorphone are also physically dependent and may experience respiratory difficulties and withdrawal symptoms after birth.

LABORATORY

Analytic Methods

A radioimmunoassay method to detect plasma levels is available but not clinically useful in the management of overdose.

Blood Levels

Two fatalities exhibited postmortem blood hydromorphone concentrations of 0.5 and 1.2 mg/L, respectively. Plasma concentrations in normal human volunteers reached an average peak of 0.022 ng/L after a single 4-mg dose.

TREATMENT

Gut Decontamination

For oral hydromorphone overdose one may use gastric lavage, activated charcoal, and cathartics with the usual precautions concerning the development of respiratory depression.

Elimination Enhancement

No data are available on the usefulness of diuresis, hemodialysis, or hemoperfusion procedures.

Supportive Measures

- Provide respiratory support and mechanical ventilation as required. Supportive treatment may include oxygen and vasopressors for the occasional overdose, which results in circulatory shock.
- Cardiac arrest or arrhythmias should be treated with usual antiarrhythmic measures outlined in ACLS protocols.
- Clonazepam may be helpful in treating myoclonus, which is occasionally seen after high doses of hydromorphone and other opioids.

ANTIDOTES

Naloxone

Naloxone is a specific antidote against the respiratory depression of hydromorphone and other narcotics. Naloxone must be used cautiously in patients known or suspected to be physically dependent on hydromorphone. Administration of a narcotic antagonist such as naloxone may precipitate a withdrawal reaction.

Question—Hydromorphone

1. Which of the following is false?

A. Hydromorphone is used for the relief of severe pain and as a cough suppressant.
B. Hydromorphone has analgesic potency 5–6 times that of morphine and 3 times that of heroin.
C. Hydromorphone is chemically related to morphine.
D. The physiology of hydromorphone resembles that of any other opiate.
E. Dialysis may be useful in treating overdoses with hydromorphone.

Tramadol

Tramadol (Ultram®) is an orally active synthetic opioid agonist analgesic marketed in Europe and in the U.S. It produces clinical analgesia as effectively as codeine, pentazocine, meperidine, and propoxyphene. Tramadol may be given by mouth, intramuscular, subcutaneous, or intravenous injection, and by suppository.

PATHOPHYSIOLOGY

Tramadol attaches to the mu receptor and blocks norepinephrine and serotonin reuptake.

PHARMACOKINETICS

Absorption

- Peak plasma levels occur at about 1.5 hours.

Distribution

- Tramadol completely penetrates the blood-brain barrier.
- Cerebrospinal fluid levels of tramadol appear to follow closely the serum elimination curve.

Elimination

- Tramadol has a plasma elimination half-life of 5–6 hours.
- It is metabolized to an active desmethyl derivative and several inactive compounds.
- Most excretion takes place through the kidneys.

CLINICAL PRESENTATIONS

Acute overdose may induce miosis, respiratory depression, seizures, hypotonicity, and acidosis. Chronic side effects include fatigue, dizziness, vertigo, headache, visual disorders, nausea, vomiting, sweating, dry mouth, constipation, premature beats, euphoria, dysphoria, hallucinations, and changed body perception. A relative absence of dependence on tramadol was evident in early clinical trials. Minimal withdrawal signs are observed in naloxone precipitation studies.

TOXIC DOSAGE/DEATH

At analgesic doses of 200 mg, vomiting, somnolence, and dizziness have been observed. A 6-month-old child was erroneously given 100 mg tramadol by suppository. Seizures, acidosis, and respiratory depression followed. The child survived with supportive therapy and naloxone.

PREGNANCY/LACTATION

Pregnancy risk factor C. Tramadol does cross the placenta.

LABORATORY

Analytic Methods

Tramadol concentrations in the cerebrospinal fluid, serum, and urine can be measured by gas chromatography-mass spectrometry.

Blood Levels

Therapeutic blood levels in adults are about 100–300 ng/mL (0.1–0.2 μg/mL). Following blood levels does not appear to be helpful in managing overdoses.

TREATMENT

Gut Decontamination

Gastric lavage with airway protection may be useful early after an overdose (within 3–4 hours). Activated charcoal and cathartics have not been studied in tramadol overdoses.

Elimination Enhancement

Dialysis has not been used to treat tramadol overdoses.

Supportive Measures

- Assisted ventilation, a source of oxygen, a central line, and fluids constitute the basic initial treatment of an overdose with tramadol.

ANTIDOTES

Administration of intravenous naloxone 10 μg/kg to a child with a tramadol overdose resulted in pupil widening and rapid restoration of alert behavior. Naloxone may need to be administered repeatedly over a 48-hour period.

Question—Tramadol

1. **Acute overdose with tramadol may cause**
   A. Miosis
   B. Respiratory depression
   C. Seizures
   D. All of the above
   E. A and B

OPIATE ANTAGONISTS

Naloxone

The patient who presents with coma, miosis, and respiratory depression frequently must be treated before knowledge of a specific causative agent or agents is obtained. Such treatment involves immediate protection of the airway, stabilization of the patient, gut decontamination, application of methods, if any, to enhance elimination, use of an antidote, and supportive treatment.

Naloxone (Narcan®), a specific antagonist with no agonist properties at all three major opioid receptor sites (mu, kappa, sigma), is effective in antagonizing symptoms that are usually due to an opiate or a close congener such as diphenoxylate or propoxyphene. Rapid administration is often life-saving. Naloxone has replaced nalorphine and levallorphan (both partial agonists) as the drug of choice in opioid poisoning. Naloxone is a synthetic congener of oxymorphone.

NALOXONE INDICATIONS WITH STRONG CLINICAL SUPPORTING EVIDENCE

- Naloxone reverses the action of opiates including heroin, morphine, methadone, codeine, pentazocine, propoxyphene, dextromethorphan, oxycodone, meperidine, alphaprodine, hydromorphone, butorphanol, and nalbuphine (Nubain®). Higher than usual dosages may be required in codeine, propoxyphene, pentazocine, methadone, and meperidine overdoses.
- Naloxone is diagnostic, and simultaneously often therapeutic in overdoses caused by a mixture of drugs or unknown drugs. Intravenous use is preferable, although intramuscular, subcutaneous, and sublingual routes may be used as required at 20–60 minute intervals. Mixed-drug overdoses may not permit a definitive reversal of symptoms after naloxone use.
- Naloxone reverses sleepiness or ventilatory compromise after administration of a therapeutic dose of morphine. It reverses peripheral vasodilatation after morphine and reverses respiratory depression but not pain relief after intrathecal injection of morphine.

NALOXONE INDICATIONS WITH PROMISING EVIDENCE, YET UNCONFIRMED BY CONTROLLED STUDIES

- Naloxone may provide temporary alleviation of hypotension in cardiogenic, septicemic, and anaphylactic shock. Doses of naloxone higher than those used in opiate overdose may be needed for patients with septic shock, because large quantities of endorphins are released in septic shock. One prospective, randomized, double-blind, placebo controlled study showed that 0.4–1.2 mg naloxone intravenously was no better than a placebo in the amelioration of hypotension in septic shock.
- There is some evidence in animals of a reversal of endotoxin-induced hypotension and possibly of hypotension resulting from bleeding, sepsis, or vasodilatation.
- Naloxone has been used as an aid in promoting weight gain (antilipolytic action) in anorexia nervosa or decreasing food consumption in obesity.
- There is some evidence that it may reverse neurologic deficits in cerebral ischemic disease, however, conflicting studies have disclosed no reversal of neurologic status after naloxone use in patients who have suffered cerebrovascular accidents.
- Naloxone may reverse the pruritus, urinary retention, and respiratory depression seen after epidural analgesia (morphine) without reversing analgesia.
- Noncontrolled observations indicate that naloxone may ameliorate long-term pruritus, asthma, urticaria, and angioedema.
- Possibly effective against (α-2 agonists such as clonidine, guanabenz and guanfacine.
- Possibly effective against imidazoline nasal sprays such as tetrahydrozoline and oxymetazoline.
- An anecdotal report suggests that intravenous naloxone, 1.6 mg, reversed the hypotension associated with a captopril overdose.
- Anecdotal evidence suggests that naloxone with activated charcoal may be useful in improving the degree of consciousness following a valproic acid overdose.

NALOXONE INDICATIONS WITH UNSUBSTANTIATED EVIDENCE

- Conflicting data have been presented on the use of naloxone in treating an ethanol overdose. Some evidence suggests that high-dose naloxone may reverse coma in suspected ethyl alcohol intoxication.
- Usefulness in senile dementia.
- Naloxone may interact with phencyclidine at the mu opiate receptors in brain controlling thermoregulatory processes.

PATHOPHYSIOLOGY

Naloxone is a semisynthetic, pure opiate antagonist derived from thebaine and is structurally similar to oxymorphone. Its presumed mechanism of action is competitive antagonism at mu, kappa, and sigma opiate receptors in the central nervous system. Mu receptors have the highest affinity for naloxone. Unlike levallorphan and nalorphine, naloxone has minimal agonist activity at clinical doses. β-endorphin actions, like those of exogenous opiates, include analgesia, cross-tolerance, physical dependence, stimulation of ADH, respiratory depression, psychomotor depression, behavioral changes, and hypotension. Naloxone reverses the effects of β-endorphins and appears to modulate the release of catecholamines presumably from chromaffin cells. Plasma epinephrine, norepinephrine, and dopamine concentrations were increased in a patient with pheochromocytoma after intravenous naloxone, 10 mg, was administered.

PHARMACOKINETICS

Absorption

- Naloxone is rapidly absorbed by the intravenous route. If this route is not feasible, the intramuscular, subcutaneous, or sublingual routes may be used. Naloxone has been used endotracheally, but this route is still investigational.
- The pKA of naloxone is 7.94. Naloxone has high lipid solubility and a high brain/serum ratio.
- From 20 minutes after injection to 2 hours, the mean serum half-life is 64 minutes.
- About 75% of naloxone given orally is absorbed in 15 minutes, with a peak plasma level reached in 30 minutes. Peak levels

are reached 15 minutes after intramuscular injection and 30 minutes after subcutaneous injection.
- The plasma half-life is two to three times longer in neonates than adults, because of the inadequately developed glucuronic acid conjugation pathway in infants.

Distribution

- Naloxone is rapidly distributed to all tissues with high concentrations found in the brain, kidney, spleen, lung, heart, and skeletal muscle.
- The apparent volume of distribution is 3 L / kg. Naloxone has a brain / serum ratio 12–15 times greater than that of morphine. Naloxone is 54% protein bound in an adult.

Elimination

- It antagonizes the action of morphine for only 45–70 minutes, but is not metabolized faster than morphine. The half-life of naloxone is around 1 hour.
- Low oral versus intravenous potency of naloxone may result from a rapid first-pass liver metabolism by glucuronidation.
- Metabolites are excreted in the urine: 24–37% of the dose in the first 6 hours, and 60% within 72 hours.

CLINICAL PRESENTATIONS

Naloxone is a pure opiate antagonist with few adverse reactions at clinical doses. Hypertension as well as atrial and ventricular dysrhythmias have been associated with the postoperative use of naloxone, mostly in patients with organic heart disease or abstinence syndrome. Postoperative sudden death has been reported in healthy young adults following intravenous naloxone. Naloxone and nalmefene can produce opioid withdrawal in dependent patients. Slow intravenous titration of naloxone to reverse the respiratory and central nervous sytem depression of opioid use avoids serious withdrawal symptoms. Naloxone may be readministered when opiate symptoms reappear until the patient is symptom-free for 2–4 hours after the last naloxone dose. Methadone overdoses require longer periods of observation.

When naloxone has been used in acutely poisoned patients, even when inadvertently given as a large overdose, there have been no reported significant adverse effects other than precipitation of opiate withdrawal. Naloxone induces a precipitation of the abstinence syndrome in patients acutely or chronically dependent on narcotics. Such patients may develop nausea, vomiting, sweating, tachycardia, elevated systolic blood pressure, and tremulousness. The postoperative reversal of narcotic depression by naloxone in one study was reported to result in hypotension and hypertension, atrial and ventricular arrhythmias, and pulmonary edema, resulting possibly from sympathetic overactivity of abstinence in an acutely dependent patient. Naloxone should be used judiciously in patients emerging from anesthesia.

TOXIC DOSAGE/DEATH

Maximal effective doses of naloxone have not been established in humans. Intravenous doses of 20 mg may produce lethargy and a sense of less well being. Some increase in systolic blood pressure and respiratory rate was noted in addition to anxiety, irritability, and depression. Parenteral doses of 24 mg/70 kg and oral doses of 3,000 mg have been given without incident.

DRUG INTERACTIONS

Hepatic microsomal drug-metabolizing enzyme inducers may shorten naloxone's half-life. Obviously, there is a decreased analgesic effect when naloxone is used concurrently with opiates. The antagonism of buprenorphine requires large doses of naloxone and is characterized by gradual onset of the reversal effects and decreased duration of action of the normally prolonged respiratory depression. The acute onset of withdrawal symptoms induced by naloxone in opiate addicts appears to be blocked by the acute action of the barbiturate methohexital.

PREGNANCY/LACTATION

In a narcotic-dependent pregnant woman, naloxone may precipitate premature labor or complete abortion. Maternal hypoxia and fetal compromise, however, are a greater risk to the mother and fetus than the use of naloxone and the possible risk of premature labor in a narcotic-dependent pregnant mother. Naloxone crosses the placenta. Pregnancy risk category B.

LABORATORY

Analytic Methods

A high-performance liquid chromatography method with electrochemical detection has a detection limit of 1 ng / mL.

Blood Levels

Plasma naloxone levels are available but are not useful in the clinical management of the opiate-poisoned patient. Peak blood levels after intravenous administration of 0.4 mg naloxone average 0.01 μg / mL in 2 minutes and decrease to 0.004 μg / mL in 5 minutes.

TREATMENT

- In reversing opiate coma, naloxone should be used with electrocardiographic monitoring in patients with known preexisting cardiac disease or in those predisposed to cardiac arrhythmias.
- Most cardiac toxicity associated with naloxone has occurred in the postanesthesia setting, and most of these patients had preexisting cardiovascular disease.
- In the face of coma and respiratory depression, naloxone should be used, regardless of the possibility of ingestion of other drugs. This is the safest method to restore normal ventilation after opiate ingestion and prevent the risk of hypoxia when used with appropriate mechanical ventilation.
- Arterial blood gases should be drawn on admission and at sufficient intervals thereafter to guide the degree of respiratory depression under treatment.
- In all comatose patients, and individuals with altered mental status, electrolytes should be obtained as a guide to hydration state and to assess anion gap. If the patient is in coma, blood glucose should be drawn before glucose is administered. Electrocardiographic monitoring should be initiated early to determine the presence of hyperkalemia or evidence of ingestion of other drugs. CAT scans should be obtained as required in the comatose patient.
- Blood alcohol levels should be drawn in all coma patients on admission. Urine may be obtained for a quick toxicology screen including tests for sedative-hypnotics or other substances that also may have been ingested or injected.

Therapeutic Dosage

- The standard dosage of naloxone for children is 0.03–0.1 mg / kg intravenously. For adults, 0.4–2.0 mg boluses are given. If there is no response, several 2.0 mg boluses up to 10 mg may be tried. If no response is observed after 10 mg of naloxone, narcotic-induced toxicity may not be present or a mixed-drug overdose may be at play.

- An intravenous drip may be helpful in treating long-acting opiates. In general, the goal is to maintain the drip at 2/3 of a dose necessary to achieve an initial response: Add 10 times this amount to 1 liter of D5W and infuse at 100 mL/hour. Half of the initial bolus should be readministered in 15 minutes.
- Naloxone (0.4 mg) may be administered via endotracheal tube if intravenous access is unavailable. The subcutaneous and intramuscular routes are alternative routes of administration.
- Certain opioid drugs (e.g., propoxyphene, pentazocine, Lomotil®, and codeine) require large naloxone doses to reverse opiate effects. At least 5 mg (0.1 mg/kg in children) should be administered in these overdoses and more should be given if a partial response is noted.
- For methadone overdoses and coma caused by other opiates, an infusion may be required for up to 48 hours. When discontinuing an infusion (usually after a 10-hour period and reassessment), patients must be observed and monitored closely for at least 2 hours. If the patient relapses into coma or respiratory depression, therapy must be reinstituted with a single bolus followed by infusion.

Questions—Naloxone

1. **Higher than usual doses of naloxone may be required for reversal of toxicity related to**
   A. Codeine
   B. Propoxyphene
   C. Lomotil®
   D. Pentazocine
   E. All of the above
2. **Numerous uses have been proposed for naloxone. Those with strong clinical supporting evidence include all of the following except**
   A. Reversing the action of opiates including heroin, morphine, and methadone
   B. To diagnose opiate use in mixed ingestions
   C. To treat septic shock
   D. To reverse sleepiness or ventilatory compromise after a therapeutic dose of morphine
   E. To treat propoxyphene overdose
3. **Which of the following regarding the clinical effects of naloxone is false?**
   A. Naloxone is a pure opiate antagonist with few adverse reactions at clinical doses.
   B. Hypertension as well as atrial and ventricular dysrhythmias have been associated with the postoperative use of naloxone, mostly in patients with organic heart disease or abstinence syndrome.
   C. Naloxone can produce opioid withdrawal in dependent patients.
   D. When naloxone has been used in acutely poisoned patients, even when inadvertently given as a large overdose, there have been no reported significant adverse effects.
   E. Naloxone, in combination with other opiate antagonists, can precipitate mania.
4. **For methadone overdoses and for severe levels of coma caused by other opiates, an infusion may be required for up to 48 hours.**
   A. True
   B. False

Naltrexone

Naltrexone (Trexan®) is structurally similar to naloxone. It has been approved as an adjunct in detoxifying from opiates, and has been used to combat ethanol dependence. Naltrexone has a high affinity for mu receptors, and has been used in functional hypothalamic amenorrheic patients to reestablish ovulation and menses. Naltrexone may be useful in regulating self-injurious behavior in autistic children. Oral naltrexone may also be useful, prophylactically, to prevent pruritus associated with epidural morphine. It may curtail abnormal sexual behavior in Tourette's syndrome, diminish seizures associated with Rett syndrome, and has been used in treating neurotic excoriations.

Naltrexone is long-acting and nonaddicting. It can be used orally and prevents the euphoriant effects of opioids. However, it does not abolish craving for narcotics and appears to be less effective than methadone maintenance in treating addiction. Furthermore, it can cause hepatic toxicity and must be carefully monitored. The long duration of naltrexone appears to be dependent on the N-cyclopropylmethyl radical, which is its main structural difference from naloxone.

PATHOPHYSIOLOGY

Naltrexone acts as a competitive inhibitor at opiate receptors. By removing the euphoria and physical withdrawal associated with opiate use, naltrexone aids in eliminating the drug-seeking behavior of the addict. However, craving is not abolished. Naltrexone is 17 times more potent than nalorphine and twice as potent as naloxone as an opioid blockade agent. Opioid receptor antagonists can decrease alcohol craving, alcohol consumption, and loss of control over drinking.

PHARMACOKINETICS

Absorption

- Naltrexone is almost completely absorbed from the gastrointestinal tract after oral administration.
- One hundred milligrams produce a peak plasma level of 44 ng/mL 1 hour after use and 2.1 ng/mL in 24 hours.

Distribution

- The apparent volume of distribution is 16 L/kg. Naltrexone is 20% bound to plasma proteins.
- Naltrexone undergoes first-pass hepatic metabolism in the liver to its major metabolite 6-β-naltrexol, which has some narcotic antagonist activity.

Elimination

- Naltrexone is slowly eliminated, with plasma levels of 2.4 ng/mL at 24 hours and 1.7 ng/mL at 72 hours. The elimination half-life of an acute single dose of naltrexone is about 10.3 hours, and that of its metabolite 6-β-naltrexol, 12.7 hours.
- Naltrexone may increase its own drug metabolism by inducing liver mixed-function oxidase enzymes, causing accumulation of drug metabolized by this system.
- Urine is the main route of elimination for naltrexone and metabolites. Sixty percent of a total dose is excreted in 48–72 hours.

CLINICAL PRESENTATIONS

One daily dose of naltrexone blocks the effects of 25 mg of intravenous heroin for 24 hours. It is nonaddicting. Unlike methadone, it does not abolish the craving for narcotics. Naltrexone, like naloxone, may precipitate acute withdrawal in subjects physically dependent on opiates. In healthy adults, 50 mg may produce fatigue, sleepiness, lightheadedness, nausea, sweating, a feeling of unreality, recurrent penile erections, and elevations of plasma luteinizing hormone.

Other reactions, suggestive of opiate agonist effects, include decreased respiratory rate, pupillary constriction, decreased oral temperature, and dysphoria. In maintenance treatment, naltrexone has induced aversive effects such as mood changes, and decreased concentration, alertness, and motor coordination. Depression and abdominal pain have also been observed.

TOXIC DOSAGE/DEATH

Patients ingesting up to 300 mg of naltrexone daily develop feelings of well-being, increased alertness, euphoria, and mild hypomania. Doses up to 800 mg of naltrexone hydrochloride per day have not produced intolerable side effects in humans.

DRUG INTERACTIONS

Interactions of naltrexone with drugs used to treat other conditions often present in patients with narcotic addiction (e.g., disulfiram, tricyclic antidepressants, lithium, phenothiazines, or other antipsychotic drugs) have not been systematically studied. Alcohol or other hepatotoxins may enhance the hepatotoxic effects of naltrexone. Drugs that alter hepatic metabolism may increase or decrease the serum concentration of naltrexone or its metabolites. Naltrexone has been used effectively with clonidine in one study to withdraw patients from methadone hydrochloride therapy.

PREGNANCY/LACTATION

There are no well-controlled studies available in pregnant women. Pregnancy risk category C.

LABORATORY

Analytic Methods

A procedure for the analysis of naltrexone in plasma and urine uses negative ion chemical ionization mass spectrometry and capillary column chromatography. Commercial assays for routine assessment of naltrexone plasma concentrations are not available.

Blood Levels

Blockade of opiate effects probably occurs at naltrexone levels of 1 ng/mL. The minimum effective plasma level of naltrexone for the treatment of opiate addiction may be < 1 ng/mL.

TREATMENT

Gut Decontamination

Since overdose reactions have not been reported, an established mode of treatment has not been proposed. Excess naltrexone ingestion may be treated with the usual measures of lavage, and activated charcoal.

Elimination Enhancement

In view of its extensive volume of distribution, naltrexone or its metabolites in overdose may not be easily removed by dialysis or hemoperfusion procedures.

Supportive Measures

- Supportive care is the mainstay of treatment, and may include oxygen, intravenous fluids, and vasopressors. One must be aware that an addict may take substantial doses of heroin or other opiates to override the effects of naltrexone.
- Naltrexone patients who are also alcoholics may be increasingly susceptible to hepatotoxic reactions.
- Reports of naltrexone ingestion after heroin administration indicate sudden induction of severe narcotic withdrawal symptoms: restlessness, fever, tachypnea, perspiration, salivation, lacrimation, rhinorrhea, mydriasis, vomiting, diarrhea, and abdominal pain with significant fluid losses. Such symptoms may continue for 2–3 days and may not be effectively controlled by low doses of morphine or methadone.
- Since naltrexone is used for narcotic addict control for periods of 6–18 months before dependence is controlled, repeated and close outpatient monitoring, including urine testing for narcotics and blood tests for hepatotoxicity is indicated.
- If severe pain occurs during naltrexone treatment, a rapidly acting analgesic can be used. Hospitalization of the patient may be necessary, as there is an increased risk of respiratory depression. Naltrexone should be discontinued 48 hours before elective surgery.
- Naltrexone recipients may develop elevated levels of serum aminotransferase (alanine transaminase). Serum aminotransferase levels should be continuously monitored during long-term treatment of the addict with naltrexone, and the drug should be discontinued if aminotransferase activity reaches three times the normal level.

Questions—Naltrexone

1. Which of the following is false?

A. Naltrexone is a unique opiate antagonist that is not structurally similar to naloxone.
B. Naltrexone has been approved as an adjunct in detoxifying from opiates, and has been used to combat ethanol dependence.
C. Naltrexone may be useful in regulating self-injurious behavior in autistic children.
D. Naltrexone is long-acting and nonaddicting.
E. Naltrexone can be used orally.

2. Regarding the physiology of naltrexone,

A. Naltrexone acts as a competitive inhibitor at opiate receptors.
B. Naltrexone is 17 times more potent than nalorphine and twice as potent as naloxone as an opioid blockade agent.
C. Opioid receptor antagonists can decrease alcohol craving, alcohol consumption, and loss of control over drinking.
D. All of the above.
E. A and B

Nalmefene

Nalmefene (Revex®) is a naltrexone derivative that is a pure opiate antagonist without agonist effects. It appears to have a longer duration of effect than naloxone and is a more potent antagonist than naloxone at all three main types of opioid receptors. Overdoses with nalmefene have not been reported, but consideration should be given to the possibility of naloxone-like catecholamine stimulation, which may induce arrhythmias and hypertension. Treatment of an overdose will probably be symptomatic and supportive. Nalmefene may last many hours and may particularly be advantageous in cases involving long-acting opiates.

Because of its prolonged duration of action, nalmefene has potential advantages over naloxone. Fewer complications are expected to occur. Less risk of renarcotization is expected in the patient who leaves the emergency department against medical advice soon after regaining consciousness. Maintenance infusion is indicated far less often, making calculation of infusion rates and monitoring of intravenous lines unnecessary in busy emergency departments.

A prolonged opiate effect may follow overdose with propoxyphene and methadone, both of which have longer half-lives than naloxone. Peak plasma levels with pentazocine, diphenoxylate, and some other drugs occur later than with heroin and much later than with naloxone. Hepatic insufficiency, renal failure, and unusually large doses of opiates can prolong opiate toxicity. Intravenous nalmefene at both 0.5-mg and 1.0-mg doses reverse opiate toxicity, rapidly, completely, and for at least 4 hours.

PATHOPHYSIOLOGY

Nalmefene is a derivative of naltrexone, which also exhibits opioid antagonist effects without producing opiate agonist effects. Nalmefene does not produce mu-opiate agonist effects in an opiate-abusing population. Nalmefene is four times as potent acutely as naloxone in antagonizing effects at the mu receptor, and more potent than naloxone in antagonizing effects at the kappa receptor. The mu receptor is "morphinelike" and mediates supraspinal analgesia, respiratory depression, miosis, physical dependency, and euphoria. Kappa receptors mediate spinal analgesia, miosis, sedation, and limited respiratory depression.

PHARMACOKINETICS

Absorption

- Unlike naloxone, with a plasma half-life of 1–2 hours, nalmefene is active after both oral and parenteral administration and has a plasma half-life of 8–9 hours, similar to that of naltrexone.
- Its serum half-life is 10–12 hours, compared with 63 minutes for naloxone.
- Although the serum half-life of nalmefene is longer than 10 hours, a 1.0-mg dose prevents respiratory depression from fentanyl challenge for only 4 hours, and a 2.0-mg dose prevents respiratory depression for up to 8 hours.

Distribution

- The volume of distribution after 0.5–2.0 mg intravenously is 9.1–11.2 L/kg.

Elimination

- Following an intravenous dose of 0.5 mg of nalmefene, the elimination half-life is 9.5 hours. After 10 mg, it is 7.8 hours and after 2.0 mg, it is 2.9 hours.

CLINICAL PRESENTATIONS

Nalmefene is occasionally associated with dizziness, lightheadedness, fatigue, agitation, irritability, muscle tension, and a "hangover feeling," which is not dose-related. Drowsiness or sleepiness is the most common drug effect observed after administration of nalmefene. Other adverse effects include myalgia, arthralgia, nausea, paranoia, and paresthesias. Oral nalmefene does not produce typical morphine-like effects and has no apparent abuse potential. Further experience may indicate that nalmefene will precipitate opiate withdrawal in dependent patients, much like naloxone.

TOXIC DOSAGE/DEATH

A single oral dose of nalmefene (50 mg) completely blocks fentanyl-induced respiratory depression, analgesia and subjective effects for up to 48 hours.

DRUG INTERACTIONS

Clearly, coadministration of opiates will decrease their efficacy.

PREGNANCY/LACTATION

Pregnancy risk factor B.

TREATMENT

Gut Decontamination

Presumably, charcoal or lavage may decrease absorption of nalmefene; however, the clinical necessity of such intervention has not been studied.

Elimination Enhancement

Dialysis has not been utilized in nalmefene overdose.

Supportive Measures

- Treatment is primarily supportive. Patients who have ingested long-acting opiates must still be monitored, as respiratory depression from these opiates may exceed the half-life of nalmefene in certain instances.

Question—Nalmefene

1. Which of the following is false?

A. Nalmefene is a naltrexone derivative that is a pure opiate antagonist without agonist effects.
B. Nalmefene appears to have a shorter duration of effect than naloxone and is a less potent antagonist than naloxone at all three main types of opioid receptors.
C. Overdose with nalmefene has not been reported, but consideration should be given to the possibility of naloxone-like catecholamine stimulation, which may induce arrhythmias.
D. Nalmefene is a derivative of naltrexone, which also exhibits opioid antagonist effects without producing opiate agonist effects.
E. Nalmefene does not produce μ-opiate agonist effects in an opiate-abusing population.

Answers

Introduction to Opiates

1. E 2. D 3. A.

Heroin

1. E 2. E 3. C 4. A 5. B 6. A
7. A 8. B

Morphine

1. E 2. A

Methadone

1. B 2. E 3. A

Diphenoxylate and Atropine

1. B 2. D 3. A 4. C

Meperidine

1. E 2. C 3. A

Propoxyphene

1. E 2. D

Codeine, Hydrocodone, and Dihydrocodeine

1. E 2. C

Pentazocine

1. B 2. A 3. A 4. A

Oxycodone

1. A 2. A

Butorphanol

1. E

Nalbuphine

1. C

Paregoric

1. B 2. A 3. A 4. B

Hydromorphone

1. E

Tramadol

1. D

Naloxone

1. E 2. C 3. E 4. A

Naltrexone

1. A 2. D

Nalmefene

1. B

SELECTED READINGS

Introductions to Opiates

1. Ling W, Wesson DR. Drugs of abuse: opiates. In: Addiction Medicine (Special Issue). West J Med 1990;152:565–572.
2. Traub SL. Clonidine for opiate withdrawal. Hosp Formul 1985;20:77–80.

Heroin

1. Goldfrank L, Weisman RS, Errick JK, Lo M-W. A dosing nomogram for continuous infusion intravenous naloxone. Ann Emerg Med 1986;15:566–570.
2. Kintz P, Mangen P, Lugnier AA, Chument AJ. Toxicological data after heroin overdose. Hum Toxicol 1989;8:587–589.
3. Smith DA, Yealy DM. Discharging heroin overdose patients after observation. Ann Emerg Med 1993;22:1638–1639.
4. Utrecht MJ, Stone AF, McCarron MM. Heroin body packers. J Emerg Med 1993;11:33–40.

Morphine

1. El Sohly NH, El Sohly MA, Stanford DF. Poppy seed ingestion and opiates urinalysis: A closer look. J Anal Toxicol 1990;14:308–310.
2. Osborne R, Joel S, Trew D, Slevin M. Morphine and metabolite behavior after different routes of morphine administration: Demonstration of the importance of the active metabolite morphine-6-glucuronide. Clin Pharmacol Ther 1990; 47:12–19.

Methadone

1. Drummer OH, Opeskin K, Syrjanen M, Cordner SM. Methadone toxicity causing death in the subjects starting on a methadone maintenance program. Am J Forens Med Pathol 1992;13:346–350.
2. Garrettson LK. Delayed onset of toxicity after methadone ingestion due to therapeutic error. Vet Hum Toxicol 1994;36:367.
3. Harding-Pink D. Methadone: One person's maintenance dose is another's poison. Lancet 1993;341:665–666.

Diphenoxylate and Atropine

1. Ahmad SR. Lomotil overdose. Pediatrics 1992;89:980–981.
2. Curtis JA, Goel KM. Lomotil poisoning in children. Arch Dis Child 1979;54: 222–225.
3. Ginsberg CM, Angle CR. Diphenoxylate-atropine (Lomotil) poisoning. Clin Toxicol 1969;2:377–382.
4. Henderson W, Psaila A. Lomotil poisoning. Lancet 1969;1:306–307.

Meperidine

1. Goetting MG. Neurotoxicity of meperidine. Ann Emerg Med 1985;14:1007–1009.
2. Hershey LA. Meperidine and central neurotoxicity. Ann Intern Med 1983; 98:548–549.

Propoxyphene

1. Jaffe JH, Martin WR. Opioid analgesics and antagonists. In: Gilman AG, Goodman LS, Rall TW, et al., eds. Goodman and Gilman's the Pharmacological Basis of Therapeutics. 7th ed. New York: MacMillan, 1985:519–520.
2. Strom J. Acute propoxyphene self-poisoning with special reference to propoxyphene cardiotoxicity and treatment. Dan Med Bull 1989;36:316–336.

Codeine, Hydrocodone, and Dihydrocodeine

1. Dawling S, Widdop B. A fatal case involving dihydrocodeine. Bull Int Assoc Forens Toxicol 1981;16(1):25–26.
2. Hart LM, Dean BS, Krenzelok EP. Massive pediatric codeine overdose with survival. Vet Hum Toxicol 1993;35:341.

Pentazocine

1. Challoner KR, McCarron MM, Newton EJ. Pentazocine (Talwin®) intoxication: Report of 57 cases. J Emerg Med 1990;8:67–74.
3. Showalter CV. T's and Blues: Abuse of pentazocine and tripelennamine. JAMA 1980;244:1224–1225.

Butorphanol

1. Butorphanol nasal spray for pain. Med Lett Drugs Ther 1993;35(909):105–106.
2. Heel RC, Brogden RN, Speight TM, et al. Butorphanol: A review of its pharmacological properties and therapeutic efficacy. Drugs 1978;16:473–505.

Nalbuphine

1. Jaillon P, Gardin ME, Lecocq B, et al. Pharmacokinetics of nalbuphine in infants, young healthy volunteers and elderly patients. Clin Pharmacol Ther 1989;46: 226–233.
2. Steve JK, Stofberg L, MacDonald G, et al. Nalbuphine analgesia in the prehospital setting. Am J Emerg Med 1988;6:634–639.

Paregoric

1. Lerner AM, Oerther FJ: Characteristics and sequelae of paregoric abuse. Ann Intern Med 1966;65:1019–1030.

Hydromorphone

1. Baselt RC. Two hydromorphone fatalities. Bull Int Assoc Forens Toxicol 1978; 14(2):20.
2. CDS: Dilaudid®-related deaths-District of Columbia 1987. MMWR 1988;37: 425–427.
3. Eisele JH Jr, Grigsby EJ, Dea G. Clonazepam treatment of myoclonic contractions associated with high dose opioids: Case report. Pain 1992;49:231–232.

Tramadol

1. Lee SR, McTavish D, Sorkin EM. Tramadol: A preliminary review of its pharmacodynamic and pharmacokinetic properties and therapeutic potential in acute and chronic pain status. Drugs 1993;46:313–347.

Naloxone

1. Kunkel DB. Narcotic antagonist update. Emerg Med 1987;19:97–108.
2. Mofenson HC, Caraccio TC. Continuous infusion of intravenous naloxone. Ann Emerg Med 1987;16:600.
3. Tenenbein M. Continuous naloxone infusion for opiate poisoning in infancy. J Pediatr 1984;105:645–648.

Naltrexone

1. Lerner AG, Sigal M, Bacolu A, Gelkopf M. Naltrexone abuse potential. J Nerv Ment Dis 1992;180:734–735.
2. Naltrexone for alcohol dependence. Med Lett Drugs Ther 1995;37(953):64–66.
3. Volpicelli JR, Alterman AI, Hayashida M, O'Brien CP. Naltrexone in the treatment of alcohol dependence. Arch Gen Psychiatry 1992;49:876–880.

Nalmefene

1. Barsan WG, Seger D, Danzl DF, et al. Duration of antagonistic effects of nalmefene and naloxone in opiate-induced sedation for emergency department procedures. Ann Emerg Med 1987;16:477.
2. Fudala PJ, Johnson RE, Heishman SJ, Henningfield JE. Evaluation of the abuse liability of nalmefene. Clin Pharmacol Ther 1991;49:167.
3. Kaplan J, Marx J. Effectiveness and safety of intravenous nalmefene for ED patients with suspected narcotic overdose: A pilot study. Ann Emerg Med 1993;22:187–190.

ACKNOWLEDGMENT

Thanks to George Bosse, MD for contributing many questions in this chapter.

CHAPTER 24
Designer Drugs

INTRODUCTION

Designer drugs are chemical substances intended for recreational use that have been modified from legitimate pharmaceutical agents. Such formulations are popular with illicit drug users because they may theoretically circumvent legal restrictions. They are often stronger and cheaper than the parent compound and can be produced by clandestine laboratories. Initially these drugs were sufficiently different from parent compounds to render them temporarily immune from the control of the U.S. Drug Enforcement Agency. Until a drug was isolated, studied, and scheduled, no laws could apply to it. Although this is no longer possible under the Controlled Substances Analogue Enforcement Act of 1986, these substances continue to appear on the street and pose a serious risk.

Designer drugs do not include new forms, or new dosing routes, of old drugs, such as cocaine used in the crystalline freebase form or "crack." They also do not include legal, although abused, alternatives to controlled substances, such as phenylpropanolamine, ephedrine, or caffeine. They do not include drug combinations either, such as "Ts and Blues" (pentazocine and tripelennamine), "speedballs" (cocaine or amphetamine and heroin), or "Star Search" (cocaine and phencyclidine).

Designer drugs create hazards not seen in other commonly abused drugs. There are few if any safety trials, so street users are unwitting investigational subjects. Chemists who produce these products, and their laboratories, are not subject to governmental controls. Contaminants may not be analyzed or removed and there is no control over potency. The clandestine drug laboratory or "clan lab" is a mini-chemical laboratory designed to make deadly, illegal drugs quickly and cheaply. Among others, clan lab chemists can produce LSD, synthetic heroin, fentanyl derivatives, mescaline hybrids, and amphetamine derivatives such as methamphetamine ("crank").

Questions—Introduction to Designer Drugs

1. Which of the following is considered a "designer drug"?
A. α-methylfentanyl or "China white"
B. Crystalline freebase cocaine or "crack"
C. Pentazocine and tripelannamine combined, or "T's and blues"
D. Cocaine and heroin or "speedball"
E. Cocaine and phencyclidine or "star search"

2. Hazards of designer drugs include
A. Lack of control of contamination
B. Lack of control over standard potency
C. Continued lack of DEA jurisdiction
D. A and B
E. All of the above

FENTANYL DERIVATIVES

Fentanyl was introduced in the United States in 1968 as an intravenous synthetic anesthetic and analgesic under the trade name Sublimaze®. It is now used for preanesthetic medication, as a primary anesthetic, and as a postsurgical anesthetic. It is about 200 times as potent as morphine and has a rapid onset and short duration of action. Overdose deaths have resulted from its use.

Overdosage with fentanyl can be treated with naloxone. Because it is so rapidly acting, patients have been found unconscious with needles and attached syringes in their antecubital vein.

Individuals having access to fentanyl in the operating room and intensive care areas of the hospital may be potential users. Fentanyl and its designer derivatives (para-fluorofentanyl, α-methylfentanyl, and 3-methylfentanyl) are often more potent than street heroin or morphine. The "rush" is perceived by addicts as qualitatively similar to that obtained with other narcotics. At an analgesic dose, there is little sedation or loss of consciousness. Tolerance and physical dependence appear to be similar to that following use of other narcotics. The antidote to fentanyl is naloxone.

Alfentanil

Ultrashort-acting (15 minutes) for minor surgical procedures, alfentanil is 20–30 times as potent as morphine. Compared with fentanyl, alfentanil has a higher degree of protein binding which is less pH-dependent. It has a lower solubility, limiting its penetration into fat and muscle, a smaller volume of distribution and a shorter elimination half-life. It has a mean distribution half-life of about 5 minutes in humans. Alfentanil has appreciable selectivity for mu receptors in the central nervous system and produces less respiratory depression than morphine or fentanyl at equally analgesic doses. About 50% of patients have nausea and vomiting.

Answers to questions in shaded boxes appear at the end of the chapter.

Alpha-methylfentanyl

α-methylfentanyl is an illicit derivative available in the streets since at least 1980 under the name "China White." Many deaths have resulted from its use. This chemical is 200 times as potent as morphine. Fentanyls may be pure white ("Persian White"), off white ("China White"), light tan ("Synthetic Heroin," "Fentanyl"), or light brown ("Mexican Brown").

Carfentanil

Carfentanil is an immobilizing agent for animals and is 3,200 times as potent as morphine.

Lofentanil

Lofentanil is long-acting and is noted for prolonged respiratory depression (as in patients suffering multiple trauma). It is 6,000 times as potent as morphine.

Sufentanil

Sufentanil is 2,000–4,000 times as potent as morphine as an anesthetic and analgesic agent for cardiac surgery (30–60 minutes in duration). It has higher lipid solubility than fentanyl and more rapid brain penetration. It can produce respiratory depression, skeletal muscle rigidity, nausea, vomiting, spasm of the sphincter of Oddi, constipation, urinary retention, tolerance, physical and psychological dependence, and bradycardia.

Pathophysiology

The fentanyl derivatives quickly cross the blood-brain barrier. In the central nervous system, they act as mu receptor agonists, leading to respiratory insufficiency or arrest, profound central nervous system depression, and/or extreme euphoria.

Pharmacokinetics

ABSORPTION

- Fentanyl is very lipophilic and reaches maximal brain concentration in 1 minute.

DISTRIBUTION

- Fentanyl and its derivatives are distributed to the brain, where it acts on the mu receptor, and then to other tissues. The distribution half-life of fentanyl is 112 minutes.
- Ten minutes after a lethal dose of 250 μg of fentanyl, 98% of a dose disappears and blood levels are less than 9 μg/mL.

ELIMINATION

- Fentanyl is metabolized to norfentanyl and despropionyl fentanyl.
- The elimination half-life of fentanyl is 10 minutes, and the beta elimination half-life after redistribution from tissues is 2–4 hours. Fifty percent is excreted in the urine and 50% into the bile.
- Secondary peaks in the plasma concentration of fentanyl and sufentanil have been observed.

Clinical Presentations

Many patients who are given fentanyl (50–75 mg), sufentanil (15 mg), or alfentanil (500 mg) begin to cough before any other drug is given. Seizure activity may be associated not only with fentanyl but also with alfentanil and sufentanil during induction of anesthesia as well as postoperatively. Respiratory arrest occurred after a single caudal epidural dose of sufentanil and bupivacaine with epinephrine, for repair of a perineal fistula. Respiratory depression with fentanyl may last up to 30 minutes.

Bradycardia, hypotension, chest wall rigidity, nausea, vomiting, hypothermia, and convulsions have been observed. Frequently, the use of illicit fentanyl analogues produces a very rapid death, and the victim may be found with a needle still in his arm. Many have also taken other drugs at the same time, such as morphine, cocaine, diazepam, amphetamine, codeine, and methadone.

Toxic Dosage/Death

More than 100 overdose deaths have been related to fentanyl and its analogs. Pulmonary edema and needle puncture sites are consistent postmortem findings. Factors that heighten the risk of death for the fentanyl user are diminished tolerance and concurrent use of ethanol. Fatal fentanyl concentrations in the blood (3.0 ng/mL) and urine (3.9 ng/mL) may be quite low. The minimal lethal dose of fentanyl is estimated at 250 μg. That of α-methylfentanyl ("China White") is 125 μg and that of fluorofentanyl is 250 μg.

Drug Interactions

Erythromycin may reduce alfentanil clearance. Alfentanil potentiates midazolam-induced unconsciousness. Regular alcohol consumption may lead to pharmacodynamic tolerance to alfentanil. Alcohol and drugs that produce respiratory or central nervous system depression may potentiate the effect of fentanyl or its analogs.

Laboratory

ANALYTIC METHODS

A radioimmunoassay method with solvent extraction is able to detect fentanyl in urine. A gas chromatography/nitrogen-sensitive detection method is sensitive in whole blood assays to 0.25 ng/mL. An alfentanil radioimmunoassay has been described. Sufentanil blood and cerebrospinal fluid concentrations are quantitated by a radioimmunoassay method. A gas chromatography-mass spectrometry method is also available.

BLOOD LEVELS

At about 34-ng/mL fentanyl in plasma, loss of consciousness has been observed. Serum or plasma levels greater than 100-ng/mL fentanyl have been measured after intravenous infusion of high doses to patients. Death was associated with a fentanyl concentration of 17.7 ng/mL. A urine screen for opioids may be negative. Blood levels in most deaths caused by α-methylfentanyl are 1–11 ng/mL. Urine levels associated with fatalities are 5–236 ng/mL and bile levels are 40–128 ng/mL.

Treatment

GUT DECONTAMINATION

The rapid effect of serious toxicity precludes the potential use of these methods in overdose.

ELIMINATION ENHANCEMENT

These methods have not been necessary, as naloxone is generally sufficient.

SUPPORTIVE MEASURES

- Administration of naloxone should not preclude immediate establishment of a patent airway, administration of oxygen, and / or controlled ventilation as indicated for hypoventilation or apnea.
- If respiratory depression is associated with muscular rigidity, a neuromuscular blocking agent may be required to facilitate assisted or controlled ventilation.
- Intravenous fluids and vasoactive agents may be required to manage hemodynamic instability.
- Fentanyl and its analogs should be used cautiously in intoxicated patients and in those given other drugs that have central nervous system respiratory depressant effects.
- Slow intravenous administration of fentanyl may help prevent muscular rigidity.

Antidotes

NALOXONE

The duration of respiratory depression following overdosage with fentanyl or its derivatives may be longer than the duration of action of an opioid antagonist. Repeated doses of naloxone may be required. It may be necessary to give up to 10 mg of naloxone by intravenous push before the need to start with a naloxone infusion becomes apparent.

Questions—Fentanyl Derivatives

1. **All of the following have known medical uses except**
   A. Alfentanil
   B. Sufentanil
   C. Lofentanil
   D. α-methylfentanyl
   E. Fentanyl
2. **Which of the following is the most potent?**
   A. Alfentanil
   B. Sufentanil
   C. Lofentanil
   D. α-methylfentanyl
   E. Fentanyl
3. **Side effects of Fentanyl and its derivatives may include**
   A. Chest wall rigidness
   B. Hypothermia
   C. Seizures
   D. A and B
   E. All of the above
4. **Factors that heighten risk of death for Fentanyl users include**
   A. Diminished tolerance
   B. Concurrent use of ethanol
   C. Parkinson's disease
   D. A and B
   E. A, B and C
5. **Treatment of a patient with Fentanyl or Fentanyl derivative overdose includes**
   A. Naloxone
   B. Gut decontamination
   C. Elimination enhancement
   D. All of the above
   E. None of the above

MEPERIDINE ANALOGUES

A serious syndrome has been identified in association with a synthetic meperidine derivative. 1-methyl-4-phenyl-1,2,3,6 tetrahydropyridine (MPTP) is a synthetic designer drug designed to act like meperidine (Demerol®). Metabolic activation by monoamine oxidase of MPTP to MPP, which acts to deplete dopamine in dopaminergic neurons, has produced a Parkinsonism-like syndrome in a number of individuals using MPTP intravenously. The activated product (MPP) selectively destroys neuronal tracts in the pars compacta of the substantia nigra. The conversion of MPTP to MPP takes place only in the presence monoamine oxidase and is prevented by monoamine oxidase inhibitors.

Clinical Presentations

MPTP induces all the major clinical signs of Parkinson's disease with the possible exception of tremor. The motor deficits induced by MPTP in primates are reversed by dopamine agonist drugs in a manner identical to that observed in humans. Repeated administration of L-dopa to MPTP-treated primates produces all of the long-term complications (dyskinesias, dystonia, "on-off" phenomena) associated with its use in the treatment of Parkinson's disease.

The motor deficits induced by MPTP in primates slowly disappear over a period of months. This contrasts with the slowly progressive nature of Parkinson's disease. The pathologic changes induced by MPTP are largely restricted to the substantia nigra. Other areas such as the locus ceruleus which die in Parkinson's disease, are spared. Lowy bodies, the pathologic marker of Parkinson's disease, are not observed in MPTP-treated primate brains.

Treatment

- Selegiline, a derivative of methamphetamine, is a selective MAO-B inhibitor whose dopaminergic effect confers efficacy in Parkinson's disease. In the United States, interest in selegiline increased after the discovery of its ability to antagonize the effects MPTP.
- Treatment recommendations otherwise resemble those of ordinary Parkinson's disease. L-Dopa and benztropine may be helpful.

Questions—Meperidine Analogues

1. **MPTP, a meperidine analogue, induces a syndrome most similar to which disease?**
   A. Alzheimer's
   B. Parkinson's
   C. Multiple sclerosis
   D. Huntington's
   E. Lou Gehrig's
2. **Treatment of MPTP effects may include**
   A. Selegine
   B. L-Dopa
   C. Benztropine
   D. All of the above
   E. None of the above

AMPHETAMINE HYBRIDS

Attempts to pharmacologically reduce undesirable side effects and abuse potential have led to the production of numerous amphetamine analogues. One of these analogues, MDMA (methylene-dioxy-methamphetamine) or methamphetamine has been nicknamed the "yuppie psychedelic" because of its popularity among students and young professionals. MDMA is a ring-substituted amphetamine derivative that is chemically related to both hallucinogens and stimulants.

Merck and Company first developed MDMA as an appetite suppressant in 1914, but it was never marketed. It is also known as "XTC," "Adam," and "MDA" and is sold as gelatin capsules or loose powder. In 1985, it was placed on Schedule I of the Controlled Substances Act. Tablets or capsules sold as "Ecstasy" may contain caffeine, ketamine, amphetamine, methamphetamine, acetaminophen, or MDEA, another amphetamine derivative.

The closely related synthetic amphetamine compound, MMDA (methoxy-methylene-dioxy-amphetamine) causes hallucinations in high doses, but MDMA produces primarily sympathomimetic effects in overdose without hallucinations. The synthetic amphetamine derivative, MDEA (methylene-dioxy-ethyl-amphetamine), is called "Eve" on the street. These products are capable of producing hyperthermia, seizures, rhabdomyolysis, coma and death in overdose. DOB (dimethoxy-bromo-amphetamine) is a brominated derivative of DOM or STP (dimethoxy-methyl-amphetamine), which itself has hallucinogenic properties similar to those of LSD.

A popular precursor for the production of illegal amphetamine derivatives is phenyl-2-propanone, a non-psychoactive substance placed in Schedule II of the Controlled Substance Act. Many clandestine laboratory operators who in the past had been producing only methamphetamine now synthesize phenyl-2-propanone either alone or in combination with methamphetamine. Another clandestine synthesis of methamphetamine uses ephedrine. Impurities found in the ephedrine reduction method may provide intelligence concerning illicit production methods, identification of samples of common origin, and the origin of possible harmful effects on the methamphetamine user. Many modifications of each method exist. The use of essential oils as precursor products, such as nutmeg oil or dill seed oil, has been contemplated in the production process of these agents.

Crystal

"Crystal," also known as "Crank," "Meth," "Speed," or "Crystal Meth" on the street refers to methamphetamines. It is a white to yellow product, easily created in amateur laboratories, which has the odor of rotten eggs; pure, it may be odorless. Crystal is snorted or used intravenously for a more intense high. Signs of addiction include irritability, nervousness, mood swings, depression, unreasonable fear, suspicion, significant weight loss, irregular sleep pattern, runny nose, neglect of work and studies, and withdrawal from family and friends. In addition to classic symptoms of amphetamine abuse (see Chapter 18, Amphetamines), ischemic stroke and thalamic infarction, as well as myocardial infarction, have been reported following the inhalational use of "Crystal Meth."

Ice

Also refers to amphetamines and methamphetamines. One form, 4-methylaminorex, is a potent anorectic and central nervous system stimulant, possessing sympathomimetic, hypotensive, and norepinephrine-potentiating properties similar to those of other amphetamines. It was first prepared in 1962 as an anorectic agent, and has been placed in Schedule I of the Controlled Substances Act. Illicit use has resulted in fatality. Another form of "Ice," also known as "Glass," originated in the Far East and arises from the synthesis of large crystals of methamphetamine with the ephedrine reduction method.

"Ice" in the form of translucent crystals is similar in appearance to rock candy or rock salt, and is a very pure form of methamphetamine. Methamphetamine powder can be injected, inhaled, smoked, or ingested. The translucent form of "Ice" is water-based, burns quickly, and leaves a milky white residue after smoking. In some places, such as Hawaii, "Ice" has surpassed cocaine as the drug of choice. It eliminates use of a needle; is longer lasting; is often odorless, colorless, and tasteless; is easy to transport; and is more expensive than cocaine, but cheaper to produce.

Ecstasy

"Ecstasy" is a popular name for the illicit drug MDMA and is widely used at dance parties or "raves." It is usually consumed orally in tablet or capsule form at a dose of about 120 mg. Its primary effect is to produce a positive mood state with euphoria, intimacy, and closeness to others. Side effects include loss of appetite, tachycardia, jaw tension, bruxism, and sweating. Effects last about 4–6 hours. It does not appear conducive to long-term heavy use because of the development of tolerance to its positive effects and exacerbation of negative effects with large doses and frequent use. There is no evidence to suggest that "Ecstasy" is addictive. "Ecstasy" use has been associated with sudden hypertensive crises with spontaneous intracerebral hemorrhage, noncardiac chest pain, hepatitis, an acute or chronic paranoid psychosis, memory impairment, arrhythmias, and death.

Pathophysiology

MDMA appears to affect serotonin release in the central nervous system. MDMA causes serotonin release but blocks uptake at serotonergic nerve terminals. Significant reductions are observed in cerebrospinal fluid levels of a presynaptic marker of serotonin. Certain animal studies on the desmethyl derivative of MDMA (MDA) show evidence of drug-induced central serotonergic nerve terminal destruction.

Clinical Presentations

Effects of "Ice" may last 2 hours to 3 days depending on the dose. Chronic abusers of "Ice" resemble chronic abusers of other amphetamines and amphetamine-like drugs. They may demonstrate delusions, paranoia, and aggressive behavior. Unfortunately, suicide and homicide are not uncommon. Tics, bruxism, and compulsive behavior are often observed. Gastrointestinal problems may include anorexia, weight loss, and malnutrition. Myocardial infarction, caudal thalamic infarcts, transient cortical blindness, systemic vasospasm, irreversible cardiomyopathy, acute pulmonary edema and death have followed its use. Withdrawal may result in abdominal cramps, gastroenteritis, headache, lethargy, dyspnea, increased appetite, and depression, occasionally terminating in suicide.

MDMA or "Ecstasy" induces euphoria, verbosity, and a feeling of closeness with others. Some who take the drug for the first time may experience paranoia, hallucinations, insomnia, tachycardia, or muscle stiffness including trismus and bruxism. There are similar characteristics of fatal "Ecstasy" ingestion and severe hyperthermia. Both may manifest with muscle rigidity, trismus, hyperthermia, sinus tachycardia, sweating, arrhythmias, cardiac arrest, tachypnea, cyanosis, metabolic acidosis, rhabdomyolysis, myoglobinuria, and disseminated intravascular coagulation.

Signs may develop several hours after "Ecstasy" ingestion. These complications occur unpredictably and require prompt action. Paranoid psychosis after chronic abuse of MDMA has been reported. Misuse of MDMA has also been associated with flashbacks, anxiety, panic attacks, suicidal depression, and insomnia. Individuals with prior psychiatric histories may have an increased susceptibility to the adverse effects of MDMA.

Toxic Dosage/Death

Usual street doses of MDMA average 50–100 mg. Anecdotal observations suggest that a dose 10–15 times the average MDMA street dose causes sympathomimetic reactions without hallucinations. Numerous deaths, some associated with trauma and some with concomitant drug use, have been associated with MDMA or MDEA in the blood.

Drug Interactions

Exaggerated sympathomimetic effects are seen when ingestion of monoamine oxidase inhibitors precedes that of other sympathomimetic agents such as amphetamine, methamphetamine, phenylpropanolamine, mephentermine, methylphenidate, ephedrine, phenylephrine, and dopamine. Ethanol is the drug most commonly associated with complications of methamphetamine. The combination of methamphetamine with ethanol results in increased cardiac work which may increase cardiac toxicity. Nicotine, cocaine, and amphetamine produce similar cardiovascular responses when combined with ethanol. The combination of methamphetamine and ethanol may produce more adverse cardiovascular or cerebrovascular events than either drug taken alone at the same dose.

Pregnancy/Lactation

Intrauterine growth abnormalities, complications of pregnancy and delivery including maternal death, and neurophysiologic and neurobehavioral abnormalities in neonates have been described with antenatal methamphetamine drug exposure. Such findings are similar to those seen after cocaine abuse. Amphetamine ingestion may present as eclampsia. Intrauterine death has followed intravenous injection of amphetamine. At birth, withdrawal symptoms may include abnormal sleep patterns, tremors, hypertonicity, a high-pitched cry, poor feeding patterns, sneezing, frantic sucking, and tachypnea. During the first year, the infant may exhibit lethargy, poor feeding, and severe lassitude. There is no evidence of an increased incidence of congenital anomalies.

Laboratory

ANALYTIC METHODS

A thin-layer chromatography method for MDMA analysis has been developed. A gas chromatography-mass spectrometry method detects 4-methylaminorex at 250 ng/mL.

BLOOD LEVELS

A 32-year-old woman ingested between 100 and 150 mg of MDMA, developed a serum level of 6500 ng/mL, and lived. A 40-year-old man ingested a single 50-mg dose, and 2 hours later, his MDMA plasma level peaked at 105.6 ng/mL.

Treatment

GUT DECONTAMINATION

Toxic amphetamine analog doses are difficult to determine. Ingestion of more than 1–2 mg/kg within an hour of presentation may warrant lavage or activated charcoal. Although amphetamines do delay gastric emptying as much as 40% and decrease motility, attempts to remove the drug from the stomach more than 4 hours postingestion probably are not efficacious. Charcoal may be effective up to 12 hours when sustained-release capsules have been ingested.

ELIMINATION ENHANCEMENT

Since amphetamine is a weak base, urinary acidification increases the excretion of unmetabolized drug and causes a decrease of the plasma half-life. The efficacy of this therapeutic maneuver on clinical outcome remains controversial however, since cardiovascular complications of forced diuresis and plasma acidification may develop. Hemodialysis and hemoperfusion have not been studied in amphetamine overdose. Despite the large volume of distribution, amphetamines can be removed via peritoneal dialysis, but the efficacy of this procedure remains questionable.

SUPPORTIVE MEASURES

- Supportive measures resemble those instituted in the treatment of common amphetamines.
- Severely intoxicated patients should receive an intravenous line, cardiac monitoring, ECG, and oxygen. Respiratory depression is uncommon in pure amphetamine intoxication, but either cardiogenic pulmonary edema or the adult respiratory distress syndrome may develop.
- Depending on clinical judgment and severity of poisoning, the laboratory examination may include complete blood count, electrolytes, calcium, phosphorus, uric acid, muscle enzymes, haptoglobin, hepatic aminotransferases, creatinine, glucose, BUN, coagulation profile, urinalysis including myoglobin, arterial blood gases, chest x-ray, ECG, cardiac monitoring, and appropriate diagnostic neurologic examinations (e.g., CAT scan) to rule out other causes of agitation.

AGITATION

- Agitation may be treated with diazepam (intravenous doses of 5–10 mg in adults or 0.1–0.3 mg/kg in children). Chlorpromazine (1 mg/kg to 25–50 mg in adults) has been recommended for severe agitation, but the added risk of seizures, hypotension, and anticholinergic excess (especially from adulterants) theoretically complicates its use. Haloperidol is probably safer.
- Droperidol has also been used successfully in amphetamine intoxications. The usual dose is 0.1 mg/kg. Slow administration of droperidol (2.5-mg/min maximum) to poisoned adults may result in the alleviation of agitation within 15 minutes.

PSYCHOSIS

- Psychosis requires hospitalization to provide a protective environment, especially since suicidal ideation may be prominent during withdrawal.
- Chlorpromazine can be instituted at dosages of 50 mg orally or intramuscularly every 4 hours. Depending on adverse effects (sedation, orthostatic hypotension) and clinical response, the total daily dose varies up to 200–800 mg divided in four to six doses.
- Haloperidol in doses of 2–5 mg orally or intramuscularly every 6 hours is an alternative. Long-term management of the habitual amphetamine user is difficult because of frequent relapses.

VITAL SIGN ABNORMALITIES

- Most patients tolerate sinus tachycardia well, but propranolol may be used to slow tachydysrhythmias in symptomatic pa-

tients. Hypotension may respond to fluid challenges, but a vasopressor may be needed. Shock is a poor prognostic sign and indicates the need for right heart catheterization to measure right-sided filling pressures and cardiac output.
- α-adrenergic blocking agents (e.g., phentolamine) have been recommended for hypertension, but they have not been proven clinically superior to intravenous sodium nitroprusside (0.5–8 μg/kg/min).
- Oral nifedipine (10 mg) is untested clinically but has a rapid onset of action (5–10 minutes sublingually, 20 minutes ingested) and potentially may be useful when elevated blood pressures require treatment acutely.
- Severe temperature elevation (i.e., over 42°C) is a poor prognostic sign. Elevated body temperature as measured by rectal probes should be treated aggressively, especially when temperatures exceed 39–40°C.
- Cooling measures include hypothermic blankets, ice baths and sedation. Chlorpromazine may reduce shivering as well as physical activity. Vital signs should be followed closely (i.e., every 15–20 minutes) and cooling measures continued until rectal temperatures are below 38.5°C.
- Diazepam followed by phenytoin is the therapy of choice for seizure activity.

Questions—Amphetamine Hybrids

1. **Which of the following is true regarding MDMA?**
   A. It was first marketed as an appetite suppressant.
   B. It produces primarily sympathomimetic effects in overdose.
   C. Effects last about 4–6 hours.
   D. Its street name is "ecstasy."
   E. All of the above
2. **Inhalation of pulverized methamphetamine has been associated with**
   A. Ischemic stroke
   B. Thalamic infarction
   C. Myocardial infarction
   D. Typical symptoms of amphetamine abuse
   E. All of the above
3. **"Ice" in the form of translucent crystals is similar in appearance to rock candy or rock salt, and is a very pure form of methamphetamine.**
   A. True
   B. False
4. **Antenatal methamphetamine drug exposure has been associated with neurobehavioral effects in the newborn which may last through the first year.**
   A. True
   B. False

METHCATHINONE

Methcathinone ("Cat") is an illicit drug commonly known by its street name "Cat." It is similar in structure and effect to methamphetamine, looks like cocaine, and produces the same euphoria as crack. A designer drug, it has been abused in the former Soviet Union since 1982, when home synthesis began in Leningrad under the name ephedrone ("Jeff"), and has been used in the rural U.S. since 1991. The recipe uses readily available, legal ingredients (e.g., ephedrine), and it is easier to make than methamphetamine. Users snort, ingest, smoke, or inject "Cat." They marginally use the drug over 15–60 minutes during binges lasting 5 days and then rest for several days. According to addicts, methcathinone is more potent and addictive than other psychostimulants.

Methcathinone can produce a variety of pharmacologic effects depending on the presence and location of substituent groups. The parent compound of this family of agents, phenylisopropylamine (i.e., amphetamine) is a psychostimulant. One of these agents, cathinone, is the active constituent of the shrub Khat, a botanical that has been abused for centuries. Others, such as aminorex and 4-methylaminorex were originally developed as potential anorectic agents by the pharmaceutical industry. Certain methoxy-substituted derivatives, for example, 1-(2,5-dimethoxy-4-methylphenyl-2-aminopropane) or "DOM" are hallucinogenic in humans. Clandestine laboratories produce methcathinone.

Pathophysiology

Methcathinone appears to act primarily in the central nervous system through dopaminergic pathways and may have active metabolites (ephedrine and phenylpropanolamine) with strong peripheral action. Effects typically last 5–10 hours, but may go on for days in large overdoses.

Clinical Presentations

Prominent findings in overdose include visual and auditory hallucinations, fever, and tachycardia, followed by periods of bradycardia and hypotension (6–12 hours) as acute symptoms resolve. "Cat" produces a euphoric high with reports of increased sexuality, creativity, and garrulousness. As dosage or time of usage increase, anxiety, disorientation, and paranoia may develop. Psychomotor activity, impulsivity, and aggression have been observed.

Other signs and symptoms may include high fevers, seizures, mydriasis, flushing, sweaty palms, upgoing Babinski reflexes, and brisk deep tendon reflexes. Withdrawal may involve cardiovascular collapse with hypotension, bradycardia, lethargy, irritability, miosis, craving for sweets, coryza, myalgias, muscle spasms, and arthralgias. Chronic use may result in paranoid psychosis, anorexia, acrocyanosis, acne, hepatomegaly, antisocial behavior, and Parkinsonism.

Toxic Dosage/Death

A specific lethal dose is not recognized. Death has been reported in Russia from cardiac arrhythmia and violent suicides.

Drug Interactions

β-blockers administered to "Cat" users with cardiac problems may leave the users susceptible to malignant hypertension and subsequent stroke.

Laboratory

ANALYTIC METHODS

Few commercial tests can detect methcathinone. Testing chronic users for suspected metabolites such as phenylpropanolamine and ephedrine may provide a clue. Such tests are not conclusive of methcathinone use because these drugs are available without prescription.

BLOOD LEVELS

As tests are largely unavailable, following blood levels in overdose is generally unhelpful.

Treatment

GUT DECONTAMINATION

As with other amphetamines, charcoal may be helpful if given within an hour of ingestion; however, this has not been proved by clinical studies.

ELIMINATION ENHANCEMENT

Hemodialysis has not been used in the treatment of significant "Cat" overdoses.

SUPPORTIVE MEASURES

- Treatment requires supportive measures similar to those used for methamphetamine or cocaine.
- The differential diagnosis after "Cat" exposure should include central nervous system infection, sepsis, thyrotoxicosis, and withdrawal from sedatives, hypnotics, or alcohol. Other similar presentations include toxic reactions to other drugs including theophylline, salicylates, nitrophenols, halogenated hydrocarbons, MDMA, LSD, mescaline, PCP, and cocaine.
- Benzodiazepines are indicated to treat patients with hallucinations, hyperactivity, seizures, or extreme agitation. Antipsychotic agents manage psychosis during the detoxification process.
- Fever generally responds to lorazepam and cooling measures. The effect of Lorazepam lasts 5–8 hours, about as long as methcathinone. Acetaminophen may be useful orally or rectally.
- Hypotension and bradycardia respond to conservative supportive therapy.

Questions—Methcathinone

1. All of the following are true of methcathinone except
   A. Its street name is "Cat."
   B. It is often made from a recipe including ephedrine.
   C. It's effects typically last 1–2 hours.
   D. Prominent findings in overdose include hallucinations and fever.
   E. Withdrawal may include cardiovascular collapse.

2. β-blockers administered to methcathinone users may leave them susceptible to
   A. Malignant hypertension
   B. Hypothyroidism
   C. Stroke
   D. A and B
   E. A and C

Answers

Introduction to Designer Drugs

1. A   2. D

Fentanyl Derivatives

1. D   2. C   3. E   4. D   5. A

Meperidine Analogues

1. B   2. D

Amphetamine Hybrids

1. A   2. E   3. A   4. A

Methcathinone

1. C   2. E

SELECTED READINGS

Fentanyl Derivatives

1. Beebe DK, Walley E. Substance abuse: The designer drugs. AFP 1991;43:1689–1698.
2. Buchanan JF, Brown CR. 'Designer drugs': A problem in clinical toxicology. Med Toxicol 1988;3:1–17.
3. Ford M, Hoffman RS, Goldfrank LR. Opioids and designer drugs. Emerg Med Clin North Am 1990;8:495–511.
4. Jerrard DA. 'Designer drugs': A current perspective. J Emerg Med 1990;8:733–741.
5. Poklis A. Fentanyl: A review for clinical and analytical toxicologists. Clin Toxicol 1995;33:439–447.

Meperidine Analogues

2. Maret G, Testa B, Jenner P, et al. The MPTP story: MDA activates tetrahydropyridine derivatives to toxins causing parkinsonism. Drug Metab Rev 1990;22:291–332.
3. Verebey K, Alrazi J, Jaffe JH. The complications of "ecstasy" (MDMA). JAMA 1988;259:1649–1650.

Amphetamine Hybrids

1. Brewster ME, Davis FT. Appearance of aminorex as a designer analogue of methylaminorex. J Forens Sci 1991;36:587–592.
2. Gurtner H. Aminorex and pulmonary hypertension. Cor Vasa 1985;27:160–171.

Methcathinone

1. Carrell S. Methcathinone: The next drug epidemic? Emerg Med News 1993;15:1–24.
2. Emerson TC, Cisek JE. Methcathinone: A Russian designer amphetamine infiltrates the rural midwest. Ann Emerg Med 1993;22:1897–1903.
3. Goldstone MS. "Cat": Methcathinone-a new drug of abuse. JAMA 1993;269:2508.
4. Young R, Glennon RA. Cocaine-stimulus generalization to two new designer drugs; Methcathinone and 4-methylaminorex. Pharmacol Biochem Behav 1993;45:229–231.

ACKNOWLEDGMENT

Thanks to Alison Deutsch, MD for contributing the questions in this chapter.

SECTION

D

Systems Toxicology

CHAPTER 25

Hematologic Toxicology

ANTICOAGULANTS

Introduction

Substances affecting blood coagulation factors include oral anticoagulants, heparin, thrombin-like defibrinating enzymes from snake venoms, plasma volume expanders; drugs that cause hepatic injury; and drugs that stimulate increased plasma coagulation factors. Overdose and poisoning from the use or misuse of these chemicals have largely been confined to the ingestion of oral anticoagulants (for human use and as rodenticides), and parenteral use of heparin.

PATHOPHYSIOLOGY

Vitamin K-dependent clotting factors include factors II, VII, IX, and X, together with proteins C and S. Factors II, VII, IX, and X are proteins that are synthesized by the liver from precursors that require vitamin K for the postsynthetic addition of gamma-carboxylic acid to glutamate residues at the ends of their molecules. In the presence of vitamin K deficiency (e.g., due to malnutrition, malabsorption or bowel sterilization by antibiotics) or vitamin K antagonists (e.g., warfarin, dicumarol, phenprocoumon, diphenadione, and rodenticides), gamma-carboxylation may not occur.

Oral anticoagulants affect vitamin K-dependent clotting factors at different rates. Factor VII (proconvertin) is the first to decrease in concentration in the plasma, followed by factors IX (Christmas factor), X (Stuart factor), and II (prothrombin). Heparin binds to antithrombin III (AT III), producing a cofactor that is an inhibitor of coagulation. AT III increases the rate at which heparin inactivates thrombin, and it also inhibits factors X, XI, and XIII. The AT III-heparin cofactor neutralizes factors VII, IX, X, XI, and XII and plasminogen. The anticoagulant action of heparin and fibrin degradation products is inhibited by protamine sulfate.

For oral anticoagulant overdosage, the one-stage prothrombin time is most useful. Factor V is usually normal during an oral anticoagulant overdose, as it is not dependent on vitamin K. Factor VIII is not made in the liver and is independent of vitamin K. For heparin use and overdose, the activated plasma thromboplastin time (PTT) is the most specific indicator of heparin action. If the prothrombin time (PT) and PTT are both prolonged, diagnostic possibilities include a circulating anticoagulant, liver disease, vitamin K deficiency, or oral anticoagulant overdose.

Questions—Introduction to Anticoagulants

1. Vitamin K-dependent clotting factors include all of the following, except
A. II
B. V
C. VII
D. IX
E. X

2. Causes of vitamin K deficiency include which of the following?
A. Malnutrition
B. Malabsorption
C. Malingering
D. All of the above
E. A and B

3. Antithrombin III inhibits the following clotting factors, except
A. X
B. XI
C. XII
D. XIII
E. B and C

4. If the prothrombin time (PT) and activated plasma thromboplastin time (PTT) are both prolonged, diagnostic possibilities include all of the following, except
A. A circulating anticoagulant
B. Idiopathic thrombocytopenic purpura
C. Liver disease
D. Vitamin K deficiency
E. Oral anticoagulant overdose

Oral Anticoagulants

WARFARIN

Oral coumarin derivative anticoagulants such as warfarin (Coumadin®) are widely used synthetic chemicals. They are used in the prophylaxis and treatment of venous thrombosis, in the prophylaxis and treatment of pulmonary embolism, in the treatment of valvular thrombi, in the treatment of atrial fibrillation and cardiomyopathy, and as an adjunct in the treatment of coronary occlusion. They are frequently employed to prevent venous thrombosis and pulmonary embolism in patients with a history of thromboembolism, in patients undergoing major surgical procedures, and in patients requiring prolonged immobilization. Moderate overdose with therapeutic oral anticoagulants is relatively frequent; however, poisoning cases are not.

Answers to questions in shaded boxes appear at the end of the chapter.

Characteristics associated with an increased risk of bleeding during long-term warfarin anticoagulation are age above 65, a history of cerebrovascular disease, stroke, gastrointestinal bleeding, heart disease, concurrent aspirin therapy, and hypertension. High-intensity warfarin therapy has also been associated with an increased risk of bleeding.

RODENTICIDES

Long-acting anticoagulants are also employed as rodenticides. Most childhood exposures to warfarin rodenticides (e.g., brodifacoum or difenacoum) are asymptomatic. Reports of poisoning with superwarfarin rodenticide coumarin anticoagulants indicate a prolonged morbidity and the necessity for aggressive therapy.

PATHOPHYSIOLOGY

Oral anticoagulants are either synthetic coumarin derivatives of 4-hydroxycoumarin (dicoumarol, phenprocoumon, warfarin potassium, warfarin sodium, acenocoumarol, and ethyl biscoumacetate), rodenticides (such as brodifacoum or difenacoum), or synthetic derivatives of indan-1, 3-dione (anisindione, diphenadione, rodenticides such as chlorphacinone). All oral anticoagulants are low-molecular-weight organic compounds and have a structure similar to that of vitamin K. The inhibition by coumarin of synthesis of vitamin K-sensitive clotting factors depends on their concentration at the site of synthesis.

The anticoagulant activity of coumarins is governed by molecular shape, solubility, rate of absorption, ease of distribution, degree of protein binding in the plasma, rate of detoxification and excretion, and presence of enantiomers of warfarin. Warfarin, as used clinically, is a racemic mixture of equal parts of R (+) and S (−) enantiomers that exist because of an asymmetric carbon atom. The S forms of both warfarin and phenprocoumon are about five times more potent in the production of hypoprothrombinemia than the R isomers.

PHARMACOKINETICS

Absorption

- Warfarin, ethylbiscoumacetate, phenprocoumon, and acenocoumarol are completely absorbed by passive diffusion in the upper gastrointestinal tract, with a bioavailability approaching 100%.
- Peak plasma concentrations of racemic warfarin sodium are reached within 1 hour.
- Absorption of coumarin anticoagulants from the gastrointestinal tract depends on gastric emptying time, gut motility, pH, and drug solubility.
- Bishydroxycoumarin absorption is slow, incomplete, and variable.

Distribution

- The volume of distribution of warfarin is 0.103 L/kg. The protein binding of warfarin is about 98–99%. Serum protein binding is a major determinant of the elimination kinetics of warfarin.
- There is, however, no correlation between prothrombin time and the concentration of free warfarin in serum. Protein binding does not appear to be the only determinant of the anticoagulant response of patients to a given concentration of warfarin.
- Other coumarins are also highly protein bound (90–99%), mostly to albumin. Protein-bound coumarins are inactive, are not metabolically transformed, and are not excreted.
- The free drug is in equilibrium with its sites of action, is metabolically transformed, and is subject to excretion through the glomerulus.

Elimination

- Coumarins are metabolized to inactive metabolites in the microsomal fraction of the endoplasmic reticulum of the liver by hepatic cytochrome P450 mixed function oxidase enzymes.
- The main metabolites are conjugated with glucuronic acid, are excreted into the bile, undergo enterohepatic recycling, and are ultimately excreted in the urine and feces.
- The elimination half-life of warfarin in normal subjects is approximately 40 hours (20–80 hours).
- The plasma half-life of acenocoumarol is 20 hours; bishydroxycoumarin, 24.0 hours; ethylbiscoumacetate, 2.5 hours; and phenprocoumon, 120–160 hours.
- The long plasma half-lives of the coumarins result from their high degree of protein binding and from the rate of biotransformation of the free fraction.

CLINICAL PRESENTATIONS

Bleeding may manifest acute toxicity. Common sites include the gums, pharynx, nose, and local lesions on the lips. Punctate hemorrhages may be seen on the mucosa of the palate and mouth. Gross hematuria may be seen. Other signs include alopecia, mydriasis, tachycardia, melena, nausea, vomiting, and diarrhea. Infrequent idiosyncratic cholestatic hepatic injury has been reported. Cutaneous reactions associated with coumarin derivatives manifest in one of four ways: ecchymosis and purpura; macular, papular, vesicular, and purpuric skin eruptions; the "purple toe" syndrome; and frank tissue necrosis. Confusion, hyperpyrexia, and urticaria may be seen as well.

Superwarfarins

The long-acting anticoagulant rodenticides are 4-hydroxycoumarin derivatives with a 4-bromo (1,1-biphenyl) side chain. Children produce abnormal prothrombin times that may not be observed until 48 hours postingestion. The occurrence of an abnormal prothrombin time may not be predicted based on a history of the amount ingested or on the presence of the characteristic green-blue product dye in or around a child's mouth. Transient abdominal pain, vomiting, or heme-positive stools may evidence acute toxicity.

Some rodenticides (superwarfarins) may have far longer action on vitamin K-dependent clotting factors than does warfarin. Fatalities have followed brodifacoum ingestion. Vitamin K1 must be administered in high doses at frequent intervals until clotting factor tests are normal (days or weeks), and the patients must be monitored for months after their test results have initially returned to normal.

Protein C and Protein S Deficiency

Protein C has anticoagulant and profibrinolytic activity. Protein S, a cofactor for protein C, potentiates protein C activity at the endothelial cell surface. Reductions in either protein C or S may be a contributing factor to thromboembolic complications. Skin necrosis associated with warfarin may be associated with an inherited heterozygous form of protein C deficiency. Lesions appear within 3–6 days of initiation of warfarin sodium therapy. Obese women around 50 years of age who are under therapy for thrombophlebitis or pulmonary thromboembolism are at the highest risk. Skin necrosis tends to occur in adipose tissue, mainly in the thighs, breasts, and buttocks.

Warfarin Abuse and Misuse

Warfarin child abuse has been reported. Surreptitious, factitious and Munchausen Syndrome types of covert oral anticoagulant ingestion have been reported as well. Oral anticoagulant drugs have been used to malinger or create factitious disease, accomplish murder, commit suicide, induce abortion, and obtain narcotics. They have also been dispensed in error or ingested by mistake. Such patients exhibit an unexplained acquired hemorrhagic diathesis associated with low prothrombin complex activity (II, VII, IX, and X). Clinical recognition of this disorder may be quite difficult and may not occur for months or years. Diagnosis is supported by finding decreased vitamin K-dependent blood clotting factors (II, VII, IX, and X) and by a good therapeutic response to vitamin K. Confirmation of diagnosis is provided by chemical detection of the drug in the patient's plasma. Methods are now available for measurement of almost all oral anticoagulant blood concentrations.

Differential Diagnosis

Prolongation of the one-stage prothrombin time may result very rarely from congenital deficiency of a blood clotting factor or, more commonly, from an acquired deficiency. Congenital deficiencies exhibit a specific factor defect that does not respond to vitamin K. Acquired deficiencies are generally due to (a) liver disease, (b) vitamin K deficiency, (c) ingestion of oral anticoagulant drugs, (d) circulating anticoagulant (as seen in hemophilia and disseminated lupus erythematosus), or (e) defibrination secondary to intravascular clotting. Coagulation defects resulting from liver diseases are often associated with reduction of the four vitamin K-dependent clotting factors (II, VII, IX, X) plus factors I, V, XI, and XIII, which do not respond to vitamin K in any amount.

DRUG INTERACTIONS

Drug interactions related to oral anticoagulant use may affect, and be affected by, a number of mechanisms including alteration of the bioavailability of vitamin K (cholestyramine), drugs that alter receptor sensitivity (estrogens, anabolic steroids, diuretics, clofibrate, thyroid function-altering drugs), drugs that affect hemostasis (aspirin, nonsteroidal antiinflammatory drugs), ulcerogenic drugs (salicylates, phenylbutazone, corticosteroids), and pharmacokinetic interactions affecting absorption, distribution, protein binding, and metabolism including effects on enantiomers and drug enzyme induction.

Sulfinpyrazone enhances the anticoagulant effect of racemic sodium warfarin. Clofibrate appears to increase the warfarin anticoagulant effect. Drugs that inhibit warfarin metabolism and increase prothrombin time include cimetidine, ciprofloxacin, enoxacin, fluoxetine, fluvoxamine, nalidixic acid, norfloxacin, paroxetine, sertraline, trimethoprim-sulfamethoxazole, and zileuton. Drugs that decrease prothrombin time when used in combination with warfarin include dicloxacillin, nafcillin, griseofulvin, disopyramide, carbamazepine, cholestyramine, aminoglutethimide, mercaptopurine, azathioprine, secobarbital, oral contraceptives, sucralfate and vitamin C.

PREGNANCY/LACTATION

Coumarin derivative exposure in the first trimester of pregnancy results in a specific malformation syndrome known as warfarin embryopathy, which is characterized by nasal hypoplasia and punctate stippled calcifications of the laryngeal cartilage, head of the ribs, transverse process of the vertebrae, or epiphyses. Ophthalmologic abnormalities are frequently observed and include optic atrophy, microphthalmia, lens opacities, and large prominent eyes. Such defects are observed in about 8% of at-risk pregnancies (exposure between 6 and 9 weeks of gestation). Early delivery and respiratory distress are seen frequently in this group.

In the second and third trimesters, deformations of the central nervous system have been observed after coumarin derivative use, resulting in mental retardation and/or blindness. Overall, the risk of central nervous system defects is about 3%. In the late third trimester, exposure to coumarin anticoagulants may result in late prenatal, perinatal, or postnatal hemorrhages. In summary, coumarin derivative use or abuse by mothers during gestation results in one-sixth of pregnancies ending with abnormal liveborn infants, one-sixth ending in abortion or stillbirth, and about two-thirds ending with a relatively normal outcome. Warfarin and other coumarin derivatives are classified as pregnancy risk factor D. Warfarin apparently does not pose a significant risk to breast-fed infants.

LABORATORY

Analytic Methods

A liquid chromatographic method can simultaneously measure the serum levels of five anticoagulant rodenticides: brodifacoum, bromadiolone, coumatetralyl difenacoum, and warfarin. A simple high-performance liquid chromatographic method has been devised to detect and quantify brodifacoum and warfarin.

Blood Levels

There is no correlation between prothrombin time and the concentration of free warfarin in serum. Abnormal and normal results follow an overdose of warfarin.

International Normalized Ratio

In an effort to standardize the results of the prothrombin time test, the World Health Organization ((WHO) introduced the International Normalized Ratio (INR). Values of INR are independent of reagents and methods and, therefore, are comparable among laboratories across the country and abroad. The INR is defined as the patient/normal prothrombin time ratio that results if the WHO primary international thromboplastin method is used to test the patient sample.

TREATMENT

Gut Decontamination

Ipecac may precipitate intracranial hemorrhage by raising intracranial blood pressure, and ipecac-induced emesis may provoke gastrointestinal bleeding. Gastric lavage should be used with suction available or by prior-cuffed endotracheal intubation in an obtunded or unconscious patient. Gastric lavage may also provoke bleeding. The efficacy of gastric emptying has not yet been established. Activated charcoal may be helpful shortly after ingestions.

Elimination Enhancement

Forced diuresis, hemodialysis, and peritoneal dialysis are not useful. Hemoperfusion has not been used. Cholestyramine, 12–16 g daily in divided doses is effective in reducing the half-life and in increasing the total clearance of oral anticoagulants. There is evidence that it may be effective in warfarin overdose, possibly by interrupting the enterohepatic recirculation of warfarin. Exchange transfusions may possibly be effective in a serious life-threatening overdose in a child, but inadequate data exist to substantiate this.

Supportive Measures

- Frequent monitoring of the coagulation time, bleeding time, and one-stage prothrombin time is necessary. Patients must be kept in a hospital under continuous observation until control of laboratory and clinical evidence of bleeding is obtained.
- When an overdose patient with prosthetic heart valves is being maintained on oral anticoagulants and continued total anticoagulation is desired, smaller doses of vitamin K (1–5 mg) can be titrated with the prothrombin time. See Antidotes below.

- In the recuperative period, iron therapy may be useful in replenishing the red blood cell mass.
- Before discharge, a psychiatric consultation should be obtained and a follow-up program for psychologic support initiated, especially for the covert ingester of anticoagulants.

Stabilization

- Patients who have overdosed on an oral anticoagulant or who have ingested an undetermined amount of drug or rodenticide should be admitted to an intensive care facility where careful follow-up with adequate laboratory testing capabilities for clotting parameters is available. The patient must be observed closely for the development of airway obstruction secondary to hemorrhage. All oral anticoagulant ingestion should cease immediately. If surreptitious ingestion is suspected, an attempt should be made to remove clandestine sources.
- Blood should be drawn for prothrombin time, complete blood count, and activated partial thromboplastin time. Prothrombin times should be performed every 12 hours for several days even if a severe prolongation is not observed in a baseline study.

Bleeding

- For active bleeding or for patients requiring emergency surgery after an oral anticoagulant overdose, exchange transfusions, whole blood, or plasma may be employed together with frequent determinations of hematocrit.
- If hemorrhage is severe, bleeding should be arrested promptly by replacing deficiencies in factors II, VII, IX, and X with whole blood or plasma (including fresh frozen plasma).
- Indications for use of such modalities as fresh frozen plasma must be tempered by appreciation of the potential risks of acquiring viral hepatitis and, possibly, AIDS.
- Vitamin K can usually reverse deficiencies in vitamin K-dependent coagulation factors II, VII, IX, and X as well as proteins C and S.

Laboratory Studies

- The laboratory test most useful for determining oral anticoagulant effectiveness is the one-stage prothrombin time test. This test correlates well with changes in factor VII concentration during the initial prothrombin test response and during its daily changes.
- Numerous abnormal test results have been associated with anticoagulant overdose. White blood cells are elevated, prothrombin time is elevated, hemoglobin and red blood cells may be decreased, bleeding time may be normal or prolonged, activated partial thromboplastin time is prolonged, stool may be positive for blood, and there are decreases in factors II, VII, IX and X.
- Fibrinogen, platelets, liver function tests and factor V level are normal.

Rodenticides

- For one-time ingestions of plain warfarin-related or superwarfarin-related rodenticides, no decontamination, no dilution, no emergency department visits, no in-hospital treatment, and no prothrombin time determinations are necessary in the absence of clinical symptoms.
- The average child eating a few mouthfuls (or a 25-g packet) of 0.005% rat bait at a single sitting is generally not at risk and no treatment is necessary.
- If a concentration of superwarfarin exceeds 0.005% or if over 25 g of a 0.005% concentration has been consumed (either acutely or over a few days in small amounts), then treatment should be begun.
- Some rodenticides (superwarfarins) may have far longer action on vitamin K-dependent clotting factors than does warfarin. Vitamin K must be administered in high doses at frequent intervals until clotting factor test results are normal (days or weeks), and the patients must be monitored for several months after their test results have initially returned to normal.
- Prothrombin times should be monitored frequently. In severe poisonings, vitamin K1 should be continued until the plasma warfarin level is in the therapeutic range (1 μg/mL) to avoid a rebound to dangerous prothrombin times.

ANTIDOTES

Vitamin K1

Phytonadione is a fat-soluble naphthoquinone derivative required for the synthesis of blood coagulation factors II (prothrombin), VII (proconvertin), IX (Christmas), and X (Stuart-Prower) in the liver. In adequate doses, vitamin K1 reverses the inhibitory action of coumarin and indandione compounds on these factors. The decision to reverse excessive warfarin anticoagulation with vitamin K1 assumes that short-term elevations in INR are associated with a significant risk of bleeding. Vitamin K1 (phytonadione) is useful in restoring the prothrombin time to normal levels and in decreasing or stopping bleeding episodes. If an overdose of an oral anticoagulant drug or an unknown dose of an oral anticoagulant pesticide has been ingested, vitamin K1 can be administered orally in doses of 10–25 mg/d for adults and 5–10 mg for children.

Vitamin K1 has a short duration of action and so must be given repeatedly. All of the human body's vitamin K1 is replaced every 2–3 hours. Intramuscular phytonadione (AquaMEPHYTON®) can be given to adults in doses of 5–10 mg and to children under 12 in doses of 1–5 mg. Doses up to 100–125 mg/day for many weeks or months may be required in a severe rodenticide overdose. Phytonadione is absorbed rapidly by the subcutaneous route. The subcutaneous route is preferable to the intravenous route unless problems are anticipated with subcutaneous absorption.

Administration of vitamin K1 parenterally to correct the INR in over-anticoagulated patients is not without risks. Rapid intravenous administration may be associated with facial flushing, diaphoresis, chest pain, hypotension, or dyspnea associated with or without anaphylaxis. Cerebral thrombosis and death have been associated with intravenous and intramuscular administration of vitamin K1. Administration of vitamin K1 may also interfere with subsequent attempts to achieve oral anticoagulation. Conservative treatment of nonbleeding patients without the use of vitamin K1 is safe and may eliminate problems associated with vitamin K1 administration. See section on Vitamin K below. Vitamin K3 (menadione) is ineffective for the treatment of warfarin and superwarfarin toxicity. It elicits a poor response and should not be used.

Coagulation Factors

Factor II/IX/X concentrate in conjunction with vitamin K1 may be used to reverse overdoses of oral anticoagulants. Both products improve the prothrombin time and partial thromboplastin time and raise depressed levels of factors II, VII, IX and X. The concentrate acts maximally at 30 minutes, except for factor VII activity. Vitamin K1 begins to correct these values, including factor VII, in 2 hours and overcorrects by 24 hours. The concentrate is more easily controlled but carries with it the risk of transmission of hepatitis and/or AIDS. Therefore, its use in oral anticoagulant reversal should be limited to correcting life-threatening hemorrhage.

Questions—Oral Anticoagulants

1. Oral coumarin anticoagulants such as warfarin are widely used in all of the following, except
A. Prophylaxis and treatment of venous thrombosis
B. Vitamin K overdose
C. Prophylaxis and treatment of pulmonary embolism
D. The treatment of atrial fibrillation and cardiomyopathy
E. As an adjunct in the treatment of coronary occlusion

2. Characteristics associated with an increased risk of bleeding during long-term warfarin anticoagulation include all of the following, except
A. Age above 65
B. History of cerebrovascular disease
C. History of diabetes mellitus
D. History of heart disease
E. Concurrent aspirin therapy

3. Most childhood exposures to warfarin rodenticides are asymptomatic.
A. True
B. False

4. All oral anticoagulants are low-molecular-weight organic compounds and have a structure similar to that of vitamin K.
A. True
B. False

5. Factors that govern the anticoagulant activity of coumarins include all of the following except
A. Molecular size
B. Molecular shape
C. Solubility
D. Rate of absorption
E. Degree of protein binding in the plasma

6. Drugs that decrease prothrombin time when used with warfarin include all except
A. Sucralfate
B. Oral contraceptives
C. Carbamazepine
D. Cimetidine
E. Dicloxacillin

7. Drugs that inhibit warfarin metabolism and increase prothrombin time include all except
A. Vitamin C
B. Ciprofloxacin
C. Paroxetine
D. Sertraline
E. Trimethoprim-sulfamethoxazole

8. For active bleeding or for patients requiring emergency surgery after an oral anticoagulant overdose, the following interventions may be helpful:
A. Exchange transfusions
B. Fresh frozen plasma
C. Vitamin K
D. Hemodialysis
E. A, B, and C

9. Intravenous Vitamin K is the safest and fastest way to reverse warfarin overdose.
A. True
B. False

10. In an effort to standardize the results of the partial prothrombin time, the World Health Organization introduced the International Normalized Ratio.
A. True
B. False

Heparin

Heparin (Calciparine®) is used for the prophylaxis and treatment of deep venous thrombosis and its extension, prophylaxis and treatment of pulmonary embolism, treatment of valvular thrombi with embolization, diagnosis and treatment of disseminated intravascular coagulation, prophylaxis and treatment of peripheral arterial embolism, prevention of coagulation in dialysis procedures, and as an anticoagulant in blood transfusions and in blood drawn for laboratory use. It has also been used to reduce lipids in idiopathic hyperlipemia.

Heparin overdose in the clinical setting occurs frequently but few poisoning cases have been reported. Overdose can usually be controlled with good supportive therapy. If bleeding is severe, protamine sulfate administered alone or together with fresh whole blood or plasma may be effective. Heparin administered surreptitiously, heparin rebound, and heparin-induced thrombosis-thrombocytopenia syndrome (HITTS) are all problems requiring immediate evaluation and care.

Heparin is an anionic sulfated glycosaminoglycan polysaccharide normally found in mast cells. Heparin is commercially available as the calcium or sodium salt. The calcium salt of heparin is prepared from porcine intestinal mucosa, and the sodium salt is prepared from either porcine intestinal mucosa or bovine lung tissue. Risk factors in heparin-induced bleeding include age greater than 60 years, females are affected more than males, median dose greater than 50 ug/kg, blood urea nitrogen greater than 50 mg/dl, heavy drinking, and concomitant intake of aspirin or other non-steroidal antiinflammatory agents.

Low-Molecular-Weight Heparins

Low-molecular-weight heparins (LMWHs) have been isolated with an average molecular weight of 4,000-6,500 daltons. They have an attenuated effect on coagulation and prolongation of the activated partial thromboplastin time compared with unfractionated heparin. An example of an LMWH product approved in the U.S. is enoxaparin injection (Lovenox®). Enoxaparins are associated with a lower rate of major bleeding episodes than standard heparins, and with moderate thrombocytopenia, fever, local irritation, pain, hematuria, erythema, and thrombolytic episodes.

PATHOPHYSIOLOGY

Coagulation factors XII, XI, IX, X, and II are cleaved during clotting to active serine esterases. These activated factors are inhibited by naturally occurring plasma protease inhibitors (antithrombin III), α-2 macroglobulin (inhibits thrombin and plasmin), α1-antitrypsin, and C1 inactivator. Antithrombin III binds to heparin, enhancing the rate at which heparin inactivates thrombin. Antithrombin III heparin also neutralizes other serine protease coagulants, factors VII, IX, X, XI, and XII, and plasminogen. In this way, heparin leads to the almost instantaneous inhibition of most of the enzymatic steps in coagulation and fibrinolysis. Heparin also inhibits platelet function, increases the permeability of vessel walls, inhibits the proliferation of vascular smooth muscle cells, inhibits delayed hypersensitivity reactions, and is involved in the regulation of angiogenesis.

PHARMACOKINETICS

Absorption

- Heparins are very acidic and are not absorbed from gastrointestinal or sublingual sites because of their large molecular size (more or less than 12,000 daltons) and polarity.
- Absorption is complete after intravenous administration, but variable after subcutaneous use. Low doses of heparin can be administered subcutaneously or into an intrafat depot. Larger doses can be administered by the continuous or intermittent intravenous route. Intramuscular heparin quite often leads to large hematomas at the site of injection.
- Anticoagulant activity begins in 20–30 minutes.

Distribution

- Heparin has a volume of distribution of 0.06 L/kg.
- Heparin is bound mainly to low-density lipoproteins, globulins, and fibrinogen.

Elimination

- Its half-life is 0.3–2 hours in normal patients and 0.5–3 hours in end-stage renal disease.
- The half-life increases with increasing dose.
- Heparin is metabolized in the liver by heparinase. The inactive metabolic products are excreted in the urine.

CLINICAL PRESENTATIONS

Overdoses of heparin result in rapid prolongation of the coagulation time and active bleeding. Examples of bleeding observed in patients receiving heparin include melena, muscular hematomas, vaginal bleeding, gingival bleeding, hematuria, ecchymoses, epistaxis, hematemesis, intracranial hemorrhage and pulmonary hemorrhage. Bleeding from puncture sites may be seen. Osteopenia and skeletal defects have been described with chronic heparin use. Necrotizing skin lesions, alopecia, hypoaldosteronism, bronchospasm, tachypnea, dyspnea, thrombocytopenia, and anemia have been reported.

Surreptitious Heparin Administration

Bleeding complications from self-administered heparin have rarely been reported. There may be a prior history of factitious disease. The prothrombin time is usually normal but may be mildly prolonged and the activated partial thromboplastin time is markedly prolonged. The thrombin time test and platelet counts are normal. All such suspected patients should be admitted to a hospital for observation and treatment. When confronted with the laboratory findings and response to treatment, patients often but not always admit to their surreptitious use of heparin.

Heparin-Induced Thrombosis-Thrombocytopenia Syndrome

Inability of heparin to control thrombosis may be due to a hypercoagulable state associated with malignancy, antithrombin III deficiency, inadequate heparin dosage, or heparin-induced thrombosis. Weisman and Tobin first described heparin as a cause of thrombosis in 1958. The heparin-induced thrombosis-thrombocytopenia syndrome (HITTS) involves platelet-fibrin thrombus formation that appears white—"the white clot syndrome." Because of platelet consumption, thrombocytopenia may result. Thrombocytopenia may occur in patients given either subcutaneous or intravenous heparin. Both bovine lung and porcine mucosal heparin may cause the syndrome.

Complications of HITTS may be thrombotic or hemorrhagic. The diagnosis is based on clinical and laboratory data. Typically, a patient on therapeutic or prophylactic heparin suddenly deteriorates 5–10 days after commencing heparin therapy and begins to require increasing doses of heparin to maintain anticoagulation. The finding of a low platelet count (as low as 5,000–29,000) is frequently seen in HITTS. Some patients may also have disseminated intravascular coagulation.

Heparin Flush Syndrome

The heparin flush syndrome indicates that iatrogenic hemorrhage can be induced by routine and unmonitored use of heparin in "flush" solutions given to "flush" arterial and venous catheters to maintain patency and vascular access. Ampules with different strengths of heparin may appear identical. Protamine sulfate rapidly halts bleeding and normalizes coagulation tests.

Heparin Withdrawal and Rebound

Within the first 24 hours of heparin discontinuation, patients not already taking aspirin or warfarin may be at increased risk for transient ischemic attack, stroke, or clinical deterioration. Heparin rebound is defined as the resurgence of anticoagulant activity in a patient whose blood heparin has been adequately neutralized with protamine. It is a potential bleeding disorder associated with cardiopulmonary bypass and either protamine sulfate or protamine chloride use.

Aldosterone Suppression

Heparin and its congeners are predictable, potent inhibitors of aldosterone production. Aldosterone suppression occurs within a few days of initiation of therapy, is reversible, and is independent of anticoagulant effect or route of administration. Decreases in aldosterone levels may occur with heparin dosages as low as 5000 U twice daily. Aldosterone suppression results in natriuresis and, less predictably, in decreased excretion of potassium. Greater than normal serum potassium levels occur in about 7% of patients, but marked hyperkalemia generally requires the presence of additional factors such as renal insufficiency, diabetes mellitus, and certain medications.

TOXIC DOSAGE/DEATH

Bleeding has occurred in infants in a neonatal intensive care unit whose indwelling umbilical artery catheters or intravenous lines were flushed with heparin instead of saline. Bleeding from puncture sites, respiratory distress, bleeding from the umbilical stump, and gross hematuria have been observed. Treatment has required exchange transfusion with fresh blood and/or protamine sulfate.

A 45-year-old man who presented with bruising, gingival bleeding, and hematuria attempted suicide by injecting himself subcutaneously with 10 ampules, each containing 25,000 units of heparin, and ingesting four hundred 5-mg tablets of warfarin. He had a previous history of four warfarin overdoses. The heparin overdose was reversed with protamine sulfate and the warfarin component was controlled with intravenous infusion of factors II, IX, and X and several intravenous injections of vitamin K1.

DRUG INTERACTIONS

Drugs that affect platelet function (e.g., aspirin, nonsteroidal antiinflammatory drugs, dipyridamole and dextran) and thrombolytic agents (e.g., streptokinase and urokinase) used with heparin may increase the risk of hemorrhage.

PREGNANCY/LACTATION

Heparin use has not been associated with fetal anomalies; however, excessive maternal deaths, fetal loss, premature deliveries, and neonatal deaths appear to be more frequent with heparin than with the coumarin derivatives. These findings may be related to the conditions being treated and not to heparin itself.

Heparin is classified as pregnancy risk category B. Heparin does not appear to cross the placenta and is not distributed into breast milk.

LABORATORY

Analytic Methods

Heparin assays may underestimate drug levels in neonatal plasma unless the neonatal antithrombin III deficiency is fully corrected in the test system. Use of standard assays may lead to overheparinization of newborn infants, thereby placing them at a higher risk of bleeding.

Blood Levels

The therapeutic plasma range of heparin is 0.2–0.6 U / mL. However, following the PTT, and not the heparin concentration, is clinically more useful in overdose. Periodic platelet counts should be obtained to detect the presence of HITTS. If the counts begin to drop or unexplained recurrent thromboembolic phenomena begin to occur, the presence of a heparin-dependent antiplatelet antibody should be suspected and heparin should be promptly discontinued.

TREATMENT

Gut Decontamination

As heparin is administered parenterally, these methods are irrelevant to the treatment of heparin overdose.

Elimination Enhancement

Dialysis procedures have not been effective in controlling heparin overdoses. Inactive metabolic products are excreted in the urine.

Supportive Measures

- Airway, breathing, and circulation must be immediately evaluated and assisted where required.
- If bleeding is minimal, administration of heparin should be stopped (short half-life). If bleeding is severe or a substantial heparin overdose has been administered, protamine sulfate may be considered and whole blood or plasma may be required. The activated partial thromboplastin time should be monitored frequently.
- Warfarin has a long latent period so is not immediately useful. Consider dextran therapy, antiplatelet drugs such as aspirin, and substitution with low-molecular-weight heparin.
- If bleeding has not been severe, patients should be hospitalized until clotting parameters are normal, patient is asymptomatic, and there is no obvious source of bleeding.
- Blood should be drawn for baseline complete blood count, platelet count, coagulation profile (bleeding time, clotting time), and activated partial thromboplastin time.
- All patients receiving heparin should have periodic platelet counts. If the counts begin to drop after the fourth day of heparin therapy or unexplained recurrent thromboembolic phenomena begin to occur, the presence of a heparin-dependent antiplatelet antibody should be suspected and heparin should be promptly discontinued. An activated partial thromboplastin time and an AT III level should be obtained.
- Platelet transfusions may be required. Treatment for HITTS includes immediate cessation of heparin therapy. The platelet count usually returns to normal in 5–6 days. If thromboemboli have already formed, additional anticoagulation is immediately required. Dextran may be useful. Intravenous immunoglobulin, 0.4 g / kg, followed by a platelet transfusion appeared to restore normal platelet counts in a patient with severe heparin-associated thrombocytopenia. Protamine sulfate has no value since the problem is not due to the anticoagulating properties of heparin, but rather to its antigenic properties.
- Posthospital care should include careful follow-up for development of heparin rebound or heparin-induced thrombosis.
- Hyperkalemia and secondary hypoaldosteronism have been observed, especially in patients with diabetes mellitus or renal insufficiency.

ANTIDOTES

Protamine

When injected, protamine sulfate, which has a pH of 6.5–7.5, acts as an effective heparin antagonist both *in vitro* and *in vivo*. It forms a stable salt by complexing with either heparin calcium or heparin sodium, which is acidic. The resulting complex is not an anticoagulant. The neutralization of heparin by intravenous injection of protamine sulfate takes about 30–60 seconds. It is used in severe overdosage or bleeding caused by heparin. When given in a dose of 50 mg (10 mg / mL) over 10 minutes, acute hypotension, bradycardia, dyspnea, transient flushing, and a feeling of warmth can be avoided. Hypersensitivity reactions may occur. The partial thromboplastin time can be used to monitor its use when blood is tested 5–15 minutes after administration.

About 1 mg of protamine sulfate neutralizes 90–115 units of heparin. If it is given within a few minutes of intravenous heparin injection, 1–1.5 mg of protamine sulfate can be used for each 100 units of heparin administered. If 1 hour has elapsed since the heparin injection, 0.5–0.75 mg of protamine sulfate can be given for every 100 units of heparin; if more than 2 hours have elapsed, 0.25–0.375 mg of protamine sulfate can be given for each 100 units of heparin.

Questions—Heparin

1. Heparin

A. Is used for the prophylaxis and treatment of deep venous thrombosis and its extension
B. Has been used to reduce lipids in idiopathic hyperlipemia
C. Is a cationic sulfated glycosaminoglycan polysaccharide normally found in red blood cells
D. All of the Above
E. A and B

2. Which of the following is false?

A. Risk factors in heparin-induced bleeding include age greater than 40 years of age, males are affected more than females, median dose greater than 100 ug / kg, blood urea nitrogen greater than 20 mg / dl, heavy drinking, and concomitant intake of nonsteroidal anti-inflammatory agents.
B. Enoxaparins are associated with a lower rate of major bleeding than standard heparins.
C. Antithrombin III binds to heparin, enhancing the rate at which heparin inactivates thrombin.
D. Heparin administered surreptitiously, heparin rebound, and heparin-induced thrombosis-thrombocytopenia syndrome (HITTS) are all problems requiring immediate evaluation and care.
E. The calcium salt of heparin is prepared from porcine intestinal mucosa, and the sodium salt is prepared from either porcine intestinal mucosa or bovine lung tissue.

3. **Heparins are basic and are not absorbed from gastrointestinal or sublingual sites because of their small molecular size and polarity.**
   A. True
   B. False
4. **Examples of bleeding observed in patients receiving heparin include**
   A. Melena
   B. Vaginal bleeding
   C. Hematuria
   D. Intracranial hemorrhage
   E. All of the above
5. **About 1 mg of protamine sulfate neutralizes 100 units of heparin.**
   A. True
   B. False
6. **Inability of heparin to control thrombosis may be due to**
   A. A hypercoagulable state associated with malignancy
   B. Antithrombin IV deficiency
   C. Heparin-induced embolus
   D. All of the above
   E. B and C

ANTI-FIBRINOLYTICS

E-Amino-N-Caproic Acid

E-amino-N-caproic acid (EACA, Amicar®) is an inhibitor of fibrinolysis that has been used for more than 20 years to control bleeding in a variety of situations including hematuria and postpartum hemorrhage. Acute renal failure, myopathy, rash, nausea, diarrhea, and prolongation of bleeding time with high doses have been reported. There have been no published reports of overdosage with EACA but the manufacturer has received reports of infusion rate errors leading to 10 to 20-fold overdoses, almost all of which were asymptomatic and resolved without sequelae.

PATHOPHYSIOLOGY

E-Amino-N-caproic acid is an antifibrinolytic agent whose action has been attributed to the inhibition of plasmin synthesis from plasminogen. Its primary action may be inhibition of activation of profibrinolysin. The minimum lethal dose is unknown. Toxicity has been associated with intravenous doses as small as 2 g. Safe use of the drug with respect to adverse effects on fetal development has not been established. Clinical studies have not been performed on breast milk excretion.

CLINICAL PRESENTATIONS

Toxic effects following therapeutic doses include nausea, vomiting, diarrhea, conjunctival hyperemia, delirium, impotence, seizures, dizziness, hypotension, and arrhythmias. Use of EACA has been associated with thrombosis of the pulmonary artery, renal artery, and cerebral vasculature. Renal and hepatic failure may follow high doses of EACA taken for long periods. Myopathy associated with weakness, fatigue, and elevated serum concentrations of creatine phosphokinase, aldolase, and aspartate transaminase have followed EACA use.

LABORATORY

Analytic Methods

Blood EACA levels may be assayed by gas chromatography.

Blood Levels

Plasma EACA concentrations greater than 130 mg/L but less than 300 mg/L are desirable. Plasma EACA concentrations are not easily measured in health care facilities.

TREATMENT

Gut Decontamination

Gastric emptying may be useful within the first several hours of ingestion of an overdose of oral EACA. There have been no clinical studies on the use of syrup of ipecac, gastric lavage, cathartics, or whole-bowel irrigation in EACA overdose.

Elimination Enhancement

E-Amino-N-caproic acid is not metabolized and is excreted largely unchanged in the urine. There are no controlled studies on the use of hemodialysis or hemoperfusion in EACA overdosage.

Supportive Measures

- In symptomatic patients with significant EACA exposure, arterial blood gases, complete blood counts, urinalysis, liver and kidney function tests, bleeding times, and fibrinolytic function tests should be monitored. Serum creatine kinase, aldolase, and lactic acid dehydrogenase determinations with urine myoglobin testing should be performed periodically.
- Hypotension is managed with intravenous fluids, Trendelenburg position and, if required, pressor amines (dopamine, norepinephrine).
- Seizures should respond to diazepam, phenytoin, and phenobarbital if necessitated.
- Patients receiving EACA should be hospitalized where monitoring of fibrinolytic activity and renal, hepatic and muscle function assays are available, and where a rapid response to thrombosis (renal, pulmonary, cerebral, and cardiac) will be able to mitigate adverse clinical effects.

Questions—E-Amino-N-caproic Acid

1. **E-amino-N-caproic acid is an inhibitor of fibrinolysis that has been used for more than 20 years to control bleeding in a variety of situations including hematuria and postpartum hemorrhage.**
   A. True
   B. False
2. **Acute renal failure, myopathy, rash, nausea, diarrhea, and prolongation of bleeding time with high doses have been reported.**
   A. True
   B. False
3. **E-Amino-N-caproic acid is an antifibrinolytic agent whose action has been attributed to the inhibition of plasminogen synthesis from plasmin.**
   A. True
   B. False

APROTININ

The basic proteinase inhibitor from bovine organs, aprotinin (Trasylol®), can only be administered intravenously, and has a half-life of about 2 hours. When it is administered at the start of cardiopulmonary bypass surgery, it appears to reduce blood loss and protect against global myocardial ischemia. Plasma concentrations of 150 KIU / mL are associated with fibrinolysis inhibition and reduction of blood loss and blood use after cardiopulmonary bypass and orthoptic liver transplantation.

A combination of high-dose aprotinin and profound hypothermia with low blood flow or circulatory arrest has been associated with disseminated intravascular coagulopathy (DIC). A dose of 625,000 KIU of aprotinin administered intravenously can lead to a decrease in arterial pressure, and metabolic acidosis. Noradrenaline, steroids, and sodium bicarbonate may be useful. Hypersensitivity reactions after repeated doses occur in approximately 10% of patients. A radioallergosorbent test (RAST) with aprotinin before repeated administration may be useful.

Questions—Aprotinin

1. **The basic proteinase inhibitor from porcine organs, aprotinin, can only be administered orally, and has a half-life of about 24 hours.**
   A. True
   B. False
2. **Hypersensitivity reactions after repeated doses of aprotinin occur in about 10% of patients.**
   A. True
   B. False

TRANEXAMIC ACID

Tranexamic acid (Cyklokapron®) may decrease the need for transfusions and factor replacement in hemophiliacs having dental extractions. It may also serve to reduce blood product usage due to blood loss following fibrinolysis during orthoptic liver transplantation.

Tranexamic acid, a synthetic lysine analog, is an antifibrinolytic agent that inhibits fibrinolysis similar to EACA by saturating the lysine binding sites at which plasminogen and plasmin bind to fibrinogen and fibrin. The elimination half-life of tranexamic acid is 2 hours, and 100% is excreted unchanged. Nausea, vomiting, diarrhea, reversible acute renal failure, disturbances of color vision, central venous stasis retinopathy, subarachnoid hemorrhage, and pulmonary thromboembolism have been observed.

Question—Tranexamic Acid

1. **Tranexamic acid, a synthetic lysine analog, is an antifibrinolytic agent that inhibits fibrinolysis similar to EACA by saturating the lysine binding sites at which plasminogen and plasmin bind to fibrinogen and fibrin.**
   A. True
   B. False

THROMBOLYTIC AGENTS

At least four thrombolytic agents have been used clinically in the U.S. These include streptokinase (SK), urokinase (UK), alteplase or recombinant tissue plasminogen activator (r-TPA), and anistreplase (APSAC). Specific agents have been used to lyse clots associated with myocardial infarction, stroke, and peripheral vascular disease. Overdose with thrombolytic agents can be associated with severe hemorrhage, which may be fatal. Bleeding may occur at puncture sites, and from the gums, gastrointestinal tract and in the central nervous system. Treatment involves the use of antifibrinolytics, cryoprecipitate, fresh-frozen plasma, whole blood, and / or platelets.

Pathophysiology

Thrombolytic agents activate the proteolytic enzyme plasminogen. Once plasminogen is activated, fibrin dissolution follows.

Clinical Presentations

Bleeding is the most common adverse event of thrombolytic therapy. The risk of bleeding is high in patients in whom invasive procedures are performed or who are given heparin concurrently or subsequently. Strokes and intracerebral bleeding have occurred. Minor bleeds have included gross hematuria, hematemesis, hematomas, and oozing from intravenous sites. Fatal hemorrhages have ranged from 0–4% in a variety of studies.

Hypersensitivity responses have been described following streptokinase and anistreplase infusion. Hypotension may follow the use of all thrombolytic agents in 10–20% of patients following either rapid infusion or high-dose infusion. Other symptoms may include serum sickness, headaches, backaches, renal dysfunction, hepatic dysfunction, nausea, vomiting, and fever. Streptokinase has been associated with the Guillain-Barré syndrome and rarely with hemolysis.

Pregnancy/Lactation

Few controlled studies on use in pregnancy and lactation have been performed with thrombolytic agents. Alteplase has been characterized as pregnancy risk factor B, and streptokinase is pregnancy risk factor C.

Laboratory

ANALYTIC METHODS

Alteplase has been assayed in human plasma using spectrophotometry, enzyme-linked immunosorbent assay, antibody radioimmunoassay, and an enzyme immunoassay.

BLOOD LEVELS

Following blood levels of these agents in routine hospital settings is generally difficult, costly, and not clinically indicated in the acute overdose situation.

Treatment

SUPPORTIVE MEASURES

- If bleeding occurs, discontinue the lytic agent and other anticoagulants. Apply pressure for 15–30 minutes to compressible bleeding sites. If bleeding occurs within 4 hours of heparin administration, consider the use of protamine sulfate.
- A fall in fibrinogen levels to less than 100 mg / mL during or after thrombolytic therapy has been associated with an increased risk of bleeding.
- If bleeding continues, cryoprecipitate (10 units) may be given. Fibrinogen levels guide further doses. Transfusion is usually not required if the level of fibrinogen is 100 mg / dL or more. If the patient continues to bleed or has fibrinogen levels greater than 100 mg / dL, 2–6 units of fresh-frozen plasma may be necessary.
- If bleeding continues after cryoprecipitate and fresh-frozen plasma are administered, obtain a bleeding time to assess platelet function. If the bleeding time is under 7 minutes, only

antifibrinolytic agents are required. E-Aminocaproic acid and tranexamic acid are available antifibrinolytic agents.
- If the bleeding time is longer than 7 minutes, an additional 10 U of platelets and antifibrinolytic drugs are recommended.

Question—Thrombolytic Agents

1. Treatment options after bleeding induced by thrombolytic agents include
 A. Application of pressure for 15–30 minutes to compressible bleeding sites
 B. Vitamin K
 C. Cryoprecipitate
 D. All of the above
 E. A and C

BLOOD AND BLOOD FORMING PRODUCTS

Citrate

Whole blood is treated with a citrate solution to prevent coagulation and for preservation. Citrate-phosphate-dextrose (CPD) has been approved by the U.S. Food and Drug Administration for blood storage up to 21 days when the blood is maintained between 1-6° C.

PATHOPHYSIOLOGY

Citrate retards glycolysis and prevents coagulation by binding ionized calcium. Sodium citrate and citric acid are used when collecting blood to chelate calcium which prevents blood clotting. Rapid infusion of blood or plasma can lead to a fall in ionized calcium.

CLINICAL PRESENTATIONS

Early signs of citrate intoxication commonly seen during hemophoresis procedures may include perioral and acral numbness and tingling, feelings of tenseness or lightness of muscles, and a sense of "twitchiness." The adverse effects of severe citrate intoxication are not inadequate coagulation but bradycardia, decreased cardiac output, and possible arrhythmia. These problems may be enhanced if cold blood is infused. Patients with severe osteoporosis (decreased calcium stores) or severe liver disease (inability to mobilize citrate to bicarbonate) may be at increased risk.

Citrate intoxication can occur in patients receiving blood at a rate greater than 1 U in 5–10 minutes. This amount may be greater than that required to bind ionized calcium and can result in hypocalcemia. Citrate also binds magnesium, and hypomagnesemia, another cause of cardiac arrhythmia (long QT syndrome, Torsade de pointes) has been reported in massively transfused patients. In general, when blood is being transfused at a rate less than 30 mL/kg/h, that is, less than 8 U/h, compensating mechanisms ensure that ionized calcium concentration remains normal.

Hypocalcemia

A deficiency of ionized calcium may increase the irritability of muscle and may induce fasciculations, tetany, seizures, or cardiac failure if the level is reduced for more than a few seconds. Ventricular fibrillation and cardiac asystole (after QT prolongation) have been the most serious cardiac complications of citrate-induced depression of ionized calcium. Arterial hypotension may be resistant to further blood transfusion or pressor agents. It may also cause some impairment of the coagulation mechanism. Acute disturbances in ionized calcium homeostasis may not be apparent from total calcium measurement. This emphasizes the need for repeated calcium measurements.

Massive Transfusions

Massive transfusion is usually described as the use of 10 U or more of whole blood or packed red cells in a 24-hour period. The definition can also be expanded to include the transfusion of more than one blood volume in 24 hours.

In children, calcium replacement has led to hypercalcemia and death. The use of calcium should be reserved for the massively transfused patient with profound liver disease or acute heart failure, two situations in which metabolism of citrate may be impaired.

TOXIC DOSAGE/DEATH

Transfusion of not more than 50 mL every 30 minutes has shown no evidence of citrate intoxication. If the rate at which citrate is infused remains below 0.5 mg/kg body weight per minute, the serum concentration of citrate ion remains below 9 mg/dL (0.5 mM/L) and the calculated ionized calcium level remains above 0.85 mM/L, which is within the normal range.

Harmful effects of citrate infusion may occur if the dosage exceeds 250 mg/kg/h. An inadvertent injection of 400 mL of citrate-phosphate-dextrose administered in a 50-minute interval led to cardiac arrest with electromechanical dissociation that responded to calcium chloride therapy. The estimated peak serum citrate level was greater than 120 mg/dL.

LABORATORY

Analytic Methods

Citrate may be measured via an enzymatic method.

Blood Levels

A toxic plasma citrate level of 50 mg/dL can result in a calculated plasma ionized calcium level of about 0.5 mM and can lead to marked depression of myocardial function. The normal range of ionized calcium is 0.9–1.6 mM (1.8–3.2 mEq/L). The total calcium level in the blood following the injection of citrate usually remains normal or may even increase.

TREATMENT

Gut Decontamination

These methods do not apply to the treatment of citrate overdose.

Elimination Enhancement

Severe hypocalcemia and citrate toxicity has been successfully managed with exchange transfusions in newborns.

Supportive Measures

- All pharmacologically active citrate solutions should be labeled boldly in color with nontoxic dye and positioned so as not to be confused with other preparations. There should be clear instructions on the bottle regarding the proper dose of citrate-phosphate-dextrose and the danger of citrate toxicity.
- When citrate is rapidly administered intravenously (or bank blood is given at a rate greater than 120 mL/min) there may be a decrease in total blood calcium. The majority of patients, however, may become hypokalemic during massive transfusion often after initial hyperkalemia. Serum potassium should be monitored in all patients who receive a massive transfusion. Monitoring is mandatory in patients with renal compromise.
- During the management of massive hemorrhage, coagulation tests and platelet counts should be monitored frequently and

aggressive correction of hypovolemia should be instituted to avoid coagulation defects associated with prolonged shock.

Hypocalcemia

- Skeletal stores of calcium are large and, as a rule, calcium salts are not needed for treatment.
- Intravenous infusion of calcium may cause disturbances in the cardiac rhythm and should be avoided if possible. There is a real danger of calcium overdosage with aggressive treatment of citrate-induced hypocalcemia.
- Cardiac monitoring and serial electrocardiograms should be followed as calcium levels normalize in overdose.

Questions—Citrate

1. **Which of the following about citrate is false?**
   A. Whole blood is treated with a citrate solution to prevent coagulation and for preservation.
   B. Citrate-phosphate-dextrose (CPD) has been approved for blood storage up to 3 months.
   C. Citrate retards glycolysis and prevents coagulation by binding ionized calcium.
   D. Sodium citrate and citric acid are used when collecting blood to chelate calcium, which prevents blood clotting.
   E. Rapid infusion of blood or plasma can lead to a fall in ionized calcium.
2. **The adverse effects of severe citrate intoxication are not inadequate coagulation but bradycardia, decreased cardiac output, and possible arrhythmia.**
   A. True
   B. False
3. **Citrate intoxication can occur in patients receiving blood at a rate greater than 1 U in 30 minutes.**
   A. True
   B. False
4. **A deficiency of ionized calcium may**
   A. Decrease the irritability of muscle
   B. Retard fasciculations
   C. Cause seizures
   D. All of the above
   E. A and B
5. **Massive transfusion is usually described as the use of _____ units or more of whole blood or packed red cells in a 24-hour period.**
   A. 5
   B. 10
   C. 15
   D. 20
   E. 25

Iron-Dextran

Iron-dextran (Imferon®) has been used in the treatment of microcytic hypochromic anemia resulting from iron deficiency, especially in those patients in whom oral administration of iron is not feasible or ineffective because of intolerance, poor absorption, gastrointestinal disease, or inability to take the oral medication. Iron-dextran preparations have been used intramuscularly or intravenously for treatment of iron deficiency anemia.

PATHOPHYSIOLOGY

Iron-dextran is a complex of ferric hydroxide with dextran of average molecular weight between 5,000–7,500 daltons. About 98% of the iron in iron-dextran is present as a stable iron-dextran complex. Imferon® contains 50 mg of elemental iron and 20 mg of dextran per milliliter.

PHARMACOKINETICS

Absorption

- Iron rapidly distributes to body tissues after intravenous administration.

Distribution

- Following rapid infusion of up to 2.5 g of iron as iron-dextran, iron accumulates in the liver, bone marrow, and spleen, and appears rapidly in circulating red cells.
- The iron-dextran is rapidly broken down in the reticuloendothelial system, and then released into a pool that exchanges freely with plasma transferrin. This is carried in the bone marrow and is imported into hemoglobin.
- During the first days of treatment with iron-dextran, serum iron concentrations may reach 50,000 μg/100 mL. When the total serum iron level is greater than 1,000 μg/100 mL, the serum turns brown.

Elimination

- Trace quantities of iron-dextran appear in the urine.
- The half-life of the complex in plasma is 2–3 days.
- Only traces of unmetabolized iron-dextran are excreted in the urine, bile, or feces.

CLINICAL PRESENTATIONS

Following an overdose with iron-dextran, muscle cramps, bilateral frontal headache, neck stiffness, opisthotonus, and photophobia may be observed. After delayed onset of 12–24 hours, arthralgias, vomiting, metabolic acidosis, bradycardia, and depressed central nervous system sensorium may be seen. The serum hemoglobin does not rise during the infusion. This results in abnormally high concentrations of free iron, which crosses into the cerebrospinal fluid and is responsible for meningitis symptoms. Poisoning with iron-dextran presents an altered clinical course compared with inorganic iron poisoning.

Hypersensitivity Reactions

Hypersensitivity reactions (immediate or delayed) follow high intravenous doses. Hypersensitivity reactions range from 1% to nearly 50% in different studies. These reactions appear to occur more frequently after large intravenous doses of iron-dextran. The most dangerous complication is an anaphylactoid (anaphylactic-like) reaction. Similar to contrast medium reactions, the anaphylactoid reaction manifests during the first few minutes of an infusion and resembles a type I (IgE-mediated) allergic reaction.

The most common hypersensitivity reaction, occurring in more than 30% of patients given dextran, is the development of arthralgias and fever within 24–48 hours of initiation of intravenous therapy. Other rare systemic hypersensitivity reactions occur 1–2 weeks after initiation of iron-dextran therapy and include lymphadenopathy, malaise, fever, elevated erythrocyte sedimentation rate, and splenomegaly. Infrequent reactions following iron-dextran use include rhabdomyolysis and systemic lupus erythematosus.

TOXIC DOSAGE/DEATH

A 32-mL dose administered intravenously has induced meningitis symptoms. A child who received 1.3 g of elemental iron intravenously as iron-dextran remained asymptomatic. A 4-

year-old who was inadvertently given 2.0 g instead of 0.3 g of iron-dextran died of sepsis.

LABORATORY

Analytical Methods

The iron-dextran complex is present in the circulation for 2–3 weeks after administration and interferes with all colorimetric iron assays. In patients receiving iron-dextran therapy, transferrin-based iron, total iron binding capacity (TIBC), total iron (except hemoglobin-iron), and dextran-bound iron levels can be measured by a colorimetric technique using dithionite.

Blood Levels

Iron-dextran may, even if administered within the previous 3 weeks, produce false-positive and abnormally elevated readings of serum iron. The total iron binding capacity may be markedly increased in response to iron-dextran therapy.

TREATMENT

Gut Decontamination

These methods do not apply to the treatment of iron-dextran overdose.

Elimination Enhancement

The drug is negligibly removed by hemodialysis. Whole blood exchange transfusion has been useful when administered early.

Supportive Measures

- Treatment of an iron-dextran overdose is symptomatic and supportive. Monitoring of serum iron and TIBC is indicated.

ANTIDOTES

Deferoxamine may decrease the side effects of iron-dextran treatment, but because the iron probably remains substantively bound to dextran, deferoxamine is probably ineffective.

Questions—Iron-Dextran

1. **Iron-dextran has been used in the treatment of microcytic hypochromic anemia resulting from iron deficiency, especially in those patients in whom oral administration of iron is not feasible or ineffective because of intolerance, poor absorption, gastrointestinal disease or inability to take oral medications.**
   A. True
   B. False
2. **Iron-dextran interferes with all colorimetric iron assays.**
   A. True
   B. False

Plasma Volume Expanders

The choice of primary agents for volume replacement is limited. Blood and blood products have limited availability and there are concerns over infectious and immunologic risks. The costs involved in obtaining, storing, crossmatching, processing, and dispersing blood and blood products continue to rise. Blood and plasma substitutes provide a cost-effective alternative to blood products.

Plasma volume expanders are used for plasma volume expansion, for antithrombotic effects, and to improve microcirculatory blood flow. Dextrans have also been studied as possibly effective modalities in the treatment of patients with myocardial ischemia, cerebral ischemia, and peripheral vascular disease and in maintaining vascular graft potency. Oral dextran sulfate may have antiretroviral activity against human immunodeficiency virus type I.

Oxygen is highly soluble in liquid perfluorocarbons, 8–10 carbon fluorinated hydrocarbons. The perfluorocarbons have been considered useful as an "artificial blood." Human hemoglobin solutions as oxygen-carrying blood substrates have been researched for 75 years. Problems have included renal toxicity due to the erythrocytic stromal components of the early hemoglobin preparation and not to the hemoglobin itself. This has led to stroma-free hemoglobin solutions with erythrocytic membrane fragments removed.

CRYSTALLOIDS

Electrolyte solutions containing sodium (crystalloids such as isotonic saline and Ringer's lactate solution) have no inherent oncotic pressure and, therefore, are relatively inefficient volume expanders. The lowered osmotic pressure favors fluid movement to the interstitial compartment, setting the stage for interstitial pulmonary edema. After intravascular infusion, these products are distributed over the entire extracellular fluid space, and only about 25% of the infused volume remains intravascular. Large volumes are required to result in effective plasma volume expansion.

COLLOIDS

Synthetic colloids are confined mainly to the intravascular space because they contain colloid osmotic particles, which, because of their size, are largely retained by normal capillary endothelial cells. The osmotic pressure exerted by these molecules across the capillary endothelium ensures that the solution is confined to the intravascular space. These colloidal macromolecules are suspended in an electrolyte solution with a sodium concentration similar to that of plasma. Three main groups of synthetic colloids include dextrans, gelatins, and hydroxyethyl starch. Human albumin solutions are also used as plasma volume expanders.

Dextrans are produced by a specially developed strain of bacterium, *Leuconostoc mesenteroides.* The molecules produced by the bacteria are very large, with molecular weights of several millions. Gelatins are prepared by hydrolysis of bovine collagen with subsequent chemical modification. Starch is the energy storage polysaccharide of plants and is analogous functionally and structurally to glycogen, the energy storage polysaccharide molecule of animals.

Starch is composed of two types of glucose polymers: amylase, a linear molecule, and amylopectin, a highly branched molecule that structurally resembles glycogen. Amylopectin is rapidly hydrolyzed enzymatically by amylase hydrolysis with a half-life of 20 minutes. In the 1960s, amylopectin was modified to make it more stable within plasma. Substituting hydroxyethyl groups to create hydroxyethyl starch did this, but its use in anemia has been disappointing.

PATHOPHYSIOLOGY

Albumin

Human albumin solutions are prepared from pooled blood, plasma, serum, or placentas obtained from healthy human donors. It is the major protein produced by the liver and its major functions include transport of a variety of substances in the blood and maintenance of osmotic pressure. The serum albumin level reflects its synthesis, degradation, and distribution. Unlike synthetic colloids, human albumin binds reversibly with anions, cations, and some substances that are active or toxic only in the free form. It has some anticoagulant properties. It may also have a role in preserving microvascular integrity. There is no convincing evidence that albumin is better than synthetic alternatives for volume replacement; nor is there clear evidence for maintaining the serum albumin concentration above a certain level.

Dextran

Dextran inhibits platelet aggregation and renders fibrin more susceptible to fibrinolytic enzymes, features that make it useful in preventing venous thrombosis. Infusion can reduce factor VIII levels, mimicking the changes of von Willebrand's disease. Dextran 70 is thus not the best choice for a plasma substitute where large volumes are needed. It also interferes with blood crossmatching, so a blood sample must be taken before a transfusion is started.

Gelatin

The colloid osmotic pressure of Haemaccel is similar to that of plasma. That of Gelofusin (succinylated gelatin) is slightly higher. These products are marketed in the United Kingdom. Their more rapid glomerular filtration leads to osmotic diuresis and a shorter half-life. Neither preparation appears to affect bleeding time or coagulation factors except through dilution.

Hydroxyethyl Starch

The particle size and colloid osmotic pressure of hydroxyethyl starch (HES) are similar to those of 5% serum albumin. Forty percent of the starch is excreted within 24 hours. The plasma half-life, about 12 days, is longer than those of other plasma substitutes. Partial thromboplastin times and factor VIII activities may be decreased.

CLINICAL PRESENTATIONS

Overzealous use of human albumin may lead to acute pulmonary edema or circulatory failure. Excess intravenous doses of dextran 40 have resulted in acute anuric renal failure, tachycardia, hypotension, hypoxia, pulmonary edema, adult respiratory distress syndrome, coagulopathy, congestive heart failure and fluid overload.

Anaphylactoid Reactions

Anaphylaxis mediated by IgG has followed the use of many colloid solutions. The incidence of anaphylactoid reactions from colloids has been estimated as 0.85% with hydroxyethyl starch, 0.14% with gelatin, 0.007% with dextran 40, 0.069% with dextran 60/75, and 0.011% with human serum albumin. The reactions can be severe and even fatal. Severe anaphylactoid reactions occur with no previous reactions to dextran given intravenously. Haemaccel, a gelatin colloid, has been associated with severe anaphylactoid reactions, some of which have resulted in death. Reactions are more likely if Haemaccel is infused rapidly and if the patient is normovolemic.

Coagulopathy

Low doses of hydroxyethyl starch have no effect on coagulation. Moderate doses transiently decrease platelet counts, prolong prothrombin and partial thromboplastin times, and decrease fibrinogen levels. Fatal disseminated intravascular coagulation and acquired von Willebrand's disease has followed infusion of hydroxyethyl starch. Low doses of dextran have not been associated with clinical bleeding, but platelet adhesiveness and plasma levels of clotting factors may be decreased. Larger doses are associated with bleeding complications.

Perfluorocarbons

Perfluorocarbons can induce a transient leukopenia, elevated liver function tests, increased pulmonary artery pressure, transient hypotension, hyperthermia, and pulmonary failure. An emulsifying agent in Fluosol is probably responsible for some of these adverse effects.

Renal Failure

Renal failure has been observed after dextran 40 but has not been reported after dextran 70. A similar result has followed infusion of gelatin, but this observation has been subject to controversy. The terms "osmotic nephrosis" and "hyperoncotic acute renal failure" have been used to describe renal failure following dextran administration.

PREGNANCY/LACTATION

Dextran in pregnant women has caused anaphylactic reactions and neonatal deaths.

DRUG INTERACTIONS

Numerous drugs bind to albumin. These include midazolam, warfarin, diazepam, dicumarol, indomethacin, salicylate, phenobarbital and theophylline. Concurrent use of these drugs may cause competition. Conditions associated with a decrease in albumin levels include age (neonate or elderly), burns, cancer, cirrhosis, enteropathy, liver abscess, malnutrition, nephrotic syndrome, pregnancy, renal failure, surgery and trauma.

TREATMENT

Gut Decontamination

These methods do not apply to the treatment of plasma volume expander overdoses.

Elimination Enhancement

Plasmapheresis has appeared to rapidly lower increased dextran levels, reduce plasma oncotic pressure, and improve glomerular filtration of urine after dextran overdoses and renal failure.

Supportive Measures

- Treatment of anaphylactoid reactions is the same as that for true anaphylaxis and may require oxygen, sympathomimetic drugs, asthmatic drugs, and volume replacement, preferably with an alternative plasma volume expander.
- Pulmonary edema is treated symptomatically and supportively with oxygen, furosemide, and other medications as required. Renal failure is treated conservatively.
- Coagulopathies are treated with multiple blood transfusions, including fresh-frozen plasma, platelet concentrates, cryoprecipitates, and packed red cells.

Questions—Plasma Volume Expanders

1. Which of the following is false?

A. Electrolyte solutions containing sodium have no inherent oncotic pressure.
B. Synthetic colloids are confined mainly to the intravascular space because they contain colloid osmotic particles, which, because of their polarity, are largely retained by normal endothelial cells.
C. Three main groups of synthetic colloids include dextrans, gelatins, and hydroxyethyl starch.
D. Dextrans are produced by a specially developed strain of bacterium, Leuconostoc mesenteroides.
E. Gelatins are prepared by hydrolysis of bovine collagen with chemical modification.

2. Human albumin solutions are prepared from
A. Pooled blood
B. Plasma
C. Placentas
D. All of the above
E. A and B

3. Albumin is the major protein produced by the liver.
A. True
B. False

4. Numerous drugs bind to albumin. These include all of the following, except
A. Midazolam
B. Warfarin
C. Citrate
D. Indomethacin
E. Theophylline

Erythropoietin

Erythropoietin (Epogen®) is a glycosylated protein that is normally produced in the kidney in response to renal hypoxia. It stimulates erythroid precursors in the marrow to increase red cell production and thus provides a simple control mechanism. The anemia of chronic renal failure is due primarily to a deficiency of renal-derived erythropoietin. The use of erythropoietin appears to improve the quality of life of hemodialysis patients.

Serious life-threatening side effects may follow the use of commercial erythropoietin (recombinant human erythropoietin). In an attempt to increase the oxygen-carrying capacity of their blood, healthy endurance athletes (e.g., runners, cyclists, and cross-country skiers) have used erythropoietin. The Medical Commission of the International Olympic Committee (IOC) has classified erythropoietin as a doping substance.

PATHOPHYSIOLOGY

Erythropoietin binds to specific receptor sites of erythroid progenitor cells causing the cells to proliferate and differentiate into morphologically recognized normoblasts. This process produces approximately 20 mL of new red blood cells each day. The mechanism of action of recombinant human erythropoietin is identical to that of natural erythropoietin.

PHARMACOKINETICS

Absorption

- Serum concentrations of erythropoietin peak about 13–18 hours after a subcutaneous dose, and bioavailability over 72 hours is 20–36%.

Distribution

- The apparent volume of distribution of epoetin alpha is about 40–90 mL/kg.

Elimination

- The half-life of recombinant human erythropoietin is 4–11 hours after intravenous use and 25 hours after subcutaneous administration. Only a few nanograms are excreted unchanged in urine.
- The role of the liver in the metabolism of recombinant human erythropoietin is unclear.

CLINICAL PRESENTATIONS

Hematocrits greater than 0.55 may be associated with encephalopathy, hypertensive seizures, vascular distension, impairment of blood flow resulting in hypoxia, and rapid clotting possibly leading to phlebothrombosis, pulmonary embolism, myocardial infarction, or stroke. The hematocrit may continue to rise for 5–10 days after the last dose of recombinant human erythropoietin is administered, thus overshooting recommended maximum levels.

In a marathon, a male runner might begin the race with a hematocrit of 42 or 43%. With an outdoor temperature of 50–55° C, he might finish with a hematocrit of 55% because of fluid loss. If the runner uses recombinant human erythropoietin he might begin the race with a hematocrit of 52–58%, and could conceivably end the race with a hematocrit in the high sixties.

TOXIC DOSAGE/DEATH

The maximum amount of epoetin alpha that can safely be administered in single or multiple doses has not been determined. Doses of up to 1500 U three times weekly for 3–4 weeks have been given without any direct toxic effects from the epoetin itself. A fatal dose has not been established.

DRUG INTERACTIONS

Aluminum intoxication during hemodialysis may cause resistance to erythropoietin by interference with heme synthesis, with accumulation of protoporphyrin. Desmopressin may contribute to the improvement in bleeding time during treatment with recombinant human erythropoietin. Theophylline appears to suppress production of erythropoietin by the kidneys, and amphotericin B may blunt the erythropoietin response to anemia.

PREGNANCY/LACTATION

Adequate and well-controlled studies during pregnancy in humans have not been done. Epoetin alpha has been placed in pregnancy risk category C. It is not known whether epoetin alpha is excreted in human breast milk.

LABORATORY

Analytic Methods

At present, there is no way to identify someone who uses the recombinant human erythropoietin. The recombinant hormone is virtually indistinguishable biochemically and immunologically from the native molecule. A radioimmunoassay is available to measure serum or plasma erythropoietin levels.

Blood Levels

Normal serum erythropoietin levels are about 10–20 U/L. No correlation appears to exist between erythropoietin concentration and hematocrit excess or blood volume in polycythemia vera patients. Serum concentrations after subcutaneous administration are about 5–10% of those found after the same intravenous dose. Peak serum levels of 1,000–3,000 U/L are measured after intravenous administration, and 32–484 U/L after subcutaneous injection.

TREATMENT

Gut Decontamination

These methods do not apply to the use or misuse of erythropoietin.

Elimination Enhancement

Elimination enhancement procedures (hemodialysis, hemoperfusion) may not be effective; however, clinical trials have not evaluated excess responses to recombinant human erythropoietin.

Supportive Measures

- If excess hematocrits are observed during routine serial hematocrit observations that accompany recombinant human erythropoietin administration, withhold the drug and perform phlebotomy to decrease the hematocrit.
- Monitoring of blood pressure, cardiac and renal function, and neurologic status are paramount in the use of recombinant human erythropoietin.

Questions—Erythropoietin

1. Which of the following about erythropoietin is false?

A. Erythropoietin is a glycosylated protein that is normally produced in the kidney in response to renal hypoxia.
B. Erythropoietin stimulates erythroid precursors in the marrow to increase red cell production.
C. The anemia of chronic renal failure is due primarily to a deficiency of erythropoietin.
D. The use of erythropoietin appears to improve the quality of life of hemodialysis patients.
E. In an attempt to prevent rhabdomyolysis after races, athletes have used erythropoietin.

2. At present, there is no way to identify someone who uses the recombinant human erythropoietin. The recombinant hormone is virtually indistinguishable biochemically and immunologically from the native molecule.

A. True
B. False

NITRATES, NITRITES, AND METHEMOGLOBINEMIA

Nitrates

INORGANIC NITRATES

These compounds, also known as saltpeter, are present in well water contaminated by runoff from nitrogen fertilizers, decaying matter, or sewage treatment plants. Certain plants (especially those grown in high-nitrate water), such as cauliflower, spinach, collard greens, and broccoli, contain high nitrate levels. Medical uses include antidiarrheal agents (bismuth subnitrate), diuretics (ammonium nitrate), and topical burn treatments (silver nitrate). Safer drugs, which do not cause methemoglobin formation, are now available for these indications. Both nitrites and nitrates are approved as food preservatives and meat-curing agents. Fertilizers contain nitrates as a source of nitrogen.

ORGANIC NITRATES

Nitroglycerin (Nitrostat®) is used to control angina and congestive heart failure. Delayed cutaneous absorption of Nitropaste allows prolonged action. Isosorbide dinitrate (Isordil®), pentaerythritol tetranitrate (Peritrate®), and erythrityl tetranitrate (Cardilate®) are also used to treat angina and congestive heart failure. Ethylene nitrate and trinitrotoluene (TNT) are used to manufacture explosives and munitions.

NITROSAMINES

High concentrations of nitrosamines occur in patients who consume food preserved with nitrates. Nitrosamines may be carcinogenic in certain animals. Nitrosamines appear naturally in untreated foods (e.g., mushrooms), cosmetics, alcoholic beverages, cigarette smoke, and gastric juice. Smoked fish, bacon, ham, and some cheeses contain trace amounts of nitrosamines. Organic nitrites are nitrosation agents, which produce nitrosamines from amino acids. Chlorogenic acids (in coffee), thiocyanate (in saliva), and formaldehyde catalyze nitrosation. Ascorbic acid, caffeine, the amino acids cysteine and histidine, glutathione, and certain synthetic oxidants inhibit nitrosation.

Nitrites

INORGANIC NITRITES

Well water contaminated by septic tanks, municipal sewage, fertilizers, and feed lots contains high inorganic nitrite levels because bacteria reduce nitrates to nitrites. Food grown in areas containing high nitrate levels also contain high nitrite levels because of the reduction of nitrates during preparation and storage (especially purees, soups, and stews).

The U.S. Department of Agriculture (USDA) originally approved nitrites as a food-coloring agent that fixed the red color in meat. Later, nitrites were found to prevent formation of *Clostridia botulinum* spores and were approved as a food preservative. Concern has been expressed about the cancer-causing potential of nitrites, since organic nitrites are nitrosation agents, which can produce the animal carcinogen, nitrosamine. Recent U.S. government studies have not linked nitrite food preservatives to cancer.

ORGANIC NITRITES

These compounds include amyl nitrite, a methemoglobin-former present in the Eli Lilly cyanide kit. Amyl nitrite is a vasodilator used for cardiac evaluation, and is also known as "poppers." Other nitrites include butyl nitrite ("Locker Room," or "Sweat"—found in room deodorizers, perfumes, and incense), isobutyl nitrite ("Rush"—found in room deodorizers, perfumes, and incense), and isoamyl nitrite, a psychedelic drug. Organic nitrites have been used as aphrodisiacs, primarily in the male homosexual community to enhance penile erection, dilate anal smooth muscle, and delay ejaculation.

Nitrite can be obtained as a prescription drug (amyl nitrite) used to treat the symptoms of angina (ampules), as liquids (in labeled bottles sold as room deodorizers), and in unlabeled bottles, which usually contain a combination of amyl, butyl, and isobutyl nitrite. The amyl nitrites have been nicknamed "poppers" because of the sound made when the glass capsules containing amyl nitrite are crushed. Nitrites have been proposed to enhance HIV transmission by their association with risky sexual behaviors and HIV infection among gay men; however, additional studies are needed to examine this issue.

Pathophysiology

The toxicity of nitrates and nitrites results from their vasodilating properties, their propensity to form methemoglobin, and individual susceptibility to these effects (e.g., methemoglobin reductase deficiency, coronary artery disease). In therapeutic doses, nitrates and nitrites produce more venodilation than arteriolar dilation. Increased venous blood pooling decreases right atrial filling pressure (termed preload), which is one of the determinants of myocardial oxygen consumption. Reduction of the oxygen requirements in patients with marginal coronary perfusion improves myocardial performance.

Nitrates also improve collateral flow in the epicardium, and this may increase oxygen delivery. Reflex increases in pulse and arteriolar constriction maintain baseline peripheral vascular resistance levels at therapeutic levels. Upright posture increases venous pooling and may result in near-syncope. Large and rapidly administered (e.g., inhaled) doses overwhelm compensatory mechanisms, and hypotension occurs in the recumbent position.

Methemoglobinemia

Agents that oxidize hemoglobin, form methemoglobin. Nitrates, nitrites and numerous other agents produce methemoglobinemia. Nitrates are weak oxidizers of hemoglobin, whereas nitrites are strong oxidizers. Aniline, which is used in dyestuff production and in the manufacture of pharmaceuticals, inks, paints, photographic developers, shoe polish, resins, varnish, perfumes, and organic chemicals is the prototype oxidizing agent. Methemoglobin-forming agents also include local anesthetics (e.g., lidocaine, phenazopyridine and benzocaine), analgesics (e.g., phenacetin), and antimicrobials (e.g., sulfonamides, dapsone and phenacetin).

The conversion of hemoglobin ($HbFe^{2+}$) to methemoglobin ($HbFe^{3+}$) reduces tissue oxygenation by two mechanisms. First, methemoglobin cannot carry oxygen or carbon dioxide, and therefore its presence reduces the oxygen-carrying capacity of the blood. Second, the presence of oxidized iron changes the heme tetramer in such a way as to reduce oxygen release in the tissues (i.e., it shifts the oxyhemoglobin dissociation curve to the left). A leftward shift increases oxygen affinity and lowers the release of oxygen to the tissues. Conditions associated with a leftward shift include alkalinity, hypothermia, stored bank blood that has reduced intracellular 2,3-diphosphoglycerate levels, fetal hemoglobin (HbF), certain familial erythrocytoses (Hb Koeln, Hb Tacoma, etc.), carbon monoxide exposure and methemoglobinemia.

Rightward shifts of the oxyhemoglobin dissociation curve reduce oxygen affinity and increase oxygen delivery to the tissues. Conditions associated with exercise cause a rightward shift and include acidity, elevated body temperature, hypoxia (altitude, pulmonary or cardiac disease), and anemia. 2,3-Diphosphoglycerate (2,3-DPG) stabilizes the deoxyhemoglobin structure by binding to hemoglobin β-chains. Such binding facilitates the dissociation of oxygen from the oxyhemoglobin molecule central cavity.

The RBC relies on glycolysis and the hexose monophosphate shunt for energy, since it lacks the tricarboxylic acid cycle and the cytochrome oxidase system. The hexose monophosphate shunt produces NADPH, which reduces excessive oxidants in the RBC. Too many oxidants cause methemoglobin formation, hemolytic anemia and Heinz body formation (e.g., G6PD deficiency). Glutathione, sulfhydryl groups, ascorbate, and catalase play minor roles in the inactivation of oxidants. Under normal conditions, the methemoglobin level is 1–2%.

Glycolysis produces NADH. NADH-dependent methemoglobin reductase (diaphorase I) catalyzes most (95%) methemoglobin produced in vivo. NADPH-dependent methemoglobin reductase (diaphorase II) reduces $< 5\%$ of endogenous methemoglobin. The hexose monophosphate shunt produces NADPH, but the lack of endogenous cofactor limits this pathway. Methylene blue acts as an exogenous cofactor. G6PD deficiency does not elevate methemoglobin levels, because the diaphorase II pathway reduces only a small amount of the normal methemoglobin load.

Rare congenital defects occur that cause clinically elevated methemoglobin levels. Hereditary autosomal dominant genes produce abnormal hemoglobins (hemoglobin M), which are more susceptible to oxidation and/or are unsuitable for reduction. Heterozygotes are cyanotic throughout life, and homozygotes do not survive. Hereditary autosomal recessive deficiency in erythrocyte NADH methemoglobin reductase (diaphorase I) produces chronically elevated methemoglobin levels. Homozygotes have methemoglobin levels ranging from 10–50% and require methylene blue and ascorbate for cosmetic purposes only. Heterozygotes are asymptomatic and acyanotic but are highly susceptible to oxidizing agents.

Sulfhemoglobinemia

The appearance of this compound in the blood results from the replacement of one nitrogen atom in the pyrrole ring of the hemoglobin molecule by one sulfur atom. Some conditions that cause methemoglobinemia also cause sulfhemoglobinemia. Oxidant drugs (e.g., phenacetin, acetanilid) and congenital problems (hemoglobin M and G6PD deficiency) produce sulfhemoglobinemia. Sulfhemoglobin normally is present *in vivo* in small quantities ($< 0.5\%$).

No mechanism for reconversion exists; therefore, this compound remains for the life of the red blood cell. Sulfhemoglobin, Heinz bodies, and hemolysis may be regarded as a continuous process of oxidative stress on the red blood cell. Sulfhemoglobin seldom occurs in concentrations large enough to produce serious hypoxia. Methylene blue is not an effective antidote. Exchange transfusion is the preferred treatment although seldom needed. Sulfhemoglobinemia produces a more intense but less symptomatic cyanosis than methemoglobinemia.

Pharmacokinetics

ABSORPTION

- Both organic nitrates and organic nitrites are readily absorbed through the skin, lungs, mucosa, and gastrointestinal tract.

DISTRIBUTION

- Peak effects depend on product formulation and route.
- For volatile nitrites, peak effects occur within 30 seconds.
- Sublingual nitroglycerin produces peak effects within 5 minutes, and dinitrates produce peak effects within 30 minutes.

ELIMINATION

- Most organic nitrates are extensively metabolized by hydrolysis to inorganic nitrites and inactive metabolites, with the exception of the long-acting cardiac nitrates (e.g., isosorbide dinitrate). Their metabolites have longer half-lives (over 8 hours) and perhaps are active.
- The duration of toxicity depends on the rate of absorption and methemoglobin formation.
- Phenylhydroxylamine may be the toxic metabolite of aniline biotransformation, which prolongs aniline-induced methemoglobinemia.

Clinical Presentations

Toxicity results from the vasodilating properties of the nitrites and nitrates and from methemoglobinemia-induced hypoxia. The cardiovascular and central nervous systems are the primary target organs. Onset of symptoms depends on the oxidizing power of the agent, the amount, and the route of delivery. Most nitrates and nitrites produce peak vasodilating effects within 30 minutes; however, inhalation of nitrites produces peak vasodilating effects within 30 seconds and clinically detectable methemoglobinemia within 15–30 minutes if inhalation continues. Oxidizing agents such as aniline that require *in vivo* conversion to an active compound may delay and significantly prolong symptomatic methemoglobinemia.

The duration of methemoglobin symptoms depends on the methemoglobin level and rarely on the presence of congenital enzyme deficiencies. Signs and symptoms of nitrite and nitrate-induced vasodilation range from headache, nausea, vomiting, postural lightheadedness, warm flushed skin, sweating, syncope, and tachycardia to hypotension, decreased peripheral vascular resistance, and cardiovascular collapse. The presence of these effects depends on methemoglobin concentration and the patient's susceptibility to hypoxia (e.g., coronary artery disease, pulmonary disease).

Clinical signs of cyanosis appear before symptoms because of the dark pigmentation of methemoglobin. Cyanosis of the lips and mucous membranes requires a methemoglobin level of only 1.5 g / dL (10% saturation in a patient with normal hemoglobin levels) compared with 5 g / dL for deoxygenated hemoglobin. A Heinz-body hemolytic anemia occurs in normal individuals exposed to methemoglobin-forming compounds or in those with a G6PD deficiency who are similarly exposed to such chemicals.

CHRONIC EFFECTS

Nitrates found in food can be converted to nitrites by bacterial action when a baby food container is left open or cooked vegetables are allowed to stand at room temperature. Infants are particularly sensitive to nitrate/nitrite toxicity. Symptoms occur rarely in adults, who may develop headaches after eating meat cured with sodium nitrites (termed "hot dog headaches"). Chronic industrial exposure to organic nitrates (e.g., ethylene nitrate gas, trinitrotoluene and nitroglycerin) has produced withdrawal symptoms in tolerant workers, some of whom developed myocardial ischemia and infarction. Nitrosamines are animal carcinogens but have not been proven carcinogenic in humans.

AMMONIUM NITRATE

Disposable ammonium nitrate cold packs are widely used in emergency departments instead of ice bags. Chronic ingestion of 6–12 g/day may cause gastritis, acidosis, osmotic diuresis, and nitrite toxicity manifested by methemoglobinemia or vasodilatation. Nitrate may be considered in the list of toxins that can decrease the anion gap, using the mnemonic BLIND (**B**romide, **L**ithium, **I**odide, **N**itrate and **D**iatrizoate sodium).

Toxic Dosage/Death

The lethal dose of organic nitrates has been estimated as 1 g. A 15-year-old who ingested 80 isosorbide mononitrate tablets (1.6 g) and 20 nitroglycerin tablets (20 mg) developed severe headache, nausea, and vomiting and recovered in 24 hours. The ingestion of 100, 0.4-mg nitroglycerin tablets over 2 days caused a fatal 7% methemoglobinemia in an elderly adult with severe cardiovascular disease.

A methemoglobin concentration of 9% was associated with the extension of a recent myocardial infarction in a cardiac patient receiving high-dose intravenous nitroglycerin. An adult who ingested 15 mL of isobutyl nitrite developed postural hypotension, tachycardia, and slurred speech with a methemoglobin level of 40%. Fatalities have occurred with larger ingestions. The mean lethal dose of aniline has been estimated as approximately 15–30 g.

Laboratory

ANALYTIC METHODS

In nitrite or nitrate poisoning, rapid tests may confirm the diagnosis. Gas chromatography may also be used to measure nitrites and nitrates.

BLOOD LEVELS

Correlation of methemoglobin levels (measured in arterial blood gas samples) with clinical symptoms depends on the presence of underlying medical disease (i.e., anemia, coronary artery disease, pulmonary function). Methemoglobin levels under 30% in healthy persons produce no or minimal symptoms (fatigue, lightheadedness, headache), whereas levels between 30–50% produce moderate depression of the cardiovascular and central nervous systems (weakness, headache, tachypnea, tachycardia, mild dyspnea). Levels between 50–70% cause severe symptoms (stupor, bradycardia, respiratory depression, convulsions, dysrhythmias, and acidosis), and levels above 70% are usually not compatible with life.

Measured oxygen saturation is reduced; however, laboratories that calculate oxygen saturation from PaO_2 levels rather than directly will report normal oxygen saturation levels in the presence of methemoglobinemia. Hence, a gap exists between calculated and measured oxygen saturation levels.

BLOOD COLOR

Methemoglobin is a dark pigment that causes venous blood to appear chocolate in color. Comparison on white filter paper of a drop of blood with a normal sample best demonstrates the presence of methemoglobinemia, but requires a methemoglobin level over 15%. Bubbling oxygen does not change the color of methemoglobin.

Treatment

GUT DECONTAMINATION

Gastric lavage and / or charcoal may be useful if significant amounts of nitrites or nitrates are ingested. Gut decontamination later than 4 hours may be effective if substances that delay gastric emptying or produce ileus are ingested. Be sure to remove clothes and wash contaminated skin.

ELIMINATION ENHANCEMENT

Theoretically, hemodialysis, forced diuresis, and hemoperfusion are not effective for pure methemoglobinemia, but may be adjunctive treatment for aniline poisoning when supportive care is inadequate. Hyperbaric oxygen has not demonstrated conclusive benefits in animal models. Exchange transfusion and / or the transfusion of packed red blood cells may be useful for methylene blue failures or for patients with known G6PD or NADPH methemoglobin reductase deficiencies. The inherent risks of the large blood volumes required in adults limit the applicability of this method.

SUPPORTIVE MEASURES

- Initial attention should be directed toward improving oxygen delivery with assisted ventilation if necessary, and 100% oxygen while intravenous methylene blue is prepared.
- A methemoglobin level should be obtained in any patient with cyanosis. Methylene blue (tetramethylthionine chloride) is the antidote of choice for serious methemoglobinemia. See Antidotes below.
- Repeat methemoglobin levels are required 1–2 hours after methylene blue therapy to assess the effectiveness of methemoglobin reduction. Be sure to correlate symptoms to methemoglobin levels, and remember that large doses of methylene blue cause a bluish skin discoloration after methemoglobin levels return to normal. If the patient fails to improve within 1 hour after methylene blue therapy, reconsider the diagnosis and review the causes of treatment failure.

- Institute cardiac monitoring, especially in patients with coronary artery or pulmonary disease.
- Hypotension should respond to Trendelenburg's position and intravenous fluids. Otherwise, dopamine may be needed.
- Evaluation of the child with "chocolate brown blood" should include a detailed history (i.e., history of similar signs in the family, drug exposure, source of drinking water, use of home remedies, diarrhea, pica, specific foods, and occupations or hobbies of family members).
- Physical examination should focus on cardiovascular and pulmonary disease, and laboratory tests may include pH, PaO_2, $PaCO_2$, quantitative methemoglobin level, G6PD screen, complete blood count, hemoglobin electrophoresis and quantitative G6PD if deficient. Quantitative NADH and NADPH methemoglobin reductase, stool culture, and/or toxicology screen may also be helpful.

Antidotes

METHYLENE BLUE

Methylene blue is administered to symptomatic patients who have been exposed to methemoglobin-forming compounds and whose methemoglobin levels exceed 20–30%. Cyanosis alone is not an indication for treatment without symptomatic evidence of hypoxia. At high levels of methemoglobin (over 70%), methylene blue reduces the methemoglobin half-life from an average of 15–20 hours to 40–90 minutes. Methylene blue acts as an electron carrier for the hexose monophosphate pathway, which reduces methemoglobin to hemoglobin. In patients with methemoglobinemia, the erythrocyte methemoglobin reductase reduces methylene blue to leukomethylene blue (colorless form), which in turn reduces methemoglobin to hemoglobin.

The usual dose of methylene blue is 1–2 mg/kg of a 1% solution (10 mg/mL) intravenously over 5 minutes. The same dose may be repeated within 1 hour if symptoms of hypoxia fail to subside. Chemicals such as aniline that produce active metabolites may require repeat doses, but limit the total dose to 7 mg/kg. Doses exceeding 7 mg/kg may produce nausea, vomiting, abdominal pain, chest pain, dizziness, diaphoresis, confusion, and cyanosis because of methemoglobin formation. The administration of ascorbic acid (100–500 mg twice daily either orally or intravenously) is harmless, but probably has a minor effect on increasing methemoglobin reduction.

Patients who ingest aniline may be less responsive to methylene blue, because the toxic intermediate, phenylhydroxylamine, may competitively block uptake of methylene blue by the erythrocytes. Methylene blue causes hemolysis in glucose-6-phosphate dehydrogenase (G6PD)-deficient patients, and exchange transfusion should be considered as an alternative to methylene blue therapy in these patients. Since methylene blue is eliminated mostly by renal excretion, the drug should be used cautiously in the presence of renal dysfunction. This drug is contraindicated as an agent to reverse methemoglobinemia if sodium nitrite is used as an antidote for cyanide poisoning.

To summarize, failure of methylene blue therapy may be seen in patients with G6PD deficiency due to low endogenous levels of NADPH, in rare patients with NADPH methemoglobin reductase deficiency who cannot activate the alternate pathway for methemoglobin reduction, and in the presence of sulfhemoglobinemia for which methylene blue is ineffective. Methylene blue failures may also be seen with excessive methylene blue doses, which produce paradoxical formation of methemoglobin, and in cases involving continuing gastrointestinal absorption or methemoglobin formation (certain drugs, such as aniline, produce cyclical formation of methemoglobin).

Questions—Nitrates, Nitrites, and Methemoglobinemia

1. Inorganic nitrates
   A. May be present in well water contaminated by runoff from nitrogen fertilizers, decaying matter, or sewage treatment plants.
   B. Have been used as antidiarrheal agents, diuretics, and thrombolytics.
   C. Have been approved as food preservatives and meat-curing agents.
   D. All of the above
   E. A and C

2. Organic nitrates
   A. Include nitroglycerin
   B. Include isosorbide dinitrate
   C. Include the explosive trinitrotoluene (TNT)
   D. All of the above
   E. A and B

3. Nitrosamines
   A. Occur in patients who consume food preserved with nitrites
   B. May be carcinogenic in certain animals
   C. Appear naturally in untreated foods such as mushrooms
   D. All of the above
   E. B and C

4. Inorganic nitrites
   A. Can contaminate well water
   B. Have been approved as food-coloring agents to fix the red color in meat
   C. Can prevent formation of *Clostridia botulinum* spores
   D. All of the above
   E. B and C

5. Organic nitrites
   A. Include methylene blue, a methemoglobin-former present in the Eli Lilly cyanide kit.
   B. Include amyl nitrite, a vasodilator used for cardiac evaluation, also known as "poppers."
   C. Include butyl nitrite used for room deodorizers, perfumes and incense.
   D. All of the above
   E. B and C

6. Agents that reduce hemoglobin, form methemoglobin.
   A. True
   B. False

7. All of the following are methemoglobin formers, except
   A. Aniline
   B. Lidocaine
   C. Carbon monoxide
   D. Dapsone
   E. Phenazopyridine

8. Regarding methemoglobin levels,
   A. Methemoglobin levels under 30% in healthy persons produce no or minimal symptoms.
   B. Levels between 10–20% produce moderate depression of the cardiovascular and central nervous systems (weakness, headache, tachypnea, tachycardia, and mild dyspnea).
   C. Levels above 50% are usually not compatible with life.
   D. A and B
   E. B and C

9. Methylene blue is administered
A. To all patients with methemoglobin in their blood
B. To symptomatic patients who have been exposed to methemoglobin-forming compounds
C. To patients with methemoglobinemia who are cyanotic
D. All of the above
E. B and C

10. Methylene blue acts as an electron carrier for the hexose monophosphate pathway, which reduces methemoglobin to hemoglobin.
A. True
B. False

11. Methylene blue itself can cause methemoglobinemia.
A. True
B. False

12. Failure of methylene blue therapy may be seen in
A. In patients with G6PD deficiency
B. In patients with NADPH methemoglobin reductase deficiency
C. In the presence of sulfhemoglobinemia
D. All of the above
E. A and B

PHENAZOPYRIDINE

Phenazopyridine hydrochloride (Pyridium®) is a synthetic azo dye used as an analgesic for problems related to the urinary tract mucosa. In overdose, phenazopyridine has produced methemoglobinemia, hemolytic anemia, and acute renal failure. Patients have usually survived with symptomatic, supportive and antidotal (methylene blue) therapy.

Pathophysiology

The most serious finding in phenazopyridine overdose is progressive oliguric renal failure. This may be due to a direct toxic effect of the drug on the renal tubules, as renal failure may occur as the only adverse effect without hemolysis. Yellow skin pigmentation in the absence of hyperbilirubinemia is probably due to deposition of azo dye in the skin and sclerae, and occurs primarily in patients with impaired renal function.

Hemolysis may follow ingestion of either phenazopyridine or aniline alone (one of the phenazopyridine metabolites). Methemoglobinemia probably follows phenazopyridine oxidation of hemoglobin iron (Fe^{2+} to Fe^{3+}). A predisposition to hemolysis and methemoglobinemia may be present in patients with glucose-6-phosphate dehydrogenase (G6PD) deficiency. Muscle damage may express itself as rhabdomyolysis and myoglobinuria.

Pharmacokinetics

ABSORPTION

- The pharmacokinetics of phenazopyridine have not been thoroughly studied. Phenazopyridine is absorbed from the gastrointestinal tract.

DISTRIBUTION

- Phenazopyridine is distributed widely to the skin, central nervous system and urinary tract.

ELIMINATION

- Renal clearance appears to be the major route of elimination of phenazopyridine.
- At least one metabolite, aniline, produces methemoglobin in humans.

Clinical Presentations

Methemoglobinemia may occur, usually with a concomitant hemolytic anemia. Hemolytic anemia may occur with and without glucose-6-phosphate dehydrogenase (G6PD) deficiency. Methemoglobinemia may follow a therapeutic dose of phenazopyridine in G6PD-deficient patients, in those with functional renal impairment, and in otherwise normal patients. Sulfhemoglobinemia has also been reported.

Nonoliguric acute renal failure usually is associated with evidence of hemolysis and methemoglobinemia. Hypersensitivity hepatitis has been reported characterized by nausea, vomiting, abdominal pain, myalgias, fever, jaundice, hepatomegaly, eosinophilia, and elevated liver enzymes. Muscle damage, rhabdomyolysis, and aseptic meningitis have also been reported.

Toxic Dosage/Death

A 15-month-old child who ingested 8.0 g survived. A 19-year-old who ingested 6.0 g was treated conservatively and survived. As little as 50 mg/kg of oral phenazopyridine has produced human toxicity, and as much as 750 mg/kg has not been lethal in previously healthy patients. As little as 600 mg/d in adults with renal impairment has caused cyanosis.

Pregnancy/Lactation

Trace amounts of phenazopyridine are believed to cross the placenta and enter the cerebrospinal fluid. It is not known if phenazopyridine is distributed into milk. Phenazopyridine is classified as pregnancy risk factor B.

Laboratory

ANALYTIC METHODS

Because of its properties as an azo dye, phenazopyridine may interfere with urinalysis based on spectrometry or color reactions. It may interfere with the phenolsulfonphthalein excretion test of renal function and with urinary glucose, steroid, and urobilinogen tests.

BLOOD LEVELS

Phenazopyridine levels have not been utilized in the management of overdoses. Methemoglobin levels may be helpful.

Treatment

GUT DECONTAMINATION

Use of induced emesis, gastric lavage, activated charcoal, or whole-bowel irrigation has not been systematically studied in phenazopyridine overdose. Supportive therapy alone has been useful.

ELIMINATION ENHANCEMENT

The role of hemodialysis or hemoperfusion has not been evaluated. Peritoneal dialysis has been used for the acute renal failure, but not specifically for phenazopyridine elimination. There are no published reports correlating the urine excretion of phenazopyridine and its metabolites and modalities used for enhancement of drug elimination.

SUPPORTIVE MEASURES

- Patients should be admitted to an intensive care facility if there is evidence of cyanosis, tachycardia, and rapid shallow respirations. An intravenous line, oxygen, and cardiac monitoring should be immediately available.
- Supportive and symptomatic measures are usually the mainstay of treatment. Almost all patients have survived with varying treatments ranging from minimal and conservative, to the use of methylene blue where indicated, gastric lavage, and intravenous fluids.
- Diminishing renal function may be evidenced by increases in serum creatinine and blood urea nitrogen, and/or with an abnormal urinalysis (proteins, sediment).
- Methemoglobinemia may be present early in the course of toxicity.
- Hemolysis (characterized by diminished hemoglobin and hematocrit, increased reticulocyte count, increased total bilirubin, anisocytosis, poikilocytosis, "bite" cells or desmocytes and/or Heinz bodies) may not occur for 24–48 hours.
- Rhabdomyolysis (characterized by myoglobinuria and elevated creatine phosphokinase) may be present.
- The urine may become deep orange-red in color.

Antidotes

METHYLENE BLUE

Intravenous methylene blue may be used for the treatment of methemoglobinemia.

Question—Phenazopyridine

1. **Which of the following is false?**
   A. Phenazopyridine hydrochloride (Pyridium®) is a synthetic azo dye used as an analgesic for problems related to the urinary tract mucosa.
   B. In overdose, phenazopyridine has produced methemoglobinemia, and encephalopathy.
   C. The most serious finding in phenazopyridine overdose is progressive oliguric renal failure.
   D. Yellow skin pigmentation in the absence of hyperbilirubinemia is probably due to deposition of azo dye in the skin and sclerae, and occurs primarily in patients with impaired renal function.
   D. Hemolysis may follow ingestion of either phenazopyridine or aniline alone (a phenazopyridine metabolites).
   E. A predisposition to hemolysis and methemoglobinemia may be present in patients with a glucose-6-phosphate dehydrogenase (G6PD) deficiency.

DIPYRIDAMOLE

Dipyridamole (Persantine®) is a vasodilator and antiplatelet agent widely used in the treatment of cerebral, peripheral, and coronary vascular disease. It has been used as an adjunct to coumarin anticoagulants in the prevention of postoperative thromboembolic complications of cardiac valve replacement. Dipyridamole has also been studied, together with thallium-201 cardiac imaging, as a test for detecting coronary artery disease in patients unable to exercise effectively.

Although patients with preexisting cardiovascular disease may develop further cardiac symptoms after normal or slightly increased doses of dipyridamole, ingestion of 5 to 7-fold overdoses of the drug have not produced serious problems related to coronary blood flow. Hypotension and tachycardia are the only cardiovascular signs that appear to follow excess ingestion of the drug. A fatality has followed use of a therapeutic dose in a patient with cardiovascular disease.

Pathophysiology

Platelet adhesion and aggregation appear to be reduced at blood dipyridamole levels above 1.5 mg/mL. Known biochemical properties of dipyridamole include inhibition of adenosine transport, inhibition of cyclic AMP and phosphodiesterase, and stimulation of prostacyclin synthesis.

Pharmacokinetics

ABSORPTION

- Oral dipyridamole is absorbed from the upper gastrointestinal tract.
- The average time to peak plasma concentrations is 70–75 minutes.

DISTRIBUTION

- Protein binding and enterohepatic recycling dominate the distribution pattern of dipyridamole. Dipyridamole is bound primarily (almost 99%) to a1-acid glycoprotein.
- The volume of distribution is approximately 2 L/kg.

ELIMINATION

- Dipyridamole is converted in the liver to the monoglucuronide conjugate and is excreted with the bile into the duodenum. In the intestine, dipyridamole glucuronide is partly reconverted to free dipyridamole. Both dipyridamole and its glucuronide are absorbed by the intestinal mucosa and returned to the liver via enterohepatic recirculation.
- Dipyridamole exhibits a decline in plasma levels that fits a two-compartment model. The alpha half-life, the initial decline after the peak concentration, is about 40 minutes. The beta half-life, the terminal decline in the plasma concentration, is approximately 10–11 hours.
- About 90% of a dose is recovered in the feces.

Clinical Presentations

At least 11 cases of overdose with dipyridamole have been reported to the manufacturer. Symptoms and signs of overdose included drowsiness, weakness, fainting, nausea, gastrointestinal distress, flushing with hypotension, and tachycardia.

Toxic Dosage/Death

Patients with unstable angina, multivessel coronary disease, and epicardial coronary collaterals appear to be at risk of dipyridamole-induced myocardial ischemia when doses of 75–100 mg are administered before planned coronary bypass surgery. A 62-year-old who ingested 5.0 g of dipyridamole developed a myocardial infarction and survived. A woman aged 17 years attempted suicide by ingesting 1.5–2.5 g of dipyridamole and survived. Chest pain may develop in 4–20% of patients who receive 200–400 mg of dipyridamole before thallium imaging. At least 8 children who have ingested overdoses up to 625 mg have survived.

Drug Interactions

Dipyridamole may inhibit platelet aggregation. Heparin given concomitantly with dipyridamole may induce bleeding. *In vitro* studies suggest that dipyridamole potentiates the anti-HIV effects of zidovudine and of dideoxycytidine in human monocyte-macrophages. Caffeine may inhibit the hemodynamic changes (increase in systolic blood pressure, pulse, pressure, and heart rate) induced by dipyridamole.

Pregnancy/Lactation

Safe use of dipyridamole during pregnancy has not been established. It has been classified as pregnancy risk category B. Few congenital abnormalities have followed administration of dipyridamole and aspirin to pregnant patients. Spontaneous abortions have been observed in some pregnancies in the first and second trimesters. Dipyridamole may, when added to a warfarin regimen during pregnancy, result in an increase in fetal wastage. Dipyridamole is distributed into breast milk. Caution should be exercised in treating nursing women.

Laboratory

ANALYTIC METHODS

A sensitive and specific high-performance liquid chromatography method is available for measuring dipyridamole in whole blood and plasma using paired ion chromatography and fluorescence detection. A fluorometric assay has also been developed.

BLOOD LEVELS

Following blood levels in overdose has not been shown to help guide therapy.

Treatment

GUT DECONTAMINATION

Activated charcoal (possibly multiple doses) may accelerate excretion of dipyridamole by interfering with its enterohepatic cycle. There is no evidence that syrup of ipecac, gastric lavage, cathartics, or whole-bowel irrigation accelerates or improves the chance of recovery.

ELIMINATION ENHANCEMENT

As dipyridamole is highly protein bound and has a high apparent volume of distribution, hemodialysis or hemoperfusion is not likely to be of benefit.

SUPPORTIVE MEASURES

- Patients who have overdosed with dipyridamole usually respond to symptomatic and supportive treatment. Attention to the airway, breathing, and circulation together with cardiac monitoring, availability of oxygen, and careful observation for incipient hypotension usually form the basis for treatment.
- Patients should be observed in the emergency department and may be discharged after 6 hours if all vital signs are within normal limits and an electrocardiogram indicates stability. Electrocardiographic changes following dipyridamole use may show ST-T wave elevations.
- Anginal symptoms and ischemic electrocardiographic changes usually resolve with sublingual nitroglycerin therapy. Severe chest pain following dipyridamole administration, which is relieved by antianginal medications, should be considered an indication of significant ischemia and treated accordingly.
- Ventricular arrhythmias, an infrequent complication, are generally transient.
- Patients presenting with suspected coronary artery disease in the setting of aortic stenosis may be at increased risk for life-threatening complications from oral dipyridamole and should be preferentially referred to cardiac catheterization.
- Accumulated data suggest that preoperative dipyridamole should not be a routine therapy in patients with unstable angina undergoing coronary bypass surgery or coronary angioplasty, especially if coronary collateral vessels are identified.
- Clinical data suggest that intravenous dipyridamole may induce severe bronchospasm in asthmatic patients. Intravenous aminophylline may be helpful in dipyridamole-induced asthma.

Questions—Dipyridamole

1. Which of the following about dipyridamole is false?

A. Dipyridamole is a vasoconstrictor and antiplatelet agent widely used in the treatment of cerebral, peripheral, and coronary vascular disease.
B. It has been used as an adjunct to coumarin anticoagulants in the prevention of postoperative thromboembolic complications of cardiac valve replacement.
C. Dipyridamole has been studied, together with thallium-201 cardiac imaging, as a test for detecting coronary artery disease in patients unable to exercise effectively.
D. Hypotension and tachycardia are the only cardiovascular signs that appear to follow excess ingestion of the drug.
E. Heparin given concomitantly with dipyridamole may induce bleeding.

Answers

Introduction to Anticoagulants

1. B 2. E 3. C 4. B

Oral Anticoagulants

1. B 2. C 3. A 4. A 5. A 6. D
7. A 8. E 9. B 10. B

Heparin

1. E 2. A 3. B 4. E 5. A 6. A

E-Aminocaproic Acid

1. A 2. A 3. B

Aprotinin

1. B 2. A

Tranexamic Acid

1. A

Thrombolytic Agents

1. E

Citrate

1. B 2. A 3. B 4. C 5. B

Iron-Dextran

1. A 2. A

Plasma Volume Expanders

1. B 2. D 3. A 4. C

Erythropoietin

1. E 2. A

Nitrates, Nitrites, and Methemoglobinemia

1. E 2. D 3. D 4. D 5. E 6. B
7. C 8. A 9. B 10. A 11. A 12. D

Phenazopyridine

1. B

Dipyridamole

1. A

SELECTED READINGS

Anticoagulants and Antifibrinolytic Agents

1. Coagulants and anticoagulants. In: McEvoy GK, ed. AHFS Drug Information 94. Bethesda, MD: American Society of Hospital Pharmacists, 1994:874–888.
2. Giddings JC, Evans BK. Drugs affecting blood coagulation and hemostasis. Int Anesthesiol Clin 1985;23(2):103–123.
3. Heparin and other anticoagulants. In: Reynolds JEF, ed.Martindale: The Extra Pharmacopoeia. 30th ed. London: Pharmaceutical Press, 1993:225–242.
4. Hirsh J. Heparin. N Engl J Med 1991;324:1565–1574.
5. Hougardy N, Machiels J-P, Ravo ETC. Heparin-induced thrombocytopenia. N Engl J Med 1995;333:1007.
6. O'Reilly RA, Aggeler PM. Covert anticoagulant ingestion: Study of 25 patients and review of world literature. Medicine 1976;55:389–399.

Thrombolytic Agents

1. Fears R. Biochemical pharmacology and therapeutic aspects of thrombolytic agents. Pharmacol Rev 1990;42:201–222.
2. Guidry JR, Raschke RA, Mortunas AE. Anticoagulants and thrombolytics. Crit Care Clin 1991;7:533–554.

Citrate

1. Bunker JP, Stetson JB, Coe RC, et al. Citric acid intoxication. JAMA 1955; 157:136–137.
2. Kruskall MS, Mintz PD, Bergin JJ, et al. Transfusion therapy in emergency medicine. Ann Emerg Med 1988;17:327–335.
3. Nolan TE, Gallup DG. Massive transfusion: A current review. Obstet Gynecol Surv 1991;46:289–295.

Iron-Dextran

1. Davidar SM, Snodgrass WR. Fatal iron-dextran poisoning: A combined iron toxicity and dextran induced immune block. Vet Hum Toxicol 1989;31:34L.
2. Harchelroad F, Rice S. Iron-dextran: Treatment or overdose. Vet Hum Toxicol 1992;34:329.
3. Reynolds JEF, ed. Martindale: The Extra Pharmacopoeia. 30th ed. London: Pharmaceutical Press, 1993:851–853.

Plasma Volume Expanders

1. Klotz V, Kroemer H. Clinical pharmacokinetic considerations in the use of plasma expanders. Clin Pharmacokinet 1987;12:123–135.
2. Mishler JM. Synthetic plasma volume expanders: Their pharmacology, safety and clinical efficacy. Clin Haematol 1984;13:75–92.
3. Moss GS, Gould SA. Plasma expanders: An update. Am J Surg 1988;155: 425–434.
4. Soni N. Wonderful albumin? Not all it is cracked up to be. Br Med J 1995; 310:887–888.
5. Vermuelen LC Jr, Ratko TA, Erstad BL, Brecker ME, Matuszewski KA, and members of the University Hospital Consortium Consensus Exercise on the use of albumin, nonprotein colloid and crystalloid solutions. Arch Intern Med 1995;155:373–379.
6. Wagner BKJ, D'Amelio LF. Pharmacologic and clinical considerations in selecting crystalloid, colloidal and oxygen-causing resuscitation fluids, part I. Clin Pharmacol 1993;12:335–46.

Erythropoietin

1. Adamson JW, Vapnek D. Recombinant erythropoietin to improve athletic performance. N Engl J Med 1991;324:698–699.
2. Canadian Erythropoietin Study Group. Association between recombinant human erythropoietin and quality of life and exercise capacity of patients receiving haemodialysis. Br Med J 1990;300:573–578.
3. Eschbach JW, Adamson JW. Guidelines for recombinant human erythropoietin therapy. Am J Kid Dis 1989;14(suppl. 1):2–8.

Nitrates, Nitrites, and Methemoglobinemia

1. Curry S: Methemoglobinemia. Ann Emerg Med 1982;11:214–221.
2. Lovejoy FH: Methemoglobinemia. Clin Toxicol Rev 1984;6(5):1–2.

Phenazopyridine

1. Gavish D, Knobler H, Gottebrer N, et al. Methemoglobinemia, muscle damage and renal failure complicating phenzaopyridine overdose. Isr J Med Sci 1986; 22:45–47.
2. Reynolds JEF. Martindale: The Extra Pharmacopoeia. 30th ed. London: Pharmaceutical Press, 1993:29.
3. Terell JR, Spruill WJ, Parish RC, Jenkins FH. Phenazopyridine-induced methemoglobinemia. Drug Intell Clin Pharm 1988;22:915.

Dipyridamole

1. Keltz TN, Gitler B, Cooper JA. Dipyridamole-induced myocardial ischemia. JAMA 1988;259:1179.
2. Ranhosky A. Dipyridamole-induced myocardial ischemia. JAMA 1987;258:203.
3. Reynolds JEF, ed. Martindale: The Extra Pharmacopoeia. 30th ed. London: Pharmaceutical Press, 1993:225–226.

CHAPTER 26

Cardiovascular Toxicology

ANTIARRHYTHMIC DRUGS

INTRODUCTION

Numerous medications have been developed to control abnormal impulse formation in the heart. These drugs are powerful and often effective, but are also characterized by a variety of side effects and profound morbidity in overdose.

Electrophysiology

Ion channels exist across cardiac cell membranes. Activation of these transport channels changes intracellular ion concentrations and membrane potential. By measuring the transmembrane potential of myocardial cells, five phases are identified that correlate to changes in the sum of potassium and sodium flux across the cell membrane. Two fundamental types of action potentials appear in myocardial cells. A fast response characterizes cells of the His-Purkinje system and normal atrial and ventricular myocardium. Slow response characterizes pacemaker cells such as cells of the sinoatrial (SA) and atrioventricular (AV) nodes. At rest (i.e., phase 4) the adenosine 5′-triphosphate (ATP)-dependent $Na+/K+$ membrane pump maintains a large sodium concentration extracellularly compared with the inside of the cell. The reverse is true for potassium ions, as this pump maintains large stores of potassium ions intracellularly compared with the extracellular space.

Because there is relatively more sodium outside the cell than potassium inside the cell, the net charge across the cell is −90 mV (inside compared with outside). Maintenance of the membrane potential is an energy-dependent process. Any disease that decreases the energy supply (e.g., ischemia) reduces the membrane potential and results in irritable myocardial cells capable of initiating dysrhythmias.

Depolarization

Pacemaker cells possess the ability to depolarize spontaneously. A gradual decrease in the outward flow of potassium occurs, which results in the movement of the transmembrane potential to the threshold firing level. Once pacemaker cells reach a threshold level, the cell depolarizes. These cells represent a tiny percentage of all the myocardial cells. Both the abundant cell-to-cell connections and the absence of faster pacemaker activity within the myocardial cells allow the pacemaker cells to direct the activity of the myocardium in a coordinated fashion.

Any electrical impulse that reaches the threshold, whether from the pacemaker cell or an aberrant source, will initiate cell depolarization. Each myocardial cell is blind to the origin of the depolarizing force, and the appearance of abnormal pacemakers causes dysrhythmias. Certain drugs reduce the propensity of abnormal cells to depolarize spontaneously and thereby suppress dysrhythmias. Antiarrhythmic agents do not reduce the incidence of dysrhythmias in every patient and, in fact, may unpredictably aggravate dysrhythmias in some patients.

Repolarization of the cell to the threshold potential restores the ability of the cell to depolarize and defines the end of the absolute refractory period. During this period, the cell will not respond to any stimulus. Only an excessive stimulus will initiate depolarization during the relative refractory period. By prolonging refractory periods, certain drugs prevent dysrhythmias.

Dysrhymogenesis

The mechanism of dysrhythmia formation is called enhanced or triggered automaticity. Drugs, ischemia, inflammation, mechanical injury, and electrolyte imbalance may alter the intrinsic firing rate (i.e., automaticity) of pacemaker cells by several mechanisms. Examples of automaticity-induced dysrhythmias include sinus tachycardia, sinus bradycardia, and ectopic beats (e.g., premature atrial and ventricular contractions). Slowed conduction in one pathway may allow the formation of a reentry circuit that triggers a tachydysrhythmia. This type of dysrhythmia requires parallel pathways connected both at top and bottom, with each pathway possessing a different conduction velocity and refractory period. Drugs that alter conduction or refractoriness may cancel this dysrhythmia.

Most serious ventricular dysrhythmias arise on the basis of reentry. In certain patients, an accessory anatomic pathway causes reentry (Wolff-Parkinson-White syndrome). Dysrhythmias may result from both altered conduction and automaticity (e.g., nonparoxysmal atrial tachycardia with 2:1 block). These dysrhythmias are complex rhythms and may result from drug toxicity (e.g., digitalis).

Torsade de Pointes is a ventricular tachycardia characterized by QRS complexes of progressively changing amplitude and contour that seem to revolve around the isoelectric line. The peaks of these complexes are successively located on one side of the baseline and then on the other. This positive, then negative polarity in the frontal plane of the electrocardiogram creates the typical "twisting-about-a-point" appearance. The diagnosis is based on the characteristic ventricular tachycardia and prolonged ventricular repolarization time, with QT intervals usually exceeding 500 milliseconds. Class I and III drugs are by far the most commonly reported drugs in association with this arrhythmia. It can be treated with overdrive pacing, magnesium, and/or isoproteronol.

Pregnancy/Lactation

Antiarrhythmic medications, with a few exceptions, generally are safe during pregnancy. Most are classified as pregnancy risk category C. Of the class IA agents, quinidine has the longest record of safe use during pregnancy. Procainamide appears to be equally safe, is well tolerated over short-term therapy (months), and has the advantage of intravenous dosing. Class IB drugs including lidocaine, appear to be relatively safe as intravenous antiarrhythmic agents. Phenytoin, on the other hand, is contraindicated because of a risk of birth defects [Food and Drug Administration (FDA) category X]. Class IC agents, which include flecainide and propafenone, appear to be relatively safe, although experience is limited.

Class II agents (β-blockers) generally are well tolerated. Cardioselective agents such as metoprolol and atenolol interfere less with peripheral vasodilation or uterine relaxation and are preferred agents. Class III agents are characterized by a delay of repolarization. Sotalol appears to be relatively safe, although there is a risk of *Torsade de Pointes*. Amiodarone, another class III drug, is associated with serious adverse effects on the fetus, including hypothyroidism, growth retardation, and premature delivery.

There are reports of maternal and/or fetal bradycardia, heart block, depression of contractility, and hypotension during treatment of fetal arrhythmias with class IV agents, the calcium-channel blockers, especially verapamil. Although classified as pregnancy risk category C, digoxin generally is safe during pregnancy. The serum concentration in the third trimester may be difficult to assess as a result of circulating digoxin-like substances that interfere with radioimmunoassay.

Treatment

- Not all dysrhythmias require treatment. Specific therapies are directed at specific dysrhythmias. Refer to ACLS guidelines for specific algorithms. Check vital signs carefully and elicit a history of ischemic symptoms (e.g., chest pain, dyspnea, diaphoresis) to determine the need for treatment.
- Because drug-induced dysrhythmias may not respond well to drug therapy while toxic levels remain, consider methods available to reduce toxic levels (e.g., serial activated charcoal, hemoperfusion) in specific situations where these measures are effective.
- Correct any electrolyte (potassium, calcium, and magnesium) and acid-base imbalance as well as hypoxia and hypovolemia.
- Consider factors that may precipitate dysrhythmias (congestive heart failure, ischemia or infarction, pericarditis, pulmonary embolism, hyperthyroidism, bradycardia with escape beats, and central lines such as pulmonary artery catheters or central venous lines that directly irritate the myocardium).
- Review the past medical history of the patient for underlying cardiopulmonary disease, and determine present medications.
- Look at the specific treatment section for each toxin, since alternate therapies may be available (e.g., sodium bicarbonate for tricyclic antidepressant-induced conduction delays). Therapeutic agents may exacerbate the toxic effect of the drug

(e.g., avoid administering a drug from the same class of antiarrhythmic drugs).

Questions—Introduction to Antiarrhythmic Drugs

1. **Which statement best characterizes the mechanism of antiarrhythmics?**
   A. They work by altering the relationship between myocardial cells and the conduction system.
   B. They produce an electrical shock to the heart like a defibrillator.
   C. They alter the conduction velocity and/or change refractory periods of parallel pathways in certain reentry circuits.
   D. They create a new arrhythmia that counteracts and cancels the arrhythmia being treated.
   E. None of the above
2. **All of the following are true regarding the characteristics of myocardial cells except**
   A. Pacemaker cells possess the ability to depolarize spontaneously
   B. Any electrical impulse that reaches its threshold will initiate cell depolarization
   C. Only ischemic myocardial cells can produce arrhythmias because they are unable to maintain the energy-dependent membrane potential
   D. Some antiarrhythmic drugs act by prolonging the relative refractory period
   E. Antiarrhythmics also can be proarrhythmic
3. **All β-blockers including sotalol are class II agents.**
   A. True
   B. False
4. **Amiodorone is in the same class as sotalol.**
   A. True
   B. False
5. **Verapamil is a class IV agent**
   A. True
   B. False
6. **Which is a fetal side effect of amiodarone during pregnancy?**
   A. Discolored teeth
   B. Macrosomia
   C. Hypothyroidism
   D. Blindness
   E. None of the above
7. ***Torsade de Pointes* can be treated with magnesium and/or isoproterenol**
   A. True
   B. False

CLASS IA DRUGS

Introduction

All class I drugs inhibit the fast sodium channel in myocardial cells and slow the maximum rate of depolarization and conduction velocity. This class is subdivided further into three groups according to their effect on action potential. Class IA drugs lengthen the action potential duration, class IB drugs shorten it, and class IC drugs produce little change in the action potential duration.

Class IA drugs are membrane-depressant compounds. Quinidine, procainamide, and disopyramide are the best-known members of this group. Drugs little used as antiarrhythmics in this class include carbamazepine and antazoline. These drugs decrease membrane responsiveness, which results in decreased conduction velocity. They also slightly prolong the action potential (increased refractoriness) and elevate the threshold for depolarization. Class IA drugs affect primarily the atria, the AV node, and the ventricles. Prolonged QT interval, bradycardia, AV block, and asystole are seen with toxicity. Drugs of class IA display greater negative inotropic effects than either class IB or class IC drugs.

Disopyramide

Disopyramide (Norpace®) is an antiarrhythmic drug that has been available since the early 1970s. Its relatively greater myocardial depression and anticholinergic properties distinguish it from other class IA antiarrhythmic drugs (e.g., quinidine, procainamide).

PATHOPHYSIOLOGY

As a class IA drug, disopyramide decreases membrane responsiveness and increases refractoriness by prolonging the action potential. Severe myocardial depression may occur, especially in patients with poor myocardial reserve. QT prolongation occurs early. Disopyramide also possesses mild anticholinergic properties.

PHARMACOKINETICS

Absorption

- Disopyramide displays good bioavailability (85%), but peak therapeutic levels may be delayed several hours because of anticholinergic properties (e.g., 2 to 2.5 hours after a therapeutic dose).

Distribution

- The volume of distribution is 40 to 80 L in an adult.
- Plasma protein binding is concentration dependent, with a small percentage (5%) occurring at high levels and relatively greater binding (65%) at concentrations below therapeutic levels.

Elimination

- The kidney excretes most of the absorbed dose of disopyramide (40% to 60%). The liver metabolizes the rest into several metabolites.
- Mono-N-dealkylated disopyramide is a major metabolite with greater anticholinergic properties than the parent compound. However, this metabolite has minimal cardiovascular effects and a mean plasma half-life in healthy subjects of 3.4 hours.
- The plasma half-life of disopyramide in healthy adults at therapeutic doses is about 6 to 8 hours.

CLINICAL PRESENTATIONS

Ingestion by healthy adults of less than 2.5 grams usually causes hemodynamically minor changes in conduction (e.g., QT and PR interval prolongation). Minor anticholinergic side effects occur, including urinary retention, blurred vision, and dry mouth. Cardiovascular collapse and apnea usually appear within several hours after a serious overdose, but the anticholinergic properties of disopyramide theoretically may delay symptoms.

Answers to questions in shaded boxes appear at the end of the chapter.

A variety of ventricular and supraventricular dysrhythmias and conduction blocks result from serious ingestions. Ventricular fibrillation and a nonresponsive myocardium are terminal events. Initial resuscitation after cardiac arrest, followed by progressive deterioration over 6 to 12 hours leading to death may occur.

TOXIC DOSAGE/DEATH

The average toxic dose in adults is approximately 1.5 grams, and the average lethal dose is about 3 grams. Serious poisoning occurs after adult ingestions exceeding 2.5 grams.

DRUG INTERACTIONS

Concomitant use with other anticholinergic drugs may exacerbate anticholinergic symptoms such as tachycardia, urinary retention, and mydriasis. Concurrent use of erythromycin may induce QTc prolongation, polymorphic ventricular tachycardia, and elevation of disopyramide serum levels. Erythromycin interferes with the hepatic N-dealkylation of disopyramide. Rifampin decreases serum levels of disopyramide when administered concurrently.

PREGNANCY/LACTATION

Pregnancy risk category C. Disopyramide may cause uterine contractions. Disopyramide and its metabolite N-monodesalkyl disopyramide have been found in breast milk.

LABORATORY

Analytic Methods

Disopyramide is quantified by gas chromatography using a flame ionization detector. Thin-layer chromatography and ultraviolet spectrophotometry also identify this compound.

Blood Levels

Toxicity generally occurs in patients with plasma disopyramide levels exceeding 9 μg/mL. In one case, a 41-year-old who ingested disopyramide developed cardiac arrest and died. Levels in postmortem blood disclosed a disopyramide concentration of 49 μg/mL and a mono-N-dealkylated metabolite concentration of 9 μg/mL.

TREATMENT

Gut Decontamination

Lavage, activated charcoal, and cathartics may be effective within the first four hours postingestion. Anticholinergic properties suggest that gut decontamination may be beneficial more than several hours after a large overdose.

Elimination Enhancement

Pharmacokinetic properties of disopyramide suggest that both hemoperfusion and hemodialysis may be effective, although experience is limited. Hemodialysis is effective in reducing the serum half-life in chronic hemodialysis patients and may be useful in cases where supportive care is not effective. One study suggests that clearance is greater with hemoperfusion than with hemodialysis, but clinical data are limited.

Supportive Measures

- Because cardiac arrest and apnea occur early in overdose, intravenous lines, cardiac monitoring, and evaluation of tidal volume and oxygenation are the first priorities.
- Use lidocaine and phenytoin (class IB) to treat ventricular dysrhythmias and avoid class IA drugs. Electrocardiographic changes include widening of the QRS and prolongation of the QT interval.
- Like quinidine, disopyramide may cause recurrent atypical ventricular tachycardia (*Torsade de Pointes*) even in conventional doses (600 mg/dL). Characteristic electrocardiographic features of *Torsade de Pointes* include QT prolongation, short bursts of ventricular tachycardia, and an undulating QRS complex that reverses every 5 to 10 beats.
- Isoproterenol or magnesium may shorten the QT interval and often abolish the ventricular tachycardia. Overdrive pacing may be necessary to terminate this dysrhythmia.
- Several cases of hypoglycemia have been associated with the therapeutic use of disopyramide.

Questions—Disopyramide

1. The following toxicities/effects have been reported with disopyramide except

A. *Torsade de Pointes* from a prolonged QTc interval
B. Uterine contractions and premature labor
C. Dry mouth, dry eyes, blurred vision, and tachycardia
D. Atrial fibrillation
E. None of the above

2. The antidote to disopyramide toxicity is

A. Lidocaine
B. Dilantin
C. Glucose
D. Hemoprofusion
E. No specific antidote

Procainamide

Procainamide (Pronestyl®) is an antiarrhythmic agent used to suppress ventricular tachydysrhythmias. Although side effects are common, overdose rarely has been reported in the literature. Its oral use is limited by the appearance of immunologic complications such as systemic lupus erythematosus (SLE) in patients on chronic oral therapy.

PATHOPHYSIOLOGY

The mechanism of action of procainamide is similar to quinidine. Toxic effects result from conduction delay and depression of myocardial contractility. Procainamide causes less hypotension and reduced systemic vascular resistance than quinidine when given intravenously. In contrast to quinidine, significant QT prolongation usually does not occur at therapeutic levels of procainamide.

PHARMACOKINETICS

Absorption

- Rapid absorption occurs after oral procainamide, and peak levels are reached within 1 hour.
- The bioavailability is approximately 85%.
- An overdose may significantly delay intestinal absorption and prolong poisoning symptoms.

Distribution

- The apparent volume of distribution is approximately 2 L/kg. Protein binding is only 15%.
- Intravenous doses must be given slowly, because the rapid initial distribution phase allows large levels to accumulate quickly at myocardial receptors.

- The plasma half-life after therapeutic doses is 3 to 4 hours. Congestive heart failure increases the plasma procainamide half-life to 5 to 8 hours.

Elimination

- At therapeutic doses, the kidney excretes most procainamide in unchanged form (40% to 70%). After an overdose, hepatic biotransformation probably is a more important elimination pathway than renal excretion.
- Hepatic acetylation produces N-acetylprocainamide (NAPA), which is an active metabolite with antiarrhythmic properties. The rate of acetylation is genetically determined and varies between individuals (i.e., fast vs. slow acetylators).
- The exact relationship between antiarrhythmic activity and plasma levels of NAPA has not been established and complicates the interpretation and therapeutic levels of the parent drug.
- Up to 15% of the intravenous procainamide therapeutic dose is metabolized to NAPA, and 81% of the NAPA dose is excreted unchanged renally.
- Congestive heart failure reduces the metabolism of procainamide; both the parent drug and metabolites accumulate in renal failure.

CLINICAL PRESENTATIONS

Side effects include gastrointestinal disturbances, headache, mild hypotension, rash, insomnia, dizziness, ataxia, hallucinations, vasculitis, weakness, and slight prolongation of the QT interval and QRS complex. Rapid intravenous injection (over 20 mg / min) exacerbates minor symptoms. An intravenous dose should always be given under careful monitoring for evidence of QRS prolongation and hypotension. A procainamide-induced systemic lupus erythematosus (SLE)-like syndrome (manifested by arthralgias, myalgias, pleurisy, and elevated antinuclear antibodies) can complicate chronic oral therapy, especially in patients who are slow acetylators.

Other side effects associated with the therapeutic use of procainamide include dysrhythmias, Raynaud's disease, agranulocytosis, giddiness, psychosis, hallucinations, delirium, a myasthenialike syndrome, thrombocytopenia, and ataxia. Serious toxic effects may include lethargy, confusion, hypotension, conduction disturbances (i.e., QRS and QT prolongation), and ventricular arrhythmias. The inability of a pacemaker to control the heart has occurred occasionally at high plasma levels. Pure red cell aplasia has followed prolonged use of sustained-release procainamide.

TOXIC DOSAGE/DEATH

A 79-year-old with cardiovascular disease and renal dysfunction survived a 19-gram procainamide ingestion despite severe hypotension, intraventricular conduction defects, and apnea.

DRUG INTERACTIONS

QT prolongation is exacerbated when used concomitantly with other class 1A agents. Respiratory failure resulting from extreme neuromuscular weakness was produced by procainamide intoxication in a patient with preexisting neuropathy caused by amiodarone. Amiodarone added to an N-procainamide regimen led to an increase in serum procainamide levels with development of occasional clinical signs of toxicity.

Cimetidine treatment appears to increase the average steady-state blood concentrations of procainamide and NAPA. Such interaction may lead to toxic procainamide levels. Trimethoprim decreases the renal clearance of procainamide and NAPA, resulting in increased plasma concentrations of both drugs and an increase in the QTc interval.

PREGNANCY/LACTATION

Pregnancy risk category C.

LABORATORY

Analytic Methods

A sensitive modified enzyme-mediated immunoassay technique (EMIT) is available for detection of procainamide and NAPA in plasma, serum, and urine.

Blood Levels

Plasma levels are only guidelines for therapy, as the interpretation of toxic levels is complicated by active metabolites. The presence of the active metabolite NAPA complicates interpretation of a true therapeutic procainamide (PA) level. Both levels (PA and NAPA) are necessary to predict accurate therapeutic concentrations. Total PA and NAPA therapeutic levels range from 5 to 25 to 30 μg/mL. NAPA appears to be less toxic than PA.

Procainamide levels up to 16 μg/mL may be required to suppress ventricular dysrhythmias. Mild toxicity may appear in the 12 to 16 μg/mL range, and serious toxicity occurs when PA levels exceed 16 μg/mL. In an overdose case, junctional tachycardia and conduction defects appeared at total procainamide and NAPA levels exceeding 42 μg/mL, and severe hypotension and lethargy, at levels greater than 60 μg/mL.

TREATMENT

Gut Decontamination

The usual measures of lavage, activated charcoal, and cathartic 4 hours postingestion are indicated unless contraindications for their use exist. Seriously poisoned patients may benefit from these measures more than 4 hours after ingestion.

Elimination Enhancement

The large volume of distribution limits measures to enhance elimination, although significant renal elimination means that dialysis is indicated in the presence of renal failure. A case report suggests the effectiveness of hemodialysis with high-clearance characteristics in removing the active metabolite NAPA.

Supportive Measures

- QT prolongation, hypotension, and QRS widening identify serious poisoning. Such patients should have intravenous (IV) lines, oxygen, and cardiac monitoring initiated in an intensive care setting.
- *Torsade de Pointes*, although usually infrequent following procainamide use, may be observed more often when there is a change in renal status and when NAPA values rise. QTc prolongation may be associated in such cases with elevated NAPA values. Measures of QT interval and QRS prolongation together with hypotension are sensitive measures of serious poisoning.
- Avoid quinidine and disopyramide. Consider pacemaker with signs of increasing AV block.

Questions—Procainamide

1. Which of the following is true concerning procainamide metabolism?

A. Procainamide is inactivated to N-acetyl procainamide by hepatic acetylation.

B. The rate of acetylation to NAPA is determined genetically.
C. Congestive heart failure increases the metabolism of procainamide.
D. Procainamide is more likely to cause significant QTc prolongation than quinidine at therapeutic levels.
E. None of the above

2. Side effects of procainamide include all of the following except
A. Thrombocytopenia
B. Psychosis
C. Renal dysfunction
D. Raynaud's disease
E. Aplastic anemia

Quinidine

Quinidine (Quinaglute®) is one of the cinchona alkaloids derived from cinchona bark. These compounds include quinine (the structural isomer of quinidine), clonidine, and cinchonine. Although it has been used medicinally since the 17th century for a variety of illnesses, the current clinical indications for quinidine are limited to the suppression of atrial and ventricular dysrhythmias.

Quinidine is a weak base. It is the dextrorotatory isomer of quinine and one of the class IA antiarrhythmic drugs, which include procainamide and disopyramide.

Pathophysiology

Quinidine produces clinical and toxic effects similar to those of procainamide. The conduction velocity decreases progressively as drug concentration rises. This is reflected by increases in the PR interval, QRS duration, and QT interval. High plasma quinidine levels cause high-grade AV block, bundle-branch block, and asystole resembling that of hyperkalemia. In contrast to procainamide, QT prolongation with quinidine occurs at therapeutic levels. Increasing potassium concentration enhances the intensity of the electrical effect.

In high doses, quinidine increases the slope of phase 4 depolarization, and this is reflected clinically by increased ventricular dysrhythmias after overdose. Intravenous quinidine depresses contractility and decreases systemic vascular resistance primarily by α-adrenergic receptor blockade. Procainamide has a similar but weaker effect. High blood levels of quinidine cause increased left ventricular end-diastolic pressure by its negative inotropic effect. Cardiovascular collapse has resulted from its depression of contractility.

PHARMACOKINETICS

Absorption

- The bioavailability of quinidine is 70% to 80% after oral use but varies among individuals and preparations.
- The sulfate salt is rapidly absorbed in 60 to 90 minutes.
- Polygalacturonate salts produce peak quinidine concentrations in 5 to 6 hours and gastrointestinal absorption of gluconate salts is intermediate (peak of 3 to 4 hours).

Distribution

- The apparent volume of distribution is 2.7 to 3.0 L/kg.
- Congestive heart failure reduces the volume of distribution by one-third, and chronic liver disease increases the volume of distribution by 30%.
- Quinidine is a basic drug that is highly bound (90%) to α-1-acid glycoprotein.
- Chronic liver disease increases the portion of unbound drug as a result of decreased protein binding, and this results in lower therapeutic levels.

Elimination

- The usual plasma half-life of approximately 7 hours after intravenous administration increases in the presence of chronic liver disease.
- Hepatic biotransformation by hydroxylation accounts for 60% to 80% of the elimination of an absorbed quinidine dose whereas the kidneys excrete 20% to 40% unchanged.
- Congestive heart failure reduces clearance by 50% compared with clearance at a urine pH of 6 to 7.
- While metabolism is highly variable between individuals, at least in cases of quinidine-induced *Torsade de Pointes*, the metabolites do not appear to contribute to the formation of dysrhythmias.

CLINICAL PRESENTATIONS

Allergic or idiosyncratic reactions are not related to plasma concentration and include drug fever, cholestatic hepatitis, SLE, asthma, anaphylaxis, thrombocytopenia, hemolytic anemia (especially in G6PD deficiency), and decreased prothrombin. Skin changes range from maculopapular eruption to thrombocytopenic purpura, cutaneous vasculitis, photosensitivity, and bullous lesions. Gastrointestinal symptoms, especially diarrhea, are the most frequent adverse reactions seen with chronic use.

Cinchonism is a toxic syndrome following prolonged, excessive use of cinchona alkaloids such as quinidine, and quinine. See Quinine section, Chapter 15, Antiparasitic and Antimalarial Drugs. This syndrome may develop at relatively low quinidine levels. Clinical manifestations include headache, fever, mydriasis, visual field and acuity changes, tinnitus, hearing loss, organic brain syndrome that varies from memory impairment to delirium, nausea, vomiting, rash, and flushed skin. Chronic organic brain syndrome may be the only symptom of cinchonism. Coma, convulsions, and cardiorespiratory arrest occur in patients with severe cinchonism.

Massive acute poisoning results in both cardiovascular and neurologic signs and symptoms. Cardiovascular effects result from delayed conduction and myocardial depression. Toxic effects often are superimposed on underlying cardiovascular disease. Increased conduction defects lead to AV block and widening of the QT, PR, and QRS complexes, idioventricular rhythm, and asystole. Conduction defects always are present in overdose, although QT prolongation may be present at therapeutic levels.

Myocardial depression and decreased peripheral vascular resistance may lead to hypotension and shock. Ventricular tachycardia and fibrillation may complicate serious overdose. "Quinidine syncope" results from bursts of polymorphous or atypical ventricular tachycardia (*Torsade de Pointes*) which may occur at therapeutic levels. Central nervous system symptoms (e.g., lethargy, delirium, convulsions, and coma) may appear without cardiovascular depression.

TOXIC DOSAGE/DEATH

The usual adult dose of quinidine sulfate is 200 to 300 mg three or four times per day. An adult who ingests 2.5 to 4.0 grams typically exhibits serious toxic effects. In one case, the ingestion of 8.0 grams of quinidine in an adult led to severe hypotension and dysrhythmias, which required overdrive pacing and an intraaortic balloon pump for control. A patient who reportedly ingested 20.0 grams survived with supportive care, in spite of hypotension and anuria. Quinine sulfate displays similar toxicity, with an average toxic dose of 4.0 grams.

DRUG INTERACTIONS

Various drugs, including amiodarone, ketoconazole, cimetidine and verapamil may increase quinidine levels. Phenytoin, phenobarbital, and rifampin may decrease quinidine levels. Quinidine may increase plasma digoxin levels. Verapamil impairs the metabolism of quinidine to 3-hydroxyquinidine and reduces the oral clearance and half-life of quinidine.

PREGNANCY/LACTATION

Pregnancy risk category C. Quinidine crosses the placenta and is excreted in breast milk. A patient at 33 weeks of gestation was administered quinidine for treatment of a fetal supraventricular tachycardia. The patient had evidence of quinidine toxicity at low to mid-therapeutic serum levels of quinidine, and markedly elevated levels of 3-hydroxyquinidine.

LABORATORY

Analytic Methods

Quinidine assay methods include fluorometry, high-pressure liquid chromatography, gas chromatography-mass spectrometry, and enzyme immunoassay techniques. Quinine does not interfere with the EMIT immunoassay method for quinidine, but will interfere with high-pressure liquid chromatography when quinine is the internal standard.

Blood Levels

The use of plasma levels to manage overdose often is not successful because of different sensitivities between laboratory methods and individual patient variation in protein binding. Therapeutic quinidine levels range from 2 to 6 μg/mL. Levels over 8 μg/mL may be associated with toxic symptoms, and levels greater than 14 μg/mL are associated with cardiac toxicity in a majority of patients.

TREATMENT

Gut Decontamination

The usual measures of lavage and activated charcoal within the first several hours (longer if sustained-release preparations are ingested) may be indicated. Repeated doses of charcoal (every 3 to 4 hours) may enhance the elimination of quinidine trapped in the acid media of the stomach.

Elimination Enhancement

Although renal excretion of unmetabolized quinidine increases in acid urine, the usefulness of acid diuresis has not been clinically evaluated. Dialysis does not remove a clinically significant amount of quinidine because of the high degree of protein binding, and should be used only in the presence of renal failure. Hemoperfusion may be useful if hepatic failure reduces metabolism.

Supportive Measures

- Serious poisoning may present early with cardiovascular collapse. Intravenous lines, oxygen, and cardiac monitoring are first priorities.
- Convulsions of severe cinchonism often are responsive to diazepam. Failure to respond to the usual anticonvulsant drugs is an indication to check serum electrolytes (particularly calcium) and glucose levels.
- Respiratory distress may result from respiratory depression, aspiration pneumonia, or the development of the adult respiratory distress syndrome (ARDS). In patients with underlying cardiovascular disease, pulmonary edema may result from depressed myocardial contractility.
- The presence of QT and QRS prolongation is an excellent marker of significant ingestion if recorded after peak plasma levels. Widening of QT and QRS intervals usually begins to occur when plasma levels exceed 2 μg/mL and definitely is evidenced at plasma levels over 8 μg/mL. A 50% increase in the QT interval or QRS complex indicates the presence of toxic quinidine levels.
- Hypotension should be treated with fluids and, if required, vasopressors. Both isoproterenol and norepinephrine have been used successfully, and a resistant case has responded to the placement of an intraaortic balloon pump. Persistent hypotension should be managed with a pulmonary catheter and arterial lines in a coronary care unit.
- Treat ventricular dysrhythmias with class IB drugs (lidocaine, phenytoin), and avoid class IA drugs (procainamide, disopyramide). Bretylium should be used with caution because of synergistic AV nodal suppression.
- When atypical ventricular tachycardia (*Torsade de Pointes*) presents, the goal is to reduce the QT interval. Isoproterenol infusion, 2 to 8 μg/min, and magnesium may be effective, but overdrive pacing (120 to 140/min) may be necessary as well. Lidocaine and procainamide are not effective and may be deleterious.

ANTIDOTES

Glucagon has a positive inotropic effect in dogs, but its clinical efficacy has not been evaluated in humans. Bretylium antagonizes quinidine-induced toxic effects on ventricular fibers, but it may enhance quinidine-induced reduction in AV conduction.

Questions—Quinidine

1. **Which of the following is true regarding quinidine's cardiovascular effects?**
   A. At high blood levels it is a positive inotrope causing lethal anterior myocardial infarction.
   B. The effect on conduction is similar to the effects of hyperkalemia including prolongation of PR, QRS, and shortening of QTc intervals.
   C. In patients with liver disease, the drug is less activated and therefore less potent.
   D. Patients with G6PD deficiency should not be given this drug.
   E. None of the above

2. **Quinidine is a class II agent.**
   A. True
   B. False

3. **A serious toxic dose of quinidine is**
   A. 300 to 600 mg/day.
   B. 600 to 1,200 mg/day.
   C. 1,200 to 2,000 mg/day.
   D. 2,500 to 4,000 mg/day.
   E. There is no toxic dose.

4. **The convulsions produced by quinidine can be treated with diazepam.**
   A. True
   B. False

CLASS IB DRUGS

Introduction

Class IB drugs include lidocaine and phenytoin (see Chapter 27, Anticonvulsant Drugs). Mexiletine and tocainide are structural analogs of lidocaine that suppress ventricular dysrhythmias when administered orally. These drugs suppress automaticity similar to other class I drugs, but they also shorten the refractory period. Both lidocaine and phenytoin shorten conduction velocity in hypoxic tissue. Unlike class IA drugs, neither lidocaine or phenytoin prolongs the QTc interval. Class IB drugs primarily affect the ventricles.

Lidocaine

Lidocaine, a synthetic cocaine derivative, is a popular parenteral antiarrhythmic and anesthetic agent. Although central nervous system manifestations such as drowsiness, dizziness, paresthesias, and euphoria may occur during intravenous use in the critical care setting, oral poisoning is rare because of a large first-pass effect. The therapeutic use of intravenous lidocaine is relatively safe even in seriously ill patients.

Massive overdoses produce convulsions, cardiovascular collapse, and asystole. Central nervous system symptoms usually precede cardiovascular poisoning characterized by myocardial depression, and suppression of intrinsic pacemakers. Oral lidocaine analogues include mexiletine and tocainide. These drugs are classified as class IB antiarrhythmics and share with phenytoin the cardiac property of shortening the action potential.

PATHOPHYSIOLOGY

Lidocaine (Xylocaine®) suppresses automaticity similar to quinidine, but also shortens refractoriness and increases conduction in hypoxic fibers. In therapeutic doses, lidocaine affects only fast channel-dependent tissue (Purkinje cells, myocardium), particularly the ischemic fibers, which display a prolonged action potential. The resultant effect of lidocaine is an improvement in the uniformity of conduction and a reduced incidence of reentry phenomena (and ectopy) without suppression of nodal tissue.

High plasma lidocaine levels depress intrinsic cardiac pacemakers and delay conduction, leading to sinus arrest and complete heart block. Both lidocaine and its metabolite monoethylglycinexylidide (MEGX) are equipotent convulsants in high dose and can produce initial sedation followed by convulsions and respiratory arrest.

PHARMACOKINETICS

Absorption

- Lidocaine possesses such poor bioavailability that therapeutic use is limited to the parenteral route, but large oral doses do cause toxic effects.
- After ingestion, the bioavailability is about 30% to 35% because of extensive first-pass hepatic extraction.

Distribution

- The apparent volume of distribution is approximately 1.3 L/kg. Congestive heart failure reduces the volume of distribution by about 30% necessitating the reduction of loading doses in congestive heart failure. Chronic liver disease increases the volume of distribution by about 40%.
- A rapid initial distribution phase (the initial plasma half-life is 10 minutes) causes a rapid reduction of plasma levels after IV bolus administrations. The maintenance infusion rate initially may not keep the patient within the therapeutic range before the bolus dose is metabolized.
- Lidocaine distributes initially into well-perfused tissue (e.g., lungs, liver, heart) and later into less well-perfused areas (e.g., skeletal muscle, adipose tissue).
- Lidocaine is 50% protein bound.

Elimination

- The liver metabolizes 95% of the lidocaine dose, chiefly by dealkylation to the metabolites glycinexylidide (half-life, 7 hours) and MEGX (half-life, 2 hours).
- MEGX possesses antiarrhythmic properties and probably contributes to toxic effects on the central nervous system.
- The kidney excretes only 5% to 10% of a dose unchanged.
- Age, myocardial infarction, congestive heart failure, and severe cirrhosis reduce clearance and increase the incidence of adverse reactions.
- The elimination half-life of therapeutic doses of lidocaine is about 2 hours.

CLINICAL PRESENTATIONS

Lidocaine causes toxic cardiovascular and central nervous system effects. Early symptoms include lightheadedness, dizziness, drowsiness, confusion, dysarthria, ataxia, hearing loss, and euphoria. Visual disturbances, agitation, and muscle fasciculations indicate more toxic plasma lidocaine levels and may portend the development of convulsions and coma. Apnea and hypotonia may occur in massive overdose. Large intravenous doses in adults (e.g., 1 to 2 grams) result in immediate asystole, apnea, and seizures.

Cardiovascular toxicity occurs primarily in massive overdose when large lidocaine doses depress myocardial contractility and delay bundle branch conduction. Case reports associate the therapeutic use of lidocaine with ARDS and methemoglobinemia. Subcutaneous injection of lidocaine in a neonate resulted in generalized tonic-clonic seizures and apnea. Symptoms of toxicity after an overdose with lidocaine may persist hours or days after the levels of lidocaine have become subtherapeutic, possibly because of metabolites.

TOXIC DOSAGE/DEATH

Oral ingestions under 7 mg/kg do not cause toxicity. A 38.7 mg/kg inadvertent adult ingestion produced acute delirium and sinus tachycardia but no serious cardiovascular or central nervous system symptoms. Two 21.2 mg/kg doses of viscous lidocaine administered 4 hours apart in an adult resulted in generalized tonic-clonic seizures, which resolved within 1 hour.

The maximum advised therapeutic intravenous dose is 2.0 to 2.5 mg/kg, but lower doses may be toxic in patients with reduced hepatic clearance (e.g., congestive heart failure, cardiogenic shock). An inadvertent administration of a 1.0-gram bolus of lidocaine in an adult resulted in apnea, convulsions, and asystole that responded to supportive measures, whereas a 2.0-gram bolus in another adult caused death despite resuscitative efforts.

DRUG INTERACTIONS

Concomitant use of propranolol or cimetidine may increase lidocaine concentrations.

PREGNANCY/LACTATION

Pregnancy risk category C. Lidocaine crosses the placenta. The American Academy of Pediatrics considers lidocaine compatible with breast feeding.

LABORATORY

Analytic Methods
Lidocaine is detected by immunoassay.

Blood Levels
Plasma lidocaine levels confirm toxicity but do not guide management. The therapeutic plasma lidocaine level is 1.5 to 3.5 μg/mL. Minor side effects of dizziness, paresthesias, and lightheadedness may appear in the upper therapeutic range. More serious side effects (twitching, visual disturbances, agitation, and seizures) occur in the 5 to 11 μg/mL range. The degree of toxicity appears to correlate better with free than with total lidocaine levels.

Postmortem lidocaine levels after overdose range from 6 to 33 μg/mL, but in most cases, the blood lidocaine level exceeds 15 μg/mL. A chemical, tris-2-butoxyethyl phosphate (TBEP), which appears in the rubber stoppers of evacuated collection tubes, displaces lidocaine from plasma proteins. The subsequent partition of lidocaine into blood cells may spuriously decrease plasma lidocaine levels as much as 25%.

TREATMENT

Gut Decontamination
Treatment should be initiated with activated charcoal within the first hours of oral ingestion. As lidocaine may induce the rapid onset of seizures, emesis is contraindicated.

Elimination Enhancement
Artificial measures are ineffective because of the extensive metabolism and large first-pass extraction of lidocaine.

Supportive Measures
- Supportive care should suffice for most overdoses in view of the short half-life of lidocaine.
- Fluids, dopamine, intubation, epinephrine, atropine, and cardiac pacing may be necessary for large doses resulting in heart block or asystole.
- The key to treatment is the early recognition of poisoning, especially in susceptible patients with shock and congestive heart failure who have reduced hepatic clearance.
- Diazepam is the drug of choice to treat seizures. Adequate ventilation and acid-base balance must be assured, because hypoxia and hypercapnia may increase cerebral penetration of the basic drug lidocaine. Avoid the use of phenytoin, because of its synergistic cardiac effects.

Questions—Lidocaine

1. All of the following are true about lidocaine's pharmacokinetics except
   A. It should be used with caution in patients with congestive heart failure because of an increase in lidocaine's volume of distribution.
   B. Liver disease decreases lidocaine's volume of distribution.
   C. Lidocaine is 50% protein bound.
   D. The liver metabolize 95% of lidocaine.
   E. Age, myocardial infarction, congestive heart failure, and cirrhosis reduce clearance and increase the incidence of adverse reactions.

2. Minor side effects in the upper therapeutic range of lidocaine include
   A. Dizziness, light headedness, and paresthesias
   B. Confusion, dysarthria, and ataxia
   C. Cough, visual disturbance, and muscle fasciculations
   D. Convulsions, coma, and apnea
   E. None of the above

CLASS IC DRUGS

Introduction

Flecainide acetate and encainide hydrochloride are antiarrhythmic drugs that slow conduction velocity similarly to other class I drugs. Flecainide is the first class IC antiarrhythmic drug marketed in the United States. Class IC drugs affect primarily the atria, the AV node, and the ventricles.

Flecainide and Encainide

Flecainide (Tambocor®) and encainide (Enkaid®) belong to a newer group of antiarrhythmic agents that produce minimal effects on repolarization. These compounds exert local anesthetic properties that depress myocardial contractility. Flecainide is the first IC antiarrhythmic released in the United States for the suppression of ventricular arrhythmias.

PATHOPHYSIOLOGY
The separate classification of class 1C drugs derives from the fact that these drugs produce little effect on the action potential duration, in contrast to class IA, which lengthens, and class IB, which shortens, this interval.

Pharmacokinetics

FLECAINIDE

Absorption
- Flecainide is well absorbed orally, with peak levels occurring about 3 hours after ingestion.

Distribution
- The apparent volume of distribution is 9 L/kg, and protein binding is approximately 50%.

Elimination
- The liver metabolizes about 50% of an absorbed therapeutic dose and the kidney excretes about 30% unchanged.

ENCAINIDE

Absorption
- Encainide also is well absorbed with an onset of action in 1 to 3 hours.

Distribution
- The protein binding of encainide is greater than 75%.

Elimination
- Encainide is extensively metabolized in the liver and its half-life is around 2.5 hours. Extensive metabolizers have an encainide half-life of 1.7 hours, producing the two active metabolites ODE and MODE.
- Nonextensive metabolizers have an encainide half-life of 9.8

hours, producing the inactive metabolite N-demethylencainide (NDE). Encainide is excreted in the urine and bile.

CLINICAL PRESENTATIONS

Like other antiarrhythmic agents, flecainide may cause proarrhythmic effects. Flecainide prolongs the AH, HV, PR, and QRS intervals as well as (to a lesser extent) the effective refractory period in the ventricular myocardium. Flecainide overdose has led to cardiorespiratory failure, ventricular fibrillation, asystole, AV block, marked prolongation of the QRS, QT, and T wave, coma, and bradycardia. Encainide may cause proarrhythmic effects, dizziness, headache, ataxia, nausea, tremors and blurred vision. Seizures, bradycardia, hypotension, and obtundation may be seen in overdose. Generalized tonic-clonic seizures may follow large ingestions of flecainide.

TOXIC DOSAGE/DEATH

A 3 to 4 gram overdose of encainide in an adult produced central nervous system (obtundation, seizures) and cardiovascular (QT prolongation, bradycardia, hypotension) effects similar to those of class IA antiarrhythmics (quinidine) and tricyclic antidepressants. A 6-month-old who ingested a single 25-mg encainide tablet developed a wide-complex sinus tachycardia (QRS, 0.16 second) and acutely decompensated with development of ventricular tachycardia in 30 minutes.

DRUG INTERACTIONS

β-Blockers may exacerbate the negative inotropic effects of encainide. Patients receiving concomitant flecainide and amiodarone have a significantly increased flecainide plasma concentration. The clearance and volume of distribution of flecainide are significantly greater in smokers than nonsmokers, though there is no difference between the two groups with respect to terminal plasma half-life or renal clearance.

PREGNANCY/LACTATION

Pregnancy risk category B. Encainide and flecainide distribute into breast milk. The risk to the suckling infant is very low. Use of flecainide during pregnancy appears to be safe.

LABORATORY

Analytic Methods

A simple, sensitive high-performance liquid chromatographic method is available to measure plasma flecainide levels. A high performance liquid chromatography (HPLC) method for the quantification of encainide and its metabolites in plasma and urine indicates limits of detection of 5 ng/mL in plasma and 25 ng/mL in urine. A reverse-phase HPLC technique is also available.

Blood Levels

The therapeutic serum range of flecainide is 200 to 1,000 ng/mL. Overdose data are limited. Plasma flecainide levels greater than 1 μg/mL probably are toxic. Atrioventricular nodal block with escape rhythm and QRS interval prolongation developed in a patient who had a flecainide plasma level of 3.0 μg/mL. Cardiac arrest developed in a patient with a postmortem blood level of 16 μg/mL. A blood concentration of 1.8 μg/mL was measured in a patient who died in acute respiratory distress and cardiogenic shock unresponsive to dopamine, dobutamine, and sodium nitroprusside.

TREATMENT

Gut Decontamination

Activated charcoal and lavage with airway protection may be helpful within the first few hours of encainide ingestion. Because encainide is readily absorbed and has a rapid onset of action, induced emesis probably is contraindicated. Gastric lavage may induce vagal stimulation and asystole. Rapid gastric emptying (within 1 hour of ingestion) may assist in removing flecainide sufficient to avoid its wide tissue distribution and cardiotoxic effects. This must be tempered by knowledge of the occasional occurrence of seizures within 2 hours of a flecainide overdose. Care must therefore be taken to protect the airway before gastric lavage.

Elimination Enhancement

Methods to enhance elimination probably do not remove significant amounts of these drugs from the blood. Hemodialysis and hemoperfusion have not proven effective in the treatment of flecainide overdose.

Supportive Measures

- Treatment is primarily supportive. Stabilization (airway, respiration, circulatory status) with oxygen, cardiac monitoring, and intravenous lines is the first priority in an intensive care facility.
- Accompanying arrhythmias are treated per ACLS protocols. Proarrhythmic effects of flecainide (e.g., sympathomimetic ventricular tachycardia) may be suppressed by high-dose amiodarone.
- Transport personnel should not delay transport until toxic signs appear, especially in infants or children in whom a single tablet may be lethal. Similarly, an adult who reports intentionally ingesting "just a minimal" dose of a rapidly and highly toxic substance deserves prompt transport for evaluation and treatment.
- Because withdrawal of encainide has led to a fatal episode of ventricular tachycardia leading to fibrillation, hospital admission should be considered for patients in whom encainide or flecainide is to be discontinued.
- Encainide exacerbates hyperglycemia in some patients. It is not known whether this is from the parent compound or its metabolites. Serum glucose levels should be monitored when encainide therapy is begun in patients with type 2 diabetes mellitus and when encainide is discontinued in patients receiving insulin therapy.
- The PR, QRS, and QT intervals may be markedly prolonged on the electrocardiogram following a flecainide overdose. Cardiogenic shock and *Torsade de Pointes* may respond to intubation, mechanical ventilation, dopamine, magnesium, and/or sodium load.

ANTIDOTES

Hypertonic sodium bicarbonate or sodium chloride may be beneficial in reversing cardiotoxic overdoses by these agents, but this has not been studied adequately. Intravenous administration of molar sodium lactate (500 mL over 30 minutes) with intravenous potassium chloride to three flecainide overdose patients resulted in an improvement in clinical status with narrowing of their QRS intervals.

Questions—Flecainide And Encainide

1. **Flecainide is a class IC agent.**
   A. True
   B. False

2. **Encainide is excreted in the urine and bile.**
   A. True
   B. False

3. **Encainide may cause proarrhythmic effects, dizziness, headache, ataxia, nausea, tremors, and blurred vision.**
   A. True
   B. False
4. **Seizures, bradycardia, hypotension, and obtundation may be seen in encainide overdose.**
   A. True
   B. False
5. **Petit mal seizures may follow large ingestions of flecainide.**
   A. True
   B. False

Propafenone

Propafenone (Rythmol®) has been marketed in the United States for the oral treatment of life-threatening ventricular arrhythmias such as sustained ventricular tachycardia. It is not recommended for treatment of less severe arrhythmias such as nonsustained ventricular tachycardias and frequent premature ventricular contractions, even if patients are symptomatic. It may have a role in treating supraventricular arrhythmias but has not been approved by the FDA for this indication.

Propafenone has been used in the United States since 1990. Overdoses have been reported following its use and fatalities have occurred. Symptomatic and supportive care is paramount in treatment of serious toxicity following propafenone poisoning. Propafenone is a class IC antiarrhythmic agent. The structure of propafenone is similar to that of many β-blockers.

PATHOPHYSIOLOGY

Propafenone is a fast sodium-channel blocker with weak β-adrenoceptor blocking activity. Its kinetics of interaction with cardiac sodium channels is similar to those of flecainide and encainide. It suppresses nonsustained ventricular arrhythmias. Its major metabolites share its sodium-channel blocking properties. Propafenone slows intraatrial and AV nodal conduction by prolonging atrial refractoriness.

PHARMACOKINETICS

Absorption

- Propafenone is well absorbed (95%) with a bioavailability of 11% to 39%, indicating an extensive presystemic clearance.
- Peak plasma concentrations of the drug and its metabolite are reached in 1 to 4 hours.

Distribution

- Propafenone has a large volume of distribution of 1.1 to 3.6 L/kg and is 97% protein bound.

Elimination

- Propafenone exhibits extensive first-pass metabolism by a hepatic oxidative pathway and is extensively metabolized into two active metabolites, 5-HP and N-depropylpropafenone
- Formation of the 5-HP metabolite is mediated by a cytochrome P450 isozyme.
- Propafenone half-life ranges from 2 to 32 hours. Extensive metabolizers have half-lives of 2 to 10 hours and poor metabolizers, 10 to 32 hours.

CLINICAL PRESENTATIONS

Signs of overdose, usually most severe within 3 hours of ingestion, include hypotension, somnolence, bradycardia, AV dissociation, and intraatrial and intraventricular conduction disturbances. Asystole also may occur. Because of its β-blocker activity, propafenone may induce reactive airway disease. Convulsions and high-grade ventricular arrhythmias have been reported.

Gastrointestinal Effects

About 20% of patients experience some mild side effects, which may include constipation, nausea, vomiting, and, rarely, diarrhea. A bitter taste is noted by 5% to 10% of patients. Rare cases of cholestatic hepatitis have been reported.

Neurologic Effects

At a plasma propafenone concentration of 900 ng/mL or higher, visual blurring, dizziness, and paresthesias may be observed. At a level of 450 ng/mL, such effects are minimal. Poor metabolizers have increased side effects. Propafenone may induce generalized myasthenic symptoms in patients with ocular myasthenia.

Cardiovascular Effects

Propafenone can cause cardiac conduction abnormalities such as new left or right bundle-branch block, AV block, and sinus node dysfunction. Propafenone may cause worsening of congestive heart failure. Conduction and myocardial depression are dose dependent and occur most often in patients with underlying heart disease. Clinically significant proarrhythmias (increase in ventricular premature contractions, conversion of nonsustained to sustained ventricular tachycardia, or new appearances of ventricular tachycardia or ventricular fibrillation) may occur in 5% of patients.

TOXIC DOSAGE/DEATH

A 57-year-old patient who ingested 1.35 grams of propafenone, a 20-year-old who ingested 4.5 grams, and a 26-year-old who ingested 6.0 grams survived. A 2-year-old ingested 180 mg, went into cardiopulmonary collapse, and recovered. Doses of 4.8 grams and 9.0 grams have been associated with fatal outcomes, however a 27-year-old who ingested 8.1 grams survived.

DRUG INTERACTIONS

Concurrent use of local anesthetics with propafenone may increase the risk of nervous system side effects. Concurrent use with other antiarrhythmic drugs may result in increased cardiac effects. Quinidine decreases propafenone clearance and its metabolic clearance. Rifampin lowers the plasma concentration of propafenone and reduces its antiarrhythmic effect.

Propafenone increases metoprolol blood levels and metoprolol β-blocking activity. Propafenone increases warfarin plasma concentration and enhances anticoagulant effect. Propafenone increases digoxin serum concentrations, requiring a reduction in digoxin maintenance dosage. The volume of distribution and nonrenal clearance of digoxin appear to be decreased.

PREGNANCY/LACTATION

Pregnancy risk category C. Both propafenone and 5-HP are detectable in newborn plasma and in maternal milk though at concentrations lower than those in maternal plasma.

LABORATORY

Analytic Methods

Plasma concentrations of propafenone and its two major metabolites are analyzed by high-performance liquid chromatography.

Blood Levels

The therapeutic plasma level of propafenone has been suggested as 0.5 to 2.0 ng/mL. Blood levels in nonsurvivors have been 7,700 ng/mL and 21,000 ng/mL. The peak plasma concentration of propafenone after a single dose of 300 mg is approximately 400 ng/mL.

TREATMENT

Gut Decontamination

As seizures may occur within 1 hour of an overdose, caution must be exercised to maintain an adequate airway with any gastric emptying attempt. Syrup of ipecac is relatively contraindicated. Activated charcoal may be useful but there is no controlled clinical evidence to support this. As plasma levels of propafenone and its active metabolites may not peak for up to 4 hours, decontamination procedures may be useful for up to 4 to 6 hours after ingestion.

Elimination Enhancement

Hemodialysis and hemoperfusion have not been useful in removing propafenone. The strong protein binding and extensive volume of distribution mitigate against such measures. Plasma exchange appeared useful in one case.

Supportive Measures

- Early recognition of poisoning is important. Hypotension, seizures, and shock may occur within 1 to 2 hours of ingestion. An intravenous line, oxygen, cardiac monitoring, and careful evaluation of tidal volume are best followed in an intensive care facility.
- Advanced cardiac life support, including atropine and pressor amines such as dopamine, and dobutamine must be available. Cardiac pacing may be necessary for heart block. A combination of bolus and infused epinephrine with temporary pacing appeared effective in one patient.
- Because a wide QRS, prolonged QT interval, and possible interference with cardiac sodium channels has been noted, sodium loading has been proposed. Molar sodium lactate was used in one overdose and the patient survived. In other cases, sodium loading with sodium bicarbonate or hypertonic saline was followed by survival. Care must be taken to prevent acute pulmonary edema secondary to sodium overload.
- Diazepam is useful in treating seizures. Phenytoin was useful in one overdose patient, however phenytoin has class IB antiarrhythmic properties and must be used with great caution in the presence of preexisting conduction defects.
- Use of other class IC drugs for treatment such as flecainide, and tocainide may exacerbate conduction problems and should be avoided.

Question—Propafenone

1. All of the following are side effects of propafenone except

A. Constipation, nausea, and vomiting
B. Visual blurring, dizziness, and parasthesias
C. Wheezing
D. Transient ischemic attacks (TIAs) and stroke
E. Bundle branch block, sinus node dysfunction, PVCs, nonsustained ventricular tachycardia, sustained ventricular tachycardia, or ventricular fibrillation

CLASS II DRUGS

Introduction

β-Blocking agents are a large group of class II antiarrhythmic drugs with wide clinical applications. Experience with massive overdose is limited. They are used therapeutically to treat hypertension, thyrotoxicosis, dysrhythmias, hyperkinetic heart syndrome, angina, sudden-death prophylaxis in postmyocardial infarction patients, essential tremor, migraine headaches, withdrawal states, and open-angle glaucoma. Individual pharmacologic variation between β-blocking drugs leads to differences in adverse reactions after therapeutic use and overdose.

This heterogeneous group of drugs shares the ability to decrease sympathetic stimulation of the heart. The toxic effects of these drugs vary considerably depending on the extent of their cardiac β-adrenergic effects, cardioselectivity, and partial agonist activity. Common adverse reactions include increased airway resistance, pulmonary edema, congestive heart failure in sensitive patients, and conduction delay and hypotension in overdose. Propranolol is the prototypical noncardioselective class II drug. Other class II members include acebutolol, alprenolol, atenolol, metoprolol, oxprenolol, pindolol, practolol, nadolol, and timolol.

β-Blockers

Propranolol (Inderal®) is the prototype β-blocking drug and has been the most common β-blocker involved in overdose. β-blocking drugs possess a high toxic-therapeutic ratio, but severe overdoses may be refractory to therapy. Serious clinical effects of overdose involve primarily the cardiovascular system (bradycardia, hypotension, cardiogenic shock, and pulmonary edema) and the central nervous system (coma, convulsions, and apnea). In severe overdose, apnea and hemodynamic compromise may appear suddenly after large ingestions of β-blockers.

PATHOPHYSIOLOGY

Class II antiarrhythmic, β-adrenoceptor-blocking agents (β-blockers) are membrane-depressant drugs that decrease the influx of sodium and calcium ions by reducing membrane-bound adenylate cyclase and cAMP. The reduction in cation transport lengthens depolarization by decreasing the amplitude and slope of the transmembrane potential. β-Blockers also reduce myocardial contractility by decreasing calcium release from the sarcoplasmic reticulum. Membrane-stabilizing activity enhances reduction in myocardial contractility in overdose in addition to producing a quinidinelike effect of QRS widening. A direct myocardial effect also leads to myocardial depression independent of β-adrenergic blockade and membrane stabilization.

Adverse reactions depend on drug affinity for β-1 and β-2 receptors. β-1 blockade activity causes decreased sinus rate, contractility, and conduction, decreased renin release, and decreased aqueous humor formation. β-2 blockade produces bronchiolar and arteriolar smooth muscle constriction, decreased insulin secretion, and decreased lipolysis and glycogenolysis resulting in decreased blood fatty acids and glucose.

β-blockers are classified as cardioselective (e.g., propranolol, practolol, atenolol, and metoprolol) based on their ability to antagonize the cardiac (β-1) but not the peripheral (β-2) receptors. However, cardioselectivity is incomplete and dose dependent and disappears at high doses. At therapeutic levels, cardioselectivity is a consideration in choosing drugs (e.g., these drugs produce less bronchospasm), but this property probably does not alter the clinical presentation of overdoses.

In addition to blocking properties, pindolol and oxprenolol possess partial agonist (sympathomimetic) properties that stimulate the heart and probably reduce toxicity in overdose. These β-blockers produce higher resting heart rates than other β-blockers, especially after large doses. Hypertension and tachycardia may occur in pindolol toxicity. Sotalol is a unique β-blocker with amiodaronelike (class III antiarrhythmic) properties that produce QT prolongation and serious ventricular dysrhythmias in overdose.

Central Nervous System Effects

Lipid solubility is an important determinant of the ability of drugs to penetrate the blood-brain barrier. β-blockers with high lipophilicity (e.g., propranolol, oxprenolol) cause depression of the central nervous system and seizures. Sudden apnea may result from central effects. Although hydrophilic β-blockers generally do not produce convulsions, seizures have been associated with sotalol overdose.

Endocrine Effects

Propranolol reduces the formation of T3 in the peripheral tissues by inhibiting membrane-bound deiodination. A β-blocker with strong membrane-stabilizing activity (i.e., alprenolol) altars thyroid hormone formation in hyperthyroidism, but other β-blockers do not.

PHARMACOKINETICS

Absorption

- β-Blocker drugs are rapidly absorbed, with a bioavailability varying between 30% and 90% because of a large first-pass hepatic extraction.
- Symptoms in propranolol overdose may appear within 30 minutes and may include the sudden onset of seizures and cardiovascular collapse. Serious symptoms often appear within 1 to 2 hours.

Distribution

- Most β-blockers, with the exception of atenolol, have volumes of distribution greater than 1 L/kg.
- Propranolol is both highly lipophilic and protein bound.
- Atenolol, metoprolol, and timolol are poorly protein bound.

Elimination

- The kidney excretes hydrophilic β-blockers (atenolol, nadolol, and practolol) and the liver metabolizes lipophilic β-blockers. Individual variation in oxidative metabolism as a result of genetic polymorphism accounts for some of the wide variation in the plasma half-life of lipophilic β-blockers (propranolol, metoprolol, timolol, and alprenolol).
- The plasma half-lives of β-blocker drugs range from 2 to 24 hours with significant prolongation occurring after serious overdose. The therapeutic half-life of propranolol averages 3.5 to 6 hours.

CLINICAL PRESENTATIONS

The appearance of adverse reactions depends on the underlying clinical state of the patient and on cardioselectivity. Side effects include hypotension, congestive heart failure, depressed SA and AV nodal conduction, bronchospasm, hypoglycemia, depression, fatigue, and Raynaud's phenomena. Overdose affects primarily the cardiovascular and central nervous systems.

Cardiovascular Effects

The hallmark of severe propranolol overdose is delayed conduction and hypotension (92% and 77%, respectively, of reported cases). First-degree AV block and bradycardia appear first. Massive overdoses cause quinidinelike widening of QRS, refractory high-grade AV block, and asystole. In severe overdose, the myocardium is unresponsive to electrical and pharmacologic stimulation. Hypotension results from decreased cardiac output and decreased renin release. Pulmonary edema occurs especially with underlying cardiac disease; cardiogenic shock may result from decreased contractility depending on cardiac reserve.

Severe hemodynamic compromise may appear early in the course of severe poisoning in patients who look deceptively well a short time before collapse. Hypertension and tachycardia are more common in partial agonist overdose (e.g., pindolol), and hypotension is unusual even in large doses. Sotalol more often is associated with serious ventricular dysrhythmias; atypical ventricular tachycardia has been reported at therapeutic levels.

Neurologic Effects

Neurologic symptoms are more common with β-blockers that possess higher degrees of membrane stabilization and lipid solubility (e.g., propranolol, oxprenolol, and metoprolol). Seizures can occur without hemodynamic compromise, but central nervous symptoms usually result from low cardiac output. Signs of conduction delay often precede the appearance of convulsions. Seizures have not been associated with hydrophilic, cardioselective β-adrenergic blockers, but have occurred following a sotalol overdose.

Lethargy, coma, amnesia, and dilated pupils may develop. Coma precedes seizures in 75% of oxprenolol cases. Respiratory depression and apnea may appear suddenly in severe overdoses (e.g., propranolol, and oxprenolol) with little warning. The presence of hypoglycemia and bronchospasm (especially with nonselective β-blockers) depends on underlying disease states.

TOXIC DOSAGE/DEATH

β-Blocking drugs generally possess a wide toxic-therapeutic margin. Both underlying cardiovascular disease and individual drug properties (e.g., cardioselectivity, lipophilicity) influence the clinical effects of a given dose. Most β-blocker-induced fatalities result from the nonselective drug propranolol, but death has occurred after the ingestion of cardioselective agents such as metoprolol and partial sympathomimetic agonists like alprenolol.

Death occurred after an 8.8 gram acebutolol overdose, whereas survival occurred with 7.6 and 9.6 gram overdoses. A 12.8-gram alprenolol ingestion resulted in death. Ingestions of 1.0 and 1.2 gram doses of atenolol by adults have produced little clinical effect except for mild bradycardia and hypotension. Hypotension and nodal rhythm have occurred after a 50-gram metoprolol overdose. Cardiac failure and bradycardia occurred in a fatal 7.5-gram overdose of metoprolol.

An adult fatality in spite of transvenous pacing was associated with a 4.48-gram ingestion of oxprenolol. High alcohol consumption and 300 mg of oxprenolol have also produced death. Survival has been reported with 3.0- and 6.0-gram doses, however. A 250-mg overdose of pindolol resulted in coma without hypotension. A 500-mg dose of pindolol produced elevated blood pressure but no other cardiac or central nervous system effects. The partial agonist activity of pindolol may contribute to the relative safety of this drug in overdose. A 5.0-gram overdose of practolol produced sinus tachycardia and a left bundle branch block. Survival occurred after a practolol dose of 9.0 grams despite severe underlying cardiovascular disease.

Clinical response following a given dose of propranolol varies. A 1.0-gram propranolol ingestion by an adult produced coma and delayed conduction, whereas a 2.0-gram ingestion in another adult caused no cardiovascular or central nervous system abnormalities. Survival has occurred after 5.0- and 8.0-gram propranolol ingestions by adults. In fatal propranolol overdose, the plasma level ranges from 4,000 to 28,000 ng/mL, whereas survival has been reported at 2,300 and 2,800 ng/mL. An adult fatality occurred after a 3.2-gram sotalol ingestion and survival has followed 2.4-gram and 8.0-gram overdoses.

DRUG INTERACTIONS

Cimetidine decreases propranolol clearance. Rifampin and phenobarbital may increase propranolol clearance. Antacids may decrease absorption of certain β-blockers.

PREGNANCY/LACTATION

Propranolol is pregnancy risk category C. It crosses the placenta and small amounts appear in breast milk. β-blockers have been widely used for the treatment of pregnancy-induced hypertension. Adverse reactions are believed to be rare and the effects on the fetus or infant are thought to be minimal.

LABORATORY

Analytic Methods

Propranolol is detected by high-pressure liquid chromatography.

Blood Levels

Propranolol blood levels confirm toxicity but do not aid immediate management. Large interpatient differences in blood levels may occur with any given dose. Therapeutic plasma levels range from 30 to 200 ng/mL.

TREATMENT

Gut Decontamination

There is no controlled clinical evidence that syrup of ipecac, gastric lavage, activated charcoal, or cathartics are of value in the treatment of overdose with this group of drugs. This group of drugs is well absorbed orally.

Elimination Enhancement

Effective extracorporeal elimination is not well documented, although pharmacokinetic parameters of atenolol, sotalol, and nadolol suggest the possible efficacy of hemodialysis and hemoperfusion. Large volumes of distribution, protein binding, and low water solubility of most β-blockers limit efforts to enhance elimination.

Supportive Measures

- Most overdoses are mild and respond to supportive care. Observe mild overdose cases at least 4 hours for the development of signs of poisoning.
- Although the onset of action is rapid, effects of massive β-blocker overdose may persist for several days despite declining plasma β-blocker levels. Watch carefully for cardiovascular or respiratory deterioration in an intensive care setting, particularly in the early hours.
- Apnea and cardiovascular collapse may appear suddenly. Hence, cardiac monitoring and intravenous lines should be established immediately.
- Be sure to obtain a rapid check of blood glucose levels in obtunded patients or administer to adults 50% dextrose solution (50 mL) intravenously, immediately. Check potassium levels in the presence of conduction defects and watch carefully for rapid deterioration of respiration or blood pressure by obtaining frequent vital signs.
- Dopamine and isoproterenol are the initial drugs of choice for hypotension and atropine may be used for bradycardia, but these agents may not be effective. Atropine doses up to 0.04 mg/kg may be necessary to abolish vagal influences on the heart at therapeutic β-blocker doses. In adult overdose, use 2 to 3 mg intravenously in 0.5 to 1 mg increments as needed.
- Sotalol toxicity may produce serious ventricular dysrhythmias, which usually are responsive to lidocaine or overdrive pacing.
- Diazepam has been effective for seizure control and is the drug of choice. Thiopental and muscle relaxants are alternative drugs for refractory seizures.
- Aminophylline and terbutaline may effectively treat bronchospasm. Albuterol may be helpful as well. Monitor the patient for dysrhythmias during and after administration of these agents.
- Treat hypotension with fluid repletion and add dopamine or norepinephrine, if necessary. Large doses of inotropic agents may be needed over several days because of the prolonged effect of β-blockade despite declining plasma β-blocker levels. Norepinephrine may be more effective than dopamine. Experience with dobutamine is limited.
- Consider the use of a pulmonary catheter and an arterial pressure line in order to assess fluid volume, contractility, and peripheral vascular resistance in patients with underlying cardiac disease and those not responding to glucagon.

ANTIDOTES

Glucagon

Glucagon is an effective antidote and should be administered early when signs of hemodynamic compromise appear. Case reports indicate the effectiveness of this non-β-adrenergic receptor agonist, which enhances cardiac contractility through increased production of cyclic AMP (cAMP). The initial dose is 50 to 100 μg/kg (5 to 10 mg for adults) intravenously followed by 70 μg/kg/hour (adult dose 1 to 5 mg/hour). Glucagon may be more effective in reversing negative inotropic effects than negative chronotropic effects, but this drug should be administered for both, since few side effects occur. Nausea and vomiting are the most frequent adverse reactions.

Glucagon probably is not effective for β-blocker-induced seizures, unless the convulsions result from hypotension. Monitor glucose, calcium, and potassium during infusion, because of the increased propensity for the development of hyperglycemia, hypokalemia, and hypocalcemia. Glucagon enhances the hypoprothrombinemic effect of dicoumarol. When it is prepared with the standard diluent, 2 mg of phenol are injected with each milligram of glucagon. Glucagon doses over 25 mg administered in the standard diluent exceed the usual intravenous maximum recommended dose of phenol (i.e., 50 mg). In such cases, other diluents should be considered (e.g., normal saline).

Isoproterenol

This drug is a nonselective β-adrenergic agonist that may be helpful in β-blocker overdose. Start at 4 μg/min in adults. Some patients may require higher dosage (as much as 10 times the usual therapeutic dose was necessary in a severe propranolol overdose case). Follow the blood pressure closely, because isoproterenol may aggravate peripheral vasodilation because of its β-2 effects at high doses. Consider glucagon and norepinephrine if patients become hypotensive because isoproterenol often is ineffective in correcting hypotension.

Prenalterol

This cardioselective β-adrenoceptor partial agonist has been used successfully to treat refractory hypotension unresponsive to glucagon, and vasopressors in massive propranolol, metoprolol, and atenolol overdoses. Prenalterol currently is not available in the United States.

Questions—β-Blockers

1. The following are therapeutic uses of β-blockers
A. The treatment of hypertension
B. The treatment of thyrotoxicosis
C. The treatment of angina
D. The treatment of essential tremor
E. All of the above

2. The following are serious clinical effects of β-blockers except
A. Hypotension
B. Heart block
C. Cardiogenic shock
D. Apnea
E. Blindness

3. The following are antidotes for β-blocker overdose
A. Glucagon
B. Isoproterenol
C. Diltiazem
D. A and B
E. None of the above

4. The following statements are true about β-blockers except
A. The severity of neurologic effects depends on the lipid solubility of the β-blocker
B. The degree of effect on bronchial smooth muscle depends on the relative affinity for β-1 versus β-2 receptors
C. The greater the β-1 selectivity, the greater the effect on the cardiovascular smooth-muscle conduction system
D. Cimetidine and rifampin decrease propranolol clearance
E. β-Blockers can cause hypoglycemia

CLASS III DRUGS

Introduction

Class III drugs effectively suppress supraventricular and ventricular dysrhythmias, including those associated with Wolff-Parkinson-White syndrome. Amiodarone is an important member of this class. Bretylium also lengthens the absolute refractory period with little effect on phase O depolarization, similar to amiodarone. Some authors include bretylium in the class II drug group because this drug decreases the effects of catecholamines by reducing epinephrine and norepinephrine release. Other members of this class include acetylprocainamide, the β-blocker sotalol hydrochloride, and experimental drugs depridil hydrochloride, and melperone.

Amiodarone and Bretylium

Amiodarone (Cordarone®) is an iodinated benzofuran derivative with a chemical structure similar to thyroxine. Recent clinical interest centers on its ability to suppress resistant supraventricular and ventricular dysrhythmias and to improve congestive heart failure. The most serious adverse reaction to its therapeutic use is the occasional development of a rapidly progressive ARDS. Acute overdose has been reported rarely.

Bretylium tosylate is a quaternary benzylammonium compound (class III antiarrhythmic) used to treat ventricular arrhythmias refractory to lidocaine. It is used in complex, life-threatening clinical settings in which many drugs often are given and its individual clinical effects may be difficult to interpret.

PATHOPHYSIOLOGY

Amiodarone prolongs the action potential of myocardial cells without altering the resting membrane potential. Consequently, the drug alters repolarization (QT prolongation) without affecting spontaneous depolarization. Because neither class I nor class II antiarrhythmic drugs possess both these properties, amiodarone is classified as a class III antiarrhythmic agent. The effect of amiodarone on thyroid metabolism remains unclear but probably involves an intracellular rather than a central or peripheral action. After a transit release of norepinephrine, bretylium inhibits further release by postganglionic nerve endings.

PHARMACOKINETICS

Absorption

- Oral absorption of amiodarone is slow, with a wide range of bioavailability (22% to 86%).
- 15% to 20% of bretylium is absorbed.

Distribution

- The volume of distribution of amiodarone is large (9 to 17 L/kg), and the elimination half-life is long (12 to 20 hours). The volume of distribution of bretylium is 3.4 to 5.9 L/kg.

Elimination

- An overdose of amiodarone displayed an elimination half-life of 31 hours.
- Duration of action of bretylium is 10 to 20 hours. Elimination half-life is 4 to 17 hours.

CLINICAL PRESENTATIONS

Serious adverse reactions to therapeutic doses of amiodarone may include a rapidly fatal ARDS, polymorphous ventricular tachycardia (*Torsade de Pointes*), hypothyroidism, and hyperthyroidism. Side effects may include photosensitivity, gynecomastia, hepatotoxicity, pulmonary fibrosis, skin pigmentation, and corneal deposits. Bretylium can cause dizziness, syncope, nausea, vomiting, respiratory depression, hypotension and bradycardia.

TOXIC DOSAGE/DEATH

An adult who ingested 8 grams of amiodarone developed diaphoresis, bradycardia, and QT prolongation that resolved over 4 days.

DRUG INTERACTIONS

Amiodarone increases digoxin levels.

PREGNANCY/LACTATION

Pregnancy risk category C. Congenital hypothyroidism has been reported when mothers have used amiodarone.

LABORATORY

Analytic Methods

Amiodarone is detected by chromatography.

Blood Levels

Blood levels do not guide management in overdose. The therapeutic range of amiodarone is 1.0 to 2.5 mg/L.

TREATMENT

Gut Decontamination

Decontamination measures such as repetitive dose charcoal may be useful beyond several hours postingestion because of the pharmacokinetics of amiodarone.

Elimination Enhancement

Dialysis is not helpful. Although bretylium is dialyzable, there is no published evidence that hemoperfusion or hemodialysis is useful in an acute overdose.

Supportive Measures

- Patients should respond to general therapeutic measures. Treatment of bretylium overdose is symptomatic. Little data on overdose is available to guide management authoritatively.

Questions—Amiodarone and Bretylium

1. **The following are class III drugs except**
   A. Bretylium
   B. Amiodarone
   C. Sotalol
   D. Pindolol
   E. None of the above
2. **The following is/are side effects of therapeutic doses of amiodarone**
   A. Photosensitivity
   B. Pulmonary fibrosis
   C. Hepatotoxicity
   D. *Torsade de pointes*
   E. None of the above

CLASS IV DRUGS

Introduction

Class IV drugs include the calcium-channel blockers. Verapamil, diltiazem, and nifedipine are considered major members of this class. These drugs have widely divergent chemical structures and multiple clinical uses. Overdoses generally are quite serious and may be refractory to aggressive treatment measures.

Calcium-Channel Blockers

This chemically diverse group of drugs inhibits calcium and sodium influx across the slow channel of cell membranes. Manganese, nickel, and cobalt were the first agents noted to inhibit slow calcium-channel conduction. The diverse molecular structures of calcium-channel blockers are consistent with differing sites and modes of action, in contrast to β-adrenergic blockers, which bind tightly to receptor sites. Receptor-binding sites exist for nifedipine. The effectiveness of other calcium antagonists may be associated with undiscovered neurotransmitter receptors that alter impulse conduction by influencing the slow calcium ion channel.

Because calcium plays a central role in electrophysiologic and mechanical properties of both cardiac and smooth muscle, these agents affect SA and AV conduction, myocardial contractility, and vasodilation. Although primarily used as antiarrhythmic and antianginal agents, other applications of calcium-channel blockers include cerebral reperfusion, dysmenorrhea, asthma, headaches, allergic reactions, esophageal spasm, and malignant hyperthermia.

Much wider variation in clinical effect, pharmacokinetic parameters, and toxicity occur in this class of drugs than with β-blockers. Verapamil (a papaverine derivative) and diltiazem (a benzothiazepine derivative) reduce cardiac nodal conduction but produce less vasodilation than nifedipine (a dihydropyridine derivative). In contrast, nifedipine produces coronary and systemic vasodilation and little impairment of cardiac conduction.

PATHOPHYSIOLOGY

These drugs reduce the influx of calcium during phase 2 and affect slow channel-dependent tissues such as the SA and AV nodes. Because the slow channel also provides the route for the calcium influx that initiates contraction, these compounds also affect myocardial and smooth-muscle contraction. Diseased fast-channel tissue also becomes more dependent on the slow channel for the initiation of impulses. Clinical effects of class IV drugs include decreased AV node conduction, arteriolar dilation, and decreased contractility. Each compound within this class varies in the extent of each of these effects. Toxicity results from negative chronotropy (bradycardia), reduced inotropy (hypotension), and conduction blockade (AV block, asystole).

Verapamil

Verapamil (Calan®) is a nonselective inhibitor of the slow channel and affects both calcium gate and channel recovery, leading to a change in cell reactivation. At high concentrations, verapamil causes alteration of the fast sodium channel. In overdose, verapamil primarily causes cardiovascular and central nervous system complications caused by hypotension and impaired cardiac conduction (AV block, bradycardia).

Nifedipine

Nifedipine (Procardia®) prevents activation of some slow channels in a more selective manner than verapamil and leaves other channels and the gating mechanism unaffected. Nifedipine actually plugs the calcium channel. In contrast to verapamil, this compound increases AV nodal conduction and shortens AV nodal refractoriness. Vasodilation and hypotension appear to be the major complications of nifedipine overdose.

Diltiazem

Diltiazem (Cardizem®) displays an intermediate action that includes slow-channel inhibition at low concentrations and fast-channel inhibition at higher ones. Diltiazem produces slowing of the AV nodal conduction equivalent to that of verapamil, but less prolongation of AV refractoriness.

PHARMACOKINETICS

Absorption

- Generally, these drugs are well absorbed, but verapamil has large first-pass hepatic extraction (70% of the therapeutic dose).
- Following oral administration of amlodipine, the bioavailability is about 50% to 88%, and peak plasma concentrations of amlodipine occur in 6 to 7 hours.

Distribution

- Calcium-channel blockers are highly protein bound and lipophilic and exhibit a large volume of distribution (over 2 L/kg).
- Amlodipine is rapidly distributed into tissue, then slowly released. Unlike other dihydropyridines, amlodipine has a high volume of distribution, about 20 L/kg.
- The protein binding of diltiazem is 80–90%.

Elimination

- Elimination of these drugs occurs almost exclusively by the liver.
- The major route of verapamil clearance is by oxidative N-demethylation to norverapamil, which possesses mild hemodynamic effects in dogs compared with the parent compound.
- Nifedipine metabolites are inactive despite primarily hepatic elimination.
- Amlodipine is subjected to extensive hepatic metabolism. Elimination half-life is 40 to 50 hours.

CLINICAL PRESENTATIONS

Because of different clinical effects on cardiac nodal conduction, myocardial contractility, and vascular smooth muscle, the three main calcium antagonists vary in their potential side effects. Manifestations of massive verapamil overdose appear to be exacerbations of therapeutic effects on conduction and contractility. Bradycardia, hypotension, and intraventricular conduction abnormalities may occur. AV dissociation, lethargy, and miosis have been reported. In overdose, signs and symptoms usually appear within 1 hour. Conduction defects worsen over the first 6 hours and may last more than 24 hours postingestion.

Central nervous system symptoms such as coma, apnea, and seizures usually are associated with poor tissue perfusion. Nonspecific symptoms of nausea, vomiting, lightheadedness, and headache also may appear. Hyperglycemia and metabolic acidosis can develop in severe verapamil overdoses. In the Wolff-Parkinson-White syndrome, verapamil may enhance conduction down accessory pathways, leading to fatal ventricular dysrhythmias.

The major toxic complication of nifedipine ingestion is hypotension, which may be associated with cardiogenic shock and an idioventricular rhythm in patients with underlying cardiovascular disease. Generally, nifedipine increases the heart rate, and arrhythmias with therapeutic doses are uncommon. Diltiazem overdose may present with bradycardia, diaphoresis, mental confusion, deterioration in renal function, slurred speech, and asystole.

The existence of a calcium antagonist withdrawal syndrome is controversial. Potentially, chronic calcium antagonist treatment may reduce intracellular calcium and increase the cellular calcium gradient. Drug withdrawal may produce increased calcium influx resulting in coronary artery spasm.

TOXIC DOSAGE/DEATH

Verapamil doses exceeding 3 grams in adults produce severe hypotension, complete AV block, bradycardia, and central nervous system depression. Ingestion of 400-mg verapamil in an 11-month-old caused coma, seizures, bradycardia, and hypotension. In an adult with chronic renal failure, 280-mg nifedipine ingestion produced profound hypotension but tissue perfusion remained adequate.

DRUG INTERACTIONS

β-blockers and calcium-channel blockers act synergistically to increase side effects. Nifedipine with β-blockade enhances hypotension in some patients. Intravenous administration of practolol and verapamil resulted in asystole in one case. Digoxin and verapamil synergistically block the AV node and must be administered cautiously together.

PREGNANCY/LACTATION

Nifedipine, nicardipine, and verapamil are capable of inhibiting uterine contractions. There may be a profound reduction in uteroplacental blood flow. All are classified as pregnancy risk category C.

LABORATORY

Analytic Methods

Verapamil and diltiazem are detected by high performance liquid chromatography.

Blood Levels

Verapamil levels confirm toxicity but usually do not aid acute management. Therapeutic levels range from 80 to 300 ng/mL. The therapeutic range of blood diltiazem concentrations is about 100–200 μg/L.

TREATMENT

Gut Decontamination

The usual measures of decontamination (i.e., charcoal and/or lavage) may be helpful in treating calcium-channel blocker overdoses within the first several hours postingestion.

Elimination Enhancement

The highly lipophilic characteristics, high protein binding, and extensive volume of distribution of calcium-channel blockers make hemodialysis, diuresis, and hemoperfusion impractical.

Supportive Measures

- Severe bradycardia, conduction block, and hypotension are the major life-threatening complications of verapamil overdose. Patients with conduction defects or signs of myocardial depression should be admitted to a monitored bed. Seriously poisoned patients should receive an intravenous line, oxygen, cardiac monitoring for 4 to 6 hours, and an electrocardiogram.
- Electrocardiographic abnormalities after verapamil overdose involve prolonged conduction (QRS, PR, and QT intervals), various degrees of AV block, and asystole. Bradycardia may be managed with atropine, and high degree AV block may require temporary pacing.
- The patient should be observed for respiratory and central nervous system depression, which usually results from shock. Hypotension may be difficult to manage, and hemodynamic monitoring (Swan-Ganz catheter) aids the proper administration of fluids and/or vasopressors (dopamine, norepinephrine).
- One case report indicated that an epinephrine infusion (0.8 μg/kg/min) was more effective than high-dose dopamine (30 μg/kg/min) in reversing hypotension. Intravenous calcium may reverse the profound hypotension as described in the antidote section.
- Other calcium-channel blockers, digoxin, β-blockers, and class I drugs should be avoided.
- Serious ventricular dysrhythmias following verapamil overdose probably reflect poor tissue perfusion and underlying cardiovascular disease rather than direct toxic effects.
- Calcium, magnesium, potassium, and sodium levels should be checked in all overdoses.

ANTIDOTES

Calcium

Calcium gluconate occasionally has been used successfully to reverse hypotension in calcium-channel blocker overdose. Calcium appears to increase conduction slightly, but there is little effect on rate. An adult dose of 10 mL of 10% calcium gluconate over 5 minutes may be used to reverse hypotension with careful monitoring of rhythm. A repeat bolus (after 10 to 15 minutes) or intravenous drip (10 to 20 mL/hour of the 10% calcium gluconate solution) may be needed to reverse hypotension. Calcium levels must be monitored carefully. Calcium chloride has been used successfully to reverse hypotension in a myocardial infarct patient who received 10 mg of intravenous verapamil.

Glucagon

Anecdotal reports have suggested that this agent may be helpful in calcium-channel blocker overdose, however controlled studies are needed to better evaluate its effect.

Questions—Calcium-Channel Blockers

1. **Which of the following conditions are treated by calcium channel blockers?**
   A. Dysmenorrhea, headache, allergic reactions, esophageal spasms and malignant hyperthermia
   B. Upper gastrointestinal bleed, esophageal reflux, hypotension, and heart block
   C. Anxiety, renal dysfunction, Bell's Palsy, and seizures
   D. Ventricular tachycardia, Q-wave myocardial infarctions, and hypoglycemia
   E. None of the above
2. **Hyperglycemia and metabolic acidosis can develop in severe verapamil overdoses.**
   A. True
   B. False
3. **Verapamil is the drug of choice in patients with Wolff-Parkinson-White syndrome because it enhances conduction down accessory pathways leading to a slowing of the heart.**
   A. True
   B. False
4. **β-Blockers and digoxin should be prescribed with caution in patients taking verapamil.**
   A. True
   B. False

DIGITALIS

Withering published the classic effects of digitalis poisoning in 1785, and yet digitalis toxicity remains a significant problem. In 1977, it was postulated that digoxin was the leading cause of unintentional death among the elderly. In 1980, digoxin was the eighth most common drug prescribed by physicians. While acute overdose is rare, as the use of cardiac glycosides has partially declined, it may be quite serious.

Digoxin (Lanoxin®) is the most commonly prescribed digitalis preparation in the United States. Digitoxin is more popular in Latin countries, Europe, and Canada. Its toxicity is significantly different because of its nonpolar structure and pharmacokinetic properties. Rarely used digitalis preparations include digitalis leaf, ouabain, lanatoside C, deslanoside, and gitalin. Cardiac-glycoside-containing plants include oleander (*Nerium oleander*), foxglove (*Digitalis purpurea*), lily of the valley (*Convallaria majalis*), yellow oleander (*Thevetia peruviana*), and red squill (*Urginea maritima*).

Pathophysiology

Digitalis compounds alter the Na+/K+ ATPase-dependent transport system, resulting in intracellular loss of potassium and intracellular elevation of sodium and calcium. These drugs increase vagal tone, enhance sympathetic tone at high levels, and sensitize the carotid baroreceptors. Physiologic effects include increased automaticity and excitability, decreased conduction velocity throughout the conduction system, increased refractoriness at the AV node, and decreased refractoriness in the atria and ventricles.

Other effects include increased force of myocardial contraction, and decreased conduction resulting in increased AV block, PR interval prolongation, and decreased heart rate. Altered impulse formation and refractoriness leading to extrasystoles and tachydysrhythmia may occur. Toxic effects result from either large intentional ingestions or chronic toxicity when predisposing factors exacerbate the clinical effects of digoxin.

Pharmacokinetics

DIGOXIN

Absorption

- Bioavailability depends on tablet dissolution. This factor is now more standardized and ranges from 50% to 80%. Patient factors that reduce absorption include coadministration of food, malabsorption syndromes, antacids, and decreased gastrointestinal motility.

Distribution

- Digoxin has a large apparent volume of distribution (adults, 7 to 8 L/kg; neonates, 10 L/kg; and infants, 16 L/kg). The volume of distribution is reduced in renal disease, hypothyroidism, and quinidine therapy and in the elderly because of loss of muscle mass.
- Most digoxin is distributed to the skeletal muscle (approximately 65% of the absorbed dose).

Elimination

- The kidney excretes 60% to 80% of digoxin unchanged.
- The terminal elimination half-life averages about 36 hours.
- Depending on the collection method, biliary excretion accounts for 8% to 30% of a therapeutic oral dose in 24 hours.

DIGITOXIN

Absorption

- Excellent absorption occurs after oral doses.
- Following an oral dose, the latency period is 1 to 2 hours and peak effects develop in 4 to 12 hours.

Distribution

- Digitoxin is highly protein bound and has a relatively small apparent volume of distribution.

Elimination

- The liver metabolizes digitoxin by removing sugar (digitoxose) to form epidigitoxigenin, which is conjugated to an inactive metabolite.
- Digoxin is a by-product of digitoxin metabolism (about 8%).
- Enterohepatic circulation likely is responsible for a long elimination half-life of about 100 hours.

Clinical Presentations

Significant clinical differences exist between single massive ingestions and chronic therapeutic overdoses of digitalis. Large, single overdoses may be quite serious. Older patients, especially with underlying disease, are at higher risk. Children often have a more benign course and tolerate much higher peak digoxin levels. Nausea and vomiting are the most consistent gastrointestinal findings in acute digitalis poisoning. Mental status changes may be present. Visual symptoms may include scotoma, blurred vision, color aberrations, photophobia, and transient blindness. Mental confusion, hallucinations, and delirium occur regularly, but convulsions are rare. Malaise, headache, weakness, and fatigue are common.

CARDIOVASCULAR EFFECTS

Cardiovascular symptoms are the most frequent effects and may be delayed up to 6 hours. In children, bradycardia and conduction delays occur commonly but endogenous pacemakers usually prevent hemodynamic compromise. Common rhythm disturbances include bradycardia, heart block, and tachydysrhythmias. Ventricular arrhythmias occur infrequently in children.

Any dysrhythmia may result from digitalis toxicity. The classic digoxin toxic rhythm is a combination of suppressant and excitatory effects (e.g., nonparoxysmal atrial tachycardia with 2:1 block). Premature ventricular extrasystoles are the most common rhythm disturbance, with premature atrial and junctional extrasystoles occurring less frequently. These extrasystoles may be multifocal or bigeminal. The most common sustained rhythms are junctional escape rhythms, followed in incidence by ectopic atrial tachycardia with some degree of AV block.

Regularization of rate in the setting of atrial fibrillation and digoxin administration suggests the development of a digitalis-toxic junctional rhythm. Further intoxication causes an increased irregular rate (enhanced automaticity), junctional tachycardia, and Wenckebach exit block. All grades of AV block can occur in digitalis toxicity and may require temporary pacing. High-grade AV block is considered a serious prognostic factor. The presence of ventricular tachycardia in this setting is associated with a 60% to 65% mortality. Hypokalemia often accompanies rhythm disturbances. Hyperkalemia may be seen in large, acute overdoses and may yield rhythm disturbances as well.

CHRONIC EFFECTS

Chronic digitalis toxicity often is minor and may be difficult to diagnose because side effects may mimic underlying disease states. Common nonspecific symptoms may include malaise, fatigue, weakness, anorexia, nausea, vomiting and headache.

Toxic Dosage/Death

A toxic oral dose is around 2 mg in adults. The lethal dose in children is 4 mg and 10 mg in adults. Ingestion of 0.05 mg/kg (e.g., one 0.5-mg tablet in a 10-kg child) is expected to produce a digoxin blood level above the upper therapeutic limit of 2 ng/mL. Although children tolerate acute digoxin ingestions better than adults do, serious sequelae of digoxin mean that any potential or suspected ingestion above this range should be treated with gut decontamination and observation in an emergency department. An 18-month-old child with a digoxin level of 48 ng/mL, 2 hours postingestion developed only transient asymptomatic conduction disturbances.

Any suicidal ingestion in a patient chronically taking digoxin should be considered a serious ingestion. Toxic effects in such patients are difficult to predict because of a variety of factors that predispose to digitalis poisoning. Death from overdose in adults results from the exacerbation of therapeutic effects. These include pump failure secondary to negative inotropic effects, conduction impairment with severe AV block, and ventricular arrhythmias from increased automaticity.

Drug Interactions

Coadministration of quinidine raises the digoxin level. Quinidine reduces the volume of distribution of digoxin by displacing digoxin from muscle-binding sites as well as decreasing nonrenal digoxin clearance. Quinidine may increase gastrointestinal side effects, but the effect on dysrhythmias is unclear. Verapamil and diltiazem, but not nifedipine, reduce the nonrenal clearance of digoxin by an average of 29% and 21%, respectively.

Verapamil coadministration raises digoxin levels. Amiodarone increases digoxin levels. Spironolactone raises the digoxin level, decreases renal and nonrenal digoxin clearance, and reduces the volume of distribution. However, at least in children, this combination probably does not increase the probability of toxic digoxin levels. Indomethacin reduces the filtration rate and thus the renal elimination of digoxin.

Pregnancy/Lactation

Digoxin crosses the placenta and may appear in breast milk. Pregnancy risk category C.

Laboratory

ANALYTIC METHODS

Radioimmunoassay and other methods may detect digoxin.

BLOOD LEVELS

Therapeutic digoxin levels are 0.8 to 2 ng/mL. Serum levels 4 hours after intravenous administration and 6 hours after oral ingestion correlate best with effect in the therapeutic setting.

Acute overdoses usually involve toxic serum levels exceeding 2 ng/mL. Levels over 15 ng/mL indicate serious intoxication. Children without cardiovascular disease tolerate levels up to 10 ng/mL and higher without serious toxicity but may have bradyarrhythmias or conduction delays. Clinical toxicity does not correlate temporally with peak plasma levels since plasma digoxin levels do not correlate well with concentrations at the receptor binding site (i.e., myocardium).

Treatment

GUT DECONTAMINATION

Gastric lavage within several hours of ingestion may be useful if there are no contraindications to its use. Charcoal may be useful as well. Serial doses of activated charcoal may reduce digoxin terminal elimination half-life, but the clinical value of this measure remains to be determined. Repetitive activated charcoal use (50 grams every 6 hours) has been suggested for digitoxin overdose, in view of its significant enterohepatic circulation. The efficacy of such therapy is not clear, and careful electrolyte balance probably is more important.

ELIMINATION ENHANCEMENT

The large volume of distribution of digitalis compounds limits the usefulness of forced diuresis, peritoneal dialysis, hemoperfusion, exchange transfer, and hemodialysis in improving clinical outcome. In a recent study, resin hemoperfusion appeared useful in a severe digitoxin overdose. Dialysis may be needed for extracellular hyperkalemia however, total body potassium levels probably are nearly normal, because potassium is released from intracellular stores, leading to intracellular hypokalemia.

SUPPORTIVE MEASURES

- Identify serious ingestions by history or cardiovascular changes early, and initiate cardiac monitoring and intravenous access. Preparation should be made early in patients with serious toxicity (i.e., manifested by initial hyperkalemia, ventricular tachycardia, and high-degree AV block) for the use of digoxin-specific Fab fragment antibodies.
- Abnormal electrolyte levels enhance digoxin toxicity. These include hypokalemia, hypomagnesemia, hyperkalemia, hypernatremia, and alkalosis. Currently, hypomagnesemia may be a more frequent contributor to digoxin toxicity than hypokalemia, because of the more widespread understanding of the hypokalemia-digoxin interaction.
- As digoxin levels are readily available, blood levels may be helpful in monitoring progress. Admit acute ingestions if the digoxin serum level is expected to exceed 2 ng/mL or if conduction disturbance or arrhythmias appear within 6 hours of observation.
- Digoxin-specific Fab fragments (see Antidotes section, below) interfere with clinical immunoassays for digitalis, and therefore such serum tests are unreliable for at least 5 to 7 days postadministration.
- Chronic toxicity usually requires hospitalization to monitor arrhythmias and correct predisposing factors. Withdraw drug, and monitor blood level and rhythm.
- Cautiously correct hypokalemia because, in the presence of bradydysrhythmia or tachydysrhythmia, elevation of the plasma potassium level may enhance conduction defects (i.e., greater than first-degree AV block). In severely hypokalemic patients, saline is the intravenous solution of choice because glucose enhances the movement of potassium intracellularly. The presence of renal failure, hyperkalemia, and depressed AV conduction (i.e., second-degree AV heart block or greater) contraindicates the use of potassium in reversing digitalis toxicity.

ARRHYTHMIAS

- Treat ventricular irritability with class II antiarrhythmics (e.g., phenytoin and lidocaine). Phenytoin is the drug of choice, because it may reverse AV nodal suppression. Propranolol is useful for tachydysrhythmias if no nodal suppression is present.
- Overdrive pacing is a therapeutic option if antiarrhythmic drugs are ineffective, but decreased fibrillatory threshold increases the risk of initiating serious dysrhythmias. Cardioversion at low energy levels is the last resort because of the potential for developing ventricular fibrillation.
- Class I antiarrhythmic drugs (procainamide, quinidine, disopyramide) are contraindicated because of depression of conduction. Clinical data on the effectiveness of bretylium are limited and controversial. The successful use of amiodarone (300 mg intravenously over 20 minutes) for intractable ventricular fibrillation has been reported.
- Treatment for symptomatic bradycardias includes atropine and a temporary pacemaker. In a patient without underlying cardiac disease, normal cardiac pacemakers usually ensure adequate cardiac output.
- Measure electrolytes carefully, especially calcium, magnesium, and potassium. Hyperkalemia often is unresponsive to insulin, sodium bicarbonate, and exchange resin (Kayexalate®) therapies. Severe hyperkalemia (over 6 mEq/L) is an indication for Fab antibody fragment administration. Elevated potassium levels are a serious prognostic sign and result from release of intracellular potassium.
- Hypokalemia often occurs in chronic toxicity. Magnesium, calcium, sodium, and phosphorus levels should be checked, because their imbalance enhances digoxin toxicity.

Antidotes

FAB FRAGMENTS

Digitalis compounds bind reversibly to cardiac receptors. Digoxin-specific antibodies (Fab fragments) reverse digitalis-induced dysrhythmias, conduction disturbances, myocardial depression, and inhibition of the sodium-potassium ATPase pump by attracting digoxin from these receptors. These antibodies are produced in sheep and are effective in adults, children, and premature infants. Papain enzymatically digests these antibodies (150,000 daltons) to improve the renal excretion of the Fab fragment digoxin complex (50,000 daltons), increase the volume of distribution, and reduce immunogenicity. Affinity chromatography further decreases immunogenicity by separating the Fab and Fc fragments. See Chapter 5, Antidotes.

Fab fragments should be used only in cases of life-threatening or potentially life-threatening overdoses. Further clinical experience is necessary to properly evaluate the risk/benefit ratio of Fab fragments in less severe forms of digitalis toxicity. Current recommendations include acute overdoses that show signs of life-threatening dysrhythmias (e.g., hyperkalemia, serious arrhythmias such as ventricular tachycardia, ventricular fibrillation, or conduction blocks unresponsive to atropine and pacemakers). Other indications include overdoses that are potentially lethal as defined by poor prognostic factors such as old age, digoxin level over 15 ng/mL, digitoxin level over 150 ng/mL.

The use of Fab fragments reverses the clinical and electrocardiographic effects of both digoxin and digitoxin toxicity within 1 hour of administration. Although total digoxin levels may increase 5 to 20 times, free serum digoxin drops to zero. Under normal conditions, the Fab fragment-digoxin complex excretion half-life is 16 to 20 hours. However, Fab fragments have reversed digitoxin toxicity in the presence of impaired renal function. These Fab fragments accelerate the excretion of digitoxin, which has a long elimination half-life in therapeutic doses (5 to 6 days).

Hypersensitivity reactions (e.g., proteinuria, anaphylaxis) have not been reported, although the immunogenic potential of foreign proteins is significant. Cardiogenic shock has occurred in patients with severe digitalis poisoning treated with Fab fragments who have preexisting heart disease. The theoretical possibility exists that Fab fragments will eliminate the beneficial effects of digoxin, leading to congestive heart failure and cardiogenic shock in patients with severe underlying cardiac disease.

Equimolar doses are recommended for neutralization of digoxin although lower doses may be equally effective. About 65 mg Fab fragments is the molar equivalent necessary to bind and neutralize 1 mg of digitoxin and the neutralization of 1 mg of dogoxin requires about 50–100 mg of Fab fragments. The dose in number of vials = the steady state digoxin level in ng/mL, x kg of body weight, ÷ 100. Four to 6 vials generally will be sufficient, except in extremely large overdoses. Administer IV over 30 minutes through a filter. A bolus injection may be used in cases of impending cardiac arrest.

Questions—Digitalis

1. Which of the following describes the mechanism of action of digoxin?

A. It decreases myocardial contractility.
B. It increases conduction through AV node.

C. It increases refractoriness in the atria and ventricles.
D. It acts by decreasing vagal tone.
E. It alters the Na+/K+ ATPase-dependent transport system.

2. The following is/are cardiovascular side effect(s) of digoxin toxicity
A. Bradycardia
B. Heart block
C. Tachydysrhythmias
D. Atrial fibrillation coarsening
E. A, B and C

3. Supportive measures of digoxin toxicity may include
A. Cautious correction of hypokalemia
B. Treat ventricular irritability with class II antiarrhythmics, such as phenytoin and lidocaine.
C. Treatment of symptomatic bradycardia with atropine and placement of a temporary pacemaker
D. Administration of Fab antibody fragments for severe hyperkalemia over 6 mEq/L
E. All of the above

ADENOSINE

Adenosine (Adenocard®) is used in the acute termination of supraventricular tachycardia. It has also been used to aid in the differential diagnosis of tachyrhythmias. It produces transient slowing of the sinus rate and delay in AV nodal conduction. It has no direct effects on ventricular tissue. Adenosine must be given intravenously, as it has an ultrashort half-life of seconds.

Pathophysiology

Adenosine decreases spontaneous depolarization (i.e., pacemaker activity) in the sinus node and conduction velocity in the AV node. Its direct negative chronotropic and dromotropic properties are the basis for its wide diagnostic and therapeutic application in patients with supraventricular tachycardia. In atrial tissue, adenosine produces a negative inotropic effect. In ventricular tissue, adenosine minimally affects the ventricular inotropic state under basal conditions.

Pharmacokinetics

ABSORPTION
- Administration is by the intravenous route.

DISTRIBUTION
- The primary clinical effect of adenosine is on cardiac tissue.

ELIMINATION
- Adenosine is fully metabolized within seconds.

Clinical Presentations

Undesirable effects include cutaneous flushing, dyspnea, chest pain, nausea, lightheadedness, headache, and dizziness in about 20% of patients. The frequency and severity of the symptoms usually are dose related. Bradycardia, transient atrial flutter or fibrillation, sinus arrest, varying degrees of AV block, and ventricular premature beats have been recorded. Adenosine rarely has been associated with transient hypotension. Prolonged bradycardia and seizures have followed its use. Proarrhythmic responses are common after bolus injection. Nonsustained polymorphic ventricular tachycardia and atrial fibrillation have been reported.

Episodes of transient asystole and heart block frequently are observed, but these usually are short-lived and resolve spontaneously without intervention. Pauses with ventricular standstill of several seconds may occur. Adenosine should not be administered in the presence of congenital or acquired prolonged QT syndrome as its negative chromotropic and dromotropic actions may induce *Torsade de Pointes*. Every patient with tachycardia should have a full 12-lead electrocardiogram before adenosine treatment.

Transient AV block can precipitate ventricular fibrillation in patients with the Wolff-Parkinson-White syndrome. Adenosine is contraindicated in patients with sick sinus syndrome, or second- or third-degree AV block unless a functioning pacemaker is in place. Overdoses have not been reported.

Toxic Dosage/Death

A fatal dose of adenosine has not been established. Idiosyncratic reactions, particularly in those with prior cardiac disease, may yield prolonged asystolic pauses.

Drug Interactions

Dipyridamole potentiates the dromotropic effects of adenosine, causing prolonged AV nodal block. Verapamil may be potentially dangerous in elderly patients with atrial flutter. If therapy is required, overdrive atrial pacing is the treatment of choice. Theophylline acts as an antagonist. Carbamazepine increases the strength of adenosine-induced heart block and asystole.

Pregnancy/Lactation

Adenosine has not been studied systematically in pregnant patients, although it has been used safely in some pregnant patients. Tachydysrhythmias during pregnancy are rare. Management of supraventricular tachycardias in pregnancy may include vagal maneuvers, β-blockade (e.g., with esmolol), and electrical cardioversion. Administration of adenosine, in one anecdotal case report, was successful in terminating a supraventricular tachycardia in a 39-week pregnant patient.

Laboratory

ANALYTIC METHODS
These methods generally are not utilized because of the rapid metabolism of the parent compound.

BLOOD LEVELS
As adenosine is fully metabolized in seconds, blood levels are unnecessary.

Treatment

GUT DECONTAMINATION
Oral overdose has not been reported. Gut decontamination would be expected to have minimal, inconsequential effects.

ELIMINATION ENHANCEMENT
Because of its short half-life, methods to enhance elimination of adenosine are not necessary.

SUPPORTIVE MEASURES

- Patients and nurses should be prepared mentally for briefly symptomatic high-grade heart blocks of several seconds' duration. External pacing should be available immediately.
- In situations of prolonged adenosine-induced chest pain in patients with ischemic heart disease, theophylline has alleviated discomfort.

Questions—Adenosine

1. What statement best characterizes adenosine's pathophysiology?
   A. It acts at β-1 receptors in the heart thereby causing slowing of tachyarrhythmias.
   B. It produces increased vagal tone to the heart slowing conduction through the AV node.
   C. It decreases spontaneous depolarization in the sinus node and conduction velocity in the AV node.
   D. It produces coronary spasm leading to ischemic slowing of the heart.
   E. None of the above

2. Which of the following are undesirable side effects of adenosine?
   A. Chest pain
   B. Seizures
   C. Dyspnea
   D. A and B
   E. A and C

ANTIHYPERTENSIVE DRUGS

INTRODUCTION

There are numerous drugs available to decrease blood pressure in acute and chronic settings. Some of these agents, such as β-blockers and calcium- channel blockers, also are utilized for their antiarrhythmic potential. Please see a complete description of these agents, above. The development of antihypertensive medication represents a vital sector of the pharmacology industry. Numerous agents have "come and gone" as new agents, with less purported adverse effects, take their place.

ANGIOTENSIN-CONVERTING ENZYME INHIBITORS

Angiotensin is a hormone that is important in the pathogenesis and pathophysiology of several common hypertensive diseases, including essential hypertension, renal hypertension, and renovascular hypertension. Its effect also is important in the pathophysiology of congestive heart failure and coronary insufficiency, and in a variety of renal diseases associated with albuminuria.

Captopril (Capoten®) and enalapril (Vasotec®) are angiotensin-converting enzyme (ACE) inhibitors that cause reduction in blood pressure in hypertensive patients. They are used with other cardioactive drugs in the management of congestive heart failure. Although side effects occur with both drugs, poisoning reports have been rare. Hypotension remains a potentially serious toxic reaction. Losartan (Cozaar®) is the first described orally active, nonpeptide, and specific angiotensin II antagonist with specificity and high affinity for type I receptors.

Pathophysiology

ACE inhibitors block the conversion of angiotensin I to angiotensin II, potent vasoconstrictors. They inhibit the ACE breakdown of bradykinin and reduce basal aldosterone secretion. ACE inhibitors work by decreasing total peripheral resistance with little change in heart rate, stroke volume, or cardiac output.

Pharmacokinetics

ABSORPTION

- Captopril's onset of action is 15 to 60 minutes.
- 60% to 75% of captopril is absorbed from the gastrointestinal tract.
- Losartan is rapidly absorbed; peak plasma concentrations are achieved within 1 hour.
- Oral bioavailability of losartan is approximately 33%.

DISTRIBUTION

- Losartan undergoes extensive first-pass hepatic metabolism to the predominant circulating form of the drug, a 5-carboxylic acid metabolite.
- Volume of distribution of captopril is 0.7 L/kg and enalapril is 1.7 L/kg.
- Protein binding of enalapril is 50% to 60%.

ELIMINATION

- The half-life of captopril is around 2 hours in a normal adult.
- 95% of captopril is excreted in the urine within 1 day.

Clinical Presentations

The principal adverse effect of ACE inhibitor overdose is hypotension, although hyperkalemia and renal failure may occur. Severe diarrhea, angioedema, myalgias, membranous glomerulopathy, bone marrow aplasia, dry mouth, arthralgias, cough, and pruritus may occur with captopril and enalapril use. Bradycardia may occur from parasympathetic stimulation.

Toxic Dosage/Death

A mixed overdose involving 300 mg of enalapril and 440 mg of enalapril has been associated with hypotension and stupor.

Drug Interactions

ACE inhibitors appear to have additive hypotensive effects with diuretics, other antihypertensive agents, nitrates, anesthetic agents, adrenergic blocking agents, β-blockers, clonidine, methyldopa, and prazosin. Hyperkalemia may occur when ACE inhibitors are used with potassium-sparing diuretics or potassium supplementation. Captopril can potentiate morphine-induced respiratory depression. Prostaglandin inhibitors such as indomethacin may blunt the response to captopril.

Pregnancy/Lactation

Defects in skull ossification, pulmonary hypoplasia, oligohydramnios, neonatal hypertension, renal failure, renal dysgenesis, anuria, and fetal death have been reported after fetal exposure during pregnancy to ACE inhibitors. Fatal acute enterocolitis in a neonate followed in utero exposure to captopril throughout pregnancy. Captopril and enalapril are pregnancy risk factor D.

Laboratory

ANALYTIC METHODS

ACE inhibitors are not evaluated routinely in hospital settings.

BLOOD LEVELS

There is no evidence that following ACE inhibitor levels in overdose helps guide management.

Treatment

GUT DECONTAMINATION

Methods of gut decontamination, including lavage and charcoal, may be helpful if initiated within a few hours of ingestion. Activated charcoal repeatedly administered may interfere with enterohepatic recirculation.

ELIMINATION ENHANCEMENT

Hemodialysis may be effective in serious poisonings if clinical deterioration continues in spite of aggressive supportive therapy. Neither losartan nor its active metabolite is removed by hemodialysis.

SUPPORTIVE MEASURES

- Treatment primarily is supportive and aimed at maintaining an adequate blood pressure. Administration of intravenous fluids to expand intravascular volume has been successful in restoring and maintaining blood pressure in several ACE inhibitor overdoses and usually is the initial choice for blood pressure support.
- If volume resuscitation is unsuccessful or not tolerated, vasopressors, including dopamine, norepinephrine, or epinephrine, may be used. Generally, position change and fluid infusion should suffice to restore pressure to pretreatment levels.
- Close monitoring of vital signs, as well as serum potassium and creatinine concentrations, must be included in the management of an ACE inhibitor overdose. Monitoring of renal function is essential.
- Home management may be instituted in patients under 6 years of age who ingest less than 4 mg/kg captopril, less than 1 mg/kg enalapril, or less than 1 mg/kg lisinopril.
- ACE inhibitor-induced cough may respond to sodium cromoglycate or other antitussive agents.

ANGIOEDEMA

- Treatment of patients with angioedema depends on the severity of the edema. The airway must be maintained and is the first and most important concern. A nasopharyngeal airway may be all that is needed, however oral or nasal intubation may become necessary as well.
- The emergency physician must be prepared for surgical intervention if the edema worsens and respiratory embarrassment ensues. If the soft tissues of the neck are too edematous for safe intubation or cricothyroidotomy, fiberoptic bronchoscopic nasal intubation or retrograde intubation over a guidewire passed through the cricothyroid membrane may be necessary.
- Fortunately, most cases of angioedema are effectively controlled with standard antiallergic drug therapy including antihistamines, epinephrine, and steroids.

Antidotes

ANGIOTENSIN II

Angiotensin II ideally is suited for treating ACE inhibitor-induced hypotension, but rarely is necessary. Angiotensin amide is pharmacologically and physiologically identical to naturally occurring angiotensin II, and has been approved by the FDA for this setting. Unfortunately, it is not widely available. Blood pressure, heart rate, and electrocardiogram are monitored continuously during angiotensin II infusion.

Questions—Angiotensin-Converting Enzyme Inhibitors

1. Which of the following is the principal adverse effect of ACE inhibitors?

A. Hypokalemia
B. Hypotension
C. Vertigo
D. Renal insufficiency and hyperkalemia
E. B and D

2. Which of the following are true concerning angioedema from ACE inhibitors?

A. Treatment of patients with angioedema depends on the severity of edema.
B. It is a dose-related phenomenon.
C. The airway must be maintained and is the first and most important concern.
D. Most cases require intubation or cricothyroidotomy.
E. A and C

CLONIDINE

Clonidine (Catapres®) has been used as an antihypertensive drug for the past 20 years. Its lowers blood pressure by stimulating presynaptic α-2 adrenergic receptors in the medulla oblongata. This stimulation inhibits sympathetic discharge and thereby decreases blood pressure. Clonidine also has been used to treat symptoms of opiate and propoxyphene withdrawal, which are felt to be manifestations of noradrenergic excess. A transdermal patch has been devised for these purposes. Transdermal application of clonidine requires a long period to achieve therapeutic drug plasma concentrations, and usually must be supplemented with oral clonidine therapy early in the treatment of hypertension and chemical withdrawal states. Deaths from clonidine rarely have been reported.

Clonidine is an imidazoline derivative similar in structure to the α-adrenergic blocking agents phentolamine, tolazoline, and guanabenz. The most common adverse effects are drowsiness and dry mouth. Acute toxicity associated with clonidine overdose may include profound hypotension, weakness, emesis, emotional lability, hyporeflexia, areflexia, lethargy, somnolence, hypothermia, symptomatic bradycardia, miosis, hypoventilation, apnea, and seizures. Symptoms may last up to 72 hours.

Pathophysiology

Clonidine acts by central stimulation of presynaptic α-2 adrenergic neuron receptors in the cardiovascular control center of the medulla oblongata and in the locus ceruleus. This stimulation inhibits sympathetic discharge, resulting in a decrease in peripheral vascular resistance, heart rate, and cardiac output. Endogenous enkephalins and endorphins also suppress these neurons. Clonidine apparently inhibits noradrenaline secretion without affecting endorphin concentrations. In addicts, this inhibiting role is relinquished to opiate drugs. In sudden withdrawal of opiates, adrenergic inhibition is lost and withdrawal symptoms ensue.

Clonidine does not have ganglionic-blocking activity. At normal doses, it does not stimulate peripheral adrenergic receptors. At high doses, rebound hypertension may occur as clonidine stimulates peripheral α-adrenergic receptors, resulting in vasoconstriction and elevation of blood pressure. Clonidine also depresses the central nervous system by reducing central nervous system noradrenergic activity.

Pharmacokinetics

ABSORPTION

- Gastrointestinal absorption is almost 75% complete after oral administration.
- There is no impairment of absorption in patients with end-stage renal disease.

DISTRIBUTION

- Hypotensive effects are produced within 30 to 60 minutes after an oral dose, peaking at 2 to 3 hours and lasting up to 8 hours.
- Protein binding of clonidine in plasma ranges from 20% to 40%.
- The apparent volume of distribution after oral administration of 0.3 mg is 3.19 to 5.56 L/kg.
- Clonidine is distributed widely to all tissues and crosses the blood-brain barrier.

ELIMINATION

- Clonidine is metabolized to six nonactive compounds, but is excreted mainly in the kidney in the unchanged form. The kidneys eliminate about 72% of clonidine within 24 hours.
- The elimination half-life after a single oral dose is about 12 to 16 hours.

Clinical Presentations

Sedation, dry mouth, drowsiness, depression, inhibition of ejaculation, constipation, orthostatic hypotension, gasping, and sighing respiration in children have been described following the therapeutic use of clonidine.

NEUROLOGIC EFFECTS

Clonidine in overdose may lead to drowsiness, sedation, respiratory depression, apnea, miosis, and coma. Initial symptoms of drowsiness can lead to unconsciousness within 30 to 60 minutes and may persist for 24 to 36 hours. Seizure activity has occurred within 8 hours of clonidine ingestion. While miosis is a common finding, mydriasis or nonreactive pupils may be seen. Centrally mediated effects of overdose may include sedation, hypothermia, hyporeflexia, and hypotonia.

CARDIOVASCULAR EFFECTS

After clonidine overdose bradycardia, hypotension, and pallor may begin within 1 to 3 hours. Hypertension may supervene secondary to enhanced peripheral α-2 adrenergic activity. Atrioventricular block has been reported. Bradycardia with hypertension may be observed at the same time. Symptoms may persist for 3 to 4 days.

WITHDRAWAL EFFECTS

Abrupt withdrawal of clonidine leads to cessation of central adrenergic inhibition and to sympathetic overacting, similar to a pheochromocytoma crisis, with anxiety, restlessness, sweating, shivering, hypertension, tachycardia, headache, and abdominal pain. Such symptoms usually appear 16 to 40 hours after withdrawal.

Toxic Dosage/Death

A therapeutic dose of clonidine ranges from 0.2 to 2 mg. Up to 5 mg/day has been used in resistant hypertensives. In adults, doses of 0.4 to 11.25 mg have been toxic. Doses up to 3.0 mg in children have been reported without fatality. Dose correlation with toxic clinical effects is not exact.

Drug Interactions

Tricyclic antidepressants may interfere with the antihypertensive action of clonidine. Clonidine is synergistic with thiazide diuretics. "Clonidine" may be confused with "klonopin" (clonazepam).

Pregnancy/Lactation

Pregnancy risk category C.

Laboratory

ANALYTIC METHODS

Clonidine may not be detected in body fluids by routine toxicology screening methods. It often is not suspected in patients who present with miosis, respiratory depression, and coma.

BLOOD LEVELS

Clonidine levels may be of confirmatory assistance in those cases of miosis, hypotension, and depressed consciousness that do not respond to naloxone. Because of delays in diagnosis, clonidine levels may not assist in the immediate management of an overdosed patient. The normal therapeutic serum level is 0.1 to 0.6 ng/mL. Plasma concentration in an adult 4 hours after ingestion of an overdose of 4.8 mg was 6.0 ng/mL. A single dose of 0.3 mg orally will produce a peak plasma concentration around 1.0 ng/mL.

Treatment

GUT DECONTAMINATION

Gastric lavage only is recommended after endotracheal intubation has been performed to protect a patient's airway. Because clonidine is absorbed rapidly, it is not useful to attempt lavage later than 4 hours after ingestion. Activated charcoal as an aqueous or sorbitol slurry can be given after lavage (adult, 60 to 100 grams and children, 30 to 60 grams).

ELIMINATION ENHANCEMENT

Extracorporeal methods are not helpful in the face of the large volume of distribution. Forced diuresis is not effective and may lead to potentiation of the hypotensive effects of clonidine. Hemodialysis use in clonidine poisoning has not been established. Peritoneal dialysis and hemoperfusion have not been studied.

Whole-bowel irrigation in one patient resulted in passage of a clonidine patch in the rectal effluent.

SUPPORTIVE MEASURES

- Because clonidine may produce respiratory depression or apnea quickly, respiratory precautions should be in place and respiratory monitoring initiated immediately. All patients should be hospitalized because clonidine has a long half-life and cardiorespiratory changes may occur many hours after an overdose has occurred. For seriously depressed respiration, endotracheal intubation and assisted ventilation will be required.
- Electrocardiographic monitoring should be instituted to watch for bradycardia and dysrhythmias. Electrocardiography usually will reveal either sinus bradycardia or conduction problems.
- Supportive care is the mainstay of treatment. In many cases, supportive treatment with atropine, to combat significant bradycardia, has been effective without other medication.
- For seizures, intravenous diazepam may be useful. The dose in adults is 10 to 20 mg given slowly, and in children, 0.1 to 0.3 mg/kg slowly.
- Hypertension during a clonidine overdose can be treated conservatively unless the hypertension is persistent or severe. In such instances, diazoxide or furosemide may be helpful. Sodium nitroprusside also may be effective in clonidine overdose because of its short half-life, but it requires continuous monitoring. Phentolamine may be effective in clonidine withdrawal.
- Bradycardia without hypotension requires no specific treatment other than close observation. Severe bradycardia responds to IV atropine sulfate; the adult dose is 0.5 to 1.0 mg and for children, 0.01 to 0.03 mg/kg repeated three to four times as necessary.
- Hypotension usually responds to intravenous fluids, 10 to 20 mL/kg. Pressors such as dopamine (10 to 20 μg/kg/min) may be required and may help reverse associated bradycardia.
- Psychiatric consult should be obtained before discharge because most adult overdoses are suicidal. In view of the long half-life of clonidine, patients should be kept under close observation for 24 hours after blood pressure, pulse, respirations, state of consciousness, and electrocardiogram have returned to normal.

Antidotes

Naloxone may reverse the cardiovascular and respiratory toxicity associated with clonidine poisoning, as well as the antihypertensive effects associated with overdose, however this has yet to be prospectively confirmed.

Questions—Clonidine

1. Clonidine

A. Stimulates α-2 receptors in the *medulla oblongata* and causes lowering of blood pressure
B. Has been used to treat opiate and propoxyphene withdrawal felt to be manifestations of noradrenergic excess
C. Symptoms of acute toxicity include hypotension, hyporeflexia, myosis, and seizures.
D. The most common adverse effects are drowsiness and dry mouth.
E. All of the above

2. Regarding clonidine overdose

A. Bradycardia, hypotension, and pallor may begin 1 to 3 hours after ingestion and hypertension may supervene secondary to enhanced peripheral α-2 adrenergic activity.
B. Overdose requires forced diuresis to prevent hypotension.
C. Overdose usually is treated over a few hours because of its short half-life.
D. Overdose never includes serious hypertension.
E. None of the above

DIURETICS

Introduction

Diuretics are used to treat congestive heart failure and to treat hepatic, renal, or pulmonary disease, when salt and water retention has resulted in edema or ascites. Diuretics generally do not affect the underlying condition causing the edema. Edema associated with right heart failure and mild to moderate left heart failure generally is treated with thiazides. The initial treatment of acute, severe, left heart failure generally is saved for furosemide or loop diuretics. Diuretics also are used to treat idiopathic hypercalciuria, hypercalcemia, anasarca, nephrotic syndrome, hypertension, and some forms of diabetes insipidus.

Overdose with diuretics is reported infrequently. The main classes of diuretics in common use include the thiazides and related compounds, loop diuretics, and potassium-sparing diuretics. Other diuretics, including carbonic anhydrase inhibitors and osmotic diuretics, have limited uses. Mercurial diuretics are used rarely today. Hypokalemia, hypochloremic acidosis, and dehydration may result from overuse or overdose. Symptoms may include dry mouth, thirst, lethargy, weakness, muscle cramping, nausea, vomiting, and excessive urination. If left untreated, symptoms may progress to confusion, convulsions, stupor, coma, and deep, rapid breathing.

Thiazides

Thiazides, such as hydrochlorothiazide (HCTZ), are ubiquitous diuretic agents used to treat mild to moderate hypertension, peripheral edema, and congestive heart failure. They also are used to control calcium homeostasis in kidney stone formers. Overdose with these agents is rare, however hypokalemia, a potential adverse effect, is common.

PATHOPHYSIOLOGY

Thiazides act at the cortical diluting segment of the nephron or early distal tubule. They decrease glomerular filtration rate and may inhibit carbonic anhydrase. They increase sodium, chloride, and potassium excretion. Magnesium, phosphate, bromide, iodide, and bicarbonate excretion also may be increased.

Hypotensive activity in hypertensive patients may occur partly by direct arteriolar dilation. Plasma renin activity and aldosterone secretion are elevated. Thiazides, perhaps by acting at pancreatic and peripheral sites, can induce hyperglycemia, and may exacerbate preexisting diabetes mellitus, or precipitate diabetes in prediabetic patients.

PHARMACOKINETICS

Absorption

- HCTZ is 60% to 80% absorbed via the oral route.
- Peak plasma level occurs in 1 to 2 hours.

Distribution

- Protein binding of HCTZ is 40%.
- Volume of distribution is 0.83 L/kg.

Elimination

- Route of elimination primarily is renal.

CLINICAL PRESENTATIONS

Overdose with thiazides may result in diuresis, lethargy, and coma in a few hours even without dehydration or electrolyte changes. The mechanism of central nervous system depression is not known. Gastrointestinal irritability may be observed. Orthostatic hypotension, pancreatitis, potentiation of parathyroid hormone activity, skin rash, photosensitivity, and thrombocytopenia have been observed.

Long-term thiazide therapy infrequently results in mild metabolic alkalosis, hypokalemia, and hypochloremia. Hypokalemia and hypomagnesemia may be associated with ventricular ectopy. Hyponatremia may be seen in older age groups. Short-term potassium supplementation that ameliorates diuretic-induced hypokalemia may induce a significant fall in blood pressure.

TOXIC DOSAGE/DEATH

A toxic or lethal dose for these agents has not been established.

DRUG INTERACTIONS

Hypokalemia, hypomagnesemia, and hypercalcemia may predispose to digitalis toxicity. Potassium depletion may prolong the action of tubocurarine chloride or gallamine triethiodide. Corticosteroids and amphotericin may exacerbate potassium loss. Thiazides can reduce lithium clearance, increase serum lithium concentrations, and result in lithium intoxication. Exacerbation of diabetes mellitus, loss of diabetic control, and increased requirements for insulin or sulfonylurea antidiabetic agents are well known consequences of thiazide use.

Thiazides can increase the hypotensive effects of other hypotensive agents and may cause severe postural hypotension in patients stabilized on guanethidine, methyldopa, or a ganglionic blocking agent. The hyperglycemic, hypotensive, and hyperuricemic effects of diazoxide can be potentiated by thiazides. Probenecid enhances the excretion of calcium, magnesium, and citrate during thiazide therapy, but does not affect excretion of sodium, potassium, ammonium chloride, bicarbonate, phosphate, and titratable acid. Thiazides increase urinary pH and may decrease urinary excretion of amphetamines and quinidine. Alcohol, barbiturates, and opiates may increase the postural hypotensive effects of the thiazides.

PREGNANCY/LACTATION

Many consider thiazides contraindicated in pregnancy because they may decrease placental perfusion. They also may provoke diabetes in pregnancy. Pregnancy risk category D.

LABORATORY

Analytic Methods

Thiazides, furosemide, and ethacrynic acid may be detected by high-pressure liquid chromatography.

Blood Levels

Diuretic blood levels are not useful and usually are not available in the management of a thiazide overdose.

TREATMENT

Gut Decontamination

Activated charcoal can be given after or without lavage (adult, 60 to 100 grams and children, 30 to 60 grams) within a few hours of presentation, however its use in diuretic overdose has not been established. Cathartics may enhance fluid loss and probably are unhelpful.

Elimination Enhancement

No systematic studies have been performed with peritoneal dialysis, hemodialysis, hemoperfusion, or exchange transfusion.

Supportive Measures

- As always, establish respirations, airway, and circulation first. Patients suspected of significant diuretic overdose should be hospitalized for continuous cardiac, electrolyte, and renal monitoring. Monitor cardiac function (electrocardiogram, pulse, blood pressure), renal function (urine output, urinalysis, serum creatinine), electrolytes, and complete blood count.
- For hypovolemic shock, establish an intravenous line and begin saline. Place the patient in Trendelenburg position. If patient is unresponsive to these measures, administer dopamine or norepinephrine as required.
- Lab tests may reveal an increase in calcium, glucose, triglycerides, uric acid, and very-low-density lipoprotein concentrations. Decreased blood levels of chloride, magnesium, potassium, and sodium may occur.
- Magnesium deficiency may be a causative factor in the production of diuretic-induced arrhythmias. Empiric magnesium administration in the face of diuretic-induced arrhythmias may be justified.
- Hemoconcentration is treated with careful fluid administration. Patients are weighed daily and the intake and output of fluids is carefully monitored.
- Potassium loss is replaced with intravenous potassium. Sodium and chloride loss is replaced, slowly, with saline. Rapid replacement with concentrated solutions of sodium chloride may be associated with serious neurological damage (e.g., central pontine myelinolysis).

Questions—Thiazides

1. Hydrochlorothiazide (HCTZ) produces

A. Hypocalcemia, hyperkalemia, hyperglycemia, and hypouricemia
B. Hypercalcemia, hypokalemia, hyperglycemia, and hyperuricemia
C. Hypocalcemia, hypokalemia, hyperglycemia, and hyperuricemia
D. Hypermagnesemia, hypokalemia, hyperglycemia, and hypouricemia
E. None of the above

2. Thiazides are

A. Unsafe during pregnancy
B. More likely to cause hypokalemia in the presence of corticosteroids and amphotericin B
C. Are used to treat diabetes mellitus
D. A and C
E. A and B

Loop Diuretics

The loop diuretics currently in use include bumetanide (Bumex®), ethacrynic acid (Edecrin®), and furosemide (Lasix®).

They are used to treat hypertension, pulmonary edema, and hypercalcemia. Few reports describe overdose with loop diuretics. Bumetanide and furosemide are sulfonamide-type diuretics that have structural similarities to the thiazides. Ethacrynic acid is a ketone derivative of aryloxyacetic acid.

PATHOPHYSIOLOGY

These agents inhibit sodium and chloride reabsorption in the ascending loop of Henle. They inhibit the chloride-binding cotransport system and enhance excretion of water, sodium, chloride, magnesium, and calcium.

PHARMACOKINETICS

Absorption

- Bumetanide is 85% to 95% absorbed via the oral route. Furosemide is 59% absorbed.
- Peak plasma level of each occurs in about 1 hour.

Distribution

- Protein binding of bumetanide is 93% to 95%. Protein binding of furosemide is greater than 98%.
- Volume of distribution of bumetanide is 0.24 to 0.35 L/kg. Volume of distribution of furosemide is 0.17 L/kg.

Elimination

- Route of elimination is primarily renal.
- 50% to 80% of these agents may be excreted unchanged.

CLINICAL PRESENTATIONS

Encephalopathy, hyperglycemia, and gynecomastia have been observed with bumetanide use. Ethacrynic acid has produced vertigo, tinnitus, and temporary or permanent deafness. Acute hypoglycemia with seizures has occurred in uremic patients receiving large doses of ethacrynic acid. Ethacrynic acid use has resulted in hyperglycemia and glycosuria when administered to both diabetic and nondiabetic patients.

Ototoxicity and gastrointestinal bleeding may follow rapid intravenous administration of ethacrynic acid and furosemide, especially in patients in renal failure. Loop diuretics may induce hepatic coma in patients in liver failure. They may lead to urinary incontinence in the elderly and precipitate acute urinary retention in those with an enlarged prostate. Bullous rashes may occur when high doses are used in renal failures.

TOXIC DOSAGE/DEATH

Toxic overdose with loop diuretics has not been described. Serious symptoms may derive from therapeutic use, drug interactions, and concomitant hepatic or renal dysfunction.

DRUG INTERACTIONS

Indomethacin, probenecid, and salicylates reduce the diuretic and natriuretic effects of bumetanide. Aminoglycoside and other ototoxic drugs may increase the risk of irreversible ototoxicity, especially in patients with decreased renal function, when used concurrently with loop diuretics. Nephrotoxic drugs may enhance the nephrotoxic effects of these drugs. Ethacrynic acid may increase the effects of antihypertensive drugs, phenothiazines, and warfarin and may decrease the effects of allopurinol by raising the uric acid level. If ethacrynic acid is taken with digitalis, the patient must be monitored to prevent hypokalemia and resultant arrhythmias. Ethacrynic acid increases lithium accumulation.

When combined with tricyclic antidepressants, ethacrynic acid may result in excessive hypotension and its effects on blood pressure-lowering action may be increased. Furosemide may decrease the effects of oral antidiabetic drugs and insulin by raising serum glucose. Salicylate toxicity may occur when used concurrently with furosemide. Use of chloral hydrate 24 hours prior to furosemide may lead to diaphoresis, flushing, and possibly hypertension.

PREGNANCY/LACTATION

Ethacrynic acid is pregnancy risk category D. Furosemide and bumetanide are pregnancy risk category C.

LABORATORY

Analytic Methods

Thiazides, furosemide, and ethacrynic acid may be detected by high-pressure liquid chromatography.

Blood Levels

Diuretic blood levels are not useful and usually are not available in the management of overdose.

TREATMENT

Gut Decontamination

Activated charcoal may be useful after the oral forms of these agents are ingested in overdose.

Elimination Enhancement

Adequate hydration is important in managing overdose with these agents. Hemodialysis has not been used primarily to treat overdose with these agents.

Supportive Measures

- See Thiazides section, above. Monitoring, in addition to other treatment, is indicated for cranial nerve VIII function.

Questions—Loop Diuretics

1. Temporary or permanent deafness can result from long-term use of ethacrynic acid.
A. True
B. False

2. Aminoglycosides, especially in patients with renal dysfunction increase the risk of irreversible ototoxicity when used with loop diuretics.
A. True
B. False

3. Loop diuretics can produce urinary incontinence in the elderly and urinary retention in those with an enlarged prostate.
A. True
B. False

Potassium-Sparing Diuretics

Potassium-sparing diuretics such as spironolactone (Aldactone®) and triamterene (Dytac®) are weak diuretics. They are used mainly because of their potassium-sparing, rather than their diuretic or antihypertensive properties. They are often prescribed in combination with thiazides. Spironolactone is a synthetic steroid aldosterone antagonist. Triamterene is a pteridine derivative structurally related to folic acid.

PATHOPHYSIOLOGY

The main site of action of these agents is at the distal tubule, but spironolactone and its active metabolite antagonize aldosterone and are especially active in the presence of high levels of circulating aldosterone. High aldosterone states include Conn's syndrome (primary hyperaldosteronism), and secondary states such as cirrhosis, nephrotic syndrome, and in edema associated with heart failure.

PHARMACOKINETICS

Absorption

- Spironolactone is 90% absorbed via the oral route. Triamterene is 30% to 70% absorbed.
- Peak plasma level of each occurs in about 3 hours.

Distribution

- Protein binding of spironolactone is 98%. Protein binding of triamterene is 67%.
- Volume of distribution of spironolactone is 0.05 L / kg. Volume of distribution of triamterene is 2.5 L / kg.

Elimination

- Route of elimination of these agents is probably renal.

CLINICAL PRESENTATIONS

Metabolic Effects

Hyperkalemia with life-threatening cardiac arrhythmias may occur, especially when potassium-sparing diuretics are used concomitantly with kaliuretic diuretics (e.g., furosemide, ethacrynic acid, or hydrochlorothiazide). Signs and symptoms of hyperkalemia may include paresthesias, muscular weakness, fatigue, flaccid paralysis of the extremities, bradycardia, shock, and electrocardiographic abnormalities. Metabolic acidosis may occur with hyperkalemia.

Cardiovascular Effects

Electrocardiographic changes of hyperkalemia include tall, peaked T waves, T-wave elevations compared with previous tracings, lowered R waves, increased depth of the S wave, widening or absence of the P wave, progressive widening of the QRS complex, prolongation of the PR interval, and / or depression of the ST segment. Cardiovascular effects secondary to electrolyte disturbances rarely occur (e.g., angina pectoris, orthostatic hypotension, palpitations, and cardiac arrhythmias).

Gastrointestinal Effects

Nausea, vomiting, anorexia, diarrhea, abdominal pain, and gastrointestinal bleeding have been associated with these agents.

Ophthalmologic Effects

Eye examination may disclose visual disturbances and increased intraocular pressure.

Endocrine Effects

Toxic effects related to the steroid-like structure of spironolactone may include painful gynecomastia, decreased libido, and relative impotence in males. Females may experience menstrual irregularities, amenorrhea, postmenopausal bleeding, and breast soreness.

TOXIC DOSAGE/DEATH

A toxic or lethal dose for these agents has not been established.

DRUG INTERACTIONS

Use of more than one potassium-sparing agent at a time may increase the risk of hyperkalemia. Captopril decreases aldosterone secretion and increases serum potassium, thus the use of a potassium-sparing diuretic with captopril may result in hyperkalemia. The risk of hyperkalemia is increased when a potassium-sparing agent is used with potassium supplements, potassium-containing medications, or other substances containing potassium (e.g., low-salt substitutes).

Although potassium-sparing agents are weak antihypertensive agents, they may produce an increased hypotensive response when used with other hypotensive agents. Potassium-sparing agents may reduce renal lithium clearance and increase the possibility for lithium toxicity. When used with digoxin, alterations in electrolytes may alter digoxin responsiveness. Spironolactone may decrease the effects of anticoagulants and salicylates may reduce the natriuretic effects of spironolactone.

PREGNANCY/LACTATION

Spironolactone is pregnancy risk category D. Triamterene is pregnancy risk category D, however the manufacturer has categorized it as risk category B. Human data are not available on breast feeding.

LABORATORY

Analytic Methods

These agents may be detected by high-performance liquid chromatography.

Blood Levels

Following blood levels in overdose is not helpful.

TREATMENT

Gut Decontamination

Lavage and / or charcoal may be helpful in large ingestions within hours of overdose, however their long-range efficacy has not been proved.

Elimination Enhancement

Persistent hyperkalemia theoretically may require dialysis.

Supportive Measures

- See Thiazides section, above. Treatment of overdose mainly is supportive. Stop use of diuretics and other sources of potassium.
- Hyperkalemia is treated with the rapid intravenous infusion of 20% to 50% glucose followed by insulin injection. A cation-exchange resin (e.g., sodium polystyrene sulfonate) may be administered orally or as a retention enema to decrease potassium.
- Continuous electrocardiographic monitoring must accompany the ongoing evaluation of electrolytes and renal and cardiovascular function.

Question—Potassium-Sparing Diuretics

1. Side effects of potassium-sparing diuretics include

A. Nausea, vomiting, abdominal pain, and diarrhea
B. Increased libido
C. Regular menstrual periods
D. Hypertension, angina pectoris, and palpitations
E. Metabolic alkalosis

Acetazolamide

Acetazolamide (Diamox®) is a carbonic anhydrase inhibitor with a sulfonamide grouping. It has been used to reduce intraocular pressure in chronic open-angle glaucoma and in selected cases of acute, congestive heart failure. It also has been used to reduce the frequency and severity of epileptic seizures, especially petit mal seizures in children and in high-altitude sickness.

PATHOPHYSIOLOGY

Acetazolamide acts on the ciliary processes of the anterior chamber of the eye, at epileptogenic foci in the central nervous system, and at the proximal convoluted tubules of the kidney. Inhibition of carbonic anhydrase results in decreased secretion of aqueous humor with concomitant decrease in intraocular pressure. Such inhibition also induces a metabolic acidosis that may contribute to the suppression of central nervous system neuron discharge.

PHARMACOKINETICS

Absorption

- Acetazolamide is absorbed rapidly from the gastrointestinal tract and reaches its peak plasma level in 2 to 3 hours.

Distribution

- Protein binding is 90% to 95%.
- Acetazolamide is distributed throughout body tissues, but principally in the red blood cells, plasma, kidneys, and, to a lesser extent, in the liver, muscles, eyes, and central nervous system.
- The apparent volume of distribution of acetazolamide is 0.2 L/kg.

Elimination

- Acetazolamide is excreted unchanged (average 90%) by the kidneys.
- It has a plasma half-life of 1.5 to 8 hours.

CLINICAL PRESENTATIONS

Signs, symptoms, and laboratory findings in acute or chronic overdosage may be similar to those found with other diuretics. These include thirst, drowsiness, nausea, vomiting, malaise, confusion, convulsions, coma, decreased serum sodium, potassium, and bicarbonate. Life-threatening idiosyncratic reactions may occur after therapeutic doses and include fatal bone marrow depression with aplastic anemia, agranulocytosis, thrombocytopenia, severe renal impairment, and liver dysfunction. Renal insufficiency may result in acetazolamide toxicity. Acetazolamide can crystallize in renal tubules, resulting in calculus production and renal colic.

A significant metabolic hyperchloremic acidosis may occur in elderly patients receiving acetazolamide for open-angle glaucoma. There is no correlation between the degree of acidosis and the dose and duration of acetazolamide therapy. Chronic metabolic acidosis may result in chronic hyperventilation, which increases pulmonary vascular resistance and decreases left-ventricular function. The fibrillation threshold, including ventricular fibrillation, may be reduced. Central nervous system toxicity also may occur.

TOXIC DOSAGE/DEATH

Acetazolamide-induced hypersensitivity caused death from cholestatic jaundice in an adult who ingested 500 mg daily for 26 days.

DRUG INTERACTIONS

Acetazolamide may enhance the effects of amphetamines, quinidine, and quinine by delaying their excretion. It may decrease the effects of aspirin and methenamine by altering urine pH. Chronic salicylate dosing competitively reduces the plasma protein binding and renal clearance of acetazolamide and thereby induces toxicity. When taken concomitantly with phenytoin, phenobarbital, or primidone, acetazolamide may precipitate an increased loss of calcium and phosphate, causing osteomalacia. When used with lithium, it may increase the risk of lithium toxicity.

PREGNANCY/LACTATION

Acetazolamide crosses the placenta and is found in the breast milk of animals. It is classified as pregnancy risk category C.

LABORATORY

Analytic Methods

Acetazolamide may be detected by high-pressure liquid chromatography.

Blood Levels

Blood levels are not easily available in most hospitals and have not been demonstrated to be useful in the management of acetazolamide toxicity. Elevated levels may be associated with inhibition of renal reabsorption of bicarbonate, especially in patients with reduced renal function. Intraocular pressure is lowered at a level of 5–10 $\mu g/mL$.

TREATMENT

Gut Decontamination

Charcoal and/or lavage may be helpful in large overdoses, especially if performed within hours of ingestion, however further studies are indicated.

Elimination Enhancement

Dialysis may remove as much as 30%, however experience in overdose does not warrant its routine recommendation.

Supportive Measures

- See Thiazides section, above. Metabolic acidosis requires careful monitoring of arterial blood gases, respiratory rate, urinary bicarbonate, sodium and potassium excretion, and cardiovascular and renal function.
- Replacement of bicarbonate may be required with constant monitoring of the above modalities to avoid sudden shifts in electrolytes.

Questions—Acetazolamide

1. Acetazolamide has been used in

A. Petit mal seizures in children
B. High-altitude sickness
C. Open angle glaucoma
D. None of the above
E. All of the above

2. All of the following may occur with acetazolamide use except

A. Life-threatening idiosyncratic effects such as thrombocytopenia, aplastic anemia, and liver dysfunction.
B. Kidney stones
C. Hyponatremia
D. Hyperkalemia
E. Metabolic acidosis

3. All of the following are treatment options in acetazolamide overdose except
A. Replacement of bicarbonate
B. Dialysis that can remove as much as 30%
C. Charcoal and or lavage may be helpful in large overdoses.
D. Close monitoring of arterial blood gases, respiratory rate, cardiovascular and renal function.
E. Volume replacement

Mannitol

Mannitol (Osmitrol®) is used to promote diuresis to prevent or treat the oliguric phase of acute renal failure after massive hemorrhage, trauma, shock, burns, transfusion reactions, or major surgery. It is used to prevent hemoglobin buildup in cardiopulmonary bypass procedures and to protect poor renal function during renal surgical procedures. It also has been used in the treatment of acute cerebral edema, to reduce increased intracranial pressure during neurosurgery, and to reduce traumatically induced edema in the spinal cord prior to surgery. Other uses include the treatment of ARDS, to reduce intraocular pressure in glaucoma, and in the dialysis dysequilibrium syndrome.

While not clinically established, mannitol has been used alone or with other diuretics to promote the urinary excretion of salicylates, some barbiturates, bromides, imipramine, and lithium. Oral mannitol has been used in paraquat intoxication. Gut lavage with mannitol and with Prussian blue has been employed in the treatment of thallium intoxication.

PATHOPHYSIOLOGY

Mannitol is an osmotic nonelectrolyte diuretic. When used intravenously, mannitol cannot cross the cell membrane, remains in equal concentration in the plasma and interstitial fluid, and, by osmotic activity, mobilizes intracellular water that migrates to the extracellular space. It is freely filterable at the glomerulus and not reabsorbed along the nephron largely. It is an alcohol with a sweet taste, chemically related to mannose, which is widely distributed in the tissue fluids of various plants. It is produced commercially from mannose and glucose.

PHARMACOKINETICS

Absorption

- Very little mannitol is absorbed after oral administration.
- After intravenous administration, diuresis occurs in 1 to 3 hours and elevated intraocular pressure will begin to decrease in 30 to 60 minutes, and persist for 4 to 6 hours.
- Elevated cerebrospinal fluid pressure may begin to fall within 15 minutes and last for 2 to 8 hours.

Distribution

- When it is administered intravenously, mannitol remains in the extracellular compartment.
- Its apparent volume of distribution is very low, 0.18 L/kg.
- Mannitol does not cross the blood-brain barrier and does not penetrate the eye.

Elimination

- Mannitol is metabolized partially to glycerin in the liver. It is filtered at the glomeruli and is not secreted by tubular cells. Over 90% are not reabsorbed by the tubules.
- The elimination half-life of mannitol is 90 minutes.
- About 79% are recovered unchanged in the urine.

CLINICAL PRESENTATIONS

Severe fluid overload may occur, leading to hypertension, congestive heart failure, peripheral edema, and pulmonary edema. Central nervous system disturbances may include confusion and lethargy out of proportion to uremia. Stupor and occasionally coma occur. Acute oliguric renal failure may occur after mannitol use. Anaphylactic reactions have been reported after the use of intravenous mannitol. Confusion, nausea, vomiting, and respiratory acidosis have been reported.

TOXIC DOSAGE/DEATH

Deaths attributed to mannitol have followed doses of 1,200 to 2,050 grams.

DRUG INTERACTIONS

Mannitol increases lithium excretion.

PREGNANCY/LACTATION

There are no data available on placental or breast-milk passage. Pregnancy risk category C.

LABORATORY

Analytic Methods

Alcohols are detected by chromatography.

Blood Levels

Mannitol blood levels are not clinically useful in overdose situations because orally, mannitol is not absorbed and intravenously, the kidneys rapidly excrete it. Indicators that are more accurate include measures of fluid balance and renal function, serum electrolytes, hemoglobin, hematocrit, glucose, and serum osmolality.

TREATMENT

Gut Decontamination

These methods are not helpful after mannitol overdose.

Elimination Enhancement

Hemodialysis is the treatment of choice in those patients who are unable to excrete the elevated osmotic load on their own (i.e., patients in renal failure). Dialysis corrects high serum osmolality and hyponatremia much faster than either peritoneal dialysis or conservative management. A rapid fall in osmolality during dialysis may create a blood-brain osmotic gradient and may be responsible for dialysis disequilibrium or brain edema.

Supportive Measures

- Control airway, breathing, and cardiac status. If respiration is impaired, assisted ventilation may be required. Hospitalize patients and place in an intensive care unit if symptomatic. Monitoring of central venous pressure via a central line may be indicated.
- An osmolar gap between measured and calculated osmolality may occur. An elevated osmolar gap also may be found with ethanol, ethylene glycol, methanol, acetone, and isopropyl alcohol.
- Sequential monitoring of serum electrolytes, osmolarity, osmolar gap, renal, cardiovascular, and central nervous system function is required until all values have returned to premannitol levels.
- There may be hyperkalemia as a result of flux of potassium from intracellular to extracellular spaces. Hypophosphatemia may occur secondary to hyperphosphaturia resulting from

inhibition of phosphate reabsorption at the level of the proximal tubule.

Questions—Mannitol

1. Which of the following are features of mannitol overdose:

A. No central nervous system effects are observed.
B. It can be characterized by an osmolar gap between measured and calculated osmolarity.
C. It crosses the blood-brain barrier.
D. Hyperkalemia and hypophosphatemia may result.
E. B and D

VASODILATORS

SODIUM NITROPRUSSIDE

Sodium nitroprusside (Nipride®) is a peripheral smooth muscle vasodilator used to treat hypertensive crises. Continuous nitroprusside infusions may produce subacute cyanide toxicity after several days of therapy. Cyanide is a metabolite of nitroprusside, and toxicity may result from rapid infusion, prolonged use where tachyphylaxis requires high doses, or renal failure. Sodium nitroprusside is a hypotensive agent structurally unrelated to any other currently available antihypertensive agents. It also may be used to reduce afterload during congestive heart failure following myocardial infarction.

Sodium nitroprusside is administered by IV infusion with a controlled infusion device, microdrop regulator, or other such device to allow precise measurement of flow rate. Cyanide and thiocyanate levels should be monitored. Thiocyanate levels should not exceed 10 mg/dL. Fatal blood cyanide levels have been reported to be 2.5 to 3.0 μg/mL. Tachyphylaxis may be indicative of the effect of cyanide on chemoreceptors.

Pathophysiology

Sodium nitroprusside produces hypotension by a direct action on vascular smooth muscle that results in peripheral vasodilatation. The drug has no direct effect on vasomotor centers, sympathetic nerves, adrenergic receptors, the myocardium, or other smooth muscle tissue such as the uterus or duodenum. Major problems relate to the production of cyanide and thiocyanate toxicity.

Pharmacokinetics

ABSORPTION

- Response to IV sodium nitroprusside is immediate with a drop in diastolic blood pressure.
- Blood pressure begins to rise when infusion is slowed and returns to pretreatment levels within 1 to 10 minutes after infusion is stopped.

DISTRIBUTION

- Few data are available on body distribution, passage through the blood-brain barrier, or distribution into breast milk.

ELIMINATION

- One of the cyanide molecules released from nitroprusside reacts with hemoglobin to form cyanmethemoglobin.
- The unstable tetracyano-compound that remains ultimately releases the other four molecules of free cyanide. These are converted in a few hours, with the aid of rhodanese present in mitochondria, to thiocyanate.
- Thiocyanate is less toxic than cyanide and is excreted in the urine largely unchanged.
- The elimination half-life of thiocyanate is approximately 3 days in normal subjects and up to 9 days in those with renal dysfunction.

Clinical Presentations

Early signs of nitroprusside toxicity include metabolic acidosis, an increase in blood lactate and in the lactate/pyruvate ratio, a narrowing of the difference of oxygen content in arterial and venous blood, or a need for higher doses of nitroprusside to maintain blood pressure control (tachyphylaxis). These signs may occur from short-term infusions (e.g., intraoperatively) and are related largely to cyanide toxicity.

CYANIDE TOXICITY

Cyanide production may produce hypotension, nausea, vomiting, sweating, headache, palpitations, bradycardia, and paroxysmal ventricular contractions leading to cardiorespiratory failure. Hyperpnea, anxiety, restlessness, agitation followed by combative behavior, stupor, convulsions, and death may be associated with elevated blood cyanide levels.

THIOCYANATE TOXICITY

Patients who receive the drug over prolonged periods or who have renal or hepatic dysfunction may develop thiocyanate toxicity. Symptoms described include muscular fatigue, nausea, vomiting, confusion, hallucinations, convulsions, coma, and death. Fatal nitroprusside toxicity also may develop in the absence of metabolic acidosis. Toxic psychosis, hyperreflexia, tinnitus, and reversible hypothyroidism also may be observed.

WITHDRAWAL EFFECTS

Abrupt withdrawal of nitroprusside in patients with severe congestive heart failure may result in an increase in systemic vascular resistance and ventricular filling pressure. Rebound hypertension after nitroprusside may be prevented by pretreatment with captopril or propranolol.

Toxic Dosage/Death

Nitroprusside toxicity appears to relate more to the rate of infusion than to the total amount administered. More than 2.7 grams has been given over a 5-day period with no problem. Doses over 3 μg/kg/min over 72 hours may be associated with toxicity, especially in patients with impaired renal or hepatic function. Monitoring of early signs of cyanide or thiocyanate toxicity is essential.

Drug Interactions

Hypotensive effects of sodium nitroprusside are additive when used with ganglionic blocking agents, general anesthetics, and circulatory depressants. Infusion of sodium nitroprusside into the bloodstream of patients containing typical amounts of secondary amines (e.g., epinephrine) or accidental mixing of sodium nitroprusside with secondary amine drugs can result in the formation of n-nitrosamines, which may pose serious long-term carcinogenic health risks.

Pregnancy/Lactation

There is evidence that nitroprusside may pass through the placenta into the fetus. Nitroprusside has been used successfully in severe preeclampsia. In pregnant patients, sodium nitroprusside is used to induce hypotension prior to vascular operations and when severe gestational hypertension is present.

Laboratory

ANALYTIC METHODS

Serum thiocyanate and cyanide are measured via a colorimetric method.

BLOOD LEVELS

During brief administration of nitroprusside in high dosage, high red blood cell cyanide levels with low thiocyanate levels evidence toxicity. The metabolism of cyanide to thiocyanate appears to occur over a few hours. Laboratory tests of blood cyanide may not predict toxicity because these do not indicate tissue cyanide concentrations. Cyanide levels associated with fatality have been reported as 2.5 to 3.0 μg/mL. Daily measurements of thiocyanate level are of most benefit during the prolonged administration of nitroprusside. Thiocyanate blood levels (therapeutic) are 6–30 μg/dL. Toxic levels usually are over 35 μg/dL.

Treatment

GUT DECONTAMINATION

These methods are unhelpful, as sodium nitroprusside is primarily an intravenous medication.

ELIMINATION ENHANCEMENT

The short half-life of sodium nitroprusside mitigates against extracorporeal methods of elimination.

SUPPORTIVE MEASURES

- Hypotension is treated by stopping the nitroprusside infusion and by beginning an infusion of intravenous fluids (normal saline). Blood pressure, pulse, respiratory rate, electrocardiogram, and urine output are monitored carefully.
- If hypotension does not respond to cessation of nitroprusside infusion and intravenous fluids, then pressor agents such dopamine or norepinephrine are indicated.
- If the respiratory rate or depth of respiration is compromised and there is evidence of central nervous system depression, endotracheal intubation with assisted ventilation may be indicated.
- Laboratory indicators of toxicity that may aid in clinical management include arterial blood, serum lactate and pyruvate, cardiac output, pulmonary artery systolic pressure, pulmonary capillary wedge pressure, central venous pressure, renal function, urinalysis, and urine output.
- Increased lactate and lactate/pyruvate ratios, decreasing arterial pH, and increasing base deficits are found after cyanide intoxication however do not aid in the prediction of cyanide toxicity.

Antidotes

There are no antidotes. For treatment of cyanide toxicity, see Chapter 45, Airborne Toxins.

Questions—Sodium Nitroprusside

1. Which of the following leads to an increased risk of cyanide toxicity from nitroprusside?
A. Liver failure
B. Renal failure
C. Slowing the rate of infusion
D. Bolusing the drug
E. B and D

2. Signs of toxicity from cyanide include
A. Nausea
B. Ventricular arrhythmias
C. Mental status changes
D. All of the above
E. None of the above

3. Thiocyanate toxicity from nitroprusside is more likely to occur in the setting of renal or hepatic dysfunction
A. True
B. False

4. Nitroprusside is used commonly in the treatment of hypotension because it reduces the afterload in patients with severe congestive heart failure following myocardial infarction.
A. True
B. False

DIAZOXIDE

Diazoxide (Hyperstat®) is a direct vascular smooth-muscle relaxant that has been used in the acute treatment of hypertensive emergencies and in hypoglycemia. Diazoxide may cause arrest of labor when used in the hypertensive crisis of eclampsia. Poisonings have been rare and other agents have largely supplanted the use of diazoxide. Overdoses can produce hypotension and hyperglycemia and generally respond to supportive management. Diazoxide is related chemically to the thiazide diuretics.

Pathophysiology

Diazoxide is a direct relaxant of arteriolar vascular smooth muscle. Diazoxide also inhibits insulin secretion by the beta cells of the pancreas, increases catecholamine release, and increases glucose concentration in the plasma.

Pharmacokinetics

ABSORPTION

- Intravenous diazoxide produces hypotensive effects in less than 5 minutes, lasting 30 minutes to 72 hours.
- Oral diazoxide produces peak blood levels in 3 to 6 hours.

DISTRIBUTION

- Over 90% are protein bound.
- The apparent volume of distribution is 0.19 to 0.25 L/kg.

ELIMINATION

- The plasma half-life of diazoxide is about 24 hours.
- It is metabolized by oxidation and sulfation, after which about 30% of the dose are excreted in the urine as unchanged drug. The metabolites are not active.

Clinical Presentations

Overdose may be characterized by prolonged hypotension, rarely with cerebral or myocardial ischemia, dizziness, and syncope. Hyperglycemia may follow oral or intravenous use and may be associated with nonketotic hyperosmolar coma and ketoacidosis. Side effects that may be associated with poisoning include sodium and water retention, angina, atrial and ventricular dysrhythmias, and electrocardiographic changes. Central nervous system toxicity may include sweating, flushing, headache, lethargy, euphoria, and anxiety. Nausea, vomiting, anorexia, abdominal discomfort, dry mouth, diarrhea, parotid swelling, and pancreatitis have been observed. Rash, leukopenia, and fever have followed its use as well.

Toxic Dosage/Death

A toxic or fatal dose has not been established.

Drug Interactions

Diuretics and hypotensive agents may increase the hyperglycemic, hyperuricemic, or hypotensive effects of diazoxide. Phenytoin may increase the metabolism (decreased effect) or decrease the protein binding (increased effect) of diazoxide. Anticoagulants may decrease protein binding and therefore increase the effect of diazoxide.

Pregnancy/Lactation

Diazoxide crosses the placenta and blood-brain barrier, but its presence in breast milk has not been determined. Fetal abnormalities may be associated with its use. Pregnancy risk category C.

Treatment

GUT DECONTAMINATION

These methods are unhelpful, as diazoxide primarily is an intravenous medication.

ELIMINATION ENHANCEMENT

In extreme overdoses, when conservative therapy has been ineffective and the clinical condition is worsening, consideration of hemodialysis and peritoneal dialysis is warranted (low volume of distribution; however, high protein binding).

SUPPORTIVE MEASURES

- Hypotensive patients initially are placed in a supine or Trendelenburg position. If the hypotension does not respond to position changes, intravenous fluids are begun. Vasopressors such as dopamine (Intropin®), 2 to 5 μg/kg/min and up or norepinephrine (Levophed®), 0.1 to 0.2 μg/kg/min may be required.
- Continuous cardiac monitoring should be instituted with central venous pressure and/or pulmonary wedge pressure monitoring if clinical symptoms do not respond to simple maneuvers.
- Intravenous fluids, restoration of electrolyte balance, and insulin may be required to control hyperglycemia. Continuous observation for at least 48 to 72 hours in a hospital is required in serious cases in view of the long half-life of diazoxide.
- Management of an overdose should include a daily blood and urine glucose, blood electrolytes, arterial blood gases, uric acid, and electrocardiographic monitoring.

Questions—Diazoxide

1. **Diazoxide overdose may be characterized by myocardial ischemia, dizziness, and syncope.**
   A. True
   B. False
2. **Diazoxide is a direct vascular smooth muscle relaxant that has been used in the acute treatment of hypertensive emergencies and in hypoglycemia.**
   A. True
   B. False
3. **The presence of anticoagulants increases the effects of diazoxide because of increased protein binding.**
   A. True
   B. False

HYDRALAZINE

Hydralazine (Apresoline®) is used to treat moderate to severe hypertension. It generally is used in patients who fail to respond to other hypertensive agents such as diuretics, adrenergic inhibitors and/or ACE inhibitors. It also is used in the treatment of congestive heart failure and to treat pregnant women with preeclampsia. Its use has been supplanted largely by a variety of newer agents.

Hydralazine poisoning rarely has been reported. It is an arteriolar smooth muscle relaxant that can cause significant hypotension and may be associated with myocardial ischemia and cardiac arrhythmias. Cardiovascular support is the primary therapeutic focus in overdose.

Pathophysiology

Hydralazine reduces peripheral resistance by direct relaxation of arterial wall smooth muscle. By reflex action, there generally is an associated increase in heart rate, stroke volume, and cardiac output.

Pharmacokinetics

ABSORPTION

- Absorption is complete (50% to 90%) from the gastrointestinal tract.
- Peak plasma levels are reached in 1 hour after ingestion and 10 to 40 minutes parenterally.

DISTRIBUTION

- The apparent volume of distribution is 3.0 to 10.6 L/kg.
- Protein binding of hydralazine is 85%.

ELIMINATION

- Extensive metabolism occurs in the gastrointestinal mucosa and liver (first-pass effect).
- The elimination half-life is 0.45 to 2.8 hours with no difference in rapid or slow acetylators.
- Metabolism in the liver is determined genetically.

Clinical Presentations

Acute toxicity may be associated with hypotension, flushing, tachycardia, headaches, nausea, vomiting, and shock. Cerebral and/or myocardial ischemia with myocardial arrhythmias may be seen in severe overdoses. Toxic effects associated with overdose also include palpitations, nasal congestion, lacrimation, muscle cramps, rash, urticaria, pruritus, leukopenia, agranulocytosis, thrombocytopenia, and peripheral neuropathy.

Chronic administration of over 400 mg of hydralazine per day has been associated with a lupus-type syndrome in 10% to 20% of patients, accompanied by an increase in circulatory antinuclear antibodies. Generally, this benign syndrome resolves without permanent sequelae.

Toxic Dosage/Death

A toxic or lethal dose of hydralazine has not been identified.

Drug Interactions

The hypotensive effects of hydralazine may be increased with diuretics or other antihypertensive agents. Effects of hydralazine also may be increased with simultaneous use of tricyclic antidepressants and monoamine oxidase inhibitors. Amphetamines may decrease the effect of hydralazine on blood pressure.

Pregnancy/Lactation

Hydralazine crosses the placenta and is found in breast milk. There have been no reports linking hydralazine with congenital abnormalities. Pregnancy risk category C.

Laboratory

ANALYTIC METHODS

Lab tests to identify hydralazine generally are not available in a hospital setting.

BLOOD LEVELS

Laboratory levels associated with overdosage have not been defined. They are not useful in the clinical management of hydralazine poisoning.

Treatment

GUT DECONTAMINATION

Lavage, activated charcoal, and / or cathartics may be useful but have not been clinically evaluated. Syrup of ipecac is contraindicated as patients may become obtunded and hypotensive.

ELIMINATION ENHANCEMENT

Peritoneal dialysis and hemodialysis have not been effective.

SUPPORTIVE MEASURES

- The first priority in hydralazine overdose is attention to the ABCs (**a**irway, **b**reathing and **c**irculation). Respirations may need to be assisted via endotracheal or nasal intubation.
- Hypotensive patients initially are placed in a supine or Trendelenburg position. If the hypotension does not respond to position changes, intravenous fluids are begun. Vasopressors such as dopamine (Intropin®) 2 to 5 μg/kg/min and up, or norepinephrine (Levophed®) 0.1 to 0.2 μg/kg/min may be required.
- Continuous cardiac monitoring should be instituted with central venous pressure and / or pulmonary wedge pressure monitoring if clinical symptoms do not respond to simple maneuvers.
- Monitor fluid balance, electrolytes, and arterial blood gases. Establish normal circulatory status.
- Avoid drugs with β-adrenergic activity (e.g., epinephrine, isoproterenol, and ephedrine), as these may induce dysrhythmias.

Question—Hydralazine

1. Toxic effects of hydralazine associated with overdose include:

A. Glomerular nephritis
B. Rash, leukopenia, agranulocytosis, thrombocytopenia
C. Lupuslike syndrome
D. Diabetes mellitus
E. Thyrotoxicosis

MINOXIDIL

Minoxidil (Rogaine®) is used to treat severe or moderately severe hypertension in patients resistant to other antihypertensive drugs such as β-adrenergic blockers and diuretics. It usually is used with a diuretic. It has also been used to treat male pattern baldness. The few reports that allude to minoxidil overdose present a rather benign picture with few symptoms. However, minoxidil has the potential for producing profound hypotension and other manifestations of serious cardiovascular compromise when taken in overdose alone or with other antihypertensive agents.

Pathophysiology

Minoxidil produces an antihypertensive effect by its ability to act as a direct vasodilator of vascular smooth muscle. The drug decreases blood pressure in the supine and standing position and induces a reflex increase in heart rate, cardiac output, and stroke volume.

Pharmacokinetics

ABSORPTION

- Minoxidil is almost absorbed completely (95%) from the gastrointestinal tract.
- Peak plasma levels are reached in 1 hour.

DISTRIBUTION

- Minoxidil is distributed widely in the tissues, with a volume of distribution of about 2.8 to 3.3 L/kg.
- Protein binding does not occur.

ELIMINATION

- The elimination half-life of minoxidil is 2.8 to 4.2 hours.
- About 90% of an oral dose of minoxidil are metabolized in the liver.
- The drug and its metabolites are excreted largely in the urine.

Clinical Presentations

Few reports of minoxidil overdose are available. The absence of any hypotensive effect after an alleged dose of 100 mg of minoxidil in a normotensive child suggests that minoxidil is a purely antihypertensive drug, unable to produce hypotension in an individual with a normal blood pressure. This observation has not been confirmed by other reports.

Adverse effects of minoxidil may include sodium and water retention, tachycardia, angina, hemorrhagic pericarditis, pericardial effusion, hypertrichosis, electrocardiographic changes (alterations in the T-wave), breast tenderness, gynecomastia, polymenorrhea, headache, and hypersensitivity reactions (such as rash, and thrombocytopenia). Prolonged hypotension lasting almost 72 hours has been observed following an initial starting dose of 10 mg.

Toxic Dosage/Death

A toxic or lethal dose of minoxidil has not been established. One patient recovered after taking 50 mg of minoxidil together with 500 mg of a barbiturate. A 2-year-old alleged to have taken 100 mg of minoxidil remained normotensive and did not demonstrate any electrocardiogram abnormalities.

Drug Interactions

Minoxidil, when used with diuretics or other antihypertensive agents, may induce a profoundly hypotensive state.

Pregnancy/Lactation

Placental passage and distribution into breast milk have not been established. Pregnancy risk category C.

Laboratory

ANALYTIC METHODS

A radioimmunoassay method is available for serum levels. Serum levels are not correlated with clinical antihypertensive activity but do confirm the presence of minoxidil.

BLOOD LEVELS

At the maximum adult dosage of 100 mg/d, peak blood levels of 1,641 and 2,441 ng/mL were observed in two patients.

Treatment

GUT DECONTAMINATION

Lavage, activated charcoal, and/or cathartics may be useful but have not been clinically evaluated. Syrup of ipecac is contraindicated, as patients may theoretically become hypotensive.

ELIMINATION ENHANCEMENT

There are no data to support the use of hemodialysis or peritoneal dialysis in the overdosed patient although minoxidil appears to be easily dialyzable.

SUPPORTIVE MEASURES

- Overdose with minoxidil has resulted in a few reports with hypertensive patients.
- Hypotensive patients initially are placed in a supine or Trendelenburg position. If the hypotension does not respond to position changes, intravenous fluids are begun. Vasopressors such as dopamine (Intropin®), 2 to 5 μg/kg/min and up or norepinephrine (Levophed®), 0.1 to 0.2 μg/kg/min may be required.
- Tachycardia or angina may be ameliorated with and by a β-blocking agent.

Questions—Minoxidil

1. Adverse effect(s) of minoxidil is/are:
A. Hemmorrhagic pericarditis
B. Electrocardiographic changes
C. Breast tenderness
D. Thrombocytopenia
E. All of the above

2. Supportive measures in minoxidil overdose include:
A. Trendelenburg, IV fluids, vasopressors in patients with hypotension
B. Treatment with β-blockers in patients with angina and/or tachycardia
C. Syrup of ipecac in patients after acute overdose
D. A and B
E. A and C

α-BLOCKERS

α-Adrenergic blockers such as prazosin (Minipress®) may be used to treat mild to moderate hypertension and generally are reserved for patients who do not respond to diet, exercise, weight reduction and therapy other antihypertensive agents such as diuretics or β-blockers. Phenoxybenzamine (Dibenzyline®) is used to control the sweating and hypertension associated with pheochromocytoma. It is not used in essential hypertension because of its tendency to produce postural hypotension and tachycardia.

Phentolamine (Regitine®) is given parenterally for both the diagnosis and treatment of pheochromocytoma. It has been used to treat vascular ischemia caused by epinephrine injection into digits and dopamine extravasation, and for the treatment of cocaine-induced hypertension and vasospasm. Yohimbine (Afrodex®) has been used as an aphrodisiac and to treat erectile dysfunction in men, but has no sanctioned uses according to the FDA.

Pathophysiology

α-1 receptors are present postsynaptically in the smooth muscles of arteries and veins and in the eye, genitourinary and gastrointestinal tracts. Catecholamine stimulation of these receptors produces smooth muscle contraction leading to vasoconstriction. α-2 receptors are present in presynaptic neurons. Norepinephrine binds to α-2 receptors in the peripheral nervous system in presynaptic areas and α-2 stimulation results in decreased norepinephrine release by the neuron.

In the central nervous system, α-2 receptors are located in the postsynaptic effector cell. Stimulation of these α-2 receptors results in decreased sympathetic outflow. α-2 receptors in the brain function in sleep control and stimulation by an α-2 agonist results in sedation.

α-1 receptor agonists include methoxamine and phenylephrine. Antagonists of α-1 receptors include prazosin, and phenoxybenzamine. Epinephrine and norepinephrine have equal potency at α-1 and α-2 receptors. Clonidine is a selective α-2 agonist and yohimbine is an α-2 selective antagonist. Phentolamine is a nonselective α-1 and α-2 antagonist. α-2 antagonism by phentolamine permits sufficient norepinephrine release to produce tachycardia, angina, and positive inotropic effects on the heart.

Pharmacokinetics

ABSORPTION

- Prazosin is 40% to 60% absorbed.
- Prazosin reaches its peak blood level in 2 to 4 hours.

DISTRIBUTION

- 92% to 97% of prazosin is protein bound.
- The volume of distribution of prazosin is 0.6 to 1.7 L/kg.

ELIMINATION

- The half life of phenoxybenzamine is 24 hours. The half-life of phentolamine is 2 to 5 hours and the half-life of prazosin is 3.8 hours.

Clinical Presentations

Overdose with α-adrenergic blockers may produce postural hypotension, dizziness, syncope, vomiting, lethargy, and shock. Nasal congestion and dry mouth has been reported. Mydriasis may be seen with phentolamine and miosis may be seen with phenoxybenzamine and prazosin overdoses. Flushing may be seen with phentolamine and piloerection may be seen with yohimbine. Urinary incontinence and priapism has been associated with prazosin.

CARDIOVASCULAR EFFECTS

Postural hypotension and tachycardia are commonly seen in this drug group. Palpitations have been reported with prazosin use. Chest pain and an intensification of angina pectoris have been reported with phenoxybenzamine. Myocardial infarction, arrhythmias and shock have been seen after parenteral use with phentolamine.

NEUROLOGIC EFFECTS

Headache, sedation, depression, dizziness, paresthesias, restlessness, and an inability to relax may be seen. A fine tremor has been associated with yohimbine.

GASTROINTESTINAL EFFECTS

Nausea, vomiting, gastritis, constipation, weight gain, and exacerbation of peptic ulcer disease have been associated with these agents.

Toxic Dosage/Death

A 19-year-old who ingested 200 mg of prazosin remained conscious and oriented. Central nervous system examination was within normal limits. A 75-year-old man who ingested 80 mg of prazosin became drowsy and mildly hypotensive. He was alert in 1 hour, walked after 48 hours, and was discharged in 1 week. His serum level on admission was 2,350 nmol/L (20 times higher than after a single dose of 5 mg). A 64-year-old who ingested 40 to 60 mg of prazosin in a suicide attempt was found comatose. Hypotension was treated with fluids and in 15 hours, he regained consciousness with a normal physical examination.

Drug Interactions

Antihypertensive medications may increase the hypotensive effects of these agents.

Pregnancy/Lactation

Prazosin, phentolamine, and phenoxybenzamine are characterized as pregnancy risk category C.

Laboratory

ANALYTIC METHODS

Blood levels for α-adrenergic blockers are available but may not be feasible in many hospitals.

BLOOD LEVELS

Blood levels are not clinically useful after an overdose. No systematic studies have been made to correlate blood levels with clinical states.

Treatment

GUT DECONTAMINATION

Emesis is not advised for α-blocker overdoses. Lavage and/or activated charcoal (adults, 50 to 100 grams and children, 15 to 30 grams in aqueous or sorbitol slurry) may be helpful, however no studies on the efficacy of these methods are available with this group of drugs.

ELIMINATION ENHANCEMENT

In view of the extensive protein binding and volume of distribution of some of the drugs in this group, it is unlikely that hemodialysis or peritoneal dialysis would be effective. No studies exist to demonstrate such efficacy.

SUPPORTIVE MEASURES

- Most cases are amenable to good supportive therapy. The first priority in α-blocker overdose is attention to the ABCs. Respirations may need to be assisted via endotracheal or nasal intubation.
- Hypotensive patients are initially placed in a supine or Trendelenburg position. If the hypotension does not respond to position changes, intravenous fluids are begun. Vasopressors such as dopamine (Intropin®), 2 to 5 μg/kg/min and up or norepinephrine (Levophed®), 0.1 to 0.2 μg/kg/min may be required.
- Continuous cardiac monitoring should be instituted with central venous pressure and/or pulmonary wedge pressure monitoring if clinical symptoms do not respond to simple maneuvers.
- Phentolamine-induced arrhythmias may be treated with lidocaine or procainamide.
- Electrolytes, urinalysis, respiratory function tests, cardiac function studies, electrocardiography, and computerized tomography may be useful.

Questions—α-Blockers

1. α-Blockers have been used clinically for:

A. The treatment of sweating and hypertension associated with pheochromocytoma
B. The diagnosis and treatment of pheochromocytoma
C. Vascular ischemia induced by epinephrine injection in digits
D. Cocaine-induce hypertension and vasospasm
E. All of the above

2. Common α-blockers include

A. Digoxin
B. Prazosin
C. Amrinone
D. Phentolamine
E. B and D

PENTOXIFYLLINE

Pentoxifylline (Trental®) is a synthetic xanthine derivative used to treat compromised vascular blood flow states. There have been conflicting reports regarding the effect of pentoxifylline on intermittent claudication. It may be useful in cerebrovascular disease and sickle cell anemia, and may improve survival of experimental skin flaps.

Pentoxifylline appears to be associated with improvement in the healing of venous ulcers of the leg, livedo vasculitis, and diabetic neuropathy. Preliminary trials indicate a potential usefulness in counteracting ARDS and diminishing symptoms of septic or hemorrhagic shock. In overdose, it may yield gastrointestinal, cardiovascular, and central nervous system symptoms. There have been no fatalities and patients typically recover within 24 hours.

Pathophysiology

An exact mechanism of action in humans has not been determined. Numerous effects have been proposed. Studies suggest that pentoxifylline increases red blood cell deformability, leading to increased blood flow and decreased whole blood viscosity. Pentoxifylline increases prostacyclin release, which may decrease microcirculatory flow disturbance in sepsis. It decreases adhesiveness of polymorphonuclear leukocytes in the endothelium, which may lead to an increase in tissue oxygenation and decreases endotoxin-induced synthesis of tumor necrosis factor, possibly the essential effector molecule in septic shock.

Pentoxifylline inhibits platelet aggregation, increases white cell deformability, and prevents an increase in pulmonary vascular permeability to proteins induced by endotoxins. It appears to modulate cachectic activity in cancer patients and inhibits phosphodiesterase, leading to relaxation of smooth muscle of the vascular wall.

Pharmacokinetics

ABSORPTION

- Pentoxifylline is rapidly absorbed.
- Maximum levels are reached 2 to 6 hours after ingestion.

DISTRIBUTION

- An apparent volume of distribution in normal subjects is 3.6 L/kg.
- There is little evidence to suggest a significant degree of plasma protein binding with pentoxifylline.

ELIMINATION

- Pentoxifylline is metabolized in the liver to a number of inactive metabolites.
- The elimination half-life is about 0.93 hour after a 100-mg intravenous infusion.
- After oral administration of a sustained-release formulation of pentoxifylline, the terminal half-life is increased to 3.4 hours with an absolute bioavailability of 20%.
- Less than 1% of the dose is excreted in the urine as unchanged compound.

Clinical Presentations

The first signs and symptoms of overdose may be observed in 4 to 5 hours. Initially, overdose of pentoxifylline may induce gastrointestinal symptoms such as nausea, vomiting, and abdominal pain. At higher dose levels, hemodynamic instability manifested by hypotension, bradycardia, and tachycardia may be observed. Central nervous system signs such as seizures, somnolence, coma, and hypothermia have been described. Agitation, sleeplessness, mydriasis, and hyperthermia may be seen as well.

Toxic Dosage/Death

Infants 1- to 2-years-old who have ingested 10 to 15 tablets of pentoxifylline have developed nausea, profuse vomiting, hypotension, sinus tachycardia, myoclonus, and seizures. A 22-year-old survived after ingesting 4 to 6 grams of pentoxifylline. She was noted to have bradycardia and first and second-degree AV block (Mobitz type II) on electrocardiogram.

A number of children and adults have ingested 10 to 80 mg/kg and survived. Hemodynamic changes may follow doses of 60 to 80 mg/kg and seizures have been observed at 75 mg/kg. A lethal dose has not been established.

Drug Interactions

There have been reports of bleeding and/or prolonged prothrombin time when pentoxifylline is used with anticoagulants or drugs that inhibit platelet aggregation. Pentoxifylline and aspirin may slow the progression of dementia resulting from cerebrovascular disease, but this has yet to be confirmed.

Pregnancy/Lactation

No systematic studies of pentoxifylline use by pregnant women have been performed. Pentoxifylline, similar to other methylxanthines, rapidly crosses into breast milk. The parent compound and metabolite are detectable 2 hours after administration to lactating females. The quantities of pentoxifylline ingested by a nursing infant are unlikely to be of clinical significance. Pregnancy risk category C.

Laboratory

ANALYTIC METHODS

High-performance liquid chromatography for pentoxifylline and its main metabolite has a limit of detection of 5 ng/mL for both compounds. A similar liquid chromatography method is useful for analyzing pentoxifylline and three of its metabolites in plasma and urine.

BLOOD LEVELS

There is no evidence that blood levels are correlated with signs and symptoms after pentoxifylline poisoning. Following a single oral dose of 400 mg, a mean pentoxifylline plasma concentration of 1,102 μg/L is reached at 1.05 hours. Following ingestion of the sustained-release formulation (400 mg), the mean peak plasma concentration was 299 μg/L at 3 hours.

Treatment

GUT DECONTAMINATION

Emesis is contraindicated as seizures may occur. Lavage and/or charcoal may be helpful but have not been systematically studied.

ELIMINATION ENHANCEMENT

Hemodialysis may be considered, but there is little experience with this modality.

SUPPORTIVE MEASURES

- Treatment is largely symptomatic and supportive and includes correction of hypotension and correction of dehydration. Signs and symptoms usually remit within 12 hours. Care must be taken to protect the airway as seizures may occur. Seizures may respond to benzodiazepines such as diazepam or lorazepam.
- Vital signs, blood sugar, serum calcium and magnesium, and the electrocardiogram should be monitored carefully. The electrocardiogram usually is normal.
- Hypotensive patients initially are placed in a supine or Trendelenburg position. If the hypotension does not respond to position changes, intravenous fluids are begun. Vasopressors such as dopamine (Intropin®), 2 to 5 μg/kg/min and up or norepinephrine (Levophed®), 0.1 to 0.2 μg/kg/min may be required.
- Continuous cardiac monitoring should be instituted with central venous pressure and/or pulmonary wedge pressure monitoring if clinical symptoms do not respond to simple maneuvers.
- Atropine has been used for bradycardia.
- Liver function tests, renal function tests, coagulation parameters, blood sugar, uric acid, complete blood count, sedimentation rates, and platelet function usually are within normal limits. There may be an increase in basal insulinemia. Blood calcium and magnesium levels may decrease.

Questions—Pentoxifylline

1. Which of the following about pentoxifylline is false?

A. Pentoxifylline is a synthetic xanthine derivative used to treat compromised vascular blood flow states.
B. Pentoxifylline appears to be associated with improvement in the healing of venous ulcers of the leg, livedo vasculitis, and diabetic neuropathy.
C. In overdose, it may yield gastrointestinal, cardiovascular, and central nervous system symptoms.
D. Studies suggest that pentoxifylline increases red blood cell deformability, leading to decreased blood flow and increased whole blood viscosity.
E. Pentoxifylline increases prostacyclin release, which may decrease microcirculatory flow disturbance in sepsis.

NITROGLYCERIN

Nitroglycerin was discovered in 1847 by Alfred Nobel and incorporated as a major component of dynamite in 1867. It initially was mixed with diatomaceous earth and later with sodium nitrate (an oxidizer) and an adsorbent combustible material such as wood pulp. In 1890 a first report of occupational health hazard after exposure to nitroglycerin described severe throbbing headaches, difficulty in breathing, weak pulse, pallor, drowsiness, weakness, diaphoresis, nausea, and vomiting. Similar symptoms were described in 1898 as "powder headache," and in 1910 as "nitroglycerin head."

Nitroglycerin is used in the manufacture of industrial explosives such as dynamite. It also is used as a coronary vasodilator for the relief of angina, for prophylaxis of angina pectoris, for the management of unstable angina, for the relief of coronary artery spasm, and for the management of acute pulmonary edema. It also is used for the management of chronic heart failure, acute myocardial infarction, and postoperative hypertension, and for the relief of esophageal spasm.

Nitroglycerin may induce a disabling syndrome characterized by throbbing headaches and hypotension experienced when workers are first exposed to this chemical. Tolerance often occurs late in the work week. Relief occurs on weekends, but serious symptoms may resume on Monday morning. When nitroglycerin is mixed with ethylene glycol dinitrate (EGDN) in the manufacture of dynamite, sudden death may occur in otherwise healthy young men. Preventive measures are crucial and treatment mainly is supportive and symptomatic.

Nitroglycerin is a highly explosive substance that is very sensitive to mechanical shock and heat. Defibrillation performed over a nitroglycerin skin patch may result in electrical arcing with a resultant flash of light and thermal injuries. In commercial explosives, its sensitivity is reduced by the addition of an adsorbent such as wood pulp and chemicals such as ethylene glycol dinitrate and ammonium nitrate.

Pathophysiology

Nitroglycerin produces smooth muscle relaxation. Although it predominantly affects vascular smooth muscle, the bronchioles, gastrointestinal tract (including the biliary system), ureters, and uterus are affected. Free radicals of nitric oxide may activate guanylate cyclase, resulting in increased synthesis of cyclic GMP. Cyclic GMP appears to reduce stored calcium and interfere with calcium-activated smooth muscle contractions.

At low concentrations, nitroglycerin is mostly a venous dilator. Localized arteriolar dilation of the face and trunk may produce a flush, and meningeal and cerebral vessel dilation may result in headache. At higher concentrations, nitroglycerin produces arteriolar vasodilation with a reduction in arterial pressure. This fall in pressure is sufficient to cause hypotension. The maximum vascular effect occurs in 5 minutes.

Vasodilation causes a fall in systolic, diastolic, and pulse pressure. The acute reaction tends to disappear after 2 to 4 days of continuous exposure because of compensatory mechanisms from an increase in vascular tone. Dilation of the coronary arteries leads to increased flow in epicardial vessels and through eccentric stenoses and collaterals. A decrease in left ventricular end-diastolic pressure enhances subendocardial blood flow.

Pharmacokinetics

ABSORPTION

- Nitroglycerin is readily absorbed through the mucous membranes, lung, and intact skin.
- When tablets are ingested or swallowed rapidly they cause little toxic effect as the drug is extracted rapidly and metabolized in the liver. Nitroglycerin poisoning therefore is rare after oral ingestion unless very large doses are involved.
- When taken sublingually or transdermally, the drug does not pass through the liver before entering the general circulation.

DISTRIBUTION

- Nitroglycerin is 60% bound to plasma proteins at plasma concentrations between 50 to 500 ng/mL.
- The apparent volume of distribution is 2.6 to 3.3 L/kg.

ELIMINATION

- Poisoning usually occurs from injection, inhalation, or absorption via mucous membranes or skin.
- The plasma half-life of nitroglycerin is minutes.
- Reactive hydrolysis in the liver leads to the formation of the free nitric oxide (NO) radical.

Clinical Presentations

Exposure to nitroglycerin among dynamite workers (and family members who have laundered their clothes) has led to headaches, flushing, palpitations, nausea, vomiting, weakness, prostration, drowsiness, diaphoresis, and dizziness. Headaches may last from hours to days. Restlessness and an inability to lie quietly are frequently present. Impaired vision, diarrhea, and abdominal pain may accompany the headache.

Tolerance develops after 3 to 4 days of exposure, but is lost after 2 days away from work. Some workers have tried to avoid the Monday headache by placing nitroglycerin under their hatbands over the weekend, sucking occasionally on a piece of dynamite, or inhaling the fumes from their work clothes. Headaches also have occurred in workers who make rocket propellants or nitroglycerin pharmaceuticals.

Nitroglycerin ointment and patches may cause local skin irritation. Eruptions of the palms and interdigital spaces and ulcers under the nails have been observed in workers handling nitroglycerin. Use of nitroglycerin sprays has lead to syncope, hypotension, and unconsciousness.

NITROPATCH EXPLOSIONS

Defibrillation performed over a nitroglycerin transdermal skin patch may result in an explosive noise, a flash of light, yellow smoke with a discoloration of the patch, superficial skin discoloration, and superficial burn injuries. The aluminized plastic in the skin patch acts as a conductor of the electrical arc between the defibrillation pad and the skin. Transdermal nitroglycerin systems should be removed before attempting defibrillation or cardioversion.

Toxic Dosage/Death

Sudden unexpected deaths have occurred after exposure to nitroglycerin and ethylene glycol dinitrate, components of dynamite since the early 1930s. All deaths occurred suddenly after a period of freedom from exposure (48 to 60 hours) before starting work again, often on a Sunday night or on Monday morning. Deaths occurred in young healthy men between the ages of about 25 to 50 years. Deaths were attributed to coronary artery disease, but coronary atherosclerosis was minimal or absent.

Drug Interactions

Serious and prolonged hypotension may follow exposure to nitroglycerin in those who are concurrently receiving calcium-channel blockers, antihypertensive agents, phenothiazines, and/or tricyclic antidepressants. Use of alcohol with nitroglycerin exposure may produce severe hypotension and collapse or may induce aberrant destructive behavior.

As noted above, nitroglycerin plus ethylene glycol dinitrate may cause death as well as Raynaud's phenomenon and peripheral neuropathy. Hallucinations, depression, mania, epilepsy, paresthesias, transient hemiparesis, and aphasia also have been observed. Hypoxia resulting from methemoglobinemia may lead to cyanosis, metabolic acidosis, coma, convulsions, and cardiovascular collapse.

Pregnancy/Lactation

No data are available on breast feeding. The use of nitroglycerin in pregnancy is limited, however it has been classified as pregnancy risk category B.

Laboratory

ANALYTIC METHODS

Nitroglycerin and its dinitrate metabolites in human plasma may be quantitated by high-performance liquid chromatography with thermal energy analyzer detection.

BLOOD LEVELS

An average plasma concentration of 2.3 ng/mL was observed 1 hour after dermal application of 45 mg of nitroglycerin as an ointment. Following nitroglycerin in overdose has not been reported.

Treatment

GUT DECONTAMINATION

Following ingestion, activated charcoal and cathartics may be useful, but there is scant clinical data to support this treatment.

ELIMINATION ENHANCEMENT

There are no definitive extracorporeal methods to help eliminate or decrease the morbidity associated with nitroglycerin.

SUPPORTIVE MEASURES

- In severe overdoses, oxygen delivery should be assured with attention to circulatory status, maintenance of an adequate airway, and assisted ventilation as required.
- Cardiac monitoring in a coronary care unit should continue for at least 48 hours, depending on the clinical status. Treatment is largely symptomatic and supportive. Patients with preexisting cardiovascular disease will require special consideration of cardiac and pulmonary function.
- Hypotension is treated by elevating the legs, administration of intravenous fluids, and if necessary, dopamine or norepinephrine. An α-adrenoceptor agonist (e.g., phenylephrine) also may be considered. Patients with normal or low pulmonary capillary wedge pressure may be particularly sensitive to the hypotensive effects of nitroglycerin.
- Methemoglobinemia up to 30% has been reported following exposure to nitroglycerin and EGDN. Methemoglobinemia is managed with methylene blue (1 to 2 mg/kg) intravenously, and oxygen. Methemoglobin levels should be repeated in 1 to 2 hours after initial therapy to assess effectiveness of methemoglobin reduction.
- Leukopenia and abnormal liver function tests have been observed.
- After skin contact with nitroglycerin, thorough washing with soap is necessary. Sodium thiosulfate (10% solution) has been used for this purpose.

Questions—Nitroglycerin

1. **Nitroglycerin**
   A. Was discovered by Alfred Nobel
   B. Is the same as dynamite
   C. Is used to produce explosions and to treat angina
   D. Has been associated with sudden death when mixed with cyclonite
   E. A and C
2. **Nitroglycerin does not** cause
   A. Disabling headaches
   B. Thready pulse

C. Hypertensive crises
D. Venodilation
E. Restlessness and weakness

3. Nitroglycerin is absorbed readily through the mucous membranes, lung, and intact skin.
A. True
B. False

4. Nitropatches can explode if bent or applied to extremely febrile patients.
A. True
B. False

VASOPRESSORS

DOBUTAMINE

Dobutamine (Dobutrex®) is used parenterally for inotropic support in the short-term treatment of adults with cardiac decompensation. Decompensation may be from depressed contractility resulting from organic heart disease or from cardiac surgical procedures. In doses that produce similar increases in cardiac output, dobutamine may produce a smaller increase in heart rate than isoproterenol, a smaller decrease in peripheral resistance, and a smaller decrease in diastolic blood pressure.

The relative value of dobutamine and dopamine in patients with congestive heart failure remains to be thoroughly established. Dobutamine may be useful in reversing hemodynamic compromise produced by early administration of β-adrenergic blocking agents in patients with myocardial infarction. Dobutamine hydrochloride is a synthetic catecholamine and an inotropic agent with modest peripheral vasodilating properties.

Pathophysiology

Dobutamine exerts its cardiovascular action through β-1 adrenergic agonist activity. It also induces α-1 adrenoceptor vasoconstriction and β-2 adrenoceptor-mediated vasodilation. Dobutamine has no action on dopamine receptors. Unlike dopamine, dobutamine does not cause release of endogenous norepinephrine.

Pharmacokinetics

ABSORPTION

- Dobutamine is inactive after oral administration because of extensive presystemic metabolism in the gastrointestinal mucosa and the liver.
- Its duration of action is less than 10 minutes.

DISTRIBUTION

- Dobutamine has an apparent volume of distribution of 0.20 L/kg in patients with low-output cardiac failure.
- In children post-open heart surgery, the volume of distribution is 3.2 L/kg.

ELIMINATION

- The plasma half-life of dobutamine is about 2 minutes.
- Dobutamine is metabolized in the liver and other tissues to an inactive compound.
- Conjugates of dobutamine are excreted mainly in the urine.

Clinical Presentations

Dobutamine excess decreases systemic vascular resistance and may cause hypotension and oliguria. Other effects may include supraventricular tachycardia, stuffy nose, hoarseness, red warm skin, anxiety, tachypnea, palpitations, chest pain, paresthesias of the upper extremities, enuresis, and urinary incontinence. Signs and symptoms usually clear within 2 hours. Commercial dobutamine solution contains sodium bisulfite, which can induce allergic-type reactions (including anaphylaxis) in sulfite-sensitive individuals (frequently seen in asthmatics).

Positive inotropic and chronotropic effects of dobutamine on the myocardium can cause hypertension, tachyrhythmias, myocardial ischemia, and ventricular fibrillation. Patients with decompensated ventricular failure who have been hemodynamically stabilized with dobutamine can develop intolerance to dobutamine withdrawal. Withdrawal can cause dyspnea, hypertension, and/or deterioration of renal function.

Toxic Dosage/Death

Few patients with dobutamine overdose have been reported. Toxic symptoms and signs usually are related to excessive cardiac β-receptor stimulation. Patients who have received 40 μg/kg/min and 70 μg/kg/min have survived. A 47-year-old who inadvertently received 130 μg/kg/min for 30 minutes survived without sequelae. A fatal dose has not been determined.

Drug Interactions

Theoretically, the cardiac effects of dobutamine may be antagonized by β-blocking agents such as propranolol, resulting in unopposed α-adrenergic effects and increased peripheral resistance. Ventricular arrhythmias have occurred in animals receiving dobutamine during halothane or cyclopropane anesthesia. There is some evidence that nitroprusside and organic nitrates may be additive to dobutamine, resulting in a higher cardiac output and a lower pulmonary wedge pressure than use of either drug alone.

Pregnancy/Lactation

Safe use of dobutamine during pregnancy has not been established. It is not known whether dobutamine crosses the placenta. Pregnancy risk category C.

Laboratory

ANALYTIC METHODS

A high-performance liquid chromatography method with electrochemical detection is available for quantitative dobutamine assays. A radioenzymatic assay also has been developed.

BLOOD LEVELS

Infusion of 2 μg/kg/min produces a serum dobutamine level of approximately 20 ng/mL in about 10 minutes. As the half-life is so short and lab turnaround time generally is lengthy, following dobutamine levels in overdose is not useful.

Treatment

GUT DECONTAMINATION

If an overdose has been ingested orally, consider use of activated charcoal, however there has been no clinical evidence to support the use of syrup of ipecac, gastric lavage, activated charcoal, or cathartics after an oral dobutamine overdose.

ELIMINATION ENHANCEMENT

Forced diuresis, peritoneal dialysis, hemodialysis, and charcoal hemoperfusion have not been evaluated in the treatment of an overdose of dobutamine hydrochloride.

SUPPORTIVE MEASURES

- Careful monitoring of vital signs is the mainstay of treatment. Dobutamine should be stopped after an overdose until the patient stabilizes, at which time it may be reintroduced at a lower dose.
- An airway should be established, a supply of oxygen ensured, and respirations monitored and supported. Vital signs, blood pressure, and, where possible, central venous pressure and pulmonary wedge pressure may be monitored.
- Patients should not be discharged or transferred until serial electrocardiograms and cardiac enzymes show no evidence of myocardial damage.
- Dobutamine withdrawal signs and symptoms have been ameliorated by hydralazine 25 mg before the first reduction in the dobutamine infusion, and every 4 hours to a maximal dose of 150 mg.
- Dobutamine, like other β-2 agonists, may produce a mild reduction in serum potassium concentrations, rarely to hypokalemic levels.

Questions—Dobutamine

1. Dobutamine exerts its cardiovascular action through β-1 adrenergic agonist activity, α-1 vasoconstriction, β-2 vasodilation, and dopaminergic stimulation.
A. True
B. False

2. All of the following about dobutamine are true, except
A. Dobutamine excess decreases systemic vascular resistance and may cause hypotension.
B. Dobutamine effects may include supraventricular tachycardia, stuffy nose, hoarseness, anxiety, tachypnea, palpitations, and chest pain.
C. Signs and symptoms usually clear within minutes.
D. Commercial dobutamine solution contains sodium bisulfite, which can induce allergic reactions.
E. Patients with decompensated ventricular failure who have been hemodynamically stabilized with dobutamine can develop intolerance to dobutamine withdrawal.

DOPAMINE AND NOREPINEPHRINE

Dopamine hydrochloride (Intropin®) is indicated for the correction of shock as a result of myocardial infarction, trauma, endotoxic septicemia, open heart surgery, renal failure, and congestive heart failure. It is useful in conditions caused by poor perfusion of vital organs, low cardiac output, and hypotension.

Dopamine is a catecholamine and pressor agent and the immediate precursor of norepinephrine. When administered intravenously it stimulates dopaminergic receptors at low doses, β receptors in higher doses, and α-adrenergic receptor sites at even higher doses. Alpha stimulation induces peripheral vasoconstriction, which may compromise the peripheral arterial circulation and can lead to gangrene.

Norepinephrine (Levophed®) also is used to treat shock and hypotension induced by drugs such as the tricyclic antidepressants and phenothiazines. Like dopamine, norepinephrine must be administered into a large vein. Few cases of accidental overdose with these agents have been reported, but tissue extravasations have required infiltration of the antidote, phentolamine. Fatalities have occurred in association with dopamine overdose. See Chapter 37, Dopaminergic Drugs, for a discussion of drugs that also stimulate dopaminergic receptors.

Pathophysiology

The effects that dopamine produces in the body are directly related to its actions on α, β, and dopaminergic receptor sites. When these receptors are stimulated, cAMP levels rise, increasing calcium transport into the cell.

The amount of dopamine determines which receptors are predominantly stimulated. Low-dose dopamine (0.5 to 1.5 μg/kg/min) results mainly in stimulation of D_1 and D_2 dopaminergic receptors. D_1 receptors are located on vascular smooth muscle and participate in renal, mesenteric, cerebral, and coronary vascular dilation. D_2 receptors are located on postganglionic sympathetic nerve endings and autonomic ganglia. D_2 agonists inhibit norepinephrine release from sympathetic nerve endings. Blood pressure remains stable or may decrease. Renal plasma flow, glomerular filtration rate, and sodium excretion usually increase.

At moderate doses (2 to 5 μg/kg/min), β-1 effects on the myocardium predominate. Myocardial contractility, heart rate, and cardiac output increase. At infusion rates greater than 5 to 10 μg/kg/min, α stimulation predominates, resulting in peripheral vasoconstriction and a rise in blood pressure. At infusion rates greater than 20 μg/kg/min, the vasoconstrictive α effect can exceed the β-1 effect.

Norepinephrine is the vasopressor of choice for drugs that cause α-blockade (e.g., phenothiazines, tricyclic antidepressants) and that inhibit dopamine β-hydroxylase (e.g., disulfiram). It is a naturally occurring catecholamine with potent α and β-1 properties, which causes both peripheral vascular constriction and increased cardiac contractility. High doses cause intense vasoconstriction, which increases blood pressure but decreases tissue perfusion. Low doses may be added to medium-range dopamine doses for refractory hypotension, but close hemodynamic monitoring is advised to assess efficacy accurately.

Pharmacokinetics

ABSORPTION

- Dopamine is inactivated after oral administration and therefore is administered only by the intravenous route.
- Steady-state plasma concentrations of dopamine are achieved in 5 to 10 minutes.

DISTRIBUTION

- As a normal plasma constituent, 99% of dopamine is conjugated to sulfate. Following IV administration, dopamine is distributed rapidly with a volume of distribution of 0.9 L/kg.
- Infants and young children appear to require larger weight-normalized dosages of dopamine to achieve effects comparable to those in adults. Dopamine does not cross the blood-

brain barrier and therefore does not affect D_1 and D_2 receptors in the central nervous system.
- The duration of action of epinephrine is 1 to 2 minutes.

ELIMINATION

- Dopamine is eliminated from the plasma with a half-life of about 9 minutes. The pharmacologic half-life of an IV bolus dose is about 2 minutes, and the duration of action is about 10 minutes.
- Dopamine and norepinephrine are metabolized extensively in the liver, partially by monoamine oxidase. Dopamine is the immediate precursor of norepinephrine.
- Less than 10% of a dopamine dose is recovered unchanged in the urine. The lungs clear about 20%.

Clinical Presentations

Patients with prior vascular disease may be subject to ischemic effects from the α vasoconstriction induced by dopamine. Such ischemic effects often begin after 24 hours of dopamine use and may progress to gangrene of an extremity. Bilateral retinal infarctions have been reported. Extravasation and infiltration of dopamine may lead to ischemia, gangrene, and amputation of an extremity. Other toxic effects include ectopic beats, conduction abnormalities, flushing, anxiety, headache, nausea, vomiting, mydriasis, and vertigo.

Toxic effects from norepinephrine may include arrhythmias, palpitations, chest pain, anxiety, nausea, vomiting, and ischemic necrosis with tissue extravasation. Headache, uterine contractions, and diaphoresis also may be seen.

Toxic Dosage/Death

Intravenous dopamine in dosages greater than 10 μg/kg/min may induce sufficient α-adrenergic stimulation to cause excessive peripheral vasoconstriction and gangrene. Infiltration of dopamine into tissues following extravasation at 5.9 and 7.0 μg/kg/min has lead to amputation of extremities. A 1-day-old, premature infant who received an overdose of 125 μg/kg/min during a 1-hour period, died within 1 hour.

Drug Interactions

Monoamine oxidase inhibitors may prolong and intensify the effects of dopamine as dopamine is metabolized by monoamine oxidase. The cardiac effects of dopamine are antagonized by β-blockers such as propranolol and metoprolol. α-blocking agents antagonize the peripheral vasoconstriction caused by high doses of dopamine.

Ventricular arrhythmias and hypertension may occur when therapeutic doses of dopamine are administered during halothane or cyclopropane anesthesia. Intravenous phenytoin infused into patients receiving dopamine may result in hypotension and bradycardia. Ergot alkaloids, tricyclic antidepressants, and guanethidine may potentiate pressor responses to dopamine. Monoamine oxidase (MAO) inhibitors, ergot alkaloids, and antihistamines may potentiate the effect of norepinephrine.

Pregnancy/Lactation

Dopamine has been placed in pregnancy risk category C. There are no adequate and well-controlled studies in pregnant women. Dopamine is unlikely to be excreted in breast milk. Norepinephrine has been classified as pregnancy risk category D.

Laboratory

ANALYTIC METHODS

Dopamine in plasma may be measured by high-performance liquid chromatography using electrochemical detection with a carbon paste electrode. A radioenzymatic assay also is available.

BLOOD LEVELS

A so-called "renal dose" of dopamine (3 μg/kg/min) corresponds to a plasma level of 57 μg/L. This is higher than the usual baseline plasma level, which affects most metabolic and cardiovascular variables.

Treatment

GUT DECONTAMINATION

As dopamine is used as an intravenous drug, these interventions are not relevant to the treatment of dopamine overdose.

ELIMINATION ENHANCEMENT

These methods have not been utilized in the management of dopamine or norepinephrine overdose.

SUPPORTIVE MEASURES

- Patients receiving dopamine and/or norepinephrine should be under careful observation in a health care facility with continued cardiac monitoring.
- Urine flow and fluid balance should be measured carefully and determinations of cardiac output and pulmonary wedge pressure are useful.
- In case of accidental dopamine or norepinephrine overdose, as evidenced by an excessive blood pressure elevation, the rate of administration should be reduced or the infusion temporarily discontinued until the patient's condition stabilizes. Additional remedial measures usually are not necessary.
- Peripheral arterial pulses and extremity color must be monitored continuously during dopamine and norepinephrine infusions, especially in elderly patients with preexisting vascular damage from arteriosclerosis, diabetes mellitus, Raynaud's disease, or frostbite.
- Intravenous chlorpromazine 10 mg as a loading dose and 0.6 mg/min drip has been used for digital ischemia following dopamine use. Further clinical trials with this medication are indicated.

Antidotes

PHENTOLAMINE

To prevent sloughing and necrosis in ischemic areas after inadvertent skin extravasation of dopamine, the affected area should be infiltrated as soon as possible with 10 to 15 mL of a saline solution containing 5 to 10 mg of phentolamine. A syringe with a fine hypodermic needle should be used, and the solution liberally infiltrated throughout the ischemic area. Sympathetic blockade with phentolamine causes immediate and conspicuous local hyperemic changes if the area is infiltrated within 12 hours.

Blood pressure must be monitored carefully following phentolamine use, and the patient observed for development of arrhythmias and tachycardia. Giving multiple small doses over a period of 1 to 2 hours may minimize the possible risk of phentolamine-induced hypotension.

Questions—Dopamine And Norepinephrine

1. **The effects that dopamine produces in the body are related directly to its actions on α, β, and dopaminergic receptor sites. Low-dose dopamine stimulates α receptors. At moderate doses, β-1 effects on the myocardium predominate. At high doses, dopaminergic effects result.**
   A. True
   B. False

2. **Which of the following about norepinephrine is false?**
   A. Dopamine is a catecholamine and pressor agent and the precursor of norepinephrine.
   B. Norepinephrine is used to treat shock and hypotension induced by drugs such as the tricyclic antidepressants and phenothiazines.
   C. Like dopamine, norepinephrine must be administered into a large vein.
   D. Multiple cases of accidental overdose with norepinephrine have been reported.
   E. Tissue extravasations of norepinephrine have required infiltration of the antidote, phentolamine.

LIPID-LOWERING DRUGS

The lipid-lowering drugs are effective in lowering serum cholesterol levels. Recent data indicates that certain lipid-lowering drugs may reduce cardiovascular morbidity or mortality. Chronic usage of certain lipid-lowering drugs may lead to gastrointestinal complaints, hepatotoxicity, skin rashes, myopathies, eye toxicity, depression, and sleep disturbance. Overdose may result in myalgias, chest pain, blurred vision, nausea, and diarrhea. Treatment is largely supportive.

Lovastatin (Mevacor®) is a metabolite derived from the fungus *Aspergillus terreus*. Simvastatin (Zocor™) is a chemical derivative of lovastatin. Pravastatin (Pravachol®) is produced by microbial transformation of compactin by *Nocardia autotropica*. Fluvastatin (Lescol®) is a synthetic mevalonolactone derivative. Bezafibrate, clofibrate (Atromid-S®) and probucol are synthetic chemicals. Acipimox is related chemically to nicotinic acid and has been used in hypertriglyceridemic states.

Pathophysiology

These drugs are categorized as fibric acids (e.g., clofibrate, gemfibrozil, fenofibrate, and bezafibrate), HMG-CoA reductase-inhibiting drugs (e.g., lovastatin, simvastatin, pravastatin, and fluvastatin), probucol, and nicotinic acid analogs (e.g., niacin and acipimox). HMG-CoA reductase-inhibiting drugs are competitive inhibitors of HMG-CoA reductase, which catalyzes the conversion of HMG-CoA to mevalonate. They primarily act in the liver, where they reduce cholesterol synthesis. This, in turn, increases the number of hepatic low-density lipoprotein receptors, resulting in an overall decrease in total blood cholesterol, low-density lipoproteins, triglycerides, and very low-density lipoprotein cholesterol.

Pharmacokinetics

Lovastatin

- Plasma concentration peaks within 2 to 4 hours.
- Only 5% of an oral dose reaches the circulation because of first-pass hepatic extraction.
- Lovastatin is detected in the cerebrospinal fluid.

Pravastatin

- Mean time to reach peak plasma concentration after a single dose is 0.9 to 1.6 hours.
- Bioavailability is 12% to 34% because of a first-pass effect.
- The volume of distribution of pravastatin is 0.54 to 0.9 L/kg. 50% of the drug is protein bound.
- Metabolites of pravastatin have 2% to 10% of the potency of the parent drug. About 80% are excreted in 24 hours. The terminal elimination half-life is 1.3 to 2.6 hours.

Acipimox

- Is readily absorbed from the gastrointestinal tract. Plasma concentration peaks within 2 hours.
- It does not bind to plasma proteins. The plasma half-life is about 2 hours.
- Acipimox is not significantly metabolized and is excreted in the urine unchanged.

Probucol

- There is no correlation between plasma levels of probucol and the degree of serum cholesterol reduction. Probucol accumulates in the adipose tissue and may persist there and in the circulation for more than 6 months. It is eliminated mainly in the bile and feces.

Clinical Presentations

Therapeutic adverse effects seen with HMG-CoA reductase-inhibiting drugs include headache, abdominal pain, diarrhea, nausea, fatigue, rash, myopathy, hepatotoxicity, depression, eye toxicity, paresthesias, neuropathy, and pancreatitis. Long-term treatment with HMG-CoA reductase inhibitors, including lovastatin and simvastatin, is a potential cause of the drug-induced lupus syndrome. Transient symptomatic hypotension and nephrotoxicity have been observed after long-term treatment with simvastatin. Contrary to initial concerns, no cataractogenesis has been observed with pravastatin, simvastatin, or lovastatin. Paresthesias and neuropathies have been described after use of simvastatin and gemfibrozil.

Two large trials suggested an increased incidence of malignant disease, particularly of the liver, gallbladder, and rectum, and an increased incidence of ectopic ventricular activity, angina, and intermittent claudication with clofibrate. Bezafibrate is related structurally to clofibrate and has been associated with cholelithiasis, a disorder frequently observed with hyperlipoproteinemia. Acute renal failure and interstitial nephritis have been reported after clofibrate treatment. Most adverse reactions reported with niacin and acipimox include transient flushing and mild gastrointestinal disturbances.

Toxic Dosage/Death

Fatal doses have not been reported with these drugs.

Drug Interactions

Skeletal muscle toxicity is observed rarely when HMG-CoA reductase inhibitors are administered alone, but is increased in patients who also are receiving cyclosporine, fibric acid derivatives, niacin, or erythromycin. Some patients who have received lovastatin in combination with gemfibrozil, niacin, or cyclosporine have developed rhabdomyolysis. The fibric acid derivatives (e.g., gemfibrozil) appear to potentiate the action of Coumadin® anticoagulants because they bind extensively to plasma albumin, which displaces other acidic drugs.

Lovastatin potentiates the effect of warfarin because it is strongly protein bound and may displace warfarin from its binding sites. Concurrent use of cimetidine, ranitidine, or omeprazole increases the serum concentration of fluvastatin. Cholestyramine decreases the bioavailability of pravastatin, but may enhance its lipid-lowering effect. Acipimox is synergistic with cholestyramine as a lipid-lowering agent.

Pregnancy/Lactation

Lovastatin and simvastatin have been placed in pregnancy risk category X. Studies in animals or human beings have demonstrated fetal abnormalities and the drug is contraindicated in women who are, or may become pregnant. An anecdotal report suggests congenital abnormalities in an infant whose mother received lovastatin in the first trimester of pregnancy. Negligible amounts of pravastatin are found in breast milk. Clofibrate is pregnancy risk category C.

Treatment

GUT DECONTAMINATION

Lavage and/or charcoal may be helpful with these agents.

ELIMINATION ENHANCEMENT

These methods have not been utilized to treat overdose with the lipid-lowering agents.

SUPPORTIVE MEASURES

- Elevations in hepatic function tests (e.g., alkaline phosphatase, transaminases) and creatine kinase have been observed after therapeutic doses of HMG-CoA reductase-inhibiting drugs.
- Torsade de Pointes following probucol use may respond to magnesium, propranolol, overdrive pacing, isoproterenol and/or cardioversion.
- Persons who have overdosed on HMG-CoA inhibitors should be observed for symptoms suggestive of myopathy (muscle tenderness, weakness, or pain), rhabdomyolysis (darkened urine), or hepatotoxicity (anorexia, abdominal pain, and jaundice).

Questions—Lipid Lowering Drugs

1. **Overdose with lipid-lowering drugs may manifest all of the symptoms below except**
   A. Seizures
   B. Chest pain
   C. Nausea, vomiting, and diarrhea
   D. Myalgias
   E. Visual disturbances

2. **Chronic toxicities of lipid lowering drugs include**
   A. Hepatic toxicity
   B. Cataracts
   C. Drug-induced lupus
   D. Gastritis/peptic ulcer disease
   E. A and C

3. **Lipid-lowering drugs potentiate the effect of Coumadin® because of protein binding.**
   A. True
   B. False

4. **Lovastatin is contraindicated in pregnancy because of the risk of fetal malformations.**
   A. True
   B. False

5. **The most important laboratory assessment of a patient overdosing with an HMG-CoA is/are**
   A. Electrocardiogram for conduction delays
   B. Creatine phosphokinase for rhabdomyolysis
   C. Liver function tests for hepatotoxicity
   D. B and C
   E. All of the above

CASE STUDY (QUESTIONS 6 AND 7)

A 52-year-old male with a history of hyperlipidemia and hypertension has been taking simvastatin for approximately 9 months for his elevated cholesterol. He presents with complaints of fatigue, nausea, and myalgias. His mild hypertension is managed with salt restriction. He is otherwise healthy. Examination is completely normal.

6. **Useful laboratory data to help define the underlying etiology would include all except**
   A. Creatine phosphokinase
   B. Rheumatoid factor
   C. Antinuclear antibody
   D. Liver function tests
   E. Blood-urea nitrogen and creatinine

7. **You discover that his creatine phosphokinase is elevated moderately at approximately 1800 U/L. He also remembers that he recently was given a medication at a walk-in clinic for "cough and congestion." Which of the medications listed below would be suspicious for a precipitating factor?**
   A. Amoxicillin
   B. Bactrim double strength
   C. Pseudoephedrine
   D. Erythromycin
   E. A and C

8. **HMG-CoA reductase-inhibiting drugs**
   A. Competitively inhibit HMG-CoA transferase
   B. Act primarily in the kidneys
   C. Increase the number of hepatic low-density lipoprotein receptors
   D. Increase low-density lipoproteins
   E. Increase very low-density lipoprotein cholesterol

9. **Long-term treatment with simvastatin is associated with all of the following, except**
   A. Drug-induced lupus syndrome
   B. Transient symptomatic hypotension
   C. Nephrotoxicity
   D. Cataractogenesis
   E. Paresthesias

10. **Skeletal muscle toxicity often is observed when HMG Co-A reductase inhibitors**
    A. Are administered alone
    B. Are given to patients also receiving cyclosporin
    C. Are given to patients also receiving erythromycin
    D. A and B
    E. B and C

11. Clofibrate has been shown to increase incidence of all of the following, except
A Renal malignancy
B. Liver malignancy
C. Rectal malignancy
D. Angina
E. Intermittent claudication

12. Fatal ingestions of lipid-lowering drugs
A. Are related to degree of hypercholesterolemia
B. Are related to cardiac function
C. Are related to history of alcoholism or liver disease
D. Have a variety of natural histories
E. Have not been reported

Answers

Introduction To Antiarrhythmic Drugs
1. C 2. C 3. B 4. A 5. A 6. C 7. A

Disopyramide
1. D 2. E

Procainamide
1. B 2. E

Quinidine
1. D 2. B 3. D 4. A

Lidocaine
1. B 2. A

Flecainide and Encainide
1. A 2. A 3. A 4. A 5. B

Propafenone
1. D

β-Blockers
1. E 2. E 3. D 4. D

Amiodarone And Bretylium
1. D 2. E

Calcium Channel Blockers
1. A 2. A 3. B 4. A

Digitalis
1. E 2. E 3. E

Adenosine
1. C 2. E

Angiotensin-Converting Enzyme Inhibitors
1. E 2. E

Clonidine
1. E 2. A

Thiazides
1. C 2. E

Loop Diuretics
1. A 2. A 3. A

Potassium-Sparing Diuretics
1. A

Acetazolamide
1. E 2. D 3. B

Mannitol
1. E

Sodium Nitroprusside
1. E, 2. D 3. A 4. B

Diazoxide
1. A 2. A 3. B

Hydralazine
1. B

Minoxidil
1. E 2. D

α-Blockers
1. E 2. E

Pentoxifylline
1. D

Nitroglycerin
1. E 2. C 3. A 4. B

Dobutamine
1. B 2. C

Dopamine and Norepinephrine
1. B 2. D

Lipid-Lowering Drugs
1. A 2. E 3. A 4. A 5. D 6. B 7. D,
8. C 9. D 10. E 11. A 12. E

SELECTED READINGS

Introduction to Antiarrhythmic Drugs

1. Ben-David J, Zipes DP. Torsade de Pointes and proarrhythmia. Lancet 1993; 341:1578–1582.
2. Campbell TJ. Proarrhythmic actions of antiarrhythmic drugs: A review. Aust NZ J Med 1990;20:275–282.

Disopyramide

1. Jaeger A, Sauder PH, Kopferschmitt J, et al. Acute disopyramide poisoning: A multicenter study of 106 cases. Vet Hum Toxicol 1982;24:285. Abstract.

Procainamide

1. Atkinson AJ, Krumlovsky FA, Huang CM, et al. Hemodialysis for severe procainamide toxicity. Clinical and pharmacokinetic observations. Clin Pharmacol Ther 1976;20:585–592.
2. Heiselman DE, Litman GI. Risk factors for procainamide-induced Torsade de Pointes. Clin Res 1986;34:7A.
3. Koch-Weser J, Klein SW. Procainamide dosage schedules, plasma concentrations and clinical effects. JAMA 1971;215:1454–1460.

Quinidine

1. Gaudreault P. Quinidine. Clin Toxicol Rev 1982;4(12):1–2.
2. Shub C. Gau GT, Sidell PM, et al. The management of acute quinidine intoxication. Chest 1978;73:173–178.

Lidocaine

1. Amitai Y, Whitesell L, Lovejoy FH Jr. Death following accidental lidocaine overdose in a child. N Engl J Med 1986;314:182–183.
2. Finkelstein F, Kreeft J. Massive lidocaine poisoning. N Engl N Med 1979;301:50.

Flecainide and Encainide

1. Levine B, Chute D, Caplan YH. Flecainide intoxication. J Anal Toxicol 1990; 14:335–336.
2. Pentel PR, Goldsmith SR, Salerno DM, et al. Effect of hypertonic sodium bicarbonate on encainide overdose. Am J Cardiol 1986;57:878–879.
3. Rosen DM, Woosely RL. Drug therapy: Flecainide. N Engl J Med 1986;315: 36–41.
4. Woosley RL, Wood AJJ, Roder DM. Encainide. N Engl J Med 1988;318:1107–1115.

Propafenone

1. Kerns W, English B, Ford M. Severe adult propafenone toxicity. Vet Hum Toxicol 1992;34:329.
2. Veale D, McComb JM, Gibson GJ. Propafenone. Lancet 1990;335:979.

β-Blockers

1. Agura ED, Wexler LF, Witzburg RA. Massive propranolol overdose: Successful treatment with high dose isoproterenol and glucagon. Am J Med 1986;180: 755–757.
2. Browning RG, Merigian KS. Acute beta blocker poisoning. Top Emerg Med 1993;15:1–14.
3. Miller A, White S. Survival following massive intravenous esmolol overdose. Clin Toxicol 1995;533:475–486.
4. Shanahan FLJ, Counihan TB. Atenolol self-poisoning. Br Med J 1978;2:773.

Amiodarone and Bretylium

1. Gibson JS, Munter DW. Intravenous bretylium overdoses. Am J Emerg Med 1995;13:177–79.
2. Goddard DJR, Whorwell PJ. Amiodarone overdose and its management. Br J Clin Pract 1989;34:184–186.
3. Martin WJ, Miller FA Jr. Amiodarone toxicity. Mayo Clin Proc 1985;60:638–639.

Calcium-Channel Blockers

1. Clark CF, Hanna TC. Calcium channel blocker toxicity. Top Emerg Med 1993; 15:15–26.
2. Jakubowski AT, Mizgala HF. Effect of diltiazem overdose. Am J Cardiol 1987; 60:932–933.
3. Ramoska EA, Spiller HA, Myers A. Calcium channel blocker toxicity. Ann Emerg Med 1990;19:649–653.
4. Watson NA, Fitzgerald CP. Management of massive verapamil overdose. Med J Aust 1991;155:124–125.

Digitalis

1. Dick M, Curwin J, Tepper D. Digitalis intoxication recognition and management. J Clin Pharmacol 1991;31:444–447.
2. Sharff JA, Bayer MJ. Acute and chronic digitalis toxicity: Presentation and treatment. Ann Emerg Med 1982;11:327–330.
3. Woolf A. Revising the management of digitalis poisoning. Clin Toxicol 1993; 31:275–276.
4. Woolf AD, Wenger T, Smith TW, Lovejoy FH Jr. The use of digoxin-specific Fab fragments for severe digitalis intoxication in children. N Engl J Med 1992; 326:1734–1744.
5. Woolf AD. Digoxin specific Fab antibody fragments. Clin Toxicol Rev 1991; 13(10):1–2.

Adenosine

1. Reed R, Falk JL, O'Brien J. Untoward reactions to adenosine therapy for supraventricular tachycardia. Am J Emerg Med 1991;9:566–570.
2. Roelke M, Yurchak PM. Adenosine and supraventricular tachycardia. N Engl J Med 1992;326: 1221.

Angiotensin-Converting Enzyme Inhibitors

1. Bauer JH, Reams GP. The angiotensin II type 1 receptor antagonists: A new class of antihypertensive drugs. Arch Intern Med 1995;155:1361–1368.
2. Hogue-Murray K, Horowitz R, Dart RC. Outcome of ACE inhibitor ingestion in children under the age of six years. ClinToxicol 1995;33:475–486.
3. Raia JJ Jr, Barone JA, Byerly WG, Lacy CR. Angiotensin-converting enzyme inhibitors: A comparative review. DICP Ann Pharmacother 1990;24:506–525.

Clonidine

1. Anderson RJ, Hart GR, Crumpler CP, et al. Clonidine overdose: Report of six cases and review of the literature. Ann Emerg Med 1981;10:107–112.
2. Conner CS, Watanabe AS. Clonidine overdose: A review. Am J Hosp Pharm 1979;36:906–11.
3. Henretig F, Wiley J, Brown L. Clonidine patch toxicity: The proof's in the poop! Clin Toxicol 1995;33:475–485.
4. Kulig K, Duffy J, Rumack BH. Naloxone for treatment of clonidine overdose. JAMA 1982;247:1697.
5. Traub SL. Clonidine for opiate withdrawal. Hosp Formul 1985;20:77–80.

Thiazides

1. Beermann G, Groschinsky-Grind M, Rosen A. Absorption metabolism and excretion of hydrochlorthiazide. Clin Pharmacol Ther 1976;19:531–537.
2. Long JW (ed). Clinical Management of Prescription Drugs. Philadelphia, Harper and Row, 1984, pp 425–442.

Loop Diuretics

1. Andreasen F, Hansen HE, Mikkelsen E. Pharmacokinetics of furosemide in anephric patients and in normal subjects. Eur J Clin Pharmacol 1978;13:41–48.
2. Ward A, Heel RC. Bumetanide. A review of its pharmacodynamic and pharmacokinetic properties and therapeutic use. Drugs 1984;28:426–464.

Potassium-Sparing Diuretics

1. Karim A. Spironolactone: Disposition, metabolism, pharmacodynamics and bioavailability. Drug Metab Rev 1978;8:151–188.
2. Pruitt AW, Winkel JS, Dayton PG. Variations in the fate of triamterene. Clin Pharmacol Ther 1977;21:610–619.

Acetazolamide

1. Heller I, Halvey J, Cohen S, et al. Significant metabolic acidosis induced by acetazolamide. Not a rare complication. Arch Intern Med 1985;145:1815–1817.
2. Kristinsson A. Fatal reaction to acetazolamide. Br J Ophthalmol 1967;51: 348–349.
3. Watson WA, Garrelts JC, Zinn PD, et al. Chronic acetazolamide intoxication. Clin Toxicol 1984/1985;22(6):549–563.

Mannitol

1. Nissenson AR, Weston RE, Kleeman CR. Mannitol. West J Med 1979;131: 277–284.
2. Smithline N, Gardner K Jr: Gaps. Anionic and osmolal. JAMA 1976;236:1594–1597.
3. Whelan TB, Bacon ME, Madden M, et al. Acute renal failure associated with mannitol intoxication. Report of a case. Arch Intern Med 1984;144:2053–2055.

Sodium Nitroprusside

1. McDowall DG, Keaney NP, Turner JM, et al. The toxicity of sodium nitroprusside. Br J Anaesth 1974;46:320–332.
2. Palmer RF, Lasseter KC. Sodium nitroprusside. N Engl J Med 1975;272:294–297.
3. Tinker JH, Michenfelder JD. Sodium nitroprusside: Pharmacology, toxicology and therapeutics. Anesthesiology 1976;45:340–354.

Diazoxide

1. Koch-Weser J. Diazoxide. N Engl J Med 1976;294:1271–1274.

Hydralazine

1. Koch-Weser J. Hydralazine. N Engl J Med 1976;295:320–323.

Minoxidil

1. Isles C, Mackay A, Barton PJM, et al. Accidental overdose of minoxidil in a child. Lancet 1981;1:97.
2. Lowe GDO. Vasodilators: Minoxidil and drugs used in peripheral vascular and cerebral disorders. Br Med J 1983:286:1262–1264.

α-Blockers

1. Lenz K, Druml W, Kleinberger G, et al. Acute intoxication with prazosin: A case report. Hum Toxicol 1985;4:53–56.
2. Mack RB. Taljaribu kila dawa isifal: Yohimbe intoxication. NC Med J 1985;46: 229–230.

Pentoxifylline

1. Garnier R, Riboulet-Delmas G, Chatenet T, Efthymiou ML. Acute pentoxifylline poisoning in children. Ann Pediatr (Paris) 1986;33:62–63.
2. Radack K, Wyderski AJ. Conservative management of intermittent claudication. Ann Intern Med 1990;113:134–146.

Nitroglycerin

1. Anon. The effects of nitroglycerin upon those who manufacture it. JAMA 1898; 31:793–794.
2. Bresler RR. Nitroglycerin reactions among pharmaceutical workers. Ind Med 1949;18:519–523.
3. Laws CE. Nitroglycerin head. JAMA 1910;54:793.
4. Rabinowitch IM. Acute nitroglycerin poisoning. Can Med Assoc J 1944;50: 199–202.

Dobutamine

1. Goethals M, Demey H. Massive dobutamine overdose in a cardiovascular compromised patient. Acta Cardiol 1984;39:373–378.
2. Majerus TC, Dasta JF, Bauman JL, et al. Dobutamine: Ten years later. Pharmacotherapy 1989;9:245–249.
3. Mutnick AH, Szymusiak-Mutnick B, Drea EJ. Dopamine versus dobutamine: Are all the facts there? Pharmacotherapy 1990;10:224–229.

Dopamine and Norepinephrine

1. Cooper BE. High-dose phentolamine for extravasation of pressors. Clin Pharm 1989;8:689.
2. Ebels TJ, Homan van der Heide JN. Dopamine-induced ischaemia. Lancet 1977; 2:762.
3. McDonald RH, Goldberg LI, McNay JL. Effects of dopamine in man: Augmentation of sodium excretion, glomerular filtration rate and renal plasma flow. J Clin Invest 1964;43:1116–1124.

Lipid-Lowering Drugs

1. McTavish D, Sorkin EM. Pravastatin: A review of its pharmacological properties and therapeutic potential in hypercholesterolemia. Drugs 1991;42:65–89.
2. Pentikainen PJ, Saraheimo M, Schwartz JI, et al. Comparative pharmacokinetics of lovastatin, simvastatin, pravastatin in humans. J Clin Pharmacol 1992;32: 136–140.
3. Smellie WAS, Lorimer AR. Adverse effects of the lipid-lowering drugs. Adverse Drug React Toxicol Rev 1992;11:71–92.

ACKNOWLEDGMENTS

Thanks to Harry Stanger, MD for preparing the majority of questions in this chapter, and to Dina Kacandes, PT for organizing and typing them. Thanks to David Huckins, MD for contributing the lipid-lowering drugs questions.

CHAPTER 27
Anticonvulsant Drugs

INTRODUCTION

The toxicity of this diverse group of chemical compounds has been well described. Experience with anticonvulsant poisoning has resulted from chronic intoxications with poorly controlled therapeutic regimens, suicidal poisonings, and accidental poisonings in children and in patients with behavioral problems. Phenobarbital overdose as a suicide vehicle is well described. The necessity for frequent use of multiple drugs often results in multiple drug interactions.

The narrow therapeutic index of these drugs may yield dosages adequate to control seizures, but not low enough to avoid toxic effects. For many of the anticonvulsants, active metabolites may be of equal or greater clinical importance than the parent compound (e.g., primidone, methsuximide, mephobarbital, and metharbital). Clinical support of patients and not overreliance on laboratory values should dictate proper treatment in all cases.

Anticonvulsant Hypersensitivity Syndrome

Phenytoin, carbamazepine, primidone, and phenobarbital can all produce an identical, multisystem hypersensitivity reaction. The onset of this reaction is usually between 4 and 12 weeks of starting the drug. A patient who develops the syndrome with one anticonvulsant may develop it with other anticonvulsant drugs, even though the drugs may be pharmacologically distinct. The initial features are mucocutaneous eruptions and fever. The cutaneous eruptions include morbilliform rashes, erythema multiforme, exfoliative dermatitis, facial edema and toxic epidermal necrolysis.

Mucosal involvement may include conjunctivitis with scarring and synechiae. Lymphadenopathy, hepatitis, eosinophilia, and lymphocytosis are frequently observed. Nephritis, bone marrow suppression, pneumonitis, and myopathy have also been reported. Management includes discontinuation of the offending agent. The reaction appears to resolve quickly after initiation of prednisolone. Treatment is otherwise symptomatic and supportive.

Paradoxical Intoxication

"Paradoxical intoxication" may follow the use of an anticonvulsant agent that, at blood levels generally above the "therapeutic" range, induce seizures without the prior presence of the usually dose-related side effects. Exacerbation of seizures in adults and children may follow treatment with phenytoin, carbamazepine, benzodiazepines, and vigabatrin.

Pseudostatus Epilepticus

Some patients who present with apparent status epilepticus may in fact have pseudostatus epilepticus, a condition that mimics status epilepticus. These "seizures" are felt to be psychogenic. Pseudostatus epilepticus seizures are also called hysterical seizures, simulated seizures, pseudoseizures, and nonorganic seizures. The patient often does not have the classic features of convulsive seizures. There may be vocalization, bizarre behavior, and preservation of consciousness despite apparent convulsions. Incontinence, tongue biting, and cyanosis may occur but are less common than in true status epilepticus.

Often there is a long history of a personality disorder. The patient may have had hysterical features, such as nonorganic paralysis and suicidal gestures. The history of epilepsy is usually highly atypical, with an unusual pattern, odd responses to treatment, and normal or "non-specific" electroencephalographic recordings. In the record there is often evidence of earlier pseudoseizures.

Pregnancy/Lactation

There is an increased incidence of congenital malformations in children born to epileptic women who have taken anticonvulsant drugs during pregnancy. If a mother has epilepsy and is taking anticonvulsant drugs, her chance of having a child with a major congenital abnormality may be as high as 6%. Several studies suggest that abnormalities are more likely if more than one anticonvulsant is used or if particularly large doses are taken.

Questions—Introduction to Anticonvulsant Drugs

1. Which of the following statements is false?
   A. Experience with anticonvulsant poisoning has resulted from chronic intoxications with poorly controlled therapeutic regimens, suicidal poisonings, and accidental poisonings in children and in patients with behavioral problems.
   B. The wide therapeutic index of these drugs may yield dosages adequate to control seizures, but not low enough to avoid toxic effects.
   C. For many of the anticonvulsants, active metabolites may be of equal or greater clinical importance than the parent compound.
   D. Phenytoin, carbamazepine, primidone, and phenobarbital can all produce an identical, multisystem hypersensitivity reaction.
   E. Cutaneous signs of anticonvulsant hypersensitivity include morbilliform rashes, erythema multiforme, exfoliative dermatitis, facial edema and toxic epidermal necrolysis.

2. "Paradoxical intoxication" may follow the use of an anticonvulsant agent that, at blood levels generally above the "therapeutic" range, induce seizures without the prior presence of the usually dose-related side effects.
   A. True
   B. False

3. Pseudoseizures
   A. Mimic status epilepticus.
   B. Are also called hysterical seizures, simulated seizures, partial complex, and nonorganic seizures. The patient often does not have the classic features of convulsive seizures.
   C. May involve incontinence, tongue biting, and cyanosis, but these symptoms are less common than in true status epilepticus.
   D. A and B
   E. A and C

PHENYTOIN

Phenytoin (Dilantin®) is used to control tonic-clonic seizures and psychomotor (grand mal and temporal lobe) seizures. It is used for the prevention and treatment of seizures occurring during and after neurosurgery, and rarely as an antiarrhythmic in digitalis-induced ventricular arrhythmias. It may be a useful intravenous adjunct in tricyclic antidepressant overdose.

Phenytoin overdose in adults occurs accidentally and during suicide attempts, and in children who inadvertently swallow commercial products often used by a relative. More frequently, phenytoin intoxication occurs during long-term treatment of an epileptic whose physical status (disease states) has recently changed or who has added a new drug to his anticonvulsant regimen. Synonyms include DPH, diphenylhydantoin, and 5,5-diphenylhydantoin. Diphenylhydantoin is related to the barbiturates in chemical structure, but has a five-membered ring. Phenytoin is a synthetic chemical.

Phenytoin overdose is debilitating and is characterized by nystagmus, ataxia, and drowsiness in the initial and mild stages. Overdose is rarely fatal and is treated by immediately discontinuing phenytoin. There is no antidote. At high doses, phenytoin's half-life is increased, but gut decontamination procedures are probably the safest and most effective method of treatment. Methods used to enhance elimination are usually ineffective.

Pathophysiology

Phenytoin stabilizes membranes protecting the sodium pump. In the brain it suppresses seizure activity. In the heart it suppresses arrhythmias induced by digitalis and tricyclic antidepressants, and decreases automaticity of the sinoauricular (SA) node. Phenytoin also increases atrioventricular (AV) conduction. Phenytoin induces cytochrome P450 mixed function oxidases and inhibits insulin release.

Pharmacokinetics

ABSORPTION

- In therapeutic doses, absorption is slow because of the limited solubility of DPH in the gastrointestinal tract.
- In overdose patients, gastrointestinal absorption of DPH may continue for as long as 60 hours even after phenytoin suspension.
- A general decrease in the rate of dissolution with increasing dose leads to sustained serum concentrations at high doses.
- Absorption may be affected by the excipients used.
- Peak concentrations may occur as late as 24 hours.

Answers to questions in shaded boxes appear at the end of the chapter.

- Peak levels after intravenous administration occur in 10 minutes.
- Steady-state levels in serum are achieved after 6–9 days of treatment.

DISTRIBUTION

- The apparent volume of distribution is about 0.5–0.8 L/kg and the apparent volume of distribution for unbound (free) phenytoin is 5–6 L/kg.
- The volume of distribution in children (overdose) is 0.78 L/kg.
- Distribution is rapid to the central nervous system and to the cerebrospinal fluid.
- Protein binding of phenytoin is 87–93%.
- There is an inverse relationship between plasma albumin level and free DPH.

ELIMINATION

- Phenytoin is excreted in the urine as unchanged phenytoin (<4%), HPPH-glucuronide (23–70%), and m-hydroxyphenytoin conjugate (5%).
- It is also excreted in the feces as unchanged drug (5%).
- At therapeutic doses, metabolism is nonlinear (first-order kinetics). At toxic doses, metabolism is linear (zero-order kinetics), governed by saturable enzyme systems in the liver.
- The therapeutic half-life is 8–60 hours and is dose-dependent with considerable intraindividual variation. For practical purposes, an average half-life of 20–30 hours can be used. The half-life in overdosed adults has ranged from 24 to 230 hours.
- Elderly patients have increased plasma clearances correlating with decreases in plasma albumin and phenytoin binding. Increased clearance and increased free fraction of phenytoin counterbalance each other and therefore the dose is usually not altered in the elderly.

Clinical Presentations

The earliest signs of overdose with phenytoin include nystagmus on lateral gaze, ataxia, and drowsiness (generally at serum levels greater than 20-30 μg/mL). Onset of symptoms is usually within 1–2 hours of ingestion and may persist for 4–5 days. As blood levels increase above 30 μg/mL, nystagmus becomes vertical, speech becomes slurred, drowsiness is more intense, ataxia and lurching gait are observed, coarse tremors of the extremities or involuntary movement become apparent, and many patients cannot walk or even stand.

With increasing dose, consciousness is lessened and the patient becomes confused, disoriented, or even hyperactive or manic. The pupils may remain normal or become dilated and reactive; deep tendon reflexes may become briskly reactive. A totally unresponsive state or respiratory depression is unusual with phenytoin intoxication. If the patient is found in coma, a search should be made for additional drug(s).

NEUROLOGIC EFFECTS

Initially nystagmus, ataxia, and drowsiness occur. Other signs may include a coarse resting tremor, bilateral ankle clonus, myoclonic movements, an increase in deep tendon reflexes, extensor rigidity, opisthotonus, and/or seizures. Lurching gait, transient hemiparesis, inability to walk, choreoathetosis, slurred speech, confusion, hallucinations, hyperactivity, and paradoxical intoxication have been described. Pupils may be normal or dilated and reactive. Nystagmus on lateral gaze is noted. Nystagmus may initially be vertical and later horizontal.

CARDIOVASCULAR EFFECTS

Cardiovascular effects are seen with rapid intravenous infusion or massive oral overdose. Signs include a decrease in heart rate, an increase in atrioventricular block, a decrease in cardiac output that can lead to congestive heart failure in those with myocardial disease, direct myocardial depression, hypotension, idioventricular rhythm, ventricular fibrillation, asystole and death.

GASTROINTESTINAL EFFECTS

Nausea and vomiting occur in large overdose. Hepatitis with fever, lymphadenopathy and leukopenia may be observed, and may lead to fatal hepatic failure.

METABOLIC EFFECTS

Hyperglycemia may be seen in both diabetic and nondiabetic patients with ketoacidosis and/or glycosuria. This may progress to fatal hyperosmolar nonketotic coma. DPH displaces thyroxine from thyroxine binding globulin, liberating free thyroxine, which is converted to triiodothyronine. The decrease in free thyroxine may lead to symptoms of hypothyroidism.

HYPERSENSITIVITY EFFECTS

Hypersensitivity reactions occur with chronic phenytoin therapy and are not generally a part of the acute overdose clinical picture. Dermatologic symptoms may include systemic lupus erythematosus or Stevens-Johnson syndrome. Chronic use of phenytoin may induce gingival hyperplasia, megaloblastic anemia, and osteomalacia with hypocalcemia.

EXTRAVASATION

Injectable phenytoin is extremely alkaline (pH 12) and irritating to soft tissues when it extravasates from an intravenous infusion. It may also precipitate when it comes into contact with blood or glucose solution, and cause venous occlusion. Phenytoin should therefore be administered with glucose-free solutions. Propylene glycol, the water-miscible vehicle used to maintain phenytoin solution, is itself reported to be a tissue irritant.

Toxic Dosage/Death

Prolonged toxicity has followed the ingestion of 1.5 grams in a 6-year-old. An adult male survived after ingesting 7.5 grams of phenytoin. Blood levels greater than 95 μg/mL (total phenytoin) have been associated with death, although one child with a level of 108 μg/mL survived an accidental overdose. Deaths have been recorded at levels of 50–70 μg/mL.

Death is rare after phenytoin overdose and when it occurs it is usually due to cardiac arrest or ventricular fibrillation. Respiratory arrest is rare. Deaths have been reported in patients who have received intravenous phenytoin. Rapid manual infusion of phenytoin and inclusion of the infusion vehicle, propylene glycol, have been suggested as factors leading to hypotension and cardiac arrhythmias.

Drug Interactions

Many drugs elevate plasma phenytoin levels and increase phenytoin's half-life. These include ethanol, methylphenidate, disulfiram, miconazole, sulfadiazine, isoniazid, ethosuximide, dicumarol, methsuximide, chlorpromazine, imipramine, valproic acid, chlordiazepoxide, prochlorperazine, carbamazepine, phenobarbital, diazepam, propoxyphene, trimethoprim, phenylbutazone, sulfamethoxazole, cimetidine, chloramphenicol and thioridazine.

Many drugs decrease plasma phenytoin levels and decrease phenytoin's half-life. These include methotrexate, digitoxin, vinblastine, carmustine, metyrapone, levodopa, dexamethasone, DDT, doxycycline, cortisol, estrogens and oral contraceptives, methadone, phenobarbital, and carbamazepine.

Pregnancy/Lactation

During pregnancy, plasma clearance is often more than doubled, causing a decrease in plasma concentrations and increased dosage. This may be observed by the second month of pregnancy and is especially increased by the third trimester. Plasma monitoring is necessary.

DPH plasma concentrations from the umbilical artery or vein are almost identical to the maternal plasma concentration. The therapeutic plasma disappearance rate of phenytoin in newborns of mothers treated with phenytoin is in the same range as adults. Phenytoin is excreted into breast milk. Methemoglobinemia, drowsiness, and decreased sucking activity have been reported. Phenytoin is classified as pregnancy risk factor D.

Teratogenic effects with phenytoin use have been observed for over 20 years. Since the risk of congenital malformations among infants exposed in utero to antiepileptic drugs is estimated to be two to three times greater than in the general population, folic acid has been recommended as an addition to the regimen of an epileptic woman who wishes to become pregnant. Vitamin K is administered to the newborn.

Physical signs of "fetal hydantoin syndrome" may include chest abnormalities, congenital breast disease, widespread hypoplastic nipples, rib/sternal abnormality, performance deficits, mental retardation, ocular hypertelorism, craniofacial abnormalities, microcephaly, broad nasal bridge, cleft lip/palate, wide fontanelle, abnormal or low-set ears, low-set hairline, epicanthal folds, broad alveolar ridge, ptosis of eyelids, metopic ridging, coloboma, short neck, coarse scalp hair, limb abnormalities, small or absent nails, altered palmar crease, hypoplasia of distal phalanges, digital thumb, dislocated hip, acne vulgaris, hernia (umbilical or inguinal), optic nerve hypoplasia, hirsutism, abnormal genitalia, neuroblastoma, melanotic neuroectodermal tumor, and/or retinoschisis.

Laboratory

ANALYTIC METHODS

Radioimmunoassay methods for phenytoin can be performed with blood obtained from a finger prick. This assay is not altered by the presence of any other anticonvulsants. Enzyme-multiplied immunoassay technique (EMIT) methods are easy to perform. Gas-liquid chromatography and high-performance liquid chromatography methods are precise, but require a skilled laboratory technician.

BLOOD LEVELS

Doses must be individually titrated to produce maximum control of seizures. Seizure control is generally effective within the total plasma level range of 10–20 μg/mL. Toxic effects are usually not seen below 15 μg/mL. However, seizures may be more effectively controlled without side effects in some patients with phenytoin blood levels over 20 μg/mL.

Nystagmus, an early sign of DPH toxicity, can be seen below 20 μg/mL, and has been observed at levels ranging from 0.6 to 32 μg/mL. Fifty percent of patients have side effects (ataxia, tremor, nystagmus, hyperreflexia, drowsiness, lethargy, and coma) at levels over 30 μg/mL. Ataxia roughly correlates with levels of 30 μg/mL, but is often not present until levels reach above 40 μg/mL. Mental changes may be seen at 40 μg/mL.

Treatment

GUT DECONTAMINATION

Absorption of phenytoin is slow and erratic. Emesis may be helpful if the overdose was recent (i.e., less than 1 hour prior to presentation); however, if the patient is increasingly obtunded, is having convulsions, has no gag reflex, or is comatose, emesis is strictly contraindicated. If emesis is contraindicated, gastric lavage may be initiated after airway protection with endotracheal intubation. Lavage can be initiated during the first 12 hours after ingestion; however its importance, when compared to charcoal alone, has not been demonstrated. The dose of activated charcoal in aqueous slurry is 50–100 grams in an adult, and 30–50 grams in a child.

Serial doses of activated charcoal may be effective. Toxicokinetic studies suggest a positive effect of multiple-dose oral activated charcoal in increasing the clearance of phenytoin. Multiple-dose activated charcoal appears to shorten the time to peak phenytoin concentration, the half-life, and the course of phenytoin intoxication.

ELIMINATION ENHANCEMENT

Charcoal hemoperfusion has produced erratic results, and it is questionable whether the risks inherent in its use (vascular trauma from catheter placement, local hematomas, air embolism, need for heparinization, hypocalcemia, thrombocytopenia, intracranial bleeding) outweigh the possible benefits that have yet to be established. Forced fluid diuresis, peritoneal dialysis, exchange transfusion, hemodialysis, and plasmapheresis are ineffective. There is little renal elimination and a danger of fluid overload.

SUPPORTIVE MEASURES

- Patients under treatment for phenytoin overdose should be monitored with serum or plasma total phenytoin levels, and serum free phenytoin levels, if available. If a patient presents with any signs or symptoms of overdose and an initial serum level greater than 30 μg/mL, phenytoin should be withdrawn for 72–84 hours before restarting. Admission phenytoin serum levels following an overdose are not a useful predictor of length of hospital stay.
- Other tests to consider include blood glucose, serum creatinine, urinalysis, aspartate and alanine transaminases, bilirubin, electrocardiogram, computed tomogram of the skull (to rule out other causes for altered mental status), and other blood levels of other drugs used concomitantly. Basal thyroid function tests may also be helpful.
- In severe cases, correct hypotension by position change (Trendelenburg), and fluid infusion to correct volume deficits, or with pressor amines (e.g., dopamine) if required. An airway must be established. Respiratory depression is unusual, but if it occurs, an artificial airway with mechanically assisted ventilation should be available.
- Treat complete heart block with intravenous atropine or a pacemaker.
- For seizures, discontinue phenytoin immediately. Diazepam, 0.1–0.3 mg/kg i.v., should be administered to a maximum of 20 mg per dose in an adult. This may be repeated in 10–20 minutes if required.
- For hyperglycemic nonketotic coma, administer fluids intravenously, inject small amounts of insulin, and carefully monitor blood glucose.
- Reinstatement of phenytoin dosage to an epileptic who has ingested an overdose may require a period of 4–6 days with

daily measurement of blood levels of phenytoin before the drug can be safely ingested once again.

Questions—Phenytoin

1. **Death due to phenytoin overdose is usually due to**
   A. Cardiac arrest or ventricular fibrillation
   B. Respiratory arrest
   C. Uncontrollable hypoglycemia
   D. Status epilepticus
   E. Massive cerebral edema
2. **All of the following cause elevated plasma phenytoin levels and increased half-life except**
   A. Miconazole
   B. Methadone
   C. Methsuximide
   D. Methylphenidate
   E. Trimethoprim
3. **Fetuses exposed to maternal phenytoin**
   A. Are at risk for methemoglobinemia
   B. May have decreased sucking activity
   C. Are at 2–3 times greater risk than the general population for congenital malformations
   D. May develop oncologic disease
   E. All of the above

CASE STUDY (QUESTIONS 4 AND 5)

A sixty-year-old male with a known seizure disorder presents with new onset slurred speech and confusion. His vital signs are notable for HR 55, and he has horizontal nystagmus and gingival hyperplasia. After a careful history, you find that he had inadvertently tripled his daily phenytoin dose for the past three days. He now has a serum level of 37 μg/mL. His last dose was one hour ago.

4. **Appropriate management includes**
   A. A single dose of activated charcoal
   B. Serial doses of activated charcoal
   C. Forced fluid diuresis
   D. Plasmapheresis once vital signs are stable
   E. Uninterrupted continuation of his maintenance phenytoin dose
5. **Additional signs of overdose may include all of the following except**
   A. Ataxia
   B. Nausea
   C. Hepatitis
   D. Hyperglycemia
   E. Thrombocytopenia

CARBAMAZEPINE

Carbamazepine (Tegretol®, CBZ) was approved in 1974 as an antiepileptic agent in the U.S. Carbamazepine is used for the treatment of complex and simple partial seizures, tonic-clonic generalized seizures (grand mal), and trigeminal neuralgia, where it is a drug of choice. Its main metabolite (CBZ-E) is also an anticonvulsant. Overdoses are seldom fatal. Supportive measures and charcoal hemoperfusion have been useful in treatment. Overdoses with carbamazepine may, because of slow absorption, lead to delayed onset of coma with compromise of respiration. There is no antidote. Carbamazepine, like meprobamate, may lead to gastric mass formation.

Pathophysiology

Carbamazepine is chemically related to the tricyclic antidepressants and is also spatially similar to phenytoin. In overdose, the tricyclic antidepressants and phenytoin share many of the effects of carbamazepine.

Pharmacokinetics

ABSORPTION

- In normal volunteers, CBZ is absorbed slowly from the gastrointestinal tract.
- Peak plasma levels are attained in 6–24 hours.
- Delayed absorption may result in unpredictable and delayed deepening of coma because of its ability to decrease gastrointestinal motility. Overdose may also be associated with production of a gastric mass with its concomitant erratic absorption pattern.

DISTRIBUTION

- The apparent volume of distribution of CBZ in the newborn is 1.52 L/kg; in children, 1.94 L/kg; and in adults, 0.82–1.20 L/kg.
- The apparent volume of distribution of CBZ-E, the major metabolite of carbamazepine, is 0.59–0.92 L/kg. The metabolites appear about as equally distributed in the body as the parent drug.
- Protein binding of CBZ is 75–80%.

ELIMINATION

- CBZ is metabolized by first-order nonsaturable kinetics.
- The liver converts CBZ to more than seven metabolites.
- Urine excretion consists of unchanged CBZ (1.2%) and metabolites (23%).
- CBZ-E is the only metabolite with anticonvulsant activity.
- Much of CBZ undergoes enterohepatic recycling and is excreted in the bile.
- The terminal half-life of CBZ varies by host.

Clinical Presentations

Patients may present with excitation and aggression. More frequently, overdose patients are obtunded with various degrees of respiratory depression and dilated, sluggish pupils. Hypothermia may be seen. Respiratory depression, irregular respirations, or apnea may occur within the first 24 hours. Nausea, vomiting, and decreased bowel sounds may be seen. Leukopenia may be seen with therapeutic use.

CARDIOVASCULAR EFFECTS

Bradycardia, hypotension or hypertension, first-degree atrioventricular block, QRS prolongation, loss of P waves, and ventricular premature beats have been described. Often the electrocardiogram is within normal limits.

NEUROLOGIC EFFECTS

Disorientation, confusion, restlessness, agitation, aggression, ataxia, dystonic posturing, and athetoid movements have been described. Drowsiness and stupor may lead to coma (may be delayed for many hours and may be cyclic). Abnormal reflexes (hyperactive, hypoactive), tremor, and encephalopathy have been observed. Dizziness, pupils sluggishly reactive to light, divergent strabismus, nystagmus, or fixed dilated pupils may be seen.

Toxic Dosage/Death

Patients have survived ingestions of 20 grams. Death has also occurred after the ingestion of 20 grams. Death after CBZ overdosage is infrequent but may result from severe cardiovascular effects, aspiration pneumonitis, severe hepatitis, or aplastic anemia. These complications have also been seen after chronic therapeutic use.

Drug Interactions

When administered concomitantly, certain drugs may induce metabolism of CBZ, and in turn may have their own metabolism affected by CBZ. These include barbiturates, hydantoins, benzodiazepines, succinimides, valproic acid, and primidone. Carbamazepine induces its own metabolism. In chronic therapy, its half-life will shorten. The half-lives of warfarin and doxycycline are shortened when administered with CBZ. The doses of these drugs may have to be increased when CBZ is added to the therapeutic regime.

Erythromycin given with CBZ may result in elevated plasma levels of CBZ. Breakthrough bleeding may occur if patients receive concomitant oral contraceptives. Propoxyphene or isoniazid tends to increase the serum level of CBZ at a given dose. Cimetidine may slightly decrease the clearance and increase the half-life of CBZ. Ranitidine appears to slightly increase the clearance and decrease the half-life of CBZ.

Pregnancy/Lactation

Carbamazepine crosses the placenta and concentrates in fetal tissues. Excretion into breast milk produces a milk:plasma ratio of approximately 1:2. Carbamazepine is classified as pregnancy risk factor C.

Laboratory

ANALYTIC METHODS

High-performance liquid chromatography is an accurate method to monitor blood levels of CBZ and CBZ-E, both of which may be monitored throughout treatment of overdosage. However, the seriousness of the toxic effects and their management is determined by the clinical status of the patient and not by the total blood levels.

BLOOD LEVELS

CBZ blood levels are ordinarily useful with therapeutic use mainly as a qualitative indication of its presence. Blood levels of CBZ in patients during long-term use range from 0.5–25 μg/mL. Levels of CBZ-E, an active anticonvulsant metabolite, range from 0.5–4.5 μg/mL. Toxic blood levels of CBZ are usually greater than 20 μg/mL. A correlation appears to exist between the blood levels of both CBZ and its chief metabolite CBZ-E, and the clinical status (e.g., coma) in an overdose patient. Maximal plasma concentration in overdose may occur as late as 72 hours after ingestion. CBZ-E usually is found in the plasma in concentrations 10–20% of those of CBZ.

Treatment

GUT DECONTAMINATION

The usefulness of emesis induction has not been established. In the obtunded patient, emesis is absolutely contraindicated. Gastric lavage with endotracheal intubation may be helpful. Gastric lavage may be ineffective due to formation of a drug mass. This may in turn be associated with a delayed rise in the blood level of CBZ. If a mass is present by an abdominal x-ray combined with gastrografin, or after a diagnostic gastroscopy, gastroscopic lavage or gastrotomy may be indicated.

Charcoal may be given up to at least 12 hours after ingestion. It can be given repetitively through the lavage tube or nasogastric tube every 2 hours until the serum level is within the therapeutic range and does not appear to be rising. The dose is 60–100 grams for adults and 30–60 grams for children. Since CBZ has a long half-life and an extensive enterohepatic cycle, repetitive administration of charcoal may be useful. Charcoal may decrease the CBZ serum half-life by as much as 50%. Proof of clinical efficacy for this procedure remains to be established, however.

ELIMINATION ENHANCEMENT

Forced diuresis is ineffective and potentially dangerous. Very small amounts of CBZ and its metabolites are excreted unchanged in the urine. Hemoperfusion may be useful for removal of both CBZ and its metabolites. It has been employed after adequate supportive care has been provided without amelioration of the clinical condition. Hemodialysis and peritoneal dialysis are not effective in overdose management. Carbamazepine is highly protein bound (75–80%). However, CBZ-E is only 50% protein bound and may be more easily removed by hemodialysis.

SUPPORTIVE MEASURES

- Establish ABC's (airway, breathing/respiration, circulation).
- If the patient is comatose, insert an endotracheal tube and connect to a source of mechanical ventilation. If hypotension exists, fluids and/or pressors may be necessary. The patient should be placed in the Trendelenburg position.
- Patients should be admitted to an intensive care facility if they are symptomatic or have ingested several grams or have high or rising plasma levels.
- The complete blood count, vital signs, electrolytes, liver enzymes, and ECG should be monitored periodically in the chronically treated patient, and for at least 24 hours after admission in the overdose patient.

Antidotes

There are no antidotes for CBZ overdose. Physostigmine salicylate has been used to diminish dystonic posturing, but has little or no effect on other signs or symptoms of CBZ poisoning. The dystonic effects are generally not life-threatening and generally resolve spontaneously.

Questions—Carbamazepine

1. Delayed absorption of carbamazepine may be due to
A. Its ability to decrease gastrointestinal motility
B. Production of a gastric mass with concomitant erratic absorption
C. Chronic exposure of intestinal mucosa to carbamazepine
D. A and B
E. A, B and C

2. Cardiovascular signs of carbamazepine overdose may include all of the following except
A. Bradycardia
B. Inverted T waves and u waves

C. Hypotension or hypertension
D. First-degree atrioventricular block
E. Normal electrocardiogram

3. Carbamazepine levels may be elevated when given with
A. Erythromycin
B. Oral contraceptives
C. Ranitidine
D. Heparin
E. Barbiturates

CASE STUDY (QUESTIONS 4 AND 5)

A nursing home patient is brought to the ER after accidentally being given 10 times her normal carbamazepine dose. She arrives with temperature 95F, HR 60, RR 10 and irregular, BP 70/50, and is obtunded.

4. Appropriate management includes
A. Endotracheal intubation and mechanical ventilation
B. Gastric lavage and abdominal x-ray with gastrografin
C. Fluids and/or pressors
D. Admission to an intensive care unit
E. All of the above

5. A reasonable method to enhance carbamazepine elimination is
A. Forced diuresis
B. Hemoperfusion
C. Hemodialysis
D. Peritoneal dialysis
E. None of the above

VALPROIC ACID

Valproic acid (Depakote®) was approved in 1978 in the U.S. for the treatment of epilepsy. Since then, reports have demonstrated mild central nervous system depression in overdose, although drowsiness and coma have also been reported. Valproic acid is also known to interact with other anticonvulsants and is generally responsive to simple supportive care. It has an unpredictable and infrequent tendency to produce hepatic necrosis or Reye-like syndrome, and acute pancreatitis.

Valproic acid and its sodium salt are synthetic chemicals unrelated to any other anticonvulsants. The valproates are used in the treatment of simple (petit mal) and complex absence seizures, and as adjuncts in patients with multiple seizure types which may include absence seizures.

Pathophysiology

Valproic acid anticonvulsant activity may be partially mediated through an increase in the inhibitory synaptic action of cerebral and cerebellar γ-aminobutyric acid (GABA). Valproic acid appears to localize in structures with the highest concentration of GABA degradative enzymes.

Pharmacokinetics

ABSORPTION

- Tablets are rapidly absorbed from the gastrointestinal tract.
- Peak levels in plasma occur from 1–4 hours after a single oral dose. After a meal, enteric coated capsules are absorbed in 1.0–4.5 hours, with peak plasma concentrations reached at 3.0–7.5 hours after ingestion.
- There is no significant first-pass elimination in the gut or liver.
- The syrup formulation is rapidly absorbed, producing peak serum levels in 15–60 minutes.

DISTRIBUTION

- The apparent volume of distribution of free drug in the plasma is about 1 L/kg and indicates some penetration and binding to intracellular structures.
- Protein binding at therapeutic concentrations is 90%. Therefore, valproic acid may compete with other drugs with high degrees of protein binding (e.g., phenytoin).
- The total serum concentrations may not reflect the amount of free drug available for therapeutic or toxic effects.
- At blood levels over 100 μg/mL, protein binding decreases, more free drug is available, and therefore the total drug concentration may decrease. Protein binding is decreased in renal insufficiency, liver cirrhosis, or hepatitis.
- Valproic acid appears to localize in structures with the highest levels of γ-aminobutyric acid (GABA) degradative enzymes. It is distributed mainly to serum, liver, lungs, spleen, skeletal muscle, kidney and gut.

ELIMINATION

- A half-life of 7–15 hours is observed in healthy normal volunteers, rising in duration with age or in epileptics on valproic acid alone.
- The half-life is the same after a single dose or after multiple doses.
- There is no autoinduction of hepatic metabolizing enzymes.
- When other antiepileptic drugs are used with valproic acid, its mean half-life is reduced.
- In children, the half-life of valproic acid alone is about 10–11 hours. When other medications are added, the half-life is reduced to about 8–9 hours.
- About 7% of a dose undergoes enterohepatic recirculation.
- Excretion occurs partially in the form of ketone bodies, which may produce a false-positive test in the urine of diabetics.

Clinical Presentations

Acute valproic acid poisoning is observed infrequently. Patients usually exhibit drowsiness and unconsciousness appears to occur only if more than 200 mg/kg has been ingested. Hypotension may occur. Respiratory arrest may occur with large overdoses. A macular, pruritic rash may be seen and transient hair loss has been reported. Nocturnal enuresis has also been reported. Valproate causes reversible proximal tubular dysfunction and Fanconi syndrome.

NEUROLOGIC EFFECTS

Patients are usually drowsy and may be apathetic, withdrawn, stuporous, confused, restless, and hyperactive. Rarely seizures, myoclonic movements, unconsciousness, or coma may be seen. Asterixis of hands and feet has been reported. Pupils may be pinpoint and sluggishly reactive.

There is little correlation between central nervous system effects such as coma, and seizures and plasma valproate levels. Encephalopathy, stupor, and coma without hepatic toxicity have been reported in adults. Children have developed a reversible dementia and apparent brain atrophy. Such patients may exhibit nontoxic valproate plasma levels, lack of fever, hyperammonemia, and normal liver function tests. Seizures occur rarely when 100-700 mg/kg valproic acid is administered daily in the treatment of epilepsy.

GASTROINTESTINAL EFFECTS

Nausea, vomiting, and diarrhea may occur. Acute pancreatitis has been reported (usually in patients receiving normal doses with therapeutic serum levels). Hepatic effects may include centrilobular necrosis and hepatic failure. Hepatotoxicity associated with valproic acid use manifests itself as three clinical syndromes: (1) asymptomatic elevations in serum concentrations of liver enzymes (fairly common); (2) hyperammonemia associated with lethargy, vomiting, stupor, or coma but generally not accompanied by hepatocellular damage; and (3) acute hepatotoxicity that may terminate fatally.

Patients may experience anorexia, muscle weakness, lethargy, and vomiting. Liver biopsy may present with a histologic picture similar to that in Reye's syndrome. Fatal liver failure has mainly been observed in children and adolescents during the first 6 months of treatment. Its frequency may be as high as 1 in 5,000 children treated with valproate.

Toxic Dosage/Death

Toxic effects are frequently associated with daily dose levels over 1,800 mg and blood levels over 100 μg/mL. Unconsciousness may occur when greater than 200 mg/kg has been ingested. Recovery has followed an ingestion of 25 grams. Death has been associated with blood levels of 1970 μg/mL, and recovery at 218 μg/mL. Plasma concentrations and observed clinical effects are not correlated closely to be of value clinically. Death results rarely from cardiac and respiratory arrest, and may be in a setting of hepatic failure.

Drug Interactions

Phenobarbital serum levels increase when valproic acid is also administered, enhancing the sedative effect. The mechanism is not known. Therefore, when phenobarbital is given with sodium valproate, the dose of phenobarbital may need to be reduced. Primidone blood levels are increased initially when administered with sodium valproate, but return to normal within 1–3 months.

Valproic acid displaces phenytoin from serum proteins, often increasing but sometimes decreasing the free phenytoin levels, and decreasing total phenytoin levels. When valproic acid and phenytoin are administered together, serum levels of phenytoin may show no change, may increase, or may decrease. When given together, blood levels (total and free) of phenytoin should be determined and dosage adjusted as required. Carbamazepine serum concentration is increased when valproic acid is added to the treatment regimen. This is largely due to an increase in the CBZ-E level.

Pregnancy/Lactation

Valproic acid is found in the placental circulation. It is dysmorphogenic in animals. Valproic acid appears in breast milk in concentrations less than 10% that in serum. Valproic acid exposure during the first trimester of pregnancy appears to be associated with an increase in neural tube defects (spina bifida). The risk of spina bifida after valproic acid use during pregnancy appears to be 1–2%.

There is no substantial evidence that valproic acid use increases the risk for major malformations above the increased risk due to maternal epilepsy. Minor facial malformations (a fetal valproate syndrome) have been described, including epicanthal folds with an infraorbital crease, flat nasal bridge, small upturned nose, long upper lip with a relatively shallow philtrum, thin upper vermilion border, and downturned angles of the mouth. Pregnancy risk category D.

Laboratory

ANALYTIC METHODS

Gas chromatography-mass spectrometry is an accurate method to determine the presence of valproic acid and its metabolites. Valproic acid is determined in the hospital clinical laboratory generally by gas chromatography. A simple, fast, sensitive, and inexpensive method has been described for routine therapeutic monitoring of both total and free valproic acid using solid-phase column extraction and gas-liquid chromatography.

BLOOD LEVELS

Serum valproate methods measure total levels (bound and free). Free valproate serum levels are not easily available in most commercial or hospital laboratories and have not been shown to be useful in the management of an overdose patient. "Therapeutic" serum concentrations are usually between 50 and 100 μg/mL and are associated with an adult daily dose of 1.2–1.5 grams. Dose and plasma concentrations are fairly well correlated. To maintain optimal serum levels when valproic acid is used with other drugs, it is often necessary to increase the dose, and give it at more frequent intervals.

Treatment

GUT DECONTAMINATION

Emesis is not advisable since the patient on admission will often be somnolent or stuporous and aspiration is possible. If the patient is comatose, is convulsing, or has lost the gag reflex, gastric lavage may be considered after endotracheal intubation. This procedure, however, may be of limited value in view of the very rapid absorption of the drug.

Activated charcoal (adults, 50–100 grams and children, 15–30 grams) may adsorb valproate but its efficacy has not been evaluated. When plasma levels of valproic acid exceed the upper therapeutic blood level of 100 μg/mL, the free drug fraction increases as binding sites become saturated. Multiple-dose activated charcoal tends to be more effective if a toxin is not extensively bound to plasma proteins. Repeated doses of activated charcoal have been used to increase the elimination of valproate despite its high protein binding.

ELIMINATION ENHANCEMENT

No systematic studies are available to support the usefulness of forced diuresis, hemodialysis, peritoneal dialysis, exchange transfusion, or hemoperfusion. The high degree of protein binding, minimal amount of unchanged drug excreted through the kidneys, and short spontaneous course to recovery with supportive treatment alone would tend to preclude the need for such measures. In view of the good recovery with supportive treatment, extracorporeal removal is of questionable benefit in valproic acid intoxication without renal failure.

SUPPORTIVE MEASURES

- If patients are stuporous, somnolent, or drowsy, but otherwise have normal vital signs and liver function tests, simple observation for 24-72 hours in a hospital may be sufficient.
- Discontinue all anticonvulsive drugs.
- Monitor serum valproate levels, other antiepileptic drugs, liver function tests, amylase, lipase, and complete blood counts, including platelets and bleeding time, in the seriously overdosed patient. Slight thrombocytopenia may be seen. The

erythrocyte sedimentation rate may be lowered and the fibrinogen level decreased. An abnormal bleeding time, partial thromboplastin time, and prothrombin time may be observed.

- Hyperammonemia may occur. Patients whose ammonia concentration after valproate use exceeds 100 μg/dL should be considered at high risk in the short term.
- Seizures should be managed with diazepam i.v. (0.1–0.3 mg/kg) to a maximum of 20 mg in an adult. This may be repeated in 10–20 minutes if required.

Antidotes

Anecdotally, naloxone has reversed coma in a few case reports.

Questions—Valproic Acid

1. All of the following regarding the pharmacokinetics of valproic acid are true except
A. Peak plasma concentrations are achieved in 3–7.5 hours after ingestion.
B. The half life is 7–15 hours in normal individuals.
C. The half life increases with multiple doses.
D. Excretion occurs partially in the form of ketone bodies.
E. When combined with other antiepileptic drugs, the half-life is reduced.

2. All of the following are true regarding the possible clinical presentation of valproic acid overdose except
A. Hypotension
B. Seizures
C. Liver failure
D. Palpable purpura
E. Vomiting

3. Regarding drug interactions of valproic acid,
A. Phenobarbital levels decrease when administered with valproic acid.
B. Carbamazepine levels increase when administered with valproic acid.
C. When given with phenytoin, the phenytoin level may increase, decrease or remain the same.
D. Primidone levels are unaffected by the administration of valproic acid.
E. B and C

CASE STUDY (QUESTIONS 4 AND 5)

An 18-year-old-male with a known seizure disorder is transported to the emergency department following an ingestion of 10g of valproic acid. He is lethargic, confused, vomiting and complaining of abdominal pain.

4. Appropriate initial intervention(s) include
A. Syrup of ipecac orally
B. Change to another anticonvulsant
C. Diazepam i.v. if seizures occur
D. All of the above
E. None of the above

5. The following method(s) to enhance the elimination of valproic acid have been proven effective:
A. Diuresis
B. Hemodialysis
C. Exchange transfusion
D. B and C
E. None of the above

BARBITURATES

Barbiturates were introduced into medical practice in 1903 after the development of barbital as a sedative-hypnotic. By the early 1970s, barbiturate overdose was a leading cause of drug-induced death. Recognition of the overdose and abuse potential of barbiturate sedatives led to their replacement by the safer and more efficacious benzodiazepines as sedatives. The result has been a greater than 50% reduction in barbiturate-induced deaths over the last 20 years. Mortality is now less than 2% in most published series of hospitalized barbiturate overdose cases. Barbiturates remain a common anticonvulsant, particularly in the pediatric and refractory adult populations.

The basic structure of all barbiturates is barbituric acid, which has no intrinsic central nervous system depressant properties. The addition of an alkyl or aryl group confers sedative properties. Barbiturate compounds are divided into four categories based on their elimination half-lives in animals. The observed clinical effect depends on absorption, redistribution from tissue stores, and the presence of active metabolites. Hence, the duration of action does not always correlate well with the elimination half-life.

Ultrashort-acting barbiturates include thiopental (Pentothal®), methohexital (Brevital®), and thiamylal (Surital®). Short-acting barbiturates include pentobarbital (Nembutal®), secobarbital (Seconal®) and hexobarbital. Intermediate-acting barbiturates include amobarbital (Amytal®), aprobarbital (Alurate elixir®), butabarbital (Butisol®) and butalbital (contained within many combination tablets such as Fiorinal®, Esgic®, and Fioricet®). Long-acting barbiturates include mephobarbital (Mebaral®), phenobarbital (Luminal®) and metharbital (Gemonil®).

Barbiturates are widely available to treat anxiety, gastrointestinal upset, pain, and sleep disorders. Long-acting barbiturates are effective anticonvulsant drugs, but diazepam and phenytoin are more commonly administered anticonvulsants in emergency department settings. Induction of anesthesia by ultrashort-acting barbiturates is an effective measure for situations such as emergency intubation. Barbiturate coma has been used in the management of hypoxic encephalopathy and trauma-induced cerebral edema. Barbiturates tend to reduce intracranial pressure and improve cerebral oxygen consumption after cranial surgery, cerebral trauma, and cardiac arrest, but cardiovascular side effects limit their usefulness.

Pathophysiology

Barbiturates are central nervous system depressants that act via inhibitory γ-aminobutyric acid (GABA) synapses in the brain. They may also depress noradrenergic activity selectively. Barbiturates abolish central respiratory drive so that respiratory depression is the usual cause of death in patients without ventilatory support. High barbiturate doses suppress skeletal, smooth, and cardiac muscle leading to depressed myocardial contractility, vasodilation, and hypotension. Reduced gastrointestinal mobility results in ileus. Biochemical effects include binding to cytochrome P450 and induction of hepatic microsomal enzymes.

Pharmacokinetics

ABSORPTION

- Long, intermediate, and short-acting barbiturates are well absorbed.
- Drug dissolution and dispersal are the rate-limiting factors for absorption.

DISTRIBUTION

- Barbiturates partition into fat in proportion to their lipid solubility.
- Ultrashort-acting barbiturates are highly lipid-soluble and distribute into the gray matter of the brain within seconds.
- Less soluble barbiturates, such as phenobarbital, accumulate relatively more slowly in the brain.
- At steady-state, the highest concentration of barbiturate in nonadipose tissue occurs in the liver and kidney.
- The apparent volume of distribution ranges from 0.6–2.6 L/kg.

ELIMINATION

- The liver biotransforms most intermediate and short-acting barbiturates.
- Short-acting barbiturates are oxidized to more polar and inactive compounds (e.g., alcohols, ketones, phenols, or carboxylic acid).
- The metabolism of long-acting barbiturates is less complete compared with other barbiturates.
- The liver hydroxylates only about 60–75% of an absorbed phenobarbital dose.
- Both mephobarbital (15% is demethylated to phenobarbital) and metharbital (demethylated to the active metabolite barbital) produce active metabolites. Metabolism is generally more rapid in children and reduced in infants and in the elderly.
- Elimination of phenobarbital follows first-order kinetics.
- The classification of duration of action does not conform to elimination half-lives.
- Liver dysfunction, renal failure, chronic use, and age affect the half-life, which ranges from an average of 1 hour (methohexital) to 86 hours (phenobarbital).

Clinical Presentations

Clinical effects result primarily from depression of the central nervous system and cardiovascular system. The onset of symptoms after ingestion depends on the type of barbiturate ingested. Victims of short-acting barbiturate overdoses develop symptoms within 15–30 minutes and these effects peak in 2–4 hours. Toxic effects of long-acting barbiturates begin at 1–2 hours and peak at 6–18 hours. Fatalities result first from cardiorespiratory arrest, and short-acting barbiturates appear more potent than other barbiturates in producing apnea. Later causes of death result from circulatory failure, pneumonia, and pulmonary and cerebral edema. The major causes of hospital mortality are pulmonary edema and aspiration pneumonia.

NEUROLOGIC EFFECTS

Mild to moderate intoxication resembles ethanol inebriation with slurred speech, ataxia, lethargy, nystagmus, headache, paresthesias, vertigo, and confusion. Pupils are constricted and reactive early in coma, but later dilate. Respiratory depression occurs early in coma, with slow or shallow respirations progressing to decreased vital capacity and minute ventilatory volume. Hypoglycemia may contribute to central nervous system depression.

CARDIOVASCULAR EFFECTS

Shock results from medullary depression and presents with a weak and rapid pulse, cyanosis, cool and clammy skin, decreased urine output, and confusion. Inhibition of vascular smooth muscle leads to a relative hypovolemia manifested by tissue hypoperfusion. Depression of myocardial contractility causes hypotension, which may be unresponsive to fluid challenges and may require placement of pulmonary pressure catheters. Hypothermia commonly occurs. Pulmonary embolism has been reported following a barbiturate overdose.

DERMATOLOGIC EFFECTS

Bullous skin lesions occur in 4–7% of barbiturate overdose cases, primarily over pressure points. These lesions are tense bullae surrounded by areas of erythema and commonly involve the fingers, malleoli, and medial aspect of the knee. They generally appear in comatose patients within 24 hours. Histological examinations show epidermal and sweat gland necrosis with a normal dermis. Bullae are not diagnostic of barbiturate intoxication since carbon monoxide, amitriptyline, methadone, and other sedative-hypnotics (e.g., meprobamate) may produce similar lesions.

ABSTINENCE SYNDROME

Like all sedative-hypnotic drugs, barbiturates produce physical dependence when taken in 3–10 times the sedative dose for 1–2 months. The abstinence syndrome can result from combination analgesic compounds which contain barbiturates. Abrupt withdrawal from prolonged barbiturate use results in anxiety, agitation, confusion, delusions, hallucinations, tremor, ataxia, and hyperreflexia. Seizures occur in up to 75% of patients on high-dose pentobarbital therapy, and morbidity results from both seizures and trauma secondary to impaired judgment.

For short and intermediate-acting barbiturates, nausea, vomiting, orthostatic hypotension, and agitation develop 12–16 hours after cessation of barbiturate use and peak in 48–72 hours with seizures and delirium. Resolution occurs in 4–7 days. Confusion, impaired memory, and disorientation may occur. Withdrawal seizures may occur prior to the onset of confusion and often are more severe than those seen in ethanolism. Visual hallucinations are common, with delusions and other types of hallucinations present less frequently. Symptoms subside 3–4 days after withdrawal and rarely persist over a week.

Toxic Dosage/Death

The generally recommended hypnotic dose of phenobarbital, secobarbital, and pentobarbital for children is 2–3 mg/kg. Average toxic doses are five times the hypnotic dose and severe toxicity may result from ten times the hypnotic dose. Potentially fatal doses are more difficult to predict since cofactors such as hepatic enzyme induction, coingested drugs, and ethanol can influence outcome. Short-acting barbiturates are somewhat more potent.

Estimated lethal adult doses have been reported as: phenobarbital, 6–10 grams; secobarbital, pentobarbital, 2–3 grams; amobarbital, butabarbital, 2–3 grams. Survival did occur in an adult who reportedly ingested 20 grams of amobarbital. Gut decontamination should be induced in all cases where the suspected ingested dose exceeds 5–6 mg/kg.

Drug Interactions

Most major interactions result from the effect of hepatic enzyme induction on the metabolism of such drugs as anticoagulants, digoxin, quinidine, tricyclic antidepressants, phenothiazines, testosterone, corticosteroids, and vitamin D or K. Barbiturates may exacerbate intermittent porphyria by increasing production of delta-aminolevulinic acid. Synergistic central nervous system depression occurs with general anesthetics, alcohols, narcotic analgesics, and other sedative-hypnotic drugs.

Pregnancy/Lactation

Barbiturates cross the placenta and are found in breast milk. Barbiturates ingested by the mother may be associated with a neonatal coagulation defect that may cause bleeding during the first 24 hours of life in the neonate. This is characterized by decreased levels of vitamin K-dependent clotting factors and prolongation of prothrombin time, partial thromboplastin time, or both.

Withdrawal symptoms can appear in neonates born to mothers who take barbiturates as anticonvulsants or as drugs of abuse. Neonatal symptoms are similar to withdrawal symptoms from opiates or other sedative-hypnotics. These include hyperactivity, restlessness, excessive crying, tremor, hyperreflexia, hypertonus, vomiting, sweating, and hyperphagia. In these infants, hyperexcitability appears at approximately 7 days (range, 2–14 days) and may last several months.

Laboratory

ANALYTIC METHODS

Barbiturates may be detected by an enzyme-multiplied immunoassay technique (EMIT) or gas chromatography-mass spectrometry.

BLOOD LEVELS

Serum barbiturate levels complement clinical judgment but are not required for management. Short-acting barbiturates are more toxic at a given level than long-acting barbiturates (e.g., mortality is 5% for short-acting barbiturate levels over 3 mg/dL and 3% for long-acting levels over 8 mg/dL).

Treatment

GUT DECONTAMINATION

Emesis is contraindicated. Because of decreased gastrointestinal mobility and delayed gastric emptying, gastric lavage with adequate airway protection may be performed with a large-bore, tube up to 6–8 hours postingestion in obtunded patients. Barbiturates are well adsorbed by charcoal. The dose of charcoal has been suggested as 10 times the ingested dose or 1 g/kg in adults.

Repeat doses of activated charcoal reduce the average serum half-life of intravenous and oral phenobarbital in human volunteers. Serial activated charcoal decreases the phenobarbital elimination half-life in the overdose setting; however, the exact role of serial charcoal has not been confirmed.

ELIMINATION ENHANCEMENT

Hemodialysis is most effective for long-acting barbiturates, which display less protein binding and lipid solubility than other barbiturates. Its use should be reserved for those patients who have ingested long-acting barbiturates and fail to respond to supportive care or who have lethal blood barbiturate levels. Hemoperfusion is more effective than dialysis for short- and intermediate-acting barbiturates. Resin hemoperfusion efficiently removes lipid-soluble barbiturates. As with hemodialysis, this measure should be reserved for the severely intoxicated patient who does not respond well to supportive care. Rebound may occur from the release of barbiturates from tissue stores and may be accompanied by clinical deterioration.

Urinary alkalinization increases phenobarbital excretion 5-10 times and also enhances metharbital excretion. Forced alkaline diuresis requires a urine flow of 3–4 mL/kg/min and a pH over 7.5. Care should be taken not to aggravate cerebral or pulmonary edema with excessive fluid loads. Alkaline diuresis is ineffective for short and intermediate-acting barbiturates. The use of alkaline diuresis requires adequate renal and cardiac function to be effective and therefore is not indicated in patients requiring vasopressor support.

SUPPORTIVE MEASURES

- Take a careful history, estimating the amount of drugs and alcohol ingested and the time of ingestion. Evaluate for trauma and signs of drug abuse. Be sure to give glucose, naloxone, and thiamine to all patients with depressed mental status.
- Respiratory arrest is the major cause of early death. Assess the patency of the airway and the adequacy of ventilation first. Appropriate corrective measures include supplemental oxygen, head tilt-chin lift, intubation, and assisted ventilation.
- Establish an intravenous line with Ringer's lactate and give a fluid challenge up to 2 L for patients who are hypotensive. Patients must be monitored for complications of alkalosis and fluid overload. These include pulmonary and cerebral edema, hypokalemia, hypomagnesemia, hypernatremia, and hypocalcemia.
- Baseline ancillary tests for moderate to severe overdoses include a complete blood count, serum electrolytes, glucose, creatinine, urine myoglobin, and chest x-ray. Order urine, blood, and toxicology screens specifically for central nervous system depressants, stimulants, and psychoactive drugs. Arterial blood gases and tidal volumes should be obtained when clinical evidence of hypocapnia or hypoxemia appears.
- EEG displays a predictable progression of changes depending on the depth of coma. In severe cases, the EEG may be isoelectric without the presence of irreversible brain damage. In patients who have become stuporous or comatose after a sedative-hypnotic or other toxic insult, and who do not have appreciable cerebral hypoxia, an EEG pattern dominated by frequencies in the alpha range is usually associated with recovery without neurologic sequelae.
- Patients who ingest long-acting barbiturates may be comatose for as long as 2–3 days. Severely intoxicated patients with significant depression of myocardial function (manifested by hypotension unresponsive to fluid challenge) require hemodynamic monitoring. Such patients may require pulmonary artery catheter and/or arterial pressure lines to guide fluid management. Consider early use of hemoperfusion and hemodialysis to hasten elimination in such patients.
- Treat bullous lesions as second-degree burns with layered dressings to protect the bullae (e.g., nonadherent dressing next to the skin surrounded by coarse gauze and a wrapping layer).

Questions—Barbiturates

1. The following clinical presentations may be seen with barbiturate overdose

A. Bullous skin lesions
B. Shock
C. Hyperthermia
D. A and B
E. All of the above

2. Regarding the abstinence syndrome of barbiturates, the following statements is (are) incorrect:

A. Seizures occur in up to 75% of patients on high dose pentobarbital therapy.
B. For short- and intermediate-acting barbiturates, effects peak in 48–72 hours.
C. Symptoms typically persist for more than 1 week.

D. Symptoms include anxiety, delusions and tremor.
E. Seizures may occur prior to the onset of confusion.

3. The neurologic presentation of barbiturate overdose may include
A. Paresthesias
B. Slurred speech
C. Early pupil dilation
D. Decreased vital capacity
E. All of the above

CASE STUDY (QUESTIONS 4 AND 5)

A 77-year-old male erroneously took 8 times his phenobarbital dose, thinking it was Tylenol. He now presents lethargic, vertiginous, and confused. He is tachycardic with absent peripheral pulses, and his extremities are cold.

4. Initial interventions include all except
A. Intravenous fluids
B. Gastric lavage
C. Activated charcoal
D. Forced alkaline diuresis
E. Airway protection

5. Regarding the management of this patient, which of the following is incorrect?
A. Serum barbiturate level is the most reliable predictor of prognosis.
B. Hemoperfusion is preferable to hemodialysis as a method to enhance elimination.
C. EEG is a reliable predictor of neurological outcome if coma were to ensue.
D. A and B
E. All of the above

PARALDEHYDE

Paraldehyde (Paral®) is a polymer of acetaldehyde that was discovered in 1820 by Weidenbusch and introduced as a hypnotic in 1884 by Cervello. By 1890, the first fatality was reported in a 20-year-old female with typhoid fever who was given 6 to 7 teaspoons of paraldehyde for her delirium and sleeplessness. She went into a coma for 4 hours and died. By 1957, at least 93 deaths had been reported.

Disadvantages of the drug include a strong characteristic odor, a disagreeable burning taste, a narrow therapeutic index, degeneration to acetic acid on storage, and a tendency to produce a serious, often fatal outcome in overdose. Severe toxic effects on the lung, right ventricle, and gastrointestinal tract are seen with misuse. Paraldehyde may yield a severe anion gap metabolic acidosis. Although its use has diminished with the advent of the benzodiazepines, paraldehyde is still marketed for its use in status epilepticus. It is a Schedule IV controlled drug in the U.S. Paraldehyde may be administered orally, intramuscularly, intravenously, and rectally.

Currently, the disadvantages mentioned above render paraldehyde unacceptable as a drug of choice in many institutions. However, it is still used by those who strictly adhere to the precautions listed above. It is used in the management of alcohol withdrawal, in preventing the development of alcohol withdrawal symptoms, to induce basal anesthesia in children (rectally administered), in some cases of refractory, idiopathic, status epilepticus, and rarely as a hypnotic or sedative.

Paraldehyde is a synthetic chemical prepared by the polymerization of acetaldehyde. It is a colorless liquid, soluble in water, and miscible with alcohol and vegetable oils. On exposure to light and air, it decomposes to acetaldehyde and is oxidized to acetic acid. It is incompatible with plastics and must be administered in glass syringes. If it has developed a brownish color or has the disagreeable pungent odor of acetic acid, it should not be used, as it may result in death.

Pathophysiology

The exact mechanism by which paraldehyde depresses the central nervous system has not been established. It may act by depressing the ascending reticular activating system.

Pharmacokinetics

ABSORPTION

- Oral absorption is approximately 95% complete and rectal absorption is about 83% complete.
- Peak levels after oral administration are reached in 30 minutes.
- After rectal administration peak levels are reached in 2.5 hours.

DISTRIBUTION

- The volume of distribution in adults is 0.89 L/Kg, similar to that in children (0.83–1.23 L/kg).
- The drug is very rapidly distributed to the blood, liver, brain, and kidney.
- Cerebrospinal fluid concentrations average 75% of serum levels.

ELIMINATION

- The half-life of paraldehyde is 3.4–9.8 hours in infants and children, and 6–13 hours in adults.
- It is believed that about 80% of paraldehyde is depolymerized in the liver to acetaldehyde, which is then oxidized to acetic acid and through the Krebs cycle to carbon dioxide and water.
- About 28% is eliminated through expired air and only 3% is excreted unchanged in the urine.
- Since paraldehyde is metabolized in the liver and excreted unchanged through the lungs, it is recommended that the rate of an intravenous drip should be decreased in the presence of pulmonary or hepatic disease.

Clinical Presentations

Abdominal pain, central nervous system depression, a severe high-anion-gap metabolic acidosis, and leukocytosis constitute the typical constellation of symptoms seen with paraldehyde poisoning. Sterile abscesses have been observed at injection sites. Pain, tissue necrosis, and sciatic nerve damage may be seen. Despite the severity of acidosis and central nervous system depression, most patients survive, though coma may develop. Hyperthermia, hypotension, cyanosis, and tachycardia may occur.

NEUROLOGIC EFFECTS

Lethargy, listlessness, ataxia and coma may occur. All may resolve within 48 hours after the drug is stopped. Confusion, disorientation, delirium, hallucinations, and hyperactive deep tendon reflexes have been reported. Pupils are usually equal and reactive to light and accommodation.

RESPIRATORY EFFECTS

Intravenous administration may lead to apnea, rapid shallow respirations, cough, cyanosis, hypotension, tachycardia, and death in minutes from massive diffuse pulmonary hemorrhages and dilatation of the right side of the heart. Typically there is a characteristic odor on the breath. Death may occur in hours from pulmonary edema. Bronchopneumonia, Kussmaul respirations, and respiratory collapse have been observed.

RENAL EFFECTS

A renal tubular defect in acidification and in conservation of bicarbonate and cation may be associated with albuminuria, increase in serum creatinine, microscopic hematuria, oliguria, or anuria. An increased anion gap metabolic acidosis, and dehydration may be observed.

GASTROINTESTINAL EFFECTS

Nausea, vomiting (with or without coffee grounds), diffuse or epigastric abdominal pain, anorexia, hepatomegaly, rectal or oral mucosal corrosion, intestinal perforation, and whitening of mouth, esophagus, and stomach mucosa (may be due to acetic acid) may be seen. Paraldehyde in high doses can produce fatty changes in the liver and a histologic picture resembling a toxic hepatitis or toxic nephritis.

HEMATOLOGIC EFFECTS

Increase in blood coagulability, general arterial thrombosis, and leukocytosis ranging from 24,000–65,000 wbc/mm^3 has been observed.

TOLERANCE

Paraldehyde may become a substitute for alcohol in alcoholism. Chronic paraldehydism may be characterized by tolerance, tremulousness, restlessness, mental anxiety, and agitation, and may be a substitution for alcoholism. Withdrawal from paraldehyde may result in delirium tremens and hallucination similar to withdrawal from alcohol. The treatment of paraldehyde withdrawal is similar to that of alcohol (i.e., sedatives, anticonvulsants, correction and monitoring of fluid, electrolytes, and carbohydrate balance).

Toxic Dosage/Death

Death has occurred after paraldehyde was given orally, rectally, intramuscularly and intravenously and is usually the result of respiratory failure. Pulmonary edema, right heart failure, and metabolic acidosis have also caused fatalities. Death has occurred from 25 grams by mouth, but one person survived 150 grams. Death has occurred after 12 mL of paraldehyde administered rectally and after 25 mL ingested orally. Patients have survived ingestion of 125 mL. The lowest lethal blood level in a study of five deaths was 543 μg/mL, whereas in another study of fatalities, the lowest concentration was 490 μg/mL.

Drug Interactions

Central nervous system depression may be additive with other similar drugs, such as barbiturates and alcohol. Disulfiram inhibits acetaldehyde dehydrogenase and may inhibit the metabolism of paraldehyde.

Pregnancy/Lactation

Paraldehyde diffuses across the placenta. A mother at term died in coma after using paraldehyde. The full-term living baby at delivery developed cyanosis and convulsions and died. Breast milk levels have not been established.

Laboratory

ANALYTIC METHODS

Bioassays of paraldehyde rely on its conversion to acetaldehyde with dilute acid and heat. Colorimetry, ultraviolet spectrophotometry, and gas chromatography each measure acetaldehyde.

BLOOD LEVELS

A single 10-mL intramuscular dose produced plasma concentrations of 77 μg/mL at 1.2 hours. Blood concentrations exceeding 200 μg/mL may be associated with periods of complete amnesia.

Treatment

GUT DECONTAMINATION

Paraldehyde is locally corrosive to the mouth and upper gastrointestinal tract, and emesis is contraindicated. There is no evidence to support the effectiveness of activated charcoal.

ELIMINATION ENHANCEMENT

Since very little paraldehyde is excreted through the kidneys, extracorporeal detoxification methods would appear to be of diminished use. Where improvement has accompanied dialysis, this may have resulted from correction of metabolic acidosis.

SUPPORTIVE CARE

- Treatment is directed toward maintenance of airway, breathing, and circulation. Supportive care is the mainstay of therapy. Patients are often critically ill and must be under constant supervision. Assisted mechanical ventilation with endotracheal intubation may be required for patients suffering from respiratory compromise.
- Helpful labs may include arterial blood gases, serum electrolytes (with estimation of the anion gap), electrocardiogram, hepatic and renal function tests, respiratory function studies, chest x-ray, cardiac function studies, complete blood count, and clotting parameters.
- Hypotension can be treated initially by placing the patient in the Trendelenburg position. Intravenous fluid may be cautiously started with great care to avoid fluid overload. Should hypotension not respond to the above measures, pressor amines (dopamine or norepinephrine) may be used. Fluid status can be monitored through a central line or Swan-Ganz catheter. Furosemide may be used if there is evidence of fluid overload. Morphine is not used since it may enhance respiration depression.
- Rectal sloughing may require local care or surgical intervention.

Questions—Paraldehyde

1. Regarding the pharmacokinetics of paraldehyde, the following statement(s) is/are true:

A. Rectal administration more rapidly achieves a peak level than oral administration.
B. Cerebral spinal fluid concentrations exceed those found in the serum.
C. Excretion through the lungs exceeds urine excretion.
D. No dose adjustment is required in the setting of liver disease.
E. B and C

2. **Clinical presentations of paraldehyde poisoning include all except**
   A. Strong odor on breath
   B. Hypothermia
   C. Coma
   D. Intestinal perforation
   E. Leukocytosis
3. **Which of the following treatment options is/are contra-indicated in paraldehyde poisoning?**
   A. Intravenous fluids
   B. Pulmonary artery catheter
   C. Morphine
   D. Induction of emesis
   E. C and D

CASE STUDY (QUESTIONS 4 AND 5)

An 18-year-old man is erroneously given a large dose of paraldehyde in an attempt to halt a seizure. He is now hypotensive, tachycardic, lethargic and vomiting.

4. **Exzpected laboratory findings include all except**
   A. Non- anion gap metabolic acidosis
   B. Leukocytosis
   C. Elevated serum creatinine
   D. Albuminuna
   E. Microscopic hematuria
5. **In the management of this patient, the following maneuver(s) is/are appropriate:**
   A. Endotracheal intubation
   B. Mechanical hypoventilation
   C. Intravenous pressor therapy
   D. Intravenous furosemide
   E. A and C

PRIMIDONE

Primidone (Mysoline®), a derivative of phenobarbital, has been used as an anticonvulsant for over 30 years. It is often used with other anticonvulsants in the treatment of epilepsy. It is used in the treatment of grand mal, psychomotor, and focal epileptic seizures. Few cases of overdose with primidone have been reported. Since phenobarbital is an active metabolite of primidone, treatment is similar to that after a phenobarbital overdose.

Pathophysiology

Primidone may be an anticonvulsant in its own right, but it also exerts its anticonvulsant properties through its metabolite phenobarbital. Central nervous system depression appears to be due to primidone alone. Primidone is 2-desoxyphenobarbital. It resembles the barbiturates to which it is chemically and pharmacologically related. Fatalities have been reported. Primidone is a synthetic chemical, prepared by reduction of phenobarbital or desulfurization of thiobarbituric acid.

Pharmacokinetics

ABSORPTION

- About 60–80% of an oral dose is absorbed from the gastrointestinal tract.
- Peak serum levels are attained in 3 hours (0.5–9 hours).

DISTRIBUTION

- The apparent volume of distribution is 0.6 L/kg.
- The product is protein bound 0–20% for primidone and phenylethylmalonamide (PEMA) and 40% for phenobarbital.

ELIMINATION

- Primidone is totally metabolized in the liver to active metabolites PEMA (large amount), and phenobarbital (small amount).
- The primidone half-life is 10–12 hours after a single dose and shorter after chronic administration.
- The half-life of PEMA is 29–36 hours, and that of phenobarbital, 4 days.
- Primidone follows first-order elimination kinetics (both metabolites).
- Primidone has an autoinducing effect on hepatic microsomal drug-metabolizing enzymes responsible for its biotransformation. Approximately 70% of a dose of primidone appear in the urine, mostly as metabolites.
- Almost no primidone appears in the urine unchanged.

Clinical Presentations

Symptoms of poisoning may include sedation, vertigo, dizziness, nausea, vomiting, ataxia, diplopia, and nystagmus. Massive crystalluria (hexagonal crystals) may occur in severe poisoning. Crystals result from precipitation of primidone in the urine at high serum levels (i.e., over 80 μg/mL).

Toxic Dosage/Death

Toxic effects may be observed at doses exceeding 1.5 grams/d. A 10-year-old who was admitted in a comatose state after an acute primidone overdosage had a serum primidone level of 95 μg/mL and a phenobarbital level of 175 μg/mL. A fatal overdosage in an adult (not under therapy with primidone) disclosed a primidone blood concentration of 65 μg/mL and a phenobarbital level of 3 mg/mL.

Drug Interactions

Primidone interactions with other drugs are similar to those of phenobarbital.

Pregnancy/Lactation

No unusual toxic effects have been reported in epileptic pregnant women taking primidone. Most pregnant women on antiepileptic drugs deliver normal infants. The effects of primidone on fetal and neonatal development have not been established. Neonatal hemorrhage with a coagulation defect resembling vitamin K deficiency has been described in newborns whose mothers took primidone and other anticonvulsants. Primidone is found in breast milk in concentrations sufficient to induce somnolence in nursing newborns.

Laboratory

ANALYTIC METHODS

Gas-liquid chromatography is the best analytical method to determine the quantity of primidone and its metabolites. Laboratory evidence of serum levels is confirmatory for the presence of primidone. Analysis for other common anticonvulsants should be pursued in a patient with clinical evidence of overdosage.

BLOOD LEVELS

The therapeutic plasma range of primidone is 5–15 μg/mL, 10–20 μg/mL of the derived metabolite, phenobarbital, and 7–10 μg/mL of phenylethylmalonamide (PEMA). At a plasma primidone concentration of 15 μg/mL, ataxia and/or somnolence may be evident.

Treatment

GUT DECONTAMINATION

The use of gastric lavage or emesis has not been studied. Activated charcoal with cathartic, although not studied, is still recommended (adults, 50–100 grams and children, 15–30 grams). No clinical studies have been performed on the pharmacokinetics of charcoal in primidone overdose.

ELIMINATION ENHANCEMENT

Fluids and supportive therapy are usually sufficient in mild to moderate primidone overdosage. Peritoneal dialysis, hemodialysis, and exchange transfusion have not been evaluated in primidone poisoning. Hemoperfusion increased the plasma clearance of primidone (normal, 30–40 mL/min) at least 200–300% in one case. It reduced the half-life of primidone from more than 12 hours to 5 hours.

SUPPORTIVE MEASURES

- Management of primidone overdosage is similar to the management of barbiturate overdose.
- Hospitalization in an intensive care facility with observation for several days may be required for the severely overdosed primidone patient.
- Monitoring of vital signs, level of consciousness, and electroencephalographic changes may be required in the severely obtunded patient.
- Serial primidone and phenobarbital levels may be helpful.

Questions—Primidone

1. **Regarding primidone pharmacokinetics, which of the following is true?**
   A. Only a small percentage of primidone is absorbed from the gastrointestinal tract.
   B. The half-life decreases with chronic administration.
   C. The liver is not a site of primidone metabolism.
   D. A large percentage of primidone is excreted in the urine unchanged.
   E. B and D
2. **Statements regarding the clinical presentation of primidone poisoning are true except**
   A. Crystalluria may result with very high serum levels.
   B. Doses as small as 100 mg/day will consistently produce toxic side effects.
   C. Primidone can be transmitted through breast milk.
   D. Symptoms may include vertigo, dizziness and nystagmus.
   E. B and C

SUCCINIMIDES

Succinimides have been used to manage absence epilepsy for over 30 years. Few reports of acute intoxication with the succinimides are available. The succinimides tend to have long elimination half-lives, are weakly protein bound, and exhibit a delayed onset of central nervous system depression, probably because of an active metabolite.

Commonly used succinimides include ethosuximide (Zarontin®), methsuximide (Celontin®), and phensuximide (Milontin®). The succinimides are synthetic chemicals. Ethosuximide is used primarily in the control of absence (petit mal) epilepsy. Methsuximide and phensuximide are also employed in the control of absence (petit mal) seizures refractory to other drugs. When used alone in mixed types of epilepsy, the succinimides may increase the frequency of grand mal seizures.

Pathophysiology

The succinimides suppress electroencephalographic activity associated with the lapses of consciousness that are common in absence (petit mal) seizures. The frequency of epileptiform attacks is reduced. This is possibly effected by depression of the motor cortex and elimination of convulsive threshold.

Pharmacokinetics

ABSORPTION

- Succinimides are completely absorbed from the gastrointestinal tract after oral administration.

DISTRIBUTION

- The apparent volume of distribution of ethosuximide is 0.9 L/kg.
- The compound is uniformly distributed throughout free body water.
- Protein binding of ethosuximide, methsuximide, and phensuximide is almost totally absent.
- One oral therapeutic dose of each of the succinimides produces a peak plasma concentration for ethosuximide in 1–7 hours, for methsuximide in 1 hour (6.8 μg), and for phensuximide in 1-hour (14 μg/mL).

ELIMINATION

- Succinimides, after absorption, are metabolized in the liver by hepatic microsomal enzymes to metabolites. Some of these are active anticonvulsants themselves (methsuximide, phensuximide).
- The elimination half-life of ethosuximide is 40–60 hours in adults, and 29 hours in children.
- Methsuximide has a half-life of 1.5 hours, normethsuximide, 28–37 hours, and phensuximide, 6 hours.

Clinical Presentations

Toxic effects of ethosuximide include lethargy, headache, fatigue, dizziness, hiccoughs, euphoria, and gastrointestinal discomfort. Idiosyncratic reactions may include systemic lupus erythematosus, eosinophilia, leukopenia, nonspecific rashes, erythema multiforme, behavior changes, and psychoses. Methsuximide may produce lethargy, ataxia, dizziness, and coma.

Toxic Dosage/Death

Since the incidence of toxic reactions to the succinimides is low, correlations of plasma concentrations of the parent drugs with toxic symptoms have not been established. Toxicity with methsuximide overdosage is more closely correlated with plasma levels of an active metabolite. Doses of 10 grams of methsuximide have been associated with toxicity.

Drug Interactions

Hepatic microsomal drug enzyme inducers are expected to enhance the rapidity of conversion of the succinimides to a metabolite. If ethosuximide is added to the therapeutic regimen of a patient receiving phenytoin, serum levels of phenytoin may increase into the toxic range. Ethosuximide does not change phenobarbital or primidone levels in patients on multiple therapy. Phenytoin increases the phenobarbital/primidone ratio by causing an increase in the blood level of phenobarbital.

Pregnancy/Lactation

No specific information is available concerning passage of succinimides through the placenta, effects on the fetus, or passage into breast milk. Ethosuximide is pregnancy risk factor C.

Laboratory

ANALYTIC METHODS

Succinimides are analyzed by flame-ionization gas chromatography and the EMIT system (also used for carbamazepine, phenobarbital, phenytoin, and primidone).

BLOOD LEVELS

After a single dose of ethosuximide, blood levels may remain elevated for up to 24 hours. Treatment may require 8–10 days to achieve a therapeutic blood level plateau. At therapeutic levels, blood levels are directly proportional to the dose. The "therapeutic" plasma levels for ethosuximide range from 40–100 μg/mL. Plasma levels over 100 μg/mL have been reported without toxic effects. Toxic effects are not closely correlated with plasma levels.

For methsuximide, therapeutic levels are less than 7 μg/mL, but plasma levels for the active metabolite, are 10–40 μg/mL (active). Cerebrospinal fluid levels are similar to those in plasma. A 1-gram dose of phensuximide produced peak plasma levels of 10–15 μg/mL.

Treatment

GUT DECONTAMINATION

Emesis may be useful if the patient is alert, is not convulsing, and is seen within an hour of ingestion; however, this has not been clinically proved. No studies are available on the efficacy of gastric lavage in succinimide overdosage. Charcoal (adults, 50–100 grams and children, 15–30 grams) may be helpful after significant overdoses. However, there is no substantive proof of efficacy for the use of activated charcoal or cathartics in succinimide poisoning.

ELIMINATION ENHANCEMENT

Forced diuresis is probably ineffective because of the limited (1–10%) renal excretion of the succinimides. Use of hemodialysis, peritoneal dialysis, and exchange transfusion for succinimide overdose has not been systematically studied. Charcoal hemoperfusion was reported to be effective in a methsuximide overdose.

SUPPORTIVE MEASURES

- Supportive measures are the mainstay of therapy, especially in view of initial apparent recovery, which may be followed by long periods of central nervous system depression.
- Hospitalize the patient in an intensive care unit if obtunded. Respiration must be established and controlled, if necessary, by mechanical assistance. Patients may be in coma for several days.
- Respiratory assistance may be required for days.
- Obtain and monitor complete blood counts and hepatic and renal function tests.

Question—Succinimides

1. Regarding the pharmacokinetics of succinimides, the following is/are incorrect:

A. They are completely absorbed from the gastrointestinal tract.
B. Protein binding plays an important role.
C. The elimination half-life is 40–60 hours in adults.
D. Peak plasma concentrations are achieved within 15 minutes after a therapeutic dose.
E. B and D

NEW ANTICONVULSANTS

Clonazepam, felbamate, gabapentin, vigabatrin, and lamotrigine are new drugs in various phases of investigation as anticonvulsants. Several are structural analogs of GABA, an inhibitory neurotransmitter. The newer anticonvulsants are generally given less often, purportedly are involved in fewer drug interactions, have wider therapeutic windows, frequently cause less sedation, and generally do not induce hepatic enzymes.

Clonazepam

Clonazepam (Klonopin®) is a synthetic benzodiazepine derivative in use as an anticonvulsant in the U.S. since 1975. It is a Schedule IV drug under the Federal Controlled Substances Act of 1970. Clonazepam has a high affinity for central benzodiazepine receptors. It is a facilitator of the γ-aminobutyric acid (GABA) system and also increases the central synthesis of serotonin.

Overdose with clonazepam may produce somnolence, confusion, ataxia, diminished reflexes, or coma. Physical or psychological dependence may follow long-term use by those who have been dependent on other drugs or by alcoholic patients. Sudden withdrawal after long-term administration may lead to dysphoria, restlessness, irritability, sleepiness, hand tremors, oral dyskinesias, muscle rigidity, and seizures. Such symptoms may occur several days after the drug is discontinued, because of its long half-life.

Depression, acute excitation, intrusiveness, and belligerence may reflect behavioral disinhibition associated with clonazepam. Anorgasmia, impaired erectile functioning, and inability to ejaculate have been observed with chronic use of clonazepam. Idiosyncratic, nonhypersensitivity-type liver damage has been reported. Respiratory, gastrointestinal, genitourinary, and hematologic dysfunction may occur during chronic use of clonazepam.

Felbamate

Felbamate (Felbatol®) is a synthetic dicarbamate related to meprobamate. It has been approved as monotherapy or adjunctive therapy for partial seizures with and without generalization in patients older than 14 years. Overdose is accompanied by mild gastric distress. The half-life is 24 hours; 25% is protein bound; elimination is 50% hepatic and 50% renal. No fatalities have been reported. Crystallunia and acute renal failure have been associated with overdose. Aplastic anemia and hepatic failure are rare sequelae.

Gabapentin

Gabapentin (Neurontin®) has been approved by the U.S. FDA for use in patients with partial (focal) seizures with or without secondary generalization. Gabapentin is structurally related to GABA, the major endogenous inhibitory neurotransmitter in the brain, but unlike vigabatrin, another GABA analog, gabapentin is not an agonist at GABA receptors; rather, it binds to a unique receptor in the brain. Overdoses are associated with lethargy, sedation, dizziness, double vision, slurred speech, and occasionally diarrhea, all of which resolve within 18 hours.

Somnolence, fatigue, dizziness, ataxia, fatigue, nystagmus, and weight gain have followed long-term use and have been observed when gabapentin was added to other antiepileptic drugs. Symptoms generally resolve within 18 hours. Doses up to 48.9 grams have been tolerated with few symptoms including moderate sedation, dizziness, fatigue, and slurred speech. There have been no reports of death following an overdose. Acute life-threatening toxicity has not been observed with doses equal to or less than 20 times the recommended human dose.

Vigabatrin

Vigabatrin (Sabril®) is a synthetic structural analog of GABA, which is an inhibitory neurotransmitter. Vigabatrin exists as a racemic mixture of two enantiomers. Only the S enantiomer is pharmacologically active. Vigabatrin appears to be most effective in partial seizures whether or not they also become generalized. Severe behavioral disturbances, drowsiness, irritability, and weight gain may be dose-dependent. Studies suggest that vigabatrin irreversibly inhibits the enzyme GABA transaminase, which itself inactivates GABA. This permits an increase in the concentration of GABA at GABA-ergic synapses in the brain. Vigabatrin is itself inactive but is converted *in vivo* to its active form by GABA aminotransferase.

Long-term use of vigabatrin is associated with drowsiness, headache, fatigue, irritability, depression, dizziness, confusion, and weight gain. These adverse effects appear to be dose-dependent. Excitation in children and hallucinations and paranoia in adults have been reported. Short temper and behavioral disturbances have been observed with doses of 3 grams/d or more. A history of psychiatric illness commonly predisposes patients to a psychotic reaction pattern. Myoclonus and visual field constriction have been seen.

As with all antiepileptic drugs, an acute exacerbation of seizures may occur after the sudden withdrawal of vigabatrin. In addition, withdrawal of vigabatrin has been followed by acute psychosis. One patient developed a psychotic episode lasting 36 hours after taking an overdose of 8–12 grams of vigabatrin during postictal confusion.

Lamotrigine

Lamotrigine (Lamictal®) is a synthetic anticonvulsant chemically unrelated to other agents currently used in epilepsy. It may produce headache, vomiting, and ataxia related to elevated plasma levels. Few patients with overdose have been reported. Treatment is symptomatic and supportive. Lamotrigine appears useful in the treatment of refractory epilepsy, partial epilepsy, and primary generalized epilepsy. Lamotrigine acts mainly by inhibiting excitatory amino acid release. It stabilizes neuronal membranes via blockade of voltage-sensitive sodium channels.

In overdose, lamotrigine induces nausea, vomiting, headache, and ataxia. Other adverse effects include dizziness, diplopia, blurred vision, somnolence, asthenia, rash (in 5% of patients), and depression. Angioedema is rarely observed. Leukopenia has been reported. First-degree heart block has been described. A few deaths have been reported after status epilepticus with disseminated intravascular coagulation and multiorgan failure. Abrupt withdrawal may lead to rebound seizures.

Questions—New Anticonvulsants

1. Which of the following about clonazepam is false?
A. Clonazepam is a benzodiazepine.
B. Clonazepam decreases serotonin production.
C. Clonazepam overdose may be associated with ataxia, confusion, and/or coma.
D. A and C
E. B and C

2. Gabapentin is structurally related to GABA, the major endogenous inhibitory neurotransmitter in the brain, but unlike vigabatrin, another GABA analog, gabapentin is not an agonist at GABA receptors, but rather binds to a unique receptor in the brain.
A. True
B. False

3. Long-term use of vigabatrin is associated with drowsiness, headache, fatigue, irritability, depression, dizziness, confusion, and weight gain.
A. True
B. False

Answers

Introduction to Anticonvulsant Drugs

1. B 2. A 3. E

Phenytoin

1. A 2. B 3. E 4. B 5. E

Carbamazepine

1. D 2. B 3. A 4. E 5. B

Valproic Acid

1. C 2. D 3. E 4. C 5. E

Barbiturates

1. D 2. C 3. E 4. D 5. A

Paraldehyde

1. C 2. B 3. C 4. A 5. E

Primidone

1. B 2. B

Succinimides

1. E

New Anticonvulsants

1. B 2. A 3. A

SELECTED READINGS

Introduction to Anticonvulsant Drugs

1. Handfield-Jones SE, Jankins RE, Whittaker SJ, et al. The anticonvulsant hypersensitivity syndrome. Br J Dermatol 1993;129:175–177.
2. Howell SJ, Owen L, Chadwick DW. Pseudostatus epilepticus. Q J Med 1989; 266:507–519.
3. Morrow JI, Routledge PA. Poisoning by anticonvulsants. Adverse Drug React Acute Poison Rev 1989;8(2):97–109.

Phenytoin

1. Booker HE, Darcey B. Serum concentrations of free diphenylhydantoin and their relationship to intoxication. Epilepsia 1973;14:177.
2. Curtis DL, Pilbe R, Ellenhorn M, et al. Phenytoin toxicity: Predictions of clinical course. Vet Hum Toxicol 1989;31:162–163.
3. Curtis DL, Pirbe R, Ellenhorn MJ, et al. Phenytoin toxicity: A review of 94 cases. Vet Hum Toxicol 1989;31:164–165.
4. Rowden AM, Spoor JE, Bertino JS Jr. The effect of activated charcoal on phenytoin pharmacokinetics. Ann Emerg Med 1990;19:1144–1147.
5. Weichbrodt GD, Elliott DR. A treatment of phenytoin toxicity with repeated doses of activated charcoal. Ann Emerg Med 1987;16:1387–1389.

Carbamazepine

1. Bridge TA, Norton RL, Robertson WA. Pediatric carbamazepine overdose. Pediatr Emerg Care 1994;10:200–263.
2. Hojer J, Malmlund H-A, Berg A. Clinical features in 28 consecutive cases of laboratory confirmed massive poisoning with carbamazepine abuse. Clin Toxicol 1993;25:449–458.
3. Seymour JF. Carbamazepine overdose: Features of 33 cases. Drug Saf 1993; 8:81–88.
4. Wason S, Baher RC, Carolan P, et al. Carbamazepine overdose: The effects of multiple dose activated charcoal. ClinToxicol 1992;30:39–48.

Valproic Acid

1. Anderson GO, Ritland S. Life threatening intoxication with sodium valproate. Clin Toxicol 1995;33:279–284.
2. Garnier R, Boudignat O, Fournier PE. Valproate poisoning. Lancet 1982;2:97.
3. Pinder RM, Borgden RN, Speight TM, et al. Sodium valproate: A review of its pharmacological and therapeutic efficacy in epilepsy. Drugs 1977;13:81–123.
4. Turnbull DM. Adverse effects of valproate. Adverse Drug React Acute Poison Rev 1983;2:191–216.

Barbiturates

1. Lindberg MC, Cunningham A, Lindberg NH. Acute phenobarbital intoxication. South Med J 1992;85:803–807.
2. Vale JA, Ruddock FS, Boldy DAR. Multiple doses of activated charcoal in the management of phenobarbitone and carbamazepine poisoning. Vet Hum Toxicol 1987;29(suppl. 2):152.

Paraldehyde

1. Beier LS, Pitt WH, Gonick HC. Metabolic acidosis occurring during paraldehyde intoxication. Ann Intern Med 1963;58:155–158.
2. Emmett M, Narins PG. Clinical use of the anion gap. Medicine 1977;56:38–54.
3. Seyffart G. Paraldehyde. In: Haddad LM, Winchester JF, eds.Clinical Management of Poisoning and Drug Overdose. Philadelphia: WB Saunders, 1983: 410–413.

Primidone

1. Brillman J, Gallagher BB, Mattson RH. Acute primidone intoxication. Arch Neurol 1974;30:255–258.
2. Gallagher BB, Baumel IP, Mattson RH, et al. Primidone, diphenylhydantoin and phenobarbital aspects of acute and chronic toxicity. Neurology 1973;23:145–149.

Succinimides

1. Browne TR, Dreifuss FE, Dyken PR, et al: Ethosuximide in the treatment of absence (petit mal) seizures. Neurology 1975;25:515–524.
2. Buchanan RA, Kinkel AW, Turner JL, et al: Ethosuximide dosage regimens. Clin Pharmacol Ther 1976;19:143–147.
3. Karch SB: Methsuximide overdose. Delayed onset of profound coma. JAMA 1973;223:1463–1465.
4. Troupin AS: The measurement of anticonvulsant agent levels. Ann Intern Med 1984;100:854–858.

New Anticonvulsants

1. Ahmad SR. Felbamate and aplastic anemia. Lancet 1994;344:465.
2. Betts T, Goodwin G, Withers RM, Yuen AWC. Human safety of lamotrigine. Epilepsia 1991;32(suppl. 2):S17–S21.
3. Brodie MJ, Porter RJ. New and potential anticonvulsants. Lancet 1990;336: 425–426.
4. Browne TR. Clonazepam. Arch Neurol 1976;3:326–332.
5. Buckley A, White JM, Dawson AH. Self-poisoning with lamotrigine. Med J Aust 1993;159:488.
6. Cohen LS, Rosenbaum JF. Clonazepam: New uses and potential problems. J Clin Psychiatry 1987;48(10, suppl):50–55.
7. Fischer JH, Barr AN, Rogers SL, et al. Lack of serious toxicity following gabapentin overdose. Neurology 1994;4:982–983.
8. Garofalo E, Koto E, Feuerstein T. Experience with gabapentin overdose: Five case studies. Epilepsia 1993;34:157.
9. Goa KL, Ross SR, Chrisp P. Lamotrigine: A review of its pharmacological properties and clinical efficiacy in epilepsy. Drugs 1993;46:152–176.
10. Jachel RA. Stevens-Johnson syndrome after treatment with felbamate. Epilepsia 1994;35:98.
11. Paljarvi L, Vapalahti M, Sivenius J, Riekkonen P. Neuropathological findings in 5 patients with vigabatrin treatment. Neurology 1990;40(suppl. 1):151.
12. Welch TR, Rumack BH, Hammond K. Clonazepam overdose resulting in cyclic coma. Clin Toxicol 1977;10:433–436.

ACKNOWLEDGMENT

Thanks to Jonathan Weinstock, MD for contributing questions in this chapter.

CHAPTER 28
Psychotropic Drugs

CYCLIC ANTIDEPRESSANT DRUGS

Introduction

Antidepressant drugs are among the most commonly encountered overdoses. These drugs include tricyclic, tetracyclic, bicyclic, and monocyclic antidepressants, as well as monoamine oxidase (MAO) inhibitors and selective serotonin reuptake inhibitors (SSRIs). See Chapter 36, Serotonergic Drugs. Of these, the tricyclic antidepressants (TCAs) are generally most toxic in overdose, with major toxicity usually noted within the first 6 hours of ingestion. About half of patients who commit suicide are depressed. Most depressed patients who commit suicide are not taking antidepressants. Therapeutic failure appears to be a greater problem with antidepressants than toxicity.

Toxicity following overdose of antidepressant drugs is most likely to be seen with the TCAs and MAO inhibitors, followed by the newer cyclic antidepressants. The older tertiary and secondary amine tricyclic compounds have been used extensively and their acute toxicity is well reported. During the past few years, the number of antidepressants under clinical investigation has expanded rapidly. Maprotiline, trimipramine, trazodone, and amoxapine are recently released compounds for which clinical data are more limited.

PATHOPHYSIOLOGY

Antidepressant agents are active at adrenergic, serotonin, dopamine, histamine H1, and muscarinic receptors. This is reflected in their toxic effects. In general, these drugs have a large volume of distribution and high protein binding, indications that extracorporeal methods of elimination may be relatively ineffective.

CLINICAL PRESENTATIONS

Although, at therapeutic dose levels, definite differences in adverse effects and pharmacokinetic parameters are observed among various tricyclic antidepressant drugs, these compounds behave similarly in overdose. Some newer tricyclic (e.g., chlorimipramine) and tetracyclic (e.g., maprotiline) compounds appear to share similar toxicity in overdose with older tricyclic drugs. Certain newer cyclic compounds appear to display different cardiovascular and central nervous systemic toxicity in overdose. Serious amoxapine toxicity results in coma and seizures with relatively few cardiovascular changes. Trazodone overdose resembles diazepam ingestion, demonstrating fewer tendencies to develop cardiotoxicity or seizures.

LABORATORY

Only the TCAs need to be identified and quantified in acute antidepressant overdose situations. Quantification of other cyclic antidepressants, MAO inhibitors, or SSRIs is not warranted. Qualitative identification of MAO inhibitors and SSRIs may be justified if these drugs are suspected of being present in combination.

Questions—Introduction to Cyclic Antidepressant Drugs

1. Which of the following statements concerning cyclic antidepressants is false?

A. Antidepressant drugs are among the most commonly encountered overdoses.

B. Most depressed patients who commit suicide are taking antidepressants.

C. Therapeutic failure appears to be a greater problem with antidepressants than toxicity.

D. Antidepressant agents are active at adrenergic, serotonin, dopamine, histamine H1, and muscarinic receptors.

E. In general, these drugs have a large volume of distribution and high protein binding, indications that extracorporeal methods of elimination may be relatively ineffective.

2. Which of the following statements concerning cyclic antidepressants is false?

A. Although, at therapeutic dose levels, definite differences in adverse effects and pharmacokinetic parameters are observed between various tricyclic antidepressant drugs, these compounds behave similarly in overdose.

B. Certain newer cyclic compounds appear to display different cardiovascular and central nervous systemic toxicity in overdose.

C. Serious amoxapine toxicity results in coma and seizures with relatively few cardiovascular changes.

D. Trazodone overdose resembles diazepam ingestion, demonstrating fewer tendencies to develop cardiotoxicity or seizures.

E. During the past few years, the number of antidepressants under clinical investigation has declined.

Cyclic Antidepressants

The tricyclic antidepressants are a group of three-ringed drugs that structurally and pharmacologically resemble the phenothiazines. Both the tricyclic antidepressants and phenothiazine compounds share similar anticholinergic, α-adrenergic blocking, and inhibitory adrenergic uptake properties. In 1948, imipramine was the first tricyclic compound synthesized and was originally intended as a hypnotic agent because of its sedative properties. Kuhn suggested the use of imipramine for endogenous depression in 1958, and soon imipramine became a popular substitute for electroshock therapy in severe depression. Amitriptyline, introduced subsequently, is equally efficacious but more sedating.

By the early 1960s, central nervous system and cardiovascular toxicity were recognized as major complications of tricyclic overdose and fatalities were recorded in both children and adults. Improvements in supportive care have reduced the overall mortality rate significantly. By 1982, tricyclic antidepressants were among the most common overdoses seen in emergency departments in the U.S. and trailed only alcohol-drug combinations and heroin in the number of drug-related fatalities.

In an effort to reduce adverse effects and to speed therapeutic action, numerous new antidepressant drugs have been developed. Other tricyclics (e.g., trimipramine), tetracyclics (e.g., maprotiline), dibenzoxazepines (e.g., amoxapine), and structurally unique antidepressants (e.g., trazodone) have been introduced into the U.S. market.

PATHOPHYSIOLOGY

The biogenic amine hypothesis suggests that depression results from a functional deficit of either serotonin or norepinephrine at central nervous system receptor sites. Some studies indicate that tricyclic antidepressants inhibit the re-uptake of synaptic norepinephrine or serotonin and thus functionally increase the amount of these neurotransmitters at critical central nervous system receptors. Tertiary amine tricyclic compounds actually reduce the production of serotonin and norepinephrine metabolites in the cerebral spinal fluid of depressed patients.

Receptor Effects

Cyclic antidepressants are competitive antagonists of muscarinic acetylcholine receptors, which constitute the predominant acetylcholine receptor class in the brain. These compounds do not alter the nicotinic acetylcholine receptors, which predominate in the spinal cord. The potency of the cyclic antidepressant antimuscarinic effects varies widely among compounds: tertiary amines (e.g., amitriptyline) > secondary amines (e.g., nortriptyline) > primary amines.

Since all tricyclic antidepressants share similar efficacy in the treatment of depression, variation in their muscarinic receptor blockade is manifested mainly by the frequency of adverse side effects (e.g., dry mouth, hesitancy, and blurred vision). In addition, these compounds possess potent antihistaminic properties. Cyclic antidepressants also block α-adrenergic and serotonin receptors. Much of the central nervous system toxicity (e.g., coma, delirium, psychosis, convulsions) seen in overdoses is

Answers to questions in shaded boxes appear at the end of the chapter.

an exaggeration of the central and peripheral anticholinergic side effects.

Cardiovascular Effects

With the exception of dibenzoxazepine and trazodone, most fatalities from cyclic antidepressant overdose result from cardiovascular effects. At least four distinct pharmacologic effects contribute to the development of dysrhythmias and cardiovascular depression:

Anticholinergic Effects. Signs include sinus tachycardia and transient hypertension. Tachycardia appears to be independent of blood pressure, since normalization of ventricular filling pressure and hypotension under hemodynamic monitoring results in little change in heart rate.

Norepinephrine Reuptake Blockade. Increased norepinephrine levels at the receptor site initially may potentiate tachycardia and hypertension as well as activate latent pacemaker cells, leading to dysrhythmias.

Stabilizing Effects. Tricyclics also stabilize myocardial membranes. Serious tricyclic antidepressant overdoses slow phase 0 depolarization and markedly impair intracardiac conduction and myocardial depression, similar to quinidine toxicity. Atrioventricular nodal conduction is depressed, suggesting a quinidine-like effect on distal conduction. Reentry dysrhythmias such as ventricular tachycardia, ventricular fibrillation, and Torsade de Pointes may occur because of prolongation of antegrade conduction.

Alpha Blockade. Tricyclics are also α-blockers. Loss of peripheral vascular resistance may lead to orthostatic hypotension that may trigger dysrhythmias. Usually, hypotension results from afterload reduction rather than decreased myocardial contractility.

Pharmacokinetics

Absorption

- Tricyclic antidepressants (TCAs) taken in large quantities exhibit altered toxicokinetics. Their absorption may be delayed by inhibition of gastric emptying and peristalsis.
- Significant enterohepatic recirculation delays final elimination of a large fraction of the drug.
- Enzymes responsible for TCA benzyl-hydroxylation can become saturated and thus reduce TCA elimination to zero-order kinetics. TCA unbound to plasma proteins may also increase because of acidemia resulting from respiratory depression after overdose.
- The peak plasma level of amitriptyline after serious overdose is between 2.0–4.5 hours after drug intake.

Distribution

- Cyclic antidepressants are highly lipophilic and possess large and variable volumes of distribution (i.e., 15–40 L/kg).
- After absorption, these drugs are rapidly distributed to tissue, where high concentrations occur in liver, kidney, lungs, and myocardium. Amitriptyline is distributed predominantly in plasma, nortriptyline in the red blood cells.
- Interpretation of TCA blood levels is clarified by assaying red blood cells and plasma. In an acute overdose, TCA antidepressant red blood cell metabolites may be the best markers of impaired intraventricular conduction.

Elimination

- Plasma concentrations of antidepressant drugs that are more than 95% metabolized are not altered by decreased renal function.
- Concentrations of drugs that are mostly excreted unchanged in the urine are greatly increased in patients with reduced renal function.
- Metabolites that account for 10% or more of the dose of the parent drug in urine are usually increased in the urine.
- Hydroxylated metabolites of antidepressant drugs are pharmacologically active. Hepatic hydroxylation is a major metabolic pathway for TCAs and other antidepressants.
- Quantities of parent drug and active metabolites may vary significantly between individuals given the same dose.
- Amitriptyline elimination half-life in overdose ranges from 15–81 hours, whereas half-lives in imipramine overdose vary between 12–21 hours.

CLINICAL PRESENTATIONS

Cardiovascular Effects

The majority of TCA overdose deaths occur before or soon after arrival at a hospital. Life-threatening arrhythmias and/or cardiac arrest usually occur in a setting of marked EKG changes, hypotension, respiratory depression, coma, or convulsions and are generally uncommon as sole events. Hypotension is common after severe TCA overdose. Hypotension often occurs independently of blood TCA concentration and prolongation of the QRS interval. Hypotension may be associated with the development of arrhythmias and pulmonary edema.

Cardiovascular toxicity with intractable myocardial depression, ventricular tachycardia, and ventricular fibrillation are common mechanisms of death. In human overdoses with fatal outcomes, mainly bradycardias are seen before death; however, tachyarrhythmias and ventricular fibrillation are the most often reported causes of death. Major arrhythmias may develop suddenly in patients who on arrival are normotensive and who have only minor electrocardiographic changes.

Electrocardiogram Effects

Potential electrocardiographic findings after cyclic antidepressant overdose include sinus tachycardia, prolonged PR, QRS and QT intervals, bundle branch block, atrial fibrillation, atrial flutter, ventricular tachycardia, Torsade de Pointes, and ventricular fibrillation. Electrocardiogram changes are usually noted early in the hospital course, and subsequent unexpected cardiac complications in TCA overdose are rare. Patients with a QRS axis greater than 90 are 3.5 times more likely to demonstrate major toxicity than those with a normal axis. Patients with a QRS interval greater than 100 milliseconds are more than 2.5 times more likely to demonstrate severe toxicity (e.g., seizures, endotracheal intubation, coma, arrhythmias requiring treatment, hypotension, or death) than those with a normal interval.

Other ECG parameters with increased likelihood of severe toxicity are sinus tachycardia greater than 120 and a prolonged QTc interval greater than 480 milliseconds. Nonetheless, ECG parameters cannot be relied on to include or exclude the diagnosis of TCA overdose, and TCA levels do not always correlate with ECG parameters. Initial clinical findings of TCA overdose are not adequately replaced by initial ECG parameters in making the diagnosis. When compared with imipramine, trazodone does not produce any PR or QRS interval prolongation.

Respiratory Effects

Tricyclic antidepressant-induced pulmonary edema can develop between 5–48 hours after ingestion. Similarities exist between the adult respiratory distress syndrome following a TCA overdose, the "heroin lung syndrome," and pulmonary injury secondary to methadone ingestion. These similarities include diffuse bilateral pulmonary infiltrates on chest x-ray, hypoxemia, noncardiogenic pulmonary edema, and postmortem findings consisting of alveolar septal thickening, lymphocytic infiltrates, and edema.

Radiographic evidence of pulmonary edema is observed in about 10% of TCA overdose patients. Patients with plasma tricyclic drug levels greater than 2000 ng/mL appear to have a greater tendency to develop bilateral alveolar infiltrates consistent with acute lung injury. A second chest film may be justified in patients with significant TCA levels even when admission films have appeared normal. Some patients with relatively low admission plasma TCA levels may go on to develop radiographic abnormalities. Fatalities involving noncardiogenic pulmonary edema underscore the potential for development of adult respiratory distress syndrome after severe TCA overdose.

Neurologic Effects

Patients with impaired drug clearance, including geriatric patients and alcoholics, may show signs of confusion, agitation, and nervousness even without prominent anticholinergic symptoms. Duration of coma tends to be short. Prolongation of coma more than 24 hours is rare and suggests complications or coingestion of central nervous system depressants. Patients with coma in TCA overdose may make a full recovery despite neurologic findings.

Acute dystonia and extrapyramidal symptoms have followed the therapeutic use of amitriptyline. Most seizures associated with cyclic antidepressant toxicity occur soon after admission, are brief, and terminate without specific anticonvulsant therapy. Even when brief, seizures may occasionally lead to hypotension, abrupt cardiovascular deterioration, and death. TCA-induced seizures appear to be associated with elevated total plasma TCA concentrations.

A significant proportion of antidepressant-related seizures occur in individuals with identifiable predisposing factors such as family history of seizures, neurologic and medical conditions, concurrent medications, and substance abuse. Seizure risk following overdose is higher for amoxapine and maprotiline than for other antidepressant drugs, but similar comparisons for bupropion, fluoxetine, and clomipramine have not been reported. Tremor, akathisia, myoclonus, dyskinesia, delirium, sedation, memory disturbances, neuroleptic malignant syndrome, and mania have been reported after therapeutic use of TCAs. Peripheral neuropathies and polyradiculopathy have followed amitriptyline overdoses.

Gastrointestinal Effects

Bowel ischemia requiring resection may follow a TCA overdose. Acute intestinal pseudo-obstruction, spontaneous cecal perforation, and fecal peritonitis may follow a TCA overdose, especially in the elderly and in those with concomitant neurologic disease. Cholestatic and hepatic reactions associated with TCAs represent an idiosyncratic hypersensitivity reaction and are generally mild and reversible. Severe hepatic injury with fulminant hepatic failure and death has been reported.

Withdrawal Effects

Withdrawal of TCAs may lead to syndromes related to cholinergic rebound. These syndromes include (a) anorexia, nausea, emesis, diarrhea, diaphoresis, myalgias, malaise, headache, chills, fatigue, and anxiety; (b) insomnia accompanied by vivid dreams; (c) akathisia or Parkinsonism; and (d) hypomania or mania. Anecdotal reports suggest that transient behavioral aberrations have followed the abrupt cessation of therapeutic use of TCAs and have included delirium after doxepin use, mania/hypomania, panic and symptoms suggestive of cholinergic hyperactivity after amitriptyline, and extreme motor activity clinically indistinguishable from akathisia after imipramine.

Amoxapine

Although amoxapine is alleged to have fewer cardiac effects than other TCAs, amoxapine overdose may be a precipitating cause of both congestive heart failure and arrhythmias. Amoxapine overdose may abolish brainstem reflexes and still lead to recovery. Corneal reflexes may return 24 hours after serious ingestion, while oculocephalic and oculovestibular responses may not return for 36–48 hours. Neuroleptic malignant syndrome has also been reported after amoxapine overdose. Amoxapine overdose is also associated with a high incidence of seizures.

Maprotiline

The combination of a high maprotiline dose together with sinus tachycardia and a pathologic electrocardiogram appears to indicate a high risk for single or multiple seizures.

Mianserin

Although cardiac arrhythmias with mianserin use are unusual, life-threatening ventricular arrhythmias including polymorphous ventricular tachycardia may follow large overdose. Pinpoint pupils, which may not respond to naloxone, have been reported in overdose.

Trazodone

Seizures and hyponatremia may follow an overdose of trazodone. Severe cardiac toxicity (sinus bradycardia, prolonged QTc interval, Torsade de Pointes, cardiac arrest), coma, and renal failure, while rare, may accompany significant overdose. Respiratory depression is most common in the presence of other central nervous system depressants, but respiratory arrest has followed 2.2 and 3.0 g of trazodone alone.

Viloxazine

Few patients have shown abnormalities on the electrocardiogram after overdose, although there have been anecdotal reports of cardiogenic shock with conduction difficulties and inferior coronary ischemia. There is one report of seizures following therapeutic use. No fatalities have been reported following overdose with viloxazine. Sedation, hypotension, anticholinergic effects, and weight gain have not usually been a problem when viloxazine has been administered in therapeutic doses. Nausea appears to occur in 20–50% of patients.

TOXIC DOSAGE/DEATH

In overdose, cases in which the sum of blood TCA parent drug and major active metabolite concentrations is more than 1.0 μg/mL, toxicity and resulting fatality are probable. Postmortem blood concentrations can be substantially higher than concentrations at the time of death. The assumption that postmortem blood concentrations mirror drug concentrations at the time of death cannot be assumed valid.

Fatal toxicity indices of some tricyclic and second-generation antidepressants suggest a somewhat greater toxicity of the older TCAs when compared with second-generation drugs of the same therapeutic class. Generally, in TCA fatalities, the ratio of parent drug to desmethyl metabolite is greater than 2 in blood as well as in tissues.

Lethal blood nortriptyline concentrations have been reported as 10–26 mg/mL. The minimum toxic dose of maprotiline is

425–750 mg. The lowest acute lethal dose of maprotiline is estimated to be 3 g, but survival has been seen with ingestions as large as 5 g. The therapeutic concentration of mianserin (plus desmethylmianserin) is 100 ng/mL, and serious toxicity has been associated with concentrations above 500 ng/mL.

Trazodone

Following ingestion of 350 mg of trazodone, a 72-year-old woman developed hyponatremia, hypertension, and seizures. A 63-year-old woman ingested 3–4.5 g of trazodone and developed lethargy, sinus bradycardia, a prolonged corrected QT interval (QTc), and Torsade de Pointes leading to cardiac arrest and death. Her serum trazodone level was 5680 ng/mL (therapeutic concentration, 1600 ng/mL). Three trazodone-related fatalities had blood trazodone concentrations ranging from 0.96–4.56 μg/mL.

DRUG INTERACTIONS

Fluoxetine significantly prolongs elimination and increases flow levels of TCAs. Toxic hepatic metabolites of acetaminophen may delay TCA elimination. The elderly have slower rates of drug elimination. All antidepressants that are not monoamine oxidase (MAO) inhibitors, and some that are, reduce seizure thresholds. Newer antidepressants, such as selective 5-hydroxytryptamine uptake inhibitors, have not yet been adequately evaluated in epileptics. Anticholinergic drugs such as antihistamines or phenothiazines may exacerbate signs of anticholinergic poisoning such as tachycardia, mydriasis and dry mucous membranes.

The combination of a TCA and a neuroleptic drug overdose may increase the plasma TCA level, may result in a greater percentage of patients with intraventricular conduction delays and first-degree atrioventricular block, and, to a lesser extent, may increase the incidence of conduction delay and ventricular arrhythmias. Three times as many patients may manifest abnormally prolonged QTc intervals when a neuroleptic drug is also ingested with a TCA. MAO inhibitors taken with certain TCAs may induce fever, muscle contractions, hypotension, metabolic acidosis, and cardiovascular collapse unresponsive to pressors and inotropes.

PREGNANCY/LACTATION

Nursing mothers treated with amitriptyline have infants with nondetectable blood levels of amitriptyline or nortriptyline and no adverse effects. In a study of 15,000 births, there was no evidence of gross congenital abnormalities in infants born to women who received TCAs during their first trimester. In the immediate postpartum period, a newborn can show effects of antidepressants received *in utero*. There are reports of infants showing signs of respiratory distress, urinary retention, myoclonus, tachycardia, and heart failure.

LABORATORY

Analytic Methods

Homogeneous enzyme immunoassays provide rapid and sensitive qualitative methods for the detection of TCAs in plasma, serum, and whole blood. The minimum detectable concentration of most of the TCAs is in the range 15–50 ng/mL. A fluorescent polarization immunoassay is useful for the rapid evaluation of TCAs. A high-performance liquid chromatography (HPLC) method provides good precision, sensitivity, and selectivity for routine confirmation of results by other methods. A reverse-phase liquid chromatography method for analysis of trazodone is sensitive to 0.1 mg/mL. Maprotiline may be detectable in serum by gas-liquid chromatography, gas chromatography-mass spectrometry, or HPLC. It is not included in routine toxic screens.

Blood Levels

In general, an alert and oriented patient with a QRS duration less than 100 milliseconds appears to be the best indicator for safe transfer to a medical or psychiatric ward, and awaiting a blood level is generally not helpful in acute overdoses. Plasma TCA concentrations in one study of 67 parents with TCA overdose were of no added value in predicting toxic complications or deciding when patients could leave the intensive care unit. It is not possible to predict outcome based on a simple amitriptyline concentration because of the wide range of concentrations of amitriptyline and amitriptyline metabolites observed between individuals.

Nonetheless, patients with plasma TCA levels greater than 450 ng/mL tend to develop cognitive or behavioral toxicity manifested by agitation, disorientation, confusion, memory impairment, fragmented speech, pacing, or decreased concentration. Postmortem blood concentrations ranged from 1.7–25.3 μg/mL in one autopsy series. Quantitative plasma concentrations are of little help in the immediate management of a TCA overdose.

TREATMENT

Gut Decontamination

Gastric decontamination in alert individuals who demonstrate an intact gag reflex should begin as early as possible, with large-volumes (at least 5 L) of gastric lavage fluid followed by charcoal administration. Pills have been recovered as late as 18 hours after cyclic antidepressant ingestion. Charcoal has been shown to decrease plasma levels. One gram per kilogram is given initially and then, if bowel sounds are present, every 2–4 hours in serious overdoses.

A multidose regimen may reduce the elimination half-life to as little as 4 hours. Repeat doses of activated charcoal may, in rare TCA overdoses, induce diminished bowel motility and produce an obstructing charcoal bezoar. Obtunded, intubated patients who have ingested TCAs should receive an initial dose of charcoal, but repetitive doses should be withheld if bowel sounds remain absent. Gastric aspiration should be performed before extubation of these patients.

Elimination Enhancement

As cyclic antidepressants are highly protein and tissue bound, hemodialysis and charcoal hemoperfusion are of little value, although hemoperfusion may have a rare role in acute refractory cardiovascular instability. One anecdotal report suggested that patients with hemodynamic collapse who are unresponsive to advanced life support measures, fluid and vasopressor therapy, may respond to femoral-femoral extracorporeal circulation, which can provide hemodynamic support until toxic cardiovascular effects abate.

Supportive Measures

- Cyclic antidepressants represent a drug group in which a patient with an acute overdose may present to the emergency department with trivial symptoms, yet may subsequently deteriorate rapidly despite maximum medical therapy.
- All patients who may have ingested more than 10–20 mg of TCAs per kilogram should immediately receive an intravenous line and cardiac monitoring. Those patients with altered mental status should receive oxygen, naloxone, glucose, and, if indicated, thiamine.

- Initial attention should be directed toward evaluation of the adequacy of ventilation. Serious toxicity usually results from ventricular dysrhythmias, hypotension, seizures, or respiratory insufficiency. As with any case of suspected overdose, the ABCs are the initial considerations, with early attention to gastric decontamination.
- A Glasgow Coma Scale score less than 8 was the most sensitive predictor of serious complications in one series of patients who overdosed on TCAs (sensitivity, 86%; specificity, 89%). This was significantly better than the QRS interval (QRS 100 milliseconds; sensitivity, 59%; specificity, 76%) as a predictor, and should be calculated in all patients with obtundation. Patients responsive to verbal stimuli on leaving the emergency department appear to be at very low risk of developing complications.
- Most patients who develop cardiovascular or central nervous system complications do so within 1 hour of admission. Few develop arrhythmias after they become alert and their electrocardiogram readings have been normal for 1 hour. Therefore, 24 hours of cardiac monitoring is considered sufficient, if no underlying cardiac disease exists.
- Other causes of anticholinergic syndrome should be considered if these symptoms are detected (tachycardia, flushing, decreased bowel sounds, mydriasis, altered mental status).
- Patients may be observed for 6 hours and discharged after a final dose of charcoal if no central nervous system depression, respiratory depression, hypotension, dysrhythmias, conduction block, or seizures persist.
- The decision to admit should be based on the presence of central nervous system depression, respiratory depression, hypotension, dysrhythmias, conduction block, and/or seizures. Most major complications develop within 6 hours of arrival. Sinus tachycardia is a nonspecific finding that probably need not alter the decision to discharge; however, persistent tachycardia demands a thorough evaluation.

Hypotension

- Intravenous access should be secured rapidly in cases of hypotension, and blood pressure should initially be supported with fluid boluses. For refractory hypotension, sympathomimetic agents such as norepinephrine may effectively counter cyclic antidepressant-induced α-blockade.
- Agents such as dopamine are less effective because of norepinephrine depletion at synaptic terminals and failure of the agent to be taken up into cells. Pure β-adrenergic agonists, such as isoproterenol and dobutamine, and even combination α- and β-adrenergic agonists like dopamine can result in unopposed β-adrenergic activity in the face of α-adrenergic blockade and may worsen hypotension and arrhythmias.
- Sodium bicarbonate has been demonstrated to increase blood pressure and should be administered concomitantly with pressors. There are anecdotal reports of success with extracorporeal bypass and an intraaortic balloon pump. Prolonged cardiac massage may even be necessary in cases of asystole, as successful recovery has occurred in both children and adults despite periods of asystole exceeding 90 minutes.
- Blockage of endogenous norepinephrine reuptake by TCAs may result in a state of catecholamine depletion. This suggests the use of direct-acting catecholamine such as norepinephrine, instead of indirect-acting agents such as dopamine, which depends on the release of endogenous catecholamines for its clinical effect. Both epinephrine and norepinephrine are effective in reversing myocardial depression during severe TCA intoxication.
- Intravenous glucagon, 10 mg followed by an infusion of 10 mg over 6 hours has resulted in a sustained rise in blood pressure following imipramine-induced hypotension. This was accompanied by shortening of the QRS interval.

Dysrhythmias

- Sodium loading may be the most important factor in reducing TCA toxicity, possibly because of overwhelming TCA-induced sodium channel blockade. Use of intravenous sodium chloride has resulted in narrowing of QRS complexes, diminished tendency to ventricular tachycardia and ventricular fibrillation, and an increase in blood pressure.
- Other drugs with membrane-stabilizing effects, namely, type IA and IC antiarrhythmic agents, may exacerbate ventricular dysrhythmias. These agents must be avoided. Phenytoin may improve conduction but has not been shown to be more effective than alkalinization and should be avoided. Lidocaine and magnesium sulfate may be used to treat TCA-induced dysrhythmias.
- In Torsade de Pointes and other ventricular dysrhythmias, magnesium is administered as a 2.0 gram intravenous bolus of magnesium sulfate. If necessary, a 2.0–4.0 gram bolus may be given 5–15 minutes later. A magnesium sulfate infusion may be given at a rate of 3–20 mg/min and continued until the QT interval is less than 500 milliseconds. Side effects of magnesium sulfate may include a flushing sensation, and mild hypotension.

Seizures

- Benzodiazepines are used to control TCA-induced seizures, providing rapid central nervous system penetration without prolonged sedation. If benzodiazepines fail to control seizure activity, phenobarbital (15–20 mg/kg) may be used as a second-line agent.
- Physostigmine, a carbamate anticholinesterase, is a nonspecific central nervous system analeptic that has been used in this setting but is relatively contraindicated due to potential side effects (i.e., cholinergic crisis, bradycardia, asystole, and death.)
- An anecdotal report suggests that when high-dose benzodiazepine therapy fails to control seizure activity in amoxapine-induced refractory status epilepticus, propofol may be effective.

ANTIDOTES

Sodium Bicarbonate

Sodium bicarbonate therapy has successfully reversed bradyrhythmias, multifocal premature ventricular ectopy, ventricular tachycardia, conduction delays, varying degrees of heart block, and hypotension. Shortening of the QRS interval to below the threshold 100 milliseconds often seen in significant TCA overdoses may be seen with its use. The exact mechanism of action is controversial as both serum pH and extracellular sodium concentrations may contribute to the beneficial effects of sodium bicarbonate on cardiotoxicity. Sodium bicarbonate is administered as an intravenous bolus of 1–2 mEq/kg followed by a continuous infusion titrated to pH. It is given immediately on the discovery of conduction abnormalities or QRS duration exceeding 100 milliseconds.

Fab Fragments

Animal studies suggest that anti-imipramine and anti-nortriptyline antibodies (Fab fragments) may help redistribute these agents and reduce target tissue concentrations. The use of equimolar amounts of Fab to neutralize TCA, as in Digibind® treatment, would appear to require excessive amounts of Fab. Titration with Fab to reduce free TCA levels may be an approach to control toxic effects of an overdose of TCA and avoid administration of excessively large amounts of protein.

Questions—Cyclic Antidepressants

1. **Which of the following statements concerning cyclic antidepressants is false?**
   A. The tricyclic antidepressants are a group of three-ringed drugs that structurally and pharmacologically resemble the benzodiazepines.
   B. Both the tricyclic antidepressants and phenothiazine compounds share similar anticholinergic, α-adrenergic blocking, and inhibitory adrenergic uptake properties.
   C. The biogenic amine hypothesis suggests that depression results from a functional deficit of either serotonin or norepinephrine at central nervous system receptor sites.
   D. Some studies indicate that tricyclic antidepressants inhibit the re-uptake of synaptic norepinephrine or serotonin and thus functionally increase the amount of these neurotransmitters at critical central nervous system receptors.
   E. Cyclic antidepressants are competitive antagonists of muscarinic acetylcholine receptors, which constitute the predominant acetylcholine receptor class in the brain.

2. **Most fatalities from cyclic antidepressant overdose result from cardiovascular effects. Which pharmacologic effect does not contribute to the development of dysrhythmias and cardiovascular depression?**
   A. Anticholinergic effects
   B. Norepinephrine re-uptake blockade
   C. α-adrenergic agonism
   D. Myocardial membrane stabilization or quinidine-like effect
   E. Loss of peripheral vascular resistance

3. **Which statement(s) about the pharmacokinetics of TCAs is/are true?**
   A. Tricyclic antidepressants (TCAs) taken in large quantities exhibit altered toxicokinetics. Their absorption may be delayed by inhibition of gastric emptying and peristalsis.
   B. Enterohepatic recirculation is not a factor in TCA overdose.
   C. TCAs unbound to plasma proteins may increase because of acidemia resulting from respiratory depression after overdose.
   D. All of the above.
   E. A and C

4. **Cyclic antidepressants are highly lipophilic and possess small volumes of distribution.**
   A. True
   B. False

5. **Which statement about the pharmacokinetics of TCAs is false?**
   A. After absorption, these drugs are rapidly distributed to tissue, where high concentrations occur in liver, kidney, lungs, and myocardium.
   B. Nortriptyline is distributed predominantly in plasma, amitriptyline in the red blood cells.
   C. In an acute overdose, TCA antidepressant red blood cell metabolites may be the best markers of impaired intraventricular conduction.
   D. Concentrations of drugs that are mostly excreted unchanged in the urine are greatly increased in patients with reduced renal function.
   E. Quantities of parent drug and active metabolites may vary significantly between individuals given the same dose.

6. **The following statements about the cardiovascular effects of TCAs are true, except**
   A. Life-threatening arrhythmias and/or cardiac arrest usually occur in a setting of marked electrocardiographic changes, hypotension, respiratory depression, coma, or convulsions and are generally uncommon as sole events.
   B. Hypertension is common after severe TCA overdose.
   C. Hypotension may be associated with the development of arrhythmias and pulmonary edema.
   D. Cardiovascular toxicity with intractable myocardial depression, ventricular tachycardia, and ventricular fibrillation are common mechanisms of death.
   E. Major arrhythmias may develop suddenly in patients who on arrival are normotensive and who have only minor electrocardiographic changes.

7. **Potential electrocardiographic findings after cyclic antidepressant overdose include**
   A. Sinus arrhythmia
   B. Prolonged PR, QRS and QT intervals
   C. Bundle branch block, atrial fibrillation and atrial flutter
   D. All of the above
   E. B and C

8. **Electrocardiogram changes are usually noted early in the hospital course, and subsequent unexpected cardiac complications in TCA overdose are rare.**
   A. True
   B. False

9. **Patients with a QRS interval greater than 100 milliseconds are more than 2.5 times more likely to demonstrate severe toxicity (seizures, endotracheal intubation, coma, arrhythmias requiring treatment, hypotension, or death) than those with a normal interval.**
   A. True
   B. False

10. **ECG parameters cannot be relied on to include or exclude the diagnosis of TCA overdose, and TCA levels do not always correlate with ECG parameters.**
   A. True
   B. False

11. **Which of the following statements is false?**
   A. Tricyclic antidepressant-induced pulmonary edema can develop hours after ingestion.
   B. Similarities exist between the adult respiratory distress syndrome following a TCA overdose, the "heroin lung syndrome," and pulmonary injury secondary to methadone ingestion.
   C. Radiographic evidence of pulmonary edema is observed in about 50% of TCA overdose patients.
   D. Patients with plasma tricyclic drug levels greater than 2,000 ng/mL appear to have a greater tendency to develop bilateral alveolar infiltrates consistent with acute lung injury.

E. Some patients with relatively low admission plasma TCA levels may go on to develop radiographic abnormalities.

12. Which of the following statements is false?
A. Patients with impaired drug clearance, including geriatric patients and alcoholics, may show signs of confusion even without prominent anticholinergic symptoms after TCA overdose.
B. Prolongation of coma after TCA overdose more than 24 hours is common.
C. Patients with coma in TCA overdose may make a full recovery despite neurologic findings.
D. Acute dystonia and extrapyramidal symptoms have followed the therapeutic use of amitriptyline.
E. A significant proportion of antidepressant-related seizures occur in individuals with identifiable predisposing factors such as family history of seizures, neurologic and medical conditions, concurrent medications, and substance abuse.

13. Seizure risk following overdose is higher for amoxapine and maprotiline than for other antidepressant drugs.
A. True
B. False

14. Withdrawal of TCAs may lead to the following symptoms, except
A. Hyperphagia, diarrhea, diaphoresis
B. Myalgias, malaise, headache
C. Chills, fatigue, anxiety
D. Insomnia
E. Hypomania or mania

15. Which of the following statements is true?
A. Gastric decontamination should never be attempted in TCA overdose.
B. Charcoal can actually increase plasma levels.
C. As cyclic antidepressants are highly protein and tissue bound, hemodialysis and charcoal hemoperfusion are of little value, although hemoperfusion may have a rare role in acute refractory cardiovascular instability.
D. Cyclic antidepressant overdose is universally treatable if recognized.
E. Alkalinization universally improves prognosis in TCA overdose.

16. In TCA overdose, pure β-adrenergic agonists, such as isoproterenol and dobutamine, and even combination α- and β-adrenergic agonists (like dopamine) can result in unopposed β-adrenergic activity in the face of α-adrenergic blockade and may worsen hypotension.
A. True
B. False

17. Which of the following statements is true?
A. Sodium bicarbonate therapy has successfully reversed bradyrhythmias and multifocal premature ventricular ectopy in TCA overdose.
B. Sodium bicarbonate therapy has successfully reversed ventricular tachycardia and conduction delays in TCA overdose.
C. Sodium bicarbonate therapy has successfully reversed varying degrees of heart block and hypotension in TCA overdose.
D. All of the above.
E. A and B

Clomipramine

Clomipramine (Anafranil®),a synthetic tricyclic antidepressant analog of imipramine, was approved in the U.S. in January 1990 for the treatment of obsessive-compulsive disorder (OCD). It may take 2–3 months before it begins to have an impact on OCD. It has been associated with death following overdose, although many patients survive after ingesting large doses.

PATHOPHYSIOLOGY

Clomipramine inhibits serotonin reuptake. This property may distinguish antidepressant drugs that are active in OCD from those that are not. Clomipramine decreases the concentration of the primary metabolite of serotonin, 5-hydroxyindoleacetic acid (5-HIAA), in the cerebrospinal fluid. The ability of clomipramine to reduce OCD symptoms may also be due to a down-regulation of serotonin receptors. Clomipramine may also cause dopamine antagonism, suppress rapid eye movement sleep, elevate plasma prolactin, and induce an increase in the heart rate and PR interval.

PHARMACOKINETICS

Absorption

- Although it is well absorbed from the gastrointestinal tract, clomipramine is subject to extensive first-pass metabolism, which decreases its oral bioavailability to about 50%.
- First-pass demethylation converts clomipramine to its primary active metabolite, desmethylclomipramine.
- Peak plasma concentrations of clomipramine occur 3–4 hours after a 150-mg dose, whereas levels of desmethylclomipramine peak after 4–6 hours.

Distribution

- The mean apparent volume of distribution is 12 L/kg (range, 7–20 L/kg).
- Clomipramine is 98% bound to plasma proteins, and its major metabolite, desmethylclomipramine, is 97% bound.

Elimination

- Clomipramine has an elimination half-life of about 39 hours.
- The elimination half-life of desmethylclomipramine has been reported to range from 4–233 days.

CLINICAL PRESENTATIONS

Side effects of clomipramine use resemble those of other TCAs. Anticholinergic effects are most frequently reported and include dry mouth, constipation, blurred vision, urinary retention, and mydriasis. Hyponatremia, excessive sweating, myoclonus, manic episodes, hyperprolactinemia, amenorrhea, anorgasmia, galactorrhea, disruption of glucose control in patients with diabetes mellitus, pancreatitis, and seizures have been reported. Clomipramine dependence may lead to anxiety attacks, perspiration, abdominal pain, and loss of efficacy following attempts to withdraw or to decrease dose.

Clinical features of overdose are similar to those observed with other TCAs. Mild intoxication generally appears within 4 hours and is characterized by dry mouth, blurred vision, dilated pupils, sinus tachycardia, extrapyramidal signs, and either drowsiness or excitation. With more severe overdose, hypotension, convulsions, coma, respiratory depression, and electrocardiographic abnormalities such as prolonged PR interval and widened QRS complex may occur. Fatalities have been reported.

TOXIC DOSAGE/DEATH

Doses up to 5 g have been ingested with complete recovery. The lowest dose of clomipramine associated with a fatality was 750 mg.

DRUG INTERACTIONS
Lithium may augment the effects of clomipramine when used in patients with obsessive and panic symptoms.

PREGNANCY/LACTATION
Clomipramine has been placed in pregnancy risk category C. Clomipramine has been detected in human milk. The American Academy of Pediatrics and other authors consider clomipramine compatible with breastfeeding. Maternal use of clomipramine during late pregnancy may lead to a full-term infant displaying a withdrawal syndrome consisting of tachypnea, intermittent hypertonia, and marked diaphoresis in the first hours of life.

LABORATORY

Analytic Methods
High-pressure liquid chromatography has been used to identify the plasma and urinary concentrations of clomipramine and its metabolites.

Blood Levels
Deaths following clomipramine overdose have been associated with blood clomipramine levels ranging from 540–6,560 ng/mL and desmethylclomipramine levels ranging from 580–9,900 ng/mL. Plasma drug concentrations are not correlated with efficacy and are not useful in treating overdose.

TREATMENT

Gut Decontamination
Gastric lavage and activated charcoal may be helpful.

Elimination Enhancement
The high degree of protein binding, together with the extensive volume of distribution, tends to preclude the potential usefulness of hemodialysis and hemoperfusion.

Supportive Measures
- Airway and circulatory support should be instituted immediately, with monitoring of vital signs, electrocardiogram, and clinical parameters. Ventilation and other life support measures may be required. Benzodiazepines or barbiturates usually stop seizures.
- Toxicologic screening of blood and urine may confirm poisoning and rule out the presence of other toxins.
- Electrocardiographic abnormalities similar to those found with other TCA overdoses may be observed with clomipramine.

ANTIDOTE
Sodium bicarbonate, as with other TCAs, may reverse cardiotoxic effects.

Questions—Clomipramine

1. Clomipramine is approved to treat
A. Tourette's disorder
B. Parkinson's disease
C. Amyotrophic lateral sclerosis
D. Obsessive-compulsive disorder
E. Schizophrenia

2. Which of the following statements is false?
A. Clomipramine inhibits serotonin reuptake.
B. Clomipramine may cause dopamine antagonism, suppress rapid eye movement sleep, elevate plasma prolactin, and induce an increase in the heart rate.
C. Clinical features of overdose are similar to those observed with other TCAs.
D. Mild intoxication generally appears within 4 hours and is characterized by dry mouth, blurred vision, pinpoint pupils, sinus bradycardia, extrapyramidal signs, and either drowsiness or excitation.
E. Fatalities have been reported after clomipramine overdose.

Venlafaxine

Venlafaxine (Effexor®) is a synthetic cyclic antidepressant useful in the treatment of depression and possibly in obsessive-compulsive disorder.

PATHOPHYSIOLOGY
Venlafaxine inhibits norepinephrine and serotonin reuptake and weakly inhibits dopamine reuptake.

PHARMACOKINETICS

Absorption
- Venlafaxine is well absorbed from the gastrointestinal tract.
- Peak serum concentrations are reached 1–2 hours after oral administration.
- Following oral administration, venlafaxine undergoes first-pass metabolism to its major active metabolite.

Distribution
- Venlafaxine is about 30% protein bound.
- The apparent volume of distribution of venlafaxine is about 6–7 L/kg.
- The volume of distribution of its major active metabolite is about 4–6 L/kg.

Elimination
- The drug is metabolized by the cytochrome P450 system in the liver, and about 1–10% is excreted in the urine as unchanged drug.
- The elimination half-life of the parent drug is about 5 hours, and that of the metabolite, 11 hours.

CLINICAL PRESENTATIONS
Adverse effects of venlafaxine resemble those of fluoxetine (Prozac®) and the other selective serotonin reuptake inhibitors. See Chapter 36, Serotonergic Drugs. Symptoms may include nausea, headache, anxiety, anorexia, nervousness, sweating, dizziness, insomnia, and somnolence. Extrapyramidal effects can occur with as little as one or two therapeutic doses of venlafaxine. Sexual dysfunction, diastolic hypertension, and weight loss may occur. Seizures have been observed. In overdose, severe central nervous system depression has been observed. All overdose patients have recovered without sequelae.

TOXIC DOSAGE/DEATH
Doses of 2.75 g have led to seizures, coma and prolongation of the QTc interval to 500 milliseconds. An adult who ingested 1.5 g became unresponsive to verbal commands and developed

sinus tachycardia. Ingestion of 2.5 g led to loss of consciousness, stupor, and sinus tachycardia in another case. A fatal dose has not been reported.

DRUG INTERACTIONS

Drugs that inhibit the cytochrome P450 system, such as quinidine, may increase serum concentrations and possibly the toxicity of venlafaxine in extensive metabolizers. Venlafaxine should not be started until at least 14 days after a monoamine oxidase inhibitor has been discontinued because of its adrenergic and serotonergic activity. Concomitant selective serotonin reuptake inhibitor (SSRI) and monoamine oxidase inhibitor (MAOI) therapy may cause hyperthermia, rigidity, myoclonus, autonomic instability, and mental status changes including agitation progressing to delirium and coma. A syndrome resembling neuroleptic malignant syndrome has been reported with concomitant TCA and MAOI therapy.

PREGNANCY/LACTATION

There are no adequate and well-controlled studies in pregnant women.

LABORATORY

Analytic Methods

Venlafaxine and its o-desmethyl metabolite are analyzed by high-performance liquid chromatography with ultraviolet detection, a method that is sensitive to as little as 10 ng/mL of both the drug and its metabolite.

Blood Levels

After ingestion of 2.75 and 2.5 g, peak plasma levels were 6.24 and 2.35 μg/mL, respectively.

TREATMENT

Gut Decontamination

Activated charcoal or gastric lavage should be considered, but the airway must be secured because of possible seizures.

Elimination Enhancement

As venlafaxine has a large volume of distribution, forced diuresis, dialysis, hemoperfusion, and exchange transfusion are unlikely to be of any benefit.

Supportive Measures

- Treatment should include maintenance of an adequate airway, oxygenation, and ventilation. Cardiac rhythm and vital signs must be monitored.
- Bicarbonate has not been used.
- Small increases in serum cholesterol have been reported.

Question—Venlafaxine

1. Which of the following statements about venlafaxine overdose is false?

A. Adverse effects of venlafaxine resemble those of fluoxetine and the other selective serotonin reuptake inhibitors.
B. Symptoms may include nausea, headache, anxiety, anorexia, nervousness, sweating, dizziness, insomnia, and somnolence.
C. Extrapyramidal effects can occur with as little as one or two therapeutic doses of venlafaxine.
D. Serious central nervous system depression has not been observed.
E. Drugs that inhibit the cytochrome P450 system may increase serum concentrations and possibly the toxicity of venlafaxine in extensive metabolizers.

MONOAMINE OXIDASE INHIBITORS

The mood-elevating properties of monoamine oxidase (MAO) inhibitors (MAOIs) were first discovered in the 1950s with use of the isoniazid derivative, iproniazid. By the 1960s, MAOI compounds such as isocarboxazid, nialamide, phenelzine, and tranylcypromine were administered to depressed patients as principal pharmacologic agents. Ultimately, cyclic antidepressant drugs have largely replaced MAOIs as the drugs of choice for endogenous depression. Interest in MAOI agents, however, has occasionally been renewed for the treatment of depression, neurotic illnesses with depressive features, and phobias. MAOI agents have been used to treat depression when tricyclic antidepressants and electroconvulsive therapy have been unsuccessful.

MAOIs block the oxidative deamination of monoamines and may produce serious drug and food interactions. Foods that contain large amounts of tyramine (i.e., over 10 g) and indirect-acting sympathomimetic drugs can cause a fatal hypertensive crisis and malignant hyperthermia syndrome in patients receiving concomitant MAOI compounds. The clinical features of MAOI overdose may be delayed 6–12 hours and include agitation, irritability, diaphoresis, tachycardia, muscle rigidity, hyperpyrexia, hypertension, and hyperreflexia. Serious reactions may involve intracranial bleeding, hypotension, coma, seizures, respiratory distress, and malignant hyperthermia, which may be fatal.

MAOIs include pargyline, iproniazid, isocarboxazid, mebanazine, nialamide, phenelzine, and tranylcypromine. Structurally these products are classified as hydrazines, hydrazides, or nonhydrazine compounds (amine or ammonia derivatives). Phenelzine is the hydrazine analogue of phenylethylamine, which is a substrate for monoamine oxidase. Isocarboxazid is a hydrazide, whereas tranylcypromine and pargyline are amines.

Selegiline, a derivative of methamphetamine, is a selective MAO-B inhibitor. Its dopaminergic effect confers efficacy in Parkinson's disease. In the U.S., interest in selegiline increased after discovery of its ability to antagonize the effects of 1-methyl-4-phenyl-1,2,3,6-tetrahydropyridine (MPTP), a "designer drug" that causes the symptoms of Parkinson's disease. Selegiline is used as an adjunct in the management of parkinsonian patients being treated with levodopa-carbidopa who exhibit deterioration in the quality of their response to this therapy.

Pathophysiology

MAO inhibitors produce their effect primarily by blocking monoamine oxidase. This results in alterations of neurotransmitter metabolism. Apparently two types of MAO receptors appear in human tissue, displaying different concentrations in different tissues and possessing different affinities for MAOI drugs (e.g., MAO-A demonstrates a preference for serotonin while MAO-B prefers phenylethylamine). In addition, MAOI compounds inhibit hepatic microsomal enzymes. Potentiation and prolongation of central neurotransmitters presumably produce mood elevation.

Several mechanisms operate during toxic states. MAO inhibition results in the elevation of brain dopamine, norepinephrine, and serotonin levels. In experimental animals, phenelzine and tranylcypromine increase the release of norepinephrine from sympathetic nerve endings. This may potentiate the effects of MAO inhibition. These drugs also possess sympatholytic properties at postganglionic nerve terminals (e.g., depletion), and this may account for late cardiovascular and central nervous system depression seen in the terminal phase of fatal overdoses.

Pharmacokinetics

ABSORPTION

- MAO inhibitor compounds are oral agents and no parenteral forms are available.
- They are rapidly and completely absorbed from the gastrointestinal tract.
- Selegiline is readily absorbed following oral administration (half-life of absorption, 0.3 hour).

DISTRIBUTION

- Plasma tranylcypromine levels peak at about 25 ng/mL, 2 hours after ingestion of a 20-mg dose.
- Selegiline is highly bound to plasma protein and has a high volume of distribution of 4.7 L/kg.

ELIMINATION

- Elimination probably occurs primarily via acetylation.
- Certain individuals (i.e., slow acetylators) may be more susceptible to toxic reactions.
- As methamphetamine and amphetamine have appeared in the plasma of a patient with a tranylcypromine overdose, these compounds may be metabolites of tranylcypromine.
- Selegiline is extensively metabolized to form methamphetamine (half-life, 20.5 hours), amphetamine and N-desmethylselegiline (half-life, 2 hours). The kidneys excrete the metabolites.

Clinical Presentations

Classical MAOIs may be associated with lethal toxicity in overdose. After a "latent" period up to 12 hours, patients may progressively develop motor uneasiness, agitation, violent motor activity with moaning and grimacing, profuse sweating, and hallucinations. Death may result from hyperthermia, which may peak as late as 24 hours post-presentation. Patients should be closely monitored for 24 hours with strict control over dietary and drug intake. Deaths have most commonly followed interaction of therapeutic MAOIs with dietary agents, tricyclic antidepressants, or sympathomimetic amines. Serious secondary events include hemolysis, rhabdomyolysis, disseminated intravascular coagulopathy, renal failure, pulmonary edema, fetal demise, and asystole.

NEUROLOGIC SYMPTOMS

Signs and symptoms of overdose may include drowsiness, dizziness, faintness, irritability, hyperactivity, agitation, severe headache, hallucinations, trismus, opisthotonus, seizures and coma, rapid and irregular pulse, hypertension, hypotension and vascular collapse, precordial pain, respiratory depression and failure, hyperpyrexia, diaphoresis, and cold, clammy skin. Therapeutic use of selegiline may lead to increased tremor, bradykinesia, falling, dystonic symptoms, dyskinesias, hallucinations, confusion, sleep disturbance, headache, dry mouth, blurred vision, orthostatic hypotension, hypertension, poor appetite, urinary retention, and diaphoresis. Hypomanic behavior may be due to the amphetamine and amphetamine metabolites of selegiline.

SEROTONIN SYNDROME

The serotonin syndrome involves the use of MAOIs with serotonin receptor drugs. See Chapter 36, Serotonergic Drugs. Patients may develop central nervous system irritability, hyperreflexia, and myoclonus. The blood pressure may be normal. Fatalities have been reported.

ABUSE

Patients with a history of substance abuse or a character disorder have abused phenelzine and tranylcypromine. Medications may be used in excessive amounts, exceeding therapeutic safety limits, often with disregard for potential or actual harmful results. Evidence of excessive dosage (irritability, anger, and teeth grinding) is often present with little evidence of tolerance to these side effects. Withdrawal symptoms may include anxiety, depression, confusion, hallucinations, tremulousness, nausea, vomiting, diarrhea, and chills.

Toxic Dosage/Death

MAOI ingestions of 2–3 mg/kg or more should be considered potentially dangerous. A phenelzine overdose of 4–6 mg/kg was fatal despite intensive supportive care. Five grams of nialamide was fatal in a 27-year-old man. A 170-mg tranylcypromine dose in an adult on a therapeutic regimen (10 mg twice daily) has been fatal. Postmortem blood tranylcypromine levels in overdose cases have been 0.25 mg/L (850-mg overdose) and 3.7 mg/L (300-mg overdose). Exposure to doses of 600 mg of selegiline may result in severe hypotension and psychomotor agitation.

Postmortem examination of MAOI-induced fatalities demonstrates nonspecific pathological findings. Autopsy abnormalities include cerebral edema, pulmonary edema, focal alveolar hemorrhage, and diffuse congestion of various organs. Histochemical examination displays a marked diminution in MAO activity, but the decrease in enzyme activity does not correlate with clinical effect.

Drug and Food Interactions

A serious drawback to the use of nonselective irreversible MAOIs is their potential for interactions that result in increased concentrations of pressor amines and, in some cases, life-threatening hypertension. This response may occur in combination with other drugs, including tricyclic antidepressants, sympathomimetic amines (e.g., pseudoephedrine and phenylpropanolamine), meperidine, and with foods rich in tyramine.

Examples of tyramine-containing foods include aged cheeses, certain beers and wines, citrus fruits, caviar, soy sauce, broad beans, snails, chicken liver, pickled herring, salami, and cream. The selective MAOI, selegiline, preferentially inhibits MAO-B and is thought to be less likely to provoke hypertensive crises with amine-rich foods or when co-prescribed with other catecholamine-enhancing drugs.

Symptoms of MAOI interactions may include a throbbing headache, hypertension, tachycardia, diaphoresis, hyperpyrexia, subarachnoid hemorrhage, and death. The impairment of microsomal enzymes by MAO inhibitor drugs potentiates and prolongs the effects of chloral hydrate, barbiturates, and other sedative/hypnotics. Hydralazine, thiazide diuretics, α-methyldopa, and guanethidine may cause hypotension or hypertension after concurrent care with MAO inhibitors. MAOI agents also possess anticholinergic properties and may seriously exacerbate the clinical effects of anticholinergic drugs such as atropine. α-blockade in the setting of MAOI-induced unopposed α sympathetic activity may cause a severe hypertensive crisis.

Ingestion of selegiline with fluoxetine by an adult led to mania, diaphoresis, and hypertension. The combination of selegiline with meperidine resulted in increased restlessness and irritability, progressing to delirium, with muscular rigidity, sweating, and hyperthermia. Combinations of selegiline with tricyclic antidepressants or serotonin reuptake inhibitors may be associated with fever, tremors, agitation, restlessness, reduced levels of consciousness, and, rarely, fatalities.

Pregnancy/Lactation

Phenelzine and tranylcypromine are pregnancy risk category C. Studies of selegiline during pregnancy or lactation have not been performed. It is not known whether selegiline is excreted in breast milk or is subject to placental transfer.

Laboratory

ANALYTIC METHODS

Methamphetamine may be assayed in the urine after selegiline use by immunoassay and gas-liquid chromatography.

BLOOD LEVELS

Plasma MAOI drug levels are not well characterized in either therapeutic or excessive doses. Plasma MAOI levels can confirm ingestion, but they neither guide clinical management nor predict clinical outcome. Drug screens typically do not detect MAOI drugs. Postmortem blood tranylcypromine levels in fatal overdose cases were 0.25 mg/L (850-mg overdose) and 3.7 mg/L (300-mg overdose).

Treatment

GUT DECONTAMINATION

MAOI doses that exceed 1 mg/kg are potentially dangerous. Patients who ingest these amounts should receive activated charcoal if they present within 4 hours of exposure. No symptoms or minimal symptoms are expected in patients within the first 4 hours because of the delayed onset of MAOI actions.

ELIMINATION ENHANCEMENT

Urinary acidification can enhance the renal elimination of tranylcypromine, but renal excretion probably accounts for only a small amount of the total drug elimination and this method is not recommended. Hemodialysis was temporally associated with clinical improvement in a case of tranylcypromine overdose, but pharmacokinetic data were not available to judge the effect of dialysis on clearance.

SUPPORTIVE MEASURES

- All patients suspected of ingesting toxic doses of MAOI drugs should be observed in a monitored setting for 24 hours because of the potential for delayed morbidity. Vital signs and cardiac rhythm should be monitored regularly.
- Patients who take MAOIs should be placed on special diets low in tyramine-containing foods. Sympathomimetic drugs, sedative/hypnotic drugs, and meperidine should be avoided. Precautions for food and drug interactions should remain in effect for 1–2 weeks postexposure.
- MAOI overdose or the concurrent ingestion of certain foods or medications with an MAOI may cause a life-threatening emergency. Patients who exhibit vital sign abnormalities should receive an intravenous line, cardiac monitor, oxygen, and assisted ventilation as needed.

HYPERTENSION

- Patients may present with seriously elevated blood pressure. The decision to lower blood pressure is a clinical judgment based on underlying cardiovascular disease, the extent of blood pressure rise, and evidence of end-organ failure (myocardial ischemia, intracranial hemorrhage, decreased visual acuity, congestive heart failure, renal failure).
- Sodium nitroprusside and intravenous phentolamine are the drugs of choice for severe hypertension in this setting. Practolol successfully reversed the vital sign abnormalities after a tranylcypromine overdose. The use of β-blockers, and theoretically unopposed α-receptor stimulation in this setting, has not been well studied.

CARDIOVASCULAR MANAGEMENT

- Hypotension, unresponsive to fluids, is preferentially treated with a direct-acting α-adrenergic agonist (e.g., norepinephrine or high-dose dopamine). In the presence of shock, hemodynamic monitoring (e.g., by pulmonary artery catheter or intra-arterial line) may be necessary to maximize right ventricular filling, cardiac output, and peripheral vascular resistance.
- Ventricular tachyarrhythmias may be treated with lidocaine, phenytoin, or procainamide. Bretylium may enhance the clinical effects of MAOIs and probably should not be administered in this setting.
- Patients who develop moderate to severe toxicity after an MAOI overdose should receive a complete blood count, serum electrolytes, serum creatinine, urinalysis, serum muscle enzymes, an electrocardiogram, and coagulation profile (prothrombin time, partial thromboplastin time, fibrinogen, and fibrin split products).

HYPERTHERMIA

- Moderately elevated temperatures may be treated with acetaminophen and external cooling. Malignant hyperthermia associated with tachycardia, tachypnea, metabolic acidosis, hypercapnia, temperatures exceeding 40° C, and muscle rigidity may develop in MAOI overdose patients.
- Intravenous dantrolene successfully reversed the malignant hyperthermia syndrome in a phenelzine overdose case. Bromocriptine is an alternative drug used in cases of malignant hyperthermia.
- Diazepam is the drug of choice to control muscle rigidity; phenytoin is an alternative. Neuromuscular paralysis with pancuronium may be necessary when excessive muscle tone contributes to respiratory failure or hyperthermia.
- The use of succinylcholine should be avoided because of its association with malignant hyperthermia.

Antidotes

There are no specific antidotes to MAOI poisoning. Phenothiazine compounds have reversed the agitation and muscle rigidity associated with MAOI overdose. However, the use of intramuscular chlorpromazine in one tranylcypromine overdose was associated with cardiac arrest.

Questions—Monoamine Oxidase Inhibitors

1. Which of the following statements is false?

A. The mood-elevating properties of monoamine oxidase inhibitors (MAOIs) were first discovered in the 1950s with use of the isoniazid derivative, iproniazid.

B. Cyclic antidepressant drugs have largely replaced MAOIs as the drugs of choice for endogenous depression.

C. MAOI agents have been used to treat endogenous depression when tricyclic antidepressants and electroconvulsive therapy have been unsuccessful.
D. Foods that contain large amounts of tyramine and cholinergic drugs can cause a fatal hypertensive crisis and malignant hyperthermia syndrome in patients receiving concomitant MAOI compounds.
E. The clinical features of MAOI overdose may be delayed 6–12 hours.

2. Which of the following statements is false regarding MAOIs?
A. Signs of overdose include agitation, irritability, diaphoresis, tachycardia, muscle rigidity, hyperpyrexia, hypertension, and hyperreflexia.
B. Serious reactions may involve intracranial bleeding, hypotension, coma, seizures, respiratory distress, and malignant hyperthermia, which may be fatal.
C. At least seven types of monoamine oxidase receptors have been identified in human tissue.
D. MAOI compounds inhibit hepatic microsomal enzymes.
E. MAO inhibition results in elevation of brain dopamine, norepinephrine, and serotonin levels.

3. MAOI compounds are oral agents, and no parenteral forms are available.
A. True
B. False

4. Which of the following statements is true concerning MAOI overdose?
A. Death may result from hypothermia, which may peak as late as 24 hours post-presentation.
B. Patients with large MAOI overdoses may be discharged in 6 hours if they do not demonstrate symptoms.
C. Deaths have never followed interaction of therapeutic MAOIs with dietary agents alone.
D. Signs and symptoms of overdose may include drowsiness, dizziness, faintness, irritability, hyperactivity, agitation, and severe headache.
E. Therapeutic use of selegiline may lead to increased tremor, hyperkinesia, falling, hypersialorrhea, blurred vision, and hypertension.

5. MAOI ingestions of ____ should be considered potentially dangerous.
A. 1 mg/kg
B. 2–3 mg/kg
C. 5 mg/kg
D. B and C
E. All MAOI ingestions should be considered dangerous.

6. Examples of tyramine-containing foods include all of the following except
A. Fresh artichokes
B. Aged cheeses
C. Certain beers and wines
D. Chicken liver
E. Pickled herring

7. Malignant hyperthermia associated with tachycardia, tachypnea, metabolic acidosis, hypercapnia, temperatures exceeding 40° C, and muscle rigidity may develop in MAOI overdose patients.
A. True
B. False

NEUROLEPTIC DRUGS

Introduction

The term "neuroleptic" refers to a potent group of drugs that therapeutically modify behavior. Also known as major tranquilizers or antipsychotic drugs, these compounds are largely responsible for a decline in institutionalized psychiatric patients. Between 1955 and 1970, the number of patients hospitalized in psychiatric facilities dropped by 67%.

Neuroleptic overdoses most commonly involve the phenothiazines. Although phenothiazines share similar anticholinergic, α-adrenergic blocking, and quinidine-like properties with tricyclic antidepressant drugs, overdoses tend to be less serious. The severe hypotension and intractable ventricular dysrhythmias that cause mortality in tricyclic antidepressant overdoses occur infrequently after neuroleptic intoxications. Periodic reports of sudden death have appeared in healthy young psychotic patients receiving phenothiazines. Patients undergoing rapid sedation for severe agitation appear particularly susceptible, and both ventricular fibrillation and respiratory depression have been associated with deaths in this setting.

Although uncommon, serious morbidity from neuroleptic ingestion usually results from cardiovascular effects like hypotension, ventricular dysrhythmias, or conduction delay. Neurotoxicity, manifested by respiratory depression, coma, seizures, or delirium, may also occur. Acute dystonic reactions may follow either a single therapeutic dose or massive ingestions and are present in about 10% of overdose cases. Rarely, the neuroleptic malignant syndrome (NMS) characterized by extrapyramidal dysfunction, hypertonicity of skeletal muscles, fluctuating consciousness, hyperthermia, and autonomic disturbances, follows the use of phenothiazines or haloperidol.

BUTYROPHENONES

Haloperidol (Haldol®) represents the most widely utilized member of this class. Haloperidol shares the three-ring nucleus of phenothiazines, but structurally haloperidol more closely resembles phenylpiperidines related to meperidine. Pharmacologically, haloperidol is similar to piperazine-related phenothiazines. Anticholinergic side effects and sedation occur less often than with aliphatic phenothiazines but extrapyramidal reactions are more common.

DIBENZOXAZEPINES

Loxapine (Loxitane®) shares toxic properties with its hydroxylated metabolite, amoxapine (Asendin®), which is marketed as an antidepressant. Clozapine (Clozaril®) is another member of the dibenzodiazepine class of antipsychotic drugs.

DIHYDROINDOLONES

Molindone (Moban®) is a dihydroindolone compound that is structurally unique among antipsychotic drugs available in the U.S.

PHENOTHIAZINES

There are three classes of phenothiazines that share a common nucleus. Piperazine derivatives cause the least sedation and hypotension and the highest incidence of extrapyramidal reactions. This group contains the most potent antipsychotic agents. In contrast, the aliphatic (Thorazine®), and piperidine derivatives are more likely to display sedation and hypotension at therapeutic doses but extrapyramidal effects are less common.

THIOXANTHENES

Replacement of the central nitrogen ring in the phenothiazine nucleus by a carbon side chain produces the thioxanthenes.

Chlorprothixene (Taractan®) and thiothixene (Navane®) are structurally similar to aliphatic and piperidine phenothiazine compounds, respectively, and share similar autonomic properties and side effects.

PATHOPHYSIOLOGY

Dopamine receptors currently are classified as D1 (stimulate adenylate cyclase) and D2 (inhibit adenylate cyclase). Neuroleptic drugs block both D1 and D2 receptors, but the significance of the ratio remains unclear. The therapeutic dose of a neuroleptic drug appears to correlate with its affinity for brain dopamine D2 receptors. Neuroleptic drugs also block a number of other receptors including H1 and H2 histamine receptors, A1 and A2 adrenergic receptors, muscarinic, and serotoninergic receptors.

Cardiovascular Effects

Dysrhythmias and hypotension are the major complications of phenothiazine overdose. The mechanism of toxicity is similar to that of tricyclic antidepressant compounds, although the dysrhythmias and hypotension tend to be less severe. Relative cardiotoxicity appears most frequently with piperidine phenothiazines (e.g., thioridazine), less frequently with aliphatic phenothiazines (e.g., chlorpromazine), and uncommonly with butyrophenones (e.g., haloperidol). Cardiotoxicity is rare with dibenzoxazepines (e.g., loxapine).

Like the tricyclic antidepressants, phenothiazine toxicity displays four specific hemodynamic and electrophysiologic effects. Anticholinergic effects result in sedation, sinus tachycardia, and delayed gastric emptying. Decreased presynaptic norepinephrine reuptake probably causes the transient hypertension seen in mild overdose. Membrane stabilization or a "quinidine-like" property depresses myocardial contractility and impairs cardiac conduction. Phenothiazines prolong the PR and QT intervals, depress ST segments, and cause flattening, inversion, and notching of the T wave. Inhibition of centrally mediated pressor reflexes produces peripheral vasodilation and orthostatic hypotension.

Neurologic Effects

Toxic doses of neuroleptics depress the reticular activating system, which is responsible for arousal. Depression of the hypothalamus produces vasodilation and contributes to orthostatic hypotension. Hypothalamic dysfunction also leads to hypothermia and occasionally to hyperthermia in overdose. Blockade of dopaminergic receptors within the mesolimbic pathway probably causes the antipsychotic effects of neuroleptic drugs. Aliphatic phenothiazines tend to be more sedating and calm hyperactive patients, whereas thioxanthenes stimulate catatonic patients. Toxic doses produce exaggerated responses of either sedation or hyperactivity. Phenothiazines lower the seizure threshold and produce spontaneous motor activity in the amygdala. Patients with a history of seizures, CNS pathology, or abnormal electroencephalograms are particularly susceptible.

Musculoskeletal Effects

Neuroleptic blockade of dopaminergic receptors disrupts the neurotransmitter balance between dopamine and acetylcholine in the striatum (nigra-neostriatal pathway). This imbalance results in extrapyramidal reactions. Excessive acetylcholinergic stimulation produces hyperkinesias (e.g., acute dystonic reactions), or akathisias characterized by muscle restlessness. Dopaminergic excess causes hypokinesias (e.g., Parkinsonian-like reactions, akinesias). The involuntary, repetitive movements of tardive dyskinesias (e.g., lip smacking, buccolingual masticatory syndrome) is postulated to result from a chronic dopaminergic receptor blockade that causes a state of denervation hypersensitivity.

PHARMACOKINETICS

Absorption

- In single therapeutic doses, chlorpromazine oral bioavailability averages 32% (range, 10–69%) relative to intramuscular doses.
- Peak concentrations of chlorpromazine occur 2–3 hours after ingestion and fall rapidly within 3–6 hours. The low oral bioavailability is due in large part to increased presystemic metabolism in the gastrointestinal lumen or intestinal wall.
- Reduced chlorpromazine plasma levels occur after chronic administration.

Distribution

- Volumes of distribution are large and average about 20 L/kg after therapeutic chlorpromazine doses.
- Most phenothiazines are highly protein bound (95–99%).
- In addition, phenothiazines accumulate in lipid tissue, and brain levels may reach concentrations ten times that of plasma.

Elimination

- Absorbed phenothiazines undergo slow liver metabolism to polar metabolites primarily by sulfoxidation and glucuronidation.
- Chlorpromazine metabolism is exceedingly complex, with more than 100 metabolites.
- Less than 1% of chlorpromazine is excreted unchanged by the kidney. As many of the metabolites are active compounds, the pharmacological half-life is difficult to calculate.
- A mean elimination half-life is approximately 18 hours (range, 6–119 hours).
- Individual differences in metabolism may account for some of the variability in therapeutic response to phenothiazines.

CLINICAL PRESENTATIONS

Numerous clinical manifestations are seen after neuroleptic use and abuse. Side effects and withdrawal phenomena may be seen. Extrapyramidal effects include dystonic reactions, Parkinsonian effects, akathisias, the "Rabbit Syndrome," and tardive dyskinesias.

Neurologic Effects

Approximately one-third of phenothiazine ingestions display no symptoms. Of those that are symptomatic, mild central nervous system (CNS) depression is the most common symptom and usually begins 1–2 hours after ingestion. The aliphatic and piperidine phenothiazines (e.g., chlorpromazine), which cause sedation in therapeutic settings, are most often associated with CNS depression in overdoses. After overdose, children appear more susceptible to the sedative properties than adults do. Prochlorperazine can cause lethargy, dysarthria, and ataxia, but serious CNS depression is rare. Stupor and coma are the major signs of neurotoxicity and indicate an attendant risk of aspiration pneumonia.

Seizures

Probably all neuroleptic drugs lower the seizure threshold. This becomes a problem when patients have taken an overdose, have underlying seizure disorders, take other proconvulsant drugs, or withdraw from sedative-hypnotic agents. The actual incidence of convulsions in pure phenothiazine ingestions is low, appearing primarily in patients already predisposed to seizure activity. Convulsions must be differentiated from acute dystonic reactions, which occur more often after prochlorperazine and haloperidol ingestions. Like its metabolite, amoxapine, loxapine ingestion can result in coma and seizures, often beginning within several hours of consumption. These convulsions may be multiple or prolonged and can lead to rhabdomyolysis.

Ophthalmologic Effects

Miosis has been suggested as a sign of serious toxicity. In one study, 72% of children comatose after phenothiazine ingestions displayed miosis. Dilated pupils may also occur and the pupillary pattern is less consistent in adults. Cataracts, retinal damage, and corneal edema may be associated with chronic phenothiazine use.

Dystonic Effects

Symptoms of acute dystonia may occur within 5 hours of ingestion and usually within the first 4 days of treatment. Phenothiazines, butyrophenones, and thioxanthenes all have produced dystonic reactions. Drugs with the least anticholinergic effects (e.g., haloperidol, prochlorperazine, trifluoperazine, and fluphenazine) exhibit the most potent extrapyramidal effects. In contrast to other extrapyramidal syndromes, one tablet is sufficient to cause acute dystonic reactions.

Dystonic reactions are more marked in infants and young adults, especially when predisposing factors such as fever and dehydration occur. Children typically present with slurred speech, dysarthria, confusion, difficulty in swallowing, lethargy, painless spasm, hypertonicity, tremors, or muscle restlessness. Prochlorperazine is the most commonly involved agent. Dystonic reactions or dyskinesias include oculogyric crisis (fixed upward gaze), torticollis (neck twisting), buccolingual movements (facial grimacing), opisthotonus (scoliosis), and tortipelvic gait (abdominal wall, pelvic, hip spasm). Symptoms may persist or recur over several days unless the patient is treated with antihistamines.

Akathisias

Hyperkinesia (motor restlessness), agitation, and insomnia occur most commonly in the early course of treatment and represent another type of extrapyramidal effect. Patients may appear agitated because they are unable to sit still. The primary complaint is a subjective feeling of inner tension, emotional unease, or anxiety. Aa many as 20% of acute psychiatric inpatients may develop akathisias, which seem dose-dependent and can continue after drug withdrawal.

Parkinsonism

The major tranquilizers can cause a syndrome resembling Parkinson's disease (i.e., shuffling gait, loss of associated movement, cogwheel rigidity, and pin-rolling tremor) usually after several weeks of therapy. Most cases appear within 72 hours of the initiation of therapy, but a persistent, drug-induced Parkinson's syndrome can develop after prolonged neuroleptic use.

Tardive Dyskinesia

This extrapyramidal reaction is the most serious side effect of prolonged phenothiazine and haloperidol treatment. Permanent dyskinesias that involve involuntary and repetitive movements may characterize this adverse reaction. The face and mouth are often involved but the limbs and trunk may also display these movements. Lip smacking, protrusion of the tongue, chewing and jaw deviations, facial grimacing, eye blinking, and furrowing of the eyebrows are typical kinetic disorders. Sleep abolishes all movements, and voluntary activity of the involved muscle group markedly reduces the frequency of involuntary repetitive movements. Dyskinesias may appear at any time during treatment but particularly occur when drug treatment is discontinued after a period of 2 years of therapy.

Rabbit Syndrome

Rabbit syndrome is a late-onset neuroleptic-induced extrapyramidal syndrome characterized by rhythmic involuntary movements of the oral and masticatory musculature that mimic the chewing movements of a rabbit. It is reversible when neuroleptic drug therapy is discontinued and responds to antiparkinsonian drug therapy. The high frequency of the perioral movements and the absence of lingual movements distinguish the rabbit syndrome from tardive dyskinesia.

Priapism

Priapism has been reported with thioridazine, triflupromazine, chlorpromazine, molindone, haloperidol, and mesoridazine. After fluphenazine use, one priapism case resolved with diphenhydramine.

Respiratory Effects

Respiratory depression requiring intubation occurs rarely, but the coingestion of sedative-hypnotic drugs and tricyclic antidepressants significantly increases the necessity of intubation. Children appear more susceptible to respiratory depression. Phenothiazine use has been associated with sleep apnea and sudden death in infants. Paradoxically, tachypnea may be noted in adult suicidal phenothiazine ingestions. Anecdotal reports describe cases of pulmonary edema developing after neuroleptic overdose. The diagnosis of phenothiazine-induced pulmonary edema should be suspected in any patient with potential access to these drugs who presents with coma and diffuse pulmonary infiltrates. Laryngeal and pharyngeal dystonias can produce life-threatening respiratory distress.

Renal Effects

Acute reversible oliguria with or without acute interstitial nephritis may follow overdoses of chlorprothixene. Rhabdomyolysis with renal failure may follow neuroleptic malignant syndrome.

Psychiatric Effects

Paradoxically, delirium may complicate phenothiazine overdose, particularly after thioridazine ingestion. Hyperkinetic behavior may be seen.

Cardiovascular Effects

Although conduction delays, hypotension, and ventricular dysrhythmias common to tricyclic overdose can be seen after phenothiazine ingestions, the severity and incidence of these complications are much less with neuroleptic overdose. Orthostatic hypotension is a common side effect of neuroleptic drugs and occurs particularly after use of the piperidine and aliphatic phenothiazines. Diastolic hypotension is the most common sign of cardiotoxicity. Intractable hypotension seen in tricyclic antidepressant overdoses appears not to be a problem in pure neuroleptic ingestions, but combined overdoses may potentiate both hypotension and malignant dysrhythmias. Paradoxically, hypertension has occurred in the setting of haloperidol, chlorpromazine, loxapine, and trifluoperazine ingestions.

Electrocardiographic Effects

Electrocardiographic changes are commonly reported with piperidine phenothiazines (e.g., thioridazine), less frequently with chlorpromazine, and uncommonly with haloperidol. Up to 50% of patients receiving thioridazine may show abnormalities such as PR or QT prolongation, mild ST segment depression, prominent U waves, or T-wave changes. Although conduction delays after phenothiazine overdose are not as well correlated with serious cardiotoxicity as is tricyclic antidepressant overdose, their presence after acute ingestion indicates the need for hospitalization and cardiac monitoring. Conduction delays are not seen in loxapine overdose where serious neurotoxicity (e.g., coma, seizures) develops without evidence of cardiotoxicity.

Dysrhythmias

The majority of phenothiazine-induced ventricular dysrhythmias occur in patients taking phenothiazines therapeutically. Like tricyclic antidepressants, prolongation of the QRS and QT intervals in the overdose setting has been associated with ventricular tachycardia. Thioridazine has been associated with persistent ventricular tachycardia, ventricular fibrillation, Torsade de Pointes, and fatal cardiac arrest.

Sinus tachycardia is the most frequent dysrhythmia seen, but its presence is not a specific indicator for the development of serious dysrhythmias. Bradycardia occurs much less frequently. Most serious ventricular dysrhythmias are associated with piperidine and phenothiazine overdoses. Dysrhythmias occur in the setting of obvious cardiotoxicity (e.g., conduction delays, tachycardia, and premature ventricular contractions) and often within several hours of admission.

Anticholinergic Effects

Decreased bowel sounds, ileus, urinary retention, syncope, skin flushing, dry mucous membranes, or salivation may occur. In addition, nausea or vomiting may complicate the clinical course.

Hypersensitivity Effects

Both haloperidol and chlorpromazine may produce diffuse urticarial reactions or a photosensitive dermatitis. In addition, chlorpromazine may cause a purple to slate-gray hyperpigmentation in light-exposed skin. Cholestatic jaundice may develop during chronic chlorpromazine therapy, characterized initially by fever, abdominal pain, malaise, morbilliform rash, pruritus, eosinophilia, anorexia, nausea, and hepatic aminotransferase elevation.

Neuroleptic Abuse

Anecdotal reports suggest that certain patients with outpatient histories of polypharmacy use and antisocial personality disorders may seek increasing doses of loxapine. These patients desire high doses of loxapine for its warm, relaxing feeling, its soporific effect, and the associated blunting of emotional pain.

Deficit Syndrome

Antipsychotic drugs such as haloperidol have been associated with a deficit syndrome characterized by sedation, extrapyramidal signs, indifference to internal and external stimuli, passivity, and reduced initiative. Some patients switched to newer antipsychotic agents such as clozapine experience an "awakening" effect. Delineation of neuroleptic-induced deficit syndrome (NIDS) from other treatment effects such as drug-induced Parkinsonism and akathisia, sedation, and depressive features of schizophrenia is still a major problem.

Neuroleptic Withdrawal

A withdrawal syndrome associated with antipsychotic drugs includes autonomic and behavioral symptoms, Parkinsonism, and withdrawal dyskinesias. The neuroleptic withdrawal syndrome has followed use of haloperidol and pimozide and the sudden cessation of amantadine. Psychotic symptoms may develop within 6 weeks of the abrupt discontinuation of treatment. This has been termed neuroleptic supersensitivity psychosis.

TOXIC DOSAGE/DEATH

Fatalities are rare in pure neuroleptic overdoses. Accidental psychotropic drug toxicity is not a major cause of poisoning-related childhood deaths. Sudden death appears to occur more commonly in agitated psychotic patients taking therapeutic doses of phenothiazines than in the overdose setting. The etiology of death in psychiatric patients is often unclear as autopsies frequently fail to reveal the cause of death. Some authors believe that causes include asphyxia during drug-induced seizures, aspiration perhaps resulting from phenothiazine-induced bulbar palsy, respiratory depression during rapid tranquilization, and ventricular fibrillation.

The toxic dose of phenothiazines is not well established because of the wide therapeutic index and synergism of other CNS depressants (e.g., antihistamines, cyclic antidepressants) commonly taken in adult overdoses. Children and infants appear more susceptible. Fatalities in infants have resulted from chlorpromazine ingestion as low as 350 mg, whereas adult death has occurred from consumption of 2 g. Survival has been associated with 10- and 17-g ingestions. Adult response to chlorpromazine ingestion is highly variable, but significant CNS depression can be expected from doses exceeding 5 g.

A 3-year-old developed coma and multiple tonic-clonic seizures but survived without sequelae after ingesting approximately 1 g of chlorprothixene. Adults have survived 8-g overdoses of chlorprothixene. Death from haloperidol ingestion has rarely been reported. Haloperidol has been implicated in pulmonary edema and sudden death during rapid tranquilization of severely agitated psychotic patients.

Loxapine overdoses appear to be similar to those from the structurally related dibenzoxazepine, amoxapine. Adult ingestions of 800 mg–2.2 g can produce coma, seizures, tachycardia, and hypertension, but not the dysrhythmias and conduction delays seen in phenothiazine and tricyclic overdose. Fatalities have occurred from 2.5-g ingestions of loxapine. Prochlorperazine causes lethargy in children at doses of 35–90 mg. Prochlorperazine has been implicated in sudden death when administered to psychotic patients at therapeutic doses.

Finally, thioridazine and its metabolite, mesoridazine, are phenothiazines commonly associated with suicidal ingestion, with fatal doses generally ranging from 1.5–8.0 g. Recovery has followed a 4-g ingestion in a 12-year-old; however, death has followed a 3-g ingestion in a 27-year-old.

DRUG INTERACTIONS

Coingestion of tricyclic antidepressants and sedative-hypnotic drugs significantly increases CNS depression and the need for intubation. Coingestion of neuroleptic drugs with tricyclic antidepressants may result in an increase in the plasma TCA level, intraventricular conduction delays, first-degree atrioventricular block, and ventricular arrhythmias. There is a higher prevalence of prolongation of the QRS duration and a threefold increase in the prevalence of QTc prolongation.

PREGNANCY/LACTATION

Haloperidol, chlorpromazine and thioridazine are all pregnancy risk category C. Contradictory findings relate both an increase in major congenital anomalies when exposure to phenothiazines occurs during the first trimester and no significant increase in severe congenital anomalies following similar exposure. Toxic effects reported in newborns include restlessness, abnormal movements, hypertonia, and an extrapyramidal syndrome, which may persist for as long as 6 months. It would appear prudent to avoid antipsychotic drugs if possible during the first trimester.

Respiratory depression and extrapyramidal reactions seen in neonates born to schizophrenic mothers receiving phenothiazines strongly suggest that these drugs cross the placental barrier.

LABORATORY

Analytic Methods

Clothiapine analysis is performed by gas chromatography with nitrogen-phosphorus detection and electron capture detection. An HPLC method for quantitation of haloperidol and reduced haloperidol has detection limits of 0.5 ng/mL in plasma and 5 ng/mL in urine. Serum concentrations of thioridazine and its metabolites are quantitated by an HPLC method. A high-performance thin-layer chromatography method is available for the quantitation of thiothixene.

Blood Levels

The relationship between serum concentrations of neuroleptics and therapeutic response is minimal. Following concentrations in overdose does not guide therapy. Blood levels of chlorpromazine, for example, do not correlate with clinical effects in part because of the large number of active metabolites. Qualitative levels will confirm ingestion but treatment is based on clinical signs and symptoms. Poor therapeutic response to chlorpromazine may occur at both low and high dosage levels. Drug serum levels between 50 and 300 ng/mL are obtained with daily chlorpromazine doses. Serum chlorpromazine levels in patients who survived 1.6- to 1.8-g ingestions ranged from 800–1,500 ng/mL.

In patients whose condition responds to haloperidol, a serum concentration of at least 5 ng/mL is associated with a positive response. The therapeutic range is about 5 to 16 ng/mL. Optimum patient response in schizophrenia was associated, in one study, with plasma haloperidol levels of 4.2–11.0 ng/mL for the first 2 weeks of treatment. Side effects generally develop in psychiatric patients whose therapeutic haloperidol levels exceed 6 ng/mL.

TREATMENT

Gut Decontamination

Up to 4–6 hours postingestion, patients may benefit from lavage or charcoal, if they have consumed more than several tablets. Tracheal protection must always be provided in obtunded patients. As seizures may suddenly develop during gut decontamination, ipecac is contraindicated. Abdominal x-ray films may help determine the adequacy of decontamination, as many phenothiazines are radiopaque.

Elimination Enhancement

High protein binding and a large volume of distribution make it unlikely that hemodialysis and forced diuresis will be useful.

Supportive Measures

- Obtunded patients should receive usual therapy with glucose, naloxone, and, if indicated, thiamine. The adequacy of respirations should be evaluated. Stuporous or comatose patients should be placed in the left lateral, head-down position and observed to prevent aspiration. Patients with vital sign or cardiac abnormalities should receive cardiac monitoring and an i.v. line.
- The primary diagnostic aim in neuroleptic overdose is to select those patients likely to develop serious toxicity from the majority of patients who require only supportive outpatient care. Usually this task is not difficult because seriously poisoned patients generally show signs of neurotoxicity or cardiotoxicity.
- Patients with a history of significant neuroleptic ingestion should receive gut decontamination, an electrocardiogram, and vital sign and cardiac monitoring. Patients with hypotension, conduction delay, or dysrhythmia should be admitted until the electrocardiogram is normal for 24 hours. Asymptomatic patients can be released after a 4-hour observation period.

Hypotension

- Hypotension is the most common sign of cardiotoxicity and usually responds to Trendelenburg position and normal saline.
- Direct-acting α-agonists (e.g., norepinephrine) are theoretical vasopressors of choice.
- Vasopressors with mixed α- and β-adrenergic function (e.g., epinephrine, dopamine) may theoretically worsen hypotension because of unopposed β-adrenergic stimulation from phenothiazine-induced α-blockade.

Dysrhythmias

- Lidocaine and phenytoin are the antiarrhythmic drugs of choice for ventricular dysrhythmias. Quinidine, procainamide, and disopyramide are contraindicated.
- Sodium bicarbonate may be used in a manner similar to its use in treating tricyclic antidepressant-induced dysrhythmias. However, its efficacy is not established in phenothiazine overdoses.
- Intractable ventricular dysrhythmias may require overdrive pacing and correction of underlying hypoxia or hypokalemia. The most appropriate treatment of thioridazine-induced arrhythmias is probably temporary pacing. This cardiac pacing may be required for days.
- With the exception of Torsade de Pointes, isoproterenol is usually contraindicated because of the exacerbation of hypotension by its β-adrenergic agonist effects.
- Physostigmine has been used for conduction delays, coma, and seizures in mixed phenothiazine and tricyclic antidepressant overdose with anecdotal success. However, serious adverse reactions such as asystole complicate the administration of physostigmine and relegate its use as a last-line drug.

Seizures

- Diazepam and phenytoin are the anticonvulsant drugs of choice. Loxapine in particular may produce recurrent and prolonged seizures.
- Temperature, oxygenation, and urine myoglobin must be followed closely in these cases.
- Persistence of seizures despite usual pharmacologic interventions may require intubation, and general anesthesia.
- Urine myoglobin and serum muscle enzyme levels should be checked in all patients with prolonged muscle rigidity or seizures.

Dystonic Reactions

- Intravenous diphenhydramine (2 mg/kg up to 50 mg over several minutes) and intramuscular benztropine mesylate (2 mg in adults) are the drugs of choice and should relieve symptoms in 5 and 15–20 minutes, respectively. Mild sedation is the main side effect.
- Follow-up treatment with an anticholinergic agent (e.g., Benadryl®, 50 mg orally three times daily) should be given over 2–3 days because of the long half-life of most major tranquilizers.
- Phenothiazines should be discontinued.

Akathisias and Parkinsonian Reactions

- These may be relieved by reducing the dose of the offending agent, or by the addition of antiparkinsonian drugs such as Artane.
- Often akathisias appear resistant to anticholinergic drugs and benzodiazepines.
- The use of low-dose propranolol suggests that β-adrenergic blockers may be efficacious.

Tardive Dyskinesia

- No drugs used for the treatment of tardive dyskinesia are uniformly safe and effective over extended periods.
- The long list of drugs used to treat tardive dyskinesia attests to their general lack of therapeutic benefits. These drugs include the serotonergic agents, such as tryptophan and cyproheptadine (Periactin®); noradrenergic agents such as lithium; the β-adrenergic receptor antagonist propranolol (Inderal®); and the α-adrenergic agonist clonidine (Catapres®).
- Trials with morphine, naloxone (Narcan®), estrogen, pyridoxine, manganese chloride, phenytoin (Dilantin®), ergoloid mesylate (Hydergine®), and papaverine have produced no or only sporadic benefits.

Thermal Dysregulation

- Hypothermia invariably is mild unless the patient has been exposed to low ambient temperatures. It is usually responsive to measures used to correct other vital signs and to passive rewarming.
- True hyperthermia represents a greater risk, and the development of the neuroleptic malignant syndrome requires prompt treatment. See Neuroleptic Malignant Syndrome below.
- In patients with hyperthermia, attention is made toward maintaining fluid and electrolyte balance and controlling seizures. Cooling blankets or ice are helpful but antipyretics probably are not.
- Phenothiazines, haloperidol, and other anticholinergic drugs should be stopped.
- The development of myoglobinuria indicates the need for alkaline diuresis to prevent acute tubular necrosis.

Questions—Introduction to Neuroleptic Drugs

1. Which of the following statements is false?
A. Neuroleptic overdoses most commonly involve the phenothiazines.
B. Although phenothiazines share similar anticholinergic, α-adrenergic blocking, and quinidine-like properties with tricyclic antidepressant drugs, overdoses tend to be more serious.
C. Periodic reports of sudden death have appeared in healthy young psychotic patients receiving phenothiazines.
D. Serious morbidity from neuroleptic ingestion usually results from cardiovascular effects like hypotension, ventricular dysrhythmias, or conduction delay.
E. B and C

2. Neurotoxic effects of phenothiazine overdose may include each of the following, except
A. Respiratory depression
B. Coma
C. Cinchonism
D. Seizures
E. Delirium

3. Acute dystonic reactions may follow either a single therapeutic dose or massive ingestions and are present in about 10% of phenothiazine overdose cases.
A. True
B. False

4. Concerning the cardiac pathophysiology of phenothiazines,
A. Anticholinergic effects result in sedation, sinus tachycardia, and delayed gastric emptying.
B. Increased presynaptic norepinephrine reuptake probably causes transient hypertension seen in mild overdose.
C. Membrane stabilization or "quinidine-like" property enhances myocardial contractility and impairs cardiac conduction.
D. Phenothiazines shorten the PR and QT intervals, depress ST segments, and cause flattening, inversion, and notching of the T wave.
E. Inhibition of centrally mediated pressor reflexes produces peripheral vasoconstriction.

5. Most phenothiazine overdoses display no symptoms.
A. True
B. False

6. After overdose, children are less susceptible to sedative properties of phenothiazines than adults.
A. True
B. False

7. Which of the following is false?
A. Probably all neuroleptic drugs lower the seizure threshold.
B. The actual incidence of convulsions in pure phenothiazine ingestions is low, appearing primarily in patients already predisposed to seizure activity.
C. Like its metabolite, loxapine, amoxapine ingestion can result in coma and seizures.
D. Miosis has been suggested as a sign of serious phenothiazine toxicity.
E. Dilated pupils may also occur.

8. Neuroleptics with the least anticholinergic effects (e.g., haloperidol) exhibit the most potent extrapyramidal effects.
A. True
B. False

9. Dystonic reactions or dyskinesias include all of the following, except
A. Oculogyric crisis (fixed upward gaze)
B. Torticollis (neck twisting)
C. Buccolingual movements (facial grimacing)
D. Hemiballismus (wild jerking motions)
E. Tortipelvic gait (abdominal wall, pelvic, hip spasm)

10. Regarding tardive dyskinesia,
A. This extrapyramidal reaction is the most serious side effect of prolonged phenothiazine and haloperidol treatment.
B. Permanent dyskinesias that involve involuntary and repetitive movements may characterize this adverse reaction.
C. The face and mouth are often involved but the limbs and trunk may also display these movements.

D. Lip smacking, protrusion of the tongue, chewing and jaw deviations, facial grimacing, eye blinking, and furrowing of the eyebrows are typical kinetic disorders.
E. All of the above.

11. Rabbit syndrome is an early-onset neuroleptic-induced extrapyramidal syndrome characterized by rhythmic involuntary movements of the oral and masticatory musculature that mimic the chewing movements of a rabbit.
A. True
B. False

12. Paradoxically, delirium may complicate phenothiazine overdose, particularly after thioridazine ingestion.
A. True
B. False

13. Which of the following is false?
A. Orthostatic hypotension is a common side effect of neuroleptic drugs and occurs particularly after use of the piperidine and aliphatic phenothiazines.
B. Intractable hypotension seen in tricyclic antidepressant overdoses appears not to be a problem in pure neuroleptic ingestions, but combined overdoses may potentiate both hypotension and malignant dysrhythmias.
C. Paradoxically, hypertension has occurred in the setting of haloperidol, chlorpromazine, loxapine, and trifluoperazine ingestions.
D. Conduction delays are not seen in loxapine overdose, where serious neurotoxicity (e.g., coma, seizures) develops without evidence of cardiotoxicity.
E. Electrocardiographic changes are rarely reported with piperidine phenothiazine (e.g., thioridazine) overdose.

Neuroleptic Malignant Syndrome

Neuroleptic malignant syndrome (NMS) is a rare and potentially fatal complication of most major neuroleptic drugs and is characterized by skeletal muscle rigidity, hyperthermia, altered consciousness (delirium or obtundation), and autonomic dysfunction (diaphoresis, pallor). This syndrome appears more often in men under 40 years of age, and predisposing factors include organic brain disease, dehydration, and physical exhaustion. The reaction is idiosyncratic and may occur after single therapeutic doses.

Neuroleptic drugs including the phenothiazines, butyrophenones, thioxanthenes, and other dopamine antagonists such as metoclopramide and Zuclopenthixol® have been associated with NMS. Non-neuroleptic agents including the tricyclic antidepressants, monamine oxidase inhibitors, anticonvulsants, and anti-parkinsonian agents have been associated with this syndrome. Lithium, in combination with a variety of agents (see Drug Interactions below) can also precipitate NMS.

Pathophysiology

NMS is presumably due to blockade of dopaminergic pathways in the hypothalamus and basal ganglia. NMS may result from dopamine depletion. Bromocriptine, a dopamine agonist, has therefore been advocated in the treatment of NMS.

Clinical Presentations

Neuroleptic malignant syndrome is characterized by a tetrad of fever, rigidity, altered sensorium, and autonomic dysfunction. Temperature typically ranges from 38.5–42° C; however, fever may not be present. The rigidity is classically described as "lead-pipe." Other signs include tremor, sialorrhea, bradykinesia, festinating gait, dystonia, chorea, trismus, opisthotonos, and dysphagia. Mental status ranges from mild confusion and agitation to lethargy, stupor, and coma. Autonomic dysfunction is manifested by tachycardia, labile blood pressure, tachypnea, urinary incontinence, respiratory stridor, diaphoresis, pallor, and cardiac arrest. Patients who present early in their course may only have a few of these features.

The most common complication is rhabdomyolysis, which results from muscle rigidity and breakdown. Other reported complications include aspiration pneumonia, pulmonary embolism, pulmonary edema, adult respiratory distress syndrome, sepsis, disseminated intravascular coagulation, seizures, myocardial infarction, peripheral neuropathy, and death. The anticholinergic properties of neuroleptic drugs and TCAs promote intestinal ileus, which may lead to necrotizing enterocolitis.

The differential diagnosis of NMS includes causes of fever, leukocytosis, and rigidity. In a patient with fever, stiff neck, and altered mentation (all commonly seen in NMS), meningitis must be ruled out. Other etiologies to consider are encephalitis, sepsis, thyrotoxicosis, heat stroke, drug overdose, delirium, malignant hyperthermia, lethal catatonia, and extrapyramidal reactions.

TOXIC DOSAGE/DEATH

Estimates of mortality from NMS range from 20–30%. Death usually occurs 3 days after the development of symptoms. Causes of death include respiratory failure, cardiovascular collapse, renal failure, arrhythmias, and thromboembolism.

DRUG INTERACTIONS

Lithium, in combination with clozapine, carbamazepine, phenelzine, chlorpromazine, anti-parkinsonian agents or doxepin can precipitate NMS.

LABORATORY

Analytic Methods

There are no diagnostic laboratory findings in NMS.

Blood Levels

Creatine kinase enzyme elevations may be substantial but hepatic aminotransferase elevation usually is small. The muscle isoenzyme of creatinine kinase may also be raised by intramuscular injection, hyperactivity, and catatonia and in medically ill patients taking neuroleptic drugs. Thus, it is not a specific indicator of NMS. Its importance in early detection of the syndrome and in other forms of neuromuscular disturbance remains doubtful.

TREATMENT

Gut Decontamination

These methods do not apply to this syndrome. Ice water lavage, in combination with other cooling measures, may aid in decreasing temperature elevations.

Elimination Enhancement

Dialysis may be necessary in the treatment of renal failure precipitated by rhabdomyolysis.

Supportive Measures

- Symptoms develop rapidly over 24–72 hours and last 5–10 days after cessation of oral neuroleptic therapy.

- Neuroleptic malignant syndrome is a life-threatening medical emergency. Patients require monitored intensive care management. Caution should be exercised when using anticholinergic and antihistaminic agents in the presence of fevers greater than 101° F.
- Treatment is generally directed against the hyperthermia and muscular rigidity. Dantrolene sodium, 1–3 mg/kg/day i.v. in four divided doses (may be increased to 10 mg/kg/day QID), also used in malignant hyperthermia, has been successfully used to diminish muscle rigidity.
- Bromocriptine, 7.5–60 mg/day in three divided doses, has been used as well. Both these agents may be started concurrently.
- Recovery from temperatures as high as 108° F after seizures, and death from temperatures of 109.5° F (complicated by acute compartment syndromes, rhabdomyolysis and acute tubular necrosis) have been reported.
- Cooling blankets, ice packs, gastric lavage, and even intraperitoneal lavage may help in decreasing severe hyperthermia.

ANTIDOTES

There are no antidotes, although dantrolene and bromocriptine (see above) may successfully reverse dangerous aspects of this syndrome.

Questions—Neuroleptic Malignant Syndrome

1. **Risk factors for neuroleptic malignant syndrome (NMS) include all of the following except**
   A. Men less than 40 years old
   B. Organic brain disease
   C. Diabetes mellitus
   D. Dehydration
   E. Physical exhaustion
2. **All of the following drugs have been associated with NMS except**
   A. Phenothiazines
   B. Diphenylhydantoins
   C. Butyrophenones
   D. Thioxanthenes
   E. Metoclopramide
3. **Neuroleptic malignant syndrome is a tetrad of**
   A. Fever, chills, neck pain and shortness of breath
   B. Fever, gastrointestinal upset, diploplia and coma
   C. Fever, rigidity, altered sensorium, and autonomic dysfunction
   D. Fever, rigidity, myoglobinuria, and myocardial ischemia
   E. Fever, hematuria, stupor, and seizures
4. **Creatine kinase enzyme elevations may be substantial but hepatic aminotransferase elevation is usually small.**
   A. True
   B. False
5. **All of the following have been used in the treatment of NMS except**
   A. Cooling blankets
   B. Bromocriptine, an ergot
   C. Dantrolene
   D. Calcium gluconate
   E. Ice water gastric lavage

Clozapine

Clozapine (Clozaril®), a member of the dibenzodiazepine class of antipsychotic drugs, was released in the U.S. in 1990 for patients with refractory schizophrenia. Its use has been limited by a 1–2% incidence of agranulocytosis and by deaths due to neutropenic sepsis. Overdose with clozapine may lead to fatalities. There is no antidote.

Clozapine is indicated in the management of severely ill schizophrenic patients who have failed to respond to other neuroleptic agents or who cannot tolerate the adverse effects produced by those agents. Because of the significant risk of agranulocytosis and seizures with clozapine, the patient should be given an adequate trial with at least two different standard antipsychotic medications before clozapine therapy is initiated.

PATHOPHYSIOLOGY

Clozapine is a "broad-spectrum" receptor antagonist at dopamine D1 and D2 receptors, α-1 and α-2 adrenoreceptors, and serotonin (5-HT2), histamine (H1), and acetylcholine (muscarinic) receptors. It differs from some of the classic antipsychotic agents in animal studies by blocking D1 more than D2 receptors, by raising plasma prolactin levels only transiently, and by its inability to induce supersensitivity in striatal dopamine systems. Clozapine may exert its effects by differentially modulating D1 and D2 receptors in the extrapyramidal, limbic, and mesocortical systems. The lower incidence of acute extrapyramidal effects with clozapine compared with other antipsychotic drugs may be due to weak antagonism of striatal dopamine D2 receptors. Tardive dyskinesia does not seem to occur, even with long-term use.

PHARMACOKINETICS

Absorption

- Following single and multiple doses, plasma concentrations of clozapine peak at 1–4 hours.
- Because of moderate hepatic first-pass metabolism, the bioavailability of orally administered clozapine ranges from 27–50%.
- A linear correlation exists between clozapine dosage and plasma clozapine concentration.

Distribution

- Clozapine is approximately 95% bound to plasma proteins *in vitro*.
- The initial distribution half-life of clozapine is 1–5 hours.
- Its apparent volume of distribution is about 5 L/kg.

Elimination

- Clozapine is extensively metabolized by N-oxidation, N-demethylation, and dehalogenation to yield pharmacologically inactive products.
- Unchanged clozapine accounts for approximately 2–5% of the excreted drug.
- The terminal elimination half-life is approximately 12 hours (range, 6–30 hours).

CLINICAL PRESENTATIONS

Symptoms of acute overdose may include drowsiness, restlessness, lethargy, areflexia, hyperreflexia, agitation, confusion, disorientation, delirium, blurred vision, mydriasis, convulsions, coma, hypotension, hypertension, arrhythmias, tachycardia, heart block, respiratory depression, hypersalivation, hypothermia, hypoactive bowel sounds, dry skin, inability to urinate, adult respiratory distress syndrome, pancreatitis, and myocarditis. Sudden death has also been reported.

Common undesirable effects following chronic use include nausea and vomiting, weight gain, transient hyperthermia, seizures, hypotension, hypertension, hypersalivation, dizziness, constipation, tachycardia, and drowsiness. Clozapine can cause neutropenia, agranulocytosis, and eosinophilia. Neuroleptic malignant syndrome has been reported following several weeks of clozapine use. Clozapine has also been associated with tardive dyskinesia and may induce obsessive-compulsive symptoms. Known causes of death include cardiac failure, aspiration pneumonia, and renal failure.

TOXIC DOSAGE/DEATH

Seizures tend to occur at clozapine doses greater than 600 mg/d. At least 11 patients have survived ingestions of more than 4.0 g and one patient survived an 11-g ingestion. However, death in adults has followed 2.0- and 3.0-g ingestions. Acute overdose of 50–200 mg of clozapine in young children has led to confusion, ataxia, muscle rigidity, nystagmus, torticollis, drooling, slurred speech, agitation, screaming, crying, and stupor. Recovery usually follows symptomatic care.

DRUG INTERACTIONS

Clozapine increases central nervous system depressant effects when used with alcohol, sedative-hypnotic agents, and opiates. Clozapine potentiates the anticholinergic effects of atropine-like drugs and may potentiate the hypotensive effects of antihypertensive drugs. Highly protein bound medications such as digoxin, heparin, phenytoin, and warfarin are displaced from their binding sites by clozapine, resulting in adverse clinical effects.

Clozapine may potentiate the myelosuppressive effects of bone marrow depressants. Such drugs may enhance the agranulocytosis following clozapine use. Smoking may decrease the serum concentration of clozapine. Cimetidine, by inhibiting the cytochrome P450 system, increases serum clozapine levels and may lead to adverse clinical effects. Phenytoin has induced a decrease in plasma clozapine concentration, and fluvoxamine elevates serum levels of clozapine.

PREGNANCY/LACTATION

Clozapine crosses the placenta. The U.S. Food and Drug Administration has placed clozapine in pregnancy risk category B. Clozapine is excreted in breast milk.

LABORATORY

Analytic Methods

A high-performance liquid chromatography method is available for clozapine.

Blood Levels

A linear relationship appears to exist between the dose of clozapine and plasma concentration. At steady-state dose levels of 300–400 mg/d, plasma concentrations of clozapine approximate 400 ng/mL. Schizophrenic patients appear to respond to plasma concentrations above 350 mg/mL. Sudden death in an adult has been associated with a plasma level of 4,460 ng/mL. Ingestion of 100–200 mg by children leads to serum clozapine levels of about 500 ng/mL.

TREATMENT

Gut Decontamination

Syrup of ipecac is not recommended in view of the possibility of sudden seizures in the clozapine overdose patient. There is no evidence that gastric lavage is effective; however, physical removal of tablets during the first hour may reduce the possibility of high plasma levels. If gastric lavage is contemplated, tracheal protection must be provided as seizures may intervene unpredictably. Activated charcoal with a single dose of cathartics may be of use, but controlled studies are not available to substantiate their efficacy.

Elimination Enhancement

In view of the extensive protein binding of clozapine and its high apparent volume of distribution, it appears that measures such as forced diuresis, peritoneal lavage, dialysis, hemoperfusion, and exchange transfusion are unlikely to be of benefit.

Supportive Measures

- Treatment is largely symptomatic and supportive. Staff should be prepared for the sudden onset of seizures, agitation, anticholinergic toxicity, and paradoxical sialorrhea.
- Patients with a history of significant clozapine ingestion should receive gut decontamination, cardiac and respiratory monitoring, and observation for at least 3 or 4 days with periodic evaluation of electrolytes and acid-base balance as metabolic acidosis may occur.
- Anecdotal reports suggest that hyponatremia may be a possible epileptogenic trigger. Severe hypoglycemia has been associated with high doses of clozapine.
- Patients receiving clozapine should have a white blood cell count each week throughout treatment and for 4 weeks after its discontinuation. Half of reported episodes of agranulocytosis occur within 3 months of starting treatment, but weekly monitoring of leukocyte counts should continue indefinitely. Agranulocytosis following clozapine use has been successfully treated with granulocyte colony-stimulating factor (G-CSF). G-CSF should be started within 48 hours of the onset of agranulocytosis.
- Clozapine alters the electroencephalogram in a majority of patients treated, with seizure frequency as high as 5–10% at doses above 600 ng/d.
- Diazepam and phenytoin are anticonvulsant drugs of choice in case of seizures. Valproic acid may also be used. Carbamazepine, which may cause agranulocytosis or aplastic anemia, is contraindicated. Temperature, oxygenation, and urine myoglobin must be followed in cases of recurrent and prolonged seizures.
- Hypotension is treated with position change, intravenous fluids, and vasopressors such as dopamine and norepinephrine. Epinephrine is contraindicated.
- Lidocaine and phenytoin are the antiarrhythmic drugs of choice for ventricular dysrhythmias. Intractable ventricular dysrhythmias may require pacing. Quinidine, procainamide, and disopyramide are contraindicated. Digitalis, sodium bicarbonate, or potassium may be required, but their effects have not been widely studied.
- Please see the section above on Neuroleptic Malignant Syndrome regarding treatment and management of this ominous syndrome.
- There has been no effective treatment for tardive dyskinesia demonstrated in controlled clinical studies.

Questions—Clozapine

1. Which of the following is false?

A. Clozapine (Clozaril®) is used to treat patients with refractory schizophrenia.

B. Its use has been limited by a 1–2% incidence of agranulocytosis and by deaths due to neutropenic sepsis.

C. It has been recommended that because of the significant risk of agranulocytosis and seizures with clozapine, the patient should be given an adequate trial with at least two different standard antipsychotic medications before clozapine therapy is initiated.
D. Clozapine appears to bind to α-2 adrenoreceptors only.
E. Tardive dyskinesia may occur with long-term use of clozapine.

2. **Clozapine may potentiate the myelosuppressive effects of bone marrow depressants.**
A. True
B. False

Haloperidol

Haloperidol (Haldol®), a butyrophenone, is a popular drug used to treat patients with psychotic disorders (e.g., schizophrenia), to treat profound agitation, to control tics and verbal utterances associated with Gilles de la Tourette's syndrome, and to manage hyperexcitable children whose condition is not responsive to other treatment modalities. Long-term use may lead to extrapyramidal side effects including tardive dyskinesia in about 30% of patients. Overdose is associated with severe extrapyramidal symptoms, hypotension, and sedation. Torsade de Pointes has also been reported.

PATHOPHYSIOLOGY

Haloperidol is felt to work by competitively blocking postsynaptic dopamine receptors in the mesolimbic system. It also possesses α-blocking and anticholinergic effects.

PHARMACOKINETICS

Absorption

- Haloperidol is well absorbed from the gastrointestinal tract, but first-pass hepatic metabolism decreases oral bioavailability to 40–75%.
- Serum concentration peaks 0.5–4.0 hours after an oral dose.

Distribution

- The volume of distribution is about 20 L/kg, consistent with the high lipophilicity of the drug.
- Haloperidol circulates in blood bound predominantly (90–94%) to plasma proteins.

Elimination

- Clearance occurs almost exclusively by hepatic metabolism.
- Renal excretion is negligible.
- Haloperidol is similar in structure to MPTP, which probably causes Parkinsonism in humans.
- The elimination half-life of haloperidol ranges from 13–35 hours.

CLINICAL PRESENTATIONS

Please see the Introduction for a complete outline of neuroleptic-induced symptoms. Accidental overdose of haloperidol in children may lead to altered consciousness, tremors, hyperreflexia, akathisia, opisthotonus, oculogyric crisis, and drooling. Most patients recover, but some may retain extrapyramidal side effects.

TOXIC DOSAGE/DEATH

A 29-month-old and an 11-month-old divided 265 mg of haloperidol and developed lethargy, hypothermia, hyperreflexia, neuromuscular rigidity, unsteady gait, and intention tremors.

DRUG INTERACTIONS

Coingestion of tricyclic antidepressants and sedative-hypnotic drugs significantly increases central nervous system depression and the need for intubation.

PREGNANCY/LACTATION

Pregnancy risk category C.

LABORATORY

Analytic Methods

Because of the high volume of distribution and the relatively low serum concentration of haloperidol, measurements are restricted to high-sensitivity methods of analysis including radioimmunoassay, gas chromatography, and high-performance liquid chromatography with electrochemical detection.

Blood Levels

Establishing a definitive relationship between serum haloperidol concentrations and therapeutic effects has been difficult. For those patients who respond to haloperidol, a serum concentration of at least 5 ng/mL is advisable to ensure a positive response. Side effects increased in incidence with plasma concentrations greater than 6 ng/mL, 12–14 hours after administration.

TREATMENT

Gut Decontamination

Syrup of ipecac is not recommended in view of the possibility of seizures in the haloperidol overdose patient. There is no evidence that gastric lavage is effective; however, physical removal of tablets during the first hour may reduce the possibility of high plasma levels. If gastric lavage is contemplated, tracheal protection must be provided as seizures may intervene unpredictably. Activated charcoal with a single dose of cathartics may be of use, but controlled studies are not available to substantiate their efficacy.

Elimination Enhancement

In view of the extensive protein binding of haloperidol and its high volume of distribution, measures such as forced diuresis, peritoneal lavage, dialysis, hemoperfusion, and exchange transfusion are unlikely to be of benefit.

Supportive Measures

- Respiratory and circulatory competence should be established immediately. Respiratory depression may require assisted ventilation.
- Hypotension and circulatory collapse are treated with intravenous fluids and pressors as necessary. Sympathomimetic vasoconstriction with β-adrenergic agonists (e.g., epinephrine) may aggravate hypotension or arrhythmias.
- Transient thrombocytosis, elevated serum transaminase levels, and electrocardiographic evidence of a prolonged QT interval have been described. Vital signs and the electrocardiogram should be monitored for signs of QT prolongation or dysrhythmias. Monitoring should continue in-hospital until the electrocardiogram is normal for 24 hours.
- Anticholinergic and antiparkinsonian medications given parenterally may relieve extrapyramidal reactions.
- Hair analysis (distal segment) for haloperidol may provide data helpful in evaluation of haloperidol regimens and compliance.

Questions—Haloperidol

1. **Uses of haloperidol include**
   A. Psychotic disorders (e.g., schizophrenia)
   B. Profound agitation
   C. To control tics and verbal utterances associated with Gilles de la Tourette's syndrome
   D. All of the above
   E. A and B
2. **Because of the low volume of distribution and the relatively low serum concentration of haloperidol, measurements are restricted to high-sensitivity methods of analysis.**
   A. True
   B. False
3. **Torsade de Pointes has been reported after haloperidol overdose.**
   A. True
   B. False

Thioridazine

Thioridazine (Mellaril®) is a phenothiazine with potent anxiolytic and antipsychotic properties. Its lengthy half-life (26–36 hours) dictates prolonged effects in overdose, and infrequent dosing intervals. The most frequent side effects are sedation and orthostatic hypotension. As with other phenothiazines, arrhythmias rarely develop in patients treated with thioridazine.

PATHOPHYSIOLOGY

Actions of thioridazine are numerous and include antagonism of cholinergic, α-1 adrenergic, dopamine (D2), histamine (H1), and serotonin-2 receptors. Its antipsychotic effect is felt to be mediated by its ability to block postsynaptic dopaminergic receptors in the mesolimbic area of the brain. At therapeutic doses, thioridazine has antiarrhythmic properties and depresses cardiac conduction, similar to quinidine. Electrocardiographic changes include a prolonged QT interval, flattening or depression of T waves, and an increase in U-wave amplitude.

PHARMACOKINETICS

Absorption

- Onset of action is 30–60 minutes.
- Thioridazine is absorbed well from the stomach and gastrointestinal tract.

Distribution

- Volume of distribution is 18 L/kg.
- Approximately 90% is protein bound.

Elimination

- Half life is 26–36 hours.
- Metabolism is primarily hepatic with up to 17% excreted via the kidneys.

CLINICAL PRESENTATIONS

The most frequent feature after an acute overdose is impairment of consciousness. Please see the Introduction to neuroleptics above for a summary of well-documented clinical possibilities. Clinical features of toxicity vary but often include progression of somnolence to a comatose state. Syncope may result within hours of ingestion. Hyperthermia may or may not be present. Both hypertensive and hypotensive syndromes have been reported.

Cardiac manifestations may include prolonged QT interval, T-wave changes, varying degrees of atrioventricular block, sinus and ventricular tachycardia (including Torsade de Pointes), and asystole. Approximately 50% of patients receiving 100–400 mg/d of thioridazine have electrocardiographic abnormalities. A direct depressant action on myocardial contractility contributes to the severe hypotension seen in severe overdoses.

TOXIC DOSAGE/DEATH

Patients have survived ingestions of 10 g of thioridazine and have died after as little as 1,500 mg/d. The lowest reported lethal dose was 900 mg. Seizures have occurred in adults who have ingested more than 2 g of thioridazine. Death follows cardiac arrhythmias, cardiac arrest, respiratory arrest, and aspiration pneumonia.

DRUG INTERACTIONS

Thioridazine may potentiate central nervous system depression when coingested with barbiturates, narcotic analgesics, antihistamines, alcohol, and other antipsychotic drugs. Anticholinergic effects may be pronounced when coingested with other anticholinergic agents such as antihistamines or anti-Parkinsonian medications. QT prolongation and the development of Torsade de Pointes may be enhanced when taken with quinidine, procainamide or disopyramide. Amiodarone may facilitate Torsade de Pointes as well.

PREGNANCY/LACTATION

Thioridazine crosses the placenta and is found in breast milk. Pregnancy risk category C.

LABORATORY

Analytic Methods

Serum concentrations of thioridazine and its metabolites are quantitated by an HPLC method.

Blood Levels

Significant overlap occurs when autopsy levels are compared with those seen in the therapeutic setting. Following blood levels in overdose is not helpful. Blood levels average 4.8 mg/L in fatal overdoses.

TREATMENT

Gut Decontamination

Gastric lavage may be useful with tracheal protection. Use of syrup of ipecac for emesis induction is not advised. Charcoal may decrease absorption. The anticholinergic effects of thioridazine may prolong gut transit time.

Elimination Enhancement

There is no evidence to support the use of extracorporeal methods of elimination such as hemodialysis, or hemoperfusion in thioridazine poisoning.

Supportive Measures

- Management of thioridazine overdose includes prevention or limitation of intestinal drug absorption, airway maintenance, and supportive care.
- Lidocaine-like agents are often ineffective in treating ventricular arrhythmias, even if electrolyte imbalance is corrected. Temporary pacing has been helpful in refractory cases.

- Treatment of ventricular tachyrhythmias associated with a prolonged QT interval should include rapid correction of metabolic and electrolyte disturbances such as hypokalemia and hypomagnesemia. Indeed, intravenous magnesium may be the drug of choice in managing Torsade de Pointes. Isoproterenol can be administered to shorten the QT interval in patients without severe coronary artery disease. Overdrive pacing may be useful as well.
- Hypotension can be explained in part by potent peripheral α-adrenergic blockade and may be managed by volume replacement and alpha agonists.
- Thioridazine in high doses may exhibit a β-adrenoceptor and a calcium channel blocking effect. Therefore, similar drugs with these properties are contraindicated in managing thioridazine overdose.

Questions—Thioridazine

1. **Actions of thioridazine are numerous and include**
   A. Antagonism of cholinergic receptors
   B. Antagonism of α-1 adrenergic receptors
   C. Antagonism of H1 histamine receptors
   D. All of the above
   E. A and B
2. **The most frequent feature after an acute overdose with thioridazine is impairment of consciousness.**
   A. True
   B. False
3. **Cardiac manifestations after an acute overdose with thioridazine may include all of the following except**
   A. Prolonged QT interval
   B. T-wave changes
   C. Diminished U-waves
   D. Varying degrees of atrioventricular block
   E. Torsade de Pointes

SEDATIVE-HYPNOTICS

Introduction

Numerous agents have been used to sedate patients, including the barbiturates (see Barbiturates in Chapter 27, Anticonvulsant Drugs), the benzodiazepines, chloral hydrate, and multiple other drugs. Many sedative agents have been abused to escape from societal pressures and stress. While some of these agents have been taken off the U.S. market as newer, safer agents have been introduced, many still may be found around the world. General treatment guidelines regarding therapeutic and overdose scenarios have been devised.

CLINICAL PRESENTATIONS

Knowledge of the exact sedative drug used is often not necessary because supportive care suffices in the vast majority of cases and no safe, effective antidotes exist in most cases. Physical signs may help differentiate the specific sedative-hypnotic drug involved. Ethchlorvynol may cause a prolonged, deep coma, hypothermia, a sweet odor on breath, hypotension, pulmonary edema, and prolonged apnea. Meprobamate may cause a deep, fluctuating coma lasting more than 24 hours, a gastric mass, hypotension, and pulmonary edema. Hyperthermia, tachycardia, paradoxical excitement, and respiratory depression characterize a methyprylon overdose.

Withdrawal

Most sedative-hypnotic drugs, including barbiturates, glutethimide, meprobamate, methyprylon, and chloral hydrate produce physical and psychological dependence when taken in 3–10 times the sedative dose for 1–2 months. Abstinence syndromes may produce major symptoms including psychosis, seizures, and death, and minor symptoms including apprehension, sympathetic hyperactivity, weakness, anorexia, sweating, insomnia, and postural hypotension. Any sedative-hypnotic drug, with the exception of the opiates, can be withdrawn with medical guidance with phenobarbital or benzodiazepines because of cross-tolerance. Co-addiction to opiates should be considered in difficult cases, as opiate withdrawal may be difficult to differentiate from sedative-hypnotic withdrawal.

LABORATORY

Blood levels can confirm ingestion of these agents, but rarely improve patient management. Because of tolerance, coingested drugs, large tissue stores, underlying medical disease, and certain active metabolites, clinical evaluation correlates better with outcome than blood levels. Ethanol and other sedative-hypnotic drugs should always be screened for when the clinical picture does not correlate with blood levels, as most central nervous system depressants have synergistic actions.

TREATMENT

Gut Decontamination

Patients who develop coma after use with these agents should only be lavaged after a cuffed endotracheal tube has been inserted to protect the airway, and the patient has been placed in the left lateral, head-down position. The initial gastric aspirate may be saved for drug analysis. Coma reduces gastrointestinal mobility and may permit effective lavage 6–12 hours after ingestion. Instillation of charcoal via a nasogastric tube may help diminish potential adverse outcomes.

Elimination Enhancement

In general, hemoperfusion clearance in sedative-hypnotic overdoses is superior to hemodialysis clearance, except for long-acting barbiturates. The decision on which measure to use depends on clinical judgment based on the occasionally available drug level and on the clinical presentation of the patient. Factors that suggest the use of hemodialysis or hemoperfusion include the failure of supportive care to maintain vital signs, the presence of underlying disease, adequate history of profound quantity of toxin, and documentation of lethal blood levels.

Supportive Measures

- Initial attention in all overdose scenarios with sedative-hypnotic agents must be to assess and stabilize the "ABCs" — airway, breathing and circulation. A clear airway must be established and ventilation maintained. All obtunded patients should receive glucose, naloxone and thiamine.
- A cuffed endotracheal tube should be inserted if gag reflex or central nervous system depression prevents adequate protection of the airway. The patient must be placed on a ventilator and arterial blood gases monitored as required.
- Coma may last for days with certain sedative-hypnotic overdoses.
- Complications such as pulmonary edema, aspiration pneumonia, bullous lesions, and withdrawal must be continuously assessed in an intensive care environment.

Cardiovascular Issues

- Intravenous access must be provided and fluids initiated.
- Hypotension is initially corrected with fluid boluses until the

systolic blood pressure reaches 100 mm Hg. Vasopressors such as dopamine may be used if fluids are insufficient.

- Patients who require vasopressors to maintain blood pressure should be hemodynamically monitored (preferably via an arterial line and pulmonary artery catheter) to guide fluid and drug management.
- Fluid balance is followed by inserting a Foley catheter to measure hourly urine volume, urine specific gravity, and urine electrolytes. Care must be taken not to give excessive fluids because of the propensity of sedative-hypnotic drugs to produce pulmonary edema in overdose.

Respiratory Issues

- After overdose with many sedative-hypnotics, respiratory arrest may occur suddenly and mental status may fluctuate. In the case of meprobamate, respiratory arrest may even occur after initial lightening of coma.
- Most deaths from sedative-hypnotic overdoses result from progressive respiratory insufficiency secondary to either adult respiratory distress syndrome (ARDS) or bacterial pneumonia.
- An elevated respiratory rate may indicate aspiration pneumonia, ARDS, pulmonary edema, and rarely, pulmonary embolus or pneumothorax.

ANTIDOTES

Except for the benzodiazepines, specific antidotes are not recognized for these drugs. Respiratory and central nervous system stimulants should not be used, as the hazards of hyperpyrexia and convulsions outweigh the benefits of these agents.

Question—Introduction to Sedative-Hypnotics

1. Which of the following statements is false?

A. Most deaths from sedative-hypnotic overdoses result from progressive respiratory insufficiency secondary to either adult respiratory distress syndrome (ARDS) or bacterial pneumonia.
B. Except for the benzodiazepines, specific antidotes are not recognized for these drugs.
C. Most sedative-hypnotic drugs, including barbiturates, glutethimide, meprobamate, methyprylon, and chloral hydrate produce physical and psychological dependence when taken in 3–10 times the sedative dose for 1–2 months.
D. Abstinence syndromes from sedative-hypnotic agents may produce major symptoms including psychosis, seizures, and death, and minor symptoms including apprehension, sympathetic hyperactivity, weakness, anorexia, dry skin, insomnia, and refractory hypertension.
E. Ethchlorvynol may cause a prolonged, deep coma, hypothermia, a sweet odor on breath, hypotension, pulmonary edema, and prolonged apnea.

Benzodiazepines

Benzodiazepines have been the most commonly prescribed drugs in the western world in part because of their efficacy, safety, and low cost. More than 10 benzodiazepines are currently marketed in the United States, each differing in their pharmacokinetic properties. Fortunately, benzodiazepines are relatively safe drugs, even in overdose. Death from pure benzodiazepine overdose is extremely rare. The discovery of benzodiazepine receptors has helped clarify the function of these drugs and explain a withdrawal syndrome associated with their use.

Benzodiazepines are predominantly used as anxiolytics. Certain benzodiazepines, such as intravenous diazepam, are highly effective as initial drugs for treating status epilepticus. Benzodiazepines are also used as sleep aids and muscle relaxants. Benzodiazepines are divided into three groups on the basis of elimination half-life. These include ultrashort-acting (e.g., midazolam), short-acting (e.g., lorazepam), and long-acting (e.g., diazepam) drugs. Acute overdose toxicity has been observed more often with the short-acting benzodiazepines, midazolam and triazolam, and the intermediate-acting flunitrazepam, than with diazepam, lorazepam, and nitrazepam. See also Clonazepam in the New Anticonvulsants section in Chapter 27, Anticonvulsant Drugs.

PATHOPHYSIOLOGY

Benzodiazepines are thought to bind in the presence of the inhibitory neurotransmitter γ-aminobutyric acid (GABA). Benzodiazepines appear to potentiate GABA-ergic transmission at a specific chloride channel complex, increasing the frequency of chloride channel opening and resulting in the inhibition of neuronal excitation. Two central benzodiazepine receptors have been identified that are located throughout the brain.

PHARMACOKINETICS

Absorption

- The gastrointestinal tract rapidly and completely absorbs most of the benzodiazepines, but absorption from intramuscular sites is erratic and delayed.
- Peak plasma levels occur 1–3 hours after ingestion.

Distribution

- The volume of distribution depends on lipid solubility. Diazepam possesses one of the highest volumes of distribution of the benzodiazepine group: chlordiazepoxide, 0.26–0.58 L/kg; triazolam, 0.8–1.3 L/kg; alprazolam, 0.97–1.17 L/kg.
- Rapid initial distribution of diazepam into tissues probably accounts for the fact that the duration of action of a single dose is much shorter than the long elimination half-life suggests.
- The benzodiazepines are highly protein bound (85–99%).

Elimination

- Half-lives for these agents include midazolam (Versed®), 2–5 hours; temazepam (Restoril®), 10 hours; triazolam (Halcion®), 1.7–3 hours; alprazolam (Xanax®), 11–14 hours; lorazepam (Ativan®), 10–20 hours; oxazepam (Serax®), 3–21 hours; chlordiazepoxide (Librium®), 5–30 hours; chlorazepate (Tranxene®), 36–200 hours; clonazepam (Klonopin®), 10–50 hours; diazepam (Valium®), 20–50 hours; and flurazepam (Dalmane®), 50–100 hours.
- Benzodiazepines are eliminated almost exclusively by metabolism. Liver biotransformation in hepatic microsomal enzymes occurs via two major pathways: demethylation and conjugation with glucuronide. Some of the subsequent metabolites are active.
- Chronic administration of diazepam, flurazepam, and chlordiazepoxide results in the accumulation of both the parent drug and active metabolites. Oxazepam and lorazepam do not accumulate as readily and produce no active metabolites.
- Elimination half-life determines the ability of a drug to accumulate but does not necessarily correlate with drug effect. The diazepam elimination half-life in high-dose abusers may range above 50 hours.

CLINICAL PRESENTATIONS

Neurologic Effects

Sedation, somnolence, diplopia, dysarthria, ataxia, and intellectual impairment are the most common benzodiazepine side effects. Even in large overdoses, symptoms are usually mild. The presence of coma should prompt a careful search for coingested drugs. The elderly and the very young are more susceptible to the central nervous system depressant action of benzodiazepines. Triazolam has been associated with anxiety between doses, rebound insomnia on ending treatment, serious paradoxical reactions such as aggression, excitation and features of psychosis, marked mental impairment, and fatal overdose.

Pulmonary Effects

Respiratory depression may rarely lead to alveolar hypoventilation, hypoxia, and metabolic acidosis. The development of pulmonary infiltrates secondary to noncardiogenic pulmonary edema is rare.

Benzodiazepine Abuse

Benzodiazepine abuse is defined as benzodiazepine use that causes impairment and dysfunction in a patient's social, occupational, emotional, psychological, or physical well-being. The impairment and dysfunction range from mild to severe and often are self-limiting. Benzodiazepine addiction is a chronic, progressive, pathologic process with biopsychosocial components that includes a compulsion to use benzodiazepines, loss of control over benzodiazepine use and continued use of the drug despite adverse consequences.

Withdrawal Effects

Long-term use of high therapeutic doses will produce most of the symptoms of long-term barbiturate or ethanol withdrawal. Chronic therapeutic doses below 40 mg of diazepam daily also will cause minor withdrawal reactions. Typically, symptoms develop 1–11 days after benzodiazepine use (average, 3–4 days) and usually are minor compared with those of ethanol and barbiturate withdrawal. Symptoms may include anxiety, insomnia, headache, muscle spasm, anorexia, vomiting, nausea, tremor, postural hypotension, and weakness.

A spectrum of affective disorders (psychosis, agitation, confusion, hallucinations, and delirium) and motor dysfunction (tremor, restlessness, myoclonic jerks, and seizures) may develop in serious cases after withdrawal from high daily doses. Seizures are rare and most commonly develop 7–8 days after withdrawal (range, 2–12 days). Rebound insomnia may occur after sudden withdrawal of short-acting benzodiazepines such as lorazepam, because of a lag in replacement of endogenous benzodiazepine compounds.

Geriatric Effects

Benzodiazepines can cause memory problems in the elderly. The ability of geriatric patients to learn new information is impaired (anterograde amnesia) with benzodiazepine therapy. Anterograde amnesia becomes more severe with increased dose, faster absorption, intravenous administration, and higher potency of the benzodiazepines. The long-term use of benzodiazepines in elderly patients commonly exacerbates underlying dementia and may cause excessive morbidity.

Elderly patients seem to be at increased risk of benzodiazepine-induced psychomotor impairment, and the impairment may gradually worsen with stable therapeutic levels. Use of alcohol and high doses of benzodiazepines and administration of other drugs such as anticholinergic agents are associated with increased sensitivity for cognitive and psychomotor effects.

TOXIC DOSAGE/DEATH

Oral doses of benzodiazepines produce sedation and ataxia but rarely cause death. Anaphylaxis is rare. A lethal dose of benzodiazepines has not been established; however, other sedative-hypnotic drugs, ethanol, and antipsychotic drugs synergistically enhance the sedation and respiratory depression properties of benzodiazepines. Intravenous diazepam is more toxic than orally administered diazepam, and rapid administration may result in apnea and hypotension, perhaps, in part, because of the parenteral vehicle, propylene glycol.

Coma with vital sign abnormalities has followed a triazolam overdose, and at least two fatal poisonings have been associated with temazepam overdose alone. Death has been reported after flunitrazepam, diazepam, nitrazepam, alprazolam, triazolam, and flurazepam. In human volunteers, diazepam produces impairment of cognitive and psychomotor tasks as early as 20 minutes before peak plasma values occur. Published tables have listed 5–20 μg / mL as toxic and over 20 μg / mL as lethal diazepam levels.

DRUG INTERACTIONS

Benzodiazepines potentiate the effect of other central nervous system depressants. Ethanol enhances diazepam absorption and thereby increases peak diazepam blood levels. Cimetidine increases the elimination half-life and reduces plasma clearance of diazepam by inhibiting hepatic microsomal enzymes, but does not affect the half-life of lorazepam or oxazepam. Absorption of clorazepate requires conversion by hydrolysis in the stomach, which may be affected by concomitant antacid therapy. The elderly have both reduced metabolism and increased sensitivity to a given dose of benzodiazepines.

PREGNANCY/LACTATION

Benzodiazepines cross the placenta and are relatively contraindicated in the first trimester. A causal relationship between teratogenicity and benzodiazepine use has not been established. High concentrations of diazepam and its active metabolites have been demonstrated for up to 12 days after birth in neonates whose mothers had received moderate (10–15 mg) to large (90 mg) doses of diazepam. Significant depression may be seen in neonates, ranging from the "floppy baby syndrome" characterized by hypotonia, respiratory depression, hypothermia, and poor reflexes, to simply lethargy and poor feeding. Seizures, prolonged hypotonia, and prolonged respiratory depression may be seen in newborns after treatment with lorazepam. Lorazepam is classified as pregnancy risk factor D.

Diazepam is excreted in the breast milk in significant amounts and may result in lethargy and poor feeding in neonates, who metabolize diazepam more slowly than adults. Benzodiazepine neonatal exposure from breast milk is about 5% of the maternal dose. Withdrawal symptoms (irritability, crying, sleep disturbance, tremors, and seizures) may occur in a neonate following exposure to a benzodiazepine *in utero* and then in breast milk. Onset of withdrawal symptoms may be delayed for 1–2 weeks. Diazepam is classified as pregnancy risk factor D.

LABORATORY

Analytic Methods

Gas chromatography-mass spectrometry methods are available to analyze chlordiazepoxide, clorazepate, diazepam, temazepam, prazepam, halazepam, alprazolam, triazolam, and midazolam benzodiazepines in the urine. Benzodiazepines are also analyzed by gas chromatography with electron capture detection. Most benzodiazepines are strongly protein bound. The analytical method must determine the free fraction rather than the total because drug clearance, distribution, toxicity and biotransformation refer to the free fraction in the blood.

Blood Levels

Benzodiazepine blood levels confirm acute ingestion but do not guide clinical management. Tolerance, drug coingestion, active metabolites, and distant tissue binding sites reduce the correlation of blood benzodiazepine level to clinical effect.

TREATMENT

Gut Decontamination

Lavage may be helpful for large ingestions when the patient presents within 2 hours of ingestion. Activated charcoal (10 times the estimated ingested dose, or 1 g/kg body weight) and cathartic within 4 hours of ingestion may be helpful as well.

Elimination Enhancement

Forced diuresis is ineffective. Hemodialysis is ineffective because of the large protein binding of benzodiazepines. Hemoperfusion has not been well studied because of the lack of indication for its use, although good extraction ratios have been obtained in one patient

Supportive Measures

- Most patients require only medical observation. Patients who are ambulating after 6–8 hours of observation may be discharged after appropriate psychiatric counseling. Most ingestions produce minor symptoms.
- Respiratory depression from coingested drugs is the main cause of death. The presence of coma unresponsive to painful stimulus should prompt a search for coingested drugs, trauma, or underlying medical disease.
- Withdrawal may be treated with the intravenous administration of 5 mg of diazepam. High-dose benzodiazepine abusers have been treated effectively with an initial diazepam dose of 40% maintenance levels followed by a daily tapering by 10%. Propranolol and clonidine may attenuate symptoms but usually do not alleviate them.
- Antidepressants, which may reduce benzodiazepine receptors in the brain, may be useful during benzodiazepine withdrawal when they are begun a few months before withdrawal. Careful observation is necessary for evidence of lowered seizure threshold by the antidepressants. Further clinical trials are necessary to evaluate the effectiveness of antidepressants in the treatment of benzodiazepine withdrawal.
- A phenobarbital substitution technique for benzodiazepine withdrawal has also been proposed. The phenobarbital substitution method uses propranolol for acute and subacute somatic complaints and symptoms.
- Phenobarbital may be used during acute benzodiazepine withdrawal and detoxification. Controlled clinical studies have not compared the relative effectiveness of phenobarbital versus chlordiazepoxide, clonazepam, or diazepam.

ANTIDOTES

Flumazenil

Flumazenil is a specific antagonist at benzodiazepine receptor sites. It is primarily indicated in the treatment of symptoms of benzodiazepine overdose. Flumazenil has little or no agonist activity in humans. Its users must be carefully monitored for respiratory and circulatory compromise. It does not obviate the need for intensive symptomatic and supportive care, which is required for the treatment of a benzodiazepine overdose. Deaths have followed its use in mixed overdoses. In coma due to multiple-drug overdose, flumazenil reverses the benzodiazepine component of central nervous system depression and may help in the diagnosis. However, because flumazenil is associated with multiple risks, it cannot be recommended for the patient with coma of unknown origin and a possibly mixed toxic ingestion.

Ventricular tachycardia, complete heart block, and death may follow flumazenil use. Seizures and acute anxiety states may be provoked in patients dependent on benzodiazepines. Acute withdrawal symptoms may be seen in the benzodiazepine-dependent patient given flumazenil in an emergency facility. Seizures are more common if the patient has taken a tricyclic antidepressant, isoniazid, cocaine, or propoxyphene in addition to the benzodiazepine. Flumazenil antagonizes the anticonvulsant properties of the benzodiazepines, leaving a medication that may be epileptogenic. Repeated doses may be required because of the short duration of action of flumazenil (1 hour).

Flumazenil should be withheld if there is a history or physical findings suggestive of seizure or if there are electrocardiographic signs of tricyclic antidepressant overdose. Flumazenil should not be used to shorten the period of observation although it may decrease the need for ventilatory support and intensive monitoring. The cardiotoxic effects of flumazenil in multiple-drug ingestions that may include a cardiogenic toxin are not known. Flumazenil should be used only if continued observation for recurrence of sedation can be ensured.

Incremental doses (0.1–0.2 mg) should be titrated to the individual patient's needs. Seizures may be precipitated in multiple-drug ingestions involving proconvulsant drugs as well as in chronic benzodiazepine users as a manifestation of a severe withdrawal reaction. Such seizures may then respond to a small dose of benzodiazepines. As a diagnostic tool in the evaluation of comatose drug overdose, flumazenil should be given as a 0.2-mg bolus intravenously, with an additional 0.1 mg/min until the patient is awake. Most patients respond to 3 mg or less. A continuous infusion of flumazenil has not been shown superior to a repeat bolus technique, often preferred for routine clinical use. An intravenous dose of 5 mg may improve consciousness in alcohol intoxication but does not improve psychomotor function.

Questions—Benzodiazepines

1. Death from benzodiazipines alone has never been reported.
   A. True
   B. False

2. Benzodiazepines are divided into three groups on the basis of elimination half-life. These include ultrashort-acting (e.g., midazolam), short-acting (e.g., diazepam), and long-acting (e.g., lorazepam) drugs.
   A. True
   B. False

3. Which of the following statements is false?
   A. Sedation, somnolence, diplopia, dysarthria, ataxia, and intellectual impairment are the most common benzodiazepine side effects.
   B. In large overdoses, symptoms are usually mild.
   C. The presence of coma should prompt a careful search for coingested drugs.
   D. The elderly and the very young are less susceptible to the central nervous system depressant action of benzodiazepines.

E. Triazolam has been associated with serious paradoxical reactions such as aggression, excitation and features of psychosis.

4. Which of the following is true concerning benzodiazepine withdrawal?
A. True benzodiazepine withdrawal has not been described.
B. Long-term use of high therapeutic doses will produce most of the symptoms of long-term barbiturate or ethanol withdrawal.
C. Typically, symptoms develop 2 weeks after benzodiazepine use.
D. Symptoms may include anxiety, diaphoresis, hypersomnia, hyperphagia and seizures.
E. Seizures are rare and most commonly develop 1 day after withdrawal

5. Which of the following statements about flumazenil is false?
A. Flumazenil is a specific antagonist at benzodiazepine receptor sites.
B. It typically obviates the need for intensive symptomatic and supportive care, which is required for the treatment of a severe benzodiazepine overdose.
C. Because flumazenil is associated with multiple risks, it cannot be recommended for the patient with coma of unknown origin and a possibly mixed toxic ingestion.
D. Ventricular tachycardia, complete heart block, and death may follow flumazenil use.
E. Seizures and acute anxiety states may be provoked in patients dependent on benzodiazepines

Chloral Hydrate

Chloral hydrate is an effective sedative-hypnotic which produces only minimal respiratory and circulatory depression in therapeutic doses. Chloral hydrate became a popular sedative after Liebreich introduced it into clinical practice in 1869. Use of chloral hydrate declined after the introduction of barbiturates in 1903. Potentiation of the sedative effects of chloral hydrate by ethanol has led to the street terms "knockout drops" and "Mickey Finns."

Chloral hydrate has been used rectally to sedate pediatric patients. Chloral hydrate, 30 mg/kg rectally every 2 hours, has been effective in treating status epilepticus in adults when conventional anticonvulsants (e.g., diazepam, phenytoin, and barbiturates) are ineffective. Less morning after "hangover" occurs with chloral hydrate than with barbiturates, and chloral hydrate exhibits little analgesic activity.

PATHOPHYSIOLOGY

Chloral hydrate is a central nervous system depressant that is structurally similar to halothane. The exact mechanism of action is unknown. Initial action may result from the parent compound but prolonged effects probably result from the active metabolite, trichloroethanol. In large overdose, chloral hydrate depresses myocardial contractility and shortens the refractory period leading to dysrhythmias. Chloral hydrate is a mucosal and skin irritant.

PHARMACOKINETICS

Absorption

- Chloral hydrate absorption is rapid and complete from the gastrointestinal tract, with peak therapeutic levels developing within 1 hour.

Distribution

- Chloral hydrate and its active metabolite trichloroethanol are highly lipid-soluble and easily penetrate all membranes. The volume of distribution of chloral hydrate is 0.6 L/kg.
- The metabolites, trichloroethanol and trichloroacetic acid, are 40% and 85% protein bound, respectively.

Elimination

- The liver metabolizes chloral hydrate almost exclusively by alcohol dehydrogenase. The major product is the active metabolite, trichloroethanol. A small amount of chloral hydrate is oxidized directly to the inactive trichloroacetic acid.
- The plasma half-life for therapeutic doses of chloral hydrate is 4–5 minutes, whereas for trichloroethanol it is 8–12 hours and for trichloroacetic acid, 67 hours.

CLINICAL PRESENTATIONS

Signs and symptoms of severe overdose are similar to those of barbiturate overdose, with respiratory depression and cardiovascular instability presenting the main threats to life. Symptoms begin with ataxia and lethargy and may progress to coma within 1–2 hours of ingestion. Pupils usually are miotic but dilate in the deeper stages of coma. The peculiar pearlike odor of chloral hydrate may help distinguish it from other sedative-hypnotics.

Cardiovascular Effects

Cardiac dysrhythmias may complicate the clinical course, particularly in severe intoxications, even without underlying cardiac disease. Multiple premature ventricular beats, multifocal ventricular tachycardia (Torsade de Pointes), ventricular fibrillation, and atrial fibrillation have been reported. There appears to be a high mortality when chloral hydrate overdose is accompanied by arrhythmias. Antiarrhythmic therapy failure may occur.

Gastrointestinal Effects

Chloral hydrate is a mucosal irritant that may cause nausea, vomiting, and abdominal pain. Gastric perforation and gastrointestinal hemorrhage followed by esophageal strictures have been reported. Jaundice, aminotransferase elevation and albuminuria may occur several days after ingestion but are rarely serious or prolonged.

Dependence

High-dose, long-term use may result in tolerance and physical dependence. Sudden withdrawal can result in a serious abstinence syndrome similar to delirium tremens (seizures and psychosis) and responds to barbiturates or other sedative-hypnotic drugs.

Pediatric Effects

Repetitive dosing of chloral hydrate in children is of concern because of the accumulation of the metabolites, trichloroethanol and trichloracetic acid. These may produce excessive central nervous system depression, predispose newborns to conjugated and unconjugated hyperbilirubinemia, decrease albumin binding of bilirubin, and contribute to metabolic acidosis.

TOXIC DOSAGE/DEATH

Adult toxicity begins at 2–3 g. Lethal levels are difficult to predict since fatalities have resulted from 3-g ingestions and survival has followed a 36-g ingestion. The reported lethal adult dose is about 5-10 g.

DRUG INTERACTIONS

Ethanol potentiates the effect of chloral hydrate, probably by inducing the formation of the active metabolite trichloroethanol because of increased NADH availability. After ethanol administration, blood trichloroethanol levels reach higher and earlier peak concentrations compared with those resulting from the consumption of chloral hydrate alone. Ethanol may also produce a disulfiram-like reaction with headache, flushing, tachycardia, and hypotension when ingested with chloral hydrate.

Other sedative-hypnotic drugs cause synergistic central nervous system (CNS) depression when administered with chloral hydrate. Triclofos (trichloroethyl phosphate monosodium) produces levels of trichloroethanol quantitatively similar to those following chloral hydrate administration and would be expected to cause synergistic CNS depression. Concurrent administration of chloral hydrate and warfarin has an unpredictable effect on the activity of coumarin and may result in excessive hypoprothrombinemia.

PREGNANCY/LACTATION

Chloral hydrate crosses the placenta and has been assigned to pregnancy risk category C. Only small amounts appear in breast milk.

LABORATORY

Analytic Methods

A gas chromatographic method with electron capture detection allows the identification and quantitation of chloral hydrate and both its metabolites, trichloroethanol and trichloroacetic acid.

Blood Levels

Blood levels for chloral hydrate confirm ingestion, but seldom guide management. The reported therapeutic level is 1.0 mg/100mL. Toxicity occurs at 10 mg/100mL and fatalities have occurred at 25 mg/100mL.

TREATMENT

Gut Decontamination

Rapid onset of action makes the use of syrup of ipecac hazardous in the lethargic patient. The immediate administration of activated charcoal with endotracheal protection is preferable to syrup of ipecac administration. Because of the corrosive properties of liquid chloral hydrate preparation, lavage tubes are relatively contraindicated and, if used, must be inserted carefully. As chloral hydrate is radiopaque, the effectiveness of decontamination measures may occasionally be confirmed with a flat plate of the abdomen; however, this may be complicated by the presence of food. Controlled studies that support or refute the use of multiple doses of activated charcoal in overdose with chloral hydrate do not exist.

Elimination Enhancement

Hemodialysis effectively removes the active metabolite trichloroethanol. Major indications for dialysis are the failure of the patient to respond to supportive care or the presence of lethal drug levels. Resin hemoperfusion also effectively removes trichloroethanol at a rate similar to that of hemodialysis. Forced diuresis is ineffective. Exchange transfusion in an infant was not useful in removing substantial amounts of trichloroethanol.

Supportive Measures

- Since chloral hydrate may cause serious arrhythmias and/or respiratory depression, all significant ingestions require careful evaluation of respiratory status, an intravenous line, oxygen, and a cardiac monitor. Hypotension is treated with fluid challenges and pressors.
- Bretylium may be an effective alternative to lidocaine and β-blocker therapy for ventricular arrhythmias. β-blockade has been helpful in suppressing arrhythmias, however.
- Watch for the development of gastrointestinal hemorrhage, hepatic and renal dysfunction, and aspiration pneumonia, as well as withdrawal symptoms.
- Baseline laboratory tests include a complete blood count, serum electrolytes, serum hepatic aminotransferases, and serum creatinine.

ANTIDOTES

There are no antidotes. Anecdotally, flumazenil has produced a dramatic response with an increased level of consciousness, verbalization, and pupillary dilation in one case. Further controlled studies are required to establish this as a specific treatment for chloral hydrate overdose.

Questions—Chloral Hydrate

1. Which of the following statements concerning chloral hydrate is false?

A. Chloral hydrate is an effective sedative-hypnotic which produces only minimal respiratory and circulatory depression in therapeutic doses.
B. Potentiation of the sedative effects of chloral hydrate by ethanol has led to the street terms "knockout drops" and "Mickey Finns."
C. Chloral hydrate has been used intranasally and intravenously to sedate pediatric patients.
D. Chloral hydrate has also been effective in treating status epilepticus in adults when conventional anticonvulsants are ineffective.
E. Less morning after "hangover" occurs with chloral hydrate than with barbiturates, and chloral hydrate exhibits little analgesic activity.

2. Chloral hydrate is a central nervous system depressant that is structurally similar to halothane.

A. True
B. False

3. In large overdose, chloral hydrate depresses myocardial contractility and shortens the refractory period, leading to dysrhythmias.

A. True
B. False

4. A peculiar vinyl-like odor helps distinguish chloral hydrate from other sedative-hypnotics.

A. True
B. False

5. The major active metabolite of trichloroethanol is

A. Trichloroacetic acid
B. Chloroform
C. Disulfiram
D. Trichloroethanol
E. Carbon disulfide

Ethchlorvynol

Ethchlorvynol (Placidyl®) was introduced in 1955 as a sedative-hypnotic that possessed a more rapid onset and shorter duration of action than barbiturates. Numerous emergency department visits and deaths were reported in the 1970s. Ethchlorvynol overdose produces a prolonged deep coma, respiratory depression, hypotension, and bradycardia. Complications may include pneumonia, cardiorespiratory arrest, peripheral neuropathy, and pulmonary edema. Ethchlorvynol has muscle-relaxant and anticonvulsant properties in addition to sedative-hypnotic properties.

PATHOPHYSIOLOGY

Ethchlorvynol is a central nervous system depressant similar to barbiturates, but its exact mechanism of action is unknown.

PHARMACOKINETICS

Absorption

- Gastrointestinal absorption occurs rapidly with onset of action in 14–30 minutes and peak levels in 1 hour. Fatty foods delay absorption.

Distribution

- Sedative effects disappear in 3–5 hours as ethchlorvynol, a highly lipophilic drug, distributes into fatty tissue stores. A rebound phase occurs at 7–10 hours as ethchlorvynol redistributes from tissue stores.
- Ethchlorvynol is 50–60% protein bound.

Elimination

- Little renal clearance of unchanged ethchlorvynol occurs and accounts for less than 10% of elimination.
- The liver metabolizes ethchlorvynol, probably by conjugation with glucuronide, although the exact pathway has not been elucidated.
- The elimination half-life after a therapeutic dose may reach 25 hours, but an overdose may prolong the half-life to over 100 hours.

CLINICAL PRESENTATIONS

The clinical picture is similar to that of barbiturate overdose with symptoms ranging from slurred speech, ataxia, nystagmus, and lethargy to coma, respiratory depression, and hypotension. Prolonged coma (many days), hypotension with relative bradycardia, pink gastric aspirate, and marked respiratory depression are characteristic of severe ethchlorvynol intoxications. Excess salivation may give the appearance of a cholinergic crisis from an organophosphate intoxication.

Hypothermia is a consistent finding. In several cases, pulmonary edema appeared immediately after intravenous injection along with a minty taste, cough, and coma. Severe chest pain may accompany dyspnea. Pneumonia and peripheral neuropathy from pressure necrosis are common complications. Like barbiturates, bullous skin lesions have been reported following ethchlorvynol ingestion.

Psychological and physical dependence may develop after chronic ethchlorvynol use. Withdrawal symptoms including agitation, confusion, tremor, hypertension, tachycardia, hallucinations, and seizures may occur. Withdrawal may appear in neonates. Symptoms reported after chronic use include ataxia, dysarthria, tremor, toxic amblyopia, and central scotomata.

TOXIC DOSAGE/DEATH

Mild to moderate intoxication begins in the 4–10 g range, depending on coingested drugs. The variable response to ethchlorvynol dosage makes the determination of lethal ingestion by history difficult. Recovery after prolonged coma was reported after ingestions of 80–125 g followed by vigorous supportive care and dialysis. Fatalities have been reported with amounts as low as 5 g alone, and with 2.5 g when ethanol was coingested.

DRUG INTERACTIONS

Ethanol increases the sedative effect of ethchlorvynol. Ethchlorvynol does not induce hepatic microsomal enzymes, and metabolism is not affected by hepatic dysfunction. This sedative-hypnotic may decrease the activity of coumarin.

PREGNANCY/LACTATION

Ethchlorvynol crosses the placenta and causes withdrawal symptoms in neonates of chronically addicted mothers. Pregnancy risk factor C.

LABORATORY

Analytic Methods

Ethchlorvynol may be measured by high-performance liquid chromatography.

Blood Levels

Serum ethchlorvynol levels confirm ingestion but seldom guide management since serum levels do not correlate well with clinical outcome. Approximate serum levels are therapeutic, 5 mg/L; toxic, 20 mg/L; lethal, 150 mg/L. Patients have survived serum levels greater than 200 mg/L with supportive care.

TREATMENT

Gut Decontamination

Obtunded patients may benefit from lavage with a protected airway as long as 8 hours postingestion. Activated charcoal may be helpful as well.

Elimination Enhancement

Although hemodialysis has reduced the half-life of ethchlorvynol, its effect on duration of coma appears minimal, perhaps because of protein binding and redistribution from large tissue stores. Resin hemoperfusion results in good extraction ratios and is superior to dialysis in ethchlorvynol removal. However, substantial rebound from tissue stores occurs and may require repeat perfusions in 6–8 hours.

Indications for resin hemoperfusion include clinical situations in which supportive measures fail, life-threatening complications that develop from prolonged coma, or blood ethchlorvynol levels that exceed 150 μg/mL. Forced diuresis is not recommended because of the limited enhancement of ethchlorvynol elimination and its propensity to produce pulmonary edema.

Supportive Measures

- Severe intoxication resembles barbiturate coma. Protection of the airway, ventilation, and circulation along with administration of glucose, naloxone, and thiamine are the first priority.
- Hypotension unresponsive to fluids may require hemodynamic monitoring. Prolonged coma is the hallmark of serious ethchlorvynol intoxication and intensive support may last days.
- Watch for development of pulmonary edema, respiratory arrest, and pneumonia.
- Baseline laboratory tests should include complete blood count, electrolytes, glucose, creatinine, and chest x-ray.

Questions—Ethchlorvynol

1. Ethchlorvynol overdose produces a prolonged deep coma, respiratory depression, hypotension, and bradycardia.
   A. True
   B. False

2. Ethchlorvynol has not been associated with fatalities.
   A. True
   B. False

3. Which of the following statements about ethchlorvynol overdose is false?
   A. The clinical picture is similar to that of barbiturate overdose with symptoms ranging from slurred speech, ataxia, nystagmus, and lethargy to coma, respiratory depression, and hypotension.
   B. Prolonged coma (many days), hypotension with relative bradycardia, pink gastric aspirate, and marked respiratory depression are characteristic of severe ethchlorvynol intoxications.
   C. Hyperthermia is a consistent finding.
   D. In several cases, pulmonary edema appeared immediately after intravenous injection along with a minty taste, cough, and coma.
   E. Like barbiturates, bullous skin lesions have been reported following ethchlorvynol ingestion.

Meprobamate

Meprobamate (Miltown®) was introduced over 25 years ago as the first modern centrally active tranquilizer lacking the peripheral autonomic side effects of phenothiazines. Initial enthusiasm was tempered by early case reports of serious overdose and addiction similar to other sedative-hypnotics. Toxic exposures to meprobamate currently are rare. Like other sedative-hypnotic drugs, meprobamate may produce lethargy, coma, and respiratory depression. Hypotension is the most serious complication of meprobamate overdose. Overzealous hydration may cause cardiac failure and pulmonary edema, as meprobamate may depress myocardial contractility. Sudden deterioration may occur after initial improvement because of release of meprobamate from drug concretions.

PATHOPHYSIOLOGY

Meprobamate acts as a central nervous system depressant to reduce sensory transmission, particularly in the thalamus. Inhibition of spinal reflexes contributes to its muscle-relaxant properties. At high doses, meprobamate depresses cardiac contractility, and this may result in hypotension without respiratory depression. In contrast to barbiturates, hypotension may appear in light stages of coma.

PHARMACOKINETICS

Absorption

- Low water solubility and stability in acid solutions may explain the propensity of meprobamate to form concretions in the stomach, and explains why most meprobamate absorption occurs in the small intestine.
- Delayed gastric emptying reduces peak plasma levels. At therapeutic doses, peak meprobamate levels are reached in 2–4 hours, but plasma levels at 8 hours may be equal to those at 4 hours because of delayed gastric emptying.

Distribution

- Meprobamate is widely distributed in body tissue with a volume of distribution of 0.75 L/kg.
- Plasma protein binding is 10–20%.

Elimination

- The kidney excretes about 10% unchanged, whereas the liver biotransforms most of the absorbed meprobamate dose to inactive hydroxy and glucuronide metabolites.
- The elimination half-life is 8–12 hours at therapeutic doses, but may be prolonged after overdose.
- Hepatic microsomal enzyme induction (e.g., in chronic ethanolism) reduces the serum half-life.

CLINICAL PRESENTATIONS

Meprobamate produces a clinical picture of central nervous system depression that is similar to that of other sedative-hypnotic drugs. Symptoms range from nystagmus, dysarthria, ataxia, and confusion, to deep coma, hypotension, apnea, and pulmonary edema. Physical signs may include dysarthria, tachycardia, ataxia, miosis or mydriasis, respiratory depression, hallucinations, seizures, dysconjugate gaze, and hypothermia. Fluctuating levels of consciousness may occur because of the presence of meprobamate masses in the stomach. Hypotension usually correlates with depth of coma, but hypotension may occur unexpectedly in early stages of coma. Cardiac arrhythmias, bradycardia, and bullous skin lesions have been reported rarely.

Meprobamate use may produce an abstinence syndrome, physical dependence, and tolerance. Abrupt withdrawal from chronic doses of as little as 1.6 g daily may produce tremor, insomnia, gastrointestinal disturbances, delirium and convulsions lasting 2–3 days. Anxiety, sweating, tremors, hyperpyrexia, seizures, and death have been associated with withdrawal from a weekly 4-g meprobamate addiction. Generally, abstinence symptoms begin 1–2 days after discontinuation.

TOXIC DOSAGE/DEATH

The usual adult therapeutic dose is 600–1,600 mg daily in three or four divided doses. Documented adult fatalities have been associated with ingestion of amounts as small as 12 g, whereas survival has occurred after a 40-g ingestion. Fatal meprobamate blood levels range from 142–342 mg/L (average, 326 mg/L) in single overdose and 43–155 mg/L in combined alcohol-meprobamate overdose deaths.

DRUG INTERACTIONS

Sedative-hypnotics, antipsychotics, opiates, and ethanol synergistically increase the central nervous system depressant effects of meprobamate.

PREGNANCY/LACTATION

Meprobamate crosses the placenta, and maternal meprobamate levels approximate those of the fetus. Meprobamate is excreted in breast milk and should not be given to lactating mothers. The use of meprobamate in pregnancy does not appear to increase the rate of fetal demise or abnormalities.

LABORATORY

Analytic Methods

A gas chromatographic method for determination of meprobamate in human plasma is sensitive to a concentration of 1 mg/L. Screening for the presence of meprobamate by thin-layer chromatography may be important, as this compound cannot be detected by high-performance liquid chromatography using ultraviolet detection.

Blood Levels
Serum meprobamate levels confirm ingestion but seldom guide management, although levels do correlate with level of consciousness in pure ingestions in nontolerant patients. Approximate serum levels include 10 mg/L (therapeutic), 80–120 mg/L (significant toxicity), and 200 mg/L (potentially lethal, deep coma). Blood levels must be interpreted with caution however, since children have regained consciousness with meprobamate levels of 144 mg/L.

TREATMENT

Gut Decontamination
Asymptomatic or mildly symptomatic patients who present more than 4 hours after ingestion require no decontamination unless sustained-release preparations are involved. Delayed gastric emptying and formation of drug masses suggest that lavage may be useful up to 12 hours after significant ingestions. Fluctuating vital signs or levels of consciousness may indicate continuous absorption from stomach drug masses and, therefore, the need for endoscopy.

Activated charcoal should be instilled either after lavage or alone. Syrup of ipecac is not recommended. The propensity of meprobamate to form concretions in the stomach has necessitated gastrotomy in a patient who deteriorated after initially responding to supportive care.

Elimination Enhancement
Hemoperfusion is indicated only after severe ingestions in patients who do not respond to supportive care, who cannot tolerate prolonged coma, or who ingest massive doses. Meprobamate blood levels greater than 100 mg/L also suggest the need for hemoperfusion. Anecdotally, continuous arteriovenous charcoal hemoperfusion was shown to remove substantial amounts of meprobamate in a patient with profound hemodynamic instability.

Although clinical experience is limited, resin hemoperfusion may also be an effective way to increase meprobamate clearance. Hemodialysis increases meprobamate elimination but less so than resin hemoperfusion. Forced diuresis is contraindicated because of the propensity of meprobamate to cause pulmonary edema. Peritoneal dialysis is less effective than hemodialysis and has no place in therapy when hemoperfusion or hemodialysis is available.

Supportive Measures
- Initial evaluation of airway, ventilation, and circulation after meprobamate overdose is similar to that required after all sedative-hypnotic overdoses. Endotracheal intubation, intravenous lines, oxygen, and cardiac monitors are used as necessary.
- Hypotension may be out of proportion to depth of coma and must be treated cautiously with fluids since the use of forced diuresis has been complicated by pulmonary edema. Patients who do not respond to fluid replacement should be treated with vasopressors such as dopamine.
- Since hypotension may appear in the early stages of coma, frequent vital signs including temperature should be taken in all obtunded patients (i.e., every 15–30 minutes until a clear trend is established, then every hour until the patient is responsive to a verbal stimulus).
- Fluctuating vital signs or coma may indicate a drug mass, and gastroscopy should be considered.
- Watch for development of pulmonary edema and aspiration pneumonia as well as withdrawal in tolerant individuals after 1–2 days.
- Marked metabolic acidosis may complicate coma. Baseline laboratory tests for severe ingestions should include a complete blood count, electrolytes, chest x-ray, and arterial blood gases.

Questions—Meprobamate

1. Which of the following statements about meprobamate is false?
A. Hypotension is the most serious complication of meprobamate overdose.
B. Overzealous hydration may cause cardiac failure and pulmonary edema, as meprobamate may depress myocardial contractility.
C. Sudden deterioration may occur after initial improvement because of a release of meprobamate from drug concretions.
D. In contrast to barbiturates, hypertension may appear in light stages of coma.
E. Low water solubility and stability in acid solutions may explain the propensity of meprobamate to form concretions in the stomach, and explains why most meprobamate absorption occurs in the small intestine.

2. Which of the following statements about meprobamate is false?
A. Meprobamate produces a clinical picture of central nervous system depression that is similar to that of other sedative-hypnotic drugs.
B. Symptoms range from nystagmus, dysarthria, ataxia, and confusion, to deep coma, hypotension, apnea, and pulmonary edema.
C. Physical signs may include dysarthria, tachycardia, ataxia, miosis or mydriasis, respiratory depression, hallucinations, seizures, dysconjugate gaze, and hypothermia.
D. Hypotension may occur unexpectedly in early stages of coma.
E. Cardiac arrhythmias, bradycardia, and bullous skin lesions are common.

Zolpidem

Zolpidem (Ambien®) is a novel, rapid-onset, short-acting hypnotic drug marketed in several European countries and the U.S. It is chemically unrelated to the benzodiazepines. In overdose it may result in coma, pinpoint pupils, and respiratory depression; it does not respond to naloxone but does respond to flumazenil. No fatalities have been reported.

PATHOPHYSIOLOGY
Imidazopyridines are thought to interact with the same GABA receptor and chloride channel complex as the benzodiazepines by high affinity with certain benzodiazepine receptors. Like the benzodiazepines, zolpidem appears to potentiate GABA-ergic transmission, thus increasing the frequency of chloride channel opening, resulting in the inhibition of neuronal excitation. Zolpidem appears to cause only sedation, and is devoid of significant myorelaxant, anxiolytic, and anticonvulsant activity.

PHARMACOKINETICS

Absorption
- After oral administration, zolpidem is rapidly and completely absorbed.

- Some first-pass biotransformation of the drug results in a bioavailability of about 70%.

Distribution

- Zolpidem is 92% bound to plasma proteins.
- The apparent volume of distribution after a 5-mg intravenous dose is 0.5 L/kg.
- Brain concentrations reach one-third to one-half of those achieved in the plasma.

Elimination

- Zolpidem is completely metabolized. Less than 1% of an administered dose is excreted unchanged in the urine. Three metabolites have been identified but have no pharmacologic activity.
- Elimination half-life is 1.5 hours.

CLINICAL PRESENTATIONS

At higher dosage, zolpidem is associated with adverse effects such as nausea and vomiting, headache, lightheadedness, dizziness, confusion, anterograde amnesia, and queasiness. Several reports have described chronic abuse, tolerance, withdrawal symptoms, and hallucinatory phenomena with zolpidem. Coma, pinpoint pupils and respiratory depression have been described in overdose. Somnolence, vertigo, and vomiting may be observed. Hand, limb, and perioral tremor, muscle twitching, myoclonic jerks, diplopia, gastric and abdominal pain, and swallowing difficulties have been reported. Seizures may follow withdrawal.

TOXIC DOSAGE/DEATH

One patient ingested 39 tablets and did not experience coma, although treatment was not begun for 6 hours. A fatal dose has not been reported.

DRUG INTERACTIONS

Potentiation of the sedative effect of zolpidem is observed when it is given in combination with chlorpromazine or imipramine. No pharmacodynamic interactions have been observed with concomitant administration of cimetidine or ranitidine.

PREGNANCY/LACTATION

The excretion of zolpidem in breast milk represents a very small percentage of an administered dose. Pregnancy risk category B.

LABORATORY

Analytic Methods

A high-performance liquid chromatographic method with fluorometric detection is available for the detection of zolpidem in body fluids (urine, serum).

Blood Levels

A peak blood level of 200 ng/mL was reached 30 minutes after oral administration of 20 mg of zolpidem. Following blood levels does not assist in managing adverse reactions.

TREATMENT

Gut Decontamination

Gastric lavage may decrease the absorption of zolpidem if it is performed within 1 hour of ingestion. Tracheal protection must be provided. Activated charcoal was used in one patient, but there are no systematic studies supporting its use.

Elimination Enhancement

Extracorporeal methods of treatment such as hemodialysis, and hemoperfusion would probably not be useful in the setting of zolpidem overdose due to high protein binding, rapid onset of action and elimination, and the availability of an effective antidote.

Supportive Measures

- Treatment is similar to that following a benzodiazepine overdose.
- Laboratory abnormalities may include increased transaminase levels, leukocytosis, a mild transient hypokalemia, and thrombocytopenia.
- Isolated intoxication with less than 100 mg of zolpidem requires no therapeutic measures other than psychiatric referral of suicidal patients. When higher doses of zolpidem are ingested, observation over a period of 12 hours is recommended for all patients with signs of intoxication.

ANTIDOTES

Flumazenil

Flumazenil, 0.04 mg/kg, rapidly reverses decreased alertness and electroencephalographic changes induced by zolpidem. In one overdose patient who ingested 300 mg of zolpidem followed by coma, pinpoint pupils, and respiratory depression, intravenous flumazenil 1 mg was followed by arousal of the patient, correction of the miosis, and normalization of the respiratory pattern and blood gas analysis. Repeated doses of flumazenil may be required.

Question—Zolpidem

1. Which of the following statements about zolpidem is false?

A. Zolpidem is chemically related to the benzodiazepines.
B. In overdose it may result in coma, pinpoint pupils, and respiratory depression; this does not respond to naloxone but does respond to flumazenil.
C. Imidazopyridines are thought to interact with the same GABA receptor and chloride channel complex as the benzodiazepines by high affinity with certain benzodiazepine receptors.
D. Zolpidem appears to cause sedation, and is devoid of significant myorelaxant, anxiolytic, and anticonvulsant activity.
E. Several reports have described chronic abuse, tolerance, withdrawal symptoms, and hallucinatory phenomena with zolpidem.

Answers

Introduction to Cyclic Antidepressant Drugs

1. B 2. E

Cyclic Antidepressants

1. A	2. C	3. E	4. B	5. B	6. B.
7. E	8. A	9. A	10. A	11. C	12. B
13. A	14. A	15. C	16. A	17. D	

Clomipramine

1. D 2. D

Venlafaxine

1. D

Monoamine Oxidase Inhibitors

1. D 2. C 3. A 4. D 5. D 6. A
7. A

Introduction to Neuroleptic Drugs

1. B 2. C 3. A 4. A 5. B 6. B
7. C 8. A 9. D 10. E 11. B 12. A
13. E

Neuroleptic Malignant Syndrome

1. C 2. B 3. C 4. A 5. D

Clozapine

1. D 2. A

Haloperidol

1. D 2. B 3. A

Thioridazine

1. D 2. A 3. C

Introduction to Sedative-Hypnotics

1. D

Benzodiazepines

1. B 2. B 3. D 4. B 5. B

Chloral Hydrate

1. C 2. A 3. A 4. B 5. D

Ethchlorvynol

1. A 2. B 3. C

Meprobamate

1. D 2. E

Zolpidem

1. A

SELECTED READINGS

Introduction to Cyclic Antidepressant Drugs

1. De Jonghe F, Swinkels JA. The safety of antidepressants. Drugs 1992; 43(suppl. 2):40–47.
2. Rudorfer MW, Manji HE, Potter WZ. Comparative tolerability profiles of the newer versus older antidepressants. Drug Saf 1994;10:18–42.
3. Seeman P, Van Tol HHM. Dopamine receptor pharmacology. Trends Pharm Sci 1994;15:264–270.

Cyclic Antidepressants

1. Dziukas LJ, Vohra J. Tricyclic antidepressant poisoning. Med J Aust 1991; 154:344–350.
2. Frommer DA, Kulig KW, Marx JA, Rumack B. Tricyclic antidepressant overdose: A review. JAMA 1987;257:521–526.
3. Newton EH, Shih RD, Hoffman RS. Cyclic antidepressant overdose: A review of current management strategies. Am J Emerg Med 1994;12:376–379.

Clomipramine

1. Clomipramine approved for severe obsessive compulsive disorder: From the FDA. JAMA 1990;263:1896.
2. Clomipramine for obsessive compulsive disorder. Med Lett Drugs Ther 1988; 30(778):102–4.
3. James WA, Lippmann SB. Clomipramine for obsessive-compulsive disorder: Prescribing guidelines. South Med J 1991;84:1242–1245.
4. Peters MD, Davis SK, Austin LS. Clomipramine: An antiobsessional tricyclic antidepressant. Clin Pharmacol 1990;9:165–178.

Venlafaxine

1. Fantasky A, Burkhart KK. A case report of venlafaxin toxicity. Clin Toxicol 1995;33:359–61.
2. Venlafaxine: A new antidepressant. Med Lett Drugs Ther 1994;36(929):49–51.

Monoamine Oxidase Inhibitors

1. Cooper AJ, O'Reilly RL. Update on the monoamine oxidase inhibitors (MAOIs). J New Dev Clin Med 1991;9:35–54.
2. Reynolds JEF, ed. Martindale: The Extra Pharmacopoeia. 30th ed. London: Pharmaceutical Press, 1993:849–850.

Neuroleptic Drugs

1. Allan MD, Greenblatt DJ, Noel BJ: Overdosage with antipsychotic agents. Am J Psychiatry 1980;137:234–236.
2. Barry D, Meyskens FL, Becker CE: Phenothiazine poisoning. A review of 48 cases. Calif Med J 1973;118:1–5.
3. Benowitz N, Rosenberg J, Becker CE: Clinical management of specific types of drug overdoses. Med Clin North Am 1979;63:276–296.
4. Casey DE. Tardive dyskinesia. West J Med 1990;153:535–541.
5. Epperly TD, McGlaughlin VG, Leok VA. Hazardous side effects of neuroleptics: Diagnosis and treatment. Geriatrics 1990;45:58–62.
6. Malprotra AK, Litman RE, Pickar D. Adverse effects of antipsychotic drugs. Drug Saf 1993;9:429–436.
7. McGuigan MA: Phenothiazines. Clin Toxicol Rev 1981;3(4):1.

Neuroleptic Malignant Syndrome

1. Bond WS. Detection and management of the neuroleptic malignant syndrome. Clin Pharm 1984;3:302–307.
2. Gelenberg AJ. Major complications of neuroleptic drug use. West J Med 1994; 160:55–56.
3. Guze BH, Baxter LR Jr: Neuroleptic malignant syndrome. N Engl J Med 1985; 313:163–166.

Clozapine

1. Beal M. Clozapine update. West J Med 1994;160:53–54.
2. Levinson B. Clozapine (Leponex) overdosage. South Afr Med J 1975;49:5.
3. Wolf LR, Otten EJ. A case report of clozapine overdose. Vet Hum Toxicol 1991;33:370.

Haloperidol

1. Dollery C, ed. Therapeutic Drugs. Edinburgh: Churchill Livingstone, 1991: H1–H4.
2. Yoshida I, Sakaguchi Y, Matsuishi T, et al. Acute accidental overdosage of haloperidol in children. Acta Paediatr 1993;82:855–880.

Thioridazine

1. Le Blaye I, Donatini B, Hall M, Krupp P. Acute overdosage with thioridazine: A review of the available clinical exposure. Vet Hum Toxicol 1993;35:147–150.

Introduction to Sedative-Hypnotics

1. Glauser FL, Smith R. Physiologic and biochemical abnormalities in self induced overdosage. Arch Intern Med 1975;135:1468–1473.
2. Jay SJ, Johanson WG Jr, Pierce AK. Respiratory complications of overdose with sedative drugs. Am Rev Respir Dis 1975;112:591–598.
3. Khantzian EJ, McKenna GJ. Acute toxic and withdrawal reactions associated with drug use and abuse. Ann Intern Med 1979;80:361–372.

Benzodiazepines

1. Busto U, Sellers EM, Naranjo CA, et al. Withdrawal reaction after long-term therapeutic use of benzodiazepines. N Engl J Med 1986;315:854–859.
2. Landry MJ, Smith DE, McDuff DR, Baughman OL III. Benzodiazepine dependence and withdrawal: Identification and medical management. J Am Board Fam Pract 1992;5:167–176.
3. O'Dowd JJ. Fatal triazolam poisoning. Br Med J 1988;297:1048.
4. Roy-Byrne PP. Benzodiazepine dependence. J Am Board Fam Pract 1992;5:245–247. Editorial.
5. Wiley J, Wiley C. Benzodiazepine ingestions in children. Clin Toxicol 1995; 33:475–486.

Flumazenil

1. Benzodiazepine antagonist approved by FDA. Clin Pharm 1992;1:287–288. Editorial.
2. Burr W, Sandham P. Death after flumazenil. Br Med J 1989;298:1713.
3. Galletly DC, Ure R, Turley A. Flumazenil: A twelve-month survey on use in a New Zealand public hospital. Anaesth Intens Care 1990;18:229–233.
4. La Fleche RF. Flumazenil. Clin Toxicol Rev 1990;12(5):1–2.
5. Votey SR. Flumazenil: A new benzodiazepine antagonist. Ann Emerg Med 1991;70:181–8.

Chloral Hydrate

1. Graham SR, Day RO, Lee R, Fulder GWO. Overdose with chloral hydrate: A pharmacological and therapeutic review. Med J Aust 1988;149:668–688.

Ethchlorvynol

1. Yell RP. Ethchlorvynol overdose. Am J Emerg Med 1990;8:246–250.

Zolpidem

1. Garnier R, Guerault E, Muzard D, et al. Acute zolpidem poisoning: Analysis of 344 cases. Clin Toxicol 1994;32:391–404.

CHAPTER 29
Endocrine Toxicology

DIABETIC DRUGS

INSULIN

Although exogenous hyperinsulinism frequently occurs after accidental injection, it may occur after surreptitious self-injection and occult malicious or factitious administration. Unfortunately, many cases of insulin overdosage are self-inflicted, often by depressed individuals intent on suicide. The incidence of hypoglycemia resulting from insulin overdose may be more common than is generally appreciated and reported cases probably are only a fraction of the number of suicide attempts actually occurring. Some cases of insulin overdose may be unrecognized in the absence of severe hypoglycemia, or they may be considered as accidental hypoglycemic episodes in patients with unstable diabetes.

Insulin is a hormone. It is a protein secreted by the β cells of the pancreatic islets of Langerhans and is composed of two chains of amino acids connected by disulfide linkages. Commercially, insulin may be produced from pork or beef pancreas or by recombinant DNA techniques. Insulin resistance has become rare, insulin antibodies have been reduced, and insulin allergy is no longer reported. Even after purification steps are taken, preparations still may contain various contaminants. Metabolic control has not been appreciably altered with the production of newer insulin products. Human insulin, which has been developed using recombinant DNA techniques, differs from porcine insulin in one amino acid and is metabolized the same way in man.

Insulins commercially available are used mostly to treat patients with insulin-dependent (type 1) diabetes mellitus. They also are used to treat adult-onset diabetics (AODM) (or non-insulin–dependent diabetes mellitus [NIDDM]), if weight reduction does not control blood sugar adequately. Both types of diabetics may require additional insulin when faced with surgery, fever, trauma, infections, renal or hepatic dysfunction, hyperthyroidism, Raynaud's disease, pregnancy, and hyperkalemia. All insulins are administered subcutaneously for usual diabetic care, but regular insulin can be given intravenously for severe diabetic ketoacidosis and coma.

Pathophysiology

Insulin stimulates carbohydrate metabolism in skeletal muscle, cardiac muscle, and adipose tissue by facilitating transport of glucose into cells. Nerve cells, erythrocytes, and cells of the intestines, liver, and kidney do not need insulin for transfer of glucose. In the liver, insulin aids in the phosphorylation of glucose to glucose-6-phosphate, which then is converted to glycogen. Insulin stimulates lipogenesis and inhibits lipolysis and free fatty acid release from adipose cells. Insulin also stimulates protein synthesis. Somatotropin, epinephrine, adrenocortical hormones, thyroid hormones, and estrogens antagonize insulin action.

Pharmacokinetics

ABSORPTION

- Insulin is absorbed rapidly from the subcutaneous (SC) site.

DISTRIBUTION

- Insulin is distributed throughout the extracellular fluids.
- Insulin preparations differ in onset, peak, and duration after SC administration.

ELIMINATION

- Insulin is metabolized 50% in the liver. It then undergoes a reduction cleavage of the two intrachain disulfide bonds by glutathione with the enzyme glutathione-insulin-transhydrogenase.
- The half-life of regular insulin administered intravenously is 20 minutes. If administered by the SC or intramuscular (IM) route, it is 2 hours.
- Insulin is reabsorbed in the proximal tubules (98%). Less than 2% is excreted unchanged.
- 60% is returned to the venous blood, and 50% to 60% is metabolized.

Clinical Presentations

Hypoglycemia symptoms depend in part on the rate at which the blood glucose falls. In acute hypoglycemia, initial symptoms are from excess adrenergic activity (tremulousness, anxiety, diaphoresis, and palpitations). This is followed by cerebral dysfunction (alterations in behavior, irritability, clouding of consciousness, and coma). Seizures occur in 10% to 20% of adults, and more frequently in children. Features of decortication or decerebration, focal abnormalities, or irreversible coma may supervene.

The skin may be cold, clammy, and pale, with profuse sweating. There may be an elevation of temperature or hypothermia. Flushing may occur and breathing may be deep and heavy, with periods of apnea. Pulmonary edema and aspiration pneumonitis have been observed. Tachycardia and palpitations from adrenergic stimulation may occur.

HYPOGLYCEMIA

The typical patient with an insulin overdose often is found in an unconscious state. Patients with intermediate or extended insulin overdosage may not develop signs and symptoms of hypoglycemia for 18 to 38 hours. With longer-acting insulin, in the first 24 hours there is a compensatory mechanism to maintain normoglycemia as glycogen stores are mobilized. When glycogen stores are exhausted, hypoglycemia becomes severe and may lead to irreversible brain and myocardial damage.

Prolonged hypoglycemia may result in behavioral disturbances, seizures, coma, and death. Serious sequelae often are related to the duration of hypoglycemia. Focal neurologic deficits may occur as a result of hypoglycemia. The duration of hypoglycemic encephalopathy, rather than quantity of insulin injected determines the severity of posthypoglycemic encephalopathy.

Hypoglycemia may develop much later than predicted for the conventional duration of action of various insulin preparations. Nondiabetics are more likely to present with decreased blood sugar and develop recurrent hypoglycemia. After insulin, the blood sugar may continue to decrease despite large, repeated doses of glucose. The most prolonged hypoglycemias occur with delayed-action insulins and with larger doses. A rapid decline from hyperglycemic to normal blood sugar levels may produce symptoms. Severe hypoglycemia may be mistaken for intracerebral disorders.

NEUROLOGIC EFFECTS

The patient may present with headaches, hysterical behavior, or depression. Drowsiness, confused behavior, violence, and restlessness may be present even after blood sugar is brought to above-normal levels with glucose therapy. The gag reflex may be absent. The patient may have no deep tendon reflex response, may have a normal response, or may be hyperreflexic. Extensor spasms may be observed. Extensor plantar reflexes may be present. After recovery, patients may be amnesic, withdrawn, and confused for an extended period.

Seizures and encephalopathy may occur and focal deficits mimicking strokes and other focal conditions may be observed. Pupils may show no reaction to light, or may be dilated. External ocular movement may be sluggish with dysconjugate gaze. Painful cramps, spasms, and twitching may be noted in the leg and other skeletal muscles.

Toxic Dosage/Death

Long-acting insulins often are used in self-poisoning. Mortality in attempted suicidal overdose with insulin has been estimated at 25%. Patients who attempt suicide with insulin may repeat the attempt using the same method. There is little correlation between insulin dose and the severity of hypoglycemia.

Clinical clues to intentional insulin overdose include a history of depression, hypoglycemia unresponsive or minimally responsive to concentrated glucose infusions, significantly elevated plasma insulin levels, low or normal C-peptide levels (with elevated insulin levels), positive insulin antibody assays (unless human insulin is abused), and erythematous injection sites.

Drug Interactions

The hypoglycemic action of insulin appears to be increased by fasting, alcohol, barbiturates, and possibly salicylates and benzodiazepines. It is decreased by epinephrine, glucagon, thyroxine, estrogens, adrenocortical hormones, and somatotropin.

Pregnancy/Lactation

Insulin requirements may increase in pregnancy. Insulin may concentrate in the placenta. No systematic studies are available in relation to its concentration in breast milk.

Laboratory

ANALYTIC METHODS

Insulin assays and fractionation (free and bound) tests are available, but their usefulness in an acute hypoglycemic episode is limited.

BLOOD LEVELS

C-peptide and insulin are secreted from the β cells of the pancreas in equimolar concentration. Exogenous insulin administration now can be more easily diagnosed by the simultaneous demonstration of low concentrations of blood glucose, high concentrations of immunoreactive insulin, and suppressed C-peptide immunoreactivity. This triad can distinguish such patients from those with insulinoma (hyperinsulinism from an islet cell insulin-producing tumor), in whom high blood levels of both immunoreactive insulin and C-peptide immunoreactivity accompany a hypoglycemic episode. Insulin levels are not correlated with severity of hypoglycemia.

Treatment

GUT DECONTAMINATION

These methods are irrelevant as insulin is given via SC or intravenous (IV) routes.

ELIMINATION ENHANCEMENT

There are no substantive studies available to support the use of extracorporeal procedures to remove insulin. Hemodialysis does not affect the elimination rate of insulin.

SUPPORTIVE MEASURES

- Airway, breathing, and circulation must be established quickly. Where required, endotracheal intubation and assisted mechanical ventilation should be instituted immediately.
- The mainstay of therapy is utilization of IV glucose (D50) to counteract the morbidity of hypoglycemia. See Antidotes section, below. Frequent monitoring of serum glucose is essential. Oral glucose cannot be relied on to maintain euglycemia.
- Potassium levels usually are within normal limits, but may be depressed. Potassium supplements may be useful for clinically important hypokalemia.
- Psychiatric follow-up is important in the care of the suicidal patient. Repeat attempts are not uncommon. The patient

should not be discharged until there is reasonable assurance the original act will not be repeated.

- Leukocytosis is observed frequently. Blood urea nitrogen, sodium, and bicarbonate levels usually are normal.
- Immunoreactive insulin levels and C-peptide immunoreactivity levels may aid in the differential diagnosis of a patient with hypoglycemia as a result of insulin administration from an insulinoma.
- Sinus tachycardia, occasional premature ventricular beats, and elevated ST segments may be seen on electrocardiogram. Frequently, the electrocardiogram is normal.

Antidotes

GLUCOSE

The comatose adult patient should be given an IV bolus of 50 mL 50% dextrose on admission with little delay. In an undiagnosed coma, naloxone and thiamine also should be given on admission. This should be followed immediately by continuous glucose infusion of 5% to 10% dextrose in water (D5W or D10W) sufficient to maintain slight hyperglycemia. Glucose administration may be required for over 5 days before the effect of insulin dosage is overcome (as demonstrated by a glucose concentration greater than 100 mg/dL on two successive occasions).

GLUCAGON

Glucagon, 1 to 2 mg IM, has a fast onset of action and mobilizes hepatic glycogen stores. However, once hepatic glycogen stores are exhausted (prolonged hypoglycemia, fasting, alcohol abuse), the effect may be variable or nil.

Questions—Insulin

1. **Which of the following is false?**
   A. Although exogenous hyperinsulinism frequently occurs after accidental injection, it may occur after surreptitious self-injection and occult malicious or factitious administration.
   B. Many cases of insulin overdosage are self-inflicted, often by depressed, suicidal individuals.
   C. Insulin overdose is easily distinguished clinically from idiopathic hypoglycemia.
   D. Insulin may be produced from pork or beef pancreas or by recombinant DNA techniques.
   E. All insulins are administered subcutaneously for usual diabetic care, but regular insulin can be given intravenously for severe diabetic ketoacidosis and coma.

2. **Insulin is a hormone secreted by the α cells of the pancreatic islets of Langerhans and is composed of two chains of amino acids connected by disulfide linkages.**
   A. True
   B. False

3. **Insulin stimulates carbohydrate metabolism in the following tissue(s) by facilitating transport of glucose into cells.**
   A. Skeletal muscle
   B. Cardiac muscle
   C. Adipose tissue
   D. All of the above
   E. A and B

4. **Signs of hypoglycemia include all of the following, except**
   A. Encephalopathy
   B. Cool, clammy skin
   C. Seizures
   D. Focal neurologic deficits
   E. Maculopapular rash

5. **Exogenous insulin administration can be diagnosed by the simultaneous demonstration of low concentrations of blood glucose, high concentrations of immunoreactive insulin, and suppressed C-peptide immunoreactivity.**
   A. True
   B. False

ORAL HYPOGLYCEMIC AGENTS

Sulfonylureas

Non-insulin–dependent diabetes mellitus, also known as AODM, accounts for 75% to 85% of patients affected with diabetes mellitus. The maintenance of good blood-glucose control aids in preventing retinopathy, nephropathy, neuropathy, and premature atherosclerosis in both insulin-dependent diabetes mellitus and NIDDM. Dietary control, weight loss, and oral hypoglycemic agents are utilized frequently in treating adult-onset diabetics.

In the mid-1960s, oral hypoglycemic agents such as tolbutamide, acetohexamide, tolazamide, and chlorpropamide were used widely. Control of dosage was difficult and overdoses were reported frequently. Dosage manipulation often led to hypoglycemia. Second-generation sulfonylureas, glyburide and glipizide, ultimately were developed. These agents are more potent than prior sulfonylureas and are associated with an increased risk of hypoglycemia.

Overdosage from oral hypoglycemic drugs and insulin in both diabetics and nondiabetics probably occurs more frequently than reported, because poison centers may not be contacted after an overdose. The hypoglycemic patient in coma may resemble patients with cerebrovascular accidents, uremia, or trauma and may, indeed, have these other diagnoses.

PATHOPHYSIOLOGY

Sulfonylureas are thought to act by a number of different mechanisms. They produce a depolarization of the pancreatic islet β cell membrane mediated by enhancement of calcium flux and cell membrane potassium ion permeability. This results in release of preformed insulin into the circulation and occurs mostly in non-insulin–dependent diabetics. Sulfonylureas may reduce basal glucose output from the liver and may increase insulin receptor binding.

Pancreatic effects are more preponderant in the acute use of sulfonylureas and depend on the presence of functioning pancreatic β cells for their effect. In chronic doses or overdose, sulfonylureas may have pronounced effects outside the pancreas, including potentiation of the effects of insulin on the liver, inhibition of hepatic gluconeogenesis in response to glucagon, stimulation of glucose uptake by muscle, and possibly an effect on insulin disposal. Indirectly, sulfonylureas may increase insulin secretion by suppressing the release of glucagon and somatostatin from α and δ pancreatic cells.

Answers to questions in shaded boxes appear at the end of the chapter.

PHARMACOKINETICS

Absorption

- Sulfonylureas are absorbed rapidly from the gastrointestinal tract.

Distribution

- Sulfonylureas are highly protein-bound.

Elimination

- Wide variation exists among the sulfonylureas in hepatic metabolism and renal clearance, factors that tend to alter the steady-state serum levels.
- Metabolites may be active, so there may be a variation between the plasma half-life of the parent drug and the degree of hypoglycemia encountered.

CLINICAL PRESENTATIONS

Coma or altered mental status generally is the most important presenting sign in the majority of patients who have ingested excessive doses of the sulfonylureas. The comatose state may be unresponsive to glucose or glucagon for many hours. Blood sugars may rise to normal or above-normal levels while the patient is still comatose. Conversely, consciousness may be associated with severe hypoglycemic levels.

Severe accidental hypoglycemia in diabetic patients may be affected by age (more in old patients), impaired renal function, impaired hepatic function, reduced food intake, weight reduction (reduces insulin resistance), drug interactions, and inadvertent errors in medication dispensed. Unpredictable adverse effects are numerous. Apnea, acute pulmonary edema, and dyspnea have been observed. Hypotension, tachycardia, and/or cardiac arrest may occur.

Neurologic Effects

The patient may be combative, trembling, or exhibit fatigue, confusion, slurring of speech, and loss of concentration. Irritability, delirium, and fainting may supervene. Neurological defects may simulate a stroke in the elderly patient. Dysarthria, monoplegia, hemiplegia, ataxia, athetoid movements, flaccidity, absence of deep-tendon reflexes, bilateral ankle clonus, and bilateral Babinski reflexes often are observed. Pupils may be normal, or fixed and dilated. They may react sluggishly to light. Diabetes insipidus, cranial nerve III palsy, motor aphasia, hemiparesis, and diminished visual acuity may be present. Seizures with or without alterations in consciousness may occur. Opisthotonos, decerebrate posturing, and death have been reported.

Dermatologic Effects

The skin may be hot and diaphoretic. Sensitivity responses rarely may include pruritic rash, urticaria, acute toxic erythema, erythema multiforme, Stevens-Johnson syndrome, and exfoliative dermatitis.

Gastrointestinal Effects

The patient may have poor appetite, history of limited food intake, nausea, vomiting, abdominal pain, and/or dyspepsia. Jaundice secondary to cholestasis may occur and recedes upon removal of the drug.

Renal Effects

Patients with prior renal disease may present with proteinuria, hyaline or granular casts in the urine, oliguria, or anuria. Dilutional hyponatremia and water intoxication resulting from inappropriate antidiuretic hormone secretion is observed with chlorpropamide and tolbutamide.

Hematologic Effects

Aplastic anemia, agranulocytosis, pancytopenia, leukopenia, and thrombocytopenia have been described. In overdose, a leukocytosis may be observed.

Disulfiramlike Effects

The ingestion of alcohol during chlorpropamide therapy has been associated with flushing. Nausea, giddiness, tachycardia, conjunctival injection, headache, and a feeling of breathlessness seen minutes after alcohol ingestion have been seen. Symptoms reach maximum intensity in 20 minutes and last one hour. Flushing also occurs rarely with tolbutamide. The reaction may be dose-dependent and has been associated with the second-generation sulfonylureas glipizide and glyburide.

TOXIC DOSAGE/DEATH

Prolonged hypoglycemic reactions may be observed after relatively low doses of sulfonylureas in patients with defective metabolism or excretion of the sulfonylureas, with decreased glycogen storage, or in conditions of prolonged and excessive insulin secretion. These conditions may be exacerbated by (1) liver damage, which may predispose to both diminished glycogen storage and slow metabolic inactivation of drugs; (2) renal damage, in which impaired sulfonylurea excretion may become critical; (3) insulinomas; (4) other drug intake (salicylates, alcohol); (5) diarrhea; (6) prior strokes; and (7) prior cardiac disorders. It is not uncommon for patients who have been maintained on a set dose for months to develop hypoglycemic symptoms requiring hospitalization.

DRUG INTERACTIONS

The binding sites on albumin for glyburide and glipizide are different from those of the first-generation agents. Therefore, displacement by coumarins, or heparin, is less likely. Alcohol interactions, as described above, may resemble those that occur following disulfiram, but they are not as common with second-generation sulfonylureas. Salicylates, sulfonamides, monoamine oxidase inhibitors, and clofibrate may exacerbate hypoglycemia.

PREGNANCY/LACTATION

Severe hypoglycemia in the newborn may develop in the first days after delivery. Sulfonylureas cross the placenta and stimulate insulin release from the fetal pancreas, however hypoglycemia develops only after delivery, when the ability of maternal glucose to cross the placenta and ameliorate such hypoglycemia is halted by birth.

LABORATORY

Analytic Methods

Plasma assays of the oral hypoglycemic agents now are available, generally with high-performance liquid chromatography, but they are clinically useful only to confirm the history of ingestion. Availability of these assays in many hospitals is limited.

Blood Levels

Management of an overdose does not rely on blood levels of the offending agent, and the clinical state is not correlated closely with such levels. Frequent measurements of blood sugar levels are important. Reliance on clinical appearance and alertness alone may not reflect the seriousness of the hypoglycemia simultaneously present. Serious hypoglycemia (blood sugar below 40 mg/dL) may be present in an asymptomatic individual and coma may be present with a normal blood sugar.

TREATMENT

Gut Decontamination

Gastric lavage and charcoal administration may be helpful within 4 hours. Airway protection is of vital importance in the obtunded or convulsing individual

Elimination Enhancement

The sulfonylureas are highly protein bound. Experience with extracorporeal removal has been limited and ineffective. There are no substantive data on the use of charcoal hemoperfusion, hemodialysis, exchange transfusion, plasmapheresis, or forced diuresis in the management of oral hypoglycemic overdosage.

Supportive Measures

- The hypoglycemic patient in coma known to have overdosed on an oral hypoglycemic agent must be subjected to the same clinical and laboratory examinations as the patient who arrives in coma from any undetermined source. Naloxone and thiamine, in addition to glucose, should be given to the comatose patient.
- Respirations must be assessed and artificially established as necessary. Endotracheal intubation, or an oropharyngeal airway may be required.
- Immediate use of IV glucose is paramount, because delay may expose the patient to unnecessary brain damage. The patient must be admitted to the hospital and monitored for at least 24 hours.
- Sodium bicarbonate, used to alkalinize the urine, appears to reduce the half-life of chlorpropamide from about 49 to about 13 hours. Use of alkalinization procedures with other sulfonylureas remains to be established.
- Monitoring of blood glucose concentrations, arterial blood gases, electrolytes, and liver and kidney function tests should be performed at frequent intervals depending on clinical status. Arterial blood gases and serum potassium levels may reflect a hypokalemic metabolic acidosis. A complete blood count may reveal moderate leukocytosis.
- Toxic screens may identify concomitant co-ingestants such as aspirin or alcohol, which may complicate the clinical presentation.
- There is little correlation between the amount of drug allegedly ingested and the depth of hypoglycemia or length of coma experienced.
- Hypotension is managed by Trendelenburg position, fluids, and pressors as required.
- Seizures may be treated with diazepam intravenously. Phenytoin may be used as required.
- The electrocardiogram may be normal, reflect prior cardiac problems, or exhibit sinus tachycardia, T-wave inversion, or changes reflecting low cellular potassium levels. Atrial dysrhythmias and ST elevations may occur.

ANTIDOTES

Glucose

Give 50 mL of 50% glucose in adults as an IV bolus immediately after withdrawing blood for analysis. At the same time, start an IV infusion of 10% glucose in water. Such infusions may require a central venous line for long-term (24 to 48 hours) use. Frequent blood glucose determinations are required even after the patient has regained consciousness, because the onset of symptoms may be delayed for over 12 hours.

Glucagon

Glucagon may aid in producing an increase in the blood sugar. Glucagon induces an increase in blood sugar and ketones, both of which are utilizable energy substrates for the central nervous system. Doses of 1 to 2 mg, IM, SC, or IV may be useful in raising blood sugar level. Glucagon efficacy requires the presence of adequate glucose stores often absent in an alcoholic. It may induce nausea and vomiting.

Diazoxide

Diazoxide is a direct inhibitor of insulin secretion. It also increases hepatic glucose output and decreases cellular glucose uptake. Oral diazoxide has been approved for hypoglycemia as a result of hyperinsulinism associated with inoperable islet cell tumors or extrapancreatic malignancy in adults.

Octreotide

Octreotide (50 mg every 12 hours, subcutaneously) may be useful in sulfonylurea overdose. It suppresses plasma insulin and C-peptide levels permitting normal plasma glucose concentrations without additional dextrose support.

Questions—Sulfonylureas

1. Which of the following is false?

A. Non-insulin–dependent diabetes mellitus (NIDDM), also known as juvenile-onset diabetes accounts for most patients affected with diabetes mellitus.
B. The maintenance of good blood glucose control aids in preventing retinopathy, nephropathy, neuropathy, and atherosclerosis in both insulin-dependent and non-insulin-dependent diabetes.
C. Dietary control, weight loss, and oral hypoglycemic agents are utilized in treating NIDDM.
D. Overdosage from oral hypoglycemic drugs and insulin probably occurs more frequently than reported, because poison centers may not be contacted after an overdose.
E. The hypoglycemic patient in coma may resemble patients with cerebrovascular accidents, uremia, or trauma and may, indeed, have these other diagnoses.

2. Sulfonylureas may reduce basal-glucose output from the liver and may increase insulin receptor binding.

A. True
B. False

3. Which of the following is false?

A. Octreotide (50 mg every 12 hours, subcutaneously) may be useful in sulfonylurea overdose.
B. The sulfonylureas are minimally protein-bound and treatment of overdose with hemodialysis has been effective.
C. Sulfonylureas cross the placenta and stimulate insulin release from the fetal pancreas, however hypoglycemia develops only after delivery, when the ability of maternal glucose to cross the placenta and ameliorate such hypoglycemia is halted by birth.
D. Salicylates and clofibrate may exacerbate hypoglycemia caused by sulfonylureas.
E. The ingestion of alcohol during chlorpropamide therapy has been associated with flushing.

4. Signs of sulfonylurea overdose include all of the following, except

A. The patient may be combative, trembling, or exhibit fatigue, confusion, slurring of speech, and loss of concentration.

B. Dysarthria, monoplegia, hemiplegia, ataxia, athetoid movements, flaccidity, absence of deep tendon reflexes, bilateral ankle clonus, and bilateral Babinski reflexes often are observed.
C. Pupils may be normal, or fixed and dilated. They may react sluggishly to light.
D. Seizures with or without alterations in consciousness may occur.
E. Pruritus, arthropathy, and sinus congestion may be seen.

5. In chronic doses or overdose, sulfonylureas may have pronounced effects outside the pancreas, including potentiation of the effects of insulin on the liver, inhibition of hepatic gluconeogenesis in response to glucagon, and stimulation of glucose uptake by muscle.
A. True
B. False

Biguanides

Biguanides represent another class of oral hypoglycemics. Phenformin, the first biguanide introduced, induced serious lactic acidosis that was often fatal (25%), and was subsequently removed from the United States market in 1977. Phenformin still is available in Europe. Metformin, a chemical relative, is available as an oral hypoglycemic alternative to the sulfonylureas.

Metformin (dimethylbiguanide) is an antihyperglycemic drug which has been used to treat NIDDM. It acts in the presence of insulin to increase glucose utilization and reduce glucose production, thereby countering insulin resistance. Metformin also is used as a lipid-lowering agent and in the treatment of obesity in patients with NIDDM.

PATHOPHYSIOLOGY

The biguanides exert their pharmacological effects by a similar basic mechanism. They induce an increase in peripheral glucose utilization, a decrease in hepatic gluconeogenesis, and a decrease in intestinal absorption of glucose, vitamin B12 and bile acids. The biguanides usually do not lower the blood sugar in a normal individual unless ethanol or another hypoglycemic agent is ingested simultaneously, or there is severe hepatic insufficiency.

PHARMACOKINETICS

Absorption

- Oral bioavailability of metformin is 50% to 60%. Absorption of metformin occurs within 6 hours.
- Phenformin is approximately 50% absorbed from the gastrointestinal tract.

Distribution

- Metformin is negligibly bound to plasma proteins. Phenformin is less than 20% protein-bound.
- The apparent volume of distribution of metformin ranges from 63 to 276 L/kg.
- Phenformin is distributed throughout the major organs.

Elimination

- The plasma elimination half-life of metformin ranges from 1.5 to 1.8 hours. It is prolonged in patients with renal impairment and is correlated with creatinine clearance.
- Phenformin is metabolized by hydroxylation in the liver, possibly governed by genetic influences.
- Phenformin is excreted 66% unchanged and about 33% as its metabolite. Its half-life in plasma is 7 to 15 hours.
- Metformin, unlike phenformin, is not metabolized but is excreted largely in unchanged form. Metformin is eliminated rapidly by renal excretion. More than 80% is excreted unchanged.

CLINICAL PRESENTATIONS

Nausea, vomiting, diarrhea, abdominal cramps, anorexia, weight loss, epigastric discomfort and pain, and hematemesis have been seen in patients with phenformin poisoning. Agitation, confusion, lethargy, seizures, extensor plantar reflexes, coma, and death have also been described. Absent corneal reflexes and fixed, dilated pupils have been observed.

Cardiovascular Effects

The patient may have rapid, deep respiratory efforts. Pulmonary hypertension has been observed after phenformin use. Tachycardia, hypotension, and myocardial infarction have been seen. Rare leukocytoclastic vasculitis has been induced by metformin.

Metabolic Effects

Lactic acidosis has been produced by all biguanides, however the incidence is by far the greatest after phenformin use. The estimated incidence of metformin-related lactic acidosis is about 1/10th to 1/20th that reported with phenformin, or 0.03 case per 1,000 patient-years. Impaired renal function is the predominant condition associated with the development of lactic acidosis. Diagnosis of lactic acidosis is made by excluding other causes of metabolic acidosis.

Laboratory findings include an anion gap metabolic acidosis, low serum bicarbonate and pH, elevated serum potassium, normal or depressed serum chloride, and an increased blood lactate and lactate/pyruvate ratio. Diabetic ketoacidosis, uremic acidosis, and drug ingestions (salicylates, paraldehyde, methanol, ethanol, ethylene glycol, and isoniazid) also may cause metabolic acidosis with a high anion gap. Biguanide-induced lactic acidosis has a serious mortality rate.

TOXIC DOSAGE/DEATH

Death from biguanide use typically is secondary to lactic acidosis. Morbidity is enhanced in older individuals, individuals with renal failure, and in those with concomitant medical problems. Death may occur even after serum bicarbonate and pH levels have been corrected, if the serum lactate level is still elevated. Overdoses of metformin (7 and 20 grams) have induced lactic acidosis. One patient recovered from a metformin overdose of 25 grams.

DRUG INTERACTIONS

Prior or concomitant ethanol intake with phenformin appears to predispose to the development of lactic acidosis. Alcohol potentiates the antihyperglycemic and hyperlactatemic effects of metformin. Cationic drugs such as amiloride, digoxin, morphine, procainamide, quinidine, quinine, ranitidine, triamterene, trimethoprim, and vancomycin, that are eliminated by renal tubular secretion, theoretically have the potential to interact with metformin by competing for common renal tubular transport systems. Drugs that produce hyperglycemia and may lead to loss of glycemic control include oral contraceptives, phenytoin, nicotinic acid, sympathomimetics, calcium-channel blocking drugs, and isoniazid.

PREGNANCY/LACTATION

Metformin is categorized as pregnancy risk category B. Insulin is considered the agent of choice during pregnancy to control gestational diabetes.

LABORATORY

Analytic Methods
Gas-liquid chromatography, high-pressure liquid chromatography, and gas chromatography–mass spectrometry are highly specific and sensitive.

Blood Levels
Blood levels of biguanides are not correlated closely with clinical symptoms of overdose. Lactic acidosis may develop without high serum phenformin levels. The plasma concentration of metformin is 1 to 2 μg/mL, 1 to 2 hours after an oral dose of 500 to 1,000 mg. Monitoring has little clinical value. There is no correlation between plasma lactate concentration and plasma metformin concentration at therapeutic drug levels.

TREATMENT

Gut Decontamination
Emesis induction with syrup of ipecac is not indicated because of biguanide-induced gastric mucosal irritation and lack of proven efficacy. Gastric lavage, activated charcoal, and cathartics may be useful but have not been systematically studied.

Elimination Enhancement
Forcing fluids may be counterproductive and result in fluid overload. Hemodialysis has been used to treat biguanide-induced lactic acidosis. Hemodialysis, in addition to rapidly removing biguanide and excess lactate, permits sodium bicarbonate to be given without risking fluid overload or hypernatremia. The use of hemoperfusion has not been evaluated in the treatment of biguanide-induced lactic acidosis.

Supportive Measures
- An airway must be established and assisted ventilation initiated with positive-end expiratory pressure if required after endotracheal intubation. Blood pressure must be monitored carefully.
- Arterial blood gases and electrolyte levels may reflect a high-anion–gap metabolic acidosis. Severe acidosis may be treated with IV sodium bicarbonate (1 to 2 mEq/kg) and repeated every 15 minutes as required. Monitoring of arterial blood gases, serum electrolytes, and the electrocardiogram (ECG) is important when administering bicarbonate. Serum potassium levels and the ECG may reflect a tendency to hypokalemia as the alkalinization process is instituted.
- Placing the patient in Trendelenburg position and cautiously using saline treats hypotension. Lactated ringers should be avoided. Dehydration and hypovolemia may require placement of a central venous line. Pressor amines (dopamine, norepinephrine) may increase lactic acid production by producing a relative hypoxemia of the skeletal muscles and should be used cautiously, with blood lactate monitoring.
- Biguanides may induce elevations in the lactate/pyruvate ratio (normally 10:1). Blood-glucose concentrations may be depressed, normal, or elevated. Early reports indicated that phenformin could produce acidosis without warning in adult patients whose blood-glucose concentrations were within normal limits and who had no glycosuria.
- Leukocytosis frequently is observed and thrombocytopenia may be present. Plasma insulin levels usually are not elevated. Renal function tests may reveal elevated creatinine and albuminuria.

ANTIDOTES

Glucose
Hypoglycemia is treated immediately with 50 mL of 50% glucose intravenously in adults or 0.5 g/kg per dose in children.

Questions—Biguanides

1. Which of the following is false?
   A. Metformin acts in the presence of insulin to increase glucose utilization and reduce glucose production, thereby countering insulin resistance.
   B. Phenformin, the first biguanide introduced, induced serious lactic acidosis that often was fatal (25%), and subsequently was removed from the United States market in 1977.
   C. The biguanides exert their pharmacological effects by a similar basic mechanism. They induce a decrease in peripheral glucose utilization, thus increasing the availability of central stores.
   D. Lactic acidosis has been produced by all biguanides, however the incidence is by far the greatest after phenformin use.
   E. Impaired renal function is the predominant condition associated with the development of lactic acidosis during biguanide use.

2. Prior or concomitant ethanol intake with phenformin appears to predispose to the development of lactic acidosis.
   A. True
   B. False

3. Blood levels of biguanides are closely correlated with clinical symptoms of overdose.
   A. True
   B. False

THYROID AND ANTITHYROID DRUGS

Thyroid Hormones

The incidence of severe reactions from thyroid hormone overdose is low. In view of the paucity of clinical reports of serious overdose with thyroid preparations, it can be assumed that a generally benign course follows thyroid overdose. Thyroid hormone overdose has been associated with relatively few symptoms, a mild thyrotoxicosis involving tachycardia, fever, and diarrhea, or rarely, a severe thyrotoxic state resembling thyroid storm. Sudden death with ventricular fibrillation in the absence of coronary artery disease rarely has been reported. Thyroid hormones are used to correct hypothyroid states and to induce clinical euthyroidism.

Thyrotoxicosis resulting from the ingestion of excessive amounts of exogenous thyroid hormone may be seen in patients receiving the medication for treatment of hypothyroidism, goiter, or nodules or in patients who ingest the hormone to reduce weight or because of personality disorders (*thyrotoxicosis factitia*). *Thyrotoxicosis factitia* can be assumed to be present when clinical hyperthyroidism is coupled with elevated levels of serum T4 and T3, depressed thyroid uptake of radioiodine, and a low or undetectable serum level of thyroglobulin in the absence of, or corrected for, the uncommon serum antithyroglobulins.

Pathophysiology

Thyroid hormones affect growth and development by influencing nuclear genome regulation of protein synthesis and growth. Thyroid hormone interacts with growth hormone. It accelerates cellular oxidation, increases energy expenditure, and leads to increased heat production and oxygen consumption. Also affected are the metabolism of lipids, carbohydrates, proteins, vitamins, and inorganic iron. Thyroid hormones potentiate the effects of catecholamines.

T3 and T4 are both metabolically active, but T3 is 3 to 5 times more potent than T4. Multiple mechanisms maintain a relatively euthyroid status in the presence of thyroid hormone overdose. Such control mechanisms include modifications of hormone serum protein binding, the volume of distribution, clearance rate, disposal rate, half-life, peripheral conversion of T4 to T3, and the number and affinity of nuclear receptors.

Pharmacokinetics

ABSORPTION

- All thyroid preparations are absorbed from the stomach in 1 to 2 hours.
- 90% to 95% of T3 and 50% to 80% of T4 is bioavailable after oral administration.

DISTRIBUTION

- T3 and T4 circulate in the blood bound to serum proteins. T3 is bound to thyroid-binding globulin (TBG), 45% to 50%; thyroid-binding prealbumin (TBPA), 1%; and albumin, 45% to 50%.
- T4 is 70% to 80% bound to thyroid binding globulin. The free hormone produces desired clinical effects. Free T4/free T3 exists in a 10:1 ratio.
- 80% to 90% of serum T3 is formed by monodeiodination of T4 in peripheral tissues within 2 to 3 days.
- Approximately 30% to 40% of T4 is converted to T3 in the peripheral tissues within 2 to 3 days.
- If initial blood levels of T4 are elevated and the patient is asymptomatic, clinical symptoms may ensue within 7 to 10 days, as T4 is converted to T3.

ELIMINATION

- T4 is eliminated 75% to 80% by deiodination. Deiodination occurs in the liver, kidney, muscle, brain, and heart. About 40% of T4 are converted to T3 within 3 days.
- 15% to 25% of T4 is conjugated with glucuronic acid in the liver and excreted in the bile; some undergoes enterohepatic recirculation. 10% to 15% is excreted in the stool and 5% to 10% in the kidney.
- The elimination of T4 decreases if protein binding is elevated (e.g., pregnancy) and increases if protein binding is decreased (e.g., nephritis, hepatic cirrhosis) or inhibited (e.g., salicylates, dicumarol).
- T3 is eliminated 75% to 80% by deiodination as well.
- Conjugation of T3 takes place in the kidney by self-conjugation. A small amount of absorbed T3 is conjugated to glucuronic acid in the liver and excreted in the bile. It also may undergo enterohepatic recirculation.

Clinical Presentations

In mild to moderate thyroid intoxications, excessive heat production, increased motor activity, and heightened sympathetic activity may induce tachycardia, fever, and diarrhea. Vomiting, restlessness, abdominal pain, and increased appetite may be observed. If thyroid hormone is chronically abused, weight loss may occur.

CARDIOVASCULAR EFFECTS

Tachycardia, palpitations, hypertension, cutaneous vasodilation, and diaphoresis may be seen. Angina, hypotension, congestive heart failure, and cardiovascular collapse rarely occur. Arrhythmias usually are supraventricular but may evolve into ventricular dysrhythmias.

NEUROLOGIC EFFECTS

Anxiety, apprehension, headache, confusion, agitation, mydriasis, and diaphoresis may be observed. Occasional weakness, tremor, acute psychosis, and coma have been reported.

THYROID STORM

Thyroid storm is a rare complication of untreated or partially treated hyperthyroidism, associated with cardiovascular, hepatic, gastrointestinal, and neurologic dysfunction. Mortality is approximately 20%. Most patients present with exaggerated signs of hyperthyroidism such as extreme agitation, emotional lability, and restlessness. Neurologic complications may include altered behavior, seizures, and choreoathetosis.

Cardinal manifestations include fever, a widened pulse pressure, flushing, sweating, cardiac dysrhythmias, tachycardia progressing to atrial flutter or fibrillation with or without congestive heart failure, and deterioration in central nervous system function. Severe diarrhea, nausea, vomiting, or jaundice may be present. Often a precipitating factor such as surgery, radioactive iodine therapy, use of an iodinated contrast medium, or intercurrent illness can be identified.

Toxic Dosage/Death

Acute ingestion of 4 mg or less of L-thyroxine (T4) by children or adults is unlikely to produce symptoms of thyrotoxicosis requiring treatment. Up to 30 mg of T4 produced few symptoms in one pediatric study.

Drug Interactions

Thyroid increases the effect of oral anticoagulants, increases the catabolism of vitamin K-dependent clotting factor, increases the need for insulin or oral antidiabetic agents in diabetes mellitus, and increases the need for digitalis in patients receiving digitalis. Cholestyramine binds thyroid hormone in the intestine and reduces thyroid hormone absorption. Anticonvulsants reduce total and free thyroxine (T4) concentrations, and propranolol decreases free triiodothyronine (T3) concentrations. Iodine-induced thyrotoxicosis has been reported after iodine supplementation.

Because of the heightened sensitivity to adrenergic stimulation seen in thyroid storm, ingestion of stimulant medications such as pseudoephedrine may be life-threatening (intracranial hemorrhage, hypertensive crises, rhabdomyolysis, seizures) in these cases.

Pregnancy/Lactation

Decreased T4 elimination occurs during pregnancy because of the increased production of thyroid-binding globulin. To compensate, thyroid gland activity is increased. Mild hyperthyroidism has little effect on the course of pregnancy, but an increased frequency of abortion, premature labor, and toxemia of pregnancy may complicate severe thyrotoxicosis. The maternal disease process may profoundly affect fetal thyroid function. Thyroxine (T4) crosses the placenta and T3 appears to cross more rapidly.

Laboratory

ANALYTIC METHODS

T3 and T4 may be measured by radioimmunoassay.

BLOOD LEVELS

Total serum T4 (normal, 4 to 12 μg/100 mL) roughly correlates with clinical thyroid activity. There appears to be little correlation between laboratory values of thyroid hormone excess and clinical state after an overdose of thyroid hormones. Abnormally elevated thyroid function tests may be found on initial examination with almost no significant signs or symptoms. However, elevated initial T4 serum levels in a levothyroxine overdose may indicate a later development of symptoms.

The clinical state may improve while laboratory values are still abnormal. Clinical toxicity may reflect tissue hormone levels, and these may lag behind serum levels. Hyperthyroxinemia without thyrotoxicosis most commonly occurs because of an increase in thyroid-binding globulin. Many signs of toxicity occur 1 to 15 days after ingestion, even while plasma hormone levels are falling.

Treatment

GUT DECONTAMINATION

The majority of pediatric T4 ingestions are not severe and may be managed on an outpatient basis. Despite marked elevations in thyroid function assays, initial therapy of acute T4 ingestions can be limited to gut decontamination by emesis and charcoal.

ELIMINATION ENHANCEMENT

Because T4 is mostly protein bound, plasmapheresis rather than charcoal hemoperfusion might be effective but its role remains to be determined. Exchange transfusion, plasmapheresis, charcoal hemoperfusion, and peritoneal dialysis may ameliorate thyroid storm.

SUPPORTIVE MEASURES

- If more than twice the recommended daily replacement dose of T4 has been ingested, begin with basic gut decontamination and obtain T4 and T3 levels 2 to 6 hours postingestion as a baseline. If the patient is asymptomatic for 6 to 8 hours, discharge from emergency facility and observe at home for 7 to 15 days to determine if delayed symptoms develop.
- After ingestion of more than 4 mg or unknown quantities of T4, an initial T4 concentration may predict delayed onset of toxicity, fever, tachycardia, hypertension, and agitation in the absence of early clinical manifestations.
- Admission should be considered for all symptomatic patients or those with T4 levels greater than 75 μg/100 mL regardless of presentation.
- In most cases, treatment with a β-blocker and observation is all that is necessary after overdose with T4. Treat sympathetic overactivity with propranolol. For adults, the oral dose is 10 to 40 mg every 4 to 6 hours. Rarely, IV propranolol, 1 to 3 mg/min with cardiovascular monitoring, may be required. Watch for hypotension. For children, the oral dose is 1 mg/kg every 6 hours. The intravenous dose, 0.01 to 0.02 mg/kg, is given over a 10-minute period for tachyarrhythmias.
- Calcium-channel blocking drugs may be useful as adjunctive therapy for thyrotoxicosis in the presence of angina, congestive heart failure, and tachyarrhythmias.

THYROID STORM

- Treatment of thyroid storm is pursued in an intensive care facility and is aimed at reducing both synthesis and peripheral conversion of T4 to T3. β-Adrenergic blockade decreases heart rate, slows cardiac dysrhythmias, and ameliorates hyperpyrexia. Propranolol and nadolol also inhibit conversion of T4 to T3 in the peripheral tissue. Propylthiouracil decreases the intrathyroid production of thyroid hormone and blocks peripheral T4-to-T3 conversion. Other agents used for blocking T4-to-T3 conversion include dexamethasone and iopanoic acid. Iodide and lithium may be used to block thyroidal secretion of hormone.
- The patient should be observed for life-threatening emergencies such as intracranial hemorrhage, hypertensive crisis, rhabdomyolysis, and seizures.
- Reduce fever to normal with cooling measures. Administer fluids, glucose, and electrolytes as required. Continue cardiopulmonary monitoring.
- Hypotension may require Trendelenburg positioning or intravenous fluids.

Questions—Thyroid Hormones

1. Which of the following is false?
- A. The incidence of severe reactions from thyroid hormone overdose is high.
- B. Thyroid hormones are used to correct hypothyroid states and to induce clinical euthyroidism.
- C. Thyrotoxicosis resulting from the ingestion of excessive exogenous thyroid hormone may be seen in patients receiving the medication for treatment of hypothyroidism, goiter, or nodules.
- D. Thyroid hormones affect growth and development by influencing nuclear genome regulation of protein synthesis and growth.
- E. Thyroid hormone increases energy expenditure and leads to increased heat production and oxygen consumption.

2. T3 and T4 both are metabolically active, but T3 is three to five times more potent than T4.
- A. True
- B. False

3. T3 and T4 circulate in the blood bound to serum proteins.
- A. True
- B. False

4. Which of the following is false?
- A. Thyroid storm is a rare complication of untreated or partially treated hyperthyroidism associated with cardiovascular, hepatic, gastrointestinal, and neurologic dysfunction.
- B. Mortality from thyroid storm approaches 80% to 90%.
- C. Most patients who present with thyroid storm demonstrate exaggerated signs of hyperthyroidism such as extreme agitation, emotional lability, and restlessness.
- D. Neurologic complications of thyroid storm may include altered behavior, seizures, and choreoathetosis.
- E. Cardinal manifestations of thyroid storm include fever, a widened pulse pressure, flushing, sweating, and cardiac dysrhythmias.

Antithyroid Drugs

Antithyroid agents are used in the management of hyperthyroidism, including the treatment of Graves' disease, in preparation of hyperthyroid patients for surgery, and as an adjunct to radioiodine therapy in hyperthyroid disease. Methimazole also has been used in the treatment of psoriasis when it may have an ameliorative effect on the immune system.

The main antithyroid agents are thiourea derivatives. The thionamides have been associated with agranulocytosis, hepatotoxicity, arthralgias, and rashes. The thiourea compounds include imidazole derivatives (carbimazole and methimazole) and thiouracils (benzylthiouracil, methylthiouracil, and propylthiouracil). Reactive metabolites of antithyroid drugs or hypersensitivity responses may be the basis for antithyroid toxicity.

The perchlorates have been associated with serious adverse effects when used as antithyroid agents and have been generally replaced by other agents. Potassium perchlorate and sodium perchlorate also are used illicitly for the preparation of explosives or fireworks.

Pathophysiology

Thioureas block the production of thyroid hormones through inhibition of thyroid peroxidase. Propylthiouracil (PTU) also inhibits the peripheral deiodination of T4 to T3. The perchlorates competitively inhibit the active transport of iodide and other anions. Reactive metabolites of propylthiouracil may be involved in hypersensitivity reactions such as agranulocytosis. Vasculitis and antineutrophil antibodies have been observed during propylthiouracil therapy.

Pharmacokinetics

ABSORPTION

- Bioavailability of carbimazole and methimazole is 90% to 100%. Bioavailability of propylthiouracil is 50% to 75%.
- Half-life of carbimazole, and methimazole is 3 to 5 hours, and PTU is 1 to 3 hours.

DISTRIBUTION

- The volume of distribution of carbimazole is 0.5 L/kg, and of PTU is approximately 30 L/kg.
- Plasma protein binding of carbimazole and methimazole is 40% and is about 80% for PTU.

ELIMINATION

- Carbimazole is converted rapidly to its active metabolite, methimazole.

Clinical Presentations

Few reports of overdose with the thioureas or perchlorates are available. Overdose of the thionamides may induce vomiting, epigastric distress, headache, fever, arthralgia, pruritus, and pancytopenia. Agranulocytosis and granulocytopenia may occur in patients taking high doses of antithyroid drugs chronically. Hepatotoxicity is a rare reaction of antithyroid drugs. Rashes may follow high doses of methimazole.

Toxic Dosage/Death

A large propylthiouracil overdose (5 to 13 grams) was associated with a benign clinical course and recovery. Acute overdose of the thionamides may be associated with minor and transient changes in thyroid hormone levels. Following 300 mg daily of propylthiouracil, an adult developed a transient hepatitis. Fatal doses for these compounds have not been determined.

Drug Interactions

No significant drug interactions have been reported. Increased sensitivity to warfarin has been observed in hyperthyroidism.

Pregnancy/Lactation

The thiourea compounds cross the placenta and are excreted in breast milk. Fetal outcome generally is satisfactory in drug-treated pregnancies. Neonatal hepatitis has followed treatment of the mother with propylthiouracil for Graves' disease.

Laboratory

ANALYTIC METHODS

A gas-liquid chromatographic method for PTU is sensitive to 5 mg/dL in urine and 1 μg/mL in blood. Methods of analysis of methimazole include high-pressure liquid chromatography, gas chromatography-mass spectrometry, and radioimmunoassay.

BLOOD LEVELS

Twelve hours following an ingestion of 5 to 13 grams of propylthiouracil, the blood level was 1 μg/mL, and the urine level, 90 mg/dL. Within 17 hours, no propylthiouracil was detected. Peak levels of methimazole are 0.2 to 2.0 μmol/L 1 to 2 hours after 60 mg carbimazole is taken orally.

Treatment

GUT DECONTAMINATION

Timely gastric lavage and activated charcoal would be expected to decrease the overall absorption of these agents however the effect of these interventions has not been studied.

ELIMINATION ENHANCEMENT

Hemodialysis has not been used to treat overdose with these agents.

SUPPORTIVE MEASURES

- Periodic follow-up should include neutrophil counts and laboratory evaluation for evidence of hepatotoxicity.
- Peripheral lymphocyte transformation may be an indicator of drug-induced liver damage.

Question—Antithyroid Drugs

1. Which of the following is false?

A. Antithyroid agents are used in the management of hyperthyroidism including the treatment of Graves' disease, in preparation of hyperthyroid patients for surgery, and as an adjunct to radioiodine therapy in hyperthyroid disease.
B. The main antithyroid agents are thiourea derivatives.
C. Propylthiouracil (PTU) inhibits the peripheral conversion of T3 to T4.
D. Reactive metabolites of propylthiouracil may be involved in hypersensitivity reactions such as agranulocytosis.
E. Vasculitis has been observed during propylthiouracil therapy.

DESMOPRESSIN

Desmopressin (DDAVP®) is a synthetic polypeptide structurally related to arginine vasopressin (antidiuretic hormone), a natural human posterior pituitary hormone. Desmopressin is used similarly to vasopressin in the diagnosis and treatment of central (hypothalamic or neurogenic) diabetes insipidus. Desmopressin is a potent antidiuretic agent. It may induce severe hypotonic hyponatremia with convulsions, especially in children. DDAVP® together with indomethacin may be useful in the treatment of resistant lithium-induced nephrogenic diabetes insipidus.

DDAVP® raises the circulating levels of factor VIII coagulant activity and von Willebrand's factor and shortens the prolonged bleeding time. It has been useful as a nontransfusional form of treatment for mild and moderate hemophilia and von Willebrand's disease. It also may be useful in other conditions with a prolonged bleeding time such as uremia, congenital platelet defects, cirrhosis of the liver, and hereditary hemorrhagic telangiectasia. DDAVP®, in a nasal spray or pill at bedtime, can decrease bedwetting in some children with primary nocturnal enuresis and decrease the severity of spinal headaches after lumbar puncture.

Pathophysiology

Desmopressin is an analog of antidiuretic hormone whose principal action is antidiuresis or oliguria. DDAVP® binds to V2 vasopressin receptors, which activate adenylate cyclase in the distal medullary nephron and which exert their effect by elevating cyclic AMP in those cells. It has little or no effect on V1 vasopressin receptors of smooth muscle and therefore, has little vasoconstrictive effect.

Pharmacokinetics

ABSORPTION

- The bioavailability following a subcutaneous dose is approximately 100%.
- Following an intranasal dose, it is only 2%.

DISTRIBUTION

- The liver and kidneys are the chief sites of metabolic inactivation of arginine vasopressin and probably that of desmopressin.

ELIMINATION

- The metabolic fate of DDAVP® is largely unknown.
- The elimination half-life ranges from 2.7 to 4.6 hours.

Clinical Presentations

Excessive administration of desmopressin may lead to the development of hypotonic hyponatremia. DDAVP® has been associated with the development of arterial thromboses and myocardial infarction in adults, and hyponatremia with convulsions in both children and adults. Adverse effects following either the intranasal or parenteral route of administration of DDAVP® generally have been infrequent and mild. Symptoms after subcutaneous injection may include headache, nausea, abdominal cramps, and vulval pain. After intranasal use, conjunctivitis, ocular edema, lacrimation, headache, dizziness, rhinitis, vulval pain, and abdominal cramps have been reported.

Risk factors for the development of hyponatremia in patients receiving DDAVP® include young age, frequent dosing, administration of hypotonic intravenous fluids, and administration of DDAVP® in the postoperative period. Excess DDAVP® in the treatment of hemophilia or von Willebrand's disease may also lead to a state of hypotonic hyponatremia with a possible increase in the severity of preexisting angina or hypertension.

Toxic Dosage/Death

Doses of 0.3 mg/kg intravenously to 2.4 mg/kg intranasally have induced hyponatremia and seizures in children and adults. No fatal dose has been established.

Drug Interactions

Carbamazepine may decrease the duration of action of desmopressin. Orally administered agents such as chlorpropamide, clofibrate, and indomethacin may prolong the action of desmopressin. The antidiuretic response to DDAVP® may be decreased in patients receiving lithium, large doses of epinephrine, demeclocycline, heparin, or alcohol.

Pregnancy/Lactation

Safe use of desmopressin during pregnancy has not been established. Desmopressin has, however, been used during pregnancy and lactation without reports of adverse effects either on the pregnant or lactating mother or on the fetus or nursing infant. There are no adequate and controlled studies to date using desmopressin in pregnant women. It is not known if desmopressin crosses the placenta. It is distributed into breast milk in low concentrations, less than 2 ng/L.

Laboratory

ANALYTIC METHODS

A radioimmunoassay, both sensitive and specific, is available to determine plasma levels.

BLOOD LEVELS

A plasma level of about 98 pg/mL is reached after intranasal administration and a level of 550 pg/mL is attained after SC use. Following blood levels is not helpful in overdose.

Treatment

GUT DECONTAMINATION

Benefit from these interventions has not been proved after oral overdoze.

ELIMINATION ENHANCEMENT

Hemodialysis has not been used primarily to treat DDAVP® overdose, but may be helpful in correcting severe electrolyte abnormalities.

SUPPORTIVE MEASURES

- Guidelines have been suggested for the use of DDAVP® in young children. Before the administration of DDAVP®, baseline electrolytes and serum osmolality should be obtained. Restrict fluids to three-fourths maintenance or less and avoid large amounts of oral or intravenous hyponatremic fluids.
- After using DDAVP®, follow serum sodium, osmolality, and urine output for 24 hours, as experience suggests that the nadir of hyponatremia occurs 9 to 20 hours after DDAVP® administration. Avoid repeat doses of DDAVP® if possible.

- Similar precautions may be advisable in older children and adults in the postoperative period, if multiple doses of DDAVP® are given, or if risk factors such as narcotics for pain relief, liver disease, or renal tubular acidosis are present.
- If hypotonic hyponatremia develops after administration of excess DDAVP®, restriction of fluids to 500 to 1,000 mL per 24 hours usually permits plasma sodium levels to return to normal within a few days. If the hyponatremia is severe, furosemide with oral salt supplementation may be useful.
- Desmopressin causes an increase in factor VIII and a mild increase in the leukocyte count.

Questions—Desmopressin

1. Which of the following is false?

A. Desmopressin (DDAVP®) is a synthetic polypeptide structurally related to arginine vasopressin (antidiuretic hormone), a natural human anterior pituitary hormone.
B. Desmopressin is used similarly to vasopressin in the diagnosis and treatment of central (hypothalamic or neurogenic) diabetes insipidus.
C. Desmopressin may induce hypotonic hyponatremia with convulsions, especially in children.
D. DDAVP® together with indomethacin may be useful in the treatment of resistant lithium-induced nephrogenic diabetes insipidus.
E. DDAVP® raises the circulating levels of factor VIII coagulant activity and von Willebrand's factor and shortens the prolonged bleeding time.

2. DDAVP® has been useful as a nontransfusional form of treatment for mild and moderate hemophilia and von Willebrand's disease.

A. True
B. False

3. Risk factors for the development of hyponatremia in patients receiving DDAVP® include all of the following, except

A. Young age
B. Frequent dosing
C. Proximate administration of hypotonic intravenous fluids
D. Administration in the postoperative period
E. Concomitant use of antibiotics

STEROIDS AND FERTILITY DRUGS

STEROIDS

Steroids are widely used in almost every area of medical practice. Steroid overdose is infrequent. Adverse effects however, from acute and chronic use, are common. Natural steroid hormones include the progestogens, estrogens, androgens, and corticoids. Synthetic derivatives of testosterone are called anabolic steroids. Inhaled synthetic corticosteroids, such as beclomethasone, budesonide, triamcinolone, and flunisolide, have been used for the topical treatment of asthma. See Chapter 32, Pulmonary Toxicology, Inhaled Steroids section. Steroids are also used topically to combat a broad array of inflammatory dermatologic conditions.

Systemic steroids are used in chemotherapeutic combinations, to treat allergic reactions and anaphylaxis, for multiple sclerosis, in birth control pills, in inflammatory bowel disease, to combat a broad array of collagen vascular diseases, to treat spinal trauma and cerebral edema, and to treat a variety of pulmonary conditions including asthma, sarcoidosis, and pulmonary hypertension. They also are used as replacement therapy in post-menopausal and surgically menopausal women, and in patients with adrenal insufficiency.

Steroids may also be abused to produce increased muscle mass and a transient feeling of well-being. Euphoria and dependence have followed the use of androgenic anabolic steroids. There are reported to be more than 1 million current or former illicit anabolic androgenic steroid users in the United States. Their use is often associated with the use of other illicit drugs, cigarettes, and alcohol. Some may have withdrawal symptoms including depression, fatigue, and craving for steroids. Some experience wide mood swings with periods of aggression.

It appears that athletes may be taking doses of androgen in 100- to 1,000-fold excess over physiologic doses to enhance performance and muscle mass. Often, several preparations are taken. Oral and parenteral forms may be used together. Anabolic steroid use in high-school students may be part of a "risk" behavior syndrome that includes increased sexual and suicidal behaviors, not wearing a passenger seat belt, riding a motorcycle without a helmet, driving after drinking alcohol, fighting, and carrying a weapon.

One steroid used as an "anti-aging" drug, dehydroepiandrosterone sulfate (DHEA), recently has become popular. DHEA is an adrenal steroid that is involved in testosterone and cholesterol synthesis. Among other things, it is touted to boost libido, strengthen immunity, fight obesity, and build muscle mass. None of these benefits have been scientifically proven. Infrequent overdoses have been reported, however side effects including androgenic changes in women, may occur.

Pathophysiology

Steroids are produced in the adrenal gland and form the backbone of numerous hormones and cholesterol. Many are controlled by the hypothalamic-pituitary axis and are modulated by adrenocorticotropic hormone (ACTH). Some, such as prednisone are "prodrugs" which are converted to an active form (ie, prednisolone is an active form of prednisone) by enzymes. Cortisone is another inactive prodrug that is converted to its active form, hydrocortisone, by an enzyme.

Pharmacokinetics

ABSORPTION

- Most steroids are well absorbed and demonstrate 80% to 100% bioavailability.

DISTRIBUTION

- The volume of distribution of these agents, (e.g., prednisolone, hydrocortisone, dexamethasone, prednisone) ranges from 0.30 to 1.20 L/kg.
- Most are 70% to 90% protein bound.

ELIMINATION

- Half-life of these agents ranges from 1.0 to 3.0 hours.
- Oral contraceptives such as ethynylestradiol and norethindrone demonstrate 7.7 hour half-lives.

Clinical Presentations

GASTROINTESTINAL EFFECTS

Exogenous estrogen therapy has been associated with a variety of infrequent epithelial liver lesions (focal nodular hyperplasia, adenoma and hepatocellular carcinoma), mesenchymal lesions (sarcomas, rhabdomyosarcomas), and mixed tumors of the liver. Nausea, vomiting, and gastric irritation are frequent side effects of oral steroid use. Hepatic effects of anabolic steroid use include abnormal liver function tests and cholestatic jaundice.

CARDIOVASCULAR EFFECTS

Oral contraceptives containing 50 mg of estrogen have been associated with an increased risk of myocardial infarctions. Additional risk factors associated with fatal myocardial infarction in women taking steroids are a history of hypertension in pregnancy, nonpregnancy-associated hypertension, hyperlipidemia, diabetes, and smoking. These risks are reduced by use of newer oral contraceptive preparations containing new synthetic progestins and/or lower doses of both estrogenic and progestogenic components. Phlebitis and hypertension also have been associated with steroid use. Estradiol implants and other steroid contraceptives may cause fluid retention, facial swelling, and pitting edema of the thighs.

ADRENAL EFFECTS

Acute adrenal insufficiency (Addisonian crisis) may follow suppression of the hypothalamic-pituitary axis caused by long-term use of steroids. Lethargy, malaise, nausea, vomiting, dizziness, headache, and varying states of consciousness may follow sudden cessation of use. Plasma cortisol levels may be depressed. Treatment includes the use of oral or intravenous corticosteroids. Adrenal insufficiency also may occur in patients who develop bilateral adrenal hemorrhage.

Increased steroids, either secondary to overproduction or exogenous use, may yield signs of Cushing's syndrome. Features of Cushing's syndrome include ecchymoses, atrophy of pelvic and shoulder girdle muscles, ulcerations and perforations of the sigmoid colon, overt diabetes, hypoproteinemia, hypokalemia, hyponatremia, hypophosphatemia, and osteoporosis.

PSYCHIATRIC EFFECTS

Psychiatric responses to steroids range from mild euphoria to psychosis. The majority of steroid psychoses have an onset within 5 days of commencing medication and may vary up to 2 to 4 weeks. The frequency of steroid-induced psychiatric disorders increases with the daily dose of medication. Affective schizophreniform and organic symptoms may be observed. Peak plasma levels of steroid medication may be related to the development of psychiatric symptoms. Mania may follow higher-than-recommended doses of beclomethasone and behavioral changes may be observed in young children after steroid inhalation therapy for asthma.

GENITOURINARY EFFECTS

High-dose topical and oral testosterone therapy has led to masculinization, including deepening of the voice. Vaginal spotting, bleeding, and secondary amenorrhea may occur.

NEUROLOGIC EFFECTS

Cerebrovascular hemorrhage, intracranial hypertension, and transient ischemic attacks have been associated with anabolic steroids.

ENDOCRINE EFFECTS

Include decreased production of luteinizing hormone (LH), follicle-stimulating hormone (FSH), and testosterone. In males, testicular atrophy, decreased sperm production, sterility, gynecomastia, hypertension, acne, and baldness may be seen with chronic steroid use. In women, hoarseness, hirsutism, menstrual irregularities, enlarged clitoris, decreased breast size, alopecia, and acne may be seen. Altered glucose tolerance and hyperinsulinism may be seen with anabolic steroid use.

MUSCULOSKELETAL EFFECTS

Osteoporosis, avascular necrosis of the hips, premature epiphyseal closure, and short stature have each been associated with chronic steroid use.

HYPERSENSITIVITY EFFECTS

Methylprednisolone may cause an anaphylactoid response characterized by sudden respiratory compromise.

DEPENDENCE

The most frequent manifestations of dependency are withdrawal symptoms including acts of physical violence, feelings of anger or hostility, manic or psychotic episodes or depression, withdrawal-related fatigue, restlessness, anorexia, and insomnia. Those who become dependent typically have used larger steroid dosages, had more cycles of use, were more dissatisfied with their body size, and had more aggressive symptoms than nondependent users.

Toxic Dosage/Death

Death from acute overdose of steroids has not been reported.

Drug Interactions

Dexamethasone and prednisone demonstrate a decreased effect with rifampin and anticonvulsants such as phenytoin and barbiturates.

Pregnancy/Lactation

Concentrations of prednisolone in breast milk do not appear to exceed 10% of the plasma concentration and it is doubtful that it may pose any danger to the nursing infant. Studies of women who have taken many steroids during pregnancy reveal that these substances have little effect on the developing fetus. Pregnancy risk category for prednisolone and prednisone is B. Certain androgenic steroids, such as danazol (see the following section), may cause virilization of the fetus during pregnancy and are given pregnancy risk category X.

Laboratory

ANALYTIC METHODS

Detection of anabolic steroids is difficult because of the availability of numerous preparations with numerous degradative products. Drug testing for anabolic steroids is performed by radioimmunoassay (RIA) and gas chromatography with mass spectrometry. Urine is screened using RIA. Steroids also may be detected by high performance liquid chromatography.

BLOOD LEVELS

Oral agents usually are detectable several weeks after discontinuation. Parenteral agents may be detectable for up to 3 months. Few laboratories offer anabolic steroid testing for individuals and following blood levels does not aid in treating clinical effects.

Treatment

GUT DECONTAMINATION

These methods have not been shown helpful in mitigating against adverse effects.

ELIMINATION ENHANCEMENT

These methods have not been used to treat steroid overdoses or adverse effects.

SUPPORTIVE MEASURES

- The treatment of complications induced by anabolic steroid use and abuse is symptomatic and supportive. Adrenal suppression is treated with intravenous hydrocortisone
- Elevations in glucose and leukocytes may frequently be seen with steroid use.
- An anecdotal report suggests that clomiphene 100 mg / d may restore follicle-stimulating hormone, luteinizing hormone, and free testosterone levels in men after recreational steroid-induced pituitary-gonadal failure.
- Treatment of anabolic steroid use in athletes is largely directed at prevention in the adolescent by education directed towards parents, teachers, and coaches.

Questions—Steroids

1. Which of the following is false?
- A. Steroids may be abused to produce increased muscle mass and a feeling of well-being.
- B. Euphoria and dependence have followed the use of androgenic anabolic steroids.
- C. Anabolic steroid use in high school students may be part of a "risk" behavior syndrome that includes increased sexual and suicidal behaviors, not wearing a passenger seat belt, riding a motorcycle without a helmet, driving after drinking alcohol, fighting, and carrying a weapon.
- D. Dehydroepiandrosterone (DHEA) is a steroid that is involved in cholesterol degradation.
- E. Exogenous estrogen therapy has been associated with a variety of infrequent epithelial liver lesions (focal nodular hyperplasia, adenoma, and hepatocellular carcinoma).

2. Systemic steroids are used in chemotherapeutic combinations, to treat allergic reactions and anaphylaxis, for multiple sclerosis, in birth-control pills, in inflammatory bowel disease, to combat a broad array of collagen vascular diseases, to treat spinal trauma and cerebral edema, and to treat a variety of pulmonary conditions including asthma, sarcoidosis, and pulmonary hypertension.
- A. True
- B. False

3. Natural steroids include all of the following, except
- A. Progestogens
- B. Estrogens
- C. Androgens
- D. Lactones
- E. Corticoids

4. Which of the following is false?
- A. Oral contraceptives have been associated with an increased risk of myocardial infarctions.
- B. Risk factors associated with fatal myocardial infarction in women taking steroids are a history of hypertension in pregnancy, nonpregnancy-associated hypertension, breast cancer, fibrocystic disease, hyperlipidemia, diabetes, and smoking.
- C. Phlebitis and hypertension also has been associated with steroid use.
- D. Estradiol implants and other steroid contraceptives may cause fluid retention, facial swelling, and pitting edema of the thighs.
- E. Acute adrenal insufficiency (Addisonian crisis) may follow suppression of the hypothalamic-pituitary axis caused by long-term use of steroids.

5. Certain androgenic steroids may cause virilization of the fetus during pregnancy and are given pregnancy risk category X.
- A. True
- B. False

DANAZOL

Danazol, an androgen, is used in the treatment of endometriosis, benign breast disease, hereditary angioedema, idiopathic thrombocytopenic purpura, and myelodysplastic syndromes. Danazol is available for oral use. It has been abused by athletes because of its presumed influence on athletic performance. Few cases of overdose have been reported. It is unlikely that serious immediate reactions will occur from a single excessive dose.

Pathophysiology

Danazol is a synthetic attenuated androgen that interferes with normal interactions between the pituitary-hypothalamic axis and the gonads. By inhibiting gonadotropin-releasing hormone and gonadotropin secretion, it suppresses menstruation, inhibits ovulation, and causes regressive changes in the vaginal smear and atrophic changes in the endometrium. It is not estrogenic or progestogenic. Danazol exhibits weak androgenic activity.

Pharmacokinetics

ABSORPTION

- Danazol is absorbed rapidly from the upper gastrointestinal tract into the enterohepatic circulation.

DISTRIBUTION

- In the peripheral circulation it binds to the sex hormone-binding globulin, displacing testosterone and estradiol.
- Free testosterone in the peripheral circulation increases.

ELIMINATION

- The half-life is about 2 to 4 hours. It is metabolized in the liver to an inactive metabolite.

Clinical Presentations

The most frequent adverse effects include mild hirsutism, decreased breast size, weight gain, menometrorrhagia, amenorrhea, altered libido, deepened voice, flushing, and acne. Like other 17-alkylated steroids, danazol may induce cholestatic jaundice, peliosis of the liver, and benign hepatic adenoma. Other toxic effects may include benign intracranial hypertension, headaches, dizziness, myalgias, and nausea.

Toxic Dosage/Death

A toxic dose has not been established and there have been no reports of death secondary to danazol use alone.

Drug Interactions

Increases in prothrombin time may occur after simultaneous use of anticoagulants with danazol.

Pregnancy/Lactation

Fetal virilization may occur when mothers use danazol during the first 12 weeks of gestation. It is suggested that danazol not be used during pregnancy and has been assigned risk category X.

Laboratory

ANALYTIC METHODS

A radioimmunoassay method can detect levels of 1.4 to 2.8 ng/mL in human plasma.

BLOOD LEVELS

Plasma levels reach a maximum of 80 ng/mL about 2 hours after a dose of 400 mg. Following blood levels does not help guide management of adverse effects.

Treatment

GUT DECONTAMINATION

Emesis induction and gastric lavage may be effective in removing the drug if patients are seen within 2 to 4 hours of ingestion, however this has not been proved. Charcoal may be helpful as well.

ELIMINATION ENHANCEMENT

Methods to enhance elimination have not been utilized with danazol use.

SUPPORTIVE MEASURES

- Diabetic patients should be monitored for possible insulin resistance.
- An anecdotal report suggests that intravenous S-adenosylmethionine (800 to 1,600 mg daily) may be useful in patients with severe drug-induced cholestasis.
- Hepatic enzymes may be elevated after doses of 400 mg or more daily.

Questions—Danazol

1. Danazol is used in all of the following, except
A. Endometriosis
B. Malignant breast cancer
C. Benign breast disease
D. Hereditary angioedema
E. Idiopathic thrombocytopenic purpura

2. Adverse effects from danazol use include all of the following, except
A. Hirsutism
B. Increased breast size
C. Amenorrhea
D. Altered libido
E. Deepened voice

FERTILITY DRUGS

Ovulation induction agents include clomiphene, bromocriptine, gonadotropin preparations, and gonadotropin-releasing hormone (GnRH) and its analogs. Each agent is associated with specific adverse effects. Although many of these adverse effects are benign and self-limited, some, in particular those effects associated with gonadotropins, may be life-threatening.

Diethylstilbestrol (DES) is a synthesized stilbene whose biological properties are similar to those of naturally occurring estrogens such as estrone and estradiol-17b. An estimated 5 to 10 million Americans received DES during pregnancy or were exposed to the drug in utero. Exposure to DES has been associated with an increased risk for breast cancer in DES mothers and an increased lifetime risk for clear cell cervicovaginal cancer in DES daughters. The association between DES exposure and testicular cancer in DES sons remains controversial. Exposure to DES also has been linked to reproductive tract abnormalities in DES sons and daughters that consist of immune system disorders and psychosexual effects.

Pathophysiology

These agents act by inducing ovulation, thereby presenting more oocytes to sperm to enhance the probability of fertilization. Many of the adverse effects related to ovulation induction agents can be predicted based on their mechanisms of action. Clomiphene is an antiestrogen, and thus its adverse effects may include hot flashes and disruption of the cervical mucus and proper endometrial maturation. As a dopamine agonist, bromocriptine often results in postural hypotension, a result of increased dopaminergic tone with exogenous gonadotropins. Its major adverse effects (e.g., multiple gestation and ovarian hyperstimulation syndrome) are related to the development of multiple follicles and exaggerated estradiol levels.

Clinical Presentations

Clomiphene (Clomid®) has been associated with hot flashes, multiple gestations, visual disturbances, cervical mucus abnormalities, and luteal phase deficiency. Most of the adverse symptoms associated with bromocriptine, such as nausea and postural hypotension, are short-lived. Gonadotropin therapy, even when used appropriately, may lead to the ovarian hyperstimulation syndrome and a high incidence of multiple gestation. Pulsatile GnRH therapy may be accompanied by adverse effects similar to those of gonadotropins, but at a far lower incidence.

Ovarian hyperstimulation syndrome is the most severe acute confirmed adverse effect related to the pharmacologic therapy of infertility. The symptoms of ovarian hyperstimulation syndrome are noted from 5 to 7 days after administration of human chorionic gonadotropin and include body weight gain, dyspnea, hypotension, oliguria, electrolyte imbalance, and increased coagulability.

Toxic Dosage/Death

A lethal or toxic dose has not been established for these agents.

Drug Interactions

There is a decreased response to clomiphene when it is used concurrently with danazol.

Pregnancy/Lactation

Clomiphene is contraindicated after conception and has been given pregnancy risk category X. Multiple congenital malformations have been associated with its use. Bromocriptine has been given pregnancy risk category B. The incidence of congenital abnormalities associated with its use during pregnancy approximates that in the general population.

Major congenital abnormalities, increased risk for spontaneous abortions, ectopic pregnancies, early cervical effacement, and premature labor have been associated with DES and its use during pregnancy is absolutely contraindicated. It has been given pregnancy risk category X.

Laboratory

ANALYTIC METHODS

An assay for clomiphene is not routinely available in hospital settings.

BLOOD LEVELS

Following blood levels does not aid in treating the adverse effects of clomiphene.

Treatment

Gut Decontamination

Gastric lavage and charcoal administration may be helpful but have not been studied in the context of fertility drug overdose or misuse.

ELIMINATION ENHANCEMENT

These methods have not been employed in the treatment of exposures to fertility drugs.

SUPPORTIVE MEASURES

- Patients with ovarian hyperstimulation syndrome are generally admitted to the hospital, where fluid intake and output are monitored. Intake should be restricted to maintain adequate output and electrolyte balance. IV fluids and not diuretics are used judiciously to maintain urine output.
- There is an increased risk of ovarian hemorrhage in patients with ovarian hyperstimulation syndrome as a result of ovarian friability. Heparin therapy should be avoided if possible. Rarely, oophorectomy may be required to control hemorrhage.
- If pregnancy does not ensue, the symptoms of ovarian hyperstimulation syndrome often regress spontaneously and rapidly, within 7 days (i.e., when menses ensue).
- The American College of Obstetricians and Gynecologists has proposed guidelines for the follow-up of women exposed to DES. In light of a slight increased risk for breast cancer, the committee recommends that women who received DES during pregnancy be encouraged to do monthly breast self-examinations, have an annual breast physical examination, and follow established recommendations for screening mammography.
- DES daughters are advised to undergo careful inspection of the cervix and vagina using Lugol (iodine) solution and palpation of the entire vaginal and cervical walls. Most cancers in women under surveillance are detected in this manner. The Committee recommends that in addition to an annual cervical pap smear, women exposed in utero to DES also should have vaginal cytologic tests and colposcopy if the results are suspicious and biopsies should be done as indicated.

Questions—Fertility Drugs

1. Which of the following is false?

A. Ovulation induction agents include clomiphene, bromocriptine, gonadotropin preparations, and gonadotropin-releasing hormone (GnRH) and its analogs.
B. An estimated 5 to 10 million Americans received diethylstilbestrol (DES) during pregnancy or were exposed to the drug in utero.
C. Exposure to DES has been associated with an increased risk for breast cancer in DES daughters and an increased lifetime risk for clear cell cervicovaginal cancer in DES mothers.
D. The association between DES exposure and testicular cancer in DES sons remains controversial.
E. Fertility drugs act by inducing ovulation, thereby presenting more oocytes to sperm to enhance the probability of fertilization.

2. Which of the following is false?

A. Clomiphene is an antiestrogen, and thus its adverse effects may include hot flashes and disruption of the cervical mucus and proper endometrial maturation.
B. As a dopamine agonist, bromocriptine often results in postural hypotension, a result of increased dopaminergic tone with exogenous gonadotropins.
C. Most of the adverse symptoms associated with bromocriptine, such as nausea and postural hypotension, last for weeks.
D. Gonadotropin therapy, even when used appropriately, may lead to the ovarian hyperstimulation syndrome and a high incidence of multiple gestation.
E. Ovarian hyperstimulation syndrome is the most severe acute confirmed adverse effect related to the pharmacologic therapy of infertility. Symptoms of ovarian hyperstimulation syndrome include body weight gain, dyspnea, hypotension, oliguria, electrolyte imbalance, hemoconcentration, and increased coagulability.

MIFEPRISTONE

Mifepristone (RU-486) when used with a prostaglandin in the first 35 days of pregnancy is an effective abortifacient. Its use in second-trimester abortion still is uncertain. It is effective in inducing labor in the presence of intrauterine death. It may be useful in Cushing's syndrome, adrenal cancer, and even glaucoma because of glucocorticoid receptor blocking. Anecdotal data also suggest its use in the treatment of meningioma. In overdose, it may be expected to induce vaginal bleeding. It is a derivative of norethisterone and is chemically related to progesterone.

Pathophysiology

Mifepristone is an antiprogesterone with abortifacient properties. Mifepristone competes with progesterone for its specific receptors and thereby antagonizes its action. It has almost no agonist activity and almost no effect on estrogen receptors in the uterus or mineralocorticoid receptors in the kidney.

Pharmacokinetics

ABSORPTION

- The bioavailability of mifepristone is about 70%.
- Plasma concentration peaks in 1 to 2 hours.

DISTRIBUTION

- The apparent volume of distribution at steady state after intravenous administration is about 26 L.
- Mifepristone is about 98% bound to plasma proteins.

ELIMINATION

- The elimination half-life is 12 to 24 hours.

Clinical Presentations

Some patients may experience excessive blood loss with or without complete expulsion of the products of conception. Other undesirable effects may include fatigue, hot flashes, gynecomastia, partial alopecia, nausea, vomiting, and abdominal pain. Cardiovascular complications also may follow mifepristone use.

Toxic Dosage/Death

A toxic dose has not been established and death from mifepristone has not been reported.

Drug Interactions

Mifepristone increases the sensitivity of the uterus to prostaglandins and the combination of these agents induces effective abortions.

Pregnancy/Lactation

Mifepristone crosses the placenta. Because of its abortifacient properties, it has been assigned pregnancy risk category X. Some pregnant patients who received mifepristone in the first 8 to 9 weeks of gestation went on to have normal pregnancies. No data are available on breast feeding.

Laboratory

ANALYTIC METHODS

A radioimmunoassay for plasma mifepristone concentrations is sensitive to 72.5 nmol/L.

BLOOD LEVELS

Blood levels do not guide therapy.

Treatment

GUT DECONTAMINATION

Timely lavage and/or charcoal use might theoretically eliminate the abortifacient potential of mifepristone, but this has not been studied formally.

ELIMINATION ENHANCEMENT

No reported uses of these methods have been associated with mifepristone use.

SUPPORTIVE MEASURES

- Obstetric consultation should be obtained and clinicians should be prepared for bleeding.
- Cortisol and thyroid-stimulating hormone levels may rise, with a decrease in thyroxine level.

Question—Mifepristone

1. **All of the following regarding mifepristone are true, except**
   A. Mifepristone (RU-486) when used with a prostaglandin in the first 35 days of pregnancy is an effective abortifacient.
   B. Mifepristone is not effective in inducing labor in the presence of intrauterine death.
   C. Mifepristone may be useful in Cushing's syndrome, adrenal cancer, and even glaucoma because of glucocorticoid receptor blocking.
   D. In overdose, mifepristone induces vaginal bleeding.
   E. Mifepristone is related chemically to progesterone.

OCTREOTIDE AND SOMATOSTATIN

Octreotide is a synthetic peptide with many uses. It is actively used to control bleeding from varices in cirrhotic patients. It is used in acromegaly after pituitary surgery if growth hormone concentrations remain elevated. It also is indicated for patients unfit for surgery or preoperatively in those with large pituitary adenomas to induce tumor shrinkage.

Octreotide may be potentially useful as an antidote for the hyperinsulinemia induced by large sulfonylurea overdose, in the treatment of thyroid-stimulating hormone-secretory adenomas, and in treating carcinoid tumors, vasoactive intestinal peptidoma, glucagonoma, and acromegaly. Octreotide may be useful in treating refractory diarrhea associated with acquired immunodeficiency syndrome (AIDS) and in reducing complications of pancreatectomy or pancreatic transplantation, such as fistula formation and acute pancreatitis. It may improve visual acuity in patients with diabetic retinopathy and macular edema.

Somatostatin is a polypeptide obtained from the hypothalamus or by synthesis. Somatostatin has been tried in the management of upper gastrointestinal hemorrhage, insulin resistance, hormone-secreting tumors, other hypersecretory disorders, and pancreatic disorders. Somatostatin is also called growth hormone release-inhibiting hormone and somatotropin release-inhibiting factor.

Pathophysiology

Octreotide is a somatostatin analog. Octreotide inhibits endocrine and exocrine gastrointestinal secretion and may be useful in the treatment of gastroenteric pancreatic tumors. Octreotide also inhibits intestinal mobility and gallbladder motility. Somatostatin inhibits the release of growth hormone from the anterior pituitary, thyrotropin and corticotropin from the pituitary, and glucagon and insulin from the pancreas. In addition, it appears to have a role in the regulation of duodenal and gastric secretions.

Pharmacokinetics

ABSORPTION

- After sc injection of 100 μg of octreotide, a peak serum concentration of about 2 μg/mL is reached in 20 to 30 minutes.

DISTRIBUTION

- The serum distribution half-life of octreotide is about 75 to 100 minutes.
- The volume of distribution is about 0.4 L/kg. About 65% are bound to plasma proteins.
- Somatostatin has a very short duration of action. Analogs have been produced to prolong its activity as well as to make its inhibitory effects more specific.

ELIMINATION

- The serum elimination half-life is 90 to 110 minutes.
- 10% to 20% of the drug is eliminated unchanged in the urine.

Clinical Presentations

The most important complications of octreotide treatment are gallstone formation and gastritis. Biliary colic, acute cholecystitis, and acute pancreatitis have followed withdrawal. Diarrhea generally is not troublesome. Avoiding mealtime administration may minimize nausea, vomiting, abdominal pain, flatulence, and steatorrhea. Congestive heart failure may worsen because of growth hormone inhibition. Hepatotoxicity has been reported in a case report. Hair loss has been observed and acute pancreatitis may be induced.

Somatostatin inhibits hydrochloric acid output, as well as pepsin, intrinsic factor, and gastric secretion. It also reduces gastrointestinal motility and splanchnic blood flow. Somatostatin use has led to life-threatening water intoxication and hyponatremia.

Toxic Dosage/Death

One patient was given 250 mg/hour of octreotide instead of 25 mg/hour intravenously for 48 hours without any side effects. A lethal dose for these agents has not been ascertained.

Drug Interactions

Octreotide prevents basal and meal-stimulated increases in gastrin caused by omeprazole.

Pregnancy/Lactation

Transplacental passage of octreotide may occur by passive diffusion. Octreotide does not seem to affect the fetus. It has been assigned pregnancy risk category B. The risk to the nursing infant is probably inconsequential.

Laboratory

ANALYTIC METHODS

A specific radioimmunoassay measures plasma octreotide concentrations.

BLOOD LEVELS

Blood levels do not guide clinical effects of octreotide or somatostatin.

Treatment

GUT DECONTAMINATION

Lavage and charcoal theoretically may be useful, but have not been studied in overdose.

ELIMINATION ENHANCEMENT

Methods to enhance the elimination of octreotide or somatostatin have not been documented.

SUPPORTIVE MEASURES

- Abdominal symptoms may indicate gallstone problems.

Questions—Octreotide and Somatostatin

1. **Which of the following uses is not associated with octreotide?**
   A. To control bleeding from varices in cirrhotic patients.
   B. To treat acromegaly after pituitary surgery if growth hormone levels remain elevated.
   C. As an antidote for the hyperinsulinemia induced by large sulfonylurea overdose.
   D. To treat thyroid-stimulating hormone-secretory adenomas and carcinoid tumors.
   E. To treat polycystic ovary syndrome.
2. **Somatostatin inhibits the release of growth hormone from the anterior pituitary, thyrotropin and corticotropin from the pituitary, and glucagon and insulin from the pancreas.**
   A. True
   B. False
3. **Important complications of octreotide treatment are kidney stone formation and sialadenitis.**
   A. True
   B. False

BISPHOSPHONATES

Bisphosphonates are used to inhibit bone resorption stimulated by parathyroid hormone, calcitriol, cytokines, and prostaglandins. Bisphosphonates have been used to treat Paget's disease, hypercalcemia of malignant disease, and vertebral crush fractures associated with osteoporosis. The main bisphosphonates are etidronate, tiludronate, clodronate, pamidronate, alendronate, and risedronate. Newer bisphosphonates include alendronate, and meridronate.

Pathophysiology

Bisphosphonates are synthetic analogs of pyrophosphate, a naturally occurring substance that inhibits the mineralization of bone. Bisphosphonates have a strong affinity for hydroxyapatite crystals and in high doses, they inhibit calcification of bone. They inhibit growth and dissolution of hydroxyapatite crystals in bone, and may impair osteoclast activity. They also diminish bone resorption and bone formation.

Pharmacokinetics

ABSORPTION

- Bisphosphonates are absorbed, excreted, and stored unchanged.
- Intestinal absorption is poor (1% to 10%) and is reduced further by concurrent ingestion of food, especially products containing calcium.

DISTRIBUTION

- Plasma clearance is rapid (half-life of about 2 hours) because of the rapid uptake of 20% to 60% of the absorbed fraction into the skeleton.

ELIMINATION

- Bisphosphonates are not metabolized. Some bisphosphonates may remain in the skeleton for life.

Clinical Presentations

The oral bisphosphonates may cause nausea, vomiting, a transient fever, leukopenia, and an increase in C-reactive protein. Pancytopenia and aplastic anemia are rare but serious complications. Rapid intravenous administration has led to renal failure. Asymptomatic hypercalcemia has been observed. Etidronate can inhibit bone mineralization when given continuously for periods greater than 6 to 12 months, resulting in bone pain and fractures. This effect is dose-dependent and reversible. This has not been described after use of alendronate, tiludronate, and pamidronate, which may even stimulate bone mineralization. Prolonged overdose may yield the nephrotic syndrome and fractures.

An overdose with etidronate may induce hypocalcemia in the first 2 days with paresthesias and carpopedal spasm. Prolonged treatment with etidronate leads to bone pain and spontaneous fractures. The chelation effects of etidronate should be reversible with intravenous calcium gluconate. No overdoses with pamidronate have been reported. Bone mineralization defects, hypocalcemia, fever, hypertension, transient taste difficulties, rickets, asthma in aspirin-sensitive asthma patients, and lymphopenia have been described.

Toxic Dosage/Death

Toxic or lethal doses have not been established for these agents.

Drug Interactions

Reduced intestinal absorption of calcium, iron, and antacids occurs with concurrent administration of bisphosphonates. Severe hypocalcemia has been reported in patients taking aminoglycosides and bisphosphonates.

Pregnancy/Lactation

Oral etidronate is pregnancy risk category B, and parenteral etidronate is pregnancy risk category C. Pamidronate is classified as pregnancy risk category C.

Laboratory

ANALYTIC METHODS

Assays for these agents routinely are not available in a hospital setting.

BLOOD LEVELS

There is little evidence of any correlation between the plasma concentration of bisphosphonates and their therapeutic effects.

Treatment

GUT DECONTAMINATION

Following an acute overdose with clodronate and the other bisphosphonates, gastric lavage may remove unabsorbed drug.

ELIMINATION ENHANCEMENT

These methods have not been reported as adjuncts to therapy of bisphosphonate overdose.

SUPPORTIVE MEASURES

- Conventional methods, including calcium supplementation, are used for the treatment of hypocalcemia. Treatment of hypercalcemia centers on adequate hydration, maintenance of high urinary sodium and calcium excretion, correction of hypophosphatemia, a low-calcium diet, furosemide, glucocorticoids, calcitonin, and bisphosphonates.
- Rarely, acute renal failure follows intravenous etidronate. Reduction in dose should be considered for patients with serum creatinine levels greater than 2.5 and should be withheld when the serum creatinine is above 5.0 mg/dL.
- Hypocalcemia, hypokalemia, hypomagnesemia, hypophosphatemia, and evidence of hepatic dysfunction have been reported with etidronate and pamidronate.

Questions—Bisphosphonates

1. Bisphosphonates are used to inhibit bone resorption stimulated by parathyroid hormone, calcitriol, cytokines, and prostaglandins.
A. True
B. False

2. Bisphosphonates have been used to treat Paget's disease, hypocalcemia of renal disease, and vertebral crush fractures associated with osteoporosis.
A. True
B. False

3. Bisphosphonates
A. Are synthetic analogs of pyrophosphate
B. Have a strong affinity for hydroxyapatite crystals and can promote calcification of bone
C. Inhibit growth of hydroxyapatite crystals in bone, and may impair osteoclast activity
D. All of the above
E. A and C

4. Clinical effects of bisphosphonates may include all of the following except
A. Nausea and vomiting
B. Fever
C. Leukopenia
D. Decrease in C-reactive protein
E. Pancytopenia and aplastic anemia

OXYTOCIN

Oxytocin (Pitocin®) is available as a synthetic octapeptide used to induce or stimulate labor, control postpartum uterine bleeding, and treat incomplete or inevitable abortion. Its antidiuretic properties can lead to water intoxication. An overdose of oxytocin in the mother may lead to hepatic and central nervous system damage, and death in the fetus. Treatment of an overdose is largely symptomatic and supportive. Oxytocin is related structurally and functionally to vasopressin (antidiuretic hormone) and is available in an injectable form and as a nasal spray.

Pathophysiology

Oxytocin is a cyclic peptide produced by the supraoptic and periventricular nuclei in the hypothalamus. It is stored in the posterior pituitary. For clinical use, it is available as a synthetic chemical compound. Oxytocin is a potent constrictor of uterine, placental, and umbilical cord vessels. Water intoxication is probably due to a combination of the antidiuretic effect of oxytocin and the large volumes of water sometimes used as a vehicle for oxytocin.

Pharmacokinetics

ABSORPTION

- Oxytocin concentration reaches a steady state in 30 to 60 minutes after intravenous administration.

DISTRIBUTION

- The apparent volume of distribution is 0.3 L/kg. Protein binding has not been detected.

ELIMINATION

- The half-life of oxytocin is about 10 minutes.
- Oxytocin is removed from plasma by the liver, kidney, and functioning mammary glands.

Clinical Presentations

Routine oxytocin administration has been associated with uterine rupture, antepartum fetal death, and prolonged neonatal hyperbilirubinemia. Water intoxication with seizures is caused by the antidiuretic effect of oxytocin and may occur if large doses are infused for long periods. Oxytocin in more than physiologic doses may be followed by a rapid transient fall in blood pressure as a result of peripheral vasodilation. Hepatic infarction, alveolar damage, subarachnoid bleed, and periventricular leukomalacia have been reported.

Toxic Dosage/Death

When doses of oxytocin exceed 20 to 50 mU/min, a decrease in urinary output is observed. Maternal antidiuretic effect probably is attained at doses of 45 mU/min or above. A single intravenous dose of oxytocin greater than 300 mU causes a drop in blood pressure within 1 minute, usually with subsequent recovery. A secondary rise in blood pressure may follow. At least four maternal deaths from hypertensive episodes, subarachnoid hemorrhage, and rupture of the uterus have been reported.

Drug Interactions

The use of oxytocin after prostaglandin for midtrimester abortion mimics the situation at term. The grand multiparous patient is at risk for uterine rupture if this treatment is used.

Pregnancy/Lactation

Exogenous oxytocin crosses the human placenta. High serum hepatic enzyme activity and coagulopathy may be observed in the fetus after maternal oxytocin overdose.

Laboratory

ANALYTIC METHODS

Radioimmunoassay methods are available for determination of oxytocin concentrations.

BLOOD LEVELS

Monitoring concentrations of oxytocin does not help in the management of overdose.

Treatment

- Treatment is primarily supportive. Monitor the blood pressure and pulse of both the mother and fetus. Administer oxygen to the mother and obtain obstetric consultation.
- Turning off the oxytocin, because of its short half-life, is the fundamental intervention needed to control most overdoses. Oxytocin must be discontinued immediately in case of uterine hyperactivity or fetal distress.
- Fetal heart, resting uterine tone, and frequency, duration, and force of contractions should be monitored when oxytocin is being used.
- Discontinuation of oxytocin, restriction of fluid intake, diuresis, correction of electrolyte imbalance, and control of seizures may manage water intoxication.

Questions—Oxytocin

1. Which of the following is false?
A. Oxytocin is used to induce or stimulate labor, control postpartum uterine bleeding, and to treat incomplete or inevitable abortion.
B. Its diuretic properties can lead to hyponatremia.
C. Oxytocin is related structurally and functionally to vasopressin and is available in an injectable form and as a nasal spray.
D. Oxytocin is produced by the supraoptic and periventricular nuclei in the hypothalamus.
E. Oxytocin is a potent constrictor of uterine, placental, and umbilical vessels.

2. Routine oxytocin administration has been associated with uterine rupture, antepartum fetal death, and prolonged neonatal hyperbilirubinemia.
A. True
B. False

3. Oxytocin in more than physiologic doses may be followed by a rapid transient rise in blood pressure due to peripheral vasoconstriction.
A. True
B. False

PROSTATE DRUGS

New drugs have been developed to combat the ubiquitous problems associated with prostatic enlargement. The first changes of benign prostatic hypertrophy (BPH) begin around age 35 years and consist of microscopic stromal nodules that occur around the periurethral glands. As men age, their levels of estrogen rise. This rise is related to both an absolute decrease in the level of testosterone production and an increased conversion of serum testosterone to estrogen in the peripheral adipose tissues. The stromal hyperplasia may trigger acinar hyperplasia.

Current pharmacotherapy for BPH is based on agents that relax the smooth muscles of the prostatic urethra, stroma, and those that deprive acinar cells of androgen. Selective blockade of androgen action at the prostatic cellular level includes the 5a-reductase inhibitors. These enzymes are required for intraprostatic conversion of testosterone to its active form, dihydrotestosterone.

Finasteride (Proscar®) is a specific competitive inhibitor of 5a-reductase. Serum DHT concentrations decrease to castration levels soon after finasteride therapy is initiated. It does not affect the hypothalamus-pituitary-testicular axis. Serum testosterone and luteinizing hormone concentrations increase only slightly. A median reduction in prostate volume of 19% has been noted within 3 months of the initiation of therapy. There is a significant decrease in symptoms of obstruction and an increase in maximum urinary flow rates.

Terazosin (Hytrin®) is a long-acting α-1 adrenoceptor antagonist, currently approved for the treatment of hypertension, which may decrease bladder outlet resistance in benign prostatic hypertrophy.

Pathophysiology

The clinical manifestations of BPH are related primarily to obstructive and irritative phenomena caused by prostatic enlargement and inflammation. Obstructive symptoms include hesitancy and straining to initiate urination, a diminished caliber and interrupted urinary stream, postmicturition dribbling, urinary frequency, nocturia, dysuria, and urgency.

The contractile properties of prostate smooth muscle are mediated by α-1 adrenoceptors. α-1 adrenergic antagonists are suited ideally for treatment of the dynamic component of bladder outlet obstruction because they can selectively reduce resistance along the bladder outlet without impairing detrusor contractility.

Pharmacokinetics

ABSORPTION

- Onset of action of terazosin is 15 minutes.

DISTRIBUTION

- Protein binding of terazosin is 90% to 95%.

ELIMINATION

- About 40% of metabolized finasteride are excreted in urine and 59% in stool.
- About 60% of terazosin are excreted in feces and 40% in urine.

Clinical Presentations

Prolonged use of finasteride may lead to a reduction in libido, ejaculatory disorders, and impotence. Terazosin overdose is associated with orthostatic hypotension, dizziness, syncope, lethargy, and shock. Urinary frequency and priapism have been associated with its use.

Toxic Dosage/Death

Toxic or lethal doses of finasteride or terazosin have not been reported.

Drug Interactions

Finasteride interacts little with other medications and may be safely used in patients taking α-blockers, β-blockers, theophylline, digoxin, sodium warfarin, diuretics, antiinflammatory agents, calcium-channel blockers, and H2 antagonists.

Pregnancy/Lactation

Women who are of childbearing age are advised not to encounter the semen of men who are taking finasteride, to avoid any effects on a developing fetus. Terazosin is pregnancy risk category C.

Laboratory

ANALYTIC METHODS

Assays for these agents are not routinely available in a hospital setting.

BLOOD LEVELS

Blood levels do not aid in the management of finasteride or terazosin overdose.

Treatment

GUT DECONTAMINATION

Lavage or charcoal may bind excessive finasteride or terazosin, however their clinical usefulness in overdose has not been ascertained.

ELIMINATION ENHANCEMENT

These methods have not been used in conjunction with finasteride. Dialysis most likely would be ineffective in terazosin overdose because of high protein binding.

SUPPORTIVE MEASURES

- Treatment of overdose is supportive with these agents. Specific drug therapy is not indicated.
- Hypotension induced by terazosin is managed with Trendelenburg's position, fluid boluses, and pressors such as norepinephrine, as required.

Questions—Prostate Drugs

1. **Current pharmacotherapy for benign prostatic hypertrophy is based on agents that relax the smooth muscles of the prostatic urethra, stroma, and those that deprive acinar cells of androgen.**
   A. True
   B. False
2. **Terazosin is a long-acting β-1 adrenoceptor antagonist, currently approved for the treatment of hypertension, which may decrease bladder outlet resistance in benign prostatic hypertrophy**
   A. True
   B. False
3. **As men age, their levels of estrogen rise. This rise is related to both an absolute decrease in the level of testosterone production and an increased conversion of serum testosterone to estrogen in the peripheral adipose tissues.**
   A. True
   B. False

METYRAPONE

Metyrapone (Metopirone®) is used in the investigation of anterior pituitary function in patients with suspected hypopituitarism, in the differential diagnosis and management of patients with Cushing's syndrome, and in the treatment of resistant edema associated with secondary hyperaldosteronism where it is used together with glucocorticoid. In overdose, it may cause gastrointestinal symptoms, signs of adrenocortical insufficiency, and fatalities. Metyrapone is a synthetic chemical product.

Pathophysiology

Metyrapone is an inhibitor of 11b-hydroxylase, a cytochrome P450 enzyme involved in the biosynthesis of cortisol and aldosterone. It also inhibits phenobarbital-induced cytochrome P450 enzymes. Metyrapone is associated with the inhibition of cortisol biosynthesis and elevation of plasma 11-deoxycortisol levels, demonstrating 11b-hydroxylase inhibition.

Pharmacokinetics

ABSORPTION

- The drug is well absorbed after oral ingestion.

DISTRIBUTION

- The plasma half-life following intravenous metyrapone ranges from 20 to 26 minutes.

ELIMINATION

- Metyrapone is metabolized in the liver. Less than 1% of a dose is excreted unchanged.

Clinical Presentations

Gastrointestinal symptoms and signs of acute adrenocortical insufficiency characterize the clinical picture of poisoning with metyrapone. Cardiac arrhythmias, hypotension, dehydration, anxiety, confusion, weakness, impairment of consciousness, nausea, vomiting, and epigastric pain may be observed. Alopecia has been reported in patients following long-term metyrapone therapy.

Toxic Dosage/Death

A 6-year-old was given 2 grams daily for 2 days and subsequently died in cardiac arrest.

Drug Interactions

In patients under treatment with insulin or oral antidiabetic agents, the signs and symptoms of acute poisoning with metyrapone may be aggravated.

Pregnancy/Lactation

There have been no studies regarding metyrapone during pregnancy or breast feeding.

Laboratory

ANALYTIC METHODS

A high-performance liquid chromatography method with ultraviolet detection is available.

BLOOD LEVELS

Metyrapone produces a peak plasma level of 2.7 $\mu g/mL$ at 1 hour. Plasma levels of metyrapone exceed 0.3 $\mu g/mL$ after doses of 750 mg every 4 hours. Following blood levels does not aid in the management of overdose.

Treatment

GUT DECONTAMINATION

Treatment of an overdose within a few hours of ingestion may benefit from gastric lavage and charcoal administration.

ELIMINATION ENHANCEMENT

Dialysis has not been utilized in overdose.

SUPPORTIVE MEASURES

- Support centers on the use of intravenous hydrocortisone, saline, and glucose as required.
- Patients should be monitored for several days with special attention to blood pressure, fluids, and electrolyte balance.

Questions—Metyrapone

1. Metyrapone is used in the investigation of anterior pituitary function in patients with suspected hypopituitarism, in the differential diagnosis and management of patients with Cushing's syndrome, and in the treatment of resistant edema associated with secondary hyperaldosteronism where it is used together with glucocorticoid.
A. True
B. False

2. Metyrapone is an inhibitor of a cytochrome P450 enzyme involved in the biosynthesis of cortisol and aldosterone.
A. True
B. False

3. Alopecia has been reported in several patients following long-term metyrapone therapy.
A. True
B. False

Answers

Insulin

1. C 2. B 3. D 4. E 5. A

Sulfonylureas

1. A 2. A 3. B 4. E 5. A

Biguanides

1. C 2. A 3. B

Thyroid Hormones

1. A 2. A 3. A 4. B

Antithyroid Drugs

1. C

Desmopressin

1. A 2. A 3. E

Steroids

1. D 2. A 3. D 4. B 5. A

Danazol

1. B 2. B

Fertility Drugs

1. C 2. C

Mifepristone

1. B

Octreotide and Somatostatin

1. E 2. A 3. B

Bisphosphonates

1. A 2. B 3. E 4. D

Oxytocin

1. B 2. A 3. B

Prostate Drugs

1. A 2. B 3. A

Metyrapone

1. A 2. A 3. A

SELECTED READINGS

Insulin

1. Bauman WA, Yalow RS. Insulin as a lethal weapon. J Forens Sci 1981;26:594–598.
2. Gorden P. Human insulin and hypoglycemia. N Engl J Med 1990;322:1007–1008.
3. Roberge RJ, Martin TG, Delbridge TR. Intentional massive insulin overdose. Ann Emerg Med 1993;22:228–234.
4. Service FJ. Hyperglycemic disorders. N Engl J Med 1995;332:1144–1152.

Sulfonylureas

1. Asmal AC, Marble A. Oral hypoglycaemic agents: An update. Drugs 1984;28:62–78.
2. Bobzien WF III. Suicidal overdoses with hypoglycemic agents. JACEP J Am Coll Emerg Physicians 1979;8:467–470.
3. Crowson TW, Kriel RL. Hypoglycemia from inadvertent use of hypoglycemic agents. Ann Intern Med 1980;92:134.
4. Lacouture PG. Oral hypoglycemics. Clin Toxicicol Rev 1984;7(3):1–2.
5. Palatnick W, Meatherall RC, Tenenbein M. Clinical spectrum of sulfonylurea overdose and experience with diazoxide therapy. Arch Intern Med 1991;151:1859–1862.
6. Peden N, Newton RW, Feely J. Oral hypoglycaemic agents. Br Med J 1983;286:1564–1567.
7. Spiller HA, Villalobos D, Krenzelok EP, et al. Prospective multicenter study of sulfonylurea ingestion in children. Clin Toxicol 1995;33:475–485 (Abstract 60).

Biguanides

1. Crofford OB. Metformin. N Engl J Med 1995;333:588–589.
2. DeFronzo RA, Goodman AM, Multicenter Metformin Study Group. Efficacy of metformin in patients with non-insulin-dependent diabetes mellitus. N Engl J Med 1995;333:541–549.
3. Paterson KR, Paice BJ, Lawson DH. Undesired effects of biguanide therapy. Adverse Drug React Acute Poison Rev 1984;3:173–182.

Thyroid Hormones

1. Lewander WJ, Lacouture PG, Silva JE, et al. Acute thyroxine ingesiton in pediatric patients. Pediatrics 1989;48:262–265.
2. Litovitz TL, White JD. Levothyroxine ingestions in children: An analysis of 78 cases. Am J Emerg Med 1985;3:297–300.
3. Singh GK, Winterborn MH. Massive overdose with thyroxine: Toxicity and treatment. Eur J Pediatr 1991;150:217–218.
4. Tunget CL, Turchen SG, Manoguerra AS, Clark RF. Determination of an acute safe exposure dose in overdoses for thyroid containing products. Vet Hum Toxicol 1993;35:348.

Antithyroid Drugs

1. Lin T-H, Kirkland RT, Kirkland JL. Clinical features and management of overdosage with thyroid drugs. Med Toxicol 1988;3:264–272.
2. Romaldini JN, Werner MC, Bromberg N, Werner RS. Adverse effects related to antithyroid drugs and their dose regimen. Exp Clin Endocrinol 1991;97:261–264.

Desmopressin

1. Desmopressin acetate. In Dollery C, ed. Therapeutic Drugs. Edinburgh: Churchill Livingstone, 1991:D37–D40.
2. Richardson DW, Robinson AG. Desmopressin. Ann Intern Med 1985;103:228–239.

Steroids

1. Beggs EJ, Atkinson HC, Gianarkis N. The pharmacokinetics of corticosteroid agents. Med J Aust 1987;146:37–41.
2. Frey BM, Frey FJ. Clinical pharmacokinetics of prednisone and prednisolone. Clin Pharmacokinet 1990;19:126–146.
3. Johnson MD. Anabolic steroid use in adolescent athletes. Pediatr Clin North Am 1990;37:1111–1123.
4. Shenfield GM, Griffin JM, Griffin JM. Clinical pharmacokinetics of contraceptive steroids: An update. Clin Pharmacokinet 1991;20:15–37.
5. Uzych L. Anabolic androgenic steroids and psychiatric-related effects: A review. Can J Psychiatry 1992;37:23–28.

Danazol

1. Donaldson VH. Danazol. Am J Med 1989;87:3(N)49N–55N.
2. Potts GO, Schane HP, Edelson J. Pharmacology and pharmacokinetics of danazol. Drugs 1980;19:321–331.

Fertility Drugs

1. Derman SG, Adashi EY. Adverse effects of fertility drugs. Drug Saf 1994;11:408–421.
2. Giusti RM, Iwamoto K, Hatch EE. Diethylstilbestrol revisited: A review of the long-term health effects. Ann Intern Med 1995;122:778–788.

Mifepristone

1. Baulieu EE. RU-486 as an antiprogesterone steroid: From receptor to contragestion and beyond. JAMA 1989;262:1808–1814.
2. Reproductive health and mifepristone. Lancet 1990;336:1480–1481. Editorial.
3. Segal SJ. Mifepristone (RU-486). N Engl J Med 1990;322:691–693.

Octreotide and Somatostatin

1. Dollery CT, ed. Therapeutic Drugs. Edinburgh: Churchill Livingstone, 1991:O1–O4.
2. Octreotide for endocrine tumours. Drug Ther Bull 1991;29(5):19–20.
3. Torres AJ, Landa I, Hernandez F, et al. Somatostatin in the treatment of severe upper gastrointestinal bleeding: A multicentre controlled trial. Br J Surg 1986;73:786–789.

Bisphosphonates

1. Compston JE. The therapeutic use of bisphosphonates. Br Med J 1994;309:711–715.

Oxytocin

1. Pauerstein CJ. Use and abuse of oxytocic agents. Clin Obstet Gynecol 1973;16:262–277.
2. Petrie RH. The pharmacology and use of oxytocin. Clin Perinatol 1981;8:35–47.

Prostate Drugs

1. Hill SJ, Lawrence SL, Lepor H. New use for alpha blockers: Benign prostatic hyperplasia. Amer Fam Phys 1994;45:1885–1888.
2. Lowe FC. Safety assessment of terazosin in the treatment of patients with symptomatic benign prostatic hyperplasia. A combined analysis. Urology 1994;44:46–51.
3. Narayan P, Indudhara R. Pharmacotherapy for benign prostatic hyperplasia. West J Med 1994;161:495–501.

Metyrapone

1. Harries-Jones R, Overstall P. Metyrapone-induced alopecia. Postgrad Med J 1990;66:584.
2. Reynolds JEF, ed. Martindale: The Extra Pharmacopoeia. 30th ed. London: Pharmaceutical Press, 1993:776.

CHAPTER 30

Gastrointestinal Toxicology

INTRODUCTION

The treatment of gastrointestinal maladies has exploded in the last 20 years. Drug treatment previously was restricted to antacids, anticholinergics, antispasmodics, cathartics, and laxatives. Recently, histamine H2-receptor antagonists (e.g., cimetidine, ranitidine, famotidine, and nizatidine) have emerged as useful products for the treatment of peptic acid disorders. Proton pump inhibitors (e.g., omeprazole), prostaglandin analogs (e.g., misoprostol), site-protective drugs (e.g., bismuth subsalicylate and sucralfate), antiemetics with prokinetic properties (e.g., metoclopramide, domperidone, and cisapride), antiinflammatory salicylates (e.g., sulfasalazine), and nonspecific antidiarrheal agents (diphenoxylate and loperamide) also are in current use.

With the exception of diphenoxylate in children (see Chapter 23, Opiates), overdose from these agents is usually not fatal, although serious multisystem effects have been observed.

ANTIINFLAMMATORY SALICYLATES

Sulfasalazine, originally developed for the treatment of rheumatoid arthritis, combines one of the first sulfonamides, sulfapyridine, with an aspirin analog, 5-aminosalicylate (5-ASA). Sulfasalazine is widely used in the treatment of inflammatory bowel disease. Its use is limited by a degree of intolerance and frequent adverse reactions, most of which were attributed to the serum sulfapyridine levels. Sulfasalazine also may be useful in treating Crohn's disease, scleroderma, and ankylosing spondylitis.

Pathophysiology

The parent drug, sulfasalazine, delivers the active component, 5-ASA, to distal disease sites. Unsplit sulfasalazine inhibits prostaglandin synthesis, prostaglandin degradation, and thromboxane synthesis, as well as interfering with neutrophil chemotaxis and scavenging radicals. The therapeutic importance of these actions is unclear. As the sulfa moiety is responsible for the toxicity of the drug and the 5-ASA moiety for its therapeutic efficacy, 5-ASA is modified to be delivered to areas of diseased bowel. Oral 5-ASA agents appear to be as effective prophylactically for ulcerative colitis as topical 5-ASA and sulfasalazine.

Pharmacokinetics

ABSORPTION

- 10% to 15% is absorbed unchanged.
- Most sulfasalazine acts topically at segments of diseased bowel.

DISTRIBUTION

- Only small amounts appear in stool or breast milk.
- Half-life is 6 to 10 hours.

ELIMINATION

- Sulfasalazine is excreted in urine after acetylation in the liver.

Clinical Presentations

While sulfasalazine generally is considered safe and nontoxic, adverse effects may include dizziness, confusion, anorexia, nausea, vomiting, hepatitis, jaundice, pneumonitis, renal failure, marrow suppression and rash. Massive sulfasalazine ingestion may be associated with seizures and ketosis. Subclinical methemoglobinemia secondary to the sulfa moiety may occur. Adverse effects associated with mesalazine, another antiinflammatory salicylate, include headache, nausea, dizziness, indigestion, muscle aches, fever, skin and cardiac hypersensitivity reactions, interstitial nephritis, pancreatitis, thrombocytopenia, and aplastic anemia.

Toxic Dosage/Death

One 23-year-old man who ingested 25 g of sulfasalazine tablets was treated with gastric lavage, activated charcoal, sorbitol, and intravenous dextrose with sodium bicarbonate. He survived with few ill effects.

Drug Interactions

Sulfasalazine may decrease digoxin absorption, the effect of anticoagulants and hypoglycemics.

Pregnancy/Lactation

Pregnancy risk category B (D at term).

Treatment

GUT DECONTAMINATION

Treatment with multiple dose activated charcoal is warranted, as little is absorbed. Cholestyramine also may reduce absorption.

ELIMINATION ENHANCEMENT

Hemodialysis has not been attempted in sulfasalazine overdoses.

SUPPORTIVE MEASURES

- Hypersensitivity reactions or anaphylactic effects caused by the sulfa moiety may be treated with antihistamines, steroids and epinephrine in severe cases.
- Blood levels have not been shown helpful in guiding therapy.
- N-acetylcysteine has been used to treat sulfasalazine-induced hepatitis, however conclusive studies to measure this intervention have not been undertaken.

Questions—Antiinflammatory Salicylates

1. **Sulfasalazine does all of the following except**
   A. Inhibits prostaglandin synthesis
   B. Decreases absorption of digoxin
   C. Inhibits cytochrome P450 oxidase activity
   D. Interferes with neutrophil chemotaxis and savaging radicals
   E. A and C

Answers to questions in shaded boxes appear at the end of the chapter.

2. **The active moiety of sulfasalazine is responsible for most of the drug's side effects.**
   A. True
   B. False

3. **Overdose of sulfasalazine**
   A. Is rarely fatal and treatment is supportive
   B. Is best treated with hemodialysis
   C. Treatment is guided by serum levels at 4 hours after ingestion
   D. May paradoxically get worse with use of activated charcoal
   E. All of the above

LOPERAMIDE

Loperamide (Imodium®) is a piperidine-derivative antidiarrheal agent. Overdoses and fatalities have occurred in infants. Overdose may lead to constipation, ileus, and neurologic symptoms including miosis, hypotonia, somnolence, and bradypnea. Naloxone is an effective antidote.

Pathophysiology

Loperamide appears to exert its antisecretory effect via opiate receptors. Unlike diphenoxylate or codeine, loperamide does not appear to exert opiate activity in humans at normal therapeutic doses.

Pharmacokinetics

ABSORPTION

- Bioavailability is about 100%.

DISTRIBUTION

- Peak plasma level is 0.75 ng/mL after 4 mg. Time to peak plasma level is around 4 hours.
- Plasma protein binding is 97%.

ELIMINATION

- Elimination half-life is 7 to 15 hours.
- About 1% is excreted unchanged.

Clinical Presentations

In overdose, disorientation, lethargy, hallucinations, inability to walk, miotic pupils, bradypnea, toxic megacolon, and coma have been observed. Nausea, abdominal cramping, dizziness, rash, and dry mouth occasionally have been reported in chronic users. One study suggests that loperamide has little abuse potential.

Drug Interactions

No specific studies on loperamide drug interactions are available. Concomitant use of narcotics increases the tendency toward bradypnea, muscular hypotonia, somnolence, and miosis.

Pregnancy/Lactation

There are no adequate studies of loperamide in pregnancy or during lactation.

Laboratory

ANALYTIC METHODS

A radioimmunoassay for loperamide is available. The loperamide antibody does not bind to structurally related drugs such as haloperidol, diphenoxylate, and difenoxin.

BLOOD LEVELS

Blood levels do not contribute to the treatment of loperamide overdose.

Treatment

GUT DECONTAMINATION

Gastric lavage should be instituted in overdose. Activated charcoal slurry, 1 g/kg, can be administered through a nasogastric tube. If vomiting has occurred spontaneously, activated charcoal slurry can be administered orally as soon as fluids are retained. 24-hour observation may not be necessary in children with small overdoses after gastric decontamination.

ELIMINATION ENHANCEMENT

Forced diuresis is not expected to be effective in loperamide overdose, as relatively little drug is excreted in the urine. There have been no studies on the use of hemodialysis or hemoperfusion in loperamide overdose.

SUPPORTIVE MEASURES

- Infants with loperamide overdose should be admitted to a pediatric intensive care facility where continuous monitoring of vital signs can be performed and where access to oxygen, intravenous fluids, and naloxone are available.
- Respiratory assistance by mechanical ventilation may be required in severe cases.
- Patients must be monitored for the recurrence of symptoms of drug overdose for at least 24 hours after the last dose of naloxone.
- The plasma potassium level should be monitored frequently in any sick infant receiving loperamide as hypokalemia may predispose to ileus in some infants.

Antidotes

NALOXONE

Naloxone is an effective antidote and may be administered if central nervous system depression occurs. Because the duration of action of loperamide is greater than that of naloxone, the patient must be watched closely and additional doses of naloxone administered as required. Vital signs should be monitored for recurrence of symptoms of drug overdose for at least 24 hours after the last dose of naloxone is administered.

Questions—Loperamide

1. **The following toxicities are reported consequences of loperamide overdose except**
   A. Ileus
   B. Constipation
   C. Mydriasis
   D. Somnolence
   E. Hypotonia

2. **Which of the following statements about loperamide is/are true except**
   A. Elimination half-life is 7 to 15 hours
   B. It exerts its antisecretory effect via opiate receptors
   C. Naloxone is not useful as an antidote
   D. Infant fatalities have been reported
   E. All of the above
3. **Loperamide**
   A. Has little abuse potential
   B. Has not demonstrated cardiac toxicity in overdose
   C. Blood levels are not helpful in managing overdose.
   D. All of the above
   E. None of the above

MISOPROSTOL

Nonsteroidal antiinflammatory drugs (NSAIDs) can cause acute upper gastrointestinal tract bleeding, primarily by inhibiting prostaglandin synthesis. Misoprostol (Cytotec®) is a prostaglandin analog. It is a water-soluble, viscous liquid that may induce fetal death and systemic symptoms. Patients have recovered from overdose with symptomatic and supportive treatment. Misoprostol has been approved for the prevention of NSAID-induced gastric ulcers in patients at high risk of complications from gastric ulcer. Misoprostol is taken for the duration of NSAID therapy.

Pathophysiology

Nonsteroidal antiinflammatory drugs inhibit prostaglandin synthesis. A deficiency in prostaglandins in the gastric mucosa may contribute to the mucosal damage caused by NSAIDs by decreasing bicarbonate and mucus secretion. Prostaglandin E1 has an antisecretory effect in gastric acid production however, it is not effective orally, has a short duration of action, and has undesirable side effects. Misoprostol is a prostaglandin E1 analog that has a greater oral activity, a longer duration of action, and a more selective effect. Unfortunately, NSAIDs still may induce gastric ulcers or gastrointestinal bleeding, even in patients receiving misoprostol therapy.

Pharmacokinetics

ABSORPTION

- Bioavailability is 88%. Time to peak plasma level is 30 minutes.
- Peak plasma level is 500 μg / mL after 400 mg is ingested orally.

DISTRIBUTION

- Volume of distribution is 12 L / kg
- Plasma protein binding is 80% to 90%

ELIMINATION

- Elimination half-life is 20 to 40 minutes.
- Active metabolites include misoprostol acid.

Clinical Presentations

In overdose, patients may experience hyperthermia, chills, shortness of breath, nausea, and abdominal cramps, but may remain alert, oriented, and coherent. Chronic misoprostol use may yield diarrhea, cramping, abdominal pain, nausea, vomiting, delirium, urinary incontinence, and headache.

Toxic Dosage/Death

A fatal dose in humans has not been established. As much as 1.6 g of misoprostol daily has been tolerated with only mild gastrointestinal discomfort. An elderly woman accidentally ingested 15, 200-mg tablets of misoprostol and recovered with supportive care.

Drug Interactions

Misoprostol does not alter the toxicokinetics of concomitantly administered ibuprofen, aspirin, or diclofenac. Misoprostol does not appear to interfere with the metabolism of drugs, such as diazepam and propranolol, by the hepatic cytochrome P450 microsomal enzyme system.

Pregnancy/Lactation

Misoprostol has abortifacient properties and is contraindicated in pregnant women. Misoprostol has been known to induce labor, however is not considered safe for inducing uterine bleeding or spontaneous abortion. It is frequently ineffective and may expose the fetus to possible risk of severe malformation. Ingestion of 400 to 600 mg orally and / or vaginally in the first trimester of pregnancy may cause a malformation consisting of localized skull defects. It is not known whether misoprostol or its acid metabolite is excreted in breast milk.

Laboratory

ANALYTIC METHODS

Misoprostol and its major active metabolite, misoprostol acid, can be estimated by radioimmunoassay with a detection limit of 23 ng / L.

BLOOD LEVELS

Blood levels of misoprostol are not useful, not easy to obtain, and not predictive of clinical course.

Treatment

GUT DECONTAMINATION

The rapid absorption of misoprostol and rapid peak plasma concentrations (30 minutes) lessens the usefulness of gastric emptying procedures. If the patient presents close to the time of ingestion or if the history is in doubt, gastric emptying with tracheal protection may be useful. Activated charcoal may be administered but there are no data to support its effectiveness.

ELIMINATION ENHANCEMENT

It is unlikely that dialysis or hemoperfusion would be useful given the high volume of distribution.

SUPPORTIVE MEASURES

- Treatment of misoprostol overdose is largely symptomatic and supportive. All overdose patients, whether pregnant or not, should be seen in an emergency care facility and be afforded access to cardiac monitoring, a source of oxygen, and an intravenous line.
- Laboratory tests should include serum electrolytes, blood urea nitrogen, creatinine, glucose, and creatine kinase. Arterial blood gases should be drawn and followed if there is evidence of acidosis or hypoxia.
- Diarrhea may be ameliorated with psyllium hydrophilic colloid.

Questions—Misoprostol

1. **Which of the following statements are true?**
   1. Misoprostol is a prostaglandin inhibitor.
   2. A deficiency in prostaglandins in the gastric mucosa may contribute to NSAID-induced mucosal damage.
   3. Misoprostol has been approved for the prevention of NSAID-induced gastric ulcers.
   4. Misoprostol is relatively safe in pregnancy.

   A. 1, 2, and 3
   B. 1, 2, and 4
   C. 1, 3, and 4
   D. 2, 3, and 4
   E. All of the above
2. **Which of the following statements regarding misoprostol overdose is/are true?**
   A. Patients may present with hyperthermia, shortness of breath, nausea, and abdominal cramps.
   B. The hepatic cytochrome P450 microsomal enzyme system is inhibited in overdose.
   C. Blood levels are not useful in management or in predicting outcome.
   D. Activated charcoal may be administered however, there is no data to support its effectiveness.
   E. A, C, and D
3. **Psyllium hydrophilic colloid has been established as an antidote for misoprostol overdose.**
   A. True
   B. False

PROTON PUMP INHIBITORS

Omeprazole (Prilosec®) is used to treat gastroesophageal reflux disease (GERD), including severe erosive esophagitis and poorly responsive symptomatic GERD. It also may be useful in some pathologic hypersecretory conditions such as Zollinger-Ellison syndrome, multiple endocrine adenomas, and systemic mastocytosis. Omeprazole has also been used for stress-induced gastric mucosal hemorrhage and in duodenal ulcer disease.

Lansoprazole (Prevacid®), a proton pump inhibitor similar to omeprazole, has been approved by the Food and Drug Administration for short-term treatment of active duodenal ulcer and erosive reflux esophagitis and for long-term treatment of chronic hypersecretory conditions, including Zollinger-Ellison syndrome.

Pathophysiology

Omeprazole is concentrated selectively in the parietal cells where it acts as a noncompetitive inhibitor of H^+/K^+ ATPase. Lansoprazole, like omeprazole, is a benzimidazole derivative that binds to H^+/K^+ ATPase at the surface of the gastric parietal cell, inhibiting the final step in secretion of hydrogen ions into the gastric lumen.

Pharmacokinetics

Omeprazole

ABSORPTION

- Bioavailability is 30% to 60%. Time to peak plasma level is 1.5 hours.
- Peak plasma level is 50 to 4,000 μg/L (after 10 to 60 mg orally)

DISTRIBUTION

- Volume of distribution is 0.3 L/kg. Plasma protein binding is 95%.

ELIMINATION

- Elimination half-life is approximately 1 hour.

Lansoprazole

ABSORPTION

- In the fasting state, about 80% of the dose of lansoprazole, compared with 50% of omeprazole, reaches the systemic circulation, where it is 97% bound to plasma proteins.
- A single dose of lansoprazole inhibits 80% to 97% of acid secretion in healthy volunteers.

DISTRIBUTION

- Plasma concentrations peak in 1 to 2 hours.

ELIMINATION

- The drug is metabolized in the liver to two main metabolites, lansoprazole sulfone and hydroxylansoprazole. Plasma half-life is about 1.5 hours.
- Lansoprazole has not been recovered from the urine in an unchanged form.

Clinical Presentations

Acute omeprazole overdose may be associated with drowsiness, diaphoresis, headache, blurred vision, and dry mouth. Symptoms typically recede within 3 hours. Chronic users may have myopathy, hemolytic anemia, gynecomastia, headache, diarrhea, abdominal pain, nausea, painful erections, fulminant hepatic failure, gastric polyposis, and/or peripheral neuropathy. Abdominal pain, nausea, and diarrhea have been reported with lansoprazole use. Headache, dizziness, skin rashes, and respiratory tract symptoms may also be observed. Suppression of acid secretion may predispose to enteric infection and may increase the endogenous generation of potential carcinogens.

Toxic Dosage/Death

Doses of up to 400 mg/day of omeprazole have been well tolerated with no serious adverse effects. There have been no reports of fatal doses for these agents.

Drug Interactions

Benzimidazole compounds, such as lansoprazole and omeprazole, partially inhibit the oxidative metabolism of drugs metabolized by the cytochrome P450 enzyme subfamily IIC, such as diazepam and phenytoin. Ataxia has been described when omeprazole is used with benzodiazepines. Catatonia has been reported with concomitant disulfiram use. There have been no reports of clinically relevant interactions between lansoprazole and propranolol, warfarin, prednisone, prednisolone, or theophylline. Sucralfate delays absorption of lansoprazole.

Pregnancy/Lactation

These agents fall within Pregnancy risk category C. No fetotoxic effects have been described.

Laboratory

ANALYTIC METHODS

These methods routinely are not available in hospital laboratories.

BLOOD LEVELS

Suppression of acid secretion is not correlated with plasma omeprazole concentration. Maximum serious lansoprazole concentrations of 0.75 to 1.15 mg/L are reached within 1.5 to 2.0 hours of oral administration.

Treatment

GUT DECONTAMINATION

The stomach may be emptied if the patient is seen within 4 hours of ingestion, however clinical studies to support this or charcoal intervention are currently lacking.

ELIMINATION ENHANCEMENT

Omeprazole is extensively protein bound and therefore is not readily dialyzable.

SUPPORTIVE MEASURES

- With lansoprazole overdose, increases have been observed in serum gastrin levels, liver enzymes, hematocrit, hemoglobin, urinary protein excretion, and uric acid levels.
- Treatment is similar to that for omeprazole.

Questions—Proton Pump Inhibitors

1. All of the following are true statements except

A. Lansoprazole and omeprazole are highly protein bound in serum.
B. Both omeprazole and lansoprazole inhibit oxidative metabolism of the P450 enzyme system.
C. Elimination half-life of lansoprazole and omeprazole is greater than 6 hours.
D. There is no antidote available for omeprazole and lansoprazole overdosage.
E. All are true.

2. In omeprazole overdose,

1. Fatality rarely, if ever, occurs.
2. Doses up to 400 mg per day of omeprazole have been well tolerated.
3. Acute toxic symptoms may include drowsiness, diaphoresis, headache, blurred vision, and dry mouth.
4. Dialysis has no role in the management of overdose.

A. 1, 2, and 3
B. 1, 2, and 4
C. 1, 3, and 4
D. 2, 3, and 4
E. All of the above.

3. Which of the following statements is not true?

A. Lansoprazole is metabolized in the kidney to two main metabolites.
B. Suppression of acid secretion may predispose to enteric infection.
C. A single dose of lansoprazole inhibits 80% to 97% of acid secretion in healthy volunteers.
D. No fetotoxic effects have been described with use of proton-pump inhibitors.
E. All are true.

ANTACIDS

Antacids generally are well tolerated, and often are considered nontoxic. However, over-the-counter remedies such as Tums® and Alka-Seltzer® contain calcium and aspirin, respectively and, in overdose, may yield serious morbidity. See Chapter 11, Salicylates. Antacid therapy is widely used prophylactically in pediatric intensive care units to prevent stress ulcers. It has been used in the medical management of gastric bleeding in newborn infants and adults. Complications in the neonatal setting have been described.

Pathophysiology

Antacids represent a broad range of substances that generally neutralize stomach acid.

Clinical Presentations

Complications of antacid therapy in the newborn infant include hypotonia, difficulty arousing, asymptomatic hypermagnesemia without hypercalcemia, and aluminum hydroxide bezoar formation. The serum magnesium level may be elevated and may be accompanied by an elevated serum calcium level. In adults, overuse of calcium carbonate, particularly in those afflicted with baseline hyperparathyroidism, may yield symptomatic hypercalcemia. Fatigue, anorexia, nausea, vomiting, elevated blood pressure, hemoconcentration, leukocytosis, metabolic alkalosis, elevated body weight, and hypokalemia all have been described.

Magnesium hydroxide or aluminum hydroxide use may cause phosphate depletion, nephrolithiasis, and ureteral obstruction. Nausea and diarrhea may occur even with therapeutic doses. Biochemical features of overuse may include hypophosphatemia, hypercalcemia, elevated plasma 1,2-dihydroxyvitamin D level, and decreased parathyroid hormone. Osteomalacia and osteitis fibrosa may also follow long-term antacid ingestion. Hypermagnesemia and elevated aluminum levels may be seen in patients with renal failure.

Toxic Dosage/Death

Specific toxic dosages of the various antacids have not been established.

Drug Interactions

Antacids may decrease the effect of digoxin, fluorides, certain nonsteroidal antiinflammatory agents, ketoconazole, and tetracycline by decreasing absorption of these agents.

Treatment

GUT DECONTAMINATION

Gut decontamination measures generally are not necessary as absorption tends to be rapid, and effects generally are well managed with supportive care alone.

ELIMINATION ENHANCEMENT

While electrolyte abnormalities theoretically may be managed with dialysis, such intervention has not been used to manage antacid use misadventures.

SUPPORTIVE MEASURES

- Diarrhea is managed effectively by discontinuing these agents and by "firming" up bowel contents with foods such as bananas or rice.

- Electrolyte abnormalities are managed via frequent serum determinations and fluid replacement.
- Hypophosphatemia may be managed with oral or intravenous supplementation.
- Hypercalcemia is managed with fluids, steroids, and other agents.
- Intravenous calcium gluconate, potassium, and glucose infusion may lead to a fall in magnesium concentration.

Questions—Antacids

1. **Complications of antacid therapy in the newborn can include all except**
   A. Aluminum hydroxide bezoar formation
   B. Hypotonia
   C. Polycythemia
   D. Hypermagnesemia
   E. Hypercalcemia
2. **Complications of antacids in adults can include all except**
   A. Hypercalcemia
   B. Porcelain gallbladder
   C. Hypophosphatemia
   D. Osteomalacia and osteitis fibrosa
   E. Nephrolithiasis

H2 RECEPTOR ANTAGONISTS

Conventional antihistamines antagonize certain histamine-induced responses. Receptors mediating antihistamine actions are known as H1 receptors. Other histamine-induced responses (e.g., gastric acid secretion) are blocked by H2 antagonists. Cimetidine and ranitidine are examples of the H2 antagonist group. Overdoses with cimetidine are not common but can be serious.

H2 receptors were discovered in 1972 and, with their discovery, came a revolution in the management of excess stomach acid secretion. The Food and Drug Administration approved the use of cimetidine in 1977 for the treatment of patients with duodenal ulcer disease, Zollinger-Ellison syndrome, and other hypersecretory states. At one point, H2 receptor antagonists became the largest selling drugs in the world.

Cimetidine

Cimetidine (Tagamet®) is used for short-term treatment of duodenal ulcer, prophylactic use to prevent duodenal ulcer recurrences in patients likely to need surgical treatment, short-term treatment of active benign gastric ulcers, and treatment of pathological hypersecretory conditions such as Zollinger-Ellison syndrome, systemic mastocytosis, and multiple endocrine adenomas.

PATHOPHYSIOLOGY

Cimetidine, a synthetic chemical, is structurally similar to histamine. It has an imidazole ring, like histamine, with a longer side chain. H1 antagonists do not have either an imidazole ring, like histamine or cimetidine, or a furan ring like ranitidine.

PHARMACOKINETICS

Absorption

- Cimetidine can be given orally, intravenously, and intramuscularly. It is completely absorbed after oral administration.
- Peak blood levels after a 300-mg dose with a meal occur in 45 to 90 minutes, and blood levels remain over 0.5 μg/mL for at least 4 hours.
- Two peaks have been reported, the first during the first 2 hours and the second in 3 to 5 hours.
- An oral dose of 300 mg raises basal gastric pH to at least 5.0 for more than 2 hours in most patients.
- Over 90% inhibition of acid secretion occurs for 4 hours after administration.

Distribution

- About 13% to 25% is plasma protein bound. The apparent volume of distribution is 1.4 to 4.3 L/kg.

Elimination

- About 15% of cimetidine is metabolized in the liver. The elimination half-life is 1.9 to 2.2 hours.
- 70% is excreted unchanged in the urine, with fecal losses accounting for approximately 10%.

CLINICAL PRESENTATIONS

Overdoses may be associated with dizziness, confusion, disorientation, and drowsiness, with or without sweating and flushing. Cardiovascular findings are rare. One large review of overdoses with up to 15 g of cimetidine revealed an absence of symptoms in 79%. There were no major medical complications and no fatalities in both children and adults. A few patients exhibited vomiting, bradycardia, and drowsiness, all of which were minor and without sequelae.

Neurologic Effects

Cimetidine penetrates the blood-brain barrier and may be associated with somnolence, confusion, restlessness, lethargy, agitation, visual hallucinations, seizures, and slurred speech. Such symptoms are seen more frequently in the elderly and very young and in those with renal or liver disease. In some cases, very high plasma cimetidine concentrations after overdosage in otherwise normal patients have not been associated with central nervous system toxicity.

Hematologic Effects

Granulocytopenia and neutropenia occasionally has been observed but may be complicated by the presence of serious underlying disease or the use of other drugs. Thrombocytopenia and aplastic anemia rarely have been observed.

Renal Effects

Transient rises in serum creatinine have been observed after therapeutic doses. An acute interstitial nephritis has followed cimetidine use but may be a hypersensitivity reaction.

Endocrine Effects

Gynecomastia, antiandrogen effects, a decrease in plasma testosterone, and a rise in serum prolactin have been observed inconsistently.

Cardiovascular Effects

The myocardium and peripheral blood vessels that possess H2 receptors. Stimulation of such receptors results in positive inotropic and chronotropic responses. Cimetidine has been associated with bradycardia, hypotension, sinus arrest, and cardiac arrest after rapid intravenous infusion. Cardiovascular toxicity is rare.

Gastrointestinal Effects

Reactions reported in the liver reflect hypersensitivity. Cimetidine can cause partial or complete healing of malignant gastric ulcers. There is no convincing evidence to support the position that cimetidine is carcinogenic. One study suggested that users of H2 antagonists appear to be predisposed to *Salmonella* infections.

TOXIC DOSAGE/DEATH

Serious drug reactions are relatively uncommon. Normal persons have ingested massive amounts of cimetidine without neurologic symptoms. 20-g ingestions of cimetidine have been well tolerated, while a 24-g ingestion in a 39-year-old resulted in death.

DRUG INTERACTIONS

Cimetidine, like other substituted imidazole compounds, inhibits the cytochrome P450 mixed-function oxidase involved in hepatic metabolism of certain drugs. It also reduces hepatic blood flow and may impede elimination of drugs such as propranolol that are metabolized in the liver. Cimetidine affects the hepatic oxidative metabolism of many drugs, but usually does not affect the conjugation reaction. It also does not appear to affect the glucuronide conjugation of drugs such as oxazepam and morphine. The propensity of cimetidine to inhibit hepatic drug metabolism probably is related to the imidazole ring in its structure, similar to other drugs with an imidazole structure that are known to be inhibitors of drug metabolism (e.g., ketoconazole, miconazole, itraconazole, metronidazole, omeprazole).

High-potency antacids inhibit the absorption of cimetidine when the two are taken together. Serum lidocaine levels rise and the volume of distribution and clearance fall when cimetidine is administered simultaneously. Increased symptoms of lidocaine toxicity may be experienced when the two are administered simultaneously. Cimetidine may prolong the effects of anticoagulants, benzodiazepines, β-blockers, digoxin, procainamide, verapamil, caffeine, carbamazepine, salicylates, metronidazole, quinidine, morphine, and theophylline and is associated with changes in the hepatic oxidative metabolism of many of these drugs. Such interactions (e.g., with benzodiazepines) may have minimal clinical importance.

PREGNANCY/LACTATION

Cimetidine crosses the placenta and is secreted in human milk. No overdose studies in pregnancy have been reported. Initial data on the use of H2-receptor antagonists (cimetidine and ranitidine) suggest that these compounds are not teratogenic in humans.

LABORATORY

Analytic Methods

A method using high-performance liquid chromatography is available.

Blood Levels

Plasma cimetidine values do not appear to correlate well with symptoms and are difficult to obtain from the average clinical laboratory. In one series of eight cimetidine overdoses in which all patients recovered, blood concentrations ranged from 18.7 to 57 μg/mL.

TREATMENT

Gut Decontamination

If not more than 4 hours have elapsed since ingestion of the drug, activated charcoal may be useful, however studies to confirm its clinical efficacy are not available.

Elimination Enhancement

There is no evidence that forced diuresis enhances excretion of cimetidine. No studies support the effectiveness of hemoperfusion or hemodialysis.

Supportive Measures

- In view of the occasional report of cardiac problems despite the apparent lack of toxicity of cimetidine, it is prudent to ascertain the airway, breathing, and circulatory status of the patient on admission and observe for seizures and dysrhythmias.
- Seizures are treated with intravenous benzodiazepines.
- Arrhythmias are treated with usual antiarrhythmic medications (e.g., atropine for bradycardias, lidocaine for ventricular arrhythmias). Limited experience with overdose treatment precludes recommendation for use of specific agents.
- Laboratory monitoring for adverse reactions to therapeutic dosage may include a complete blood count including platelets, liver and renal function tests, and prothrombin times if an oral anticoagulant is also taken. Significant laboratory abnormalities after overdose with cimetidine have not been reported.
- Clinical symptoms may also dictate electrocardiogram (ECG) monitoring or endocrine assays.

Questions—Cimetidine

1. Which of the following statements are true about cimetidine pharmacokinetics?

1. Over 90% inhibition of acid secretion occurs for 4 hours after ingestion.
2. Approximately 90% is plasma bound to protein.
3. 70% is excreted unchanged in the urine.
4. The elimination half-life in man is approximately 2 hours.

A. 1, 2, and 3
B. 1, 2, and 4
C. 1, 3, and 4
D. 2, 3, and 4
E. All of the above

2. The following toxicities have been reported with cimetidine overdose except

A. Seizures
B. Somnolence
C. Visual hallucinations
D. Pancreatitis
E. Elevation in serum creatinine

3. Which of the following statements about cimetidine are true?

1. There are no antidotes available for cimetidine.
2. Cimetidine crosses the placenta and is secreted in human milk.
3. Cardiovascular toxicity is unusual.
4. Plasma cimetidine levels do not correlate well with symptoms of toxicity.

A. 1, 2, and 3
B. 1, 2, and 4
C. 1, 3, and 4
D. 2, 3, and 4
E. All of the above

Ranitidine

Ranitidine inhibits gastric acid secretion with potency four to eight times that of cimetidine. Its structure is similar to that of histamine, but has a furan instead of an imidazole ring. Unlike cimetidine, it has little affinity for androgen receptors and does not bind substantially to the hepatic cytochrome P450 mixed function oxidase enzyme system.

PATHOPHYSIOLOGY

Ranitidine (Zantac®) is an H2 receptor antagonist that acts on the gastric parietal cell to inhibit gastric acid secretion.

PHARMACOKINETICS

Absorption

- Ranitidine is well absorbed after ingestion, with a bioavailability of 48%.
- Absorption is not influenced by food.

Distribution

- Peak plasma concentrations occur from 1.0 to 4.2 hours after ingestion. Small amounts appear in cerebrospinal fluid. The volume of distribution is 1.5 L/kg, similar to that of cimetidine.
- The serum half-life after oral administration is 2 to 3 hours and 1.87 hours after intravenous (IV) administration.
- In older age groups, critically ill patients, and those with liver disease, the half-life is prolonged two to threefold.

Elimination

- Ranitidine is metabolized in the liver by "first-pass" kinetics.
- Up to 30% is metabolized to nitrogen oxide, sulfuric oxide, and desmethyl derivatives.
- After intravenous use, 50% to 70% is excreted unchanged by the kidney.

CLINICAL PRESENTATIONS

Only minor side effects have been reported, but experience is limited. These include headache, malaise, dizziness, constipation, nausea, and skin rash, all of which resolve or subside despite continued therapy. Transient hepatic transaminase increase has been noted, and a hypersensitivity type of hepatitis has been observed. Ranitidine apparently produces a higher incidence of hepatic hypersensitivity reactions than cimetidine, although hepatotoxicity from either H2 blocker is uncommon.

Unlike cimetidine, ranitidine does not decrease basal testosterone levels and has no antiandrogenic activity. There has been less confusion and mental depression reported than with cimetidine and no interstitial nephritis has thus far been reported. Agranulocytosis has been reported following ranitidine use. At least five reports have indicated that ranitidine may be associated with thrombocytopenia. There have been additional anecdotal reports of cardiac arrest, granulocytopenia, bone marrow hypoplasia, mania, chest pain, confusion, and pancreatitis.

TOXIC DOSAGE/DEATH

A toxic dose has not been identified. Patients have survived extremely large doses.

DRUG INTERACTIONS

Ranitidine does not inhibit drug metabolism or interfere with androgenic function. Cimetidine, with an imidazole ring structure, binds and inhibits hepatic cytochrome P450. Ranitidine, with a furan ring structure instead, retains potent H2 receptor blocking activity but binds cytochrome P450 with much less affinity. Ranitidine has been reported to interact with warfarin, midazolam, metoprolol, benzodiazepines, fentanyl, nifedipine, and acetaminophen, but may be preferred to cimetidine when warfarin also is being administered. Ranitidine does not inhibit theophylline clearance, in contrast to cimetidine.

PREGNANCY/LACTATION

Ranitidine is distributed into breast milk. A pattern of fetotoxicity has not been identified.

LABORATORY

Analytic Methods

A reverse-phase, high-performance liquid chromatography method is available for determination of ranitidine in whole blood and plasma.

Blood Levels

A plasma concentration of 36 to 94 ng/mL produces a 50% inhibition of gastric acid secretion maintained 6 hours after ingestion of 150 mg.

TREATMENT

Gut Decontamination

If not more than 4 hours have elapsed since ingestion of the drug, activated charcoal may be useful, however studies to confirm its clinical efficacy are not available.

Elimination Enhancement

Ranitidine is poorly dialyzable.

Supportive Measures

- Treatment of overdose is similar to that for cimetidine.

Questions—Ranitidine

1. Compared to cimetidine, which of the following are true of ranitidine?

1. It has much lower affinity for androgen receptors.
2. Unlike cimetidine, it is not secreted into breast milk.
3. In contrast to cimetidine, ranitidine does not inhibit theophylline clearance.
4. It binds to cytochrome P450 with much less affinity.

A. 1, 2, and 3
B. 1, 2, and 4
C. 1, 3, and 4
D. 2, 3, and 4
E. All of the above

2. The following toxicities have been reported with ranitidine except

A. Headache, malaise, and dizziness
B. Agranulocytosis
C. Transaminase elevation
D. Hypotestosteronemia
E. Rash

3. Ranitidine

1. Is 4 to 8 times more potent than cimetidine in inhibiting gastric acid secretion
2. Is poorly dialyzable
3. Overdose is treated effectively with steroids
4. Is metabolized by "first pass" kinetics in the liver

A. 1, 2, and 3
B. 1, 2, and 4
C. 1, 3, and 4
D. 2, 3, and 4
E. All of the above

Famotidine

Famotidine (Pepcid®) is an H2 receptor antagonist that rarely has been reported in overdose. Rare cardiac, hematologic, central nervous system, and muscle dysfunction requires that patients who overdose be observed. Symptomatic and supportive therapy suffices in most cases.

PATHOPHYSIOLOGY

Famotidine is another H2 receptor antagonist that decreases gastric acid production at the parietal cell by competing with histamine.

PHARMACOKINETICS

Absorption

- Bioavailability is 40% to 50%. Time to peak serum level is 1 to 3 hours.
- Onset of action occurs within 60 minutes and half-life is around 3 hours, generally longer than other H2 blockers.

Distribution

- Volume of distribution is 1.1 L/kg. 15% to 20% is protein bound.

Elimination

- 35% is metabolized by the liver.
- Elimination as unchanged drug occurs in urine.

CLINICAL PRESENTATIONS

Adverse effects following usual therapeutic doses of famotidine may include hypertension, thrombocytopenia, fever, vasculitis, bradycardia, second-degree atrioventricular block, rhabdomyolysis, and mental confusion. Mental confusion also has been reported with cimetidine and ranitidine. Hyperprolactinemia may be observed with famotidine therapy.

TOXIC DOSAGE/DEATH

A well-established toxic dosage has not been identified. There have been no reported deaths from famotidine alone.

DRUG INTERACTIONS

Famotidine may decrease chlorpromazine absorption.

PREGNANCY/LACTATION

Pregnancy risk category B. Famotidine does distribute into breast milk.

LABORATORY

Analytic Methods

Famotidine may be detected by gas chromatography-mass spectroscopy.

Blood Levels

Serum concentration of 13 ng/mL inhibits 50% of gastric acid production. Following blood levels in overdose has not been studied.

TREATMENT

Gut Decontamination

Unabsorbed material can be removed, if clinically indicated, by gastric lavage if the patient is seen within the first few hours of an oral ingestion. Activated charcoal may be of some benefit in hastening excretion.

Elimination Enhancement

Hemodialysis may be useful, particularly in elderly, anuric patients, although definitive studies to confirm this intervention are still necessary.

Supportive Measures

- Treatment of overdose is similar to that for cimetidine. Patients should be monitored for 24 hours for cardiac arrhythmias, development of rhabdomyolysis, and the possible onset of thrombocytopenia.
- Mental confusion may be treated symptomatically.
- Following release, the patient should have platelet counts periodically for 1 week to determine if thrombocytopenia has developed.

Questions—Famotidine

1. Which of the following statements about famotidine are true?
   1. It decreases parietal cell gastric acid production by competing with histamine.
   2. It is secreted in human milk.
   3. Hyperprolactinemia may be observed with famotidine therapy.
   4. It has a longer serum half-life than cimetidine, ranitidine and nizatidine.

   A. 1, 2, and 3
   B. 1, 2, and 4
   C. 1, 3, and 4
   D. 2, 3, and 4
   E. All of the above.

2. Which of the following concerning famotidine overdose is false?
   A. Management is similar to cimetidine overdose
   B. Hemodialysis may be useful particularly in the elderly
   C. Cardiac toxicity has been described including bradycardia and second-degree AV block
   D. The most common neurotoxicity is seizure
   E. There is no antidote

3. Which of the following are known adverse effects of famotidine at therapeutic doses?
   1. Hypertension
   2. Thrombocytopenia
   3. Mental confusion
   4. Rhabdomyolysis

   A. 1, 2, and 3
   B. 1, 2, and 4
   C. 1, 3, and 4
   D. 2, 3, and 4
   E. All of the above.

Nizatidine

Nizatidine (Axid®) is a specific and potent H2 receptor antagonist. Gastric acid suppression induced by 100 mg of nizatidine is equal to that induced by 300 mg of cimetidine.

PATHOPHYSIOLOGY

Nizatidine is an H2 receptor antagonist that decreases gastric acid production at the parietal cell by competing with histamine.

PHARMACOKINETICS

Absorption

- Nizatidine bioavailability is nearly 100%.

Distribution

- The volume of distribution is 0.5 to 1.2 L/kg. Protein binding is about 30%.

Elimination

- The half-life is 1.3 hours, similar to those of cimetidine and ranitidine.

CLINICAL PRESENTATIONS

Sweating, urticaria, somnolence, and hepatic toxicity (similar to cimetidine or ranitidine) have been reported. Nizatidine, like cimetidine and ranitidine, occasionally may exhibit negative chronotropic effects. Chest pain has been reported. Leukocytosis, mild thrombocythemia, and eosinophilia have been observed after therapeutic use.

TOXIC DOSAGE/DEATH

Studies with up to 250 mg IV indicated no serious side effects or coagulation abnormalities. No effects were observed on pulse, blood pressure, or ECG. LD50 has been estimated at 80 mg/kg.

DRUG INTERACTIONS

Nizatidine may decrease chlorpromazine absorption. Nizatidine does not interfere with the hepatic metabolism of drugs such as oral anticoagulants and theophylline.

PREGNANCY/LACTATION

Pregnancy risk category C.

TREATMENT

Gut Decontamination

Unabsorbed material can be removed, if clinically indicated, by gastric lavage if the patient is seen within the first few hours of an oral ingestion. Activated charcoal may be of some benefit in hastening excretion.

Elimination Enhancement

Hemodialysis has not been utilized or studied in nizatidine overdose.

Supportive Measures

- Treatment is similar to other H2 receptor antagonists.
- A complete blood count with platelets is recommended.
- Urticaria may be treated with antihistamines.
- ECG and monitor if presentation is associated with chest pain.

Questions—Nizatidine

1. The following statements about nizatidine are true
1. It is more potent than cimetidine in suppressing gastric acid secretion
2. Its serum half-life is similar to that of cimetidine
3. Like cimetidine, it interferes with metabolism of drugs such as theophylline.
4. Like famotidine, it may decrease absorption of chlorpromazine.

A. 1, 2, and 3
B. 1, 2, and 4
C. 1, 3, and 4
D. 2, 3, and 4
E. All of the above.

2. Which of the following statements about nizatidine overdose are true?
1. There is no known antidote.
2. Activated charcoal may be of some benefit.
3. Treatment is largely supportive.
4. Patients presenting with somnolence should be dialyzed.

A. 1, 2, and 3
B. 1, 2, and 4
C. 1, 3, and 4
D. 2, 3, and 4
E. All of the above.

PROKINETIC DRUGS

A number of prokinetic agents enhance gastrointestinal motor function and accelerate transit by acting on a group of receptors shown to affect gut function. These drugs may aid patients who demonstrate gut hypomotility conditions. Such disease states include esophageal reflux with inefficient clearance of gastric acid, poor gastric emptying after surgery or in diabetes, small bowel hypomotility or pseudo-obstruction, and slow colonic transit in some patients with constipation.

Cisapride

Cisapride represents the third generation of prokinetic agents. It is unique in that it does not have antidopaminergic properties, but exerts its effect by increasing the release of acetylcholine from postganglionic nerve endings of the myenteric plexus. It is not an antiemetic, nor does it increase prolactin release.

Domperidone

Domperidone blocks the inhibitory effect of dopamine on gut motility. It has no central nervous system effects, but produces an increase in prolactin secretion (breast enlargement, nipple tenderness, galactorrhea, and menstrual irregularities). Domperidone has been associated with cardiac arrhythmias, seizures, and sudden death when used intravenously. Parenteral use of this product has been discontinued.

Metoclopramide

Metoclopramide (Reglan®) reduces the inhibitory effect of dopamine in gut motility but it passes through the blood-brain barrier and, in about 10% to 30% of patients, may induce extrapyramidal signs (ranging from a Parkinsonlike syndrome to tremors and agitation). It induces prolactin secretion and is an antiemetic. A number of reports of overdose have appeared.

Pathophysiology

CISAPRIDE

Cisapride increases gastric motility by enhancing the release of acetylcholine from postganglionic neurons in the gut. It does not produce dopaminergic inhibition of either the gastrointestinal tract or central nervous system. Cisapride is a serotonin (5-HT4) agonist and may stimulate 5-HT4 receptors in the right atrium, which may account for tachycardia following its use.

DOMPERIDONE

Domperidone is a peripherally acting dopamine antagonist. It has no important effects within the central nervous system. Domperidone inhibits gastric relaxation and enhances central contractions probably through antagonism of dopamine receptors in the gastrointestinal tract.

METOCLOPRAMIDE

Metoclopramide blocks 5-hydroxytryptamine (5-HT3) receptors in the gastrointestinal tract when administered in high doses. Its prokinetic action is believed to reflect its agonist effects on a putative 5-HT4 receptor. Metoclopramide also enhances acetylcholine release and sensitizes muscarinic receptors in the gastrointestinal tract. It stimulates gastric emptying without increasing gastric acid secretion. Metoclopramide antagonizes the inhibitory effect of dopamine receptors located in the smooth muscle of the gastrointestinal tract. It also exerts an antidopaminergic effect within the central nervous system, resulting in extrapyramidal adverse effects.

Pharmacokinetics

CISAPRIDE

Absorption

- Onset of action after oral ingestion is 0.5 to 1.0 hours.

Distribution

- Volume of distribution is 2.5 L/kg and 98% is protein bound.

Elimination

- 7- to 10-hour half life.
- Elimination is via urine and stool.

METOCLOPRAMIDE

Absorption

- Onset of action after oral ingestion is within 30 to 60 minutes.

Distribution

- Volume of distribution is 3.5 L/kg.
- 30% protein bound.

Elimination

- 4- to 7-hour half-life
- Elimination essentially is as unchanged drug in urine and stool.

Clinical Presentations

CISAPRIDE

Cisapride generally is well tolerated. Undesirable effects include abdominal cramping, borborygmi, diarrhea, somnolence, fatigue, tachycardia, palpitations, hypertension, premature beats, and parkinsonian tremors. Extrapyramidal symptoms are rare but a dystoniclike reaction has been reported. There are no reports of acute overdose following cisapride use.

DOMPERIDONE

Ventricular arrhythmias, hypokalemia, cardiac arrest, and sudden death have been reported following intravenous domperidone in high doses. The manufacturers have withdrawn the parenteral preparation from general use. Seizures also followed high-dose intravenous domperidone in patients receiving cisplatin. Domperidone produces few dystonic reactions because of its low penetration through the blood-brain barrier. Dopamine receptors in the pituitary, however, are blocked, resulting in prolactin excess with resulting breast tenderness, galactorrhea, gynecomastia, and menstrual irregularities. Neuromuscular malignant syndrome also has followed domperidone use.

METOCLOPRAMIDE

Excessive doses in children may produce opisthotonos, increased muscle tone, oculogyric crisis, torticollis, facial grimacing, agitation, diplopia, trismus, nystagmus, strabismus, crying, seizures, cyanosis of the extremities, conjugate deviation of the eyes, and cogwheel rigidity. Most patients develop symptoms within 36 hours of starting treatment with metoclopramide. Methemoglobinemia, tardive dyskinesia, and neuroleptic malignant syndrome also have been seen with metoclopramide use. Dystonic reactions with sudden death after high-dose intravenous use have been described. A withdrawal syndrome with akinesia and akathisia also may be seen. This may persist for months and may be refractory to therapy.

Toxic Dosage/Death

A few deaths related to metoclopramide have been reported following acute dystonic reactions to the drug. Bradycardia and total heart block have followed intravenous use. No lethal dose of metoclopramide has been reported. Doses of 360 and 800 mg have been followed by survival with minimal supportive care. Death followed ventricular fibrillation in an adult administered a 200-mg intravenous dose of domperidone.

Drug Interactions

CISAPRIDE

Cisapride prevents a delay in gastric emptying associated with administration of morphine. It results in a decrease in plasma ranitidine levels. Cisapride has been associated with life-threatening ventricular arrhythmias, including Torsade de Pointes, when used in combination with ketoconazole, a potent inhibitor of the cytochrome P450 enzyme system.

METOCLOPRAMIDE

Metoclopramide has been reported to decrease the half-life of aspirin, cimetidine, cyclosporine, diazepam, digoxin, levodopa, mexiletine, morphine, acetaminophen, and tetracycline. With digoxin and quinidine, there may be a slight decrease in absorption.

Pregnancy/Lactation

Metoclopramide crosses the placenta and is distributed into breast milk. Domperidone crosses the placenta. Cisapride crosses the placenta and is found in human breast milk.

Laboratory

ANALYTIC METHODS

Levels of cisapride and its major metabolite in biological fluids are measured by high-performance liquid chromatography. Concentrations of unchanged domperidone in plasma and urine have been determined by radioimmunoassay. A rapid liquid chromatographic method is available for the determination of metoclopramide in human plasma. The method compares favorably with high-performance liquid chromatography methods.

BLOOD LEVELS

Low-dose-therapy plasma levels of metoclopramide usually are less than 0.2 $\mu g/mL$, but plasma concentrations of 0.5 to 1.5 $\mu g/mL$ are measured after high-dose intravenous therapy.

Treatment

GUT DECONTAMINATION

There is no published evidence to support the use of gastric emptying procedures, activated charcoal, cathartics, or whole-bowel irrigation following overdose with this group of drugs. Absorption is rapid, and syrup of ipecac may induce emesis at the same time that the patient has seizures, predisposing the patient to an aspiration pneumonitis. If gastric emptying procedures are to be attempted, tracheal protection is advised.

ELIMINATION ENHANCEMENT

Activated charcoal and extracorporeal procedures such as hemodialysis or hemoperfusion have not been used following overdose with prokinetic drugs. The high apparent volumes of distribution of all of the drugs in this group and their high protein binding would tend to mitigate against the use of these elimination procedures. Toxicokinetic studies indicate that cisapride is not cleared by hemodialysis.

SUPPORTIVE MEASURES

- Maintenance of the airway, support of respirations, and cardiovascular integrity are vital in sustaining life following a prokinetic drug overdose.
- Extrapyramidal signs following metoclopramide overdose should be followed in a hospital facility where an intravenous line, cardiac monitoring, and oxygen are available. Withdrawal of metoclopramide usually is followed by amelioration of symptoms. Diphenhydramine, 25–50 ng IV may be helpful as well.
- Seizures are treated with diazepam, if necessary.
- Few arrhythmias have been reported with domperidone therapy since the parenteral preparation was withdrawn from distribution.
- In cases of methemoglobinemia, discontinue metoclopramide and give methylene blue, if clinically indicated.
- Muscle rigidity and fever of neuroleptic malignant syndrome following metoclopramide use have responded to intravenous dantrolene 2 mg/kg, immediate discontinuation of the causal drug, temperature reduction, and other supportive measures.
- Obtain and follow serial electrolytes. Hypokalemia has been associated with cardiac arrhythmias and sudden death following intravenous use of domperidone.

Questions—Prokinetic Drugs

1. Which of the following statements regarding prokinetic drugs are true?

1. Metoclopramide, domperidone, and cisapride are prokinetic drugs that increase gastric motility by blocking dopaminergic receptors in the gastrointestinal motor system.
2. Neuroleptic malignant syndrome has been a reported toxic reaction with use of the prokinetic drugs metoclopramide and domperidone.
3. Unlike metoclopramide, cisapride has no antiemetic properties.
4. Prolactin levels are commonly elevated with use of metoclopramide and domperidone.

A. 1, 2, and 3
B. 1, 2, and 4
C. 1, 3, and 4
D. 2, 3, and 4
E. All of the above.

CASE STUDY (QUESTIONS 2 AND 3)

A 35-year-old woman with ovarian cancer is rushed to the emergency department shortly after receiving metoclopramide intravenously prior to chemotherapy with an acute dystonic reaction, irritability, and restlessness.

2. Which of the following are appropriate measures for initial management?

A. Endotracheal intubation
B. Dantrolene
C. Diphenhydramine
D. Methylene blue
E. None of the above.

3. The above patient responds to treatment with improvement in her symptoms but shortly thereafter has recurrence of dystonia and has a grand mal seizure. Appropriate treatment includes

1. Careful neurologic examination
2. Maintenance of airway, support of respirations, oxygen, IV, and cardiac monitoring
3. Diazepam
4. Hemodialysis

A. 1, 2, and 3
B. 1, 2, and 4
C. 1, 3, and 4
D. 2, 3, and 4
E. All of the above.

SUCRALFATE

Sucralfate (Carafate®) is an aluminum salt used to treat duodenal ulcers.

Pathophysiology

This salt forms a pastelike protective barrier when combined with stomach acids over inflamed ulcers.

Pharmacokinetics

ABSORPTION

- Onset of action occurs within 1 to 2 hours.
- Less than 5% is absorbed.

DISTRIBUTION

- Acts locally at ulcer sites

ELIMINATION

- It is not metabolized and elimination is mostly via the fecal route.

Clinical Presentations

Toxicity generally is minimal. In overdose, it may be associated with abdominal pain, nausea, and vomiting. In uremic patients, it may induce aluminum toxicity with encephalopathy and bone pain. Rash, constipation, and occasional bezoars have been reported. Bone biopsies may show osteomalacia after a few years of treatment.

Toxic Dosage/Death

A toxic dosage has not been established. Death from sucralfate alone has not been reported.

Drug Interactions

Sucralfate decreases the bioavailability of digoxin, quinidine, theophylline, tetracycline, cimetidine, phenytoin, warfarin, thyroxine, ciprofloxacin, and norfloxacin possibly because of chelation with an aluminum ion that is released on dissociation of the sucralfate molecule. Use of cimetidine may increase the gastric pH and lead to an increase in aluminum absorption.

Pregnancy/Lactation

Pregnancy risk category B.

Treatment

GUT DECONTAMINATION

There is no published evidence to support the use of gastric emptying procedures, activated charcoal, cathartics, or whole-bowel irrigation following overdose with this drug.

ELIMINATION ENHANCEMENT

Activated charcoal and extracorporeal procedures such as hemodialysis or hemoperfusion have not been used following overdose with sucralfate. Deferoxamine, a chelator, may enhance aluminum excretion in severe cases. Clinical importance of deferoxamine in this setting, however, has not been proved.

SUPPORTIVE MEASURES

- Treatment of an overdose includes withdrawal of sucralfate and is largely symptomatic.
- Use of cimetidine is contraindicated as it may increase gastric pH and lead to an increase in aluminum absorption.

Questions—Sucralfate

1. Which of the following statements about sucralfate are true?

1. It is a magnesium salt used for treatment of duodenal ulcers.
2. Uremic patients are especially sensitive to toxicity.
3. Death from sucralfate overdose has not been reported.
4. There is no antidote for sucralfate overdose.

A. 1, 2, and 3
B. 1, 2, and 4
C. 1, 3, and 4
D. 2, 3, and 4
E. All of the above.

2. Sucralfate decreases the bioavailability of which of the following drugs?

1. Digoxin
2. Quinidine
3. Theophylline
4. Cimetidine

A. 1, 2, and 3
B. 1, 2, and 4
C. 1, 3, and 4
D. 2, 3, and 4
E. All of the above.

BISMUTH SUBSALICYLATE

Bismuth subsalicylate (BSS)(Pepto-Bismol®) is used to soothe gastric irritation with a protective coating action. It also is used to control diarrhea and relieve abdominal cramping. See Chapter 11, Salicylates, and Chapter 47, Metals.

Pathophysiology

The salicylate moiety provides an antisecretory effect and bismuth exhibits antimicrobial and antacid properties. It is believed to work against diarrhea by binding to bacterial toxins, and by normalizing fluid movement via an antisecretory mechanism.

Pharmacokinetics

ABSORPTION

- The salicylate in BSS is almost entirely available and is essentially absorbed in the small intestine.

DISTRIBUTION

- BSS is nearly completely hydrolyzed in the stomach to form bismuth oxychloride and salicylic acid.

Elimination

- BSS undergoes chemical dissociation to bismuth salts.

Clinical Presentations

Adverse effects may be comparable to the toxic profile of other salicylates in severe overdoses. Elderly patients who ingest large amounts of Pepto-Bismol® daily may develop agitation, confusion, lethargy, disorientation, slurred speech, and acute pulmonary edema. Such patients may develop a mixed respiratory alkalosis and metabolic acidosis. Encephalopathy may occur after large or repetitive doses. Bariumlike contrast densities may be seen on abdominal plain film. Bismuth may cause nephrotic syndrome. Darkening of the tongue and stool are notable side effects.

Toxic Dosage/Death

One death, involving the ingestion of 66 bismuth subsalicylate tablets by a 36-kg patient, resulted in a salicylate dose of 187 mg/kg. This may be compared with the recommended dosing schedule of 2 tablets four times a day, which would deliver 11.6 mg of salicylate/kg/day to a 70-kg man.

Drug Interactions

Unfortunately, a recommended dose (15 mL up to eight times per 24 hours) when added to an antiinflammatory dose regimen of aspirin, may yield serious salicylate intoxication. Caution is advised in the administration to patients taking medication for anticoagulation.

Pregnancy/Lactation

Pregnancy risk category C (D in the 3rd trimester).

Laboratory

ANALYTIC METHODS

Gas chromatography and high-performance liquid chromatography can detect salicylates.

BLOOD LEVELS

One adult dose of Pepto-Bismol® liquid (30 mL of original strength) provides 25 mg of salicylate; one adult dose of Pepto-Bismol® tablets (2 tablets) provides 204 mg of salicylate, similar to the salicylate dose delivered by one regular-strength aspirin (249 mg of salicylate). Maximum-Strength Pepto-Bismol® liquid contains 460 mg salicylate per dose. 60 mL of Pepto-Bismol® leads to a peak salicylate concentration of 40.1 μg/mL in 1.8 hours.

Treatment

GUT DECONTAMINATION

There is no published evidence to support the use of gastric emptying procedures, activated charcoal, cathartics, or whole-bowel irrigation following overdose with BSS.

ELIMINATION ENHANCEMENT

Extracorporeal procedures such as hemodialysis or hemoperfusion have not been used following overdose with BSS but may be useful in treating significant salicylate overdoses.

SUPPORTIVE MEASURES

- Discontinuation of drug and supportive measures are the mainstay of treatment.
- Monitor for bleeding and follow renal function.
- Monitor salicylate levels in extreme cases (Chapter 11, Salicylates, for management issues).

Questions—Bismuth Subsalicylate

1. The following statements regarding bismuth subsalicylate are true except

A. It is used to control diarrhea and abdominal cramping.
B. The salicylate moiety provides an antisecretory effect.
C. The bismuth moiety provides antimicrobial and antacid properties.
D. Darkening of the tongue and stool are common side effects.
E. Overdose can lead to a metabolic imbalance characterized by mixed respiratory acidosis and metabolic alkalosis.

2. Bismuth subsalicylate overdose

1. Is associated with a toxic profile similar to that of aspirin
2. Requires early and frequent doses of activated charcoal
3. Can lead to nephrotic syndrome
4. Can be fatal

A. 1, 2, and 3
B. 1, 2, and 4
C. 1, 3, and 4
D. 2, 3, and 4
E. All of the above.

Answers

Antiinflammatory Salicylates

1. C 2. B 3. A

Loperamide

1. C 2. E 3. D

Misoprostol

1. A 2. E 3. B

Proton Pump Inhibitors

1. C 2. E 3. A

Antacids

1. C 2. B

Cimetidine

1. C 2. D 3. E

Ranitidine

1. C 2. D 3. B

Famotidine

1. E 2. D 3. E

Nizatidine

1. B 2. A

Prokinetic Drugs

1. D 2. C 3. A

Sucralfate

1. D 2. E

Bismuth Subsalicylate

1. E 2. C

SELECTED READINGS

Antiinflammatory Salicylates

1. Dunn, R. Sulfasalazine and seizures. Clin Tox 1998;36(7):759–760.
2. Heard, K, O'Malley, G, Dart, R, Smith, M. Is sulfasalazine toxic? Clin Tox 1998; 36(7):757–8.
3. Minocha A, Dean HA, Mayle JE. Acute sulfasalazine overdose. Clin Toxicol 1991;29:543–51.

Loperamide

1. Bhutta FL, Tahir KI. Loperamide poisoning in children. Lancet 1990;335:363.
2. Hart LM, Dean BS, Krenzelok EP. Loperamide overdose in children: Is it as bad as Lomotil? Vet Hum Toxicol 1992;34:332.
3. Sandhu BF, Tripp JH, Candy DCA, Haries JT. Loperamide: Studies on its mechanism of action. Gut 1981;22: 658–662.

Misoprostol

1. Arns PA. Misoprostol. Am J Med Sci 1991;301:133–137.
2. Garris RE, Kirkwood CF. Misoprostol: A prostaglandin E1 analogue. Clin Pharm 1989;8:627–644.
3. Grober DJ, Meier KH. Acute misoprostol toxicity. Ann Emerg Med 1991;20: 549–551.

Proton Pump Inhibitors

1. Ferner RE, Allison TR. Omeprazole overdose. Hum Exp Toxicol 1993;12: 541–542.
2. Holt S, Howden CW. Omeprazole: Overview and opinion. Dig Dis Sci 1991; 31:385–393.
3. Jackson MP, Wood JP. Omeprazole. Br Med J 1991;303:1200–1201.
4. Lansoprazole. Med Lett Drugs Ther 1995;37(953): 63–64.

Antacids

1. Brand JM, Greer FR. Hypermagnesemia and intestinal perforation following antacid administration in a premature infant. Pediatrics 1990;85:121–124.
2. Carmichael KA, Fallon MD, Dalinka M, et al. Osteomalacia and osteitis fibrosa in a man ingesting aluminum hydroxide antacid. Am J Med 1984;76:1137–1140.

Cimetidine

1. Colin-Jones DG, Langman MJS, Lawson DH, et al. Safety of cimetidine. Br Med J 1985;291:1721–1722.
2. Krenzelok EP, Litovitz T, Lippold KP, McNally CF. Cimetidine toxicity: An assessment of 881 cases. Ann Emerg Med 1987;16:1217–1221.
3. Mangini RJ. Clinically important cimetidine drug interactions. Clin Pharm 1982; 1:433–440.

Ranitidine

1. Feely J, Warmsley KG. H2 receptor antagonists: Cimetidine and ranitidine. Br Med J 1983;286:695–697.
2. Lima MA. Hepatitis associated with ranitidine. JAMA 1984;252:3253.
3. Zeldis JB, Friedman LS, Isselbacker KJ. Ranitidine: A new H2 receptor antagonist. N Engl J Med 1983;309:1368–1373.

Famotidine

1. Ahmad S. Famotidine and cardiac arrhythmia. DICP Ann Pharmacother 1991; 25:315.
2. Norwood J, Smith TM, Stein DS. Famotidine and hyperpyrexia. Ann Intern Med 1990;112:632.

Nizatidine

1. Nizatidine (AXID). Med Lett Drugs Ther 1988;30(772):77–78.

Prokinetic Drugs

1. Ahmad SR, Wolfe SM. Cisapride and Torsade de pointes. Lancet 1995;345:508.
2. Brogden RN, Carmine AA, Heel RC, et al. Domperidone: A review of its pharmacologic activity, pharmacokinetics and therapeutic efficacy in the treatment of chronic dyspepsia and as an antiemetic drug. Drugs 1982;24:360–400.
3. Cisapride: More selective than metoclopramide. Drug Ther Bull 1990;28(23): 89–90.
4. Low LCK, Goel KM. Metoclopramide poisoning in children. Arch Dis Child 1980;55:310–312.
5. Reynolds JC, Putnam PE. Prokinetic agents. Gastroenterol Clin North Am 1992; 21:567–596.

Sucralfate

1. Anderson W, Weatherstone G, Ved C. Esophageal medication bezoar in a patient receiving enteral feedings and sucralfate. Am J Gastroenterol 1989;8: 205–206.
2. Min DI, D'Elia JA. Sucralfate-associated aluminum toxicity in a patient with renal failure: Treatment with deferoxamine. Clin Pharm 1992;11:636–639.

Bismuth Subsalicylate

1. Pickering LK, Feldman S, Ericsson CD, Cleary TG. Absorption of salicylate and bismuth from a bismuth subsalicylate containing compound (Pepto-bismol). J Pediatr 1981;99:654–656.
2. Sainsbury S. Fatal salicylate toxicity from bismuth subsalicylate. West J Med 1991;155:637–639

ACKNOWLEDGMENTS

Thanks to Richard Levy, MD for contributing the questions in this chapter.

CHAPTER 31
Immunotoxicology

INTRODUCTION

Immunotoxicology encompasses the interactions of foreign substances with the immune system and assesses the importance of these interactions in terms of risk to human or animal health. Numerous chemicals and drugs have produced immunologic disturbances in experimental animals and humans. Functional components of the immune response include the leukocyte subsets: T-lymphocytes, B-lymphocytes, natural killer lymphocytes, and mononuclear phagocytes. Clinical effects of immunotoxic substances may be manifested as an enhanced but inappropriate immune response, or as a failure to mount an appropriate immune response. The principal effects induced by immunotoxic substances are immunosuppression, autoimmunity, and hypersensitivity.

Immunotoxicity, or an immunotoxic effect, is defined as an adverse or inappropriate change in the structure or function of the immune system following exposure to a foreign substance of either synthetic or natural origin. Foreign substances include industrial, agricultural, and household chemicals, drugs, and food additives. Conditions known to alter reactivity to substances, in addition to genetic factors, are age, presence of concurrent disease, nutritional status, hormone levels, diurnal variation in drug disposition or sensitivity, environmental factors that induce or inhibit drug metabolism, smoking, and efficiency of repair mechanism.

Clinical Presentations

Immunologic hypersensitivity is an overreaction of the immune system to a substance and is probably the most prominent form of immunotoxicity seen in patients. This reaction is an exaggerated response to an antigenic stimulus in which there is a reduced threshold to an antigen. Terms used to describe types of hypersensitivity include anaphylaxis, atopy, and allergy. Occupational exposure to chemicals and other xenobiotics is an important cause of hypersensitivity reactions. Many chemicals can induce asthma, for example. Workers can become sensitized after exposure to concentrations of chemicals well below the statutory exposure limits.

The diagnosis of hypersensitivity myocarditis is considered when new electrocardiographic changes, mildly elevated enzyme levels, cardiomegaly, or unexplained tachycardia is noted in a patient who has an ongoing allergic reaction to a drug. Biopsy of the myocardium may confirm the diagnosis. Histology may reveal diffuse interstitial infiltrates rich in eosinophils, with or without cellular necrosis. Methyldopa, the sulfonamides, and penicillin have caused most cases of hypersensitivity myocarditis as a result of drugs.

Laboratory

Numerous laboratory tests may help the clinician gauge the immunologic health of an individual. The World Health Organization's Immunology Section has recommended eight immunologic tests as an initial screening for patients with suspected immune dysfunction: (1) a complete blood count with differential cell count; (2) quantitative protein electrophoresis; (3) humoral mediated immunity immunoelectrophoresis; (4) quantitation of IgG, IgM, IgA, and IgE; (5) isoantibody titers; (6) cell-mediated immunity; delayed hypersensitivity skin testing; (7) autoimmunity, autoantibody titers; and (8) C3 and C4 levels. A goal-directed, stepwise approach to diagnosis may not require this complete screening panel in all cases.

Some practitioners of traditional and alternative medicine may use the laboratory to support therapeutic regimens based on unique and scientifically unproven concepts. Numerous tests, such as those for antimyelin and antibenzene antibodies, have not been subjected to careful prospective studies involving determinations of sensitivity and specificity when correlated with definitive diseases.

Questions—Introduction to Immunotoxicology

1. The principal effect(s) of immunotoxic substances are
A. Immunosuppression
B. Autoimmunity
C. Hypersensitivity
D. All of the above
E. None of the above

2. Which of the following tests does the World Health Organization Immunology Section not recommend as an initial screening for patients with suspected immune dysfunction?
A. Complete blood count
B. Quantitation of IgG and IgM
C. Delayed hypersensitivity skin testing
D. Antimyelin antibodies
E. Quantitation of IgA and IgE

3. A patient with an ongoing allergic drug reaction and hypersensitivity myocarditis may have the following findings.
A. New electrocardiographic changes
B. Cardiomegaly
C. Elevated cardiac enzymes levels
D. All of the above
E. None of the above

IMMUNOTHERAPY

Immunotherapy involves the use of antibodies, or antibody fragments, for therapeutic purposes. Antibodies are complex glycoproteins synthesized by B-lymphocytes and plasma cells and are classified as immunoglobulin G (IgG), M (IgM), E (IgE), D (IgD) or A (IgA). IgG is the main circulating immunoglobulin and the one generally employed therapeutically. Each molecule has two class-specific heavy chains and two light chains arranged to provide two binding sites. IgG can be cleaved by enzymes into Fab (antibody fraction) fragments and Fc (constant fraction) components.

Historically, antibodies raised in horses were frequently associated with severe, and sometimes fatal, side effects. Risks of immunotherapy have been reduced by the production of antibodies in sheep rather than horses and the use of Fab fragments rather than intact IgG. Antibodies are raised against small molecules, such as drugs, by covalently coupling them to a carrier protein. This has widened the possibilities for using antibodies in immunotherapy.

Antibodies raised in animals are called polyclonal because they are the products of many different clones of the B-lymphocyte. Each clone produces antibodies directed against different sites (epitopes) on the antigen to which they bind with different strengths (affinities). Monoclonal antibodies are formed using hybridomas consisting of B-lymphocytes fused with cancer cells. These are bound to an epitope with the same affinity, but may be less effective than polyclonal counterparts.

Fab fragments usually are used in immunotherapy because of their greater diffusion in body compartments and the higher renal clearance of the toxin-antibody conjugate compared with IgG. Certain target toxins frequently have been mentioned in this growing field of toxicology.

Arsenic

The low molecular weight, high volume of distribution, antigenicity, and high potency of arsenic compounds provide a model for studying the therapeutic application of antibodies. Arsenate antibodies have been produced in mice and preliminary animal studies indicate a modest effect on arsenic-induced mortality. Additional studies are required to define the usefulness of immunotherapy for poisoning with this metal.

Colchicine

Colchicine binds to tubulin and blocks mitosis in metaphase. The half-life of the tubulin-colchicine complex is about 36 hours. Colchicine exerts multiorgan toxicity. The severity and mortality rates are dose related. Treatment at present is based on decontamination by early gastric lavage and aggressive supportive measures. Supportive measures include maintaining electrolyte balance, correction of shock, hematologic and coagulation disturbances, and the prevention of sepsis. Despite aggressive therapy, mortality is high.

Anticolchicine antibodies may be able to detach colchicine from its target organs before cellular damage has occurred. Use of anticolchicine antibodies ultimately may be indicated in patients who have ingested more than 0.8 mg/kg. Unfortunately, conventional therapy is not effective because of the high volume of distribution and low circulating blood concentration of colchicine. Animal studies with antibodies have shown promise, however human data are lacking.

Digoxin

Digitalis compounds bind reversibly to cardiac receptors. Digoxin-specific antibodies (Fab fragments) reverse digitalis-induced dysrhythmias, conduction disturbances, myocardial depression, and inhibition of the sodium-potassium ATPase pump by attracting digoxin from these receptors. These antibodies are produced in sheep and are effective in adults, children, and premature infants.

Answers to questions in shaded boxes appear at the end of the chapter.

Oleander

Preliminary studies in oleander-intoxicated dogs with antidigoxin-Fab fragments suggest that large doses of Fab may be effective in the treatment of dysrhythmias and hyperkalemia. Further studies are required to confirm these observations in humans.

Phencyclidine

There is no known specific antagonist to the actions of phencyclidine (PCP). The drug is lipophilic and has extensive extravascular distribution and low renal clearance. These toxicokinetic criteria render it a good candidate for immunotherapy. It may be possible to use high-affinity PCP-specific Fab to produce both a redistribution and an inactivation of the drug through high-affinity binding. Whether Fab will be effective in actually reversing clinical toxicity remains to be determined.

Tricyclic Antidepressants

Toxic dose levels of tricyclic antidepressants (TCAs) are higher than those of digoxin or colchicine. Reversal of TCA toxicity may require a large amount of Fab fragments. Currently under development are antibodies directed predominantly against the tricyclic ring that can recognize both the TCA molecule and its active demethylated metabolite. Animal studies with anti-TCAs appear to demonstrate neutralization of the TCA function in the vascular compartment with reduction of TCA distribution into the heart.

Questions—Immunotherapy

1. **IgG can be cleaved enzymatically into the following components:**
   A. Fab fragment
   B. Fc fragment
   C. Fg fragment
   D. A and B
   E. A and C
2. **Immunotherapy involving Fab fragments has been used successfully in humans to treat overdoses with which of the following:**
   A. Tricyclic antidepressants
   B. Colchicine
   C. Digoxin
   D. Arsenic
   E. Ciguatera toxin
3. **The antigen-binding site is found on which portion of the IgG glycoprotein?**
   A. Fc fragment
   B. Fab fragment

IMMUNOSUPPRESSION

Introduction

Immunosuppression reflects a generalized decrease in immune responsiveness that may result in an increased incidence of infectious disease or neoplasms such as lymphoma, leukemia, and certain other cancers. Pharmaceuticals, abused drugs, pesticides, and other chemicals may destroy or inhibit innate and acquired resistance mechanisms in both humans and animals. Use of immunosuppressant drugs in transplant patients may be associated with an increase in the posttransplantation incidence of neoplasms, infections, and certain neurologic complications.

The most frequently used immunosuppressive drugs fall into four basic categories: alkylating agents, glucocorticosteroids, antimetabolites, and natural products. Alkylating agents (e.g., cyclophosphamide) disrupt cell functions, particularly mitosis, and are highly toxic to rapidly proliferating cells, such as lymphoid cells. Glucocorticosteroids alter phagocytosis and depress T- and B-lymphocyte function. Antimetabolites (e.g., azathioprine) act chiefly by inhibiting DNA synthesis. Natural products, such as cyclosporine, appear to act through modulation of mechanisms regulating immune responsiveness.

Questions—Introduction to Immunosuppression

1. **There is an increased incidence of the following cancers when immunosuppression is required after organ transplantation.**
   A. Gastric
   B. Lymphoma
   C. Pancreatic
   D. Leukemia
   E. B and D
2. **Antimetabolites include**
   A. Cyclophosphamide
   B. Prednisone
   C. Azathioprine
   D. Cyclosporine
   E. Reverse transcriptase

Azathioprine

Azathioprine (Imuran®) is an immunosuppressant used for the prevention of kidney allograft rejection in conjunction with other immunosuppressive treatments including radiation therapy, corticosteroids, and cytotoxic agents. It also has been used in the treatment of rheumatoid arthritis and in inflammatory bowel disease. Its principal toxic effect in long-term use is bone marrow depression. Overdose has been associated with nausea, vomiting, diarrhea, leukopenia, and liver function abnormalities.

PATHOPHYSIOLOGY

Azathioprine inhibits DNA synthesis and, as a purine antimetabolite, exerts its effect on activated lymphocytes, which require purines during their proliferative phase. It inhibits both cellular and humoral responses, but does not interfere with phagocytosis or interferon production. It is a nonspecific cytotoxic agent. It is metabolized to mercaptopurine, which is felt to give azathioprine its immunosuppressant effect.

PHARMACOKINETICS

Absorption

- Azathioprine is well absorbed from the gastrointestinal tract and has an oral bioavailability of approximately 60%.

Distribution

- Azathioprine is cleared rapidly from the blood. Azathioprine and mercaptopurine are approximately 30% bound to serum proteins, both appear dialyzable, and both cross the placenta.

Elimination

- Orally administered azathioprine is rapidly divided to form 6-mercaptopurine.
- 6-Mercaptopurine undergoes extensive intestinal and hepatic metabolism along three major competing routes.
- Less than 2% of azathioprine and 20% to 40% of 6-mercaptopurine are excreted as unchanged drugs in the urine. The elimination half-life of azathioprine is approximately 12 to 15 minutes, and that of 6-mercaptopurine is approximately 30 minutes to 4 hours.

CLINICAL PRESENTATIONS

Therapeutic use may lead to bone marrow depression, leukopenia, anemia, thrombocytopenia, and bleeding. Other effects include hepatic dysfunction manifested by elevated serum bilirubin, alkaline phosphatase, and transaminases, and hepatic reno-occlusive disease. Additional adverse reactions may include infections, drug fever, rash, urticaria, hypersensitivity vasculitis, nausea, vomiting, diarrhea, and possibly an increase in non-Hodgkin's lymphoma when used in conjunction with corticosteroids in rheumatoid arthritis.

TOXIC DOSAGE/DEATH

A toxic overdose of 7.5 g was ingested by a renal transplant patient which resulted in mild vomiting, a transient fall in the leukocyte count, and a rise in serum bilirubin and transaminases with ultimate recovery. The manufacturer has knowledge of an overdose of 850 mg, which resulted in no symptoms or laboratory abnormalities.

DRUG INTERACTIONS

Allopurinol inhibits the principal metabolic pathway of azathioprine, the oxidative metabolism of mercaptopurine by xanthine oxidase. This may lead to toxic accumulation of azathioprine with concomitant bone marrow depression.

PREGNANCY/LACTATION

Azathioprine is teratogenic in animals. Wherever possible, its use in pregnant women should be avoided. One retrospective analysis of 16 pregnancies in 14 women receiving azathioprine for inflammatory bowel disease revealed no congenital abnormalities or subsequent health problems in their children. This suggests that termination of pregnancy is not mandatory for those who conceive while taking the drug. Neither azathioprine nor its metabolites have been detected in appreciable quantities in breast milk.

LABORATORY

Analytic Methods

An enzymatic endpoint method may be used to detect individuals with low thiopurine methyltransferase who have excessive immunosuppression when taking azathioprine.

Blood Levels

Following blood levels of azathioprine has not been shown to be helpful in overdose. Measurement of the red blood cell concentration of 6-thioguanine nucleotides may predict bone marrow toxicity.

TREATMENT

Gut Decontamination

It is unlikely that early gastric emptying will reduce the rapidly absorbed 6-mercaptopurine metabolite. There is no evidence for the usefulness of gastric emptying, activated charcoal, or whole-bowel irrigation. Nonetheless, if an attempt is made within the first 30 minutes to 1 hour, gastric emptying might theoretically reduce the likelihood of bone marrow depression or hepatotoxicity following an overdose.

Elimination Enhancement

There are no published experiences to confirm the use of hemodialysis.

Supportive Measures

- All patients who overdose on azathioprine should be monitored for airway patency, breathing difficulties, and circulatory stability.
- An area of the body that has been exposed to azathioprine should be thoroughly washed with soap and water. Personnel involved in a spill should wear protective clothing, and special care should be taken to decontaminate a spill area.
- Patients should be periodically monitored for the development of hepatotoxicity (serum bilirubin, alkaline phosphatase, and hepatic transaminases) and bone marrow depression (including red blood cell, platelet, and white cell counts, and red cell 6-thioguanine nucleotide level), if possible.

Questions—Azathioprine

1. Azathioprine is metabolized to the following compound
- A. Mercaptopurine
- B. Adenine
- C. Guanine
- D. Cytosine
- E. Thymine

2. The following have been proven useful in the treatment of an azathioprine overdose
- A. Gastric emptying
- B. Charcoal
- C. Whole bowel irrigation
- D. None of the above
- E. All of the above

3. Azathioprine is useful in the treatment of all the following conditions except
- A. Rheumatoid arthritis
- B. Inflammatory bowel disease
- C. Renal transplantation
- D. Congestive heart failure
- E. Allograft rejection

Cyclosporine

Cyclosporine is an immunosuppressive medication that is used before and after organ transplants to suppress an undesirable immune response. Other possible uses for cyclosporine being investigated include psoriasis, refractory atopic dermatitis, uveitis, rheumatoid arthritis, nephrotic syndrome, Crohn's disease, aplastic anemia, primary biliary cirrhosis, lichen planus, asthma, autoimmune hemolytic anemia, and myasthenia gravis. Overdose with cyclosporine has been reported following suicide attempts or inadvertent errors. Parenteral overdoses may lead to fatalities with renal failure, especially in neonates.

PATHOPHYSIOLOGY

Cyclosporine is produced by *Tolypocladium inflatum Gams* or *Cylindrocarpon lucidum Booth.* It is one of several biologically active antibiotics produced by these fungi. The predominant immunologic effect of cyclosporine is the inhibition of T-lymphocyte proliferation. Its use is not associated with myelosuppression. Cyclosporine decreases the production and secretion of interleukin-2 and interferon.

PHARMACOKINETICS

Absorption

- Cyclosporine exhibits a two to threefold interindividual variation in its absorption and elimination. Peak blood and plasma concentrations generally occur in about 2.5 hours. Peak serum concentrations in patients who have received an overdose may be delayed as late as 6 hours after ingestion of the drug.
- Following oral administration, cyclosporine is largely metabolized on first pass through the liver.
- The bioavailability of orally administered drug is only about 35%. Part of this relatively poor oral bioavailability may be a result of substantial metabolism by the cytochrome P450 system.

Distribution

- The unbound fraction of cyclosporine varies between 1.0% to 2.4% (i.e., 97.6% to 99% is protein bound, mainly to lipoproteins). The apparent volume of distribution is 1.2 L/kg.
- About 50% of cyclosporine in whole blood are bound to erythrocytes. Because of the preferential distribution of cyclosporine and its metabolites into red blood cells, blood levels generally are higher than plasma levels.

Elimination

- The elimination half-life after an oral cyclosporine dose of 350 mg is 8.9 hours and after a 1,400-mg dose, the half-life is 11.9 hours.
- Elimination occurs predominantly by metabolism in the liver to form 18 to 25 metabolites. Metabolites of cyclosporine possess little immunosuppressive activity.
- Cyclosporine is metabolized extensively in the liver by cytochrome P450IIIA oxidase.
- Only 0.1% of a dose is excreted unchanged.

CLINICAL PRESENTATIONS

Clinical responses to cyclosporine overdose vary widely. Healthy persons or those with stable renal function exhibit little or no signs of toxicity. In one case, an adult was given 5 g of cyclosporine by error, and suffered few toxic effects. Other patients have experienced nausea, vomiting, diarrhea, a feeling of drunkenness, a burning sensation in the mouth, altered taste, hyperesthesia of the hands, a burning sensation in the feet, sore gums, flushing of the face, a sensation of increased abdominal girth, foot swelling, stomach upset, abdominal pain with mild hepatotoxicity, anxiety, perspiration, sinus tachycardia, hypertension, headache, and drowsiness.

Premature infants and neonates have developed hypotension, wheezing, pallor, tachycardia, cyanosis, metabolic acidosis, respiratory depression, and renal failure. Death from overdose has been reported. Chronic use has been associated with numerous, multiorgan effects.

Neurologic Effects

Tremor, burning palmar and plantar paresthesias, headache, flushing, depression, confusion, and somnolence may occur with chronic use. Hypertension (particularly in children), concomitant methylprednisolone therapy, hypomagnesemia, infection, hemorrhage, or cerebral infarction may trigger seizures. Cyclosporine use in patients undergoing transplantation may induce fever, seizures, altered mental status, cortical blindness, and speech and motor disturbances. Reversible changes in the cerebral white matter have been observed on magnetic resonance imaging.

Dermatologic Effects

Hypertrichosis of the face, arms, shoulders, and back develops in at least 50% of renal transplant recipients given cyclosporine.

Gastrointestinal Effects

Anorexia, bloating, nausea, or vomiting may occur. Acute pancreatitis has been reported. Cholestasis with hyperbilirubinemia and elevated transaminase levels is observed frequently.

Endocrine Effects

Hyperglycemia, increased serum prolactin, decreased testosterone levels, and gynecomastia in men has been observed.

Renal Effects

Cyclosporine causes at least a 20% reduction in renal function in almost all patients, usually reversed in 2 weeks on discontinuation of therapy. Other drugs may enhance cyclosporine-induced nephrotoxicity. Acute nephrotoxicity may occur within 7 days of initiation of therapy, and subacute toxicity may appear in 7 to 60 days with evidence of tubular and glomerular dysfunction. Chronic irreversible renal insufficiency may appear after 30 days.

TOXIC DOSAGE/DEATH

Oral overdoses of up to 150 mg/kg (10 to 30 times the recommended values) have led to few overt signs and symptoms (vomiting, drowsiness, headache, and episodic hypertension). One adult ingested 25 g over 8 days and survived. Two adults and one child received 5.0 g of cyclosporine, each by error, and lived. An adult woman took 7.5 g in a suicide attempt and exhibited few symptoms. The highest recorded total dose is approximately 10 g. Death has been reported in a premature neonate who received 178 mg/kg intramuscularly.

DRUG INTERACTIONS

Cyclosporine increases the volume of distribution, half-life, and renally eliminated fraction of digoxin. Cyclosporine potentiates vecuronium blockade and prolongs recovery time. To avoid drug interactions with plasticizers in intravenous solution bags, cyclosporine is dispensed from glass bottles. Cyclosporine may induce myopathies with abnormal electromyograms. Colchicine and lovastatin added to a cyclosporine regimen may enhance muscular toxicity.

PREGNANCY/LACTATION

Cyclosporine crosses the placenta and is distributed into milk.

LABORATORY

Analytic Methods

High-pressure liquid chromatography has been the only specific method available to measure the parent drug, whereas radioimmunoassay measures the parent drug and some of its metabolites. Most medical centers prefer to monitor cyclosporine by radioimmunoassay, despite the lack of specificity, because it is more easily performed. Cyclosporine concentrations measured by radioimmunoassay appear to correlate better with nephrotoxicity than those measured by HPLC.

Blood Levels

The relatively minor clinical picture of toxicity following oral cyclosporine overdose and the absence of a definite correlation between blood levels and clinical severity mitigate against dependence on the blood level for guidance and for the use of strenuous decontamination methods. Reported blood cyclosporine concentrations vary widely because of the heterogenicity of patients, analytical methods, and sampling times.

Neurotoxicity and possibly nephrotoxicity usually correlate with raised blood levels of cyclosporine metabolites. Clinicians can administer cyclosporine by continuous intravenous infusion during the first few days after transplantation, then orally by twice-daily doses, to achieve plasma cyclosporine concentrations of 75 to 150 ng/mL. It appears safe to maintain a trough plasma cyclosporine concentration of about 75 to 150 ng/mL, however, this does not necessarily guarantee safety from nephrotoxicity.

TREATMENT

Gut Decontamination

It is doubtful whether cathartics, or activated charcoal, in single or multiple doses, will be useful, but a controlled clinical trial has not been performed. In patients with preexisting altered renal function, it may be worthwhile to take measures to reduce the absorption of the drug, such as emesis induction and gastric lavage, although there are little data to support their usefulness. Certainly, prolonged vomiting following induction of emesis may precariously alter fluid balance in a renally compromised patient.

Elimination Enhancement

Cyclosporine is highly protein bound and has a high volume of distribution. It is unlikely that hemodialysis, plasmapheresis, and charcoal hemoperfusion will be effective.

Supportive Measures

- Cyclosporine overdose patients should be admitted to a health-care facility where vital signs and renal function can be carefully monitored.
- Healthy subjects, or patients with stable renal function, usually exhibit minor or no signs of toxicity and can be discharged within 24 hours of disappearance of signs and symptoms.
- Premature neonates have been subject to the few overdoses of cyclosporine reported in the infant age group. They appear to be at high risk of sustaining metabolic acidosis and renal failure.
- Lab tests in overdose patients should include serial renal function tests, evaluation of fluid balance and electrolytes, and measurement of arterial blood gases.
- Patients with stable renal function can be treated supportively. Renal function usually is not affected by the overdose but is more closely related to the underlying condition of the patient.
- Magnetic resonance imaging (MRI) and computed tomography (CT) scans may demonstrate symmetric, nonenhancing cortical and/or white matter changes. Both clinical and imaging changes may be reversible.

Questions—Cyclosporine

1. Cyclosporine is metabolized by the following hepatic enzyme(s)
A. N-acetyl transferase
B. P450 system
C. Xanthine oxidase
D. Alcohol dehydrogenase
E. Rhodanase

2. The predominant immunologic effect of cyclosporine is on
A. Plasma cell proliferation
B. T-cell proliferation
C. B-cell proliferation
D. Macrophages
E. Polymorphonuclear leukocytes

3. Evaluation of patients with cyclosporine overdose incudes all of the following except
A. Serial renal function
B. Arterial blood gas
C. Electrolytes
D. Cyclosporine level
E. Monitoring fluid balance

4. Symptoms of a cyclosporine overdose may include
A. Tremor
B. Seizures
C. Nausea
D. Flushing
E. All of the above

5. Cyclosporine has been known to have interactions with all the following medications except
A. Digoxin
B. Lovastatin
C. Vecuronium
D. Famotidine
E. Plasticizers

CYTOKINES

Cytokines are soluble factors that act as supportive, cytotoxic, or immune modulators. More than 30 peptides have been purified and sequenced and the coding genes cloned. The cytokines are divided into five main groups. These include (1) interferons (α, β, and γ), originally recognized by their ability to protect cells from viral infection; (2) interleukins (1-9), diverse immunoregulatory factors named in historical sequence; (3) hematopoietic colony-stimulating factors (erythropoietin, granulocyte-macrophage colony-stimulating factor, granulocyte colony-stimulating factor, and macrophage colony-stimulating factor), structurally dissimilar, but related in controlling hematopoiesis; (4) tumor necrosis factors (α and β), structurally related proteins with cytotoxic activity in vitro; and (5) assorted growth factors (e.g., platelet-derived growth factor), named according to the cell system in which their activity was discovered.

Granulocyte and Macrophage Stimulating Factors

Hematopoietic colony-stimulating factors include granulocyte colony-stimulating factors (G-CSF) and granulocyte-macrophage colony-stimulating factors (GM-CSF). Neutrophil counts rise in a dose-proportional fashion in response to recombinant G-CSF in patients who are neutropenic after cancer chemotherapy. Treatment comprises discontinuation and monitoring for an increase in white blood cells.

CLINICAL PRESENTATIONS

Granulocyte-macrophage colony stimulating factors (GM-CSF) may lead to fever, arthralgias, myalgias, a capillary leak syndrome with generalized edema, pleural and pericardial effusions, erythroderma, and, at high doses, thromboses at the site of venous catheters. Intravenous boluses and short infusions of

GM-CSF are more likely to produce adverse effects. Effects are dose related. A syndrome of flushing, hypotension, tachycardia, dyspnea, nausea, and vomiting with arterial oxygen desaturation may occur after the first injection and is reversed by oxygen and intravenous fluids.

G-CSF toxic effects include bone pain, hypotension, and renal dysfunction at the highest doses. Other adverse reactions include dyspnea, malaise, nausea, fever, rash, sinus tachycardia, headache, and chills, reversible after discontinuation. G-CSF has led to stimulation of multiple myeloma growth.

Interferons

Interferons have been used in the treatment of hairy-cell leukemia, multiple sclerosis, chronic myelogenous leukemia, Kaposi's sarcoma, malignant melanoma, renal-cell carcinoma, cutaneous T-cell lymphoma, and bladder cancer. They are not active alone against breast, colon, lung, and prostate cancers. Interferons may reduce hepatic microsomal cytochrome P450 activity. A reduction in clearance and a prolongation of the half-life of theophylline have been observed. Management of toxicity is largely symptomatic and supportive.

PATHOPHYSIOLOGY

Interferons, in high doses, can inhibit both B- and T-cell proliferation and can decrease humoral and cellular immune responses. At lower doses, interferons stimulate the immune system by increasing the cytocidal activity of natural killer cells, macrophages, and T-lymphocytes. Interferons may produce a flulike syndrome with fever, malaise, and myalgias.

CLINICAL PRESENTATIONS

Toxic effects appear to be similar for all interferons (α, β, and γ). These include a flulike syndrome of fever, chills, arthralgias, myalgias, and headache. Chronic side effects include fatigue, anorexia, nausea, vomiting, diarrhea, suppression of blood counts, elevation of hepatic enzymes, and central nervous system and cardiovascular toxicity. Toxicity is usually dose related and often is enhanced when interferon is given intravenously or administered to older patients.

Central nervous system toxic effects such as anxiety, agitation, somnolence, altered cognitive function, seizures, coma, and electroencephalographic abnormalities have been observed. Toxic cardiovascular effects include cardiac arrhythmias, cardiomyopathy, myocardial ischemia, acute myocardial infarction, and hypo- or hypertension. High intravenous doses may lead to some prolongation of the prothrombin time and partial thromboplastin time. Interferon alpha has induced reversible acute renal failure.

Interleukins

Various interleukins activate neutrophils and macrophages, stimulate T-cells, support T-cell growth and expansion, promote hemopoietic progenitors, activate B-cells to proliferate into plasma cells, promote proliferation of eosinophils, and stimulate B-cells to produce antibodies.

CLINICAL PRESENTATIONS

Non-life–threatening and life-threatening toxic effects are common with interleukin-2 use. Hypotension (transiently responsive to fluid administration), increase in heart rate and cardiac output, and decrease in systemic peripheral resistance have been observed. A capillary leak syndrome contributes to the hypotension. Other cardiovascular toxic effects include a decrease in left ventricular stroke work and ejection fraction, ventricular and supraventricular arrhythmias, myocardial ischemia, infarction, and death (if underlying coronary artery disease is present). Anuria, pulmonary edema, and adult respiratory distress syndrome have been observed.

Acute neuropsychiatric toxicity often is observed and includes severe behavioral changes, cognitive changes, disorientation, and confusion. These resolve within 48 to 72 hours of discontinuation of interleukin-2. Coma and seizures have been observed. Rarely, an acute fatal leukoencephalopathy has been reported.

Anecdotal reports also have associated interleukin-2 with the nephrotic syndrome, pancreatitis, thrombocytopenia, elevated adrenocorticotropic hormone, cortisol, epinephrine and norepinephrine levels, hypothyroidism, and an increase in the incidence of hypersensitivity to iodine-containing radiographic contrast media.

Questions—Cytokines

1. At low dose, interferon's effects on the immune system is/are
A. Inhibit B- and T-cell proliferation
B. Decrease the humoral response
C. Increase activity of natural killer cells
D. Decrease killer T cell production
E. Increase B-cell proliferation

2. Interleukins
A. Activate neutrophils and macrophages
B. Stimulate T-cells and support T-cell growth and expansion
C. Promote hemopoietic progenitors
D. Activate B-cells to proliferate into plasma cells
E. All of the above

INTRAVENOUS IMMUNE GLOBULIN

Intravenous immune globulin (IVIG) has been used increasingly to treat a variety of debilitating conditions. Immunomodulatory uses include immune thrombocytopenic purpura (ITP), Kawasaki's disease, Guillain-Barré syndrome, chronic inflammatory demyelinating neuropathy, and acquired hemophilia. It also is used as replacement therapy in a variety of immune deficiency states.

The ideal IVIG preparation contains structurally and functionally intact immunoglobulin molecules with normal biologic half-lives and a normal proportion of immunoglobulin subclasses. The preparation ideally contains high levels of the antibody or antibodies relevant to its proposed use. There should be no contamination with vasomotor peptides, endotoxins, or infectious agents, particularly viruses.

Commercial IVIG consists primarily of IgG, although trace quantities of IgA, IgM, IgE, and other serum proteins are present. Intravenous immune globulin is prepared from plasma derived from many donors. All IVIG preparations in the United States are manufactured with stabilizing agents, are acidified, and are recommended for infusion over several hours. Subcutaneous and intramuscular administration may be useful as well.

Pathophysiology

In patients with immune deficiency, the major effect of IVIG seems to be replacement of deficient immunoglobulins. In immune regulatory disorders, and/or reticuloendothelial blockade, an increase in suppressor T-cells or natural killer cells, and/or a decrease in antibody synthesis may be mediated by antibodies in the immunoglobulin preparation. The mode of action of IVIG in bacterial and viral infections is not known, but most likely involves antibacterial or antiviral antibodies in the preparation. Infused antibodies may also block recognition of infected cells by cytotoxic T-lymphocytes, thus preventing immune-mediated cell damage.

Pharmacokinetics

ABSORPTION

- Peak serum immunoglobulin levels measured immediately after intravenous administration correlate with dose.

DISTRIBUTION

- By 24 hours, serum immunoglobulin levels are 70% to 80% of peak levels and decrease to about 50% by 72 hours.
- Baseline levels of immunoglobulins are usually reached 21 to 28 days after infusion with IVIG.

ELIMINATION

- The elimination half-life of most immunoglobulin preparations is 18 to 32 days, similar to that of native IgG. The half-life of IgG is dependent on the half-lives of the individual IgG subclasses.

Clinical Presentations

HYPERSENSITIVITY EFFECTS

Allergic reactions have been observed after IVIG use. Manifestations may include abdominal pain and chest tightness. Individuals with IgA deficiency often may have IgG antibodies to IgA, and may develop an anaphylactic reaction to IVIG. If the IVIG preparation contains aggregates with anticomplementary activity, vasomotor symptoms may develop including chills, nausea, flushing, chest tightness, and wheezing. Hemolysis and thrombosis rarely have been reported.

GASTROINTESTINAL EFFECTS

Symptomatic hepatitis and elevated hepatic transaminase levels probably reflect contaminated lots of IVIG. The current consensus is that IVIG preparations do not transmit non-A, non-B hepatitis and no cases of hepatitis B have followed the use of IVIG.

NEUROLOGIC EFFECTS

Transient headaches, vomiting, altered consciousness with chills and fever, meningitis, and aseptic meningitis have been reported following use of IVIG.

DERMATOLOGIC EFFECTS

Some patients have developed alopecia within 1 to 4 weeks of IVIG treatment. The alopecia resolved within 4 months.

PULMONARY EFFECTS

Hypotension with respiratory failure and bronchospasm is very rare after IVIG use.

RENAL EFFECTS

Reversible renal dysfunction rarely has followed the use of IVIG. Acute renal failure can follow the use of IVIG in patients with prior evidence of impaired renal function.

ABUSE

Overrapid infusion of IVIG has produced an intense tingling, electric "buzz" sensation, lasting up to 5 minutes, followed by shivering, sweating, myalgias, and bronchospasm.

Toxic Dosage/Death

Use of IVIG 400 mg/kg/d for 5 days resulted in a reversible rise in serum creatinine when IVIG was administered to nephrotic patients.

Pregnancy/Lactation

Administration of IVIG during pregnancy has resulted in the birth of healthy infants.

Treatment

- Reducing the rate or the volume of infusion can often alleviate adverse reactions.
- Hydrocortisone, 1 to 2 mg/kg intravenously, may decrease adverse reactions in persons with previous side effects such as fever, chills, headache, hypertension, and chest pain. It can be given 30 minutes before IVIG infusion.
- Patients who experience an anaphylactic reaction to IVIG should be given symptomatic and supportive treatment with epinephrine, assurance of an airway and adequate respiration, cardiac monitoring, and oxygen as required.

Questions—Intravenous Immune Globulin

1. Commercial IVIG contains all of the following classes of immunoglobulins except
A. IgA
B. IgD
C. IgE
D. IgG
E. IgM

2. The elimination half-life of immunoglobulins is
A. 12 to 24 hours
B. 24 to 72 hours
C. 10 to 12 days
D. 18 to 32 days
E. 1 hour

3. IVIG has been used to treat all of the following diseases except
A. ITP
B. Kawasaki's disease
C. Guillain-Barré syndrome
D. Bell's Palsy
E. Chronic inflammatory demyelinating neuropathy

4. Treatment of anaphylactic reactions to IVIG is supportive and may include the following
A. Epinephrine
B. Cardiac monitoring
C. Airway management
D. All of the above
E. None of the above

5. The use of IVIG has resulted in the transmission of hepatitis B.
A. True
B. False

AUTOIMMUNITY

Autoimmunity results from a breakdown in the immune system's ability to distinguish "self" from "nonself." In the autoimmune reaction, the body mounts an immune response against some of its own normal components. These immune responses are mounted by antigens of "self" (autoantigens), and may be humoral responses (i.e., production of autoantibodies directed against autoantigens) and/or cell-mediated immune responses (i.e., development of delayed-type hypersensitivity reactions to autoantigens that are mediated by "self"-reacting T-lymphocytes).

An autoimmune disorder is one in which the immune system reacts to an endogenous antigen with subsequent injury to the tissues. The course is characterized by abnormalities of the immune response, chronic inflammation, and autoantibody formation. These disorders often are associated with human leukocyte antigens (HLA) related to a complex of genes known as the major histocompatibility complex and are of importance in graft rejection after organ transplantation.

Pathophysiology

Antireceptor antibodies can induce a number of autoimmune diseases by depressing (myasthenia gravis, insulin-resistant diabetes) or stimulating (Graves' disease) receptor function. Autoantibodies also are involved in morbid conditions when they are deposited, via the circulation, or formed *in situ* into immune complexes as in systemic lupus erythematosus (SLE), glomerulonephritis, periarteritis nodosa, Wegener's granulomatosis, and mixed connective-tissue disease. These diseases are relatively resistant to cyclosporine, but are sensitive to corticosteroids and alkylating agents such as cyclophosphamide.

T-cell–mediated autoimmune diseases include insulin-dependent diabetes mellitus, uveitis, psoriasis, atopic dermatitis, primary biliary cirrhosis, and rheumatoid arthritis. These diseases are very sensitive to cyclosporine and corticosteroids, but are relatively resistant to alkylating agents. Some diseases are sensitive to immunosuppressive agents where there are no immunoglobulin deposits in glomeruli and no clear immunologic abnormalities. This group includes the idiopathic nephrotic syndrome, inflammatory bowel diseases including Crohn's disease and ulcerative colitis, aplastic anemia, lichen planus, and polymyositis.

Clinical Presentations

Symptoms related to autoimmune disorders may include joint swelling and pain, erythema, swollen glands, unusual fatigue, and swelling of the hands and feet. Various other clinical disease states have been associated with chemically induced autoimmunity.

GLOMERULONEPHRITIS

Glomerulonephritis may be mediated by immune complexes. A membranous nephropathy may follow penicillamine use. It is associated with granular deposits of IgG and complement along capillary walls. Chronic mercury intoxication can cause a membranous nephropathy. Cadmium and gold may cause glomerular disease as well.

HEMOLYTIC ANEMIA

An autoimmune hemolytic anemia may be associated with red blood cell antibodies. Methyldopa, procainamide, and chlorpropamide have been associated with this malady.

HEPATITIS

Autoimmune hepatitis has been associated with methyldopa, halothane, isoniazid, nitrofurantoin, fenofibrate, and papaverine.

SYSTEMIC LUPUS ERYTHEMATOSUS

Numerous chemicals and drugs have been identified that induce autoimmunity. Systemic lupus erythematosus (SLE) has been associated with hydralazine, penicillamine, procainamide, and many other agents. Hydralazine and procainamide-induced SLE usually is milder than the native disease. Drug-induced lupus typically has little renal or central nervous system involvement.

MYASTHENIA GRAVIS

Long-term (months to years) penicillamine use has resulted in myasthenia gravis, which improves after the drug is withdrawn. Autoantibodies develop to acetylcholine receptors. The disease is similar but less severe than idiopathic myasthenia gravis. It tends to present more frequently with ocular manifestations.

PEMPHIGUS

This bullous dermatologic disease has been associated with penicillamine and captopril. Circulating autoantibodies to the basement zone are found in penicillamine-induced bullous pemphigoid. Termination of treatment is followed by a decrease in autoantibody titers and clinical improvement.

SCLERODERMA

Progressive systemic sclerosis (scleroderma) is a collagen-vascular disease with antinuclear antibodies formed to extractable nuclear antigens, the nucleolus, and the centromere. Sclerodermalike syndromes have been associated with vinyl chloride, silicosis, vibrations, the toxic oil syndrome, bleomycin and tryptophan.

THROMBOCYTOPENIA

An autoimmune thrombocytopenia associated with antiplatelet antibodies has been associated with carbamazepine, gold therapy, and interferon.

THYROID DISEASE

Autoimmune thyroid disease has been associated with numerous chemicals and drugs including dietary iodine, polybrominated biphenyls, polychlorinated biphenyls, lithium, anticonvulsant therapy, penicillamine, and amiodarone.

Treatment

At least six classes of agents have been widely used as immunosuppressive agents to treat autoimmune disease. These include (1) corticosteroids; (2) antimetabolites (azathioprine, methotrexate); (3) alkylating agents (cyclophosphamide, chlorambucil); (4) cyclosporine; (5) other agents such as intravenous γ-globulins and antilymphocyte globulins; and (6) newer agents such as tacrolimus and anti-CD3 antibodies. Unfortunately, several problems are related to their use. These include an insufficient rate of response, occurrence of relapse at cessation of treatment, persistent risk of direct drug toxicity, and immunosuppression.

Questions—Autoimmunity

1. **Which of the following diseases is associated with antibodies that stimulate receptor function?**
   A. Myasthenia gravis
   B. Graves disease
   C. Insulin-dependent diabetes
   D. Loeffler's syndrome
   E. Hypertension
2. **T-cell–mediated autoimmune diseases are sensitive to all of the following agents except**
   A. Cyclosporine
   B. Corticosteroids
   C. Alkylating agents
   D. All of the above
   E. None of the above
3. **Hemolytic anemia has been associated with the following drug(s)**
   A. Methyldopa
   B. Procainamide
   C. Chlorpropamide
   D. All of the above
   E. None of the above
4. **Procainamide has been associated with the following autoimmune disease(s)**
   A. Hemolytic anemia
   B. Systemic lupus erythematosus
   C. Insulin resistant diabetes
   D. B and C
   E. A and B
5. **Sclerodermalike syndrome has been associated with the following agent(s)**
   A. Vinyl chloride
   B. Silicosis
   C. Toxic oil syndrome
   D. Tryptophan
   E. All of the above

SPECIFIC IMMUNOTOXICANTS

In addition to the topics outlined above, numerous agents have been associated with immunologic responses. While by no means exhaustive, the following list identifies certain agents that have been studied for their immunologic potential.

Aluminum

Exposure to aluminum has produced abnormal T4/T8 ratios because of a disproportionate increase in the T8 cells. This has been associated with B-cell lymphoma in adult workers.

Beryllium

In chronic beryllium disease, beryllium acts as an antigen, stimulating local proliferation and accumulation in the lungs of beryllium-specific CD4-positive (helper/inducer) T-cells.

Cadmium

Glomerulonephritis and renal tubular lesions may follow cadmium use. IgG glomerular deposits in the basement membrane, suppression of antibody formation in animals, as well as both impairment and enhancement of growth of animal tumors indicate that cadmium may deter segments of the immune system but augment others.

Ciprofloxacin

Ciprofloxacin has been associated with a serum sickness type of reaction in an adult, classified as a leukocytoclastic vasculitis. Tests for antinuclear antibodies, rheumatoid factor, cryoglobulins and Coombs' test were negative. Tests for circulatory immune complexes were positive and skin biopsy showed a small-cell vasculitis.

Contrast Media

Lymphocytes from patients sensitive to amidotrizoate cross-react to structurally related ionic contrast media. Nonionic contrast agents do not induce proliferation of the lymphocytes. Ionic radiographic contrast agents may be antigenic in humans.

Formaldehyde

Formaldehyde may induce chronic antigenic stimulation in patients who have multiple subjective health complaints. Certain laboratory findings, including the development of antiformaldehyde antibodies (IgE, IgM, IgG), analyses of helper/suppressor T-ratios, and an increase in antigen memory cells, suggest this association.

Hydralazine

Hydralazine may facilitate induction of serious nephritic or systemic reactions with autoantibody production. Hydralazine-associated nephritis in humans is associated with antinuclear antibodies (ANA), but not with antibodies to DNA.

Insulin

Routine administration of insulin results in the production of antiinsulin IgG antibodies. A high serum concentration of total immunoreactive insulin, the presence of insulin autoantibodies, and fasting hypoglycemia characterize the insulin autoimmune syndrome.

Lead

Lead modulates the immune response *in vivo,* by inhibiting macrophage development, activating B-cells, and both inhibiting and enhancing T-cell subsets. Lead involvement in immune-mediated nephritis has been suggested. In one study, children with measurable blood-lead concentrations showed no associated significant effects on major immunoglobulin concentrations, C3, or total complement.

Mercury

Membranous nephropathy with immunofluorescent deposits of finely granular IgG/IgM and C3 complement has followed use of creams containing inorganic mercury. T-cell–dependent autoimmune phenomena are induced by mercuric chloride in animals.

Nickel

Nickel and nickel compounds can induce both dermal and pulmonary disease. Lung and nasal cancer, asthma, and nasal septal necrosis have followed nickel exposure. Nickel may enhance tumor progression by inhibiting natural killer cell activity and may cause allergic contact dermatitis.

Pesticides

There is little evidence that occupational or environmental exposure to pesticides has led to clinically significant immunosuppression and, therefore, to an increased risk of developing infections or cancer. Hypersensitivity reactions to pesticides generally are low.

Phenobarbital

Phenobarbital has induced a hypersensitivity state consisting of tubulointerstitial nephritis, an exfoliative dermatitis, and hepatitis. Immunoglobulins (IgG, IgA, and IgM) were decreased and total complement activity (CH50) was low.

Polyaromatic Hydrocarbons

Halogenated polyaromatic hydrocarbons (PAHs) include polychlorinated biphenyls (PCBs), phenols, chlorinated dibenzo-p-dioxins, dibenzofurans, hexachlorobenzene, pentachlorophenol, and polybrominated biphenyls (PBBs). Human studies have not convincingly disclosed any significant immunologic health effects after exposure to these agents.

Toluene

Preliminary studies suggest that pulmonary hypersensitivity and contact sensitivity to toluene diisocyanate may be diagnosed by determination of toluene diisocyanate-specific antibodies. Additional studies are needed.

Questions—Specific Immunotoxicants

1. The following agent(s) have been associated with pulmonary findings
A. Beryllium
B. Nickel
C. Toluene
D. All of the above
E. None of the above

2. Ciprofloxacin-associated leukocytoclastic vasculitis is associated with the following positive test results
A. Coombs test
B. Circulatory immune complexes
C. Antinuclear antibody (ANA)
D. Rheumatoid factor
E. Haptoglobin

3. Renal involvement has been seen with all of the following heavy metals except
A. Cadmium
B. Mercury
C. Nickel
D. Lead
E. All of the above

4. Occupational exposure to pesticides has led to clinically significant immunosuppression
A. True
B. False

5. Chronic formaldehyde exposure has been associated with the following laboratory findings
A. Positive ANA
B. Positive antiformaldehyde antibodies
C. Positive rheumatoid factor
D. Positive Coombs' test
E. Positive urinary leukocyte esterase

HUMAN ADJUVANT DISEASE AND SILICONE IMPLANTS

Thousands of breast implants are performed each year in the United States, and more than a half million augmentation mammoplasties using silicone implants were performed between 1959 and 1979. Connective tissue diseases may develop in individuals who have had various materials, including silicone, implanted. There have been no controlled clinical trials to clearly support a connection. The term "human adjuvant disease" has been proposed to describe such connective tissue disorders. The term "adjuvant" means assistance or help. An "immunologic adjuvant" is a substance that nonspecifically increases or changes the characteristics of the immune response to an antigenically unrelated antigen.

Numerous materials have been used for breast augmentation and other plastic procedures. Early use of paraffin, processed petroleum, and liquid silicone often induced severe local inflammatory and general immunologic tissue responses. After 1950, organosilicone polymers mostly supplanted these materials.

Silicone

Silicone is any organic compound in which all or part of the carbon atoms has been replaced by silicon. Silicones can be synthesized into liquids, gels, or rubberlike (elastomer) products.

Silicone Elastomers

Dimethylpolysiloxane is polymerized into long chains as an elastomer. Elastomeric silicone has been used in the production of heart valves, prosthetic finger joints, arteriovenous shunts for dialysis patients, and ventricular shunts for hydrocephalus. Silicone elastomer envelopes may be filled with saline or gels. No connective tissue diseases have been reported following these uses. The form (gel-filled implant) or the amount of silicone used may be a contributing factor.

Silicone Gel

The elastomer polymer is cross-linked to produce the gel.

Silicone Liquid

Glucoselike dimethylpolysiloxane polymer chains without fillers have been used as liquid silicone.

Silicone Polymers

Silicone polymers (polydimethylsiloxane), as used in implant surgery, are composed of polymer, filler, and catalyst.

Silicone Shells

Silicone mammary implant shells for both gel- and saline-filled implants consist of dimethylpolysiloxane polymer with 30% silicone dioxide filler. The silicone dioxide is fused to the silicone polymer by a chemical process. It is possible that silicone dioxide projections will be sheared off from the surface.

Pathophysiology

It has been theorized that adjuvants may potentiate the immune response by enhancing antigen localization, enhancing antigen presentation, and activating lymphocytes.

Clinical Presentations

Characteristics of human adjuvant disease have been proposed. These include autoimmune diseaselike symptoms that develop in individuals usually years after plastic surgery with foreign substances. Symptoms related to autoimmune disorders include joint swelling and pain, skin redness or swelling, swollen glands, unusual fatigue, and swelling of the hands and feet.

It has been proposed, but not definitively proven, that this disease is associated with injection into the breasts or other areas, with silicone, paraffin, or related substances that possibly have adjuvant effects. Autoantibodies may be detected by serologic testing. In some patients, there may be improvement in symptoms after removal of the foreign substance. Infection, malignancy, or other comorbid conditions that may mimic these symptoms must be excluded.

Connective tissue diseases, such as systemic lupus erythematosus (SLE), progressive systemic sclerosis (scleroderma), mixed connective-tissue disease, rheumatoid arthritis, Hashimoto's thyroiditis, Sjogren's syndrome, and morphea, have been reported following the use of silicone products or paraffin for breast augmentation. Disease may occur months to years after the original injection or implant. Raynaud's phenomenon, arthralgias, dry mouth, swollen stiff fingers, liver dysfunction, and jaundice have been described. Whether silicone or other adjuvants are directly or indirectly responsible for these symptoms has not been conclusively proven in the medical literature.

On February 20, 1992, the Food and Drug Administration recommended that silicone gel-filled breast implants be available only to women enrolled in clinical protocols. They recommended that any woman who requires breast reconstruction, following mastectomy or injury, be allowed to participate in clinical protocols if alternative reconstruction methods are not suitable. They also recommended that women who already have silicone breast implants should not consider having them removed unless there are problems. Women should be alert to symptoms that may signal implant rupture, capsular contracture, or autoimmune or connective-tissue disorders. Symptoms may include changes in the firmness, size, shape, or color of the breasts, as well as any pain or tenderness.

Treatment

- Treatment of human adjuvant disease is symptomatic and supportive. Mild discomfort may respond to nonsteroidal antiinflammatory drugs. Steroids may be of value depending on clinical judgment. Surgical consultation should be obtained if there are obvious capsular breaks, contracture, or asymmetry of implants.
- If connective tissue disease or human adjuvant disease has been diagnosed, consideration should be given to the removal of silicone implants, however this procedure may not be effective in lessening symptoms of the connective tissue disease. Again, it has not been conclusively shown that silicone or any other implantable material has been responsible for the development of the symptoms associated with connective tissue diseases.
- Patients should have a full immunohematologic workup including erythrocyte sedimentation rate, immunoglobulin levels, complement C3 and C4 levels, fluorescent ANA levels, and, if positive, tests for extractable nuclear antigen, ribonucleoprotein, Smith and rheumatoid factors.
- Histopathologic and immunopathologic examinations done from biopsied tissue may be helpful.
- Periodic medical examinations are recommended to detect breast cancer or implant rupture. Women with implants should have regular mammography examinations to detect breast cancer, if recommended for their age group.
- Breast cancer is not induced by silicone implants, however manual detection of lumps may be complicated by the presence of implants.
- For now, the Food and Drug Administration recommends that surgeons should not implant silicone gel breast implants, and that saline-filled implants can be used when breast implants are medically necessary.

Questions—Human Adjuvant Disease and Silicone Implants

1. Adjuvants may enhance the immune system by
   A. Enhancing antigen localization
   B. Enhancing antigen presentation
   C. Activating lymphocytes
   D. All of the above
   E. None of the above

2. Silicone elastomers have been used for the following products without any known association with connective tissue disease.
   A. Heart valves
   B. Prosthetic finger joints
   C. Arteriovenous shunts
   D. Ventricular shunts
   E. All of the above

3. The Food and Drug Administration currently recommends that silicone gel-filled breast implants not be used.
   A. True
   B. False

4. Symptoms consistent with rupture of a breast implant include of the following except
   A. Change in color of the breasts
   B. Change in the firmness of the breasts
   C. Pain
   D. Fever
   E. Asymmetry

5. The Food and Drug Administration recommends that all silicone gel-filled breast implants be removed from all patients that have had them implanted.
   A. True
   B. False

Answers

Introduction To Immunotoxicology

1. D 2. D 3. D

Immunotherapy

1. D 2. C 3. B

Introduction To Immunosuppression

1. E 2. C

Azathioprine

1. A 2. D 3. D

Cyclosporine

1. B 2. B 3. D 4. E 5. D

Cytokines

1. C 2. E

Intravenous Immune Globulin

1. B 2. D 3. D 4. D 5. B

Autoimmunity

1. B 2. C 3. D 4. E 5. E

Specific Immunotoxicants

1. D 2. B 3. C 4. B 5. B

Human Adjuvant Disease and Silicone Implants

1. D 2. E 3. A 4. D 5. B

SELECTED READINGS

Introduction To Immunotoxicology

1. Anderson JA, Adkinson NF Jr. Allergic reactions to drugs and biologic agents. JAMA 1987;258:2891–2899.
2. De Shazo RD, Lopez M, Salvaggio JE. Use and interpretation of diagnostic immunologic laboratory tests. JAMA 1987;258:3011–3031.

Immunotherapy

1. Brooks BO, Sullivan JB Jr. Immunotoxicology. In: Sullivan JB Jr, Krieger GR, eds. Hazardous Materials Toxicology: Clinical Principles of Environmental Health. Baltimore: Williams & Wilkins, 1991:190–214.
2. Burrell R. Human immune toxicity. Mol Aspects Med 1993;14:1–81.
3. Scherrmann J-M, Terrien N, Urtizberea M, et al. Immunotoxicotherapy: Present status and future trends. Clin Toxicol 1989;27:1–35.

Introduction To Immunosuppression

1. Identifying and controlling immunotoxic substances: Background paper. Congress of the United States, Office of Technology Assessment, Landrigan PC, Chairman. Washington, DC: U.S. Government Printing Office, April 1991.
2. Rossi SJ, Schroeder TJ, Hariharan S, Finst MR. Prevention and management of the adverse effects associated with immunosuppressive therapy. Drug Saf 1993;9:104–131.
3. Walker RW, Brochstein JA. Neurologic complications of immunosuppressive agents. Neurol Clin 1988;6:261–278.

Azathioprine

1. Carney DM, Zukoski CF, Ogden DA. Massive azathioprine overdose: Case report and review of the literature. Am J Med 1974;56:133–136.
2. Lawson DH, Lovatt GE, Gurton CS, Hennings RC. Adverse effects of azathioprine. Adverse Drug React Acute Poison Rev 1984;3:161–171.

Cyclosporine

1. Avellano F, Monka C, Krupp PF. Acute cyclosporin overdose: A review of present clinical experience. Drug Saf 1991;6:226–276.
2. Kokado Y, Takahara S, Ishibashi M, Sonoda T. An acute overdose of cyclosporin. Transplantation 1989;47:1096–1097.
3. Shannon M. Cyclosporin. Clin Toxicol Rev 1993;15(1):1–2.

Cytokines

1. Fent K, Zbinden G. Toxicity of interferon and interleukin. Trends Pharm Sci 1987;8:100–105.
2. Galvani DN. Cytokines, biological function and clinical use. J R Coll Physicians Lond 1988;22:226–231.
3. James DG. Which immunomodulator? Br J Clin Pract 1991;45:52–56.

Intravenous Immune Globulin

1. Berkman SA, Lee ML, Gale RP. Clinical uses of intravenous immunoglobulin. Ann Intern Med 1990;112:278–292.
2. Dwyer JM. Manipulating the immune system with immune globulin. N Engl J Med 1992;326:107–116.
3. Misbah SA, Chapel HM. Adverse effects of intravenous immunoglobulin. Drug Saf 1993;9:254–262.
4. Wordell CJ. Use of intravenous immune globulin therapy: An overview. DICP Ann Pharmacother 1991;25:805–817.

Autoimmunity

1. Back J-F. The new era of immunosuppressive therapy in autoimmune disease. Transplant Proc 1991;23:3319–3321.
2. Comdemi JJ. The autoimmune diseases. JAMA 1987;258:2920–2929.
3. Hess E. Drug-related lupus. N Engl J Med 1988;318:1460–1462.
4. Spears CJ, Batchelor JR. Drug-induced autoimmune disease. Adv Nephrol 1987;16:219–230.

Specific Immunotoxicants

1. Gleichmann E, Kimber I, Purchase IFH. Immunotoxicology: Suppressive and stimulatory effects of drugs and environmental chemicals on the immune system. Arch Toxicol 1989;63:257–273.

Human Adjuvant Disease And Silicone Implants

1. Baldwin CM Jr, Kaplan EN. Silicone-induced human adjuvant disease? Ann Plast Surg 1983;10:270–273.
2. Byron MA, Venning VA, Mowat AG. Post-mammoplasty human adjuvant disease. Br J Rheumatol 1984;23:227–229.
3. Fock KM, Feng PH, Tey BH. Autoimmune disease developing after augmentation mammoplasty: Report of 3 cases. J Rheumatol 1984;11:98–100.
4. Osebold JW. Mechanisms of action by immunologic adjuvants. JAMA 1982; 181:983–987.
5. Sanchez-Guerrero J, Colditz GA, Karlson EW, Silicone breast implants and the risk of connective tissue diseases and symptoms. N Engl J Med 1995;332:1666–1670.

ACKNOWLEDGMENTS

Thanks to George Stedman, MD for contributing the questions in this chapter.

CHAPTER 32
Pulmonary Toxicology

INTRODUCTION

Ahlquist first developed the concept of α and β subgroups of adrenoceptor agonists in 1948. Isoprenaline (isoproterenol) was the first selective β-adrenoceptor agonist and was developed in the 1940s. Metaproterenol was later developed as an orally active agent. In the mid-1960s β-adrenoceptors were further classified as β-1 or β-2.

The force and rate of contraction of cardiac muscle were considered to be mediated by β-1 receptors, and relaxation of the bronchial and uterine smooth muscle appeared to be mediated by β-2 receptors. This stimulated research for more selective β-2 adrenoceptor agonists, which led to isoetharine, albuterol, and terbutaline. Some of these β-2 agonist drugs are useful in the treatment of asthma (e.g., albuterol and terbutaline), and others are used as tocolytic agents in the treatment of premature labor (e.g., ritodrine and isoxsuprine). At high doses, skeletal muscle tremor and cardiac stimulation limit the use of all these drugs.

β-2 AGONISTS

The primary therapeutic effect of most β-2 adrenoceptor drugs is related to their use as bronchodilators in the treatment of bronchial asthma, chronic bronchitis, and bronchospastic states. Many β-2 adrenoceptor agonists have been used to inhibit uterine contractions in premature labor.

Pathophysiology

β-2 adrenoceptor agonists produce effects on smooth muscle and skeletal muscle. These include bronchodilatation, relaxation of uterine muscle, and some vasodilating effect on peripheral vasculature. With binding at these sites, ATP is converted to cyclic AMP, which, in turn, activates protein kinase. Certain proteins then are phosphorylated, which increases bound intracellular calcium. The reduced availability of intracellular calcium inhibits actin-myosin linkage, leading to relaxation of smooth muscle.

β-2 agonists have an antiallergic effect on mast cells, causing inhibition of release of bronchoconstriction mediators including histamine, neutrophil chemotactic factor, and prostaglandin. The cyclic AMP system probably acts as the second messenger in regulating the mast cell response.

β-2 adrenergic stimulation also promotes an intracellular shift of potassium from serum, possibly via stimulation of Na-K ATPase. This may lead to a temporary decrease in both elevated and normal potassium concentrations. Both intravenous and inhaled β-2 adrenergic agonists may cause a decrease in serum potassium concentrations. Stimulation of nonpulmonary β-2 receptors may lead to an increase in heart rate, prolongation of the QTc interval, nonspecific T-wave changes, skeletal muscle tremor via β-2 receptor sites on skeletal muscle, and a slight increase in blood glucose and fatty acids.

Pharmacokinetics

β-agonists are administered orally, by inhalation, and by subcutaneous, intramuscular, and intravenous injection. Their bioavailability is dependent on their mode of administration.

ABSORPTION

- Following oral administration, most β-2 agonists are well absorbed.
- Despite extensive absorption, the systemic bioavailability of oral β-agonists is very low as a result of extensive sulfation of the drugs in the liver and possibly in the wall of the small intestine. Therefore, the oral dose of β-agonists needs to be 5 to 10 times greater than the parenteral dose.
- For relief of bronchospasm, β-2 agonists can be administered directly to the lungs by inhalation via pressurized metered-dose inhalers or as a spray generated by a nebulizer. With a nebulizer, about 10% to 20% is absorbed. The lungs absorb more of the dose and less is swallowed.
- After aerosol administration, the proportion of an administered dose recovered in the urine as unchanged drug and metabolites is up to 80% for albuterol, 69% for isoprenaline, and about 50% for terbutaline.
- Most of an inhaled dose is deposited on the pharynx after inhalation and is swallowed. About 3% of an oral inhaled dose reaches the lungs. First-pass metabolism is avoided with oral inhalation.
- After aerosol administration, the time to maximum plasma drug concentration is approximately 2 to 4 hours, comparable to that following oral administration and consistent with swallowing most of an inhaled dose.
- Plasma concentrations of terbutaline peak more rapidly (within 15 to 30 minutes) after subcutaneous administration than after oral use. Systemic bioavailability of subcutaneous terbutaline is about 100%.

DISTRIBUTION

- The plasma protein binding of most β-agonists is about 10%.
- Tissue distribution is large (from 1 to 29 L/kg).

ELIMINATION

- β-agonists are eliminated by metabolism and renal excretion of unchanged drug.
- Metabolism of resorcinol derivatives (terbutaline, albuterol, fenoterol, xamoterol, prenalterol, pirbuterol, and orciprenaline) is by sulfate conjugation.
- Renal excretion is the major route of elimination of parenterally administered β-agonists.

Clinical Presentations

Characteristic features of β-2 adrenoceptor agonist poisoning include nausea, tachycardia, tremor, hyperglycemia, and hypokalemia. The skin may be warm with evidence of diaphoresis. Other symptoms may include agitation, hand tremor, apprehension, dizziness, vomiting, headaches, and dilated pupils. Rarely, rhabdomyolysis, lactic acidosis, renal failure, leukemoid reaction, and hypoglycemia have been observed.

Cardiovascular effects of overdose may include precordial pressure or chest pain, angina pectoris, hypotension, and electrocardiographic changes. β-2 agonists can provoke myocardial ischemia by acute reduction of diastolic blood pressure or by precipitation of cardiac rhythm disturbances. β-2 agonists in overdose may induce prolongation of the QTc interval, atrial fibrillation, atrial premature beats, right bundle-branch block, and nonspecific ST-T wave changes. Sinus tachycardia is the most frequent electrocardiographic abnormality seen and may be a reflex reaction secondary to peripheral vasodilation. Ventricular tachycardia may be precipitated by aerosolized terbutaline in patients with preexisting coronary artery disease.

Continued dependence on albuterol tablets taken in high doses may lead to toxic or paranoid psychosis. Psychological dependence on β-agonists, manifested by numerous daily (i.e., greater than 50) inhalations of albuterol, has been documented in asthmatics because they "need" it and want to "feel good." Long-term tolerance may develop to bronchodilator action, tremor, tachycardia, prolongation of the QTc interval, hyperglycemia, hypokalemia, and vasodilator response.

Toxic Dosage/Death

ALBUTEROL

160 to 200 mg albuterol ingestions in adults have yielded significant tachycardia, skeletal muscle irritability, hypokalemia, and agitation; however, survival has been uniform with supportive care. A survey of 40 children revealed ingestions of albuterol between 5 and 240 mg in which all responded well to supportive measures. Another survey revealed 112 children under the age of 12 who ingested up to 96 mg of albuterol. They were observed at home (0.6 mg/kg ingested) or in a health-care facility (0.3 to 6.3 mg/kg) and all recovered with minimal intervention.

TERBUTALINE

Palpitations, chest pain, tremor, tachycardia, hypertension, and electrocardiogram (ECG) changes reflecting myocardial ischemia have been observed in adults ingesting 10 times the usual dose. Tremor and tachycardia may persist 1 to 2 days.

DEATH

An increase in the death rate from asthma in the United Kingdom during the 1960s was associated with the use of inhalers delivering high-potency isoproterenol, a relatively nonselective β agonist. Similar association with death after increasing the number of canisters or metered-dose inhalations per month has been observed with albuterol. Factors that may contribute to such deaths may include regular versus acute use for attacks only, hypokalemia, unsupervised use, and the induction of paradoxical bronchospasm by products that may contain propellants, emulsifying agents, preservatives (e.g., benzalkonium chloride and sulfites) or contaminants.

Drug Interactions

Treatment with diuretics augments the hypokalemia that occurs with β-2 agonists. Use of orally inhaled β-2 agonists with other oral sympathomimetics produces additive sympathomimetic effects. Administration of a β-agonist by any route other than oral inhalation (e.g., intravenous, subcutaneous) together with theophylline may lead to deleterious cardiovascular effects. β-2 agonists should be administered with caution to patients being treated with monoamine oxidase inhibitors or tricyclic antidepressants because the action of the β-2 agonist on the vascular system may be potentiated. β-Receptor antagonists, especially those without β-1 receptor selectivity, inhibit β-receptor agonists.

Pregnancy/Lactation

Pregnancy does not appear to significantly influence the toxicokinetics of β-2 agonists. Any of the inhaled β-agonist bronchodilators may be useful for the management of asthma during pregnancy. The Food and Drug Administration (FDA) has placed albuterol in pregnancy risk category C. The rates of perinatal mortality, congenital malformations, preterm delivery, and delivery of low-birth-weight infants are not increased in pregnant women using β-2 adrenergic agonists for asthma. There are no differences in Apgar scores, rates of complications of labor or delivery, or postpartum bleeding.

Case reports of spontaneous abortion and death (from arrhythmia) in pregnant patients receiving terbutaline have been published. When β-2 agonists are administered for the treatment of premature labor, fetal tachycardia may be seen, with hyperglycemia, hypotension, and a respiratory distress syndrome in infants delivered after the failure of tocolytic therapy. Placental transfer is rapid.

After oral terbutaline administration to the mother, milk concentrations of the drug may be similar to or greater than plasma concentrations. Nursing infants exhibit no clinical signs of β-adrenoceptor stimulation. Few data are available on other β-adrenoceptor drugs.

Laboratory

ANALYTIC METHODS

Plasma concentrations of fenoterol can be assayed by high-pressure liquid chromatography separation with ultraviolet spectrum monitoring. Albuterol can be assayed by a gas chromatography-mass spectrometry method. A method combining immunoaffinity chromatography with high-performance liquid chromatography also is available. Terbutaline has been determined in the serum and plasma by thin-layer fluorometry, liquid chromatography with electrochemical detection and gas chromatography-mass spectrometry.

BLOOD LEVELS

Lung function improvement, plasma cAMP concentration, and increases in skeletal muscle tremor and heart rate appear to correlate with plasma concentrations of albuterol, terbutaline, ritodrine, and rimiterol. Peak pharmacologic effects occur later than peak plasma drug concentration. For a given plasma concentration of β-2 agonist, there is a large interpatient variation in bronchodilation, tremor, and heart rate responses. There also is considerable intrapatient variability reflecting the development of tolerance during continuous treatment.

The approximate serum terbutaline concentration required to produce bronchial muscle relaxation is 2 ng/mL. Bronchodilator effects correlate with plasma levels when measured by forced expiratory volume and cAMP. The normal therapeutic concentration of terbutaline is 2 to 6 ng/mL.

Treatment

GUT DECONTAMINATION

When the patient is seen within the first 4 to 6 hours, gastric lavage may be useful, although patients with little evidence of cardiovascular abnormality, tremor, hyperglycemia, or hypokalemia probably will do well with observation only. There are no data to support the use of activated charcoal in these patients; however, it may be helpful after oral overdoses.

ELIMINATION ENHANCEMENT

A high volume of distribution and often high plasma protein binding make the use of extracorporeal techniques such as hemodialysis and hemoperfusion of little potential value. In the rare instance of rhabdomyolysis with acute renal failure, hemodialysis may be required.

SUPPORTIVE MEASURES

- Selective β-2 adrenoceptor drugs may be relatively innocuous in overdose in younger age groups. In children, ingestions of 0.6 mg/kg or less require observation only.
- For ingestions greater than 0.6 mg/kg, consideration should be given to direct medical evaluation and gastrointestinal decontamination. In these patients, observation in an emergency department for 4 to 6 hours and attention to normal heart rate, absence of tremor, normal blood sugar, and normal potassium level are sufficient for discharge if the patient is otherwise asymptomatic.
- Patients who are in older age groups or who present with symptoms of chest pressure, chest pain, or arrhythmias should be placed on a cardiac monitor with a source of oxygen available.
- An ECG should be obtained in all significant β-agonist exposures. Monitor oxygen status and obtain serial arterial blood gases and creatine kinase levels with cardiac enzyme fractions.
- Watch electrolytes, especially potassium, carefully. Hypokalemia following β-2 agonist therapy has been associated with cardiac arrhythmias. Hypokalemia usually reverts to normal spontaneously. If the serum potassium level, also reflected on ECG, is seriously depressed, consider slow administration of potassium chloride, with repeat serum potassium levels and serial ECGs.
- Follow blood sugars in serious cases. Hyperglycemia may be a result of the glycolytic effect of β-2 adrenoceptor agonists on hepatic glycogen stores.
- β-blockers may be used to treat supraventricular arrhythmias, or tremor, but must be used with great care in asthmatic patients.
- If an overdose of terbutaline has been administered to a pregnant patient in labor, pulmonary edema may be precipitated. Oxygen, intravenous diuretics, and fluid restriction may be required.
- Check creatine phosphokinase, renal function and phosphorous as terbutaline may rarely cause rhabdomyolysis with acute renal failure and hypophosphatemia.

Antidotes

There is no specific antidote for β-2 adrenoceptor agonist overdoses although the use of β-blocking agents (e.g., propranolol 0.01 mg/kg) may improve tremor, tachycardia, and hypokalemia in certain cases. Although there is danger in the use of such drugs in the presence of asthma, and some have advocated a more cardioselective β-blocker, such as metoprolol, there is scant evidence that this group of drugs materially enhances recovery.

Questions-β-2 Agonists

1. Which of the following is false?
- A. The primary therapeutic effect of most β-2 agonists relates to their use as bronchodilators.
- B. Many of the β-2 adrenoceptor agonists have been used to stimulate uterine contractions in premature labor.
- C. β-2 adrenoceptor agonists produce effects on smooth muscle and skeletal muscle.
- D. β-2 agonists have an antiallergic effect on mast cells, causing inhibition of release of bronchoconstriction mediators including histamine, neutrophil chemotactic factor, and prostaglandin.
- E. β-2 adrenergic stimulation promotes an intracellular shift of potassium from serum.

2. Despite extensive absorption, the systemic bioavailability of oral β-agonists is very low because of extensive sulfation of the drugs in the liver and possibly in the wall of the small intestine. Therefore, the oral dose of β-agonists needs to be 5 to 10 times greater than the parenteral dose.
- A. True
- B. False

3. Which of the following is true?
- A. Characteristic features of β 2-adrenoceptor agonist poisoning include nausea, tachycardia, tremor, hyperglycemia, and hypokalemia.
- B. Other symptoms may include agitation, hand tremor, apprehension, dizziness, vomiting, headaches, and dilated pupils.
- C. Rarely, rhabdomyolysis, lactic acidosis, renal failure, leukemoid reaction, and hypoglycemia have been observed.
- D. Cardiovascular effects of overdose may include precordial pressure or chest pain, angina pectoris, hypotension, and electrocardiographic changes.
- E. All of the above.

4. β-2 agonists can provoke myocardial ischemia by
- A. Acute reduction of diastolic blood pressure
- B. Precipitation of cardiac rhythm disturbances
- C. Inducing cardiomyopathy
- D. All of the above
- E. A and B

5. Cardiac effects of β 2-agonist overdose may include
- A. Shortening of the QTc interval
- B. Atrial fibrillation
- C. Ventricular tachycardia
- D. A and C
- E. B and C

INHALED STEROIDS

Inhaled corticosteroids, such as beclomethasone, budesonide, triamcinolone, and flunisolide, have been used for the topical treatment of asthma. At low dose, corticosteroids are largely free of adverse effects. For more severe asthma, where higher doses are required, there may be some suppression of the hypothalamus-pituitary-adrenal axis. Behavioral changes have been observed in children. Treatment of excessive dosage is symptomatic. No fatalities have been reported.

Pathophysiology

Substitution at the 17a ester portion of cortisol has resulted in a group of very potent steroids (e.g., beclomethasone, betamethasone, and budesonide) that are effective when applied topically for skin diseases and when inhaled for asthma. The antiasthmatic potency of an inhaled steroid is approximately proportional to its potency as an antiinflammatory agent.

Pharmacokinetics

ABSORPTION

- Systemic availability of budesonide is 11% after oral administration and 73% after inhalation, which points to an extensive first-pass metabolism probably in the liver.

Answers to questions in shaded boxes appear at the end of the chapter.

- Plasma protein binding is 88%, similar to that reported for other glucocorticosteroids.

DISTRIBUTION

- Budesonide has an apparent volume of distribution of 4.2 L/kg.

ELIMINATION

- The plasma elimination half-life of budesonide is about 2 hours in adults. This can be compared with half-lives of 1.5 to 2.0 hours for flunisolide and 15 hours for beclomethasone.
- About 70% of a dose is excreted in the urine.

Clinical Presentations

There are anecdotal reports of skin thinning and spontaneous, easy bruising, striae, acneiform eruptions, and contact dermatitis, especially in the elderly who have used high doses for long periods. Growth retardation has been observed with inhaled beclomethasone and with budesonide. Aggressiveness, bed wetting, hyperactivity, and episodes of severe temper may be observed in young asthmatic children after budesonide inhalation therapy. Acute psychosis also has been described.

Rarely, Cushing's syndrome, adrenal suppression, dysphoria, oral candidiasis, nausea, headache, dry throat, gas, pruritus, rash, impaired taste, diarrhea, constipation, and heartburn have followed the use of inhaled corticosteroids.

Toxic Dosage/Death

At inhaled doses of 200 to 400 mg of budesonide, young children develop adverse behavior problems. No dose associated with fatality has been reported.

Drug Interactions

Risk factors for development of corticosteroid inhalation-induced dysphoria include the use of oral corticosteroids and concomitant use of theophylline, calcium antagonists, and nitrates.

Pregnancy/Lactation

Very large doses of inhaled corticosteroids may be teratogenic, but the risks to mother and fetus if asthma is uncontrolled may be greater.

Laboratory

ANALYTIC METHODS

A sensitive radioimmunoassay has been developed for detection of budesonide in plasma.

BLOOD LEVELS

Inhalation of 1 mg of budesonide leads to a peak plasma level of 2.3 ng/mL in about 1 hour.

Treatment

GUT DECONTAMINATION

Charcoal theoretically may decrease available corticosteroid in oral overdose, however its efficacy has not been described.

ELIMINATION ENHANCEMENT

No indication for additional elimination methods is recognized in the literature.

SUPPORTIVE MEASURES

- Treatment is symptomatic and supportive. Cessation of use of the corticosteroid is indicated.
- A slight transient depression of plasma cortisol levels has been observed, together with an increase in neutrophils, decrease in lymphocytes, and fall in eosinophils.
- An increase in serum cholesterol and insulin levels also has been reported; however, this has not been associated with overt hypoglycemic symptoms.

Questions—Inhaled Steroids

1. Inhaled corticosteroids include all of the following except

A. Beclomethasone
B. Budesonide
C. Triamterene
D. Triamcinolone
E. Flunisolide

2. Clinical effects of inhaled steroids may include all of the following except

A. Skin thinning, easy bruising, and striae
B. Growth stimulation
C. Aggressiveness, bed wetting, and hyperactivity
D. Acute psychosis
E. Cushing's syndrome

XANTHINES

Theophylline

Theophylline is a member of the xanthine family, which has been used since the 1930s as a treatment for asthma. It is structurally related to caffeine. Theophylline effects include improved ventilatory response to hypoxia, a dose-dependent augmentation of diaphragmatic contractility, and increased oxygen saturation during sleep. Despite its positive effect as a bronchodilator, its narrow therapeutic index may yield significant toxicity because of age-related or drug-induced changes in theophylline clearance. Theophylline and β-adrenergic agonists induce similar clinical (vomiting, tachycardia, tremulousness, agitation, wide pulse pressure, and hypotension) and laboratory (hypokalemia, hyperglycemia, lactic acidosis) effects after overdose.

Theophylline toxicity typically presents after inadvertent overmedication in its chronic form, or as a large intentional ingestion in its acute form. Clinical presentation and treatment differs by type. Hypotension, hypokalemia, and low serum bicarbonate, for example, are seen frequently in large single, but not chronic, overdoses. Serious complications may occur at lower theophylline levels, such as the 40 to 70 μg/mL range, in chronic toxicity, as compared with acute ingestions, where these complications are associated with levels over 100 μg/mL.

PATHOPHYSIOLOGY

In addition to promoting diaphragmatic contractility, theophylline promotes mucociliary clearance, aids cardiac function, lowers pulmonary artery pressure, and exhibits antiinflammatory effects. Theophylline, a phosphodiesterase inhibitor, increases tissue levels of cyclic AMP, a potentially epileptogenic substance. Increasing cAMP levels inhibit the IgE-induced release of mediators of smooth muscle constriction.

Theophylline also is an adenosine receptor antagonist and may cause seizures by antagonizing the depressant effect of adenosine in the cerebral cortex. Theophylline stimulates catecholamine release, leading to elevated plasma epinephrine and norepinephrine. The hypercatecholamine effects of theophylline intoxication include possible mediation of hyperglycemia, hypercalcemia, metabolic acidosis, prolongation of the QT interval on ECG, and may be a cause of tachyarrhythmias.

PHARMACOKINETICS

Absorption

- Theophylline is well absorbed orally. Dissolution appears to be the rate-limiting step for absorption. Sustained-release preparations differ markedly in their absorption and to a lesser extent in their bioavailability.
- Therapeutic doses in uncoated tablets or liquids reach peak levels within 1 to 2 hours.
- The gastrointestinal tract absorbs liquid and suspension formulations more rapidly than capsules.

Distribution

- The volume of distribution of theophylline remains relatively constant, ranging from 0.2 to 0.7 L/kg. Liver cirrhosis increases and obesity decreases the volume of distribution at therapeutic doses, whereas age, sex, chronic pulmonary disease, and smoking have little effect.
- In plasma, protein binding of theophylline at therapeutic concentrations is approximately 50%.
- Peak levels after the ingestion of sustained-release preparations occur within 1 to 24 hours (mean, 11 hours). Regular formulations produce peak levels 2 to 8 hours (mean, 5 hours) postingestion.
- Smoking reduces half-life, presumably through enzyme induction by components of cigarette smoke.
- Secondary elevations of theophylline levels and subsequent clinical toxicity may result from the development of sustained-release tablet bezoars.
- Sustained-release preparations increase the duration of drug levels by increasing the absorption half-life rather than altering clearance. These formulations may vary in the completeness, rate, or consistency of absorption.

Elimination

- A cytochrome in the P450 system is responsible for most theophylline metabolism in humans.
- In adults, about 10% of a dose of theophylline is excreted unchanged in the urine.
- Major metabolic pathways in the adult involve demethylation and oxidation, which produce methylxanthine and methyluric acids.
- In the neonate, 50% is excreted unchanged. In the neonate, all the metabolic pathways of theophylline observed in adults are only partially developed. In premature infants, theophylline has a half-life 9 times that of children 1 to 4 years old.
- In premature infants, theophylline is methylated partially to caffeine, which can itself be toxic.
- Pregnancy reduces theophylline protein binding (11% vs. 23%) and increases the volume of distribution (31 L vs. 37 L) and elimination half-life (262 minutes vs. 389 minutes). Increased clearance of unbound drug, however, may offset these effects.
- At therapeutic doses, blood levels follow first-order kinetics, but in overdose, mixed first- and zero-order (Michaelis-Menten) kinetics prevail.
- Overdose may produce a biphasic elimination pattern with a slow initial phase due either to continued absorption or to saturation of metabolic pathways.

CLINICAL PRESENTATIONS

The risk for major toxicity in cases of acute theophylline intoxication is predicted best by peak serum theophylline concentration. Acute theophylline intoxication, defined as peak serum theophylline concentration of 30 mg/L or greater, is influenced by method of intoxication. Patients with chronic theophylline intoxication have a greater risk for major toxicity (seizures or cardiac arrhythmias associated with hemodynamic instability) at lower serum theophylline concentrations than those with acute intoxication.

The risk for major toxicity in cases of chronic overmedication cannot be predicted by peak serum theophylline concentration. Age greater than 60 years has the greatest diagnostic accuracy in identifying patients at highest risk, but age does not provide the same degree of prognostic accuracy in cases of chronic overmedication as the peak serum theophylline concentration does in cases of acute intoxication.

Neurologic Effects

Tremulousness and agitation are present in almost 50% of seriously intoxicated patients. Seizures in both children and adults may occur at therapeutic or only mildly toxic levels. Intractable seizures also may occur in severe intoxications and can lead to permanent neurologic sequelae. The seizures usually are generalized. Seizures may result in rhabdomyolysis, hypothermia, and hypoxia. Patients with a preexisting seizure disorder or other neurologic conditions such as meningitis, head trauma, and cerebrovascular accident are particularly vulnerable to seizures. In chronic overmedication, seizures may be the initial sign of toxicity. Theophylline induces cerebral vasoconstriction and ischemia. Coma is an uncommon sign of theophylline intoxication. Ataxia and visual hallucinations have been reported in pediatric theophylline overdoses.

Cardiovascular Effects

Theophylline-induced cardiotoxicity may be a result of its direct action on cardiac membrane depolarization, antagonism of the cardioprotective effects of endogenous adenosine, stimulation of plasma catecholamine activity, and the resultant increase in myocardial oxygen demand. Cardiotoxic effects may occur in patients with theophylline intoxication and in patients whose levels are within therapeutic range.

In patients with serum theophylline concentrations greater than 30 mg/L, sinus tachycardia and complex atrial and ventricular ectopy are common. Sustained supraventricular and ventricular tachyrhythmias are uncommon. Ventricular tachycardia appears to be a rare complication that tends to occur in the setting of advanced age, underlying heart disease, and/or very high serum theophylline concentrations. Ventricular fibrillation and cardiac arrest may follow self-poisoning, which results in a serum theophylline concentration greater than 100 mg/L.

Muscular Effects

Muscle aches are a common complaint. Acute compartment syndrome may occur rarely following rhabdomyolysis that has been reported in theophylline poisoning. It also can follow repeated seizures, exacerbated by hypokalemia, hypotension, and limb compression.

Hypersensitivity Effects

Asthmatic patients may experience a delayed hypersensitivity reaction to the ethylenediamine component of theophylline. Cross-reactivity may occur with chemically related agents including certain antihistamines, triethanolamine-containing creams, and hydroxyzine.

Gastrointestinal Effects

Nausea and vomiting are the most common symptoms of toxicity. Abdominal pain occurs less frequently, and rarely the clinical picture resembles acute pancreatitis. In chronic repeated overmedication, the gastrointestinal symptoms appear less than after single intentional ingestions.

Metabolic Effects

In acute theophylline poisoning, β-2 adrenergic stimulation appears to be an important mediator of hypokalemia and hyperglycemia. Hypokalemia may be a result of potassium loss following protracted vomiting, but it may occur in the absence of vomiting. An intracellular shift of potassium follows the catecholamine-induced stimulation of membrane-bound sodium-potassium ATPase. These factors may be contributory mechanisms in the production of hypokalemia. Potassium shifts, and not potassium depletion, usually are the cause of hypokalemia.

TOXIC DOSAGE/DEATH

In adults and young children, 1 mg/kg of theophylline raises serum theophylline levels approximately 2 μg/mL. Hence, ingestions over 10 mg of theophylline per kilogram are potentially toxic. Recovery has occurred following single acute ingestions with serum theophylline levels as high as 204 μg/mL.

DRUG INTERACTIONS

Theophylline is particularly susceptible to drug interactions as 90% of its elimination is via metabolism in the P450 system. Its clearance increases or decreases when numerous other drugs are administered. Drugs such as contraceptives, allopurinol, caffeine, erythromycin, and cimetidine decrease theophylline clearance while phenobarbital and phenytoin promote the metabolism of theophylline. Furosemide, propranolol, hydrocortisone, and influenza immunization reportedly delay theophylline metabolism.

PREGNANCY/LACTATION

Theophylline use during pregnancy is not associated with an increased risk of stillbirth. Association of some rare cardiovascular anomalies with theophylline exposure in animals and in one human study suggests that theophylline may be a cardiovascular teratogen. For the fetus with prenatal exposure to theophylline, fetal echocardiography may be useful in detecting any possible severe cardiac defect. Theophylline levels in breast milk and maternal blood concentrations follow similar kinetics. Theophylline is classified as pregnancy risk category C.

LABORATORY

Analytic Methods

High-performance liquid chromatography is the standard of measurement. A commercially available theophylline assay obtained by fingerstick is able to measure theophylline concentrations within the range of 0.4 to 30 μg/mL. The method correlates well with high-performance liquid chromatography.

Blood Levels

After acute single ingestions, minimal toxicity occurs between peak theophylline levels of 20 to 40 μg/mL, moderate toxicity at 40 to 100 μg/mL, and severe toxicity at more than 100 μg/mL. A blood concentration of 5 to 10 mg/L typically provides a useful therapeutic level. Individual variation exists and the severity of intoxication should not be judged by laboratory values alone.

Chronic overmedication causes poisoning at lower serum theophylline levels than acute overdoses. Seizures and serious dysrhythmias frequently appear in chronic overmedication cases at theophylline levels between 40 and 70 μg/mL. Patients under 40 years of age tend to develop serious dysrhythmias when theophylline levels exceed 50 μg/mL while older patients may display serious rhythm disturbances at levels above 35 μg/mL.

TREATMENT

Gut Decontamination

Gastric lavage may be used in patients suspected of ingesting more than 10 mg/kg of theophylline who present within 1 or 2 hours of overdose. Emesis is absolutely contraindicated in patients with coma, seizures, and an absent gag reflex, and may delay more definitive therapy with charcoal. Multiple-dose activated charcoal should be administered in doses of 1 g/kg in all cases of acute and chronic theophylline toxicity. As serum theophylline diffuses across gastrointentinal (GI) mucosa, the use of charcoal is justified even in cases representing intravenous intoxication. One dose of activated charcoal is followed by a second dose in 4 hours. If doses are vomited, they should be repeated.

Oral activated charcoal is considered the treatment of choice in acute theophylline overdose with sustained-release theophylline tablets and in infants. In about 25% of patients who have taken overdoses of sustained-release theophylline, a further rise in serum theophylline concentration may occur despite conventional therapy with gastric lavage followed by the administration of activated charcoal. Vomiting in acute sustained-release theophylline toxicity may be protracted and may limit the use of activated charcoal in patients with severe acute theophylline poisoning. If vomiting is resistant to an antiemetic and the delivery of activated charcoal by nasogastric tube, the patient may be paralyzed and ventilated if absolutely necessary.

Elimination Enhancement

Hemoperfusion and hemodialysis effectively enhance theophylline clearance and, on the basis of case studies, are the elimination procedures of choice when indicated. Indications for hemoperfusion and hemodialysis include intractable seizures, persistent hypotension unresponsive to fluids and vasopressors, and uncontrollable dysrhythmias. In patients with acute ingestions, theophylline levels exceeding 80 μg/mL suggest the use of hemoperfusion or hemodialysis. For those with intractable vomiting, this threshold may be lowered to 60 μg/mL. In patients with chronic overmedication, serum theophylline levels greater than 40 to 50 μg/mL may indicate the need for hemoperfusion or hemodialysis.

The early use of hemoperfusion or hemodialysis is necessary if serum theophylline levels in the moderately toxic range are rising quickly after the ingestion of sustained-release preparations. Extracorporeal drug removal by hemoperfusion or hemodialysis performed before the onset of seizures or arrhythmias may alter the clinical course of intoxication. There are risks with hemoperfusion, especially in the elderly and the very young. Patients must be observed for hypotension, hypocalcemia, platelet consumption, and bleeding diathesis.

Charcoal hemoperfusion may cause thrombocytopenia, hypoglycemia, and complications associated with the extracorporeal circulation such as hemorrhage, infection, hemolysis, and air embolism. Charcoal hemoperfusion probably is more effective than resin hemoperfusion. Unfortunately, it is not universally available, it has not been shown to reduce morbidity or mortality in late severe toxicity, and its prophylactic role before severe manifestations is yet to be assessed. All interventions continue until the serum theophylline concentration decreases to below 100 μmol/L (20 mg/L) and all serious signs of toxicity abate.

Hemodialysis should be considered when hemoperfusion is indicated but unavailable. Hemodialysis is less effective than hemoperfusion. Peritoneal dialysis is effective in severe intoxication when hemodialysis is unavailable. Forced diuresis is not effective. Exchange transfusion in isolated cases of severe theophylline intoxication in newborns may be helpful.

Whole-bowel irrigation has been used successfully in patients who have ingested both sustained-release and conventional preparations. It may be useful in patients with rapidly increasing serum theophylline concentrations that persist even after multiple doses of activated charcoal or extracorporeal removal. It can be used in combination with activated charcoal. There is, however, no clinical evidence that whole-bowel irrigation provides additional benefit over activated charcoal alone in sustained-release theophylline poisoning.

Supportive Measures

- Monitor cardiac rhythm and obtain an ECG. Lidocaine may be used in cases of ventricular irritability. β-Adrenergic blockade by propranolol or esmolol may be of benefit in the management of supraventricular irritability, especially in the nonasthmatic patient and also, possibly, in the asthmatic patient with severe hypokalemia or cardiac arrhythmias.
- Adenosine may be effective in treating supraventricular irritability in theophylline poisoning.
- Potassium is repleted as necessary. Generally, only mild repletion with 5 to 10 mEq KCl per hour is required. Monitor serum magnesium, phosphate, calcium, potassium, acid-base balance, and theophylline levels until a peak is confirmed.
- Serum theophylline concentrations should be drawn and repeated hourly while they are increasing. Always be aware that serious toxicity from sustained-release preparations may develop hours after the initial presentation, because serum theophylline levels following overdose of sustained-release preparations can peak more than 12 hours after ingestion.
- Monitor urine myoglobin and serum creatinine and creatine kinase levels to detect evidence of rhabdomyolysis. Treatment of rhabdomyolysis and myoglobinuria requires hydration and maintenance of a high urine output.
- Persistent vomiting after a theophylline overdose may preclude the ability to administer activated charcoal. A slow infusion of ondansetron may control vomiting. Metoclopramide and ranitidine also may be useful.
- Prolonged hypotension following theophylline overdose may require higher than conventionally recommended doses of vasopressors to prevent the development of serious sequelae.
- Diazepam and phenobarbital are the drugs of choice for treatment of theophylline-induced seizures. Dilantin generally is ineffective. Anesthesia may be required in refractory cases.
- Intensive-care unit (ICU) admission is suggested in cases of moderate or severe clinical toxicity. Criteria to consider for possible ICU admission include theophylline concentration greater than 50 mg/L in acute poisonings, and greater than 40 mg/L in cases of chronic overmedication, in patients less than 6 months or greater than 60 years of age, or in patients with chronic illness.
- Endoscopic removal of sustained-release theophylline bezoars may be necessary when theophylline levels continue to rise after adequate gut decontamination.

ANTIDOTES

Adenosine effectively reverses supraventricular irritability caused by theophylline.

Questions—Theophylline

1. Which of the following is false?

A. Theophylline is structurally related to caffeine.
B. Theophylline effects include improved ventilatory response to hypoxia, a dose-dependent augmentation of diaphragmatic contractility, and increased oxygen saturation during sleep.
C. Theophylline and β-adrenergic agonists induce dissimilar clinical effects in overdose.
D. Theophylline toxicity typically presents after inadvertent overmedication in its chronic form, or as a large intentional ingestion in its acute form.
E. Hypotension, hypokalemia, and low serum bicarbonate are seen frequently in large single, but not chronic, theophylline overdoses.

2. Serious complications may occur at lower theophylline levels, such as the 40 to 70 μg/mL range, in chronic toxicity, as compared with acute ingestions where these complications are associated with levels over 100 μg/mL.

A. True
B. False

3. Physiologic effects of theophylline include

A. Promoting diaphragmatic contractility
B. Mucociliary clearance
C. Some antiinflammatory effects
D. All of the above
E. A and B

4. Theophylline, a phosphodiesterase inhibitor, increases tissue levels of cyclic AMP, a potentially epileptogenic substance.

A. True
B. False

5. Theophylline also is an adenosine receptor antagonist and may cause seizures by stimulating the depressant effect of adenosine in the cerebral cortex.

A. True
B. False

6. The hypercatecholamine effects of theophylline intoxication include all except

A. Hyperglycemia
B. Hypercalcemia
C. Respiratory acidosis
D. Prolongation of the QT interval
E. Tachyarrhythmias

7. The risk for major toxicity in cases of acute theophylline intoxication is best predicted by

A. Heart rate
B. Age
C. Method of administration
D. Peak serum theophylline concentration
E. Blood pressure

8. Patients with chronic theophylline intoxication have a greater risk for major toxicity (seizures or cardiac arrhythmias associated with hemodynamic instability) at higher serum theophylline concentrations than those with acute intoxication.

A. True
B. False

9. Concerning theophylline-induced seizures
A. Seizures in both children and adults may occur at therapeutic or only mildly toxic levels.
B. The seizures usually are generalized.
C. Seizures may result in rhabdomyolysis, hypothermia, and hypoxic injury.
D. Patients with a preexisting seizure disorder or other neurologic conditions such as meningitis, head trauma, and cerebrovascular accident are particularly vulnerable to seizures.
E. All of the above.

10. Concerning theophylline-induced cardiotoxicity
A. Theophylline-induced cardiotoxicity may be the result of its direct action on cardiac membrane depolarization, antagonism of the cardioprotective effects of endogenous adenosine, stimulation of plasma catecholamine activity, and the resultant increase in myocardial oxygen demand.
B. Cardiotoxic effects may occur in patients with theophylline intoxication and in patients whose levels are within therapeutic range.
C. Sustained supraventricular and ventricular tachyrhythmias are uncommon.
D. All of the above
E. A and B

11. Which of the following is false?
A. Theophylline is particularly susceptible to drug interactions as 90% of its elimination is via metabolism in the P450 system
B. Oral contraceptives promote the metabolism of theophylline.
C. Erythromycin decreases theophylline clearance.
D. Cimetidine decreases theophylline clearance.
E. Phenobarbital promotes the metabolism of theophylline.

12. The following methods are indicated in the treatment of theophylline overdose except
A. Gastric lavage
B. Multiple-dose activated charcoal
C. Hemoperfusion
D. Hemodialysis
E. Syrup of ipecac

Caffeine

Caffeine is chemically related to other xanthines such as theophylline. Caffeine has been part of the daily diet of millions of people for many years. Its consumption goes back to the origins of tea in China about 6,000 years ago. It is frequently ingested in food, beverages, or proprietary medications. It may be considered the most widely used of all mind-altering drugs.

Hundreds of chemicals have been identified in coffee, some of which may have deleterious pharmacologic significance (e.g., chlorogenic acid, which may be present in greater quantities than caffeine). Caffeine has been the most intensively studied chemical and largely accounts for the stimulatory properties of the beverage that have led to its popularity. Caffeine is an ingredient in more than 60 over-the-counter medications including allergy and cold medications, analgesics, appetite suppressants, menstrual products, and stimulants. Prescription drug products also may contain caffeine.

PATHOPHYSIOLOGY

Methylxanthines, such as caffeine, inhibit phosphodiesterase and cause cyclic AMP to accumulate. This results in nonspecific α and β stimulation of the sympathetic nervous system and release of epinephrine from the adrenal medulla. Caffeine induces stimulation of the cerebral cortex, medulla, and spinal cord. It increases vigilance and decreases motor reaction time in response to both visual and auditory stimuli. It does not significantly reverse the depressant effects of ethanol on the central nervous system.

More nondrinkers than heavy drinkers of coffee report sensitivity to the sleep-altering effects of caffeine. Heightened feelings of alertness or anxiety are influenced by individual variations in sensitivity or acquired tolerance to the drug. A relationship between caffeine and nicotine use is common. Drinking decaffeinated coffee also leads to an increase in cigarettes smoked by normal volunteers. Caffeine may increase systolic blood pressure. It typically decreases heart rate initially, then increases it for up to 2 hours. Plasma epinephrine, norepinephrine, and plasma renin activity are increased. Caffeine increases the respiratory rate in non–caffeine-using subjects. Orally administered caffeine results in bronchodilator effects similar to those of oral theophylline.

Caffeine increases the metabolic rate. Caffeine does not alter plasma glucose levels in normal healthy persons or in caffeine-habituated persons, but may cause an increase in blood glucose in caffeine-naive individuals. A linear relationship exists between plasma caffeine levels and gastric secretion of acid and pepsin. Acute ingestion of caffeine produces mild increases in urine volume and sodium excretion. Tolerance quickly develops. Diuretic effects of methylxanthines result primarily from a decrease in tubular reabsorption of sodium and water. Potassium excretion is not increased with therapeutic doses of caffeine.

PHARMACOKINETICS

Absorption

- Caffeine is absorbed readily from the gastrointestinal tract. Peak plasma levels occur in 45 minutes to 2 hours.
- A 250-mg dose yields peak plasma concentrations between 5 and 25 μg/mL with 15% protein binding.

Distribution

- Caffeine is distributed rapidly into body water with an apparent volume of distribution of 1 L/kg.

Elimination

- Caffeine is metabolized in the liver to 3,7- (theobromine), 1,3- (theophylline), and 1,7- (paraxanthine) dimethylxanthines. These, together with small amounts of unchanged caffeine, are excreted in the urine, saliva, semen, and breast milk, and are found in umbilical cord blood.
- The half-life of caffeine is increased in patients with alcoholic liver disease, after cimetidine and oral contraceptives, during pregnancy, and in neonates and newborns.
- The half-life in normal adults is 3.0 to 7.5 hours; in preterm infants at birth, 65 to 103 hours; in term infants at birth, 82 hours; in 3- to 4-month-old infants, 14.4 hours; and in 5- to 6-month-old infants, 2.6 hours.

CLINICAL PRESENTATIONS

Gastrointestinal Effects

GI effects occur early and consist of nausea, vomiting, and abdominal cramps, with occasional hematemesis. Heartburn may result from reflux esophagitis. No relation between coffee or caffeine and gastric or duodenal ulcer has been established. Coffee enemas used as part of alternative treatment programs for cancer therapy may produce polymicrobial enteric septicemia and have been considered responsible for severe electrolyte imbalance leading to death.

Neurologic Effects

Symptoms such as agitation, irritability, and restlessness may lead to tonic posturing, rigidity, fluctuating coma, and convulsions. Convulsions may be epileptiform or associated with reflex hyperexcitability. Cerebral edema and death rarely have been reported without convulsions. Neuromuscular effects may include hypertonicity, hypotonicity, and muscle fasciculations. In neonates, caffeine overdosage may result in hyperirritability, opisthotonus, hypertonicity, hypotonicity, ocular deviation (upward), rigidity, and purposeless lip movements.

Cardiovascular Effects

Cardiovascular effects include sinus tachycardia, premature beats, systemic hypertension, ventricular fibrillation, and cardiopulmonary arrest. Initially, the patient may have a slow pulse and normal blood pressure. As blood levels rise within the first 30 minutes, the blood pressure begins to rise about 15/10 mm Hg, peaking about 2 hours after ingestion. Cerebral vascular resistance may increase. In a habitual drinker, sudden cessation of coffee drinking may provoke the pain of cerebral vascular dilatation, and a caffeine withdrawal headache is experienced. Many studies have concluded that no association exists between coffee consumption and myocardial infarction.

Metabolic Effects

Caffeine overdose may be associated with hypokalemia. Hyperglycemia also may occur. Caffeine appears to increase urinary calcium output and has been implicated as a risk factor for osteoporosis. Ingestion of over 2.5 cups of coffee per day may be associated with an increased risk of hip fracture.

Dependence

Caffeine tends to produce a pattern of subjective effects that varies as a function of dose. Although low doses, in the range of 20 to 200 mg, generally produce mild, positive, subjective effects (e.g., increased feelings of well-being, alertness, energy), higher doses, in the range of 200 to 800 mg, can produce negative effects (e.g., nervousness, anxiety), especially in volunteers who usually are caffeine abstinent. Previous studies have shown that subjects can be intoxicated with the excessive use of caffeine and that caffeine can produce a withdrawal syndrome when subjects stop habitual use.

The most common symptom of caffeine withdrawal is headache. Caffeine withdrawal headache generally occurs 12 to 24 hours after the last dose of caffeine and usually resolves within 2 to 4 days. Other features of caffeine withdrawal include drowsiness, impaired concentration, anxiety, depression, and flulike symptoms. Caffeine withdrawal can include impairments in psychomotor performance, irritability, rhinorrhea, confusion, diaphoresis, blurred vision, and craving for caffeine.

TOXIC DOSAGE/DEATH

There is little evidence that a modest dose of coffee (200 mg caffeine) is arrhythmogenic even among patients with known life-threatening arrhythmias. A large prospective study of 51,529 men in the United States 40 to 75 years of age does not support the hypothesis that either coffee or caffeine consumption increases the risk of coronary heart disease or stroke. The oral dose of caffeine that is toxic to humans has not been well established. Few cases of acute caffeine poisoning have been reported in the literature.

Adverse effects begin to appear when approximately 0.5 to 1.0 g of caffeine, equivalent to 10 cups of coffee, is ingested by an adult. This produces a plasma concentration of at least 30 μg/mL. In children, oral doses of about 80 to 100 mg/kg have produced severe symptoms. Deaths have been reported after oral doses of 5.3 g in a child and 6.5 g in an adult. The acute lethal dose of caffeine in adults appears to be approximately 5 to 10 g (equivalent to 75 cups of coffee, 125 cups of tea, or 200 cola beverages) orally or intravenously.

DRUG INTERACTIONS

Coadministration of caffeine and phenylpropanolamine appears to produce an additive increase in blood pressure. Verapamil may inhibit caffeine elimination. Phenytoin appears to increase the clearance of caffeine and reduce its half-life. Animal studies suggest that caffeine potentiates the acute toxicity of both cocaine and amphetamine. Cimetidine may inhibit caffeine clearance, while smoking appears to stimulate caffeine clearance. Caffeine appears to enhance the analgesic efficacy of acetaminophen, and acetaminophen appears to reduce caffeine toxicity at high serum caffeine levels.

PREGNANCY/LACTATION

The weight of evidence suggests that ingesting more than 300 mg per day of caffeine during pregnancy may cause intrauterine growth retardation, decreased birthweight, and possibly spontaneous abortion. Few adverse pregnancy outcomes have been reported in women who consume less than 300 mg/day of caffeine during pregnancy. No solid conclusions can be made regarding the safety of caffeine at lower levels. Caffeine is pregnancy risk category B.

Infants exposed to high maternal levels of caffeine for the majority of the pregnancy may develop irritability, jitteriness, and vomiting in the immediate newborn period. Caffeine is excreted in breast milk and is found in umbilical cord blood. The half-life of caffeine is prolonged in pregnancy. In 1980, the FDA advised pregnant women to avoid or limit use of caffeine-containing foods and drugs.

LABORATORY

Analytic Methods

A high-performance liquid chromatography method is available for determination of dimethylxanthine metabolites of caffeine in human plasma. Ultraviolet spectrophotometry measures caffeine, but clinical laboratory usefulness in caffeine poisoning treatment has not been established.

Blood Levels

Some correlations of caffeine blood levels and clinical effects appear to exist. The mean peak plasma caffeine 1 hour after consumption of two cups of strong coffee is about 5.3 μg/mL. Seizures occur with caffeine levels ranging from 79 to 199 μg/mL. Arrhythmias other than sinus tachycardia may be seen with levels greater than 180 μg/mL. Deaths have occurred with caffeine levels from 106 to 180 mg/mL. Patients with levels from 190 to 200 μg/mL have survived.

TREATMENT

Gut Decontamination

If caffeine has been ingested within 4 hours in amounts over 15 mg/kg, activated charcoal probably is useful. Watch for spontaneous vomiting and convulsions.

Elimination Enhancement

Resin hemoperfusion may be helpful in particularly severe cases. Charcoal hemoperfusion may be useful in patients with a potentially lethal ingestion who are exhibiting life-threatening complications such as cardiac arrhythmias or severe central nervous system toxicity.

Supportive Measures

- Airway, breathing, and circulation must be addressed initially. Seizures are treated with diazepam, 5 to 10 mg intravenously, slowly in adults, and may be repeated. Children's dose is 0.1 to 0.3 mg/kg.
- In caffeine poisoning there may be an elevated white blood cell count, hyperglycemia (over 200 mg/dL), glycosuria, ketonuria, and significant hypokalemia.
- Intravenous glucose may lead to quick recovery in children with acute caffeine poisoning, as glucose is known to antagonize the excitatory effect of caffeine and theobromine in the nervous system.
- β-Blockers such as esmolol may be useful in diminishing caffeine-induced arrhythmias.
- Adenosine may effectively eliminate supraventricular tachyarrhythmias in many instances.

Questions—Caffeine

1. Which of the following about caffeine is false?
A. Methylxanthines inhibit phosphodiesterase and cause cyclic AMP to accumulate.
B. Caffeine inhibits stimulation of the cerebral cortex, medulla, and spinal cord.
C. It increases vigilance and decreases motor reaction time to both visual and auditory stimuli.
D. It does not significantly reverse depressant effects of ethanol on the central nervous system.
E. Caffeine is excreted in breast milk.

2. Clinical effects of caffeine overdose include each of the following except
A. Nausea, vomiting, and abdominal cramps
B. Seizures
C. Hypertonicity, hypotonicity, and muscle fasciculations
D. Sinus tachycardia, premature beats, systemic hypertension, ventricular fibrillation, and cardiopulmonary arrest
E. Hyperkalemia

3. More nondrinkers than heavy coffee drinkers report sensitivity to caffeine's sleep-altering effects.
A. True
B. False

4. Which of the following is false?
A. Coadministration of caffeine and phenylpropanolamine appears to produce an additive increase in blood pressure.
B. Verapamil may increase caffeine elimination.
C. Phenytoin appears to increase the clearance of caffeine and reduce its half-life.
D. Cimetidine may inhibit caffeine clearance.
E. Smoking appears to stimulate caffeine clearance.

Answers

β-2 Agonists

1. B 2. A 3. E 4. E 5. E

Inhaled Steroids

1. C 2. B

Theophylline

1. C 2. A 3. D 4. A 5. B 6. C
7. D 8. B 9. E 10. D 11. B 12. E

Caffeine

1. B 2. E 3. A 4. B

SELECTED READINGS

β-2 Agonists

1. Burrows B, Lebowitz MD. The beta-agonist dilemma. N Engl J Med 1992; 326:560–561.
2. Gomolin I, Ingelfinger JA. Terbutaline overdose. N Engl J Med 1979;300:143.
3. Nelson HS. B-adrenergic bronchodilators. N Engl J Med 1995;333:499–506.
4. Sears MR, Taylor DR, Print CG, et al. Regular inhaled β-agonist treatment in bronchial asthma. Lancet 1990;336:1391–1396.
5. Spiller HA, Ramoska EA, Henretig FM, Joffe M. A two-year retrospective study of accidental pediatric albuterol ingestions. Pediatr Emerg Care 1993;9:338–340.
6. Woolcock AJ. Beta-agonists and asthma mortality: What have we learned? What questions remain? Drugs 1990;40:653–656.

Inhaled Steroids

1. Barnes PJ. Pulmonary disorders. In: Melmon KL, Morrelli HF, Hoffman BB, Nierenberg DW, eds. Clinical Pharmacology: Basic Principles in Therapeutics. 3rd ed. New York: McGraw Hill, 1992:198–202.
2. Boe J, Skoogh BE. Is long term treatment with inhaled steroids in adults hazardous? Eur Respir J 1992;5:1037–1039.
3. Toogood JH. Complication of topical steroid therapy for asthma. Am Rev Respir Dis 1990;141(suppl.):89–96.

Theophylline

1. Britt A, Burkhart KK. Theophylline toxicity. Top Emerg Med 1992;15:72–77.
2. Cooling OS. Theophylline toxicity. J Emerg Med 1993;11:415–425.
3. Parr MJ, Anaes FC, Day AC, et al. Theophylline poisoning: A review of 64 cases. Intens Care Med 1990;16:394–398.
4. Shannon M, Lovejoy FH Effect of acute versus chronic intoxication on clinical features of theophylline poisoning in children. J Pediatr 1992;121:125–130.
5. Shannon M, Lovejoy FH Hypokalemia after theophylline intoxication: The effects of acute vs chronic poisoning. Arch Intern Med 1989;149:2725–2729.
6. Shannon MW, Lovejoy FH, Woolf A. Acute complications and predictions of major toxicity after theophylline overdose. Vet Hum Toxicol 1992;34:328.

Caffeine

1. Dietrich AM, Mortensen ME. Presentation and management of an acute caffeine overdose. Pediatr Emerg Care 1990;6:296–298.
2. Glass RM. Caffeine dependence. What are the implications? JAMA 1994;272: 1065–1066.

CHAPTER 33
Veterinary Toxicology

Many who attempt suicide with veterinary agents are employed in the veterinary profession. Accidental human exposures to a variety of potential toxins have occurred after ingestions of veterinary foods or drugs and after exposures to organophosphorous insecticides used for veterinary purposes. Veterinary pharmaceuticals that have been involved in human poisoning include those commonly used for veterinary euthanasia, nonsteroidal antiinflammatory drugs (e.g., equine phenylbutazone), antibiotics (e.g., penicillin), antiprotozoans (e.g., monensin), etamphylline, and clenbuterol (added to animal feed). Most states do not require child-resistant packaging for prescription veterinary medicines.

Hazard Classes

The National Animal Disease Center has classified veterinary agents according to risk assessment for laboratory and professional workers. Class 1 agents represent no or minimal hazards under ordinary conditions of handling. Class 2 agents may produce disease of varying degrees of severity from accidental inoculation or injection or other means of cutaneous penetration, but which are contained by ordinary laboratory techniques. Class 3 agents involve special hazards that require special conditions for containment. Class 4 agents require the most stringent conditions for containment because they are extremely hazardous to laboratory personnel or may cause serious epidemic disease in animals.

Autoinoculations

Self-inoculations of veterinary vaccines and medications may induce physical tissue injury, direct toxicity, stimulation of host immune response, or infection. Such self-inoculations usually occur when an inadequately restrained animal gives a sudden jerk during a vaccination procedure.

PHYSICAL INJURY

Physical injury by needlestick may penetrate nerves, blood vessels, or tendons. If the needle has previously passed through animal tissue or another nonsterile field, it may introduce foreign bodies, infectious material, or both. Oil adjuvants in veterinary vaccines may induce vasospasm and ischemia, which can lead to loss of digits.

IMMUNE RESPONSE

If a veterinary vaccine is accidentally self-inoculated by an individual previously exposed to the same vaccine, a hypersensitivity reaction may develop within hours, characterized by pain, redness, swelling, chills, and fever. Recovery generally occurs within days. Local irritation may undergo necrosis for months.

INFECTION

Autoinoculations may develop into infections. The organisms at highest exposure risk include *Brucella* species, *Mycobacteria* species, and *Leptospira* species.

Clinical Presentations

ACEPROMAZINE

Acepromazine, a phenothiazine structurally similar to chlorpromazine, is used as an aid in controlling intractable animals. Overdoses in humans present with central nervous system (CNS) dysfunction ranging from coma and sedation to extrapyramidal symptoms and seizures. Cardiovascular effects may include sinus tachycardia, ventricular arrhythmias, intraventricular conduction delays, hypotension, miosis, hypothermia, hyperthermia, and pulmonary edema.

AMITRAZ

Amitraz is active against mites on fruit trees and kills mange mites on livestock and ticks on cattle. It is an acaricide and insecticide intended for use on animals and plants. It is usually formulated in a xylene preparation. When humans are exposed to Amitraz, they manifest symptoms and signs of both xylene and Amitraz exposure. Fatalities have been reported.

The main metabolite of Amitraz exhibits monoamine oxidase-inhibiting properties at high doses. The hydrolyzed metabolic product is a relatively weak methemoglobin former in dogs, and presumably in humans. Amitraz appears to be a central α-2 adrenoceptor agonist whose action results in diminished peripheral sympathetic tone with a lowering of blood pressure and heart rate. Peripherally, it exhibits both α-1 and α-2 adrenoceptor agonist activities resulting in some elevation of blood pressure. The xylene present in Amitraz formulations is more likely to induce CNS depression.

Clinical signs and symptoms after human exposure to Amitraz may include drowsiness, loss of consciousness, confused mental state, agitation, weakness, headache, vomiting, and malaise. Absent bowel sounds, miosis or mydriasis, abdominal pain, and hyperactive deep tendon reflexes have been observed in children. Human exposure to Amitraz formulations may terminate fatally. In animals, Amitraz induces bradycardia and hypotension within 1–5 hours. Common signs and symptoms in animals include CNS depression with episodes of hyperexcitability, hypotension, bradycardia, hypothermia, hypoglycemia, and in some cases hemoconcentration.

Xylene in humans may, after acute exposure, induce CNS depression with ataxia, impaired motor coordination, nystagmus, stupor, and coma. Ingestion may cause a burning sensation of the mouth, possible blistering of the mucosa, substernal and abdominal pain, nausea, vomiting, diarrhea, headache, dizziness, sedation, and incoordination. The early toxic effects of Amitraz formulations are probably due to xylene.

AZAPERONE

Azaperone is a butyrophenone used as a sedative for animal handling. Recovery has followed an adult ingestion of 2 g, confirmed by thin-layer chromatography and mass spectrometry, in 2 days.

BARBITURATES

Ingestion or injection of veterinary euthanasia preparations containing pentobarbital has caused death. Barbiturate solutions used in veterinary euthanasia frequently contain glycols such as propylene glycol. Toxic doses of propylene glycol can cause hyperosmolarity, acidosis, and CNS depression and may contribute to the toxicity of these solutions.

BAYO-N-OX-1

This quinoline derivative is used as a feed additive for the prevention of bacterial enteritis in pigs. Pig breeders have experienced allergic contact dermatitis and photocontact dermatitis.

BERENIL

Berenil is used in veterinary medicine for the treatment of trypanosomiasis and babesiosis. Because it may cause brain damage in dogs and asses, and pyelonephritis in horses and camels, its use in humans has not been recommended. When it has been used in humans, it has induced toxic reactions.

Berenil is structurally related to pentamidine. Toxic, reversible effects may include paralysis, coma, and numbness of the legs. Other signs and symptoms include fever, numbness, pain in the feet, paralysis, nausea and vomiting. Guillain-Barré syndrome has also been reported.

CARISOPRODOL

An adult became dependent on a veterinary carisoprodol product that she ordered over the counter through a veterinary mail-order outlet. Federal law does not restrict such sales from states that permit them.

CLENBUTEROL

Clenbuterol, a veterinary and human β-agonist, is used illicitly in animal feeding to induce regression of body lipids, muscle growth, and weight gain. Ingestion by 195 patients of bovine liver contaminated with clenbuterol led to muscle tremors, palpitations, tachycardia, nervousness, and myalgias lasting about 60 hours. Symptoms may also include dizziness, nausea, vomiting, fever, and seizures and appear to cease spontaneously in 48 hours.

CLOSANTEL

Eleven Lithuanian women lost their eyesight after closantel, a veterinary antihelminthic, was inadvertently prescribed for a gynecologic condition. The eyesight later returned, but eye pain persisted. Vacuolation of the optic nerve has been described. Plasmapheresis and activated charcoal may enhance elimination. High-dose corticosteroids may be helpful.

ETAMPHYLLINE

Etamphylline overdose has led, within 45 minutes, to nausea, weakness of the lower limbs, a coarse tremor, restlessness, hyperventilation, hypertension, olfactory hallucinations, seizures, cyanosis, and sinus tachycardia.

FLUNIXIN MEGLUMINE

Ingestion of flunixin meglumine (Banamine granules) for the relief of arthritic pain has led to Cheyne-Stokes respirations, coma and hypertension. The patient recovered within days.

METHIMAZOLE

Methimazole, illicitly used in animal feeding as a weight enhancer, has been associated with congenital scalp aplasia.

ORGANOPHOSPHATES

A veterinary technician who was splashed with an organophosphorous carbamate mixture developed headache, nausea, vomiting, diarrhea, and difficulty in breathing. These signs and symptoms remained for 4 days.

PENICILLIN

Consumption of cat food with high levels of penicillin by an 11-month-old child led to nausea, vomiting, fever, and death.

PHENYLBUTAZONE

Signs of equine phenylbutazone intoxication in humans may include melena and gastric bleeding. Pallor and ecchymosis were observed in one patient who ingested equine phenylbutazone and subsequently died of aplastic anemia. Hypertension, seizures, renal and hepatic dysfunction, respiratory failure, and coma have also been observed.

SODIUM MONENSIN

In one cluster of cases, seven people ate flour contaminated by sodium monensin used as an additive in chicken feed. They developed abdominal pain, nausea, vomiting, weakness, muscle cramps, and joint pains. Two patients died within 15 days.

SPIRAMYCIN

This macrolide antibiotic, used by chick breeders, has induced asthma and dermatitis.

T-61

T-61 has been used for veterinary euthanasia in Germany since 1962 and in the United States since 1963. T-61 contains embutramide (a general anesthetic), mebezonium iodide (a neuromuscular blocker), and tetracaine (a local anesthetic) in a dimethylformamide (a hydrocarbon) solvent. Injections of T-61 have led to seizures, coma, respiratory arrest, cyanosis of the mucous membranes, decreased deep tendon reflexes, sinus bradycardia, hypotension, and constricted, nonreactive pupils. Pulmonary infiltrates, fever, dizziness, epigastric pain, vomiting, jaundice, a flapping tremor, renal failure, and hepatic fetor have also been observed.

TILMICOSIN

Exposures to this veterinary antibiotic have largely occurred after accidental needlesticks. Local symptoms (pain at site) predominate. Patients who experience nausea, vomiting or respiratory difficulty within 30 minutes should be evaluated in a hospital. Treatment is supportive.

XYLAZINE

Xylazine is a veterinary sedative, analgesic, and skeletal muscle relaxant effective in a wide range of domestic and wild animals. Xylazine, a 1,3 thorazine, shares pharmacologic properties with a number of structurally related drugs including the phenothiazines, tricyclic antidepressants, and clonidine. Xylazine acts on α-2 adrenoceptors that control central neuronal dopamine and norepinephrine storage.

Human overdose may cause pronounced bradycardia, significant CNS and respiratory depression, electrocardiographic abnormalities, including possible ventricular arrhythmias, and transient hyperglycemia. Phenothiazines, tricyclic antidepressants, and clonidine may also produce bradycardia, CNS depression, and electrocardiogram abnormalities.

A toxic or fatal dose has not been identified.

Toxic Dosage/Death

ACEPROMAZINE

A 19-year-old veterinary assistant attempted suicide by ingesting 1.25 g of acepromazine. She became lethargic, was treated with ipecac, charcoal, and a cathartic, and was discharged in 36 hours. A 2-year-old who ingested 75–100 mg of acepromazine developed marked sedation, tachycardia, and evidence of poor perfusion. The child recovered within 6 hours.

BARBITURATES

A veterinarian was found dead after ingesting 1.5 g of a veterinary euthanasia preparation containing pentobarbital in a 50% propylene glycol base, and ethanol. Death has followed the use of Socumb, used for veterinary euthanasia, containing pentobarbital, 360 mg/mL. An individual survived after ingesting 50 mL of sodium pentobarbital with 15 mL of T-61.

CLENBUTEROL

Clenbuterol, a veterinary and human β-agonist, may accumulate in the liver where it may subsequently poison humans who ingest it. Some farmers have added clenbuterol to animal feed and have died after inhaling it.

DETOMIDINE

Detomidine hydrochloride is an α-2 adrenergic agonist similar to clonidine and xylazine and is used as a veterinary sedative. The dose of detomidine required for anesthesia in horses is 40–80 mg/kg i.m. or i.v. An intramuscular injection of 50 mg in a 36-year-old man, together with butorphanol, led to sedation and signs of opiate poisoning that responded to naloxone.

ETAMPHYLLINE

A 15-year-old ingested her dog's heart tablets, containing approximately 12 g of etamphylline camsylate, a xanthine compound similar in action to theophylline. She survived.

FLUNIXIN MEGLUMINE

An adult who ingested 250 mg of flunixin meglumine was found in coma, regained consciousness in 24 hours, and survived.

ORGANOPHOSPHATES

In 1991, the Veterinary Medicine Directorate of the United Kingdom received 135 reports of adverse reactions following exposure to organophosphorous compounds in veterinary medicines. Accidental self-injection was the most frequently reported history.

PENICILLIN

An 11-month-old child with a prior history of eating cat food ate cat food with a high penicillin content and died with a hypersensitivity-type myocarditis.

PHENYLBUTAZONE

Phenylbutazone is probably the most frequently used nonsteroidal antiinflammatory agent in equine medicine. Racetrack personnel who take it for muscle aches and bruises often refer to it as "Bute." One adult race horse track worker who ingested equine phenylbutazone (1 g/tablet) for 3 months survived; however, a jockey who ingested 2 g of equine phenylbutazone for 3 days died. A greyhound handler who ingested 17 g of phenylbutazone over 24 hours survived.

RADIATION

Epidemiologic data suggest that female veterinarians who perform five or more radiographic examinations per week may be at an increased risk for spontaneous abortion.

SODIUM MONENSIN

Ingestion of the antiprotozoal chicken food additive sodium monensin by seven people (following its mistaken addition to wheat flour) led to severe abdominal pain, nausea, vomiting, weakness, muscle cramps, and joint pains. Two of the seven died within 15 days.

T-61

In one suicide attempt, a 20-year-old female injected 12 mL intramuscularly and survived. Fifty mL intramuscularly has caused death in children. A 37-year-old was found dead approximately 20–30 minutes after ingesting about 100 mL of T-61. An adult who ingested 15 mL of T-61 with about 3.25 g of sodium pentobarbital survived.

TILMICOSIN

Tilmicosin is a veterinary antibiotic. The Ontario Regional Poison Information Centre has collected 36 reports of accidental human exposure, most of whom were exposed to less than 1 mL from needle punctures.

Treatment

SUPPORTIVE MEASURES

- Treatment protocols depend on individual effects and agents. Treatment of hypersensitivity reactions will usually include an antihistamine and steroid.
- Infections should respond to symptomatic and supportive therapy and to antibiotics in relevant cases (e.g., tetracycline for *Brucella*). Veterinary surgeons who handle vaccines and are self-inoculated by strains of bacteria or viruses should be screened by periodic skin tests and agglutination titers where applicable.
- Accidental self-inoculations, especially into the hand, require immediate attention as early incision and irrigation of the injected area may be required. Tetanus status must also be assessed.
- Laboratory studies useful after self-inoculation of autoinfective biologic products should include blood cultures, cultures of the wound site, an initial agglutination titer, and serial titers. Serum aminotransferases, creatine kinase, and lactic acid dehydrogenase levels should be obtained to follow hepatic function and muscle status.

Amitraz

- Initial attention should be directed toward evaluation and support of ventilation, with oxygen and endotracheal intubation provided as required. Cardiac monitoring is advisable because of the possibility of cardiac arrhythmias.
- Unconscious patients should be hospitalized, monitored, and admitted to an intensive care unit. Patients may not be fully conscious for several days after ingestion.
- A baseline chest x-ray and follow-up films within 6–24 hours may provide an indication of aspiration pneumonitis from xylene.
- Patients should be admitted to a hospital where a complete blood count, liver function tests, blood and urine glucose and ketone levels, and a serum creatinine concentration can be obtained. Glycosuria, ketonuria, increased serum aminotransferases and alkaline phosphatase, and a neutrophil leukocytosis have been observed.
- Symptomatic and supportive care should be used to ameliorate hypotension (intravenous fluids) and bradycardia (atropine). Patients should be monitored for hypothermia.

Barbiturates

- Patients who have overdosed on veterinary euthanasia products should be hospitalized in an intensive care facility after emergency evaluation to ascertain adequate respiratory, airway, and circulatory status. Oxygen and cardiac monitoring should be available. Endotracheal intubation with mechanical ventilation may be required.
- The treatment of pentobarbital poisoning consists mainly of symptomatic and supportive care. If pentobarbital solution has been ingested, gastric lavage with endotracheal protection and administration of activated charcoal may be useful.
- After massive overdoses of pentobarbital, following continued deterioration despite supportive care, charcoal hemoperfusion may be effective, although this procedure is usually more effective for elimination of the longer-acting barbiturates. See Chapter 27, Anticonvulsant Drugs.

Organophosphates

- Prompt showers and removal of contaminated clothing should be performed while preparations are made for specific therapy. Therapy is primarily supportive in conjunction with atropine and oxime therapy in serious cases. See Chapter 48, Pesticides.

Phenylbutazone

- Overdoses of equine phenylbutazone require symptomatic and supportive treatment. Gastric irritation may be ameliorated with H2 receptor antagonists.
- Aplastic anemia may require bone marrow transplants.
- Hemodialysis is probably ineffective due to high protein binding and low water solubility. The value of hemoperfusion remains controversial, although it has been recommended for severe phenylbutazone poisoning.

T-61

- Seizures are controlled with diazepam. Musculoskeletal paralysis can be reversed with anticholinesterase agents such as pyridostigmine.
- Embutramide can produce respiratory arrest from its CNS depressive actions.
- Decontamination of the gastrointestinal tract with gastric lavage, under tracheal protection, and activated charcoal may be useful.

Xylazine

- Supportive measures include endotracheal intubation as needed, ventilatory assistance, control of hypotension with intravenous fluids, position change, bladder catheterization, central venous pressure monitoring, and cautious use of vasopressors such as dopamine.
- Acid-base status, glucose and electrolytes must be monitored and corrected as needed.
- Serious overdoses require extended clinical observation and cardiac monitoring for possible myocardial infarction and ventricular arrhythmias. Lidocaine may be used for ventricular arrhythmias. Atropine or dopamine is used for hypotension and bradycardia.
- Nitroprusside may be useful for paradoxical hypertension.

Questions—Introduction to Veterinary Toxicology

1. Prescription veterinary medicines

A. Are required to be in child-resistant packaging in all states
B. Are more commonly used in suicide attempts by veterinarians than by others
C. Consisting of nonsteroidal antiinflammatory drugs are safe in humans
D. Are not classified by risk to people, only to animals
E. None of the above

2. Veterinary agents that are extremely hazardous to laboratory personnel are

A. Class 1
B. Class 2
C. Class 3
D. Class 4
E. Not distinguished from other agents

3. Self-inoculations of veterinary vaccines and medications may cause

A. Physical tissue injury
B. Direct toxicity
C. Stimulation of host immune response
D. Vasospasm and ischemia
E. All of the above

4. Acepromazine overdose

A. Presents with central nervous system dysfunction
B. Has primarily liver toxicity
C. Is often preceded by human addiction
D. Is associated with frequent optic nerve damage
E. All of the above

5. All of the following are true about closantel except

A. Use in humans has been associated with loss of eyesight.
B. This blindness has been permanent, accompanied by eye pain.
C. Vacuolation of the optic nerve has been described.
D. Plasmapheresis may be helpful.
E. High-dose corticosteroid may be helpful.

6. Human use of equine phenylbutazone

A. Is associated with melena and gastric bleeding
B. Has not been associated with death
C. Is associated with olfactory hallucinations
D. Has long been used for veterinary euthanasia
E. All of the above

7. Clenbuterol

A. May cause symptoms that last 48 hours
B. May cause death
C. Has been ingested and inhaled
D. May accumulate in the liver
E. All of the above

8. Which of the following veterinary medicines has been used illicitly by humans to treat muscle aches?

A. Tilmicosin
B. Closantel
C. Phenylbutazone
D. Spiramycin
E. All of the above

9. Amitraz is used

A. For veterinary euthanasia
B. For arthritic symptoms in horses
C. To kill mites on fruit trees and livestock
D. To kill ticks on humans
E. None of the above

10. Signs of human exposure to amitraz include

A. Abdominal pain
B. Agitation
C. Absent bowel sounds
D. Confusion
E. All of the above

11. Berenil is used in animals to treat

A. Guillain-Barré Syndrome
B. Trypanosomiasis and babesiosis
C. Foot pain
D. Seizures
E. Folliculitis

Answers to questions in shaded boxes appear at the end of the chapter.

12. Treatment of berenil ingestion by humans
  A. Should include an offer of antidote with explanation of risks
  B. Should be guided by serum levels
  C. Should not include lavage and charcoal
  D. Routinely includes hemodialysis
  E. None of the above

13. Xylazine is structurally related to
  A. Phenothiazines
  B. Tricyclic antidepressants
  C. Clonidine
  D. All of the above
  E. None of the above

Answers

Veterinary Toxicology

1. B	2. D	3. E	4. A	5. B	6. A	7. E
8. C	9. C	10. E	11. B	12. E	13. D	

SELECTED READINGS

Veterinary Toxicology

1. Cordell WH, Curry SC, Furbee RB, Mitchell-Flynn DL. Veterinary euthanasia drugs as suicidal agents. Ann Emerg Med 1986;15:939–943.
2. Geller RJ. Human effects of veterinary biological products. Vet Hum Toxicol 1990;32:479–80.
3. Hoen E, Hodgkin C, Mikevicious D. Harmful human use of donated veterinary drugs. Lancet 1993;342:308–309.
4. Miller CD, Songer JR, Sullivan JF. A twenty-five year review of laboratory-acquired human infections at the National Animal Disease Center. Am Ind Hyg Assoc J 1987;48:271–275.
5. Woodward KN, Gray AK. Adverse reactions in humans following occupational exposure to veterinary drugs. Hum Exp Toxicol 1990;9:326.

ACKNOWLEDGMENT

Thanks to Alison Deutsch, MD for contributing the questions in this chapter.

SECTION

E

Receptor Toxicology

CHAPTER 34
Anticholinergic Drugs

INTRODUCTION

Anticholinergic agents are frequently used in the treatment of peptic ulcer disease and irritable bowel syndrome. Atropine is used to treat symptomatic bradycardia, and as an antidote for organophosphate and other cholinergic poisonings. See Chapter 5, Antidotes and Chapter 48, Pesticides. Anticholinergic toxins are also found in a number of botanicals. See Jimsonweed and Anticholinergic Plants in Chapter 57, Wild Plants, Mushrooms and Mycotoxins.

Atropine and scopolamine are used as preoperative medications to inhibit salivation and diminish excessive secretions of the respiratory tract. Genitourinary tract problems such as uninhibited contractions and reflex neurogenic bladder have been treated with atropine, and oxybutynin. The antimuscarinic agents are also potent bronchodilators. Benztropine and trihexyphenidyl are used in the management of Parkinson's disease and to treat drug-induced extrapyramidal reactions.

Pathophysiology

Antimuscarinic drugs competitively inhibit muscarinic effects of acetylcholine. They are also known as parasympatholytic, atropinic, atropine-like, or anticholinergic agents. Atropine is the prototype antimuscarinic agent. Antimuscarinic agents are classified on the basis of their source (natural, semisynthetic, or synthetic) or their cationic structure (tertiary amine or quaternary ammonium compounds). Atropine, hyoscyamine, and scopolamine are natural tertiary amines.

Clinical Presentations

Peripheral symptoms of overdose may include dilated and unreactive pupils, blurred vision, hot, dry, and flushed skin, dry mucous membranes, difficulty in swallowing, diminished or absent bowel sounds, urinary retention, tachycardia, hyperthermia, hypertension, and tachypnea. Central nervous system (CNS) manifestations may resemble acute psychosis and include disorientation, incoherence, confusion, hallucinations, delusions, paranoia, disturbed speech, periods of hyperactivity, anxiety, abnormal motor behavior, and restlessness.

In severe overdoses, CNS depression, circulatory collapse, and hypotension may be observed. Death from respiratory failure, hyperthermia (especially in children) or cardiac depression may follow coma and skeletal muscle paralysis. Electrocardiographic abnormalities may include widening of the QRS complex, prolongation of the QT interval, ST segment depression, ventricular arrhythmias, premature beats, sinus tachycardia and supraventricular tachycardia.

Treatment

GUT DECONTAMINATION
Gastric lavage with a cuffed endotracheal tube, activated charcoal, and saline cathartics have been used and may be helpful.

ELIMINATION ENHANCEMENT
Hemodialysis or peritoneal dialysis is not useful.

SUPPORTIVE MEASURES
- Treatment of overdose is largely symptomatic and supportive. Patients should be hospitalized and closely monitored with continuous electrocardiographic monitoring. Fluids are administered and shock treated as required.
- Hyperthermia is treated with cold packs, cooling devices, or sponging with tepid water.
- Diazepam may be used to control excitement, delirium, or manifestations of acute psychosis. Phenothiazines should not be used because they may also have anticholinergic effects.
- Maintenance of an adequate airway, respiratory assistance, and urinary catheterization are vital aspects of patient management.

Antidotes

PHYSOSTIGMINE
The use of physostigmine is controversial. Physostigmine may induce seizures, bronchospasm, or asystole. It has been used in patients with extensive delirium or agitation, repetitive or long-lasting seizures, unstable supraventricular tachycardia, or hyperthermia unresponsive to mechanical cooling. The usual therapeutic adult dose is 2 mg intravenously. If there is no response, 1–2 mg can be given every 20 min until reversal of toxic antimuscarinic effects occurs, or until adverse cholinergic effects develop. The usual intravenous pediatric dose of physostigmine recommended by the manufacturer is 0.02 mg/kg.

Physostigmine should not be used to treat cardiac conduction defects or ventricular tachyarrhythmias. Excessive doses of physostigmine may produce cholinergic toxicity manifested by bradycardia, increased salivation, diarrhea, seizures, or respiratory arrest. Physostigmine can cause life-threatening bronchoconstriction, bradycardia, and seizures. These effects may respond to intravenous administration of atropine (0.5 to 1 mg intravenously).

Questions—Introduction to Anticholinergic Drugs

1. **All of the following are peripheral symptoms of anticholinergic overdose except**
   A. Blurred vision
   B. Increased secretions
   C. Urinary retention
   D. Tachycardia
   E. Hypertension
2. **The following are central nervous system manifestations of anticholinergic overdose except**
   A. Hallucinations
   B. Speech disturbance
   C. Hemiballismus
   D. Disorientation
   E. Anxiety
3. **Treatment of anticholinergic overdose may include**
   A. Gastric lavage
   B. Hemodialysis
   C. Peritoneal dialysis
   D. All of the above
   E. None of the above
4. **Physostigmine**
   A. Should be given as a single dose, not repeated doses
   B. Is dosed for children and adults identically
   C. Has no toxicity
   D. Is usually given in repeated doses until reversal of effects occurs
   E. All of the above

ATROPINE AND HOMATROPINE

Atropine

Atropine and hyoscine are alkaloids that are produced by the roots, leaves, and beans of plants of the Solanaceae family. Deadly nightshade (Atropa belladonna) and hyoscyamine are examples of solanaceous alkaloids. These alkaloids can be synthesized, but plant extraction is less expensive. Duboisia myoporoides is now the main source, in addition to Atropa belladonna and Datura stramonium (jimsonweed). These plants have been regarded as poisonous for centuries. Linnaeus named the deadly nightshade shrub "Atropo belladonna" after Atropos, eldest of the three fates, whose duty was to cut the thread of life.

Atropine toxicity may result after sensitivity to a therapeutic dose, after medical personnel have administered erroneous or excessive amounts, after pharmacy error, or after voluntary administration. Occasionally atropine toxicity will manifest after covert use (i.e., "factitious atropine syndrome"), after excessive use of atropinic eyedrops by elderly patients, and occasionally after overexuberant use in the treatment of organophosphate or carbamate poisonings.

Atropine sulfate has numerous uses. It is used in ophthalmic preparations to induce mydriasis and cycloplegia, and especially after glaucoma surgery to maintain a dilated pupil and prevent posterior synechiae. Atropine is also used in the diagnosis and treatment of sinus node dysfunction; in the evaluation of coronary artery disease during atrial pacing; in sinus bradycardia induced by drugs with cholinergic effects; in advanced cardiac life support for bradycardia accompanied by hypotension; by inhalation in the treatment and prevention of asthma, bronchitis, and chronic obstructive pulmonary disease; and for symptomatic relief of Parkinson's disease.

Homatropine

Homatropine hydrobromide is a tertiary amine antimuscarinic agent used in eyedrops to produce mydriasis and cycloplegia for refraction, and in the management of acute inflammatory conditions of the uveal tract. It is a short-acting mydriatic and cycloplegic agent. Mydriasis reaches a maximum in 10–30 min and may last from 6 hours to 4 days. Cycloplegia reaches a maximum in 30–90 min and lasts 10–48 hours.

Pathophysiology

Atropine competitively inhibits the muscarinic effects of acetylcholine. Atropine prevents acetylcholine from exerting its usual action on effector cells but does not diminish the production of acetylcholine. It acts at autonomic effectors innervated by postganglionic cholinergic nerves, or on smooth muscles that do not contain cholinergic innervation. Central nervous system effects of atropine and related drugs result from central antimuscarinic actions.

Pharmacokinetics

ABSORPTION

- The bioavailability of atropine is about 95%. Time to peak plasma level is about 13 min after intramuscular administration and 1 hour after an oral dose.

DISTRIBUTION

- The volume of distribution of atropine is 2–4 L/kg.
- Plasma protein binding is 50%.

ELIMINATION

- Elimination half-life is 2–4 hours.
- Twenty to 50% of atropine is excreted unchanged.

Clinical Presentations

Atropine is the prototype anticholinergic drug. The so-called "anticholinergic syndrome" that follows atropine use is associated with numerous drugs including the cyclic antidepressants, phenothiazines, and antihistamines. The overdose patient may exhibit thirst, parched throat and lips, slurred speech, dilated pupils with no reaction to light or accommodation, blurred vision, visual hallucinations, restlessness, delusions of place and identity, agitation, amnesia, delirium, incoherence, flushed and hot skin, rapid pulse, bladder distension, ataxic gait, hyperpyrexia, hyperreflexia, and seizures.

Signs and symptoms of "atropinism" may follow use of atropine by any route (eye, oral, intramuscular, intravenous, or inhalation). Those with Down's syndrome have an increased sensitivity to atropine. Seizures without prior evidence of hallucinations or delirium have followed the use of atropine in adults and children. Homatropine eyedrops have caused confusion, hallucinations, disorientation, restlessness, photophobia, incoherent speech, abnormal gait, rapid respirations and pulse, a flushed face, and dilated pupils. No fatalities have been reported after homatropine use.

Answers to questions in shaded boxes appear at the end of the chapter.

Toxic Dosage/Death

Atropine in toxic amounts leads to drowsiness, stupor, convulsions, and coma. A fatal dose may be as low as 1.6 mg and as high as 100 mg in children. Recovery in an adult has followed ingestion of 1 g. Deaths reported after atropine administration have usually been in children and are frequently associated with severe hyperpyrexia.

Drug Interactions

Atropine may exert additive effects when used with other drugs that have anticholinergic effects such as anti-Parkinson's drugs, benztropine, orphenadrine, trihexyphenidyl, phenothiazines, amantadine, meperidine, tricyclic antidepressants, glutethimide, quinidine, disopyramide and antihistamines. The combination of atropine and succinylcholine, though commonly used in children, has been observed to increase the occurrence of skeletal muscle rigidity with malignant hyperthermia. Atropine may decrease the effects of pilocarpine eyedrops, reducing their ability to lower intraocular pressure in the treatment of glaucoma. An interaction between monoamine oxidase inhibitors and atropine may exaggerate the response to normal doses of atropine or atropine-like drugs.

Pregnancy/Lactation

Atropine has been used as a premedication in obstetric anesthesia, as a test of fetoplacental insufficiency, and in the diagnosis of fetal asphyxia. There is evidence of rapid placental transfer of atropine. Nursing infants have not been known to be adversely affected when mothers are using atropine. Pregnancy risk factor C.

Laboratory

ANALYTIC METHODS

A gas chromatography-mass spectrometry method for the rapid quantitation of atropine in blood has a limit of detection of atropine to about 10 ng/mL.

BLOOD LEVELS

Plasma levels confirm a clinical diagnosis but do not guide management, which must be based on clinical evaluation. There is little correlation between the dose of atropine, the plasma or serum concentration, and observed clinical effects. Pharmacologic effects have been observed at blood levels of 2–3 ng/mL.

Treatment

GUT DECONTAMINATION

Emesis may be useful after substantial ingestions if initiated within minutes of ingestion (the peak blood level of atropine is 1 hour), and if there is no evidence of obtundation, coma, or convulsions. Any advantage of emesis versus lavage and/or charcoal has not been proven. Gastric lavage with endotracheal intubation should be performed as soon as possible if the patient is obtunded and is unable to protect his airway. Activated charcoal (50–100 g in adults and 15–30 g in children) may be administered as aqueous slurry with saline cathartics or with sorbitol; however, the safety and efficacy of cathartics have not been established in the treatment of atropine toxicity.

ELIMINATION ENHANCEMENT

Enhancement of elimination of atropine by extracorporeal means has not been evaluated but is not likely to be effective in view of the large volume of distribution. In cases of overdoses reported to date, recovery has been achieved without use of these procedures.

SUPPORTIVE MEASURES

- Patients may be conscious on admission but may lapse into coma with profound respiratory depression. The airway should be maintained by endotracheal intubation where necessary. Electrocardiogram and vital signs should be continuously monitored.
- Toxicity from ingested doses may not correlate well with the suspected amount ingested. Treatment should be provided in a hospital intensive care facility with adequate respiratory assistance available.
- A quiet dark room with avoidance of unnecessary stimuli and with padding of bedsides may be useful for agitated subjects. Reassurance and diazepam can be employed as indicated.
- The clinician must rule out other causes of dilated pupils such as angle-closure glaucoma, cerebral aneurysm, brain tumor, and subdural or subarachnoid hemorrhage.
- Cooling measures should be instituted in hyperpyrexic patients.
- Concomitant use of drugs with anticholinergic properties such as phenothiazines, antihistamines, tricyclic antidepressants, disopyramide, and procainamide should be avoided.
- Blood studies may show a leukocytosis. The fasting blood sugar is usually normal but may be decreased. Urinalysis is generally normal unless there are complications such as convulsions or hyperthermia.
- An electrocardiogram may show sinus tachycardia, ST-segment elevations, diphasic T waves, prolonged QT interval, ventricular tachycardia, and ventricular fibrillation.
- Bladder catheterization may be required for urinary retention.

Antidotes

PHYSOSTIGMINE

Physostigmine may be useful when atropine overdose causes coma, arrhythmias, hallucinations, severe hypertension, or seizures. Reversal of these and other anticholinergic findings can be expected within minutes if there has not been any other central nervous system damage or exposure to a combination of drugs. Patients should be observed carefully for evidence of physostigmine toxicity (seizures, asystole, hypotension, hypersalivation, and bradyrhythmias). Physostigmine is relatively contraindicated in the presence of asthma, gangrene, or mechanical obstruction of the gastrointestinal or urogenital tract.

Questions—Atropine and Homatropine

1. **Deaths reported after atropine overdose administration**
   A. Have only occurred after more than 1000 mg were taken
   B. Have usually been in the elderly
   C. Are frequently associated with hyperpyrexia
   D. Are frequently associated with hypothermia
   E. None of the above
2. **All of the following may exert additive anticholinergic effects when used with atropine except**
   A. Phenothiazines
   B. Penicillin

C. Amantadine
D. Tricyclic antidepressants
E. Quinidine

3. The combination of atropine and succinylcholine
A. Is rarely used in children
B. May increase the occurrence of skeletal muscle rigidity with hyperthermia
C. Has no toxicity
D. Often causes hypoglycemia
E. All of the above

4. Atropine overdose may be treated with
A. Induced emesis
B. Gastric lavage
C. Activated charcoal
D. All of the above
E. None of the above

5. Plasma levels of atropine
A. Confirm clinical diagnosis of atropine overdose
B. Guide management of atropine overdose
C. Correlate with the dose of atropine given
D. Correlate with the clinical effects of atropine overdose
E. Are uniformly unreliable

6. Signs and symptoms of atropine overdose include
A. Thrombocytosis
B. Hyperglycemia
C. Prolonged QT interval
D. Constricted pupils
E. Hyponatremia

7. Physostigmine may be useful when atropine overdose causes
A. Coma
B. Arrhythmia
C. Hallucinations
D. Seizures
E. All of the above

8. Physostigmine toxicity includes
A. Hypertension
B. Seizures
C. Tachycardia
D. Pulmonary edema
E. Muscle breakdown

9. Physostigmine is contraindicated in patients with
A. Asthma
B. Gangrene
C. Gastrointestinal obstruction
D. Genitourinary obstruction
E. All of the above

BENZTROPINE

Benztropine (Cogentin®) is used for the symptomatic treatment of Parkinsonism. It is also used for the treatment of drug-induced extrapyramidal symptoms except for tardive dyskinesia, which may be exacerbated by its use. See Chapter 5, Antidotes. It has been investigated for use in the control of bedwetting by schizophrenic patients. Overdose may produce an anticholinergic poisoning syndrome, which can be present for days and may end fatally.

Pathophysiology

Benztropine mesylate is a synthetic tertiary amine antimuscarinic antiparkinsonian agent that resembles both atropine and diphenhydramine in chemical structure. It exhibits anticholinergic, antihistaminic, and local anesthetic properties. Benztropine exerts its effects by blocking central and peripheral muscarinic cholinergic receptor sites.

Pharmacokinetics

The toxicokinetics of benztropine have not been systematically studied. Data on its bioavailability, half-life, apparent volume of distribution, and clearance are not available.

Clinical Presentations

Adverse reactions to benztropine include dryness of the mouth, blurred vision, mydriasis, nausea, nervousness, tachycardia, and skin rash. In high doses or in particularly susceptible patients, benztropine may produce mental confusion or excitement, weakness, inability to move muscle groups, urinary retention, constipation, numbness of the extremities, listlessness, depression, vomiting, paralytic ileus, hyperthermia, heat stroke, and visual hallucinations. Choreoathetoid movements, agitation, picking at bed sheets, rapid incoherent speech, and auditory and visual hallucinations have been observed. Coma may be observed. Anticholinergic toxicity may last up to 8–9 days.

Toxic Dosage/Death

A 20-year-old who ingested 70 mg of benztropine plus an unknown amount of amitriptyline recovered. A 35-year-old man who received 12 mg of benztropine daily for 3 weeks recovered as well. At least two fatal cases have been reported: a 30-year-old observed taking a handful of benztropine 1.5 hours before death, and another patient who ingested an undocumented amount.

Drug Interactions

Administration of benztropine with other drugs having anticholinergic effects may increase the risk of adverse anticholinergic effects. If benztropine is administered with phenothiazines or tricyclic antidepressants, paralytic ileus, hyperthermia, or heat intolerance may occur and can be fatal.

Pregnancy/Lactation

Safe use of benztropine during pregnancy and lactation has not been established. Pregnancy risk factor C.

Laboratory

ANALYTIC METHODS

A quantitative gas chromatography-mass spectrometry assay is available for determination of benztropine in human urine and plasma.

BLOOD LEVELS

Serum benztropine levels, if they can be obtained, may have some correlation with the clinical course, but are generally not helpful in the acute setting. Therapeutic serum levels have not been established. Patients receiving 4 mg/d exhibited plasma levels of 19–125 ng/mL. Postmortem blood benztropine concentrations of 700 ng/mL have been reported after ingestion of an unknown amount.

URINE

Urine levels of 5.3–123 ng/mL were observed after four patients ingested 4 mg/d.

Treatment

GUT DECONTAMINATION

Syrup of ipecac is not advised in view of the possibility of seizures and obtundation. There is no evidence that activated charcoal adsorbs benztropine. The time to reach peak blood levels is not available. Lavage may be theoretically helpful as many as 12 hours after ingestion, as anticholinergic effects may slow bowel transit time.

ELIMINATION ENHANCEMENT

There are no data on the apparent volume of distribution of benztropine. It may be assumed to be large, similar to other anticholinergic products such as cyclic antidepressants. There has been no experience with active elimination methods such as forced diuresis, peritoneal dialysis, hemodialysis, and hemoperfusion.

SUPPORTIVE MEASURES

- Patients should be evaluated for intact airway, respiration (including tidal volume), and circulatory status. Although there have been no reports of sudden hemodynamic instability, fatalities have occurred within 1.5 hours of ingestion.
- Patients should be treated with oxygen, naloxone, glucose, and, if indicated, thiamine if there is evidence of altered mental status. Arterial blood gases should be drawn in obtunded patients and electrocardiographic monitoring instituted.
- The electrocardiogram may indicate sinus tachycardia without evidence of QRS or QTc prolongation. Patients who are admitted should receive cardiac monitoring until they are symptom-free for 24 hours.
- Urinalysis is generally normal unless there are complications such as convulsions or hyperthermia. The patient should be observed for evidence of rhabdomyolysis (urine myoglobin, serum creatine kinase).
- The bladder should be catheterized in cases of urinary retention.
- Hyperthermia usually resolves with conservative measures (cooling blankets, ice bags).
- Hypertension may appear early in the course of poisoning. It is usually mild and requires no special treatment.

Antidotes

PHYSOSTIGMINE

Physostigmine use should be reserved for the rare unstable patient, as most patients with benztropine overdose require only supportive care. If there is a serious danger of agitation and hallucinations without a history of gangrene, asthma, ulcerative colitis, cardiovascular disease, or seizures, then physostigmine may be considered. See the Introduction above.

Questions—Benztropine

1. Benztropine is used for

A. Drug-induced extrapyramidal symptoms
B. Tardive dyskinesia
C. Bedwetting in children
D. Psychosis
E. Treatment of anticholinergic poisoning

2. In high doses or susceptible patients, benztropine may produce

A. Mental confusion
B. Weakness
C. Urinary retention
D. Hypernatremia
E. All of the above

3. Patients with benztropine overdose should be treated with

A. Oxygen, as they are often hypoxemic
B. Glucose, as they are often hypoglycemic
C. Thiamine if they have altered mental status
D. Naloxone
E. None of the above

DICYCLOMINE

Dicyclomine (Bentyl®) is used in functional disturbances of the gastrointestinal tract such as irritable bowel syndrome. It has also been used for infantile colic and to increase bladder capacity in patients with uninhibited bladder contractions that result in incontinence. Dicyclomine overdose has been reported mainly in young children who have ingested products containing dicyclomine together with other drugs. Signs and symptoms of overdose are treated as an anticholinergic poisoning with symptomatic and supportive treatment. Sudden death has been observed.

Pathophysiology

Dicyclomine hydrochloride is a competitive antagonist at muscarinic cholinergic neurons.

Pharmacokinetics

ABSORPTION

- Dicyclomine is rapidly absorbed after oral administration, with a peak plasma concentration noted 1.5–2.0 hours after an oral dose.

DISTRIBUTION

- The apparent volume of distribution of dicyclomine is about 3.65 L/kg.

ELIMINATION

- Approximately 80% of a dose is eliminated in the urine and 10% in the feces.
- The half-life of the drug in the initial distribution phase is about 1.8 hours, and the half-life in the terminal elimination phase is about 9–10 hours.

Clinical Presentations

Serious toxicity has been described in very young children, although there are few reports of ingestion of dicyclomine alone.

Signs and symptoms in overdoses that terminate fatally include restlessness, disorientation, ataxia, myoclonic and tonic-clonic seizures, flushed facies, fever, agitation, dilated pupils, coarse nystagmus, vomiting, and cardiac and respiratory arrest.

Survivors of overdose may demonstrate dilated pupils, an intoxicated appearance, dry mouth, smacking of the lips, agitation, confusion, nervousness, vomiting, drowsiness, flushed facies, toxic delirium, hallucinations, hot dry skin, tachycardia, apnea, cyanosis, and rigidity. Reported cases of apnea, seizures, and coma following dicyclomine use have occurred within 30 minutes of administration.

Toxic Dosage/Death

A 2-year-old who ingested 90 mg exhibited slightly dilated pupils, appeared slightly intoxicated, and survived. A 2-year-old ingested 200 mg of dicyclomine and survived. A 15-month-old ingested 300 mg of dicyclomine and survived. The maximum human doses of dicyclomine hydrochloride recorded were 600 mg by mouth in a 10-month-old child and approximately 1500 mg in an adult, each of whom survived.

An 18-month-old who ate a bottle full of dicyclomine tablets developed signs of anticholinergic toxicity and respiratory and cardiac arrest, and died. A 3-year-old ingested 100 Bendectin® tablets, developed signs of restlessness, disorientation, ataxia and tonic-clonic seizures, and later died in cardiorespiratory arrest.

Drug Interactions

Dicyclomine is an anticholinergic drug and will probably interact in an additive manner with other drugs whose site of action is the muscarinic cholinergic receptor. Agents that may increase certain actions or side effects of anticholinergic drugs include amantadine, class I antiarrhythmic agents, antihistamines, antipsychotic agents (e.g., phenothiazines), benzodiazepines, monoamine oxidase inhibitors, narcotic analgesics (e.g., meperidine), nitrates and nitrites, sympathomimetic agents, and tricyclic antidepressants.

Pregnancy/Lactation

Dicyclomine has not been associated with a significant increase in teratogenic congenital limb defects. The U.S. Food and Drug Administration has placed dicyclomine in pregnancy risk category B.

Laboratory

ANALYTIC METHODS

Dicyclomine may be detected in blood by gas chromatography using nitrogen-selective or flame ionization detection. A capillary gas chromatography method using nitrogen-selective detection is adequate for analyzing plasma concentrations as low as 5 ng/mL.

BLOOD LEVELS

Blood concentrations of dicyclomine may be roughly correlated with toxic symptoms, but are not correlated with dose ingested and can be used only as an indication of ingestion and not necessarily as a guide to severity of disease. A 2-year-old found unresponsive had a blood dicyclomine concentration of 505 ng/mL. Another 2-month-old child was discovered apneic and died with a blood dicyclomine concentration of 221 ng/mL.

Treatment

GUT DECONTAMINATION

Syrup of ipecac is not advised in view of the possibility of seizures and obtundation. There is no evidence that activated charcoal is helpful; however, it is still advised in large overdoses. Lavage may be theoretically helpful as well, many hours after ingestion, as anticholinergic effects may slow bowel transit time.

ELIMINATION ENHANCEMENT

There has been no experience with active elimination methods such as forced diuresis, peritoneal dialysis, hemodialysis, and hemoperfusion.

SUPPORTIVE MEASURES

- Treatment of dicyclomine overdose is largely symptomatic and supportive and should follow the guidelines for treatment of poisoning with other anticholinergic agents.

Antidotes

PHYSOSTIGMINE

Physostigmine use should be reserved for the rare, unstable patient, as most patients with dicyclomine overdose require only supportive care. If there is a serious danger of agitation and hallucinations without a history of gangrene, asthma, ulcerative colitis, cardiovascular disease, or seizures, then physostigmine may be considered. See the Introduction above.

Questions—Dicyclomine

1. Dicyclomine has been
   A. Used in irritable bowel syndrome
   B. Shown to cure infant colic
   C. Commonly used to treat stool incontinence
   D. Used to treat extrapyramidal symptoms of Parkinsonism
   E. None of the above

2. Dicyclomine toxicity
   A. Is most common in the elderly
   B. Is usually due to isolated ingestion of dicyclomine
   C. Occurs within a well-defined range of ingested doses
   D. Is most common in depressed adolescents
   E. None of the above

3. Symptoms of dicyclomine toxicity include all of the following except
   A. Seizures
   B. Cyanosis
   C. Rigidity
   D. Increased secretions
   E. Apnea

4. Dicyclomine side effects may be increased by concomitant use of the following except
   A. Antihistamines
   B. Antiarrythmics
   C. Antipsychotics
   D. Antidepressants
   E. Antibiotics

5. Treatment of dicyclomine overdose may include
A. Urine drug levels to correlate with dose ingested
B. Serum drug levels to correlate with dose ingested
C. Syrup of ipecac to induce emesis
D. Lavage, up to several hours after ingestion
E. None of the above

IPRATROPIUM

Ipratropium bromide (Atrovent®) is used as a bronchodilator for maintenance treatment of bronchospasm associated with chronic obstructive pulmonary diseases, including bronchitis and emphysema. Ipratropium has also been useful in organophosphate insecticide poisoning when given intratracheally. Overdose may follow excessive use of metered-dose inhalers for bronchospasm. Symptoms are short-lived and often remit spontaneously without any measures other than symptomatic and supportive treatment. One possible fatality has been described.

Pathophysiology

The predominantly central distribution of cholinergic nerves and muscarinic receptors in the airways contrasts with the more peripheral distribution of β-adrenergic receptors. Ipratropium is a competitive antagonist of the muscarinic acetylcholine receptor. By blocking cholinergic receptors present on most cells, it inhibits the release of cyclic guanosine monophosphate, which in turn inhibits the release of bronchoconstrictive mediators, such as antihistamine.

Pharmacokinetics

ABSORPTION

- After it is inhaled, ipratropium starts to act within 15 min.
- Activity peaks in 30–120 minutes, and is sustained for 3–4 hours.

DISTRIBUTION

- Ninety percent of the inhaled drug remains in the upper airways.
- The volume of distribution of ipratropium bromide is approximately 5 L/kg.
- Ipratropium does not cross the blood-brain barrier.

ELIMINATION

- Most ipratropium is excreted unchanged in the feces.
- Its half-life is similar to that of atropine, about 3 hours.
- Fifty percent appears unchanged in the urine after intravenous administration.

Clinical Presentations

Large doses of ipratropium can lead to cough, a metallic or bitter taste, dry mouth, buccal ulceration, blurred vision, paralytic ileus, and bladder neck obstruction. Paradoxical bronchoconstriction may occur. At least one case of drug abuse and five possible cases of overdose have been reported since the product was first marketed in 1987. Several elderly patients have developed shortness of breath and increased bronchospasm after several weeks of therapy.

Toxic Dosage/Death

One elderly patient who used the product 6 or more times per day developed shortness of breath and increased bronchospasm, and recovered. A 66-year-old woman suspected of overusing Atrovent® developed hypoxia secondary to status asthmaticus, went into cardiac arrest, and died.

Drug Interactions

Acute angle-closure glaucoma has been reported in elderly patients receiving combined nebulized ipratropium bromide and salbutamol. Use with terbutaline sulfate inhalers has led to pharyngeal blistering. Ipratropium may have an additive effect on bronchodilation when used with albuterol for the emergency treatment of acute severe asthma.

Pregnancy/Lactation

It is unknown whether placental transfer or excretion into human milk occurs. No adequately controlled studies have been conducted in pregnant women. Pregnancy risk category B.

Laboratory

ANALYTIC METHODS

There is no reliable method for the measurement of ipratropium in body fluids. Few clinical laboratories have the facilities to measure blood ipratropium levels. A radioreceptor assay can detect urine levels to 5 ng/mL and plasma levels to 500 ng/mL.

BLOOD LEVELS

Blood levels have not been studied in overdose. There is little evidence that blood levels are clinically useful.

Treatment

GUT DECONTAMINATION

These methods have not been studied in the setting of ipratropium overdose.

ELIMINATION ENHANCEMENT

Measures to enhance elimination of ipratropium have not been used in patients with suspected overdose. Hemodialysis and hemoperfusion would probably be ineffective in view of the extensive volume of distribution.

SUPPORTIVE MEASURES

- Patients who have used ipratropium excessively will probably respond to symptomatic and supportive care combined with cessation of drug use.
- Intraocular pressure may increase after ipratropium bromide use.
- Patients developing side effects after excessive use often recover within 24 hours of cessation of ipratropium use.

Questions—Ipratropium

1. Ipratropium is used in
A. Asthma
B. Bronchitis
C. Emphysema
D. Organophosphate poisoning
E. All of the above

2. **Inhaled ipratropium**
   A. Reaches its peak activity at 15–45 min
   B. Has activity which is sustained for up to 2 hours
   C. Does not cross the blood-brain barrier
   D. Is mostly excreted in urine, whether inhaled or given intravenously
   E. All of the above

3. **Large doses of ipratropium can cause**
   A. Bladder neck obstruction
   B. Bronchoconstriction
   C. Paralytic ileus
   D. Cough
   E. All of the above

4. **Ipratropium use**
   A. Has caused optic nerve damage in the elderly
   B. Is safe in pregnancy but not breastfeeding
   C. Is safe in breastfeeding but not in pregnancy
   D. Has been associated with pharyngeal blisters
   E. All of the above

OXYBUTYNIN

Oxybutynin (Ditropan®) is a smooth muscle antispasmodic agent used mainly in patients with urinary incontinence due to detrusion irritability or detrusion hyperreflexia. Following an overdose, it may lead to a series of anticholinergic effects involving the central nervous system, eyes, skin, and heart. There have been no reported fatalities.

Pathophysiology

Oxybutynin hydrochloride is a direct smooth muscle relaxant with weak antimuscarinic properties. It exerts atropine-like anticholinergic actions. It also possesses local anesthetic and analgesic effects. Oxybutynin has no antinicotinic effects at skeletal neuromuscular junctions or autonomic ganglia.

Pharmacokinetics

ABSORPTION

- Oxybutynin is rapidly absorbed from the gastrointestinal tract.
- The absolute systemic availability is about 6%.

DISTRIBUTION

- The apparent volume of distribution is 0.5–1.2 L/kg.

ELIMINATION

- Oxybutynin is rapidly metabolized in the liver. The half-life of oxybutynin is 2 hours.
- Very little oxybutynin is excreted unchanged in the urine.

Clinical Presentations

Oxybutynin overdose may produce central nervous system symptoms including restlessness, tremor, irritability, disorientation, seizures, delirium, hallucinations, psychotic behavior, dilated pupils, dry skin and mouth, and urinary retention. Cardiovascular symptoms may include flushing, tachycardia, hypertension, hypotension, and circulatory failure. Fever, nausea, and vomiting may also occur. Severe overdose may lead to paralysis, respiratory failure, and coma.

Oxybutynin may aggravate signs and symptoms of hyperthyroidism, coronary heart disease, congestive heart failure, cardiac arrhythmias, hiatal hernia, hypertension, tachycardia, and prostatic hypertrophy. In patients with ulcerative colitis, it may enhance induction of paralytic ileus or toxic megacolon. In areas of high environmental temperature, oxybutynin may decrease sweating and induce fever and heat stroke.

Toxic Dosage/Death

A 34-year-old who ingested 100 mg of oxybutynin became drowsy, hallucinated, and later became comatose. She recovered by the third day. Overdose fatalities have not been reported.

Drug Interactions

Alcohol or other sedatives may increase the drowsiness observed with oxybutynin. Antihistamines, tricyclic antidepressants, phenothiazines, and atropine may enhance the anticholinergic effects of oxybutynin.

Pregnancy/Lactation

Oxybutynin has not been studied in pregnant or lactating women. The U.S. Food and Drug Administration has assigned the drug to pregnancy risk category B.

Laboratory

ANALYTIC METHODS

A radioreceptor assay is available. The product and its metabolites have been studied by gas chromatography and mass spectrometry. A preferred method uses reverse-phase high-performance liquid chromatography.

BLOOD LEVELS

An average plasma concentration of about 8 ng/mL is reached less than 1 hour after oral ingestion of 5 mg. Levels of 20–50 ng/mL may follow a 5-mg dose. Blood levels after an overdose have not been reported. Plasma analysis may be useful to confirm presence, but not to guide treatment of oxybutynin after an overdose.

Treatment

GUT DECONTAMINATION

Emesis induction is not advised in patients who are precomatose, having seizures, or in a psychotic state. Activated charcoal may be useful, but has not been specifically studied. Overdose patients with oxybutynin benefit from gastric lavage if they are seen with 2 hours.

ELIMINATION ENHANCEMENT

Measures to enhance the elimination of oxybutynin have not been used in patients with suspected overdose.

SUPPORTIVE MEASURES

- Treatment is largely symptomatic and supportive. Airway patency should be ascertained at all times. Assisted ventilation may be required if paralysis of respiratory muscles occurs.
- In patients with severe intoxication, thiopental or chloral hydrate may be necessary to combat extreme excitement. Restlessness and delirium can generally be treated with diazepam. Phenothiazines can lead to additive anticholinergic effects and should be avoided.

- Intravenous fluids may be necessary because of potential dehydration from vomiting and fever.
- Fever is treated with cooling measures.
- An electrocardiogram may reveal sinus tachycardia and/or ventricular premature beats.

Antidotes

PHYSOSTIGMINE

Physostigmine use should be reserved for the rare unstable patient, as most patients with oxybutynin overdose require only supportive care. If there is a serious danger of agitation and hallucinations without a history of gangrene, asthma, ulcerative colitis, cardiovascular disease, or seizures, then physostigmine may be considered. See the Introduction above.

Questions—Oxybutynin

1. Oxybutynin is used primarily to treat
   A. Fecal incontinence
   B. Urinary incontinence
   C. Distal muscle hyperreflexia
   D. Diarrhea
   E. Constipation

2. Oxybutynin is
   A. Available systemically as only a small percentage of what is taken
   B. Metabolized rapidly in the liver
   C. Excreted in a small proportion in the urine
   D. Absorbed rapidly in the gastrointestinal tract
   E. All of the above

3. Oxybutynin overdose may cause
   A. Paralysis
   B. Hypertension
   C. Hypotension
   D. Fever
   E. All of the above

4. Oxybutynin is known to aggravate all of the following conditions except
   A. Hyperthyroidism
   B. Coronary heart disease
   C. Cellulitis
   D. Congestive heart failure
   E. Cardiac arrhthymias

5. Patients with oxybutynin overdoses
   A. Should have serum levels measured to guide treatment
   B. Benefit from gastric lavage up to 1 day after ingestion
   C. May require assisted ventilation
   D. Do not benefit from physostigmine use
   E. Are at high risk for mortality

SCOPOLAMINE

Scopolamine or hyoscine is a naturally occurring belladonna alkaloid and anticholinergic agent. Its peripheral action resembles that of atropine. Scopolamine is used by anesthesiologists as a premedicant and to control postoperative nausea. It is commonly used transdermally to treat motion sickness. Each scopolamine patch (Transderm Scop®) contains 1.5 mg of scopolamine and is programmed to deliver 0.5 mg scopolamine over 3 days.

Reports of accidental poisoning with transdermal scopolamine have resulted from misinterpretation of prescribing information. Patients have applied transdermal patches at intervals more frequent than the recommended 3 days or applied multiple transdermal systems at once. Side effects have included hallucinations, fever, confusion, and disorientation. Treatment of scopolamine overdose is largely symptomatic and supportive.

Pathophysiology

Scopolamine acts by antagonizing acetylcholine competitively at cholinergic postganglionic nerve endings. Its action on the iris, ciliary body, and certain secretory glands (salivary, bronchial, sweat) is more potent than that of other belladonna alkaloids. Cardiac muscle, exocrine glands, and smooth muscles of the gastrointestinal tract are also affected. Blood pressure increases, pulse rate may decrease, pupils become dilated, and hallucinations may occur. Scopolamine crosses the blood-brain barrier, and enters the central nervous system.

Pharmacokinetics

ABSORPTION

- When the transdermal patch is applied, an initial primary dose of 140 μg is provided. The remainder is released at 5 μg/h.

DISTRIBUTION

- The apparent volume of distribution in animals is 1.6–3.7 L/kg.

ELIMINATION

- Half-life is about 50 min.
- The percentage of administered dose excreted as unchanged scopolamine is 1.7–5.9%.

Clinical Presentations

Symptoms following transdermal use include drowsiness, dry mouth, reduced concentration, confusion, and hallucinations. Severe scopolamine toxicity presents with flushed, hot skin, dilated fixed pupils, blurred vision, cardiac arrhythmias, and convulsions. Without treatment, these conditions may terminate fatally. Disorientation, memory disturbances, dizziness, restlessness, difficulty urinating, rashes, erythema, acute narrow-angle glaucoma, and dry, itchy, or red eyes may be seen.

When transdermal scopolamine has been used longer than 3 days, dizziness, nausea, vomiting, headache, and disturbance of equilibrium have occasionally followed withdrawal of its use. Occasionally, restlessness, hallucinations, and delirium may follow the use of scopolamine in the elderly. Headache may also accompany the use of transdermal scopolamine.

Toxic Dosage/Death

A toxic psychosis has been described in a 6-year-old child who wore the patch for 12 hours.

Drug Interactions

Alcohol or other sedatives may increase the drowsiness observed with scopolamine. Antihistamines, tricyclic antidepressants, phenothiazines, and atropine may enhance the anticholinergic effects of scopolamine.

Pregnancy/Lactation

The U.S. Food and Drug Administration has placed the transdermal scopolamine patch in pregnancy risk category C. Controlled studies have not been performed in pregnant women or during lactation. Scopolamine crosses the placenta.

Laboratory

ANALYTIC METHODS

A radioreceptor assay has been described for analysis of blood scopolamine levels. The lower detection limit is 0.08 nmol/L in plasma.

BLOOD LEVELS

Following ingestion of 0.6 mg scopolamine or use of buccal scopolamine 0.6 mg, peak levels of about 1.2 nmol/L scopolamine are obtained in about 1 hour. Free scopolamine levels of 890 pg/mL in plasma and 113 ng/mL in urine confirmed scopolamine intoxication in a 6-year-old child.

Treatment

GUT DECONTAMINATION

There is no experience confirming the efficacy of charcoal in conjunction with transdermal patch or other scopolamine ingestion.

ELIMINATION ENHANCEMENT

There are no data to support the use of hemodialysis or hemoperfusion, which are in any case not likely to be useful in enhancing elimination of scopolamine because of its extensive volume of distribution.

SUPPORTIVE MEASURES

- Symptoms associated with the use of the transdermal patch generally subside within 24–36 hours.
- The patch or patches should be removed carefully. After a patch is applied or removed, the hands should be thoroughly washed to remove any residual scopolamine. Any adhesive remaining on the hands after application or removal of the patch may contain scopolamine. Subsequent touching of the eye may produce mydriatic effects.
- More than 90% of unilateral dilated pupils occur on the same side as the patch. The diagnosis of scopolamine contamination can be confirmed by prompt and extensive constriction of the pupil on instillation of 0.5–1.0% pilocarpine hydrochloride in the affected eye.
- Patients infrequently require admission to a hospital. Physostigmine is rarely required.

Questions—Scopolamine

1. Scopolamine can cause
A. Increased secretions
B. Vertigo
C. Hallucinations
D. Hypothermia
E. All of the above

2. Scopolamine effects may be enhanced by
A. Antihistamines
B. Tricyclic antidepressants
C. Phenothiazines
D. Atropine
E. All of the above

3. The scopolamine patch
A. Has no known side effects
B. Should be used for 3 hours at a time
C. Should be used for no more than 3 days at a time
D. Can be used safely by simultaneously applying 4 patches for one-fourth the prescribed time
E. Delivers an initial dose of 5 mg

4. The toxicity of a scopolamine patch
A. Usually subsides within 2–3 days
B. Usually subsides within 2–3 hours
C. Usually indicates the need for hospital admission
D. Should be treated with gut decontamination
E. None of the above

TRIHEXYPHENIDYL

Trihexyphenidyl (Artane®) is used in the treatment of Parkinson's disease and to ameliorate drug-induced extrapyramidal effects. It may be useful in the prevention or treatment of nerve gas poisoning in chemical warfare. The effects of overdose with trihexyphenidyl are typical of anticholinergic drug toxicity. Complete recovery usually occurs in 3–4 days, but symptoms and signs may continue for up to one month. Treatment is symptomatic and supportive.

Pathophysiology

Trihexyphenidyl hydrochloride is a synthetic, tertiary amine, antimuscarinic agent, with anticholinergic effects after overdose.

Pharmacokinetics

ABSORPTION

- Trihexyphenidyl hydrochloride is almost completely absorbed from the gastrointestinal tract.

DISTRIBUTION

- Peak plasma levels are reached about 1 hour after an oral dose.

ELIMINATION

- Trihexyphenidyl is eliminated by first-order kinetics with a half-life of about 4 hours.
- About one-half of an oral dose is excreted in the urine within 72 hours.

Clinical Presentations

Symptoms of anticholinergic overdose may include confusion, hallucinations, dry mouth, dilated pupils, blurring of vision, tachycardia, and fever. Paranoid psychosis may be seen in the elderly. Cognitive impairment may persist after acute intoxication. Antiparkinsonian drugs can be abused by some patients to achieve pleasurable effects ranging from mild euphoria with increased sociability at lower doses, to toxic psychosis with disorientation and hallucinations at higher doses.

Long-term abuse (6–20 mg/d) can lead to memory and cognitive impairments. Following prolonged use of trihexyphenidyl hydrochloride, withdrawal can lead to anxiety, irritability, persecutory ideas, insomnia, headache, excessive perspiration, and tachycardia. Most patients have recovered after 2–4 days; however, symptoms may persist for weeks.

Toxic Dosage/Death

Ingestion of 180 mg of trihexyphenidyl hydrochloride has resulted in symptoms of anticholinergic overdose. The patient recovered within several weeks. Another patient ingested 300 mg of trihexyphenidyl with suicidal intent, developed evidence of anticholinergic toxicity, and recovered in 1 week. No deaths following overdose with trihexyphenidyl have been described.

Drug Interactions

Concomitant use of other drugs with anticholinergic profiles may exacerbate the anticholinergic syndrome produced by trihexyphenidyl in overdose.

Pregnancy/Lactation

Pregnancy risk factor C.

Laboratory

ANALYTIC METHODS

Gas-liquid chromatography is used to assay trihexyphenidyl hydrochloride in body fluids.

BLOOD LEVELS

Monitoring blood levels in overdose does not guide management.

Treatment

GUT DECONTAMINATION

Gastric lavage and/or charcoal may be helpful.

ELIMINATION ENHANCEMENT

These methods have not been reported in conjunction with trihexyphenidyl overdose.

SUPPORTIVE MEASURES

- Treatment is generally symptomatic and supportive. Patients with serious overdoses should be admitted to a hospital for continuous electrocardiographic and cardiac monitoring.
- Withdrawal symptoms may respond to cessation of drug use and benzodiazepines.

Antidotes

Physostigmine is rarely required.

Questions—Trihexyphenidyl

1. Trihexyphenidyl is used
A. To treat Parkinson's disease
B. To lessen drug-induced extrapyramidal effects
C. To prevent nerve gas poisoning
D. To treat nerve gas poisoning
E. All of the above

2. Trihexyphenidyl overdose
A. Usually causes symptoms which resolve in 3–4 days
B. Usually causes symptoms which last more than 1 month
C. Causes predominantly cholinergic symptoms
D. Has been known to cause death
E. None of the above

3. Cognitive impairment may occur
A. After acute intoxication with trihexyphenidyl
B. After long-term abuse but not acute exposure to trihexyphenidyl
C. After acute but not long-term exposure to trihexyphenidyl
D. Only with paranoid psychosis resulting from trihexyphenidyl abuse
E. None of the above

4. Withdrawal after prolonged use of trihexyphenidyl can lead to all of the following except
A. Anxiety
B. Insomnia
C. Dry, irritated skin
D. Irritability
E. Headache

5. Overdose of trihexyphenidyl
A. Has been described as causing death
B. Does not require serum levels to guide management
C. Always indicates hospital admission
D. Generally requires physostigmine treatment
E. All of the above

Answers

Introduction to Anticholinergic Drugs

1. B 2. C 3. A 4. D

Atropine and Homatropine

1. C 2. B 3. B 4. D 5. A 6. C
7. E 8. B 9. E

Benztropine

1. A 2. E 3. C

Dicyclomine

1. A 2. E 3. D 4. E 5. D

Ipratropium

1. E 2. C 3. E 4. D

Oxybutynin

1. B 2. E 3. E 4. C 5. C

Scopolamine

1. C 2. E 3. C 4. A

Trihexyphenidyl

1. E 2. A 3. A 4. C 5. B

SELECTED READINGS

Introduction to Anticholinergic Drugs

1. Reynolds JEF, ed. Martindale: The Extra Pharmacopoeia. 30th Ed. London: Pharmaceutical Press, 1993:418.

Atropine and Homatropine

1. Miller JJ. Symposium on atropine toxicity therapy. J Nerv Ment Dis 1956; 124:260–264.
2. O'Connor PS, Mumma JV. Atropine toxicity. Am J Ophthalmol 1985;99: 613–614.
3. Shutt LE, Bowes JB. Atropine and hyoscine. Anesthesia 1979;34:476–490.
4. Tyson WJ. Toxic effects of atropine drops. Br Med J 1889;2:921.
5. Weinstock FJ. Dilated fixed pupils from atropine. JAMA 1974;229:267–268.
6. Welbourn RB, Buxton JD. Acute atropine poisoning: Review of eight cases. Lancet 1948

Benztropine

1. Fahy P, Arnold P, Curry SC, Bond R. Serial serum drug concentrations and prolonged anticholinergic toxicity after benztropine (Cogentin) overdose. Am J Emerg Med 1989;7:199–202.
2. Perry PJ, Wilding DC, Juhl RP. Anticholinergic psychosis. Am J Hosp Pharm 1978;35:725–727.
3. Stern TA. Continuous infusion of physostigmine in anticholinergic delirium. J Clin Psychiatry 1983;44:463–464. Case Report.

Dicyclomine

1. Garriott JC, Rodriguez R, Norton LE. Two cases of death involving dicyclomine in infants: Measurement of therapeutic and toxic concentrations in blood. Clin Toxicol 1984;22:455–462.
2. Weissbluth M, Christoffel KK, Todd Davis A. Treatment of infantile colic with dicyclomine hydrochloride. J Pediatr 1984;104:951–955.
3. Wise GW, Green VA. Toxicant cases: Bendectin ingestion. Action 1974;2:5.

Ipratropium

1. Cugell DW. Chemical pharmacology and toxicology of ipratropium bromide. Am J Med 1986;8(suppl. 5A):18–22.
2. Gross MJ. Ipratropium bromide. N Engl J Med 1988;319:486–494.

Oxybutynin

1. Banerjee S, Routledge PA, Pugh S, Smith PM. Poisoning with oxybutynin. Hum Exp Toxicol 1991;10:222–226.

Scopolamine

1. Price NM, Schmitt LG, McGuire J, et al. Transdermal scopolamine in the prevention of motion sickness at sea. Clin Pharmacol Ther 1981;29:414–419.
2. Saxena K, Saxena S. Scopolamine withdrawal syndrome. Postgrad Med 1990; 87:63–66.
3. Wilkinson JA. Side effects of transdermal scopolamine. J Emerg Med 1987;5: 389–392.

Trihexyphenidyl

1. Enchava D. Trihexyphenidyl overdose: Clinical presentation and management. Vet Hum Toxicol 1993;35:370.

ACKNOWLEDGMENT

Thanks to Alison Deutsch, MD for contributing the questions in this chapter.

CHAPTER 35
Antihistamines

INTRODUCTION

Antihistamines are predominantly H1 receptor blockers. For practical purposes, H1 antagonists are often divided into first-generation, or relatively sedating medications, and second-generation, relatively non-sedating medications. The latter group includes drugs introduced since 1981, of which terfenadine, astemizole, and loratadine are the best known.

Antihistamines were first synthesized in 1942 and have been used clinically for almost 50 years. They are available as prescription and over-the-counter products for the treatment of allergy symptoms, as "cold" remedies, and as sleep medications. Over-the-counter sleep preparations (e.g., Sominex®, Nytol®, and Sleepeze®), which formerly contained other products, now, after FDA review, all contain diphenhydramine as their sole ingredient.

Accidental or intentional ingestion and overdose are common. Doxylamine succinate is an antihistamine often used as a sleeping aid which produces signs and symptoms of anticholinergic toxicity in overdose. Fatalities and rhabdomyolysis have been reported. Hydroxyzine is an antihistaminic drug with anxiolytic properties which, in overdose, also produces anticholinergic effects including sinus tachycardia, seizures, and flushing of the skin. Reports of poisoning with hydroxyzine include coma and death. Treatment is symptomatic and supportive.

Antihistamines, H1 receptor blocking agents, are structurally similar to histamine and are substituted ethylamines. They are classified by the chemical group, which joins two aromatic rings to an ethylamine moiety. Examples include an ethylenediamine group (as in tripelennamine), alkylamines (as in chlorpheniramine), a phenothiazine nucleus (as in chlorpromazine), a piperazine nucleus (as in chlorcyclizine), or ethanolamine derivatives (as in diphenhydramine). Some second-generation H1 antagonists do not fit readily into any of the traditional classes. For example, terfenadine, astemizole, loratadine, ketotifen, and levocabastine all have diverse chemical structures.

SEDATING H1 RECEPTOR ANTAGONISTS

Sedating H1 blockers are used as cold remedies, antiallergy medications, premedication for surgery, antinauseants, for motion sickness, for treatment of dystonic reactions, and as anti-Parkinson medication. Many, especially doxylamine and diphenhydramine, are used as sleep aids. In combination with antitussives and decongestants, antihistamines may provide temporary relief of cough and cold symptoms. Hydroxyzine is used in the symptomatic management of anxiety and tension associated with psychoneuroses. It is also used for the management of pruritus and as a sedative before and after general anesthesia.

Pathophysiology

Diphenhydramine is an H1 receptor antagonist noted for its sedative and anticholinergic properties as seen after both therapeutic use and overdosage. Its sedative effects are frequently seen in adults and may lead to severe central nervous system (CNS) depression, coma, and death. The antihistamines do not inhibit histamine release, antibody production, or antigen-antibody interaction. They do antagonize the effects of histamine on receptor sites. Doxylamine is an antihistamine drug with hypnotic, anticholinergic, and local anesthetic properties. Hydroxyzine has CNS-depressant, anticholinergic, antispasmodic, local anesthetic, antihistaminic, sedative, and antiemetic effects.

Pharmacokinetics

ABSORPTION

- Diphenhydramine is rapidly absorbed after an oral dose. Maximum blood and tissue levels are achieved 2 hours after an oral dose and 1 hour after a parenteral dose.
- Doxylamine is also easily absorbed from the gastrointestinal tract.
- The absorption of hydroxyzine by the gastrointestinal tract is also rapid following oral administration. The plasma absorption half-life of hydroxyzine is about 1 hour.
- Sedative effects of hydroxyzine may persist 2–6 hours following administration of a single dose.

Distribution

- Diphenhydramine is 98% protein bound. It has a large first-pass effect and at least half is metabolized in the liver to diphenylmethane before it reaches the general circulation.
- The apparent volume of distribution of diphenhydramine is 3–7 L/kg.
- The apparent volume of distribution of doxylamine is 2.5 L/kg.
- The apparent volume of distribution of hydroxyzine in young adults is 16.0 L/kg, and in those over 65 years of age is 22.5 L/kg.

ELIMINATION

- The serum half-life of diphenhydramine is 4–10 hours.
- Metabolites in the urine include glutamine and glucuronide-conjugated and unconjugated diphenylmethoxyacetic acid. Less than 2% of diphenhydramine is excreted unchanged in the urine.
- The elimination half-life of doxylamine is 10.1 hours. Doxylamine is excreted in the urine as unchanged doxylamine (60%), nordoxylamine, and dinordoxylamine.
- The hydroxyzine elimination half-life is 3–20 hours. It is eliminated by hepatic metabolism.
- The mean elimination half-life of hydroxyzine in older adults may be as high as 29.3 hours.

Clinical Presentations

Impaired consciousness is the most common symptom in diphenhydramine overdose. Psychotic behavior similar to catatonic stupor may be observed. Adults usually present with CNS depression, which may lead to coma and/or seizures. Topical antihistamine lotions may induce acute anticholinergic toxicity in young children.

Signs of peripheral anticholinergic toxicity include arrhythmias, tachycardia, urinary retention, decreased gastrointestinal motility, dryness of mouth, thickening of bronchial secretions, and blurry vision. Impaired consciousness, seizures, tachycardia, mydriasis, and psychosis may characterize acute doxylamine overdose. Rhabdomyolysis with impairment of renal function and acute renal failure have been observed.

In children, the most frequent adverse effects related to antihistamine exposure include drowsiness, vomiting, lethargy, mydriasis, hyperactivity, irritability, flushing, ataxia, nausea, diarrhea, tachycardia, slurred speech, and stupor. Children and young adults may present with fixed dilated pupils and CNS stimulation manifested by excitement, tremors, disorientation, hyperactivity, hallucinations, hyperpyrexia, and tonic-clonic seizures.

Toxic Dosage/Death

An adult ingested 5 g of diphenhydramine (80 mg/kg) and developed hyperpyrexia, status epilepticus, coma, and cardiac arrhythmias. The patient survived with supportive treatment. A toxic dose of doxylamine for children of more than 1.8 mg/kg has been reported. Rhabdomyolysis was observed in an adult who ingested 2.25 g of doxylamine. Coma, grand mal seizures and cardiorespiratory arrest have characterized fatal doxylamine intoxication. Children appear to be at a high risk for cardiorespiratory arrest. The manufacturer states that 1–2 g of hydroxyzine in adults produces drowsiness and lethargy, which may progress to coma.

Drug Interactions

Diphenhydramine may potentiate the sedative effects of alcohol, sedative-hypnotics, and narcotics. Anticholinergic effects may enhance similar effects due to tricyclic antidepressants, anti-Parkinson drugs, and antipsychotics, particularly in the elderly. Caution is indicated if a monoamine oxidase inhibitor is being used simultaneously. Hydroxyzine may potentiate the action of CNS depressants such as opiates, barbiturates, other sedatives, anesthetics, and alcohol. Additive anticholinergic effects may occur when hydroxyzine is administered with other anticholinergic agents. Hydroxyzine may inhibit and reverse the vasopressor effects of epinephrine.

Pregnancy/Lactation

Diphenhydramine is minimally secreted into breast milk. No effects have been seen in infants of nursing mothers taking diphenhydramine. Maternal use has been associated with a neonatal abstinence syndrome consisting of tremors and diarrhea. No effects on the human fetus have been shown in prospective studies of mothers treated with diphenhydramine during pregnancy, although one retrospective study pointed to an increase in cleft palates in children born to mothers who took the drug in the first trimester of pregnancy. There are no adequate studies on the effects of hydroxyzine in pregnancy.

Laboratory

ANALYTIC METHODS

When available, gas chromatographic procedures seem to be accurate. Sensitive and specific doxylamine detection and quantitation may be achieved with gas chromatography/mass spectrometry.

BLOOD LEVELS

Blood levels of antihistamines are not performed by the average commercial clinical laboratory and are not useful in clinical overdosage.

Treatment

GUT DECONTAMINATION

Syrup of ipecac should not be administered because seizures may intervene and lead to serious aspiration pneumonitis. Gastric lavage with prior endotracheal intubation may be performed if a clinically significant ingestion has occurred. Gastric lavage may be useful in the first 12 hours after ingestion as anticholinergic effect may slow gastrointestinal motility. Activated charcoal may be administered, but there are scant data to support its efficacy.

ELIMINATION ENHANCEMENT

Since the liver largely metabolizes diphenhydramine, fluid diuresis is unhelpful. As a result of the large volume of distribution, high protein binding, and rapid clearance from the serum, hemodialysis, hemoperfusion, and exchange transfusion are not likely to enhance removal. Hemoperfusion may be tried in patients whose liver clearance is compromised.

SUPPORTIVE MEASURES

- Immediate control of airway, breathing, and circulation must be the first priority. Respiratory assistance via intubation may be required.
- If there are few anticholinergic symptoms (e.g., heart rate less than 110), no skin flushing, normal active bowel sounds, and the patient is awake without seizures or muscle jerks, then consider discharge after 12 hours.
- Obtain chest x-rays if there has been a gastric lavage, any respiratory difficulties, or seizures.
- Seizure precautions must be undertaken, especially in the pediatric patient. Seizures will usually respond to intravenous diazepam. Anticonvulsants, which are CNS depressants, should be avoided.
- Electrocardiographic changes may include a wandering pacemaker, prolonged QT interval, nonspecific ST-T change, and left bundle-branch block. Continual ECG monitoring is essential. No patient is out of danger until the ECG is normal and remains so for at least 12–24 hours.
- Avoid antiarrhythmics such as quinidine and disopyramide, which may exacerbate conduction problems induced by the antihistamines.
- Rarely, an antihistamine overdose may produce clinically significant myocardial pump failure. Norepinephrine or metaraminol may be used if a vasopressor is needed in patients receiving hydroxyzine. Epinephrine should not be used.
- Phenothiazines should be avoided since they may enhance anticholinergic effects already induced by the antihistamines.
- In all suspected cases of doxylamine overdose, the patient should be observed for evidence of rhabdomyolysis. Laboratory tests should include a determination of creatine kinase.
- Urinary catheterization is required in cases involving urinary retention.

Antidotes

PHYSOSTIGMINE

Physostigmine may be given intravenously (0.5 mg in children and up to 2 mg in adults given over 5–7 minutes every 40–60 minutes until reversal of symptoms), if there appears to be a life-threatening complication such as supraventricular tachycardia in a patient with coronary artery disease, hypertension, or severe agitation. Conduction delays contraindicate the use of physostigmine. Additional indications may include myoclonic seizures. Coma may be temporarily reversed (for about 30 minutes), but the drug should not be given simply to keep a patient awake.

Care must be taken to prevent severe physostigmine toxicity such as seizures, asystole, hypotension, hypersalivation, and bradyarrhythmias, which may supervene. The drug is contraindicated in those with asthma, gangrene, or mechanical obstruction of the gastrointestinal or urogenital tract. Doses may be cautiously repeated until cholinergic symptoms, such as increased bronchial secretions, appear. The drug is metabolized in 30–60 minutes. Atropine in doses one-half those of physostigmine can be administered to reverse cholinergic effects such as bronchial constriction.

Question—Sedating H1 Receptor Antangonists

1. Antihistamines are included in many over-the-counter medications, including
A. Cold and allergy medications
B. Sleep aids
C. Anti-motion sickness / anti-nausea medications
D. All of the above
E. A and B only

2. The most common presentation in patients with significant diphenhydramine overdose is
A. Nausea and vomiting
B. Impaired consciousness / lethargy
C. Palpitations or syncope
D. Seizures
E. Rhabdomyolysis

3. A toxicity unique to doxylamine among the antihistamines is
A. Prominent anticholinergic effects
B. Seizures
C. Mydriasis
D. Coma
E. Rhabdomyolysis

4. Typical anticholinergic signs which can be seen in antihistamine overdose include all of the following except
A. Urinary retention
B. Vomiting and diarrhea
C. Dilated pupils
D. Dry mucus membranes
E. Tachycardia

5. Contraindications to the use of physostigmine for antihistamine overdose include all except
A. Non–life-threatening symptoms
B. Conduction delays on EKG
C. Serious tachyarrhythmias
D. Mechanical bowel or urinary obstruction
E. Asthma

CASE STUDY (QUESTIONS 6 AND 7)

A 22-year-old college student is found unresponsive in her room with an empty bottle of Benadryl (25-mg tablets) at the bedside. On arrival to the emergency department her friend states that the patient has been depressed recently and is seeing a psychiatrist. She last saw the patient several hours earlier, so she is unsure when her friend ingested the pills. On exam, the patient is obtunded, the BP is 108/74, pulse is 125, and pupils are dilated.

6. In spite of the fact the ingestion may have occurred several hours earlier, gastric lavage may still be indicated because
A. Antihistamines slow gastric emptying
B. Other serious coingestants cannot be excluded
C. The patient is exhibiting significant symptomatology
D. All of the above
E. Gastric decontamination is not indicated

7. Interventions at this stage should include all except
A. Physostigmine 1 mg i.v. over 1 minute
B. Urinary catheterization

Answers to questions in shaded boxes appear at the end of the chapter.

C. EKG, toxicologic screen, constant EKG monitoring
D. Airway control
E. Activated charcoal via nasogastric or orogastric tube

NON-SEDATING H1 RECEPTOR ANTAGONISTS

Non-sedating histamine H1 receptor antagonists include terfenadine (Seldane®), astemizole (Hismanal®), loratadine (Claritin®), and fexofenadine (Allegra®). Terfenadine and astemizole are no longer marketed in the U.S. due to potential cardiotoxic effects; however, they may still be found around the world. All of these drugs have toxic effects similar to those of other antihistamines. The H1 receptor antagonists are synthetic chemicals. Terfenadine, astemizole, Fexofenadine and loratadine have been used in the systematic treatment of allergic rhinitis, chronic rhinitis, and chronic urticaria.

Pathophysiology

TERFENADINE

Terfenadine is a selective histamine H1 receptor antagonist that does not exhibit substantial anticholinergic, antiadrenergic, or antiserotonergic effects. It preferentially binds to peripheral rather than central histamine H1 receptors. Terfenadine is structurally related to haloperidol. The butanol moiety of the terfenadine molecule is considered responsible for the lack of central nervous system (CNS)-depressant effects associated with terfenadine.

ASTEMIZOLE

Astemizole is a long-acting selective histamine H1 receptor antagonist without substantial central and autonomic nervous system effects. Binding at the H1 receptors by astemizole persists for 3 days. Such inhibition of histamine H1 receptors occurs predominantly in the periphery. Astemizole penetrates the CNS poorly, which may account for its lack of sedative effects. Astemizole is structurally related to tricyclic antidepressants, known provokers of Torsade de Pointes. Stimulation of cardiac histamine receptors (H1 and H2) increases cyclic AMP, producing both increased inotropic and chronotropic effects.

LORATADINE

Loratadine is a selective peripheral histamine H1 receptor antagonist that has no substantial cerebral and autonomic nervous system effects. Loratadine is a piperidine and is structurally related to cyproheptadine (Periactin®). It is also chemically similar to the tricyclic antidepressants imipramine (Tofranil®), nortriptyline (Pamelor®), and doxepin (Sinequan®).

FEXOFENADINE

Fexofenadine is a metabolite of terfenadine. It is a selective peripheral histamine H1 receptor antagonist that does not have the same cardiotoxic drug interaction profile as terfenadine.

Pharmacokinetics

ABSORPTION

- All of these compounds are well absorbed. Astemizole, for example, is absorbed within 1 hour.

DISTRIBUTION

- Terfenadine and astemizole are highly protein bound. Loratadine is 97–99% bound to plasma proteins.
- The volume of distribution of astemizole is 250 L/kg.
- A volume of distribution of terfenadine has not been determined.
- Neither the parent drug of terfenadine nor the metabolites penetrate the blood/brain barrier.

ELIMINATION

- More than 99% of an absorbed dose of terfenadine is metabolized through hepatic metabolism by the cytochrome P450 system.
- Elimination of terfenadine occurs via the fecal route (60%) and in the urine.
- Astemizole is extensively metabolized in the liver. Desmethylastemizole is an active metabolite of astemizole.
- Loratadine is extensively metabolized in the liver to a minor active metabolite.
- The elimination half-life of loratadine is 7.8–15 hours.
- The apparent half-life of astemizole is about 20–60 hours, and that of the metabolite is 18–20 days. In astemizole overdose, the serum elimination half-life may be as long as 2 weeks.
- The alpha (distribution) half-life of terfenadine is 3–4 hours, and the beta (elimination) half-life is 20.3 hours.

Clinical Presentations

Increased levels of terfenadine, and astemizole, caused by overdose or impairment of metabolism, block the cardiac potassium current by a mechanism similar to that of quinidine-induced arrhythmia. This block delays repolarization and causes a prolonged QT interval and morphologic changes that define Torsade de Pointes, or polymorphic ventricular tachycardia. Reasons for increased concentration of drug that may induce Torsade de Pointes are intentional overdose, a decrease in metabolism due to liver disease (e.g., as in cirrhosis), or drug interactions.

Headache, nausea, confusion and seizures have followed overdoses with terfenadine. Somnolence, depression, apathy, confusion, agitation, anxiety, paresthesias, tremor, insomnia, and depersonalization have been reported after use of astemizole and terfenadine. Syncope may precede the onset of severe arrhythmias.

Accidental astemizole ingestion in young children is particularly dangerous because only a few tablets may cause significant toxicity, routine measures to prevent absorption seem to have limited effect, and the worst cardiac effects can appear late and last a long time. All children who ingest more than 10 mg of terfenadine or astemizole or who are less than 1 year old should be referred to a health care facility.

Toxic Dosage/Death

A fatal dose for the non-sedating antihistamines has not been established. Delayed consequences such as hypotension and ventricular tachyarrhythmia (Torsade de Pointes) may occur 5–7 hours after significant (e.g., 200 mg) astemizole ingestion. Astemizole has been taken off the market in the U.S. but may still be available around the world. QT prolongation, ventricular arrhythmias, serious drug reactions, and death may occur in children who ingest as little as 10 mg of astemizole. A patient who ingested 900–1,200 mg of terfenadine developed Torsade de Pointes and survived.

Drug Interactions

Symptomatic life-threatening ventricular arrhythmias have been reported from concomitant use of terfenadine or astemizole with ketoconazole, an antifungal agent. Ketoconazole can be associated with prolongation of the QT interval in healthy individuals or when used with terfenadine. Ketoconazole and itraconazole inhibit the metabolism of terfenadine, resulting in reduced clearance of terfenadine and its active metabolite. Any drug that inhibits hepatic metabolism such as erythromycin, ciprofloxacin, cimetidine, or disulfiram may impair the clearance of terfenadine.

Patients with impaired hepatic function, or who are receiving ketoconazole or macrolide antibiotics (including erythromycin), or who have conditions or medications that may lead to QT prolongation (e.g., hypokalemia, congenital QT syndrome, procainamide, quinidine, disopyramide) may experience QT prolongation, Torsade de Pointes, and/or ventricular tachycardia in addition to cardiac arrest and death at recommended terfenadine and astemizole doses. Astemizole is contraindicated in patients with hepatic dysfunction or electrolyte abnormalities such as hypokalemia and hypomagnesemia or in those ingesting diuretics with potential for the induction of electrolyte abnormalities.

Pregnancy/Lactation

Terfenadine and astemizole are classified as pregnancy risk category C drugs. Controlled clinical studies in pregnant or lactating women are not available for terfenadine, or astemizole. Loratadine is excreted into breast milk.

Laboratory

ANALYTIC METHODS

A high-performance liquid chromatography method on a reversed-phase column with ultraviolet detection can detect astemizole and its metabolite. A radioimmunoassay technique can also analyze astemizole plus its hydroxylated metabolite. A gas chromatography method and radioimmunoassay are available to detect terfenadine.

BLOOD LEVELS

Following blood levels of these agents in overdose does not guide management.

Treatment

GUT DECONTAMINATION

Decontamination of the gastrointestinal tract is achieved with gastric lavage and activated charcoal. Absorption of these agents is generally quite rapid, and the clinical efficacy of these methods is still uncertain.

ELIMINATION ENHANCEMENT

Astemizole and other non-sedating H1 blockers are not significantly removed by hemodialysis. There is limited experience with hemoperfusion.

SUPPORTIVE MEASURES

- Always consider astemizole-induced toxicity in the differential diagnoses of prolonged QTc interval, ventricular tachyarrhythmias, syncope, and seizures. If dizziness, palpitations, syncope, or seizures occur, use of the drug should be discontinued immediately and the patient should be hospitalized for cardiac monitoring.
- In ventricular arrhythmias following astemizole overdose or overdose of other related drugs, it appears logical to avoid drugs known to prolong the QTc interval or to cause Torsade de Pointes (e.g., amiodarone, quinidine, procainamide, disopyramide and sotalol).
- For symptomatic patients, standard life support measures and treatment of arrhythmias are instituted as required. Electrolytes must be normalized.
- Electrocardiographic abnormalities are an absolute indication for admission to an intensive care unit. QTc intervals should be monitored and the patient should not be discharged from the hospital until the QTc interval is normal.
- If necessary, lidocaine or propranolol may be used to control ventricular dysrhythmias.
- In children, seizures are treated with diazepam 0.3 mg/kg, administered every 5 minutes to a total dose of 10 mg. Adults may receive 10 mg of diazepam every 15 minutes up to 30 mg. This may be followed by intravenous phenytoin 15 mg/kg in children over a period of at least 20 minutes, or in adults 15 mg/kg at 50 mg/min.

TORSADES DE POINTES

- For Torsade de Pointes, magnesium sulfate (20%), 2 g every 2–3 minutes, is administered. If there is no response in 10 minutes, this regimen is repeated and followed by a continuous infusion of 5–10 mg/min for 2 hours, followed by 30 mg/min for 90 minutes, twice a day.
- The serum magnesium level must be monitored. Magnesium is given slowly with electrocardiographic monitoring and calcium gluconate available.
- Torsades de Pointes may also require temporary overdrive cardiac pacing at 100–120 beats/min in serious intoxications, isoproterenol, and/or direct-current cardioversion.

Questions—Non-sedating H1 Receptor Antagonists

1. The most important serious side effect/toxicity of non-sedating antihistamines is
A. Central nervous system depression
B. Cardiotoxicity/arrhythmias
C. Seizures
D. Hepatotoxicity
E. Nephritis

2. An electrocardiogram finding typical of terfenadine toxicity is
A. Bradycardia
B. Tachycardia
C. Conduction block
D. Prolongation of the QT interval
E. None of the above

3. Drugs that affect the metabolism of terfanadine include all of the following except
A. Erythromycin
B. Ketaconazole
C. Cimetidine
D. Itraconazole
E. Penicillin

4. The antiarrhythmic drug of choice in ventricular arrhythmias induced by terfenadine is procainamide or other Type I antiarrhythmics.
A. True
B. False

CASE STUDY (QUESTIONS 5 AND 6)

A 46-year-old male presents to the emergency room after a brief syncopal episode. He is otherwise healthy with no significant cardiac history or risk factors. He reports no preceding illness except for "some cough and congestion" starting last week that is now improved after his physician started him on terfenadine and "some antibiotic." His vital signs, exam and labs are normal except that his EKG has some prolongation of the QT interval.

5. Appropriate disposition and instructions at this point would be
   A. Drink plenty of fluids and finish the current antibiotic.
   B. Stop all medications and return if any further syncopal episodes occur.
   C. See the primary physician in the morning for reevaluation.
   D. Admit to the hospital for further evaluation.
   E. Admit to the ICU for constant cardiac monitoring.

6. While in the E.R., the patient has another near syncopal episode and his monitor shows a wide complex tachycardia with variable morphology. He remains awake but his BP drops from 142/82 to 92/56 while the arrhythmia persists. Appropriate treatment would be
   A. Carotid massage
   B. Adenosine 6 mg i.v. push
   C. Magnesium sulfate 20%, 2 g slow i.v. push
   D. Load with 1 g of i.v. procainamide at 50 mg/min
   E. Immediate defibrillation at 360 joules

Answers

Sedating H1 Receptor Antagonists

1. D 2. B 3. E 4. B 5. C 6. D
7. A

Non-sedating H1 Receptor Antagonists

1. B 2. D 3. E 4. B 5. E 6. C

SELECTED READINGS

Sedating H1 Receptor Antagonists

1. Koppel C, Ibe K, Tenczer J. Clinical symptomatology of diphenhydramine overdose: An evaluation of 136 cases in 1982 to 1985. Clin Toxicol 1987;25:53–70.
2. Koppel C, Tenczer J, Ibe K. Poisoning with over the counter doxylamine preparations: An evaluation of 109 cases. Hum Toxicol 1987;6:355–359.
3. Reynolds JEF, ed. Martindale: The Extra Pharmacopoeia. 30th ed. London: Pharmaceutical Press, 1993:938–939.

Non-sedating H1 Receptor Antagonists

1. Kelloway JS, Pongowski MA, Schoenwetter WF. Additional causes of Torsade de pointes. Mayo Clin Proc 1995;70:197–200.
2. Nightingale SL. US Food and Drug Administration warnings issued on nonsedating antihistamines, terfenadine and astemizole. JAMA 1992;268:705.
3. Non-sedating antihistamines. Aust Adverse Drug React Bull, May 1991;10.
4. Sorkin EM, Heal RC. Terfenadine: A review of its pharmacodynamic properties and therapeutic efficacy. Drugs 1985;29:34–56.
5. Woodward JK. Pharmacology and toxicology of nonclassical antihistamines. Cutis 1988;42:5–9.

ACKNOWLEDGMENT:

Thanks to David Huckins, MD for contributing the questions in this chapter.

CHAPTER 36

Serotonergic Drugs

INTRODUCTION

The treatment of depression began with the use of electroconvulsive therapy in the 1930s. Heterocyclic antidepressants and monoamine oxidase inhibitors followed in the 1950s, lithium in the 1960s, and carbamazepine, a mood-stabilizing anticonvulsant, in the 1970s. To find agents with fewer side effects, drugs were produced that could increase the concentration of serotonin (5-hydroxytryptamine or 5-HT) at the synapse.

Serotonergic dysfunction has been implicated in illnesses such as depression, anxiety, obsessive-compulsive disorder, sleep and eating disorders, schizophrenia, Alzheimer's dementia, personality disorders, alcoholism, autism, pain, aggression, and impulse disorders. A new class of drugs with antidepressant actions has been developed that selectively block the reuptake of serotonin into presynaptic neurons. Selective serotonin uptake inhibitors include fluoxetine, sertraline, paroxetine, fluvoxamine, and citalopram.

Pathophysiology

Serotonin or 5-HT is a regulatory neurotransmitter with general inhibitory effects. It is synthesized from l-tryptophan, which crosses the blood-brain barrier. Serotonin does not cross the blood-brain barrier. The central nervous system absorbs l-tryptophan and then synthesizes 5-HT in the cell. The cell bodies of the serotonergic system are concentrated in the raphe or midline section of the brainstem. This network is the largest chemical system in the mammalian brain.

Four major types of serotonin receptors have been identified (types 5-HT1, 5-HT2, 5-HT3, and 5-HT4). The 5-HT1 group is further divided into subtypes A, B, C, D, and E. The 5-HT2 group is also subdivided into subtypes A and B. The 5-HT3 receptors are found both in the peripheral and in the central nervous systems. Antagonists of peripheral 5-HT3 receptors such as ondansetron are used in the treatment of nausea and vomiting.

The selective serotonin reuptake inhibitors (SSRIs) do not bind to any specific neuroreceptor systems but produce antidepressant effects through selective blockade of serotonin uptake. These agents undergo extensive metabolism to clinically inactive compounds, possess relatively large volumes of distribution, and are highly bound to plasma proteins. Their elimination half-lives range from 15–26 hours.

Serotonergic Drug Withdrawal

Vertigo, lightheadedness, nausea, emesis, fatigue, and myalgias may follow the abrupt or gradual withdrawal of paroxetine, sertraline, or fluoxetine. Symptoms lessen after cautious reintroduction of the drug and gradual tapering downward. No chronic neurologic deficits have been observed.

Questions—Introduction to Serotonergic Drugs

1. Which of the following statements is false?
   A. Only one major type of serotonin receptor has been identified.

B. The selective serotonin reuptake inhibitors (SSRIs) undergo extensive metabolism to clinically inactive compounds, possess relatively large volumes of distribution, and are highly bound to plasma proteins.
C. Abrupt or gradual withdrawal of paroxetine or sertraline may be followed by vertigo, lightheadedness, severe nausea, emesis, fatigue, and myalgias.
D. Serotonin or 5-HT is a regulatory neurotransmitter with general inhibitory effects.
E. Serotonin does not cross the blood-brain barrier.

2. Serotonergic dysfunction has been implicated in the following illnesses
A. Depression, anxiety, obsessive-compulsive disorder
B. Sleep and eating disorders
C. Schizophrenia, Alzheimer's dementia, personality disorders
D. Alcoholism, autism, pain, aggression, and impulse disorders
E. All of the above

3. A class of drugs with antidepressant actions has been developed that selectively block the reuptake of serotonin into presynaptic neurons. These include
A. Fluoxetine
B. Meprobamate
C. Haloperidol
D. Maprotiline
E. Desmopressin

THE SEROTONIN SYNDROME

The serotonin syndrome is most commonly the result of the interaction between serotonergic agents and monoamine oxidase inhibitors (MAOIs). The 5-HT receptors responsible for producing the serotonin syndrome are located in the lower brainstem and spinal cord. The serotonin syndrome has been reported in patients with unipolar and bipolar depression, obsessive-compulsive disorder, eating disorders, and Parkinson's disease. Sternbach first reported the syndrome in 1991.

Pathophysiology

Tricyclic antidepressants, MAOIs, 5-HT reuptake inhibitors, antidepressants, electroconvulsive therapy, and 5-HT1A receptor agonists appear to enhance 5-HT neurotransmission in the brainstem and spinal cord. These drugs are capable of increasing the availability of serotonin in the central nervous system.

Clinical Presentations

Clinical features may include altered mental status, agitation, restlessness, confusion, incoordination, hypomania, coma, seizures, altered muscle tone, myoclonus, hyperreflexia, shivering, rigidity, tremor, autonomic instability (i.e., hypertension or hypotension, tachycardia or profuse sweating), hyperpyrexia, and diarrhea. The serotonin syndrome most commonly occurs within 2 hours of the first dose of the precipitating agent and resolves within 6–24 hours of removal of the offending agent.

Toxic Dosage/Death

Death may follow the use of fluoxetine and an MAOI within hours. At least 3 deaths have probably occurred secondary to the use of tranylcypromine after withdrawal of fluoxetine.

Drug Interactions

Drug interactions most commonly reported concerning the serotonin syndrome are those between l-tryptophan and the MAOIs, with or without concomitant lithium. Fluoxetine in conjunction with MAOIs or l-tryptophan is the second most frequent drug combination associated with the serotonin syndrome. Because of the long-lasting serotonergic activity of the MAOIs and serotonin uptake inhibitors, depressed patients who have been switched from fluoxetine to an MAOI without a drug interval of at least 5 weeks are susceptible to the serotonin syndrome

Combinations of tricyclic antidepressants such as clomipramine, trazodone, and imipramine with MAOIs may induce the serotonin syndrome. The MAOI-meperidine interaction represents central serotonergic overactivity and may include muscle twitching, fever, hyperreflexia, diaphoresis, hypotension, hypertension, coma, and death. Patients receiving MAOIs who need opiates should be given morphine, which does not block serotonin reuptake.

Dextromethorphan blocks neuronal uptake of 5-HT and has been implicated in the serotonin syndrome when used with an MAOI. Similarly, pentazocine with fluoxetine has led to lightheadedness, anxiety, nausea, upper extremity paresthesias, diaphoresis, flushing, ataxia, tremulousness, and hypertension. Combinations of trazodone or buspirone, and paroxetine have induced the syndrome.

Treatment

SUPPORTIVE MEASURES

- When the offending agents are removed, the syndrome often resolves on its own within 24 hours. Artificial ventilation for respiratory insufficiency, anticonvulsants for seizures, clonazepam for myoclonus, and nifedipine for hypertension may be useful.
- Cooling blankets and benzodiazepines are used for hyperthermia.
- If these measures are not effective, propranolol or methysergide, both 5-HT1A-receptor antagonists, may be of limited benefit.
- Some have advocated elective paralysis with a nondepolarizing agent and mechanical ventilation for MAOI overdose or interaction patients with a core temperature greater than 39°C.
- Cyproheptadine may be helpful.

Questions—The Serotonin Syndrome

1. Which of the following statements is false?
A. The serotonin syndrome is most commonly the result of the interaction between serotonergic agents and monoamine oxidase inhibitors (MAOIs).
B. The 5-HT receptors responsible for producing the serotonin syndrome are located in the motor strip.
C. The serotonin syndrome has been reported in patients with unipolar and bipolar depression, obsessive-compulsive disorder, eating disorders with depression, and Parkinson's disease.
D. Clinical features of the serotonin syndrome may include altered mental status, agitation, restlessness and confusion.
E. The serotonin syndrome most commonly occurs within 2 hours of the first dose of the precipitating agent and resolves within 6–24 hours of removal of the offending agent.

2. **Drug interactions implicated in the serotonin syndrome include each of the following except**
   A. Fluoxetine in conjunction with MAOIs
   B. Combinations of tricyclic antidepressants, such as imipramine, with MAOIs
   C. Combinations of trazodone or buspirone and paroxetine
   D. Fluoxetine and phenytoin
   E. Dextromethorphan and an MAOI

BUSPIRONE

Buspirone (BuSpar®) is used for the management of anxiety disorders. It may be useful in the treatment of maladaptive behavior and anxiety in developmentally disabled persons, the premenstrual syndrome, Tourette's syndrome, and anxiety in HIV-infected drug users. Preliminary observations indicate its possible usefulness in tardive dyskinesia, smoking, and obsessive-compulsive disorder (when used with fluoxetine). Further confirmation of these additional uses is required. Buspirone may have advantages over tricyclic antidepressants in treating depression in patients with severe heart disease, including minimal orthostatic hypotension and lack of intraventricular conduction prolongation.

Pathophysiology

Buspirone hydrochloride is an anxiolytic agent that appears to have a high affinity for 5-HT1A receptors and D2 dopamine receptors in the central nervous system. Buspirone has no affinity for the γ-aminobutyric acid (GABA)-benzodiazepine receptor site. It has no affinity for α-1, α-2, or β-adrenergic receptors. It has no effect on norepinephrine uptake, and no effect on cholinergic receptors. It induces no euphoric effect but has been subject to abuse. Buspirone hydrochloride is a member of a new class of structurally unique molecules, the azaperones.

Pharmacokinetics

ABSORPTION

- After oral administration, the drug is rapidly and completely absorbed in the gastrointestinal tract, but first-pass metabolism reduces its mean bioavailability in humans to 4%.

DISTRIBUTION

- The apparent volume of distribution is approximately 5.3 L/kg after intravenous administration.
- Buspirone is approximately 95% bound to plasma proteins.

ELIMINATION

- Following extensive hepatic metabolism, less than 1% of buspirone is excreted unchanged.
- Its elimination half-life averages 2–4 hours.
- Buspirone is metabolized to 5-hydroxybuspirone (HB) and 1-pyrimidinylpiperazine (1-PP).
- 1-PP is an α-2 adrenergic receptor antagonist and may induce hypertensive responses in some panic disorder patients. 1-PP reaches levels four times higher than buspirone after a 20-mg dose of buspirone and may have pharmacologic activity.

Clinical Presentations

Adverse effects following buspirone use include dizziness, drowsiness, headache, fatigue, nervousness, insomnia, and lightheadedness. Muscle tremors, lower motor restlessness, tardive dyskinesia, exacerbation of spasmodic torticollis, stiffness, and dystonia have been observed. Manic states have followed buspirone use, but the mechanism of mania development has not been elucidated. Buspirone is minimally toxic in overdose. Clinical symptoms may include nausea, gastrointestinal distress, hypotension, lightheadedness, and loss of consciousness.

Toxic Dosage/Death

Doses up to 2.4 g/day were administered during early trials. Akathisia, tremor, and rigidity were observed. Acute overdose with up to 300 mg of buspirone has resulted in drowsiness in approximately one-half of patients studied. One fatality followed ingestion of 450 mg of buspirone with other drugs (alprazolam, diltiazem, alcohol, and cocaine). Fatal doses of buspirone alone have not been established.

Drug Interactions

Buspirone given with a monoamine oxidase inhibitor may induce a rise in blood pressure. With trazodone, an elevation in alanine transaminase has been observed. Buspirone raises the plasma level of haloperidol when both are given together. Buspirone with fluoxetine may have an additive effect in the treatment of obsessive-compulsive disorder. Fluoxetine may antagonize the anxiolytic action of buspirone.

Pregnancy/Lactation

There are no adequate and controlled studies using buspirone in pregnant women. The extent of distribution of buspirone and its metabolites into human milk is not known. Buspirone is classified as pregnancy risk category B.

Laboratory

ANALYTIC METHODS

A high-pressure liquid chromatography method is available for buspirone determinations. An assay is also available for the active metabolite, 1-PP.

BLOOD LEVELS

Mean maximal plasma concentrations of 1–6 ng/mL occur within 40–90 minutes and appear to be dose-related. Blood levels in overdose patients have not been evaluated.

Treatment

GUT DECONTAMINATION

Gastric lavage within 1–2 hours may be helpful. Charcoal may be helpful as well.

ELIMINATION ENHANCEMENT

Methods to enhance elimination are probably not necessary in a buspirone overdose. Diuresis, hemodialysis, and hemoperfusion have not been studied in this context. The extensive volume of distribution of buspirone tends to preclude the efficacy of these therapeutic measures.

SUPPORTIVE MEASURES

- Treatment of overdose with buspirone involves symptomatic and supportive care. Blood pressure, pulse, and respirations should be monitored.

- The patient should be observed for the development of extrapyramidal signs or for evidence of behavior disturbances such as panic and mania.
- Careful observation of the patient for 24 hours with electrocardiographic determinations and liver function tests is indicated in those depressed patients who may also have ingested other drugs.

Questions—Buspirone

1. Which of the following statements about buspirone is false?

A. Buspirone (BuSpar®) is used for the management of anxiety disorders.
B. It may be useful in the treatment of maladaptive behavior and anxiety in developmentally disabled persons, the premenstrual syndrome, Tourette's syndrome, and Guillain-Barré.
C. Buspirone may have advantages over tricyclic antidepressants in treating depression in patients with severe heart disease, including minimal orthostatic hypotension and lack of intraventricular conduction prolongation.
D. Buspirone hydrochloride is an anxiolytic agent that appears to have a high affinity for 5-HT1A receptors and D2 dopamine receptors in the central nervous system.
E. Buspirone has no affinity for the γ-aminobutyric acid (GABA)-benzodiazepine receptor site.

2. Clinical effects of buspirone may include all of the following except

A. Dizziness, drowsiness, headache, and fatigue
B. Nervousness, insomnia, and lightheadedness
C. Muscle tremors, amnesia, paralysis
D. Lower motor restlessness, tardive dyskinesia, and exacerbation of spasmodic torticollis
E. Manic states

CYPROHEPTADINE

Cyproheptadine (Periactin®) is a serotonin antagonist that has the actions and uses of antihistamines and is largely used to treat allergic reactions. It has been used for appetite stimulation, Cushing's syndrome, carcinoid syndrome, migraines, acromegaly, hyperprolactinemia, and for antidepressant-induced anorgasmia. Cyproheptadine has also been used to treat essential blepharospasm, and anecdotal reports indicate some improvement in tardive dyskinesia, in akathisia and in the serotonin syndrome. Initial studies indicate that cyproheptadine may reverse the resistance of Plasmodium falciparum to chloroquine.

Pathophysiology

Cyproheptadine is an H1-receptor antagonist and a serotonin (5-HT2) antagonist. It also may have antimuscarinic and calcium channel blocker activity. Cyproheptadine is structurally and pharmacologically related to azatadine, another H1-receptor antagonist.

Pharmacokinetics

ABSORPTION

- Cyproheptadine appears to be well absorbed following oral administration.
- Following a single dose of radiolabeled drug in fasting healthy adults in one study, plasma concentrations of radioactivity peaked 6–9 hours after administration.

DISTRIBUTION

- Low plasma levels of cyproheptadine and metabolites in humans after an oral dose are consistent with extensive distribution of the drug and its metabolites.

ELIMINATION

- The drug appears to be completely metabolized principally to the quaternary ammonium glucuronide conjugate.
- Cyproheptadine is not excreted unchanged in the urine, but is excreted as metabolites.

Clinical Presentations

At therapeutic doses, cyproheptadine has a sedative effect. Central nervous system depression, hallucinations, ataxia, seizures, and death have followed overdose. Symptoms in children who accidentally ingested excessive doses of cyproheptadine include somnolence, excitation, hallucinations, ataxia, tachycardia, muscle twitching, gastric distress, mydriasis, and facial erythema. Symptoms appear rapidly after ingestion and do not last longer than 6–12 hours.

Toxic Dosage/Death

At least 20 deaths have been reported in infants or children. Fatal doses appear to range from 25 to 250 mg/kg. A 3-year-old child who ingested 12 mg of cyproheptadine developed a staggering gait, disorientation and akathisia. A 7-year-old who ingested 16 mg developed a toxic psychosis. No life-threatening effects have been observed in children after doses of 0.3–6.5 mg/kg.

Drug Interactions

Monoamine oxidase inhibitors prolong and intensify the anticholinergic effects of antihistamines, including cyproheptadine.

Pregnancy/Lactation

Controlled studies with cyproheptadine have not been performed during pregnancy or lactation. Cyproheptadine is classified as pregnancy risk category B.

Laboratory

ANALYTIC METHODS

Analysis in plasma, serum and urine has been performed by a gas-liquid chromatographic method sensitive to 3 ng/mL. A high-performance liquid chromatography method with nitrogen-sensitive detection distinguishes cyproheptadine from its desmethyl metabolite.

BLOOD LEVELS

Peak plasma levels reach 30 μg/L after therapeutic use. Following blood levels in overdose has not been studied.

Treatment

GUT DECONTAMINATION

Vomiting usually occurs spontaneously, but cyproheptadine may also be removed by gastric lavage. Charcoal may be helpful as well.

ELIMINATION ENHANCEMENT

There is no clinical evidence to justify the use of hemodialysis or hemoperfusion after cyproheptadine overdose. It is not likely that these measures would be useful in light of its extensive volume of distribution.

SUPPORTIVE MEASURES

- Treatment of cyproheptadine overdose is largely symptomatic and supportive and is similar to the treatment given to patients who have been poisoned with other H1-receptor antagonists. Patients with hypotension, hallucinations, or seizures should be admitted to the hospital.
- Seizures may be treated with diazepam, phenytoin, and/or phenobarbital. Hypotension may require treatment with saline, Trendelenburg position and/or pressor agents.
- Patients should be observed for at least 24 hours until there is no further evidence of ataxia, seizures, and hallucinations, and there is no evidence of electrocardiographic abnormality.

Questions—Cyproheptadine

1. Which of the following statements is false?

A. Cyproheptadine (Periactin®) is a serotonin agonist that has the actions and uses of antihistamines and is largely used to treat allergic reactions.
B. It has been used for appetite stimulation, Cushing's syndrome, carcinoid syndrome, migraines, acromegaly, hyperprolactinemia, and for antidepressant-induced inorgasmia.
C. Cyproheptadine has also been used to treat essential blepharospasm.
D. Initial studies indicate that cyproheptadine may reverse the resistance of Plasmodium falciparum to chloroquine.
E. Cyproheptadine may have antimuscarinic and calcium channel blocker activity.

2. Which of the following statements is true?

A. At therapeutic doses, cyproheptadine has a mood enhancing effect.
B. Symptoms take hours to appear after cyproheptadine overdose.
C. Hemodialysis or hemoperfusion are effective after cyproheptadine overdose.
D. Cyproheptadine is poorly absorbed following oral administration.
E. Deaths have been reported from cyproheptadine use.

FLUOXETINE

Fluoxetine (Prozac®) is used for the treatment of depression. Limited numbers of patients have shown evidence of effectiveness in the treatment of obsessive-compulsive disorder, eating disorders including bulimia and anorexia nervosa, obesity, bipolar disorders, cataplexy, diabetic neuropathy, panic disorders, agitated dementia, premenstrual syndrome, fetishes, trichotillomania, pathologic jealousy, and problematic behaviors associated with autism.

Fluoxetine appears to be minimally toxic in doses up to 1.5 g. Symptoms may include drowsiness, tremor, nausea, vomiting, and tachycardia. When fluoxetine is ingested with alcohol, hypertension, tachycardia and a decreased level of consciousness may be observed. The incidence of overdose is low in relation to the extensive worldwide use of this product. About half of overdose patients are asymptomatic.

Pathophysiology

Fluoxetine is a selective inhibitor of serotonin uptake at the presynaptic neuronal membrane. It appears to have minimal or no effect on the reuptake of norepinephrine or dopamine, and does not exhibit anticholinergic, antihistaminic, or α-1 adrenergic blocking activity at the usual therapeutic dosage. Fluoxetine is an aromatic ring phenylpropylamine derivative and a bicyclic antidepressant.

Pharmacokinetics

ABSORPTION

- Fluoxetine is well absorbed from the gastrointestinal tract. At least 60–80% of an oral dose is absorbed.
- Within 4–8 hours, peak blood levels of 15–55 ng/mL are reached.

DISTRIBUTION

- Fluoxetine binds extensively to plasma proteins (about 95%).

ELIMINATION

- Fluoxetine is metabolized largely by N-demethylation to the active metabolite, norfluoxetine.
- Less than 5% of fluoxetine is excreted in the urine unchanged. About 10% of norfluoxetine is excreted in the urine unchanged and about 73% is excreted as unidentified metabolites.
- Fluoxetine has elimination half-lives of 1–4 days after a single dose and 2–7 days after multiple doses.
- The potency and selectivity of serotonin reuptake inhibition of the principal metabolite, norfluoxetine, are similar to those of the parent drug. Norfluoxetine has an elimination half-life of 7–15 days following either single or multiple doses.

Clinical Presentations

Fluoxetine in overdose produces minor symptoms, which are usually not serious or life-threatening. Common effects include drowsiness, tachycardia, nausea, vomiting, and tremor. Infrequent effects include euphoria, headache, sore throat, agitation, lightheadedness, seizures, and dry mouth. Rare prolongation of the bleeding time with petechiae may be accompanied by a normal platelet count. Platelet dysfunction may not respond to platelet therapy. Reversible hair loss has been reported. About 50% of patients reported to have taken an overdose remained asymptomatic. Patients generally recover quickly without sequelae.

A number of adverse effects have been associated with fluoxetine. These include serum sickness manifested by fever, rash, arthralgias, lymphadenopathy, and skin eruptions which generally resolve in 1–2 weeks. Seizures beginning 3–5 days after initiation of fluoxetine have been reported. Other effects include narrow-angle glaucoma, stuttering that interferes with speech and sleep, rhabdomyolysis following combined drug overdose with alcohol, and exacerbation of multiple sclerosis. Other effects include cardiac dysrhythmias in the elderly, chest discomfort associated with bradycardia, dizziness, pressure in the throat, shortness of breath associated with supraventricular tachycardia and hypotension, eye tics with hearing impairment, and other extrapyramidal symptoms. Mania, violence and fluoxetine abuse have also been reported.

ELECTROCARDIOGRAM

Bradycardia, supraventricular tachycardia, and atrial fibrillation may be observed. Infrequent reports of atrial flutter and atrioventricular block have followed fluoxetine use. Rare prolongation of the PR interval, left bundle-branch block, and left anterior hemiblock have been observed. Electrocardiographic abnormalities are usually observed in fluoxetine overdoses with coingestants and may include junctional rhythms, low-voltage and nonspecific T-wave changes, ventricular tachycardia, premature ventricular contractions, supraventricular tachycardia, premature atrial contractions, trigeminy, right bundle-branch block, and first-degree heart block.

SYNDROME OF INAPPROPRIATE SECRETION OF ANTIDIURETIC HORMONE

Fluoxetine is a possible cause of the syndrome of inappropriate secretion of antidiuretic hormone (SIADH), particularly in the elderly. Within a few weeks of beginning fluoxetine treatment, some patients may experience drowsiness, confusion, and lightheadedness. Laboratory findings may include depression of serum sodium and chloride values with depressed serum and urine osmolality. There appears to be a relationship between serotonin uptake blockers, which include tricyclic antidepressants and monoamine oxidase inhibitors, and SIADH.

SUICIDAL IDEATION

Several initial studies suggested that patients appeared to develop suicidal ideation while on fluoxetine. The U.S. Food and Drug Administration reviewed all the data on suicide and fluoxetine, including an extensive review of 1,765 patients who received fluoxetine for depression. They concluded that fluoxetine does not cause suicidal ideation or violent behavior in depressed patients. The report suggests that patients treated with fluoxetine should be monitored closely in the early stages of treatment during which time the risk of suicide is highest. Whether the drug increases hostility or aggression remains an open question.

WITHDRAWAL

Agitation, inability to concentrate, and insomnia have been reported within 48 hours of discontinuation. A 32-year-old man who had received fluoxetine for 6 months developed an acute dystonic reaction involving the neck, back and upper extremities 2 days after stopping fluoxetine therapy. Diaphoresis, tremulousness, tongue movements, and increased motor tone were observed. All symptoms resolved 45 minutes after an intramuscular administration of diphenhydramine.

Toxic Dosage/Death

Serious toxic effects do not usually appear until doses exceed 1.5 g. The mean overdose in asymptomatic patients in one study was 341 mg, and symptomatic patients had ingested a mean dose of 544 mg. Children who ingested an average of 1.76 mg/kg fluoxetine had minor symptoms such as sleepiness, hyperactivity, and diarrhea. When fluoxetine is ingested in doses greater than 500 mg with ethanol, a rise in blood pressure, tachycardia and a decreased level of consciousness may be seen.

Deaths involving fluoxetine are generally in conjunction with other agents. These include diphenhydramine and carbon monoxide, meperidine, clonidine, acetaminophen, pargyline, fluphenazine, lorazepam, diphenhydramine alone, propranolol, ethanol, and maprotiline. An estimated lethal dose of fluoxetine of 1–2 g has been suggested; however, this requires confirmation. Fluoxetine levels of patients who have died have varied but are usually greater than 1300 ng/mL.

Drug Interactions

Fluoxetine may induce toxic drug interactions by several mechanisms. When fluoxetine is ingested with alcohol, toxic effects are frequently observed. Common findings include depressed consciousness, tachycardia, drowsiness, tremor, nausea, vomiting and other gastrointestinal symptoms. Patients usually recover without sequelae. Serious effects seen with methamphetamine, diphenhydramine, and meprobamate include seizures. Respiratory arrest and unresponsiveness have been associated with tricyclic antidepressants, and dystonic reactions have been seen with haloperidol.

Pregnancy/Lactation

Fluoxetine is classified as pregnancy risk category B. Nursing mothers should be warned that fluoxetine and its active metabolite are excreted into breast milk.

Laboratory

ANALYTIC METHODS

Quantitation of fluoxetine and norfluoxetine in human plasma can be performed using gas chromatography with an electron-capture detector. A reverse-phase high-performance liquid chromatography method with ultraviolet detection is also available

BLOOD LEVELS

Fluoxetine levels are often not readily available in community hospitals and are of limited value in treatment of an overdose. Drug concentrations do not correlate well with toxicity whether fluoxetine is ingested alone or with other drugs. Chronic therapeutic dosing results in serum fluoxetine concentrations ranging from 47–469 ng/mL, and norfluoxetine concentrations range from 52–446 ng/mL. Two reviews indicate that there is little evidence of toxicity unless the combined fluoxetine and norfluoxetine level is greater than 1390–2,000 ng/mL. Seizures are usually correlated with combined levels greater than 3,000 ng/mL.

Treatment

GUT DECONTAMINATION

As fluoxetine reaches peak blood levels slowly (i.e., over 4–8 hours), gastric emptying may be helpful if patients present hours after significant overdoses. Emesis induction should not be performed if the patient is lethargic, having seizures, or has a depressed gag reflex. Gastric lavage in such patients should be performed after prior cuffed endotracheal intubation. Activated charcoal may be administered via nasogastric tube or orally in the alert patient.

ELIMINATION ENHANCEMENT

The large apparent volume of distribution and plasma protein binding of fluoxetine indicate that removing substantial amounts of fluoxetine or norfluoxetine after an acute ingestion, by hemodialysis, hemoperfusion, forced diuresis, peritoneal dialysis, or exchange transfusion, would most likely not be effective. Whole-bowel irrigation has not been evaluated in fluoxetine overdose. Serum alkalinization, often used for tricyclic antidepressant poisoning, has not been shown to be of value in a fluoxetine overdose.

SUPPORTIVE MEASURES

- Acute fluoxetine overdose involves primarily symptomatic and supportive care. Airway patency, an adequate source of oxygen, and careful monitoring of ventilation are the initial focus of management. Cardiac monitoring and an intravenous line should be instituted on admission.

- Vital signs and hemodynamic status must be closely monitored as patients may simultaneously ingest other drugs such as tricyclic antidepressants. A 12-lead electrocardiogram provides a more accurate status of cardiac rhythm abnormalities.
- Where patients are entirely asymptomatic, have no evidence of significant electrocardiographic changes, and no cardiovascular irritability, consider discharge from the emergency department after an observation period of 6–8 hours.
- Treat cardiac dysrhythmias with standard antiarrhythmic agents. Continuous electrocardiographic monitoring is indicated.
- As blood levels of fluoxetine may be detectable 4 weeks after an overdose or after discontinuation of therapy, do not initiate therapy with monoamine oxidase inhibitors, tricyclic antidepressants, and other drugs known to adversely interact with fluoxetine for at least 5 weeks.
- Agitation, tremulousness, diaphoresis, insomnia, and inability to concentrate may indicate fluoxetine withdrawal symptoms. Intravenous diphenhydramine 50 mg often relieves such symptoms.
- Transaminase levels may be infrequently elevated in patients who develop an acute hepatitis while receiving chronic fluoxetine treatment. Observe patients for platelet dysfunction and bleeding.

OBSERVATION CRITERIA

- If a high dose (e.g., 1,500 mg) of fluoxetine has been ingested, admit the patient for observation, even if asymptomatic, for 24 hours. If the patient is symptomatic (e.g., seizures, altered mental status, and/or dysrhythmias), admit to an intensive care facility for at least 24 hours. If fluoxetine was ingested with alcohol or other coingestants, admit to an intensive care facility after gastric decontamination, activated charcoal, and specific treatment directed at the most lethal agent.
- Monitor suicidal patients closely, especially in the early stages of treatment. Assess clinical evidence of severity of depression, suicidal ideation, aggressive ideation or behavior, agitation, or akathisia. Depressed or suicidal patients may require admission to a psychiatric unit after psychiatric evaluation.
- Intravenous diazepam is the drug of choice for treatment of seizures that do not remit spontaneously. If seizures recur after diazepam, use phenytoin or phenobarbital.

EXTRAPYRAMIDAL SYMPTOMS

- Discontinue fluoxetine if akathisia is noted. Akathisia can be treated with propranolol 60 mg/d. If β-blockers are contraindicated, treat with oral diphenhydramine 50 mg twice daily.
- Discontinue fluoxetine if Parkinsonian symptoms occur. Administer antiparkinsonian drugs as indicated if symptoms are severe.
- Discontinue fluoxetine if an acute dystonic reaction occurs. For a mild reaction, give 50 mg diphenhydramine by mouth three times a day for 1 week. For a severe reaction, give 50 mg diphenhydramine intravenously, hospitalize and observe.

SYNDROME OF INAPPROPRIATE SECRETION OF ANTIDIURETIC HORMONE

- Within 48 hours of discontinuation of fluoxetine, serum sodium and serum chloride levels usually return to normal. If hyponatremia is mild and attributable to fluoxetine, discontinue the drug and restrict total fluid intake.
- This may be combined with oral sodium chloride supplementation if required.
- If hyponatremia is symptomatic or sufficiently severe to pose the threat of seizures (usually less than 120 mEq/L), hypertonic (3%) saline may be infused carefully and slowly.

Questions—Fluoxetine

1. Which of the following regarding fluoxetine is false?

A. Fluoxetine is a possible cause of the syndrome of inappropriate secretion of antidiuretic hormone (SIADH), particularly in the elderly.
B. Laboratory findings may include depression of serum sodium and chloride values with elevated serum and urine osmolality.
C. There appears to be a relationship between serotonin uptake blockers, which include tricyclic antidepressants and monoamine oxidase inhibitors, and SIADH.
D. The U.S. Food and Drug Administration concluded that fluoxetine does not cause suicidal ideation or violent behavior in depressed patients.
E. Agitation, inability to concentrate, and insomnia have been reported within 48 hours of discontinuation of fluoxetine.

2. Which of the following statements is true?

A. Fluoxetine has been used for the treatment of depression, obsessive-compulsive disorder, eating disorders including bulimia and anorexia nervosa, obesity, bipolar disorders, cataplexy, diabetic neuropathy, panic disorders, agitated dementia, premenstrual syndrome, fetishes, trichotillomania, pathologic jealousy and problematic behaviors associated with autism.
B. Fluoxetine in overdose appears to be extremely toxic in low doses.
C. When fluoxetine is ingested with alcohol, hypotension, bradycardia and a decreased level of consciousness may be observed.
D. The incidence of overdose is high in relation to the extensive worldwide use of this product.
E. About 1–3% of overdose patients are asymptomatic.

3. Concerning the pathophysiology of fluoxetine,

A. Fluoxetine is a selective inhibitor of serotonin secretion at the presynaptic neuronal membrane.
B It appears to have minimal or no effect on the reuptake of norepinephrine or dopamine, and does not exhibit anticholinergic, antihistaminic, or α-1 adrenergic blocking activity at the usual therapeutic dosage.
C. Fluoxetine is an aromatic ring phenylpropylamine derivative and a tricyclic antidepressant.
D. Serum alkalinization, often used for tricyclic antidepressant poisoning, has been shown to be of value in a fluoxetine overdose.
E. The small apparent volume of distribution and low plasma protein binding of fluoxetine indicate that removing substantial amounts of fluoxetine or norfluoxetine after an acute ingestion by hemodialysis would most likely be effective.

ONDANSETRON

Ondansetron (Zofran®) is used for the prevention of nausea and vomiting associated with emetogenic cancer chemotherapy including high-dose cisplatin. It appears to be less effective with moderately emetic chemotherapy such as cyclophosphamide,

5-fluorouracil, and Adriamycin, but is effective in ifosfamide-induced nausea and vomiting.

Ondansetron also appears to be effective in decreasing postoperative nausea, radiation-induced emesis, and nausea and vomiting occurring during the terminal stage of cancer. Ondansetron has been useful in the treatment of vomiting associated with theophylline overdose, and an anecdotal report indicates a potential use in hyperemesis gravidarum. Few reports of overdose have been published.

Pathophysiology

Ondansetron is a selective 5-HT3 antagonist. It blocks serotonin peripherally and centrally in the chemoreceptor trigger zone.

Pharmacokinetics

ABSORPTION

- The oral bioavailability of ondansetron is 60%.

DISTRIBUTION

- The protein binding of ondansetron is about 70–76%.
- The apparent volume of distribution of ondansetron is large, about 1.8 L/kg.

ELIMINATION

- Ondansetron is cleared from the body almost entirely by metabolism with 5–10% of a dose excreted unchanged in the urine.
- Ondansetron has a terminal plasma half-life of 3.0–3.5 hours.

Clinical Presentations

Clinical presentations following suspected overdoses of ondansetron have included fever, rash, pruritus, and restlessness, which were treated with diphenhydramine and resolved within 12 hours. Adverse effects may include extrapyramidal symptoms, head jerking, akathisia, headaches, diarrhea, and seizures. Anaphylactoid and anaphylactic reactions may occur and are characterized by urticaria, angioedema, hypotension, bronchospasm, and dyspnea.

Toxic Dosage/Death

Individual doses as large as 145 mg (1.5 mg/kg) and a total daily dose of 252 mg have been tolerated after intravenous administration. The patient who received 252 mg experienced an itchy nose, vague restlessness, and hot flashes. A fatal dose has not been established.

Drug Interactions

Ondansetron does not appear to induce or inhibit the cytochrome P450 drug-metabolizing enzyme system. Hepatic cytochrome P450 drug-metabolizing enzymes metabolize ondansetron. Inducers or inhibitors of these enzymes may change the clearance and half-life of ondansetron.

Pregnancy/Lactation

Safe use of ondansetron during pregnancy or lactation has not been established. Ondansetron is classified as pregnancy risk category B.

Laboratory

ANALYTIC METHODS

Plasma concentrations can be assayed using high-performance liquid chromatography produced with solid-phase extraction and ultraviolet detection.

BLOOD LEVELS

A relationship between serum concentrations and efficacy has not been clearly established. Plasma levels may not necessarily reflect drug activity at the target receptors. Peak plasma concentrations averaging about 30 ng/mL follow an oral dose of 8 mg and are reached in 1 hour.

Treatment

GUT DECONTAMINATION

While gastric lavage and/or charcoal may be helpful after rare oral ingestion, these methods have not been studied.

ELIMINATION ENHANCEMENT

Methods to enhance elimination such as hemodialysis and hemoperfusion are unlikely to be of value because of the high protein binding and large volume of distribution of ondansetron.

SUPPORTIVE MEASURES

- Treatment of ondansetron overdose is largely symptomatic and supportive.
- Mild transient elevations of the serum lactate dehydrogenase level occur.

Question—Ondansetron

1. Which of the following statements is false?

A. Ondansetron (Zofran®) is used for the prevention of nausea and vomiting associated with emetogenic cancer chemotherapy.

B. It appears to be less effective with moderately emetic chemotherapy such as 5-fluorouracil, cyclophosphamide, and Adriamycin, but is effective in ifosfamide-induced nausea and vomiting.

C. Ondansetron is not effective in decreasing postoperative nausea, radiation-induced emesis, and nausea and vomiting occurring during the terminal stage of cancer.

D. Ondansetron has been useful in the treatment of vomiting associated with theophylline overdose, and an anecdotal report indicates a potential use in hyperemesis gravidarum.

E. Few reports of overdose have been published.

PAROXETINE

Paroxetine (Paxil®) is used in the treatment of depression, including severe depression and depression associated with symptoms of anxiety. Paroxetine is a selective serotonin reuptake inhibitor (SSRI) that has few anticholinergic side effects. Paroxetine hydrochloride is a phenylpiperidine derivative that is structurally distinct from other SSRIs. Overdoses have been relatively nontoxic.

Pathophysiology

Paroxetine selectively inhibits serotonin reuptake in brain neurons. It exerts its antidepressant action through an increased concentration of the neurotransmitter at the synaptic cleft, thereby enhancing serotonergic transmission. At higher concentrations, the SSRIs inhibit the reuptake of norepinephrine and, to a lesser degree, dopamine. Paroxetine has a low affinity for α-adrenoceptors, dopamine (D2), histamine (H1), and serotonin (5-HT2) receptors, and therefore has little ability to cause central and autonomic side effects.

Pharmacokinetics

ABSORPTION

- When ingested orally, paroxetine is readily absorbed from the gastrointestinal tract.
- There is a marked first-pass effect both in the gut wall and in the liver.

DISTRIBUTION

- The apparent volume of distribution of paroxetine is 13 L/kg.
- Paroxetine is 95% protein bound.

ELIMINATION

- Paroxetine is eliminated primarily by hepatic metabolism to glucuronide- and sulfate-conjugated metabolites that are inactive. The elimination half-life is 24 hours.
- The urinary excretion of unchanged paroxetine is less than 2% of a daily dose.

Clinical Presentations

Adverse effects during clinical trials included nausea, headache, somnolence, dry mouth, asthenia, insomnia, sweating, constipation, dizziness, tremor, and akathisia (also seen with the other SSRIs, fluoxetine and sertraline). In patients with bipolar disorders, paroxetine may be associated with a 2% rate of mania. Extrapyramidal reactions are more common with paroxetine than with other SSRIs. Dizziness, sweating, nausea, insomnia, tremor, and confusion appear to be more common with withdrawal from paroxetine than with withdrawal from other SSRIs.

Toxic Dosage/Death

An overdose of 850 mg has been well tolerated. Patients have recovered fully without seizures or loss of consciousness. In one series of pediatric exposures, ingestion of 120 mg or less by children less than 5 years of age led to favorable outcomes with gastrointestinal decontamination and minimal symptomatic care. No fatalities have been reported after overdose.

Drug Interactions

Paroxetine appears to have a low potential to cause toxicokinetic interactions with other drugs. Experience with other SSRIs suggests that a clinical serotonin syndrome may occur in combination with MAOIs. There are no reported interactions with lithium. Paroxetine is an inhibitor of an isozyme of cytochrome P450.

Pregnancy/Lactation

There have been no controlled clinical trials of paroxetine during pregnancy or lactation. All offspring have been reported to be healthy in cases in which the pregnancies proceeded to term. Paroxetine is classified as pregnancy risk category B.

Laboratory

ANALYTIC METHODS

A high-performance liquid chromatography method for quantitation is available.

BLOOD LEVELS

Paroxetine at 30–40 mg/d does not induce significant changes in heart rate, blood pressure, or electrocardiographic parameters. No significant effects are observed on the electroencephalogram at therapeutic doses. There is little correlation between paroxetine plasma concentrations and clinical or adverse effects. Serum levels at steady state are 10–110 ng/mL. There is no evidence of a relationship between serum levels and antidepressant effect. Plasma concentrations peak at 0.8–65 ng/mL in approximately 5 hours.

Treatment

GUT DECONTAMINATION

There are no data to substantiate the use of activated charcoal in paroxetine overdose; however, it may be useful. If the patient is seen within 5 hours of ingestion, gastric emptying may lessen peak blood levels.

ELIMINATION ENHANCEMENT

The high degree of protein binding and large volume of distribution suggest that hemodialysis or other extracorporeal methods would be inefficient in removing a significant amount of drug from the body.

SUPPORTIVE MEASURES

- Treatment of a paroxetine overdose is symptomatic and supportive. Few anticholinergic symptoms are observed.
- Patients should be hospitalized after significant overdoses. Most do not experience a loss of consciousness, and few changes in heart rate (except for an occasional sinus tachycardia), blood pressure, or electrocardiographic parameters should be expected.
- Paroxetine causes a small decrease in hemoglobin level, hematocrit, and white blood cell level.
- All overdose patients should be observed for 6 hours. Special attention should be given to other drugs ingested simultaneously. If the patient is symptom-free, has no evidence of seizures or cardiac abnormalities (normal electrocardiogram), has normal vital signs and is alert, consideration can be given to discharge within 12 hours after psychiatric counseling.
- Hyponatremia has followed its use in the elderly, in whom it may be due to the syndrome of inappropriate secretion of antidiuretic hormone.

Questions—Paroxetine

1. Which of the following statements is false?

A. Paroxetine is used in the treatment of depression, including severe depression and depression associated with symptoms of anxiety.

B. Paroxetine is a selective serotonin reuptake inhibitor (SSRI) known for its anticholinergic side effects.

C. Paroxetine hydrochloride is a phenylpiperidine derivative that is structurally distinct from other SSRIs.

D. Overdoses have been relatively nontoxic.
E. At higher concentrations, the SSRIs inhibit the reuptake of norepinephrine and, to a lesser degree, dopamine.

2. **Which of the following statements concerning paroxetine is true?**
A. Paroxetine has a high potential to cause toxicokinetic interactions with other drugs.
B. Experience with other SSRIs suggests that a clinical serotonin syndrome has not occurred in combination with MAOIs.
C. There are numerous reported drug interactions with lithium.
D. Paroxetine does not affect the cytochrome P450 system.
E. Paroxetine has a low affinity for α-adrenoceptors, dopamine (D2), histamine (H1), and serotonin (5-HT2) receptors and therefore has little ability to cause central and autonomic side effects.

RISPERIDONE

Risperidone (Risperdal®) appears to be a useful antipsychotic drug in the treatment of "negative" symptoms of chronic schizophrenia (e.g., emotional withdrawal, scarcity of speech, and affective blunting). Risperidone is an antipsychotic agent with antagonist action on dopamine (D2) and serotonin (5-HT2) receptors. Overdoses induce electrolyte changes (e.g., hyponatremia and hypokalemia) and reversible changes in QTc and QRS intervals, and follow a benign course.

Pathophysiology

Risperidone is a benzisoxazole derivative. It is a centrally acting potent serotonin (5-HT2) and catecholamine antagonist. It also exhibits dopamine (D2) antagonism and has an affinity for cholinergic muscarinic receptors. It is a potent LSD antagonist. Classic anti-dopamine antipsychotic compounds treat the "positive" symptoms of schizophrenia (e.g., hallucinations, delusions and thought disorders) effectively, but not the "negative" inactive symptoms (e.g., emotional withdrawal, blunted affect, and poverty of speech). Risperidone, perhaps because of its serotonin antagonism, seems to treat the positive and the negative symptoms simultaneously while lessening extrapyramidal symptoms. Risperidone also has α-1 and α-2 noradrenergic activity and is antihistaminic.

Pharmacokinetics

ABSORPTION

- Risperidone is rapidly absorbed after oral administration.
- Plasma risperidone concentration peaks in 2 hours.
- Absorption is consistent with some first-pass metabolism.

DISTRIBUTION

- Risperidone is rapidly distributed and has an apparent volume of distribution of 1–2 L/kg.
- Risperidone is 88% bound to plasma proteins.

ELIMINATION

- About 4–30% of risperidone is excreted in the urine unchanged.
- The terminal half-life is about 34 hours for 9-hydroxyrisperidone, an active metabolite, and 2–4 hours for risperidone in extensive metabolizers.

Clinical Presentations

Few cases of risperidone overdose have been reported. An anecdotal case report described auditory hallucinations, electrocardiogram changes (QRS and QTc prolongation), hyponatremia, and hypokalemia. Abnormalities appear to resolve over a 12-hour period. Chronic use leads to blurred vision, vertigo, postural dizziness, impaired concentration, decreased appetite, and erection and ejaculation disturbances. Risperidone, like clozapine, can precipitate or exacerbate obsessive-compulsive symptoms in patients with schizophrenia.

Toxic Dosage/Death

Tachycardia, drowsiness, slurred speech, altered consciousness, hypertension, tremors, agitation, and extrapyramidal effects were observed among six patients who ingested 5–270 mg. Symptoms lasted 6 hours. An adult who ingested 240 mg of risperidone was treated symptomatically and recovered in 24 hours. High doses of risperidone may cause extrapyramidal effects. Neuroleptic malignant syndrome, which may be fatal, has also been described.

Drug Interactions

Drugs that produce postural hypotension (e.g., tricyclic antidepressants, antipsychotic agents, and alcohol) may exacerbate this effect with risperidone. Excess sedation may occur with concomitant administration of antihistamines. Difficulties may also be expected with concurrent administration of dopamine agonists (e.g., for Parkinsonism).

Pregnancy/Lactation

The safe use of risperidone during pregnancy or lactation has not been established.

Laboratory

ANALYTIC METHODS

Radioimmunoassay and high-performance liquid chromatography are preferred for the analysis of risperidone and its metabolites in blood and urine.

BLOOD LEVELS

Following risperidone concentrations in overdose has not been studied.

Treatment

GUT DECONTAMINATION

Gastric lavage within 2–3 hours of ingestion followed by activated charcoal may lessen absorption and decrease both the duration and severity of toxic symptoms. Management is similar to that for tricyclic antidepressant overdose.

ELIMINATION ENHANCEMENT

These methods have not been utilized or studied after risperidone overdose.

SUPPORTIVE MEASURES

- Cardiac and electrolyte monitoring is indicated for at least 24 hours after significant overdoses.
- Anticholinergic agents can be used to treat extrapyramidal symptoms.
- Prolongation of the QTc and QRS intervals may be seen. No clinically significant electrocardiographic changes have been seen with doses up to 25 mg/d.
- Hypokalemia and hyponatremia have been associated with risperidone overdose.
- Risperidone can induce an increase in prolactin levels that is reversed on drug withdrawal.

Questions—Risperidone

1. **Which of the following statements is false?**
   A. Risperidone appears to be a useful antipsychotic drug in the treatment of "positive" symptoms of chronic schizophrenia (e.g., emotional withdrawal and affective blunting).
   B. Risperidone is an antipsychotic agent with antagonist action on dopamine (D2) and serotonin (5-HT2) receptors.
   C. Overdoses induce electrolyte changes (e.g., hyponatremia and hypokalemia) and reversible changes in QTc and QRS intervals, and follow a benign course.
   D. Risperidone is a centrally acting potent serotonin 5-HT2 and catecholamine antagonist.
   E. Risperidone is a potent LSD antagonist.
2. **Which of the following is true concerning risperidone?**
   A. Risperidone is poorly absorbed after oral administration.
   B. Plasma risperidone concentration peaks in 5 minutes.
   C. Absorption is consistent with some first-pass metabolism.
   D. All of the above
   E. A and B

SERTRALINE

Studies with sertraline (Zoloft®) suggest that it is effective in the treatment of depression and obsessive-compulsive disorder. Animal studies suggest that sertraline might be helpful in the pharmacologic treatment of obesity and reduction of alcohol craving. Sertraline is a selective 5-HT reuptake inhibitor antidepressant that, in overdose, appears to have a low risk of toxicity. Patients are largely treated symptomatically and supportively.

Pathophysiology

Sertraline is a naphthylamino compound that is structurally dissimilar to other antidepressants. It is a selective 5-HT reuptake inhibitor that does not have cardiovascular, anticholinergic, antidopaminergic, convulsant, or monoamine oxidase-inhibiting effects. Sertraline does not cause significant reuptake blockade of dopamine or norepinephrine. Sertraline, through inhibition of 5-HT release, may cause β-adrenoceptor downregulation.

Pharmacokinetics

ABSORPTION

- Sertraline is absorbed readily through the gastrointestinal tract. Its absolute bioavailability has not been determined in humans.
- Sertraline displays first-order kinetics.

DISTRIBUTION

- Plasma protein binding is approximately 98% to both albumin and a1-acid glycoprotein.
- Distribution following oral administration of sertraline is biphasic with a prolonged absorption phase. The elimination phase begins 12–16 hours following the dose.
- The volume of distribution has not been determined in humans but is more than 20 L/kg in rats and dogs. Both sertraline and its metabolites extensively distribute to tissues outside the blood.

ELIMINATION

- Sertraline undergoes extensive metabolism. The elimination half-life of sertraline is 24 hours.
- The clinically active desmethyl metabolite is eliminated more slowly than the parent drug, with a half-life of approximately 66 hours.
- Unchanged sertraline is not detected in the urine.

Clinical Presentations

Adverse effects of sertraline may include nausea, dry mouth, diarrhea, male sexual dysfunction, tremor, akathisia, dyspepsia, and chest pain. Systolic blood pressure may rise within 8 hours of a dose. Sertraline has been associated with an abrupt change in mood from depression to hypomania, a reaction that is seen with other antidepressants. It has also been associated with hypernatremia, the syndrome of inappropriate antidiuretic hormone secretion, and the serotonin syndrome. Extrapyramidal effects similar to those seen with other serotonin reuptake inhibitors have been observed after sertraline use. Tachycardia, hypertension, hallucinations, coma, tremors, and hyperthermia have been reported in overdose. Paradoxical sedation has also been described.

Toxic Dosage/Death

Up to 4.5 g has been tolerated without profound toxicity. A 23-year-old who ingested an overdose of 700–1,000 mg and a 28-year-old who ingested 2.1 g received gastric lavage and recovered fully with no sequelae. In a U.S. series of 6 cases of overdose, all experienced lethargy and four had sinus tachycardia. All recovered within 24 hours of gastric lavage, activated charcoal, and supportive care. A fatal dose has not been established.

Drug Interactions

Because of its extensive protein binding, sertraline may cause a shift in plasma concentrations of tightly protein-bound drugs. Sertraline appears to induce hepatic microsomal enzymes. Patients receiving a serotonin reuptake inhibitor in combination with a monoamine oxidase inhibitor may develop serious, sometimes fatal, reactions called the serotonin syndrome. Signs and symptoms may include hyperthermia, rigidity, myoclonus, autonomic instability, agitation, delirium, and/or coma.

Pregnancy/Lactation

Sertraline has not been subject to controlled studies during human pregnancy or lactation. Sertraline is classified as pregnancy risk category B.

Laboratory

ANALYTIC METHODS

A gas chromatography-mass spectrometry method is available for quantitation of plasma concentrations. This analytical procedure may not be available in hospital clinical laboratories.

BLOOD LEVELS

Ingestion of approximately 1.0 g led to a plasma concentration of about 245 ng/mL. Toxic plasma levels are greater than 200 ng/mL. There is no indication that blood levels are clinically useful in guiding treatment or that they correlate with the severity of overdoses.

Treatment

GUT DECONTAMINATION

Activated charcoal and/or gastric lavage may be helpful within hours of overdose. No controlled studies have compared these measures in sertraline overdose.

ELIMINATION ENHANCEMENT

Because of the large volume of distribution and extensive protein binding of sertraline, forced diuresis, dialysis, hemoperfusion, and exchange transfusion are not likely to be of benefit.

SUPPORTIVE MEASURES

- Unstable patients should be hospitalized and monitored via cardiac monitor. An airway should be established and maintained, and adequate oxygenation and ventilation ensured.
- Sertraline may rarely cause a transient elevation in hepatic transaminase levels.
- Patients should remain under observation for at least 48 hours after an overdose, as an active metabolite has a half-life of several days.
- Sertraline at doses of 50–400 mg/d has no effect on the QTc, PR, or PR intervals.

Questions—Sertraline

1. Which of the following statements is false?
  A. Studies with sertraline (Zoloft®) suggest that it is effective in the treatment of depression and obsessive-compulsive disorder.
  B. Animal studies suggest that sertraline might be helpful in the pharmacologic treatment of obesity and reduction of alcohol craving.
  C. Sertraline is a selective 5-HT reuptake inhibitor antidepressant that, in overdose, appears to have a high risk of toxicity.
  D. Patients are largely treated symptomatically and supportively after sertraline overdose.
  E. Sertraline is a selective 5-HT reuptake inhibitor that does not have cardiovascular, anticholinergic, antidopaminergic, convulsant, or monoamine oxidase-inhibiting effects.

2. Which of the following statements is true?
  A. Adverse effects of sertraline may include nausea, dry mouth, diarrhea, male sexual dysfunction, tremor, akathisia, dyspepsia, and chest pain.
  B. Sertraline has been associated with hyponatremia, the syndrome of inappropriate antidiuretic hormone secretion, and the serotonin syndrome.
  C. Extrapyramidal effects, unlike those seen with other serotonin reuptake inhibitors, have not been observed after sertraline use.
  D. Coma has not been reported in sertraline overdose.
  E. Paradoxical mania has also been described.

SUMATRIPTAN

Sumatriptan (Imitrex®) is used subcutaneously or orally for the acute treatment of migraine and cluster headaches. Few overdoses have been reported; however, sumatriptan has been associated with coronary vasospasm, chest pain, hypertension, ventricular arrhythmias, and ST wave changes on the electrocardiogram. No fatalities have been reported after an overdose. Sumatriptan chemically resembles 5-hydroxytryptamine and is a synthetic chemical product.

Pathophysiology

Cerebral vasodilation contributes to the severity of migraine headaches. 5-HT receptors on blood vessels, predominantly subclass 5-HT1, are vasoconstrictive. Those on the temporal arteries are 5-HT2. Sumatriptan, a 5-HT antagonist, stimulates 5-HT receptors on blood vessels, redistributes blood flow within the brain, and reduces headaches. Sumatriptan is a highly selective agonist at 5-HT1 subtypes. It is almost devoid of activity at 5-HT2 and 5-HT3 receptors.

Pharmacokinetics

ABSORPTION

- The bioavailability of sumatriptan after subcutaneous injection is 96% and is 14% after oral administration.

DISTRIBUTION

- The apparent volume of distribution is about 2.4 L/kg.
- The plasma protein binding of sumatriptan is low (14–20%).

ELIMINATION

- Most of the drug is eliminated as metabolites (80%). The principal metabolite is an indoleacetic analog, which appears to have no activity.
- The half-life is about 2 hours with single dosing, but longer after repeat oral dosing.

Clinical Presentations

The most common adverse effects of sumatriptan are an unpleasant taste or an injection site reaction. Most side effects are minor and resolve within 30 minutes. Tingling, a warm or hot sensation, dizziness, malaise, chest tightness and pressure, and fatigue may occur. There have also been reports of asthma and ventricular arrhythmias, and sumatriptan is contraindicated in patients with Prinzmetal's angina. Sumatriptan may cause a rise in blood pressure and coronary vasoconstriction.

It may cause flow-limiting coronary artery stenosis resulting in myocardial ischemia and infarction. The drug is contraindicated in patients with symptomatic ischemic heart disease when either angina or ischemia has been documented previously. No association between chest complaints and electrocardiographic changes has been observed. Sumatriptan probably potentiates α-adrenoceptor-mediated vasoconstriction. Sumatriptan has induced stroke after a 6-mg subcutaneous injection in a patient with sagittal sinus thrombosis.

Toxic Dosage/Death

There are few reports of overdose with sumatriptan. Three cases of accidental overdose with sumatriptan (up to twice the recommended daily dose) led to few symptoms except for severe burning on the forehead of one patient. During clinical trials, volunteers received single doses as high as 16 mg without serious adverse effects. Doses of 100–200 mg/kg in animals have resulted in seizures, tremor, inactivity, erythema of the extremities, reduced respiratory rate, cyanosis, ataxia, mydriasis, injection site reactions and paralysis. A fatal dose has not been determined.

Drug Interactions

Sumatriptan should not be used in patients receiving MAOIs, lithium, or serotonin reuptake inhibitor antidepressants. Its vasoconstrictive effects may be additive to those of ergotamine and the catecholamines.

Pregnancy/Lactation

Safe use of sumatriptan in pregnancy has not been established. There are no data on its excretion in breast milk. Sumatriptan is classified as pregnancy risk category C.

Laboratory

ANALYTIC METHODS

Sumatriptan and its principal metabolites are determined in plasma, urine, and other biological fluids by reverse-phase high-performance liquid chromatography.

BLOOD LEVELS

Plasma concentrations after intravenous use (3 mg, 15-minute infusion) peak at 76.8 ng/mL. After an oral 100-mg dose, the plasma level peaks at 53.8 ng/mL in 1.5 hours. Following sumatriptan levels in overdose has not been studied.

Treatment

GUT DECONTAMINATION

While charcoal and/or lavage may be helpful after overdose, formal studies are lacking.

ELIMINATION ENHANCEMENT

There are no data on the use of hemodialysis, hemoperfusion, or peritoneal dialysis in relation to the serum concentrations of sumatriptan.

SUPPORTIVE MEASURES

- Following a significant overdose, supportive and symptomatic treatment should be provided.
- The blood pressure and electrocardiogram should be monitored for at least 12 hours.
- Vasodilatory therapy may be required. If sumatriptan induces symptoms suggestive of angina, for example, nitrites may be helpful.
- T-wave abnormalities and ST elevations may be seen.

Questions—Sumatriptan

1. Which of the following statements is false?

A. Sumatriptan is used subcutaneously or orally for the treatment of migraine and cluster headaches.
B. Few overdoses have been reported; however, it has been associated with coronary vasospasm, chest pain, hypertension, ventricular arrhythmias, and ST wave changes on the electrocardiogram.
C. Fatalities have been reported after an overdose.
D. All of the above
E. A and C

2. Which of the following is true?

A. Sumatriptan chemically resembles 5-hydroxytryptamine and is a natural chemical product.
B. Sumatriptan, a 5-HT agonist and dopaminergic antagonist, stimulates 5-HT receptors on blood vessels, redistributes blood flow within the brain, and reduces headaches.
C. Sumatriptan is not selective at 5-HT1 subtypes.
D. Safe use of sumatriptan in pregnancy has not been established
E. Following sumatriptan levels in overdose is well established.

Answers

Introduction to Serotonergic Drugs

1. A 2. E 3. A

The Serotonin Syndrome

1. B 2. D

Buspirone

1. B 2. C

Cyproheptadine

1. A 2. E

Fluoxetine

1. B 2. A 3. B

Ondansetron

1. C

Paroxetine

1. B 2. E

Risperidone

1. A 2. C

Sertraline

1. C 2. A

Sumatriptan

1. C 2. D

SELECTED READINGS

Introduction to Serotonergic Drugs

1. 5-HT blockers and all that. Lancet 1990;336:345–346. Editorial.
2. Cowen PJ. A role for 5-HT in the action of antidepressant drugs. Pharmacol Ther 1990;46:43–51.
3. Hesketh PJ, Gandara DR. Serotonin antagonists: A new class of antiemetic agents. J Natl Cancer Inst 1991;83: 613–620.
4. Mills KC. Serotonin toxicity: A comprehensive review for emergency medicine. Top Emerg Med 1993;15:54–73.
5. Van Harten J. Clinical pharmacokinetics of selective serotonin reuptake inhibitors. Clin Pharmacokinet 1993;24:203–220.

The Serotonin Syndrome

1. Henry JA. Serotonin syndrome. Lancet 1994;343:607.
2. Sporer KA. The serotonin syndrome: Implicated drugs, pathophysiology and management. Drug Saf 1995;13:94–104.
3. Tueth MJ. The serotonin syndrome in the emergency department. Ann Emerg Med 1993;22:1369.

Buspirone

1. Balster RL. Abuse potential of buspirone and related drugs. J Clin Psychopharmacol 1990;10:31S–37S.
2. Goetz CM, Krenzelok EP, Lopez G, Borys D. Buspirone toxicity: A prospective study. Ann Emerg Med 1990;19:630.
3. Tiller JWG, Burrows GD, O'Sullivan BT. Buspirone overdose. Med J Aust 1989;150:54–55.

Cyproheptadine

1. Bharucha BA, Kalawala TY, Pandya AL, et al. Cyproheptadine poisoning. Indian Pediatr1987;24:165–169.
2. McEvoy GK, ed. AHFS Drug Information 94. Bethesda, MD: American Society of Hospital Pharmacists, 1994:16–17.
3. Reynolds JEF, ed. Martindale: The Extra Pharmacopoeia. 30th ed. London: Pharmaceutical Press, 1993:935–937.

Fluoxetine

1. Borys DJ, Setzer SC, Ling LJ, et al. Acute fluoxetine overdose: A report of 235 cases. Am J Emerg Med 1992;10:115–120.
2. Gram LF. Fluoxetine. N Engl J Med 1995;332:960–961.
3. Jenkins J, Shannon MW, Woolf A. Fluoxetine intoxication: Clinical course and serum concentrations. Vet Hum Toxicol 1990;32:348.
4. Stokes PE. Fluoxetine: A five year review. Clin Therap 1993;15:216–243.

Ondansetron

1. Finn A. Toxicity and side effects of ondansetron. Semin Oncol 1992;19(4, suppl. 10):53–60.
2. Markham A, Sorkin EM. Ondansetron: An update of its therapeutic use in chemotherapy induced and postoperative nausea and vomiting. Drugs 1993; 45:934–952.

Paroxetine

1. Boyer WF, Feighner JP. An overview of paroxetine. J Clin Psychiatry 1992; 53(2,suppl.):3–6.
2. Caley CF, Weber SS. Paroxetine: A selective serotonin reuptake inhibiting antidepressant. Ann Pharmacother 1993;27:1212–1222.
3. Van Harten J. Clinical pharmacokinetics of selective serotonin reuptake inhibitors. Clin Pharmacokinet 1993;24:203–241.

Risperidone

1. Heather GS, Vicas IMO. Risperidone overdose: A case series. Vet Hum Toxicol 1994;36:371.
2. Livingston MG. Risperidone. Lancet 1994;343:457–460.

Sertraline

1. Kassner J, Woolf A. Sertraline HCl: A new antidepressant. Vet Hum Toxicol 1992;34:343.
2. Myers LB, Dean BS, Krenzelok ER. Sertraline (Zoloft®): Overdose assessment of a new antidepressant. Vet Hum Toxicol 1993;35:341.

Sumatriptan

1. Bateman DN. Sumatriptan. Lancet 1993;3241:221–224.
2. Hillis WS, MacIntyre PD. Sumatriptan and chest pain. Lancet 1993;341:1564–1565.
3. Neighbor ML. Sumatriptan: A new treatment of migraine. West J Med 1993; 159:597–598.

CHAPTER 37
Dopaminergic Drugs

INTRODUCTION

Dopamine agonists directly stimulate dopamine receptors. In Parkinson's disease (idiopathic or drug-induced), presynaptic neurons in the substantia nigra degenerate. By acting at postsynaptic dopamine receptors of the striatum, dopaminergic agonists bypass degenerating presynaptic neurons and act independently of the synthetic dopaminergic enzyme system. Agonists have long half-lives. They do not increase the level of dopamine itself and are specific to subpopulations of dopamine receptors. They are devoid of properties related to norepinephrine and serotonin. See Chapter 26, Cardiovascular Toxicology, for a complete discussion of the vasopressor dopamine.

The blockade of certain dopaminergic receptors by dopaminergic antagonists represents the central mechanism by which many antipsychotic medications work. See Chapter 28, Psychotropic Drugs. Extrapyramidal symptoms and acute dystonic reactions are mediated via dopaminergic receptor (specifically D2) blockade. Neuroendocrine effects such as prolactin release are also mediated via central dopaminergic receptors.

Pathophysiology

The substantia nigra and ventral tegmental nuclei are composed of dopaminergic neurons with branches distributed to the corpus striatum, limbic nuclei, and frontal cortex. Eight pharmacologically distinct dopamine receptors have now been identified through molecular cloning techniques (D1, D1A, D1B, D2A, D2B, D2C, D3, and D4). D1 receptors activate adenyl cyclase and increase intracellular levels of cyclic AMP. D2 receptors exert an inhibitory effect on adenyl cyclase and may be linked to additional second messenger systems.

In the early 1980s two receptor subtypes, DA1 and DA2, were identified as being involved in regulating the cardiovascular system. DA1 receptors are found in the central nervous system, some vascular beds, the kidney, and sympathetic ganglia. Stimulation of postsynaptic DA2 receptors leads to vasodilation in renal, mesenteric, coronary, and cerebral blood vessels. Presynaptic DA2 agonists diminish the release of noradrenaline at sympathetic nerve endings, resulting in a reduction of vascular resistance.

Neuroleptic-induced Deficit Syndrome

Classic antipsychotic drugs that induce blockade of central dopamine (D2) receptors have been associated with a deficit syndrome characterized by impairment of cognitive, social, and affective function when administered to schizophrenic patients. Symptoms include sedation, indifference to internal and external stimuli, passivity, and reduced initiation. Use of drugs such as clozapine, sulpiride, remoxipride, and risperidone can lead to an "awakening" characterized by the lifting of a "physical straitjacket" which is probably extrapyramidal in nature. This may be followed by physical and physiologic stimulation associated with akathisia, a decreased need for sleep, and intellectual and emotional arousal.

Questions—Introduction to Dopaminergic Drugs

1. Which of the following statements is false?

A. The substantia nigra and ventral tegmental nuclei are composed of dopaminergic neurons with branches distributed to the corpus striatum, limbic nuclei, and frontal cortex.
B. Eight pharmacologically distinct dopamine receptors have now been identified through molecular cloning techniques.
C. D1 receptors activate adenyl cyclase and decrease intracellular levels of cyclic AMP.
D. DA1 and DA2 are involved in regulating the cardiovascular system.
E. Stimulation of postsynaptic DA2 receptors leads to vasodilation in renal, mesenteric, coronary, and cerebral blood vessels.

2. Which of the following statements is true?

A. Classic antipsychotic drugs that induce blockade of peripheral dopamine receptors have been associated with a deficit syndrome characterized by impairment of cognitive, social, and affective function when administered to schizophrenic patients.
B. Symptoms of neuroleptic induced deficit syndrome include sedation, passivity, and reduced initiation.
C. Use of drugs such as clozapine, sulpiride, remoxipride, and risperidone can lead to an "awakening" characterized by the lifting of a "physical straitjacket" which is probably extrapyramidal in nature.
D. All of the above.
E. B and C

BROMOCRIPTINE

Bromocriptine (Parlodel®) is an ergot derivative with potent dopaminergic agonist activity. Bromocriptine is used for the treatment of hyperprolactinemia, suppression of puerperal lactation, cyclic benign breast disease, acromegaly, Parkinsonism, and neuroleptic malignant syndrome. Bromocriptine has also been used to treat the manic phase of manic-depressive psychosis in patients in whom the use of phenothiazines or lithium carbonate is contraindicated. It has been used to reverse cocaine craving. Few reports of overdose are available. See the Ergots and Derivatives section in Chapter 57, Wild Plants, Mushrooms, and Mycotoxins.

Pathophysiology

The ergot alkaloids are indole alkaloids. They have a four-ringed structure known as ergoline, of which there are two types: the lysergic acid derivatives and the clavines. The lysergic acid derivatives are usually either amides or cyclic peptides. Bromocriptine belongs to the cyclic peptide group of lysergic acid derivatives.

Bromocriptine is a dopamine (D2)-receptor agonist that activates postsynaptic dopamine receptors. It inhibits prolactin secretion at both the pituitary and the hypothalamus. In acromegaly, it inhibits growth hormone release. Bromocriptine has central effects like those of L-dopa, induces arterial and venous relaxation, increases gastric acid, and inhibits furosemide-induced aldosterone increase.

Pharmacokinetics

ABSORPTION

- Between 40–90% of the drug is absorbed from the gastrointestinal tract.
- Peak plasma levels of 8–12 ng/mL are observed about 100 minutes after doses up to 100 mg.

DISTRIBUTION

- The volume of distribution is 1–4 L/kg. Plasma protein binding is 96%.
- Following a dose of 50 mg, plasma levels peak in 2-3 hours.
- Bromocriptine easily crosses the blood-brain barrier.

ELIMINATION

- The main site of bromocriptine metabolism is the liver.
- The main route of elimination of its metabolites is biliary. Less than 0.1% is excreted unchanged.
- The plasma half-life is about 15 hours.

Clinical Presentations

The most commonly reported side effects of bromocriptine use are nausea, vomiting, dizziness, postural hypotension, nasal congestion, constipation, and mood changes. With doses more than 20 mg, hallucinations, fatigue, erythromelalgia (tender red edematous feet), digital vasospasm, bladder disturbances, and alcohol intolerance have been reported. Dyskinesia, diplopia, ergotism, and aggravation of angina have been reported. Pleural effusions have been seen in Parkinson's patients after long-term treatment, and hyperthermia may follow discontinuation of therapy. Symptoms of overdose include drowsiness, dizziness, postural hypotension, hallucinations, nausea, and vomiting.

Toxic Dosage/Death

Toxic effects may be seen after ingestion of 50 mg, although nausea and orthostatic hypotension are commonly observed at the initiation of treatment. Most side effects are dose related and can occur at doses exceeding 10 mg. No dangerous effects have been reported in adults taking up to 225 mg or infants taking up to 7.5 mg in overdose. A fatal dose has not been determined.

Involuntary movements, chorea, orofacial dyskinesias, and dystonic posture of the trunk and limbs may appear after doses of 90–180 mg. Withdrawal of bromocriptine therapy is associated with reversal of its beneficial effects, including a return of hyperprolactinemia, return of excess growth hormone secretion, exacerbation of Parkinson's disease, and hyperthermia.

Drug Interactions

The bioavailability of bromocriptine is increased by the concomitant intake of erythromycin. Interaction of bromocriptine with other prolactin secretagogues such as the neuroleptics, tricyclic antidepressants, rauwolfia alkaloids, and estrogens may be observed. Alcohol may reduce tolerance to bromocriptine, and bromocriptine may decrease tolerance to alcohol. Lack of efficacy may occur when patients are treated with dopamine antagonists such as the phenothiazines, butyrophenones, metoclopramide, prochlorperazine, methyldopa, and reserpine.

Answers to questions in shaded boxes appear at the end of the chapter.

Pregnancy/Lactation

Bromocriptine is a pregnancy risk category B drug. No adverse effects of bromocriptine secreted in breast milk have been reported. There does not appear to be an increased incidence of spontaneous abortion or birth defects.

Laboratory

ANALYTIC METHODS

Radioimmunoassay methods have a detection limit of about 0.2 μg/L.

BLOOD LEVELS

The plasma concentration of bromocriptine that inhibits prolactin excretion is about 0.7 μg/L. Following blood levels in overdose has not been studied.

Treatment

GUT DECONTAMINATION

Patients seen within 1–2 hours of ingestion may benefit from gastric lavage. Charcoal may be helpful, but there is no evidence to prove its efficacy.

ELIMINATION ENHANCEMENT

There is no evidence that extracorporeal methods of elimination enhancement are useful in treating an overdose.

SUPPORTIVE MEASURES

- Patients should be observed for the development of hypertension or shock and treated symptomatically.
- Bromocriptine has been associated with transient increases in levels of serum transaminases, creatine kinase, alkaline phosphatase, uric acid, and blood urea nitrogen.

Questions—Bromocriptine

1. Bromocriptine (Parlodel®) is an ergot derivative with potent dopaminergic agonist activity which is used for all of the following except
   A. Hyperprolactinemia
   B. Cyclic benign breast disease
   C. Acromegaly
   D. Addison's Disease
   E. Parkinsonism

2. Which of the following statements is true?
   A. Bromocriptine belongs to the cyclic peptide group of lysergic acid derivatives.
   B. Bromocriptine is a dopamine (D2)-receptor antagonist that activates postsynaptic dopamine receptors.
   C. It stimulates prolactin secretion at both the pituitary and the hypothalamus.
   D. In acromegaly it stimulates growth hormone release.
   E. Bromocriptine inhibits arterial and venous relaxation.

3. Symptoms of bromocriptine toxicity include all of the following except
   A. Nausea, vomiting, dizziness, postural hypotension, constipation, and mood changes
   B. Hallucinations, fatigue, digital vasospasm, bladder disturbances, and alcohol intolerance
   C. Dyskinesia, diplopia, and angina
   D. Pleural effusions have been seen in Parkinson's patients after long-term treatment, and hyperthermia may follow discontinuation of therapy.
   E. Anticholinergic signs such as hyperpyrexia.

BUPROPION

Bupropion (Wellbutrin®) is an antidepressant that was originally introduced in 1985. It was withdrawn from the market in 1986 after clinical experience indicated an increased rate of seizures in bulimic patients. Subsequently, after an extensive survey indicated a convulsion rate of only 0.4%, it was re-released in 1989. In overdose, bupropion seems to lack cardiovascular toxicity but it does manifest significant neurologic toxicity. It has caused deaths in overdose.

Bupropion is used for the treatment of depression and smoking cessation. Other potential uses include attention-deficit hyperactivity disorder in adults and children, reduction of cocaine use, in "rapid cycling" bipolar patients, and chocolate craving.

Pathophysiology

Bupropion is an antidepressant phenylbutamine of the amino ketone class chemically unrelated to tricyclic, tetracyclic, or other known antidepressant agents. Bupropion is not a monoamine oxidase inhibitor, exerts no effect on 5-hydroxytryptamine uptake, and minimally alters the reuptake of norepinephrine at presynaptic sites. It is a weak inhibitor of dopamine reuptake, but its mechanism of action has not been clarified.

Pharmacokinetics

ABSORPTION

- Absorption of bupropion from the gastrointestinal tract is rapid.
- First-pass metabolism and enterohepatic circulation occur.

DISTRIBUTION

- The mean half-life for the rapid distribution phase ranges from 1.2–1.4 hours.
- The volume of distribution is 1.4–3.2 L/kg.
- *In vitro* studies show that about 80% of bupropion is bound to plasma proteins.

ELIMINATION

- The elimination half-life of bupropion is 10–14 hours.
- Bupropion is metabolized mostly by side-chain oxidative cleavage in the liver.
- Less than 1% of a bupropion dose is excreted unchanged.
- The major metabolites of bupropion have substantially longer half-lives (up to 43 hours) than the parent compound.

Clinical Presentations

Healthy volunteers using up to 375 mg/d experienced dizziness, nausea, vomiting, and miosis. At overdoses of 850–4200 mg during the clinical development of bupropion, a few patients had mild sinus tachycardia, and 3 patients experienced hypokalemia. Bupropion can lower the seizure threshold. In overdose, seizures have been noted in approximately one-third of patients. Coma and seizures have been reported after ingestions of 600–6500 mg.

Frequent adverse effects include edema, nonspecific rashes, nocturia, ataxia, incoordination, seizures, myoclonus, dyskinesia, dystonia, mania, hypomania, increased libido, hallucinations, decrease in sexual function, depression, stomatitis, and flulike symptoms. A depressant effect on cardiac conduction tissue is minimal. Menstrual irregularities have also been described.

Toxic Dosage/Death

A 57-year-old woman who ingested 9.0 g of bupropion, 300 mg of tranylcypromine, and an unspecified amount of aspirin experienced a tonic-clonic seizure, was treated with intravenous diazepam 10 mg, and recovered without further sequelae. Overdoses of 900 to 3,000 mg of bupropion have led to vomiting, confusion, hypokalemia, and nonspecific ST-T changes. One patient who ingested approximately 17.5 g of bupropion, 25 mg of alprazolam, and 200 mg of clonazepam became confused, developed slurred speech, and recovered in 3 days.

The estimated seizure incidence for bupropion increases about tenfold between 450–600 mg/d. The risk of seizures is associated with dose and the presence of predisposing factors such as prior head trauma, prior seizure(s), central nervous system tremor, and/or concomitant medication that also lowers seizure threshold. An ingestion of 16.5 g of bupropion led to uncontrolled seizures, bradycardia, reduction in ejection fraction, congestive heart failure, and fatal cardiac arrest in one patient, and lethal doses may be less than 10 g.

Drug Interactions

Bupropion can lower the seizure threshold. Precautions are indicated when bupropion is used concurrently with neuroleptics, xanthines, and other epileptogenic compounds because ictal thresholds may be synergistically depressed. Abrupt discontinuation of ethanol, benzodiazepines, and sedatives during bupropion therapy may precipitate seizure activity. Bupropion should also be avoided in physiologic states associated with lowering of ictal thresholds, such as hyponatremia.

Carbamazepine, cimetidine, phenobarbital, and phenytoin are hepatic drug-metabolizing enzyme inducers and may affect the clinical activity of bupropion when administered together. Monoamine oxidase inhibitors, such as phenelzine, may enhance bupropion toxicity. Bupropion has dopamine reuptake-blocking activity. When bupropion is used with amantadine, which facilitates the release of presynaptic dopamine, dopaminergic overdrive may be associated with delirium. Caution is also advised with concomitant use of L-dopa.

Pregnancy/Lactation

There have been no adequate and well-controlled clinical studies in pregnant or lactating women. Safe use during pregnancy and lactation has not been established. Bupropion accumulates in breast milk in concentrations much higher than in maternal plasma. Pregnancy risk category B.

Laboratory

ANALYTIC METHODS

A specific radioimmunoassay with a sensitivity limit of 1 ng/mL is available. A liquid chromatography method with dual-wavelength ultraviolet detection has been developed.

BLOOD LEVELS

High plasma concentrations of bupropion metabolites may be associated with a poorer outcome. There are, however, insufficient data available to relate blood levels of bupropion to the clinical course after ingestion. The optimal therapeutic range is 50–100 ng/mL. In two fatal cases, blood levels of 4.0 and 4.2 mg/L were reported.

Treatment

GUT DECONTAMINATION

The usual measures for gut decontamination should be employed. Syrup of ipecac is contraindicated in view of the possibility of seizures or myoclonus following an overdose of bupropion. If the patient is stuporous or comatose, intubation followed by gastric lavage may be of value in the first 12 hours after ingestion. Activated charcoal, after tracheal protection, may adsorb drug from the gastrointestinal tract and perhaps interfere with its enterohepatic circulation.

ELIMINATION ENHANCEMENT

The usefulness of diuresis, dialysis, or hemoperfusion would tend to be minimal in view of the large volume of distribution. No clinical experience with these modalities in bupropion overdose has been published.

SUPPORTIVE MEASURES

- Patients should be hospitalized after a bupropion overdose. Modalities for seizure treatment should be prepared and available, as should an intravenous line, oxygen, and cardiac monitoring.
- Initial attention should be directed towards the adequacy of ventilation with arterial blood gases. If the patient is stuporous or comatose, oxygen, naloxone, glucose, and thiamine should be administered. Protection of the airway via endotracheal intubation should be performed as necessary and mechanical ventilation should have top priority.
- Seizures usually respond to intravenous diazepam. Phenytoin is a second-line drug and phenobarbital may also be used. If necessary, intubation and neuromuscular blockade with a nondepolarizing neuromuscular blocking agent and thiopental anesthesia may be required. Continuous electroencephalographic and hemodynamic monitoring is helpful in determining the effectiveness of therapy.
- Recurrent seizures indicate the need to monitor urine myoglobin, serum creatinine and creatine kinase levels to detect evidence of rhabdomyolysis.
- Hypokalemia usually results from the intracellular transport of potassium rather than depletion of body stores. Therefore, only mild repletion of extracellular potassium is usually necessary.
- Electrocardiographic abnormalities including a left bundle-branch block have followed extensive overdoses.

Questions—Bupropion

1. Which of the following statements about bupropion is false?

A. Bupropion is an antidepressant that seems to lack cardiovascular toxicity but it does manifest significant neurologic toxicity.
B. Bupropion has caused deaths in overdose.
C. Bupropion has been used for the treatment of depression, smoking cessation and attention-deficit hyperactivity disorder.

D. Bupropion is chemically related to the monoamine oxidase inhibitors, and should not be taken with tyramine-containing foods.
E. Its mechanism of action has not been entirely clarified.

2. Which of the following statements is true?
A. Monoamine oxidase inhibitors, such as phenelzine, may compete with bupropion because of their chemical similarity.
B. Bupropion can lower the seizure threshold.
C. Taking other neuroleptics when bupropion is being used does not pose any added risk.
D. Bupropion may be helpful in treating hyponatremia.
E. When bupropion is used with amantadine, a serotonin-like syndrome has been described.

3. Symptoms of bupropion toxicity include all of the following except
A. Dizziness, nausea, vomiting
B. Miosis
C. Seizures
D. Edema, nonspecific rashes, enterocolitis
E. Nocturia, ataxia, incoordination

OTHER DOPAMINERGIC DRUGS

Levodopa

Levodopa (Dopar®) is an indirect dopamine agonist by virtue of its peripheral and central conversion to dopamine. It is used primarily in the treatment of Parkinson's disease. Dopaminergic toxic effects include nausea, vomiting, hypotension, cardiac arrhythmias, behavioral changes, and abnormal involuntary movements. Acute overdose was reported in a 61-year-old man following an ingestion of 100 g of levodopa. He experienced hypertension initially, followed by hypotension for a few hours, mild nausea, and severe anorexia that gradually resolved over 1 week. He reportedly had insomnia for about 1 week, confusion for 2 days, and agitation for 3–4 days.

Carbidopa-levodopa

Carbidopa-levodopa (Sinemet®) is also used to treat Parkinson's disease. In overdose, it may lead to convulsions, agitation, paranoia, or mania. Carbidopa is a decarboxylase inhibitor that prevents peripheral destruction of levodopa. A 57-year-old woman ingested 15–17 tablets of carbidopa-levodopa 10/100 tablets (carbidopa 150 mg and levodopa 1,500 mg) together with carisoprodol, ibuprofen, and hydrocodone-acetaminophen. She became obtunded and developed choreiform movements, hypoventilation, myoglobinuria, and an increase in her creatine kinase level. She was treated supportively with pancuronium and was discharged without symptoms after the eighth day. Withdrawal of levodopa or carbidopa-levodopa has resulted in neuroleptic malignant syndrome (NMS) with hyperpyrexia, which may be fatal.

TREATMENT

- Treatment of these agents in overdose is primarily symptomatic and supportive.

ANTIDOTES

The decarboxylation of levodopa to dopamine is catalyzed by the pyridoxine-dependent enzyme l-amino acid decarboxylase. Pyridoxine has been used to reverse the dyskinesias and choreoathetosis of levodopa.

Questions—Levodopa and Carbidopa-levodopa

1. Which of the following statements about levodopa is false?
A. Levodopa is an indirect dopamine agonist by virtue of its peripheral and central conversion to dopamine.
B. It is used primarily in the treatment of Parkinson's disease.
C. Dopaminergic toxic effects include vomiting, hypertension, dilated pupils, and diarrhea.
D. Cardiac arrhythmias, behavioral changes, and abnormal involuntary movements have been associated with its use.
E. Anorexia and insomnia may be associated with levodopa use.

2. Which of the following statements about carbidopa-levodopa is false?
A. Carbidopa-levodopa is used to treat Parkinson's disease.
B. In overdose it may lead to convulsions, agitation, paranoia, or mania.
C. Carbidopa enhances dopamine release and synergistically improves the effect of levodopa.
D. Withdrawal of levodopa or carbidopa-levodopa has resulted in neuroleptic malignant syndrome (NMS) with hyperpyrexia, which may be fatal.
E. Signs of toxicity can include obtundation and choreiform movements.

Pergolide

Pergolide (Permax®) is a synthetic ergoline derivative that acts as a dopamine agonist in the treatment of Parkinson's disease and hyperprolactinemia. A fatal dose has not been established. Oral absorption is more than 60%. The plasma half-life is 15–42 hours. Pergolide has an extensive volume of distribution (about 20 L/kg) and exhibits plasma protein binding of 90%. Overdoses have resulted in hallucinations, involuntary movements, palpitations, hypotension, and premature ventricular beats.

TREATMENT

Gut Decontamination
Activated charcoal may be useful.

Elimination Enhancement
There is no experience with hemodialysis or hemoperfusion.

Supportive Measures
- Management of an overdose is largely symptomatic and supportive. The patient's airway is protected as necessary and cardiac function is monitored.
- Nausea may respond to an antiemetic (e.g., domperidone).

Sulpiride

Sulpiride (Sulpitil®) is an antidepressant and antipsychotic agent which exerts its antipsychotic action via selective blockade of central dopamine D2 receptors. Although this mechanism of action was believed to preclude any association with extrapyramidal side effects, drug-induced Parkinsonism, tardive dystonia, akathisia, and tardive dyskinesia have followed its use.

PHARMACOKINETICS

Absorption

- Sulpiride is absorbed from the gastrointestinal tract but has a low bioavailability (about 37%).
- Following oral administration of 100 mg, peak serum concentrations of up to 180 ng/mL are observed in 3–6 hours.

Distribution

- Sulpiride has a volume of distribution (after intravenous use) of 2.7 L/kg.

Elimination

- There is very little first-pass metabolism by the liver after oral administration.
- About 70% of the dose is recovered as unchanged drug in the urine.
- The elimination half-life is about 7 hours.

CLINICAL PRESENTATIONS

Coma has followed ingestion of sulpiride. Overdoses may result in restlessness, extrapyramidal symptoms, agitation, confusion, and hypertension. Symptoms may last several hours. No special hematologic, biochemical, or electrocardiographic abnormalities have been observed.

TOXIC DOSAGE/DEATH

Patients have survived doses up to 20 g. In one study involving 20 patients who overdosed, there were no deaths. At least one fatality involving sulpiride has been reported.

LABORATORY

Analytic Methods

A high-performance liquid chromatography assay is available.

Blood Levels

Blood levels may be useful in confirmation of drug presence, but will not likely be used in gauging the severity of poisoning or guiding the management of patients.

TREATMENT

Gut Decontamination

Although charcoal and/or lavage may be helpful, there is little evidence to support their use.

Elimination Enhancement

These methods have not been reported as being helpful in the management of sulpiride overdose.

Supportive Measures

- Management of sulpiride overdose is largely symptomatic and supportive with appropriate care of coma (glucose, naloxone, thiamine, oxygen, endotracheal intubation) in an intensive care unit.
- Parkinsonism symptoms may be managed with appropriate medication as indicated.

Tiapride

Tiapride, an atypical neuroleptic agent, is a selective dopamine D2-receptor antagonist with little propensity for causing catalepsy and sedation. Tiapride demonstrates antidyskinetic activity reflecting antidopaminergic actions and anxiolytic activity mediated by mechanisms that are poorly understood.

Tiapride facilitates management of alcohol withdrawal. Tiapride ameliorates psychological distress, improves abstinence, reduces drinking behavior, and, in the short-term, facilitates reintegration within society. The potential risk of tardive dyskinesia at the dosage employed (300 mg/d) requires evaluation and necessitates medical supervision.

PATHOPHYSIOLOGY

Tiapride is a selective adenyl cyclase-independent dopamine D2-receptor antagonist that lacks affinity for dopamine D1 receptors. Tiapride does not appear to cause physical or psychological dependence. It does not possess antiepileptic properties, but does not lower the epileptogenic threshold. In common with other dopaminergic antagonists, tiapride causes hyperprolactinemia, although the effects of prolonged tiapride administration on circulating prolactin levels have not been assessed.

PHARMACOKINETICS

Absorption

- Bioavailability of tiapride is about 75% after oral or muscular administration.

Distribution

- Peak plasma tiapride concentrations are achieved within 0.4–1.5 hours when given by oral or muscular administration, and steady state occurs 24–48 hours after initiating three-times-daily administration.
- The drug is rapidly distributed and does not bind appreciably to plasma proteins.

Elimination

- Tiapride is eliminated mainly by renal excretion, principally in the unchanged form.
- The elimination half-life is approximately 3–4 hours.

CLINICAL PRESENTATIONS

The most frequently reported adverse events are drowsiness, extrapyramidal syndromes, dizziness, and orthostatic hypotension. There have been a few reports of tardive dyskinesia in elderly patients undergoing long-term therapy. For patients undergoing acute alcohol withdrawal with tiapride, the most serious event appears to be neuroleptic malignant syndrome.

TREATMENT

- There is little experience to guide management of tiapride overdose.

Question—Other Dopaminergic Drugs

1. Which of the following statements is false?

A. The most frequently reported adverse events with tiapride use are drowsiness, extrapyramidal syndromes, dizziness, and orthostatic hypotension.
B. Tiapride facilitates management of alcohol withdrawal.
C. Sulpiride is an antidepressant and antipsychotic agent, which exerts its antipsychotic action via selective blockade of peripheral serotonin receptors.
D. Coma has followed ingestion of sulpiride.
E. For patients undergoing acute alcohol withdrawal with tiapride, the most worrisome serious event appears to be neuroleptic malignant syndrome.

Answers

Introduction to Dopaminergic Drugs

1\. C 2. E

Bromocriptine

1\. D 2. A 3. E

Bupropion

1\. D 2. B 3. D

Levodopa and Carbidopa-levodopa

1\. C 2. C

Other Dopaminergic Drugs

1\. C

SELECTED READINGS

Introduction to Dopaminergic Drugs

1. Creese I, Sibley DR, Leff S, Hamblin M. Dopamine receptors: Subtypes, localization and regulation. Fed Proc 1981;40:147–152.
2. Lader MH. Neuroleptic-induced deficit syndrome. J Clin Psychiatry 1993;54: 493–500.
3. Rosenkrantz RP, McClelland DL. An historical perspective of dopamine and its analogs. Proc West Pharmacol Soc 1990;33:15–19.
4. Sibley DR, Monsma FJ Jr. Molecular biology of dopamine receptors. Trends Pharmacol Sci 1992;13:61–69.

Bromocriptine

1. Thorner MO, Flackiger E, Calne DB. Bromocriptine: A clinical and pharmacological review. New York: Raven Press, 1989.
2. Vance ML, Evans WS, Thormer MO. Bromocriptine. Ann Intern Med 1984; 100:78–91.

Bupropion

1. Friel PN, Logan BK, Fligner CL. Three fatal overdoses involving bupropion. J Anal Toxicol 1993;17:436–438.
2. James WA, Lippmann S. Bupropion: Overview and prescribing guidelines in depression. South Med J 1991;84:222–224.
3. Spiller HA, Ramoska EA, Krenzelok EP, et al.: Bupropion overdose: A 3 year multicenter retrospective analysis. Am J Emerg Med 1994;12:43–45.

Levodopa and Carbidopa-levodopa

1. Hoehn MM, Rutledge CO. Acute overdose with levodopa. Neurology 1975; 25:792–794.
2. Sporer KA. Carbidopa-levodopa overdose. Am J Emerg Med 1991;9:47–48.

Pergolide

1. Arky RT, Medical Consultant. In: Physicians' desk reference. 48th ed. Montvale, NJ: Medical Economics, 1994.
2. Langtry HD, Clissold SP. Pergolide: A review of its pharmacological properties and therapeutic potential in Parkinson's disease. Drugs 1990;39:491–501.

Sulpiride

1. Kintz P, Tracqui A, Parent Y, et al. Fatal sulpiride intoxication. Bull Int Assoc Forens Toxicol 1994;24:37.
2. Mielke DH, Gallant DM, Roniger JJ, et al. Sulpiride: Evaluation of antipsychotic activity in schizophrenic patients. Dis Nerv Syst 1977;38:569–571.
3. Miller LG, Jankovic J. Sulpiride induced tardive dyskinesia. Mov Disord 1990; 5:83–84.

Tiapride

1. Peters DH, Faulds D. Tiapride: A review of its pharmacology and therapeutic potential in the management of alcohol dependence syndrome. Drugs 1994;47: 1010–1073.

PART III

The Home

CHAPTER 38

Household Products

INTRODUCTION

Household cleaning products account for approximately 5–10% of annually reported toxic exposures, with soaps, detergents, bleaches, and corrosive cleaning agents being the most common. Over 90% of toxic exposures to household cleaning products occur at home in children under 5 years of age and usually at a time when the product is in use rather than in storage. Fortunately, two-thirds of such exposures generally result in no symptoms. Mild gastrointestinal symptoms and mucosal irritation most often occur in the remainder of exposures, with symptoms generally lasting less than 24 hours. Death and disability are rare except in deliberate adult ingestions. Selected laundry products, automatic dishwasher detergents, certain household cleaners (e.g., oven cleaner), and corrosive cleaners (e.g., toilet bowl cleaners) are caustic enough to produce serious mucosal injuries. See Chapter 42, Acids, Bases, and Gastroesophageal Issues.

CLEANING PRODUCTS

Antiseptics and Disinfectants

The term "antiseptic" refers to a chemical agent that destroys or inhibits microorganisms on living tissue and has the effect of limiting or preventing the harmful results of infection. Numerous antiseptics are available. They include quaternary ammonium preservatives in ophthalmic solutions, topical lotions, and others. Allergic contact dermatitis and hypersensitivity may occur from these agents. One antiseptic, benzalkonium chloride, is used in eye drops and contact lens solutions. Allergic dermatitis, stomatitis, and allergic conjunctivitis have resulted from its use. Cetrimide, a cationic surfactant, is another antiseptic which may cause contact dermatitis and chemical peritonitis.

The term "disinfectant" refers to a chemical agent that destroys microorganisms but not usually bacterial spores. Liquid disinfectants may contain acids, alkalis, alcohol, pine oil, phenol, or cationic detergents such as quaternary compounds (e.g., Zephiran). Combination cleaners with pine oil (see Chapter 46, Hydrocarbons) and phenol are the most toxic compounds in this group. In some disinfectants, the vehicle is more toxic than the germicide (e.g., Lysol® contains 79% ethanol).

Disinfectants include ethanol, isopropyl alcohol, and ethyl alcohol-methyl alcohol mixtures. See Chapter 17, Alcohols, Glycols and Disulfram. Other disinfectants include aldehydes (e.g., formaldehyde, glutaraldehyde), cationic surfactants (e.g., benzalkonium chloride, cetrimide, cetylpyridinium chloride, domiphen bromide), and chlorhexidine and chlorine-releasing substances (e.g., sodium hypochlorite, chloramine, chlorinated lime, bichlorodimethylhydantoin, halazone, oxychlorosene, and sodium dichloroisocyanurate).

Questions—Antiseptics and Disinfectants

1. Pine oil-containing disinfectants are particularly toxic agents.
A. True
B. False

2. Antiseptic agents destroy microorganisms while disinfectant agents kill bacterial spores.
A. True
B. False

CHLORHEXIDINE

Chlorhexidine is a disinfectant that is generally used topically. It has been associated with methemoglobinemia. Skin, gastric, eye, hepatic, neurologic, and cardiac reactions have been reported when chlorhexidine was ingested, inhaled, or used topically. There have been no fatalities. Chlorhexidine may be effective against some Gram-positive and Gram-negative bacteria, some viruses, and some fungi. It is inactive against bacterial spores.

Pathophysiology

Chlorhexidine is commercially available as the acetate, the gluconate, and the hydrochloride. A 0.05% aqueous solution is used as a wound disinfectant, as eye irrigation, and for storage and disinfection of clean instruments. It is available as a cream, lozenge, dusting powder, ear drops, mouthwash, swab, spray, solution, gel, and irrigant. Trade names include Chlorsept® and Hibiclens®. Chlorhexidine is a synthetic chemical.

Pharmacokinetics

Absorption

- Chlorhexidine gluconate 4% is strongly adsorbed on the skin surface and may not be removed by 70% isopropyl alcohol.

Distribution

- Neonates exhibited blood levels of 53–607 ng/mL 1 hour after a chlorhexidine wash.

Elimination

- Parachloraniline, a decomposition product, has not been detected in the urine of animals or humans.

Clinical Presentations

A newborn who ingested chlorhexidine developed cyanotic spells and sinus bradycardia, which responded to atropine. The neonate improved with cessation of bradycardia after 6 days. Babies accidentally fed chlorhexidine 0.05% with cetrimide 1% developed superficial erythema and edema of the lips, mouth, and tongue that appeared to be due to caustic burns. One baby developed acute pulmonary edema with prominent oral frothing. Urticaria, pruritus, rash, occupational asthma, dyspnea, and anaphylactic shock have followed topical use of chlorhexidine. Chlorhexidine gluconate 4% may produce corneal damage (bullous keratopathy, epithelial defects, and corneal opacification) when applied to the eyes.

Gastrointestinal Effects

Repeated ingestion of chlorhexidine gluconate 4% by an adult led to numerous episodes of vomiting. Fiberoptic gastroscopy may show multiple erosions in the stomach and duodenum with an active atrophic gastritis. High aminotransferase blood levels and a diffuse fatty degeneration and lobular hepatitis of the liver have followed ingestion of chlorhexidine by an adult.

Toxic Dosage/Death

Numerous exposures have been reported. Chlorhexidine gluconate 4% used as a mouthwash and swallowed may not cause

Answers to questions in shaded boxes appear at the end of the chapter.

significant morbidity. An 89-year-old inadvertently ingested 30 mL of 4% chlorhexidine gluconate, remained asymptomatic, and survived. Ingestion of 30 g (150 mL) of chlorhexidine gluconate led to hepatotoxicity in an adult patient.

Pregnancy/Lactation

Chlorhexidine sprayed on a mother's breast may inadvertently be fed to a child.

Laboratory

Analytic Methods

Serum chlorhexidine may be analyzed by a high-performance liquid chromatography.

Blood Levels

Serum concentrations of chlorhexidine in a newborn 120 hours after oral exposure to chlorhexidine breast spray were 11 pg/L.

Treatment

Gut Decontamination

Avoid gastric lavage for fear of rupturing ulcerated areas. Charcoal has not been studied in this setting. Milk feedings may be helpful; however, further studies are needed.

Elimination Enhancement

There are no data to support the use of elimination enhancement procedures for chlorhexidine poisoning.

Supportive Measures

- Treatment is largely symptomatic and supportive. Ingestions should be treated as caustics. See Chapter 42, Acids, Bases and Gastroesophageal Issues.
- Corneal defects should be treated symptomatically and with antibiotic ointments.
- When chlorhexidine gluconate was inadvertently used as a humidifying fluid in premature baby incubators, parachloraniline, known to be a decomposition product of chlorhexidine, induced methemoglobinemia in infants. Methemoglobinemia is treatment with methylene blue if clinically indicated.
- Airway hyperresponsiveness should be treated by removal from the offending site and pulmonary function evaluation with appropriate symptomatic treatment.

Questions—Chlorhexidine

1. Chlorhexidine may be effective against all of the following except

A. Some Gram-positive bacteria
B. Some Gram-negative bacteria
C. Some bacterial spores
D. Some viruses
E. Some fungi

2. Which of the following may be helpful in treatment of chlorhexidine poisoning?

A. Gastric lavage
B. Milk feeding
C. Serum concentration to guide management
D. All of the above
E. None of the above

CRESOLS

Lysol® disinfectant is a mixture of cresol (50%) in saponified linseed oil, potassium hydroxide, and water. It is a yellowish or brownish liquid of syrup consistency and is strongly alkaline. Cresols are used as antiseptics, disinfectants, insecticides, resins, and plasticizers. Ingestion leads to corrosive effects and systemic toxicity of the vascular system, liver, kidneys, and pancreas.

Pathophysiology

The cresols are alkyl derivatives of phenol. Their bactericidal potency is about three times that of phenol. Like phenol, cresol is a derivative of coal tar. Cresols may be converted to gluconol and catechol, which give a characteristic dark color to the urine.

Clinical Presentations

All isomers of cresol can cause skin and eye burns. Renal impairment, hepatotoxicity, central nervous system disturbances and cardiovascular disturbances have also been observed. Coma, often associated with hypothermia, may come on quickly and last for over 12 hours. Acute pancreatitis may be seen. Death after some days may follow acute renal failure.

Dermatologic Effects

Following skin contact, a burning sensation, erythema, skin peeling, localized anesthesia, and occasional darkening of the skin have been seen. A hypersensitivity response may be observed. Burns and scalding with cresol are potentially lethal. Burns after ingestion may be seen on the lips, gums, tongue, cheeks, pharynx, and tonsils. Stricture rarely forms in the gastrointestinal tract. Blisters, followed by a painful sloughing of mucous membrane, may occur. Hoarseness or aphonia may develop.

Hematologic Effects

Methemoglobinemia, Heinz body formation, and massive intravascular hemolysis may follow ingestion of Lysol®. Lysol® poisoning has been associated with incomplete abortions, shock, tachycardia, leukocytosis, hemolysis, fever, central nervous system irritability, respiratory embarrassment associated with pulmonary edema and/or oil emboli, local tissue necrosis with uterine hemorrhage, and anemia.

Abuse

Lysol® Disinfectant Spray contains the relatively harmless component o-phenyl-phenol (0.1%) and ethyl alcohol. Consumption has become a problem on Native American reservations where the product has been mixed with orange juice and drunk by children.

Toxic Dosage/Death

The lethal dose of Lysol® is about 60–120 mL, although lesser amounts have been associated with death. Ingestions of 4–120 ml of 25–50% cresol generally cause nausea within minutes. About 20 mL of a 90% cresol solution accidentally poured over an infant's head resulted in chemical burns, cyanosis, unconsciousness, and death within 4 hours. Intrauterine injection of Lysol® as an abortifacient has led to shock, coma, and death within 2 hours due to pulmonary oil embolism.

Laboratory

Analytic Methods

A thin-layer chromatography method is able to identify phenols and cresol isomers. A high-performance liquid chromatography method with UV detection is able to analyze phenols, cresol, and xylenols in workplace air.

Blood Levels

Cresol blood concentrations of 120 mg/mL followed the rapid death (4 hours) of a 12-month-old infant, which followed the spilling of a 90% cresol solution on the baby's head. Ingestion by an adult of 25 g of cresol led to dyspnea, tachycardia, and hypotension. In 24 hours the serum total phenols were 90 mg/mL (over 10 mg/mL may have serious prognostic significance). Hemodialysis for 8 hours did not significantly alter phenol concentrations.

Treatment

Gut Decontamination

Charcoal may be useful following ingestion of cresols.

Elimination Enhancement

These methods have not been described as successful adjuncts to the treatment of cresol overdoses.

Supportive Measures

- Skin contact should be immediately washed with large volumes of water, then bathed with polyethylene glycol, propylene glycol or glycerol, vegetable oil, or soap and water.
- Patients may require resuscitation procedures, ventilatory support, and volume replacement.

Antidotes

Methylene blue is used to treat methemoglobinemia.

Questions—Cresols

1. All of the following statements about cresols are true except
A. They are yellowish or brownish liquids of syrup consistency.
B. They are used as antiseptics, disinfectants, insecticides, resins, and plasticizers.
C. They are strongly acidic.
D. Their bactericidal potency is about three times that of phenol.
E. Cresol is a derivative of coal tar.

2. Clinical effects of cresol exposure may include
A. Burns and scalding
B. Leukopenia
C. Pancreatitis
D. A and B
E. A and C

3. Treatment of cresol skin contact may include washing with large volumes of water followed by bathing with propylene glycol or vegetable oil.
A. True
B. False

ETHYLENE OXIDE

Ethylene oxide is a colorless gas with a distinctive, sweet, etherlike odor, which is used to sterilize medical instruments, particularly those made of heat-labile materials. It is also used in the production of ethylene glycol, polyesters, and detergents and is regulated by the U.S. Occupational Safety and Health Administration (OSHA) as a carcinogen. Ethylene oxide is typically supplied in compressed gas cylinders that contain 88% freon and 12% ethylene oxide, or in single-dose cartridges of 100% ethylene oxide. Workers in central supply, dental operations, and surgical suites are at risk of potential exposure.

The typical source of ethylene oxide exposure in the hospital environment is through the operation of sterilizing equipment. Unless good engineering controls and good work practices are used, workers may encounter relatively high concentrations of ethylene oxide over relatively brief periods. Data suggest the need to control short-term peak exposures to ethylene oxide.

Pathophysiology

Ethylene oxide is a mutagen and animal carcinogen and probably a human carcinogen. It is a highly reactive epoxide and alkylating agent.

Clinical Presentations

Exposure to high levels of ethylene oxide may result in skin lesions, mucous membrane irritation, nausea, vomiting, headache, convulsions, and death. Contact with ethylene oxide-sterilized equipment or wrapping that has not been adequately aerated to remove residual ethylene oxide may cause severe burns with large blisters and peeling skin. Healing may leave hyperpigmentation.

Data on chronic exposure to ethylene oxide suggest an increased tendency to cognitive decline, a reversible sensorimotor neuropathy of the distal axonopathy type and certain neuropsychologic deficits suggestive of central nervous system dysfunction. Further studies will be required to define these deficits. A study of 18,254 workers exposed to ethylene oxide at 14 plants producing sterilized medical supplies suggests a trend toward an increase in hematopoietic cancer with increasing lengths of time since first exposure.

Toxic Dosage/Death

Although ethylene oxide has an odor threshold of about 400-ppm, exposure at 200 ppm may cause irritation of the eyes and upper respiratory system. Brief exposure to more than 1,000 ppm produces chest pain, cough, dyspnea, headaches, nausea, vomiting, weakness, gait disturbances, and ataxia. Whether ethylene oxide is carcinogenic or teratogenic in humans remains to be determined.

Pregnancy/Lactation

Ethylene oxide is a possible human teratogen and should be avoided if possible by the pregnant individual.

Treatment

Gut Decontamination

Emesis is not advised and there is little clinical experience with charcoal and lavage.

Elimination Enhancement

These methods have not been utilized to treat exposures of ethylene oxide.

Supportive Measures

- The U.S. National Institute for Occupational Safety and Health (NIOSH) has proposed engineering controls for ethylene oxide. Sterilizers should be enclosed either in a mechanical access room or a cabinet, and the enclosure should be exhausted to a dedicated ventilation system. Sterilizing operations should be centralized and access to sterilizer rooms should be restricted.

- Workers should use protective gloves and splash-proof goggles and / or a face shield when changing ethylene oxide supply cylinders. If good engineering controls are used a respirator should not be necessary. When cleaning up liquid spills that contain ethylene oxide, workers should wear protective outer clothing and dispose of or launder it immediately afterward.
- A positive-pressure, self-contained breathing apparatus should be available for emergencies and should be stored in an area away from the sterilizer and the ethylene oxide supply location.
- Immediate treatment for ethylene oxide exposures includes movement to fresh air and oxygen if necessary. Monitor complete blood count and do serial neurologic exams.

Questions—Ethylene Oxide

1. Ethylene oxide is used to
   A. Clean bathrooms
   B. Sterilize medical instruments
   C. Sterilize teeth before dental procedures
   D. Decrease skin hyperpigmentation
   E. None of the above

2. Data on chronic exposure to ethylene oxide suggest
   A. No effects on cognitive abilities
   B. Reversible sensorimotor neuropathy of the distal axonopathy type
   C. Trends toward an increase in hematopoietic cancer
   D. A and B
   E. B and C

FORMALDEHYDE

Formaldehyde is a commonly used disinfectant, tissue preservative, and feedstock for synthetic chemical processes. Formaldehyde is ubiquitous in our environment as a contaminant of smoke and in photochemical smog. Industrial uses include the manufacture of urea formaldehyde foam, paint pigment, and plastic molding. Formaldehyde processes produce wrinkle-free, crease-resistant textiles. It is used as a disinfectant, antiseptic, deodorant, tissue fixative and embalming agent. Synonyms for formaldehyde include formalin, methyl aldehyde, and methylene oxide.

Formaldehyde is also found in plastics, dyestuff, fertilizers, paper, and in the foundry and tanning industries. Particleboard, gas appliances, and carpeting may release formaldehyde vapor indoors. Moisture and heat may cause decomposition of formaldehyde-containing products into formaldehyde vapor. Release of these vapors in mobile homes has been associated with headache and pulmonary and dermal irritation. Except after thermal degradation in fires, polyurethane foam does not release formaldehyde vapor.

Formaldehyde is a major byproduct of combustion processes, including tobacco smoking. It is produced in both mainstream and sidestream smoke. Tobacco cigarettes and marijuana have been dipped in formaldehyde ("amp") before smoking because of its alleged hallucinogenic effect. Encephalopathy, rhabdomyolysis, and coma have followed as little as two "amp"-dipped cigarettes.

Urea formaldehyde foam insulation (UFFI) consists primarily of polymers of urea and formaldehyde in combination with numerous other chemicals. Free formaldehyde may be released during the initial reaction and through decomposition depending on temperature, humidity, and acid content of the foam. The adverse health effects of UFFI remain controversial.

Pathophysiology

Formaldehyde is a mild sensory irritant and potent sensitizer. Some people are more sensitive to formaldehyde than others.

Clinical Presentations

Respiratory Effects

Formaldehyde is a respiratory irritant capable of reducing FEV1 in individuals with hyperreactive airway disease acutely. Although the concentration generally is too low to cause symptoms in home environments, low-dose formaldehyde exposure from UFFI may cause headache, rhinitis, and dyspnea. At exposure levels of 1–4 ppm, formaldehyde is a strong mucous membrane irritant, producing burning and lacrimation.

For sensitive individuals, formaldehyde is a potent allergen, causing asthma and dermatitis. Cough, chest pain, dyspnea, and wheezing may occur in individuals exposed to 5–30 ppm. There is no evidence that prolonged exposure to formaldehyde causes irreversible chronic obstructive pulmonary disease. An epidemiologic study of morticians exposed to formaldehyde did not demonstrate any significant increased incidence of bronchitis or reduced pulmonary function.

Gastrointestinal Effects

After oral ingestion, patients present early with severe corrosion of the gastrointestinal tract and systemic effects. Inflammation and ulceration of the mouth, esophagus, and stomach result in severe abdominal pain, diarrhea, and vomiting, which may progress to strictures.

Carcinogenic Effects

Formaldehyde is a mutagen and animal carcinogen, but its relationship to occupational cancer is unclear. British studies including thousands of workers in the formaldehyde industry failed to detect significant increases in nasal or lung cancer. An increased incidence of cancer of the buccal cavity and multiple myeloma was detected. Concern over the irritant effects and carcinogenic potential of formaldehyde vapor has led to a proposed ban on the use of urea formaldehyde foam insulation. In sum, despite widespread use, epidemiologic data have not clearly demonstrated that formaldehyde is a human carcinogen.

Hypersensitivity Effects

Repeated exposure to formaldehyde may cause some persons to become sensitized. Sensitization may occur days, weeks, or months after the first exposure. Sensitized individuals will experience eye or upper respiratory irritation or an asthmatic reaction at levels of exposure that are too low to cause symptoms in most people. Reactions may be quite severe with swelling, itching, wheezing, and chest tightness.

Neurologic Effects

Disturbances in memory, mood, equilibrium, and sleep, in addition to headache and fatigue, have been reported in occupational and non-occupational exposure to formaldehyde. Severe acidosis results from rapid conversion of formaldehyde to formic acid. Coma, hypotension, renal failure, and apnea may complicate severe ingestions.

Toxic Dosage/Death

Both death and survival from 4-ounce formalin ingestions have been reported in adults. The probable mean lethal adult dose is 1–2 ounces. Death may occur within 3 hours. Survival past 48 hours usually means recovery. Odor is not a reliable warning for the presence of formaldehyde. Many people experience pulmonary irritation below 1 ppm.

Laboratory

Analytic Methods

An analytic procedure has been developed that permits the specific quantitation of formaldehyde and glutaraldehyde in one sample by high-performance liquid chromatography separation.

Blood Levels

Blood levels do not guide management of acute exposures or overdose.

Treatment

Gut Decontamination

Dilution with milk or water in alert patients as a first aid measure may reduce corrosive effects at the scene. Use of nasogastic tubes to perform lavage is generally discouraged given the corrosive nature of formaldehyde. There is little evidence to support the use of activated charcoal to absorb formate or formaldehyde.

Elimination Enhancement

Severe acidosis and deteriorating vital signs are indications for considering dialysis, but the literature does not contain adequate case studies to guide treatment.

Supportive Measures

- Monitor electrolytes, fluids, acid-base, and kidney function closely.
- Watch for signs of gastrointestinal hemorrhage and perforation after oral ingestion, with serial vital signs, abdominal examinations, and complete blood counts.
- Check blood methanol levels and treat accordingly in formalin ingestions.
- Local exhaust ventilation should be installed over workstations where formalin or specimens preserved in formalin are being used.
- Skin and eye contact with formaldehyde should be avoided. Appropriate protective gloves should be used whenever hand contact is possible.

Questions—Formaldehyde

1. Formaldehyde may be found in
A. Tissue preservatives
B. Fertilizers
C. Paper
D. All of the above
E. None of the above

2. Which of the following has a clear association with formaldehyde exposure?
A. Irreversible chronic obstructive pulmonary disease
B. Lung cancer
C. Chronic bronchitis
D. Reduced pulmonary function
E. None of the above

3. The mean adult lethal dose of formaldehyde ingestion is closest to
A. 0.1–0.2 ounces
B. 1–2 ounces
C. 10-20 ounces
D. 12 ounces
E. 120 ounces

GLUTARALDEHYDE

Glutaraldehyde is commonly used as a sterilizing agent in medical facilities. It is effective as a disinfectant against many microorganisms and viruses, including the HIV viruses, and is usually harmless to medical equipment. Glutaraldehyde is a strong nasal and ocular irritant.

Pathophysiology

Cross-linking of the peptidoglycan in the bacterial cell wall with intermolecular bonding between teichoic acid chains and glutaraldehyde may cause a partial sealing and contraction of the outer cell envelope.

Clinical Presentations

Glutaraldehyde may cause skin irritation, cracking or bleeding, eye irritation, throat discomfort, nasal discomfort, chest tightness, palpitations, cough, and headache. It is a contact irritant and sensitizer. A significant number of embalmers have positive patch test reactions to glutaraldehyde. Mucous membrane irritation may predispose the patient to epistaxis.

Oral ingestions may cause severe gastrointestinal distress. Proctitis has been reported after the use of glutaraldehyde as a disinfectant of flexible sigmoidoscopes. Within hours of an examination, patients may have acute tenesmus and bloody diarrhea. Occupational contact dermatitis is frequently observed in health care personnel after exposure to glutaraldehyde. Hand eczema may be prevalent. Glutaraldehyde can cause occupational asthma, palpitations and tachycardia.

Toxic Dosage/Death

Glutaraldehyde has a pungent odor with a threshold recognition of 0.04 parts per million by volume in air. Eye and respiratory irritation are noted at a level of 0.3 ppm.

Pregnancy/Lactation

Glutaraldehyde may produce fetotoxicity in animals.

Laboratory

Analytic Methods

A high-performance liquid chromatography method enables quantitation of formaldehyde and glutaraldehyde.

Blood Levels

Following blood levels is not helpful in overdose.

Treatment

Gut Decontamination

Dilution with milk or water may be helpful. The use of charcoal is probably not effective in reducing absorption.

Elimination Enhancement

The literature does not contain adequate case studies to guide treatment.

Supportive Measures

- Workers should avoid breathing glutaraldehyde vapors. They should also be provided with and be required to wear splash-proof safety goggles where there is any possibility of contaminating the eyes with glutaraldehyde.
- If clothing becomes contaminated with glutaraldehyde, it should be promptly removed and not reworn until the glutaraldehyde has been removed.
- Skin that becomes contaminated with glutaraldehyde should be washed immediately.
- Eye exposure is treated with copious irrigation with saline.

Questions—Glutaraldehyde

1. **Glutaraldehyde is effective as a disinfectant against many microorganisms and viruses, excluding the HIV viruses.**
   A. True
   B. False
2. **Which of the following may be helpful in the treatment of glutaraldehyde poisoning?**
   A. Dilution with milk or water
   B. Charcoal to reduce absorption
   C. Blood levels to guide treatment
   D. Elimination enhancement
   E. None of the above
3. **Which of the following statements is false?**
   A. Glutaraldehyde may cause skin irritation, cracking or bleeding, eye irritation, throat discomfort, nasal discomfort, chest tightness, cough, and headache.
   B. Glutaraldehyde is a contact irritant and sensitizer.
   C. A significant number of embalmers have positive patch test reactions to glutaraldehyde.
   D. Proctitis has been reported after the use of glutaraldehyde as a disinfectant of flexible sigmoidoscopes.
   E. Unlike formaldehyde, glutaraldehyde does not cause occupational asthma.

GENTIAN VIOLET

The dye gentian violet was introduced as an antiseptic in 1890 and has been used for almost 100 years. No serious side effects have been reported when gentian violet is used externally. When used as a vermifuge, gentian violet may act as a direct irritant of the gastrointestinal mucosa. It is added routinely to banked blood in different countries in Latin America. No serious side effects have been observed in the more than 100,000 patients transfused with this blood.

Gentian violet is used to control fungal infections, to treat the umbilical cord of newborns, and for the prevention of infection in burn patients. It is a blood additive used to prevent transmission of Chagas' disease by blood transfusion. It is also used as a mycostatic agent in poultry feed, as a biologic stain in the Gram reaction, and as a dye for silk, wood, cosmetics, and food. There have been no reports of oral or intravenous overdose. A preparation known as Bonney's Blue, which contains gentian violet, has long been used as a skin marker by surgeons.

Pathophysiology

Gentian violet has been found to be a potential carcinogen in animals. However, there have been no reports of cancer following human exposure to this product. A photodynamic action of gentian violet, apparently mediated by a free radical mechanism, has been described in bacteria and *trypanosoma cruzi.*

Clinical Presentations

Gentian violet may cause irritation or sensitivity reactions such as anaphylaxis and ulceration of mucous membranes. Esophagitis, laryngitis, or tracheitis may result from swallowing a solution of gentian violet. Laryngeal obstruction has followed prolonged use of the drug in the treatment of oral candidiasis. Apple packers, wood pulp workers, and dye manufacturers may develop nosebleeds from exposure to dust from gentian violet used as markers. Accidental injection of gentian violet through the urethra resulted in severe hemorrhagic cystitis in one case.

Toxic Dosage/Death

One patient received 34 liters of gentian violet-treated blood in 74 reported transfusions within a 6-month period and another patient received 4 liters of such blood at one time. No toxic effects were seen in either case. Ingestion of 6.8 mg/kg of gentian violet by a septicemic adult led to gastrointestinal irritation. No fatal dose has been reported.

Treatment

Gut Decontamination

As overdoses have not been reported, these methods have not been studied in overdose.

Elimination Enhancement

As overdoses have not been reported, these methods have not been studied in overdose.

Supportive Measures

- Treatment of the toxic effects of gentian violet administration is symptomatic and supportive.

Questions—Gentian Violet

1. **Serious side effects have been observed in more than 100,000 patients transfused with blood to which gentian violet has been added.**
   A. True
   B. False
2. **Benefits of gentian violet include all of the following except**
   A. Its ability to control fungal infections
   B. Its use in treating the umbilical cord of newborns
   C. Its use in prevention of infection in burn patients
   D. Its known safety in bladder irrigation
   E. Its use in preventing transmission of Chagas' disease by blood transfusion

HEXACHLOROPHENE

Hexachlorophene was developed in 1939 and was quickly recognized as an effective bacteriostatic agent, particularly against Gram-positive bacteria. By the 1950s, hexachlorophene was a constituent of a variety of cosmetic products, including shaving creams, soaps, shampoos, deodorants, and feminine hygiene agents. Because hexachlorophene is poorly soluble in water and remains on the skin after rinsing, the compound became a popular germicidal agent for surgical care. By the 1960s, case studies documented dermal toxicity after chronic application to both damaged and normal skin, as well as acute toxicity from accidental ingestions. Typically, symptoms involved gastrointestinal distress, lethargy, fever, jitteriness, convulsions, and, in severe cases, coma and death.

In 1972, 204 French children developed neurologic toxicity resulting in 36 deaths when a baby talcum powder was contaminated with 6.5% hexachlorophene. The U.S. FDA subsequently required that all hexachlorophene-containing products be sold as prescription drugs. The use of hexachlorophene on newborn infants remains controversial.

Pathophysiology

The exact mechanism of toxicity is unclear. Neurologic symptoms in neonates after acute exposure probably result from cerebral edema. Pathologic lesions consist of spongiform changes confined to myelinated white matter. Characteristic empty vacuoles formed by splitting and separation of myelin lamellae give this lesion the name vacuolar encephalopathy. Vacuolization of the white matter is not a lesion unique to hexachlorophene toxicity, however; it is also produced by a number of drugs and chemicals, including isoniazid, triethyl tin, cuprizone, and phenelzine.

Pharmacokinetics

Absorption

- Hexachlorophene toxicity may occur via the dermal and gastrointestinal routes.

Distribution

- Only small amounts of hexachlorophene penetrate intact skin of full-term neonates and children.

Elimination

- Hexachlorophene is both metabolized by the liver to glucuronide conjugates and excreted by the kidney unchanged, but the kinetics in humans have not been well studied.
- The elimination half-life in neonates washed daily with 3% hexachlorophene ranged from 6.1–44.2 hours and followed first-order kinetics.

Clinical Presentations

The signs and symptoms of toxicity depend on the length and type of exposure, as well as the age of the patient. Gastrointestinal distress and encephalopathy may characterize hexachlorophene toxicity after oral use. Cardiac dysrhythmias, apnea, and cardiac arrest may occur as the final event 48-60 hours after ingestion in large overdoses.

Gastrointestinal Effects

Within several hours of large ingestions, patients may develop nausea, vomiting, and diarrhea, which may progress to dehydration and hypotension.

Neurologic Effects

Neurologic signs may include lethargy, facial twitching, fever, blurred vision, blindness, hyperreflexia, seizures, and coma and may peak within 12–18 hours. Topical applications may produce nausea, vomiting, irritability, diplopia, hypertonicity, anorexia, and weakness. In severe cases, papilledema, retinal hemorrhages, convulsions, coma, and death may occur. Three percent hexachlorophene emulsion application has been associated with vacuolar encephalopathy of the brainstem reticular activating system.

Dermatologic Effects

Infants exposed to 6.3% hexachlorophene-contaminated diaper talc developed an erythematous, ulcerative groin rash.

Toxic Dosage/Death

Gastrointestinal distress occurs after ingestion of as little as 10–20 mg/kg. An ingestion of 250 mg/kg by a 6-year-old retarded child resulted in hypotension, convulsions, and death. Fatalities have occurred after the acute ingestion of hexachlorophene by adults and the chronic dermal application of 3% hexachlorophene emulsion to neonates with burns and severe ichthyosis. Full-term neonates washed daily with 3% hexachlorophene develop blood levels generally below 0.1 μg/mL (range, up to 0.65 μg/mL). Deaths have been reported in infants with blood levels of 3–16 μg/mL, and survival has occurred in adults with levels between 23–74 μg/mL. Generally, clinical effects do not correlate well with blood hexachlorophene levels, and no safe level has been determined for premature infants.

Pregnancy/Lactation

Hexachlorophene crosses the placenta in mice and accumulates in neural tissue. One epidemiologic study of women exposed occupationally to hexachlorophene suggested an increased incidence of congenital abnormalities.

Treatment

Gut Decontamination

Patients who ingest hexachlorophene in doses larger than 10–20 mg/kg may benefit from lavage. Activated charcoal does not absorb hexachlorophene.

Elimination Enhancement

Peritoneal dialysis did not remove significant amounts of hexachlorophene after an accidental ingestion. Hemoperfusion and activated charcoal are potential therapeutic modalities, but neither has been tested clinically.

Supportive Measures

- Seizures and respiratory depression are immediate life-threatening problems. Diazepam is the drug of choice for seizure control. Follow arterial blood gases and respiratory rate closely in severe poisonings.
- Hypotension may result from dehydration and may respond to fluid and electrolyte replacement.
- Severely poisoned patients should be monitored in an intensive care setting to watch for the potential development of dysrhythmias, hypotension, and apnea.

Questions—Hexachlorophene

1. All of the following statements are true regarding neurologic effects of hexachlorophene toxicity except

A. Signs and symptoms depend on length and type of exposure.
B. In severe cases, death may occur.
C. Topical applications may produce nausea and vomiting.
D. Neurologic symptoms peak at 3–4 days.
E. All of the above are true

2. Hexachlorophene

A. Is found in Hibiclens®
B. Is highly soluble in water so is easily rinsed
C. Can only be obtained with a prescription
D. A and B
E. A and C

HYDROGEN PEROXIDE

Hydrogen peroxide is a popular household disinfectant, also used to clean out earwax, as a gargle, in toothpaste, and as a bloodstain remover. It has also been used for removal of inspissated meconium and during roentgenography of abdominal viscera. It has been recommended as a disinfectant for tonometer tips, ophthalmic instruments, and certain contact lenses to prevent the transmission of viruses, especially human immunodeficiency virus.

Most hydrogen peroxide exposures involve common household strength (3%) and are usually benign. Ingestion of concentrations greater than 10%, however, can result in disastrous sequelae. Deaths following ingestion are rare. Low concentrations of hydrogen peroxide, 3–9%, are used in the treatment of otitis externa and as a mouthwash or gargle. Hydrogen peroxide has been applied in root canals of teeth and has been used as a vaginal douche solution. More potent solutions (20-30%) are used as hair-bleaching and tooth-bleaching agents.

Pathophysiology

At the cellular level, hydrogen peroxide induces DNA damage. A "snow white" color (mucosal whitening and frothy oxygen bubbles) is seen when hydrogen peroxide is applied to blood and on the colonic mucosa after topical application, secondary to penetration into epithelial interstices and capillaries.

Clinical Presentations

Hydrogen peroxide decomposes to water and oxygen. When used in closed spaces or under pressure, liberated oxygen cannot escape. Systemic oxygen embolization and surgical emphysema have been reported after ingestion and radiologic use. The diagnosis of hydrogen peroxide ingestion is suggested by white foam issuing from the mouth, nose, and/or anus. Clinical presentations may include shock, acute coronary insufficiency, respiratory arrest, status epilepticus, cerebrovascular accident, or sepsis. After colonic use, x-rays may reveal gas in the mesenteric, gastric, splenic, or portal venous systems, with or without gastric and duodenal distension.

After ingestion, gastric distension may occur. Gastritis, duodenitis and colitis have been reported. Pneumoretroperitoneum has been described. Oxygen embolization in the small intestinal veins and lymphatics may occur during irrigation of the ileum with 1% hydrogen peroxide. Hydrogen peroxide (1%) used as lavage for meconium ileus in an infant caused mesenteric and portal vein gas embolism and death. Colitis may follow the use of hydrogen peroxide enemas. Excess use of hydrogen peroxide with or without the use of sodium bicarbonate and salt as a mouth rinse may be abrasive to soft tissues of the gums.

Use of 3% hydrogen peroxide to disinfect soft contact lenses may lead to stinging, tearing, hyperemia, blepharospasm, edema, and corneal damage. Ingestion of household-strength peroxides is mildly irritating to the mucous membranes and may result in spontaneous emesis or mild abdominal bloating. Ingestions of industrial-strength peroxides can result in severe burns of the oropharynx and gastrointestinal tract, with the possibility of rupture of a hollow viscus secondary to the liberation of oxygen. The foam may cause obstruction of the respiratory tract and may result in mechanical asphyxia. Respiratory failure has been the alleged cause of death in fatalities reported after oral ingestion of industrial-strength (over 10%) hydrogen peroxide.

Toxic Dosage/Death

A specific toxic or lethal dose has not been identified.

Laboratory

Analytic Methods

Hydrogen peroxide levels are generally not available in hospital labs.

Blood Levels

Following hydrogen peroxide levels does not help guide management of exposures.

Treatment

Gut Decontamination

Gastric lavage is not recommended, as hydrogen peroxide may be corrosive. Activated charcoal, cathartics, or other gut decontamination procedures have not been shown to be useful after ingestion of industrial-strength hydrogen peroxide.

Elimination Enhancement

There are no procedures that routinely enhance the elimination of hydrogen peroxide.

Supportive Measures

- Hydrogen peroxide poisoning is generally treated with symptomatic and supportive measures.
- Early aggressive airway management is critical because respiratory failure and arrest appear to be the proximate cause of death. The patient may require endotracheal intubation. An IV line, oxygen, and cardiac monitor should be available. Arterial blood gases should be obtained. Seizures, potentially secondary to embolization, may require diazepam.
- Careful esophagogastroduodenoscopy is recommended soon after admission for significant ingestions. Antacids may be used for gastric burns, following endoscopy.
- Laparotomy may be required where there is evidence of air in the gastrointestinal tract.

Questions—Hydrogen Peroxide

1. Common household-strength hydrogen peroxide
A. Is usually a 3% concentrate
B. Usually results in life-threatening ingestions
C. Is used as a disinfectant and to clean out earwax
D. A and B
E. A and C

2. Treatment of hydrogen peroxide ingestion includes
A. Serum levels to guide management
B. Gastric lavage
C. Elimination enhancement
D. All of the above
E. None of the above

PHENOLS

Phenolics were among the first disinfectants used in hospitals. Certain detergent disinfectants belong to the phenol group, including phenol, para-tertiary butylphenol, and para-tertiary amylphenol. They are generally used for a wide range of bacteria, but they are not effective against spores. Phenolics are widely used on floors, walls, furnishings, glassware, and instruments. Phenol has also been used for "face peels" by plastic surgeons and in nerve blocks.

Pathophysiology

Phenolic compounds are characterized by the substitution of hydroxyl groups for one or more hydrogen groups on a benzene ring. Chemically related substances include cresol, creosote (oily mixture of phenolic and aromatic compounds), and hydroquinone. Eugenol is a phenolic compound that is present in clove cigarettes and possesses less irritant and central nervous system depression properties than phenol. Phenol does not uncouple oxidative phosphorylation like dinitrophenol and pentachlorophenol and does not cause a heat exhaustion-like syndrome.

Pharmacokinetics

Absorption

- Phenol is absorbed rapidly through the lungs and through the skin.
- The lungs of human volunteers absorbed 60–80% of an inhaled phenol dose in one study.

Distribution

- Dilution of phenol may increase absorption and may increase toxicity.

Elimination

- The urine may be dark because of an oxidation product of phenol metabolism.
- Most absorbed phenol is biotransformed by the liver to ethereal and glucuronide sulfates.
- Some phenol is excreted unchanged in the urine. The kidney rapidly excretes conjugated phenol metabolites, with elimination almost complete by 24 hours.

Clinical Presentations

Severe toxicity causes rapidly profound central nervous system depression with coma and respiratory arrest. An excitatory phase may be seen early. Convulsions may complicate the course of poisoning and have appeared as long as 18 hours after ingestion. Hypotension and ventricular tachycardia that require vasopressor and antiarrhythmic therapy, respectively, can occur. Chronic exposure to phenol may cause diarrhea, sore throat, pharyngeal sores, and dark urine.

Renal failure, fever, hypertension, adult respiratory distress syndrome, laryngeal edema, and death can follow cutaneous absorption of phenol. Cardiac arrhythmias have frequently been seen after cutaneous application. Use of throat spray (Chloraseptic®) containing phenol 1.5% may induce local throat burning, acute dyspnea, lethargy, vomiting, stridor, loss of consciousness, angioedema, rash, glossitis, and contact dermatitis.

Toxic Dosage/Death

Children have died after the application of 5% phenol compresses. A 10-year-old boy developed ventricular dysrhythmias following application of 6 mL (2.5 g) phenol to a giant hairy nevus on the skin. The lethal oral dose is estimated between 10–30 g, although an adult survived a 26.7-g ingestion without permanent sequelae. Fatalities have occurred after ingestions of as little as 2 g of pure phenol and 4.8 g.

Laboratory

Analytic Methods

A microtechnique for quantifying phenol in plasma uses gas chromatography-mass spectrometry and is sensitive to 0.1 mg/L.

Blood Levels

Following blood levels does not guide management in overdose. Urinary phenol levels above 81 mg/L suggest excessive exposure in workers. Postmortem plasma phenol concentrations after poisoning have ranged from 27–130 mg/L.

Treatment

Gut Decontamination

Because of the rapid onset of symptoms, possible increased phenol absorption with dilution, and the potential for development of seizures, activated charcoal (1 g/kg) is preferable to lavage or syrup of ipecac. *In vitro* studies indicate that activated charcoal efficiently absorbs phenol.

Elimination Enhancement

Hemodialysis probably does not increase removal significantly, but *in vitro* studies suggest that charcoal hemoperfusion effectively removes free phenol.

Supportive Measures

- The management of severe exposures initially focuses on establishment of a patent airway, confirmation of breathing and hemodynamic support. Intubation and/or pressors may be required after large overdoses.
- Metabolic acidosis can complicate severe phenol toxicity, but whether the acidosis is a primary or secondary event is not clear. The urine may be dark because of an oxidation product of phenol metabolism.
- When working with phenol, workers should be provided with and required to use protective clothing, gloves, face shields, splash-proof safety goggles, and other appropriate protective clothing necessary to prevent any possibility of skin or eye contact with solid or liquid phenol or liquids containing phenol.
- If there is any possibility that the clothing has been contaminated with phenol, a worker should change into uncontaminated clothing before leaving the work area and the suspect clothing should be stored in closed containers until it is discarded or until provision is made for removal of the phenol. The worker laundering or cleaning such clothes should be informed of phenol's hazardous properties.
- Skin that becomes contaminated with phenol should be immediately washed with soap or mild detergent and rinsed with water.

Questions—Phenols

1. Phenol is used for all of the following except

A. Disinfecting against bacteria and spores
B. Face peels
C. Clove cigarettes
D. Nerve blocks
E. Instrument cleaning

2. Symptoms of phenol toxicity may include

A. Central nervous system excitation
B. Central nervous system depression
C. Hypertension
D. Hypotension
E. All of the above

Soaps and Shampoos

SOAPS

Soaps are sold as personal hygiene bars or liquids, although some handwashing and dishwashing products appear as soap flakes. To promote wetting and emulsification, heavy-duty soaps contain inorganic builders (e.g., phosphates, carbonates, silicates, sodium citrate, and aluminosilicates). These agents alter pH and inactivate hard-water minerals (e.g., calcium) which interfere with the cleaning properties of the soap. Hand soaps and light-duty laundry soaps generally are "unbuilt" (contain no builders), while heavy-duty laundry soaps usually are "built" (contain builders). Minerals in hard water combine with soaps to form insoluble precipitates (scum), which may impart an undesirable grayish color to clothes.

SHAMPOOS

Most soap-based shampoos have been replaced by nonionic and anionic surfactants. Some liquid shampoos contain alkyl sodium sulfate, which has more mucosal irritant properties than nonionic surfactants. Most additive agents such as selenium, salicylic acid, and resorcinol in antidandruff preparations, and preservatives, fragrances, and coloring agents are not present in concentrations high enough to contribute to systemic toxicity, but some of the agents may produce an allergic dermatitis.

Dry shampoos may contain methanol or isopropanol. Industrial-strength rug shampoos and carpet-cleaning products may contain potentially toxic compounds, especially when the products are not properly diluted. These compounds include sodium carbonate, sodium perborate, sodium phosphate, ammonia compounds, borax, pine oil, trichloroethylene, tetrachloroethylene, naphtha, naphthalene, kerosene, petroleum solvents, alkyl benzene sulfonate, and alkyl-aryl sodium sulfonate.

PATHOPHYSIOLOGY

Soaps are salts of fatty acids produced by the action of alkali on fats. Shampoos are irritants.

CLINICAL PRESENTATIONS

Soaps are mild gastrointestinal and mucous membrane irritants, which occasionally produce nausea, vomiting, diarrhea, and abdominal pain. Some deodorant bars contain photosensitizing agents (e.g., biocides, perfumes, and detergents). Most ingredients (e.g., hexachlorophene) are present in concentrations too low to produce toxicity.

Household shampoos usually produce only mild gastrointestinal tract irritation. Rug shampoos may cause a respiratory illness characterized by cough, headache, sore throat, dyspnea, fatigue, nausea, and other gastrointestinal complaints. See Chapter 46, Hydrocarbons, for clinical presentations of hydrocarbon-containing shampoos.

TREATMENT

Gut Decontamination

Emesis, lavage and charcoal are unnecessary in pure soap ingestions. Symptomatic treatment, including milk or water dilution and several hours of observation for spontaneous vomiting, usually suffices in most household shampoo exposures. Heavy-duty or industrial-strength solution exposures may require further treatment (e.g., lavage) if highly toxic substances are involved (see specific treatment sections under individual toxins).

Elimination Enhancement

These methods are unnecessary as overdoses are mild and symptoms are self-limited.

Supportive Measures

- Irrigate symptomatic ocular exposures with saline (water is an acceptable alternative if saline is unavailable). Minor ocular irritation may benefit from a soothing agent (e.g., a vasoconstrictor solution containing naphazoline). Local ophthalmic anesthetic agents (e.g., tetracaine) should not be prescribed for outpatient use.
- Administer clear liquids and an antiemetic as needed for gastrointestinal symptoms.

Questions—Soaps and Shampoos

1. All of the following may follow ingestion of soap except
- A. Nausea
- B. Vomiting
- C. Diarrhea
- D. Lower tract gastrointestinal bleeding
- E. Abdominal pain

2. Which of the following statements is true?
- A. Household shampoos usually produce gastrointestinal (GI) and respiratory symptoms.
- B. Household shampoos usually produce predominantly respiratory symptoms.
- C. Rug shampoos usually produce predominantly GI symptoms.
- D. Rug shampoos usually produce GI and respiratory symptoms.
- E. None of the above

Detergents

Detergents contain synthetic, organic, surface-active agents called surfactants, which are derived from petroleum product precursors. In contrast, soaps are the natural products of fatty acids. Surfactants are designed to lower the surface tension of water and thereby reduce the insoluble precipitates formed by soaps and hard water. Surfactant classification is based on molecular changes required to increase water solubility.

Detergents may contain a variety of additives (e.g., bleaches, bacteriocidal agents, enzymes, perfumes, colorants, whitening agents, softeners) but their concentrations are generally too low to produce primary irritation. These additives may, however, cause contact dermatitis.

Liquid detergents are similar to granular detergents but exist as aqueous or hydroalcoholic solutions. Alcohol concentrations are too low to cause toxicity except in large ingestions. The toxicity of liquid detergents is considered lower than that of detergent granules, although larger amounts may be ingested. Liquid dishwashing detergent (*not* laundry or electric dishwashing detergents) has been recommended as a substitute emetic when syrup of ipecac is unavailable.

AMPHOTERIC SURFACTANTS

These compounds contain both anionic and cationic surface-active molecules and occur more commonly in industrial cleaning products.

ANIONIC SURFACTANTS

The surface-active property of these compounds resides in negatively charged ions. Examples include sodium, potassium, and ammonium salts of fatty acids and sulfonated and phosphorylated hydrocarbons (e.g., alkyl sodium sulfate, sodium lauryl sulfate). Anionic compounds are the most common surfactants used in commercial detergents. Anionic surfactants are irritants, with the major exception of electric dishwasher products, in which builders enhance alkalinity.

CATIONIC SURFACTANTS

Cationic surfactants use quaternary ammonia compounds with positively charged surface-active moieties (e.g., benzalkonium chloride). Commercial application includes use in disinfectants, industrial and institutional products, fabric softeners, antistatic compounds, and swimming pool algicides. Concentrated cationic solutions (10–15%) are caustic, and even dilute solutions (0.1–0.5%) may produce significant mucosal irritation. Large ingestions may produce central nervous system symptoms.

NONIONIC SURFACTANTS

This group includes electrically neutral medium- to long-chain polyether sulfates, alcohols, or sulfonates (e.g., alkyl-aryl polyether sulfates). They appear in heavy-duty laundry liquids, nonphosphate granular products, and many low-sudsing laundry products. Most household products contain either anionic or nonionic surfactants. Nonionic surfactants produce less local irritation than anionic surfactants.

Pathophysiology

Manufacturers add inorganic "builders" to detergents to improve their wetting and emulsifying properties. Hard-water minerals such as calcium inhibit these properties. Most heavy-duty detergents contain builders and include inorganic salts such as phosphates, carbonates, silicates, sodium citrate, and aluminosilicates. Environmental concerns have led to the production of low-phosphate, biodegradable detergent products. Complex phosphate-containing detergents produced before 1965 decomposed slowly in surface water and sewage plants. Their presence in environmental water produced sudsing and eutrophication (enhanced algae production) in lakes.

Increasing concentrations of nonphosphate builders, especially silicates and carbonates, produce more irritating formulations. Although trisodium phosphate is more biodegradable, its presence significantly enhances product causticity (e.g., electric dishwasher detergent). Most builders help adjust the pH of detergent solutions toward acceptable ranges except in specific products (e.g., electric dishwasher detergents).

Clinical Presentations

Most exposures to household cleaning products do not result in symptoms. Symptomatic patients most often have gastrointestinal complaints such as nausea, vomiting, and diarrhea. Granular laundry detergents, liquid laundry detergents, and liquid dishwashing agents produce more nausea, vomiting, and diarrhea than fabric softeners or soaps. Abdominal pain is uncommon except in automatic dishwashing detergents. Symptoms typically resolve within 24 hours.

In contrast to anionic or nonionic detergents, cationic detergents produce systemic toxicity and, in rare circumstances, death. Concentrations above 1% are mucosal irritants that may produce gastrointestinal distress. Systemic symptoms may include apprehension, restlessness, confusion, muscle weakness, respiratory paralysis, and hypotension.

Most laundry products are mild mucosal irritants and can produce a mild chemical conjunctivitis as well as gastrointestinal irritation. Sensitizing halogenated sulfones can form in liquid dishwashing solutions containing the anionic surfactant alkyl ether sulfate. The resulting product causes an allergic contact dermatitis. Cationic detergents are more potent irritants than anionic or nonionic detergents. High (20%) concentration cationic detergents possess the potential to produce esophageal and gastric erosion as well as perforation and peritonitis. Automatic dishwasher detergents may produce significant ocular and oropharyngeal burns and esophago-gastric erosions.

Toxic Dosage/Death

Death has occurred after intentional ingestion of a low-phosphate detergent. The fatal adult dose of cationic detergents is estimated to be between 1–3 g.

Treatment

Gut Decontamination. Most detergent and soap ingestions require only dilution with water or milk. Patients should be observed at home several hours in the upright position for spontaneous vomiting. Cationic detergents such as quaternary ammonium compounds (e.g., benzalkonium chloride) generally require gut decontamination (emesis, dilution, lavage) except when a small amount has been ingested (less than a swallow), the concentration is less than 1%, or the time since ingestion exceeds several hours.

Ingestion of agents containing greater than 5–10% cationic detergents should be treated as caustic ingestions (immediate dilution plus esophagoscopy as needed). Transient contact with cationic detergent requires only dilution. Large cationic detergent ingestions may be treated with charcoal, although no clinical studies have demonstrated clear effectiveness.

Elimination Enhancement

These methods have not been used to treat the effects of these agents.

Supportive Measures

- Dilution, support and observation are generally sufficient.
- Copiously irrigate all eye exposures with saline for 20 minutes. Be sure to retract the eyelids to search for granules. Each patient should receive an eye examination, including fluorescein staining to detect corneal abrasions.
- Hypocalcemia and tetany are rare complications of phosphate-containing detergent ingestions.
- Published evidence that weak soap solutions bind quaternary ammonium compounds to prevent absorption is lacking. Since most soaps now contain anionic surfactants, the recommended use of soap for these ingestions is not practical.

Questions—Detergents

1. **Most exposures to household cleaning products**
   A. Do not result in symptoms
   B. Result in moderate gastrointestinal symptoms
   C. Result in moderate respiratory symptoms
   D. Result in symptoms lasting 24-48 hours
   E. None of the above
2. **Treatment of detergent or soap ingestions may include all of the following except**
   A. Dilution with water
   B. Dilution with milk
   C. Maintenance of upright position for spontaneous vomiting
   D. Gut decontamination
   E. Elimination enhancement

Bleaches

Most household bleaches (e.g., Clorox®) contain less than 5% sodium hypochlorite and may cause mucosal irritation if ingested. Commercial chlorine bleaches may be significantly more concentrated and more caustic. Granular bleaches are considered more toxic because the granules prolong mucosal contact and because solid bleaches tend to be more concentrated. Commercial bleaches contain other agents (e.g., sodium peroxide, sodium perborate, sodium carbonate, and oxalic acid), and proper therapy requires accurate identification. See Chapter 42, Acids, Bases and Gastroesophageal Issues.

PATHOPHYSIOLOGY

Bleaches are bases and may cause liquefaction necrosis after prolonged significant exposures. Household products, generally below pH 12.5, are mild to moderate mucosal irritants.

CLINICAL PRESENTATIONS

Mixing hypochlorite solutions with acid (such as toilet bowl or tile cleaner) results in release of chlorine gas. The combined use of calcium hypochlorite and trichloro-s-triazinetrione, both chlorinating agents, may induce an explosive release of chlorine gas. When ammonia interacts with hypochlorite-containing products, a combination of monochloramine and dichloramine, fumes known as chloramine are produced.

Gastrointestinal Effects

Products with a pH below 12.5 generally do not cause serious burns after transient exposures. However, moderately alkaline liquids (e.g., bleaches with a pH of 11–12) may produce deep, partial-thickness chemical burns after large, intentional ingestions. Bleaches produce a high percentage of nausea, vomiting, and abdominal pain when taken by mouth. Industrial-strength hypochlorite bleaches (15–20% solutions) may induce caustic injuries. Sodium peroxide decomposes in the stomach by releasing oxygen and may cause gastritis. Sodium perborate is metabolized to peroxide and borate, which has moderate mucosal-irritating properties and systemic effects. Esophageal irritation depends on volume ingested, viscosity, gastric content, pH concentration, pyloric tonicity, and duration of contact.

Pulmonary Effects

Sodium hypochlorite solutions may release small amounts of hypochlorous acid and chlorine gas, but usually the concentrations of these toxic gases are too low to cause damage. Mixing solutions of ammonia and sodium hypochlorite produces monochloramine and dichloramine fumes. Chloramine fumes in a confined bathroom may result in a chemical pneumonitis. Prolonged inhalation of chloramine fumes can produce obstructive pulmonary deficits, chest infiltrates, and acute pulmonary edema.

Dermatologic Effects

Skin, eye, and esophageal irritation depend on volume, viscosity, pH concentration, and duration of contact. Generally, products with a pH below 12.5 do not cause serious burns, but failure to remove bleaches with a pH of 11–12 may produce partial-thickness chemical burns. A desquamating erythematous rash, which progresses to exfoliation ("boiled lobster" syndrome), characterizes severe, acute boric acid toxicity after sodium perborate ingestions.

Neurologic Effects

Sodium perborate ingestion has been associated with convulsions, hypotension, restlessness, agitation, and delirium progressing to apnea and coma.

TREATMENT

Gut Decontamination

Immediate dilution with water or milk has been recommended as the first-aid procedure of choice for suspected caustic ingestion; however, the efficacy and rationale for this maneuver remain somewhat controversial. Exposure to products such as industrial-strength hypochlorite solution and perborate should be evaluated as a potential caustic exposure. Charcoal is probably not helpful. Lavage may be dangerous after ingestion of industrial-strength bleaches.

Elimination Enhancement

Methods to enhance elimination do not help in the treatment of these exposures.

Supportive Measures

- Observation, support and dilution with clear liquids or milk are generally all that is required after mild household bleach exposures.
- Decontaminate both skin and eyes with copious saline irrigation. Be sure to remove all contaminated clothing (e.g., diapers in chlorine bleach exposure). Check all exposed eyes for corneal abrasions with fluorescein staining.
- Chlorine exposures require evaluation of acid-base and respiratory status. Treatment of bleach exposures with acid solutions may cause heat and exothermic reactions and is not advised.
- Pulmonary edema may occur up to 24 hours after chloramine exposure. Patients who are well 24 hours after exposure may be discharged. Persistent hypoxemia can be associated with a high mortality. Intravenous fluids should be given with great caution. Fluid overload is very dangerous in these patients, and diuretics such as furosemide may be useful as indicated.
- Corticosteroids are controversial in the patient with pulmonary edema, and clinical studies evaluating their efficacy are lacking. The patient with persistent hypoxemia may require positive end-expiratory airway pressure (PEEP), in addition to supplemental oxygen.
- Nebulized sodium bicarbonate may ameliorate respiratory symptoms by neutralizing the acid found when chlorine gas encounters water in the airways. This may result in an exothermic reaction. Patients should be carefully monitored before and after this procedure. Few clinical studies have confirmed this approach. It is not known if such therapy is safe or effective for severe toxicity (e.g., pulmonary edema and respiratory compromise).

Questions—Bleaches

1. Symptoms of bleach ingestion may include all of the following except

A. Deep partial-thickness burns
B. Gastritis
C. Chemical pneumonitis
D. Convulsions
E. Coma

2. Immediate dilution with water or milk has been recommended as the first-aid procedure of choice for suspected caustic ingestion; however, the efficacy and rationale for this maneuver remain somewhat controversial.

A. True
B. False

Pine Oil and Turpentine

Liquid household cleaners contain more toxic constituents (e.g., acids, glycol ethers, petroleum distillates, pine oil) than synthetic detergents. Pine oil is a mixture of highly lipophilic, unsaturated, cyclic hydrocarbons that is one-fifth as toxic as turpentine in animals. Pine-scented household cleaners contain small amounts of pine oil and have minimal toxicity compared with Pine Sol® (20–35% pine oil). See Chapter 46, Hydrocarbons.

Turpentine is a natural solvent composed of pine oils, camphenes, and terpenes. The volatile components of turpentine (α-pinene, β-pinene, and δ-3-carene) are significant pulmonary aspiration hazards.

PATHOPHYSIOLOGY

Turpentine is a central nervous system depressant and mucous membrane irritant, and possesses high volatility with low viscosity.

CLINICAL PRESENTATIONS

Pine Oil

Pine oil produces primarily gastrointestinal irritation (hemorrhagic gastritis, substernal chest pain, nausea, vomiting, diarrhea) and central nervous system depression (weakness, respiratory failure, hypothermia). The most common symptoms reported in one survey were somnolence, gastroenteritis, agitation, delirium, headache, ataxia, and weakness. Renal failure may occur, but death is rare. The lungs excrete pine oil constituents, resulting in a characteristic violetlike odor.

Turpentine

Turpentine is a local irritant, central nervous system depressant, and pulmonary aspiration hazard. It is similar to other volatile oils such as camphor, sassafras, eucalyptus, and wintergreen; however, acute turpentine toxicity is less severe than that of these volatile oils. Casual exposures may produce mucosal irritation, mild respiratory tract inflammation, and urinary tract irritation. In large intentional doses, coma and convulsions may occur. Pulmonary aspiration of turpentine may produce a hemorrhagic pulmonary edema. The ingestion of turpentine has been associated with the onset of thrombocytopenic purpura in several children.

TOXIC DOSAGE/DEATH

The suggested adult lethal dose of pine oil is 60–120 g, although survival without sequelae after an ingestion of 400–500 g has been reported. As little as 15 mL of turpentine may produce symptoms in children, and 120–180 ml is a potentially lethal adult dose.

TREATMENT

Gut Decontamination

Most accidental ingestions of household cleaners (including hydrocarbons) require only dilution with milk or water to reduce mucosal-irritant properties. Turpentine ingestions should be treated like toluene exposures, and gut decontamination measures should only be used when the ingestion exceeds approximately 2 mL/kg. Patients who ingest more than several swallows of concentrated pine oil products (e.g., Pine Sol®, which contains 20–35% pine oil) should be lavaged provided their gag reflex is intact or their airway is protected. Emesis may be helpful in large ingestions and when patients present within 30 minutes of exposure; however, this intervention remains controversial after pine oil and turpentine ingestions.

Elimination Enhancement

These methods have not been utilized in the treatment of overdose with these agents.

Supportive Measures

- Be sure to check product contents to determine the appropriateness of decontamination measures. Treatment is generally symptomatic and supportive. Delirium may be treated with benzodiazepines.
- Aspiration pneumonitis is treated with oxygen, antibiotics and blood gas determinations. Admission is generally warranted. See Chapter 46, Hydrocarbons, regarding the treatment of hydrocarbon aspiration.

Questions—Pine Oil and Turpentine

1. Pine oil poisoning
A. Produces primarily pulmonary irritation
B. Frequently causes somnolence and headache
C. Often causes renal failure or death
D. Results in a characteristic rose-like odor
E. None of the above

2. Turpentine poisoning
A. Can cause urinary tract irritation
B. Can cause hemorrhagic pulmonary edema
C. Can lead to thrombocytopenic purpura
D. A and B
E. A, B and C

3. Most accidental ingestions of household cleaners require only dilution with milk or water to reduce mucosal-irritant properties.
A. True
B. False

PERSONAL PRODUCTS

Cosmetics

The cosmetic industry selects from more than 5,000 different ingredients. Cosmetics and personal care products constituted the third most frequently involved category of human exposures reported to poison centers in 1997. Cosmetics contain moisturizers, preservatives, antioxidants, antimicrobials, thickeners, solvents, emulsifiers, coloring agents, and pH adjusters. Many of these ingredients are discussed elsewhere (see individual chapters). Some properties of major cosmetic classes include the following:

BATH PREPARATIONS

Bubble bath usually contains mildly toxic anionic and nonionic surfactants along with alcohols and preservatives. The presence of trisodium phosphate builders enhances causticity. Bath salts may contain borax, which causes boric acid poisoning in large ingestions in addition to mucosal irritation. Bath oils contain vegetable and mineral oils. Volatile essential oils may produce systemic complaints after large ingestions.

COLOGNES

Toxicity depends on ethanol concentration, which may range from 50–95%.

CONDITIONERS

These products contain synthetic cationic surfactants, perfumes, and alcohols.

DENTAL PRODUCTS

Toothpaste, tooth powders, and tooth liquids contain nontoxic constituents such as calcium phosphates, alumina, abradants, and anionic surfactants. Fluoride concentrations are generally too small to contribute to acute toxicity. Mouthwashes and breath fresheners usually contain alcohol, flavoring, and sweeteners. Toxicity depends on the ethanol content. Denture cleaners contain bicarbonates, borates, phosphates, and carbonates, some of which may be caustic. The methyl methacrylate constituent of acrylic denture material may produce a contact dermatitis in health care professionals.

DEODORANTS

The aluminum and zinc included in deodorants for their antiperspirant properties have limited toxicity because of packaging and formulations.

HAIR COLORATION

Permanent hair colors contain an oxidizer, which usually is 6% hydrogen peroxide, and a dye intermediate. Semipermanent hair colors (for covering gray) contain propylene glycol, isopropanol, fatty acids, fragrance, alkanolamines, and dyes. Some formulations contain lead.

HAIR STRAIGHTENERS

May contain highly caustic sodium hydroxide with a pH as high as 13. Ingestion by children has resulted in drooling, vomiting, lip swelling, redness, and blisters.

HAIR WAVING

Waving lotions possess thioglycolic acids and ammonia sulfides. Most wave neutralizer solutions contain hydrogen peroxide, sodium bromate, or sodium perborate in mildly acidic solutions. Some permanent wave fixatives contain mercuric chloride, which has caused severe mercury poisoning in an adult. Bromate salts can be extremely toxic and may cause deafness and renal failure.

MAKEUP PRODUCTS

Because they usually contain innocuous ingredients and are sold in small packages, these compounds are generally nontoxic, except for local hypersensitivity reactions.

NAIL POLISH AND REMOVERS

Nail polish contains hydrocarbon solvents such as xylene, toluene, and acetone, alcohols such as methanol, and ethanol, plasticizers, and resins such as nitrocellulose. The chief ingredients of nail polish remover are solvents such as acetone or ethanol.

PERFUMES

Toxicity depends on ethanol concentration, which may range from 50–95%.

Clinical Presentations

Most accidental cosmetic exposures result in no symptoms or minor gastrointestinal upset. Systemic symptoms are unusual. Skin care products, hair preparations, and facial makeup are often associated with contact dermatitis. Fragrances, preservatives (such as quaternium-15, formaldehyde, imidazolidinyl urea, and parabens), p-phenylenediamine, and glycerol monothioglycolate are the most frequent skin sensitizers.

Ethanol

Perfumes, colognes, mouthwashes, and toilet water may contain substantial amounts of ethanol and produce intoxication. Hypoglycemia may complicate ethanol intoxication, especially in children.

Potassium Bromate

This clear, odorless and tasteless compound is an extremely toxic agent that can produce nausea, vomiting, diarrhea, deafness, acute renal failure, hypotension, central nervous system depression, and hemolysis. Gastrointestinal symptoms usually begin within one-half hour of ingestion. Both the otic symptoms and renal impairment may be permanent. Renal biopsies indicate primarily tubular damage, which can progress to interstitial fibrosis and glomerular sclerosis.

Sodium Perborate

This compound decomposes to sodium borate and peroxide and produces less toxicity than potassium bromate. Cutaneous manifestations after oral ingestion are characterized by a "boiled lobster" appearance with a desquamating, erythematous rash commonly over the buttocks, scrotum, palms, and soles. This rash may progress to exfoliation. Central nervous system symptoms may range from irritability, restlessness, and headache to coma and convulsions in severe cases. Anorexia, nausea, vomiting, and diarrhea are common, and severe cases may display hematochezia. Acute renal tubular necrosis occurs in moderate to severe cases and may result in renal failure.

Volatile Oils

Also called essential oils, examples include sage, eucalyptus, turpentine, pine, pennyroyal, and cinnamon. These colorless liquids contain cyclic hydrocarbons, ethers, alcohols, esters, and ketones. Essential oils are moderate mucosal irritants, which can lead to gastrointestinal distress and salivation. Concentrated formulations of essential oils can produce convulsions in adults and central nervous system depression. Chemical pneumonitis result from aspiration, but high viscosity limits toxicity to a chemical lipoid pneumonia. See Chapter 55, Herbal Medicines, Volatile Oils and Plant Dermatitis.

Laboratory

Analytic Methods

Various methods apply to individual agents.

Blood Levels

Potassium bromate exposures are potentially quite serious. Toxicity does not correlate with serum bromide levels. Blood levels in most cosmetic overdoses are unhelpful in guiding management.

Treatment

Gut Decontamination

Most ingestions of cosmetics do not require any form of gut decontamination. Cationic surfactants, perborate, and substantial essential oil ingestions may benefit from lavage and/or charcoal if taken shortly after presentation; however, proof that these interventions substantially alter outcome is lacking.

Elimination Enhancement

The role of early dialysis in the prevention of nephrotoxicity and ototoxicity after potassium bromate exposure remains unproved.

Supportive Measures

- Since most cosmetics are nontoxic, only supportive care and perhaps dilution are required.

- Potassium bromate exposures are potentially quite serious. Lavage may be helpful if the patient presents within a few hours of ingestion. Lavage with 2% sodium bicarbonate solution has been advocated, as has the intravenous administration of 10–50 ml of 10% sodium thiosulfate at a maximum rate of 3 mL/min, to reduce bromate to the less toxic bromide ion. (An alternative intravenous solution is 100–500 mL of 1% sodium thiosulfate.)
- All symptomatic patients after potassium bromate ingestion should be observed in the hospital for the development of renal and/or otic damage.
- Ethanol exposures may be associated with hypoglycemia, particularly in children. Glucose should routinely be checked after pediatric perfume, cologne and toilet water ingestions.

Questions—Cosmetics

1. Which of the following products is incorrectly matched?
A. Bath salts–Mucosal irritation
B. Hair dyes–Lead content
C. Deodorants–Mercuric chloride content
D. Makeup products–Local hypersensitivity reactions
E. Perfumes–50-95% ethanol concentration

2. Which of the following personal product ingredients is incorrectly matched?
A. Ethanol–Intoxication may be complicated by hypoglycemia
B. Hydrogen peroxide–Large ingestions may produce mild gastritis
C. Potassium bromide–Can produce permanent renal damage
D. Sodium perborate–Can produce permanent deafness
E. Volatile oils–Can produce seizures and central nervous system depression

Tobacco Products

Nicotine is a highly toxic alkaloid, which is the principal pharmacologically active component in cigarettes and cigars. It is ubiquitous around the world and is found in measurable quantities in smokers as well as nonsmokers. Poisoning occurs in children who ingest cigarettes, snuff, and nicotine gum, and less often industrially in the tobacco and insecticide industries. Poisoning may also occur in adults who smoke or chew tobacco, and in those involved in the processing and extraction of tobacco (green tobacco sickness). Tobacco pouches may release varying amounts of nicotine. They are mistakenly considered a safe alternative to more conventional tobacco products, although there is cumulative evidence of production of oral cancer.

The nicotine content of the plants *Nicotiana tabacum* (cultivated tobacco) and *Nicotiana rustica* ranges from 1-6%. Blending of tobacco typically results in a tobacco nicotine content of 1–2%. In the 1950s, plain, short cigarettes contained 30 to 40 mg of tar and 2.1 mg of nicotine. The king-size filter tips of the 1960s contained less than 20 mg of tar and less than 1.7 mg of nicotine. By the 1980s, cigarettes contained 15 mg of tar and 1.3 mg of nicotine. Smokers have compensated for lower nicotine contents by consuming more cigarettes. Of the available nicotine, 10–50% is absorbed during mouth puffing and 80–100% during deep lung inhalation. A single cigarette puff delivers approximately 0.05–0.15 mg of nicotine.

Cigarette smoking is the number one public health problem in the United States and is the single largest preventable cause of disease and death. Each year, more than 350,000 premature deaths are attributed to smoking, including 170,000 deaths from coronary heart disease, 130,000 deaths from cancer, and 50,000 deaths from obstructive lung disease. These figures do not include fetal and neonatal deaths caused by smoking during pregnancy or hundreds of deaths caused by fires attributed to cigarette smoking.

Depending on the region, a significant number of male high school and college students regularly use snuff or chewing tobacco. Such products contain at least three types of chemical carcinogens: benzopyrene, polonium 210, and nitrosamines. Chronic snuff use commonly leads to oral leukoplakia, which is a premalignant lesion. Moderate use of smokeless tobacco causes a four to sevenfold increase in the risk of oral cancer.

Nicotine gum has been approved by the FDA for prescription use as an aid in smoking cessation. Each piece of gum contains nicotine bound to an ion-exchange resin in a sugar-free, flavored gum base, with a bicarbonate buffer. Chewing one piece for 20–30 minutes releases 90% of the nicotine.

PATHOPHYSIOLOGY

Initially, and only briefly, nicotine is stimulating to the autonomic nervous system ganglia and neuromuscular junction. The most prominent effects relate to stimulation of the adrenal medulla, central nervous system, cardiovascular system via release of catecholamines, gastrointestinal tract via parasympathetic stimulation, salivary and bronchial glands, and the medullary-vomiting center. There is subsequent blockade of autonomic ganglia and the neuromuscular junction transmission, inhibition of catecholamine release from the adrenal medulla, and central nervous system depression.

PHARMACOKINETICS

Absorption

- The oral mucosa, respiratory tract, gastrointestinal tract (except the stomach), and skin absorb nicotine readily. In an alkaline medium, there is an increase in the small amount of nicotine absorbed in the stomach.
- Nicotine from gum is absorbed through the buccal mucosa.

Distribution

- Nicotine undergoes a large first-pass effect during which the liver metabolizes 80–90%.
- The apparent volume of distribution in animals is approximately 1.0 L/kg, whereas in one clinical study it was 2.0 L/kg in smokers and 3.0 L/kg in nonsmokers.
- Peak serum levels of nicotine are attained in 15–30 minutes while chewing nicotine gum, much longer than the time to peak after smoking a cigarette (2 minutes).

Elimination

- Nicotine and its metabolites are excreted in the urine.
- At a pH of 5.5 or less, 23% is excreted unchanged. At a pH of 8, 2% is excreted in the urine.
- The plasma terminal half-life of nicotine is 2–2.2 hours.
- Cotinine is the major metabolite of nicotine. It has a half-life of 10–20 hours.

CLINICAL PRESENTATIONS

Nicotine is an exceedingly lethal poison, but few deaths have been reported from its use alone. Serious toxicity resulting from ingestion of cigarette tobacco is rare. Symptoms of nicotine alkaloid poisoning may develop within 15 minutes. The onset of symptoms is much more rapid after the ingestion of liquid nicotine (e.g., insecticides, teas) compared with nicotine-containing organic material (plant parts). Death may occur within 5 minutes of ingestion of concentrated nicotine insecticides.

Gastrointestinal Effects
Gastrointestinal signs and symptoms occur first and include mouth and throat burning followed by profuse salivation, nausea, vomiting, abdominal pain, and occasionally diarrhea.

Neurologic Effects
Headache, confusion, dizziness, agitation, restlessness, and incoordination develop initially after serious nicotine overdoses. Within 30 minutes, in severe poisonings, convulsions and coma occur. Cholinergic signs initially include diaphoresis, salivation, lacrimation, increased bronchial secretions, and miosis. Later, mydriasis may be seen. Neuromuscular symptoms include hypotonia, decreased deep tendon reflexes, weakness, fasciculations, and muscle paralysis, including respiratory muscles. Subarachnoid hemorrhage is 5.7 times more common in smokers than in nonsmokers. The risk of subarachnoid hemorrhage in women who smoke and take oral contraceptives is 22 times that in women who do not smoke and do not use oral contraceptives.

Respiratory Effects
Initial tachypnea, but later dyspnea, decreased respiratory rate, and cyanosis may be seen with nicotine poisoning. Respiratory arrest may occur within minutes. Cigarette smoking is the major cause of chronic obstructive lung disease in the U.S. in both men and women.

Cardiovascular Effects
A transient increase in blood pressure followed by hypotension, bradycardia, paroxysmal atrial fibrillation, or cardiac standstill may be observed after nicotine poisoning. Cigarette smoking is associated with accelerated coronary artery disease, sudden cardiac death and hypertension.

Carcinogenic Effects
Cigarette smoking is a major cause of cancer of the lung, larynx, esophagus, and oral cavity and a contributing factor in causing cancer of the urinary bladder, kidney, and pancreas in both men and women. Approximately 30% of deaths from cancer have been attributed to smoking. Other data suggest that the risk of developing cancer increases as a result of passive inhalation of smoke.

Green Tobacco Sickness
This entity occurs in workers who do not smoke but who work with wet, uncured tobacco. They may experience nausea, vomiting, and/or prostration.

Addiction
Need for oral gratification and other psychological problems may result in withdrawal symptoms including anxiety, impaired concentration and memory, depression, hostility, sleep disturbances, and increased appetite. Correlations between smoking and alcoholism have been observed. Psychological and physical habituation to smoking is a complex and largely insoluble problem for most smokers. Nicotine gum and transdermal nicotine may reduce cigarette craving.

Nicotine Gum
Nicotine gum may aggravate coronary heart disease, vasospastic disease, hypertension, peptic ulcers, diabetes, hyperthyroidism, and esophagitis. It is contraindicated in smokers who have had a recent myocardial infarction, who have life-threatening arrhythmias, severe or worsening angina, temporomandibular joint disease, or who are pregnant.

Cigarette Ingestions
Children ingesting less than 2 cigarettes or less than 6 cigarette butts may experience vomiting within 20 minutes. Lethargy or irritability is observed infrequently and completely resolves. The absence of vomiting predicts a favorable outcome. Cigarette ingestions in children rarely require specific treatment. Ingestions of more than 2 whole cigarettes or 6 butts are potentially toxic and should be referred to the emergency department regardless of symptoms. Decontamination of the mouth with water and administration of ipecac have been recommended before transport to the emergency department.

TOXIC DOSAGE/DEATH
Nicotine is highly toxic. Two to five mg may cause nausea and 40–60 mg may be lethal; however, survival has followed ingestions of 1–4 g. Four to eight mg orally may produce serious symptoms in nonhabituated individuals.

DRUG INTERACTIONS
By enhancing the production of drug-metabolizing enzymes, cigarettes alter the metabolism of caffeine, glutethimide, propranolol, theophylline, imipramine, lidocaine, pentazocine, phenacetin, and warfarin. Smoking cigarettes appears to have no effect on the clearance of alcohol, chlordiazepoxide, chlorpromazine, diazepam, meperidine, nortriptyline, or phenytoin.

PREGNANCY/LACTATION
Nicotine passes into breast milk in small quantities, which are not clinically significant. Heavy smoking (more than 20 cigarettes per day) may alter the supply of milk and cause vomiting in the infant. There is a greater danger to the infant from "second-hand smoking" (i.e., inhaling smoke from others). Cigarette smoking increases the risk of pneumonia, bronchitis, and sudden infant death syndrome.

Pregnant smokers deliver babies who are lighter and smaller. The risk of spontaneous abortion, fetal death, and neonatal death increases as does the frequency of abruptio placentae, placenta previa, early or late bleeding during pregnancy, premature and prolonged rupture of membranes, and preterm delivery.

The term "fetal tobacco syndrome" is applied to an infant when the mother smokes five or more cigarettes per day throughout the pregnancy, the mother has no evidence of hypertension during pregnancy and the newborn has symmetrical growth retardation at term (37 weeks or more). The parameters of retardation are defined by a birth weight less than 2,500 g and a ponderal index (weight in grams × 100/length in cm) greater than 2.32.

LABORATORY

Analytic Methods
A rapid high-pressure liquid chromatography assay is available.

Blood Levels
Plasma nicotine levels correlate well with absorbed dose and can provide a means of evaluating occupational exposure to nicotine, but the short half-life of nicotine in plasma requires that blood be drawn shortly after exposure. Prior smoking may affect levels. After cigarette smoking, typical nicotine levels are 18.3–22 ng/mL. A 2-mg stick of nicotine gum produces blood levels of nicotine equivalent to smoking one-half cigarette in 1 hour.

Cotinine in plasma, saliva, and urine appears to have a clear dose-response relationship to passive smoke exposure. Urine cotinine is used as an index to nicotine exposure in tobacco harvesters. Nicotine concentrations in the urine are not useful in the management of overdose since they fluctuate greatly with changes in pH and urine flow.

TREATMENT

Gut Decontamination

If vomiting has not occurred following liquid nicotine ingestion, remove stomach contents by gastric lavage with tracheal protection. Induction of emesis is not advised since seizures or coma may intervene. Children who ingest more than one cigarette should receive activated charcoal and medical observation for at least several hours.

Elimination Enhancement

Hemodialysis and hemoperfusion have not been evaluated in acute nicotine poisoning.

Supportive Measures

- Immediate establishment of an airway, monitoring of breathing patterns and maintenance of circulation are essential in serious overdose cases. Mechanically assisted ventilation should be readily available for respiratory depression.
- Preparations for possible seizures or rapid progression to coma must be initiated in serious overdose cases by establishment of an intravenous line, supplemental oxygen, cardiac monitoring, and direct observation. Artificial ventilation procedures and oxygen may be required.
- Wash exposed skin with nonabrasive, nonalkaline soaps and cool water.
- Seizure activity and agitation can be controlled with diazepam.
- Bronchial secretions, excess salivation, and diarrhea may be ameliorated with atropine.
- Preventive measures for occupational exposure to nicotine include adequate ventilation, chemical goggles, mechanical filter respirators, rubber gloves, aprons, and boots.

Questions—Tobacco Products

1. Nicotine is readily absorbed by all of the following except
   A. Oral mucosa
   B. Stomach
   C. Respiratory tract
   D. Small intestine
   E. Skin

2. All of the following statements about cigarette ingestions in children are true except
   A. Ipecac has been recommended before transport to the emergency room.
   B. Lethargy or irritability is observed infrequently and completely resolves.
   C. Cigarette ingestions in children rarely require specific treatment.
   D. Ingestions of more than one whole cigarette or butt are potentially toxic and should be referred to the emergency department regardless of symptoms.
   E. The absence of vomiting predicts a favorable outcome.

3. Infants of smokers are in greater danger from nicotine passed into breast milk than from second-hand smoke.
   A. True
   B. False

Hobbies, Arts and Crafts

Millions of people throughout the world are involved in hobbies, arts, and crafts that may subject them to a large variety of toxic and other health hazards. Numerous hobbies involve chemicals. Hobby and craft exposures largely parallel those in industry. Numerous dermatologic and respiratory complaints may follow exposures to various arts and crafts materials. Teratogenic, mutagenic, and carcinogenic problems may also follow certain exposures.

After participating in hobbies, symptomatic patients should be asked (a) to list all solids, liquids, and gases used in the activity; (b) what processes were used; (c) the number of hours per week, and the number of years of exposure to the activity; (d) the work environment (outdoors or indoors, small closed room or ventilated area, alone or with others); (e) leisure time activities; and (f) smoking habits.

VENTILATION

The phrase, "use with adequate ventilation" appears on many product labels, and requires definition. There are two types of ventilation to control toxic contamination. These include "dilution ventilation" and "local exhaust ventilation."

Dilution ventilation involves bringing clean air into a room where work is performed and mixing it with "contaminated air." The diluted, and safer concentration, is then exhausted via fan to the outside world. This type of ventilation is adequate when working with small amounts of solvents or gases that are not very toxic. For example, a window exhaust fan is adequate dilution ventilation for oil painting where a cup of turpentine is used per day. Similarly, dilution ventilation is adequate for photographic darkrooms. Dilution ventilation is not adequate for work involving large amounts of solvents, such as those involved in printing with silk screens, or for highly toxic solvents, like those in lacquer thinners. Dilution ventilation is also inadequate for dusts.

Local exhaust ventilation uses hoods, spray booths, etc. to capture contaminants where they are generated, before they can get into general room air. The contaminants are then exhausted to the outside through ducts. Local exhaust ventilation is preferred in situations where highly concentrated solvents are being used, or where small amounts are considered particularly dangerous.

CLINICAL PRESENTATIONS

Neurologic Effects

Neurotoxins associated with hobbies may include mercury, manganese, carbon disulfide, organophosphates, and plasticizers. Plasticizers are substances used to improve the working properties of resins in fiberglass sculpture. Isolated peripheral neuropathies have been associated with methyl butyl ketone (MBK), aerosols, polyester resins, and lead. Organic solvents such as toluene and xylol may cause central nervous system problems. Printmakers and silk screen printers volatilize these solvents as sprays, potentiating their toxicity. Neurotrauma from the use of hammers and chisels can cause vibration syndrome and carpal tunnel syndrome.

Ophthalmologic Effects

The eyes can be a site of trauma and toxicity from almost all art forms. Ultraviolet light and heat exposure can cause cataracts, retinal damage, and superficial punctate keratopathy ("welder's conjunctivitis").

Cardiovascular Effects

Cardiotoxic heavy metals may be contained in paints. Barium, cobalt, and many of the organic solvents such as toluol, methyl chloroform, and methylene chloride are direct cardiac toxins.

Respiratory Effects

Respiratory tract irritants affect different sites based on particle size and solubility. Highly lipid-soluble dusts and fumes cause more systemic injury and minimally lipid-soluble substances produce more local effects. Substances that are more water-soluble will remain in the upper respiratory tract and the skin. Less water-soluble substances will affect the lower respiratory tract. Irritants include nitrogen dioxide (welding gas, carbon arc, etching, and enameling), chromium gas (from etching acid), hydrogen chromide (heating, plastics, and polyvinyl chloride), caustic dusts (lime, dichromate, soda ash, and potassium), and antiskinning agents (eugenol and clove oil).

Iron oxides, aluminum, and barium sulfate may cause pneumoconiosis. Pulmonary fibrosis may be caused by silica, coal, talc, scrap stone, and asbestos. Asthma is exacerbated by wood and bone dust, fibers, reactive dyes, formaldehyde, turpentine, polyurethane, isocyanates, and aluminum oxide. Hypersensitivity pneumonitis is caused by wood dusts and heavy metals.

Hepatic Effects

Clinical hepatitis may be caused by chlorinated hydrocarbons, phenol, ethyl alcohol, nitrobenzene, cadmium, styrene, arsenic, toluene, lead, and xylene. Manganese may cause pathologic hepatic changes.

Renal Effects

Direct renal toxins include oxalic acid, cadmium, turpentine, ethylene glycol, and mercury. A large number of other chemicals are associated with numerous forms of nephrotoxicity.

Dermatologic Effects

The grinding of fiberglass-reinforced sculptures produces particles that can cause an intensely pruritic rash. Plaster and cement contain lime, which can produce a severe dermatitis. Other causes of dermatitis include photographic developers, exotic woods, soaps, metals such as nickel drying agents, and solvents.

Hematologic Effects

Polyvinyl chloride, nitrates, and other photographic developers may cause cyanosis. Lead, cadmium, benzene, and naphthalene can cause hemolytic anemia.

Carcinogenic Effects

Teratogens and carcinogens include chromium, zinc, and arsenic. Chromium, a documented carcinogen, may be inhaled when metal sculptors grind or weld chromium-plated steel (used in car manufacturing). Cadmium is also a carcinogen. Artists may be subject to increased rates of leukemia, cancers of the bladder, colon, rectum, kidney, and brain. Colon cancer deaths appear to be elevated among male painters and sculptors. Known or suspected carcinogens to which artists may be exposed include 2-naphthylamine, polychlorinated biphenyls, benzidine, formaldehyde, asbestos, benzene, dioxane, and methylene chloride.

PREGNANCY/LACTATION

Many substances used by arts, crafts, and hobby enthusiasts may be mutagens (e.g., lead, formaldehyde, and trichloroethane). Women in their childbearing years should be counseled regarding exposure to materials that may pass the placental barrier and possibly lead to birth defects (e.g., lead, cadmium, azo dyes, benzene, chlorinated hydrocarbon solvents, toluene and xylene). Breast-feeding during use of such materials may expose the infant to toxic substances in the mother's milk supply.

TREATMENT

- Numerous recommendations have been devised regarding general safety when working with hobbies, arts and crafts. Most reflect common sense and respect for potential injury.
- Protect against fire. Do not smoke or keep open flames, sparks, or static electricity near flammable liquids or gases. Store flammable and combustible liquids in safety cans and keep only amounts on hand needed for a few days. Never store toxic substances in cans or jars, which can be mistaken for foodstuffs.
- Large amounts of flammable and combustible liquids should be stored in a flammable storage cabinet. Smoke alarms and proper, functioning fire extinguishers are mandatory. If ordinary combustibles, flammable liquids, and electrical equipment are used, have a Class ABC fire extinguisher. Know how to use the fire extinguisher. If flammable liquids are used, exhaust systems must be explosion-proof.
- Clean up carefully. Always clean up spills immediately. For dusts, wet mop or vacuum. Do not sweep as this may stir up dust. For clay and other highly toxic dusts, the vacuum cleaner should be equipped with a special (HEPA) filter.
- Dispose of art materials safely. Do not pour solvents down the sink. Small amounts, generally less than a pint, can be disposed of safely by evaporation inside a local exhaust hood or outdoors. For larger amounts, contact a waste disposal service. Nonpolluting materials dissolved in water can be poured down the sink one at a time with lots of water. Acids and alkalis should be neutralized carefully.
- Maintain good personal work practices. Do not eat, drink, or smoke in an art studio. Wash chemical splashes off the skin with lots of water immediately. In case of eye contact, rinse with water for at least 20 minutes and see a doctor. An eyewash fountain is recommended. If concentrated acids and alkalis are being used, have an emergency shower available. Do not wash hands with solvents if possible. Soap and water is preferable. To remove oil paints, use baby oil, soap and water. Have a first aid kit available.
- Wear proper personal protective clothing and equipment. Wear special work clothes (smocks, hair covering, etc.) and wash these items separately from other clothing. Use the right type of gloves, goggles, hearing protectors, respirators, etc. Make sure they are approved for the chemicals being used and that they fit properly. Respirators should be approved by the National Institute for Occupational Safety and Health (NIOSH) for specific contaminants in the workspace.
- Avoid physical and electrical hazards. Put machine guards on all machinery if possible. Do not wear loose clothing, or wear long hair or necklaces around machinery. Keep equipment and electrical wiring in good repair. Ground electrical equipment and do not overload wiring.
- Seek medical assistance if symptoms may be associated with any hobbies, arts or crafts.

Question—Hobbies, Arts and Crafts

1. Irritants include all of the following except
A. Nitrogen dioxide
B. Modeling clay
C. Chromium gas
D. Hydrogen chromide
E. Eugenol

Non-toxic Ingestions

Many household products cause no symptoms in the doses encountered in most accidental ingestions. A "non-toxic ingestion" is one which occurs after an individual consumes a nonedible product that usually does not produce symptoms. The designation requires that certain criteria be met. These include absolute identification of the product, ingestion of a single product, and lack of symptoms. An accurate history of quantity ingested helps define the exposure as non-toxic. Qualifications exist for many categories, so the extent of symptoms may depend on actual circumstances (e.g., specific product, quantity, and host).

NON-TOXIC SUBSTANCES

Numerous non-toxic household products, chemicals, drugs, plants, and building materials have been identified. Co-ingestion of numerous substances may complicate the classification of an ingestion as "non-toxic." Certain agents, while non-toxic in small doses, can be toxic or even deadly in large enough doses. Cases must be considered on an individual basis. Some relatively non-toxic products include the following:

ADHESIVES

Rubber, plastic, and airplane glues contain aromatic hydrocarbons, which produce central nervous system depression in doses over 1 mg/kg. Cyanoacrylate adhesives (e.g., Crazy Glue®) produce rapid adhesion by combining with amino and carboxylic acid groups in collagen. These links may dissolve with ethanol, acetone, and various oils. Mineral oil soaks effectively destabilize the covalent bond between skin and adhesive, which is especially helpful near eyelids. Ingestion does not cause systemic toxicity and cyanide is not released.

BABY PRODUCTS

Baby products are generally nontoxic, but inhalation of baby powder can produce aspiration pneumonitis or chronic talc pneumoconiosis.

COSMETICS

These products usually cause no symptoms except some mild mucosal irritation. The ethanol, aromatic hydrocarbons, and perborates present in these products may produce systemic toxicity. Most creams, lotions, suntan preparations, bath salts, and dental care preparations are nontoxic. Bubble bath products may produce cystitis.

INKS

Black and blue inks are nontoxic, but some red, green, and purple inks contain aniline dyes, which in large doses cause methemoglobinemia. Similarly, red and orange dyes may contain p-nitroaniline, which in large doses may be hazardous.

MARKERS

Pencil lead is graphite, which is nontoxic. Indelible markers produce local irritation but no systemic toxicity. Ballpoint pens contain carbitol and diethyl glycol, which require large doses to produce toxicity. Chalk is nontoxic.

PAINTS

Hydrocarbon solvents and toxic pigments are the primary constituents of concern. Water-based paints are generally innocuous in doses less than 5 mL/kg. Outdoor paints (especially bridge paints) contain higher lead concentrations than indoor paints, but chronic ingestion is required to produce lead toxicity.

PESTICIDES

Many household and garden weed killers and pesticides are relatively harmless in small amounts (e.g., less than a swallow). The amount ingested and concentration of ingredients in slug/snail pellets (e.g., metaldehyde) and antkillers (e.g., arsenic) usually are too small to cause toxicity. Pyrethrins are relatively nontoxic (toxic dose 1–2 g/kg) but may produce hypersensitivity reactions. Warfarin also has low toxicity in single ingestions. However, each pesticide must be identified because some formulations are exceedingly dangerous (e.g., 20% paraquat concentrate, and "superwarfarins").

SCHOOL SUPPLIES

Most modeling clays, water-soluble pastes, glues, and school paints are nontoxic. Water colors and poster paints contain resin gums (gamboge), which are mucosal irritants and cathartics.

TOBACCO

Usually, the nicotine in cigarettes and cigars absorbed after an accidental ingestion by a child (i.e., less than one cigarette) is too small to produce convulsions or respiratory depression, but vomiting is common. Dehydration may result from protracted vomiting. Matches contain potassium chlorate, but a child would have to consume 10–20 books of matches before significant methemoglobinemia appears.

MISCELLANEOUS AGENTS

The following substances are generally non-toxic in small doses, but may be toxic in large doses or in certain formulations or sizes (e.g., larger batteries may be more dangerous than others). **A:** Adhesives, A&D ointment, Ajax cleaner, Air fresheners, Aluminum foil, Antacids, Antibiotic ointments, Antiperspirants, Ashes (wood, fireplace); **B:** Baby products, Baby wipes, Ballpoint pen pinks, Bathtub floating toys, Batteries (some), Bath oil (castor oil and perfume), Bleach (less than 5%), Body conditioners, Bubble bath soaps (detergents); **C:** Calamine lotion, Candles, Cat food, Caulk, Caps (for toy pistols), Chalk (calcium carbonate), Charcoal and charcoal briquettes, Cigarettes (less than one), Cigarette ashes, Clay (modelling), Colognes (depending on alcohol content), Contraceptive pills (without iron), Comet Cleanser, Corticosteroids and their ointments, Cold packs (a swallow), Crayons (marked AP, CP, CS-140), Crayola Markers, Crazy Glue® (cyanoacrylate), Cyclamate; **D:** Dehumidifying packets (silica or charcoal), Deodorants, Detergents (phosphate type, anionic), Disposable diapers, Dishwashing liquid soaps (not automatic electric dishwasher liquids); **E:** Erasers, Etch-A-Sketch®, Eye Makeup; **F:** Fabric softener, Felt tip markers and pens, Fertilizer (nitrogen, phosphoric acid, and potash), Fingernail polish, Fish bowl additives, Fluoride (as caries preventive); **G:** Glade Plug-ins®, Glitter, Glues and pastes, Glowsticks/jewelry, Golf ball core, Grease, Gypsum; **H:** Hair products (conditioner, shampoos, not Lindane®), Hand lotions and creams; **I:** Indelible markers, Ink (blue, black), Iodophor® disinfectant; **K:** Kaolin®, Kitty litter; **L:** Lanolin, Latex paint, Laxatives, Lipstick, Lotrimin® cream, Lubricants, Lysol® Disinfectant Spray (70% ethanol); **M:** Magic Markers®, Makeup (eye, liquid facial), Mascara (domestic), Matches (book type, 3 books), Massengill® disposable douches, Miracle Gro® Plant Food, Mineral oil; **N:** Newspaper, Nutrasweet®; **P:** PAAS® Easter egg dyes (after 1980), Paints (indoor latex acrylic), Preparation H® suppository/ointment, Pencil lead (graphite), Perfumes, Petroleum jelly (Vaseline®), Photographs, Plastics, Plaster (non-lead containing), Play-doh®, Polaroid picture coating, Porous tip ink marking pens, Prussian blue (ferricyanide), Putty; **R:** Rouge, Rust, Rubber cements, Rug cleaners/shampoos (most); **S:** Saccharin, Sachets (essential oils), Shampoo (liquid), Shaving creams, Shoe polish, Silica gel, Silly Putty®, Soaps and soap products, Soil Shackles, Starch, Sunscreen and tan preparations, Sweetening agents; **T:** Teething rings (fluid may have bacteria), Thermometers (mercury, phthalate alcohol), Toilet water (depending on alcohol content), Toothpaste (even fluoride); **V:** Vaseline®, Vitamins (even fluoride excluding iron); **W:** Warfarin (single dose), Watercolor paints, Windex® Glass Cleaner with ammonia D; **Z:** Zinc oxide, Zirconium oxide.

Questions—Non-toxic Ingestions

1. Crazy Glue® bonds can be dissolved with

A. Hibiclens®
B. Acetone
C. Elbow grease
D. All of the above
E. None of the above

2. Which of the following pairs is incorrectly matched?

A. Baby talc inhalation–Pneumoconiosis
B. Bubble bath–Cystitis
C. Aniline dyes–Thrombocytosis
D. Outdoor paints–Lead toxicity
E. Gamboge–Mucosal irritation

Pica

Pica derives from the Latin for magpie, a bird of fickle appetite that will steal and consume almost anything. The term encompasses the eating of clay, laundry starch, ashes, sand, coffee grounds, oyster shells, matches, ice, newspapers, and cigarette butts. Patients usually conceal the problem from the physician. Risk factors for pica development include family disorganization, poor nutrition, poverty, cultural traits and mental retardation. Inquisitive children may ingest paint chips or toys covered in dusts from old paint (which may contain lead). Cissa is a craving for unusual or unwholesome articles of food, for example, unusual longings during pregnancy.

FOOD PICA

Food pica is a common symptom of iron deficiency. The patient compulsively eats one kind of food such as celery, potato chips, carrots, peanut butter, sunflower seeds, parsley, soda crackers, pickles, orange juice, chocolate ice cream, lettuce, Life Savers®, chewing gum, or pretzels. These foods are rarely a good source of iron, are often brittle, and tend to be crunchy.

GEOPHAGY

Geophagy is the deliberate consumption of earth substances, and is classified as a form of pica. It groups together aberrant behaviors such as the consumption of starch, ice, paint, cigarette butts, and burnt matches. Geophagy is widespread in the animal kingdom and is common among primates, including chimpanzees. It has been implicated both as a cause and a result of particular nutritional deficiencies in humans and is practiced all over the world. It is not restricted to disadvantaged people. Australian aborigines have used clay for stomach discomfort and diarrhea. An abdominal x-ray may show clay opacities. Pica for ice (pagophagia) may resolve after iron therapy.

PAPER PICA

Pica for paper is not uncommon, especially in the mentally retarded, and can cause intestinal obstruction, intestinal perforation, and occasional lead poisoning. Glossy paper, produced by the addition of varnish (commonly ethyl cellulose) may lead to a paper bezoar. Mercurial compounds used in the pulp and paper industry may lead to mercury poisoning in paper pica.

Question—Pica

1. Which of the following Pica subtypes is matched correctly?

A. Food pica–Mercury poisoning
B. Paper pica–Iron deficiency
C. Geophagy–Limited to humans
D. Pagophagia–Iron deficiency
E. None of the above

Boron Compounds

Borax has been known as a cleaning agent since the days of the Greek and Roman empires and has long been used as a food preservative in Europe and America. Boric acid was introduced in 1702 as a sedative, analgesic, and antispasmodic. Lister first employed boric acid as an antiseptic in 1875, and it has since been used in the form of solutions, medicated powders, skin lotions, ointments, toothpaste, mouth washes, water softeners, topical astringents, and antiseptics.

Boric acid is a colorless, odorless compound commercially available as granules, crystals, and white powder. Boric acid solutions have been used for irrigation of the bladder, pleural cavity, lower bowel, skin ulcers, abscesses, inflamed joints, and inflamed mucous membranes. Boric acid may be found in roach powders, contact lens solutions and soaps.

Borate poisoning may follow ingestion, parenteral injection, enemas, and lavage of cavities. Toxicity has been produced by excessive topical use in surgical wounds, burns, ulcers, and diaper dermatitis. Pentaborane is a highly volatile, liquid boron hydride which is an active reducing agent. Sodium perborate, an oxidizer in tooth powders and toothpaste, is 7.03% boron by weight. Fatalities have resulted from accidental administration of boric acid to infants.

PATHOPHYSIOLOGY

Borates are central nervous system depressants and gastrointestinal irritants.

PHARMACOKINETICS

Absorption

- Boron is absorbed readily from abraded, denuded, or irrigated skin.
- It is well absorbed from the stomach.

Distribution

- Boric acid is distributed throughout the body, especially to the brain, liver, and kidneys.

Elimination

- After a single dose, 50% is excreted via the kidneys during the first 24 hours and the remainder is excreted over 5–7 days.

CLINICAL PRESENTATIONS

Gastrointestinal Effects

Persistent nausea, vomiting, and diarrhea in children has led to acute dehydration, shock, and coma. Death resulting from circulatory collapse rarely occurs after boric acid ingestion. Nausea, vomiting, diarrhea, epigastric pain, hematemesis, and blue-green discoloration of both feces and vomitus characterize adult boron intoxication.

Dermatologic Effects

Erythema with desquamation in 1–2 days, and exfoliation (generalized or localized to the hands, feet, or face) may occur (the "boiled lobster" syndrome). Erythema may be prominent on the buttocks and scrotum. Acute skin changes may develop after boric acid ingestion or applications of boric acid powder.

Neurologic Effects

Hyperexcitability, irritability, restlessness, opisthotonus, tremors, convulsions, delirium, coma, weakness, lethargy, headaches, excitement, and depression have been reported.

Renal Effects

Renal toxicity after borate use may present with oliguria, anuria, and/or renal tubular necrosis.

Pentaborane Poisoning

Poisoning from pentaborane gas may yield respiratory irritation and convulsions. Elevated aminotransferase levels and rhabdomyolysis with an elevation in creatine kinase may be seen. Psychiatric symptoms of stress and minimal brain dysfunction may persist for weeks.

TOXIC DOSAGE/DEATH

Single borate ingestions are frequently asymptomatic. Children have ingested 10–20 g with no adverse signs or vomiting only. A 28-year-old who ingested 297 g in a suicide attempt spontaneously vomited in 1 hour and survived. The fatal dose in 5 infants was 4.5–14.0 g, and as little as 1 g has been fatal. Fatalities have been reported after 15–30 g ingestions in adults.

LABORATORY

Analytic Methods

Most laboratories are not equipped to do accurate blood boron or boric acid levels. Tumeric acid strips can detect borates in urine; however, false positives can occur.

Blood Levels

Serum and urine borate levels reflect the fact that exposure has occurred, but they do not correlate well with the clinical state. Symptoms of toxicity generally occur when blood levels exceed 20–150 $\mu g/mL$, although blood levels of 56 and 147 $\mu g/mL$ have produced mild irritability, diarrhea, and perianal erythema in neonates.

TREATMENT

Gut Decontamination

Activated charcoal has not been shown to be of value and probably does not adsorb boron well. If the patient is brought in within a few hours after ingestion, activated charcoal (adults, 60–100 g and children, 30–60 g) may follow gastric lavage, but its value is still not defined.

Elimination Enhancement

Diuresis may be useful if the kidneys are able to excrete the borates before they have irreversibly damaged the renal tubular epithelium. Although peritoneal dialysis and hemodialysis may remove some borates, there have been no systematic studies documenting the clinical effectiveness of these modalities.

Supportive Measures

- Assess and correct any abnormalities found in airway, breathing, and circulation.
- Dehydration may lead to electrolyte abnormalities and should be corrected with normal saline. Pressor agents may be useful but have not been studied. Elevated blood urea nitrogen and serum creatinine levels reflect renal damage. Liver function tests (aspartate and alanine aminotransferases) may be elevated.
- For seizures, administer diazepam intravenously (adult up to 10 mg initially and children, 0.1–0.3 mg/kg slowly). For skin exposures, wash exposed areas several times with mild soap and water. For eye exposures, irrigate copiously with water for at least 20 minutes. If irritation or pain persists, obtain an ophthalmologic consultation. For inhalation exposures, move to fresh air and check for respiratory distress.

Questions—Boron Compounds

1. **Adult boron intoxication is characterized by all of the following except**
   A. Nausea
   B. Epigastric pain
   C. Orange discoloration of feces and vomitus
   D. Hematemesis
   E. Diarrhea
2. **Erythema with desquamation in 1–2 days may follow boron ingestion. This has been called**
   A. The "red man" syndrome
   B. The "boiled lobster" syndrome
   C. Erythema universalis
   D. Erythema boronica
   E. Erythema nodosum

Mothballs and Deodorizers

Mothballs contain either paradichlorobenzene or naphthalene compressed into a solid ball, occasionally with added essential oils and fragrances. Naphthalene is more toxic than paradichlorobenzene, exhibiting more hematologic (e.g., hemolytic anemia, methemoglobinemia) and nervous system effects. Camphor (see Chapter 39, Over-the-counter Products) was used as a mothball ingredient until the 1980s. The presence of camphor may produce serious central nervous system effects such as seizures and coma.

Cake deodorizers for garbage pails, diaper pails, and bathrooms often contain paradichlorobenzene, which is relatively nontoxic in small doses. Paradichlorobenzene has replaced the more toxic naphthalene in most deodorizers and mothballs, although "old-fashioned" preparations may still contain naphthalene. Paradichlorobenzene is also used in the manufacture of certain resins, in the pharmaceutical industry, and as a general insecticide in farming.

Wick deodorizers contain water, agar gel, perfume, and surfactants, which are nontoxic. Amyl and butyl nitrites have been marketed as room deodorizers ("Locker Room," and "Sweat"), which may be abused as adjuncts to sexual intercourse. Nitrites may produce vasodilation, hypotension, and methemoglobinemia.

PATHOPHYSIOLOGY

The oxidative metabolite of naphthalene, alpha-naphthol, can produce hemolysis and methemoglobinemia, particularly in newborn infants and G6PD-deficient patients. Paradichlorobenzene is a mucosal irritant.

PHARMACOKINETICS

Absorption

- Routes of paradichlorobenzene toxicity include inhalation, ingestion, and dermal exposure.
- Humans absorb naphthalene by pulmonary, gastrointestinal, and cutaneous routes.

Distribution

- Naphthalene is found in the urine within a few days of ingestion. Naphthalene and its metabolites may be retained in adipose tissue.
- Paradichlorobenzene has been found in human blood, fatty tissue, and breast milk following inhalation exposure.

Elimination

- The major route of paradichlorobenzene elimination appears to be in the urine.
- 2,5-Dichlorophenol is the major urinary metabolite of paradichlorobenzene.

CLINICAL PRESENTATIONS

Paradichlorobenzene is a mild mucosal irritant capable of producing a sensitizing dermatitis and rhinitis. Exposures to paradichlorobenzene vapors have been associated with renal dysfunction, aplastic anemia, and hepatotoxicity, but the exact contribution of paradichlorobenzene in these cases remains unclear. Methemoglobinemia, hyperchromic anemia, and acute hemolytic anemia have also been described. Ingestion of this compound is common in children but symptoms rarely develop.

Naphthalene may produce delayed (1–3 days) hemolytic anemia in G6PD-deficient patients. Nausea, vomiting, abdominal pain, headache, confusion, and hemolytic anemia may follow inhalation of naphthalene. Renal toxicity, vertigo, listlessness, lethargy, and death may follow ingestion.

PREGNANCY/LACTATION

Hemolytic anemia and jaundice have developed in neonates following *in utero* exposure.

LABORATORY

Analytic Methods

Turpentine dissolves paradichlorobenzene mothballs within 60 minutes; however, naphthalene mothballs are only moderately soluble. This differential dissolution rate may provide a method of identifying the more toxic naphthalene. Heating paradichlorobenzene yields a green color and naphthalene yields no color. 1-Naphthol is analyzed by spectrophotometry, thin-layer chromatography, and gas chromatography.

Blood Levels

Following blood levels of these agents after an overdose does not guide management.

Urine

1-Naphthol is found in the urine of industrial workers exposed to naphthalene.

TREATMENT

Gut Decontamination

Lavage is indicated after large amounts of paradichlorobenzene (several mothballs or a whole cake). Ingestion of a single naphthalene mothball requires gut decontamination in a small child presenting within 2 hours of exposure. Activated charcoal may be useful.

Elimination Enhancement

These methods are not generally utilized in the treatment of paradichlorobenzene ingestions. Dialysis may be required after substantial hemolysis from naphthalene ingestions. Exchange transfusion may also be required.

Supportive Measures

- Irrigate exposed skin or eyes copiously with saline and check for corneal abrasions with fluorescein staining. Antiemetics and demulcents such as antacids may be helpful.
- Hemolysis may require blood transfusion, packed red blood cell transfusions, alkaline diuresis, or exchange transfusion, particularly in infants.
- An abdominal radiograph indicates that paradichlorobenzene is strongly radiopaque, but products containing naphthalene are radiolucent.

Questions—Mothballs and Deodorizers

1. The major component of modern mothballs is camphor.
A. True
B. False

2. Naphthalene does not cause
A. Methemoglobinemia
B. Hemolysis
C. Nausea and vomiting
D. G6PD–deficiency
E. Confusion

3. Heating paradichlorobenzene yields no color and naphthalene yields a green color.
A. True
B. False

Answers

Antiseptics and Disinfectants

1. A 2. B

Chlorhexidine

1. C 2. B

Cresols

1. C 2. E 3. A

Ethylene Oxide

1. B 2. E

Formaldehyde

1. D 2. E 3. B

Glutaraldehyde

1. B 2. A 3. E

Gentian Violet

1. B 2. C

Hexachlorophene

1. D 2. D

Hydrogen Peroxide

1. E 2. E

Phenols

1. A 2. E

Soaps and Shampoos

1. D 2. D

Detergents

1. A 2. E

Bleaches

1. C 2. A

Pine Oil and Turpentine

1. B 2. E 3. A

Cosmetics

1. C 2. D

Tobacco Products

1. B 2. D 3. B

Hobbies, Arts and Crafts

1. B

Non-toxic Ingestions

1. B 2. C

Pica

1. D

Boron Compounds

1. C 2. B

Mothballs and Deodorizers

1. B 2. D 3. B

SELECTED READINGS

Antiseptics and Disinfectants

1. Handbook of pharmaceutical excipients. Washington, DC: American Pharmaceutical Association; London. The Pharmaceutical Society of Great Britain, 1986; pp. 27–28.
2. Reynolds JEF. Martindale: The extra pharmacopoeia. 13th ed. London: The Pharmaceutical Press, 1993; pp. 781–805.

Chlorhexidine

1. Emerson D, Pierce C. A case of a single ingestion of 4% Hibiclens. Vet Hum Toxicol 1988;30:583.

Cresols

1. Arthurs GJ, Wise CC, Coles GA. Poisoning by cresol. Anaesthesia 1977;32: 642–643.
2. Green MA. A household remedy misused—fatal cresol poisoning following cutaneous absorption (a case report). Med Sci Law 1975;15:65–66.

Ethylene Oxide

1. Salinas E, Sasich L, Hall DH, et al: Acute ethylene oxide intoxication. Drug Intell Clin Pharm 1981;15:384–385.
2. Currier MF, Carlo GL, Poston PL, et al: A cross sectional study of employees with potential occupational exposure to ethylene oxide. Br J Ind Med 1984; 41:492–498.

Formaldehyde

1. Bartone NF, Grieca RV, Henn BS: Corrosive gastritis due to ingestion of formaldehyde. JAMA 1968;203:50–51.
2. Harris JC, Rumack BH, Aldrich FD: Toxicology of urea formaldehyde and polyurethane foam insulation. JAMA 1981;245:243–246.
3. Wartew GA: The health hazards of formaldehyde. J Appl Toxicol 1983;3: 121–126.

Glutaraldehyde

1. Binding N, Witting U. Exposure to formaldehyde and glutaraldehyde in operating theatres. Int Arch Occup Environ Health 1990;62:233–238.
2. Nethercott JR, Holness DL, Page E. Occupational contact dermatitis due to glutaraldehyde in health care workers. Contact Dermatitis 1988;18:193–6.

Gentian Violet

1. Docampo R, Moreno SNJ. The metabolism and mode of action of gentian violet. Drug Metab Rev 1990;22:161–178.
2. Drinkwater P. Gentian violet—is it safe? Aust NZ J Obstet Gynaecol 1990; 30:65–66.

Hexachlorophene

1. Herskowitz J, Rosman NP: Acute hexachlorophene poisoning by mouth in a neonate. J Pediatr 1979;94:495–496.
2. Hexachlorophene today. (Editorial) Lancet 1982;1:87–88.
3. Mullick FG: Hexachlorophene toxicity—Human experience at the Armed Forces Institute of Pathology. Pediatrics 1973;51:395–399.

Hydrogen Peroxide

1. Cina SJ, Downs CU, Conradi SE. Hydrogen peroxide: a source of lethal oxygen embolism. Am J Forensic Med Pathol 1994;15(1):44–50.
2. Giberson TP, Kern JD, Pettigrew DW III, Eaves CC Jr, Haynes JF Jr. Near-fatal hydrogen peroxide ingestion. Ann Emerg Med 1989;18:778–779.
3. Sleigh JW, Linter SPK. Hazards of hydrogen peroxide. Br Med J 1985;291:1706.

Phenols

1. Brancato DJ: Recognizing potential toxicity of phenol. Vet Hum Toxicol 1982; 24:29–30.
2. Soares ER, Tift JP: Phenol poisoning: Three fatal cases. J Forensic Sci 1982;27: 729–731.

Soaps, Shampoos, Detergents, Bleaches

1. Edwards JN, Jenkins HC, Volans GN: Hazards of household cleaning products. Hum Toxicol 1982;1:403–409.
2. Temple AR, Veltri JC: Outcome of accidental ingestions of soaps, detergents and related household products. Vet Hum Toxicol 1979;21(suppl):31–32.

Pine Oil and Turpentine

1. Koppel C, Tenczer J, Tennesmann U, et al: Acute poisoning with pine oil—Metabolism of monoterpenes. Arch Toxicol 1981;49:73–78.
2. McGuigan MA: Turpentine. Clin Toxicol Rev 1985;8(1):1–2.

Cosmetics

1. Adams RM, Maibach HI. A five year study of cosmetic reactions. J Am Acad Dermatol 1985;13:1062–1069.

Tobacco Products

1. Benowitz N. Cigarette smoking and nicotine addiction. Med Clin North Am 1992;76:415–537.
2. Blanchard J. Nicotine. I. Clin Toxicol Rev 1993;15(1):1–2.
3. Lavoie FW, Harris TM. Fatal nicotine ingestion. J Emerg Med 1991;9:133–136.

Hobbies, Arts and Crafts

1. Babin A. Center for Safety in the Arts. Art Hazards Information Center. Health and Safety Resources for the Arts. Hazards News 1992;15:4–7 Art.
2. Glasbrenner K. Maladies may be linked to artists' material. JAMA 1984;251: 1391–1395.
3. Lesser SH, Weiss SJ. Art hazards. Am J Emerg Med 1995;13:451–458.
4. Pike S. Hazards from hobbies, arts and crafts. Proc Fourth Annual Southwestern Poison Symposium. Scottsdale, AZ. Arizona Poison and Drug Information Center, November 2, 1984, 34–49.

Non-toxic Ingestions

1. Comstock EG. Morbidity due to non-poisoning. J Occup Med 1978;20:755–758.
2. Henry J, Wiseman H. ABC of poisoning. Non-poisons. Br Med J 1984;289: 240–241.
3. Mofenson H, Greensher J. The non-toxic ingestion. Pediatr Clin North Am 1970;17:583–590.

Pica

1. Crosby WH. Pica. JAMA 1976;235:2765.

Boron Compounds

1. Linden CH, Hall AH, Kulig KW et al. Acute ingestions of boric acid. Clin Toxicol 1986;24:269–279.
2. Litovitz TL et al. Clinical manifestations of toxicity in a series of 784 boric acid ingestions. Vet Hum Toxicol 1986;28:505 (abstract).

Mothballs and Deodorizers

1. Hibbs BF, Donahue JM, Normandy MJ. Naphthalene. Toxicological profile. Draft Agency for Toxic Substances Disease Registry, October, 1993.
2. Winkler JV, Kulig K, Rumack BH. Mothball differentiation: Naphthalene from paradichlorobenzene. Ann Emerg Med 1985;14:30–32.

ACKNOWLEDGMENT

Thanks to Alison Deutsch, MD for contributing the questions in this chapter.

CHAPTER 39
Over-the-Counter Products

INTRODUCTION

Over-the-counter products, while seemingly benign to the public at large, can cause serious morbidity and even death. Camphor, a ubiquitous ingredient of many cold remedies and emollients, can cause refractory seizures. Fluorides and vitamins, also generally believed to be benign, can cause deadly consequences ranging from hypocalcemia to liver disease. Even water and salt, ingested improperly, can lead to dangerous consequences.

BAKING SODA

Inadvertent substitution of baking soda (sodium bicarbonate powder) for powdered formula may lead to obtundation, convulsions, persistent neurologic abnormalities, or cardiorespiratory arrest associated with hypernatremia.

Pathophysiology

The approximate volume of gas produced from the chemical reaction of 1 teaspoon of sodium bicarbonate (12 g) using Avogadro's and Charles' Law is 3.4 liters. With a large meal and aerophagy (while attempting to belch), this may approach the 4 L that has been calculated as necessary for gastric rupture. The rapidity of pressure buildup probably also plays a large part. People with a full feeling after overeating are advised not to ingest anything, regardless of whether it has the potential for gas production. If, in spite of this admonition, sodium bicarbonate were ingested, it would be advisable to use one-half of a level teaspoon, rather than a larger dose.

Clinical Presentations

Baking powder is composed of 30% sodium bicarbonate with cornstarch, sodium aluminum sulfate, calcium acid phosphate, and calcium sulfate. The main effect of ingestion and chronic abuse is hypokalemic hypochloremic metabolic alkalosis. Other metabolic abnormalities, including hypernatremia and hypocalcemia, are possible. Transient albuminuria, neuromuscular irritability, including hyperreflexia, and elevations in blood urea nitrogen have been observed. The presence of hypernatremia with metabolic alkalosis and an elevated urine pH suggests the possibility of ingestion of exogenous alkali. Hyperglycemia may be present as well.

The maximum recommended dose of baking soda for an adult is eight half-teaspoons over a 24-hour period. The diagnostic triad for spontaneous rupture of the stomach includes surgical emphysema of the neck and a distended abdomen following sudden abdominal pain. Radiography often is unhelpful. A perforated peptic ulcer rarely is bigger than 1.5 cm, whereas gastric ruptures may be 5 cm long. The lesser curvature of the stomach is the usual site of rupture.

Sodium bicarbonate (3 to 4 tbsp per day) may be ingested by patients with anorexia nervosa to dampen their appetites. This may be associated with recurrent hypokalemic metabolic alkalosis. Features of Munchausen's syndrome may accompany such abuse (50 to 150 g per day).

Treatment

GUT DECONTAMINATION

Gut decontamination is contraindicated as this may increase the potential for gastric rupture.

ELIMINATION ENHANCEMENT

These methods have not proved to be helpful in baking soda ingestions.

SUPPORTIVE MEASURES

- Follow and monitor serum sodium, electrolytes, pH, and volume status.
- Early surgery in cases of gastric rupture is important with thorough peritoneal lavage. Postoperative intraabdominal sepsis can be deadly.

- In infants, rehydration with oral electrolyte solutions may be useful in cases of mild metabolic alkalosis from bicarbonate ingestion. Intravenous correction of electrolytes may be necessary as well.
- "Rebound hyperkalemia" may require weeks to normalize.
- Acetazolamide promotes renal excretion of both sodium and bicarbonate; however, this is accompanied by a risk of volume depletion.

Questions—Baking Soda

1. **As 1 tsp of sodium bicarbonate can theoretically produce 3.4 L of gas, the volume necessary for gastric rupture is approached.**
   A. True
   B. False
2. **Chronic ingestion of baking soda is associated with all of the following except**
   A. Hypokalemic hypochloremic metabolic alkalosis
   B. Hyperreflexia
   C. Hypernatremia and hypocalcemia
   D. Albuminuria
   E. Elevations in blood urea nitrogen
3. **Which of the following is true or indicated for the treatment of baking soda ingestion?**
   A. Gut decontamination within 4 hours of ingestions
   B. Repeated doses of activated charcoal often are helpful
   C. Serum potassium levels may need to be followed over several weeks
   D. Oral rehydration is never sufficient treatment
   E. None of the above

BROMIDES

Bromides were formerly used as sedative-hypnotic drugs and distributed for both over-the-counter (OTC) and prescription drug use. The bromide salt now has been largely removed from OTC products, but still is available in prescription drugs and as part of the antihistamine molecule brompheniramine. Bromide intoxication now is rarely observed. Methyl bromide is a fumigant insecticide and is used in some fire extinguishers and refrigerants. Ethylene dibromide is a scavenger of lead in leaded fuels and a fumigant insecticide. Bromide intoxication has followed pyridostigmine bromide intoxication.

Pathophysiology

Allegedly, bromide is a central nervous system depressant. Newer, more specific drugs have superseded its antiepileptic action.

Pharmacokinetics

ABSORPTION

- Oral bioavailability is complete (averaging about 96% in one study).

DISTRIBUTION

- Bromides are distributed throughout the body similarly to chloride, except in the red cell.
- The apparent volume of distribution of bromides is 0.41 L/kg.

ELIMINATION

- Bromides are excreted by selective reabsorption in the renal tubular filtrate, preferentially to chloride. Body chloride thus is lowered.
- Total body clearance is 20 to 33 mL/kg/day.
- Its half-life is approximately 12 days after oral administration and 9.5 days after intravenous (IV) administration. With chloride loading, the bromide half-life is 3 days. Mannitol diuresis reduces the half-life to 37 hours.
- With hemodialysis, the half life is 1 to 2 hours.

Clinical Presentations

Acute poisoning is rare. Large amounts of ingested bromide produce gastric irritation and emesis. Therapeutic effects often coincide with toxic effects. In large single oral doses, bromides may cause gastric irritation and emesis. Initially, bromides induce sedation, but they may produce headache, irritability, agitation, delirium, memory loss, decreased appetite, dysarthria, hallucinations, acne-like rash, stupor, and coma. Ataxia and generalized hyperreflexia may be observed.

Toxic Dosage/Death

The therapeutic dose in adults is 3 to 5 g. Fatal dose has been estimated as 10 to 20 g.

Drug Interactions

Bromides taken with other sedatives may yield extreme lethargy.

Pregnancy/Lactation

Three cases of fetal abnormalities have been described in the fetuses of mothers who took large doses of bromides during pregnancy. Fetal effects may include microcephaly and cardiac abnormalities.

Laboratory

ANALYTIC METHODS

Quick colorimetric tests on filter paper have been developed for bedside determination of significant bromide presence.

BLOOD LEVELS

Serum bromide levels over 50 mg/dL may be associated with toxic symptoms, but the correlation is not consistent. Levels below 50 mg/dL usually are not associated with symptoms. Seriously disturbed mental status appears when serum bromides are 150 mg/dL or greater. Correlation of neurologic symptoms and signs with blood levels of bromide is inexact.

Treatment

GUT DECONTAMINATION

If the patient has ingested over 5 g of organic bromide compounds, has not vomited, and has no evidence of convulsions, coma, or loss of gag reflex, syrup of ipecac, activated charcoal, and cathartics may be helpful. If these conditions are present, gastric lavage, after endotracheal intubation, is indicated in severe overdoses. Confirmation of efficacy has not been proved.

ELIMINATION ENHANCEMENT

Hemodialysis can reduce bromide half-life substantially. Forced saline diuresis may be helpful in eliminating excessive bromide burdens as well.

Answers to questions in shaded boxes appear at the end of the chapter.

SUPPORTIVE MEASURES

- Confirm integrity of airway, breathing, and circulation.
- Forced saline diuresis may be helpful. Use normal saline IV or 0.45% sodium chloride in 5% dextrose in water. Hydration, and diuresis, can be augmented with a diuretic such as furosemide, 1 mg/kg to 40 mg, to obtain a urine flow of 3 to 6 mL/hour.
- Saline with diuretic is administered until the serum bromide level is below 50 mg/dL and the patient has relief of symptoms.
- In chronic cases, sodium chloride can be given orally, 9 to 12 g/day (2 to 3 g, three to four times daily) as a saline solution or in bouillon. Continue until the serum bromide level falls below 100 mg/dL and symptoms disappear, generally in 1 to 4 weeks. Acneiform rashes may take as long as 6 months to disappear.
- Supportive measures include symptomatic treatment for confusion or delirium.
- Serum electrolyte studies may include a pseudodecreased anion gap. Elevated serum chloride often is the first clue to the diagnosis because of the apparent, but not true, elevation of serum chloride, as some laboratory tests do not differentiate chloride from bromide ion.
- The electroencephalogram (EEG) may exhibit a generalized slowing.

Questions—Bromides

1. **Acute bromide poisoning**
   A. Occurs frequently because of its presence in over-the-counter drugs
   B. Produces gastric irritation and emesis
   C. Causes initial sedation
   D. A and B
   E. B and C
2. **Fetal abnormalities have not been reported in the fetuses of mothers who ingest large amounts of bromides.**
   A. True
   B. False
3. **Treatment of bromide overdose may include all of the following except**
   A. Syrup of ipecac
   B. Activated charcoal
   C. Urine acidification
   D. Hemodialysis
   E. Forced saline diuresis

CAMPHOR

Camphor has been used for centuries as an antipruritic and topical rubefacient, abortifacient, aphrodisiac, contraceptive, cold remedy, suppressor of lactation, and antiseptic. For decades, camphor intoxication has been reported in the medical literature and in many instances has involved the accidental ingestion of camphorated oil, mistaken for castor oil or other patent medications, notably cough and cold preparations.

Camphorated oil has been classified by the Food and Drug Administration (FDA) as "not generally recognized as safe," and has been declared illegal to manufacture or ship. Camphor, on the other hand, remains an ingredient in over 950 currently available products listed in the Poisindex® System. Such preparations have no scientifically established place in clinical therapeutics. Camphor is a cyclic ketone of the hydroaromatic terpene group, with a penetrating characteristic odor and a pungent, aromatic taste. It currently is produced synthetically.

In 1983, the FDA ruled that the concentration of camphor in medicinal products must not exceed 11%. Camphorated oil in concentrations of up to 20% still is stocked in many Canadian drug stores. Camphor is absorbed rapidly when taken orally, but a considerable amount also can be absorbed via inhalation or through intact skin. Typically, symptoms begin 5 to 90 minutes after ingestion of a toxic dose. The onset of seizures can be sudden and may be followed by postconvulsive depression and coma. Death may result from respiratory depression or complications of status epilepticus.

Pathophysiology

Camphor is a rubefacient that has irritating effects on the upper gastrointestinal tract and is both excitative and depressant to the central nervous system. Its action has been postulated to be intraneuronal on the oxidation cycle at a phase above the cytochrome b level of the cytochrome oxidase system.

Pharmacokinetics

ABSORPTION

- Camphor in liquid form is absorbed rapidly through the skin, mucous membranes, and gastrointestinal tract. Food may interfere with absorption.
- Symptoms of intoxication usually appear within 5 to 90 minutes.

DISTRIBUTION

- Measurable serum levels occur 15 minutes after ingestion of approximately 0.5 to 1.0 g.
- It is distributed widely in tissues and easily crosses the placental barrier.

ELIMINATION

- Camphor is metabolized to a "campherol," conjugated with glucuronic acid in the liver, and excreted in the urine as an inactivated compound.
- It is not clear whether camphor toxicity can be attributed to the parent compound, a metabolite (secondary alcohols including borneol and isomers of hydroxycamphor), or both.

Clinical Presentations

Symptoms begin within 5 to 90 minutes after ingestion and initially consist of a burning feeling in the mouth and throat, vomiting, and a feeling of warmth. An odor of camphor on the breath may be present. Urinary retention, albuminuria, and anuria have been described in nonfatal cases. Death may be caused by respiratory depression or may follow status epilepticus.

GASTROINTESTINAL EFFECTS

Spontaneous nausea and vomiting occur in almost all patients. Symptoms may be delayed for several hours if food is present in the stomach. Mild, transient elevations of aspartate aminotransferase and lactic dehydrogenase have been reported. More severe intoxications may result in hepatic failure.

NEUROLOGIC EFFECTS

Confusion, vertigo, restlessness, delirium, and hallucinations may occur. Increased muscular activity, tremors, and jerky movements may progress quickly to seizure activity followed, in some cases, by postconvulsive depression and coma. Neuronal necrosis has been reported.

OPHTHALMOLOGIC EFFECTS
Strabismus, dilated pupils, and amblyopia have been observed. Camphor is an eye irritant.

Toxic Dosage/Death

Camphor in liquid form is quite toxic, with a probable human lethal dose of 50 to 500 mg/kg. The ingestion of 2 g generally produces dangerous effects in adults and quantities as small as 1 g have proved fatal in children. The successful recovery of an adult patient who ingested 42 g of camphor has been reported. For perspective, 20 g of Vicks VapoRub® contains about 1 g of camphor and 10 mL of Campho-Phenique® contains about 1 g of camphor. Clinically significant camphor toxicity generally is not manifested below 30 mg/kg and is uncommon below 50 mg/kg. The ingestion of solid camphor "moth balls" has produced serious symptoms and death.

Pregnancy/Lactation

Camphor poisoning during pregnancy has been reported. In one case, fetal death occurred, but it was not determined that the death was from camphor alone. Camphor can cross the placenta. Camphor is categorized as pregnancy risk category C.

Laboratory

ANALYTIC METHODS
Methods to quantify camphor levels generally are not available in hospital laboratories.

BLOOD LEVELS
Camphor blood levels generally are not available. A level of 1.95 mg/dL, 7 hours after ingestion, was associated with convulsions in one case.

Treatment

GUT DECONTAMINATION
Because camphor is absorbed rapidly and may be associated with sudden convulsions and aspiration secondary to impaired consciousness, syrup of ipecac is strictly contraindicated. In the presymptomatic or early symptomatic stages, gastric lavage with appropriate tracheal protection may be used, but its efficacy, compared with charcoal alone, has not been proven. Activated charcoal is marginally effective in adsorbing camphor; however, no study has demonstrated its effectiveness as a decontaminant in cases of camphor poisoning.

Oils, alcohols, and other lipophilic substances enhance intestinal absorption and are contraindicated. Some have suggested that if the maximum possible ingested dose of camphor is less than 10 mg/kg, patients be observed at home. If between 10 and 30 mg/kg has been ingested, activated charcoal plus a saline cathartic may be given. For ingestions over 30 mg/kg, observation in an emergency facility is mandatory.

ELIMINATION ENHANCEMENT
Diuresis is ineffective in assisting the removal of camphor. While hemodialysis and resin hemoperfusion may reduce blood camphor levels, their clinical efficacy is unproved.

SUPPORTIVE MEASURES
- Severe symptoms may arise very rapidly. Emergency transportation to a medical facility is warranted if there is any question concerning quantity ingested. Airway, breathing, and circulation should be assured in all cases before specific therapy is initiated. Endotracheal intubation must be initiated if necessary.
- Patients must be admitted for monitoring and treatment when serious central nervous system, hepatic, renal, eye, or skin problems exist. Seizures may be treated effectively with intravenous benzodiazepines such as diazepam (adults, 5 to 10 mg and children, 0.1 to 0.3 mg/kg) with the addition of phenytoin if protracted.
- Recovery usually is complete within 24 to 48 hours postingestion but more prolonged recovery periods have been reported. One death occurred 4 days following ingestion.
- Minor "taste" or "swallow" ingestions of camphor-containing products cause only minor symptoms of oral and gastrointestinal irritation and can be safely handled at home.
- The vast majority of camphor ingestions will remain asymptomatic and can be observed at home if the amount ingested is known to be less than 1 g in an adult. If the ingestion exceeds 1 g, observation in a health care facility is recommended.
- If the patient exhibits marked symptoms of central nervous system excitation or is seen more than 1 hour after ingestion, blood and urine samples should be obtained to monitor hepatorenal function.
- Liver function tests are indicated after chronic camphor exposure.
- Exposed skin should be washed copiously with soap and water. Exposed eyes should be irrigated copiously with water continuously for 20 minutes. If there appears to be anything other than eye irritation (e.g., pain, photophobia), an ophthalmology consult should be obtained.

Questions—Camphor

1. **Camphor is absorbed rapidly when taken orally, but**
   A. Is absorbed in minimal amounts via inhalation
   B. Is absorbed in minimal amounts via skin absorption
   C. Does not produce symptoms until over 4 hours after exposure
   D. Usually is absorbed even faster when taken with food
   E. None of the above
2. **Which of the following is the most common gastrointestinal side effect of camphor overdose?**
   A. Mild, transient elevations of lactic dehydrogenase
   B. Spontaneous nausea and vomiting
   C. Mild, transient elevations of aspartate aminotransferase
   D. Hepatic failure
   E. None of the above
3. **Camphor toxicity**
   A. Has not been reported during pregnancy
   B. Is uncommon below 50 mg/kg
   C. Is uncommon below 10 mg/kg
   D. Has not been serious when a result of camphor "moth ball" ingestion
   E. Has not been reported to be fatal
4. **As symptoms of camphor toxicity can arise rapidly, syrup of ipecac should be given quickly.**
   A. True
   B. False

EXCIPIENTS

Drug dosage forms contain many substances in addition to the active drug. Such substances are known as excipients. Excipients may include diluents, binders, lubricants, disintegrators, colors, flavoring agents, surfactants, solubilizing agents, antioxidants, aerosol propellants, preservatives, antibacterials, thickening, suspending, and binding agents, solvents, perfumes, fats, and oils. Excipients may provide hidden hazards in many drug products. A well-known excipient, Rhodamine B, is a red dye. Occupational exposure may cause skin and mucous membrane irritation.

Coloring Agents and Rhodamine B

AMARANTH (FD&C YELLOW NO. 2)

Amaranth has been associated with generalized pruritus, urticaria, angioedema, and may be a theoretical carcinogen.

BRILLIANT GREEN

Brilliant green has been associated with eczema, and may cross-react with gentian violet and malachite green.

CARMINE

Carmine may cause allergic alveolitis.

CONGO RED

Congo red is used to test for amyloidosis and for achlorhydria. Its use may cause anaphylactic shock, substernal pain, cold sweat, visual impairment, and/or vomiting. Congo red can be fatal after intravenous use. Use of Congo red or Evans blue as pharmaceutical colorants is not permitted by the FDA.

ERYTHROSINE (FD&C RED NO. 3)

Erythrosine is an iodinated fluorescein derivative, which may interfere with thyroid function in large doses. It has been associated with increased protein-bound iodine values and depressed iodine uptake.

EVANS BLUE

Evans blue is used for blood volume estimations and to outline lymphatics. Allergic contact dermatitis and generalized urticaria have been linked to this agent.

GENTIAN VIOLET

Gentian violet may cause sensitization and anaphylactic reactions.

PATENT BLUE V

Patent blue V is a potential sensitizer.

PONCEAU (FD&C RED NO. 4)

Ponceau has been associated with chest heaviness.

RHODAMINE B

Rhodamine B is used commonly as a coloring agent in lipsticks. The FDA restricts its concentration to less than 6%. Rhodamine B also is used to check for fuel leaks in M-1 tanks and other military vehicles by adding a small quantity into diesel fuel and observing for the appearance of red coloring on the outside of the fuel tank. Other uses include as a dye for fabrics, an analytical reagent for metals, a tracing agent in water pollution studies, and a color marker in herbicidal sprays. Rhodamine B also is known as FD&C Red No. 19. It is very soluble in water with a bluish-red color. Rhodamine B presents as green crystals or a reddish-violet powder.

Acute exposure to aerosolized rhodamine can lead to burning of the eyes, excessive tearing, nasal burning, nasal itching, chest pain and tightness, rhinorrhea, cough, dyspnea, burning of the throat, headache, and nausea. Symptoms typically resolve in 4 to 24 hours. Rhodamine B is considered a possible carcinogen.

SUNSET YELLOW (FD&C YELLOW NO. 6)

Sunset yellow has been associated with allergic purpura after ingestion of colored foods.

TARTRAZINE (FD&C YELLOW NO. 5)

Tartrazine may cause hyperactivity in children. Pharmacologically, this dye may cause histamine release from basophils.

Questions—Coloring Agents

1. **Which of the following coloring agents is associated with the incorrect side effect?**
   A. Evans blue—Generalized urticaria
   B. Ponceau—Chest heaviness
   C. Sunset yellow—Possible interference with thyroid function
   D. Gentian violet—Sensitization and anaphylactic reactions
   E. Congo red—Visual impairment
2. **Rhodamine B**
   A. Can lead to burning of the eyes and excessive tearing
   B. Causes symptoms that typically resolve in 2 to 4 hours
   C. Is considered a possible carcinogen
   D. A and B
   E. A and C

Surfactants and Solubilizing Agents

Anionic surfactants such as sodium lauryl sulfate may be a direct skin irritant at high concentrations. One percent may cause development of contact dermatitis with burning, redness, tightening of skin, leathery texture, painful fissures, and lamellar exfoliation. Two percent in a dentifrice resulted in a case of painless oral desquamation. Eczematous patients often use another anionic surfactant, triethanolamine, found in lotions and creams. A 5% concentration may produce an irritant toxic reaction, allergic eczema, or contact dermatitis.

Nonionic surfactants such as polyoxyethylene sorbate esters (Tweens or polysorbates), sorbitan monostearate and monooleate (Spans), and sorbitan sesquioleate may cause contact allergy. They generally are weak sensitizers, are considered low toxicity, and are used widely in pharmaceuticals. Bullous eruptions and edema associated with sorbitan monolaurate have been described. Cremophor EL or polyethoxylated castor oil is another nonionic surfactant frequently used as a solubilizing agent. Possible anaphylaxis and hyperlipidemia have been associated with this agent. This product has been linked with anaphylactic reactions in association with some anesthetic agents (Taxol) and vitamin K preparations in Australia.

Aliphatic alcohols and esters used in the formulation of creams rarely are associated with hypersensitivity reactions. Stearyl and cetyl alcohols cause rare allergic urticarial reactions. Use of glycerol monostearate also results in rare allergic symptoms.

Question-Surfactants and Solubilizing Agents

1. **Which of the following surfactants has been associated with anaphylaxis?**
   A. Polyoxyethylene sorbate esters
   B. Cremophor EL or polyethoxylated castor oil
   C. Sodium lauryl sulfate
   D. Sorbitan monostearate
   E. Triethanolamine

Aerosol Propellants

Aerosol propellants are used frequently in pharmaceuticals such as bronchodilators, steroids, and dermatological preparations. They are used also to propel cosmetics and various toiletries. Halogenated hydrocarbons often constitute over 80% of the contents of an aerosol can and may include trichlorofluoromethane (Freon 11), dichlorodifluoromethane (Freon 12), carbon tetrafluoride (Freon 14), chloroform, or even halothane.

Fluorocarbon propellants are anesthetic and cardiotoxic. Freon 11, inhaled at 5% concentration, sensitizes the myocardium to epinephrine. A 6% concentration may result in apnea and areflexia. A 10% concentration can produce cardiac arrhythmias. Deaths resulting from cardiovascular collapse after arrhythmias have been reported after inhalation of Freons 11 and 12. Accidental inhalation of an aerosol deodorant containing propane, n-butane, and isobutane has been associated with ventricular tachycardia and seizures in a child. Aerosol propellants also can produce hallucinogenic effects and contact dermatitis, and contribute to ozone layer destruction.

Question—Aerosol Propellants

1. **Aerosol propellants can cause**
   A. Hallucinations
   B. Cardiotoxicity
   C. Contact dermatitis
   D. All of the above
   E. B and C

Preservatives and Antibacterials

Preservatives and antibacterials are added to products to maintain sterility and to prevent spoilage by bacteria or fungi in nonsterile medications. Preservatives are used to prevent microbial spoilage of food and drug preparations. Sterilization refers to the total removal or destruction of all living microorganisms. Sterility usually is produced by heat or radiation methods.

BENZALKONIUM CHLORIDE

Benzalkonium chloride is the preservative most commonly present in nebulizer solutions. It is used for its bactericidal properties and is present in albuterol, beclomethasone, metaproterenol, and ipratropium bromide nebulizer solutions. It also is used in eye drops and contact lens solutions. Allergic dermatitis, stomatitis, and allergic conjunctivitis have been associated with this agent. Ingestion may lead to fatalities. Patch tests may be positive.

PATHOPHYSIOLOGY

Benzalkonium chloride is a caustic mixture of alkyldimethylbenzyl ammonium chlorides. Benzalkonium chloride may cause bronchoconstriction by releasing spasmogenic mediators from mast cells within the bronchial wall and stimulating cholinergic and noncholinergic nerves to produce bronchoconstriction.

CLINICAL PRESENTATIONS

Ingestion of benzalkonium chloride in concentrations of 10% or more may produce corrosive lesions of the palate, hypopharynx, esophagus, and stomach. Nausea, vomiting, diarrhea, dyspnea, confusion, hypotension, hypoxemia, renal insufficiency, restlessness, seizures, coma, muscle weakness, pulmonary edema, and methemoglobinemia have been observed. Greyish-white membranes may form in the mouth, hypopharynx, and stomach. Death may follow within minutes to hours and may be a result of circulatory failure, respiratory insufficiency, muscle weakness, and central nervous system depression.

Bronchoconstriction may occur in patients with reactive airway disease such as bronchial asthma and may be dose related. Responses to benzalkonium chloride, although rapid in onset, are prolonged and may continue to affect the airway after lung function has returned to baseline.

TOXIC DOSAGE/DEATH

Use of benzalkonium chloride for antisepsis of the skin should be limited to 1:1000 or 1:750 dilution. Caustic oral action may occur with a preparation diluted to 1:2000 or 1:5000. A 77-year-old male who swallowed 50 mL of a 10% aqueous solution of benzalkonium chloride died; however, a 70-year-old woman who ingested 40 mL of a 33.3% aqueous solution of benzalkonium chloride survived. Human fatalities have been described following oral doses of 100 to 400 mg/kg, or parenteral doses of 5 to 15 mg/kg.

TREATMENT

Gut Decontamination

Endotracheal intubation and esophagoduodenoscopy are performed if required prior to gastric lavage under appropriate anesthesia. Following esophagoscopy in the case of second-degree burns, a large-bore nasogastric tube may be inserted in an attempt to prevent strictures and to lavage the stomach. In the setting of more extensive burns, esophagogastrectomy may be life-saving. The nasogastric tube may be left *in situ* and used for enteral feeding.

Elimination Enhancement

Experience with these methods has not been described in the literature.

Supportive Measures

- Treatment of benzalkonium chloride ingestion is mainly symptomatic and supportive and follows guidelines for the treatment of caustic products including early esophagoscopy.
- Asthmatic patients should be hospitalized in an intensive care facility with access to intravenous lines, cardiac monitoring, and oxygen. Treatment must be directed toward rehydration, parenteral nutrition, and supplemental oxygen.
- Local treatment for mouth and hypopharynx burns includes tepid water sponging around the mouth, acetaminophen orally, antibiotics, and intravenous fluids until oral intake is resumed.
- When clinically indicated, expansion of circulatory blood volume, vasoactive drugs, supplemental oxygen, and treatment of seizures should be instituted promptly.
- A complete blood count, methemoglobin determination, glucose, creatinine, lactic acid dehydrogenase, bilirubin, aminotransferases, and arterial blood gases should be performed periodically. Chest x-ray and electrocardiogram (ECG) should

be obtained early. A leucocytosis and elevations in uric acid and aminotransferases may occur.

- If solutions stronger than 1:3000 enter the eyes, irrigate the eyes with water for 15 to 20 minutes.
- Benzalkonium chloride may cause a false elevation of serum sodium and potassium as measured with some ion-selective electrodes.

BENZYL ALCOHOL

Benzyl alcohol is a preservative and local anesthetic. It is used as a preservative in newborn medications such as bacteriostatic saline, heparin, phenobarbital, pancuronium, AquaMEPHYTON®, and neonatal trace metal solutions. Preterm infants may develop a "gasping syndrome" characterized by gradual neurologic deterioration, severe metabolic acidosis, a striking onset of gasping respirations, hematologic abnormalities, skin breakdown, hepatic and renal failure, hypotension, and cardiovascular collapse.

CETRIMIDE

Cetrimide (atrimonium bromide) is a cationic surfactant used as an antiseptic. Contact dermatitis and sterile chemical peritonitis have been associated with this agent. Oral cetrimide may lead to irritation of the gastrointestinal mucosa, vomiting, and depolarization at cholinergic neuromuscular junctions. Respiratory paralysis, hypotension, and coma may cause death. At least two deaths secondary to cetrimide ingestion have been reported. Cetrimide ingestion is treated as a caustic agent. There is no specific antidote to cetrimide.

CHLORBUTOL

Chlorbutol (chlorbutanol) is used as a preservative in some European preparations of heparin (benzyl alcohol is used more often in the United States). This agent may have significant hypotensive, respiratory depressant, sedative, and cumulative effects. Chlorbutanol is related structurally to trichloroethanol, the active metabolite of the hypnotic sedative chloral hydrate. In Australia, it is available as an OTC sleep aid. Death after ingestion of chlorbutol by an adult was associated with whole blood chlorbutanol concentrations of 64 μg/mL analyzed by gas chromatography.

CHLOROACETAMIDE

Chloroacetamide is a preservative used in cosmetic creams. Toxic effects may include contact dermatitis and allergic contact eczema.

CHLOROCRESOL

Chlorocresol is a phenolic antibacterial preservative, which may cause contact dermatitis and eczema.

DEQUALINIUM

Dequalinium may cause allergic reactions, genital ulcerations, and necrosis.

FORMALDEHYDE POLYMERS

Formaldehyde polymers are used as preservatives, antifungal and antibacterial agents in cosmetics, and topical pharmaceuticals. These agents actually may release formaldehyde and cause skin and respiratory sensitization.

MERCURIALS

Phenylmercuric acetate, phenylmercuric nitrate, nitromersol, thiomersal, mercurochrome, mercurobutol, and merthiolate are chemicals used as preservatives in eye drops, eye ointments, vaccines, and other products. They also are used in skin disinfection, treatment of skin infections, contraceptive jellies, and hemorrhoidal treatments. A thiomersal-preserved contact lens gel contact left residual mercury in the cornea and aqueous humor in one case. Contact sensitization may occur. Eye drops with phenylmercuric nitrate may leave a melanoid pigmentation on the lens.

PARABENS

Parabens or parahydroxybenzoate esters include methyl, ethyl, propyl, butyl, and benzoyl esters of p-hydroxybenzoic acids, and are preservatives in pharmaceuticals, cosmetics, and foods. Contact allergies, contact dermatitis, bronchospasm, pruritus, rash, nausea, and vomiting may develop following use of these compounds. Cross-reaction to benzocaine and procaine has occurred.

QUATERNARY AMMONIUM ANTISEPTICS

These are preservatives used in ophthalmic solutions and topical lotions. Allergic contact dermatitis and hypersensitivity may occur with these agents.

SORBIC ACID

Sorbic acid is an antimicrobial used in topical preparations. It is a weak sensitizer, which may cause contact sensitivity and eczema.

TRICLOSAN

Triclosan is a chlorinated phenol used as an antimicrobial in cosmetic products. Contact sensitivity has been reported with this agent.

Questions—Preservatives and Antibacterials

1. **Benzalkonium chloride**
   A. Ingestion may produce corrosive lesions of the palate, hypopharynx, esophagus, and stomach
   B. Has been observed to cause pulmonary edema and methemoglobinemia
   C. Typically is followed by death in 2 to 3 days after ingestion
   D. A and B
   E. B and C

2. **Which of the following preservatives is matched with its correct associated side effect?**
   A. Phenylmercuric nitrate—Melanoid pigmentation on the lens
   B. Parabens—Gasping syndrome
   C. Benzoyl alcohol—Hypotension
   D. Chlorbutol—Cross reaction to benzocaine
   E. All of the above

Thickening, Suspending, Binding And Solvent Agents

These agents keep solids suspended in mixtures. Starches are used in manufacturing tablets and may cause problems in patients with celiac disease (gluten enteropathy). Acacia and tragacanth may cause sensitivity reactions and angioneurotic edema. Polyvinylpyrrolidone (PVP, povidone) is a suspending agent used in skin and hair sprays to produce a firm film and in injectables such as penicillin, cortisone, procaine, and insulin to delay absorption. PVP may cause lung lesions, pseudotumors at injection sites, polyneuropathy, and deposits of PVP in organ systems. Carboxymethylcellulose may cause an allergic contact dermatitis.

Ethylenediamine is used in the manufacture of aminophylline preparations and as a preservative in some creams. Products containing ethylenediamine include many brands of rubber gloves and other rubber products, shellacs, insecticides, waxes, and dyes. It is a potent sensitizer. Antihistamines of the ethylenediamine group (e.g., antazoline, pyrilamine) provoke reactions if taken by sensitized individuals. Cross-sensitivity between ethylenediamine and ethylenediamine tetraacetic acid (EDTA) may occur. Ethylenediamine-induced delayed hypersensitivity has been described. In addition, various solvents are used to suspend and dissolve various pharmaceutical and other products.

ALCOHOLS

At least 500 pharmaceutical agents contain ethanol. Most are oral preparations. Some such as diazepam, trimethoprim-sulfamethoxazole, digoxin, and phenytoin are parenteral. Intravenous nitroglycerin may contain 0.06 to 0.14 mL ethanol/mg nitroglycerin and can produce somnolence, slurred speech, and snoring respirations.

DIMETHYL SULFOXIDE

Dimethyl sulfoxide is a penetrating solvent for some topical medicaments. Nausea, vomiting, abdominal cramps, chills, chest pains, and drowsiness have been reported as well as erythema, itching, garlic odor on the breath, and transient hemolysis. See Chapter 46, Hydrocarbons.

POLYETHYLENE GLYCOLS

These low-molecular-weight liquid, polymeric alcohols are used as solvent vehicles in topical pharmaceuticals, shampoos, cosmetics, contraceptive gels, and other products. Mixtures of higher polyethylene glycols (PEGs) such as carbowax are ingredients in formation of suppositories and pessaries. Urticaria and delayed allergic eczematous reactions may occur. Burn patients have died with acute renal failure after use of polyethylene glycol burn creams.

PROPYLENE GLYCOL

Propylene glycol is used as a vehicle for oral, injectable, and topical preparations. The compound may be absorbed and may produce a rise in serum osmolality. Contact dermatitis, erythematous edematous plaques, and contact hypersensitivity may occur.

Questions—Thickening, Suspending, Binding and Solvent Agents

1. Polyvinylpyrrolidone (PVP) may cause all of the following except
A. Lung lesions
B. Pseudotumors at injection sites
C. Polyneuropathy
D. Thrombocytopenia
E. Deposits in organ systems

2. Suppositories and pessaries may contain which of the following ingredients?
A. Propylene glycol
B. Polyethylene glycol
C. Dimethyl sulfoxide
D. Polyvinylpyrrolidone
E. None of the above

Lubricants, Fats and Oils

Lubricants are used to prevent compressed tablets from sticking to surfaces during the manufacturing process. Common examples include magnesium stearate, talc, liquid paraffin, stearic acid, and boric acid. Talc also is used to coat tablets. Talc retinopathies have been associated with drug abuse. Although talc is similar chemically to asbestos and may contain traces of asbestos, no firm relationship between talc and neoplasia has been established. Talc is a lubricant in surgical gloves and may induce granuloma formation. Starch also may cause granuloma formation.

Lanolin is used in ointment bases, creams, soaps, toiletries, leather manufacture, polishes, and shoe creams. Hypersensitivity may result from its aliphatic alcohols. There is a high incidence of lanolin allergy among eczema patients. Oleomas (paraffinomas or oleogranulomas) rarely occur in the gastrointestinal tract after paraffin use. They may occur in skin after injection of mineral or vegetable oil as parenteral drug vehicles, or accidentally with high-pressure grease guns. Hypersensitivity from petrolatum (soft paraffin) is extremely rare.

Questions — Lubricants, Fats And Oils

1. Which of the following may cause granuloma formation?
A. Talc
B. Liquid paraffin
C. Starch
D. Magnesium stearate
E. A and C

2. Talc retinopathies have been associated with drug abuse.
A. True
B. False

3. Oleomas occur in the gastrointestinal tract after paraffin use
A. Usually
B. Always
C. Rarely
D. Never
E. None of the above

Flavoring and Sweetening Agents

ACESULFAME

Acesulfame, also known as acesulfame K, has been approved for use in chewing gum, dry drink mixes, gelatin, puddings, and nondairy creamers. It is about 200 times sweeter than sugar and is not metabolized or broken down for use by the body. Acesulfame has some structural resemblance to saccharin and may bind to the same receptor.

ANISEED OIL

Aniseed oil, also called anise, may cause mucous membrane and skin sensitivity.

ASPARTAME

L-Aspartyl-L-phenylalanine methyl ester is a nutritive sweetener approved by the FDA in 1981 that provides 4 kcal/gram, and is 180 to 200 times sweeter than sucrose. Although 10% is converted to methanol, this has not proved to be a problem in clinical use. Aspartame elevates plasma phenylalanine levels. One liter of soft drink sweetened with aspartame can contain up to 400 mg of aspartame. Patients with urticaria after use of aspartame have been reported.

Data accumulated to date appear to indicate that the majority of individuals, including pregnant women and children, who consume less than 50 mg / kg / d of aspartame, do not experience adverse effects. One study indicated that migraine sufferers may experience an increase in frequency of migraines after aspartame ingestion. Anecdotal reports of accidental ingestion of large numbers of Equal® tablets (25 to 100) by small children suggest that it has not caused adverse effects.

CYCLAMATE

Excessive doses of the artificial sweetener cyclamate may induce diarrhea, a photosensitivity reaction, erythematous rash, renal tubular acidosis, and hypokalemia. Cyclamate may be cocarcinogenic in animals and is banned in the United States. Cyclamate may cause occasional hypersensitivity and urticaria relieved by diphenhydramine, pruritus, wheezing, and exacerbation of symptoms of systemic lupus erythematosus.

FRUCTOSE

Sucrose is metabolized in the liver to fructose. Fructose may be fatal in infants with fructose intolerance and dangerous in patients with fructose-1, 6-diphosphatase deficiency.

LACTOSE

While pharmacologically inert, and nontoxic, lactose malabsorption may involve as many as 5% to 10% of the British population. Those intolerant of lactose may have abdominal cramps, diarrhea, flatulence, distention, and sometimes vomiting.

LICORICE

Licorice root (7% glycyrrhizic acid) is a steroidal glucoside. Long-term ingestion of 1 g or more daily of glycyrrhizic acid can result in severe metabolic disturbances. Hypokalemia may be severe and require potassium chloride by central venous catheter. Toxic effects of licorice ingestion may include rare hyperprolactinemia, amenorrhea, headache, and hyperaldosteronism with hypokalemia and low plasma renin. Other clinical effects may include salt and water retention with edema, hypertension, congestive heart failure, weakness, tetany, loss of libido, and myoglobinuria.

The mineralocorticoid activity of licorice results from the inhibition of an enzyme that normally inactivates cortisol. By preventing the inactivation of cortisol, licorice increases the glucocorticoid concentration in mineralocorticoid-responsive tissues. Consequently, glucocorticoids occupy the mineralocorticoid receptors and produce a mineralocorticoid response, as evidenced by increased sodium retention and hypertension.

MONOSODIUM GLUTAMATE

Monosodium glutamate (MSG) may cause a constellation of adverse clinical symptoms that has been termed the "Chinese Restaurant Syndrome." Flushing, headache, and chest pain have been associated with ingestion of this agent.

PEPPERMINT OIL

Peppermint oil contains menthol and various terpenes. Atrial fibrillation, swelling of tongue, lips, and gingival mucosa, urticaria, flushing, and headache all have been associated with its use.

SORBITOL

This sugar alcohol may cause flatulence, diarrhea, and abdominal distention. In dialysis solutions, it may cause vomiting, hypertension, and coma.

SUCROSE

Liquid medicines, particularly those intended for children, often are formulated as sucrose-based syrups. Total sugar content may be as high as 80%. Adverse effects include complication of diabetes management and increased dental caries.

Question—Flavoring and Sweetening Agents

1. Which of the following tend to cause mucous membrane and skin sensitivity?
A. Anise
B. Acesulfame
C. Aspartame
D. Cyclamate
E. A and D

2. Which of the following are associated with licorice toxicity?
A. Headache
B. Amenorrhea
C. Hyperprolactinemia
D. B and C
E. All of the above

3. All of the following are associated with peppermint oil ingestion except
A. Atrial fibrillation
B. Lip and tongue swelling
C. Diarrhea
D. Urticaria
E. Flushing

4. Ingestions of a large number of Equal® tablets by children have resulted in no adverse effects.
A. True
B. False

FLUORIDES

Fluoride is a halogen element with unique properties. In toxic quantities, it can alter calcium availability to tissues, effect changes in blood clotting parameters, cause severe cardiac dysfunction, alter bone and tooth structure, and lead to death. It is used for prophylaxis against dental caries, in insecticides, in certain rodenticides, and as a dietary supplement. It also is used in swine anthelminthics, the petroleum industry in hydrofluoric acid, in timber preservation, glass etching, toothpaste, phosphate, aluminum, and magnesium production, and is potentially useful in treating and preventing osteoporosis.

PATHOPHYSIOLOGY

Fluoride ions have a strong affinity for calcium ions, altering calcium within the bloodstream, impairing calcium / phosphorus homeostasis, and effecting tissue changes secondary to diminished calcium levels in the heart, muscle, and clotting mechanisms. Fluoride ions in gastric juice react with acid locally to form the highly irritating hydrofluoric acid, which accounts for many of the gastrointestinal adverse effects that are a feature of fluoride poisoning.

Fluoride interferes with collagen formation and acts directly on muscle and nerve tissue to cause neurologic disturbances. Fluorides interfere with enzymes involved in anaerobic glycolysis, cholinesterase function, and enzymes that contain magnesium or zinc that are involved in tissue respiration. Fluorides may act directly on vasomotor smooth muscle tone of blood vessels.

PHARMACOKINETICS

Absorption

- Sodium fluoride is almost 100% absorbed through the stomach and small intestine.
- Absorption may be retarded if calcium salts, milk, or antacids are taken simultaneously.
- Fluoride inhaled as a result of industrial exposure is absorbed mainly through the respiratory tract in either gaseous or particulate form.
- Gaseous fluoride is almost all hydrogen fluoride, has a high aqueous solubility, and is absorbed in the upper respiratory tract.
- On the skin, fluoride deposits may cause hydrofluoric acid burns.

Distribution

- Peak levels of fluorides in the serum are reached in 30 minutes, after which the fluoride is distributed throughout the intracellular and extracellular water.
- Deposition occurs mostly in teeth, bone, thyroid, aorta, and kidney.
- In sufficient doses, 50% of absorbed fluoride is taken up by bone. Plasma contains about 72% of whole blood fluoride.
- Fluoride occurs as a free ion and is not protein bound.
- Bone and teeth contain 112 to 310 mg/kg and brain, lung, liver, and kidney contain 0.2 to 0.8 mg/kg.

Elimination

- 50% of fluorides appear in urine within 24 hours. Six to 10% is found in the feces, 13% to 23% in sweat (may be up to 50% depending on temperature and humidity), and the remainder in bone.
- The therapeutic half-life of fluorides is 2.0 to 9.0 hours; however, in end-stage renal failure the half-life can be as high as 2 years.
- The urine concentration of fluorides (normal) ranges from 0.2 to 1.1 mg/L.

CLINICAL PRESENTATIONS

Acute toxicity may occur within minutes. Chronic fluorosis generally develops after prolonged (10 to 20 years) exposure to industrial dusts, insecticides, or water where fluorides exceed 4 ppm. This is especially true in workers involved in the production of aluminum, steel, or glass.

Gastrointestinal Effects

Small amounts produce a metallic, bitter taste. Larger amounts may result in acute burning in the mouth and a sore tongue. Nausea, vomiting, and diarrhea may occur soon after ingestion and are accompanied by sialorrhea, hematemesis, and epigastric cramping abdominal pain. These symptoms may persist for 24 hours.

Respiratory Effects

Respiration first is stimulated, then depressed. Laryngeal and pulmonary edema may be observed. When severe overdoses occur, symptoms develop within 30 minutes and death can supervene within 2 to 4 hours. If the victim survives the first 24 hours, the prognosis is good. Sulfur hexafluoride (SF_6) may cause acute pulmonary edema. Sulfur tetrafluoride (SF_4) has an odor similar to sulfur dioxide. The toxicity of SF_4 has been compared with that of phosgene. Shortness of breath, chest tightness, productive cough, nose and eye irritation, headache, nausea, and vomiting may follow exposure.

Bone Effects

The only toxic effect of fluoride on teeth occurs when excessive doses are taken during the formative period of the teeth, which is from birth to age 8 to 10 years. If a young child ingests over 1.5 to 2.0 mg/day, a white lacy fluorosis occurs. At 3 mg or more per day, a brown stain occurs. Sodium fluoride increases spinal bone mass, but does not appear to prevent vertebral fractures in patients who already have had vertebral fractures. There still is little evidence that sodium fluoride increases cortical bone mass. Bone that forms with fluoride therapy does not appear to have normal strength and appears to be qualitatively inferior. Sodium fluoride does not appear to be an effective or safe treatment for postmenopausal osteoporosis.

Neurologic Effects

Tetany, carpopedal spasm, positive Chvostek sign, and hyperreflexia are associated with depression in serum calcium. Headaches, paresthesias, visual disturbances, optic neuritis, convulsions, and central nervous system depression may result from the direct effect of fluoride ion on nervous tissue. Patients may have nonspecific symptoms such as headaches, nausea, diminished appetite, or vague back pains and stiffness.

"Neighborhood" Fluorosis

"Neighborhood" fluorosis has been described in families residing near a source of fluoride emission from industrial plants. This nonskeletal fluorosis manifests with fatigue, arthralgias, myalgias, severe headaches, nausea, vomiting, epigastric pain, diarrhea, nasal irritation, and conjunctival irritation.

TOXIC DOSAGE/DEATH

The therapeutic dose of sodium fluoride is 0.25 to 0.5 mg/day orally, and this produces a therapeutic blood level of 0.4 to 2 μg/dL. The lethal dose is 5 to 10 g (70 to 140 mg/kg) orally. Less than 1 g of sodium fluoride by mouth has caused severe poisoning; however, 6 g given over 9 days intravenously has been tolerated. Ingestion of as little as a spoonful of glass etching cream (ammonium bifluoride 20% and sodium bifluoride 13%) can lead to life-threatening risk of injury.

Excessive fluoridation of water may cause teeth alterations. 1 ppm produces no effects, 1.5 to 2 ppm results in yellowish-brown mottling of enamel and over 2.5 ppm leads to roughening of the surface and dark discoloration of enamel. It is recommended that no supplemental fluorides be given to infants or children where the fluoride content of the drinking water is over 0.7 ppm. Unfortunately, overfluoridation of drinking water has resulted in mass intoxication.

DRUG INTERACTIONS

Complexation of fluoride ion with calcium-containing products has been referred to above.

PREGNANCY/LACTATION

Fluoride may appear in breast milk. There appears to be a physiologic plasma-milk barrier against fluoride in the newborn, in contrast with another halogen, bromine, which rapidly accumulates in milk. Normal fluoride metabolism is not altered in pregnant women.

LABORATORY

Analytic Methods

A fluoride-specific, ion-specific potentiometer electrode method is available for measurement of fluoride ion.

Blood Levels

Blood levels for fluorides are useful, but only within the first hour after ingestion because of their rapid absorption. When either blood or urine is obtained, treatment cannot wait for delays in obtaining and processing of samples. Urine levels may be more useful but must be obtained within the first hours after exposure. Levels in some cases may remain elevated for days. Blood fluoride levels may be normal or slightly elevated in chronic exposures. A lethal fluoride level is estimated at 3 mg/L. Urine fluoride values as high as 320 μg/mL have been reported in cases of fatal ingestion.

TREATMENT

Gut Decontamination

If fluoride insecticides have been ingested recently, gastric lavage followed by milk has been suggested. Charcoal probably is ineffective. In noninsecticide fluoride ingestions, treatment guidelines vary depending on the amount ingested. If less than 8 mg/kg of elemental fluoride has been eaten, give milk and observe at home for at least 6 hours. Refer to a health care facility if any symptoms, such as nausea, vomiting, diarrhea, abdominal pain, lethargy, fatigue, or weakness develop. Whether to induce emesis with syrup of ipecac in this group of patients is somewhat controversial.

If more than 8 mg/kg of elemental fluoride has been ingested, gastric lavage, milk, and referral to a health care facility are recommended. In cases where an unknown amount is ingested, if asymptomatic, give milk, observe at home for at least 6 hours, and refer to a health care facility if any symptoms develop. If symptomatic, give milk and refer immediately to a health care facility.

Elimination Enhancement

Peritoneal dialysis and hemodialysis are unnecessary in the presence of normal renal function. Consider hemodialysis in patients with significant toxicity and evidence of renal failure.

Supportive Measures

- Treatment in a health care facility includes cardiac monitoring and support of vital signs.
- Maintain airway (endotracheal intubation if inadequate tidal volume), and evaluate blood pressure frequently, as shock may supervene rapidly. Keep patient warm, treat shock vigorously with isotonic saline in 5% glucose to restore blood volume, and enhance renal excretion of fluorides. Pressor amines may be required.
- Keep close observation on intake and output. Monitor for any development of pulmonary edema.
- Monitor and treat alterations in serum electrolytes, calcium, and magnesium levels.
- Whole blood and ionized calcium levels will be depressed in serious overdoses within minutes and may remain depressed for 4 to 24 hours. Blood levels of potassium may be decreased or increased and magnesium levels often are decreased.
- ECGs may show prolongation of Q-T intervals, peaked T-waves (hyperkalemia), or arrhythmias (including ventricular fibrillation). Cardiovascular collapse may be related to the propensity of fluoride ion to bind calcium and magnesium ions intracellularly and extracellularly.
- Lidocaine for arrhythmias and temporary pacemakers may be necessary. Administer milk, or aluminum or magnesium-based antacids to bind fluoride in alert patients.
- Leukocytosis and fever may be secondary to the known ability of fluoride to activate superoxide production and arachidonic acid release from neutrophils. Clotting factors may be altered.
- X-ray of the long bones may show evidence of fluorohydroxyapatite deposition in chronic cases.

ANTIDOTES

Where evidence of hypocalcemic or normocalcemic tetany is present, calcium gluconate (10 mL of a 10% solution) is slowly injected intravenously to avoid tachycardia. Calcium chloride (5% to 20%) given intravenously in doses of 5 to 10 mL slowly may be useful if calcium gluconate is not available, but if used repeatedly in an acidotic patient or in a patient with renal insufficiency it may induce systemic acidosis.

Questions—Fluorides

1. Absorption of fluoride
   A. Is almost 100% through the large intestine
   B. May be slowed if milk is taken simultaneously
   C. Is not possible via inhalation
   D. Through the skin is uncomplicated
   E. None of the above

2. Fluoride toxicity affects all of the following systems except
   A. Bone
   B. Respiratory system
   C. Ophthalmologic
   D. Neurologic system
   E. Gastrointestinal system

3. Chronic exposure to fluoride is incompatible with normal serum fluoride levels.
   A. True
   B. False

4. Treatment of fluoride toxicity may include
   A. Drinking milk
   B. Hemodialysis
   C. Careful monitoring of calcium and potassium
   D. A and C
   E. All of the above

IODINE

Iodine is used as an antiseptic and still may be found in home medicine cabinets. In the hospital setting, iodine frequently is used to clean skin before minor laceration repairs and in the operating room before surgery. Acute ingestion of iodine can result in corrosive injury of the gastrointestinal tract and renal damage. Cardiopulmonary collapse secondary to circulatory failure, edema of the epiglottis, and aspiration pneumonia may cause death.

Iodine toxicity may arise from dietary supplements, oral drugs (e.g., potassium iodide), topical medications (antiseptics), injected iodinated contrast media, and intentional excess iodine ingestion, symptoms may include corrosive gastroenteritis, ventricular irritability, large tender salivary glands, hyperthyroidism, hemolytic anemia, metabolic acidosis, seizures, and acute renal failure. Death has been reported after iodine use.

Iodophors are loose complexes of elemental iodine attached to a high-molecular-weight carrier. They generally enhance the bactericidal activity of iodine. Povidone-iodine (Betadine®) is found commonly in emergency departments and operating rooms.

Pathophysiology

Elemental iodine is a topical antiseptic effective at concentrations equal to or over 0.5 ppm. Iodophors, solutions of complex iodine-containing anionic and nonionic detergents, contain low free-iodine levels in the range of 0.8 to 1.2 ppm. Betadine prep solution (10% povidone-iodine) is an iodophor of iodine, polyvinyl-pyrrolidone (PVP), and detergent. Betadine surgical scrub is 7.5% povidone-iodine.

Metabolic acidosis, hyperchloremia, hypernatremia, hyperosmolarity, and renal failure have been associated with elevated serum iodine concentrations. The metabolic acidosis may be due to the acidic pH (2.43) of the povidone-iodine or to the consumption of bicarbonate by the combination of free iodine with serum sodium bicarbonate. Hyperchloremia probably represents spurious elevations in the serum chloride from interference with the assay by iodine.

Pharmacokinetics

ABSORPTION

- Iodine may result in poisoning by (a) the oral ingestion of iodine or its alcoholic solution; (b) the oral ingestion of the salts of iodine, which occasionally result in iodism; (c) the inhalation of fumes into the upper and lower respiratory tracts; (d) absorption of the tincture from a cyst into which it has been injected; and (e) the absorption of alcoholic solutions or povidone-iodine solutions applied to the skin or to body cavities.
- The occlusive nature of an ointment or the greater absorption of a povidone-iodine solution would be expected to enhance iodine absorption.

DISTRIBUTION

- Iodine is converted in the intestine before it is absorbed.
- Iodide is actively transported into thyroid tissue.

ELIMINATION

- Both iodine and iodide are excreted in the urine.

Clinical Presentations

Metabolic acidosis, hyperchloremia (iodide concentrations can falsely elevate serum chloride measurements), hypernatremia, hyperosmolarity, diminished anion gap, and renal failure may follow excessive absorption of iodine from topical iodine-containing preparations. Clinical hypothyroidism, hyperthyroidism, changes in sensorium manifested by agitation, confusion, hallucinations, stomatitis, and diarrhea have been observed. Hypotension, tachycardia, cyanosis, and shock are consistent with iodine toxicity.

Early clinical signs of acute systemic iodine/iodide toxicity may stem from the stimulation of exocrine gland secretions producing rhinorrhea, conjunctivitis, and cough. A high anion-gap metabolic acidosis (lactic acid-mediated), acute respiratory distress, and congestive heart failure may intervene.

Toxic Dosage/Death

The minimum lethal dose of iodine in humans is unknown. The fatal dose of iodine has been reported as 2 to 4 g of free iodine or 1 to 2 ounces of strong iodine tincture. A 74-year-old woman absorbed about 800 mL of one-quarter-strength Betadine® solution, developed a cardiac arrest and died. A 72-year-old male who had a povidone wash twice daily for 6 months for decubitus ulcers developed thyrotoxicosis. Very-low-birth weight infants subjected to 10% povidone-iodine solutions for insertion of intravenous cannulae and blood gas determinations have developed hypothyroidism.

Pregnancy/Lactation

Studies on the use of iodine-containing solutions as antiseptics or disinfectants in pregnant or lactating women have not been performed. Iodides cross the placenta and are excreted in breast milk.

Laboratory

Analytic Methods

Serum may be analyzed for iodine and iodine moieties by using the known iodine-catalyzed reduction of ceric ammonium sulfate by arsenious oxide. Serum chloride determinations may result in false elevations in serum chloride levels. In the presence of elevated iodine concentrations, a silver halide precipitation assay may be used for an accurate measurement of serum chloride concentration.

BLOOD LEVELS

There are no studies of clinical correlations with serum iodine determinations, and the actual concentration at which toxic symptoms may occur is unknown. The extent of iodine skin absorption appears to be related to the size of the area of application. Serum iodine concentrations ranged from 590 to 1400 μg/dL after application of povidone-iodine ointment to burns of 0% to 15% total body surface area, from 910 to 2390 μg/dL in 15% to 30% total body surface area (TBSA) burns, and from 1200 to 4900 μg/dL in over 30% TBSA burns.

Treatment

GUT DECONTAMINATION

Emesis is contraindicated. Charcoal does not adsorb iodine and has not been shown helpful after iodine ingestion. Milk every 15 minutes has been suggested to manage stomach irritation. Gastric lavage is contraindicated if there is evidence of esophageal damage. Administration of starch (25 g in 500 mL water) followed by sodium thiosulfate (15%) may convert iodine to relatively harmless iodide.

ELIMINATION ENHANCEMENT

There are no studies on the use of modalities such as extracorporeal methods (hemodialysis, hemoperfusion) in the treatment of antiseptic iodine excess.

SUPPORTIVE MEASURES

- Patients who have developed symptoms of iodine overdose should be seen in a hospital facility to be evaluated for evidence of metabolic acidosis, anion gap abnormalities, hyper- or hypothyroidism, and renal failure.
- Maintenance of the airway, and circulatory stabilization are the mainstays of therapy. Fluid and electrolyte balance must be monitored.
- Iodine toxicity may be associated with elevated serum aminotransferase levels, hyperbilirubinemia, neutropenia, and hypoxemia. Povidone-iodine added to a urine sample may be a cause of factitious hematuria (false-positive dipstick).
- Elevated iodine levels have been reported following application of povidone-iodine to intact skin and umbilical cords of normal infants, during continuous mediastinal irrigation, after

peritoneal irrigation, and in burn patients treated topically with povidone-iodine.

SKIN CONSIDERATIONS

- Skin contaminated with excess povidone-iodine should be washed with soap and water.
- Starch may be applied to ascertain that all of the iodine has been removed (note the blue color).
- If skin burns develop, observe for metabolic acidosis, renal failure, and altered mental status.
- To prevent skin contact with solids or liquids containing iodine, workers should be provided with and required to use personal protective equipment such as gloves, face shields, and any other appropriate protective clothing deemed necessary.
- If there is any possibility that clothing has been contaminated with solid iodine or liquids containing iodine, a worker should change into uncontaminated clothing before leaving the work area.
- Workers who handle solid iodine or liquids containing iodine should wash their hands thoroughly with soap or mild detergent and water before eating, smoking, or using toilet facilities.
- Eye exposures are irrigated for 15 minutes with water.

Questions—Iodine

1. **Iodine toxicity causes**
   A. Corrosive injury of the gastrointestinal tract
   B. Headaches
   C. Diarrhea
   D. A and B
   E. A and C
2. **Elevated serum iodine levels typically have been associated with**
   A. Metabolic acidosis
   B. Hyperchloremia
   C. Hypernatremia
   D. All of the above
   E. None of the above
3. **Serum iodine determinations are known to correlate well with clinical symptoms.**
   A. True
   B. False

LAXATIVES

Laxatives are ubiquitous products that are available as liquids, tablets, gums, powders, granules, suppositories, and enema dosage forms. Many millions of dollars are spent in the United States on more than 500 laxative preparations sold as OTC cathartic preparations. They work in different ways to promote stool evacuation and, while generally safe in prescribed situations, may cause significant morbidity when abused. Purging or catharsis is employed by most individuals at some time during their lifetime in an attempt to "clean" the gastrointestinal tract. However, the surreptitious ingestion of laxative drugs is a common etiology to account for severe chronic diarrhea in individuals who have had extensive investigations that fail to reveal a diagnosis.

Bulk Laxatives

Bulk-forming laxatives absorb water in the intestine and swell the stool into an easily passed soft mass. Each dose is taken with an 8-ounce glass of liquid. Although bulk agents generally are regarded as the safest form of laxative, users should be aware that the products can interfere with absorption of certain drugs, including aspirin, digitalis, antibiotics, and anticoagulants. People with the genetic disorder phenylketonuria should not take any sugar-free bulk laxative containing phenylalanine. Bulk laxatives include FiberCon®, Metamucil®, and Serutan®.

Although bran is considered a bulk agent, the FDA has said that bran cereals marketed solely as food products will not be subject to laxative regulations. Many bulk-laxative products contain water-soluble gums such as karaya, methylcellulose, plantago seed, psyllium, and polycarbophil. Psyllium hydrophilic mucilloid, a nonproteinaceous gum composed of a mixture of polysaccharides, is derived from the seeds or husk of the plant *Plantago ovata.* Psyllium seed hypersensitivity (e.g., asthma, allergic rhinitis, and anaphylaxis) has been observed in nurses dispensing the product or pharmaceutical workers involved in its manufacture. Anaphylaxis has followed oral ingestion of a psyllium-containing cereal. Water-soluble gums taken without adequate water can cause choking.

Carbon Dioxide Releasers

Carbon dioxide-releasing suppositories produce carbon dioxide in the bowels. The gas pushes stubborn stools toward elimination.

Combinations

Some products contain a combination of laxatives. These drugs may carry a higher risk of side effects.

Enemas

Enemas introduce fluid and various stimulants to the lower gastrointestinal tract to promote elimination of feces. Enemas may include lubricants such as mineral oil, and various ingredients including glycerin, sodium phosphate, Kayexalate and sorbitol.

Hyperosmotics

Hyperosmotic laxatives mimic the action of saline laxatives, but pose less risk of salt depletion. OTC hyperosmotics such as glycerin are available for rectal use only. A physician must prescribe oral hyperosmotics. Overuse of hyperosmotics can cause diarrhea.

Lubricants

Lubricant laxatives "grease" stools, facilitating elimination. Mineral oil and mineral-oil emulsions are the most common forms of lubricants. Among them are Agoral Plain® and Fleet Mineral Oil Enema®.

Saline Laxatives

Saline laxatives draw water into the bowel, thereby promoting easier passage of stools. Loss of body salts is a key risk of long-term use of these products. Among laxatives in this group are Milk of Magnesia, Citrate of Magnesia, and Epsom Salts.

Stimulants

Stimulant laxatives agitate or excite intestinal walls, causing waves of muscular contractions that expel fecal matter. Product names include Carter's Little Pills®, phenolphthalein, Dulcolax®, Ex-Lax®, Feen-A-Mint®, and Fletcher's Castoria®.

Stool Softeners

Stool softeners or emollients soften hard stools by enabling them to absorb more liquids. Brands include Colace®, Dialose®, Regutol®, and Surfak®.

Pathophysiology

Stimulant drugs alter fluid and electrolyte absorption, producing net intestinal fluid accumulation. Increased concentrations of cyclic AMP occurring in colonic mucosal cells may alter permeability and lead to net fluid accumulation and laxative action. Phenolphthalein also acts directly or reflexly to increase the activity of the small intestine.

Pharmacokinetics

ABSORPTION

- Up to 15% of a therapeutic dose of phenolphthalein is absorbed and eliminated by the kidney, most of it in conjugated form.
- Phenolphthalein acts mainly on the colon about 6 hours after ingestion.

DISTRIBUTION

- The urine becomes pink or red after phenolphthalein use if it is sufficiently alkaline (pH 7 or more).

ELIMINATION

- Some absorbed phenolphthalein also is excreted in the bile, and the resulting enterohepatic cycle may contribute to prolongation of the laxative effect.

Clinical Presentations

The major findings in a laxative-abuse patient include chronic diarrhea, vomiting, abdominal pain, lassitude, thirst, weakness, edema, bone pain resulting from osteomalacia, and weight loss. Findings may disclose a protein-losing enteropathy, steatorrhea, and pathologic colon changes associated with featureless radiologic findings, acid-base abnormalities, and hypokalemia. Such patients do not comply readily with treatment recommendations.

Metabolic problems may be secondary to chronic potassium depletion, a toxic effect on the nerve supply to the colon, or an injury to the liver. These patients may undergo extensive diagnostic workups including sigmoidoscopy, barium enema studies, rectal biopsies, upper gastrointestinal series, and computed tomography (CT) scans. Various agents, including senna, phenolphthalein, and sodium phosphate enemas have been abused by the above groups. These agents also may be accidentally misused or given to inadvertent recipients such as children.

LAXATIVE ABUSE

At least three well-recognized groups of individuals have been identified who abuse or misuse laxatives. Some become unwitting victims of laxative abuse. These individuals begin by taking laxatives regularly to relieve constipation and note that continued use of laxatives over years leads to increasing degrees of constipation. In turn, these individuals resort to stronger laxative purges, which may result in permanent distension and functional impairment of the colon.

The second group consists mostly of younger women with eating disorders, such as anorexia nervosa or bulimia. The third group consists predominantly of older women, without a known eating disorder, who are surreptitious laxative abusers, do not tell their physicians of their laxative use, deny its use when confronted, and experience symptoms after laxative use as a means of gaining attention. They are categorized as chronic, factitious (Munchausen type) laxative abusers.

PHENOLPHTHALEIN

Phenolphthalein is a stimulant laxative similar in many respects to bisacodyl, another diphenyl methane derivative. Child abuse has led to multiple "illnesses" associated with diarrhea and hospitalizations. Children who acutely ingest 1 g or less of a phenolphthalein-containing product are at minimal risk for developing dehydration. Phenolphthalein sensitization may be manifested by rash, pruritus, palpebral edema, fever, joint pains, diarrhea, colic, hypotension, seizures, paresis, coma, and even death. Hypersensitivity reactions have led to death.

PHOSPHATES

Adult-sized sodium phosphate enemas administered to constipated children may cause hypocalcemic tetany associated with elevated serum phosphate and decreased serum calcium. Calcium supplementation and hydration can reverse this state. Hazards of phosphate enemas administered rectally include hypocalcemia, hyperphosphatemia, hypokalemia, tetany, rectal necrosis, perforation, and death. Clinical features of hypocalcemia other than tetany may include weakness and fatigue with psychiatric manifestations of anxiety, depression, and irritability.

Extrapyramidal movement disorders, abdominal pain, urinary frequency, and muscle cramps may be seen. Arrhythmias with QT and ST prolongation are early cardiac manifestations. As hypocalcemia progresses, tetany, seizures, psychosis, bronchospasm, laryngospasm, heart failure, or hypotension may develop. Because of these serious effects, sodium phosphate enemas may lead to fatal poisoning, especially in infants.

POLYSTYRENE

Sodium polystyrene (Kayexalate®) in sorbitol enemas may lead to catastrophic colonic complications such as extensive transmural necrosis and infarction. Kayexalate crystals may be found adherent to the mucosa. Data suggest that sorbitol should not be included in Kayexalate® enemas given for hyperkalemia in renal transplant patients.

SENNA

Escherichia coli and other intestinal bacteria split Sennoside, the major substrates of senna leaf and fruit, to rhein anthron in the intestine. Anthraquinones such as rhein anthron in rhubarb have been incriminated in liver disease. Tetany associated with hypokalemia and hypocalcemia has been associated with chronic ingestion of excessive quantities of senna. Osteomalacia and arthropathy also have followed senna abuse. The clubbing may be reversible. Pericentral vein hepatic necrosis and hepatitis may follow senna abuse.

Toxic Dosage/Death

Toxic doses of phenolphthalein are generally greater than 100 mg. Doses associated with fatalities have been 1.8 g, and 0.65 to 1.3 g. Ingestion of a box of Ex-Lax® has led to fatalities.

Pregnancy/Lactation

Phenolphthalein is pregnancy risk category C.

Laboratory

ANALYTIC METHODS

Phenolphthalein concentration in the serum may be determined by thin-layer chromatography detected under ultraviolet light, and by a red color in the urine and feces.

BLOOD LEVELS

Serum phenolphthalein levels of 0.4 μg/L were observed in a chronic laxative abuser who developed coma and fever.

Treatment

GUT DECONTAMINATION

There is little indication for the use of activated charcoal. Children usually will not require gastric decontamination. They should be encouraged to consume extra fluids.

ELIMINATION ENHANCEMENT

Peritoneal dialysis was employed in an adult with a lactic acidosis and pulmonary edema after phenolphthalein overdose. The patient recovered. There is little clinical data on the use of extracorporeal methods to hasten elimination of phenolphthalein.

SUPPORTIVE MEASURES

- Treatment is largely symptomatic and supportive. Attention should be drawn towards volume and electrolyte repletion as needed.
- Treatment of patients with laxative abuse often is unsuccessful. If the patient is amenable, psychiatric intervention may require long-term inpatient psychiatric care.
- J-waves, typical of hypothermia, may be seen on ECG after phenolphthalein overdose. Metabolic acidosis may be present with lactic acidosis.
- Myoglobin in serum and urine, increased creatine phosphokinase, hypoglycemia, and elevated aminotransferases have been seen with laxative abuse.
- Electrolyte disturbances, particularly hypocalcemia, hypokalemia, and hypomagnesemia, all may be seen and should be adjusted accordingly.
- Urine color may be red-orange in individuals who use phenolphthalein. If a specimen of stool is alkalinized with sodium hydroxide and turns bright red, this generally indicates the presence of phenolphthalein and may suggest surreptitious use in certain cases. A deep purple Clinitest reaction with stool also suggests the possibility of phenolphthalein.

Questions—Laxatives

1. Bulking agents
A. Are the safest form of laxative
B. Interfere with the absorption of many medications
C. May include psyllium hydrophilic mucilloid
D. All of the above
E. None of the above

2. Glycerin is categorized as which kind of laxative?
A. Bulking agents
B. Carbon dioxide releasers
C. Enemas
D. Hyperosmotics
E. Lubricants

3. A key risk of chronic Milk of Magnesia use is
A. Malabsorption
B. Loss of body salts
C. Hypersensitivity reaction
D. Extrapyramidal movements
E. All of the above

4. The only well-described group of individuals who abuse or misuse laxatives is younger women with eating disorders.
A. True
B. False

5. Phenolphthalein can turn urine
A. Black
B. Purple
C. Red
D. Green
E. Blue

POISON LOOK-ALIKES

Numerous look-alike and sound-alike drugs often confuse inquisitive children, seeking candy, or well-meaning physicians who prescribe comparable-sounding medications. Certain iron preparations look like M&M® candy. Some look-alike drugs, often containing OTC stimulants such as caffeine and pseudoephedrine, intentionally resemble legitimate drugs (complete with imprint codes), and are advertised to college students by mail order as legal stimulants. They may be illegally sold, without usual ingredient or caution labeling, to teenagers who think the pills are street drugs such as "speed." They are known on the street by the same names as their controlled substance counterparts: black beauties, dexies, bennies, and others.

Fatal overdoses from caffeine-containing look-alike drugs have been reported. The FDA has given notice that OTC products containing caffeine, phenylpropanolamine, and ephedrine or combinations of any two of these are not allowed on the market. Despite the attempt to block the distribution and manufacture of look-alikes, such products continue to appear in forensic laboratories, in police confiscations, and as sources of overdoses.

SALT

Salt (sodium chloride) overdose is a serious poisoning, relatively infrequent in occurrence, difficult to manage, and frequently fatal. It is a toxicologic emergency. The most severe hypernatremia in adults has been seen as a result of salt emetics, bicarbonate administration during cardiac arrest, saline abortion, and accidental or voluntary ingestion of salt. Fortunately, with the lessened use of table salt as an emetic, this poisoning is seen less than before. Hypernatremia may follow amniotic fluid embolism during a saline-induced abortion. A small quantity of salt (1 to 2 tbsp) may produce profound hypernatremia and a rapidly progressive and fatal clinical course in the pediatric population.

Salt poisoning also has followed excessive intake of seawater, addition of salt instead of sugar to infant formulas, and excessive accidental intake by children or adults. It has followed forced feeding of children, a form of child abuse, and the use of hypertonic saline for gastric lavage. Too-rapid administration of normal saline (or hypertonic saline) with a rapid rise in plasma sodium concentration during treatment of hyponatremia, may lead to central pontine myelinolysis.

Pathophysiology

Sodium is the primary extracellular cation (140 mEq/L in the vascular and extracellular compartments and 10 mEq/L in the intracellular compartment). It is absorbed rapidly after oral intake. Rapid osmolar change is detected by osmoreceptors in the hypothalamus, leading to release of antidiuretic hormone. Increase in osmolality leads to stimulation of the thirst center, which in turn leads to an increase in fluid intake. Central nervous system damage occurs in salt poisoning because of cellular dehydration in brain cells following acute osmotic shift of intracellular fluids to the extracellular space. Cell shrinkage in the brain leads to distended cerebral vessels and may result in subarachnoid, subdural, and intravascular hemorrhage.

Pharmacokinetics

ABSORPTION

- Salt is freely soluble in water and slightly soluble in alcohol.
- The normal total body sodium is approximately 2,000 mEq, which accounts for about 90% of the osmolarity of the extracellular fluid.

DISTRIBUTION

- Increased intake of sodium chloride is distributed in the body to the extracellular fluid, resulting in an increase in the plasma sodium concentration and an increase in the total body sodium level.
- Because sodium contributes to about 90% of the osmolality of the extracellular fluid, an increase in plasma sodium will increase the plasma osmolality. As this occurs, the extracellular fluid becomes hypertonic, causing a shift of water from the intracellular to the extracellular space.
- The apparent volume of distribution of salt is 0.6 L/kg.

ELIMINATION

- Sodium chloride is excreted by the kidneys through the glomerulus and reabsorbed at the proximal tubule at the rate of about 1,000 mEq/h.

Clinical Presentations

When patients experience hypernatremia, skin loses its turgor, mucous membranes become dry, and muscles weaken. There is increased thirst and decreased appetite. With dehydration comes a rise in body temperature and a metabolic acidosis. In babies, the anterior fontanelle becomes flat. The brain volume decreases, leading to an increase and then a decrease in deep tendon reflexes, muscle rigidity, an increase in irritability, lethargy, opisthotonos, seizures, coma, and death resulting from circulatory collapse or central nervous system damage.

If the patient survives, there may be residual neurologic damage. Gastric mucosal irritation with vomiting and gastrointestinal ulceration have been reported. In slower courses, patients may develop pulmonary edema, tachypnea, tachycardia, and congestive heart failure. Hypotension, which manifests itself early in the course, may be refractory to fluid replacement.

Toxic Dosage/Death

Prior case reports of salt poisoning in the literature have demonstrated lethal dosages as low as 0.75 g/kg body weight, but generally have been estimated to be 3 g/kg body weight. An ingestion of 0.5 to 1 g/kg is toxic to most patients. In reports of severe hypernatremia resulting from salt or hypertonic saline intake, patients with serum sodium levels over 170 mmol/L have not survived. Death can be expected from severe osmolality values between 400 and 500 mOsm/kg. The mortality rate among adult patients with sodium levels over 160 mmol/L is 60%. Even in those who survived, severe central nervous system sequelae occurred.

Laboratory

ANALYTIC METHODS

Sodium is measured via an ion-specific electrode.

BLOOD LEVELS

The normal range for sodium is 135 to 146 mEq/L. Acute salt poisoning has been observed when serum sodium concentrations are over 170 mEq/L and usually is fatal in adults when the serum concentration is over 185 mEq/L. Recovery has occurred, in a chronic case, with a sodium concentration as high as 274 mEq/L.

Treatment

GUT DECONTAMINATION

Acute ingestions of salt may result in vomiting, and nausea without vomiting also may be evident. Syrup of ipecac may be useful in inducing emesis if the patient is seen within 30 minutes to 2 hours after ingestion, is alert, has not been convulsing, is not obtunded, has an active gag reflex, and is symptomatic following an excess ingestion of sodium chloride. Activated charcoal does not adsorb sodium and is not useful.

ELIMINATION ENHANCEMENT

The aim of treatment in salt overdose is to lower plasma or serum sodium and, thereby, to eliminate potential central nervous system damage. Intravenous 5% dextrose in water is used within the first 12 hours of ingestion. Rates of infusion will depend on the amount of diuresis, the change in serum osmolarity, and the neurologic status. Generally, the goal is to lower serum sodium by 10 mEq/L/d. In severe salt poisoning, especially with renal impairment, there is a possibility of inducing pulmonary edema, congestive heart failure, cerebral edema, and seizures if reduction in serum sodium with hydration occurs too rapidly.

If the hypernatremia is long-standing, a solution containing 25 to 50 mEq of sodium per liter should be used. If the serum sodium is over 180 mEq/L, there is no response to conservative therapy, and there is evidence of renal insufficiency, hemodialysis may be useful. Peritoneal dialysis was shown to be useful in lowering the serum sodium in a child who did not respond to conservative therapy in whom the serum sodium was between 185 and 200 mEq/L. Peritoneal dialysis is slow and may require over 24 hours of continuous exchanges to effect clinical improvement. Hemofilters have been developed that are suitable for use in infants and children. Continuous arteriovenous hemodiafiltration may be a useful alternative in the management of hypernatremia, particularly in the presence of renal failure.

SUPPORTIVE MEASURES

- Airway must be maintained by endotracheal intubation if necessary. Continuous cardiovascular monitoring should be instituted (ECG, pulse, and blood pressure) in severe cases.

- Treat hypotension with intravenous fluids and dopamine or norepinephrine, if required.
- Treat seizures with intravenous diazepam. If seizures cannot be controlled easily, phenytoin may be used.
- The exact rate at which hypernatremia should be corrected is unknown. In general, plasma sodium should be lowered gradually over 48 to 72 hours. Typically, half the deficit should be replaced over the first 12 to 24 hours and the remaining deficit should be replaced over the second 24- to 48-hour period.
- Slower rates are recommended in elderly patients: half the deficit should be replaced over 24 hours. Suggested rates of decrease of plasma Na range from 0.5 mEq/hour in chronic hypernatremia to 2 mEq/hour in acute hypernatremia. Many suggest 1 mEq/hour.
- It is imperative that treatment be actively instituted as soon as possible because central nervous system changes may occur within a few hours or less. Clinical evaluation of the patient is more important than calculations determined to establish the probable serum sodium level.
- Laboratory findings associated with sodium chloride excess include an increased serum and osmolarity, an increase in urine and plasma osmolarity, and a decrease in blood calcium (may cause tetany and seizures). Decreased serum potassium may be evident after fluid correction.

Questions—Salt

1. Central pontine myelinolysis may be avoided by
A. Sufficiently rapid sodium correction
B. Sufficiently slow sodium correction
C. Use of hypertonic saline for gastric lavage
D. All of the above
E. None of the above

2. Symptoms of hypernatremia may include all of the following except
A. Increased deep tendon reflexes
B. Decreased deep tendon reflexes
C. Hypotonic muscles
D. Seizures
E. Coma

3. Treatment of salt intoxication may include all of the following except
A. Syrup of ipecac
B. Activated charcoal
C. Hemodialysis
D. Peritoneal dialysis
E. Careful monitoring of rate of sodium change

TOXIC OIL AND EOSINOPHILIA-MYALGIA SYNDROMES

Toxic Oil Syndrome

In May 1981, the first cases of what would later be called the toxic oil syndrome occurred in Madrid, Spain, and surrounding suburbs. Hundreds and later thousands of individuals suddenly developed an acute mycoplasmalike pneumonitis. Approximately 2% to 3% of patients died of acute respiratory insufficiency. Patients failed to respond to standard antibiotics and exhibited signs and symptoms in multiple organ systems including fever, lymphadenopathy, nausea, vomiting, arthralgias, myalgias, and pruritic exanthems.

By June 1981, it had been established that all patients with this syndrome had ingested varying quantities of industrial rapeseed oil that had been marketed as olive oil. Rapeseed oil is required by Spanish law to be denatured with 2% aniline. Some distributors of olive oil took this rapeseed oil, removed the aniline by denaturing, and mixed it with other seed oils or olive oils. The oil then was sold as olive oil. Within 1 to 2 weeks of ingesting this oil, the patients developed the syndrome. The Spanish government removed all illegally marketed oil. By this time, over 20,000 patients were affected and over 200 died. The cause of toxic oil syndrome remains obscure.

By mid-August, many of these patients returned with signs and symptoms of a collagen vascularlike illness with widespread, crippling, progressive myalgias. They began to lose muscle and cutaneous sensation. Their skin became diffusely or focally sclerodermoid. Their mucous membranes dried, and they began losing hair. About 10% with the initial illness developed neurologic abnormalities.

Eosinophilia-Myalgia Syndrome

L-tryptophan was introduced in the United States in 1974 as a dietary supplement without prescription. Other uses included insomnia, the premenstrual syndrome, depression, and weight loss. The average patient dose of tryptophan ranged from 1 to 5 g/day. In 1989, three patients presented with an unexplained acute illness characterized by intense myalgias and eosinophilia. A nationwide outbreak of the disease, termed the eosinophilia-myalgia syndrome (EMS), was subsequently recognized. Case-control studies confirmed an unequivocal epidemiologic association between the EMS and the use of L-tryptophan. Despite discontinuation of L-tryptophan use, a substantial proportion of patients developed a protracted course dominated by manifestations of cutaneous and neuromuscular involvement.

By August 1992, 1,571 cases of the EMS had been reported to the Centers for Disease Control (CDC), and it was suggested that the actual number might be considerably higher. Eighty-five percent of affected patients developed symptoms between July 1989 and February 1990. One-third of the patients required hospitalization, and 38 deaths from neurologic, cardiac, and pulmonary complications, in addition to secondary infections attributable to the EMS, have been reported.

Pathophysiology

In 1991, investigators in Japan reported the discovery of a trace contaminant in L-tryptophan that bears a structural similarity to an impurity found in implicated rapeseed oil from Spain, which was isolated from samples of oil consumed by persons in whom the toxic oil syndrome (TOS) developed. This raises the possibility that EMS and TOS have a common etiologic trigger.

Clinical Presentations

TOXIC OIL SYNDROME

Clinical characteristics of TOS include the intake of cooking oil sold in bulk, other cases among relatives, and an interstitial-alveolar pattern on chest x-ray during the first 4 months. Eosinophilia (500 eosinophils/mL), myalgia, or rash during the first 4 months also is seen. Other findings include pulmonary hypertension, hepatic disease, scleroderma, sicca syndrome, polyneuropathy, joint contractures, Raynaud's disease, muscle cramps, and chronic lung disease.

TOS appears to share features of progressive systemic sclerosis (PSS). Features similar to both these conditions include dermal sclerosis, dermal edema, Raynaud's syndrome, dysphagia, hypopigmentation, esophageal hypomotility, pulmonary hypertension, right-sided heart failure, and inflammatory myositis. Common laboratory features include eosinophilia, antinuclear antibodies, hypergammaglobulinemia, organ-specific autoantibodies, and endovasculitis on biopsy examination.

Differences between TOS and PSS exist, however. Patients with TOS have an acute toxic syndrome; patients with PSS have an insidious onset. Patients with TOS develop pulmonary hypertension but never pulmonary fibrosis. Patients with TOS develop a peripheral neuropathy, which is rare in scleroderma. The skin changes in TOS develop primarily in areas of neuromuscular injury, do not involve acral sites, and are reversible with time.

EOSINOPHILIA-MYALGIA SYNDROME

CDC criteria for EMS include an eosinophil count greater than 1,000 cell/mm^3, generalized myalgias of severity sufficient to affect a patient's ability to pursue his or her daily activities, plus one or more of the following: exclusion of trichinosis by serologic tests performed at an appropriate interval after onset of symptoms, a muscle biopsy specimen that does not show trichinosis but does show inflammatory eosinophilic infiltrates, and/or absence of an infection or neoplasm that could account for eosinophilia or generalized myalgias.

Eighteen to 24 months after the onset of illness, most symptoms and physical findings in most patients with EMS resolve or improve. Cognitive changes may be worse in one-third of patients. Prednisone may be helpful in the acute phase of illness; however, no treatment was proven valuable in the management of the later phase of the syndrome.

EOSINOPHILIA-MYALGIA SYNDROME and TOXIC OIL SYNDROME COMPARED

TOS and EMS have major similarities. Both demonstrate certain vascular changes, pulmonary changes, skin pathology, skeletal muscular lesions, peripheral nerve changes, and cardiac abnormalities. The pathologic lesions in TOS are much more severe than in EMS, indicating that the etiologic agent in TOS is more potent or that its cation is more extensive and/or intensive than that of EMS. Over time and with further examination, the more chronic changes seen in TOS may be found in EMS.

Similarities between TOS and EMS have been summarized by the World Health Organization (WHO). The organs affected by TOS and EMS are similar: skin, muscles, lungs, nervous system, and fasciae. Early constitutional symptoms (such as malaise, fatigue, and fever) also are similar. The two syndromes share certain features, including alopecia, pruritus, xerostomia, pulmonary hypertension, and cutaneous papules. Similarities in laboratory results include marked eosinophilia, elevated aldolase with normal creatine phosphokinase, and x-ray findings of pulmonary interstitial infiltrates. Both syndromes show a similar pattern of cutaneous and deep-tissue involvement, although the severity may vary.

Differences between TOS and EMS have been noted as well. Early and often severe lung involvement is virtually universal in TOS, but is less prevalent and/or less severe in EMS. Early elevation of immunoglobulin E (IgE) levels (in about 50% of TOS cases) generally is not seen in EMS cases. The two syndromes affect different populations. This reflects different exposure patterns to the toxic agents, particularly in relation to socioeconomic class, gender, and age. Hyperglycemia and elevated triglyceride levels found in the intermediate stage of TOS have not been reported in EMS.

Pregnancy/Lactation

In pregnant women, hypersensitivity or toxicity to prescription or nonprescription medications, including L-tryptophan, should be considered in the differential diagnosis of maternal eosinophilia. The maternal use of tryptophan may result in newborn eosinophilia. In one patient who had ingested two 500-mg tablets of L-tryptophan daily from the fourth month of gestation until delivery, a full-term live infant was delivered with an eosinophilia and no other remarkable symptoms. No specific malformations have been associated with exposure to TOS during pregnancy.

Laboratory

ANALYTIC METHODS

A single high-performance liquid chromatographic peak was most predictive of L-tryptophan lots associated with EMS cases.

BLOOD LEVELS

Blood levels have not been helpful in identifying either EMS or TOS.

Treatment

GUT DECONTAMINATION

Both syndromes involve insidious development of symptoms and do not represent acute overdose situations. Charcoal and lavage would not be helpful.

ELIMINATION ENHANCEMENT

These methods have not been studied as aids to management in either EMS or TOS.

SUPPORTIVE MEASURES

TOS

- Treatment of TOS is primarily supportive and guided by individual symptoms.
- Steroids may be helpful during the early phase of the disease.
- Penicillamine has been associated with some symptomatic improvement.
- Elevated aminotransferase and alkaline phosphatase levels are seen in most patients with TOS.
- Positive signs on chest radiography observed in TOS include Kerley A and B lines and diffuse interstitial or alveolo-interstitial infiltrates with or without effusion. Despite complete radiographic resolution of acute bilateral interstitial pulmonary infiltrates, cardiomegaly may develop in 63% of patients.
- Antinuclear antibody was positive in almost all patients late in the first year. Rheumatoid factor, C-reactive protein, cryoglobulins, anti-DNA, and anti-ENA (extractable nuclear antigen) are negative; C3 and C4 are normal. IgG level is high during the first 2 months.

EMS

- Some patients experience a gradual spontaneous improvement of symptoms.
- Prednisone 10 to 100 mg/day may relieve myalgias, pulmonary manifestations, and cutaneous involvement in some patients. Exacerbation of myalgias may occur when prednisone therapy is tapered or discontinued. Some clinical recovery in the resolution of pulmonary symptoms occurs with steroids.
- Plasma exchange, IV methotrexate, and hydroxychloroquine have been used in a limited number of severely ill patients, and conclusions cannot be made on their efficacy.

- Nonsteroidal antiinflammatory drugs and steroids have not been associated with long-term improvement in symptoms.
- Cyproheptadine has been successful in relieving muscle cramps in some patients.

Questions—Toxic Oil and Eosinophilia-Myalgia Syndromes

1. **Symptoms of eosinophilia myalgia syndrome include**
   A. Eosinophil count over 1,000 cells/mm^3
   B. Mild myalgias
   C. Improvement of most symptoms by 24 hours
   D. A and B
   E. A and C
2. **Early and often severe lung involvement is more common in toxic oil syndrome than in eosinophilia-myalgia syndrome.**
   A. True
   B. False
3. **Steroids may be helpful in toxic oil syndrome but not in eosinophilia-myalgia syndrome.**
   A. True
   B. False
4. **Eosinophilia-myalgia syndrome has been associated with**
   A. L-Tryptophan
   B. D-Tryptophan
   C. Rapeseed oil
   D. Homogentisic acid
   E. Valine
5. **The predominant initial symptoms of toxic oil syndrome involved**
   A. The hematologic system
   B. The pulmonary system
   C. The gastrointestinal system
   D. The dermatologic system
   E. The neurologic system

VITAMINS

Introduction

The public and certain physicians have long considered vitamins as relatively harmless and innocuous in high doses for use in numerous conditions including learning disabilities, prevention of cancer, and even the treatment of schizophrenia. Doses taken and suggested often have been significantly higher than the recommended dietary allowances suggested by the Food and Nutrition Board of the National Academy of Sciences.

Large overdoses of water-soluble vitamins, such as pyridoxine (vitamin B6), vitamin C, and niacin (nicotinic acid) are excreted readily in the urine, yet have been associated with toxic problems when taken for long periods. Fat-soluble vitamins (A, D, E, and K) are stored in various tissues and are more likely to cause adverse effects when taken in excess. See Vitamin K in Chapter 25, Hematologic Toxicology. Folate (a B-complex vitamin) is discussed in Chapter 44, Chemotherapeutic Drugs, and Folinic Acid (Leucovorin®) is found in Chapter 5, Antidotes.

Acute overdoses of multivitamin preparations often are seen, usually without serious sequelae, but because as much as 15 mg of elemental iron can be found in a multivitamin tablet, toxic levels can be reached easily. Unfortunately, many vitamin tablets look like candy to children and are inadvertently ingested in overdose.

Niacin

Niacin (nicotinic acid) is used to treat pellagra. Primary niacin deficiency is rare in the United States. A secondary deficiency may be found in alcoholics, dietary cultists, and the malabsorption syndrome. Niacin, not niacinamide, may be useful in reducing blood lipid levels (lowers rate of synthesis of low-density lipoprotein and apoprotein B) in hyperlipoproteinemias. It has a doubtful use as a vasodilating agent. Its usefulness in psychiatry is not established.

PATHOPHYSIOLOGY

Niacin inhibits the synthesis of very low-density lipoproteins. It acts as a coenzyme involved in lipid metabolism, respiration, and glycogenolysis.

PHARMACOKINETICS

Absorption

- Niacin is well absorbed in the gastrointestinal tract. Peak serum concentration after oral dose occurs in 45 minutes.

Distribution

- Niacin is converted to niacinamide in the liver.

Elimination

- Excretion is primarily via urine. Half-life is 45 minutes.

CLINICAL PRESENTATIONS

Niacin releases histamine and may cause severe flushing, pruritus, and gastrointestinal disturbances. It may aggravate asthma, activate peptic ulcers, impair glucose tolerance, and cause hyperuricemia. High doses of niacin (over 4 g/day) may be associated with lactic acidosis, a cystoid maculopathy, myopathy, and fulminant hepatic failure. Hepatic toxicity may be more severe following sustained-release nicotinic acid than after an unmodified nicotinic acid preparation in equivalent therapeutic doses.

TOXIC DOSAGE/DEATH

Death has not been reported following pure niacin overdose. One report describes atrioventricular block in an adult following ingestion of 15 500-mg niacin tablets (7,500 mg), which responded to symptomatic treatment. Severe life-threatening hyperglycemia has been described following 3-g-per-day doses of niacin.

DRUG INTERACTIONS

Niacin potentiates the effect of ganglionic blocking agents and, when used together in hypertensive patients, can result in orthostatic hypotension.

PREGNANCY/LACTATION

Pregnancy risk category A [C if used in doses exceeding the recommended daily allowance (RDA) recommendations].

TREATMENT

Gut Decontamination

Niacin overdose may be managed with syrup of ipecac, charcoal and/or lavage; however, clinical efficacy of these interventions has not been proved.

Elimination Enhancement

Dialysis has not been employed in niacin overdose.

Supportive Measures

- Stop use immediately. Aspirin may counteract the flushing experienced with niacin use. Ibuprofen also may be effective.
- Symptoms usually will resolve spontaneously over several hours without sequelae.

Questions—Niacin

1. All of the following are true about niacin except
   A. Peak serum concentration occurs 45 minutes after an overdose.
   B. It is converted to niacinamide in the kidneys.
   C. Excretion primarily is via urine.
   D. It releases histamine, which may cause severe flushing.
   E. Death has not been reported following pure niacin overdose.

2. Management of niacin overdose may include
   A. Aspirin
   B. Syrup of ipecac
   C. Continued low dose used to prevent withdrawal
   D. A and B
   E. B and C

Retinoids

Retinoids are vitamin A derivatives that are used in the treatment of hyperkeratotic dermatoses, psoriasis, and acne. While used mainly for the treatment of skin diseases, they may be useful in lymphoproliferative conditions, certain forms of leukemia, and extracutaneous malignancies. There are now over 1,500 synthetic retinoids and three major oral retinoids marketed in the United States and Europe. These include retinol (vitamin A), isotretinoin (Accutane®), and etretinate.

Systemic administration of these compounds has been associated with mucocutaneous side effects, ocular toxicity, liver toxicity, and abnormal serum lipid profiles. The teratogenic effects of all retinoids limit their use in women of childbearing potential. Chronic toxic effects include skeletal abnormalities including diffuse idiopathic hyperostosis and premature epiphyseal closure. Overdoses with isotretinoin have been reported followed by minor symptoms and no deaths.

PATHOPHYSIOLOGY

The actions of retinoids on the skin are similar to those of Retin-A® and include inhibition of inflammation, keratinization, and cell growth.

PHARMACOKINETICS

Absorption

- Peak plasma concentrations of etretinate occur about 4 hours after intake of a single dose.
- After oral administration, about 40% of etretinate is absorbed from the gut.
- About 98% of etretinate is bound to plasma proteins.
- Peak blood concentrations of isotretinoin occur in 2 to 4 hours. After oral administration, peak serum concentrations of acitretin are noted in 3 to 5 hours.

Distribution

- The apparent volume of distribution of isotretinoin is 1.54 L/kg.

Elimination

- Isotretinoin has a half-life of 1 day. Acitretin, itself a metabolite of etretinate has a half-life of 50 hours. Etretinate is lipophilic and has a half-life of about 10 hours.
- After multiple doses during long-term treatment, the terminal elimination half-life of etretinate in plasma may be 100 days.
- Etretinate can be detected in serum in low levels for more than 2 years after a course of therapy has been discontinued.

CLINICAL PRESENTATIONS

Overdose of oral isotretinoin has led to abdominal discomfort, headaches, irritability, vomiting, mild tachycardia, tachypnea, hypertension, facial flushing, dizziness, and ataxia. All symptoms resolve quickly without residual effects. No fatalities have been reported following an overdose. Chronic use of isotretinoin has been associated with a number of undesired effects that generally are mucocutaneous, dose dependent, and reversible with discontinuation of the drug.

Depression has followed etretinate use (100 mg/day). Two potential ocular side effects are corneal deposits and papilledema secondary to pseudotumor cerebri. Dry eye has been observed. Immune complex vasculitis has followed isotretinoin and etretinate therapy. Isotretinoin and etretinate have been associated with skeletal abnormalities after both long-term and short-term therapy. Retinal function disturbances have followed long-term use of the synthetic retinoids. Olfactory and taste disturbances may persist after isotretinoin therapy ceases.

Chronic use of Retin-A® may be hepatotoxic. Etretinate has been implicated in reversible serum aminotransferase elevations, acute hepatitis, and chronic active hepatitis. The main metabolite of etretinate, acitretin, may induce a severe hepatotoxic reaction with progression to liver cirrhosis.

TOXIC DOSAGE/DEATH

A fatal dose for the retinoids in humans has not been established. Isotretinoin, 350 to 1600 mg, has been taken in overdose with minimal effects.

DRUG INTERACTIONS

In the presence of raised concentrations of liver enzymes, abstinence from alcohol is advised when concurrently taking isotretinoin. Simultaneous administration of etretinate with vitamin A may increase toxic effects. Concomitant treatment of etretinate with tetracycline and corticosteroids may increase the risk of hypertension. Drugs that increase serum lipids should be used with caution in patients receiving etretinate. Phenytoin or barbiturate blood levels may be altered. Special care should be used in epileptics receiving both drugs.

PREGNANCY/LACTATION

Isotretinoin first was marketed in the United States in 1982. Within a year, the FDA received reports of birth defects and spontaneous abortions after exposure to isotretinoin during the first trimester of pregnancy. By 1983, case reports of affected infants began to appear in the literature establishing isotretinoin as a potent human teratogen. Warnings were sent to physicians in 1984.

Teratogenicity has been associated with both isotretinoin (oral, cream) and etretinate. Defects have included external ear malformations, cleft palate, micrognathia, heart defects, ventricular septal defects, aortic arch malformations, and some brain malformations. Fetal malformation has followed 4 months to 1 year after the last dose of etretinate. Limb reduction defects have followed maternal use of isotretinoin in the first trimester of pregnancy. Both isotretinoin and etretinate carry pregnancy category X labeling.

Women who are pregnant or who may become pregnant while taking the drug should not use isotretinoin or etretinate. Pregnancy should be ruled out before treatment begins. This precaution may be accomplished best by obtaining a negative pregnancy test no more than 2 weeks prior to the beginning of therapy and starting therapy on the second or third day of the patient's next menstrual period. An effective form of contraception should be used for at least 1 month before therapy begins.

Women who have received isotretinoin should continue using an effective form of contraception for 1 month after discontinuing treatment. New measures include provision for signed informed consent; extensive education initiatives aimed at physicians, patients, and pharmacists; further studies (e.g., to evaluate alternative dosage regimens); and a follow-up survey ascertaining patient awareness, disease status, contraception use, and any pregnancy that occurs and outcomes.

The period during which pregnancy must be avoided after treatment is discontinued has not been determined for women who have received etretinate. Since isotretinoin has a half-life of only 1 day, after 1 month off therapy and the completion of one full menstrual cycle, women may safely become pregnant. This must still be confirmed by controlled clinical studies. Female patients should be counseled on the risk of major birth defects associated with first-trimester exposure to isotretinoin or etretinate. Should a pregnancy occur during treatment (or after treatment, in the case of etretinate), the woman should consult her physician about the management of her pregnancy.

LABORATORY

Analytic Methods

A reverse-phase, high-performance liquid chromatography method is available for retinoic acid and its metabolites.

Blood Levels

Seven and 20 days following ingestion of 350 mg of isotretinoin, only insignificant levels of isotretinoin have been found. However, 2 to 5 ng/mL of the 4-oxo metabolite of isotretinoin may be seen.

TREATMENT

Gut Decontamination

Emesis or gastric lavage may be helpful in documented overdoses without evidence of obtundation from other drugs or comorbid conditions. Administer activated charcoal as well.

Elimination Enhancement

Dialysis is not helpful in the management of retinoid overdoses.

Supportive Measures

- Ophthalmic examination of patients on long-term etretinate should be done with special attention to color vision and dark adaptation.
- Patients on chronic long-term therapy with retinoids should be evaluated by x-ray for any retinoid-induced bone change.
- Lipid or hepatic enzyme abnormalities are not observed following isotretinoin overdose. Infrequent elevation of liver function values after chronic use is transient and totally reversible on withdrawal of the drug.
- Thrombocytopenia may follow use of retinoids. Monitoring of the platelet count during therapy may be advisable. Hypertriglyceridemia has been observed.

Questions—Retinoids

1. Systemic administration of retinoids has been associated with all of the following except
A. Mucocutaneous side effects
B. Ocular toxicity
C. Renal toxicity
D. Liver toxicity
E. Abnormal serum lipid profiles

2. Overdose of oral isotretinoin has led to all of the following except
A. Headache
B. Vomiting
C. Hypertension
D. Tachycardia
E. Death

3. Teratogenicity has been associated with all of the following except
A. Oral isotretinoin
B. Isotretinoin cream
C. Etretinate
D. Decreased calcium deposits in myocardium
E. None of the above

Vitamin A

Vitamin A is a fat-soluble vitamin. Lack of vitamin A causes night blindness, thinning of the skin, keratinization of mucous membranes, defective bone modeling, swelling of Kupffer cells, and increased clotting time. Recommended uses, although largely unsubstantiated, have included the treatment of acne, psoriasis, minimal brain dysfunction, and other neuropsychiatric conditions.

PATHOPHYSIOLOGY

Toxicity is caused by unbound vitamin A. It may occur at low serum vitamin A concentrations in patients with a low retinol-binding protein (e.g., malnutrition, liver disease, and hyperlipoproteinemias).

PHARMACOKINETICS

Absorption

- Vitamin A is absorbed from the intestine as retinyl esters.
- Peak serum levels are found 4 hours after a therapeutic dose.

Distribution

- 90% of vitamin A is stored in the liver from which it is mobilized as the free alcohol, retinol.
- 95% is carried bound to plasma proteins, the retinol-binding protein.

Elimination

- Half-life is about 9 hours. 50% is eliminated in the feces and 20% is eliminated in the urine.

CLINICAL PRESENTATIONS

Headache, nausea, vomiting, and irritability have been observed after excessive consumption of animal liver, or one dose of 1,500,000 international units (IU). After 350,000 IU, infants age 3 to 7 months developed vomiting, irritability, bulging fontanelles and elevated cerebrospinal fluid pressures. In children, administration of more than 50,000-600,000 IU/day for months has resulted in hepatosplenomegaly, hypoplastic anemia, leukopenia, sparse coarse hair, clubbing, and advanced skeletal maturation.

In adults, toxic effects may occur after ingestion of 25,000 IU / day for 8 months. Signs may include papilledema, diplopia, headaches, pseudotumor cerebri, weakness, fatigue, pain in bones and joints, anoxexia, headaches, muscle stiffness, weight loss, polyuria, polydipsia, urinary frequency, dry skin, desquamation, pruritus, hair loss, hepatomegaly, splenomegaly, and nasal and oral bleeding.

TOXIC DOSAGE/DEATH

The lowest reported intakes causing toxicity have occurred in persons with liver function compromised by drugs, viral hepatitis, or protein-energy malnutrition. Especially vulnerable groups include children, with adverse effects occurring with intakes as low as 1,500 IU / kg / day and pregnant women, with birth defects associated with maternal intakes as low as about 25,000 IU / day.

In one case, a 28-year-old woman ingested 1.3 million units of vitamin A as a remedy for sunburn. She experienced nausea, vomiting, intense headache, and blurring of vision. Papilledema was noted on the physical examination. The symptoms gradually subsided over the next 3 days. Exfoliation began on the fourth day and lasted 2 weeks. The patient recovered. A 62-year-old man ingested 8 mL of preparation containing 500,000 units / mL of vitamin A. Symptoms included nausea, severe headache, and blurring of vision. Exfoliation of the skin began on day 3. The patient recovered completely.

PREGNANCY/LACTATION

The association between vitamin A itself and human teratogenicity is unclear. Women in their reproductive years should be informed that the excessive use of vitamin A shortly before and during pregnancy could be harmful to their babies and that a bioaccumulation of vitamin A from continuous high doses is a concern. Women of childbearing potential should consult with their physicians concerning birth control before consuming these products. Doses lower than 10,000 IU probably are not teratogenic.

LABORATORY

Analytic Methods

Vitamin A is detected by high-pressure liquid chromatography.

Blood Levels

Therapeutic vitamin A levels are 65 to 275 unit / mL in serum and 300 μg / g in liver. Peak serum levels of vitamin A retinyl esters are found 4 hours after a therapeutic dose. However, blood levels are not a useful guide in clinical vitamin A overdose. The portion of vitamin A retinyl ester found in the plasma in normal individuals is 0.1% to 4.7% and in hypervitaminosis A, it rises to 67%.

TREATMENT

Gut Decontamination

Induce emesis or gastric lavage as indicated in severe, documented overdoses without evidence of obtundation from other drugs or comorbid conditions. Some have recommended gastrointestinal emptying with syrup of ipecac when the amount ingested is 12,000 units / kg or more. This corresponds to an ingestion of 180,000 units in a 15-kg child, and an ingestion of 840,000 units in a 70-kg adult. Administer activated charcoal as well.

Elimination Enhancement

Dialysis is not helpful in the management of vitamin A overdose.

Supportive Measures

- Assess airway, breathing, and circulatory functions. Monitor vital signs, fluids, electrolytes, and central nervous system status.
- Reduce documented increased intracranial pressure with mannitol or steroids via consultation with neurosurgery or neurology. Mannitol is administered 0.25 g / kg IV and repeated every 5 minutes as required. It can be increased to 1 g / kg per dose if symptoms and / or papilledema persist. Watch plasma osmolality.
- Steroids may be helpful. The initial dose of dexamethasone is 0.15 mg / kg IV and maintenance dose is 0.25 mg / kg / day, divided every 4 to 6 hours for 5 days. Taper over the following 5 days.
- There may be an increase in hepatic transaminase enzymes. Hypercalcemia occurs in 25% to 33% of cases, especially in adolescents and adults. Clotting times may be abnormal. There may be hypoprothrombinemia with prolonged prothrombin time.
- X-rays of bones may reveal cortical hyperostosis of long bones, retardation of growth, premature closure of epiphysis, and hypomineralization or hypermineralization.

Questions—Vitamin A

1. Toxic effects of vitamin A in adults may include
A. Hypotonia
B. Pseudotumor cerebri
C. Weight gain
D. Increased hair growth
E. All of the above

2. Those with liver compromise are particularly sensitive to vitamin A toxicity.
A. True
B. False

VITAMIN B6

Vitamin B6 is composed of pyridoxine, pyridoxal, and pyridoxamine. These are metabolically interrelated and collectively are called pyridoxine. Pyridoxine deficiency syndrome is rare except in combination with other vitamin B complex deficiencies (e.g., alcoholism, malabsorption syndromes). Pyridoxine has been used for infants with hyperirritability and epileptiform convulsions during the first week of life, to prevent pyridoxine-responsive sideroblastic anemias, and to prevent or treat peripheral neuritis caused by isoniazid, cycloserine, hydrazine-containing mushrooms, penicillamine, and other drugs. Its use in the treatment of premenstrual syndrome, especially in high doses, has not been substantiated by controlled studies. Another use is prevention of oxalosis in adults and children with type I primary hyperoxaluria.

As an antidote, pyridoxine may prevent isoniazid-induced seizures and subsequent lactic acidosis. It is recommended that pyridoxine be given to any symptomatic patient with isonicotinic acid hydrazide poisoning or any asymptomatic patient suspected of ingesting 80 mg / kg of isoniazid or more. Pyridoxine is a cofactor in the metabolism of toxic intermediaries of ethylene glycol and may enhance the elimination of these toxic products. It should be given to anyone with a known or suspected ingestion of ethylene glycol. See Chapter 5, Antidotes.

PATHOPHYSIOLOGY

Pyridoxine is a water-soluble B-complex vitamin involved in the transamination of amino acids and conversion of tryptophan to niacin. This vitamin appears to be essential in the synthesis of γ-aminobutyric acid (GABA) within the central nervous system. Isoniazid-induced seizures are thought to result from decreased GABA levels as a consequence of isoniazid inhibition of brain pyridoxal-5-phosphate activity.

PHARMACOKINETICS

Absorption

- Pyridoxine is well absorbed in the jejunum.

Distribution

- Volume of distribution is approximately 0.07 to 0.17 L/kg. Protein binding is 0%.

Elimination

- Excretion is primarily via the urine. The half-life of pyridoxine is 2 to 3 weeks.

CLINICAL PRESENTATIONS

Ingestion of 6 g daily for prolonged periods (2 months or more) has resulted in severe peripheral neuropathies with ataxia, perioral numbness, and clumsiness of the hands and feet with profound loss of position and vibration sense. Recovery may be complete within 6 months to 3 years. Women taking high doses of pyridoxine (50 to 300 mg daily) for premenstrual syndrome have developed sensory neuropathies, with burning, shooting, and tingling pains, paresthesias, clumsiness, ataxia, and perioral numbness. Areflexia and encephalopathy have been reported in infants after excessive doses. Nausea and allergic reactions have been reported.

TOXIC DOSAGE/DEATH

Most individuals can consume up to 20 mg/day without problems. Pyridoxine usually is nontoxic even in large doses. Several years of daily doses ranging from 500 mg to 2 g led to a progressive sensory neuropathy that improved after discontinuation of the vitamin in one case. Sixteen patients with a pure sensory central-peripheral distal axonopathy were described after long-term use of pyridoxine in doses of 0.2 to 5 g/day. Improvement followed discontinuation.

DRUG INTERACTIONS

Pyridoxine (25 mg/day) can antagonize levodopa and decrease its effectiveness in Parkinson's disease. Anticonvulsant effects of barbiturates and phenytoin are opposed by pyridoxine. Pyridoxine may enhance amiodarone-induced photosensitivity.

PREGNANCY/LACTATION

One mother ingested pyridoxine, 50 mg/d, during the first 7 months of a full-term pregnancy. A girl, born by normal vaginal delivery, had a near-total amelia of her left leg at the knee. Interestingly, the sensory neuropathy following pyridoxine abuse is similar to that seen with thalidomide administration. Pregnancy risk category A (C if dose exceeds the daily RDA recommendation).

LABORATORY

Analytic Methods

Pyridoxine is detected by high-pressure liquid chromatography.

Blood Levels

Blood levels do not aid in the treatment of overdose situations. A broad range of 25 to 80 ng/mL is accepted as normal.

TREATMENT

Gut Decontamination

Pyridoxine overdose may be managed with charcoal and/or lavage; however, clinical efficacy of these interventions has not been proved.

Elimination Enhancement

Dialysis has not been employed in pyridoxine overdose.

Supportive Measures

- Management essentially is supportive. Stop pyridoxine immediately. Follow with careful neurologic evaluations.

Question—Vitamin B6

1. **High-dose chronic ingestion of vitamin B6 mainly affects which system?**
   A. Renal
   B. Neurologic
   C. Cardiac
   D. Endocrine
   E. Gastrointestinal

VITAMIN C

Vitamin C (ascorbic acid) is used in the prevention and treatment of scurvy. Scurvy is rare in the United States but still prevalent in developing countries. Most susceptible are the elderly, the chronically ill, alcoholics, and dietary cultists. Vitamin C may facilitate wound healing and recovery from extensive burns or trauma (doses 300% to 500% higher than RDAs may be useful). It has been used to acidify urine as well.

PATHOPHYSIOLOGY

Vitamin C is essential in collagen formation and is involved in certain oxidation-reduction reactions. Ascorbic acid therapy may place the erythrocytes of premature infants at risk of oxidative damage. The significance of these findings remains to be determined.

PHARMACOKINETICS

Absorption

- Vitamin C is a well-absorbed, water-soluble vitamin. Absorption is dose dependent.

Distribution

- Oxidized and hydrolyzed in the liver.

Elimination

- Excretion is primarily via urine. Half-life is 45 minutes.

CLINICAL PRESENTATIONS

Vitamin C in overdosage may be associated with diarrhea and gastitis may predispose to renal oxalate calculi. Development of acute renal failure secondary to tubular obstruction from calcium oxalate crystals has been described. Vitamin C increases iron adsorption and may be dangerous in patients with hemochromatosis, thalassemia, or sideroblastic anemia. Ascorbic acid has induced hemolysis in patients with glucose-6-phosphate dehydrogenase deficiency.

TOXIC DOSAGE/DEATH

Ascorbic acid in large doses (4 to 8 g) may result in a diminution of uric acid excretion, which may in turn precipitate an acute gouty arthritis in predisposed individuals. Esophageal and stomach irritation may occur with large doses.

DRUG INTERACTIONS

A decreased effect of Coumadin® may be seen when used concurrently with vitamin C. As vitamin C acidifies urine, there may be an increased elimination of phencyclidine (PCP) or amphetamine when taken together. High-dose vitamin C appears to increase plasma ethinyl estradiol in women taking oral contraceptives. This theoretically may increase the risk of cardiovascular disease in such patients; however, this has not been proven.

PREGNANCY/LACTATION

Large doses are relatively contraindicated during pregnancy. Pregnancy risk category A (C if used in doses exceeding RDA recommendations).

LABORATORY

Analytic Methods

Vitamin C is detected by spectrophotometry.

Blood Levels

High doses of ascorbic acid may interfere with tests that check for blood in the stool (which will be falsely negative). Tests for urine sugar (ChemStrip G) can be falsely lowered, whereas Clinitest gives a falsely high result. Monitoring vitamin C levels is not helpful in overdoses.

TREATMENT

Gut Decontamination

Vitamin C overdose may be managed with charcoal and/or lavage; however, clinical efficacy of these interventions has not been proved. Dilution may be indicated as well.

Elimination Enhancement

Dialysis has not been employed in vitamin C overdose.

Supportive Measures

- Stop use immediately. Symptoms usually will resolve over several hours without sequelae.
- Hydration is necessary to prevent renal oxalate deposition in significant overdoses.

Questions—Vitamin C

1. **Vitamin C may cause**
   A. Constipation
   B. Polycythemia
   C. Decreased effect of warfarin
   D. Urine alkalinization
   E. Decreased plasma ethinyl estradiol in women taking oral contraceptives
2. **High dose ascorbic acid may interfere with stool blood tests.**
   A. True
   B. False

Vitamin D

Vitamin D is a fat-soluble vitamin. Lack of vitamin D, due to dietary restriction, defective absorption, or hepatic or renal abnormalities, causes hypocalcemia, hypophosphatemia, and rickets in infants and children. Osteomalacia may result in adults. Vitamin D is used to prevent rickets and osteomalacia and to regulate calcium and phosphorus metabolism in the intestine, bone, and possibly kidney, together with calcitonin and parathyroid hormone. Renal osteodystrophy, hepatic rickets, hypoparathyroidism, and vitamin D-resistant rickets may be useful indications for vitamin D.

PATHOPHYSIOLOGY

Vitamin D stimulates calcium and phosphate absorption from the small intestine. Excess vitamin D results in hypercalcemia, hypercalciuria, decreased fecal fat, and accelerated deposits of calcium in soft tissues such as the renal tubules, myocardium, arterial wells, and alveolar septa of lung.

PHARMACOKINETICS

Absorption

- Vitamin D is absorbed through the duodenum and jejunum.
- Peak serum vitamin D concentration occurs approximately 12 hours after a single oral dose and returns to basal levels within 72 hours.

Distribution

- Small amounts are stored in adipose tissue and muscle.
- Transport in circulation is effected by a specific carrier protein, transcalciferol.

Elimination

- It is inactive until it is hydroxylated in the liver to 25-hydroxyvitamin D.
- Further hydroxylation in the kidney forms 1,25-dihydroxyvitamin D.

CLINICAL PRESENTATIONS

Hypercalcemia, hypercalciuria, muscle weakness, apathy, headache, anorexia, nausea, vomiting, constipation, bone pain, ectopic calcification, proteinuria, hypertension, and cardiac arrhythmias may occur with hypervitaminosis D. Arrhythmias may occur with hypercalcemia. Pancreatitis has been reported in overdose. Chronic hypercalcemia may lead to generalized vascular calcifications, nephrocalcinosis, and rapid deterioration of renal function.

TOXIC DOSAGE/DEATH

In children, a toxic dose is 10,000 IU/day for 4 months or 200,000 IU/day for 2 weeks. In most cases, 25,000 to 60,000 IU/day for 1 to 4 months will cause toxicity. In one study, infants given more than 1,800 units of vitamin D daily did not grow as well as infants given 340 units daily. In adults, 60,000 IU/day or more for several weeks or months will cause signs and symptoms of hypervitaminosis D. When vitamin D intoxication is found in a patient who is not taking a pharmaceutical preparation of vitamin D, a careful search for another exogenous source (fortified milk, for example) is warranted.

DRUG INTERACTIONS

Vitamin D activity may be reduced in patients simultaneously taking anticonvulsants (hydantoins, barbiturates). Glutethimide is known to induce synthesis of hepatic microsomal enzymes and may alter vitamin D metabolism in the liver.

PREGNANCY/LACTATION

Pregnancy risk category A (D if doses exceed RDA recommendations). Massive doses (10,000 IU/kg) may be teratogenic.

LABORATORY

Analytic Methods
Vitamin D is measured by competitive protein binding/solid-phase chromatography.

Blood Levels
Serum 25-hydroxyvitamin D measurements are a good indicator of exposure to vitamin D from dietary sources and synthesis of the vitamin by the skin. Normal vitamin D and 25-hydroxyvitamin D serum levels are 10 to 50 ng/mL. Toxicity is associated with serum 25-hydroxyvitamin D greater than 500 ng/mL and free 1,25-dihydroxyvitamin D greater than 80 pg/mL.

TREATMENT

Gut Decontamination
If an excessive amount is taken, charcoal and/or gastric lavage may decrease substrate.

Elimination Enhancement
Peritoneal dialysis and hemodialysis may be used in patients with compromised renal function to decrease elevated calcium levels.

Supportive Measures
- Severe hypercalcemia is treated with prednisone, 1 mg/kg/day, calcitonin (salmon, 4 to 8 units/kg every 6 hours), and mithramycin (50 μg/kg). Saline infusion is used to improve glomerular filtration and reduce renal tubular reabsorption of calcium. Caution must be exercised in patients with cardiac or renal compromise.
- Cardiac arrhythmias resulting from hypercalcemia may be treated with small doses of potassium under continuous cardiac monitoring.
- Serum calcium, phosphorus, alkaline phosphatase, complete blood count, and renal and hepatic function should be monitored. Hypercalciuria, elevated serum phosphorus, elevated blood urea nitrogen, and hypochromic anemia may be evident.
- Cholestyramine orally (8 g twice daily) may aid in decreasing hypercalcemia. Calcium concentrations are frequently greater than 11 mg/100 mL and alkaline phosphatase levels may be depressed.
- X-rays of bones in patients with chronic hypervitaminosis D may show periosteal thickening and increased intensity of mineralization. Metastatic calcifications may be present in kidneys, blood vessels, lungs, adrenal glands, cerebral membranes, and muscles.

Questions—Vitamin D

1. Excess vitamin D can cause
   A. Hypocalcemia
   B. Hypocalciuria
   C. Increased fecal fat
   D. Decreased calcium deposits in myocardium
   E. None of the above

2. Vitamin D activity may be increased in patients taking barbiturates.
   A. True
   B. False

Vitamin E

Vitamin E is a fat-soluble vitamin. Inadequate vitamin E in neonates may cause hemolytic anemia and shortened red blood cell survival time. Thrombocytosis and platelet hyperaggregability also may occur in infant vitamin E deficiency. Vitamin E is used to supplement deficiency states such as malabsorption syndromes with steatorrhea (e.g., celiac disease, tropical sprue, and gastrointestinal resections).

Other conditions with prolonged malabsorption of fats include cystic fibrosis, hepatic cirrhosis, biliary obstruction, and excessive ingestion of mineral oil. Vitamin E possibly may be effective in reducing oxygen-induced damage to the lungs in bronchopulmonary dysplasia and in the eyes in retrolental fibroplasia (in neonates). Vitamin E also may reduce intracerebral hemorrhage in premature infants.

PATHOPHYSIOLOGY
Eight tocopherols with vitamin E activity occur naturally. α-Tocopherol is the most important, constituting about 90% of the total tocopherols in animal tissues. Available data appear to show that vitamin E is the major lipid antioxidant in biological membranes.

PHARMACOKINETICS
Vitamin E is 50% to 80% absorbed, transported by lipoproteins, and stored in adipose tissue, liver, and muscle.

CLINICAL PRESENTATIONS
In 1984, the CDC reported an illness in premature infants who developed ascites plus some or all of the following: hepatosplenomegaly, jaundice, azotemia, and thrombocytopenia. All had received E-Ferol and the outbreaks ceased when E-Ferol was discontinued. With the withdrawal of E-Ferol from the market, there is no IV form of tocopherol. Only oral preparations of tocopherol or tocopherol acetate are available. Other signs of vitamin E excess include rash, erythema multiforme, high cholesterol, hypertriglyceridemia, and blurry vision.

TOXIC DOSAGE/DEATH
Long-term use of 400 to 800 IU/day may result in nausea, muscular weakness, fatigue, headache, and blurred vision. Doses of 2,000 to 12,000 IU/day have been reported to cause gonadal dysfunction, creatinuria, and gastrointestinal upset, which disappear within a few weeks when excessive doses are discontinued. Data on these effects are not established.

DRUG INTERACTIONS
Excessive use of vitamin E may deplete vitamin A stores and antagonize vitamin K function (inhibition of prothrombin production). Vitamin E may increase the effect of oral anticoagulants.

PREGNANCY/LACTATION
Pregnancy risk category A (C if dose exceeds RDA standards).

LABORATORY

Analytic Methods
A high-performance liquid chromatography method is available for determination of vitamin E levels in serum and plasma.

Blood Levels
Elevated vitamin E levels (normal levels are 0.5 to 2.0 mg/dL) may be observed after high doses of vitamin E. Levels above 3 to 4 mg/dL probably should be avoided. If the recommended

pharmacologic dose of 100 mg/kg/d for retrolental fibroplasia is used, plasma levels must be monitored on a weekly basis.

TREATMENT

Gut Decontamination
In overdoses, charcoal and lavage may be helpful; however, this has not been confirmed.

Elimination Enhancement
These methods have not been applied in the management of vitamin E overdose.

Supportive Measures
- Treatment should include discontinuation of large doses of vitamin E and evaluation of laboratory parameters. Treatment essentially is supportive.
- Abnormalities in prothrombin time and clotting time have been observed. Careful hematologic evaluations for hemolysis and platelets should be performed in neonates receiving vitamin E in large doses.

Questions—Vitamin E

1. **Vitamin E at RDA standards is pregnancy category**
   A. A
   B. B
   C. C
   D. D
   E. X
2. **Long-term use of vitamin E has been associated with all of the following except**
   A. Blurred vision
   B. Fatigue
   C. Gonadal dysfunction
   D. Gastrointestinal upset
   E. Death

WATER INTOXICATION

Water intoxication is an infrequent clinical event that follows excessive parenteral or enteral water administration by medical personnel, malicious forcing of water on a child, repeated immersion (as in infant swimming lessons), and voluntary ingestion of ice water to control toothache. It may occur inadvertently during marathon runs, after drug testing (individuals drink massive quantities of water to dilute the urine enough to drive drug levels down), or as a manifestation of psychosis (as in psychogenic polydipsia).

Psychogenic Water Intoxication

In 1938, Barabal documented the first case of water intoxication in a patient with schizophrenia. In 1974, Raskind reported a fatality from self-induced water intoxication. Self-induced water intoxication is a condition found almost exclusively (80%) in patients with psychiatric disorders. The two most important pathogenic factors are primary polydipsia (also referred to as compulsive water drinking or psychogenic polydipsia) and an inappropriate antidiuretic state.

Compulsive water drinking (CWD) refers to continuous or habitual drinking of greater than normal quantities of water, and psychogenic polydipsia refers to the consumption of excessive quantities in a relatively short period; the latter is more likely to lead to intoxication. Signs of water intoxication include restlessness, weakness, nausea, vomiting, diarrhea, polyuria, muscle fasciculations, hypotonia, seizures, and coma.

Syndrome of Inappropriate Antidiuretic Hormone (SIADH)

Certain conditions are associated with the inappropriate secretion of high levels of antidiuretic hormone. Essential features of SIADH include hyponatremia with hypoosmolality of serum, continued renal excretion of sodium despite hyponatremia, absence of clinical evidence of dehydration, urine less than maximally dilute (i.e., urine is hypertonic relative to plasma), and normal renal and adrenal function. Among the factors reported to be associated with SIADH are: stress, smoking, head injury, psychotropic drugs (e.g., amitriptyline, fluphenazine, haloperidol, chlorpromazine, and thiothixene), anticonvulsants (e.g., carbamazepine), diuretics, anticancer drugs, and various medical disorders (notably malignant tumors).

SIADH is similar to psychogenic polydipsia in that serum sodium, osmolality, and blood urea nitrogen are low, due to the extracellular fluid expansion that is secondary to excess renal water retention. Consequently, the urine of SIADH patients is concentrated, with high osmolality, while that of patients with psychogenic polydipsia is dilute, because of the high volume throughout.

Pathophysiology

For water intoxication to occur, there must be a rapid decline in extracellular solute concentrations (osmolality) creating a concentration gradient generally between extracellular fluid and cell water and a gradient between the vascular fluid of the brain and the rest of the brain fluids in particular. The brain is affected differently because, unlike other tissues, tight junctions (i.e., the blood-brain barrier) bind the endothelial cells of the cerebral blood vessels.

When an osmolal gradient is produced, relief of the gradient in the brain cannot be achieved quickly by rapid diffusion of sodium and chloride ions from the extracellular fluid brain, but must be equilibrated by movement of water molecules into both the extracellular fluid and cells of the brain. The brain picks up disproportionately more water than other organs. Such swelling may cause seizures, but only if the dilution occurs over a few hours. If the change is gradual, enough sodium chloride diffusion occurs, keeping the respective volumes constant and preventing seizures. The rate of change is more important than the degree of hyponatremia in precipitating seizures.

Clinical Presentations

In infants, acute symptomatic hyponatremia includes generalized tonic-clonic seizures, hypothermia, and respiratory insufficiency. Hyponatremic seizures are prolonged and respond poorly to usual anticonvulsant doses. Hyponatremic seizures typically occur at serum sodium concentrations lower than 125 mmol/L. Hyponatremia should be strongly considered in infants presenting with their first seizures in which evidence of another cause is lacking.

Early features of water intoxication in adults include headache, blurred vision, polyuria, vomiting, tremor, and worsening psychosis. More severe features include muscle cramps, ataxia, delirium, stupor, coma, and convulsions. Major motor seizures are the most common feature of self-induced water intoxication in patients with psychiatric illness and have been reported in about 80% of reported cases. Self-induced water intoxication should be included in the differential diagnosis of seizures of recent onset, especially in psychiatric patients in hospitals.

Central pontine myelinolysis may occur with rapid increase in sodium associated with the treatment of water intoxication. Clinical manifestations may include decreasing level of consciousness, behavioral changes, spastic quadriplegia, and pseudobulbar palsy. Patients with hyponatremia less than 105 mmol/L appear to be at greater risk of developing the complications associated with rapid correction of hyponatremia than are patients with higher sodium concentrations.

Laboratory

ANALYTIC METHODS

Sodium is measured by ion-specific electrode.

BLOOD LEVELS

The serum sodium in clinically relevant cases usually is rapidly reduced within a few hours to less than 125 mmol/L. Urine-specific gravity usually is quite low. Urine toxic screen usually will fail to reveal substances capable of causing seizures, respiratory failure, or hyponatremia, but may be relevant in drug-induced SIADH. Imaging studies of the brain usually show no evidence of trauma, structural abnormalities, or gross cerebral edema.

Treatment

GUT DECONTAMINATION

As water is readily absorbed, these methods serve no role in water intoxication.

ELIMINATION ENHANCEMENT

While dialysis may effectively reduce total body water burden, this method generally is not employed in the treatment of water intoxication.

SUPPORTIVE MEASURES

- Treatment of self-induced water intoxication depends on recognition, restriction of fluids in the early stages, and furosemide.
- SIADH associated with polydipsia can be treated with the antidiuretic hormone demeclocycline (600 to 1,200 mg/day) or lithium carbonate (900 to 1,200 mg/day).
- One study suggested that naloxone injections appeared to attenuate compulsive drinking in psychiatric patients with psychosis, intermittent hyponatremia, and polydipsia; however, this has yet to be independently confirmed.
- When chronic hyponatremia (e.g., secondary to diuretic therapy, or SIADH) is asymptomatic, there is no indication for emergency treatment. Treatment should be directed at the underlying cause.
- When the condition is symptomatic, treatment should be designed in relation to the severity of the clinical manifestations. If these are mild (e.g., lethargy, confusion), treatment should consist of removal of the primary cause and water restriction.
- In more serious cases of symptomatic patients with acute hyponatremia, hypertonic saline administration of at least 1 mmol/L/hour may suffice. Great care must be taken during administration, as rapid correction with hypertonic saline may yield pontine myelinolysis.
- Oral potassium loading (when the serum concentration of potassium is decreased or low normal) increases the serum concentration of sodium through an increase in intracellular osmolality.
- Acute hyponatremia may occur secondary to iatrogenic fluid overload in the postoperative period or excessive ingestion of fluids as a result of a psychiatric disturbance. Acute correction to a target sodium concentration of 120 to 130 mmol/L by means of water restriction and infusion of calculated amounts of saline should be carried out.
- Increase in serum concentration of sodium should be limited to 10 mmol/L per day. Twice-normal saline generally is adequate and tends to avoid major acute changes in serum osmolality induced by greater concentrations. Serum electrolytes should be measured at 2- to 3-hour intervals.

Questions—Water Intoxication

1. Most cases of water intoxication are in patients with psychiatric disorders.
   A. True
   B. False

2. SIADH and water intoxication are similar in that
   A. Serum sodium is low in both
   B. Serum osmolality is high in both
   C. Blood urea nitrogen is low in both
   D. A and B
   E. A and C

Answers

Baking Soda

1. A 2. B 3. C

Bromides

1. E 2. B 3. C

Camphor

1. E 2. B 3. C 4. B

Coloring Agents

1. C 2. E

Surfactants and Solubilizing Agents

1. B

Aerosol Propellants

1. D

Preservatives and Antibacterials

1. D 2. A

Thickening, Suspending, Binding Solvent Agents

1. D 2. B

Lubricants, Fats and Oils

1. E 2. B 3. C

Flavoring and Sweetening Agents

1. E 2. E 3. C 4. A

Fluorides

1. B 2. C 3. B 4. E

Iodine

1. E 2. D 3. B

Laxatives

1. D 2. D 3. B 4. B 5. C

Salt

1. B 2. C 3. B

Toxic Oil and Eosinophilia-Myalgia Syndromes

1. A 2. A 3. B 4. A 5. B

Niacin

1. B 2. D

Retinoids

1. C 2. E 3. D

Vitamin A

1. B 2. A

Vitamin B6

1. B

Vitamin C

1. C 2. A

Vitamin D

1. E 2. B

Vitamin E

1. A 2. E

Water Intoxication

1. A 2. E

SELECTED READINGS

Baking Soda

1. Del Beccaro M, Robertson WO. Baking soda poisoning. Vet Hum Toxicol 1988;30:164–165.
2. Downs NM, Stonebridge PA. Gastric rupture due to excessive sodium bicarbonate ingestion. Scott Med J 1989;34:534–535.
3. Holloway M, Wason S. Baking soda: a potentially fatal home remedy. Vet Hum Toxicol 1990;32:371.

Bromides

1. Carney MWP. Five cases of bromism. Lancet 1971;2:523–524.
2. Hanes F, Yates A. An analysis of four hundred instances of chronic bromide intoxication. South Med J 1938;31:667–671.
3. Trump DL, Hochberg MC. Bromide intoxication. Johns Hopkins Med J 1976;138:119–123.

Camphor

1. Alsop JA. Camphor toxicity from accidental ingestions. Vet Hum Toxicol 1993;35:346.
2. Siegel E, Wason S. Camphor toxicity. Ped Clin North Am 1986;33:376–379.
3. Skoutakis VA, Koumbourlis TC. Camphor intoxication: diagnosis and management. Clin Toxicol Consult 1981;4:131–136.

Coloring Agents

1. Bell T. Colourants and drug reactions. Lancet 1991;338:55–56.
2. Dine DJ, Wilkinson JA. Acute exposure to rhodamine B. Clin Toxicol 1987;25:603–607.
3. Smith JM, Dodd TRP. Adverse reactions to pharmaceutical excipients. Adverse Drug React Acute Poisoning Rev 1982;1:93–142.

Excipients

1. Golightly LK, Smolinske SS, Bennett ML, Sutherland EW III, Rumack BH. Pharmaceutical excipients adverse drug effects associated with "inactive" ingredients in drug products. Parts I and II. Med Toxicol 1988;3:128–135; 209–240.
2. Napke E, Stevens DGH. Excipients and additives. Hidden hazards in drug products and in product substitution. CMA J 1984;131:1449–1452.

Fluorides

1. Augenstein WL, Spoerke DG, Kulig KW, et al. Fluoride ingestion in children: a review of 87 cases. Pediatrics 1991;88:907–911.
2. Yolken R, Konecny P, McCarty P. Acute fluoride poisoning. Pediatrics 1976;50:90–93.

Iodine

1. d'Auria J, Lipson S, Garfield JM. Fatal iodine toxicity following surgical debridement of a hip wound: case report. J Trauma 1990;30:353–355.
2. dela Cruz F, Brown DH, Leikin JB, Franklin C, Hryhorczuk DO. Iodine absorption after topical administration. West J Med 1987;146:43–45.
3. Pennington JAT. A review of iodine toxicity reports. J Am Diet Assoc 1990;90:1571–1581.

Laxatives

1. Buchanan N, Cane RD, Glantz R, Hunt JA. Phenolphthalein poisoning. S Afr Med J 1976;50:1060–1061.
2. Lantner RR, Espiritu BP, Zumerchik P, Tobin MS. Anaphylaxis following ingestion of a psyllium-containing cereal. JAMA 1990;264:2534–2536.
3. Mrvos R, Swanson-Bierman B, Dean BS, Krenzelok AP. Acute phenolphthalein ingestion in children. A retrospective review. J Pediatr Health Care 1981;5:147–151.
4. Shepard KV. Cleansing enemas after sodium polystyrene sulfonate enemas. Ann Intern Med 1990;112:711.

Poison Look-Alikes

1. Aronson AJ. National Coordinator for OTC Look-Alike Drugs. Letter correspondence to all toxicologists, pathologists, coroners, medical examiners from the Food and Drug Administration. Rockville, MD, Public Health Service, Department of Health and Human Services, Nov 21, 1984.
2. Pruitt AW, Anyan WR Jr, Hill RM, et al. Committee on Drug 'look-alikes.' Pediatrics 1983;72:256–257.

Salt

1. Addleman M, Pollard A, Grossman RF. Survival after severe hypernatremia due to salt ingestion by an adult. Am J Med 1985;78:176–178.
2. Cassorla FG, Gill JR Jr, Gold PW, Rosen SW. Nosocomial hypernatremia. N Engl J Med 1985;313:229.
3. Raya A, Giner P, Aranequi P, Guerrero F, Vazquez G. Fatal acute hypernatremia caused by massive intake of salt. Arch Intern Med 1992;152:640–646.

Toxic Oil and Eosinophilia-Myalgia Syndromes

1. Alonso-Ruiz A, Calabozo M, Perez-Ruiz F, Mancebo L. Toxic oil syndrome. A long-term follow-up of a cohort of 332 patients. Medicine 1993;72:285–295.
2. Bronchide MH. Toxic oil syndrome. N Engl J Med 1984;310:1260-1261.
3. Duffy J. Eosinophilia-myalgia syndrome. Mayo Clin Proc 1992;67:1201–1202.
4. Hedberg K, Urbach D, Slutsker L, Matson P, Fleming D. Eosinophilia-myalgia syndrome. Natural history in a population-based cohort. Arch Intern Med 1992;152:1889–1892.

Vitamins

1. Davidson RA. Complications of megavitamin therapy. South Med J 1984;77: 200–203.
2. Herbert V. The vitamin craze. Arch Intern Med 1980;140:173–176.
3. Issenman RM, Slack R, MacDonald L, et al. Children's multiple vitamins: Overuse leads to overdose. CMA J 1985;132:781–784.
4. Toxic effects of vitamin overdosages. Med Lett Drug Ther 1984;26(issue 667):73–74.

Niacin

1. Toxic effects of vitamin overdosage. Med Lett Drug Ther 1984;26(667):73–74.

Retinoids

1. Accutane risks evaluated. Strong precautions needed. FDA Drug Bull 1990; 20(2):5–6.
2. CDC: Birth defects caused by isotretinoin-New Jersey. JAMA 1988;239:2362–2365.
3. David M, Hodak E, Lowe NJ. Adverse effects of retinoids. Med Toxicol 1988; 3:273–288.
4. Nightingale SL (FDA). Isotretinoin restrictions. JAMA 1988;260:315.
5. Sutton JD. Overdose of isotretinoin. J Am Acad Dermatol 1983;9:600.
6. Teelmann K. Retinoids: toxicology and teratogenicity to date. Pharm Ther 1989;40:29–43.

Vitamin A

1. Fossler MJ. The acute toxicity of vitamin A. Toxalert. Maryland Poison Center 1991;8:(3):1.
2. Hall JG: Vitamin A teratogenicity. N Engl J Med 1984;311:797.
3. La Mantia RS, Andrews CE. Acute vitamin A intoxication. South Med J 1981; 74:1012–1114.
4. Wason S. Vitamin A. Clin Toxicol Rev 1982;5(3):1–2.

Vitamin B6

1. Dalton K. Pyridoxine overdose in premenstrual syndrome. Lancet 1985;1:1168–1169.
2. Schaumburg H. Sensory neuropathy from pyridoxine abuse. N Engl J Med 1984;310:198.
3. Toxic effects of vitamin overdosage. Med Lett Drug Ther 1984;26(667):73–74.

Vitamin C

1. Toxic effects of vitamin overdosage. Med Lett Drug Ther 1984;26(667):73–74.

Vitamin D

1. Davies M, Adams PH. The continuing risk of vitamin D intoxication. Lancet 1978;2:621–623.
2. Goldman JM, Ahn Y-H, Wheeler MF. Vitamin D and hypercalcemia. JAMA 1985;254:1719.
3. Ko MLB, Liberman MM, Salzmann M. Chronic vitamin D overdosage: a reminder. Arch Dis Child 1991;66:1002.
4. Toxic effects of vitamin overdosage. Med Lett Drug Ther 1984;26(666):73–74.

Vitamin E

1. Hittner HM. Vitamin E toxicity. Pediatrics 1984;74:565–569.
2. Phelps DL. E-Ferol: What happened and what now? Pediatrics 1984;74:1114–1115.
3. Toxic effects of vitamin overdosage. Med Letter Drug Ther 1984;26(667):73–74.

Water Intoxication

1. Arieff A. Managing hyponatremia. Br Med J 1993;307:305–308.
2. Cooney JA. Compulsive water drinking, water intoxication and alcohol abuse. Irish J Psycholog Med 1991;8:22–25.
3. Ferrier IM. Water intoxication in patients with psychiatric illness. Br Med J 1985;291:1594–1595.
4. Vercammen M, Ramet Sacre L. Water intoxication in infants: report of twin brother case and review of the literature. Vet Human Toxicol 1987;29(Suppl 2):28–30.

ACKNOWLEDGMENTS

Thanks to Alison Deutsch, MD, and Liesa Lessard, MEd, for contributing questions to this chapter. Thanks to Jennifer Schonwald, MS, and Liesa Lessard, MEd, for help in typing and organizing this chapter.

CHAPTER 40
Cold Remedies

INTRODUCTION

Any visit to a local pharmacy will reveal hundreds of over-the-counter (OTC) cold remedies. Cold remedies, ranging from pseudoephedrine to dextromethorphan, may cause adrenergic crisis in overdose, and numerous side effects at therapeutic doses. Antihistamines (see Chapter 35, Antihistamines) are ubiquitous. Many are found in combination with other cold remedies and the majority of them are found OTC.

EPHEDRINE AND PSEUDOEPHEDRINE

Overdose with sympathomimetic OTC cold remedies may be associated with signs of adrenergic stimulation including tachycardia, hypertension, cardiac dysrhythmias, or atrioventricular block. The ubiquitous sympathomimetics ephedrine (Efedron®) and pseudoephedrine (Sudafed®) are optical isomers with both α- and β-adrenergic activity that are used as nasal decongestants and in bronchodilators.

Pathophysiology

Both products are weak bases. They act like phenylpropanolamine, stimulating adrenergic receptors as well as releasing neuronal norepinephrine. They raise heart rate (β-2 activity) as well as blood pressure, and cause bronchodilation (β-1 effect). Amounts up to 60 mg (ephedrine) and 180 mg (pseudoephedrine) do not cause a rise in blood pressure.

Pharmacokinetics

ABSORPTION

- These substances are well absorbed via the gastrointestinal route.

DISTRIBUTION

- The normal apparent total body clearance and volume of distribution for pseudoephedrine is approximately 250 to 300 mL/min and 2.0 L/kg, respectively.

ELIMINATION

- The serum half-life of pseudoephedrine is 7 hours. This is reduced to 1.9 hours in urine pH of 5.6, and 21 hours in urine pH 7.4.
- Ephedrine has a half-life of 2.7 to 3.6 hours (serum half-life in acid urine). Both are well absorbed after oral administration and excreted largely unchanged in the urine.
- A small amount of pseudoephedrine is excreted as the active metabolite norpseudoephedrine, and less than 10% of ephedrine is excreted as norephedrine.

Clinical Presentations

Overdoses are rare, but these drugs may induce cardiovascular and central nervous system stimulant effects. Intracerebral hemorrhage after pseudoephedrine overdose has occurred in the face of normotension. Severe headache, nausea, vomiting, diaphoresis, hypertension, tremulousness, dizziness, and epigastric pain have been reported. Sinus tachycardia with nonspecific S-T changes and hyperthermia, as in other adrenergic overdoses, may be seen. Pseudoephedrine overdoses can be as severe as other sympathomimetic ingestions and may cause agitation, rhabdomyolysis, and seizures.

Chronic overuse of ephedrine may induce a vasculitis of the central nervous system. Ephedrine has a high abuse potential. Following ingestion of excess ephedrine, both ischemic and hemorrhagic stroke have been observed. One study of pure pseudoephedrine effects in children revealed frequent drowsiness especially in doses over 120 mg. Children who ingest 120 mg or less generally develop no significant symptoms, regardless of any treatment.

Toxic Dosage/Death

The ephedrine concentrations in three fatalities with caffeine/ephedrine combinations were 3.49, 7.85, and 20.5 mg/L. Pseudoephedrine concentration in a case of fatal overdose was 19 mg/L.

Drug Interactions

These drugs should not be used in patients taking monoamine oxidase (MAO) inhibitors. Use with β-adrenergic agents or other sympathomimetics may be cumulative.

Pregnancy/Lactation

These drugs are categorized as pregnancy risk category C. They do distribute into breast milk.

Laboratory

ANALYTIC METHODS

Ephedrine, pseudoephedrine, and their metabolites are analyzed in plasma and urine by gas chromatography.

BLOOD LEVELS

A single oral dose of 60 mg of pseudoephedrine produces an average peak plasma concentration of 0.21 mg/L at 3 hours.

Treatment

GUT DECONTAMINATION

Lavage and activated charcoal may be effective in sympathomimetic overdoses if given within a few hours of ingestion.

ELIMINATION ENHANCEMENT

Hemodialysis does not appear to be useful in removal of pseudoephedrine because of its high volume of distribution.

SUPPORTIVE MEASURES

- Hemodynamic dysfunction (hypertension, tachyarrhythmias, and palpitations) and central nervous system dysfunction (tremors, agitation) may respond to careful propranolol administration. Propranolol is a β-blocker. Watch for aggravation of hypertension resulting from unopposed α-agonist effects when using β-blockers.
- Labetalol given intravenously over a few hours also may be used to curtail extreme hypertension, as may sodium nitroprusside.
- Treatment of overdose is similar to that for phenylpropanolamine. Agitation generally responds to reduced sensory input and may require haloperidol or benzodiazepines. Hyperthermia may require the use of a cooling blanket. Monitor for cardiac dysrhythmias.
- Treat symptomatic bradycardia with atropine and ventricular ectopy (without atrioventricular block) with lidocaine or propranolol. Avoid quinidine, procainamide, and disopyramide.
- Heart block in hemodynamically unstable patients may require cardiac pacing.

Questions—Ephedrine and Pseudoephedrine

1. Ephedrine and pseudoephedrine at higher than prescribed doses may

A. Raise heart rate
B. Raise blood pressure
C. Cause bronchodilation
D. A and B
E. A, B and C

2. Overdose of ephedrine or pseudoephedrine may cause all of the following except

A. Central nervous system vasculitis
B. Intracerebral hemorrhage
C. Hyperthermia
D. Rhabdomyolysis
E. Seizures

3. All of the following may be seen with pseudophedrine overdose except

A. Cyanosis
B. Headache
C. Tremor
D. Diaphoresis
E. Vomiting

4. Treatment of ephedrine or pseudoephedrine overdose may include
A. Lavage and activated charcoal if given within a few hours of ingestion
B. Careful propranolol administration
C. Haloperidol or benzodiazepines
D. Cardiac pacing
E. All of the above

EPINEPHRINE

In addition to its use in dire code situations, numerous epinephrine preparations are available as OTC preparations. Epinephrine (Primatene® Mist) is used widely in the treatment of pediatric and severe asthma. Nebulized racemic epinephrine is used to relieve respiratory distress in patients with upper airway edema caused by endotracheal intubation or in laryngotracheobronchitis (croup). It also may be used in treating anaphylaxis from any etiology.

Advanced Cardiac Life Support guidelines recommend epinephrine doses equivalent to a maximum of 2.8 μg/kg/minute. An intravenous (IV) bolus dose of 15 μg or more is considered high-dose epinephrine therapy and has been utilized increasingly in various resuscitation scenarios. Recent studies suggest that there does not appear to be any difference in the overall rate of return of spontaneous circulation, survival to hospital admission, survival to hospital discharge, or neurologic outcome between patients treated with a standard dose of epinephrine (0.2 mg/kg body weight) and those treated with a high dose.

The optimal doses of epinephrine in cardiac arrest are somewhat controversial. The standard IV bolus dosage of epinephrine is 1.0 mg every 3 to 5 minutes in code situations. The endotracheal dose of epinephrine should be at least 2 to 2.5 times larger than peripheral IV dosing.

Pathophysiology

Epinephrine and norepinephrine are relatively nonselective and stimulate α-1 and α-2 receptors with roughly similar potency. Epinephrine, in addition to its α effects, also stimulates β-1 and β-2 receptors. In overdose, β-adrenergic stimulation increases heart rate, cardiac output, and myocardial oxygen consumption and may produce cardiac arrhythmias. α-Adrenergic stimulation results in increased peripheral vascular resistance. Cumulative effects can lead to life-threatening systemic hypertension.

Pharmacokinetics

ABSORPTION

- Epinephrine is well absorbed rapidly by all routes.
- Onset of action is 1 minute by inhalation, 3 to 5 minutes by subcutaneous administration.

DISTRIBUTION

- Epinephrine does not cross the blood-brain barrier.

ELIMINATION

- Monoamine oxidase and catechol-o-methyltransferase metabolize epinephrine. It is contraindicated, therefore, in patients on MAO inhibitors.

Clinical Presentations

Numerous adverse effects have been described in oral overdose. High oral doses administered to babies resulted in (1) shock manifested by pallor, poor peripheral circulation, and tachycardia, (2) distension of the abdominal wall associated with dilated and edematous loops of small bowel on abdominal x-ray films, (3) initial leukocytosis with neutrophilia and thrombocytosis, followed by leukopenia, neutropenia, and thrombocytopenia within 48 to 72 hours, (4) transient hyperglycemia, hyperkalemia, and metabolic acidosis, (5) progressive respiratory insufficiency requiring mechanical ventilation within 4 to 24 hours, and (6) very high catecholamine levels in gastric aspirates. Bradycardia, pulmonary edema and respiratory failure also have been described in babies.

In adults, oral epinephrine has little physiologic effect, because of its rapid deactivation by conjugation in the gut mucosa and subsequent hepatic inactivation by catechol-o-methyltransferase. Nonetheless, diarrhea, abdominal cramping pain, and transient systemic adrenergic stimulation have been described.

Accidental injection of epinephrine into a finger may cause severe ischemia. A painful, pale, cool finger, demonstrating poor capillary refill, can last for several hours in this scenario. In one case, accidental intraarterial injection of epinephrine led to unconsciousness, hypotension, and ventricular tachycardia with marked pallor of the arm. Phentolamine 5 mg injected through the same arterial catheter led to rapid return of perfusion to the arm.

Symptoms of pallor, cyanosis, headache, diaphoresis, hypertension, tachycardia, myocardial ischemia, premature ventricular contractions (PVCs), bigeminy, precordial chest discomfort, palpitations, numbness, paresthesias, and abdominal pain may develop within seconds to minutes after excessive injection of epinephrine. Metabolic acidosis, hypotension, and pulmonary edema may have a delayed onset.

Toxic Dosage/Death

An IV dose of 3 mg has been reported as fatal, while other patients have survived IV doses as large as 30 mg.

Drug Interactions

As epinephrine is metabolized by monoamine oxidase, it is contraindicated in patients taking MAO inhibitors. Epinephrine may cause increased cardiac irritability if administered concomitantly with inhalational anesthetics.

Pregnancy/Lactation

Epinephrine is characterized as pregnancy risk category C. It crosses the placenta and does appear in breast milk.

Laboratory

ANALYTIC METHODS

High-performance liquid chromatography with electrochemical detection and a radioenzymatic thin-layer chromatographic method are available for assay of epinephrine and norepinephrine.

Blood Levels

Following blood levels in overdose does not help guide therapy.

Treatment

GUT DECONTAMINATION

Charcoal or emesis has not been shown to be valuable in the treatment of epinephrine overdose.

ELIMINATION ENHANCEMENT

Clinical experience has not shown any proven benefit from hemodialysis.

SUPPORTIVE MEASURES

- Treatment is directed at ameliorating tachycardias, shock, cardiac arrhythmias, systemic hypertension, pulmonary edema, and lactic acidosis. Cardiac monitoring is mandatory.
- IV phentolamine is useful in the treatment of epinephrine-induced hypertension. A short-acting β-blocker such as esmolol can be useful for a severe tachycardia. Labetalol has been effective as well, but there is the potential for incomplete α-blockade in the face of a more complete β-blockade.
- Adrenergic blocking agents and vasodilators should be used with caution because of the frequent biphasic hypertensive-hypotensive nature of epinephrine overdose.
- Shock and recovery of ventricular function may require aggressive supportive care, possibly including sodium nitroprusside, dobutamine, balloon pump, and noradrenaline.

DIGITAL INJECTION

- Topical nitroglycerine has been tried in these cases, but may not restore perfusion.
- Locally infiltrated phentolamine 1.5 mg (0.3 mL Regitine®) may cause hyperemia, renewed warmth, and normal capillary refill within 5 minutes. Local injection of 0.5 mg phentolamine with 1 mL of 2% lidocaine also may be effective in restoring circulation.

Questions—Epinephrine

1. Epinephrine
   A. Has only α-adrenergic properties
   B. Has α- and β-adrenergic properties
   C. Does not affect the same receptors that norepinephrine affects
   D. In overdose, has only β-adrenergic activity
   E. In overdose, has only α-adrenergic activity

2. All of the following are true about epinephrine except
   A. Absorption is rapid regardless of the route of administration.
   B. It crosses the blood-brain barrier.
   C. Onset of action is faster when given via inhalation versus subcutaneously.
   D. It is contraindicated in patients on MAO inhibitors.
   E. In overdose, it can produce cardiac arrhythmias.

3. High oral doses of epinephrine in infants
   A. Cause symptoms because of deactivation by conjugation in gut mucosa
   B. Cause circulatory, gastrointestinal, hematological, and metabolic changes
   C. Cause no respiratory symptoms
   D. Have the same effects at the same doses that they have in adults
   E. None of the above

4. Treatment of epinephrine overdose may include
   A. Amelioration of tachycardia, shock, and arrhythmia
   B. IV phentolamine
   C. Esmolol to treat severe tachycardia
   D. Serial electrocardiograms and cardiac monitoring
   E. All of the above

5. When a digit is injected accidentally with epinephrine,
   A. The finger often becomes red, warm, and edematous.
   B. Topical nitroglycerine is 95% effective in restoring perfusion.
   C. Local infiltration of phentolamine should be considered.
   D. Symptoms of poor perfusion can last no more than a few minutes
   E. None of the above

PHENYLPROPANOLAMINE

Phenylpropanolamine (PPA) has been a commonly used nasal decongestant and weight-control medication. PPA has been found in most OTC diet pills either alone or in combination with caffeine, vitamins, methylcellulose, benzocaine, fructose, lecithin, and grapefruit extract. More than 50 products have been actively sold OTC. PPA also has been found in decongestant formulations and in "look-alike" drugs, which have become popular as legal substitutes for amphetamines.

PPA is a synthetic sympathomimetic compound with action similar to ephedrine and the amphetamines, and with the same potential adverse effects. Serious adverse effects of PPA have become increasingly apparent within the past few years. Serious toxic effects usually are induced at doses considerably higher than those used therapeutically. Because a significant incidence of strokes recently has been associated with PPA, the FDA has curtailed its use in the U.S. PPA remains a ubiquitous cold remedy around the world, however.

Pathophysiology

PPA primarily is an indirect α-adrenergic agonist releasing norepinephrine at postganglionic sympathetic nerve terminals. It also has direct α-agonist properties and has a lesser degree of β-agonist activity. Its efficacy as an appetite suppressant may result from increased norepinephrine concentrations in some brain areas, but this has not been established. It causes elevation of blood pressure by α-mediated vasoconstriction of peripheral vessels.

Nasal decongestion is a result of direct α vasoconstriction of the mucosal blood vessels. The elevation in blood pressure usually is associated with a reflex bradycardia mediated by baroreceptors, and this can result in postural hypotension. An antihistamine or anticholinergic may block this effect.

Pharmacokinetics

ABSORPTION

- Oral therapeutic doses of PPA are absorbed rapidly, with maximal therapeutic effect in 1 to 3 hours.
- Nasal decongestion may occur within 30 minutes after 25 mg PPA is administered orally.

DISTRIBUTION

- Animal studies indicate that distribution occurs widely into many tissues, including the cerebrospinal fluid and brain. No studies in man are available.

ELIMINATION

- PPA is eliminated 80% to 90% unchanged in the urine. Small amounts of the drug are metabolized slowly in the liver to an active metabolite.
- In acid urine, the elimination half-life is 2.7 to 3.4 hours. However, because urine pH usually is in the range of 5.5 to 7.0, acidification procedures usually are unnecessary.

Clinical Presentations

Problems with PPA typically arise in children under 5 years of age who accidentally ingest it, in teenagers who buy a look-alike that they think is amphetamine, in adults who try to accelerate weight loss by taking more than two or three capsules at once, and in patients who have hypertension, cardiac disease, hyperthyroidism, or diabetes as an underlying disease.

Hypertension is the most common and most serious toxic effect of PPA. If tachycardia is seen in a patient with a toxic reaction to PPA, it usually is a result of other concomitantly ingested drugs such as caffeine, ephedrine, or an antihistamine. Death from adult respiratory distress syndrome (ARDS) has been reported. Acute renal failure and rhabdomyolysis have been described. An increased incidence of cerebrovascular accidents has also been associated with PPA use.

CARDIOVASCULAR EFFECTS

A low therapeutic index is a unique and dangerous property of PPA. Over 85 to 100 mg orally can produce severe hypertension in adults. Serious reactions in children may occur at lower doses. Sequelae of severe hypertension can include hypertensive encephalopathy and intracerebral hemorrhage and occasionally are fatal. Chest pain, ventricular arrhythmias, or other electrocardiogram (ECG) abnormalities (e.g., atrioventricular conduction block) may be seen. In general, reflex bradycardia is seen in conjunction with hypertension. Ischemic effects involving the coronary, renal, cerebral, and visceral vascular beds have been reported.

NEUROLOGIC EFFECTS

In high doses, PPA causes toxic effects similar to those of amphetamines: anxiety, agitation, and psychotic behavior. Some patients develop an organic brain syndrome with confusion and disorientation, acute memory loss, and aphasia. Seizures have occurred, particularly when PPA is combined with caffeine. Of the many well-documented intracerebral hemorrhages caused by PPA there seems to be no correlation of dose or blood pressure with incidents of hemorrhage. Some patients have reportedly had strokes after one or two tablets. The measured blood pressure, though usually elevated, often is not dramatically high. In general, central nervous system symptoms resolve within 6 hours; however, psychotic symptoms may last for days.

Toxic Dosage/Death

In overdose, the peak toxic reaction usually is seen within 2 to 3 hours after ingestion. In adults, no significant effect on blood pressure or heart rate is usually seen after ingesting 25 to 75 mg. Moderate agitation and dizziness may be seen with 50 to 75 mg. An increase in diastolic blood pressure may be seen in generally normotensive subjects with 85 mg. Toxic dose is considered 100 mg. Children appear more sensitive to the central nervous system stimulant effects of PPA and other sympathomimetics. Headaches and seizures in children may occur with as little as 50 mg or with 10 to 25 mg PPA in combination with caffeine.

Drug Interactions

PPA and caffeine administered together may lead to severe life-threatening and occasionally fatal hypertensive reactions. PPA with caffeine results in significantly elevated caffeine levels. In patients receiving MAO inhibitors, severe hypertension may develop after ingestion of PPA. PPA itself produces hypertension with a reflex bradycardia that limits blood pressure rise. This protective effect may be antagonized by concomitant administration of drugs that increase heart rate, such as atropine, caffeine, or antihistamines. However, this generally does not occur at therapeutic doses. Similar caution should be observed if the patient is receiving tricyclic antidepressant or ganglionic blocking agents.

Pregnancy/Lactation

PPA toxicity has not been studied in pregnancy or in the lactating female.

Laboratory

ANALYTIC METHODS

A stereospecific high-performance liquid chromatography assay for the enantiomers of phenylpropanolamine in human plasma has been developed that is sensitive to as little as 10 $\mu g/L$ of each enantiomer. Qualitative tests of urine for PPA with thin-layer chromatography may be available in some clinical laboratories. The enzyme multiplied immunoassay technique (EMIT) does not differentiate between amphetamines and PPA. Gas chromatography distinguishes PPA from amphetamines.

BLOOD LEVELS

Serum levels of PPA generally are not available. Toxic levels have not been established.

URINE

Drug screening of urine or gastric contents should be performed if a patient who is reluctant to give information has ingested a look-alike pill he or she believes to have been an amphetamine.

Treatment

GUT DECONTAMINATION

Treatment may include syrup of ipecac emesis after small ingestions at home; however, this may preclude careful evaluation of blood pressure at a health care facility. With any loss of consciousness, gastric lavage may be initiated after endotracheal intubation. After gastric evacuation, activated charcoal (adults, 50 to 100 g and children, 30 to 60 g) should be administered orally or via nasogastric tube. A repeat dose of activated charcoal 4 hours after the first may be useful for many sustained-release products.

ELIMINATION ENHANCEMENT

Maintenance of adequate urine output is essential. If the urine is acidic, excretion of PPA is rapid, with a half-life of 3 hours. Acidification may promote myoglobinuric renal failure and generally is discouraged. Hemoperfusion may be useful in renal failure but has not been adequately studied. There is no evidence for usefulness of forced diuresis, hemodialysis, or peritoneal dialysis.

SUPPORTIVE MEASURES

- Establish integrity of the airway, breathing, and circulation and establish an IV line. Establish baseline vital signs. Serial blood pressure readings should be taken where hypertension has developed, and 24-hour monitoring should be instituted if diastolic pressure remains high.
- If blood pressure is elevated, or there are signs of myocardial ischemia, tachyarrhythmias, or bradyarrhythmias, begin ECG monitoring immediately. Treat severe hypertension with IV nitroprusside or phentolamine. IV nitroprusside acts rapidly and can be carefully titrated. Start with 1 μg/kg/minute IV infusion and adjust to control blood pressure. Average dose is 3 μg/kg/minute. Phentolamine, an α-blocker, may be used for hypertension as well.
- Tachycardia may be treated with IV propranolol. Symptomatic or severe bradycardia may be treated with atropine. Ventricular tachycardia and premature ventricular contractions are treated with lidocaine.
- Monitor urine output and obtain baseline chest x-ray in severe cases.
- Blood urea nitrogen, serum creatinine, and serum myoglobin should be obtained. ECG, creatine kinase, and MB isoenzymes should be obtained in the face of hypertension or chest pain.
- Obtain urine pH and check for proteinuria, hemoglobinuria, and myoglobin.
- Obtain a computed tomography scan immediately in any patient with sudden onset of severe headache, headache associated with vomiting, neurologic deficits, abnormal mental status, or headache that persists after blood pressure lowering. Seizures may be treated with diazepam.
- Central nervous system effects such as agitation, disorientation, increased motor activity, hallucinations, hyperventilation, and tachypnea are treated symptomatically.

Questions—Phenylpropanolamine

1. Which of the following incorrectly describes the presumed actions of phenylpropanolamine?
   - A. Elevates blood pressure by α-mediated vasoconstriction
   - B. Suppresses appetite by increased brain norepinephrine
   - C. Decongests nasal passages by vasodilation of mucosal vessels
   - D. Causes reflex bradycardia associated with hypertension
   - E. All of the above are correct

2. In therapeutic usage, phenylpropanolamine
   - A. Has maximal therapeutic effect at 4 to 7 hours, regardless of the route of administration
   - B. Has maximal therapeutic effect in 1 to 3 hours if given orally
   - C. Is mostly hepatically metabolized
   - D. Is not metabolized hepatically at all
   - E. Is known to distribute into spinal fluid and brain

DEXTROMETHORPHAN

The primary use for dextromethorphan is as an antitussive (Robitussin® DM) for the short-term symptomatic relief of mild cough associated with the common cold or uncomplicated respiratory tract infection. It is nearly equal in efficacy to codeine as an antitussive. Dextromethorphan use is reported to poison centers with reasonable frequency. Most ingestions occur in the pediatric population under 6 years of age.

Dextromethorphan has not been reported to produce physical dependence or fatalities, although it may be abused. Dextromethorphan is the d-isomer of the codeine analog and narcotic analgesic levorphanol. Unlike the l isomer, it has no analgesic or addictive properties. Approximately 50 OTC products containing dextromethorphan hydrobromide as their principal cough suppressant are sold in the United States.

Pathophysiology

Dextromethorphan is a cough suppressant that probably acts centrally, similar to codeine. Neurotoxicity by endogenous excitatory amino acids such as glutamate has been implicated as a mechanism for central neuronal cell loss after hypoxia and ischemia. Blockage of synaptic transmission and antagonism of specific postsynaptic glutamate receptors may be protective. Dextromethorphan is a potent N-methyl-D-asparate (NMDA) receptor antagonist and appears to protect against hypoxic-ischemic damage in animal models of brain injury. Dextromethorphan is known to decrease responsiveness of NMDA receptors and may be useful in the treatment of heroin addicts.

Pharmacokinetics

ABSORPTION

- Dextromethorphan is absorbed orally.

DISTRIBUTION

- It is converted quickly in the liver to an O-demethylated product, dextrorphan.

ELIMINATION

- The glucuronide and sulfate ester conjugates of dextromethorphan, together with 3-hydroxy-N-morphinan and traces of unmetabolized dextromethorphan, are excreted in the urine.
- O- and N-demethylation, followed by subsequent conjugation, are the main metabolic pathways.
- Less than 2.5% of a dose is excreted unchanged in the urine within 24 hours.

Clinical Presentations

Symptoms of acute dextromethorphan toxicity include central nervous system effects (hyperexcitability and restlessness, lethargy, ataxia, slurred speech, and tremors); ophthalmologic effects, including nystagmus and variable pupillary changes; diaphoresis; and hypertension. Complex partial seizures may occur after use of long-acting dextromethorphan. The drug has been subjected to abuse by teenagers who describe an acute euphoria after consumption, with intense craving and dysphoria on withdrawal.

Many of the effects of intoxication may be caused by its active metabolite, dextrorphan. Dextromethorphan hydrobromide can potentially cause bromide poisoning manifested by headache, apathy, irritation, slurred speech, psychosis, tremulousness, ataxia, hallucinations, coma, weight loss, and acneiform rash. Symptoms of possible overuse in children include urticaria, restlessness, lethargy, nystagmus, ataxia, tachycardia, and blood pressure elevation.

Toxic Dosage/Death

Unusual behavior, respiratory depression, and neurologic abnormalities have appeared after 360 mg of dextromethorphan (in Robitussin® DM) in a 2-year-old. A Food and Drug Administration review panel found that doses as high as 100 times the therapeutic level were not associated with fatalities.

Drug Interactions

Dextromethorphan is a high-affinity substrate for certain P450 enzymes and competitively inhibits P450-mediated metabolism. Over 30 drugs are substrates for the same enzyme. Dextromethorphan is a specific inhibitor of serotonin uptake and increases central nervous system serotonin levels. Combined use of dextromethorphan and MAO inhibitors may result in the serotonin syndrome. Dextromethorphan is incompatible with penicillins, tetracyclines, salicylates, and phenobarbital.

Laboratory

ANALYTIC METHODS

A high-performance liquid chromatography assay is available for the simultaneous determination of dextromethorphan, dextrorphan, 3-hydroxymorphinone, and 3-methoxymorphine in plasma and urine. Although dextromethorphan is structurally similar to opioids, the ingestion of a single normal, or twice normal, dose of dextromethorphan is not likely to produce a falsely positive 6-hour urine opioid EMIT screen.

BLOOD LEVELS

Postmortem examination of two fatalities following ingestion of an unknown quantity of dextromethorphan revealed serum levels of 9.2 and 3.3 ng/mg, respectively.

Treatment

GUT DECONTAMINATION

Gastric decontamination should be considered after acute ingestions of over 10 mg/kg. Activated charcoal or gastric lavage may be preferable to syrup of ipecac; however, there are no controlled clinical data to support the usefulness of any gut decontamination.

ELIMINATION ENHANCEMENT

The use of extracorporeal procedures or forced dialysis cannot be recommended as the distribution of dextromethorphan has not been studied and conservative therapy generally is sufficient.

SUPPORTIVE MEASURES

- Dextromethorphan overdose patients should be examined in an emergency facility initially to evaluate airway, breathing, and circulation. Some patients (unusual behavior, respiratory depression) will require admission to an intensive care unit while most can be observed in an emergency facility for 4 to 6 hours if they remain asymptomatic.
- Patients with minor symptoms such as restlessness, ataxia, or urticaria can be discharged with appropriate supervision.
- Ethanol and acetaminophen levels may be helpful as a variety of dextromethorphan products contain these substances.

Antidotes

NALOXONE

Some authors recommend administration of naloxone 0.4 to 2.0 mg IV in an adult with repetition of the dose every 2 to 3 minutes as needed to a total dose of 10 mg. Symptomatic patients who respond to naloxone should be observed for at least 4 to 6 hours. Continuous IV infusion of naloxone may be required when long-acting preparations of dextromethorphan have been involved. Some cases of dextromethorphan overdose have anecdotally not responded to naloxone therapy.

Questions—Dextromethorphan

1. All of the following are true about dextromethorphan except

A. Dextromethorphan probably acts peripherally on cough receptors.
B. Neurotoxicity by endogenous excitatory amino acids has been implicated as a mechanism for central neuronal cell loss after hypoxia and ischemia.
C. Dextromethorphan is a potent NMDA receptor antagonist.
D. Dextromethorphan is known to decrease responsiveness of NMDA receptors.
E. It may be useful in the treatment of heroin addicts.

2. Symptoms of dextromethorphan toxicity include all of the following except

A. Hyperexcitability and restlessness
B. Nystagmus and variable pupillary changes
C. Cold, dry skin
D. Complex partial seizures
E. Hypertension

3. A child presenting with urticaria, restlessness, lethargy, and nystagmus may have these symptoms from dextromethorphan overuse.

A. True
B. False

4. Dextromethorphan is incompatible with all of the following except

A. Penicillins
B. Cephalosporins
C. Tetracyclines
D. Salicylates
E. Phenobarbital

5. The ingestion of a twice-normal dose of dextromethorphan

A. Will produce a false-positive urine opioid EMIT screen in 6 hours
B. Is not likely to produce a falsely positive 6-hour urine opioid EMIT screen
C. Will produce a falsely positive 6-hour urine opioid EMIT screen in children under 6 years
D. Will produce a falsely positive 6-hour urine opioid EMIT screen if coingested with acetaminophen
E. None of the above

EYE AND NOSE DROPS

Numerous OTC eye and nasal preparations are available in the United States. Imidazoline derivatives include naphazoline, tetrahydrozoline, oxymetazoline, and xylometazoline. Tetrahydrozoline (THZ) is an α-adrenergic agent with vasoconstrictor and decongestant properties, widely available without prescription for relief of pink-eye in a 0.05% concentration.

THZ is found in Murine Plus®, Visine®, and Soothe Eye®. THZ generally is safe for use in the eye without serious side effects. In overdose, patients may exhibit miosis, mydriasis, palpitations, hypertension, hypotension, bradycardia, pallor, cyanosis, diaphoresis, anxiety, insomnia, tremor, agitation, hallucinations, seizures, lethargy, obtundation, and coma. Treatment is supportive.

Pathophysiology

Imidazolines act peripherally and centrally as α-2-adrenergic agonists. Neo-Synephrine® (phenylephrine) is an α-adrenergic sympathomimetic receptor stimulant structurally similar to ephedrine and epinephrine.

Clinical Presentations

Overuse of oxymetazoline hydrochloride, phenylephrine hydrochloride, and ephedrine hydrochloride may cause profound α-adrenergic stimulation and lead to hypertension, cardiomegaly, seizures, and congestive heart failure. The clinical picture may be confusing with periods of hyperactivity alternating with episodes of cardiopulmonary and central nervous system depression. Signs and symptoms depend on whether peripheral or central α-2 adrenergic receptor stimulation predominates.

After topical ocular instillation of phenylephrine, systemic absorption may occur. A 2.5% solution of Neo-Synephrine® contains 1.2 to 2.0 mg per drop. Cardiovascular effects such as acute hypertension are more likely to follow use of the 10% ocular solution of Neo-Synephrine®, but have occurred within 30 minutes after topical administration of the 2.5% preparation.

Naphazoline (Privine®, Clear Eyes®, Naphcon®, and VasoClear®) and oxymetazoline (Afrin®, Neo-Synephrine®), both sympathomimetics, also may cause central nervous system depression when accidentally ingested or administered intranasally to children. Oxymetazoline as well as other sympathomimetic nose sprays can produce tachycardia, hypertension, and flushing.

Although THZ is a sympathomimetic agent, it can produce central nervous system depression. Cases of lethargy and obtundation have been described in children. Miosis, bradycardia, hypotension, and vasomotor collapse all have been observed.

Treatment

GUT DECONTAMINATION

Rapid onset of depressed consciousness following use of the topical imidazolines makes use of syrup of ipecac inadvisable. Activated charcoal may be useful if administered shortly after ingestion; however, efficacy data are not available.

ELIMINATION ENHANCEMENT

Such methods have not been studied in overdose.

SUPPORTIVE MEASURES

- Drug screening and specific drug analytic methods are not helpful. Provide airway protection and ventilatory support to the patient with depressed consciousness.
- Complications such as hemodynamic instability, respiratory insufficiency, and seizures respond to traditional measures. Atropine sulfate may be used to treat bradycardia.
- Diazepam may be used for seizures.

Antidotes

No specific antidote exists for these agents. Naloxone (0.01 to 0.1 mg/kg IV in children and 2.0 mg IV in adults) has been suggested in imidazoline overdoses because the imidazoline derivatives show central α-receptor stimulation properties and naloxone may be effective at these sites. Additional data are required to confirm the usefulness of naloxone.

Questions—Eye And Nose Drops

1. Tetrahydrozoline in overdose may cause
   A. Miosis
   B. Palpitations
   C. Hypertension
   D. Hypotension
   E. All of the above

2. Cardiovascular effects such as acute hypertension have followed use of the 10% ocular solution of Neo-Synephrine®), but not administration of the 2.5% preparation.
   A. True
   B. False

Answers

Ephedrine and Pseudoephedrine

1. E 2. A 3. A 4. E

Epinephrine

1. B 2. B 3. B 4. E 5. C

Phenylpropanolamine

1. C 2. B

Dextromethorphan

1. A 2. C 3. A 4. B 5. B

Eye and Nose Drops

1. E 2. B

SELECTED READINGS

Ephedrine and Pseudoephedrine

1. Clark RF, Curry SS. Pseudoephedrine dangers. Pediatrics 1990;85:389–391.
2. Rose SR, Gorman RL, Oderda GM, Klein-Schwartz W. Prospective evaluation of pseudoephedrine ingestion. Vet Hum Toxicol 1988;3:359.
3. Wezorek C, Kurta D, Dean B, Krenzelok E. Pediatric pseudoephedrine ingestions. A retrospective study. Vet Hum Toxicol 1991;33:362.

Epinephrine

1. Brown CG, Martin DR, Peper PE, et al. A comparison of standard dose and high dose epinephrine in cardiac arrest outside the hospital. N Engl J Med 1992;327:1051–1055.
2. Hall AH, Kulig NN, Rumack BH. Intravenous epinephrine abuse. Ann J Emerg Med 1987;5:64–65
3. Karch SB. Coronary artery spasm induced by intravenous epinephrine overdose. Am J Emerg Med 1989;7:485–488.
4. Maguire WA, Reisdorff EJ, Smith D. Epinephrine-induced vasospasm reversed by phentolamine digital block. Am J Emerg Med 1990;8:46–47.

Phenylpropanolamine

1. Brown CR. Phenylpropanolamine-an ongoing problem. Clin Toxicol Update 1987;9(2):5–8.
2. Prisant LM, Carr AA. Over-the-counter drugs that may increase blood pressure. Postgrad Med 1989;86:205–208.
3. Veltri JC, Bradford DC, Dring T, Kassner S, et al. Acute exposure to phenylpropanolamine: An analysis of 5447 cases reported to poison control centers from 1984-1987. Postmarket Surveill 1992;6:95–106.

Dextromethorphan

1. Fisher DD. Dextromethorphan. Clin Toxicol Rev 1991;13(4):1–2.
2. Schneider SM, Michelson EA, Baucek CD, Ilkhanipour K. Dextromethorphan poisoning reversed by naloxone. Am J Emerg Med 1991;9:237–238.
3. Wolfe TR, Caravati EM. Massive dextromethorphan ingestion and abuse. Am J Emerg Med 1995;13:174–176.

Eye and Nose Drops

1. Fraunfelder FT, Meyer SM. Systemic reactions to ophthalmic drug preparations. Med Toxicol 1987;2:287–293.
2. Higgins GL III, Campbell B, Wallace K, Talbot S. Pediatric poisoning from over-the-counter imidazoline-containing products. Ann Emerg Med 1991;20: 655–658.
3. Knauerhase TP. Topical imidazoles. Clin Toxicol Rev 1990;12(12):1–2.

ACKNOWLEDGMENT

Thanks to Alison Deutsch, MD for contributing the questions in this chapter.

CHAPTER 41
Food Toxicology

INTRODUCTION

Diarrhea kills about four million people in developing countries each year. Daily, over 10,000 children die worldwide from dehydration associated with diarrhea. It remains a problem in developed countries as well. In the United States, it has been estimated that 5-year-old children experience 20 million episodes of diarrhea each year, leading to several million doctor visits, 200,000 hospitalizations, and about 400 deaths. In clinical practice, up to 10% of ambulatory visits result from diarrheal illness. Most hospitalizations and deaths from diarrhea occur in the first year of life.

In the United States, despite many improvements in water treatment, sanitation, education, and medical care, diarrhea remains one of the most common pediatric illnesses. Sources of food poisoning include microbial toxins (e.g., bacteria, parasites, and viruses), the plant kingdom (e.g., solanine, oleander, pokeweed, and mushrooms), chemical toxins (e.g., monosodium glutamate, cadmium, mercury, tri-o-cresyl phosphate, and nitrosamines), and marine biotoxins.

Historical Clues

The history is quite important in identifying etiologic agents of foodborne illness. The patient interview should focus on identifying the source of the poisoning and evaluating the severity. Numerous factors such as travel history, medications and drugs, occupational exposures, illness in companions, sexual orientation, and water supply information may be helpful. Of course, a complete food history is mandatory whenever patients present with nausea, vomiting and/or diarrhea.

DRUGS

A thorough drug history is mandatory, as drug reactions frequently cause gastrointestinal symptoms. Antibiotics are particularly common offenders, in addition to quinidine and digoxin. Any recently implemented drug regimen should be a suspected cause of gastrointestinal distress. Most antibiotic-induced diarrheas are benign, but severe abdominal pain, localized tenderness, and hematochezia may indicate antibiotic-associated pseudomembranous colitis. Although clindamycin and lincomycin were originally implicated in this disease, other antibiotics may produce this syndrome as well.

FOOD

A thorough food history for the preceding 48 to 72 hours is necessary and should include the method of food preparation and refrigeration facilities. Bacterial contaminants often do not change the smell, taste, or appearance of the food. Certain foods commonly are associated with documented outbreaks. Although infrequent, even well-prepared foods such as pasteurized milk may transmit pathogens (e.g., *Yersinia enterocolitica*). *Salmonella,* mycobacteria, *Brucella, Campylobacter, Yersinia,* and *Listeria* can contaminate raw milk and milk products (e.g., cheese). Norwalk virus and *Vibrio* species can produce illness after consumption of contaminated raw shellfish. The most common milk-borne enteric pathogens are *Campylobacter jejuni, Campylobacter fetus, Salmonella,* and *Y. enterocolitica.*

ILLNESS IN COMPANIONS

Associated illness in other individuals who were in close contact tends to imply a foodborne illness. The history should include workers, family, friends, and sexual contacts. Oral, anal, and genital contact may cause the spread of *Shigella, Salmonella, Campylobacter, Giardia,* and *Entamoeba histolytica,* as well as that of *Streptococcus* and *Gonococcus,* particularly in homosexual men.

TRAVEL

Although some intestinal parasites are endemic in the United States (e.g., *Giardia* in mountain areas), certain agents are associated with travel to foreign countries. Almost one-half of travelers to Mexico develop diarrhea, and enterotoxigenic *Escherichia coli* accounts for up to 70% of these cases. To date, enterotoxigenic *E. coli* is the most frequent cause of traveler's diarrhea in all countries studied.

WATER SUPPLY AND COMMON SOURCES

Questions regarding a common water supply and other sources may yield significant clues. Sources may include a contaminated water supply, day-care centers, barnyard animals (e.g., *Salmonella, Campylobacter, Yersinia, Giardia,* and *Cryptosporidium*), pets (e.g., *Salmonella*), mass catering (e.g., *Clostridium*), and Chinese restaurants (e.g., monosodium glutamate, Bacillus-contaminated fried rice). Waterborne agents include enterotoxigenic *E. coli, Campylobacter, Shigella,* Norwalk virus, *Giardia, Salmonella,* and *Vibrio* species.

Clinical Presentations

Constitutional symptoms (e.g., malaise, weakness, and lightheadedness) may be related to dehydration or to the invasive organism. *Salmonella* can cause an enteric fever syndrome after entering the blood through the distal small bowel. Local infections may develop, particularly in susceptible hosts (e.g., *Salmonella osteomyelitis* in patients with sickle cell disease). *Yersinia* infections can produce a clinical bacteremia as well as polyarthritis, arthralgias, and erythema nodosum.

NONINFLAMMATORY DIARRHEA

Grouping the causes of infectious diarrhea into inflammatory and noninflammatory may help distinguish among pathogens. Although this classification aids the clinical workup, exceptions do occur. Acute infectious diarrheas typically resolve within 1 week. Persistent diarrhea lasting more than 1 week indicates a chronic medical condition, drug reaction, or parasitic infection.

Many viral, parasitic, and bacterial organisms produce a secretory type of diarrhea characterized by high-volume, watery stools that typically do not contain mucus, blood, or leukocytes. Nausea, vomiting, and low-grade fever occur, but the more toxic constitutional symptoms seen with inflammatory diarrheas usually are absent. Abdominal pain, if present, is a diffuse, crampy, periumbilical pain that is poorly localized.

Often these organisms produce toxins (e.g., enterotoxigenic *E. coli*), and typically these agents localize in the proximal portion of the small intestine, in contrast to the inflammatory diarrhea-producing organisms, which invade the distal small intestine and colon. Agents associated with noninflammatory diarrhea include *Vibrio cholerae, Rotavirus, Giardia lamblia* and *Aeromonas.*

INFLAMMATORY DIARRHEA

These organisms invade the mucosa of the ileum and colon, and produce a diarrheal illness characterized by hypogastric pain, fever, constitutional complaints, and frequent small-volume, bloody, or mucoid stools. Rectal inflammation may lead to tenesmus, urgency, and pain relieved by defecation. Fecal leukocytes usually are present.

Examples of agents associated with inflammatory diarrhea include *Salmonella,* which can produce both invasive and toxin-induced secretory diarrhea. *Shigella* cause an initial secretory diarrhea followed by a classic invasive diarrhea. Invasive pathogenic *E. coli* causes a syndrome clinically similar to that induced by *Shigella,* with an initial secretory diarrhea developing into the passage of mucus and pus. *Entamoeba histolytica,* a parasite, causes a typical invasive diarrhea confirmed by identification of organisms on stool examination.

VOMITING

Most pathogens that cause the abrupt onset of vomiting within 8 hours of exposure produce preformed toxins. *Staphylococcus aureus* is a classic example. *Bacillus cereus* causes prominent vomiting within 1 to 5 hours and/or severe diarrhea. Acute ingestion of large doses of most heavy metals (e.g., zinc, copper, arsenic, and cadmium) causes a severe hemorrhagic gastritis within several hours. Hepatotoxic mushrooms cause delayed vomiting (more than 6 hours), but early vomiting occurs with the co-ingestion of gastrointestinal irritant mushrooms.

The initial phase of parvovirus infection causes prominent vomiting, but symptoms usually occur 36 to 72 hours postexposure. Raw red beans, solanine in green potatoes, scombrotoxin in certain fish, and the dinoflagellates of paralytic shellfish poisoning cause vomiting and other symptoms with a short incubation period (up to several hours).

PERITONITIS

Severe gastroenteritis may cause signs of mild peritonitis, but hyperactive bowel sounds usually are present. *Y. enterocolitica* can produce inflammation of the ileum and a mesenteric lymphadenitis in older children that mimics appendicitis. *Salmonella* and *Campylobacter* also can produce a clinical picture similar to appendicitis.

NEUROLOGIC EFFECTS

Certain neurologic symptoms have been associated with certain foodborne illnesses. Children hospitalized with *Shigella* may experience seizures before they develop diarrhea. *Clostridium botulinum* poisoning may be associated with cranial nerve and bulbar palsies, followed by descending paralysis. Scombroid fish produce a histaminelike substance that can cause headache and dizziness. Ciguatera poisoning is associated with paresthesias and a hot-cold sensation reversal.

Paralytic shellfish poisoning is associated with a neurotoxin produced by dinoflagellates, which produces paresthesias, dysphagia, dysarthria, and respiratory paralysis. Tetrodotoxin in the puffer fish causes paresthesias, lightheadedness, and a feeling of impending doom after consumption of contaminated parts. Fatalities may occur from respiratory depression. Guillain-Barré syndrome has been associated with *Campylobacter* poisoning.

COMPLICATIONS

The presence of blood in the stool generally indicates inflammatory diarrhea. An invasive diarrhea may cause bacteremia that seeds the meninges or joints. Fever (over 102°F) is uncommon in enterotoxin-induced diarrheas (e.g., labile or heat-stable *E. coli, Clostridium perfringens,* or *Vibrio parahaemolyticus*), but is frequent in diarrheas produced by more-invasive organisms (e.g., *Salmonella, Campylobacter,* and *Shigella*) and viruses. Rarely, toxic shock syndrome may be preceded by staphylococcal food poisoning.

Laboratory

FECAL LEUKOCYTES

The presence of more than two methylene blue-stained leukocytes per high-power field indicates an abnormal number of fecal leukocytes. Although the presence of fecal leukocytes suggests mucosal invasion, one study showed that sensitivity is up to 90% in shigellosis but slightly less in *Campylobacter* and *Salmonella* infections. Fecal leukocytes are uncommon in secretory diarrhea, giardiasis, and viral infections and are variable in *Yersinia, Entamoeba histolytica,* and *Vibrio parahaemolyticus* infections. In amebiasis, fecal leukocytes usually are more mononuclear than polymorphonuclear. Both regional enteritis and ulcerative colitis also produce fecal leukocytes.

OVA AND PARASITES

Examination of stools for ova and parasites is indicated in high-risk cases (e.g., travelers and homosexuals), in cases of diarrhea lasting longer than 1 week, and in the presence of positive tests for fecal leukocytes. Three freshly voided daily morning specimens in preservative are needed for proper screening. A negative stool examination does not exclude giardiasis, because the diagnostic yield on three specimens does not exceed 50%. Concentrating procedures, duodenal aspirates, and even small-bowel biopsy may be necessary to confirm or exclude giardiasis.

STOOL CULTURES

Indications for stool cultures include persistent (over 5 days) or excessive diarrhea (more than 8 stools per day), evidence of invasive diarrhea (e.g., occult blood and/or presence of fecal leukocytes), immune compromise in hospitalized patients, recent foreign travel, or consumption of raw shellfish, meat, or milk.

STOOL OSMOLALITY

The osmolality of freshly assayed diarrheal stool samples ranges from 280 to 330 mOsm. Improper stool storage (i.e., storage at room temperature) raises the osmolality because of continuing bacterial metabolism. Secretory diarrhea frequently produces a negative stool osmolal gap (measured stool osmolality minus twice the sodium plus potassium concentrations), whereas osmotic-induced diarrhea (e.g., lactulose, and sorbitol) results in large osmolal gaps (i.e., greater than 200 mOsm). An osmolal gap less than 100 mOsm does not distinguish between secretory and osmotic-induced diarrhea.

Treatment

SUPPORTIVE MEASURES

- Restoration of fluid and electrolyte balance is the primary therapy of gastroenteritis.
- Most patients with gastroenteritis do not become seriously dehydrated and can be maintained on balanced electrolyte and glucose solutions, potable fruit juice, caffeine-free soft drinks, and salted crackers. Small frequent feedings and clear, hypotonic liquids are helpful. Alcohol and caffeine-containing beverages should be avoided.
- Because dairy products aggravate diarrhea in some patients, milk and other dairy products should be avoided initially. As the patient improves, advancement to a high-carbohydrate, low-fat BRATT (i.e., **B**ananas, **R**ice, **A**pples, **T**ea or **T**oast) diet may firm up stool.

ORAL HYDRATION

- Oral therapy has become the mainstay of the World Health Organization's efforts to decrease diarrhea morbidity and mortality, and diarrheal disease control programs have been established in more than 100 countries worldwide. Proper nutrition for children with diarrhea is viewed as an important adjunct to therapy, whereas antibiotics and other drugs play only a limited role.
- The treatment of acute diarrhea (rather than persistent diarrhea lasting 2 weeks or longer) is aimed primarily at watery diarrhea rather than bloody diarrhea (dysentery). Oral rehydration therapy (ORT) encompasses two phases of treatment: (1) the rehydration phase, in which water and electrolytes are given as oral rehydration solution (ORS) to replace existing losses and (2) the maintenance phase, which includes both replacement of ongoing fluid and electrolyte losses and adequate dietary intake.
- ORS can be used to treat diarrhea regardless of the patient's age, causative pathogen, or initial sodium values. Many physicians continue to prescribe a variety of clear liquids to treat patients with diarrhea instead of an appropriately composed ORS. Clear fluids can cause osmotic diarrhea and electrolyte imbalance, and often contain inadequate sodium bicarbonate and excess sugar for appropriate replacement of stool losses.

INTRAVENOUS HYDRATION

- Patients with orthostatic changes (i.e., a pulse rise of 15 to 20 going from a lying to a standing position or a decrease of 20 mm Hg in the systolic blood pressure) or hypotension benefit from intravenous (IV) fluids with 5% dextrose in Ringer's lactate or saline.
- Serum electrolytes and creatinine may be helpful in cases of moderate to severe dehydration (i.e., orthostatic changes) or in patients receiving cardiac medications.
- Signs of shock indicate fluid deficits exceeding 10%. These patients should receive rapid fluid infusions (1 to 2 L in adults and 20 to 30 mL/kg in children).

ANTIBIOTICS

- Most gastroenteritides are self-limited diseases that require only supportive care.
- Antibiotics are reserved for specific indications. These include all patients infected with *E. histolytica, V. cholerae,* and *G. lamblia;* all symptomatic patients infected with *Shigella;* and severe, protracted cases in susceptible hosts who are infected with *Salmonella, Campylobacter,* and *Clostridium difficile.*
- Antibiotics may promote a carrier state in patients infected with *Salmonella* and *Campylobacter.*
- Prophylactic antibiotics can prevent traveler's diarrhea, but risks may outweigh benefits.

ANTIPERISTALTIC AGENTS AND SECRETION INHIBITORS

- Use of adsorbents (e.g., kaolin-pectin), antimotility agents (e.g., loperamide), antisecretory drugs, or toxin binders (e.g., cholestyramine) is a common practice in many developed and developing countries. Available data do not demonstrate their effectiveness in reducing diarrhea volume or duration. Stool water losses are unchanged, and electrolyte losses may increase.
- Reliance on antidiarrheal agents shifts the therapeutic focus away from appropriate fluid, electrolyte, and nutritional therapy; can interfere with oral therapy; and can unnecessarily add to the economic cost of the illness.
- Little evidence exists to support the use of nonspecific drug therapy in children, and much information exists to the contrary. These drugs should be avoided in children under 2 years of age and discontinued if symptoms persist over 48 hours.
- The use of antimotility agents is controversial in secretory diarrhea because of uncertainty concerning the importance of the natural effect of diarrhea on the clearance of toxins.
- Pepto-Bismol® (bismuth subsalicylate) can decrease the frequency of stool production in traveler's diarrhea, but stool output remains similar over the first 4 hours. Pepto-Bismol® contains large amounts of salicylate. 60 mL of Pepto-Bismol® contains the equivalent of two regular adult (325-mg) aspirins. High salicylate concentrations in Pepto-Bismol® have important implications for children and for patients with aspirin sensitivity, concurrent salicylate use, and bleeding disorders.
- Children absorb over 90% of the calculated amount of salicylate in bismuth subsalicylate after both single and multiple doses. Hypercalcemia may develop after the administration of large doses of Pepto-Bismol® tablets in susceptible patients.
- Kaolin and pectin appear to increase stool consistency but do not decrease abdominal cramps, stool frequency, or the duration of illness.
- Activated charcoal is not helpful in the treatment of diarrhea.

HOSPITALIZATION

- Indications for hospitalization include moderate to severe dehydration. This is defined as more than 5% dehydration in infants or persistent orthostatic changes in adults despite 1 to 2 L of fluid replacement. Adults whose blood pressure stabilizes after fluid therapy and who are not in a toxic condition may be discharged after fluid administration.
- Other indications for hospitalization include febrile patients (102 to 103°F) who appear seriously ill, persons in whom botulism or paralytic shellfish poisoning is suspected, and in susceptible hosts (e.g., sickle cell disease, elderly diabetics, and neonates) who manifest any difficulty in maintaining fluid and/or electrolyte balance.
- Specific follow-up should be provided to patients so that they have a referral if symptoms do not clear in 1 week or if complications develop.

PREVENTION

- Since there are no antidotes, prevention of serious foodborne contamination is the best measure. Follow public health procedures for equipment and food handling. Avoid contamination of food after cooling by separating areas and utensils for raw and cooked food.
- Avoid abnormal-looking or abnormal-smelling food. Most contaminated foods look normal, however.
- Boil home-canned food for 20 minutes if there is any question about proper processing. In general, reheated food must reach boiling temperature throughout.
- Keep foods frozen until used, and defrost meat and poultry thoroughly before cooking. Foods that contain *Salmonella* and *C. perfringens* require thorough heating to destroy the organisms. Food should be eaten within 1 hour of cooking.
- Immediately refrigerate leftovers at temperatures below 40 C.

Questions—Introduction to Food Toxicology

1. The most frequent cause of traveler's diarrhea is
A. *Giardia*
B. *Entamoeba histolytica*
C. *Escherichia coli*
D. *Campylobacter*
E. *Shigella*

2. Which foodborne illness is associated with the correct neurologic sequelae?
A. *Shigella*—headache and dizziness
B. *Clostridium botulinum*—cranial nerve and bulbar palsies
C. Ciguatera—seizures
D. Scombroid fish—hot/cold sensation reversal
E. All of the above

3. Fecal leukocytes are common in
A. *Shigella* infections
B. *Giardiasis*
C. Viral enteritides
D. Secretory diarrhea
E. None of the above

MICROBIAL FOODBORNE ILLNESS

BACTERIAL FOODBORNE ILLNESS

Bacteria account for approximately 70% of cases of food poisoning. *Staphylococcus* is the most common cause of foodborne bacterial illness and *Salmonella, Campylobacter,* and *Shigella* are the most frequent causes of infectious diarrhea in the United States. Ingested toxins are the next most frequent cause. Bacterial food poisoning (with the exception of botulism and cholera) exhibits a short incubation period and usually is mild and self-limited, lasting 1 to 3 days. These illnesses may occur in epidemics and lead to fatal outcomes, especially infants, young children, the elderly, and immunologically compromised patients.

Bacillus Cereus

B. cereus is an aerobic, spore-forming, motile, gram-positive rod that is ubiquitous in soil. Common sources for food poisoning are fried rice, powdered milk, and dried fruit. Diagnosis is made by culturing a contaminated food source. *B. cereus* causes two recognized forms of foodborne gastroenteritis. The first is an emetic syndrome resembling that caused by *S. aureus,* characterized by an incubation period of 1 to 6 hours.

The second is a diarrheal illness characterized by an incubation period of 6 to 24 hours. Fever is uncommon with either syndrome. A highly stable toxin that survives high temperatures and exposure to trypsin, pepsin, and pH extremes mediates the emetic syndrome. The diarrheal syndrome is mediated by a heat- and acid-labile enterotoxin that is sensitive to proteolytic enzymes.

TREATMENT

- This mild, self-limited disease requires supportive treatment only.

Questions—Bacillus Cereus

1. The syndrome typically associated with *Bacillus cereus* infection
A. May include emesis but usually not diarrhea
B. May include diarrhea but not emesis
C. May include an early emetic syndrome or a later-onset diarrheal illness
D. Usually includes fever
E. C and D

Campylobacter

Campylobacter species are found in a large number of animals, including chickens, turkeys, pigs, cattle, sheep, goats, dogs, cats, horses, and rodents. Unchlorinated water as well as raw cow and goat milk transmit *Campylobacter* diarrheal disease. Human-to-human transmission is rare, although an asymptomatic carrier state does exist. Sick pets and contaminated food and water are the most common sources. Both *Giardia* and *Campylobacter* species are frequent contaminants of surface water in Rocky Mountain parks.

PATHOPHYSIOLOGY

Campylobacter is one of the three most common causes of diarrhea in the world along with *rotavirus* and *Shigella* (*E. coli* is more common in underdeveloped countries). *Campylobacter fetus* subspecies *jejuni* and *intestinalis* are the principal human intestinal pathogens. Recent DNA homolog studies have demonstrated that *C. fetus* subspecies *jejuni* actually represents two organisms, *Campylobacter jejuni* and *Campylobacter coli. Campylobacter* causes invasion of the mucosal wall and production of an enterotoxin.

Recently the presence of *Campylobacter pyloridis* on the gastric mucosa has been associated with gastritis, duodenitis, and duodenal ulceration. This organism colonizes the stomach in over 70% of patients with gastric ulcers. The resolution of gastritis by treatment with bismuth subsalicylate suggests that *C. pyloridis* may contribute to the development of gastritis. *Campylobacter* species produce a heat-labile choleralike enterotoxin that increases cyclic AMP and causes profuse diarrhea and cramping.

CLINICAL PRESENTATIONS

The onset of symptoms ranges from 1 to 8 days. Patients develop watery or bloody diarrhea together with fever, malaise, abdominal pain, and headache. In adults, *Campylobacter* illness may be clinically indistinguishable from shigellosis, but children under 5 with shigellosis frequently have high fevers (over 38°C). *Campylobacter* illness may resemble inflammatory bowel diseases. *C. jejuni* has increasingly been associated with immune-mediated disorders, including Guillain-Barré syndrome, reactive arthritis, Reiter's syndrome, and acute glomerulonephritis.

Answers to questions in shaded boxes appear at the end of the chapter.

Rarely, acute anterior uveitis, myalgias, hemolytic-uremic syndrome, erythema nodosum, and urticaria have been reported after *Campylobacter* infections. The average duration is 3 to 4 days, but symptoms of illness may persist in an immunocompromised patient.

Fatalities have resulted from *C. jejuni* and *C. fetus* infections. The latter are commonly associated with bacteremia, cellulitis, and osteomyelitis in immunocompromised patients. Neurological complications of *Campylobacter enteritis* may include seizures, subdural empyema, meningoencephalitis, subarachnoid hemorrhage, stroke, and encephalopathy. *C. jejuni* septicemia affects patients at the extremes of life as well as immunocompromised patients, although mortality occurs primarily in the latter group. Up to 30% of these septic patients have no symptoms of gastroenteritis.

LABORATORY

Analytic Methods

Dark-field microscopy of the stool may reveal characteristic curved gram-negative nonsporing, thin, motile rods (Campylobacter means "curved rod" in Greek). Gram stains should be counterstained with carbolfuchsin. Blood cultures are appropriate in immunocompromised or toxic patients. Sigmoidoscopy demonstrates an edematous, hyperemic mucosa with shallow gray-based aphthous ulcers.

TREATMENT

- Without treatment, *C. enterocolitis* usually resolves in 7 to 10 days. Fluids often are the only treatment necessary. Opiates and anticholinergics may lengthen intestinal transit time.
- Erythromycin or clarithromycin shorten the excretion of the organism. Their effectiveness in reducing symptoms when administered over the first 5 days of illness is questionable. Erythromycin may not provide adequate coverage for *C. fetus septicemia* or *Campylobacter pyloridis* infections. Ciprofloxacin, and/or ampicillin with or without an aminoglycoside are alternatives when the organism is sensitive to these drugs.
- Graded compression ultrasonography of the right lower abdominal region may show mural thickening of the terminal ileum and cecum.

Questions—Campylobacter

1. **All of the following are associated with *Campylobacter* infection except**
   A. Botulism
   B. Guillain-Barré Syndrome
   C. Reactive arthritis
   D. Reiter's syndrome
   E. Acute glomerulonephritis
2. **All of the following medications may play a role in the treatment of *Campylobacter* except**
   A. Erythromycin
   B. Ciprofloxacin
   C. Aztreonam
   D. Ampicillin
   E. Clarithromycin

Clostridium Perfringens

C. perfringens produces a noninflammatory diarrheal disease. This ubiquitous organism commonly contaminates meat, meat products, gravy, and poultry. Two percent to 5% of normal subjects harbor this organism. Apparently, heat-stable spores survive cooking, reproduce in the gastrointestinal tract, and then form toxins. Five major types (A–E) occur; type C causes necrotizing colitis. *C. difficile* has been associated with pseudomembranous colitis. See Chapter 13, Antibiotics and Antituberculous Drugs.

CLINICAL PRESENTATIONS

The incubation period is approximately 12 hours (range, 6 to 24 hours), and the duration is approximately 24 hours (range, 12 to 48 hours). Vomiting and fever are uncommon. Characteristically, watery diarrhea occurs with occasional abdominal pain and nausea. The diagnosis is based on culture of food source. An enzyme-linked immunosorbent assay is a useful epidemiological tool for detection of enterotoxin.

A protein-losing enteropathy and intravascular hemolysis (usually associated with underlying malignancy) have been reported in *C. perfringens* infections. Systemic distribution of *C. perfringens* type A has been suggested as a possible cause of sudden infant death syndrome in the immunologically vulnerable infant.

TREATMENT

- Treatment is supportive, because this organism usually causes a mild illness lasting 24 to 36 hours.

Question—Clostridium Perfringens

1. **The most common symptom(s) after *Clostridium perfringens* include**
   A. Vomiting
   B. Watery diarrhea
   C. Fever
   D. A and B
   E. B and C

Escherichia Coli

E. coli is the most common facultative anaerobe in the healthy human intestine. Pathogenic *E. coli* are complex, invasive, and toxin-producing organisms that cause multiple distinct syndromes. Biochemical and serologic markers distinguish invasive and toxin-producing strains, which are difficult to identify clinically. Except for pathogenic strains that produce the hemolytic-uremic syndrome, most pathogenic *E. coli* strains require adhesion to gut receptors to produce disease.

Although a heat-labile enterotoxin derived from *E. coli* is the most common cause of traveler's diarrhea, site and season may predispose the traveler to diarrhea associated with other causative bacteria. These infections are most commonly acquired through ingestion of contaminated food and water, but may be transmitted by person-to-person contact. Many beaches around the world are now contaminated with sewage and fecal microorganisms.

CLINICAL PRESENTATIONS

Pathogenic strains of *E. coli* produce multiple clinical syndromes. Infantile enteropathogenic *E. coli* (EPEC) and enteroinvasive *E. coli* (EITC) produce an inflammatory or dysentery-like picture. The dysentery-like syndrome resembles *Campylobacter, Yersinia,* and *Shigella* infections. Enterotoxigenic *E. coli* (ETEC) produces a secretory, choleralike illness and enterohemorrhagic *E. coli* causes hemorrhagic colitis and hemolytic-uremic syndrome. The cholera type mimics *Vibrio* and *Bacillus cereus*-induced diarrheas.

Enteroadherent *E. coli* (EAEC) is a less-well-defined category that is associated with traveler's diarrhea. Hemolytic-uremic syndrome has been associated with *E. coli* 0157:H7 enteric infections and is characterized by microangiopathic hemolytic anemia, thrombocytopenia, and renal dysfunction. Toxin-mediated damage to the endothelial cells of the glomerular capillaries and small renal arterioles probably initiates the hemolytic-uremic syndrome. The diarrheal phase of illness usually precedes the appearance of hemolysis.

LABORATORY

Analytic Methods

Stool culture identifies the presence of *E. coli* strains, but differentiation between invasive and toxigenic strains requires expensive animal testing, which is not routinely cost-effective. The sorbitol fermentation reaction is an effective screening procedure for patients with hemorrhagic colitis or hemolytic-uremic syndrome, because the *E. coli* 0157:H7 is a sorbitol-negative strain compared with the other *E. coli* organisms.

TREATMENT

- Prophylactic antibiotic treatment for travelers' diarrhea is reserved for the medically compromised patient. Trimethoprim-sulfamethoxazole, doxycycline, and quinolones, such as ciprofloxacin, are effective.
- Pepto-Bismol®, 60 mL four times daily, reduces the incidence of travelers' diarrhea significantly.
- Some travelers substitute Pepto-Bismol® tablets, which contain 350 mg of calcium carbonate in addition to the 300 mg of bismuth subsalicylate. Hypercalcemia is a potential risk under certain conditions (e.g., dehydration, renal insufficiency and use of vitamin D preparations). These tablets also contain significant quantities of absorbable salicylate.
- Travelers can protect themselves by drinking bottled beverages or purified water. Boiling is the most reliable way to purify water. Alternatively, 5 drops of Tincture of Iodine can be added per quart (or liter) of clear water 30 minutes before drinking.
- Travelers should not consume ice, uncooked food, unpasteurized milk, and fruit that cannot be peeled. Portable water filters may offer some protection, but have not been extensively tested.

Questions—Escherichia Coli

1. **Hemolytic-uremic syndrome due to *Escherichia coli* 0157:H7 includes**
   A. Thrombocytosis
   B. Thrombocytopenia
   C. Renal dysfunction
   D. A and B
   E. B and C
2. **Stool cultures cannot distinguish between invasive and toxigenic strains of *E. coli***
   A. True
   B. False

Listeria Monocytogenes

L. monocytogenes is a ubiquitous, facultative, intracellular bacterium appearing in streams, sewage, soil, domestic and wild animals, fowl, and humans. Carrier rates in man approximate 5% in healthy adults and are higher in special risk groups. *Listeria* can penetrate the placenta and produce intrauterine infections. *L. monocytogenes* can remain in pasteurized milk even after proper processing. Epidemics of listeriosis have resulted from consumption of cabbage, cheese, pasteurized milk, and raw vegetables. *L. monocytogenes* causes disease primarily in pregnant women, neonates, and immunocompromised patients. Resistance to infection depends mostly on cell-mediated immunity, although humoral factors may contribute. *Listeria* produces no toxins.

CLINICAL PRESENTATIONS

In healthy adults and children, *L. monocytogenes* produces a mild flulike syndrome, with gastrointestinal symptoms and myalgias resolving in several days. Meningitis and/or sepsis characterized by nausea, vomiting, headache, and fever develops in immunocompromised patients. Perinatal infections can cause either perinatal meningitis or intrauterine fetal demise. Diagnosis is based on cultures of blood, cerebrospinal fluid, and amniotic fluid.

TREATMENT

- In susceptible patients, listeriosis can be a life-threatening disease that requires hospitalization and antibiotics (e.g., ampicillin and gentamicin).
- Pregnant patients should be treated with antibiotics (e.g., ampicillin and/or erythromycin) in consultation with an obstetrician. Healthy patients usually require only symptomatic treatment.

Questions—Listeria Monocytogenes

1. ***Listeria* can cause infections in**
   A. The placenta
   B. The cerebrospinal fluid
   C. The blood
   D. All of the above
   E. None of the above
2. **Infections due to Listeria occur most often in which of the following groups?**
   A. Healthy newborns
   B. Healthy children
   C. Healthy adults
   D. A and B
   E. B and C

Salmonella

Salmonella are ubiquitous organisms, especially in animal intestines. Eggs, meat, poultry products, and milk (especially unpasteurized) are common sources. Because the organism is heat labile and destroyed by stomach acid (pH 2.0), large numbers of organisms usually are required to cause infection. Drug-resistant *Salmonella* organisms from animals fed antimicrobials are a serious cause of concern in human salmonellosis. *Salmonella enteritis* infection has been associated with the consumption of raw eggs. Raw milk products (e.g., unpasteurized goat's milk cheese) have been associated with outbreaks of *S. enterica* infection.

Pet turtles, iguanas, and snakes may harbor *Salmonella* organisms toxic to humans, especially children. *Salmonella arizonae,* an opportunistic pathogen in compromised patients [e.g., acquired immunodeficiency syndrome (AIDS)], is commonly found in reptiles. Rattlesnake powder or meat is a common Mexican folk remedy used to treat cancer, diabetes, arthritis, skin disorders, and other ailments. Spices and shellfish also may serve as a vehicle of infection. *Salmonella* organisms produce an inflammatory diarrhea by invading the mucosa, and may penetrate the bowel wall, causing septicemia.

CLINICAL PRESENTATIONS

At least four clinical syndromes characterize *Salmonella* infections. *Salmonella gastroenteritis* has an 8- to 48-hour incubation period and is followed by 2 to 5 days of loose, watery diarrhea that may contain blood or mucus. A second clinical syndrome involves bacteremia with focal extraintestinal infection. This form is seen in infants, sickle cell disease patients, the elderly, and immunosuppressed patients (AIDS). The bacteremia usually is transient and does not alter clinical outcome, but both septicemia and meningitis can develop, particularly in infants less than 3 months of age. Watery diarrhea may precede septic arthritis by 5 to 15 days, making the diagnosis difficult.

Enteric fever is a subacute disease characterized by an incubation period of about 1 week, active invasion of gut lymphoid tissue during the second week, and establishment of bacteremic foci in the gut during the third week. Symptoms include fever, headaches, myalgias, anorexia, nausea, cough, and/or sore throat. Symptoms may progress to fulminant sepsis or localized infection in the gastrointestinal tract, urinary tract, respiratory tract, or musculoskeletal system. A fourth clinical syndrome or asymptomatic carrier state also occurs. Indiscriminate use of antibiotics encourages this state, and antibiotics lengthen the course of intestinal shedding.

TREATMENT

- Stool cultures establish the disease state, and sensitivities help select the antibiotic. Blood and urine cultures during the active phase of enteric fever may be positive.
- Antibiotics should not be prescribed in mild disease. Antibiotics are given selectively to bacteremic and high-risk individuals (e.g., patients with sickle cell disease and AIDS, the elderly, and infants).
- Chloramphenicol is effective if no sensitivity test is available. Either ampicillin or trimethoprim-sulfamethoxazole is indicated if sensitivity on culture confirms their effectiveness. Multiple-drug–resistant strains of *Salmonella typhimurium* have been reported.

Questions—Salmonella

1. *Salmonella* infections may be acquired from
   A. Turtles
   B. Raw milk products
   C. Goats
   D. All of the above
   E. B and C

2. The following should be treated with antibiotics if *Salmonella* infection is documented except
   A. Healthy patients with bacteremia
   B. Healthy patients with mild gastrointestinal symptoms
   C. Sickle cell patients with mild gastrointestinal symptoms
   D. Infants with Hemoccult negative stool
   E. Elderly patients with Hemoccult negative stool

Shigella

Shigella may be found in fruits, vegetables, and milk. Person-to-person transmission may occur via the oral-anal route in homosexuals. Fifty percent of cases occur in children under 4, with peak incidence at 2 years of age. *Shigella sonnei* and *Shigella flexneri* account for most reported cases. Intraepithelial cell replication by *Shigella* causes destruction of mucosa. In addition, both an enterotoxin and a neurotoxin are elaborated, but their exact roles are not known.

CLINICAL PRESENTATIONS

Classically, this organism requires an incubation period of 1 to 3 days before the onset of large, watery stools. This is followed in 24 hours by bloody diarrhea and constitutional complaints. Children may have seizures, but the role of a neurotoxin is unclear. Bacteremia caused by *Shigella* species may be more common than realized, because the optimal time for recovery of these organisms from the blood is the first 24 hours of illness. The incidence of shigellemia apparently does not correlate with the severity of symptoms in mild to moderately ill patients. Potential systemic complications of bacteremia include meningitis, pyelonephritis, osteomyelitis, and otitis media.

Death has been reported. Risk factors for poor outcome include age less than 1 year, lack of breast feeding in patients 1 to 2 years of age, hypothermia, severe malnutrition, severe dehydration, altered consciousness, abdominal distension, thrombocytopenia, hypoproteinemia, hyponatremia, hypoglycemia, renal failure, and bacteremia. Additionally, intestinal perforation, toxic megacolon, seizures, encephalopathy, hemolytic-uremic syndrome, and pneumonia are complications that can lead to death during shigellosis.

TREATMENT

- Fecal leukocytes are present in up to 90% of *Shigella* cases. Stool cultures are important in determining sensitivities. Nucleic acid hybridization techniques using both radiolabeled DNA and nonradioactive DNA probes have been developed recently to detect various pathogens, including *Shigella.*
- Trimethoprim-sulfamethoxazole is generally effective. Confirmed cases in symptomatic patients are treated with antibiotics.
- Multiple-drug resistance has caused decreased susceptibility to tetracycline and ampicillin in developing countries. Nalidixic acid, and the newer quinolones show evidence of effectiveness. There is a need for more data on the safety of quinolones before they can be routinely administered to children.

Question—Shigella

1. The risk factors for poor outcome in patients with *shigella* infection include
   A. Hypothermia
   B. Thrombocytopenia
   C. Hyponatremia
   D. Hypoproteinemia
   E. All of the above

Staphylococcus Aureus

S. aureus probably is the most common cause of bacterial foodborne illness. All previously cooked, proteinaceous food (e.g., ham, shrimp, potato salad, egg salad, and natural cream-containing baked goods) may be reservoirs. Imitation cheeses and synthetic cream filling can support the growth of *Staphylococcus* organisms at room temperatures.

Preformed heat-stable enterotoxins (A-F) produce the gastroenteritis. Staphylococcal toxins form at temperatures between

68 and 112°F; the optimum temperature is 95 to 99°F. The toxin is detectable 4 to 8 hours after the incubation begins. Enterotoxin A is the most common type. There is a strong correlation between *S. aureus* strains producing enterotoxin F and toxic shock syndrome.

CLINICAL PRESENTATIONS

The illness has a short incubation period (average, 4 hours), with a range of 1 to 6 hours and a mean duration of 20 hours. Vomiting, nausea, diarrhea, and abdominal pain are present in descending order of frequency. Vomiting frequently is severe, whereas diarrhea is mild. A subjective feeling of fever occasionally occurs, but fever usually is absent. Rarely, the symptoms of gastroenteritis may progress rapidly to pallor, cyanosis, and hypotension as a result of toxic shock.

Staphylococcal food illness generally is a clinical diagnosis that usually is seen in an office setting. The number of staphylococcal organisms in food does not always accurately establish the source, because environmental conditions modulate colony numbers after ingestion. About 1 mg toxin/100 grams of food will induce clinical symptoms. A radioimmunoassay and enzyme-linked immunosorbent assay can detect as little as 0.1 to 1.0 ng toxin/gram of food, but may not be able to distinguish between biologically active and inactive toxin.

TREATMENT

- The illness is a mild, self-limited disease that requires supportive treatment only.

Questions—Staphylococcus Aureus

1. **Which is the most frequent symptom associated with *Staphylococcus aureus* infection?**
   A. Diarrhea
   B. Hematochezia
   C. Vomiting
   D. Abdominal pain
   E. All are equally frequent.
2. ***Staphylococcus aureus* gastrointestinal infection usually causes a mild, self-limited disease that requires supportive treatment only.**
   A. True
   B. False

Vibrio Cholerae

V. cholerae causes a prototypical toxin-mediated secretory diarrhea. The heat-labile enterotoxin, choleragen, attaches to intestinal epithelial cells, causing activation of adenyl cyclase and increases intracellular conversion of ATP to cyclic AMP. Additionally, both vasoactive intestinal polypeptide and prostaglandins directly enhance adenyl cyclase activity. The net effect is the stimulation of active chloride secretion throughout the intestinal tract and the inhibition of sodium chloride absorption in the small bowel and proximal colon.

Numerous epidemics have occurred in India (i.e., Madras and Calcutta) and Bangladesh in the 1990s (*V. cholerae* type 0139). Hundreds of deaths have been reported. An epidemic of cholera that began in Peru in January 1991 led to over 533,000 cases of cholera and 7,400 deaths in 19 countries in South America. Cholera cases have been reported in 14 states in the United States. Sporadic cases of *V. cholerae* have been reported in Texas and Louisiana since 1973. Raw oysters and crabs are the most common sources of foodborne epidemics. Infections are most common during the summer and early fall. Diagnosis is based on stool cultures.

CLINICAL PRESENTATIONS

Adults may lose up to 1 liter of isotonic fluids per hour in an explosive watery diarrhea that is noninflammatory. Severe cholera produces an elevated anion gap metabolic acidosis because of hyperproteinemia, lactic acidemia, and hyperphosphatemia; the serum chloride changes little.

TREATMENT

- The diagnosis of cholera should be considered in patients with watery diarrhea who have recently (i.e., within 7 days) returned from cholera-affected countries.
- Antibiotic treatment decreases the duration of illness, the requirements for fluid replacement, and the period of *Vibrio* excretion. Replacement of fluid and electrolyte losses is important initially, together with the use of tetracycline, 250 mg four times daily, for 5 days pending sensitivity results. The 0139 serotype is sensitive to tetracycline but resistant to cotrimoxazole.
- Adults with severe gastroenteritis, dehydration, and shock should receive Ringer's lactate solution or saline, with added potassium chloride. The IV solution is administered at a rate of 110 mL/kg body weight over 4 hours, with 2 L being given during the first 30 minutes.
- One study suggested that nicotinic acid, 2 g/day orally, reduces secretory diarrhea in severe cholera.

Prevention

- Field trials of oral cholera vaccines appear promising. Parenteral vaccinations yield limited, short-term protection.
- The rapid spread of the *V. cholerae* 0139 epidemic in southern Asia, even among adults previously exposed to *V. cholerae* 01, suggests that preexisting immunity to *V. cholerae* 01, whether the result of natural infection or cholera vaccine, offers little or no protection.
- Crabs must be boiled 10 to 14 minutes or steamed 30 minutes to kill *Vibrio* organisms. Avoid contaminated water, ice, fruit, vegetables, and raw or undercooked seafood in endemic areas.
- Persons traveling in cholera-affected areas should not eat food that has not been cooked and should only drink beverages that are carbonated or made from boiled or chlorinated water.

Questions—Vibrio Cholerae

1. **The most common sources of foodborne epidemics of *Vibrio cholera* are**
   A. Turtles and frogs
   B. Snakes
   C. Uncooked chicken
   D. Raw oysters and crabs
   E. Exotic fish
2. **No cholera epidemics have occurred since the 1950s.**
   A. True
   B. False

Vibrio Parahaemolyticus and Vibrio Vulnificus

Shellfish-associated outbreaks of gastroenteritis may be associated with *Vibrio* species, *Salmonella typhi*, *Campylobacter* species, hepatitis A, and Norwalklike viruses. *V. parahaemolyticus* and *V. vulnificus* contaminate seafood and shellfish and cause disease among coastal communities. *V. parahaemolyticus* probably is both invasive and toxin producing, although a toxic mechanism is not entirely clear. Most *V. parahaemolyticus* infections occur during the summer months. In Japan, *V. parahaemolyticus* causes between 20% and 30% of all cases of food poisoning, perhaps because of the large consumption of raw fish.

V. vulnificus is a marine organism that can cause wound infections in healthy persons or septicemia in immunosuppressed patients. Raw oysters are a frequent source of *V. vulnificus* infections. Risk factors for septicemia include underlying liver disease, hematopoietic disorders, chronic renal insufficiency, immunosuppressive agents, and alcoholism. Patients who develop sepsis secondary to *V. vulnificus* frequently do not demonstrate gastrointestinal symptoms.

CLINICAL PRESENTATIONS

The incubation period for *V. parahaemolyticus* ranges from 4 to 96 hours, and the duration is approximately 3 days (range, 1 to 10 days). *V. parahaemolyticus* produces predominantly a large-volume watery diarrheal illness. Abdominal pain and vomiting are less common. Diagnosis is confirmed by stool culture.

Healthy persons are unlikely to develop septicemia after ingesting food contaminated with *V. vulnificus*. Any person with a risk factor for septicemia should never eat raw seafood, especially raw oysters. One review of *V. vulnificus* sepsis revealed: fever (94%), chills (91%), skin lesions (64%), nausea (58%), vomiting (16%), diarrhea (40%), and hypotension (37%).

TREATMENT

- *V. parahaemolyticus* infections require only supportive treatment and no antibiotics.
- There are limited *in vivo* data on the treatment of *V. vulnificus septicemia,* but tetracycline appears efficacious. Shellfish-borne *Vibrio* infections can be prevented by cooking seafood thoroughly, keeping from cross-contamination after cooking, and eating it promptly. Cooked seafood is best stored at 60°C (140°F) or greater, or 4°C (39.2°F) or below.
- Patients with liver disease and those who are in any way immunocompromised (including AIDS) should be warned of the dangers of eating raw seafood.

Question—Vibrio Parahaemolyticus and Vibrio Vulnificus

1. *Vibrio parahaemolyticus* and *vulnificus* infections
A. Usually are from farm animals
B. Do not cause wound infections
C. Usually occur in summer months
D. A and B
E. B and C

Yersinia Enterocolitica

Y. enterocolitica is an invasive gram-negative coccobacillary organism that may produce mesenteric lymphadenitis, septicemia, and peritonitis. This disease is rare in the United States. Both wild and domestic animals harbor this organism. It contaminates the food chain because of its frequency in farm animals. Outbreaks have followed the ingestion of tofu and both unpasteurized and pasteurized milk. The organism can replicate at refrigerator temperatures.

Y. enterocolitica, using deferoxamine produced by *Streptomyces pilosis,* as a siderophore, can transfer iron across its membranes for its metabolic needs. Iron loading increases the virulence of *Y. enterocolitica.* Iron overload and deferoxamine therapy are independent predisposing factors for systemic infections with *Y. enterocolitica.*

CLINICAL PRESENTATIONS

Patients under 5 years of age generally develop a self-limited gastroenteritis with variable amounts of diarrhea and fever. A dysenterylike picture may be characterized by fever (93%), abdominal pain (86%), diarrhea (83%), vomiting (41%), sore throat (22%), rash (22%), bloody stools (20%), and joint pain (15%). Older children often develop mesenteric adenitis and ileitis, which mimics appendicitis.

Adults may develop bacteremia, hepatic abscess, Reiter's syndrome, glomerulonephritis, polyarthritis, arthralgias, or erythema nodosum. Intestinal perforation, peritonitis, and gangrene of the small bowel have been reported after *Y. enterocolitica* infections. Diagnosis by stool culture requires a special culture technique of cold enrichment. Serologic examination of paired sera also helps establish the diagnosis.

TREATMENT

- This disease usually is self-limited. Tetracycline is reserved for severe, protracted cases. Trimethoprim-sulfamethoxazole also is effective.
- Raw chitterlings, an ethnic food often prepared for holiday meals, is an important vehicle for transmitting *Y. enterocolitica* infections.

Question—Yersinia Enterocolitica

1. *Yersinia* infection may produce
A. Mesenteric lymphadenitis
B. Septicemia
C. Peritonitis
D. A and B
E. All of the above

VIRAL GASTROENTERITIS

Viruses invade microvilli of intestinal epithelial cells and cause a transient "tropical spruelike" malabsorption syndrome. Clinically important viruses include rotavirus, parvovirus, and enteric adenovirus. No apparent increase in intestinal secretions follows viral infections. Usually, viral gastroenteritis is a diagnosis of exclusion based on the clinical presentation and a history of an epidemic. Identification of virus in the stool by electron microscopy or detection of viral antigens in the stool confirms the diagnosis, but these tests usually are unnecessary for clinical purposes.

Rotavirus is the major cause of nonbacterial gastroenteritis and causes epidemic outbreaks especially in young children (6 to 24 months). Transmission occurs by the oral-fecal route, with viral shedding common among asymptomatic infants. The incidence of rotavirus infections peaks during the winter months and occurs uncommonly in the summer. Astroviruses are a common cause of viral gastroenteritis in children, producing clinical findings similar to those caused by rotavirus infection. They appear to be associated with illness more frequently than the enteric adenoviruses and are associated with almost half as many illnesses as rotavirus infection.

Parvovirus (e.g., Norwalk agent and Hawaiian agent) is a highly contagious agent that causes illness in older children and adults. This virus produces a noninflammatory diarrhea in epidemics. No animal reservoirs are known, but waterborne sources of the disease occur frequently and raw oysters have been implicated in an outbreak of gastroenteritis. Several enteric adenovirus serotypes can cause a mild gastrointestinal disease in young children. Enteroviruses probably are not an important source of gastroenteritis.

Clinical Presentations

Rotavirus and adenovirus produce intestinal disease, often in an epidemic setting, with a 24- to 72-hour incubation period. Vomiting begins abruptly and then resolves. Four to 7 days of watery, foul-smelling diarrhea generally follow. A simple rapid immunoassay test is available to detect rotavirus as a cause of diarrheal epidemics. Fecal leukocytes and erythrocytes are seen rarely.

Parvovirus gastroenteritis in adults is characterized by a 24- to 36-hour incubation period followed by the abrupt onset of diarrhea, nausea, malaise, and mild abdominal cramps. Nonspecific symptoms (e.g., myalgias) often accompany the illness. No blood appears in stools.

Treatment

- Every child should be evaluated for signs of dehydration. Small children should be placed on a clear, caffeine-free, hypotonic fluid diet devoid of milk (e.g., cola, ginger ale, apple juice) and supplemented with balanced electrolyte solutions (e.g., Pedialyte®) as needed.
- Older children and adults may benefit from the BRATT diet (**B**ananas, **R**ice, **A**pples, **T**ea, and **T**oast). The severity of symptoms and dehydration determine the need for hospitalization.

Question—Viral Gastroenteritis

1. The major cause of nonbacterial gastroenteritis is
A. Parvovirus
B. Astrovirus
C. Rotavirus
D. Norwalk Virus
E. All of the above are equally common.

PROTOZOA AND OTHER GASTROINTESTINAL PARASITES

Amebiasis

The trophozoite of amebiasis invades the colon, producing punctate, yellowish-white ulcers, and colitis. Oral-fecal transmission occurs with the cyst spreading disease most commonly through contaminated water. Male homosexuals and travelers are at highest risk of acquiring the disease. Most infections are subclinical.

CLINICAL PRESENTATIONS

Disease caused by these organisms typically occurs in three forms. An explosive, acute invasive diarrhea associated with fever, bloody diarrhea, abdominal cramps, and tenesmus may follow exposure. A chronic, low-grade diarrhea characterized by bloating, foul-smelling, blood-streaked diarrhea, malaise, and weight loss may be seen. And third, hepatic abscess, characterized by a mild prodrome followed by right upper quadrant tenderness, fever, and malaise may occur. The abscess may rupture into the pleural space.

Amebiasis should be suspected in any patient with invasive diarrhea and relevant risk factors (i.e., travel, and homosexuality). Techniques for identification of trophozoites and cysts include fresh stool examination, rectal biopsy, and sigmoidoscopy. Sigmoidoscopy provides direct visualization of punctate lesions. Serologic tests also are available.

TREATMENT

- Metronidazole is the drug of choice (750 mg every 8 hours for 5 to 10 days). Administration of this antibiotic results in an 85% to 90% cure rate. The combination of iodoquinol (650 mg every 8 hours for 21 days) and metronidazole is recommended by some authors.
- Dehydroemetine dihydrochloride is reserved for severe cases because of its cumulative skeletal and cardiac muscle toxicity.
- Observe enteric isolation precautions and look for evidence of hepatic abscess if clinically indicated.

Questions—Amebiasis

1. Those at highest risk of acquiring amebiasis are
A. Travelers
B. Homosexuals
C. Children
D. A and B
E. B and C

2. Treatment of amebiasis usually is
A. Supportive care only
B. Metronidazole
C. Dehydroemetine dihydrochloride
D. Computed tomography scan to identify hepatic abscesses
E. None of the above

Cryptosporidiosis

The protozoan *Cryptosporidiosis parvum* has emerged in the past decade as a cause of severe diarrhea in immunodeficient patients and as a cause of failure to thrive, malnutrition, persistent diarrhea, and impaired delayed skin hypersensitivity in immunocompetent patients, particularly children in developing countries.

Cryptosporidiosis is a zoonosis or infectious disease characterized by animal-to-human transmission. Infectious Cryptosporidium oocytes may be found in the stools of immunologically compromised persons as well as in sporadic healthy individuals, travelers to Russia, animal handlers, and homosexual men. *Cryptosporidiosis* occurs mostly in infants who are not breast fed, suggesting a protective role for humoral immunity. Cryptosporidium infections appear frequently in animals, especially in pigs, calves, lambs, and goats.

Oocytes attach to the microvillous border of epithelial cells in the small intestine. With invasion, a mild villous atrophy may develop, but intracellular invasion does not occur. The oocytes can survive for extended periods. Transmission occurs via the oral-fecal route by direct contact, and indirectly via food, water, or fomites. The incubation period is 5 to 10 days.

CLINICAL PRESENTATIONS

Watery diarrhea, weight loss, and anorexia characterize this illness. Fever, chills, and vomiting appear uncommonly. Acute pancreatitis has been associated with infections by the Cryptosporidium parasite. The duration of illness is typically 10 to

14 days, but infection in immunocompromised patients causes a prolonged, debilitating, chronic diarrhea. *Cryptosporidiosis* should be considered in the differential diagnosis of traveler's diarrhea.

Studies with human immunodeficiency virus (HIV)-positive patients suggest that pulmonary cryptosporidiosis should be considered in all immunoincompetent patients with lung symptoms. Toxic megacolon resulting from cryptosporidiosis may be found in AIDS patients and can be fatal in AIDS patients as well.

TREATMENT

- This self-limited, enteric illness usually resolves without therapeutic intervention.
- Feces from infected persons should be considered infectious and enteric precautions taken.
- Identification of oocytes in stools requires a three-step stool examination with iodine stain, acid-fast stain, and Sheather's sugar flotation for Cryptosporidium oocytes. Positive anticryptosporidial antibodies appear within 2 weeks of onset of diarrheal disease.
- Contrast radiographic studies and other routine laboratory tests such as complete blood count and liver function tests are not helpful in establishing the diagnosis.
- There is no specific therapy for cryptosporidiosis. Symptomatic patients are treated with IV fluids, electrolyte management, and nonspecific antidiarrheal agents.

Questions—Cryptosporidiosis

1. All of the following are true of *cryptosporidiosis* except
   A. Infections are in humans not in animals.
   B. Infections are more often in bottle-fed than breastfed infants.
   C. Its oocytes may be found in stools of travelers to Russia.
   D. Transmission is oral-fecal.
   E. Incubation is 5 to 10 days.

2. Treatment of *Cryptosporidiosis* consists of
   A. Supportive care only
   B. Metronidazole
   C. Albendazole
   D. Quinacrine hydrochloride
   E. None of the above

Giardia Lamblia

G. lamblia are protozoal parasites that favor the duodenum and small intestine. Ingested cysts reproduce in the small bowel. Newly formed trophozoites superficially invade the mucosa and cause a malabsorption syndrome. Fecal-oral transmission between humans occurs. Waterborne sources provide a reservoir, but the extent of animal-to-human transmission is unclear.

Patients at risk are travelers (e.g., St. Petersburg, Russia), the elderly with gastric surgery and with hypoalbuminemia, backpackers (especially in the Rocky Mountains and Sierra Nevada region), and homosexuals; however, the large reservoir in the human population makes disease more common in persons without the above risks.

CLINICAL PRESENTATIONS

The clinical picture resembles a subacute abdominal malabsorption syndrome with bloating, crampy abdominal pain, excessive flatus, abdominal distension, and light, foul-smelling stools. Vomiting is unusual. The incubation period is 1 to 2 weeks, and the diagnosis should be suspected when diarrhea persists over 2 weeks. Trophozoites in loose stool or cysts in formed stool are seen in most cases. In highly suspicious cases with negative stools, duodenal aspiration or biopsy may be required to confirm the diagnosis.

TREATMENT

- Quinacrine hydrochloride (100 mg every 8 hours for 7 days) is the drug of choice and has a 95% cure rate; however, others recommend metronidazole (250 mg every 8 hours for 7 days).

Question—Giardia Lamblia

1. Symptoms of *Giardia* typically include all of the following except
   A. Bloating
   B. Abdominal pain
   C. Vomiting
   D. Excessive flatus
   E. Foul-smelling stool

Microsporidiosis

Microsporidia are being increasingly recognized as important opportunistic pathogens in HIV infection. Microsporidiosis also has been described in immunocompetent hosts. Diseases caused by the different microsporidia include diarrhea, keratoconjunctivitis, hepatitis, myositis, kidney and urogenital infection, ascites, cholangitis, and asymptomatic carriage.

Knowledge of the epidemiology of microsporidiosis in humans is limited, but as with cryptosporidiosis, microsporidiosis is probably a common, self-limited or asymptomatic infection in immunocompetent hosts. Most likely, these are waterborne pathogens, and the environmental reservoirs need to be identified. Six *microsporidian genera* have been associated with human disease.

CLINICAL PRESENTATIONS

The major syndrome associated with microsporidiosis is diarrhea and wasting. This condition usually is caused by *Enterocytozoon bieneusi* (more than 90% of cases in the United States) and occasionally by *Septata intestinalis* (although in Europe this organism may be a more frequent cause of diarrhea than is *E. bieneusi*). Several studies have been done on the association between microsporidiosis and diarrhea. In HIV-infected patients evaluated for diarrhea, the prevalence of microsporidiosis has ranged from 10% to 40%.

The small intestine has provided the highest diagnostic yield, but organisms have been seen in colon biopsy specimens. The inability to detect toxin in most stool specimens obtained more than 3 days after toxin ingestion indicates that toxin is absorbed, degraded, or excreted by this time.

TREATMENT

- Therapy with albendazole (400 mg twice daily) eliminates *Encephalitozoon* (*Septata*) *intestinalis* infection and its symptoms.
- Diarrhea is markedly reduced in patients with *E. bieneusi* infection who receive albendazole treatment. In such treated patients, however, the organism can still be seen in biopsy specimens, and relapse is common when treatment is stopped.

Questions—Microsporidiosis

1. **Microsporidiosis causes**
   A. Diarrhea
   B. Keratoconjunctivitis
   C. Hepatitis
   D. Cholangitis
   E. All of the above
2. **Treatment of microsporidiosis includes**
   A. Trimethoprim
   B. Quinacrine hydrochloride
   C. Albendazole
   D. Metronidazole
   E. None of the above

BOTULISM

According to lethality studies in animals, botulinum toxin, by weight, is the most potent natural poison in the world. Three types, (foodborne, wound, and infant) plus one unclassified variety, result from infection with *Clostridium botulinum* organisms. In foodborne (classic) botulism, a preformed heat-labile toxin binds irreversibly to the neuromuscular junction and impairs presynaptic release of acetylcholine. Nerve conduction is blocked and this results in profound weakness. There are seven immunologically distinct toxins (A-G). Three types commonly cause human toxicity (A-primarily Western states, B-primarily Eastern states, E-Northern Lakes, Alaska).

Botulinum toxin type A has been of therapeutic value in the treatment of a variety of neurologic and ophthalmologic disorders. The Food and Drug Administration (FDA) recently approved botulinum toxin (Oculinum®) as a therapeutic agent in patients with strabismus, blepharospasm, and other facial nerve disorders, including hemifacial spasm. The toxin exerts its paralytic action by rapidly and strongly binding to presynaptic cholinergic terminals. It becomes internalized and inhibits the exocytosis of acetylcholine and decreases the frequency of acetylcholine release.

FOODBORNE BOTULISM

Home-canned foods are the most common source of foodborne botulism. Sources include canned olives, asparagus, tomatoes, beets, mushrooms, fish, peppers, and onions. Toxin formation is unlikely below a pH of 4.5 or in the presence of nitrites. Clostridium spores are ubiquitous in soil and are relatively heat resistant. Spores can survive several hours of boiling and can form toxin in food that was initially cooked and then held at ambient temperature for 16 hours without recooking.

Clinical Presentations

Clinical symptoms appear 24 to 36 hours after ingestion of the toxin (range, 6 hours to 8 days). Systemic complaints and gastrointestinal symptoms appear first and include weakness, malaise, lightheadedness, sore throat, and nausea. Dry mouth is almost universally present. In one type A botulism outbreak, three of the following four symptoms were present in all patients admitted to an emergency department: generalized weakness, diplopia, dry mouth, and difficulty in speaking. Gastrointestinal symptoms are absent in one-third of foodborne botulism cases. When gastrointestinal symptoms appear, constipation is the most frequent complaint.

Neurologic symptoms usually appear within 3 days of generalized symptoms but may be delayed for up to 1 week. Cranial nerves (III, VI, IX, X, XI) are affected first, with diplopia, ptosis, blurred vision, and lateral rectus palsy developing most commonly. Fixed pupils are a late sign. Both dysarthria and dysphagia often are present. A bilateral descending symmetrical weakness follows the onset of bulbar symptoms. Laboratory analysis of blood, gastric contents, and food can confirm the presence of neurotoxin.

Treatment

- Basic treatment involves supportive care and prevention of disease progression. Lavage, emesis, and charcoal may be used if ingestion is recent (e.g., within 24 hours).
- Supportive care includes careful observation for respiratory failure. Decreased vital capacity is the most sensitive indicator of respiratory compromise. Patients with vital capacity less than 30% predicted should be electively intubated. Respiratory failure usually occurs soon after oculomotor nerve weakness (cranial nerve III palsy).
- Aminoglycosides and polymyxins are contraindicated because they enhance neuromuscular blockade. Tensilon® (edrophonium bromide) does not reverse botulism (classic or infant). It is useful in myasthenia gravis, a disease that exhibits postjunctional receptor insufficiency. A Tensilon® challenge test should be done to exclude myasthenia gravis.
- Every patient with suspected botulism should have serum, stool, and, when possible, gastric aspirate specimens submitted for toxin assay and anaerobic culture. However, botulism may be incorrectly excluded if the diagnostic process depends too heavily on laboratory testing.
- Save suspected food items, stool samples, and the patient's serum in a refrigerated environment for later analysis.
- A pressure cooker must be used to home-can vegetables safely because it can reach temperatures necessary to kill botulism spores (212°F or 100°C for 10 minutes). Jams and jellies can be safely home-canned without a pressure cooker because their high sugar content will not support the growth of *C. botulinum*. Boiling food for 10 minutes before eating generally destroys any toxin present.

Antidotes

ANTITOXIN

Equine antitoxin neutralizes blood-based toxin and prevents progression of the disease but does not reverse existing neurologic deficits. Use of this product requires testing for horse serum sensitivity, because allergic reactions occur in up to 20% of patients. The trivalent antitoxin form (ABE) is most frequently administered and is most effective against type E.

BOTULISM IMMUNE GLOBULIN

Human-derived botulism immune globulin (BIG) is being studied. It is hoped that treatment with BIG will substantially shorten both the duration of illness and the cost of hospital stay for affected infants.

GUANIDINE

Guanidine has been used as adjunctive therapy for cranial nerve palsies in mild cases where it may enhance acetylcholine release, but its effectiveness has not yet been substantiated. The administration of guanidine does not reverse respiratory paralysis. Side effects may include nausea, epigastric distress, diarrhea, tremors, twitching, hypoglycemia, rash, and paresthesias. The FDA has not approved guanidine for general use.

Questions—Foodborne Botulism

1. **Symptoms of foodborne botulism**
   A. Usually include dry mouth
   B. Usually appear one week after ingestion
   C. Often include dysarthria and dysphagia
   D. A and B
   E. A and C
2. **All of the following are true of treatment for botulism except**
   A. Lavage may be useful if ingestion is recent.
   B. Emesis may be useful if ingestion is recent.
   C. Charcoal may be useful if ingestion is recent.
   D. Tensilon® may be useful to reverse botulism.
   E. Equine antitoxin may be useful to reverse existing neurologic deficits.

WOUND BOTULISM

Wound botulism results from production and absorption of toxin in a contaminated wound. It is a rare, life-threatening complication of trauma and IV drug abuse. Only 27 cases of wound botulism were reported in the medical literature between 1943 and 1982. Neurologic symptoms develop 4 to 14 days after infection, and gastrointestinal symptoms usually are absent. Patients present with cranial nerve weakness and descending paralysis without sensory involvement. Symptoms can lead to respiratory failure and last for months. The syndrome is usually associated with type A botulinum toxin formation.

Clinical Presentations

An influenzalike syndrome with myalgias, pharyngitis, fever, and chills occurs after a 1- to 3-day incubation period. The most commonly reported symptoms include shortness of breath, dysphagia, dysphonia or dysarthria, diplopia, poor accommodation, and dry or sore throat. The most common signs on physical examination include descending paralysis, respiratory insufficiency, and diplopia. Temperature elevation above 38°C is an inconsistent finding.

Botulism should be suspected in patients with acute onset of flaccid paralysis with ophthalmoplegia, ptosis, or other cranial nerve dysfunction, particularly when the paralysis is descending, symmetric, and associated with a normal cerebrospinal fluid protein level. A history of drug injection or a food history that does not identify a probable source for foodborne botulism should prompt consideration of wound botulism and elicitation of a thorough history and physical examination for evidence of cellulitis or abscess.

A meticulous physical examination is necessary because wounds containing *C. botulinum* may be small and initially unnoticed. The differential diagnosis includes foodborne botulism, infant botulism, the Eaton-Lambert syndrome, hypermagnesemia, and aminoglycoside toxicity, especially when associated with compatible electromyographic data.

Treatment

- A detailed history and physical examination are the main keys to diagnosing wound botulism and initiating treatment. The diagnosis is supported by electromyography.
- Wound cultures and serum assays for botulinum toxin are confirmatory. Other laboratory findings are nonspecific. Initial treatment decisions should not necessarily await neurologic test results.
- Antibiotics have not been shown to be effective in treating or preventing wound botulism.
- Surgical debridement of the wound and intensive respiratory care are the most important aspects of therapy. The appearance of the wound may not be clinically helpful.
- The efficacy of the use of botulism antitoxin in the treatment of wound infection has not been firmly established.
- A diagnosis of myasthenia gravis, and not botulism, is supported by improvement in muscle function after the administration of edrophonium (Tensilon®).

Questions—Wound Botulism

1. **Symptoms of wound botulism**
   A. Usually begin with cranial nerve weakness and descending paralysis
   B. Usually develop 4 to 14 hours after infection
   C. Last no more than 2 weeks
   D. A and B
   E. A and C
2. **Treatment of wound botulism should include**
   A. Wound cultures and serum assays
   B. Antibiotics
   C. Surgical debridement
   D. A and B
   E. A and C

INFANT BOTULISM

Traditional teaching dictates that foodborne botulism results from the ingestion of preformed toxin. In a few cases, production of the toxin apparently continues *in vivo*, as in the syndrome of infant botulism. Predisposing factors in these cases include antibiotic therapy, intestinal surgery, and gastric achlorhydria. Infant botulism is the most common type of botulism recognized in the United States.

Spores colonize the intestine and produce the toxin *in vivo*. Usually, botulinum toxin type A or B, and rarely type F, is involved. In contrast to classic botulism, which is intoxication from preformed toxin, infant botulism is an infection that produces the toxin subsequently. About 20% of cases are traceable to infants who have been fed honey, whereas the other 80% of sources are unknown. *C. botulinum* is not found in breast milk.

Clinical Presentations

At least three clinical presentations of infant botulism have been described. These include a moderate to severe paralysis requiring immediate hospitalization, a generalized weakness characterized as failure to thrive, and fulminant paralysis with sudden death, resembling the sudden infant death syndrome (SIDS). The classic presentation is a 2- to 4-month-old child with constipation, poor sucking, lethargy, and a weak cry ("floppy child"). Ptosis, ophthalmoplegia, and mydriasis are present. Neurologic examination reveals symmetric weakness without sensory abnormalities.

Treatment

- Treatment is similar to that for foodborne disease, except that mortality usually is low.

- Botulism antitoxin is not recommended in infants because of its substantial side effects and lack of effect on the toxin-producing organisms in the gut. Watch closely for progression of symptoms, especially respiratory depression. Antibiotics have not proven to be effective.
- Botulinum toxin may appear in the feces in infant botulism, in contrast to classic botulism, where the toxin usually, but not always, is found exclusively in the blood.
- Electromyograms indicate a defect in acetylcholine release at the neuromuscular junction.
- Laboratory tests such as electrolytes, complete blood count, calcium, magnesium, cerebrospinal fluid, chest x-ray, and electrocardiogram (ECG) are normal.
- A positive edrophonium test in a weak infant neither excludes infant botulism nor diagnoses congenital myasthenia gravis.

Questions—Infant Botulism

1. Predisposing factors to infant botulism include
A. Antibiotic therapy
B. Intestinal surgery
C. Gastric achlorhydria
D. All of the above
E. None of the above

2. Most cases of infant botulism are traced to ingestion of honey.
A. True
B. False

3. The classic presentation of infant botulism includes a child who
A. Is 12 to 14 months old
B. Has profuse diarrhea
C. Has new-onset hyperactivity
D. Screams meaninglessly
E. None of the above

MARINE FOODBORNE ILLNESS

Marine foodborne illness may be caused by microbes (see *Vibrio Parahaemolyticus* and *Vibrio Vulnificus* section, above) or toxins. Marine biotoxins are classified as orally acquired parenteral toxins (injected by teeth or spines), or crinotoxins (secreted directly into the water). Subclassification of fish containing oral toxins includes ichthyosarcotoxic fish, which contain a poison within their flesh (e.g., scombroid and ciguatera fish poisoning), ichthyohemotoxic fish, which have poisonous blood, and ichthyotoxic fish, which contain poison in their gonads.

Bacteria survive well in seafood and can double in number every 15 minutes between temperatures of 40 to 120°F. Fish that have been caught should be packed in ice before being transported home. Groceries should not be left on the car seat on a hot day and at home, the fish should be refrigerated immediately. Fresh fish or shellfish should not be held more than 1 to 2 days before being cooked. Cooking or placing shellfish in clean, running water greatly reduces, but does not eliminate, the chance of poisoning.

BLUE-GREEN ALGAE

Toxic freshwater blue-green algal species grow in small bodies of stagnant water and slow-moving streams. These primitive algal species possess no nuclear membrane and contain endotoxins that are released during decomposition. Grazing animals are affected more often than humans are, because the disagreeable color and odor discourage human consumption. Exposures have occurred as a result of consumption of contaminated water while swimming in contaminated lakes. No human deaths have been definitely linked to blue-green algal toxins. Workers at risk include teachers of water sports, cleaners and maintainers of canals and rivers, water quality testers, and fish farmers.

Most algal poisoning in Canada is associated with *Anabaena flos-aquae,* which contains a potent neurotoxin that causes rapid postsynaptic neuromuscular blockade and respiratory depression. Blooms of *A. flos-aquae* are responsible for toxic symptoms in the northeastern United States and contain saxitoxin, the neurotoxin responsible for paralytic shellfish poisoning. Microcystin or "fast death factor" is a lethal, low-molecular-weight polypeptide released by *Microcystis aeruginosa* upon decomposition. This algal species also contains a dialyzable, heat-stable, hepatotoxic pentapeptide.

Clinical Presentations

Local irritant effects (e.g., swelling, conjunctivitis and earache) as well as allergic reactions (e.g., rhinitis and pruritic maculopapular rash) can develop after both blue-green and marine algal exposures. Gastroenteritis beginning within 3 to 5 hours of ingestion, manifested by diarrhea, abdominal cramps, nausea, and vomiting may appear, similar to amebic dysentery, but it resolves within 1 to 2 days. Consumption of water contaminated by *M. aeruginosa* has produced significant liver transaminase elevations.

Treatment

- Workers at risk should be monitored for eye, skin, pulmonary, and gastrointentinal (GI) (especially liver) problems.
- Chronic copper poisoning may result from treatment of the local water supply with copper sulfate, an algicide. Symptoms related to this may be wrongly ascribed to blue-green algae.

Question—Blue-Green Algae

1. Symptoms of blue-green algae exposure include
A. Conjunctivitis
B. Gastroenteritis
C. Pruritic maculopapular rash
D. All of the above
E. None of the above

CIGUATERA

Ciguatera poisoning results from the ingestion of fish that are endemic to tropical reefs and contain a toxin known as ciguatoxin. Small reef fish ingest the dinoflagellate *Gambierdiscus toxicus,* which probably produces the toxic agent. Large reef fish that prey on smaller fish are the most likely source of ciguatera-type fish poisoning. The fish most commonly involved in ciguatoxin poisoning are bottom dwellers such as barracuda, grouper, red snapper, and amberjack. This type of marine poisoning accounts for more than half of all foodborne outbreaks related to fish in the United States.

Ciguatoxin possesses cholinergic and anticholinesterase activity, but these mechanisms do not account for its toxicity. In animal models, ciguatoxin partially inhibits the action potential, perhaps by blockade of calcium sites that regulate passive sodium permeability. The sodium-potassium ATPase pump is not affected by ciguatoxin. Maitotoxin, scaritoxin, and several other polyethers may contribute to ciguatera intoxication. The toxin is heat stable, acid stable, lipid soluble, tasteless, and odorless, so that one cannot identify tainted fish before consumption.

Clinical Presentations

Watery diarrhea, vomiting, and abdominal cramps begin 1 to 6 hours (range, minutes to 30 hours) after ingestion of ciguatoxin-containing fish. This is followed by prominent neurologic symptoms such as paresthesias, dysesthesias, and headache. Hypersalivation, blurred vision, odontalgia, dysphagia, tremor, athetosis, and ataxia may occur. Generalized symptoms include weakness, myalgias, pruritus, arthralgias, dizziness, and a desquamative or erythematous rash. Hypotension, bradycardia, and reversible T-wave changes on the ECG develop rarely. Abdominal symptoms usually resolve in 1 to 3 days.

Neurologic symptoms usually are the most bothersome and lingering complaints. Paresthesias, described as uncomfortable tingling sensations, most often develop in the extremities, oral cavity (sensation of loose tooth), and pharynx. The most characteristic hallmark is paradoxical dysesthesias, often labeled as temperature reversal, which most often manifests as cold objects feeling hot, burning, or painful to the touch. Neurologic complaints may persist as long as 6 months.

Paradoxical sensory discomfort probably is due to an exaggerated and intense nerve depolarization occurring in peripheral myelinated and nociceptor fibers. Fatalities rarely occur and result from respiratory depression and seizures. The most serious symptoms appear in patients previously exposed to ciguatoxin and include hypotension and bradycardia. Symptoms of protracted pruritus, weakness, hiccoughs, and paresthesias may persist for months, or may recur during periods of stress.

Treatment

- Treatment is purely supportive. Emetics, charcoal, and cathartics may be administered within several hours of exposure if the patient has not vomited spontaneously.
- Diagnosis is based on the clinical presentation of abrupt gastrointestinal and neurologic symptoms after ingestion of bottom-dwelling reef fish. Bioassays and radioimmunoassay methods have been developed but rarely are used clinically. Presently, there is no available blood test that confirms ciguatera poisoning in man.
- Magnesium-containing cathartics possess the theoretical disadvantage of augmenting the calcium channel blockade. Fluid losses should be replaced, and patients who present with significant volume depletion or those who are severely symptomatic should be admitted.
- Anecdotal case studies suggest that persistent dysesthesias and pruritus may respond to amitriptyline (25 mg twice daily). Tocainide® may improve chronic neurologic symptoms.
- Rare cases of coma and cerebral edema caused by ciguatera fish poisoning responded well to mannitol infusion. Mannitol may shorten morbidity and hospital stays by improving headache, malaise, pruritus, irritability, and other manifestations of acute ciguatoxin poisoning.
- Mannitol is a strong diuretic and may present a potential hazard to a patient dehydrated from vomiting and diarrhea. Assess and correct fluid and electrolyte balance before mannitol is given. If the patient has been symptomatic for 24 hours or more, mannitol may be less effective.
- Dopamine, plasma expanders, and calcium gluconate may be useful for shock.
- Steroids, opiates, and barbiturates are not effective on ciguatera, and alcohol consumption may exacerbate symptoms.

Questions—Ciguatera

1. All of the following fish are commonly involved in ciguatoxin poisoning except

A. Barracuda
B. Salmon
C. Grouper
D. Red snapper
E. Amberjack

2. The symptoms of ciguatera poisoning

A. Are most serious in patients previously exposed to the toxin
B. May last for months or recur in stressful periods
C. Often lead to death
D. A and B
E. A and C

DOMOIC ACID

An outbreak of an acute illness occurred in 1987 in Canada following ingestion of mussels contaminated with domoic acid. The source of domoic acid in the Canadian outbreak appears to have been *Nitzschia pungens,* a pennate phytoplankton diatom present in extensive blooms in the Cardigan River estuary. Domoic acid is a natural, heat-stable, water-soluble neuroexcitatory amino acid produced by microscopic algae (phytoplankton) known as *Nitzschia pseudoserita.* Another outbreak followed ingestion of shellfish on the Pacific Northwest Coast in 1991.

Okadaic acid and domoic acid are the parent structures of marine toxins produced by the phytoplankton that are responsible for diarrhea, shellfish poisoning, and amnesic shellfish poisoning. Domoic acid impersonates the normal neurotransmitter glutamic acid, resulting in neuronal damage. It is considered a natural "excitotoxin," an agent that overstimulates but does not destroy cells.

Clinical Presentations

Immunocompromised individuals are most susceptible. Gastrointestinal symptoms such as vomiting, abdominal cramps, and diarrhea occur within the first 24 hours. This is followed in 48 hours by unusual neurologic abnormalities including headache, short-term memory loss, confusion, disorientation, abnormal eye movements, mutism, grimacing, seizures, myoclonus, and coma. Additional signs included profuse respiratory secretions, fever, hemodynamic instability, hiccups, cardiac arrhythmias, and piloerection. Chronic manifestations included an amnesic syndrome. At least 3 patients have died from domoic acid poisoning.

Treatment

- Diagnosis is based on the abrupt onset of gastrointestinal symptoms and the later development of neurologic symptoms following ingestion of mussels or related marine animals.
- Patients should be hospitalized in an intensive care unit where neurologic dysfunction may be immediately evaluated and treated. Respiratory intubation and mechanical ventilation may be required. Tachycardia and pulmonary edema should be treated appropriately.

- CT scans may be normal. Electroencephalogram may demonstrate generalized, slow wave activity. Neuropathologic studies show neuronal necrosis and loss, most pronounced in the hippocampus, amygdala, and parts of the thalamus.
- Mussels can be tested for the presence of domoic acid by a mouse bioassay and high-performance liquid chromatography. The relative preservation of intellect and higher cortical functions distinguishes the mussel-induced intoxication syndrome from Alzheimer's disease.
- Sacks of mussels are now labeled with respect to time and place of harvesting. Before commercial distribution, mussels are tested for the presence of domoic acid.

Question—Domoic Acid

1. Domoic acid is produced by
A. Microscopic algae (phytoplankton)
B. Mussels
C. Shellfish
D. B and C
E. None of the above

PARALYTIC SHELLFISH POISONING

Specific neurotoxic species of the dinoflagellate genus *Gonyaulax* bloom between May and October. Their red color yields the appearance of a red tide, which become visible when the concentration of dinoflagellates exceeds 20,000/mL. The dinoflagellates appear in nearly all the oceans of the world. Bivalve shellfish (e.g., mussels, clams and scallops) concentrate the neurotoxin during periods of red tides.

Shrimp, abalone, and crab do not feed on this plankton and therefore do not cause this type of food poisoning. Mussels present the greatest hazard. Ingestion of saxitoxin leads to muscle weakness by a curarelike effect resulting from blockage of sodium conductance. The neurotoxin is colorless, odorless, and heat stable. The estimated lethal dose in humans is 0.3 to 1.0 mg. A single contaminated mussel may contain up to 50 lethal doses.

Clinical Presentations

Diarrhea, vomiting, nausea, abdominal pain, and paresthesias of the face develop within 30 minutes and are followed in severe cases by muscle paralysis, weakness, dysphagia, salivation, and ataxia. Symptoms typically occur 30 minutes after eating a mollusk or crab. Paresthesia usually is noted first. Tingling, numbing, or burning sensations begin over the lips and tongue, and spread over the face, scalp, and neck to the fingertips and toes. Sensory exam and proprioception are distorted, and the patient becomes ataxic and incoordinated.

Speech is incoherent and aphasia may develop. The patient feels faint and weak and often complains of headache and "tightness" in the throat and chest. Salivation and perspiration may be profuse. The pulse becomes weak and thready. The deep tendon reflexes are markedly diminished, and the superficial reflexes are absent. Symptoms can grow progressively worse and may culminate in respiratory paralysis and death. The first 12 hours are critical, but if the patient survives this period, the prognosis is favorable.

Treatment

- Diagnosis is based on the clinical presentation. Watch carefully for signs of respiratory depression and admit symptomatic patients for observation for 24 hours.
- Gut decontamination may be helpful if spontaneous vomiting does not occur within several hours of exposure.

Questions—Paralytic Shellfish Poisoning

1. The greatest hazard of paralytic shellfish poisoning is from
A. Shrimp
B. Abalone
C. Mussels
D. Crab
E. All are equally hazardous.

2. Symptoms of paralytic shellfish poisoning typically occur 30 minutes after ingestion.
A. True
B. False

SCOMBROID

If scombroid fish are inadequately preserved, bacteria break down endogenous histidine in the fish tissue to form high levels of histamine and the toxic substance saurine. The toxin is tasteless, odorless, and heat stable. Ingestion of contaminated scombroid fish produces the disease.

Scombroid families include the saurie, needlefish, kingfish, wahoo, and albacore in addition to the tuna, Bonita, skipjack, and mackerel. Other dark-meat fish not belonging to the Scombroidea, which have been implicated in scombroid fish poisoning include the amberjack (yellowtail or Kahala), mahi mahi (dolphin fish), bluefish (*Pomatomus saltatrix*), kahawai, anchovy, herring, and Australian ocean salmon. In Hawaii, the fish most frequently implicated is mahi mahi.

Clinical Presentations

Within minutes to hours after ingesting affected fish, the patient develops signs and symptoms of a severe histamine-mediated reaction. These include diffuse erythema of the face resembling sunburn, giant urticaria, pruritus or a hot burning sensation, dizziness, throbbing headache, nausea, vomiting, abdominal cramps and diarrhea, and, in severe cases, bronchospasm, respiratory distress, and hypotension. Toxic effects on the myocardium may include a rapid weak pulse, palpitations, and the development of arrhythmias, usually supraventricular. The symptoms generally are self-limited and subside in 8 to 10 hours.

Treatment

- Treatment is entirely supportive. Diagnosis is based on the clinical presentation. For epidemiological studies, serum histamine levels may be ordered.
- The efficacy of decontamination (syrup of ipecac, activated charcoal, cathartics) in this setting is unknown, but theoretically it has value within the first several hours of ingestion when spontaneous emesis does not occur.
- Antihistaminic agents, including intravenous diphenhydramine and cimetidine, may be helpful.
- Fluids and bronchodilators are administered as needed.
- Scombrotoxin is heat stable, so cooking (drying, heating, smoking) will not alter the poisoned fish, nor will freezing, salting, or marinating fish that are already contaminated. Pre-

vention of scombroid poisoning requires proper handling and storage of fish (rapid refrigeration).

Questions—Scombroid

1. Which of the following fish has been implicated in scombroid fish poisoning?
A. Yellowfish
B. Mahi Mahi
C. Bluefish
D. Anchovy
E. All of the above

2. Diagnosis of scombroid poisoning is based on serum histamine levels.
A. True
B. False

SEA HARES

Sea hares are a group of marine gastropod mollusks belonging to the order Aplysiomorpha. In Fiji, the animal is known as "veata" (*Dolabella auricularia*). The sea hares are known to concentrate bromine. Fractions of the sea hare digestive glands have been characterized as brominated sesquiterpenes. Sea hare poisoning may be a form of subacute bromine intoxication.

Clinical Presentations

Poisoning may lead to vomiting, tachypnea, tremor, diarrhea, limb pain, tingling, restlessness, muscle fasciculations, disturbed coordination, fever, and hallucinations. Recovery occurred in one patient after 6 days with some residual perioral muscle twitching.

Treatment

- Sodium or ammonium chloride therapy may have a theoretic basis for use, but has not been tried.

Question—Sea Hares

1. Sea hares are known to concentrate
A. Chlorine
B. Bromine
C. Saxitoxin
D. Tetrodotoxin
E. Ammonium chloride

TETRODOTOXIN

Puffer fish belong to one family of the order Tetraodontiformes. Other families in this order also contain poisonous species including *Canthigaster cinctus* (sharp-nosed puffers), *Mola-mola* (sunfish, headfish), and *Diodon holocanthus* (porcupine fish). A nonprotein, heat-stable neurotoxin (tetrodotoxin) concentrates in the ovaries, kidneys, and intestines of the puffer fish. Tetrodotoxin is produced internally, and concentrations vary during the year.

This toxin possesses local anestheticlike properties that disrupt sodium conductance by physically blocking the fast sodium channel during cell depolarization, similar to saxitoxin. Tetrodotoxin is slightly less neuroactive than saxitoxin, but its effects are more prolonged. Saxitoxin produces less hypotension and vomiting than tetrodotoxin. Toxic ingestions of tetrodotoxin result in a mortality approaching 60%. Tetrodotoxin equally and reversibly affects myelinated nerve fibers along the entire length of the axon by lowering conduction of sodium currents at nodes of Ranvier.

Puffer fish muscle during the nonreproductive season is nontoxic and is considered a delicacy in Japan. Salamanders such as the California newt and the Eastern salamander (*Ambystoma punctatum*) also possess tetrodotoxin in sufficient quantities to cause death. Other species known to contain tetrodotoxin include the goby (*Gobius cringer*), atelopid frogs of Costa Rica, and the blue-ringed octopus (*Hapalochlaena maculosa*).

Clinical Presentations

Paresthesias begin shortly after ingestion (10 to 45 minutes), and vomiting is common. Lightheadedness, paresthesias, feelings of doom, and weakness are early symptoms. An ascending paralysis develops, with respiratory depression as a preterminal event (6 to 24 hours postingestion). Cardiac dysrhythmias (bradycardia, asystole, and depressed AV node conduction) may occur.

Salivation, muscle twitching, diaphoresis, pleuritic chest pain, dysphagia, difficulty in speaking, and convulsions may occur. Hypotension, bradycardia, depressed corneal reflexes, and fixed, dilated pupils indicate a serious poisoning. A rare "locked-in" syndrome has been described in which the patient appears completely flaccid but remains conscious. A sociological investigation has implicated the use of tetrodotoxin as the cause of zombiism in Haitian voodoo culture, but this observation has been challenged.

Treatment

- Treatment is supportive and diagnosis is based on the clinical presentation. Bradycardia and hypotension in a patient suffering from mild intoxication may respond to atropine, intravenous fluids, and oxygen. Hypotension may be reversed with catecholamines.
- Decontamination and endoscopic removal of the fish, if feasible, may be vital if performed quickly. All patients should be admitted.
- While not universal, intravenous edrophonium (10 mg) or intramuscular neostigmine (0.5 mg) has been effective in restoring motor strength.

Questions—Tetrodotoxin

1. All of the following are common symptoms of tetrodotoxin poisoning except
A. Vomiting
B. Paresthesias
C. "Locked-in" syndrome
D. Lightheadedness
E. A and C

2. Treatment of tetrodotoxin poisoning includes
A. Atropine and fluids for bradycardia and hypotension
B. Endoscopic removal of fish if feasible
C. Observation for 6 hours of asymptomatic patients
D. A and B
E. A and C

FOOD SENSITIVITY

INTRODUCTION

For centuries, chemicals have been added to food to improve appearance, edibility, and safety. Reasons for the inclusion of food preservatives in food include improvement of nutritional content, color, and flavor as well as extension of shelf life, food stability, and reduction of toxic organisms. Methods of food preservation include drying, freezing, addition of salt, addition of chemical preservatives or sugar, heat, ionizing radiation, refrigeration, fermentation, and packaging.

In 1938, the Food, Drug, and Cosmetic Act gave the FDA authority over any chemicals in food considered unsafe for human consumption. By 1958, the Food Additive Amendment required food companies to demonstrate the safety of any new additive. The generally-recognized-as-safe (GRAS) list concerns those products on the market before 1958. Throughout the 1970s, the FDA initiated reviews to determine which additives should remain on the GRAS list.

Food preservatives protect foods from the destructive effects of their own enzymes (discoloration, overripening too fast), from bacteria and fungi (food spoilage), and from the environment (heat, humidity, and oxygen can make foods dry, soggy, or rancid). Emulsifiers prevent the separation of oil and aqueous phases in food and humectants (e.g., glycerol, sorbitol) prevent desiccation. Preservatives such as salt, vinegar, nitrates, sugar, and hops have been used in food storage for centuries. More recently, food preservatives have included benzoic acid, propionic acid (cakes), sulfur dioxide (dried fruit), sorbic acid, and sodium metabisulfite.

Certain individuals may develop chemical food intolerance or food-aversion reactions to food additives based on immunological, pharmacological, and psychological mechanisms. Food aversion includes both psychological food intolerance, in which disguised food causes no reaction, and complete food avoidance for psychological reasons.

Clinical Presentations

True food allergy involves both IgE-mediated allergic reactions and other chemical mechanisms (e.g., pharmacological, pseudoallergic, enzyme deficiency, and / or local irritation). Anaphylactic reactions occur from 30 minutes to 2 hours after ingestion. There usually is a history of atopy and ingestion of known food allergens (e.g., peanuts, egg, fish and / or walnuts). Allergy skin tests or radioallergosorbent tests to the foods are positive. About 10% to 15% of the general population is at risk and fatalities have been reported.

Clinical manifestations of food sensitivity may include urticaria, angioedema, rhinitis, asthma, eczema, headache, and gastrointestinal symptoms. The mechanism of intolerance to food additives is not known. Less common reactions to food include sensitivity to caffeine-containing products (headache, vomiting, tachycardia), Chinese restaurant syndrome (monosodium glutamate), bitter lemon purpura (quinine-induced thrombocytopenic purpura), and favism (hemolytic anemia in G6PD-deficient patients).

Questions—Introduction to Food Sensitivity

1. **What percentage of the general population is at risk for food allergy?**
   A. Less than 5%
   B. 10% to 15%
   C. 40% to 50%
   D. 75%
   E. More than 75%
2. **Clinical manifestations of food sensitivity include**
   A. Eczema
   B. Headache
   C. Angioedema
   D. A and B
   E. All of the above

CANTHAXANTHIN

Canthaxanthin is a carotenoid pigment with an orange-red color, but unlike β-carotene, it possesses no vitamin A activity. Listed as GRAS, canthaxanthin is used as a food coloring and is added to animal feed to enhance the color of egg yolks and skin of chicken and flesh of rainbow trout. It also has been taken orally by humans to produce a sun tan and is used as a yellow-orange colorant in soft drinks, candy, fruit, lemonade, and yogurt.

Clinical Presentations

A retinopathy has been associated with canthaxanthin use consisting of fine dustlike golden particles in the layer of nerve fibers close to the maculae and in the paramacular region. These particles have appeared in the eyes of about 12% to 14% of patients who have ingested total doses of 37 to 60 grams. The retinopathy may appear at lower doses in patients who have focal disease of the pigment epithelium, ocular hypertension, or are using β-carotene concurrently. Visual loss has been reported. Electroretinogram tests have indicated some abnormalities.

A 20-year-old woman who ingested "tanning" pills containing an unknown amount of canthaxanthin developed aplastic anemia and died. While definite canthaxanthin causation of aplastic anemia has not been established, it was implicated by association in this case. Hepatitis and generalized urticaria also have been described following canthaxanthin use.

Treatment

- Treatment is symptomatic and supportive.

Questions—Canthaxanthin

1. **Canthaxanthin**
   A. Is an orange-red carotenoid pigment
   B. Possesses no vitamin A activity
   C. Is associated with retinopathy but not visual loss
   D. A and B
   E. All of the above
2. **Canthaxanthins may be found in tanning pills.**
   A. True
   B. False

MONOSODIUM GLUTAMATE

Monosodium L-glutamate (MSG) was proposed as the cause of the Chinese restaurant syndrome in 1968. MSG is a widely used food additive that causes a symptom complex after ingestion of Chinese and other foods. Dried foods, processed meats, canned foods other than plain vegetables and fruit, frozen dinners, and gourmet specialties are all suspect. It frequently is present in wonton soup. MSG is GRAS by the FDA, and no limitation is placed on its use as a food additive.

Pathophysiology

Glutamate is a possible neurotransmitter. Glutamate fed to immature animals appears to destroy central nervous system neurons in the hypothalamus. No evidence linking MSG to serious long-term medical problems in the general population has been found. When glutamate that has been bound within a protein is released during breakdown of the protein molecule "free glutamate" is formed. Some foods such as ripe tomatoes and Parmesan cheese contain high levels of naturally occurring free glutamate.

Clinical Presentations

A burning sensation, facial pressure, and chest pain are the most constant findings. Tightness and numbness of the neck and face, and headache also may be noted when susceptible individuals consume a meal containing MSG on an empty stomach. A sensation of tightness and pressure may be noted over the malar areas, occasionally extending into the zygomatic and retro-orbital regions.

Anecdotal reports of supraventricular and ventricular tachycardia have followed ingestion of Chinese food; however, association with MSG has not been confirmed definitively. A sensation of pressure over the precordium or substernal area, occasionally radiating to the axillae or neck, has been referred to as chest pressure after MSG consumption. Dizziness, nausea, and vomiting may develop as well.

Toxic Dosage/Death

Some individuals can develop short-term reactions after consumption of about 1 to 3 grams or more per meal of MSG or related "free glutamates." 200 mL of wonton soup alone has been sufficient to provoke an attack. At least one subject ingested 25 grams of MSG without symptoms.

Treatment

- No decontamination measures have been reported and no antidotes exist.
- An ECG and cardiac evaluation is required if chest pain persists. Alert patient to avoid foods with MSG.
- Specifically request that your meal be prepared without MSG if you have a history of sensitivity.

Questions—Monosodium Glutamate

1. The FDA limits MSG use to prevent Chinese restaurant syndrome.
A. True
B. False

2. When MSG toxicity is suspected,
A. Symptoms usually include a burning sensation and facial and chest pain.
B. Ventricular tachycardia usually develops.
C. Decontamination measures have been shown to diminish symptoms.
D. A and B
E. A and C

SULFITES

Sulfite food preservatives include sulfur dioxide, potassium metabisulfite, sodium sulfite, sodium metabisulfite, sodium bisulfite, and potassium bisulfite. In acid foods, sodium metabisulfite releases sulfur dioxide. These agents decrease the oxidation of oils and fats by ambient oxygen and slow the development of rancidity. They may produce sensitivity reactions in susceptible individuals, especially asthmatics. The first recognized sulfite-induced allergic reaction occurred in 1976.

Studies have suggested that as many as 5% of the 9 million asthmatics in the United States may be sulfite sensitive. These reactions also may involve nonasthmatic individuals. An exact cause-and-effect relationship in fatal cases associated with sulfite exposure has not been confirmed. Packaged sulfited foods, alcoholic beverages, and prescription drugs are required to be labeled.

Sources

Sulfite additives are found in processed beverages and foods, including fruit juices, soft drinks, wines, beers, cider vinegar, potato chips, dried fruits, and vegetables. The antibrowning properties of sulfites enhance their usefulness in preventing spoilage of commercially prepared or displayed fresh foods, such as ingredients of salad bars, dips, seafood, fruits, vegetables, cole slaw, frozen or dried potatoes, avocado salad, and guacamole.

Sulfur dioxide is a common air pollutant that also is released during the nebulization of many bronchodilators, including isoproterenol hydrochloride, metaproterenol sulfate, isoetharine hydrochloride, and racemic epinephrine. Sulfites appear in parenteral steroid and antibiotic preparations, parenteral cardiovascular drugs, intravenous infusions, peritoneal dialysis solutions, local anesthetics, radiocontrast dyes, and other medications.

Pathophysiology

Although ingestion of food containing sulfiting agents can result in type I immediate hypersensitivity reactions in normal, nonasthmatic individuals, reactions have occurred without evidence for an IgE-mediated mechanism in asthmatics. Bronchial challenge or mere sniffing may evoke a response.

Clinical Presentations

Symptoms may include sudden generalized flushing, faintness, syncope, nausea, diarrhea, wheezing, shortness of breath, cyanosis, rapid pulse, and cold, clammy skin. Urticaria, angioedema, and abdominal distress may be seen within minutes of exposure. Acute asthma attacks, respiratory arrest, loss of consciousness, anaphylactic shock and death may occur.

Toxic Dosage/Death

The total amount of sulfites delivered depends on concentration, duration, and frequency of use as well as delivery method.

Bronchoconstriction can develop in asthmatics exposed to concentrations of sulfur dioxide as low as 1.0 ppm. The 0.3% metabisulfite level in a bronchodilator and 0.9 mg sodium bisulfite in a lidocaine solution can produce symptoms of bronchospasm. Metabisulfite effects from bronchodilator use appear to be dose dependent.

Treatment

- The usual therapy for anaphylactic and bronchoconstriction reactions is applicable here, with special care to avoid epinephrine suspended in a sulfiting agent. Paradoxical bronchoconstrictive reactions may occur when bronchodilator solutions containing bisulfite are employed.
- Cromolyn sodium, atropine, doxepin, and oral cyanocobalamin have been found useful in the treatment of sulfite reactions in uncontrolled studies.
- The FDA has initiated a program to encourage restaurants to notify customers of the sulfite content of foods served. Restaurant managers should be requested to state whether a dish contains sulfites.

Question—Sulfites

1. Sulfites appear in
A. Parenteral steroid preparations
B. Peritoneal dialysis solutions
C. Radiocontrast dyes
D. All of the above
E. None of the above

TARTRAZINE

By 1959, tartrazine (FD&C Yellow No. 5) was implicated in three adult cases of urticaria. Subsequently, persons with known sensitivity to dyes manifested by urticaria, rhinitis, and/or asthma were cautioned against using any medication or products containing tartrazine. In 1976, a survey indicated that more than 1,100 drugs contained this agent. In 1979, the FDA required the presence of tartrazine to be listed in the ingredient labeling.

Pathophysiology

Cross intolerance of tartrazine with aspirin was identified in 1975. Between 10% and 40% of persons sensitive to aspirin also are sensitive to tartrazine. Doses as small as 0.1 mg can provoke urticaria, but tartrazine is not an inhibitor of prostaglandin synthesis. IgE-mediated immune responses are not involved in adverse reactions to tartrazine. IgE antibodies may be associated with a hypersensitivity response, but there are no clinically available skin or laboratory tests to predict predisposition to tartrazine sensitivity. A pharmacologic mechanism suggested for food additive intolerance may involve the ability of dyes to cause histamine release from basophils.

Clinical Presentations

Urticaria, mild rhinitis, severe asthma, and systemic anaphylaxis may occur. In some tartrazine- and aspirin-intolerant individuals, indomethacin, phenylbutazone, fenoprofen, and ibuprofen may provoke an asthmatic response.

Treatment

- If an overdose of tartrazine-containing tablets is ingested, stabilization of the patient (airway, breathing, circulation) and gut decontamination (syrup of ipecac-induced emesis, gastric lavage, activated charcoal, and cathartics as indicated) may be useful.
- Treat severe respiratory symptoms symptomatically (e.g., 0.3 mL epinephrine 1:1,000 subcutaneously in adults). Repeat the dose within 15 to 20 minutes in adults if symptoms continue.
- Some medications used to treat allergic reactions may contain sodium metabisulfite and theoretically may worsen an acute reaction.
- Urticaria usually does not require treatment, but tartrazine-free antihistamines may be employed for symptomatic relief.

Questions—Tartrazine

1. Tartrazine is
A. A potent poison found in bottom-dwelling fish
B. A potent poison carried by shellfish
C. Red dye
D. Yellow dye
E. None of the above

2. There is a cross intolerance in many people between tartrazine and
A. Tylenol
B. Aspirin
C. Codeine
D. Ibuprofen
E. None of the above

Answers

Introduction to Food Toxicology

1. C   2. B   3. A

Bacillus Cereus

1. C

Campylobacter

1. A   2. C

Clostridium Perfringens

1. B

Escherichia Coli

1. E   2. A

Listeria Monocytogenes

1. D   2. A

Salmonella

1. D   2. B

Shigella

1. E

Staphylococcus Aureus

1. C   2. A

Vibrio Cholerae

1. D   2. B

Vibrio Parahaemolyticus and Vibrio Vulnificus

1. C

Yersinia Enterocolitica

1. E

Viral Gastroenteritis

1. C

Amebiasis

1. D 2. B

Cryptosporidiosis

1. A 2. A

Giardia Lamblia

1. C

Microsporidiosis

1. E 2. C

Foodborne Botulism

1. E 2. D

Wound Botulism

1. A 2. E

Infant Botulism

1. D 2. B 3. E

Blue-Green Algae

1. D

Ciguatera

1. B 2. D

Domoic Acid

1. A

Paralytic Shellfish Poisoning

1. C 2. A

Scombroid

1. E 2. B

Sea Hares

1. B

Tetrodotoxin

1. C 2. D

Introduction To Food Sensitivity

1. B 2. E

Canthaxanthin

1. D 2. A

Monosodium Glutamate

1. B 2. A

Sulfites

1. D

Tartrazine

1. D 2. B

SELECTED READINGS

Bacterial Foodborne Illness

1. CDC. Bacterial enteritis. MMWR 1990;39:3.
2. CDC. The management of acute diarrhea in children: Oral rehydration, maintenance and nutritional therapy. MMWR 1992;41:1–20.
3. DuPont HL, Ericsson CD. Prevention and treatment of traveler's diarrhea. N Engl J Med 1993;328:1821–1827.
4. Ericsson CD, DuPont HL. Traveler's diarrhea: Approaches to prevention and treatment. Clin Infect Dis 1993;16:616–626.
5. Guerrant RL, Bobak DA. Bacterial and protozoal gastroenteritis. N Engl J Med 1991;325:327–340.
6. Swerdlow DL, Ries AA. Cholera in the Americas. Guidelines for the clinical. JAMA 1992;267:1495–1499.

Viral Gastroenteritis

1. Blacklow NR, Cukor G. Viral gastroenteritis. N Engl J Med 1981;204:397–406.
2. CDC. Viral gastroenteritis. 1990;39:6.
3. Cukor G, Blacklow NR. Human viral gastroenteritis. Microbiol Rev 1984;48:157–179.

Protozoa and Other Gastrointestinal Parasites

1. Current VL, Carcia LS. Cryptosporidiosis. Clin Microbiol Rev 1991;4:325–358.
2. Weiss LM And now microsporidiosis. Ann Intern Med 1995;123:954–956.
3. Wofsy C. Cryptosporidiosis and isosporiasis. AIDS Clin Care 1991;3(4):25–27.
4. Wolf MS. Giardiasis. N Engl J Med 1978;298:319–321.

Botulism

1. Burmingham MD, Water FG, Mecham C. Wound botulism. Ann Emerg Med 1994;24:1184.
2. CDC. Foodborne botulism-Oklahoma, 1994. MMWR 1995;44:200–201.
3. CDC. Wound botulism-California, 1995. JAMA 1996;275:95–96.
4. Hikes DC, Manoli A II. Wound botulism. J Trauma 1981;21:68–71.
5. Schmidt RD, Schmidt TW. Infant botulism. A case series and review of the literature. J Emerg Med 1992;10:713–718.

Marine Foodborne Illness

1. Eastaugh J, Shepherd S. Infectious and toxic syndromes from fish and shellfish consumption. A review. Arch Intern Med 1989;149:1735–1740.
2. Gellert GA, Ralls J, Brown C, Huston J, Merryman R. Scombroid fish poisoning underreporting and prevention among non-commercial recreational fishers. West J Med 1992;157:645–647.
3. Glavin GB, Bose R, Pinsky C. Infections and toxic syndromes from fish and shellfish consumption. Arch Intern Med 1990;150:2425.
4. Juranovic LR, Park IL. Foodborne toxins of marine origin. Ciguatera. Rev Environ Contam Toxicol 1991;117:51–52.
5. Saavedra-Delgado AM, Metcalfe DD. Seafood toxins. Clin Rev Allergy 1993; 11:241–260.
6. Swift AEB, Swift TR. Ciguatera. Clin Toxicol 1993;31:1–29.

Food Sensitivity

1. Herbert V. Canthaxanthin toxicity. Am J Clin Nutr 1991;53:573.
2. La Roche & Co, Basle, Switzerland. In: Toxicological evaluation of certain food additives and contaminants. Geneva: WHO Food Additives Series 26, 1990; 45–73.
3. Sogn D. The ubiquitous sulfites. JAMA 1984;251:2986–2987.
4. Zautcke JL, Schwartz JA, Mueller EJ. Chinese restaurant syndrome: a review. Ann Emerg Med 1986;15:1210–1213.

ACKNOWLEDGMENTS

Thanks to Alison Deutsch, MD for contributing the questions in this chapter and thanks to Liesa Lessard, MEd, for her help in typing and organizing this chapter.

PART

IV

Chemical Products

CHAPTER 42

Acids, Bases, and Gastroesophageal Issues

INTRODUCTION

Most toxic acid-related emergencies result from accidental exposure to such household products as toilet bowl and metal cleaners. Although acid ingestions are less common than alkali ingestions, the morbidity (33% of reported acid ingestions developed strictures) and mortality (18%) are worse for acid ingestions. This more severe toxicity may reflect the more intentional nature of acid ingestions, since severe pain often limits casual childhood exposures. General parameters to consider in acid exposures are listed below. Specific acids are considered thereafter.

ACIDS

Introduction

Numerous acid products are available in hardware stores and pharmacies. Hydrochloric acid and sulfuric acid are the most common agents ingested. Toilet bowl cleaners may contain 10–80% sulfuric acid, or 10–25% hydrochloric acid. Drain cleaners may contain up to 95–99% sulfuric acid. Metal cleaners and anti-rust compounds contain phosphoric acid (5–80%), oxalic acid (1%), hydrochloric acid (5–25%), sulfuric acid (10–20%), or chromic acid (5–20%). Gun bluing products contain selenious acid. Soldering fluxes include zinc chloride (10–35%) and hydrochloric acid (up to 40%). Automobile battery fluid contains sulfuric acid (25–30%).

Industrial uses for acid products are numerous. Chromic anhydride (99.9%) is a strong inorganic acid whose commercial uses include plating, chemical and dyestuff manufacturing, photography, cement manufacturing, and leather tanning. Hydrochloric or muriatic acid is used in its dilute (less than 10%) form as a bleaching agent, and in its concentrated form (36%) in dye and chemical synthesis, metal refining, and the plumbing industry. Nitric acid used for engraving is 63% pure. Other commercial users of nitric acid include soda makers, metal refiners, electroplaters, and fertilizer manufacturers. Phosphoric acid (85–90%) is involved in metal cleaning, rust proofing, and superphosphate production. The dilute 10% solution is used as a disinfectant.

Chemical, munitions, and fertilizer manufacturers use up to 95–98% sulfuric acid. More dilute sulfuric acid (25–30%) is used in machinery and batteries. Concentrated acetic acid (60%) solutions are used in hat making, printing, dyeing, and rayon manufacturing. Dilute solutions (6–40%) are used in disinfectants and hair wave neutralizers. Formic acid (up to 60%) is used by airplane glue makers, cellulose formate workers, and tanning workers. Oxalic acid is used in the tanning, blueprint paper, chemical synthesis, cleaning iron, and leather industries. Carbolic acid (phenol) is used as a disinfectant and by the dye, pharmaceutical, and plastics industries.

PATHOPHYSIOLOGY

Strong acids produce coagulation necrosis characterized by the formation of a coagulum (eschar). This results from the desiccating action of acid on proteins in superficial tissue. The coagulum limits the penetrating ability of acids compared with the liquefaction necrosis of alkali ingestions where continuing penetration produces injury after exposure ceases. Three pathophysiological phases characterize both acid and alkali ingestions:

Acute Inflammatory Phase

This phase begins within the first 4–7 days of exposure. Vascular thrombosis and cellular necrosis reach a maximum in the first 24–48 hours, with destruction of the columnar epithelium, submucosa, and muscularis. The necrotic mucosa sloughs by the 3rd or 4th day and an ulcer forms.

Latent Granulation Phase

Fibroplasia begins about the middle of the first week and fresh granulation tissue fills the sloughed area of mucosa. Collagen starts to replace the granulation tissue by the end of the first week. Perforation is most likely during this phase, which lasts 2 weeks after injury.

Chronic Cicatrization Phase

The formation of excessive scar tissue around the submucosa and the muscularis produces contractures. This dense fibrous tissue begins to form 2–4 weeks after injury, at a rate that may be either rapid or slowly progressive. The primary goal of management is to prevent this relentless complication.

The distal stomach (antrum and pylorus) is the most frequently injured gastrointestinal site. Fluid propulsion physiology in the esophagus predicts the location of major damage. Stomachs that contain food prior to ingestion have predominantly pyloric damage and lesser curvature damage. In empty stomachs, the lesser curvature is more upright and contracted so that prolonged acid contact occurs in the antrum and midgastric regions. Chronic stricture formation may result in pyloric obstruction, antral stenosis, or an hourglass-type deformity.

Esophageal injury occurs in 6–20% of acid ingestions and usually in association with major gastric damage. Esophageal injury is usually mild and responds to supportive care. Limited esophageal damage in acid ingestion probably results from rapid esophageal transit and limited penetrating ability rather than from any special protective properties of the columnar epithelium.

RISK FACTORS

Substance Type

Generally, substances with a pH below 2 are strong corrosives. However, pH is not the only determinant of severity; lemon juice has a pH around 2 and is minimally irritating. Factors increasing corrosive properties of an acid include its concentration, molarity, and complexing affinity for hydroxyl ions. The more concentrated the solution, the greater the probability of serious injury regardless of other factors. Higher-molarity sulfuric acid (18 M) produces more damage compared with the stronger hydrochloric acid at lower molarity (12 M). In addition, the greater the amount of base required to neutralize the acid, the greater the tissue damage.

Volume

Large volumes increase the area of injury as well as predisposing to emesis, which reexposes gastrointestinal tissue to damage.

Contact Time

Areas of slowing in the gastrointestinal tract such as the cricopharyngeus muscle, pyloric sphincter, diaphragmatic hiatus, and aortic arch increase contact time and predispose to corrosive damage. Increased viscosity and high specific gravity reduce esophageal contact time but speed the acid to the stomach, where prolonged contact may occur. Crystals tend to produce intense localized upper esophageal lesions, whereas liquid preparations produce circumferential, and distal lesions.

Stomach Contents

Preexisting stomach fluid dilutes corrosion and washes crystals off the mucosa. A full stomach is less susceptible to injury and the corrosive effect is more diffuse and superficial.

CLINICAL PRESENTATIONS

Initial symptoms reflect the corrosive properties of strong acids. These include severe pain associated with dysphagia, drooling, vomiting, hematemesis, substernal and abdominal pain, and melena. The presence of oropharyngeal burns suggests, but does not confirm, gastric involvement. For alkali burns, esophageal damage may be present without oropharyngeal burns.

Gastrointestinal Effects

Perforation is the most common serious initial clinical manifestation and may progress to peritonitis and shock without therapy. Increasing abdominal pain, persistent vomiting, direct and indirect rebound, and a tense abdominal wall suggest perforation. Serious acid ingestions are at highest risk for perforation within the first 72 hours. Septicemia, hypovolemia, and shock complicate early gastric perforation.

Late gastric perforation and abscess formation may occur during the latent period (up to 2 weeks). Small-bowel involvement occurs in roughly 20% of acid exposures, whereas acute esophageal perforation from acid ingestions has not been reported. Pyloric obstruction is the most common long-term sequela and may begin within 3–4 weeks of ingestion. Progressive weight loss, anorexia, bloating, early satiety, and vomiting suggest pyloric obstruction. Case studies suggest that acid ingestions, similar to alkali ingestions, may increase the risk of cancer.

Respiratory Effects

Upper airway obstruction secondary to laryngeal edema represents a serious potential complication of acid ingestion manifested by tachypnea, air hunger, inspiratory stridor, dyspnea, and cyanosis. Aspiration of corrosive material produces a severe aspiration pneumonitis. Most acids are respiratory irritants and produce varying degrees of tracheobronchitis and, in high concentrations, adult respiratory distress syndrome. Household bleaches (sodium hypochlorite) produce chlorine gas when mixed with acids and chloramine gas when mixed with ammonia. These respiratory irritants can cause upper respiratory tract irritation. Ammonia, hydrochloric acid, hydrofluoric acid, and chlorine also are potent upper airway irritants that produce mucosal edema and inflammation.

Dermatologic Effects

Symptoms generally result from direct contact with aqueous solutions, and the extent of injury depends on the concentration and duration of contact. Injuries range from erythema and vesicle formation to penetrating ulcers. The coagulative necrosis of acid burns tends to limit penetration to initial contact. Hydrogen fluoride is an exception because the fluoride ions bind to tissue calcium. Signs of hydrogen fluoride exposure range from initial erythema, blanching, and edema to vesicles and deep penetrating ulcers, which may extend to bone.

Symptoms of hydrogen fluoride poisoning depend on concentration and may be delayed. For solutions less than 20%, pain may be delayed up to 24 hours. Hydrogen fluoride solutions of 20–50% produce pain apparent in 1–8 hours. Immediate symptoms appear after exposure to solutions over 50%. Certain acids may present with characteristic lesions. For example, chronic exposure to chromic acid exposure produces circular ulcers (a chrome hole), and exposure to nitric acid causes disfiguring spots.

Metabolic Effects

Systemic toxicity may occur in severe acid exposures, including acidosis, hemolysis, hyponatremia, and shock, as a direct result of acid absorption. Hydrogen fluoride exposure has the potential to produce acute fluoride toxicity, resulting in dysrhythmias attributable to hypocalcemia and hyperkalemia, renal failure, tetany, and respiratory arrest. Fatal fluoride poisoning has occurred after cutaneous hydrofluoric acid exposure. Oxalic acid exposure may produce hypocalcemia, oxaluria, and renal damage.

TREATMENT

Gut Decontamination

Emesis by syrup of ipecac is contraindicated because of reexposure of the esophagus to corrosive material. Charcoal has no place in acid management because it is ineffective and obscures the endoscopic field. Most authors advise against lavage with a soft rubber catheter, and no clinical trials support its use; however, some authors recommend the use of lavage within 1 hour of ingestion because most esophageal acid injuries are superficial, and gastric intubations have not caused complications. The removal of ingested acids such as hydrogen fluoride may outweigh the risk of perforation.

Immediate dilution (milk or water) within 30 minutes of ingestion is widely recommended for oral ingestions despite the fact that tissue injury occurs rapidly, especially with liquid acids. Do not attempt to neutralize acid with weak bases, as an exothermic reaction may extend corrosive injury. Since reexposure of mucosa to acid is harmful, be careful to avoid further vomiting and limit fluids to one or two glasses in an adult.

Elimination Enhancement

Specific acids may require methods to enhance elimination.

Supportive Measures

- Airway problems may arise from laryngeal edema and inhalation exposure. Treat with 100% oxygen initially. Respiratory distress may require cricothyroidotomy if excessive swelling contraindicates oral intubation.
- Intravenous lines should be established immediately in all cases where there is evidence of circulatory compromise. Patients should not be fed orally until endoscopy has confirmed the extent of injury in severe cases.
- An upright chest x-ray may detect free peritoneal air when a perforation is suspected. Chest x-ray may detect inhalation injury but often is normal initially. An abdominal series is helpful to detect ileus and free peritoneal air. Barium swallow and an upper gastrointestinal series detect gastric-outlet obstruction weeks after exposure.
- Patients who are symptomatic or have oropharyngeal burns should be endoscoped. Insufficient data exist to guide the judgment of which asymptomatic patients should receive endoscopy. Optimally, endoscopy is performed within 24–48 hours of ingestion. The extent of the procedure usually is limited to the first area of ulceration to prevent the complication of perforation. Since signs and symptoms are not reliable indicators of potential complications, endoscopy helps diagnose the severity of injury.
- Antibiotics should be reserved for documented infections.

- The administration of steroids is highly questionable in humans since no clinical study supports their use. Although steroid therapy delays stricture formation in animals when given within 48 hours of injury, steroids have been implicated in the obscuration of developing peritoneal signs after acid ingestion.
- Follow fluid and electrolyte balances carefully (including calcium, phosphorus, and protein levels in hydrogen fluoride and oxalic acid poisoning). Significantly symptomatic patients should receive a complete blood count with differential, electrolytes, creatinine, and urinalysis.
- Once discharged, patients who ingest acid should be followed for the development of gastric-outlet obstruction. Patients should return if signs of obstruction develop (progressive anorexia, weight loss, early satiety, or nausea). A routine upper gastrointestinal series 3–4 weeks after exposure detects early contractures.

Skin Considerations

- Skin lesions require copious saline irrigation and removal of any contaminating fragments.
- Hydrogen fluoride burns may benefit from cool benzalkonium chloride (Zephiran®) or 25% magnesium sulfate (Epsom Salts®) soaks. Prolonged exposure to hydrogen fluoride concentrations greater than 20% often requires intradermal 10% calcium gluconate infiltrated with a 30-gauge needle into subcutaneous skin at the rate of 0.5 mL/cm^2 of skin area. Intra-arterial calcium gluconate via an intra-arterial line and infusion pump may be helpful in resistant hydrogen fluoride burn cases. See the section regarding Calcium Gluconate in Chapter 5, Antidotes.
- Consider nail debridement if subungual injury occurs.
- Treat chemical burns as thermal burns with nonadherent gauze and wrapping. Deep second-degree burns may benefit from topical silver sulfadiazine.

Eye Exposures

- After eye exposure to acid, immediately irrigate with sterile saline for at least 20–30 minutes. Copious irrigation of acid injuries requires retraction of the eyelids so that the conjunctival cul-de-sacs are well washed.
- Use anesthetic agents (proparacaine, tetracaine) and retractors as necessary. Be sure to remove all particulate matter. Do not use neutralizing solutions or any other additives. Several liters of saline are required. As long as the lids are retracted, simple intravenous tubing is all that is required to adequately decontaminate the eye.
- Caustic eye injuries require a thorough examination, preferably with a slit lamp, to detect the extent of corneal injury after decontamination. The examination should include visual acuity, extraocular motility, examination of the eyelids, conjunctiva, and sclera, pupillary reactions, anterior chamber depth, staining of corneal surfaces with fluorescein to detect abrasions and ulcerations, and examination of the retina and posterior chamber with an ophthalmoscope.
- Cycloplegic drops (1% cyclopentolate for short-term use or 5% homatropine for longer use), antibiotic drops, vasoconstrictive agents, or artificial tears may be indicated depending on the severity of symptoms. Steroid eye drops should be given only with the approval of a consulting ophthalmologist.
- Although most acid exposures are less severe than alkali exposures, hydrogen fluoride exposure is an exception. All such exposures should be treated as alkali exposures and an ophthalmologist should be consulted immediately after decontamination.

Questions—Introduction to Acids

1. Which of the following does not describe the actions of strong acid on tissue?
A. Acid desiccates proteins in superficial tissue.
B. Desiccation by acid produces a coagulum (eschar).
C. The coagulum (eschar) limits acid penetration.
D. Later liquefaction necrosis enhances penetration.
E. Acute inflammation begins within the first 4–7 days.

2. The goal(s) of managing an acid exposure is/are to
A. Prevent fibroplasia and granulation
B. Prevent perforation
C. Stop vascular thrombosis and cellular necrosis
D. Prevent contractures from excessive scar formation
E. All of the above

3. Clinical presentations of various acid exposures can include which of the following?
A. Abdominal pain, persistent vomiting, rebound
B. Tachypnea, dyspnea, stridor, cyanosis
C. Skin erythema and vesicles
D. Acidosis, hemolysis, hyponatremia
E. All of the above

4. Which of the following treatments for acid exposure is correct?
A. Neutralize acid with a weak base.
B. Dilution within 30 minutes of ingestion using milk or water
C. Emesis using syrup of ipecac
D. Lavage using a soft rubber catheter
E. Give charcoal.

5. Which of the following is not a proper supportive measure for acid exposure?
A. Copiously irrigate skin lesions with saline.
B. Use steroids.
C. Establish i.v. lines.
D. Follow fluid and electrolyte balance.
E. Use 100% oxygen initially and protect the airway.

Acetic Acid

Acetic acid ingestion may result in gastrointestinal burns, bleeding, and volume depletion. Acetic acid is widely used for the production of vinyl plastics, acetic anhydride, acetone, acetanilide, acetylchloride, ethyl alcohol, ketone, methyl ethyl ketone, acetate esters, and cellulose acetates. It is also used alone in the dye, rubber, pharmaceutical, food preserving, textile, and laundry industries and is used in the manufacture of Paris green, white lead, tint rinse, photographic chemicals, stain removers, insecticides, and plastics. Acetic acid is a colorless liquid with a pungent vinegar-like odor. Glacial acetic acid contains 99% acid. Synonyms include ethanoic acid, methane carboxylic acid, vinegar acid, and pyroligneous acid.

PATHOPHYSIOLOGY

Acetic acid, like other acids, acts by coagulation necrosis.

CLINICAL PRESENTATIONS

Ingestion may result in penetration of the esophagus, hematemesis, hemolysis, diarrhea, shock, disseminated intravascular coagulation, and hemoglobinemia followed by anuria. Acetic acid vapor may produce irritation and damage of the eyes, nose,

Answers to questions in shaded boxes appear at the end of the chapter.

throat, and lungs. Contact with concentrated acetic acid may lead to severe skin damage and eye damage sufficient to cause a loss of sight. Repeated or prolonged exposure to acetic acid may cause skin darkening, erosion of the exposed front teeth, and chronic inflammation of the nose, throat, and bronchi. Pneumonia, pulmonary edema, and reactive airways dysfunction syndrome (RADS) may follow acute inhalation overexposure. Chronic exposure may result in pharyngitis and bronchitis.

TREATMENT

Gut Decontamination

Activated charcoal, emesis, and lavage play no role in the treatment of acetic acid ingestion.

Elimination Enhancement

Exchange transfusion may be considered in the face of significant intravascular hemolysis.

Supportive Measures

- Supportive measures follow general treatment protocols for acids (see above).
- Assess local injury (mouth, pharynx) following ingestion.
- Consider replacement of intravascular volume and coagulation factors, diuretics, and prompt correction of acidosis.
- Workers who work with glacial acetic acid should have personal protective equipment; protective clothing, gloves, and goggles should be worn.
- Eye fountains and showers should be available in areas of potential exposure.

Questions—Acetic Acid

1. Which of the following is true of acetic acid exposure?
A. Ingestion may cause esophageal penetration.
B. Vapor may produce damage of the eyes, nose, throat.
C. Liquid splashed on the eyes may cause loss of sight.
D. Prolonged exposure can cause skin darkening.
E. All of the above

2. Which of the following is not true of supportive measures for acetic acid exposure?
A. Assess mouth and pharynx following ingestion.
B. Consider replacement of intravascular volume.
C. Workers using glacial acetic acid need to use protective gear.
D. Promptly correct acidosis.
E. There are specific antidotes for acetic acid exposure.

Formic Acid

Formic acid ingestions are unusual in their ability to cause death after prolonged (several weeks) acid-induced gastrointestinal damage. Other complications include severe metabolic acidosis, intravascular hemolysis, and disseminated intravascular coagulation. Accidental ingestions usually do not lead to fatalities since the pungent taste of the chemical usually precludes an ingestion of a lethal dose. It is nevertheless a problem when used deliberately for suicide.

The accumulation of formic acid accounts for most of the metabolic acidosis that follows methanol ingestion and probably correlates better with clinical toxicity than do serum methanol levels. See Chapter 17, Alcohols, Glycols, and Disulfiram. In Europe, formate is a well known, if relatively infrequent, vehicle for suicide. Formic acid skin burns may cause systemic toxicity.

Formic acid is used as a component of proprietary descaling agents and in stain-removing fluids. It is also used in dyeing wool, electroplating, coagulating latex rubber, regenerating old rubber, and dehairing and tanning leather. It is used for the manufacture of acetic acid, airplane dope, allyl alcohol, cellulose formate, phenolic resins, and oxalate and in the textile, insecticide, refrigeration, and paper industries.

PATHOPHYSIOLOGY

Formic acid directly damages clotting factors, leading to an increase in bleeding time and hemorrhage. It directly corrodes gastrointestinal tissue via coagulation necrosis and destroys normal histology down to muscularis mucosa. Hematemesis may lead to hypovolemia. Formic acid has a direct hemolytic effect on red blood cells. Hemolysis plus the effect of formic acid on renal parenchyma may lead to acute renal failure. Necrotic tissue fragments probably trigger disseminated intravascular coagulation. Formic acid is well absorbed and has an elimination half-life of 2.5 hours.

CLINICAL PRESENTATIONS

Formic acid exposures may be characterized by burning pain in the mouth and pharynx, salivation, edematous mucosa, and ulcerations of the buccal mucosa and pharynx. Mydriasis and hyperemic conjunctivae may be seen. Gastrointestinal effects include nausea, vomiting, abdominal pain, upper gastrointestinal bleeding, abdominal rigidity, and/or pancreatitis. Hemorrhagic esophagitis and gastritis, with or without sloughed mucosa, may be seen. Hepatotoxicity may occur.

Dermatologic effects may include erythema, blisters, cutaneous purpura, and bruising around sites. Depression, drowsiness, weakness, coma, and death have all been reported. Muscle contractions may be seen in severe cases. Respiratory effects include shortness of breath, aspiration pneumonitis, bilateral coarse rhonchi, adult respiratory distress syndrome (ARDS), and respiratory arrest. Formic acid may also cause diuresis, anuria and acute tubular necrosis.

Tachycardia, bradycardia, hypertension, hypotension, central cyanosis, and asystole have been reported. Methemoglobinemia, intravascular hemolysis, and disseminated intravascular coagulation may be seen. Metabolic acidosis and respiratory acidosis also have been reported with formic acid use.

TOXIC DOSAGE/DEATH

Ingestions of less than 10 g in which children recovered have led to superficial oropharyngeal burns. Ingestions of 5–30 g in adults may cause minor superficial oropharyngeal burns, abdominal pain, dyspnea, and dysphagia. A few patients may exhibit hematemesis, pneumonitis, or esophageal stricture. Fatalities are usually not seen in this group. Ingestion of 30–45 g of formic acid usually leads to hematemesis, hepatotoxicity, ulcerations, hemorrhage, and gastrointestinal perforation. Some patients experience reversible disseminated intravascular coagulation or acute renal failure, and many will develop esophageal strictures. Occasional deaths have been reported in this dose range.

In those who ingest 45–200 g, reversible disseminated intravascular coagulation, pneumonitis, acute renal failure, and esophageal stricture may be observed in the few who recover. Most develop corrosive perforations of the abdominal viscera, gastrointestinal hemorrhage, and in some cases acute renal failure. Death occurs at this dose level in the majority of patients within 36 hours of ingestion.

LABORATORY

Analytic Methods

Formic acid serum concentrations are quantitated enzymatically using formate dehydrogenase with spectrophotometric measurements.

Blood Levels

The formic acid concentration 2 hours after ingestion of about 100 g (200 mL 50% formic acid) is 348 μg/mL. Ingestion of 50 mL of formic acid led to a serum formic acid level of 180 μg/mL in 6 hours in one case.

TREATMENT

Gut Decontamination

Immediate dilution with milk but not with alkalis, which may cause a local exothermic reaction, may be useful. Emesis with syrup of ipecac, or gastric lavage, or the use of a nasogastric tube is contraindicated. Activated charcoal has not been used and could enhance mucosal irritation in addition to its possible penetration through a mucosal perforation. It has no place in acid management and obscures the endoscopic field.

Elimination Enhancement

Renal failure may require dialysis. Peritoneal dialysis may be preferable to hemodialysis since heparin used with hemodialysis may increase gastrointestinal bleeding. Intravascular hemolysis may respond to exchange transfusion.

Supportive Measures

- Patients who have ingested formic acid should be hospitalized for treatment in an intensive care facility. Airway problems may arise from laryngeal edema. The patient should be monitored for cardiorespiratory function. A supply of 100% oxygen should be available.
- Intravenous lines should be inserted and central venous pressure measurements should be taken periodically to ensure circulatory stability.
- Diazepam may be used for sedation provided tracheal protection is in place.
- Lidocaine application may be useful for mouth lesions.
- Gastroscopy may (in the first 24 hours) discern severe lesions of the esophagus, stomach, and duodenum.
- Coagulation studies may yield an increase in prothrombin time, accelerated partial thromboplastin time, and fibrin degradation products. The hematocrit and fibrinogen levels may be within normal limits, however.
- Other laboratory abnormalities encountered include elevations in the lactic acid dehydrogenase, aminotransferases, amylase, glucose, lactate, and creatinine. There may be an increase in free hemoglobin, methemoglobin, and the white blood cell and platelet counts.
- Arterial blood gases may reflect severe metabolic acidosis.
- The chest x-ray may be normal or exhibit bilateral patchy consolidation or a "shock lung."
- The role of cimetidine and steroids is not clear.
- Follow fluid intake and output and electrolytes, especially potassium, in the presence of hemolysis. Formic acid poisoning can bring the bicarbonate level to zero.
- Sodium bicarbonate may be indicated for severe metabolic acidosis. Correction of acidemia and urinary alkalinization are used to decrease lipophilicity of formic acid and enhance urinary elimination of formate. Urinary alkalinization may increase hemoglobin solubility and decrease the rate of acute tubular necrosis.
- Intravenous furosemide (20 mg every 4 hours) may prevent renal tubular reabsorption of formate in the urine.
- High-dose i.v. folinic acid (1 mg/kg bolus followed by 6 doses of 1 mg/kg at 4-hour intervals until clinical improvement) may enhance formate degradation by the liver.

ANTIDOTE

There is no specific antidote for formate poisoning.

Questions—Formic Acid

1. The consequences of ingesting formic acid can include
A. Intravascular hemolysis
B. Severe metabolic acidosis
C. Disseminated intravascular coagulation
D. Death several weeks after ingestion due to gastrointestinal damage
E. All of the above

2. How much formic acid ingestion generally results in death?
A. Less than 10 g
B. 5–30 g
C. 30–45 g
D. 45–200 g
E. None of the above

3. Which of the following is not an appropriate treatment for formic acid ingestion?
A. Immediate dilution with milk
B. Give activated charcoal
C. Exchange transfusion for intravascular hemolysis
D. Dialysis for renal failure
E. Pentoneol dialysis

4. Supportive measures for formic acid ingestion include
A. Hospitalization in the intensive care unit
B. Establish i.v. access and send blood tests
C. Protect the airway, intubating if necessary
D. Carefully follow fluid intake and output
E. All of the above

5. Which supportive measure for formic acid ingestion is not correct?
A. Steroids are generally helpful.
B. Use sodium bicarbonate for severe metabolic acidosis.
C. Urinary alkalinization can enhance elimination of formate.
D. Intravenous furosemide may prevent renal tubular reabsorption of formate.
E. High-dose i.v. use of folinic acid may enhance hepatic degradation of formate.

Hydrofluoric Acid

Concentrated hydrofluoric acid (90%) is used as an anhydrous catalyst for high-octane gasoline, removal of sand from metal casing, petroleum refining, antimony fluoride extraction, and synthesis of pharmaceuticals and germicides. Dilute solutions (10–20%) are used in tanning, frosting, and metal etching processes. Hydrogen fluoride burns are a hazard in the semiconductor industry in which this acid is used as an "etchant" for chip manufacturing.

Significant ingestion of hydrofluoric acid may lead to death within 1–7 hours. Ingestions of relatively dilute solutions of hydrofluoric acid may be rapidly fatal. Patients may present with hematemesis, hypovolemic tetanic convulsions, upper airway obstruction, severe hypocalcemia, acidosis, shock, and coma. Myocardial irritability and subsequent life-threatening cardiac arrhythmias may be due to binding of potassium, magnesium, and calcium ions.

PATHOPHYSIOLOGY

In cases of hydrofluoric acid exposure, the fluoride anion (not the hydrogen ion) produces liquefaction necrosis by combining with calcium and magnesium in tissues. Fluoride ions may have a direct toxic effect on the central nervous system, leading to stupor, coma, and respiratory failure.

CLINICAL PRESENTATIONS

Significant hypocalcemia may follow dermal exposure of a 50% or greater hydrofluoric acid concentration to 1% of body surface area, any dermal exposure to more than 5% of body surface area, inhalation of vapors from a 60% or greater concentration of acid solution, or any ingestion of hydrofluoric acid solutions. Hemorrhagic gastritis, hypocalcemia, pulmonary edema, and metabolic acidosis may occur.

TOXIC DOSAGE/DEATH

One mouthful of rust remover led to severe hypocalcemia, acidosis, and fatal asystole in 90 minutes. Survival has been reported in one case following ingestion of 2 ounces of a rust-removal agent containing 12% hydrofluoric acid.

TREATMENT

Gut Decontamination

Ingestion at home may be treated immediately with milk to dilute the acid and perhaps bind some of the fluoride ion. If spontaneous vomiting has not occurred and the time between ingestion and treatment is less than 90 minutes, consider gastric lavage. Addition of 10% calcium gluconate to the lavage fluid may provide some free calcium to bind the fluoride. There are no data or guidelines for the amount of lavage fluid used for decontamination of the stomach. Syrup of ipecac is not advised. After decontamination, monitor the patient for signs of airway compromise, gastric perforation, gastric hemorrhage, and systemic toxicity.

Elimination Enhancement

Dialysis may be required to remove excess serum potassium and fluoride.

Supportive Measures

Burns

- All patients should be admitted to a burn unit or intensive care unit if the total extent of the burns is greater than 2–3% body surface area, or if there is significant respiratory distress. Administer 1 g (10 mL) of 10% calcium gluconate i.v. if immediate serum calcium levels are not available and exposure is greater than 5% body surface area.
- Hydrofluoric acid burns of the skin require immediate and copious irrigation with water, preferably under a shower or faucet for at least 15–30 minutes. Cleansing and debridement follow as necessary.
- For exposures to hydrofluoric acid concentrations less than 20%, liberal and frequent application of a 2.5% calcium gluconate gel may be the topical therapy of choice. A 2.5% calcium gluconate gel is formulated by mixing 3.5 g of calcium gluconate powder USP with 150 mL (5 ounces) of a water-soluble lubricant such as K-Y Jelly.
- An occlusive barrier (e.g., vinyl gloves or plastic wrap) may secure the gel, and repeated application may be administered as often as necessary to eliminate pain.

Acidosis

- Correct systemic acidosis with sodium bicarbonate guided by arterial blood gas measurements. Cardiac arrhythmias secondary to electrolyte imbalance, acidosis, or hypoxia should be identified and corrected.
- Obtain frequent calcium, magnesium, phosphorus, and potassium levels.
- A prolonged QT interval on ECG may represent hypocalcemia in this setting.
- Watch for fluoride-induced hyperkalemia as a cause of arrhythmias. Hypotension should be managed with volume expansion and vasopressors as required.

Eye Exposure

- Eye exposures should be treated by immediate and copious irrigation for at least 30 minutes. Local ophthalmic anesthetic drops will increase patient comfort and compliance with prolonged irrigation. The pH of the eye fluid should be periodically checked with litmus paper and irrigation continued until it is normal. Assess visual acuity after the eye irrigation is completed.
- Obtain an ophthalmologic consultation. Repeated instillation of 1% calcium gluconate eye drops combined with conventional treatment of acid eye burns is effective in hastening recovery from hydrofluoric acid-induced corneal erosion.

Inhalation

- Inhalation exposure and injury are treated by removing the victim from the source and into fresh air, accompanied by decontamination of clothes and skin.
- Monitor the patient for laryngeal edema, pneumonitis, pulmonary edema, pulmonary hemorrhage, and systemic toxicity.

ANTIDOTES

Calcium

Skin lesions resulting from exposure to hydrogen fluoride concentrations over 20% usually require intradermal injection of 10% calcium gluconate (0.5 mL/cm^2 of skin, with a 30-gauge needle). Frequently, hydrofluoric acid burns occur on the fingers, where intradermal calcium injections are hazardous. For these areas, the intraarterial infusion of 10 mL of 20% calcium gluconate (180 mg calcium) in 40 mL of normal saline over 4 hours has been recommended.

Calcium chloride infusion (10 mL of a 10% solution mixed in 40–50 mL 5% dextrose) is also an effective treatment for concentrated hydrofluoric acid burns of the fingers. These patients should be admitted to an intensive care unit (ICU) for arterial pressure wave monitoring. The injured extremity is checked for residual pain and tenderness at the end of 4 hours. If tenderness persists, then another infusion is given. Serum calcium, magnesium, phosphorus, PT, and PTT are obtained 1 hour after completion of the infusion.

Ingestions that induce hypocalcemia (manifested by a prolonged QT interval, positive Trousseau's or Chvostek's sign) and hypomagnesemia may require multiple intravenous doses of calcium gluconate and magnesium sulfate over a period of many hours. Repeated cardioversions (for ventricular fibrillation) may be required until normal calcium and magnesium levels and cardiac stability are achieved.

Questions—Hydrofluoric Acid

1. Hydrofluoric acid is used in which of the following processes?
A. Catalyst for high-octane gasoline
B. Synthesis of pharmaceuticals and germicides
C. Tanning, frosting, and metal etching
D. Etchant in semiconductor chip manufacturing
E. All of the above

2. Significant hypocalcemia may follow which of the following hydrofluoric acid exposures?
A. Inhalation of vapors from less than 50% concentration
B. Any ingestion of hydrofluoric acid solutions
C. 1% dermal exposure to less than 50% concentration
D. 1% dermal exposure to more than 50% concentration
E. B and D

3. Supportive measures for hydrofluoric acid burns include
A. Admission to a burn unit or intensive care unit if more than 3% of body surface area is involved
B. Immediate i.v. administration of 1 g of 10% calcium gluconate if exposure is greater than 5% of body surface area
C. Immediate and copious water irrigation of the exposed areas
D. Application of 2.5% calcium gluconate gel on areas exposed to acid concentrations of less than 20%
E. All of the above

4. Hydrofluoric acid ingestion can cause
A. Significant hypercalcemia
B. Significant hypocalcemia
C. Significant hypermagnesemia
D. Significant hypomagnesemia
E. B and D

Monochloroacetic Acid

Monochloroacetic acid (MCA) is corrosive and stronger than acetic acid. It is extremely toxic via dermal and inhalational routes. MCA is used in the production of carboxymethyl cellulose, phenoxyacetates, pigments, and drugs. It is also used as a wart remover and herbicide.

PATHOPHYSIOLOGY

MCA reacts with sulfhydryl groups of essential enzymes. MCA can produce severe local reactions of the skin, eye, or respiratory tract. MCA inhibits the tricarboxylic acid cycle and prevents the conversion of citrate to isocitrate. MCA is readily absorbed after ingestion and after skin contact.

CLINICAL PRESENTATIONS

Splashes of 80% MCA solution on the skin can lead to epidermal and superficial skin burns. Within a few hours, features of systemic poisoning may occur. These include disorientation, agitation, cardiac failure, and coma. Severe metabolic acidosis, rhabdomyolysis, renal insufficiency, and cerebral edema with uncal herniation can lead to death. Oral exposure has led to refractory ventricular tachycardia, pulmonary edema, acidemia, and death in 8 hours. Other manifestations of poisoning may include malaise, vomiting, cardiovascular shock, and seizures. Vomiting and diarrhea are common early signs.

Central nervous system features include excitability with disorientation, delirium, and seizures followed by central nervous system depression and coma with cerebral edema. Severe myocardial depression with shock and electrocardiographic changes of a nonspecific nature are observed. Progressive renal failure, hypokalemia, and severe metabolic acidosis may be observed. Hypocalcemia may be delayed for 1–2 days. Acetylating agents such as MCA may cause a bullous dermatitis with extensive desquamation.

LABORATORY

Analytic Methods

A gas chromatography-mass spectrometry method for determining MCA in plasma was developed from a gas chromatography method used for measuring MCA in industrial wastewater.

Blood Levels

Four hours after a skin splash of 80% MCA on 25–30% of the body surface, an adult exhibited an MCA concentration of 33 μg/mL. Following an inadvertent administration of 5–6 mL of an 8% MCA wart remover, a 5-year-old died and exhibited a postmortem MCA level of 100 μg/mL.

TREATMENT

Gut Decontamination

After ingestion, emesis should be induced at the accident site, despite the risk of corrosive damage, to lessen the inception of severe systemic poisoning.

Elimination Enhancement

MCA is found in plasma in fairly high concentrations. Hemodialysis may be of benefit if commenced at an early stage.

Supportive Measures

- After exposure to liquid MCA, urgent skin decontamination and removal of contaminated clothing are indicated. If greater than 1% of body surface is exposed, hospitalization is required.
- Intervention may include fluid therapy and correction of acid-base and electrolyte disturbances (such as hypokalemia). Alkalinization of urine to prevent myoglobin deposition in the renal tubules may be required in rhabdomyolysis.
- Inotropic support with dopamine or dobutamine is indicated for hemodynamic compromise.
- Controlled hyperventilation may be required to prevent and treat cerebral edema.
- Laboratory abnormalities may include hypokalemia, high creatine kinase, and high aspartic and amine aminotransferase concentrations. Hypocalcemia may be delayed for 1–2 days.

ANTIDOTES

Ethanol and glyceryl monoacetate have been advocated both for fluoroacetate poisoning and for MCA poisoning, but there is little clinical evidence to support their use. MCA is bound to glutathione and other sulfhydryl-containing substances. N-acetylcysteine (Mucomyst®) could be tried as a sulfhydryl donor; however, there is no clinical experience with this product in MCA poisoning.

Questions—Monochloroacetic Acid

1. Clinical presentations of MCA exposure may include
A. Severe metabolic alkalosis
B. Progressive hyperkalemia
C. Severe metabolic acidosis
D. Severe myocardial excitation
E. Hypercalcemia

2. The following is/are true of MCA poisoning
A. Hypocalcemia may be delayed for 1–2 days.
B. Hemodynamic compromise may necessitate inotropic support.
C. MCA is bound to glutathione and sulfhydryl-containing substances.
D. Cerebral edema and uncal herniation can occur.
E. All of the above

Oxalic Acid

Oxalic acid is used as an analgesic reagent and in the manufacture of dyes, inks, bleaches, paint removers, varnishes, wood and metal cleaners, dextrin, cream of tartar, celluloid, oxalates, tartaric acid, purified methyl alcohol, glycerol, and hydrogen cyanide. It is also used in the photographic, ceramic, metallurgic, rubber, leather, engraving, pharmaceutical, paper, and lithographic industries. Oxalate is also called ethanedioic acid.

Oxalic acid is a colorless, odorless powder or granular solid. Oxalates are present in sorrel and rhubarb, where its content is high in the leaves and low in the stalk. It occurs in plants in a partly insoluble form as acid oxalate and free oxalic acid and partly in insoluble form as calcium oxalate.

PATHOPHYSIOLOGY

Target organs for oxalic acid poisoning include the skin, eyes, respiratory system, and kidneys. Oxalic acid has a corrosive effect on the digestive tract. Once absorbed it reacts with calcium in plasma, and insoluble calcium oxalate tends to precipitate in organs such as the kidneys, blood vessels, heart, lungs, and liver. This reaction may also lead to hypocalcemia. An estimated 66% of renal calculi and 75% of bladder calculi are composed of calcium oxalate. Hypercalciuria secondary to hyperparathyroidism, sarcoidosis, renal tubular acidosis, hypervitaminosis D, or hyperoxaluria may cause such stones.

CLINICAL PRESENTATIONS

Oxalic acid has a corrosive action on the skin, eyes, and mucous membranes that may result in irritation. Local prolonged contact to the extremities may result in localized pain, cyanosis, and possibly gangrenous changes secondary to localized vascular damage. Chronic exposure may lead to chronic inflammation of the upper respiratory tract. Vomiting, diarrhea, coma, respiratory depression, kidney failure, liver failure, metabolic acidosis, hypocalcemia and death have all been seen in extreme cases of oxalate ingestion.

TOXIC DOSAGE/DEATH

The lethal dose of oxalic acid for adults is 15–30 g, although amounts as low as 5 g have been fatal. The U.S. Occupational Safety and Health Administration (OSHA) TWA standard is 1 mg/m^3 with a short-term exposure limit of 2 mg/m^3. Immediate danger to life and health follows an exposure of 500 mg/m^3.

TREATMENT

Gut Decontamination

Oral dilution with water or milk is usually sufficient. Charcoal, lavage or emesis is generally unnecessary unless large quantities of plant material have been ingested within an hour of presentation. Gastric lavage with calcium gluconate may be helpful; however, great caution must be exercised, as hypercalcemia may develop.

Elimination Enhancement

Dialysis may be required in cases of renal failure.

Supportive Measures

- The presence of increased urinary oxalate crystals may be useful in the evaluation of oral poisoning.
- Serum calcium should be monitored. Hypocalcemia is treated with calcium gluconate supplementation.
- Oxalate levels may be obtained, but generally do not guide therapy.
- Ingestion of oxalic acid from sorrel or rhubarb may lead to extensive renal damage and death. In severe cases, admission to an intensive care unit to support hydration and electrolyte status is warranted. Electrocardiographic monitoring and serum calcium determinations should be initiated.
- In ocular exposures, irrigate immediately for 15 minutes with copious amounts of water or saline.
- Skin exposures require flushing with water promptly.

Questions—Oxalic Acid

1. Immediate danger to life and health follows which of the following oxalic acid exposures?
A. 50 mg/m^3
B. 100 mg/m^3
C. 200 mg/m^3
D. 300 mg/m^3
E. 500 mg/m^3

2. Which of the following is not true of oxalic acid exposure?
A. Oxalate levels generally guide therapy.
B. Serum calcium should be monitored.
C. Dialysis may be required.
D. Ingestion of rhubarb may lead to extensive renal damage.
E. Skin exposures must be promptly flushed with water.

BASES

Ingestion of alkali corrosives, such as household substances with pH ranging from 7–14, is more common and usually more serious than acid ingestion because of deeper, more intense irritant effects. Fortunately, the number of alkali ingestions in the U.S. has decreased as a result of lower product alkali concentrations, safety packaging, and increased public awareness. Prior to 1965, most lye ingested was of granular composition, which tended to produce limited esophageal injury and occasional delayed esophageal (rarely gastric) strictures. Pain on ingestion commonly limited children's exposure to a few crystals. Liquid lye, which was introduced in 1967, allows greater injury both to the esophagus (because of high viscosity, which causes prolonged contact) and to the stomach. The majority of corrosive ingestions occur accidentally in children. Adult ingestions tend to be more serious because of their intentional nature.

Numerous alkaline formulations line grocery store and hardware store shelves. Sodium hypochlorite (e.g., Clorox®) household bleach products usually contain 3–6% concentrations and have a pH up to 11. Some bleaches (e.g., Purex®) contain silicate (15–17%) and sodium carbonate (60%) and have a pH around 10.5. Household bleaches may produce erosions but rarely penetrate the submucosa to cause esophageal strictures. Granular and commercial bleaches may contain higher concentrations of hypochlorite or carbonate, leading to greater tissue destruction.

Sodium or potassium hydroxide drain cleaners clear plugged drains and cut grease buildup. Red Devil Drain Opener and Lye® (96–100% sodium hydroxide) has a pH of 14. Crystalline Drano® (57% sodium hydroxide) has a pH of 14. Liquid Drano® (10% sodium hydroxide) and Liquid Plum'r (5% sodium hydroxide) also have a pH of 14. Some drain cleaners have been reformulated to contain 1,1,1-trichloroethane, which is a hydrocarbon rather than a caustic. Oven cleaners also contain sodium hydroxide.

The ammonium hydroxide concentration in household ammonia ranges from 3–10%. Weaker 3% solutions are mild irritants, but higher concentrations may be significantly corrosive. Volatile ammonia solutions can produce inhalation injuries and systemic symptoms. An 8.8% ammonia solution has a pH of 12.5. Automatic dishwasher detergents contain builders (e.g., sodium tripolyphosphate, sodium metasilicate, sodium silicate, and sodium carbonate) that produce corrosive lesions (pH 10.5–13).

Clinitest® tablets, still used by some diabetics to detect glucose in urine, contain copper sulfate, citric acid, sodium hydroxide, and sodium carbonate. Unfortunately, they look like many other drugs, such as aspirin, and may occasionally be accidentally ingested. Injury occurs both by direct corrosive action and by an exothermic heat reaction. Commonly damaged sites include the proximal esophageal mucosa and, occasionally, the gastric and duodenal mucosa.

Cement can produce full-thickness chemical burns after prolonged skin contact (e.g., cement spilled inside a boot). Other alkaline corrosive products include potassium permanganate, nonphosphate detergents (sodium carbonate), metal cleaners (but usually not metal polishes, which are ammonia compounds), paint removers, washing powders, and some home concoctions purportedly used to determine the sex of the fetus from the mother's urine.

PATHOPHYSIOLOGY

Alkali corrosives damage the gastrointestinal tract by liquefaction necrosis in which the saponification of fats and solubilization of proteins allow deep penetration into tissues. In contrast to acids, which cause a coagulation necrosis with the formation of protective eschars, alkalis cause continuing damage after exposure because of their ability to penetrate tissue and produce continuing vascular thrombosis and necrosis. Superficial dilution has less effect in alkali injury because of this penetrating ability. Determinants of severity dictate whether alkali burns extend to adjacent viscera.

Areas of involvement depend on the type of product (granules, liquid) and the corrosive nature of the product (pH, viscosity, concentration, etc.) Solid lye products produce primarily upper esophageal and oropharyngeal injury seen as deep irregular burns. Serious injury occurs in about one-third of patients who ingest solid lye products. Stricture formation is common and involvement may lead to perforation. Perforation leads to mediastinitis or peritonitis and sepsis. Distal gastric injury is uncommon.

Liquid lye ingestions may cause serious esophageal injury without evidence of oropharyngeal involvement. A higher incidence of serious esophageal injury appears after liquid rather than solid lye ingestions. Household bleaches rarely produce more serious injury than mucosal erosions, and esophageal strictures usually do not occur.

Determinants of severity include pH, viscosity, concentration and volume ingested, contact time, premorbid conditions of the stomach, and exothermic reactions. The critical pH range within which esophageal ulceration occurs is 12–12.5, although most cases of deep ulceration producing stricture involve lye solution with a pH of 14. Studies in animals indicate that increasing viscosity increases the severity of injury at a given pH and concentration.

Large volumes increase the amount reaching the stomach and predispose to emesis and repeat exposure of the stomach to corrosive. Increased contact time, particularly by the embedding of particles or tablets or a slow passage of liquids over areas of anatomical narrowing, adds to the injury. The water and citric acid in Clinitest® tablets combine with sodium hydroxide to generate heat. Tissue damage results from the intense heat of hydration.

CLINICAL PRESENTATIONS

Acute Inflammatory Phase

An acute inflammatory phase occurs within the first 3–4 days. Edema, erythema, vascular congestion, thrombosis, and necrosis characterize this phase. This phase peaks within 48 hours.

Latent Granulation Phase

A latent granulation phase occurs within 4–14 days. Fibroplasia starts, granulation tissue fills after mucosal sloughing, and collagen deposition follows. The esophageal wall is weakest during this phase and represents a significant hazard for perforation.

Chronic Cicatrization Phase

A chronic cicatrization phase may occur within several weeks to years. Scar tissue replaces the defect, which can lead to symptomatic esophageal obstruction.

Esophageal Burns

Symptoms of esophageal burns include dysphagia, odynophagia, spontaneous vomiting, and abdominal pain. Most patients with esophageal injury complain of pain, but symptoms may not localize to the area of greatest mucosal injury, perhaps because of the loss of nerve endings. Whether or not all patients with significant esophageal injury have symptoms has not been resolved. Signs of chemical injury may include drooling, inability to swallow, erythema and ulceration of the oropharynx, hematemesis, and occasionally shock and respiratory distress. Severe signs indicate severe injury, but not all patients with significant esophageal damage have external signs of injury.

Extensive alkali mucosal burns present as gray or gray-black pseudomembranes covering the buccal mucosa or palate. Approximately one-third of patients with oral burns have significant esophageal injury, whereas 2–15% of patients with esophageal injuries have no oral burns. Automatic dishwasher detergents often produce esophageal and gastric erosion without evidence of oral burns, although esophageal strictures are rare. Clinitest® tablet ingestions differ from liquid alkali ingestions in the higher frequency of accidental adult ingestion. Compared with other alkali exposures, esophageal strictures are relatively more proximal and less severe.

Complications of alkali burns represent the greatest hazard to the patient, and each patient should be examined carefully for adverse consequences of alkali exposure. Acute complications may include gastrointestinal hemorrhage manifested by melena, hypotension, shock, and hematemesis. Upper airway obstruction may cause aphonia, dyspnea, stridor, cyanosis, or hoarseness. Perforation of the esophagus leading to mediastinitis may present with fever, substernal chest pain radiating to the back, severe abdominal pain with abdominal wall rigidity and rebound, Hamman's crunch, and subcutaneous air. Gastric perforation is rare in alkali ingestions.

Chronic Effects

Chronic complications may include esophageal obstruction secondary to strictures. These patients may experience progressive dysphagia, weight loss, and anorexia. Scarring of the posterior cricoarytenoid muscle may result in airway obstruction secondary to vocal cord paralysis. This is a late, relatively rare complication. Squamous cell carcinoma of the esophagus complicates 1–4% of lye ingestions, with a mean onset of about 40 years. The risk of esophageal cancer is estimated to be increased about 1,000 times, 25 years after significant exposures.

TREATMENT

Gut Decontamination

Catharsis and emesis are absolutely contraindicated. Diluents remain a controversial intervention. Milk and water may be helpful in dislodging solid lye particles. Although diluents are commonly recommended, their value in liquid ingestions is less clear since vomiting may reexpose the esophagus to alkali. No more than one to two glasses of diluent should be given to an adult, as emesis may reexpose viable tissue to corrosive. Dilution more than 1 hour after injury probably is not efficacious. Neutralizing agents should never be given since the exothermic heat reaction enhances injury. Activated charcoal does not absorb alkali and obscures the endoscopic visual field. Gastric lavage should not be used in alkali ingestions.

Elimination Enhancement

These methods have not been shown to aid in the treatment of alkali ingestions.

Supportive Measures

- Carefully assess the airway in all individuals, and intubate patients with significant respiratory compromise. Respiratory distress is uncommon but presents occasionally because of soft tissue edema. Unless intubation can be accomplished under direct visualization, a cricothyroidotomy or tracheostomy may be necessary (blind nasotracheal intubation in this setting is contraindicated). Oxygen is given as indicated.
- The chest x-ray is usually unremarkable. Search for signs of perforation (free subdiaphragmatic air, mediastinal emphysema), and examine lung parenchyma for signs of aspiration.
- Withhold all oral feedings initially and carefully assess fluid and electrolyte balances.
- Watch for development of complications such as esophageal perforation, sepsis, mediastinitis, and upper gastrointestinal hemorrhage in severe ingestions by serial examinations and vital signs.
- The use of a nasogastric tube as a stent and for nutrition is controversial, and such a tube should be passed only during endoscopy. Some authors recommend early surgical intervention and use of an intraluminal stent in patients with second- or third-degree esophageal burns because perforations that require surgical repair may be missed.
- The use of early surgical intervention (esophagogastrectomy with colonic disposition) to prevent subsequent fistulas, abscesses, and strictures requires evaluation of the amount of tissue necrosis.
- Intraluminal splinting with Silastic tubes, penicillamine, and lathyrogens (prevent formation of covalent collagen crosslinks) to reduce stricture formation are under investigation.
- Patients should be instructed to seek medical attention if they develop any dysphagia.
- The presence of shock suggests perforation and mandates intravenous fluid administration.
- Alkali injuries to the eye and skin should be irrigated copiously for at least 20–30 minutes with saline. Alkali injuries to the eye are ophthalmologic emergencies and require ophthalmologic consultation after copious irrigation.
- Hospitalized patients should receive a complete blood count, electrolytes, creatinine, type and cross for several units of blood, and a Hemoccult test for blood in stool. Metabolic acidosis is rare without the concomitant presence of shock, but has been reported.

Esophagoscopy

- Since signs and symptoms do not correlate well with the location or severity of injury, esophagoscopy is an important adjunct in evaluation of the presence and extent of injury. When flexible fiberoptic scopes are used within the first 48 hours, the risk of perforation is small. The exact timing of esophagoscopy within the first 48 hours depends on availability, edema, and the patient's general condition.
- The issue of whether or not to pass the first site of injury is controversial. The risk of potential perforation versus the necessity of finding more serious lesions, which would indicate the use of steroids, must be considered. Esophageal findings are classified into superficial, transmucosal, and transmural.
- Definite indications include the presence of oral burns, and symptomatic patients. The use of esophagoscopy for asymptomatic patients is controversial and requires consideration of time lapsed since ingestion, type of corrosive involved, and extent of exposure. Accidental ingestion of household bleach does not require endoscopy, but intentional, symptomatic ingestion of more than 1 mL/kg may benefit from endoscopy.
- Contraindications to esophagoscopy include upper airway obstruction, signs and symptoms of perforation, and more than 48 hours since exposure.

Esophagograms

- This procedure is not as reliable as esophagoscopy in the early evaluation of esophageal injury, but may be used if more than 48 hours have passed since exposure. Diffuse blurred esophageal margins (mucosal ulceration or sloughing) and linear streaks (deep necrotic ulcers) indicate esophageal injury. Gaseous dilation and retention of contrast suggest impending perforation.
- A routine 3-week postinjury barium swallow is suggested for evaluation of stricture formation unless symptoms dictate an earlier study. An upper gastrointestinal series is useful for evaluating the pylorus and duodenum when endoscopy is not helpful. The routine series is necessary to identify complications such as scarring and outlet obstruction at the end of the first month.
- Water-soluble contrast media should be used whenever perforation is a possibility.

Steroids

- The potential use of steroids is based on studies in animals that show that corticosteroids given within the first 48 hours reduce subsequent stricture formation. Steroids should be avoided if perforation is likely or there is a history of peptic ulcer disease or active infection.
- The development of strictures appears to be related to the severity of injury. Steroids do not appear to be needed for first- and second-degree injuries and are ineffective and possibly dangerous for third-degree injury in humans.
- While still controversial, steroids should not be used routinely in caustic ingestions, but may be effective in patients with

dyspnea, stridor, hoarseness, or other evidence of respiratory compromise. Steroids in such cases may decrease laryngotracheal edema and may lessen respiratory dysfunction.

- Although data on animals suggest the need for prophylactic antibiotics in steroid-treated animals, no controlled human studies confirm the effectiveness of antibiotics in reducing the infectious complications of steroid therapy. Several authors recommend withholding antibiotics until signs of perforation or secondary infection exist.

Questions—Bases

1. **Which of the following is not true of alkaline formulations?**
   A. Most lye ingested prior to 1965 was granular.
   B. Liquid lye causes the same amount of injury as granular lye.
   C. Household bleach products have a pH up to 11.
   D. Drain cleaners have a pH of 14.
   E. Cement on the skin can cause a full-thickness burn.
2. **The critical pH range within which esophageal ulceration occurs is**
   A. 8–9
   B. 9–10
   C. 10–11
   D. 11–12
   E. 12–12.5
3. **Which of the following statements is not true of bases?**
   A. Increased viscosity increases the severity of injury at a given pH.
   B. Water and citric acid in Clinitest® tablets combine with sodium hydroxide to generate heat.
   C. Liquid lye can cause esophageal injury without evidence of oropharyngeal involvement.
   D. At 22.5%, sodium hydroxide causes complete necrosis of the esophagus within 2 minutes.
   E. Increased contact time adds to injury.
4. **Which of the following statements is true concerning alkali ingestion?**
   A. Three-fourths of patients with oral burns have significant esophageal injury.
   B. One-third of patients with oral burns have significant esophageal injury.
   C. Forty-five percent of patients with esophageal injuries have oral burns.
   D. Twenty-five percent of patients with esophageal injuries have oral burns.
   E. A and D
5. **Complications of alkali burns may include which of the following?**
   A. Gastrointestinal hemorrhage
   B. Perforation of the esophagus
   C. Upper airway obstruction
   D. Esophageal strictures
   E. All of the above
6. **Which of the following is not true of the use of diluents in alkali ingestion?**
   A. Milk and water may be helpful to dislodge solid lye particles.
   B. Dilution more than 1 hour after ingestion probably does not help.
   C. The volume of diluent must be large.
   D. Neutralizing agents must not be used.
   E. Catharsis and emesis are contraindicated.
7. **All of the following are clinical presentations of alkali ingestion except**
   A. Dysphagia, odynophagia, vomiting, and abdominal pain
   B. Most patients with esophageal injury complain of pain.
   C. Drooling, inability to swallow, ulceration of the oropharynx
   D. All patients with esophageal injury have external signs.
   E. Occasionally shock and respiratory distress
8. **Which of the following is not true of aspects of the workup of alkali ingestion?**
   A. Respiratory distress is uncommon.
   B. Chest x-ray usually is remarkable for pathology.
   C. One must carefully assess fluid and electrolyte balance.
   D. Alkali injuries to the eye are ophthalmologic emergencies.
   E. Shock suggests perforation.
9. **All of the following are contraindications to esophagoscopy after alkali ingestion except**
   A. Upper airway obstruction
   B. Signs and symptoms of perforation
   C. More than 48 hours since exposure
   D. Shock
   E. None of the above

Case Study (Questions 10 and 11)
A 2-year-old female is brought to the emergency room after the cap from a bottle of Liquid Plum'r is found in her hand and the bottle is discovered spilled nearby. The child is crying and drooling. Examination of the oropharynx is negative.

10. **Which of the following is true with respect to the child's presentation?**
    A. She could have not drunk any of the Liquid Plum'r.
    B. She could have ingested the Liquid Plum'r.
    C. The absence of oropharyngeal lesions does not mean that she has no esophageal lesion.
    D. The drooling may or may not be a significant sign.
    E. All of the above
11. **Workup of the child should include all of the following except**
    A. Obtain vital signs, establish i.v. access, and obtain blood work
    B. Admit the child to the hospital
    C. Consider early esophagoscopy
    D. Allow the child to eat in order to dilute the possible ingestion
    E. After discharge consider a 3-week follow-up to assess for any stricture formation.

BATTERIES

Electronic miniaturization has produced rapid growth in the use of small disc batteries to power hearing aids, calculators, watches, and cameras. Often smaller than a dime, these batteries represent a significant ingestion hazard for children less than 5 years. Fortunately, most disc batteries pass through the gut without producing symptoms. However, impaction of batteries in the esophagus and intestines has led to necrosis, perforation, and rare deaths.

To produce electricity, the disc battery is composed of an anode, a cathode, and an electrolyte-soaked paste that separates the two. A nickel-plated steel can covers the cathode; a brass-plated top covers the anode. A plastic grommet separates the cathode and anode and seals the battery. The three main battery types are alkaline (manganese dioxide cathode, zinc anode), silver oxide (silver oxide cathode, zinc anode), and mercuric oxide (mercuric oxide cathode, zinc anode). Mercuric oxide enhances longevity but increases the potential toxicity of mercury poisoning.

Battery formulations contain varying amounts of heavy metals (lithium hydroxide, nickel hydroxide, manganese dioxide, oxides of mercury, zinc, silver and cadmium) as well as alkaline corrosives. Disc batteries range from 8–25 mm (a dime is 17 mm and a quarter is 23 mm). Size is an important determinant of esophageal impaction since most esophageal perforation case studies to date involved disc batteries larger than 18 mm (the size of an American penny). Disc battery ingestions that most often require intervention are larger manganese batteries (21–23 mm) and mercury batteries.

PATHOPHYSIOLOGY

All severe complications to date involved disc battery impaction with subsequent tissue necrosis. An alkaline camera battery may potentially cause a fatal esophageal perforation characterized by liquefaction necrosis. Tracheoesophageal fistula has occurred after impaction in the esophagus. The mechanism of mucosal erosion probably is multifactorial. Alkaline electrolyte material (40–45% potassium hydroxide) found within these batteries may cause liquefaction necrosis.

Spontaneous leakage from the seal area of the battery may occur after gastric acid bathes the casing. The generation of hydroxide at the anode surface may contribute to necrosis. The electrolyte-rich fluids of the gastrointestinal tract provide a suitable medium for the passage of current between the anode and cathode. Pressure necrosis from impaction may contribute as well.

Mercury toxicity has been a potential concern because inorganic mercury is present in certain disc batteries. Despite the fact that many retrieved disc batteries have been corroded, pitted, or split, only one case of slightly elevated mercury levels has been reported in an asymptomatic patient. Mercuric oxide has corrosive effects but is poorly soluble and slowly absorbed. Gastric acid may further limit absorption by reducing inorganic mercury to metallic mercury, which has minimal potential for absorption.

CLINICAL PRESENTATIONS

The presence of gastrointestinal signs and symptoms suggests necrosis and perforation, since most free-floating disc batteries pass spontaneously without symptoms. Patients with impacted esophageal batteries may present with fever, dysphagia, vomiting, tachypnea, and odynophagia. Intermittent abdominal pain, guarding, tenderness, and vomiting may occur after perforation.

Split disc batteries may produce black, nonmelanotic stool, mild gastrointestinal tract bleeding, vomiting, anorexia, and lassitude. Symptoms of mercury toxicity have not been reported after disc battery ingestions. Black stools most often reflect elemental mercury precipitate rather than gastrointestinal bleeding. The typical transit time of an ingested battery ranges from 14 hours–7 days.

TREATMENT

Gut Decontamination

Syrup of ipecac or other emetics are ineffective and unsafe as the battery may become lodged in the esophagus. There does not appear to be any indication for activated charcoal.

Elimination Enhancement

Whole gut lavage and other methods of elimination enhancement are unnecessary in the treatment of battery ingestions.

Supportive Measures

- An initial roentgenogram should be obtained promptly to determine battery location. Battery size and symptom occurrence cannot be used reliably to detect every patient with a button cell lodged in the esophagus.
- Glucagon 0.05 mg/kg intravenously may be used to relax the esophagus. The usual side effects of glucagon are diarrhea, nausea, and vomiting, which could lead to aspiration when a distal esophageal foreign body is present. Administering the glucagon slowly, over 1 minute can minimize these effects.
- Batteries lodged in the esophagus should be removed immediately. Burns due to esophageal lodgment have occurred as early as 4 hours after ingestion, and perforation has occurred as soon as 6 hours after ingestion. Removal should be done with endoscopy. Neither Foley nor magnetized catheter removal of batteries lodged in the esophagus is highly successful.
- An attempt should be made to identify the battery diameter and chemical system by determining the imprint code of a duplicate battery, by measuring the battery compartment within the product, or by checking product or battery instructions and packaging. Most button cells are 7.9 mm or 11.6 mm in diameter. If the battery can be determined to be one of these sizes, identification of the chemical system is rarely necessary (unless fragmentation or free radiopaque material is documented on roentgenogram).
- Batteries that have passed beyond the esophagus need not be retrieved unless the patient manifests signs or symptoms indicative of injury to the gastrointestinal tract (hematochezia, abdominal pain with tenderness, etc.). Minor gastrointestinal symptoms such as a few episodes of vomiting generally do not necessitate battery removal.
- Stool discoloration alone, in the absence of evidence of gastrointestinal blood or other signs or symptoms, should not prompt battery retrieval. Large-diameter cells, which fail to negotiate the pylorus, will require retrieval.
- Patients with batteries beyond the esophagus can continue normal activity and diet, with outpatient observation. If the patient remains asymptomatic, follow-up roentgenograms are necessary only to confirm battery passage so that patient monitoring and parental consternation can cease. Preferably, battery passage can be confirmed by inspection of all stools.
- More frequent follow-up roentgenograms should be considered, but are by no means mandatory, if a 15.6-mm diameter mercuric oxide cell is ingested (due to the greater likelihood that these cells will split in the gastrointestinal tract). Roentgenograms may be obtained on these patients once or twice weekly.
- If a battery with a diameter of 15 mm or greater is ingested by a child less than 6 years of age, and has not passed within

48 hours, it is unlikely that it will pass, and may require endoscopic retrieval.

- When mercuric oxide cells are ingested, blood and urine mercury levels are necessary only if the cell is observed to split in the gastrointestinal tract or radiopaque droplets are evident in the gut. Chelation therapy need not be initiated in asymptomatic patients unless toxic mercury levels are documented.
- Button batteries lodged in the external auditory canal or nasal cavity must be removed promptly because of their potential to produce dermal necrosis, nasal perforation, or destruction of ossicles. Saline solutions and drops should be avoided prior to removal since these liquids may increase local currents. After removal, the area may be irrigated to remove debris.

Questions—Batteries

1. The following statements are true of battery ingestion except
   A. Batteries represent a significant ingestion hazard for children of all ages.
   B. Most disc batteries pass through the gut without problems.
   C. Impaction of a battery can lead to necrosis and perforation.
   D. Mercuric oxide battery ingestion increases the potential toxicity of mercury poisoning.
   E. Disc batteries range in size from 8–25 mm.

2. Most esophageal perforations due to battery ingestion are cause by batteries that are
   A. 8–10 mm in diameter
   B. 10–12 mm in diameter
   C. 12–17 mm in diameter
   D. 18–25 mm in diameter
   E. None of the above

3. Which of the following is not true of the problems caused by battery ingestion?
   A. All severe complications are associated with tissue necrosis.
   B. The associated tissue necrosis is of the coagulation type.
   C. Tracheoesophageal fistulas have occurred.
   D. Pressure necrosis can occur.
   E. Mercury toxicity is not a significant concern.

4. The typical transit time of a battery ranges from
   A. 4 hours to 5 days
   B. 10 hours to 10 days
   C. 14 hours to 7 days
   D. 14 hours to 10 days
   E. 18 hours to 12 days

5. Supportive measures after battery ingestion include all of the following except
   A. Obtain x-rays to determine the location.
   B. Use glucagon 0.05 mg/kg for esophageal relaxation.
   C. Immediately remove batteries lodged in the esophagus.
   D. Attempt to determine the battery diameter.
   E. Admit all children no matter where the battery is in the GI tract.

MEDICATION-INDUCED ESOPHAGEAL INJURIES

Medication-induced esophageal injury (MIEI) was first described in 1970. Numerous medications have been reported to induce esophageal injury. These include antibiotics such as tetracycline, doxycycline, trimethoprim-sulfa, ampicillin, dicloxacillin, and erythromycin. Other culprits include aspirin, sulindac, dietary fiber, and potassium chloride.

Risk factors for MIEI include abnormal esophageal transit, habit of drug ingestion (e.g., reclining after drug ingestion), form of drug (e.g., anhydrous pill), and taking drugs with little or no fluid. Structural or motility abnormalities increase the risk of esophageal obstruction. These include strictures, Schatzki's rings, esophageal tumors, hiatal hernias, extrinsic compression, and esophagitis. Older age, male gender, left atrial enlargement, ingestion of sustained-release formulations, and prior esophageal structural abnormality may be risk factors for stricture development.

PATHOPHYSIOLOGY

Proposed mechanisms of injury by drugs in medication-induced esophageal injuries include a caustic or acidic effect, hyperosmotic effect, heat production, gastroesophageal reflux, impaired esophageal clearance of acid, and accumulation of drug within the basal squamous epithelium.

CLINICAL PRESENTATIONS

MIEI must be suspected in all patients who present with unexplained esophageal symptoms. Symptoms may include heartburn, vomiting, odynophagia, retrosternal pain, dysphagia, weight loss, abdominal pain, hematemesis, fever, and dehydration. The most common site of MIEI is the mid-esophagus at the level of the aortic arch or the area adjacent to the left atrium. The proximal third of the esophagus is involved in 26% of pill-induced esophageal strictures; 52% are found in the middle third, and 22% of patients experience distal-third injuries.

TREATMENT

Gut Decontamination

Antacids may be soothing. Emesis and charcoal have no role in MIEI.

Elimination Enhancement

These methods play no role in MIEI.

Supportive Measures

- Preventive care is of paramount importance. Patients should remain standing at least 90 seconds after taking all medications. Tablets should be swallowed with at least 100 mL of fluid. Large tablets should preferably be oval and not round. Patients who are bedridden or have difficulty swallowing should be given liquid medication if possible.
- The diagnosis of MIEI can often be suspected by the clinical history alone. Flexible fiberoptic endoscopy is probably the most reliable method for diagnosing MIEI, but endoscopic findings are not by themselves diagnostic. Ulcers at the mid-esophageal region are a clue to MIEI.
- Definitive endoscopic evidence of MIEI must include debris of the drug at the ulcer base, but this is not common. Material may be removed with normal saline irrigation, suction, and forceps. Repeat esophagoscopy is suggested 7–10 days later.
- Symptom resolution and endoscopic healing are generally evident in 3 days–6 weeks.
- Single contrast barium swallow is not sufficiently sensitive in detecting esophageal ulcers, but double contrast barium swallows may be useful.

Questions—Medication-induced Esophageal Injuries

1. Which of the following is not true of medication-induced esophageal injury (MIEI)?
A. Numerous medications can produce such injury.
B. The malady was first described in 1960.
C. Risk factors can include abnormal esophageal transit, and taking drugs without water.
D. Structure abnormalities increase the risk.
E. Tetracycline can cause MIEI.

2. The proposed mechanisms of MIEI include
A. Caustic or acidic effect
B. Hyperosmotic effect
C. Heat production
D. Gastroesophageal reflux
E. All of the above

3. Which of the following is not true of the clinical presentation of MIEI?
A. Symptoms may include heartburn, nausea, vomiting, dysphagia.
B. One can note weight loss.
C. Twenty-six percent of cases of pill-induced stricture involve the proximal third of the esophagus.
D. The most common site is the proximal esophagus above the aortic arch.
E. Twenty-two percent of cases of pill-induced stricture involve the distal third of the esophagus.

AVERSIVES

A number of aversive agents have been used to deter ingestions of dangerous substances. These have included quassin, brucine, bitter aloes, sucrose octaacetate and sucrose benzoate. Denatonium benzoate, which may be the bitterest substance available, was discovered in 1958. It is marketed as Bitrex®. It is an inert odorless material that can be detected by taste at 10 ppb and is recognizably bitter at 50 ppb. The product is now used as an alcohol denaturant, in windshield washes, for oil and tallow denaturing, as an animal repellent, in anti-nailbiting formulations, in finger paints, as a bird-repellent seed dressing, and in rodenticides. It is used in some liquid detergents in the U.S. The role of denatonium benzoate in preventing serious poisoning has yet to be defined.

Questions—Aversives

1. Aversive agents are used for
A. Enhancing medication efficacy
B. Preventing ingestion of dangerous substances
C. Counteracting the effect of medications
D. Counteracting adverse attitudes toward medications
E. None of the above

2. Which of the following is not true of denatonium benzoate?
A. It may be the bitterest substance available.
B. It was discovered in 1958.
C. It is inert and odorless.
D. It has the brand name of Bitrex®.
E. It has a clearly defined role in serious poisoning.

BEZOARS

Bezoars are intraintestinal masses composed of accumulated ingested drugs or other materials. The word bezoar means antidote, and it is believed to derive either from the Hebrew word *beluzaar*, the Arabic word *bedzehr*, or the Persian word *padzahr*. Bezoars were, at various times, thought to cure a variety of ailments, neutralize poisons, and rejuvenate the aged.

Concretions represent medications that form a gastric mass. Medications reported to cause bezoars or concretions include aluminum hydroxide, aspirin, bromide, calcium phosphate, cholestyramine, cyanocobalamin (vitamin B12), iron, meprobamate, nifedipine, sodium polystyrene sulfonate, sucralfate, theophylline (sustained-release), and vitamin C. Of these, aluminum hydroxide, aspirin (coated/buffered), calcium combinations, cyanocobalamin, iron, sucralfate and some vitamins have been reported to be radiopaque. Those reported not to be radiopaque include meprobamate, nifedipine, theophylline, bromide, cholestyramine and sodium polystyrene sulfonate.

PATHOPHYSIOLOGY

Phytobezoars

These bezoars consist of vegetable products or concretions of citrus fruit. Persimmons, fruit stones, raisins, grape skins, oranges, peaches, apples, bran, figs, husks of oats or psyllium, and peanuts are the foods most commonly found. This group constitutes as many as 40% of all bezoars. They are largely afflictions of adult males and are more frequent following the increased incidence of gastric resection and vagotomy for peptic ulcer disease.

Trichobezoars

These are concretions of human or animal hairs, or synthetic or natural fibers, which are usually found in the stomach or small intestine. Patients frequently are young women between the ages of 15 and 20 years with long hair who are often mentally retarded, have psychiatric problems, or engage in trichotillomania. Mixed bezoars are combinations of hair and vegetable matter.

Lactobezoars

These are undigested milk concretions generally reported within the first year of life. These are associated with feedings of incorrectly prepared powdered formula, ingestion of undiluted concentrated formula, and ingestion of certain infant formulas.

CLINICAL PRESENTATIONS

Patients often present with an epigastric mass, abdominal pain, nausea, vomiting, hematemesis, weight loss, lethargy, diarrhea, or constipation. Severe vomiting may occur in cases of gastric outlet obstruction. Anemia, halitosis, anorexia, flatulence, and presence of foreign material in the vomitus may also occur. There may be no symptoms as well. Complications may include bleeding, obstruction with metabolic abnormalities, perforation complicated by peritonitis, and gastrocutaneous or colocutaneous fistulas.

TREATMENT

Gut Decontamination

Gastric dilatation and intraluminal gastric mass with irregular surface contours separate from the gastric mucosa may be seen on contrast study of the upper gastrointestinal tract. Gastroscopy with biopsy, echography, and analysis of stool contents are also useful. Esophageal bezoars may be visualized by endoscopy. Emesis and charcoal serve no role.

Elimination Enhancement

These methods are irrelevant in the treatment of concretions per se. Individual agents such as aspirin; however, may require dialysis in severe cases.

Supportive Measures

- Esophageal bezoars are treated with bougienage, endoscopy and manipulation.
- Gastric bezoars are treated with endoscopy. Irrigation of the stomach with 0.9% sodium chloride solution or papain (e.g., meat tenderizer) has yielded inconsistent results. Caution must be exercised in using Adolph's Meat Tenderizer® in view of a report of hypernatremia and confusion in a 65-year-old patient following its use for treatment of a phytobezoar.
- Limited experience suggests that acetylcysteine may enhance dissolution of gastric mucous, which may encase cellulose bezoars.
- Small bowel bezoars may require enterotomy in severe cases.
- Surgery may be useful when bleeding, obstruction, or perforation has occurred. If a large bezoar is present, gastrotomy, enterotomy, or bowel resection may be the treatment of choice.

Questions—Bezoars

1. **Bezoars, i.e., intestinal masses, can be**
   A. Vegetable products
   B. Concretions of hair, fibers, etc.
   C. Undigested milk concretions
   D. All of the above
   E. None of the above
2. **Which of the following is not true of the clinical presentation of bezoars?**
   A. All patients are symptomatic.
   B. There can be severe nausea and vomiting.
   C. Anemia and weight loss can occur.
   D. One can have diarrhea or constipation.
   E. Complications can include gastrocutaneous or colocutaneous fistulas.

Answers

Introduction to Acids

1. D 2. E 3. E 4. B 5. B

Acetic Acid

1. E 2. E

Formic Acid

1. E 2. D 3. B 4. E 5. A

Hydrofluoric Acid

1. E 2. E 3. E 4. E

Monochloroacetic Acid

1. C 2. E

Oxalic Acid

1. E 2. A

Bases

1. B 2. E 3. D 4. B 5. E 6. C
7. D 8. B 9. D 10. E 11. D

Batteries

1. A 2. D 3. B 4. C 5. E

Medication-induced Esophageal Injuries

1. B 2. E 3. D

Aversives

1. B 2. E

Bezoars

1. D 2. A

SELECTED READINGS

Acids

1. Caravati EM. Acute hydrofluoric acid exposure. Am J Emerg Med 1988;6: 143–150.
2. El Saadi MS, Hall AH, Hall PK, et al. Hydrofluoric acid dermal exposure. Vet Hum Toxicol 1989;31:243–247.
3. Friedman EM, Lovejoy FH. The emergency management of caustic ingestions. Emerg Med Clin North Am 1984;2:77–80.
4. Klein-Schwartz W, Oderda GM. Management of corrosive ingestions. Clin Toxicol Consult 1983;5:39–55.
5. Penner GE. Acid ingestion: toxicology and treatment. Ann Emerg Med 1980; 9:374–379.
6. Rajan N, Rabim R, Kumar SK. Formic acid poisoning with suicidal intent: a report of 53 cases. Postgrad Med J 1985;61:35–36.
7. Upfal M, Doyle C. Medical management of hydrofluoric acid exposure. J Occup Med 1990;32:726–731.
8. Woolf A. Oxalates. Clin Toxicol Rev 1993;16:1–2.

Bases

1. Friedman EM, Lovejoy FH. The emergency management of caustic ingestions. Emerg Med Clin North Am 1984;2:77–86.
2. Howell JM, Dalsey WC, Hartsell FW, et al. Steroids for the treatment of corrosive esophageal injury. A statistical analysis of past studies. Am J Emerg Med 1992; 10:421–425.
3. Moore WR. Caustic ingestions: pathophysiology, diagnosis, and treatment. Clin Pediatr 1986;25:192–196.
4. Thompson JN. Corrosive esophageal injuries. I. A study of nine cases of concurrent accidental caustic ingestion. Laryngoscope 1987;97:1060–1068.

Batteries

1. Litovitz T, Schmitz BF. Ingestion of cylindrical and button batteries: an analysis of 2382 cases. Pediatrics 1992;89:747-757. Commentary by K. Kulig in AACT Update 1992;5(4):1–2.
2. Litovitz TL. Button battery ingestions: a review of 56 cases. JAMA 1983;249: 2495–2500.

Medication-induced Esophageal Injuries

1. Bott S, Prokash C, McCallum RW. Medication-induced esophageal injury. Survey of the literature. Am J Gastroenterol 1987;82:758–763.
2. Ovartlarnporn B, Kulwichit W, Hiranniramol S. Medication-induced esophageal injury. Report of 17 cases with endoscopic documentation. Am J Gastroenterol 1991;86:748–750.
3. Perry PA, Dean BS, Krenzelok EP. Drug-induced esophageal injury. Vet Hum Toxicol 1988;30:349.

Aversives

1. Hansen SR, Janssen C, Beasley VR. Denatonium benzoate as a deterrent to ingestion of toxic substance: toxicity and efficacy. Vet Hum Toxicol 1993; 234–236.
2. Sibert JR, Frude N. Bittering agents in the prevention of accidental poisoning: children's reaction to denatonium benzoate (Bitrex). Arch Emerg Med 1991; 8:1–7.

Bezoars

1. Andrus CH, Ponsky JL. Bezoars: classification, pathophysiology and treatment. Am J Gastroenterol 1988;83:476–478.
2. DePiro JT, Bowden TA Jr. Treatment of gastric bezoars. Clin Pharm 1989; 8:181–182.

ACKNOWLEDGMENT

Thanks to Blake L. Powell, MD, JD for contributing the questions in this chapter.

CHAPTER 43
Anesthetic Agents

INTRODUCTION

Anesthetic agents may be administered intravenously, intramuscularly, rectally, orally, or by inhalation. They may be given locally, regionally, via the epidural space, or topically. They have become a ubiquitous part of modern medical practice, and a number of relevant issues have arisen surrounding their use.

Drug abuse among hospital personnel, especially anesthesia personnel, is a serious, ongoing problem. Alcohol, narcotics, barbiturates, tranquilizers, and nitrous oxide have been implicated in numerous deaths. Drugs that tempt the abuser can be stolen readily from anesthesia services. These include nitrous oxide, halogenated anesthetics, opiates, barbiturates, tranquilizers, and ketamine.

Death may follow accidental overdose or suicide. Everyone associated with the clinical use of these agents must be made aware of their potential for abuse and the potential of sudden death during abuse. Access to these drugs should be restricted to anesthetists for their immediate use. Cylinders and containers should be labeled to indicate that a suffocation hazard may exist.

A relation between exposure to anesthetics and the incidence of chronic diseases such as cancer, leukemia, and liver and kidney disease has not been firmly demonstrated. Immunologic disturbances may be found in anesthetic personnel chronically exposed to high occupational concentrations of nitrous oxide and halothane.

Toxic Dosage/Death

Anesthesia has been associated with a low mortality in recent years, but it is still associated with significant morbidity. Human error remains an important factor in the causation of anesthesia faults, near accidents, and accidents. A number of terms have been devised to aid in describing anesthetic errors.

Aspiration of gastric contents with a pH of 3.5 or less into the lungs may follow vomiting and regurgitation during general anesthesia. Pulmonary inflammation, destruction of the alveolar lining, and transudation of fluid into the alveolar space occur rapidly. This syndrome continues to be a cause of maternal mortality after cesarean section. The patient may become tachypneic, hypoxic, and febrile. The leukocyte count may rise, and the chest x-ray may suddenly change from normal to a complete white-out within 8 to 24 hours. Acid aspiration prophylaxis, consisting of an H2 receptor antagonist such as ranitidine, may be helpful.

A "fault" is a procedure that has resulted (or could have resulted) in injury or harm to a patient, while this injury or harm (or chance thereof) could have been prevented by another procedure. An "accident" represents any event except a fault or a complication that has resulted in harm or injury to a patient. A "near accident" is an event that could have developed into a fault, a complication, or an accident but that was prevented by chance or by a previously unplanned intervention. A "complication" represents harm or injury to a patient occurring as a result of a known risk of a treatment or a diagnostic procedure.

Pregnancy/Lactation

Mortality during anesthesia does not appear to be different in pregnant women from that of women who are not pregnant. There is also no good evidence to suggest that any particular anesthetic technique will induce preterm labor. Any drug that readily passes into the central nervous system can generally reach the fetus. Intravenous sedatives that have an effect on the central nervous system can generally cross the placenta. Water-soluble drugs that are highly ionized, such as muscle relaxants, do not cross the placenta to any great extent. A U.S. Center for Disease Control (CDC) study has suggested an increased risk for hydrocephalus and eye defects in babies born to mothers exposed to first-trimester general anesthesia.

Atracurium and curare cross the placenta poorly. Benzodiazepines cross the placenta. See Chapter 28, Psychotropic Drugs. Uterine muscle is relaxed by enflurane. Uterine response to oxytocin is maintained during enflurane use, if high inspired concentrations (over 2.5–3.0%) are not employed. Etomidate is considered safe and effective induction during cesarean section.

Fentanyl derivatives may cause maternal delay in gastric emptying, rigidity of the chest wall, and difficulty with ventilation during anesthesia induction. Neonatal rigidity of the chest wall has been seen. No teratogenic abnormalities have been seen with the use of narcotics. The U.S. Food and Drug Administration (FDA) has placed fentanyl in pregnancy risk category C. Fentanyl is excreted in human milk and is not recommended for use in nursing women.

Halothane produces dose-dependent relaxation of uterine muscle in both pregnant and nonpregnant women. During labor and delivery it may cause uterine atony accompanied by increased blood loss. Isoflurane induces uterine relaxation. Placental transfer is rapid with ketamine. Nitrous oxide also crosses the placenta and at least one large prospective study has shown the safety of nitrous oxide in early pregnancy.

Pancuronium, succinylcholine and propofol cross the placenta. Vecuronium does not cross the placenta as readily as pancuronium. No adverse effects on infants have been identified with propofol use; however, more study is required. Thiopental is transferred from the human maternal circulation into placental tissue during the first trimester of pregnancy and at term.

Laboratory

ANALYTIC METHODS

The vapors of anesthetic gases such as enflurane, halothane, and isoflurane can be monitored with charcoal tubes. Nitrous oxide can be monitored with a direct-reading infrared analyzer or by passive dosimeters. Records of all collected air samples should be kept, and results should be noted in the medical records of corresponding workers.

BLOOD LEVELS

Following blood levels is generally unhelpful in treating anesthetic complications, although confirmation at autopsy may be helpful in certain cases.

Treatment

GUT DECONTAMINATION

These methods are generally not utilized in treating anesthetic complications.

ELIMINATION ENHANCEMENT

These methods are generally not utilized in treating anesthetic complications.

SUPPORTIVE MEASURES

- Operating room workers can protect themselves from excess exposure by properly connecting the scavenging equipment, turning the gas off when the breathing system is disconnected from the patient, and ensuring that all patients have properly fitting masks.
- Workers exposed to anesthetic gas should have complete medical histories on file. These should include family, genetic, and occupational histories and the outcome of all pregnancies of female workers and of the wives of male workers.
- Baseline data should be obtained on the hepatic, renal, and hematopoietic systems. Exposed workers should be monitored periodically for liver and kidney function.

Antidotes

Please see individual agents below regarding specific antidotal therapies.

Questions—Introduction to Anesthetic Agents

1. Which of the following associations with anesthetics has been firmly demonstrated?
A. Cancer
B. Leukemia
C. Liver disease
D. Kidney disease
E. None of the above

2. Which term is correctly defined?
A. Fault: Injury to a patient occurring as a result of a known risk of a treatment
B. Accident: Procedure that resulted in harm that could have been prevented
C. Near accident: Event that could have developed into a fault, a complication, or an accident but that was prevented by chance
D. Complication: Any event, except a fault, that has resulted in harm or injury to a patient
E. None of the above

3. Which of the following statements about pregnancy and anesthetics is true?
A. Mortality during anesthesia differs significantly in pregnant women from that of women who are not pregnant.
B. There is no good evidence to suggest that any particular anesthetic technique will induce preterm labor.
C. There is no relationship between a drug's ability to pass into the central nervous system and its ability to reach the fetus.
D. Atracurium and curare cross the placenta easily.
E. None of the above

MALIGNANT HYPERTHERMIA

Malignant hyperthermia (MH) is a rare, inherited, life-threatening disorder of skeletal muscle calcium regulation that is associated with a hypermetabolic state. It is most often initiated by volatile anesthetic agents and is estimated to occur in 1 in 15,000 general anesthetics. Children less than 5 years of age have comprised about half of all MH cases. Males account for about three-fourths of all reported MH fatalities.

Genetically predisposed individuals may suffer from MH after being exposed to drugs such as skeletal muscle relaxants (succinylcholine, decamethonium, gallamine, d-tubocurarine), all inhalational anesthetics, and local anesthetics (mainly amide-type such as lidocaine, mepivacaine, and bupivacaine). A variety of other drugs have been implicated, but data suggest they rarely precipitate an MH crisis but rather exacerbate a preexisting one. Stress, high temperatures, emotional excitement, severe muscle exercise, and infections have been associated with malignant hyperthermia.

Pathophysiology

The sarcoplasmic reticulum of the muscle cell normally takes up calcium during muscle relaxation and releases calcium to the myoplasm during contraction. Although not entirely elucidated, MH is believed to occur following a decrease in calcium uptake by the sarcoplasmic reticulum. The subsequent increase in myoplasmic calcium initiates a number of aerobic and anaerobic metabolic processes, which result in heat, carbon dioxide, and lactic acid production.

Clinical Presentations

The management of MH depends largely on early recognition of this syndrome by careful and routine monitoring during anesthesia. The anesthesiologist should entertain the diagnosis if any of numerous signs occur. These include unexplained tachycardia, unexplained cyanosis and tachypnea, rigidity after succinylcholine administration, or failure of the masseters to relax for intubation. The rigidity may present at any time or may never occur.

Later indications include marked hyperthermia, increased end-tidal CO_2, and increased mixed venous CO_2. The normal anesthetized patient does not become hyperthermic if the room temperature is below 25.5°C. Any rise in temperature of more than 0.5°C in 15 minutes should be regarded as possible malignant hyperthermia. Fever is a late sign and carries a poor prognosis if therapy has not yet been started. Other signs include hypotension, complex arrhythmias, respiratory and/or meta-

Answers to questions in shaded boxes appear at the end of the chapter.

bolic acidosis, electrolyte disturbances, hyperkalemia, hypercalcemia, rhabdomyolysis, disseminated intravascular coagulation, renal failure, and pulmonary edema.

MH shares some traits with neuroleptic malignant syndrome (NMS); however, the two can be distinguished. MH occurs within minutes of starting anesthesia and NMS usually develops over a longer period. MH is a genetic disorder and NMS has no specific genetic component. Succinylcholine and general anesthetics may be a triggering factor for MH, whereas patients with NMS who have been given succinylcholine and general anesthesia generally have no toxic effects. Neuroleptic analgesia has been used successfully in patients who are susceptible to MH.

Toxic Dosage/Death

Death may follow conversion of an ectopic ventricular arrhythmia into ventricular fibrillation, acute disseminated intravascular coagulopathy, acute pulmonary edema, acute myoglobinemia, renal failure, or cerebral edema with brain death.

Laboratory

ANALYTIC METHODS

Several invasive screening tests for MH susceptibility have been developed and standardized. Muscle biopsy specimens are exposed to halothane alone, caffeine alone, or halothane and caffeine together. Halothane and caffeine contracture tests appear somewhat indicative of MH susceptibility, but in view of the relative rarity of the MH reaction, the practicability of these tests as a screening method is questionable. Further refinements of MH tests are required before general acceptance and routine use can be validated. Detection of clinical episodes of MH continues to remain the responsibility of the anesthetist during a surgical procedure.

BLOOD LEVELS

There are no identifiable blood levels that help in identifying or managing this syndrome.

Treatment

GUT DECONTAMINATION

These methods are not applicable to the treatment of malignant hyperthermia. Ice water lavage may help decrease the core temperature, but does not reduce the causative potential toxin in any way.

ELIMINATION ENHANCEMENT

These methods are not immediately applied to the treatment of MH. However, dialysis following rhabdomyolysis may be required.

SUPPORTIVE MEASURES

- Certain questions may be useful in identifying persons who may need further counseling regarding the possible presence of the MH trait. Inquiries regarding family members who have had unusual anesthetic experiences may be helpful. Inquiries regarding unexplained CPK elevation, unusual muscle cramping, and caffeine intolerance may be helpful as well.
- Anesthesia for susceptible patients may involve pretreatment with dantrolene, depending on the likelihood of MH. The patient may be premedicated with fentanyl, droperidol, or both. Local or regional anesthesia is preferred. Propofol may be safe for induction. If general anesthesia is necessary, thiopental, fentanyl, and droperidol may be used.
- Acute-phase treatment involves immediately discontinuing all volatile inhalation anesthetics and succinylcholine, and hyperventilation with 100% oxygen.
- Hyperkalemia is common and may be treated with bicarbonate, intravenous glucose, and insulin (10 units of regular insulin with 50 mL of 50% glucose). Life-threatening hyperkalemia may also be treated with calcium administration (e.g., 2–5 mg/kg of calcium chloride).
- Bicarbonate may also be administered to correct profound metabolic acidosis as guided by blood gas analysis. In the absence of blood gas analysis, 1–2 mEq/kg should be administered.
- Actively cool the hyperthermic patient. Cooled saline may be used, in addition to cooling blankets, ice pack application, and ice water lavage. Monitor closely since vigorous treatment may lead to hypothermia.
- Dysrhythmias will usually respond to treatment of acidosis and hyperkalemia. If they persist or are life-threatening, standard antiarrhythmic agents may be used, with the exception of calcium channel blockers, which may cause hyperkalemia and cardiovascular collapse in this setting.
- Determine and monitor end-tidal CO_2, arterial, central, or femoral venous blood gases, serum potassium, calcium, clotting studies, and urine output.
- Ensure urine output of greater than 2 mL/kg/hr. This may require furosemide and/or mannitol in severe cases. Consider central venous or PA monitoring because of potential fluid shifts and hemodynamic instability.

Antidotes

DANTROLENE

Dantrolene (see also Chapter 12, Muscle Relaxants and Chapter 5, Antidotes) appears to decrease calcium release from the sarcoplasmic reticulum and lowers intracellular calcium levels. Administration of dantrolene early in an MH episode generally halts progression of the syndrome. A starting dose of 2.5 mg/kg with sterile distilled water is given intravenously. Each vial of dantrolene also contains mannitol. Dantrolene may be repeated every 5–10 minutes until a total dose of 10 mg/kg is given if symptoms persist. Continue dantrolene for 3 days after the episode to prevent recurrence. The oral dosage is 1–2 mg/kg/day in divided doses.

Questions—Malignant Hyperthermia

1. Which of the following has been associated with malignant hyperthermia?
A. Succinylcholine
B. Lidocaine
C. High environmental temperatures
D. Emotional excitement
E. All of the above

2. Any rise in temperature of the patient undergoing anesthesia of more than 0.5°C in 15 minutes should be regarded as possible malignant hyperthermia.
A. True
B. False

3. **Which of the following is a true distinction between neuroleptic malignant syndrome and malignant hyperthermia?**
   A. MH occurs within minutes of anesthesia and NMS usually develops over a longer period.
   B. MH is a genetic disorder and NMS has no specific genetic component.
   C. Succinylcholine and general anesthetics may be a triggering factor for NMS, whereas patients with MH who have been given succinylcholine and general anesthesia generally have no toxic effects.
   D. A and B
   E. A and C

4. **Treatment of malignant hyperthermia may include**
   A. Gut decontamination
   B. Ice water lavage
   C. Measurement of blood levels to help in identifying or managing this syndrome
   D. Prophylactic treatment for hypokalemia
   E. All of the above

5. **Which of the following is false regarding use of dantrolene in MH?**
   A. It appears to decrease calcium release from the sarcoplasmic reticulum.
   B. Administration of dantrolene early generally halts progression of the syndrome.
   C. A starting dose of 25 mg/kg with sterile distilled water is given intravenously.
   D. Dantrolene may be repeated every 5–10 minutes until a total dose of 10 mg/kg is given if symptoms persist.
   E. Dantrolene may be continued for 3 days after the episode to prevent recurrence.

INHALATION ANESTHETICS

Inhalation anesthetics are widely used because of their ability to induce anesthesia rapidly, their relative ease of control, and their ease and safety of recovery. The most widely used inhalation anesthetics are nitrous oxide, halothane, enflurane, sevoflurane, and isoflurane. Their anesthetic action is related to their partial pressure in the brain, which is more directly reflected by their alveolar partial pressure.

The wrong vaporizer for a given agent, or a vaporizer connected in series, rather than parallel, can produce overdosage. Accidental overdosage can also result from confusion regarding the "ON/OFF" rotation direction of certain controls or unfamiliarity with different equipment. Operating room personnel illicitly abusing halothane have left vaporizers on. Certain anesthetic agents, particularly nitrous oxide, have been abused as well. See the section on Inhalation Abuse in Chapter 45, Airborne Toxins.

Pathophysiology

Pharmacologically active products of biotransformation generally cause the toxicity of inhalation anesthetics. Other mechanisms for toxicity include anesthetic protein interactions and anesthetic tissue interactions. Halothane, enflurane, and isoflurane have all been involved in serious and fatal overdose reactions. Dose-related respiratory depression follows direct effects on the medullary respiratory centers, thoracic respiratory muscles, and diaphragm.

Pharmacokinetics

ABSORPTION

- The uptake and distribution of an inhalation anesthetic depends on the inhaled concentration, pulmonary ventilation, solubility in blood, cardiac output, and tissue uptake.

DISTRIBUTION

- Concentration gradients developed during general anesthesia in descending order are delivered, inspired alveolar, arterial, and brain.

ELIMINATION

- Nitrous oxide is eliminated through the lungs.

Clinical Presentations

There is little evidence that enflurane, halothane, or isoflurane represent a hazard to the staff of operating areas that are well ventilated with scavenging devices. High occupational exposure may lead to hepatic microsomal drug metabolizing enzyme induction.

CYCLOPROPANE

Death has very rarely been reported after overdose with cyclopropane.

DESFLURANE

As with isoflurane, the use of desflurane may result in increases in brain volume or intracranial pressure. Its use in the neurosurgical patient should therefore be carefully considered. Desflurane with controlled ventilation and constant $PaCO_2$ can cause cardiovascular depression. Cardiac output is well maintained.

ENFLURANE

High levels of inorganic fluoride have not been toxic. Enflurane prolongs the QTc interval without altering the QRS, PR, or QT intervals. Rare fatal hepatic necrosis may follow repeated enflurane anesthesia. Clinical, biochemical, and histologic features of enflurane anesthesia-associated hepatitis are similar to those seen with halothane-related hepatitis. Seizures without loss of consciousness may follow enflurane use.

HALOTHANE

Halothane-associated hepatitis presents as one of two clinical syndromes occurring most often in adult patients. These syndromes may develop after uneventful anesthesia and surgery, with no apparent time-dose relationship. One syndrome is characterized by moderate increases in the aminotransferase concentration and occasional transient jaundice. There is a low morbidity. It may occur after an initial exposure to halothane, and its incidence may be up to 20%.

The second syndrome occurs in one of 35,000 anesthetics, is associated with repeated exposure to the drug administered frequently at short intervals, and is associated with the development of fulminant hepatic failure with high mortality. Halothane administered to adults does not appear to significantly alter the PR or QRS intervals, but does increase the QT and QTc intervals.

ISOFLURANE

Hepatotoxicity is usually not seen in isoflurane anesthesia unless there is severe hypoxia present. Isoflurane use can cause increased intracranial pressure. Isoflurane anesthesia does not appear to significantly change the QRS, PR, or QT intervals, but significantly prolongs the QTc interval. Isoflurane may rarely be associated with malignant hyperthermia.

NITROUS OXIDE

Anesthesia with nitrous oxide in normal humans for 2–4 hours has induced tachypnea, tachycardia, increased systemic blood pressure, atrioventricular junctional rhythm, acute cardiovascular failure, mydriasis, diaphoresis, and occasional clonus and opisthotonus. Repeated abuse of nitrous oxide may induce bone marrow depression. Careful hematologic evaluation, including folate and vitamin B12 blood levels, may be indicated.

Signs of severe vitamin B12 and folic acid deficiency after a single operative exposure to nitrous oxide are rare. The prolonged use of nitrous oxide (i.e., for days) may result in aplastic anemia, neuronal degeneration, megaloblastic changes, and death. It may depress respiration and circulation and increase muscle tone, resulting in increasing dose requirements for muscle relaxants.

Toxic Dosage/Death

The U.S. National Institute for Occupational Safety and Health (NIOSH) has recommended exposure limits for numerous anesthetic gases. Death from these agents is quite unusual. Intravenous and oral halothane exposures have been survived; however, a 3-mL mixture of halothane and methohexital given intravenously was fatal to a 20-year-old woman who died with acute pulmonary edema. Ingestion of 35 mL of halothane by an adult has ended fatally as well. Ingestion of 150 to 200 mL of halothane by an adult led to coma and survival. A 48-year-old patient survived an ingestion of 250 mL of halothane after a coma of 36 hours.

Inhalation of 10.2% isoflurane has led to cyanosis and shock. Ingestion of 80 mL of isoflurane by a 37-year-old man terminated fatally. Inhalation of 250 mL of enflurane led to the death of a 29-year-old female. Exposure to 50–70% nitrous oxide for 3 hours may decrease hepatic methionine synthase activity and may result in aplastic anemia and death.

Drug Interactions

Isoflurane has caused a significant increase in the action of atracurium and vecuronium. Nalbuphine reduces isoflurane requirements. Isoflurane appears to inhibit enflurane metabolism in humans. Nitrous oxide may reduce the therapeutic benefits and increase the side effects of methotrexate therapy. AV dissociation may be observed when epinephrine with lidocaine is used in a patient receiving nitrous oxide.

Ventricular irritability has been observed in adults undergoing halothane-induced anesthesia when epinephrine or lidocaine has also been administered. Halothane administered to children with up to 10 mg/mL of epinephrine by infiltration appears to be a relatively safe combination in normocarbic and hypocarbic pediatric patients without congenital heart disease. Children appear less susceptible to the more serious ventricular arrhythmogenic effects of epinephrine.

Nitrous oxide added to steady-state halogen-oxygen anesthesia may increase mean arterial pressure, right atrial pressure, and systemic vascular resistance. Cardiac arrest has followed halothane use with verapamil and fenfluramine. Halothane may potentiate neuromuscular blocking drugs.

Pregnancy/Lactation

Inhalation anesthetics usually present no hazard to the nursing infant. Lactating mothers who need surgery usually tolerate these agents well by not nursing for 12 to 24 hours, by which time virtually all anesthetic agents are gone from maternal blood. Please see the Introduction to this chapter for relevant information about specific agents.

Laboratory

ANALYTIC METHODS

By measuring and monitoring the alveolar partial pressure (by mass spectrometry), the anesthesiologist is able to control the depth of anesthesia.

BLOOD LEVELS

Blood levels are not utilized in treating overdoses with these agents.

Treatment

- Following the discovery of an overdose of an inhalation anesthetic, immediate measures should include discontinuation of the anesthetic, applying principles of cardiopulmonary resuscitation as indicated, and flushing the anesthetic circuit with 100% oxygen.
- Continuous cardiac monitoring, a supply of oxygen, and intravenous lines should be established. If the patient has not been provided with an endotracheal tube, this should be put in place immediately. Mechanical ventilation should be provided as indicated.
- Oxygen and positive end-expiratory pressure ventilation may ameliorate hypoxia.
- Blood is drawn for arterial blood gases, liver enzymes, B12 blood level, and creatinine, as well as electrolytes.
- β-2 adrenergic antagonists (e.g., salbutamol), oxygen, and mechanical ventilation may be administered for bronchospasm.
- Seizures can be treated with intravenous diazepam and phenytoin if required.
- Pulmonary edema may respond to oxygen, and furosemide. Continuous cardiac monitoring and serial arterial blood gases will be indicated.
- Avoid central nervous system or respiratory depressants.
- A surgical procedure may need to be discontinued if an adverse effect occurs during surgery. If the anesthesiologist and surgeon agree, a procedure may proceed with another anesthetic. This should be carefully weighed with the risk of enhancing hemodynamic stability in an already compromised patient.

Questions—Inhalation Anesthetics

1. Which of the following statements is true?

A. High occupational exposure may lead to hepatic microsomal enzyme induction.
B. Nitrous oxide is eliminated through hepatic metabolism.
C. Much evidence confirms that enflurane, halothane, and isoflurane each represent a hazard to the staff of operating areas, even if the areas are well ventilated with scavenging devices.
D. Neither halothane nor isoflurane has been involved in serious or fatal overdose reactions.
E. All of the above

2. Which of the following inhaled anesthetics is inaccurately described?
- A. Desflurane may result in increases in brain volume or intracranial pressure.
- B. Enflurane prolongs the QTc interval without altering the QRS, PR, or QT intervals.
- C. Halothane-associated hepatitis presents as one of two clinical syndromes occurring most often in adult patients.
- D. Isoflurane is often associated with malignant hyperthermia or hepatotoxicity.
- E. Repeated abuse of nitrous oxide may induce bone marrow depression.

3. There are no recommended exposure limits for any anesthetic gases.
- A. True
- B. False

4. Regarding halothane-associated hepatitis,
- A. It presents as one of two clinical syndromes occurring most often in pediatric patients.
- B. One syndrome is characterized by moderate increases in the aminotransferase concentration and occasional transient jaundice.
- C. The second syndrome occurs in one of 35,000 anesthetics, is associated with repeated exposure to the drug administered frequently at short intervals, and is associated with the development of fulminant hepatic failure with high mortality.
- D. All of the above
- E. B and C

INTRAVENOUS AND TRANSDERMAL ANESTHETICS

The first effective intravenous anesthetic induction agent, hexobarbital, was introduced into clinical practice in Germany in 1932. Thiopental, introduced in 1934 in the United States, remains a widely used intravenous induction agent.

Droperidol is a synthetic butyrophenone derivative similar in chemical structure to haloperidol. It is frequently administered together with fentanyl as a neuroleptic. Droperidol is a powerful antiemetic often used to treat opiate-induced vomiting. It exhibits extrapyramidal side effects and may cause hypotension due to its central nervous system and α-adrenergic blocking properties. Etomidate is a γ-aminobutyric acid (GABA)-mimetic. It is a short-acting, nonbarbiturate sedative-hypnotic agent that lacks analgesic properties, and is used largely for induction.

Fentanyl and fentanyl derivatives are powerful opiate analgesics frequently used in anesthesia. Illicit production of these agents constitutes a designer drug problem in certain addicts. See Chapter 24, Designer Drugs. The U.S. Food and Drug Administration approved a Fentanyl Transdermal System (FTS, Duragesic®) in 1991. FTS can provide up to 72 hours of analgesia with each application and can maintain predictable plasma concentrations with chronic dosage. Excess absorption of fentanyl from this system may result in symptoms of an opioid overdose.

Ketamine, a synthetic chemical, is used as a general anesthetic during surgery. Ketamine was developed because of dissatisfaction with its chemical relative, phencyclidine, as a surgical anesthetic drug. See Chapter 22, Phencyclidine. Street use of ketamine by injection was first observed in San Francisco and Los Angeles in 1971. In his 1976 film, *Family Plot,* Alfred Hitchcock depicted a kidnap victim sedated with ketamine.

Propofol is a synthetic, intravenous, sedative-hypnotic anesthetic that may, in overdose, or after inadvertent intraarterial injection, induce cardiovascular and respiratory depression. Propofol is safe in those who are susceptible to malignant hyperthermia. Propofol has successfully controlled seizures in status epilepticus.

Pathophysiology

Doses of nonopioid drugs can be injected as a bolus intravenously to induce anesthesia, or administered by continuous infusion for partial or complete maintenance of anesthesia. Fentanyl is a potent opioid analgesic that interacts with the opioid μ-receptor and may cause profound respiratory depression. Please see Chapter 23, Opiates for additional details.

Ketamine analgesia is mediated partially by the opioid μ-receptor. Ketamine interacts with sigma and phencyclidine binding sites. The sigma and phencyclidine component may mediate the dysphoria induced by ketamine. Ketamine's sites of action, NMDA (N-methyl-d-aspartate) receptors, play a major role in the transmission of sensory information. Phencyclidine and ketamine are noncompetitive NMDA antagonists. They bind to a site that is distinct from NMDA. Ketamine is 10–50 times less potent than phencyclidine in blocking NMDA-mediated neurotoxicity, seizures, and physiologic effects and in substituting for phencyclidine in drug discrimination paradigms.

Clinical Presentations

Involuntary movements and hypertonus are seen with all intravenous agents when given to the unpremedicated patient. The incidence varies among agents. Thiopental has an incidence of about 8%, and muscle movements following etomidate use may occur in as many as 95% of patients. The rate is about 30–35% with methohexital, and 14% following propofol use. The incidence depends on the dose of drug administered and whether premedication was used.

All of the intravenous hypnotic agents used for the induction of anesthesia can cause pain on injection and postoperative venous sequelae. Incidences of such sequelae are low when veins of the antecubital fossa are employed, but rise by four- or five-fold when injections are made into the dorsum of the hand. Accidental injection of intravenous agents directly into an artery may result in marked sequelae. Red cell hemolysis and platelet aggregation may occur, leading to intravascular thrombosis. Severe tissue necrosis may result in amputation of affected tissue.

ALFENTANIL

Alfentanil is a structural analog of fentanyl that is about one-fourth as potent as fentanyl and has one-third the duration of action. It appears to have a relative lack of adverse cardiovascular effects. Alfentanil used for rapid sequence intubation produces less muscular rigidity than fentanyl.

DROPERIDOL

In patients who are hypovolemic or who are receiving vasodilator therapy, droperidol can induce profound hypotension. Arrhythmias and respiratory side effects are minimal. Droperidol has no analgesic effect. Overdose may lead to reversible Parkinsonism.

ETOMIDATE

Overdose with etomidate may result in prolonged deep unconsciousness. Hyperventilation may be followed by apnea in 30% of patients receiving etomidate.

FENTANYL
Fentanyl is about 50–100 times more potent than injectable morphine. It can be given intravenously or by the transdermal route. Most adverse effects reported with the use of the transdermal system are common to opioid analgesics. Other effects include localized itching and erythema. Adverse reactions include nausea, vomiting, constipation, dry mouth, somnolence, confusion, and sweating. Seizures, hypotension, and death have followed fentanyl use.

KETAMINE
Ketamine induces sedation, immobility, amnesia, and analgesia. It produces an unusual trancelike cataleptic state, where the patient appears to be "dissociated" from his environment, but not necessarily asleep. The patient can have profound analgesia and be awake with his eyes open or unconscious. Ketamine maintains anesthesia and analgesia while preserving pharyngeal reflexes and respiratory function. It is subject to drug abuse and may result in death.

Ketamine induces an increase in heart rate, cardiac output, and blood pressure. Cardiac dysrhythmias are uncommon. Ketamine maintains functional residual capacity, induces bronchodilation, stimulates salivary and tracheobronchial secretions, and causes mild respiratory depression. Laryngospasm and stridor have been reported in children. Apnea may be observed.

LOFENTANIL
Lofentanil is 20 times more potent than fentanyl and has a duration of action about 20 times that of fentanyl.

METHOHEXITAL
Cough, hiccup, and laryngospasm are seen in high frequency with intravenous anesthetics, mainly with methohexital. Hyperventilation may occur after induction with etomidate and methohexital.

PROPOFOL
Signs of propofol toxicity may include apnea, bradycardia, hypotension, hypertension, and perioperative myoclonia.

SUFENTANIL
Sufentanil is highly lipophilic and distributes rapidly and extensively. Respiratory depression, delayed gastric emptying, and increased intrabiliary pressure may occur. Physical dependence occurs with prolonged usage. Muscle rigidity may follow intravenous infusion.

Toxic Dosage/Death

Two hours after a heating pad was applied to a fentanyl transdermal system (FTS), pinpoint pupils and shallow respirations were observed, all of which responded rapidly to i.v. naloxone in one case.

Drug Interactions

Ketamine and propofol should not be mixed with other drugs. Muscle relaxants (e.g., atracurium, vecuronium), other anesthetic agents, opiates, and benzodiazepines enhance the respiratory depression and hypotension following use of fentanyl. Ketamine potentiates the effect of neuromuscular blocking agents in a dose-dependent manner. The elimination half-life and blood levels of ketamine are increased by concomitant administration of diazepam or halothane. Alcoholics tend to be resistant to ketamine anesthesia. Concurrent use of ketamine with aminophylline may decrease the seizure threshold and an acute hypertensive crisis, pulmonary hypertension, and pulmonary edema have been seen in a patient with a history of cocaine abuse.

Pregnancy/Lactation

Please see the Introduction section above for specific agents. Ketamine is pregnancy risk factor B.

Laboratory

ANALYTIC METHODS
A radioimmunoassay method is sensitive and specific for fentanyl. Like phencyclidine, ketamine can be measured by gas chromatography / mass spectometry.

BLOOD LEVELS
Following use of a 125-mg / hr patch, fentanyl levels plateau in the range of 2.5 to 3.5 ng / mL. Blood levels in cases of ketamine overdose are not significantly different from control cases and are not helpful in the management of ketamine intoxications. A blood level of 27 μg / mL was found in a patient who had self-administered about 1 g by the intramuscular route. Following the fatal administration of 900 mg of ketamine, a blood level of 7 μg / mL was observed.

Treatment

GUT DECONTAMINATION
These methods are generally not applicable to overdose with intravenous agents.

ELIMINATION ENHANCEMENT
These methods are generally not applicable to overdose with intravenous agents.

SUPPORTIVE MEASURES
- After fentanyl overdose, ensure that a patent airway is established and administer oxygen. Use assisted or controlled ventilation as indicated with an oropharyngeal airway or endotracheal tube as required. Use cooling measures for hyperthermia. Remove transdermal patch if present.
- Naloxone is indicated for signs and symptoms suggestive of an opioid overdose. The duration of hypoventilation following an overdose may be longer than the effects of the narcotic antagonist's action. Additional treatment is symptomatic.
- For severe and persistent hypotension, consider hypovolemia and manage with appropriate parenteral fluid therapy.
- Akathisia from droperidol can be treated with anticholinergics such as benztropine or diphenhydramine, dopamine agonists such as amantadine, or with β-blockers such as propranolol. Discontinuation of droperidol may lead to reversal of akathisia within 72 hours.
- Oxygen, intravenous fluids, and cardiac monitoring should be available after propofol overdose. Patients should be continuously monitored for early signs of significant hypotension and / or bradycardia, and for respiratory depression.
- For cardiovascular depression after propofol use, increase the rate of intravenous fluid administration, elevate lower extremities, and use pressor agents and atropine as required.

Ketamine
- Ketamine adverse reactions or overdosage treatment is largely symptomatic and supportive. If respiratory depression, depressed level of consciousness, or stridor is present, establish prompt airway control and ventilatory support.

- Seizures are treated with benzodiazepines as required.
- Treat emergence reactions with reassurance, a quiet dimly lit room, and benzodiazepines (orally for mild reactions and intravenously for severe reactions). Benzodiazepines decrease the severity of dreams, hallucinations, and illusions.
- Perform routine toxicologic screening in a suspected attempted suicide overdose, as polydrug use is often a possibility.
- Glycopyrrolate or atropine may be used to reduce excessive tracheobronchial secretions.
- Serious cardiovascular stimulation can be blocked by α- and β-adrenoceptor antagonists, and by verapamil. Benzodiazepines may also be useful in this setting.
- Discharge from the emergency department after treatment with benzodiazepines and a short period of observation. Persistent alterations in mental status require assessments for other causes of central nervous system impairment.
- Treat dystonic reactions with intravenous diphenhydramine or benztropine.
- Ketamine produces consistent changes in the electroencephalogram, including a reduction in α-wave activity, while beta-, delta-, and theta-wave activity are increased.

Antidotes

Naloxone counteracts fentanyl-induced hypoventilation. However, because of its short half-life (30–80 minutes) compared with fentanyl, repeated administration of naloxone may be required with careful monitoring for recurrence of pain. See Chapter 23, Opiates, and Chapter 24, Designer Drugs.

Questions—Intravenous and Transdermal Anesthetics

1. Hexobarbital is the most widely used intravenous induction agent.
A. True
B. False

2. Which of the following anesthetics is inaccurately described?
A. Droperidol is a powerful antiemetic often used to treat opiate-induced vomiting.
B. Etomidate is a short-acting, nonbarbiturate sedative-hypnotic agent that lacks analgesic properties.
C. Propofol is particularly dangerous in those who are susceptible to malignant hyperthermia.
D. Fentanyl can be used via a transdermal patch that provides up to 72 hours of analgesia with each application.
E. All of the above are accurate.

3. Which of the following drugs is the most potent?
A. Alfentanil
B. Fentanyl
C. Lofentanil
D. Morphine
E. All are equally potent.

4. Treatment of intravenous fentanyl overdose may include
A. Gut decontamination
B. Elimination enhancement
C. Serial urine levels
D. Naloxone
E. All of the above

5. All of the following are associated with ketamine except
A. A "dissociated anesthesia" characterized by profound analgesia, amnesia, and catalepsy
B. Bronchoconstriction with decreased salivation
C. A feeling of floating, vivid dreams, hallucinations, and delirium
D. Acute dystonic reaction
E. Snorting by recreational users

6. Treatment of ketamine overdose may include
A. Blood levels to guide management
B. Elimination enhancement
C. Gastric decontamination if any amount of ketamine has been ingested
D. Seizures treated with benzodiazepines as required
E. Discharge from the emergency department after treatment with benzodiazepines and 24 hours of observation

LOCAL AND SPINAL ANESTHETICS

Local anesthetic overdose may follow intravenous administration, inadvertent spinal or epidural administration, excessive local injection, or inadvertent intraarterial injection. Subdural injection of a local anesthetic may be followed by unduly prolonged blockade. Toxic reactions may include cardiovascular collapse, respiratory depression or arrest, seizures, arrhythmias, and death. Treatment is supportive and symptomatic. Methemoglobinemia may be treated with methylene blue.

Pathophysiology

Local anesthetics reversibly block the generation and conduction of impulses through sensory, motor, and autonomic fibers. The blockade of peripheral nerves usually progresses in the following order: peripheral vasodilation and skin temperature elevation, loss of pain and temperature sensation, loss of proprioception, loss of touch and pressure sensation, and motor paralysis.

Pharmacokinetics

ABSORPTION

- The onset of action of bupivacaine is 2–10 minutes, and the onset of action of prilocaine and procaine is 2 minutes.

DISTRIBUTION

- Bupivacaine is 82–96% protein bound, etidocaine is 94–96%, lidocaine is 62%, mepivacaine is 60–85%, and prilocaine is 70%.
- The volume of distribution of bupivacaine is 0.4–1.0 L/kg, etidocaine is 1.9 L/kg, lidocaine is 2.16 L/kg, and mepivacaine is 1.2 L/kg.

ELIMINATION

- The half-life of bupivacaine is 1.5–6 hours, lidocaine is 0.7–2 hours, and mepivacaine is 2 hours.

Clinical Presentations

Complications common to local anesthetic blocks include local anesthetic toxicity, neurologic complications, block failures, total spinal anesthesia, and medication errors. Local effects refer to effects on local tissue, for example, nerve or muscle. Systemic effects account for the majority of toxic effects of local anesthetics. They most frequently occur following accidental intravascular injection of local anesthetics.

HYPERSENSITIVITY EFFECTS

Allergic reactions to local anesthetics are rare and usually associated with ester compounds. Idiosyncratic reactions, such as vasovagal syncope or hysterical reactions, are unusual and unpredictable.

NEUROLOGIC EFFECTS

A general pattern of increasing central nervous system signs and symptoms is discernible when local anesthetics are given by intravenous infusion. In ascending order they may include numbness of the tongue and mouth, lightheadedness, tinnitus, visual disturbances, slurred speech, muscular twitching, irrational conversation, loss of consciousness, seizures, coma, apnea, and death. Permanent neurologic injury in regional anesthesia may be secondary to trauma, infection, ischemia, or compression, or may be idiopathic in origin. Neurologic complications of spinal anesthesia can include paraplegia from hematoma or abscess, arachnoiditis, local nerve trauma, and headache.

SPINAL EFFECTS

Total spinal anesthesia may follow when a large quantity of local anesthetic drug intended for the epidural space reaches the subarachnoid space or when an excessive quantity of local anesthetic drug is given during spinal anesthesia. It may follow retrobulbar blocks, brachial plexus anesthesia, and sympathetic blocks. There may be a rapid onset of flaccidity, apnea, unconsciousness, and circulatory collapse. Inadvertent intrathecal administration of various agents may result in hypotension, metabolic acidosis, hyperkalemia, seizures, contrast media in cerebral ventricular and subarachnoid spaces, loss of lower extremity function, cyanosis, and coma.

CARDIOVASCULAR EFFECTS

High serum levels of local anesthetics may decrease impulse generation in nodal pacemaker tissue, alter conduction, and reduce myocardial contractility. Some agents may also produce ventricular arrhythmias and can cause profound vasodilation. Myocardial depression and peripheral vasodilation can lead to cardiovascular collapse, which may be resistant to conventional methods of resuscitation. The more potent, lipid-soluble, longer-acting local anesthetics (bupivacaine and etidocaine) may be more cardiotoxic than less-potent agents such as lidocaine. The serum concentration that induces cardiovascular collapse, compared with the production of seizures, is narrower for the potent local anesthetics. Complications of spinal and epidural anesthesia include bradycardia, heart block, and, rarely, cardiac arrest.

HEMATOLOGIC EFFECTS

Prilocaine is an aniline derivative. One of its metabolic products oxidizes hemoglobin to methemoglobin. Lidocaine may also precipitate methemoglobinemia.

Toxic Dosage/Death

Lidocaine, 1 g intravenously, has caused apnea and asystole. Deaths can follow paracervical anesthesia in first-trimester abortions and have occurred after lidocaine overdose produced seizures and cardiopulmonary arrest.

Drug Interactions

Spinal and epidural anesthesia may cause conduction blockade when used with local anesthetic agents. Physiologic effects may include venous pooling and decreased venous return, causing decreased cardiac output, and hypotension.

Pregnancy/Lactation

Local anesthetics may reduce sympathetic tone in the fetus, decrease maternal blood pressure and cardiac output, and reduce placental perfusion. They may directly vasoconstrict placental vessels, cross the placenta, and act on fetal cardiac and neural tissue directly. The advantages of regional analgesia and anesthesia for labor and delivery include provision of good analgesia, decreased catecholamine secretion, stabilization of the cardiovascular system, prevention of the hypo- and hyperventilation cycle, and lack of depression of the fetus and newborn.

Regional anesthesias commonly used for labor and delivery include paracervical, pudendal, epidural, and spinal blockade. Contraindications to regional anesthesia include patient refusal, infection at the planned site of needle insertion, sepsis, active neurologic disease, and inherited or acquired bleeding diathesis. Relative contraindications include volume depletion, severe anemia, fetal distress, previous difficulty with regional anesthesia, and emotional or psychiatric aberration.

Regional anesthesia is being used with increasing frequency in the pregnant population. This group of patients may be at increased risk for development of local anesthetic toxicity. Physiologic factors may increase the volume of distribution, alter the metabolic state, and reduce the cardiopulmonary reserve of the parturient. Venous engorgement increases the risk of inadvertent i.v. injection, especially in the case of epidural anesthesia. Hypoglycemia and plasma cholinesterase deficiency found in the pregnant patient may predispose patients to toxicity from ester anesthetics.

Spinal anesthesia in obstetrics differs from spinal anesthesia in nonpregnant patients, as smaller doses of local anesthetic are needed in pregnancy. The spread in cerebrospinal fluid is less predictable. Hypotension, spinal headache, and opioid side effects such as respiratory depression are more common in pregnant patients than in general surgical patients. The fetus may be affected adversely by maternal hypotension or inappropriate vasopressors. Technical difficulty in finding the subarachnoid space may be greater in pregnancy because of increased lumbar lordosis.

Laboratory

ANALYTIC METHODS

Bupivacaine, chloroprocaine, etidocaine, lidocaine, mepivacaine, prilocaine, and procaine are analyzed by gas chromatography.

BLOOD LEVELS

Blood levels are not easy to obtain in the acute, overdose setting, and are generally not helpful in managing ill effects. High blood levels of bupivacaine may be associated with dizziness, ringing in the ears, hypotension, seizures, and ventricular tachycardia. Toxic reactions to bupivacaine usually do not occur at plasma levels below 4 μg/mL. Ten μg/mL appears to be the minimum blood concentration of lidocaine at which toxic manifestations (including seizures) may occur. Ingestion of lidocaine solutions intended for topical anesthesia has led to serum levels of 7.3–12 μg/mL with toxic signs and symptoms. A serum level of 19 μg/mL followed an accidental intravenous injection of 1,200 mg of lidocaine. Asystole and grand mal seizures were observed.

Plasma mepivacaine concentrations of 4.4–8.6 μg/mL following caudal administration of 5.5–9.4 mg/kg have been associated with apprehension, confusion, muscular twitching, nausea, and vomiting. The toxic threshold for blood mepivacaine is about 6.3 μg/mL. Following a dose of 864 mg of prilocaine, postmortem prilocaine concentrations of 13 μg/mL in blood, and 69 μg/mL in urine were obtained. The patient died in the dentist's chair within 1 hour.

Treatment

GUT DECONTAMINATION

These methods are generally not applicable.

ELIMINATION ENHANCEMENT

Use of diuretics, hemodialysis, or hemoperfusion in local anesthetic overdose cannot be recommended.

SUPPORTIVE MEASURES

- Resuscitation equipment to manage changes in ventilatory and cardiac status must be available in settings where local and spinal anesthetics are routinely used. Continuous monitoring of neurologic and cardiac systems will provide early warning of an inadvertent intravenous injection of a local anesthetic, or of elevated blood levels.
- When bupivacaine is used epidermally, it should always be injected slowly, there should be a high suspicion of the possibility of accidental intravenous injection, and the drugs, equipment, and knowledge required for resuscitation should be immediately available.
- Most seizures caused by local anesthetics are self-limited, unless a massive i.v. overdose is given. Maintain an adequate airway and ventilate the patient with 100% oxygen. Maintain a normal acid-base balance with hydration, hyperventilation, or bicarbonate administration if necessary. Acidosis decreases the protein binding of local anesthetics, increasing levels of free drug and therefore toxicity.
- If seizures persist, diazepam (10 mg), thiopental (50 to 100 mg), or midazolam (2 mg) may be useful. It may be necessary to administer succinylcholine if manual ventilation is to be effective in a seizure patient.
- Hypotension is managed with position change, intravenous fluids, and in severe cases, pressors.
- Bradycardia is managed with atropine.
- Ventricular tachycardia or fibrillation may follow the use of certain anesthetics, particularly bupivacaine. Electrical cardioversion, and/or bretylium (5 mg/kg i.v. up to a maximum of 10 mg/kg) may be helpful in these settings. Cardiopulmonary bypass has been effective in the resuscitation of one patient with bupivacaine-induced cardiac arrest.
- Total spinal anesthesia is managed with ventilation and circulatory support.
- Atrioventricular cardiac pacing was successful in the treatment of a cardiac arrest following a 2-g accidental administration of lidocaine into a cardiopulmonary bypass circuit. In general, however, acute lidocaine toxicity is best managed with nonspecific supportive therapy.

Antidotes

There are no antidotes for local anesthetics. The rare case of prilocaine or lidocaine-induced methemoglobinemia is treated with methylene blue.

Questions—Local and Spinal Anesthetics

1. Contraindications to regional anesthesia include all of the following except
A. Patient refusal
B. Infection at the planned site of needle insertion
C. Pregnancy
D. Active neurologic disease
E. Inherited or acquired bleeding diathesis

2. High blood levels of bupivacaine may be associated with all of the following except
A. Dizziness
B. Ringing in the ears
C. Seizures
D. Hypertension
E. Ventricular tachycardia

NEUROMUSCULAR BLOCKING AGENTS

Muscle relaxants are classified according to the mechanism by which they decrease the effects of acetylcholine. They are either depolarizing or nondepolarizing (competitive). Neuromuscular blockers in overdose, both depolarizing and nondepolarizing, may lead to prolonged skeletal muscle paralysis, hyperkalemia, histamine release, hypotension, cardiac arrest, and death.

Atracurium, gallamine, pancuronium, succinylcholine, and vecuronium are synthetic products. Metocurine is semisynthetic, and tubocurarine is extracted from plants of the genus *Chondodendron.* Succinylcholine includes two molecules of linked acetylcholine. Pancuronium and vecuronium are steroidal neuromuscular blockers that are structurally similar to corticosteroids.

Pathophysiology

Neuromuscular blocking agents inhibit the effects of acetylcholine on nicotinic receptors. Succinylcholine is a short-acting depolarizing blocker that is structurally similar to acetylcholine. It is called "depolarizing" because it produces muscle depolarization like acetylcholine. The bradycardia on first injection of succinylcholine may be caused by stimulation of parasympathetic ganglia or cardiac muscarinic receptors in the SA node. Succinylcholine has been associated with anaphylaxis. It may disrupt mast cells and cause release of histamine. Flushing, bronchospasm, hypotension, and other anaphylactoid reactions may follow a normal dose of 1 mg/kg.

The nondepolarizing muscle relaxants exert their effect at the neuromuscular junction by competitive inhibition of acetylcholine at the nicotinic receptor. Most nondepolarizing muscle relaxants have two positively charged quaternary ammonium groups that attach to the negatively charged cholinergic receptor. Muscle relaxants usually act directly on tissue mast cells and release histamine without antibody or complement activation. The histamine release is related to the dose and rate of administration of the muscle relaxant. Severe reactions may lead to circulatory collapse.

Pharmacokinetics

ABSORPTION

- Neuromuscular blockers are rapidly distributed within minutes.

DISTRIBUTION

- In general, muscle relaxants are moderately protein bound, and have a low apparent volume of distribution. Individual variation occurs among agents.

ELIMINATION

- Nondepolarizing agents have an elimination half-life of several hours.
- Succinylcholine is rapidly metabolized, mainly by plasma pseudocholinesterase to succinylmonocholine and choline. Succinylmonocholine has about one-twentieth the activity of succinylcholine and is a nondepolarizing blocking agent.
- Succinylmonocholine may accumulate and cause apnea in patients with impaired renal function.
- Approximately 2–10% of succinylcholine is excreted unchanged in the urine.

Clinical Presentations

HYPERSENSITIVITY EFFECTS

Depolarizing and nondepolarizing neuromuscular blockers may rarely be associated with life-threatening anaphylactic reactions manifested by circulatory collapse, bronchospasm, and skin flushing. Skin tests are positive in about one-third of cases. Evidence appears to suggest a direct action of succinylcholine on susceptible mast cells without IgE mediation. Succinylcholine and tubocurarine may lead to an increase in plasma histamine levels in normal patients during anesthesia. Anaphylactoid reactions have been reported with vecuronium.

NEUROLOGIC EFFECTS

Fasciculations, muscle pain, malignant hyperthermia, myoglobinuria, increased intragastric pressure, and increased intraocular pressure may be observed with succinylcholine use. An abnormal sensitivity to nondepolarizing muscle relaxants is a feature of myasthenia gravis and is manifested by prolonged neuromuscular block. Vecuronium-induced prolonged paralysis has been associated with renal failure and higher plasma concentrations of a potentially active metabolite.

Poisoning by curariform blocking agents is characterized by complete paralysis of skeletal muscles beginning with the small, rapidly moving muscles of the ears, fingers, and toes, followed by those of the face and neck, then spreading to the extremities and finally the diaphragm and intercostal muscles. Consciousness may be unaffected. Death is caused by hypoxia secondary to respiratory paralysis.

METABOLIC EFFECTS

Succinylcholine-induced hyperkalemia may be seen in a number of circumstances. These include massive burns or muscle trauma, lower motor neuron disease, (including traumatic degeneration, demyelinating disease such as Guillain-Barré and poliomyelitis), upper motor neuron disease (including spinal cord transection, cerebrovascular accidents, and encephalitis), and tetanus. Following succinylcholine depolarization in normal patients, a slight increase in plasma potassium ion concentration may be observed.

NEUROMUSCULAR EFFECTS

Long-term use of nondepolarizing neuromuscular blocking agents, especially vecuronium and pancuronium, may produce prolonged weakness. Two patterns of neuromuscular dysfunction are observed. One involves prolonged neuromuscular blockade after termination of treatment, resulting in prolonged weakness. This is felt to result from an accumulation of neuromuscular blocker metabolites. The other is a myopathy, which may include flaccid paralysis, and mild to severe weakness with proximal muscles often weaker than distal muscles. Cognition, sensation, and cranial nerves are normal and recovery may take weeks to months. The creatine phosphokinase is normal or elevated.

RESPIRATORY EFFECTS

Prolonged periods of apnea may follow succinylcholine use in those patients with genetically determined atypical pseudocholinesterase or in those who have received cholinesterase inhibitors.

CARDIOVASCULAR EFFECTS

Atracurium use may result in an increase in mean arterial pressure and heart rate that does not require treatment. Overdosage with atracurium may increase the risk of histamine release.

Toxic Dosage/Death

Inadvertent gallamine administration (30 mg) into the subarachnoid space of an adult has been tolerated. Pancuronium, 105 mg administered to a 79-year-old man, resulted in ultimate death from circulatory shock. An adult committed suicide by self-injection of pancuronium bromide (1 mg/mL). A fatal dose of pancuronium has been reported as 10 mg i.v.

A patient who accidentally received pipecuronium bromide 520 mg/kg (about 11 times the effective dose) demonstrated paralysis for 70 hours. Neostigmine and pyridostigmine administration failed to reverse the blockade. An intravenous dose of 30 mg of tubocurarine stops breathing in most adults within 2–3 minutes. Two cases of accidental overdose were given 80 mg and 100 mg respectively and recovered.

A 9.7-kg, 23-month-old child with Down's Syndrome received 37 mg of vecuronium in 1 hour intravenously. Hemodynamic studies remained unchanged over the next 24 hours. The dose given was a five-fold overdose of the manufacturer's recommended infusion rate.

Drug Interactions

Drugs that interfere with muscle relaxation may exert themselves proximal to the neuromuscular junction in the central nervous system or in the bloodstream, at the neuromuscular junction, or distal to the junction at the muscle cell membrane. At the neuromuscular junction, interactions may take place at the nerve terminal, in the synaptic cleft, or at the postsynaptic membrane. Numerous drugs have been identified that may interact with the effects of nondepolarizing relaxants.

ANESTHETIC AGENTS

Ketamine potentiates tubocurarine but not pancuronium. Midazolam potentiates vecuronium-induced blockage. Chronic tricyclic antidepressant administration may predispose a patient given pancuronium to ventricular tachycardia.

ANTIBIOTICS

Antibiotics such as the aminoglycosides (e.g., amikacin, streptomycin, gentamicin, kanamycin, and tobramycin) and the polypeptides (e.g., polymyxins A, B, and C) not only potentiate nondepolarizing relaxants, but also produce neuromuscular blockade on their own. The tetracyclines have weak neuromuscular blocking properties alone, but also potentiate nondepolarizing relaxants.

ANTICONVULSANTS
Patients on long-term phenytoin therapy may be resistant to pancuronium and vecuronium but not to atracurium. Phenytoin may cause a 50% reduction in the duration of neuromuscular blockade. Phenytoin appears to have prejunctional effects similar to the nondepolarizing relaxants. Patients receiving carbamazepine may be resistant to pancuronium. Recovery times from pancuronium and vecuronium may be 65% shorter in patients receiving carbamazepine.

CARDIOVASCULAR DRUGS
Furosemide, 1 mg/kg, facilitates recovery of pancuronium-induced blockade. However, large doses of furosemide may antagonize pancuronium-induced blockade in neurosurgical patients. β-blockers block the acetylcholine-binding site at the postsynaptic membrane. They may aggravate or unmask myasthenia gravis and induce a myasthenic syndrome. Procainamide aggravates myasthenia gravis and induces weakness in healthy subjects. Quinidine augments the block caused by nondepolarizing relaxants. Verapamil and nifedipine potentiate the neuromuscular blocking effect of d-tubocurarine, pancuronium, atracurium, and vecuronium.

CORTICOSTEROIDS
Pancuronium-induced blockade may be diminished in patients on long-term steroid therapy. Corticosteroids may also enhance the potential for paresis when administered with a steroidal neuromuscular blocking agent such as pancuronium and vecuronium.

CYCLOSPORINE
Cyclosporine comes in a Cremophor solvent. Cremophor alone may potentiate the neuromuscular blocking effect of vecuronium and atracurium.

LITHIUM
Lithium may potentiate pancuronium blockade and may induce a myasthenic reaction. Lithium reduces the synthesis and release of acetylcholine at the nerve terminal.

MAGNESIUM
Magnesium potentiates the neuromuscular blockade of pancuronium and vecuronium. The dose of vecuronium should be reduced in patients receiving magnesium sulfate infusions. Magnesium decreases the presynaptic release of acetylcholine, reduces the sensitivity to acetylcholine of the postsynaptic membrane, and decreases the excitability of the muscle fiber membrane.

METHYLXANTHINES
Aminophylline and theophylline antagonize pancuronium. Aminophylline may inhibit the ability of pancuronium to induce neuromuscular blockade.

Pregnancy/Lactation

Please see the Introduction section above for specific agents. Numerous agents, including atracurium, gallamine, pancuronium, d-tubocurarine, and succinylcholine cross the placenta.

Laboratory

ANALYTIC METHODS
A high-performance liquid chromatography assay is available for atracurium. Total (free plus bound) concentrations of gallamine in plasma are measured by a fluorometric assay. Ion-pair extraction and fluorometry perform analyses of pancuronium in blood, serum, and urine. Analysis of succinylcholine in urine has been accomplished by thin-layer chromatography and quantitation gas chromatography. A sensitive radioimmunoassay for tubocurarine employs a tritium label. A liquid chromatography assay with ultraviolet detection has also been described.

BLOOD LEVELS
An adult who committed suicide by intravenous injection of 10 mg of pancuronium exhibited postmortem blood and urine levels of 1.6 and 1.5 $\mu g/mL$, respectively.

Treatment

GUT DECONTAMINATION
These methods are not utilized in the treatment of neuromuscular blocker overdose.

ELIMINATION ENHANCEMENT
These methods are not utilized in the treatment of neuromuscular blocker overdose.

SUPPORTIVE MEASURES
- Immediately ascertain that a patent airway exists and administer assisted ventilation as required. Maintain a supply of oxygen to the patient, as well as a cardiac monitor and intravenous lines.
- If signs of malignant hyperthermia develop, prompt treatment is required (see the earlier section on Malignant Hyperthermia).
- Since there is no agent available to reverse the activity of succinylcholine, continue ventilatory support until muscular paralysis subsides.
- Where cardiovascular support is required, consider proper patient positioning, fluid administration, and the use of vasopressors.
- If the reversal of neuromuscular blockade is inadequate because of severe debilitation, carcinomatosis, or concomitant drugs that have depressed respiration or affected neuromuscular blocking ability, symptomatic treatment is indicated and manual or mechanical assisted ventilation should be instituted until there is adequate recovery.
- Hyperkalemia induced by succinylcholine may be managed with bicarbonate, insulin and glucose, or calcium in serious scenarios.
- Anaphylaxis is managed with fluid support, antihistamines, epinephrine, pressors as required, and steroids.

Antidotes

Neuromuscular blockade spontaneously reverses when relaxants diffuse away from their sites of action. Depolarizing agents like succinylcholine are noncompetitive and cannot be reversed pharmacologically in most cases. Agents that inhibit the enzyme acetylcholinesterase, such as edrophonium, neostigmine, and pyridostigmine, may increase available acetylcholine and may accelerate recovery.

All of these agents, like acetylcholine itself, have nicotinic and muscarinic effects. Muscarinic stimulation, which may lead to salivation, bradycardia, tearing, miosis, and bronchoconstriction, can be minimized by prior administration of an anticholinergic drug such as atropine or glycopyrrolate. 4-Aminopyridine increases the release of acetylcholine presynaptically and may be helpful.

Questions—Neuromuscular Blocking Agents

1. **Neuromuscular blockers in overdose may lead to all of the following except**
   A. Prolonged skeletal muscle paralysis
   B. Hypokalemia
   C. Histamine release
   D. Hypotension
   E. Cardiac arrest
2. **Which of the following statements is not true?**
   A. Certain neuromuscular blockers may cross the placenta.
   B. Nondepolarizing agents have an elimination half-life of several hours.
   C. Succinylcholine may accumulate and cause apnea in patients with impaired renal function.
   D. Anaphylactoid reactions have been reported with vecuronium.
   E. All are true.
3. **All of the following may antagonize the effects of neuromuscular blockade except**
   A. Phenytoin
   B. Azathioprine
   C. Ketamine
   D. Theophylline
   E. Aminophylline
4. **Neuromuscular blocking agents inhibit the effects of acetylcholine on nicotinic receptors.**
   A. True
   B. False

TOPICAL ANESTHETICS

Topical anesthetics may cause toxicity when applied to the skin where normal barriers have been disrupted, as on abrasions, lacerations or burns. Toxicity may also follow application to the mucous membranes, as may inadvertently happen with TAC (tetracaine, adrenaline, and cocaine), or during bronchoscopy. Symptoms may include seizures, cardiovascular and respiratory depression, bronchospasm, visual abnormalities, hemodynamic instability, and death. Treatment is generally supportive and symptomatic.

Numerous over-the-counter products contain varying amounts of benzocaine, which, after excessive use, can cause methemoglobinemia. Anbesol®, Vagisil®, and Lanacane® products may contain up to 20% benzocaine. Methemoglobinemia is treated with methylene blue. TAC is still widely used to topically anesthetize small lacerations. EMLA® cream contains lidocaine 2.5% and prilocaine 2.5% and is used as a pretreatment for needle punctures.

Pathophysiology

Blood levels of a local anesthetic arising from topical anesthesia of the trachea may equal those obtained by intravenous injection. Systemic toxic reactions may occur. Salivary secretions may dilute the anesthetic and prevent adequate contact with mucous membranes. Most topical drugs require 3–5 minutes before anesthesia begins, and anesthetic action typically lasts 20–30 minutes.

Pharmacokinetics

ABSORPTION

- Absorption of these agents is generally quite limited by intact skin; however, absorption is enhanced by occlusion (as with EMLA® cream), or disruption of the epidermis.
- Absorption may be quite rapid via the mucous membranes.
- Lidocaine when introduced rectally is readily absorbed and when administered to a baby may induce convulsions.
- When lidocaine is applied to the mucous membranes, blood levels may simulate those resulting from intravenous injections. Similarly, peak blood levels are attained quickly after application to mucous membranes of the tracheobronchial tree.

DISTRIBUTION

- The volume of distribution of lidocaine is 1.6 L/kg. Protein binding of lidocaine is 60%.

ELIMINATION

- The elimination half-life of lidocaine is 2–10 hours. Certain metabolites of lidocaine may be active.

Clinical Presentations

BENZOCAINE

Methemoglobinemia has followed the topical use of benzocaine and Cetacaine. The methemoglobinemia is frequently not described in drug package inserts. Topical sprays and ointments containing 14–20% benzocaine often cause dose-dependent methemoglobinemia. Benzocaine absorbed from mucous or pulmonary membranes oxidizes blood hemoglobin in proportion to the absorbed dose.

Infants and children are more susceptible than adults to methemoglobinemia because fetal hemoglobin is more easily oxidized to methemoglobin, newborns have lower levels of NADH-methemoglobin reductase, catalase, and glutathione peroxidase, and the dosage usually is greater per kilogram body weight. Benzocaine sprays, gels, and ointment should be avoided in infants and in patients with anemia or other diseases in which reduced oxygen transport may be of special concern.

DIBUCAINE

A 2-year-old who ingested dibucaine staggered, seized, became cyanotic, vomited, developed a cardiorespiratory arrest, and died.

HEXYLCAINE

A 32-month-old child who received an adult dose (3.5 mL) of hexylcaine 5% to facilitate bronchoscopy developed apnea, dilated pupils, and seizures. Supportive treatment was successful for recovery. An adult became apneic and experienced seizures after swallowing 10 ml of hexylcaine.

LIDOCAINE

Severe and even lethal intoxications have followed local application to mucous membranes. Visual disturbances, dizziness, confusion, seizures, and cardiorespiratory arrest have occurred. Following topical administration of lidocaine to the nasal mucosa, severe methemoglobinemia may result in patients who have the heterozygous form of NADH-methemoglobin reductase deficiency. Death has rarely followed a hypersensitivity reaction to topical lidocaine 10% spray. Lidocaine lowers the seizure threshold. Oral lidocaine in children may be followed by a delay of minutes to hours with sedation, agitation, and seizures requiring adequate resuscitation.

TAC

Misuse of TAC (i.e., tetracaine, adrenaline and cocaine) may result in seizures or death. Absolute contraindications to TAC application include lacerations of mucosal surfaces, digits, glans of the penis, nasal alae, and ear lobes, and extensively abraded skin. Relative contraindications include underlying seizure or cardiac dysrhythmic disorders.

TETRACAINE

Dizziness, difficulty in speaking, tonic-clonic seizures, and a transient facial paresis have been observed. Topical ocular anesthetic abuse may result in keratitis and persistent epithelial defects with possibly permanent corneal damage and visual loss. The management of patients with suspected or known use or abuse of topical ocular anesthetic agents revolves initially around discontinuation of the anesthetic agent. Counseling, confiscation of the anesthetic, and admission for observation may be useful. Supportive treatment may permit healing of epithelial defects.

Toxic Dosage/Death

LIDOCAINE

Topical lidocaine cream applied to 60% of the body (25 g of lidocaine base) twice daily caused visual disturbances, dizziness, confusion, seizures, and a cardiorespiratory arrest. Suggested maximum doses of lidocaine for topical anesthesia of the pharynx, larynx, and trachea in a healthy 70-kg adult is 200 mg. Doses of lidocaine of up to 8.5 mg/kg have proved safe when administered over a period longer than 15 minutes. A 5-month-old boy developed status epilepticus after a 7.5-mg/kg/dose administered as a 2% solution over 5 days. Manual application of 2% viscous lidocaine to the gums of an 11-month-old led to seizures.

TAC

As noted above, the use of topical anesthetics on mucosal or denuded surfaces may predispose in some cases to serious adverse reactions. TAC in amounts greater than 5 mL applied repeatedly or to contraindicated areas of the body (mucosal surfaces or burned skin) has resulted in seizures and fatality. If the cocaine in TAC is completely absorbed, 590 mg may be lethal. The recommended maximum dose of cocaine for orotracheal use in a healthy adult is 100 mg and for tetracaine is 50 mg. As little as 2 mL of TAC solution used on the buccal mucosa in a 5-year-old led to a seizure. Fatalities have followed one TAC application to the mucosal lip in a 7-month-old. Ten mL of TAC applied to multiple surface burn areas has led to seizures in 2 or 3 minutes.

TETRACAINE

Two patients who gargled with 4–5 mL of 5% tetracaine survived; however, a 75-year-old patient who gargled with 4 mL of a 0.5% solution died. Tetracaine 0.5% ophthalmic ointment has produced corneal damage.

Drug Interactions

Succinylcholine should be used with caution with ester-type topical anesthetics, because it can stop tonic-clonic activity, but mask ongoing central nervous system seizure activity. Both ester anesthetics and succinylcholine use pseudocholinesterase for metabolism. Hypotension, neuromuscular block, apnea, and seizure activity may be worsened or prolonged when the two are used concomitantly.

Laboratory

ANALYTIC METHODS

Methodology for the determination of cocaine and tetracaine blood levels (e.g., in TAC) is available. See Chapter 19, Cocaine.

BLOOD LEVELS

Treatment of topical agent overdose is primarily guided by clinical judgment, and confirmed by laboratory studies if available. Blood levels may be of value in following the course of lidocaine toxicity. Therapeutic serum concentrations of lidocaine for use as an antiarrhythmic are 1–5 μg/mL. Toxic manifestations first appear at a serum lidocaine concentration of 5 μg/mL. Early symptoms (5–10 μg/mL) are dizziness, drowsiness, tinnitus, and perioral paresthesias. More severe symptoms (at concentrations of 10–20 μg/mL) include disorientation, delirium, convulsions, and coma. Cardiorespiratory arrest supervenes above 20 μg/mL.

Following TAC use in a 7-month-old infant, the postmortem plasma cocaine level was 11.9 μg/mL and the blood tetracaine level 1 μg/mL. Blood levels in 11 patients lethally overdosed with cocaine ranged from 0.1 to 20.9 μg/mL. A 2-year-old who ingested dibucaine ointment died with a dibucaine blood level of 1.3 μg/mL.

Treatment

GUT DECONTAMINATION

Charcoal may help decrease systemic levels of oral or topical (mucous membrane) lidocaine and its metabolites; however, clinical relevance of this intervention requires further study. Topical anesthetics on the skin can be washed off briskly with repeated soap and water washings. Gastric lavage may be performed after endotracheal intubation; however, the possibility of seizures should alert the clinician to use gastric lavage only in large, recent ingestions.

ELIMINATION ENHANCEMENT

There is little evidence to support the use of diuresis, hemodialysis, or hemoperfusion after a toxic reaction induced by a topical anesthetic.

SUPPORTIVE MEASURES

- Evaluate airway, breathing, and circulation in all patients as topical anesthetics can, in sufficient quantities, induce seizures, cardiovascular depression, respiratory depression, or bronchospasm. Cardiac monitoring, intravenous lines and oxygen should be available.
- Give naloxone, glucose, and thiamine to all obtunded patients.
- Dopamine is the drug of choice for cardiovascular collapse in topical anesthetic toxicity because of its inotropic effect on the heart.
- Seizures following lidocaine use may be treated with a benzodiazepine (e.g., lorazepam, diazepam, or similar anticonvulsant agents).
- Preventive measures are of great importance in diminishing the toxicity of topical anesthetics. When topical anesthetics are applied to the oral mucosa, an attempt should be made

to have the patient expectorate any excess to diminish absorption.
- Two-percent viscous Xylocaine® is not recommended by the manufacturer for teething discomfort.
- Recommendations have been made to avoid use of TAC on mucosal or denuded surfaces.

Antidotes

Severe methemoglobinemia following topical anesthetic use (e.g., lidocaine, benzocaine) is rapidly reversed by intravenous methylene blue (1–2 mg / kg in a 1% solution administered over 5 minutes).

Questions—Topical Anesthetics

1. Topical use of benzocaine has been followed by methemoglobinemia, though it is not frequently described in package inserts.
A. True
B. False

2. Relative contraindications to TAC use include
A. Age under 6 years old
B. Laceration over arteries
C. Underlying seizure disorder
D. Atrial septal defect
E. None of the above

Answers

Introduction to Anesthetic Agents

1. E 2. C 3. B

Malignant Hyperthermia

1. E 2. A 3. D 4. B 5. C

Inhalation Anesthetics

1. A 2. D 3. B 4. E

Intravenous and Transdermal Anesthetics

1. B 2. C 3. C 4. D 5. B 6. D

Local and Spinal Anesthetics

1. C 2. D

Neuromuscular Blocking Agents

1. B 2. E 3. C 4. A

Topical Anesthetics

1. A 2. C

SELECTED READINGS

Introduction to Anesthetic Agents

1. Barash PG, Cullen BF, Stoelting RK, eds. Handbook of clinical anesthesia. Philadelphia: JB Lippincott, 1991.
2. Beecher HK, Todd DP. A study of the deaths associated with anaesthesia and surgery based on a study of 599,548 anaesthesias in 10 institutions 1948-1952 inclusive. Ann Surg 1954;140:2–35.
3. Cohen MM, Duncan PG, Pope WDB, et al. A survey of 112,000 anesthetics at one teaching hospital (1975-1983). Can Anaesth Soc J 1986;33:22–31.
4. Gravenstein JS, Kory WP, Marks RG. Drug abuse by anesthesia personnel. Anesth Analg 1983;62:467–472.
5. Wood PR, Soni H. Anaesthesia and substance abuse. Anaesthesia 1989;44: 672–680.

Malignant Hyperthermia

1. Addonizio G, Susman VL, Roth SD. Neuroleptic malignant syndrome. Review and analysis of 115 cases. Biol Psychiatry 1987;22:1004–1020.
2. Caroff SN, Mann SC, Rosenberg H, et al. The relationship between malignant hyperthermia and neuroleptic malignant syndrome. Anesthesiology 1989; 70:172–173.
3. Strazis KP, Fox AW. Malignant hyperthermia. A review of published cases. Anesth Analg 1993;77:297–304.
4. Tomarken JL, Britt BA. Malignant hypothermia. Ann Emerg Med 1987;16:1253–1265.
5. Zuckerberg AL. A hot mnemonic for the treatment of malignant hyperthermia. Anesth Analg 1993;77:1077–1086.

Inhalation Anesthetics

1. Barash PG, Cullen BF, Stoelting RK. Handbook of clinical anesthesia. Philadelphia: JB Lippincott, 1991, pp. 148–158.
2. Elliott RH, Strum L. Hepatotoxicity of volatile anesthetics. Br J Anaesthesia 1993;70:339–48.
3. Halsey MJ. Drug interactions in anaesthesia. Br J Anaesth 1987;59:112–123.
4. Wrigley SR, Jones RM. Inhalational agents—an update. Eur J Anaesthesiol 1992;9:185–201.

Intravenous and Transdermal Anesthetics

1. Barash PG, Cullen BF, Stoelting RK. Handbook of clinical anesthesia. Philadelphia: JB Lippincott, 1991.
2. Grandins A. Ketamine. Clin Toxicol Rev 1994;16(1):1–2.
3. Haas DA, Harper DG: Ketamine. A review of its pharmacologic properties and use in ambulatory anesthesia. Anesth Prog 1992;39:61–68.
4. Reich DL, Silvay G. Ketamine. An update on the first twenty-five years of clinical experience. Can J Anaesth 1989;36:186–197.
5. Wood M. Intravenous anesthetic agents in Wood M, Wood AJJ: Drugs and Anesthesia. Pharmacology for Anesthesiologists. Baltimore: Williams and Wilkins 1990;206–207.
6. Zech DFJ, Grand SUA, Lynch J et al. Transdermal fentanyl and initial dose finding with patient controlled analgesia in cancer pain. A pilot study with 20 terminally ill cancer patients. Pain 1992;50:293–301.

Local and Spinal Anesthetics

1. Cardiotoxicity of local anesthetic drugs. Lancet 1986;2:1192–1194 (editorial).
2. Dershowitz M. Local anesthetics. In: Firestone LL, Lebowitz PW, Cook CE, eds. Clinical anesthesia procedures of the Massachusetts General Hospital. 3rd ed. Boston: Little, Brown, 1988, pp. 185–198.
3. Voulgaropoulos DS, Johnson MD, Covina BG. Local anesthetic toxicity. Sem Anesth 1990;9:8–15.
4. Weiss LD, Generalovich T, Heller MB, et al. Methemoglobin levels following intravenous lidocaine administration. Ann Emerg Med 1987;16:323–325.

Neuromuscular Blocking Agents

1. Argov Z, Mastaglia FF. Disorders of neuromuscular transmission caused by drugs. N Engl J Med 1979;301:409–413.
2. Gooch JL. Prolonged paralysis after neuromuscular blockade. Clin Toxicol 1995;33:419–26.
3. Miller RD. Neuromuscular blocking agents. In: Smith et al, eds. Drug interactions in anesthesia. Philadelphia: Lea and Febiger, 1981; pp. 249–269.
4. Ostergaard D, Engbaek J, Viby-Mogensen J. Adverse reactions and interactions of the neuromuscular blocking drugs. Med Toxicol Adverse Drug Exp 1989; 4:351–368.
5. Wood M. Neuromuscular blocking agents. In: Wood M, Wood AJJ, eds. Drugs and anesthesia. Pharmacology for anesthesiologists. 2nd ed. Baltimore: Williams & Wilkins, 1990; pp. 271–318.

Topical Anesthetics

1. Bonadio WA. TAC: a review. Pediatr Emerg Care 1989;5:128–130.
2. DiFazio C. Local anesthetics. Action, metabolism and toxicity. Otolaryngol Clin North Am 1981;14:515–518.
3. Duffin RM, Olson RJ. Tetracaine toxicity. Ann Ophthalmol 1984;16:836–837.
4. Wehner D, Hamilton GD. Seizures following topical application of local anesthetics to burn patients. Ann Emerg Med 1984;13:456–458.

ACKNOWLEDGMENT

Thanks to Alison Deutsch, MD for contributing the questions in this chapter.

CHAPTER 44
Chemotherapeutic Drugs

INTRODUCTION

There are over 60 anticancer drugs in active general use, as well as a number of investigational drugs available for special use. Anticancer drugs are generally characterized as alkylating agents, antimetabolites, natural products, hormone inhibitors, or other miscellaneous products. Within each group of cytotoxic drugs, the toxic effects exhibited by one member of the class are not easily translated to others of the same group.

When cancer chemotherapeutic agents are administered in overdose (e.g., orally or by injection) or at the wrong site (e.g., intrathecally instead of intravenously), predictable (e.g., bone marrow suppression) and unpredictable (e.g., brain damage after inadvertent intrathecal use) toxic reactions may follow. Most overdoses with cytotoxic drugs are managed without antidotes. Protective measures for the patient and health care personnel who handle cytotoxic drugs have often been inadequate.

Pathophysiology

The clinical toxicity of antineoplastic drugs is known to be particularly centered in rapidly dividing cells: in the bone marrow, gut mucosa, hair follicles, and germinal epithelium of the testes, thymus, and fetus. In addition, some cytotoxic agents are photosensitizing (e.g., fluorouracil), but this is uncommon. Severe toxicity may also be caused by local irritation and ulceration resulting from extravasation of cytotoxic drug into the tissues outside a vein. Many antineoplastic agents exhibit a direct irritant effect on the skin, eyes, mucous membrane, and other tissues.

Antineoplastic drugs induce vomiting through a multiafferent neural reflex arc. Three major afferent limbs have now been identified. These include a humoral pathway consisting of chemical mediators that affect the chemoreceptor trigger zone (CTZ) in the brain stem, a peripheral pathway activated by direct stimulation of nerve endings in the gastrointestinal tract, and a cerebral cortical pathway activated by stimuli (sights, odors, or memories) associated with past episodes of emesis. Disrupting this reflex arc is the key to the prevention of chemotherapy-induced vomiting.

Clinical Presentations

The chemotherapeutic drugs are meant to be cytotoxic. While neoplastic cells remain the intended target, numerous organs and organ systems may be adversely affected by usual antineoplastic doses, and in overdose.

CARCINOGENIC EFFECTS

The most common secondary malignancy in survivors of initial chemotherapy for Hodgkin's disease and ovarian cancer, as well as other tumors, is acute nonlymphocytic leukemia with two predominant subgroups: acute myelomonocytic leukemia and acute erythroleukemia. Risks of leukemia appear to be highest within the first 3 to 5 years after completing initial therapy.

Risk factors for secondary neoplasias include the agent initially used (alkylating agents have been associated with the highest risk for the subsequent development of leukemia), the cumulative dose given, the drug schedule, possibly altered immunity, a history of radiotherapy, and possibly the age of the patient. The prognosis for secondary leukemia is poor. Secondary neoplastic changes in the gastrointestinal tract and other organs have also been reported. Bladder cancer has been associated with cyclophosphamide use. Nonalkylating agents have also been linked to secondary cancer development. These include cisplatin, etoposide, hydroxyurea, mitomycin, doxorubicin, dacarbazine, interleukin-2, prednimustine, mitoxantrone, tamoxifen, bleomycin, and others.

CARDIAC EFFECTS

Cytotoxic chemotherapy, particularly with the anthracyclines (e.g., doxorubicin, daunorubicin), and less often cyclophosphamide, may be associated with acute or delayed cardiotoxicity. Heart failure from dose-related cardiomyopathy is the most clinically important manifestation of anthracycline cardiotoxicity. A higher risk is also found in patients with underlying coronary, vascular or myocardial disease, hypertension, or cardiac irradiation. Cardiotoxicity with doxorubicin is dose-related and usually develops after a cumulative dose of over 500 mg/m^2. The cardiac changes caused by cancer therapy may progress for 1–15 years after treatment and lead to functional changes (echocardiographically detectable abnormalities of left ventricular afterload and contractility) that are often initially asymptomatic. Cardiac function may continue to deteriorate after doxorubicin treatment is discontinued.

EXTRAVASATION EFFECTS

Extravasation of cytotoxic drugs refers to the unintentional instillation or leakage of these agents into the perivascular and subcutaneous spaces during their administration. Cytotoxic drugs that cause local irritation after extravasation include carmustine, cyclophosphamide, dacarbazine, streptozotocin, teniposide and thiotepa. Vesicant cytotoxic drugs that may cause tissue necrosis and local ulceration after extravasation include actinomycin D, cisplatin, daunorubicin, doxorubicin, fluorouracil, mitomycin, mitoxantrone, mechlorethamine, mithramycin, vinblastine, and vincristine.

FERTILITY EFFECTS

Alkylating agents and procarbazine are especially toxic to the terminal epithelium of the testis. Single-dose alkylating agents produce dose-dependent impairment of spermatogenesis, and combination chemotherapy regimens such as mechlorethamine, vincristine, procarbazine, and prednisone (MOPP) may cause permanent infertility in 90% of patients. Lower risks of permanent infertility are associated with other combinations of chemotherapy regimens such as doxorubicin, bleomycin, vinblastine, dacarbazine (ABVD) or cisplatin, vinblastine, and bleomycin. There is no effective method to protect the testis from the effects of chemotherapy. Sperm banking prior to chemotherapy can be considered.

GASTROINTESTINAL EFFECTS

Almost every chemotherapeutic agent whether used orally or parenterally is capable of inducing nausea and vomiting. Chemotherapeutic agents have been classified according to their emetogenic potential. Chemotherapy-induced nausea and vomiting may be severe enough to prevent patients from completing curative courses of treatment. Chemotherapeutic drugs with high emetogenic potential include cisplatin, dacarbazine, cyclophosphamide, cytarabine, carmustine, streptozotocin, pentostatin, mechlorethamine, and lomustine. Relatively high doses of numerous other agents are quite emetogenic as well.

GENITOURINARY EFFECTS

Bacille Calmette-Guérin (BCG) vaccine has been associated with epididymitis and granulomatous pyelonephritis. Bleomycin, mitotane, and cyclophosphamide may cause hemorrhagic cystitis. Busulfan causes azoospermia, and finasteride, leuprolide, and goserelin cause impotence.

HEMATOLOGIC EFFECTS

Bone marrow depression and other hematologic consequences are common after chemotherapeutic drug use. Among others, bone marrow depression has been associated with altretamine, amsacrine, azacitidine, busulfan, carboplatin, chlorambucil, cisplatin, cladribine, cyclophosphamide, cytarabine, dacarbazine, dactinomycin, daunorubicin, doxorubicin, etoposide, fludarabine, 5-fluorouracil (5-FU), gemcitabine, hydroxyurea, idarubicin, ifosfamide, interferon, levamisole, mechlorethamine, melphalan, mercaptopurine, methotrexate, mitomycin, mitoxantrone, paclitaxel, pentostatin, procarbazine, teniposide, thioguanine, thiotepa, trimetrexate, vinblastine, and vincristine.

HEPATIC EFFECTS

Liver damage following use of androgen-receptor antagonists has been reported. Hepatitis (cytotoxic and cholestatic) and fulminant hepatic failure may follow the steroidal antiandrogens (e.g., cyproterone acetate, megestrol acetate) and the nonsteroidal antiandrogens (e.g., nilutamide, flutamide). Hepatotoxicity has also been associated with methotrexate, mitomycin, plicamycin, diethylstilbestrol, carmustine, and others.

HYPERSENSITIVITY EFFECTS

Certain antineoplastic agents (e.g., L-asparaginase, cisplatin, melphalan, mechlorethamine, and teniposide) produce hypersensitivity reactions often enough to be a clinical problem. Others (e.g., cyclophosphamide, doxorubicin, daunorubicin, methotrexate, and procarbazine) do so only occasionally. Bleomycin induces an occasional hyperpyrexic reaction with findings similar to anaphylaxis. Doxorubicin causes a "flare" or localized urticaria in the area of drug injection. Hypersensitivity reactions caused by Taxol® were a major concern in early studies with this agent. This may have been due to the Cremophor EL® vehicle (polyoxyethylated castor oil) used in drug formulation. Other drugs formulated with this vehicle (e.g., cyclosporine, teniposide, intravenous vitamin K, and didemnin) have also caused hypersensitivity reactions.

NEUROLOGIC EFFECTS

Neurologic symptoms and signs arise at some point during the treatment of many patients with malignancies. Peripheral neuropathies have been associated with amsacrine, carboplatin, cisplatin, cytarabine, etoposide, procarbazine, suramin, Taxol®, teniposide, vincristine and vindesine. Cranial neuropathies may be seen with chlorambucil, steroids, fludarabine, 5-flourouracil (5-FU), laetrile, procarbazine, cisplatin and vincristine. Encephalopathy may be seen with the nitrosureas, ifosfamide, L-asparaginase, hexamethylmelamine, 5-FU, and alkylating agents. Central nervous system depression may follow mitotane, pentostatin, asparaginase, and altretamine.

OPHTHALMOLOGIC EFFECTS

Numerous toxic ocular effects have been related to cancer chemotherapy. Toxic retinopathy has followed chlorambucil, cisplatinum, mitotane, nitrosureas, procarbazine, tamoxifen and tilorone. Conjunctivitis may follow doxorubicin, cyclophosphamide, cytosine arabinoside, 5-FU, methotrexate and nitrosureas. Cataracts may follow use of busulfan, steroids, dibromomannitol, mitotane and nafoxidine.

ORAL EFFECTS

Unfortunately, painful oral effects are common after use with certain chemotherapeutic agents. Stomatitis may follow bleomycin, amsacrine, vinblastine, vinorelbine, procarbazine, thioguanine, hydroxyurea, idarubicin, daunorubicin, doxorubicin, and dactinomycin use. Cheilitis has been associated with isotretinoin and tretinoin use. Oral ulcerations may be seen with floxuridine, mechlorethamine, mercaptopurine, 5-FU, and cytarabine. Among others, mucositis may be seen with etoposide, trimetrexate, and thiotepa.

PULMONARY EFFECTS

Drugs representing all groups of cytotoxic agents may induce lung disease affecting the parenchyma or vasculature (pulmonary emboli). Factors associated with an increased risk of drug-induced pneumonitis include total dose, age, oxygen therapy (with bleomycin, cyclophosphamide, mitomycin, nitrosureas), radiation therapy to the lungs, combination drug use with increased toxicity, and preexisting pulmonary disease. Drug-induced pulmonary toxicity most frequently presents with dyspnea, nonproductive cough, fatigue, and malaise over a period of weeks or months. Hypersensitivity drug-induced lung disease develops within hours. Fever, chest pain, and rales are often present. Although a basilar or diffuse reticular nodular pattern may be present on radiologic examination and a restrictive ventilatory defect with diminished carbon monoxide diffusing capacity may be observed, ultimately a lung biopsy is necessary for diagnosis.

RADIATION EFFECTS

Recall radiation reactions (i.e., a reaction at a previously sensitized area), and radiosensitization reactions (i.e., enhanced sensitivity of an area to doses of radiation) may occur when antineoplastic drugs and other agents interact with radiotherapy. Radiosensitization responses may develop following concomitant chemotherapy and radiotherapy or in instances where radiotherapy is given before chemotherapy (i.e., radiation recall). Cytotoxic drugs that enhance toxic reactions to radiotherapy include actinomycin D, aminoglutethimide, bleomycin, cyclophosphamide, doxorubicin, fluorouracil, hydroxyurea, melphalan, vincristine, and tamoxifen. The usual effect of radiation–chemotherapeutic agent interactions on the skin is erythema followed by desquamation. More severe cases may be associated with painful vesicles, oozing, necrosis and painful ulceration.

RENAL EFFECTS

Certain chemotherapeutic agents have been associated with a range of adverse renal effects. Among others, these include cisplatin, amsacrine, asparaginase, dacarbazine, pentostatin, aldesleukin, gallium nitrate, ifosfamide, lomustine, mitomycin, and streptozotocin. The syndrome of inappropriate antidiuretic hormone (SIADH) may follow the use of cyclophosphamide, vincristine and ifosfamide.

TUMOR LYSIS SYNDROME

Tumor lysis syndrome occurs in patients who harbor rapidly growing tumors that are highly sensitive to chemotherapy or radiation. It is characterized by the development of hyperkalemia, hyperphosphatemia, hyperuricemia, and hypocalcemia. Electrolyte imbalances can lead to life-threatening complications such as cardiac dysrhythmias, severe neuromuscular dysfunction, and acute renal failure. Prior existence of renal insufficiency, hyperuricemia, or electrolyte imbalance places the patient at high risk of a potentially fatal outcome. Those with elevated white blood cell counts and large tumors are at additional risk.

VASCULAR EFFECTS

Antineoplastic agents may induce a heterogeneous group of disorders ranging from asymptomatic arterial lesions to hepatic veno-occlusive disease (e.g., cyclophosphamide, dacarbazine, urethane, mitomycin, azathioprine, and thioguanine) to a lethal thrombotic microangiopathic syndrome. The latter may follow treatment with cisplatin, mitomycin, bleomycin, or vinca alkaloids.

Toxic Dosage/Death

Maximally tolerated doses of anticancer drugs in adults and children are carefully monitored during therapy. High-dose toxicity following antineoplastic drug use often manifests itself in signs and symptoms that frequently are not similar to those found after ordinary therapeutic use. Frequent central and peripheral nervous system manifestations, as well as hepatotoxic changes, may be observed. Blood levels largely parallel dosages, but significant differences are observed within a specific drug group. Deaths occur more frequently in high dose ranges.

Drug Interactions

Numerous potential drug interactions are recognized among the chemotherapeutic agents. Concomitant use of the anthracyclines with etoposide, vincristine, bleomycin, busulfan, mitomycin C, cisplatin and cyclophosphamide can worsen cardiotoxicity. Cisplatin-induced nephrotoxicity can reduce bleomycin clearance. Furosemide may reduce the urinary excretion of cisplatin, producing higher peak plasma concentrations. Mannitol may neutralize cisplatin's effect. Increased bone marrow depression may be noted when cyclophosphamide is used with allopurinol or phenobarbital.

Tetrahydrouridine increases the half-life of cytarabine. Doxorubicin increases effects of radiation and decreases the gastrointestinal absorption of oral digoxin. Concomitant use of etoposide with vindesine and warfarin displaces warfarin from its albumin binding sites. Methotrexate increases the effectiveness and toxicity of 5-fluorouracil (5-FU). Thymidine decreases the renal clearance of 5-FU and cimetidine may increase 5-FU peak concentrations. Disulfiram may decrease ifosfamide-induced bladder damage. Allopurinol enhances the hematotoxicity of 6-mercaptopurine.

Pregnancy/Lactation

The simultaneous occurrence of cancer and pregnancy is uncommon, but cancer remains among the chief causes of maternal and fetal morbidity and mortality. As there is an increasing trend for women to delay childbearing, there may be a more frequent co-occurrence of cancer and pregnancy in the future. There are few, if any, human studies of transplacental passage of antineoplastic agents, but many antineoplastic agents have qualities necessary to cross the placenta and enter the fetal circulation. These include low molecular weight, high lipid solubility, a nonionized state, and low plasma protein binding.

Cytotoxic drugs may induce an all-or-none phenomenon. Either a spontaneous abortion or a normal fetus may follow use of these agents, but during the first trimester chemotherapy may also lead to an increased fetal risk of congenital malformations. In the second and third trimesters these drugs usually do not cause significant malformations, but they can impair fetal growth and development and result in microcephaly, mental retardation, and impaired learning behavior. Late effects of maternal cytotoxic drug therapy that need further studies include physical growth, intellectual and neurologic development, gonadal function and reproductive capacity, transplacental mutagenesis of germ-line tissue, transplacental carcinogenesis, and second-generation teratogenesis.

It is prudent to advise lactating mothers who are receiving cytotoxic drugs to refrain from breastfeeding their infants. Since most drugs enter breast milk by diffusion of the un-ionized form of a drug, the relative concentration of the drug in milk and plasma, i.e., the milk to plasma (M/P) ratio, will depend on its relative ionization in milk and plasma, the lipid solubility of the un-ionized moiety, and the relative protein binding of the drug in milk and plasma. Methotrexate, cisplatin, cyclophosphamide, doxorubicin, and hydroxyurea are all readily detectable in serum after use, and have been assayed in breast milk. The infants of two nursing mothers who received high doses of cyclophosphamide experienced bone marrow suppression.

Laboratory

ANALYTIC METHODS

There are few indications for routine drug-level monitoring of cytotoxic drugs with the exception of high-dose methotrexate regimens. Methotrexate is measured by an enzyme-multiplied immunoassay technique (EMIT).

BLOOD LEVELS

Blood levels generally are not useful as a guide to the clinician who administers and guides chemotherapy.

Treatment

GUT DECONTAMINATION

Overdose with many antineoplastic drugs induces seizures at an early stage. Syrup of ipecac is not recommended. If gastric lavage is contemplated, prior adequate protection of the airway must be ensured. The use of gastric emptying procedures as well as activated charcoal and cathartics for cytotoxic drug overdose has not been evaluated by controlled clinical studies.

ELIMINATION ENHANCEMENT

There is a paucity of evidence to support the use of any extracorporeal treatment methods (e.g., hemodialysis, hemoperfusion, peritoneal dialysis, or exchange transfusion) in the treatment of antineoplastic drug overdose. High volumes of distribution, high protein binding values, extensive metabolite formation, and limited clinical experience with the use of the above procedures in patients with cytotoxic agent overdose caution against use of these procedures at present. Hemodialysis may be helpful in managing profound electrolyte abnormalities after the tumor lysis syndrome.

SUPPORTIVE MEASURES

- Drug doses to be administered should be recalculated by each individual involved in patient care. The pharmacist should

perform cross-checking of proper and complete labeling of the syringe, and its accuracy should be double-checked by the nurse and physician prior to administration.
- The clinical follow-up of patients who have received a cytotoxic drug will require, in most instances, careful hematologic studies performed frequently over the first four weeks and periodically thereafter. This may include peripheral blood counts, bone marrow analyses, and other tests related to the blood and blood-forming organs.
- Similarly, renal and liver function tests are also followed.
- Since the gastrointestinal tract and central nervous system are often sites of clinical toxicity following chemotherapy, adequate use of investigative procedures for study of these organ systems (e.g., x-ray, computer tomography, nuclear magnetic resonance, endoscopy, spinal fluid studies) must be immediately available in those medical centers that are involved in the care of cancer patients.

PREVENTION

- Prevention of overdose is paramount. Guidelines have been developed to preclude the danger of overdosage with any injected chemotherapeutic agent. All personnel involved in handling chemotherapeutic agents should be fully knowledgeable of the potential dangers.
- Charts of normal doses of chemotherapeutic agents should be available in all nursing stations and wherever drugs are prepared or administered.
- All chemotherapeutic doses should be fully calculated and recorded in the chart by a member of the hematology—oncology service. The dose should be written in mg/kg or an equivalent SI concentration, total dose, and volume.
- Only an experienced physician who can check the dose and concentration before it is administered should give chemotherapy.
- Stock only small dose vials of vincristine, for example, (10 mL = 1 mg) or other injectables where possible. This greatly reduces the opportunity to give a massive overdose.

OVERDOSE

- Cytotoxic drugs administered in overdose by the oral route (inadvertent or self-induced) seldom result in an immediate life-threatening emergency.
- All patients suspected of ingesting toxic doses of cytotoxic drugs must have a careful hematologic analysis.
- If the patient is asymptomatic after 8 hours, discharge may be considered. Because of delayed evidence of myelosuppression, the patient should be followed weekly with blood counts for at least 4 weeks.
- Similar periodic follow-up is indicated for cardiovascular evaluation following overdose (usually intravenous) with the anthracyclines. These patients should be followed weekly, then monthly in view of the frequently delayed onset of cardiotoxicity.
- Patients who exhibit vital sign abnormalities should receive an intravenous line, cardiac monitor, oxygen, and assisted mechanical ventilation as needed. Attention must be directed toward assessment of the adequacy of ventilation and blood pressure and correction of abnormalities.

CONJUNCTIVITIS

- Ocular exposures are treated with profuse irrigation with normal saline and ophthalmologic consultation as needed.
- Conjunctivitis may be ameliorated with antibiotic drops or ointments.

ELECTROLYTE DEPLETION

- Hyponatremia, hypokalemia, hypocalcemia, and hypomagnesemia may be seen in overdose (e.g., Actinomycin D).
- Electrolyte depletion may accompany nausea, vomiting and diarrhea often exhibited by chemotherapy patients.
- Replacement therapy (intravenous electrolytes) should be accompanied by cardiac and respiratory monitoring, including periodic arterial blood gas determinations.

ENCEPHALOPATHY

- Periodic electroencephalography (EEG), lumbar puncture for cerebrospinal fluid analysis, computerized tomography, and nuclear magnetic resonance studies may be required to rule out other causes of encephalopathy.
- Possible "CSF washout" and rehabilitation may be required. See the section on Intrathecal Antineoplastic Overdose below.

EXTRAVASATIONS

- Whenever possible, administer vesicants through a central line. This is particularly important if the vesicant is ordered as a continuous infusion and a peripheral site cannot be continually monitored.
- To ensure patency of a peripheral i.v., it is best to administer a vesicant through a recently started i.v.. Avoid sites in the dorsum of the hand and near joints, as these sites are more susceptible to permanent damage because of the close proximity to arteries and tendons.
- Administer vesicants by slow i.v. push into the side-arm port of a running i.v. of a compatible solution. Assess a peripheral site continually for signs of redness or swelling. Verify patency of the i.v. site by aspirating blood return before vesicant infusion and during the infusion.
- Ask the patient to report any sensations of burning or pain at the infusion site. Some investigators suggest delaying the administration of antiemetics until after vesicant administration. The antiemetics often have a sedative effect and the patient may be unable to report any sensations at the infusion site.
- On extravasation, stop the injection of the cytotoxic drug infusion immediately. Do not remove the needle. Disconnect the intravenous administration set. An attempt should be made to aspirate the extravasated drug from the needle or cannula (by way of the needle). Aspiration of the surrounding tissues is usually ineffective in removing any more of the extravasated drug.
- Instill any appropriate antidote through the needle and into the surrounding tissues, infiltrating the area where the extravasation has occurred, then remove the needle or cannula.
- Mark the border with indelible ink and photograph to provide a baseline for later comparison and for medicolegal documentation. Apply cold compresses for 20–40 minutes to the site of extravasation for all drugs except the vinca alkaloids.
- Apply dressings to the site, elevate the arm, and apply 1% hydrocortisone cream (injections of hydrocortisone may be contraindicated in the case of vinca-alkaloid agents, and it may be appropriate to use hyaluronidase ointment instead).
- The patient is asked to return at weekly intervals unless local irritation or necrosis is not anticipated. Advise patient on follow-up care, telling patient of relevant symptoms and signs.
- Local corticosteroid injections, with or without sodium bicarbonate and with or without intravenous hydrocortisone, have been used for doxorubicin toxicity. Dimethylsulfoxide (DMSO) has also been used to limit local doxorubicin ulceration.

- Hyaluronidase and normal saline have proved useful in animals in limiting the effects of the extravasation of vinca alkaloid vesicants.
- Sodium thiosulfate has been reported useful after mitomycin or mechlorethamine extravasation.

FEVER

- Fevers are common after numerous chemotherapeutic agents. Sources may include infections, intrinsic neoplasia, and the chemotherapeutic agents themselves.
- Blood, urine, sputum, or other sources of cultures should be repeatedly obtained to rule out specific bacterial or other infections.
- Intravenous antibiotics are vital in leukopenic patients.
- Reverse isolation procedures may be indicated.

HEMATOLOGIC EFFECTS

- Thrombocytopenia may be treated with platelet transfusions in severe cases.
- Anemia is treated with red blood cell transfusions.

HEMORRHAGIC CYSTITIS

- Mesna is a uroprotectant for cyclophosphamide and ifosfamide-induced hemorrhagic cystitis. Mesna is administered in doses of 1500 mg / m^2 / day intravenously and orally.
- Toxic effects following its use may include abdominal discomfort and vomiting, both of which may tend to reflect its disagreeable taste orally. Doses of over 85 mg / kg intravenously have resulted in vomiting and diarrhea.

HYPERSENSITIVITY REACTIONS

- Treatment should include immediate cessation of an infusion, close monitoring, diphenhydramine (mild reactions) or epinephrine, and i.v. fluids for anaphylaxis.
- Aminophylline and / or β-agonists may be used to relieve bronchospasm.

INTRATHECAL ANTINEOPLASTIC OVERDOSE

- "Cerebral washout" or cerebrospinal fluid (CSF) drainage is required as soon as possible after an inadvertent intrathecal injection of methotrexate (MTX) (most commonly) or other agents.
- Initially, the lumbar puncture is repeated and CSF drainage to gravity is instituted. Drainage of 30 mL of CSF within the first 15 minutes after an intralumbar overdose may remove nearly 95% of injected MTX. Drainage 2 hours after injection may remove less than 20% of the dose.
- CSF drainage alone is insufficient to treat a massive MTX overdose, since toxic amounts are still present in CSF after the procedure is completed. With MTX overdoses of more than 100 mg, CSF drainage must be accompanied by ventriculolumbar perfusion.
- Pentobarbital and / or phenytoin may be given intravenously to prevent seizures.
- Coma will require intubation with mechanical ventilating support. Maintain careful fluid balance to avoid any cerebral edema by checking intake and output carefully. Cerebral edema may be ameliorated by mannitol. Steroids are not drugs of choice here as they have not been shown to prevent MTX-induced encephalopathy or myelopathy.
- Twenty-four hours after the intrathecal overdose, rescue with thymidine. Thymidylate salvage from cytotoxic effects of MTX has been used in a dose of 8 g / m^2 / day by continuous intravenous infusion. Thymidine is an investigational drug for this use.
- Consider alkalinization of the urine to promote urinary excretion of MTX. There are no controlled clinical studies, however, to support this procedure in MTX overdose.
- Leucovorin (folinic acid) intravenously may be given at an unusually high dose (1,000 mg) to facilitate its passage across the blood-brain barrier. It is then continued intravenously until the MTX blood and CSF levels are within the nontoxic range.

NAUSEA AND VOMITING

- Dehydration is treated with intravenous fluids with careful attention to urine output and central venous pressure as indicated.
- Phenothiazines (e.g., prochlorperazine), butyrophenones (droperidol), and metoclopramide all have substantial antidopaminergic activity and are widely used as antiemetic agents.
- A potent antiemetic "cocktail" can be prepared with metoclopramide (particularly useful with cisplatin use), steroids (e.g., Decadron®, methylprednisolone), and lorazepam (reduces anxiety, produces sedation or amnesia).
- Occasional extrapyramidal reactions may be managed with an antihistamine such as diphenhydramine 25–50 mg intravenously in adults.
- Serotonin receptors appear to be principal mediators of the emetic reflex and are found in the central nervous system and gastrointestinal tract. Ondansetron is as effective as metoclopramide in preventing the acute nausea and vomiting that occurs within 24 hours of chemotherapy.
- In the delayed phase of nausea and vomiting (days 2 through 6), results with both ondansetron and metoclopramide appear less effective, and metoclopramide may be useful.
- Ondansetron has been used in doses of 8 mg intravenously (acute phase) followed by 1 mg per hour for 24 hours, and in children in doses of 5 mg / m^2 once intravenously. Delayed-phase doses suggested in adults are 8 mg three times daily and in children are 2–4 mg every 8 hours.
- Adverse reactions to ondansetron include headache, constipation, elevation of liver enzymes, and infrequent anaphylactoid reactions. Treatment for ondansetron overdose is largely supportive.
- The efficacy and usefulness of other antiemetic modalities such as ginger root, acupuncture, cyclizine, and rectal thiethylperazine in the prevention and treatment of chemotherapy-induced emesis remain to be established.
- Dronabinol (δ-9-tetrahydrocannabinol; THC; Marinol®) may be effective for patients who have failed to respond adequately to conventional antiemetics. Dry mouth, sedation, orthostatic hypotension, ataxia, dizziness, and dysphoria have been observed (see Chapter 21, Marijuana and Cannabinoids).

ORAL MUCOSITIS

- Use parenteral sources of nutrition and local therapy for oral lesions.
- One randomized, double-blind, placebo-controlled study suggested that topical application of 1 milliliter of vitamin E oil, 400 IU / mL, applied topically to all lesions twice a day for 5 days is effective in the therapy of chemotherapy-induced mucositis.

PREGNANCY ISSUES

- If the condition of a mother with cancer deteriorates, and if a cure or amelioration of a neoplastic process is a realistic goal, then she can be treated as indicated with cytotoxic drugs regardless of the trimester. Harmful effects at any period of pregnancy are not inevitable.

- If there is no hope for cure or even significant palliation, the primary goal may become protection of the fetus from the harmful effects of antineoplastic drugs or radiation and the delivery of a healthy infant.
- Throughout the decision-making period, it is prudent for the clinician to interact with a team consisting of the patient's obstetrician, family physician, oncologist, pediatrician, neonatologist, and other ancillary consultants.
- Single and combination chemotherapy may be administered during the second and third trimester with a relatively low risk of teratogenicity. Delivery can be planned when maternal blood counts are optimal. Long-term follow-up of the fetus so exposed is indicated.
- Drugs that may be relatively safe during the first trimester include alkylating agents given alone and vinblastine alone.

SEIZURES

- Caution must be exercised with those drugs known to induce early seizures.
- Intravenous diazepam remains the initial drug of choice.
- Airway precautions (endotracheal intubation) must be exercised if the patient has evidence of respiratory difficulty or presents in a state of diminished consciousness.

SKIN

- Skin exposures are treated with soap and water.
- Vesicant exposures should be flooded with saline (e.g., doxorubicin).
- See extravasation and hypersensitivity effects for additional treatment options.

SYNDROME OF INAPPROPRIATE ANTIDIURETIC HORMONE

- SIADH is treated with fluid restriction and careful attention to fluid and electrolyte balance.
- ADH assay may help confirm the diagnosis.

TUMOR LYSIS SYNDROME

- The predominant electrolyte abnormality will usually determine the clinical course. Hypocalcemia leads to muscle cramps, tetany, ventricular dysrhythmias, confusion, and convulsions. Hyperuricemia leads to nephropathy, oliguria, or hematuria. Hyperphosphatemia results in hypocalcemia and renal failure because of the production of high levels of calcium phosphate that precipitate in the kidney. Hyperkalemia is known to be associated with life-threatening ventricular arrhythmias and sudden death.
- Hyperuricemia, electrolyte abnormalities, and renal function abnormalities should be aggressively treated prior to initiation of antineoplastic therapy.
- Allopurinol in doses up to 500 mg/m^2 body surface area is instituted for amelioration of hyperuricemia, and high-flow intravenous fluids and urinary alkalinization are of value until uric acid levels are normalized.
- Serum electrolytes, creatinine, blood urea nitrogen, uric acid, calcium, phosphorus, and lactic acid dehydrogenase should be monitored until stable and thereafter up to 3–5 days.
- Hemodialysis may be considered in severe cases. Suggested criteria that may be followed to initiate hemodialysis, or to reduce rapidly rising volume overload associated with symptomatic hypocalcemia, include serum potassium 6 mEq/liter or above, serum uric acid 10 mg/dL or above, and serum phosphorus 10 mg/dL or above.

Antidotes

There are few antidotes useful in the amelioration of antineoplastic drug overdoses. Mesna (Mesnex® injection), a uroprotectant, may diminish the hemorrhagic cystitis of cyclophosphamide and ifosfamide. Folinic acid (leucovorin, citrovorum factor) is used to mitigate methotrexate toxicity, but is of unproven value in vincristine toxicity. Methylene blue may be useful in reversing ifosfamide-associated encephalopathy.

Chemoprotectants for 5-FU have been directed at the formation of a metabolite of 5-FU, 5-fluorouridylate triphosphate (5-FUTP), which is incorporated into RNA and interrupts further RNA synthesis. Allopurinol, through its metabolite oxypurinol, may permit doubling of the 5-FU infusion dose. This has not, however, produced significantly enhanced clinical 5-FU response rates. More active 5-FU combinations with leucovorin or levamisole are under trial.

DEXRAZOXANE

The U.S. Food and Drug Administration has approved dexrazoxane (Zinecard®) for protection against cardiac toxicity from doxorubicin (Adriamycin® and others) in women with metastatic brain cancer. Dexrazoxane is started 30 minutes before doxorubicin. They are usually given at a 1:1 ratio, 500 mg/m^2 of dexrazoxane for every 40 mg/m^2 of doxorubicin.

LEUCOVORIN

Leucovorin (folinic acid) can replenish and substitute for the endogenous reduced-folate cofactor that methotrexate diminishes. It replenishes intracellular reduced-folate pools and prevents methotrexate-induced cytotoxicity via blockade of thymidine synthesis. Little antidotal activity is possible unless leucovorin is administered within 48 hours of methotrexate. Other attempts at site protection (asparaginase, thymidine) are not yet clinically proven. See Chapter 5, Antidotes.

Questions—Introduction to Chemotherapeutic Drugs

1. Which of the following statements about chemotherapeutic drugs is false?

A. Certain antineoplastic agents (e.g., L-asparaginase, cisplatin, melphalan, mechlorethamine, and teniposide) produce hypersensitivity reactions often enough to be a clinical problem.
B. Hepatitis (cytotoxic and cholestatic) and fulminant hepatic failure may follow steroidal antiandrogens (e.g., megestrol acetate) and nonsteroidal antiandrogens (e.g., nilutamide).
C. Alkylating agents and procarbazine are toxic to the terminal epithelium of the testis.
D. Factors associated with an increased risk of drug-induced pneumonitis include total dose, age, oxygen therapy, co-existing lung cancer, sex, radiation therapy to the lungs, combination drug use with increased toxicity, and diabetes mellitus.
E. The tumor lysis syndrome occurs in patients who harbor rapidly growing tumors that are highly sensitive to chemotherapy or radiation. It is characterized by the development of hyperkalemia, hyperphosphatemia, hyperuricemia, and hypocalcemia.

2. Anticancer drugs are generally characterized as

A. Sulfate scavengers
B. Alkylating agents

Answers to questions in shaded boxes appear at the end of the chapter.

C. Antimetabolites, natural products, hormone inhibitors
D. All of the above
E. B and C

3. **Within each group of cytotoxic drugs, the toxic effects exhibited by one member of the class are not easily translated to others of the same group.**
A. True
B. False

4. **Clinical toxicity of antineoplastic drugs is known to be particularly centered in rapidly dividing cells. These include cells in each of the following, except**
A. Bone marrow
B. Gut mucosa
C. Hair follicles
D. Thyroid
E. Thymus

5. **Antineoplastic drugs induce vomiting through a multi-afferent neural reflex arc. These afferent limbs include**
A. Chemical mediators that affect the chemoreceptor trigger zone (CTZ) in the occipital cortex
B. A pathway activated by direct stimulation of nerve endings in the gastrointestinal tract
C. A cerebral cortical pathway activated by stimuli associated with past episodes of emesis
D. All of the above
E. B and C

6. **The most common secondary malignancy in survivors of initial chemotherapy for Hodgkin's disease and ovarian cancer is**
A. Testicular cancer
B. Acute myelomonocytic leukemia
C. Non-Hodgkin's lymphoma
D. Mycosis fungoides
E. Breast cancer

7. **Risk factors for secondary neoplasias following chemotherapy use include all except**
A. The agent initially used
B. The cumulative dose given
C. The stage of cancer that a chemotherapeutic agent is given
D. The drug schedule
E. A history of radiotherapy

SPECIFIC ANTINEOPLASTIC AGENTS

Overdoses with cytotoxic drugs must be evaluated in light of the numerous complexities surrounding antineoplastic treatment. These include the use of prior recent treatment regimens, the use of multiple chemotherapeutic agents simultaneously, and the presence of multiple system dysfunctions deriving from acute or chronic disease processes. There is also a paucity of clinical experience with antineoplastic overdoses, and the occasional use of unusual routes (e.g., intrathecal) for an instillation of what are frequently investigational agents.

Some clinical experience, however, to provide some ideas regarding the diagnosis and treatment of some of these cytotoxic drugs is now available. It cannot be assumed that experience with one member of a chemical or biologic cytotoxic drug class provides complete insight into the diagnosis and treatment of overdose with another member of the same class. Specific toxic associations and doses associated with overdose are presented below. The list is by no means exhaustive.

Actinomycin-D

Actinomycin-D is an example of an anti-tumor antibiotic. Overdose may result in seizures, hyponatremia, hypovolemia, hypocalcemia, hypomagnesemia, thrombocytopenia, oral mucositis, diarrhea, and fever.

Asparaginase

L-Asparaginase (Elspar®) is an immune modulator which has been associated with central nervous system toxicity, manifested by lethargy, somnolence, and coma. It has also been associated with pancreatitis, coagulation defects, thrombosis, renal damage and hepatotoxicity. "Asparagine rescue" infusions have been used to reverse serious drug-induced brain dysfunction syndromes, but this observation must be confirmed by other studies.

Bleomycin

Bleomycin (Blenoxane®) inhibits the synthesis of DNA. It is used to treat squamous cell carcinomas, lymphomas, sarcomas and testicular carcinomas. Life-threatening bleomycin lung toxicity (manifested by pneumonitis and pulmonary fibrosis) may be reversible when large doses of corticosteroids (up to 80 mg prednisolone daily for 10 days with gradual tapering) and azathioprine (150 mg/day) are administered. Other manifestations of delayed toxicity include rash and hyperpigmentation, stomatitis, hemorrhagic cystitis and alopecia.

Chlorambucil

Chlorambucil (Leukeran®) is a nitrogen mustard alkylating agent. Therapeutic doses of chlorambucil in both adults and children range from 0.1 to 0.2 mg/kg/day. At total doses of 4 to 6 mg/kg in adults, myoclonus and seizures may occur. Dosages of 1.5–6.8 mg/kg may be associated with lethargy, irritability, myoclonus, vomiting, abdominal pain, ataxia, seizures, and coma.

Cisplatin

Cisplatin (Platinol®) inhibits DNA synthesis by forming DNA cross-links and denaturing the double helix. Acute overdose with cisplatin may result in renal failure, hepatic failure, deafness, ocular toxicity (including detachment of the retina), significant myelosuppression, intractable nausea and vomiting, neuritis and/or death. No antidotes have been established for cisplatin overdose. Hemodialysis is not useful in eliminating platinum from the body, but plasmapheresis lowers the plasma platinum concentration. Management is based on supportive and symptomatic treatment.

At least three error types have caused inadvertent overdose. These include mistaking the total dose to be divided over several days for the daily dose, administering cisplatin when the patient was to have received carboplatin, and writing the wrong cisplatin dose. The present literature states that "Caution should be exercised to prevent inadvertent overdosage with Platinol® (cisplatin)." No proven antidotes have been established for cisplatin overdose.

Cyclophosphamide

Cyclophosphamide (Cytoxan®) is a nitrogen mustard alkylating agent. Patients have died after toxic doses and have suffered from residual cardiac damage. Common types of delayed toxicity include bone marrow depression, alopecia, hemorrhagic cystitis, sterility, pulmonary infiltrates and fibrosis, hyponatremia, leukemia, bladder cancer, and SIADH.

Doxorubicin

Doxorubicin (Adriamycin PFS®) inhibits an enzyme involved in DNA cleavage and inhibits DNA and RNA synthesis by intercalating between DNA base pairs. The risk of cardiotoxicity with doxorubicin increases with total dose. Cardiomyopathy may be fatal. Encephalopathy, dysuria, gait disturbances, an abnormal electroencephalogram, absent tendon reflexes, coma, seizures, mydriasis, myelotoxicity, mucositis, and elevated cerebrospinal fluid protein levels have been observed.

Etoposide

Etoposide (VePesid®) is a natural epidophyllotoxin. Overdose may lead to a decrease in leukocyte counts, T-lymphocytes, and blast transformation. Delayed toxicity may manifest as rash, alopecia, peripheral neuropathy, mucositis, and/or leukemia.

5-Fluorouracil

An overdose of 5-fluorouracil (Adrucil®, 5-FU), a pyrimidine analogue, may cause nausea, vomiting, diarrhea, gastrointestinal ulceration, bleeding, and bone marrow depression. Life-threatening cardiotoxicity manifested by atrial and ventricular arrhythmias, congestive cardiac failure, myocardial ischemia, and sudden death has followed the use of 5-fluorouracil. It is difficult to predict which patients will be affected.

Flutamide

Flutamide (Eulexin®) is an androgen blocker. Clinical trials with doses up to 1,500 mg per day for periods up to 36 weeks have yielded gynecomastia, breast tenderness, and some increases in the SGOT. The dose of flutamide associated with symptoms of overdose or considered to be life-threatening has not been established.

Hydrazine

Hydrazine overdose has lead to ataxia, lateral nystagmus, loss of vibration sense, and paresthesias. Hydrazine is also hepatotoxic in animals and may induce seizures.

Ifosfamide

Ifosfamide (Ifex®) is a nitrogen mustard alkylating agent. Therapeutic doses of ifosfamide range from 1.2 to 2.5 g/m^2/day intravenously. The maximum tolerated dose reported has been 17 g/m^2 given by continuous intravenous infusion over 120 hours with mesna uroprotection in one study and 16 g/m^2 with mesna protection in another patient. Dose-limiting renal toxicity has been observed at 18 g/m^2. Duration of myelosuppression, frequency and severity of mucositis, and renal tubular acidosis appear to be dose-dependent. There are no antidotes for ifosfamide or its metabolites. Dialysis may be considered in view of the favorable toxicokinetics (low apparent volume of distribution), but no studies are available yet to confirm this.

Lomustine

Lomustine (CeeNU®) is a nitrosurea alkylating agent, which is usually administered in doses of 100–130 mg/m^2 orally every 4–6 weeks. Overdose may lead to pancytopenia. Pulmonary fibrosis, renal damage and leukemia have been associated with its use. Treatment is supportive.

Melphalan

Melphalan (Alkeran®) is a nitrogen mustard alkylating agent. Therapeutic doses of melphalan have ranged from 0.15 to 0.25 mg/kg/day, with doses of 2.0–2.5 mg/kg used on occasion. Reversible bone marrow suppression, diarrhea, a reversible nephropathy, and moderate oral ulcerations have been observed. Symptomatic treatment appears to be the mainstay of treatment following a melphalan overdose. In view of its high protein binding and other toxicokinetic properties, hemodialysis or hemoperfusion may not be effective. There are no antidotes.

Mercaptopurine

6-Mercaptopurine (Purinethol®, 6-MP) is a purine analogue. In overdose, dizziness, headache, abdominal pain, and a rise in serum bilirubin may be seen. Characteristic hepatotoxic features after 6-mercaptopurine ingestion are a combination of intrahepatic cholestasis and parenchymal cell necrosis. Hepatotoxic reactions are most common when daily doses exceed 2.5 mg/kg. These effects are usually reversible on discontinuation of the drug. However, elevation of serum bilirubin may forewarn of impending cholestasis, which can be fatal. Treatment is supportive.

Methotrexate

The therapeutic use of methotrexate (Folex®, MTX), a folic acid antagonist, as an antineoplastic agent generally involves doses of 20–80 mg/m^2 intravenously and intramuscularly, 0.5 to 2 mg/kg orally, and/or 10–15 mg/m^2 intrathecally. High doses of over 20 mg/kg have been used, as well as 35–150 mg/kg intravenously with citrovorum factor (folinic acid) rescue. Overdose may lead to pancytopenia and mucositis. Prompt leucovorin rescue and charcoal hemoperfusion appear useful in bringing down the plasma methotrexate concentration.

Intrathecal methotrexate may induce at least three types of toxic reactions. The most common is a chemical arachnoiditis, generally mild, that occurs soon after instillation of the drug and resolves within several days (occasionally the clinical and cerebrospinal fluid findings may resemble bacterial meningitis). A second category includes spinal cord and/or nerve damage. Reversible and/or ascending paraplegia may develop and can result in death. Patients may also develop encephalopathy, dementia, seizures, coma, and death. The toxicity of intrathecal MTX may be related in part to preservatives such as benzyl alcohol. See treatment guidelines in the Introduction section of this chapter.

Mitoxantrone

Mitoxantrone (Novantrone®) is an anthraquinone related chemically to the anthracyclines. Overdoses have led to death with severe leukopenia, thrombocytopenia, and infection.

Procarbazine

Procarbazine (Matulane®) inhibits DNA and RNA synthesis and may damage DNA directly. The major manifestations of overdose with procarbazine that would be anticipated are nausea, vomiting, diarrhea, hypotension, tremors, convulsions, and coma. Procarbazine use is subject to serious hematotoxic and hepatotoxic effects. Supportive therapy is the mainstay of treatment.

Vincristine

Vincristine (Norcristine®) is an example of a vinca alkaloid. Vinca alkaloids bind to microtubular proteins and cause metaphase arrest. Following vincristine overdose, fever, nausea, and vomiting usually begin in the first 24 hours and resolve within 1 week. There may be progressive development of peripheral neuropathy during the first week, associated with diminished deep tendon reflexes, particularly in the lower extremities, followed by paresthesias in 10–14 days, and muscle weakness and disturbed gait in 2–3 weeks. Slow recovery may occur over 30–45 days.

Inappropriate antidiuretic hormone secretion may begin 3–7 days after injection, and is frequently associated with seizures that do not appear to be directly related to associated hyponatremia. Sensory disturbances may begin during the first week, progress to lethargy and disorientation by the second week, and resolve over the next 2–4 weeks. Bone marrow depression is characterized by leukopenia with a nadir at 10 days and complete recovery within 3 weeks.

Gastrointestinal disturbances usually begin 4–72 hours after an injection, and may be followed by abdominal pain, ileus, and constipation within 9–13 days. Cranial nerve palsies, especially ptosis, and autonomic dysfunction may occur after 2–3 weeks, and improve over 4–8 weeks. Alopecia and early hypertension may be observed. Most instances of inadvertent intrathecal administration of vincristine have resulted in ascending paralysis and death in several weeks.

Leucovorin does not appear to significantly alter toxicity following a vincristine overdose. Plasmapheresis was used to treat a vincristine overdose in an 18-year-old patient who received ten times the intended dose of vincristine in error. Vincristine is highly bound to plasma proteins and cannot be dialyzed.

Vindesine

Vindesine is another vinca alkaloid. Vindesine overdose (45 mg instead of 4.5 mg) has been associated with generalized muscle pain, tinnitus, diarrhea, sleeplessness, a burning sensation in the mouth, and hiccups. Patients usually respond to supportive treatment.

Questions—Specific Antineoplastic Agents

1. Heart failure from dose-related cardiomyopathy is the most clinically important manifestation of anthracycline cardiotoxicity.
A. True
B. False

2. Which of the following associations does not exist?
A. Bleomycin–Lung toxicity
B. Cis-platinum–Renal toxicity
C. Doxorubicin–Heart toxicity
D. Mercaptopurine–Liver toxicity
E. Procarbazine–Thyroid toxicity

3. All of the following statements are true about vincristine except
A. Vincristine is an example of a vinca alkaloid.
B. Vinca alkaloids bind to microtubular proteins and cause metaphase arrest.
C. There may be progressive development of peripheral neuropathy during the first week, associated with increased deep tendon reflexes, particularly in the lower extremities, followed by paresthesias in 3–4 weeks, and muscle weakness and disturbed gait in 1–2 months.
D. Inappropriate antidiuretic hormone secretion may begin 3–7 days after injection, and is frequently associated with seizures that do not appear to be directly related to associated hyponatremia.
E. Bone marrow depression is characterized by leukopenia with a nadir at 10 days and complete recovery within 3 weeks.

4. All of the following statements are true about methotrexate except
A. Methotrexate is a folic acid antagonist.
B. High doses may be used with citrovorum factor (folinic acid) rescue.
C. Overdose may lead to pancytopenia and mucositis.
D. Prompt leucovorin rescue and hemodialysis appear useful in bringing down the plasma methotrexate concentration.
E. Intrathecal methotrexate may cause a chemical arachnoiditis, spinal cord damage, and / or encephalopathy.

5. All of the following statements are true about cis-platinum except
A. Cisplatin inhibits DNA synthesis by forming cross-links and denaturing the double helix.
B. Acute overdose with cisplatin may result in renal failure, hepatic failure, deafness, significant myelosuppression, intractable nausea and vomiting, neuritis and / or death.
C. No antidotes have been established for cisplatin overdose.
D. Hemodialysis is useful in eliminating platinum from the body, but plasmapheresis does not lower the plasma platinum concentration.
E. Management is based on supportive and symptomatic treatment.

Answers

Introduction to Chemotherapeutic Drugs

1. D 2. E 3. A 4. D 5. E 6. B
7. C

Specific Antineoplastic Agents

1. A 2. E 3. C 4. D 5. D

SELECTED READINGS

Chemotherapeutic Drugs

1. Boivin J-F: Second cancers and other late side effects of cancer treatment. A review. Cancer 1990;65:770–775.
2. Council on Scientific Affairs. Guidelines for handling parenteral antineoplastics. JAMA 1985;253:1590–1592.

3. Doll DC, Ringenberg Q, Yarbro JW. Antineoplastic agents and pregnancy. Semin Oncol 1989;16:337–346.
4. Drugs of choice for cancer chemotherapy. Med Lett Drugs Ther 1995;37: 251–252.
5. Dundee JW, Yang J, Ghaly RG. Vomiting and chemotherapy. Lancet 1990; 535-541.
6. Flotre M, Borenstein M, Blair TMH, eds. Evaluation and management of oncologic emergencies. Emerg Med Rep 1991;12(2):11–16.
7. Foot ABM, Hayes C. Audit of guidelines for effective control of chemotherapy and radiotherapy induced emesis. Arch Dis Child 1994;71:475–480.
8. Nicholson HO. Cytotoxic drugs in pregnancy. J Obstet Gynecol Br Comm 1968;75:307–312.
9. Nicolson M, Leonard RCF. Adverse effects of cancer chemotherapy. An overview of techniques for avoidance of minimisation. Drug Safety 1992;7:316–322.
10. Schneider SM, Distelborst CW. Chemotherapy-induced emergencies. Semin Oncol 1989;16:572–578.

CHAPTER 45
Airborne Toxins

INTRODUCTION

The lungs are a vulnerable target for chemicals because of their high exposure to air (approximately 10,000 L / day), high exposure to blood and cardiac output (about 7,000 L / day), and large surface area. The five major cell populations of the lung include the type I and type II alveolar epithelial cells, capillary endothelial cells, alveolar macrophages, and interstitial cells. These cells form the basic structures underlying gas exchange in the lung. Two other cell types (Clara cells and neuroendocrine cells) are of interest to the toxicologist because they appear to play important roles in xenobiotic metabolism and carcinogenesis.

Alveolar Macrophages

Alveolar macrophages join in the defense against hostile pathogenic organisms. When they are compromised by toxic inhalants, they may increase susceptibility to infectious diseases. They also are involved in the development and pathogenesis of chronic lung diseases such as silicosis and asbestosis. They may work in collaboration with polymorphonuclear leukocytes.

Alveolar Type I Cells

These epithelial cells comprise 8% of the parenchymal cell population and cover over 90% of the alveolar surface. Possibly, because of their relative lack of cytoplasmic organelles and the long distance between their cytoplasmic processes and cell nucleus, they are vulnerable to inhaled and blood-borne toxic agents. Type I cells expose the largest percentage of their epithelial surface to toxic agents.

Alveolar Type II Cells

The type II epithelial cell produces surfactant and may replace damaged type I cells. They cover 7% of the alveolar surface, but represent 16% of the total cell population.

Capillary Endothelial Cells

Capillary endothelial cells represent the largest single cell population in the lung, comprising 30% of all human lung cells. They form the first line of defense against blood-borne toxic agents.

Clara Cells

Clara cells, or nonciliated bronchiolar cells, have a substantial agranular cytoplasmic reticulum. They function as the primary secretory cell type in the conducting airway of the centriacinar region (terminal bronchioles). The Clara cell replicates itself, or it may develop into a ciliated cell. It is the primary site of cytochrome P-450 monooxygenase activity within the lungs.

Interstitial Cells

Fibroblasts, lymphocytes, interstitial macrophages, mast cells, pericytes, and plasma cells constitute the lung cells that occupy the interstitial space and represent approximately 37% of all lung cells. When pulmonary epithelial cells react to toxic chemicals, there may be a subsequent increase in fibroblast number and an increase in collagen production, resulting in interstitial pulmonary fibrosis. This may follow toxic lung damage induced by airborne substances, including oxidant gases, dusts, and fibers (e.g., silica, asbestos) or following blood-borne agents such as antineoplastic drugs.

Neuroendocrine Cells

Neuroendocrine cells also are known as APUD cells (**a**mino **p**recursor **u**ptake and **d**ecarboxylase) or Kulchitsky cells. They are found in the mucosa lining the airways or in the pulmonary parenchyma. These cells proliferate when exposed to hyperoxia.

Questions—Introduction to Airborne Toxins

1. Which of the following is an incorrect match?
- A. Alveolar macrophages—Involved in the development and pathogenesis of chronic lung disease such as silicosis and asbestosis
- B. Alveolar type I cells—Cover over 90% of the alveolar surface
- C. Capillary endothelial cells—Represent the largest single cell population in the lung
- D. Clara cells—The primary site of cytochrome P-450 monooxygenase activity within the lungs
- E. Interstitial Cells—APUD or Kulchitsky cells

2. All of the following are correct except
- A. Alveolar macrophages defend against hostile pathogenic organisms
- B. Type I alveolar cells are particularly vulnerable to inhaled toxins
- C. Neuroendocrine cells are the most common cell types in the lung
- D. Type II alveolar cells produce surfactant
- E. Capillary endothelial are major line of defense for blood-borne toxins

INDOOR AIR POLLUTION

Problems associated with indoor air quality (IAQ) have been reported in newly constructed or remodeled buildings. Some new buildings are sealed and energy-efficient with few or no open windows. Outside air may only be provided through a recirculated air-conditioning system. These buildings are known as "sick buildings."

Answers to questions in shaded boxes appear at the end of the chapter.

Sick Building Syndrome

Sick Building Syndrome (SBS) refers to a constellation of symptoms frequently reported by those who work in "sick buildings" and includes nasal, eye, and mucous membrane irritation, lethargy, dry skin, headaches, nausea, and sensitivity to odors. Other terms for the SBS have included "tight building syndrome," "closed building problem," "new building syndrome," "indoor air pollution," and "building-associated illness." No objective findings or laboratory tests are diagnostic of SBS in symptomatic individuals.

An "outbreak" of SBS is considered an excessive reporting of one or more such symptoms by the occupants of a "sick building." "Work-related" refers to the occurrence of symptoms after coming to work, worsening of symptoms during work, and the disappearance of symptoms after leaving work. Preexisting medical conditions or exposure to known occupational toxins must be ruled out in making the distinction of "sick building syndrome."

Sick Hospital Syndrome

Between 40% and 50% of operating room and recovery room personnel may have acute symptoms such as fatigue, headache, dizziness, lightheadedness, nausea, drowsiness, cough, and skin irritation from exposure to nitrous oxide, ethylene oxide, and halogenated anesthetics. Germicidal agents, including isopropyl alcohol, glutaraldehyde, and parachlorophenol, have been implicated. Airborne transmission of infectious agents such as rubella, chickenpox, and *Legionella* may contribute.

Mass Psychogenic Illness

The rapid spread of symptoms whose basis lies in psychosocial factors may be a confounding factor in defining a building-specific syndrome. So-called "mass psychogenic illness" may be similar to those symptoms typically reported in the sick building syndrome. Odors are the most common triggering event. The threshold for detection of chemical odor often is well below air concentrations associated with any toxicity. Workers may believe that odors signal dangerous indoor air pollution. Workers may be alarmed if they believe that environmental contaminants may cause damaging long-term effects, particularly cancer or birth defects. Concerns are increased if the source, often an offensive odor, is unknown.

Pathophysiology

Environmental tobacco smoke, irritant gases, respirable fibers, dusts, particulates, and volatile organic compounds (VOCs) may contribute to the development or exacerbation of bronchiolitis, chronic bronchitis, and emphysema by direct effects on elastic fibers, connective-tissue repair, and alteration of protease inhibitors. Research is required to establish a definite correlation between chronic indoor oxidant exposure (nitrogen dioxide, sulfur dioxide, ozone) and chronic obstructive pulmonary disease (COPD) development.

Tobacco smoke and cleaning / renovation activities continue to be prominent sources of respirable particulates. Controlled studies of such contaminants and COPD have not been performed. Gases such as nitrogen dioxide, sulfur dioxide, and ozone are known irritants, but whether they cause irritation at concentrations commonly found in indoor air remains to be determined. Most dusts and fibers are irritating to the eyes and mucous membranes.

Clinical Presentations

No specific etiology has been discovered for sick building syndrome, although there have been associations with certain closed building ventilation systems and with a variety of indoor air pollutants. Numerous potential pollutants may circulate through indoor airspace.

MICROBES

Human respiration releases water vapor, carbon dioxide, and microbes into the air. Humidity, certain temperatures, and appropriate physical and nutritional substrates may enhance microbial growth. Airborne exposure to *Legionella pneumophila* may lead to Legionnaires' disease, a progressive pneumonia associated with confusion, vomiting, and diarrhea. Sources of this organism may include air conditioning and cooling towers, evaporative condensers, showerheads, drinking water, and streams.

HUMIDIFIER FEVER

Microbial contaminants of humidifiers, vaporizers, or saunas often are associated with a variant of hypersensitivity pneumonitis (HP) called humidifier fever (HF). Symptoms of HP and humidifier fever may be similar. Microbial toxins cause HF, and HP has been linked to actinomycetes, fungi, and organic dusts. Fever is observed more in HF than in HP. Symptoms of HF often begin in the first 4 to 6 hours after beginning the workweek and subside during the week. These may include headache, polyuria, weight loss, and joint pain. The etiologic agents of HF have not been defined.

HVAC SYSTEMS

Heating, ventilation, and air-conditioning (HVAC) systems can be a source of indoor air contaminants such as combustion products, bio aerosols, fibers, and particulates. HVAC systems, insulation, fabrics, ceiling tiles, and carpets also may be substrates for microbial growth. Man-made mineral fibers (MMMF), including fiberglass, glass wool, and rock wool, are used extensively in HVAC ducting. Any repair activities that disrupt the integrity of the duct-lining materials may introduce MMMF into indoor air. Lighting, vibrations, and noises also can intensify indoor air pollution problems.

VOLATILE ORGANIC COMPOUNDS

Indoor volatile organic compounds (VOCs), such as formaldehyde, airborne alcohols, aldehydes, aliphatic, aromatic and halogenated hydrocarbons, and ketones, may be associated with mucosal irritation. Massive exposure to VOCs may result in reactive airways dysfunction syndrome (RADS), characterized by bronchial hyperresponsiveness. Many VOCs arise from building materials and interior furnishings. Common materials leading to problems in IAQ include paints, adhesives, caulks, carpeting, other flooring products, glazing compounds, and insulation materials. Particulates and fibers from asbestos and fiberglass insulation also may contribute to indoor air pollution problems.

RESPIRATORY IRRITANTS

Persistent lung diseases such as cancer, emphysema, fibrosis, and chronic bronchitis may be a result of inhaled gases or particulates. Environmental tobacco smoke, radon, asbestos, organic particulates, and VOCs may exert individual and additive effects on the initiation of human cancer. The association between indoor air and induction of cancer has not been demonstrated by controlled studies.

ODORS

Odors are more annoying to people who work in clean environments such as offices than to those who work in dirty environments such as print shops or garages. Odor-induced bronchospasm in asthmatics may follow exposure to tobacco smoke, perfumes, and colognes. Most IAQ complaints in nonindustrial environments are triggered by chemical levels 100- to 1,000-fold below published standards affecting performance and health. Investigation of IAQ problems requires a personal interview and clinical histories of the individuals involved, walk-through environmental surveys, environmental monitoring (if required), inspection of HVAC systems, and communication of results.

Treatment

SUPPORTIVE MEASURES

- Approaches to diminish the incidence of sick building syndrome include a complete history and physical examination, temporary removal of an individual from the workplace, correction of building problems, and delaying occupancy of a new building for several weeks while ventilation is maintained at 100% outside air.
- Repair of roof leaks and checking for water contamination in the HVAC systems is required. Frequent replacement of air conditioning filters, recognition of an SBS outbreak, and banning of cigarette smoking may be helpful.
- Indoor air pollution concentrations can be kept below levels that produce illness by excluding or removing sources of contamination, diluting room air with cleaner air (ventilation), removing contaminants from the air (filtration), and providing local exhausts.
- Prevention of excessive indoor microbial contamination requires appropriate HVAC installation, operation, and maintenance. Clean outdoor air makeup, appropriate humidity control, filtration to limit intrusion of outdoor bioaerosols, and dedicated housekeeping and maintenance protocols, may be helpful.
- Prevention may be enhanced by using low-VOC–emitting materials, supplies, and equipment, and by assuring adequate ventilation. Appropriate housekeeping and air filtration usually are effective in reducing airborne concentrations of dusts, particulates, and fibers. Selection of materials with low odor levels plus adequate ventilation and housekeeping usually are effective in eliminating unacceptable odors.

Questions—Indoor Air Pollution

1. Sick building syndrome
   A. May be diagnosed with a single laboratory test
   B. Also has been called tight building syndrome
   C. Is associated with nasal, eye, and mucous membrane irritation
   D. All of the above
   E. B and C

2. Sick hospital syndrome may be a result of anesthetic gases, ethylene oxide, isopropyl alcohol, and/or infectious agents.
   A. True
   B. False

3. The most common triggering event in mass psychogenic illness is
   A. A truly sick co-worker
   B. Annoying sounds
   C. Annoying odors
   D. New carpeting
   E. Illegal drug use

4. Indoor volatile organic compounds (VOCs) include
   A. Hydrocarbons
   B. *Legionella pneumophila*
   C. Radon
   D. All of the above
   E. A and B

OUTDOOR AIR POLLUTION

Photochemical Smog

The acute and chronic effects of various forms of air pollution can be deadly. In 1955, for example, during a week-long heat wave in Los Angeles, more than 247 deaths occurred per day because of the atmospheric and geographic conditions. A strong temperature inversion layer reduced the mixing height of pollutants and increased pollutant concentrations to deadly levels.

High temperatures, sunlight, and the emission of hydrocarbons from automobile exhausts can produce large amounts of photochemical smog. Minimal wind conditions can produce stagnant air, which intensifies concentration of smog. Generally, these episodes are short-term and sporadic. Aesthetically, fine mists produced from hydrocarbons, sulfur dioxide, and nitrogen oxides cause visibly dirty air, and chemical oxidizing may cause pervasive odors.

Direct acute health effects of photochemical smog are difficult to establish. Eye irritation is frequent. Excess mortality is less easily demonstrated, because there are cyclical variations in various pollutant levels, and other factors (e.g., season, high temperatures, rapid temperature changes, holidays, day of week). Photochemical smog may increase the risk of asthmatic attacks in a small number of susceptible patients, reduce pulmonary function after long-term exposure, cause mucous membrane irritation and cough, and interfere with athletic performance.

Nonphotochemical Smog

High levels of carbon monoxide, sulfur oxides, and particulate matter occur frequently in the northeastern United States and parts of Europe. The high density of cities increases the background concentration of pollutants. In 1936, in the Meuse Valley in Belgium, high sulfur dioxide emissions from coal-burning plants combined with light winds to produce several thousand cases of pulmonary irritation and 65 deaths.

In 1948, in Donora, Pennsylvania, high concentrations of particulate matter and sulfur dioxide emissions from industrial smoke caused a severe pollution episode with at least 20 excess deaths. Almost half of the city residents developed conjunctival and upper respiratory irritation along with gastrointestinal symptoms. In 1952, in London, high particulate matter and sulfur dioxide concentrations in the absence of air movement produced over 4,000 excess deaths.

By law, the United States government sets ambient air quality standards at levels that provide an adequate margin of safety to protect health. These standards are based on threshold values established from animal experiments, experimental human exposures, and epidemiologic studies. Such threshold values do not represent no-effect values, as they are set to reduce detectable health effects to those levels "normally" seen in a general population. Sensitive individuals, such as those with chronic cardiopulmonary disease, may sustain adverse effects at or below these levels.

Clinical Presentations

The effect of air pollution depends on pollutant concentration, specific pollutants, duration of exposure, and presence of underlying cardiopulmonary disease. Both acute symptoms and aggravation of chronic disease may result from exposure, but the complex variables involved in large epidemiologic studies make the detection of injury and the establishment of limits on exposure difficult.

Particular susceptibility to urban air pollution occurs in premature infants, the newborn, the elderly, those with chronic cardiac and pulmonary disease, hypersensitive individuals, and heavy cigarette smokers. Suggested toxic effects of pollution include impaired expiratory flow rate, airway inflammation, increased cough and sputum production, reduced resistance to pulmonary infections, decreased exercise tolerance in cardiac patients, unfavorable electrocardiogram (ECG) changes, impaired oxygen transport, transient eye irritation, and excess death rates. Exercise performance is definitely reduced.

ACID RAIN

In recent years, acidity of rain and snow has increased sharply over the Northeastern United States and Canada, Western Europe, and Scandinavia. The normal pH of precipitation (5.6) is a result of naturally occurring sulfur dioxide and hydrogen sulfide (e.g., from volcanoes), which are oxidized and hydrolyzed to sulfuric acid. Nitrogen oxides are converted similarly to nitric acid. The increasing release of sulfur and nitrogen oxide from burning fossil fuels has changed precipitation in certain areas from neutral solutions 200 years ago to dilute acidic solutions today. The most extreme reported case was the presence of rain at a pH of 2.4 (i.e., the pH equivalent of vinegar) in Scotland in 1974.

Although human health effects have not been documented, damage to forests and lakes has been obvious. Potential human effects include the inhalation of nitrogen and sulfur oxides, as well as the mobilization of trace elements from the soil (e.g., lead, mercury, and aluminum). Efforts at control have been frustrated by the fact that damage occurs at great distances from the source of pollutants. Ironically, the building of large smokestacks has reduced local pollution but increased the transport of pollutants to distant areas where acid rain forms.

ALDEHYDES

Examples of aldehydes are acrolein and formaldehyde. Pulmonary irritation and bronchospasm may follow significant exposures.

CARBON MONOXIDE

High concentrations impair oxygen transport, which may affect cardiac patients on smoggy days. Generally, no ill effects occur in healthy individuals at existing levels.

HYDROCARBONS

There probably are no adverse health effects at ambient air concentrations, but these compounds combine with primary pollutants and sunlight to form oxidants and mists.

NITROGEN OXIDES

Interstitial edema, epithelial proliferation, and, in high concentrations, fibrosis and emphysema develop after heavy nitrogen dioxide exposures. At current pollution levels, nitrogen oxides are less toxic than ozone, and short-term exposures probably do not contribute to cardiorespiratory disease. See Nitrogen Oxides section, below.

OZONE

This chemical causes eye irritation and bronchitis, aggravates COPD, and perhaps increases the risk of acute and chronic pulmonary disease, mutagenesis, and fetotoxicity. Ozone damages tissue by rapidly oxidizing thiol-containing compounds and unsaturated fatty acids. Symptoms of respiratory irritation and decreased forced expiratory volume occur at exposures above 0.3 ppm, but strenuous exercise causes these effects to develop at lower ozone levels. See Ozone section, below.

SULFUR DIOXIDE

Sulfates and sulfur dioxide, together with particulate matter and photochemical pollutants, aggravate chronic pulmonary disease and increase the risk of acute and chronic respiratory illness. These compounds impair pulmonary mucociliary clearance, primarily in those patients with preexisting pulmonary disease, probably because of hydrogen ion deposition on the bronchial lining. Sulfur dioxide has been responsible for major air pollution disasters. In high-exposure communities, smokers and nonsmokers have a higher incidence of persistent cough and sputum production compared with controls in low-exposure communities.

Questions—Outdoor Air Pollution

1. **Which of the following is false?**
   A. Outdoor air pollution can be deadly.
   B. High temperatures, sunlight, and the emission of hydrocarbons from automobile exhausts can produce photochemical smog.
   C. Sulfur dioxide, nitrogen oxides, and carbon monoxide cause visibly dirty air.
   D. All of the above
   E. A and C
2. **High levels of sulfur dioxide emissions from coal-burning plants have caused numerous deaths in neighboring communities.**
   A. True
   B. False
3. **Which of the following is false?**
   A. The normal pH of precipitation is slightly acidic.
   B. The increasing release of sulfur and nitrogen oxide from burning fossil fuels has changed precipitation in certain areas from neutral solutions to dilute acidic solutions today.
   C. Rain actually has been measured as having a pH less than three in certain areas.
   D. Despite the presence of acid rain, damage to forests and lakes has not been recorded.
   E. C and D

CARBON DIOXIDE

Carbon dioxide, a major endproduct of cellular respiration, may act as an asphyxiant in certain settings, and potentially cause death. Asphyxiants produce hypoxia by displacing oxygen from the environment. Other asphyxiants include nitrogen gas, methane, and other low-molecular-weight hydrocarbons. Numerous fatalities have occurred after individuals have entered fermentation vats, wells, and silos where air has been replaced by carbon dioxide. Deaths and cerebral damage have been associated with accidental hypercapnia following the use of carbon dioxide in anesthesia. In 1986, carbon dioxide was blamed as the cause of death of about 1,700 people in Cameroon, West Africa, when a massive release of gas occurred from Lake Nyos, a volcanic crater lake.

Most commercially available carbon dioxide is recovered from industrial processes in which it is generated as a byproduct. It is present in natural gas wells and is a product of fuel combustion and of fermentation. Carbon dioxide is used in the carbonation of beverages, as a propellant in aerosols, and as dry ice for refrigeration.

Pathophysiology

Carbon dioxide exerts a key influence on the control of respiration and cerebral circulation. Carbon dioxide dissolves in serum and forms carbonic acid. It induces graded increases in respiratory minute volume and ventilatory rate. Increased carbon dioxide levels may result in respiratory acidosis. It acts peripherally, both as a vasodilator and as a vasoconstrictor, and is a powerful cerebral vasodilator.

At high concentrations, it exerts a stimulating effect on the central nervous system, while excessive levels exert depressant effects. Carbon dioxide is a colorless, odorless, noncombustible gas that is soluble in water. It normally is present in the atmosphere at a concentration of approximately 0.03% (300 ppm). It is a normal body constituent arising from cellular respiration.

Clinical Presentations

Acute exposure to 6% to 10% carbon dioxide may decrease vascular resistance, increase renal blood flow, and increase cerebral blood flow. It also increases systolic and diastolic blood pressure, pulse rate, and respiratory muscle volume with sweating and hyperpnea. Exposure to 10% to 20% carbon dioxide may induce myoclonic twitching, dilated pupils, and restlessness. At 17% for 20 to 50 seconds, throat irritation, tachypnea, dimness of vision, dizziness, and unconsciousness may supervene. Chronic hypercapnia in patients suffering from pulmonary disease may cause headache, somnolence, mental confusion, lassitude, irritability, and unconsciousness.

Toxic Dosage/Death

Concentrations of 20% to 30% result in unconsciousness and convulsions within 1 minute of exposure. Exposure to concentrations of 75,000 ppm (7.5%) for 15 minutes has resulted in headache, dizziness, restlessness, and dyspnea. Neurologic signs, including eye flickering, myoclonic twitches, dilated pupils, and restlessness, have followed exposure to 100,000 to 150,000 ppm of carbon dioxide for 15 minutes.

Treatment

GUT DECONTAMINATION

These methods play no role in reversing the ill effects of carbon dioxide.

ELIMINATION ENHANCEMENT

These methods also play no role in reversing the ill effects of carbon dioxide.

SUPPORTIVE MEASURES

- Initial management of severe symptoms following carbon dioxide inhalation requires immediate removal from the source, establishment of an adequate oxygen supply, and careful attention to airway, breathing, and circulation.
- Near-fatal carbon dioxide embolism during laparoscopy and hysteroscopy has been successfully treated with cardiopulmonary bypass.
- Exposures to 7.5% carbon dioxide for 15 minutes may lead to a decrease in total eosinophils, increase in blood sugar, and increase in arterial $PaCO_2$ and pH.

Question—Carbon Dioxide

1. Which of the following is false?
   A. Asphyxiants produce hypoxia by displacing oxygen from the environment.
   B. Asphyxiants include nitrogen gas, methane, and carbon dioxide.
   C. In 1986, carbon dioxide was blamed as the cause of death of about 1,700 people in Cameroon, West Africa, when a release of gas occurred from Lake Nyos, a volcanic crater lake.
   D. Death from carbonated beverages has been reported.
   E. Exposure to 10% to 20% carbon dioxide may induce myoclonic twitching, dilated pupils, and restlessness.

CARBON DISULFIDE

Although acute carbon disulfide toxicity is relatively rare, chronic carbon disulfide toxicity was well known in the French and German rubber industry by the late 1800s. Early American industrial exposure resulted in severe debilitating central nervous system symptoms including irritability, mania, tremors, hallucinations, and memory loss. Recent concern centers on chronic industrial exposures, which may cause neuropsychiatric changes, peripheral neuropathies, and accelerated atherogenic changes. Carbon disulfide is primarily a synthetic product that produces disturbances in trace mineral balance in humans. Minute amounts are found in coal and crude oil.

Carbon disulfide is a man-made product. It has a sweet, aromatic odor resembling that of decaying cabbage. Most poisonings occur in the viscose rayon manufacturing industry. Commercial applications include use as a chemical intermediate for adhesives, a grain and soil fumigant, a solvent in the rubber and rayon industries, a grease remover, a corrosion inhibitor, and an insecticide. Carbon disulfide also is a metabolite of disulfiram and may be responsible for some of the adverse effects associated with that agent.

Pathophysiology

Carbon disulfide reacts with a variety of compounds in the body, including pyridoxamine (a member of the vitamin B6 complex), cerebral monoamine oxidases, and dopamine decarboxylase. Carbon disulfide binds to microsomal enzymes, reducing their activity, and produces a centrilobular hepatic necrosis. Carbon disulfide also may interfere with copper and zinc metabolism by acting as a chelating agent. Chronic exposure to carbon disulfide can result in permanent axonal neuropathy.

Pharmacokinetics

ABSORPTION

- Carbon disulfide is well absorbed through the lungs, and serious toxicity has resulted from ingestion.

DISTRIBUTION

- Peak blood concentrations appear 2 hours after inhalation.
- The liver and fat tissue store concentrated carbon disulfide.

ELIMINATION

- The plasma elimination half-life is about 1 hour.
- The body metabolizes between 80% and 90% of the absorbed dose; the lungs excrete all except a small fraction of the rest.
- Disulfiram is metabolized to carbon disulfide.

Clinical Presentations

DERMATOLOGIC EFFECTS

Local contact results in erythema and pain because carbon disulfide is a potent fat solvent. Prolonged contact produces vesiculation and chemical burns. Severe chemical burns of the cornea result from direct contact with the eyes.

NEUROLOGIC EFFECTS

Acute inhalation produces rapid onset of both local irritation and central nervous system symptoms ranging from pharyngitis, nausea, vomiting, dizziness, fatigue, headache, mood changes, lethargy, and blurred vision to agitation, delirium, hallucinations, convulsions, coma, and death. Carbon disulfide is a potent neurotoxin. Peripheral neuropathies, cranial nerve dysfunction, and neuropsychiatric changes are common in chronic carbon sulfide poisoning victims. Impaired psychomotor function and higher cortical function, as well as neurasthenic symptoms (i.e., mood swings, irritability, headache, nausea, fatigue, malaise, memory loss), characterize the neurologic illness associated with excessive carbon disulfide exposures.

CHRONIC EFFECTS

Chronic long-term exposures (e.g., in rayon workers) may result in elevated blood cholesterol, retinopathy (e.g., microaneurysms, optic neuropathy), peripheral neuropathy, decreased glucose tolerance, reduced serum thyroxine levels, and parkinsonism. Increases in atherosclerosis, coronary artery disease, deaths, suicide rates, personality changes, and hypertensive disease have been suggested, but not confirmed, by epidemiologic studies.

Toxic Dosage/Death

Exposure to a time-weighted average of 11 ppm results in headache and dizziness. Exposure to 20 ppm results in sleep disturbances, fatigue, nervousness, anorexia, and weight loss. Long-term exposure to levels in excess of 20 ppm may result in atherogenic and diabetogenic changes. Most acute carbon disulfide fatalities result from ingestion. 15 mL may be fatal to an adult.

Laboratory

ANALYTIC METHODS

An iodine-azide test for urinary metabolites of carbon disulfide is used to assess industrial exposure.

BLOOD LEVELS

Blood levels do not guide management of overdose.

Treatment

- Lavage and charcoal use after very recent ingestion of toxic quantities may be helpful, but such interventions have not been shown to be uniformly reliable.
- Initial management of severe inhalational poisoning requires careful attention to airway, breathing, and circulation. Otherwise, treatment involves removal from source and symptomatic care.
- Electromyography and nerve conduction studies are sensitive methods for the early detection of carbon disulfide peripheral neuropathy.
- The Santa Ana Dexterity Test, tests of simple reaction time, and Wechsler Adult Intelligence Scale (WAIS) subtests on block design, digit symbols, and digit span have been suggested as accurate measures of carbon disulfide-induced neuropsychiatric dysfunction. Patients must be matched to age-appropriate controls.

Questions—Carbon Disulfide

1. Carbon disulfide
A. Is used in the viscose rayon manufacturing industry
B. Is used as a grain and soil fumigant
C. Is used as a grease remover
D. Is used as a lubricant in the computer industry
E. A, B and C

2. Carbon disulfide
A. Can cause severe debilitating central nervous system symptoms including irritability, mania, tremors, hallucinations, and memory loss
B. May cause neuropsychiatric changes and peripheral neuropathies
C. May cause accelerated atherogenic changes
D. All of the above
E. A and B

3. Carbon disulfide
A. Reacts with pyridoxamine (a member of the vitamin B6 complex)
B. Binds to microsomal enzymes and produces a centrilobular hepatic necrosis
C. Can cause a permanent axonal neuropathy
D. All of the above
E. None of the above

4. Carbon disulfide is a metabolite of _____ and may be responsible for some of the adverse effects associated with that agent.
A. Sulfur dioxide
B. Carbon tetrachloride
C. Disulfiram
D. Methanol
E. Sulfuric acid

CARBON MONOXIDE

Carbon monoxide (CO) is the leading cause of poisoning deaths in the United States. Roughly two-thirds of fatalities occur in fire victims. Most accidents from CO poisoning result from the incomplete combustion of carbon-containing material with inadequate ventilation. Automobile exhaust contains up to 9% CO, and catalytic converters substantially reduce CO levels to below 1%. About two-thirds of deaths occur in cars. Because of lack of ventilation, automobile exhaust can leak into a car and slowly overcome passengers. Lethal CO levels can occur in a closed garage within 10 minutes. Expressway CO levels may approach 25 to 100 ppm.

About one-third of CO deaths involve faulty heating equipment. Although natural gas contains no CO, improperly vented gas water heaters or kerosene space heaters cause CO poisoning. Charcoal grills, hibachis, and Sterno® all give off CO when used for heating in closed spaces (e.g., in campers, garages, and caves). Kerosene space heaters may produce subtle symptoms of carbon monoxide poisoning, which may be misdiagnosed as pneumonia, myocardial infarction, cholecystitis, epilepsy, or viral syndrome. Typically, patients present in winter with headache, nausea, vomiting, weakness, decreased cognitive function, new-onset angina pectoris, or exacerbation of chronic cardiopulmonary disease.

CO is the most frequent cause of immediate fire deaths, and CO poisoning should be suspected in every fire victim. CO levels in fires may reach 10%, which can raise carboxyhemoglobin levels in active firefighters without respiratory protection to 75% within 1 minute. CO victims may continue to suffer both severe and subtle long-term neurologic sequelae. As many as 15% to 40% of victims of serious, nonfatal CO poisoning develop neuropsychiatric symptoms including personality changes and memory impairment, which can appear after apparent recovery. Despite extensive clinical experience, treatment remains somewhat controversial.

Methylene chloride, a constituent of paint and varnish removers, is converted *in vivo* to CO. Use of these removers for 3 hours may lead to carboxyhemoglobin levels of 5% to 10%. The use of paint remover in a poorly ventilated space has been reported to cause myocardial infarction and death in patients with preexisting cardiovascular disease.

Pathophysiology

HEMATOLOGIC EFFECTS

CO toxicity results from impaired oxygen delivery and utilization, which lead to cellular hypoxia. CO affects several different sites within the body, but the exact contribution of each pathophysiological effect remains unclear. Carboxyhemoglobin (COHb) impairs the release of oxygen from hemoglobin by increasing oxygen binding to hemoglobin. The result is a shift of the oxyhemoglobin dissociation curve to the left, which reduces unloading of oxygen in tissues. Leftward shift also can be caused by methemoglobinemia, hypothermia, alkalosis, and contrast media. The resultant myocardial depression and hypotension cause ischemia and potentiate the hypoxia induced by impaired oxygen delivery.

NEUROLOGIC EFFECTS

Severe CO poisoning produces anatomic changes in the central nervous system including cerebral edema, hemorrhagic focal necrosis, venodilation, petechiae, and perivascular infarcts. Bilateral necrosis of the globus pallidus is a characteristic lesion of CO toxicity. Other vulnerable areas of the cerebral gray matter include the substantia nigra, hippocampus, cerebral cortex, and cerebellum. These histopathological changes are indistinguishable from other causes such as hypoxia, cardiorespiratory arrest, hypoglycemia, and cyanide poisoning.

CARDIOVASCULAR EFFECTS

The heart is particularly vulnerable to CO poisoning because of its high oxygen requirements. The normal cardiac oxygen extraction ratio is 75% compared with 25% for most other tissues. Increasing levels of COHb reduce this level, leading to ischemia. Patients with preexisting cardiac disease are particularly vulnerable because of their inability to increase coronary artery perfusion to compensate for reduced oxygen extraction.

Pharmacokinetics

ABSORPTION

- The lungs rapidly absorb CO, which avidly combines with hemoglobin at 230 to 270 times greater affinity than oxygen.
- Methylene chloride is well absorbed by the lung. Toxicity has resulted from oral ingestion.
- Methylene chloride can be absorbed by intact skin, but probably not in quantities sufficient to cause systemic toxicity.

DISTRIBUTION

- About 85% of absorbed CO combines with hemoglobin. The remainder attaches to myoglobin and blood proteins.

ELIMINATION

- Elimination occurs exclusively through the lungs. The half-life of COHb in room air is 3 to 4 hours depending on minute ventilation.
- Administration of 100% oxygen shortens the half-life to 30 to 50 minutes. Hyperbaric oxygen (100% oxygen at 2.5 atm) further reduces the half-life to as little as 15 to 25 minutes.
- The COHb half-life after methylene chloride exposure is more than two times longer because of continuing endogenous conversion to carbon monoxide.
- The body metabolizes between one-quarter and one-third of the absorbed dose of methylene chloride to CO and the rest to carbon dioxide.

Clinical Presentations

The effects of CO are protean and occasionally mimic other diseases. CO poisoning affects primarily the organs most susceptible to hypoxia (e.g., heart, brain), but symptoms can develop in almost every organ. Subacute toxicity may be misdiagnosed as flulike syndrome consisting of headache, dizziness, nausea, malaise, decreased exercise tolerance or gastroenteritis, especially in children. Chest pain, palpitations, visual disturbances, difficulty concentrating, and syncope are common complaints associated with chronic occult carbon monoxide exposures.

DERMATOLOGIC EFFECTS

Patients may develop bullae that are indistinguishable from those produced by coma or sedative-hypnotic drugs. Bullae tend to occur over pressure areas. Alopecia and sweat gland necrosis is reported rarely. The appearance of bullae appears to be related to the severity of toxicity. Cherry-red skin (e.g., lips, mucous membranes) is characteristic of nonsurvivors, because the high COHb levels required to produce this appearance usually are not compatible with life.

CARDIOVASCULAR EFFECTS

Patients with cardiovascular disease are particularly sensitive to CO cardiotoxicity and may develop exertional angina at COHb levels as low as 5% to 10%. Sudden death has occurred in workers with severe arteriosclerotic heart disease when their COHb levels exceeded 20%. Occasionally, myocardial infarction, conduction defects, premature ventricular contractions, and atrial fibrillation may occur, especially in patients with preexisting atherosclerotic disease. Hypotension results from myocardial depression, even in healthy patients, when COHb levels exceed 60%. Chronic low-level exposure, as seen with heavy cigarette smokers, may accelerate atherosclerosis.

ACUTE NEUROLOGIC EFFECTS

Symptoms reflecting cerebral hypoxia range from headache, lethargy, agitation, and confusion to coma, trismus, muscle spasm, hyperreflexia, and convulsions. A frontal bandlike headache (less often occipital and diffuse) is the most characteristic sign but may be absent after toxicity from high carbon monoxide levels. "Warehouse worker's headache" follows use of propane-fueled forklifts in enclosed warehouses. Common complaints include headache, nausea, and lightheadedness. Syncope and loss of consciousness may occur.

DELAYED NEUROLOGIC EFFECTS

Delayed neurologic sequelae may include visual loss, dementia, retardation, constructional apraxia, temporospatial disorientation, memory loss, dysphasia, personality changes, concentration deficits, and frank psychosis. Parkinson's disease is very rare. In one study, delayed neurological sequelae occurred in 11.8% of patients hospitalized for CO poisoning, and the mean onset of symptoms was 22 days postexposure (range, 2 to 40 days). The most frequent symptoms are mental deterioration, incontinence, gait disturbance, and mutism. Cerebellar signs (e.g., intention tremor) are unusual.

Characteristically, those patients experiencing delayed neurologic sequelae are middle-aged or older. The level of consciousness on admission appears to correlate loosely with subsequent development of gross neuropsychiatric sequelae. Degree of recovery is variable, with up to 75% resolving after 1 year, but memory deficits and gait disturbances may remain. Patients who do not lose consciousness after carbon monoxide exposure may develop delayed neurologic sequelae.

SENSORY EFFECTS

Retinal venous engorgement and peripupillary hemorrhage occur occasionally in both acute and subacute CO exposures. Their presence should alert the physician to the possibility of CO poisoning. CO decreases light sensitivity and dark adaptation. Cochlear and brain stem hypoxia may lead to central hearing loss and vestibular dysfunction (e.g., nausea, vomiting, vertigo), with vestibular symptoms usually more prominent than auditory loss.

PULMONARY EFFECTS

Respiratory complications of CO poisoning include aspiration pneumonia, adult respiratory distress syndrome (ARDS), and pulmonary edema. CO poisoning usually does not produce hyperventilation. Pulmonary edema may result from the direct effects of CO on capillary membranes or the secondary effects of hypoxia on the heart or alveolar membranes.

HEMATOLOGIC EFFECTS

Several cases of hemolytic anemia have been reported after severe CO poisoning. Thrombocytopenic purpura with respiratory dysfunction has been reported.

MUSCULAR EFFECTS

Rhabdomyolysis, acute renal failure, and neuropathies (e.g., ulnar palsy) occur rarely. Myonecrosis may be massive, leading to edema, compartment syndrome, and acute renal failure.

Toxic Dosage/Death

Atmospheric CO levels of 50, 100, and 200 ppm produce average COHb levels of 8%, 16%, and 30%, respectively. Perceptible clinical effects occur with 2-hour exposures to concentrations as low as 100 ppm. An 8-hour exposure to 250 ppm methylene chloride caused the carboxyhemoglobin level to exceed 8%. Severe, acute methylene chloride exposures have resulted in COHb levels as high as 50%.

CO toxicity is increased by numerous factors, including decreased barometric pressure (e.g., high altitude), increased alveolar ventilation (e.g., activity), high metabolic rate (e.g., children, pets, birds), preexisting cardiovascular and cerebral vascular disease, reduced cardiac output, anemia, and hypovolemia.

Postmortem COHb levels usually exceed 50%, but concentrations detected during autopsy may fall below lethal levels. Reasons for unexpectedly low postmortem COHb levels include rapid onset of intoxication, individual ability to tolerate hypoxia (e.g., cardiopulmonary disease), concomitant presence of other drugs, effects of resuscitation attempts, and sample accuracy.

Pregnancy/Lactation

The fetus is particularly vulnerable to CO poisoning because of increased accumulation in fetal blood (10% to 15% higher than maternal levels) and lower initial fetal PaO_2. Furthermore, the fetal hemoglobin dissociation curve lies to the left of the adult curve, resulting in greater tissue hypoxia at similar COHb levels. Acute nonlethal maternal intoxication may result in fetal demise or permanent neurologic sequelae (e.g., cerebral palsy). Prolonged exposure to low doses (5% to 10% COHb in smoking mothers) is associated with smaller babies and elevated neonatal mortality.

Laboratory

ANALYTIC METHODS

PaO_2 is normal after CO exposure, but the oxygen saturation expressed as a percentage is decreased. Some laboratories calculate oxygen saturation rather than measure it with an oximeter. Therefore, reliability depends on which laboratory method is used. $PaCO_2$ may be normal or reduced. Metabolic acidosis is a feature of CO poisoning and reflects both ischemia and hypoxia.

Pulse oximetry is a noninvasive method used to monitor oxygen saturation. It is relatively easy to perform, painless, rapid in its response, and accurate when arterial oxygen saturations are greater than 65%. In CO poisoning, pulse oximetry gives higher readings than true oxyhemoglobin levels and fails to alert the physician to potentially lethal hypoxia. COHb absorbs light almost identically to oxyhemoglobin and the oximeter responds to COHb as if it were oxyhemoglobin.

BLOOD LEVELS

Endogenous production of CO results from metabolism of the protoporphyrin ring during hemoglobin catabolism and produces a normal blood COHb level of 0.4% to 0.7%. Hemolytic anemia raises endogenous CO production and may increase COHb levels to 4% to 8%. Tobacco smokers have chronically elevated COHb levels. Consumption of one pack per day produces 5% to 6% COHb levels, and consumption of 2 to 3 packs/day results in 7% to 9% COHb levels.

Clinical features correlate only roughly with COHb levels and may vary substantially based on duration of exposure, tissue distribution, time of measurement in relation to oxygen therapy, and patient susceptibility. COHb levels can be used to document exposure, estimate severity, and help determine efficacy of treatment, but relying on COHb levels alone will result in treatment errors because of the above-mentioned variation among patients.

Treatment

GUT DECONTAMINATION

Emesis, lavage, and charcoal play no role in the treatment of CO poisoning.

ELIMINATION ENHANCEMENT

Oxygen (100%) should be delivered through a tight-fitting mask or an endotracheal tube as necessary. Continue 100% oxygen therapy until the COHb level falls below 15% to 20%. Oxygen reduces the COHb half-life from 5 to 6 hours to one-half to 1 hour. Hyperbaric oxygen further reduces COHb half-life to 20 to 30 minutes (see Antidotes, below).

SUPPORTIVE MEASURES

- Immediate removal from the contaminated environment, control of airway, support of breathing with ventilation, 100% oxygen, and the institution of intravenous lines and cardiac monitoring are the initial priorities. The decision to admit must correlate symptoms, individual susceptibility, and peak carboxyhemoglobin levels.
- Although somewhat controversial, certain patients generally should be admitted for observation and oxygen therapy. These include pregnant patients with COHb levels over 10% and patients with cardiovascular disease whose COHb levels exceed 15%.
- Other individuals to admit include asymptomatic patients with COHb levels over 25%, patients with a history of unconsciousness, abnormal neuropsychiatric examination, or ischemiclike chest pain, and patients with reduced body temperatures, metabolic acidosis, chest x-ray abnormalities, myoglobinuria, hypoxia, or an abnormal ECG.
- All patients with a history of CO exposure should have their cardiac and respiratory status monitored. Baseline ECG and cardiac enzymes are recommended after significant exposures. Ischemic changes may range from ST depression and T-wave flattening or inversions, to ST elevation indicative of myocardial infarction. Dysrhythmias range from frequent premature ventricular contractions to atrial fibrillation and ventricular tachyarrhythmias. Sinus tachycardia is the most common abnormality.
- Abnormal ECG findings are common (diffuse slow waves, low voltage) and parallel the progression of hypoxic encephalopathy. The predictive value of the ECG is questionable, because a patient with a critically abnormal ECG may completely recover.
- Chest x-rays usually are normal on admission, but may ultimately reveal a ground-glass appearance, perihilar haze, peribronchial cuffing, and intra-alveolar edema.
- Other toxic inhalants, such as cyanide, and methemoglobin formers, should be considered in patients who do not respond promptly to therapy. Concomitant trauma and hypoxic encephalopathy also should be considered.
- Watch for the development of cerebral edema with serial neurologic exams, computed axial tomography (CAT) scans, and funduscopic examination. Positive CAT scan results predict severe neurologic sequelae within 24 hours (e.g., low-density globus pallidus lesions), but not all patients with neurologic impairment have abnormal CAT scans.
- Obtain a neurologic consultation when the diagnosis of cerebral edema is suspected. Corticosteroids have been used, although their efficacy in CO exposures has not been proven.
- Elevated intracranial pressure is treated with hyperventilation, head elevation, and mannitol (0.25 to 1 g/kg of a 20% solution over 30 minutes).
- Metabolic acidosis should not be treated aggressively unless the acidosis itself contributes to toxicity (i.e., generally below pH 7.1). Acidosis increases the unloading of oxygen in tissues, and therapy has a theoretical advantage in CO poisoning where the dissociation curve shifts leftward.
- Initial laboratory tests should include a complete blood count, glucose, creatinine, cardiac enzymes, urinalysis, carboxyhemoglobin, arterial blood gases, ECG, and chest x-ray. Clinical judgment determines the necessity of cyanide and methemoglobin levels. Muscle necrosis may result in elevated serum creatine kinase, lactate dehydrogenase levels, and myoglobinemia.

Antidotes

HYPERBARIC OXYGEN

In human volunteers, hyperbaric oxygen (HBO) reduces the blood COHb elimination half-life from 250 minutes at room air, and 47 minutes at 100% oxygen, to 22 minutes at 2.5 atmospheres. Interestingly, women demonstrate 25% faster half-lives at all these levels. The incidence of permanent neuropsychiatric complications from CO exposure, including personality changes and memory impairment, ranges widely in numerous studies, depending in part on treatment and severity on presentation. Numerous case reports attest to the effectiveness of HBO in preventing such sequelae even when delayed up to 16 hours. Seriously poisoned patients, identified by computerized tomography (CT) as having low-density lesions in the globus pallidus, have poor outcomes despite administration of hyperbaric oxygen.

While controversial, hyperbaric oxygen therapy may be useful in CO poisoning in symptomatic patients or if the COHb level is greater than 25%, or greater than 15% in a pregnant patient. It also may be helpful in methylene chloride poisoning, cyanide and hydrogen sulfide poisoning, and in severe cases of methemoglobinemia. It may possibly be useful in carbon tetrachloride poisoning and has been suggested for treatment of severe brown recluse spider envenomation (*Loxosceles reclusa* bites). Current data do not support the transfer of potentially unstable patients for long distances unless better intensive care sites are available.

Specific recommendations in pregnant patients remain controversial. Some recommend that pregnant patients be treated when COHb levels exceed 20% or when fetal monitoring shows signs of distress. More conservative recommendations suggest hyperbaric oxygen therapy when COHb levels are greater than 15% in a pregnant female at any time during exposure. If fetal distress occurs within 12 hours of initial treatment, additional HBO treatments may be considered.

Individual responses to CO levels vary, and predicting who will develop severe neurologic sequelae (e.g., demyelination) is unclear. Subtle neurologic or psychological sequelae may be a common long-term problem, but prior available tests have not been sensitive to these changes. Complications of HBO therapy include decompression sickness, rupture of tympanic membranes, sinus damage, cerebral gas embolism, oxygen toxicity, potentiation of pneumothorax, and transport complications. Seriously poisoned patients require a compression chamber large enough to support an intensive care setting with ventilators and cardiac monitoring.

Questions—Carbon Monoxide

1. Which of the following statements is correct?

A. Natural gas contains approximately 22% carbon monoxide (CO).
B. Most CO deaths occur in automobiles.
C. Charcoal grills, hibachis, and Sterno pose a negligible risk of CO indoors.
D. The highest incidence of CO intoxication occurs in Spring.
E. None of the above are correct.

2. Which are true with respect to methylene chloride.
A. It is toxic by ingestion but not by inhalation.
B. Carbon monoxide production occurs through combustion of the compound.
C. Blood testing should include carboxyhemoglobin determination.
D. Methylene chloride levels are helpful in the acute management of intoxication.
E. All of the above are correct.

3. With respect to carbon monoxide (CO) intoxication
A. Higher levels of CO exposure are required to produce toxicity in pregnancy.
B. The fetus is protected because of the nature of fetal blood.
C. Fetal hemoglobin in the neonate protects against CO intoxication.
D. Acute nonlethal maternal intoxication may result in fetal demise.
E. All of the above are correct.

4. With respect to carbon monoxide (CO) poisoning, all of the following are correct except
A. CO replaces oxygen in the hemoglobin leading to a relative anemia.
B. Carboxyhemoglobin causes a left-shift in the oxyhemoglobin dissociation curve.
C. CO toxicity primarily targets areas of low metabolic activity in the body.
D. CO binds to cytochrome oxidase *in vitro*, but this is of unknown significance.
E. CO saturates myoglobin in three times higher concentration than skeletal muscle.

5. A leftward-shift in the oxyhemoglobin dissociation curve can be detrimental by reducing oxygen unloading to the tissues. This leftward shift is caused by all of the following except
A. Methemoglobinemia
B. Hypothermia
C. Acidosis
D. Carbon monoxide
E. Cyanide

6. Carbon monoxide (CO) poses several challenges with respect to laboratory diagnosis of the intoxication. Which of the following is true regarding CO measurements?
A. Pulse oximetry accurately reflects oxygen saturation in the setting of CO poisoning.
B. Heavy smokers will have normal carboxyhemoglobin levels in the blood even in the setting of toxicity.
C. A co-oximeter usually gives inaccurate measurements of carboxyhemoglobin in the blood.
D. Oxygen saturation often is calculated rather than measured in arterial blood-gas laboratory analysis, and can be falsely reassuring.
E. Metabolic alkalosis is the usual laboratory finding in severe CO intoxication.

7. When available, hyperbaric oxygen therapy should be employed in each of the following carbon monoxide-intoxicated patients except
A. A patient who has suffered from a seizure
B. A patient with altered mental status and a carboxyhemoglobin saturation of 40%
C. An asymptomatic pregnant woman with a carboxyhemoglobin level of 28%
D. A 40-year-old man with a carboxyhemoglobin level of 22%
E. An 8-year-old female who was unconscious for 40 minutes.

8. Which of the following is true?
A. In human volunteers, hyperbaric oxygen reduces the blood carboxyhemoglobin elimination half-life from 600 minutes at room air, and 90 minutes at 100% oxygen, to 10 minutes at 2.5 atm.
B. In human volunteers, hyperbaric oxygen reduces the blood carboxyhemoglobin elimination half-life from 50 minutes at room air, and 7 minutes at 100% oxygen, to 2 minutes at 2.5 atm.
C. In human volunteers, hyperbaric oxygen reduces the blood carboxyhemoglobin elimination half-life from 250 minutes at room air, and 47 minutes at 100% oxygen, to 22 minutes at 2.5 atm.
D. In human volunteers, hyperbaric oxygen reduces the blood carboxyhemoglobin elimination half-life from 250 minutes at room air, and 47 minutes at 2.5 atmospheres, to 22 minutes at 5 atm.
E. In human volunteers, hyperbaric oxygen reduces the blood carboxyhemoglobin elimination half-life from 2 hours at room air, and 30 minutes at 100% oxygen, to 10 minutes at 2.5 atm.

CYANIDE AND NITRILES POISONING

Cyanide

Acute cyanide toxicity may result from medicinal uses (e.g., Laetrile), industrial exposures, genocide, and suicide attempts (especially in chemists). Under normal conditions, cyanide appears in the blood of healthy individuals because of vitamin B12 metabolism and environmental factors such as food and smoking. Symptoms can occur within seconds of hydrogen cyanide (HCN) inhalation, within minutes of ingesting cyanide salts, and may be delayed up to 12 hours after ingestion of cyanogenic glycosides, nitriles, or thiocyanates.

Cyanide is one of the most rapidly acting lethal poisons and is well known to the public after such homicidal disasters as the Jonestown massacre and the cyanide-Tylenol® deaths. Commercial cyanide applications include electroplating, extraction of gold and silver ores, metal processing, photographic processes, production of synthetic rubber, chemical synthesis, manufacture of plastics, pesticide and rodenticide control, dehairing of hides, and laboratory processes. The most commonly employed method of illicit manufacture of phencyclidine (PCP) uses potassium cyanide.

Continuous nitroprusside infusions may produce subacute cyanide toxicity after several days of therapy. Cyanide is a metabolite of nitroprusside, and toxicity may result from rapid infusion, prolonged use where tachyphylaxis requires high doses, or renal failure. Chronic cyanide exposure is associated with ataxic neuropathy from chronic cassava consumption, tobacco amblyopia from smoking, and Leber's optic atrophy from a congenital metabolic defect in cyanide metabolism. Cyanide exists as a gas or the liquid hydrogen cyanide (HCN), which also is known as prussic acid. Common salts of cyanide ion (CN) are potassium, sodium, and calcium.

Cyanogenic glycosides are present in significant concentrations in a variety of plants and plant parts. Naturally occurring enzymes in plant parts, such as fruit pits, hydrolyze these glycosides and release HCN. Hydrolysis of amygdalin (the active ingredient in Laetrile) results in HCN. β-Glucosidase, which is present in the gastrointestinal tract, will convert amygdalin to HCN in the human gut. Sources of common cyanogenic glycosides include bitter almonds and apricot seeds, which have high levels of amygdalin, and peach, plum, pear, and apple pits, which have smaller amounts. Prunasin, a metabolite of cherry laurel, dhurrin, sorghum, and linamarin, found in cassava and certain lima beans yield hydrocyanic acid.

Polyurethane and polyacrylonitrile, which commonly are used in modern plastic furniture, release HCN on combustion. Natural products such as silk and wool also release cyanide during fires. Cyanide toxicity may be an important contributor to tissue hypoxia in severe smoke inhalation injuries. Although CO poisoning commonly accounts for most fire deaths, significantly elevated cyanide levels have been reported in survivors of severe smoke inhalation. Each cigarette liberates between 150 and 200 mg of HCN, and smokers have high thiocyanate levels. Tobacco amblyopia may be secondary to cyanide in cigarette smoke.

Nitriles

Nitriles are used in plastic production, as chemical intermediates, as solvents, as lubricating oil additives, and in resin synthesis. Acrylonitrile is the most commonly used aliphatic nitrile compound. Other commercially important nitriles include the less toxic acetonitrile (methyl cyanide) and the more toxic propionitrile. Acute toxicity in this group resembles cyanide poisoning, with deaths reported from acute acetonitrile inhalation.

Acetonitrile is used as a solvent remover of acrylic sculptured nails that are bonded to the natural nail with cyanoacrylic glues. The diagnosis of acetonitrile poisoning is difficult. Conventional toxicology panels do not detect it. The delayed onset of symptoms (3 to 12 hours) does not suggest typical cyanide intoxication.

Enough acetonitrile is contained in a one-ounce sculptured nail glue removal bottle for several fatal doses. The bottles do not have child-resistant lids. Diagnosis of acetonitrile ingestion involves differentiating nail polish remover (acetone) from nail glue remover (acetonitrile). Initial symptoms of acetonitrile ingestion are indistinguishable from those of acetone and common alcohols. In the absence of cyanide level determinations, lethargy, vomiting, seizures, and the lack of normal venous blood hemoglobin desaturation may be clues to cyanide toxicity. Acetonitrile poisoning is included in the differential diagnosis of anion gap and osmolar gap metabolic acidosis.

The major use of acrylonitrile is in the production of acrylic (e.g., blankets, carpets) and modacrylic (e.g., wigs, furs) fibers by copolymerization with agents such as vinyl chloride and methyl methacrylate. Other industrial applications include manufacture of plastics, and the chemical production of acrylamide, adiponitrile, and a fumigant. Acrylonitrile decomposes to cyanide during pyrolysis and is heavier than air. As such, it presents a significant hazard during fires.

Pathophysiology

CYANIDE

Cyanide binds to heme iron in the cytochrome a-a3 complex with greatest affinity for oxidized iron (Fe^{3+}). This complex inhibits the final step of oxidative phosphorylation and halts aerobic metabolism. The patient essentially suffocates from an inability to use oxygen. The diversion of carbohydrate metabolism from pyruvate to lactate production results in accumulation of lactic acid. Other enzymes are even more sensitive to cyanide than cytochrome oxidase.

In minimal lethal doses, cyanide affects primarily the central nervous system. Cyanide initially stimulates peripheral chemoreceptors, causing increased respirations. It also promotes slowing of the heart by stimulating carotid body receptors. The electrical activity of the brain may stop while the heart is still beating. No specific pathologic changes characterize cyanide toxicity.

NITRILES

Acetonitrile is an organocyanide that is slowly metabolized to inorganic cyanide in a reaction forming hydrogen cyanide. The major toxicity of acetonitrile is a result of the *in vivo* formation of cyanide as a metabolite. Although cyanide is released from the hepatic biotransformation of acrylonitrile, acute toxicity results primarily from the whole molecule. Detoxification of reactive groups may lead to liver toxicity.

Pharmacokinetics

Cyanide

ABSORPTION

- Rapid absorption generally occurs. Inhalation of high cyanide gas concentration results in symptoms within seconds.
- Hydrochloric acid in the stomach causes the release of HCN, which is absorbed rapidly as the cyanide ion (CN).
- Absorption occurs across mucous membranes and intact skin.

DISTRIBUTION

- Cyanide is concentrated in red blood cells.
- The volume of distribution of CN is approximately 1.5 L/kg.
- About 60% of CN in plasma are protein bound.

ELIMINATION

- Cyanide is metabolized by at least four pathways. The enzyme rhodanese converts the majority of cyanide (80%) in the presence of thiosulfate to thiocyanate, which the kidney excretes.
- The rate-limiting step is the amount of thiosulfate. Rhodanese is present in high concentrations in the liver and kidney (especially mitochondria), but the supply of thiosulfate is limited.
- Alternate pathways include the conversion of hydroxocobalamin (vitamin B12a) in the presence of HCN to the nontoxic cyanocobalamin (vitamin B12).
- Only small amounts of cyanide are excreted in the lung and sweat, where they produce a bitter almond odor.

Nitriles

ABSORPTION

- Acrylonitrile is readily absorbed through the stomach, skin, and lungs with most acute exposures resulting from inhalation.
- Cutaneous absorption of acrylonitrile (about 1%), occurs through contaminated leather and rubber because of excellent penetrating properties.

DISTRIBUTION

- After absorption, most acrylonitrile is converted to cyanide, which is then transformed to thiocyanate.

ELIMINATION

- Around half of an oral dose of acrylonitrile is excreted as seven urinary metabolites.
- The presence of hydrogen cyanide in smoke indicates that plasma levels of thiocyanate and cyanide are higher in smokers than in nonsmokers.
- Elimination half-lives following an ingestion of 5 mL of 98% acetonitrile is 32 hours for acetonitrile and 15 hours for cyanide.

Clinical Presentations

The diagnosis of cyanide toxicity is difficult because of the lack of pathognomonic signs. Classic signs of bright red venous blood, profound metabolic acidosis, and bitter almond breath often are absent. A hypertensive, bradycardiac, acyanotic, and tachypneic patient suggests cyanide poisoning, especially when the patient subsequently develops central nervous system and cardiovascular depression. Cyanide should be included in the differential diagnosis of rapid onset of coma, and whenever coma and metabolic acidosis appear together.

Signs and symptoms of acute cyanide poisoning reflect cellular hypoxia and are often nonspecific. Onset of symptoms depends on dose, route, and duration of exposure. Inhalation produces the most rapid and serious exposures, resulting in flushing, headache, tachypnea, and dizziness within 30 seconds, progressing to irregular stridorous breathing, coma, seizures, and death within 10 minutes. Oral exposures are less rapid because of slower entry into the circulation and passage of cyanide through the portal system, where the liver detoxifies some cyanide by the first-pass effect.

NEUROLOGIC EFFECTS

The central nervous system is the most sensitive target organ of cyanide poisoning, with early stimulation followed by central nervous system depression. Early symptoms include lightheadedness, giddiness, tachypnea, nausea, vomiting, feeling of neck constriction and suffocation, confusion, restlessness, and anxiety. Initial tachypnea results from direct stimulation of carotid body chemoreceptors followed by respiratory depression. Severe cyanide poisonings progress to stupor, coma, opisthotonus, convulsions, fixed dilated pupils, and death.

CARDIOVASCULAR EFFECTS

Depression of the cardiovascular system requires cyanide doses higher than those necessary for depression of the central nervous system. Initial tachycardia occurs followed by bradycardia. Dysrhythmias and hypotension often precede peripheral vascular collapse. The ECG may display striking ischemic changes. Pulmonary edema may complicate severe intoxications.

DERMATOLOGIC EFFECTS

In serious poisonings, the skin is cold, clammy, and diaphoretic. Cyanosis may be a late finding, because poor tissue utilization of oxygen results in elevated venous oxygen levels. Venous blood may be bright red.

CHRONIC EFFECTS

The most common symptoms of a long-term cyanide exposure are headache, dizziness, nausea, vomiting, and a bitter or almond taste. Chronic cyanide exposure has been associated with ataxic neuropathy from chronic cassava consumption, tobacco amblyopia from smoking, and Leber's optic atrophy from a congenital metabolic defect in cyanide metabolism. Nitroprusside use may result in subacute thiocyanate toxicity.

LEBER'S OPTIC ATROPHY

Leber's hereditary optic atrophy probably results from inborn errors of metabolism that produce low urinary and plasma thiocyanate levels in the presence of normal liver rhodanese levels. The suspected inborn metabolic deficiency limits the ability of the patient to detoxify cyanide by conversion to thiocyanate.

TOBACCO AMBLYOPIA

Visual abnormalities of tobacco amblyopia are associated with heavy smoking and vitamin B12 deficiency. This disease is similar to the retrobulbar neuritis associated with pernicious anemia. Central scotomata develop with occasional temporal pallor of the optic disk.

TROPICAL NEUROPATHY

The signs and symptoms of tropical ataxic neuropathy have been linked with chronic cassava consumption and elevated thiocyanate levels. These patients apparently are not deficient in vitamin B12. Hydroxocobalamin is not as efficacious in treating tropical ataxic neuropathy as it is in treating Leber's hereditary optic atrophy. Segmental demyelination leads to a peripheral sensory neuropathy, optic atrophy, ataxia, and deafness. Stomatitis, and scrotal dermatitis may be present.

NITROPRUSSIDE

Nitroprusside infusions given at rates of over 4 μg/kg/minute can produce toxic cyanide concentrations in 5 to 10 hours. Lactic acidosis and venous hyperoxemia may not be present for several hours after nitroprusside administration, making the diagnosis of nitroprusside-induced cyanide toxicity difficult. Patients with renal insufficiency also are at risk for developing thiocyanate toxicity, which may be manifested by confusion, hyperreflexia, seizures, coma, and death. CN in cyanomethemoglobin is inactive, although it is measured as part of the elevated blood cyanide levels seen during nitroprusside infusions. Simultaneous infusion of thiosulfate reduces toxicity.

NITRILES

Following acetonitrile exposure, the earliest symptoms are nausea and vomiting. A latent period, during which cyanide is produced in the liver, may last up to 12 hours. Symptoms do not appear until enough cyanide has been produced to exhaust endogenous stores of thiosulfate or to overwhelm the rhodanese pathway. Patients may ultimately exhibit signs and symptoms of cyanide intoxication, including lethargy, seizures, respiratory depression, and death. Other symptoms may include headache, abdominal cramps, weakness, hyporeflexia, urinary frequency, stupor, shock, hypothermia, and bradycardia. There may be a rapid progression to coma, lactic acidosis, and respiratory arrest as a result of damage of brain stem neurons controlling respiratory drive.

Other signs and symptoms may include painful blisters, sweating, rashes, conjunctivitis, metabolic acidosis with a decreased arteriovenous oxygen gradient, tachycardia, decreased cardiac output, hypotension, depressed ST segments, varying degrees of atrioventricular block, an erratic supraventricular rhythm, ventricular fibrillation, and tachypnea. Vertigo, mental deterioration, weakness, anorexia, and weight loss may be observed with chronic acetonitrile exposures. Chronic cyanide poisoning may be associated with thyromegaly, altered B12 and folate metabolism, personality changes, extrapyramidal syndromes, optic atrophy, demyelinating syndromes, and psychosis.

Acute acrylonitrile inhalation may produce headache, sneezing, mucous membrane irritation, chest discomfort, nausea, vomiting, diarrhea, lightheadedness, weakness, and apprehension, with severe exposures resulting in asphyxia and cardiovascular collapse. The clinical syndrome also resembles cyanide poisoning. Liver dysfunction may develop and is characterized by jaundice, malaise, anorexia, and leukocytosis. Cutaneous exposure may produce a chemical burn that is exacerbated by prolonged contact with contaminated rubber or leather. Substantial evidence in animals incriminates acrylonitrile as a carcinogen, although evidence in humans is more limited.

Toxic Dosage/Death

INHALATION

Cyanide gas is a rapid-acting poison producing symptoms in seconds and death in minutes. The threshold of bitter almond odor (genetically determined and absent in 20% to 40% of the population) is 0.2 to 5.0 ppm. Slight symptoms (e.g., headache) develop after several hours of exposure to 18 to 36 ppm. Death probably occurs in 1 hour at 100 ppm, and 300-ppm exposures prove fatal within several minutes.

INGESTION

Cyanide is a potent oral poison producing symptoms in minutes and death in minutes to hours. One teaspoon of 20% liquid HCN has been fatal. The lethal adult dose of HCN is 50 mg. The lethal oral adult dose of cyanide salts [e.g., potassium cyanide (KCN)] is 200 to 300 mg, and the calculated lethal dose of KCN in children is 1.2 to 5 mg/kg. A lethal dose for cyanogenic plant ingestions cannot be predicted because of variations in HCN content, extraction methods, and metabolism.

NITROPRUSSIDE

Higher-than-recommended doses and prolonged infusion produce symptoms of thiocyanate poisoning. Recommended limits are 1 to 1.5 mg/kg for 1 to 3 hours, and 0.5 mg/kg/hour for treatment exceeding 48 hours. Toxicity also results from rapid infusion and the presence of renal failure.

NITRILES

Ingestion of 5 mL of acetonitrile may be fatal in a small child. A 26-year-old who swallowed 40 g of acetonitrile experienced seizures, vomiting, acidosis, shock, and coma following a 3-hour latency period. The patient recovered after treatment with Dicobalt EDTA and hydroxocobalamin.

Laboratory

ANALYTIC METHODS

Although microdiffusion techniques using the Conway cell generally require 2 to 4 hours, a modification of the procedure allows a semiquantitative reading after 10 minutes of diffusion in an emergency. The Lee-Jones test is a quantitative cyanide rapid spot test performed on gastric aspirate. A paper test for cyanide in blood at blood-cyanide concentrations of over 1.0 mg/liter is sensitive to a concentration of 0.2 mg/L of cyanide in whole blood. Preliminary studies suggest its potential usefulness in determination of the presence of over 0.5 mg/liter of cyanide after an acute cyanide poisoning or after exposure to fire. Gas chromatography/mass spectrometry can confirm the presence of acetonitrile.

BLOOD LEVELS

Blood cyanide levels are useful in confirming toxicity, but therapeutic interventions usually must be made before the level is available. Documentation of human cyanide levels is sparse. Correlation of symptoms to whole blood cyanide levels may be misleading, because the effect of cyanide depends on the intracellular concentration at the cytochrome oxidase binding sites, the duration of poisoning and perhaps the route of toxicity. Levels lower than 0.2 μg/mL usually cause no symptoms. At concentrations between 0.5 and 1.0 μg/mL, the patient is conscious and flushed with tachycardia. Stupor and agitation appear between 1.0 and 2.5 μg/mL. Levels over 2.5 μg/mL are associated with coma and are potentially fatal.

Treatment

GUT DECONTAMINATION

Because of the rapid onset of cyanide toxicity, gut decontamination should follow antidote therapy. Gastric lavage, charcoal, and cathartics may be used after antidote therapy if less than 2 hours has passed since ingestion.

ELIMINATION ENHANCEMENT

Hemodialysis and hemoperfusion are ineffective against cyanide. Use of hyperbaric oxygen has been suggested, but few data on humans exist to recommend its use in cyanide toxicity. Hemodialysis and hemoperfusion may return thiocyanate concentrations to subtoxic levels. Hemodialysis may be considered for severely poisoned patients because severe symptoms can persist for several days and administration of antidotal therapy may be limited by sodium content in some patients.

SUPPORTIVE MEASURES

- Rapid support of respiration and circulation is essential to successful treatment of cyanide intoxication. Immediate attention should be directed toward assisted ventilation, administration of 100% oxygen, insertion of intravenous lines, and institution of cardiac monitoring.
- Obtain an arterial blood gas immediately and correct any severe metabolic acidosis (pH below 7.15). Oxygen (100%) should be used routinely in moderate or severely symptomatic patients even in the presence of a normal PaO_2, since 100% oxygen increases oxygen delivery, may reactivate cyanide-inhibited mitochondrial enzymes, and potentiates the effect of thiosulfate.
- All patients must be followed for at least 24 to 48 hours. Watch for the development of pulmonary edema and aspiration pneumonia in comatose patients.
- Changes noted on the ECG during cyanide intoxication are nonspecific and reflect cellular hypoxia. Tachycardia and nonspecific ST-T wave changes appear first. AV block, a short Q-T interval, and an obliterated ST interval also can occur.
- Later, the ECG may exhibit signs of progressive hypoxia with bradycardia and nodal or idioventricular rhythm, followed by atrioventricular block and a slow agonal rhythm. A striking ST elevation may be present, especially in patients with underlying cardiovascular disease.
- Electrical activity in the basal ganglia, hypothalamus, and midbrain is depressed before similar depression in pons and medullary activity. Clinical parkinsonism as a result of cyanide exposure may be associated with bilateral lucencies in the putamen and external globus pallidus.
- Laboratory tests that suggest cyanide intoxication include a serum lactate level of more than 10 mmol/L, an elevated serum anion gap, and evidence of the arterialization of venous blood (decreased peripheral oxygen extraction), which may be determined by the simultaneous determination of arterial and venous oxygen saturations. Arterial-venous oxygen difference often is diminished because of the decreased tissue utilization of oxygen.

Antidotes

Cyanide binds to ferric ion, interferes with cytochrome oxidase, and reduces cellular respiration. Nitrites, exogenously given in cases of cyanide poisoning, induce methemoglobin formation, which, in turn, attracts cyanide off cytochrome oxidase. Thiosulfate enhances renal elimination of cyanide by forming thiocyanate when combined with cyanomethemoglobin.

Reaction 1: Hemoglobin-Fe^{2+} + sodium nitrite → methemoglobin-Fe^{3+}

Reaction 2: Methemoglobin-Fe^{3+} + cyanide/cytochrome oxidase complex → cyanide-methemoglobin-Fe^{3+} + cytochrome oxidase (free)

Reaction 3: Cyanide-methemoglobin-Fe^{3+} + thiosulfate → hemoglobin-Fe^{2+} + thiocyanate (less toxic, easily eliminated renally)

NITRITES

Although included in the Cyanide Antidote Kit (produced by Eli Lilly), amyl nitrite perles are questionably effective, as they produce very low methemoglobin levels. Intravenous sodium nitrite, also in the kit, produces a methemoglobin level of 25%, which must be reduced in the presence of anemia.

Because of potentially adverse effects and the fact that patients have survived with supportive care only, nitrites should not be given indiscriminately. In all cases of moderate to severe cyanide poisoning, nitrites should be given along with thiosulfate. Mildly symptomatic patients who are alert may be given supportive care, unless their mental status deteriorates or they develop a metabolic acidosis. Nitrites produce both hypotension and methemoglobinemia. Cyanosis appears at 15% methemoglobin levels, but symptoms usually do not appear until the level reaches 30% to 40%. The lethal methemoglobin level is 70%.

The therapeutic goal in treating cyanide poisoning is 20% to 30% methemoglobinemia. Although the use of methylene blue to reverse excessive methemoglobinemia is recommended in the package insert, its use is extremely hazardous in this setting. Oxygen saturation and methemoglobin levels must be monitored closely. Nitrites must be used with caution in patients with cardiovascular or cerebral vascular disease. Headache, nausea, hypotension, and syncope can occur after nitrite use.

AMYL NITRITE

Amyl nitrite perles are designed to produce 3% to 5% methemoglobinemia while an intravenous line is established for intravenous (IV) sodium nitrite. As a temporizing measure, the patient inhales the vapors until the sodium nitrite is ready. Because of the variability in methemoglobin production and the potential for cardiovascular collapse, this step may be omitted if sodium nitrite is readily available and the patient is not in extremis. Adequate ventilation and oxygenation are more important than administration of amyl nitrite.

Amyl nitrite perles are first crushed in gauze and given to patients to inhale for 15 seconds. A fresh perle is used every 3 minutes. Children under 25 kg require reduced doses based on hemoglobin—contact your local poison center for specifics. In adults, sodium nitrite (10 mL of 3% solution) is given intravenously over 2 to 5 minutes. Subsequently, 25% sodium thiosulfate (1.65 mL/kg up to 50 mL) is administered intravenously over 10 minutes. Use 1.65 mL/kg in children.

SODIUM NITRITE

Sodium nitrite, 10 mL of a 3% solution (i.e., 300 mg), is administered intravenously slowly over 4 minutes to produce a 20% methemoglobin level in adults. Children should receive 0.33 mL of the 3% solution per kilogram initially at an infusion rate of 2.5 mL/min, up to a maximum of 10 mL. Administer sodium nitrite doses to children on the basis of body weight, because fatal methemoglobinemia has occurred in children. Time permitting, adjustments also should be made for hemoglobin concentrations.

SODIUM THIOSULFATE FOR CYANIDE POISONING

Rhodanese, an enzyme located in the mitochondria, catalyzes the irreversible transfer of a sulfone donor from thiosulfate to cyanide, which produces the nontoxic thiocyanate. Because thiosulfate does not penetrate cells well, large doses are required and the detoxification rate is slow. Thiosulfates are given with nitrites for confirmed cyanide poisoning and are available in Eli Lilly's cyanide antidote kit. Thiocyanate levels greater than 10 mg/dL may cause vomiting, arthralgias, muscle cramps, and psychosis. Renal failure enhances thiocyanate toxicity by decreasing thiocyanate excretion.

A 25% solution of thiosulfate is administered intravenously after nitrites are given. The adult dose is 50 mL (12.5 g) intravenously at a rate of 3 to 5 mL/min. The pediatric dose is 1.65 mL/kg up to 50 mL. If symptoms reappear or persist within 1 hour, readminister sodium nitrite and sodium thiosulfate at 50% of the initial dose. Always check methemoglobin levels.

SODIUM THIOSULFATE FOR NITRILE POISONING

IV sodium thiosulfate is the drug of choice for treatment of acetonitrile poisoning. Low-sodium-content IV solutions should be used. Nitrites may exacerbate hypotension and seem to be of dubious value. 4P-methyl-aminophenol also has been used, however its role in acetonitrile poisoning remains to be determined. Antidotes are recommended in seriously poisoned patients who fail to respond immediately to standard supportive measures.

HYDROXOCOBALAMIN

This compound combines with cyanide to form cyanocobalamin (vitamin B12), which the kidney excretes. This drug is not approved in the United States for the treatment of cyanide poisoning, although studies in animals suggest that hydroxocobalamin is safe and effective. Limited human experience precludes a specific dosage recommendation for cyanide poisoning, although 50 times the ingested cyanide dose has been recommended.

DICOBALT EDTA

Cobalt compounds chelate cyanide and cause no methemoglobinemia. This compound is available in France and Great Britain, but not in the United States. Occasional vomiting and rare anaphylactic reactions may occur. Patients have developed facial edema, retrosternal chest pain, diaphoresis, ventricular tachycardia, and laryngeal edema requiring intubation after IV administration of Dicobalt EDTA (edetate) for cyanide poisoning.

Questions—Cyanide And Nitrile Poisoning

1. Which of the following plants and fruits have cyanogenic seeds?

A. Plums
B. Pears
C. Apples

D. Apricots
E. All of the above

2. Which of the materials listed does not release cyanide upon combustion?
A. Cotton
B. Polyacrylonitrile
C. Silk
D. Wool
E. Polyurethane

3. Which of the following describes the metabolic derangements seen in cyanide poisoning?
A. Increased oxygen consumption and lactate production, with decreased ATP production
B. Decreased oxygen consumption, increased lactate, and increased ATP production
C. Increased oxygen consumption, increased lactate, and decreased ATP production
D. Decreased oxygen consumption, decreased lactate, and decreased ATP production
E. Decreased oxygen consumption, increased lactate, and decreased ATP production.

4. Antidotes, which may be useful in cyanide poisoning, include all of the following except
A. Methylene blue
B. Amyl nitrite
C. Sodium nitrite
D. Hydroxocobalamin
E. Sodium thiosulfate

5. Which of the following are NOT typically associated with intoxication by the nitriles?
A. Gastritis and upper gastrointestinal hemorrhage
B. Headache, stupor, and weakness
C. Abdominal cramps, nausea and vomiting
D. Tachypnea and tachycardia
E. Sweating, blisters, and rashes

6. Which of the following is true regarding nitrile compounds such as acetonitrile?
A. The parent compound is much more toxic than the metabolite.
B. Antidotes to cyanide may be useful in the treatment of oral ingestion.
C. Blood cyanide levels are the basis for the acute management of toxicity.
D. This class of compounds is used widely in silk production.
E. None of the above

HYDROGEN SULFIDE

Hydrogen sulfide is a toxic gas associated with the "rotten egg" smell of homemade "stink bombs." In the workplace, it is a leading cause of sudden death. Its excellent olfactory warning properties are lost at high concentrations, leading to insidious exposures and serious toxicity. Toxicity and fatalities have been reported in poorly ventilated spaces after agitation of liquid manure tanks, after addition of sulfuric acid to a drain and hydrochloric acid to a well, after the cleaning of a propane tank, and after entry of victims and rescuers into areas containing fish meal. The most important determinants of clinical toxicity are gas concentration and duration of exposure. Pulmonary edema is a common complication of serious toxicity, whereas upper respiratory tract irritation, keratoconjunctivitis, and nonspecific complaints (e.g., headache, nausea, and dizziness) can develop at lower exposure levels.

Natural sources include subterranean emissions from caves and volcanoes, and bacterial decomposition of sulfur in soil and the gastrointestinal tract. The decay of organic sulfur-containing products (e.g., fish, sewage, manure, septic tanks) and pouring of acid on sewage, liberate hydrogen sulfide. Other toxic gases released from a decomposing environment include carbon monoxide, sulfur dioxide, carbon dioxide, methane, ammonia, and certain amines. Commercial exposures involve hydrogen disulfide as the manufacturing by-product of viscose rayon (along with carbon disulfide). It has been associated with silk production, petroleum and tanning processes, paper mills, damp mines, geothermal energy and hot sulfur springs, roofing asphalt tanks, the burning of wool, hair, meals, and hides, the production of heavy water for nuclear reactors, metal refining, and the vulcanization of sulfur-containing rubber.

Pathophysiology

The addition of dilute sulfuric or hydrochloric acid to iron sulfide or the reaction of hydrogen with elemental sulfur produces hydrogen sulfide gas. Although the exact mechanics of toxicity are unknown, hydrogen sulfide produces both local irritation and cellular asphyxia, probably by binding to the iron in cytochrome oxidase a3. Like cyanide, hydrogen sulfide probably is an intracellular toxin that inhibits cytochrome oxidase by disrupting electron transport. Hydrogen sulfide is a somewhat more potent inhibitor of the cytochrome oxidase system than cyanide. The resulting switch to anaerobic metabolism causes lactate accumulation and metabolic acidosis. At lower doses, hydrogen sulfide is a mucous membrane and respiratory irritant (200 ppm), but at high doses (1000 ppm), it causes direct respiratory depression. Death usually results from respiratory arrest and hypoxia.

Pharmacokinetics

ABSORPTION

- Hydrogen sulfide is primarily a respiratory toxin, because cutaneous absorption is negligible.

DISTRIBUTION

- Inorganic sulfides are present in the body only in small quantities (0.05 mg/L).

ELIMINATION

- The toxicokinetics of hydrogen sulfide have not been studied in man. In animals, excretion of hydrogen sulfide by the lungs is minimal after parenteral administration.
- Elimination occurs via oxidation to sulfate, methylation, and reaction with metalloproteins or disulfide-containing proteins.
- Detoxification of hydrogen sulfide occurs rapidly (85% of a lethal dose per hour in animals), with the red blood cell and liver mitochondria being the primary sites.
- Hydrogen sulfide poisoning does not produce sulfhemoglobin.

Clinical Presentations

In high doses, the central nervous system is the primary target organ, with symptoms of irritation of the eyes and respiratory tract developing on prolonged exposure. Local irritant properties result in rhinitis, pharyngitis, bronchitis, pneumonia, and pulmonary edema. Dyspnea, cyanosis and hemoptysis may occur. Keratoconjunctivitis may occur.

NEUROLOGIC EFFECTS

Central nervous system depression may result in headache, lethargy, vertigo, horizontal or vertical nystagmus, and coma. The combination of vomiting and central nervous system depression may lead to aspiration pneumonia. Symptoms of severe exposure include loss of consciousness, dizziness, nausea, vomiting, headache, sore throat, conjunctivitis, weakness, and convulsions.

CARDIOVASCULAR EFFECTS

Cardiac symptoms may include dysrhythmias, myocardial depression, conduction defects, and abnormal ventricular repolarization.

CHRONIC EFFECTS

Headache, weakness, nausea, vomiting, and weight loss occur in chronic exposures and may appear for several months after acute exposure. Long-term adverse effects are unusual in victims promptly resuscitated. Chronic exposure to at least 0.6 ppm of hydrogen sulfide for almost 1 year produced truncal ataxia, choreoathetosis, and dystonia with bilateral lucent areas in the basal ganglia in a 20-month-old child. Removal from the source of the gas resulted in clinical recovery with resolution of the basal ganglia abnormalities.

Toxic Dosage/Death

On exposure to levels exceeding 1,000 ppm, victims rapidly develop coma, respiratory paralysis, and hypoxia. Death then occurs, unless the victim is quickly removed from the exposure and effective artificial ventilation is established. Most fatalities occur at the scene. Patients who have vital signs on arrival usually survive, provided severe hypoxic encephalopathy is not present.

An odor is detectable at 0.2 to 0.3 ppm, and a definite odor appears at 20 to 30 ppm, but olfactory paralysis develops between 100 and 150 ppm. Between 150 and 300 ppm, respiratory tract and eye irritation is prominent (e.g., blepharospasm, keratoconjunctivitis, blurred vision, colored halos around lights), accompanied by mucous membrane irritation, bronchitis, and pulmonary edema. Severe systemic toxicity develops above 500 ppm (headache, nausea, vomiting, weakness, disorientation, and coma within 30 minutes of exposure).

Above 700 ppm, cardiorespiratory arrest occurs and death becomes imminent. Autopsies demonstrate nonspecific findings such as visceral congestion, scattered petechiae, and hemorrhagic pulmonary edema. A sulfide smell may be present on the slicing of tissue. Most but not all autopsy cases demonstrate pulmonary edema.

Laboratory

ANALYTIC METHODS

A specific ion electrode in combination with Conway microdiffusion cells has been developed to detect elevated sulfide ion in blood.

BLOOD LEVELS

Waiting for blood levels or guiding potential treatment on hydrogen sulfide concentrations is dangerous and unwarranted, as patient demise may be rapid. Sulfide ion levels measured soon after hydrogen sulfide-induced death ranged from 1.70 to 3.75 mg/L. Postmortem confirmation of toxic levels is complicated by the rapid endogenous destruction of the sulfide ion, formation of sulfide from protein degradation postmortem, and deterioration of the sulfide ion in storage.

Treatment

GUT DECONTAMINATION

These methods are unhelpful after hydrogen sulfide exposure.

ELIMINATION ENHANCEMENT

Hyperbaric oxygen may be helpful. See Antidotes, below.

SUPPORTIVE MEASURES

- Immediate supportive care is the most important phase of treatment, because most fatalities occur at the scene. Rescuers must cautiously enter areas that potentially contain hydrogen sulfide. Closed areas (e.g., inside storage tanks) require self-contained breathing apparatus, safety lines, and outside observation. After protection of the rescuer, the most important priority is the establishment of adequate ventilation and circulation.
- The victim must be moved to a well-ventilated area. Would-be rescuers have lost consciousness while applying mouth-to-mouth resuscitation. 100% oxygen must be applied as soon as possible.
- Violent seizures have required the use of general anesthetics (i.e., succinylcholine) to complete intubation.
- Skin decontamination is not necessary due to poor cutaneous absorption.
- If nitrites are used (see Antidotes), check methemoglobin levels.
- All seriously poisoned patients should have chest x-rays and arterial blood gases to search for evidence of aspiration pneumonia and pulmonary edema. Early widening of the alveolar-arterial oxygen gradient suggests the development of pulmonary edema or pneumonia.
- CAT scan may reveal bilateral symmetric lucent areas within the cerebral hemispheres, which probably correspond to the lentiform nucleus. Such lesions are consistent with focal brain lesions produced by hypoxia or hypotension.

Antidotes

NITRITES

Nitrites produce methemoglobin, which attracts sulfide from cytochrome oxidase and reactivates aerobic metabolism. Sulfmethemoglobin undergoes rapid spontaneous detoxification in the body. The use of nitrites in serious cases may be effective only at the exposure site. The lifetime of sulfide in oxygenated blood is short, and induction of methemoglobin more than 10 to 15 minutes postexposure may not aid the victim.

The use of an antidote must not delay the establishment of adequate ventilation and oxygenation. The dosages of nitrites are similar to those used in cyanide poisoning. An amyl nitrite perle is broken and inhaled for 30 seconds every minute while an IV line is established. This step should be omitted until good oxygenation is present. Adults should receive 300 mg of sodium nitrite (10 mL of a 3% solution) over 4 minutes intravenously similar to cyanide poisoning. No absolute guidelines are available for the use of nitrites in hydrogen sulfide poisoning in the hospital setting, because most hospital inpatients survive with supportive care only and nitrites have inherent toxicity. Thiosulfate is not required, because the body spontaneously detoxifies sulfmethemoglobin.

HYPERBARIC OXYGEN

Several anecdotal case studies suggest that hyperbaric oxygen may be useful for severe hydrogen sulfide toxicity. Although patients who continue to show symptoms after standard therapy may benefit from HBO therapy, the clinical efficacy of this modality remains to be determined.

Questions—Hydrogen Sulfide

1. **Which of the following statements regarding hydrogen sulfide is correct?**
   A. The primary route of absorption is dermal.
   B. Hydrogen sulfide is primarily secreted by the lungs.
   C. Sulfhemoglobin formation accounts for the majority of toxicity.
   D. At high doses (1,000 ppm) hydrogen sulfide causes respiratory depression
   E. Sources include combustion of iron, steel, and aluminum

2. **With respect to the treatment of hydrogen sulfide poisoning, all of the following are correct except**
   A. Nitrites are useful up to 24 hours after exposure.
   B. Methemoglobin is used to remove hydrogen sulfide from the cytochromes.
   C. Parts of the standard cyanide treatment kit also are useful in this poisoning.
   D. Sodium thiosulfate is not useful in this intoxication.
   E. Early intubation is often required with serious intoxications.

INHALANT ABUSE

The inhalation of substances provides a rapid, easy route for recreational drugs (e.g., nicotine, opiates, cannabis, Jimson weed). In the 1800s, surgical anesthetics such as chloroform and ether were abused. Indeed, the recreational use of nitrous oxide, another anesthetic, persists today. A "solvent-sniffing epidemic" was observed in California in the late 1950s and quickly spread across the United States by the middle 1960s. Solvent abuse still exists. The low cost of solvents provides an inexpensive chemical high, mostly in the adolescent age group.

Numerous products and volatiles may be abused by inhalation. Popular substances include typewriter correction fluids such as trichloroethane and trichloroethylene, glues, paint thinners, gasoline, methanol, various nitrites ("poppers"), cyclohexane and nitrous oxide. Substances that have been associated with fatalities include butane, adhesive solvents, cleaning agents, aerosols, and fire extinguishers. Fluorocarbon propellants, benzene, trichloroethane, gasoline, toluene, and hydrocarbons have been implicated in numerous sudden deaths after inhalant abuse in which no obvious cardiac or pulmonary pathology existed. See also Chapter 46, Hydrocarbons.

Various methods are used to enhance the inhalant effect. Methods include "sniffing," or inhaling directly over an open container, "bagging," or holding an open bag or container over the head, and "huffing," or pouring material on a cloth that is held over the mouth. These methods concentrate the vapors to potentially lethal levels. Abuse may occur in industry where workers intentionally overexpose themselves to vapors. Deaths may result from direct toxic effects, however asphyxia, aspiration, and trauma may account for deaths as well.

Pathophysiology

Heavy exercise or stress has been associated with several of these deaths, and some authors have proposed that these inhalants sensitize the myocardium to endogenous catecholamines. Hypoxia, hypercarbia, and acidosis may exacerbate these effects. Hydrocarbons sensitize various animal models to epinephrine-induced ventricular fibrillation, but the exact mechanism remains unclear. Respiratory depression contributes significantly to sudden death.

Clinical Presentations

Multiorgan effects characterize inhalant abuse. Abusers may use one or more intoxicants together or on separate occasions. Optic atrophy, persistent cerebellar ataxia, dysequilibrium, and an organic brain syndrome are long-term sequelae reported after chronic solvent abuse.

NEUROLOGIC EFFECTS

Some acute effects are similar to those of alcohol intoxication, including slurred speech, diplopia, ataxia, euphoria, blurred vision, and CNS depression. Disorientation to time and place and visual hallucinations occur commonly, in contrast to ethanol intoxication. Recovery is rapid after solvent abuse, with symptoms resolving in an average of 30 minutes (range up to 2 hours). Headaches develop less commonly than after ethanol intoxication. Coma and seizures may occur.

RENAL EFFECTS

Glue and paint thinner sniffing, and toluene inhalation in particular, produce a variety of serious renal abnormalities. Type I distal renal tubular acidosis (RTA) with normal anion gap, acidosis and severe hypokalemia can occur. Glue sniffing can cause selective proximal tubular dysfunction with Fanconi's syndrome (increased aminoaciduria, glycosuria, phosphaturia, calciuria, uricosuria). Trichloroethylene and toluene inhalation can produce acute renal tubular necrosis.

GASTROINTESTINAL EFFECTS

Trichloroethylene inhalation and toluene inhalation can also produce a transient but severe centrilobular hepatic necrosis. Halothane has been reported to produce sudden death, a hypersensitivity hepatitis, and fatal acute yellow atrophy in abusers.

SPECIFIC TOXINS

Specific toxins have been associated with specific target organs. Although not exhaustive, the following list elucidates some of these associations. Also see Chapter 46, Hydrocarbons.

Acetone

Heavy exposure to acetone vapor causes initial central nervous system excitement followed by lethargy, stupor, and coma.

Benzene

Headache, dizziness, euphoria, delirium, agitation, convulsions, coma, liver and renal dysfunction, aplastic anemia, leukemia, and sudden death may follow use of benzene.

Correction Fluids

Inhalation of typewriter correction fluids such as trichloroethane and trichloroethylene may lead to vomiting, dizziness, coma, cerebral edema, and sudden death due to cardiac arrhythmias.

Cyclohexane

Narcosis has been observed after cyclohexane inhalation.

Gasoline

Heavy abusers have developed organic lead encephalopathy, arrhythmias, ataxia, delirium, tremor, and narcosis. 15 to 20 breaths of gasoline vapor produces a 5- to 6-hour intoxicated state characterized by giddiness, dizziness, ataxia, excitement, confusion, restlessness, and hallucinations that resemble ethanol-induced CNS changes. The most consistent neurologic signs are abnormal jaw jerk, gait abnormalities, hyperactive deep tendon reflexes, and intention tremor. Chronic intentional sniffing or huffing can result in death.

Halogenated Hydrocarbons

Carbon tetrachloride, trichloroethylene and trichloroethane can produce euphoria, nausea, vomiting, headache, seizures, tremor, coma, acute renal/hepatic failure, neuropathy, dysrhythmias, and sudden death.

Hexane

Chronic hexane glue sniffers can develop a polyneuropathy, similar to the insidious symmetric stocking-glove sensorimotor neuropathy seen in workers in glue factories that use hexane.

Methanol

Central nervous system depression, nausea, vomiting, shortness of breath, photophobia, and/or decreased visual acuity follows inhalation of methanol. Blood methanol and formic acid levels are often elevated.

Nitrites

Isobutyl, butyl, and amyl nitrites can cause mild methemoglobinemia, cyanosis, and hypotension.

Nitrous Oxide

Short- and long-term inhalation of nitrous oxide produces bone marrow depression, megaloblastic hematopoiesis, and subacute combined degeneration of the spinal cord. Nitrous oxide appears to inactivate vitamin B12, impair DNA synthesis, increase serum folate, and reduce serum methionine levels. Nitrous oxide concentrations over 50 ppm reduce dexterity, cognition, motor and audiovisual skills. Whipped cream dispensers charged with nitrous oxide can produce fatalities, hypoxia, bone marrow depression, brain-cell death, and peripheral neuropathy.

Nitrous oxide abuse by the dental profession has caused corticospinal tract and posterior column signs resembling the subacute combined degeneration of the spinal cord seen in vitamin B12 deficiency. The polyneuropathy is more sensory than motor and presents with paresthesias of hands and feet, Lhermitte's sign, loss of balance, weakness, ataxia, impotence, and sphincter disturbances.

Toluene

Adult toluene abuse presents as three syndromes: muscle weakness, gastrointestinal distress, and neuropsychiatric syndrome. Muscle weakness syndrome, characterized by gait disturbance and quadriparesis, results from hypokalemia, hypophosphatemia, hypocalcemia, and metabolic acidosis. Dysrhythmias, probably secondary to electrolyte imbalance, and rhabdomyolysis may occur. Type I distal renal tisular acidosis has been associated with toluene abuse.

Gastrointestinal distress (e.g., abdominal pain, nausea, vomiting, and hematemesis) occurs, perhaps secondary to the accumulation of the metabolite benzoic acid, which is a gastric irritant. The neuropsychiatric syndrome involves headache, dizziness, vertigo, syncope, sensorimotor neuropathy, cerebellar signs, hallucinations, lethargy, and coma.

Xylene

Central nervous system excitation, ataxia, mucous membrane irritation, nausea, and vomiting may be seen. Chronic abuse results in hepatic and renal dysfunction as well as cerebral and cerebellar degeneration.

Laboratory

ANALYTIC METHODS

Gas chromatography of blood samples provides diagnostic information on the solvents involved in abuse but usually does not guide therapy.

BLOOD LEVELS

Toluene blood levels above 2.5 $\mu g/mL$ are associated with seriously ill patients and levels above 50 $\mu g/mL$ probably are fatal. Toluic acids are the main metabolites of xylene, and their presence in the urine indicates xylene exposure. Hippuric acid (a metabolite of toluene) is a naturally occurring substance in the urine, but a hippurate/creatinine ratio exceeding one indicates recent (several days) toluene exposure.

Treatment

- Since sudden death results from dysrhythmias, initial support involves assisted ventilation, intravenous lines, and a cardiac monitor. Rescuers should be aware that mouth-to-mouth resuscitation can allow transfer of inhalants to the rescuer.
- Remove the offending agent that is producing the adverse consequences.
- Perform a detailed physical and medical evaluation to assess the possible existence of additional toxicity. The mainstay of the treatment is to confront the usual denial of the drug use and to establish a commitment to recovery.
- Involvement in 12-step programs such as Alcoholics Anonymous or Narcotics Anonymous may be useful to maintain abstinence from these agents.
- Visual evoked potentials, brainstem auditory evoked potentials, and somatosensory evoked potentials may be abnormal at an early stage of neurologic damage in inhalant abusers.
- Screen for electrolyte imbalance (e.g., calcium, potassium, phosphate) and acid-base disturbances in chronic solvent abusers.
- Transient toxic hepatitis usually clears within several days. Acute tubular necrosis may occur.
- Chronic solvent abusers may be addicted to other drugs. Observation for withdrawal symptoms and neuropsychiatric care may be warranted.
- Check serum lead and free erythrocyte protoporphyrin levels in gasoline sniffers (lead is no longer found in US gasoline, however old containers or international patients may increase this possibility).

Questions—Inhalant Abuse

1. Which of the following occur commonly after acute inhalant abuse?
   A. Disorientation to time and place
   B. Seizures
   C. Hypersensitivity hepatitis
   D. Severe hypokalemia
   E. All of the above

2. Which of the following abused inhalants is incorrectly matched with associated symptoms?
   A. Acetone—Central nervous system excitement, then depression
   B. Benzene—Aplastic anemia
   C. Correction fluid—Cerebral edema
   D. Gasoline—Acute renal/hepatic failure
   E. Hexane—Polyneuropathy

3. Which of the following statements regarding nitrous oxide inhalent abuse is false?
   A. It appears to inactivate vitamin B12
   B. Short-term inhalation has not led to bone marrow depression
   C. Concentrations over 50 ppm reduce dexterity, cognition, motor, and audiovisual skills
   D. Whipped cream dispensers charged with nitrous oxide can produce fatalities
   E. None of the above

4. Adult toluene abuse can present as a muscle weakness syndrome
   A. Characterized by gait disturbance or quadriparesis
   B. Resulting from hypokalemia, hypophosphatemia, hypocalcemia, and metabolic acidosis
   C. Exacerbated by hypoxia
   D. All of the above
   E. A and B

5. Which of the following is the best answer with respect to inhalant abuse?
   A. "Bagging" refers to holding an open bag or container over the head.
   B. "Huffing" refers to pouring material on a cloth that is held over the mouth.
   C. "Sniffing" refers to inhaling directly over an open container.
   D. Many hydrocarbons are thought to sensitize the myocardium to catecholamines, particularly those that are halogenated.
   E. All of the above are correct.

6. Which of the following anomalies characterizes chronic toluene abuse?
   A. Hyperkalemia
   B. Renal tubular acidosis
   C. Severe hypercalcemia
   D. Muscle hypertrophy in the lower extremities
   E. All of the above

OCCUPATIONAL LUNG DISEASE

Introduction

Because the lungs continuously sample their environment by exchanging 8–12 liters of air per minute, occupational lung disease is a significant hazard in workplaces contaminated by inorganic dusts, biological aerosols, toxic chemicals, or respiratory carcinogens. Numerous occupational toxins can cause a broad array of pulmonary problems. Bronchospasm may follow the use of hundreds of agents. Asbestos can cause mesothelioma and lung cancer. Organic dusts can cause a febrile respiratory illness, and numerous environmental substances and toxins can cause hypersensitivity pneumonitis in sensitive individuals.

Mechanisms of injury in occupational lung disease are many. Occupational asthma is the most prevalent occupational lung disease in developed countries. About 250 agents, including diisocyanates in the plastics industry, wood dusts in the construction trade, metals, drugs in the pharmaceutical industry, and laboratory animals can cause occupational asthma.

PATHOPHYSIOLOGY

Many agents produce similar reactions and the same agent may cause different reactions depending on dose, susceptibility, and underlying disease. Various agents are irritants and can cause alveolitis, bronchiolitis obliterans, and bronchitis. Other agents yield immunologic compromise. Byssinosis, caused by the inhalation of cotton or hemp dust, yields bronchial edema and plugging by an immunologic mechanism. Farmer's lung, felt to be caused by various fungi, and berylliosis is felt to be caused by immunologic mechanisms. Fibrogenesis also represents a serious mechanism of injury. Silica, asbestos, and coal dust promote fibrotic changes and pulmonary limitation.

Large volumes have been written in an effort to list the several thousand agents that can cause occupational lung disease. Few pathognomonic features identify specific occupational lung diseases. Pulmonary reactions such as bronchitis and hypersensitivity pneumonitis are caused by both environmental and nonenvironmental factors. Hence, the occupational history remains the most important means of diagnosing the presence of occupational lung disease. Routine screening should include a list of current and past jobs, questions about exposure to fumes, chemicals, and dusts, as well as the temporal relation of disease to jobs and coworkers.

LABORATORY

Pulmonary function tests with spirometry provide information about maximal lung volumes and flow rates. Typical volumes, when compared with normal population values, help define obstructive and restrictive patterns. Since lung volumes affect flow rate, the forced expiratory volume (FVC) and FEV1 (forced expiratory volume in 1 second)/FVC ratio define obstructive and restrictive defects.

Obstructive defects demonstrate normal lung volume (FVC) and low flow rates (FEV1/FVC ratio). Peak flow is reduced and flow rates at mid- and low-lung volumes are markedly decreased. Obstructive patterns cause increased airway resistance to flow, which results in air trapping and elevated lung volumes. Chronic bronchitis and emphysema produce irreversible airway obstruction as a result of mucosal edema, inflammatory fibrosis, and focal destruction of septa. Asthma produces reversible airway obstruction defined by at least a 10% response to bronchodilators.

Normal flow rates (FEV1/FVC) and low lung volumes (FVC) characterize restrictive lung disease. Restriction means reduced lung volumes. Interstitial fibrosis (e.g., asbestosis, aluminosis) produces restrictive defects, as do pleural scarring, rib cage abnormalities, and muscle dystonias. Restrictive diseases decrease elastic recoil and increase the work of breathing. Complex pneumoconiosis often combines obstructive and restrictive effects, complicating the interpretation of pulmonary function tests.

Lung diffusing capacity measures the capacity of the lung to transfer carbon monoxide to the blood. It is a complex measurement that depends on a number of anatomic variables including alveolar surface area, perfusion, capillary membrane integrity, ambient carbon monoxide levels, and hemoglobin-carrying capacity. The lung diffusing capacity is useful in measuring the severity of interstitial lung disease. Severe impairment occurs when diffusion values fall less than 40% of normal.

Questions—Introduction to Occupational Lung Disease

1. The most prevalent occupational lung disease in developed countries is
A. Hypersensitivity pneumonitis
B. Occupational asthma
C. Mesothelioma
D. Lung cancer
E. None of the above

2. The most important means of diagnosing the presence of occupational lung disease is
A. Underlying disease
B. Pathognomonic features which identify specific occupational lung diseases
C. Occupational history
D. Age of the patient
E. Sex of the patient

3. Farmer's Lung is felt to be a result of
A. Enterovirus
B. Wheat fibers
C. Various bacteria
D. Various fungi
E. None of the above

Asthma, Bronchitis and Reactive Airways Dysfunction Syndrome

ASTHMA

Two categories of asthma in the workplace are occupational asthma and work-aggravated asthma. Occupational asthma is characterized by variable airflow limitation, bronchial hyperresponsiveness, or both, resulting from conditions in a particular work environment, and not to stimuli outside the workplace. Work-aggravated asthma represents preexisting or concurrent asthma that is aggravated by irritants or physical stimuli in the workplace. Occupational asthma may develop in a person with preexisting asthma or concurrent asthma after a workplace exposure.

The presence or absence of a latency period can distinguish two types of occupational asthma. Occupational asthma with latency is the most common type. This develops after a period of exposure that may vary from a few weeks to several years. Occupational asthma with latency includes all instances of immunologic asthma, although the immunologic mechanism has not yet been identified for some agents. Occupational asthma without a latency period follows exposure to high concentrations of irritant gases, fumes, or chemicals on one or several occasions.

BRONCHITIS

Bronchitis results when respiratory irritants induce upper airway edema and hypersecretion, which produce cough, dyspnea, and pain. This syndrome is defined clinically by the presence of a productive cough without localized bronchopulmonary disease for at least 3 months of the preceding 2 years. Both chronic bronchitis and emphysema produce pathologically similar end-stage lung disease, however chronic bronchitis initially does not affect the alveolar septa.

Typically, long-term sequelae do not develop after acute bronchitis. However, bronchiolitis obliterans or fibrotic destruction of peripheral respiratory bronchioles is a well-known complication of nitrogen dioxide exposure (termed silo-filler's disease). The contribution of the workplace to the formation of chronic bronchitis is complicated by numerous host factors that modulate respiratory-tract response. These include smoking, air pollution, toxic dust exposure, individual susceptibility such as α1-antitrypsin deficiency, and the concentration of irritants.

REACTIVE AIRWAYS DYSFUNCTION SYNDROME

RADS differs from typical occupational asthma because of the absence of a preceding period of sensitization and the onset of illness after a single, first-time exposure. Subsequent inflammatory processes may alter the threshold of receptors in the bronchial mucosa.

Clinical criteria for the diagnosis of RADS include a documented absence of preceding respiratory complaints, the onset of symptoms after a single, specific exposure, and exposure to a gas, smoke, fume, or vapor that was irritating and present in high concentration. The onset of symptoms occurs within 24 hours of the exposure and persists for at least 3 months. Symptoms include cough, wheezing, and dyspnea, and resemble asthma. In fact, pulmonary function testing may show airflow obstruction and methacholine challenge test may be positive.

PATHOPHYSIOLOGY

Occupational asthma is the variable airway narrowing that results from exposure to dusts, fumes, or vapors in the workplace environment. Resistance to pulmonary airflow lies primarily in the central airways, 2 mm and larger in diameter (80% to 90% of total resistance). Gas exchange occurs in the terminal bronchioles and alveoli, which account for approximately 10% of total airway resistance. Exposure to certain agents produces mucous secretions, mucosal edema, and bronchial smooth muscle constriction. This results in reversible or partially reversible increases in airway resistance.

In bronchitis, hyperplasia of mucus-producing cells in response to particulate or chemical irritation produces excessive sputum. Epithelial changes reduce ciliary transport and ultimately lead to obstructive changes in the small airways, where inflammatory changes occur from the inability to clear secretions.

Increased airway resistance in asthma results from immunological responses (e.g., IgE-mediated release of chemical bronchoconstrictors), pharmacologically induced responses (i.e., no sensitization required), direct irritation by toxic fumes and gases (e.g., sulfur dioxide), and reflex bronchoconstriction. The immunologic or allergenic responses have classically been divided:

Type I Responses

Type I responses are immediate hypersensitivity reactions characterized by allergic and anaphylactic reactions. Sensitized individuals have circulating IgE antibodies, which are produced in response to specific antigens (allergens). These antibodies bind to mast cell or basophil receptors, which then release bronchoconstrictive factors such as histamine, serotonin, and leukokinins. Examples of individuals subject to occupational IgE-mediated asthma include animal handlers (dander), antibiotic workers (antibiotic sensitivity), detergent workers (*Bacillus subtilis*), chemical workers (azo dyes), plastic workers (phthalic anhydride), organic dust-exposed workers (castor beans, grains, spices), and platinum workers (complex platinum salts).

Type II Responses

Type II responses are direct cytotoxic reactions in which the antibody forms an immune complex on cell surface receptor sites. In this type of reaction, cell-bound antigens initiate cell destruction via K (killer) cells with or without complement. Drug-induced hemolytic anemias are an example of type II reactions.

Type III Reactions

Type III reactions, or Arthus reactions, cause inflammation by forming soluble, circulating antibodies that activate complement and release chemotactic factors. The hypersensitivity pneumonitis of organic dusts, serum sickness, and arthritis are examples.

Type IV Reactions

Type IV reactions are the classic delayed hypersensitivity reactions of cell-mediated immunity, in contrast with the above three reactions of humoral immunity, which require antibody production. Graft rejection and tumor immunity are examples of type IV reactions. Cell-mediated immunity may play a limited role in some types of asthma.

CLINICAL PRESENTATIONS

Symptoms of reversible airway obstruction include wheezing, chest tightness, cough, dyspnea, and decreased exercise tolerance after exposure, which improves after removal of the agent. Symptoms of RADS include cough, wheezing, and dyspnea and resemble asthma. Some substances (e.g., low-molecular-weight compounds) induce a late asthmatic reaction. These workers complain of nocturnal symptoms rather than immediate symptoms after exposure during working hours.

Improvement of symptoms over weekends, holidays, and vacations, in addition to recurrence of symptoms on resumption of work, suggests occupational asthma. Reversible airway obstruction is best measured by a reduction in the FEV1. A 10% to 15% improvement after bronchodilator therapy suggests reversible disease.

TOXIC DOSAGE/DEATH

Various allergens may precipitate these syndromes. Specific amounts may vary from individual to individual. Ceiling exposure limits to numerous irritant gases and chemicals have been proposed.

PREGNANCY/LACTATION

Asthma occurs in 0.5% to 1.5% of pregnant patients and may yield significant morbidity, and even mortality, to both mother and fetus. Treatment guidelines generally resemble those of the nonpregnant patient, however theophylline may cross the placenta and some have advised that it be avoided because of possible adverse fetal effects. Steroids and β-agonists are felt to be generally safe during pregnancy. Epinephrine is categorized as pregnancy risk category C.

LABORATORY

Analytic Methods

In cases of occupational asthma in which allergic factors are important (e.g., high-molecular-weight compounds), intradermal and prick skin tests may help identify specific causes. Specific antibodies may be demonstrated against low-molecular-weight compounds conjugated to proteins by a radioallergosorbent test (RAST) or enzyme-linked immunosorbent assay (ELISA), but these tests generally are less sensitive than skin testing. Positive skin tests and RAST assays indicate sensitization rather than disease and may be present in asymptomatic workers.

Spirometry and methacholine or histamine challenges (nonspecific bronchial provocation tests) are sensitive tests for the presence or absence of bronchospasm. Serial measurements of FEV1 over the workday and evening detect reactions to workplace chemicals and biological agents. Specific bronchial provocation tests to suspected workplace substances may be helpful as well.

Blood Levels

Blood levels do not help identify or manage these syndromes.

TREATMENT

Gut Decontamination

These methods are unhelpful in the management of these illnesses.

Elimination Enhancement

These methods also have not been shown helpful in treating asthma, bronchitis, or RADS.

Supportive Measures

- The ideal treatment for patients with occupational asthma with a latency period is removal from exposure. Most people with occupational asthma have to be retrained for a job with another employer in a different field.
- Any patient with occupational asthma who returns to the same job should have close medical follow-up. Worsening of asthma should lead to immediate removal from exposure.
- Pharmacologic treatment is similar to the treatment of patients with other forms of asthma. These primarily include epinephrine in pronounced cases, corticosteroids, and β-agonists.

Questions—Asthma, Bronchitis and Reactive Airways Dysfunction Syndrome

1. Which of the following is correctly described?

A. Occupational asthma represents preexisting or concurrent asthma that is aggravated by irritants or physical stimuli in the workplace.
B. Work-aggravated asthma is characterized by variable airflow limitation, bronchial hyperresponsiveness, or both, resulting from conditions in a particular work environment, and not to stimuli outside the workplace.
C. Bronchitis results when a patient has a period of localized bronchopulmonary disease for at least 3 months of the preceding 2 years.
D. Reactive Airways Dysfunction Syndrome (RADS) includes a documented absence of preceding respiratory complaints, the onset of symptoms after a single, specific exposure, and exposure to a gas, smoke, fume, or vapor that was irritating and present in high concentration.
E. None of the above

2. Occupational asthma is the variable airway narrowing that results from exposure to which of the following in the workplace environment?

A. Dusts
B. Fumes

C. Vapors
D. All of the above
E. None of the above

3. Which of the following is incorrectly described?
A. Type I responses are immediate hypersensitivity reactions characterized by allergic and anaphylactic reactions
B. Type II responses are those in which sensitized individuals have specific antigens which bind mast cell receptors causing release of bronchoconstrictive factors
C. In Type III reactions, soluble, circulating antibodies are formed that activate complement and release chemotactic factors
D. Type IV reactions are classic delayed hypersensitivity reactions of cell-mediated immunity
E. None of the above

4. Occupational asthma may improve over weekends, holidays, and vacations.
A. True
B. False

Hypersensitivity Pneumonitis

Hypersensitivity pneumonitis (HSP) is an immunologically induced inflammation of the lung parenchyma resulting from the repeated inhalation of a variety of etiologic agents, including organic dusts and simple chemicals. Numerous agents including thermophilic actinomycetes from moldy grains, bird allergens in psittacosis, cork and coffee dusts, various anhydrides, animal furs, numerous fungi, and isocyanates have been implicated. In the acute form, respiratory symptoms such as cough, sneezing, and dyspnea, and systemic symptoms such as fever, chills, myalgias, and malaise resemble the flu. Recovery occurs after removal from causative antigen or antigens.

PATHOPHYSIOLOGY

Hypersensitivity pneumonitis or extrinsic allergic alveolitis is an immunological pulmonary parenchymal disease that affects the bronchioles and alveoli. Although it appears that these infiltrative diseases are linked to type II and type III reactions, the exact mechanism remains unclear. IgE levels are usually not elevated. Hypersensitivity pneumonitis may develop in both atopic and nonatopic individuals.

CLINICAL PRESENTATIONS

Both systemic and respiratory symptoms may occur. In the acute form, influenzalike symptoms often predominate, consisting of chills, fever, sweating, myalgias, lassitude, headache, and nausea that begin 2 to 9 hours after exposure. Symptoms may peak between 6 to 24 hours, and last from hours to days. Respiratory symptoms such as cough and dyspnea are common but not universal.

A subacute form may appear gradually over days to weeks, is marked by cough and dyspnea, and may progress to severe dyspnea with cyanosis, leading to urgent hospitalization. The chronic form has an insidious onset over a period of months, with increasing cough and exertional dyspnea. Fatigue and weight loss may be prominent symptoms. Typically, signs and symptoms disappear within days, or weeks if the causative agent is no longer inhaled.

TOXIC DOSAGE/DEATH

The amount of allergen required to induce hypersensitivity pneumonitis varies among individuals.

PREGNANCY/LACTATION

Like asthma and bronchospastic disease, the treatment of hypersensitivity pneumonitis in pregnancy is similar to the treatment of nonpregnant individuals.

LABORATORY

Analytic Methods

Pulmonary function tests exhibit a restrictive pattern with decreases in the FVC and FEV1, but minimum alteration in the FEV1/FVC ratio. The most common response displays maximum reductions of FVC and FEV1 at approximately 6 hours post-inhalation. The diffusing capacity and arterial oxygen tension (especially after exercise) are also decreased.

Blood Levels

The attempted demonstration of antibody against suspected antigens by precipitin reactions in agar is an important part of the diagnostic workup. Precipitins are not demonstrable in all patients, and available antigens are not standardized.

TREATMENT

Gut Decontamination

These methods are unhelpful in the management of this illness.

Elimination Enhancement

These methods also have not been shown helpful in treating hypersensitivity pneumonitis.

Supportive Measures

- Chest x-rays usually are normal but may show increased bronchovascular markings, tiny nodules, or a reticulonodular pattern. Continuous exposure to etiologic agents may produce irreversible interstitial fibrosis (e.g., farmer's lung) and honeycombing.
- To make a definitive diagnosis in patients without sufficient clinical criteria, lung biopsy may be indicated, especially to rule out other diseases requiring different treatment. Open lung biopsy usually will provide adequate material, whereas transbronchial biopsy may not. Lung biopsy indicates a granulomatous-type disease.
- After acute exposure, peripheral blood neutrophilia and lymphopenia are common. Eosinophilia is not expected. Mild elevations in erythrocyte sedimentation rate, C-reactive protein, rheumatoid factor, and in immunoglobulins may be present occasionally, reflecting acute or chronic inflammatory changes. Antinuclear antibodies or other autoantibodies seldom are detected.
- Routine use of inhalational challenge is not recommended, especially in patients with forms of the disease other than simple, acute, recurrent, or transient attacks.
- Removal of the causative agent from the patient's environment, or of the patient from the incriminated inhalant, should be followed by improvement in most acute cases within days, weeks, or months and helps confirm the diagnosis.

Questions—Hypersensitivity Pneumonitis

1. Hypersensitivity pneumonitis is best described as
A. An infectious phenomenon
B. Immunologically-induced inflammation
C. A severe response to a new exposure of an occupational toxin

D. Always being caused by mold-exposure
E. None of the above

2. **Respiratory symptoms such as cough and dyspnea are universally found in hypersensitivity pneumonitis.**
A. True
B. False

3. **Treatment of hypersensitivity pneumonitis includes**
A. Blood levels to demonstrate antibody against suspected antigens
B. Gut decontamination
C. Elimination enhancement
D. All of the above
E. None of the above

Pneumoconioses

INTRODUCTION

Dusts are ubiquitous in occupational and familiar settings. Numerous varieties may be responsible for a huge cross-section of acute and chronic pulmonary illnesses. Pneumoconioses develop from the deposition of dust particles in the lungs. The pulmonary response to inhaled dust and particles depends on their physical characteristics (e.g., size, chemical composition, surface geometry, shape), chemical reactivity, respiratory rate and pattern, intensity of exposure (e.g., concentration, duration), and host factors (individual susceptibility, cigarette smoking, underlying disease states).

Organic dust toxic syndrome (ODTS) is a nonallergic, noninfectious, febrile respiratory illness caused by organic dust from moldy silage, hay, or other agricultural products. It also is known as pulmonary mycotoxicosis because the organic dust consists largely of microbial hyphae and spores. Exposure may occur when farm workers are involved in the dusty activity of transferring moldy silage.

Fibrogenic Dusts

Physiological changes from these agents commonly are greater than the radiograph or exposure suggests. Common agents include silica (silicosis), diatomaceous earth, asbestos (asbestosis, mesotheliomas, pulmonary and peritoneal cancer), alumina abrasives (Shaver's disease), and aluminum (aluminosis).

Mineral Dusts

Inorganic agents produce varying degrees of pulmonary fibrosis, and obstructive and restrictive lung changes, depending on the intensity of exposure and the toxicity of the specific agent. Benign pneumoconioses from iron (siderosis), barium (baritosis), tin (stannosis), perlite, carbon black, and antimony cause few, if any, physiological abnormalities.

Mixed Dusts

Mineral rock dust exposures rarely involve a single dust. Clay, calcium oxides, slate, fuller's earth, mica, aluminum silicates, and graphites all have been implicated in varying degrees of pulmonary dysfunction. Biologically active rock dusts can be identified by rock type.

Organic Dusts

These agents produce reversible airway disease (i.e., occupational asthma) and both acute and chronic allergic disease (e.g., hypersensitivity pneumonitis or extrinsic alveolar alveolitis). Plant dusts, animal dander, microbes, and proteolytic enzymes are examples.

PATHOPHYSIOLOGY

The deposition of particles depends on a combination of physical forces that move particles (e.g., turbulence) and airway anatomy. Particles between 5 and 30 μm are deposited in the nasopharyngeal region by impaction. Spherical particles between 0.5 and 5 μm reach the alveoli and terminal bronchioles. Nonspherical particles flow in response to their mean aerodynamic diameter. Nonrectilinear fibers, such as chrysotile (the most common asbestos fiber), have a diameter that increases in proportion to their deviation from rectilinearity. An increased respiratory rate during exercise increases both particle impaction in the upper airways and sedimentation in the lower airways.

Particle clearance depends primarily on the health of the mucociliary system, which is impaired by COPD and chronic bronchitis. Pulmonary macrophages phagocytize particles and clear them mostly through the lymph system. These entrapped particles may dissolve and enter the blood or lymph system.

Parenchymal damage depends on the toxicity of the inhaled particles. In benign pneumoconiosis, phagocytosis of inert substances may produce no symptoms despite large depositions (e.g., coal). Storage of these inert particles in alveolar macrophages, pulmonary lymphatics, and hilar lymph nodes may produce no significant structural or functional alterations.

CLINICAL PRESENTATIONS

Clinically, patients with pneumoconiosis experience an insidious onset of dyspnea. Pulmonary function tests show both obstructive and restrictive changes. Obstructive changes usually result from decreased lung elasticity caused by focal and diffuse destruction of small airways around dust deposits. Ventilation/perfusion mismatching causes hypoxemia, especially during exercise. Patients with simple silicosis, coal-worker's pneumoconiosis (CWP), and mixed-dust pneumoconiosis generally demonstrate mild degrees of obstruction. Those with complicated pneumoconiosis (e.g., progressive massive fibrosis) often have combination defects (obstructive, restrictive, and diffusion abnormalities).

Certain dusts produce primarily interstitial fibrotic disease (e.g., acute berylliosis, aluminosis, and asbestosis) rather than the focal nodular lesions seen in simple pneumoconiosis. See Beryllium section in Chapter 47, Metals. Fibrotic lesions appear out of proportion to the presence of dust-laden macrophages. Restrictive changes occur most often in pneumoconioses such as asbestosis and aluminosis, which cause diffuse interstitial fibrosis.

Symptoms of organic dust toxic syndrome may include chills, malaise, myalgia, a dry cough, dyspnea, headache, and nausea after a heavy organic dust exposure. ODTS is similar to acute farmer's lung and other forms of hypersensitivity pneumonitis in that both exhibit increased numbers of neutrophils in the bronchoalveolar lavage, both may be more common in nonsmokers, and both have a latency period of 4 hours or more. They differ in that the chest x-ray in ODTS does not show infiltrates, severe hypoxemia does not occur, and there are no known sequelae of physiologic significance.

TOXIC DOSAGE/DEATH

Variable amounts of dust may precipitate variable presentations among individuals.

LABORATORY

Analytic Methods

Prior sensitization to antigens in the ODTS usually does not occur (i.e., serology-allergen panel usually is negative).

Blood Levels
Occupational and exposure history, not any specific blood or lab tests, are most important in identifying etiologic agents.

TREATMENT

Gut Decontamination
These methods are not relevant as exposure, by definition, involves the lungs.

Elimination Enhancement
These methods are irrelevant as well.

Supportive Measures
- β-Agonist therapy may help reverse elements of reversible illness and steroids have been used with variable success depending on specific agents.

Questions—Introduction to Pneumoconioses

1. Which of the following dusts is incorrectly described?
   A. Fibrogenic dusts generally cause physiologic changes that are greater than the x-ray suggests.
   B. Fibrogenic dusts include silica and asbestos.
   C. Mineral dusts produce varying degrees of pulmonary fibrosis, obstructive and restrictive lung changes, depending on the intensity of exposure and the toxicity of the specific agent.
   D. Organic dusts include carbon black and antimony.
   E. Mixed dusts have been implicated in varying degrees of pulmonary dysfunction.

2. Which of the following is true regarding organic dust toxic syndrome?
   A. The chest x-ray does not show infiltrates.
   B. Severe hypoxemia often occurs.
   C. There are no known sequelae of physiologic significance.
   D. A and B
   E. A and C

SILICOSIS
Silicosis results from the inhalation of crystalline or free silica, usually in the form of quartz. Workers at risk include sandblasters, miners, tunnelers, silica millers, abrasives and flour workers, ceramics workers, glassmakers, and quarry and foundry workers. Three criteria are required to make the diagnosis of silicosis. These include an appropriate history of exposure, radiologic findings consistent with silicosis, and the absence of a likely alternative explanation for the clinical and radiologic findings.

Crystalline silica forms in the earth's crust. Free silica refers to pure crystalline silicon dioxide. The medically important crystalline phases of silicon dioxide are known as alpha quartz, cristobalite, and tridymite. Among these, alpha quartz is the most common mineral of commercial importance. It is a major constituent of igneous rocks such as granite and pegmatite, but it also is found in sandstone, slate, and shale. Cristobalite and tridymite are formed from quartz at high temperatures and have a restricted geologic distribution.

PATHOPHYSIOLOGY
It is important to distinguish among the terms silicon (the element), silica (the minerals), silicates (the minerals), and silicone (a man-made synthetic polymer). Silica and silicon dioxide exist in nature in amorphous and crystalline forms. Amorphous silica includes natural and synthetic glasses, including the glasses in mineral wool, and fume silica. Amorphous silica is much less toxic than crystalline silica although it is not biologically inert. Silicates are less fibrogenic than silica when inhaled into the lungs, but cause characteristic lesions after heavy prolonged exposure.

CLINICAL PRESENTATIONS

Chronic Silicosis
Chronic silicosis represents the most common form, and results from low-to-moderate exposure for more than 20 years. Typical radiographic findings are nodular opacities, usually predominating in the upper lung zones. Typically, discrete silicotic nodules form, without interstitial fibrosis. In the early stages of simple silicosis, there usually are no symptoms and signs. When findings are present, they usually are attributable to concomitant cigarette smoking or industrial bronchitis. As the disease progresses, decrements in pulmonary function become more apparent and are greater in smokers than nonsmokers. Enlargement of the hilar lymph nodes is common, with peripheral (eggshell) calcification in 5% to 10% of cases. This pattern is not pathognomonic for silicosis, but is highly suggestive if there is a history of exposure.

Once silicosis begins, it continues to progress even in the absence of ongoing exposure. Complicated or conglomerate silicosis, caused by the coalescence of silicotic nodules, usually in the upper lung zones, is diagnosed when the radiographic opacities are greater than 1 cm in diameter. This condition, referred to as progressive massive fibrosis, produces a restrictive pattern of pulmonary function, with decreased gas transfer, and eventually may result in cor pulmonale.

Acute Silicosis
Acute silicosis or silicoproteinosis progresses rapidly, may develop after only a few years of very intense exposure to free silica, and may be seen in sandblasters. Acute silicosis resembles idiopathic alveolar proteinosis histologically. X-rays of the chest reveal diffuse air-space disease, and the findings may mimic those in pulmonary edema. Progressive restriction and impairment in gas transfer can lead to extreme dyspnea, cor pulmonale, and death within several years.

Accelerated Silicosis
Accelerated silicosis is a less-well-defined entity that is intermediate between chronic silicosis and acute silicoproteinosis. The features of accelerated disease are identical to those of chronic silicosis but are more rapidly progressive, requiring only 4 to 8 years of exposure.

Silicotuberculosis
Mycobacterial infection must be ruled out whenever a patient with silicosis has radiographically evident progression or deterioration in respiratory function. An increased risk of tuberculosis and atypical mycobacterial infections in patients with silicosis is well recognized. Before the introduction of effective therapy, tuberculosis was the most important cause of death in workers with silicosis. *Aspergillus* species and other species also may colonize tuberculous or ischemic cavities in patients with silicosis.

TOXIC DOSAGE/DEATH
Progressive respiratory failure and death may occur in silicosis. Specific "doses" of silica responsible for silicosis in susceptible individuals have not been identified, however length of time

spent working with silica may distinguish the syndromes outlined above.

LABORATORY

Analytic Methods

The laboratory findings in patients with silicosis are nonspecific and specific analytic methods are not recognized.

Blood Levels

A moderate elevation in the angiotensin-converting-enzyme concentration and various immunologic abnormalities are common. Positive antinuclear-antibody titers are found in approximately one-third of these patients. An increased prevalence of rheumatoid factor and elevated levels of immunoglobulins and immune complexes also have been found.

TREATMENT

Gut Decontamination

There is no evidence that gut or other decontamination measures after silica exposure will help avert the eventual production of silicosis.

Elimination Enhancement

These methods play no role in treating silicosis.

Supportive Measures

- Treatment is supportive and depends on the extent of illness. Severe cases may require chronic oxygen therapy. The use of steroids and bronchodilators may yield variable responses.
- All patients with silicosis should be tested annually for tuberculosis with purified protein derivative (PPD) and any induration of 10 mm or more should be considered positive. A positive PPD test, symptoms, or radiographic changes suggesting tuberculosis require the examination of acid-fast smears and cultures for mycobacteria.
- Sputum cultures in patients with silicotuberculosis may not be consistently positive. Patients with positive smears or cultures should be treated initially with four drugs and for a year with at least two bactericidal agents.

Questions—Silicosis

1. Patients with silicosis often have unremarkable chest radiographs.
   A. True
   B. False

2. Which of the following is false regarding silicosis?
   A. Once chronic silicosis begins, it continues to progress even in the absence of ongoing exposure.
   B. Acute silicosis progresses rapidly and may develop after only a few years of very intense exposure to free silica.
   C. The features of accelerated disease are identical to those of chronic silicosis but are more rapidly progressive, requiring only 4 to 8 years of exposure.
   D. Chronic silicosis represents the most common form.
   E. None of the above

3. All of the following are associated with silicosis except
   A. Moderate decrease in the angiotensin-converting-enzyme concentration
   B. Positive antinuclear-antibody titers
   C. An increased prevalence of rheumatoid factor
   D. Elevated levels of immunoglobulins
   E. Elevated levels of immune complexes

ASBESTOS-RELATED DISEASE

Asbestos was, and is, a ubiquitous urban environmental contaminant. For years asbestos was used indiscriminately as a fire-retardant and was found commonly around home heating pipes, furnaces, and tiles. Despite public awareness of detrimental outcomes after prolonged exposure, much asbestos remains in the environment. Some studies of exposed urban dwellers who develop asbestosis indicate that a majority of these individuals have asbestos bodies within their lungs.

It has been estimated that as many as 65,000 Americans may have asbestosis, and that perhaps one-third of these will develop malignant pleural carcinomas (mesothelioma). Asbestos is a family of fibrous, silicate materials composed of three types of fibers. These include chrysotile, which accounts for 90% of commercial production, amosite, and crocidolite. All three fiber types can cause pleural thickening and the fibrotic lung disease asbestosis, but the etiologic role in the production of mesotheliomas by amosite and crocidolite is unclear.

PATHOPHYSIOLOGY

Exposure-response studies suggest a relationship between retained asbestos fiber size in the lung and specific disease predilection. Asbestosis has been associated with fibers with lengths of 2 mm and diameters of 0.15 mm. Mesothelioma has been associated with fibers with lengths of 5 mm and diameters of 0.1 mm. Lung cancer has been associated with fibers with lengths of 10 mm and diameters of 0.15 mm. Considerable cross-over may exist.

CLINICAL PRESENTATIONS

Asbestosis

Interstitial pulmonary fibrosis results from asbestos exposure. Radiologic evidence generally is not present until at least 5 years postexposure. Usual clinical symptoms are dyspnea, cough (with or without sputum), fatigue, weight loss, and chest pain. The primary physiological defect is restrictive lung disease and impaired gas diffusion. Obstructive disease may occur in asbestosis, but the effect of host factors (e.g., smoking) as an etiology needs to be delineated.

The presence of rales, restrictive lung disease, radiologic findings of interstitial lung disease, and an asbestos exposure history strongly suggests asbestosis. Open-lung biopsy can detect discrete foci of fibrosis associated with accumulations of asbestos bodies, but the lack of uniform and persistent asbestos body distribution has resulted in controversy over the sensitivity and necessity of this procedure. The histopathological diagnosis is complicated by the fact that neither the presence of interstitial fibrosis nor of asbestos bodies alone confirms the diagnosis of asbestosis. Generally, the presence of two or more asbestos bodies per square centimeter of nontumorous lung tissue, and chronic fibrosis in small conducting airways and septa, indicates asbestosis.

Pleural Thickening

A substantial portion of workers exposed to heavy concentrations of asbestos over long periods will develop pleural inflammatory fibrosis and plaques. Such changes may impair pulmonary function. Asbestos bodies rarely occur in these plaques. Pleurisy is the most common asbestos-related symptom during the first two decades of exposure. Plaques typically are bilateral, symmetric, and localized areas of pleural thickening and are highly suggestive of asbestos exposure when other causes such as infection, trauma, or surgery are excluded. Diaphragmatic calcification may be seen. Pleural plaques rarely appear before 15 years postexposure and usually are seen 30 years postexposure. Pleural plaques probably are not premalignant.

Cancer

It has been estimated that about 20% to 40% of patients with asbestosis will develop lung cancer. Mesothelioma is a rare pleural or peritoneal carcinoma that definitely has been associated with asbestos exposure. Chest pain is the first symptom of mesothelioma and radiologic evidence of pulmonary fibrosis often is not present. The histopathological diagnosis of mesothelioma is difficult and requires incisional biopsies of the pleural or peritoneal masses. Smoking probably does not predispose to the progression or development of asbestos-related disease, however smoking greatly increases the risk of bronchogenic carcinoma in asbestos workers (5- to 50-fold). Several preliminary studies have indicated that there appears to be an increased number of deaths from colon cancer in asbestos workers. The incidence of esophageal cancer appears to be increased as well.

TOXIC DOSAGE/DEATH

Progressive respiratory failure and death may occur in asbestosis. Specific "doses" of asbestos responsible for asbestosis or mesothelioma in susceptible individuals have not been identified, however an increased length of time spent working with asbestos may increase the likelihood of developing these diseases.

LABORATORY

Analytic Methods

Patients with asbestosis may demonstrate restrictive lung disease with spirometric testing.

Blood Levels

There are no specific blood levels or other tests available to make the diagnosis or guide management of these conditions.

TREATMENT

Gut Decontamination

There are no studies to demonstrate that lavage or charcoal is helpful after asbestos exposure.

Elimination Enhancement

These methods are not utilized in treating asbestosis.

Supportive Measures

- Radiographic findings in asbestosis are nonspecific. Small, irregular opacities involving the lower lung field are commonly noted, but in the absence of an exposure history, asbestosis may be difficult to distinguish clinically or radiographically from other pulmonary fibrotic disorders.
- Periodic chest x-rays are necessary to assess the possibility of lung cancer in asbestos-exposed patients, especially in smokers.
- Periodic pulmonary function testing may guide progression of disease.
- Bronchodilators, steroids, and oxygen therapy may be helpful in individual cases.

Questions—Asbestos-Related Disease

1. Asbestos has been removed almost completely from the environment.
A. True
B. False

2. Which of the following regarding asbestosis is true?
A. Radiologic evidence generally is not present until at least 1 year postexposure.
B. The primary physiological defects are restrictive lung disease and impaired gas diffusion.
C. Usual clinical symptoms are dyspnea, fatigue, weight loss, and chest pain.
D. A and B
E. B and C

3. Which of the following is true regarding asbestos exposure?
A. It is associated with lung cancer.
B. It is associated with mesothelioma.
C. Smoking predisposes one to the progression of asbestos-related disease.
D. A and B
E. All of the above

BYSSINOSIS

Byssinosis is an occupational lung disorder most commonly observed in textile workers and caused by the inhalation of cotton, flax, or hemp dust. Initially, workers may have chest tightness and shortness of breath on the first day of the workweek, called "Monday chest tightness." This typically is accompanied by a moderate and reversible decrease in ventilatory function. These symptoms subside as the week continues.

After many years of exposure, symptoms typically worsen and may persist throughout the workweek, as well as in the absence of work exposure. Both obstructive and restrictive pulmonary dysfunction develops. An endotoxin, known to be a component of Gram-negative bacteria that colonize cotton plants, is a possible causative agent of byssinosis. Treatment is symptomatic.

Questions—Byssinosis

1. The initial symptoms of byssinosis are
A. Cough
B. Hemoptysis and hematemesis
C. Chest tightness and shortness of breath
D. Restrictive pulmonary function
E. All of the above

2. Byssinosis, an occupational lung disorder, is most commonly observed in
A. Textile workers
B. Retail clothing salespersons
C. Marijuana smokers
D. All of the above
E. None of the above

RESPIRATORY TRACT IRRITANTS

Introduction

Respiratory tract irritants may affect the mucous membranes, upper and lower respiratory tract, and lung parenchyma. Irritant gases are divided into two categories based on water solubility. Highly soluble gases such as ammonia, aldehyde gases, hydrogen chloride, and others are adsorbed onto the upper respiratory tract and have their primary effects there. Gases with lower water solubility such as phosgene, nitrogen dioxide, chlorine, and isocyanates evade this first line of defense and have their primary effect on the lower respiratory tract. Any irritant gas at sufficiently high concentration may be a factor in producing pulmonary edema.

Ammonia

Ammonia is a colorless gas with pungent warning properties. Fertilizer manufacturing accounts for almost 80% of current production. Serious exposures result from leakage of pressurized liquid ammonia during transportation or industrial accidents. Wool, silk, nylon, and melamine release ammonia during combustion. Ammonia sprays may be employed in cases of criminal assault during which victims are temporarily immobilized by ammonia solution squirted into their eyes.

The ammonium hydroxide concentration in household ammonia ranges from 3% to 10%. Weaker 3% solutions are mild irritants, but higher concentrations may be significantly corrosive when ingested. Volatile ammonia solutions can produce inhalation injuries and systemic symptoms. An 8.8% ammonia solution has a pH of 12.5. See Bases section in Chapter 42, Acids, Bases, and Gastroesophageal Issues.

Ammonia inhalants are mild stimulants used to treat syncope, weakness, or threatened collapse and are common components of first-aid kits. Each glass ampule, enclosed in a fiber mesh, may contain 0.33 mL of a mixture of 18% ammonia and 36% alcohol. When the aromatic ammonia "smelling salts" are bitten into by children, vomiting, drooling, dysphagia, cough, and oral pharyngeal burns may ensue. Treatment is symptomatic. Endoscopy is reserved for those children with clinical evidence of upper airway involvement such as stridor, dysphagia, or drooling.

PATHOPHYSIOLOGY

Ammonia is a highly water-soluble, intensely irritating, alkaline gas that produces liquefaction necrosis in high concentrations.

PHARMACOKINETICS

Absorption

- Ammonia is not well absorbed by the gastrointestinal route.

Distribution

- Ammonia is water-soluble.

Elimination

- Ammonia is metabolized in the liver to urea and glutamine.

CLINICAL PRESENTATIONS

Mild-to-moderate inhalations produce headache, cough, bronchospasm, nausea, vomiting, pharyngeal and retrosternal pain, and conjunctivitis. Severe inhalation produces laryngospasm, signs of upper airway obstruction such as stridor, hoarseness, and difficulty in speaking, and, in excessively high doses, pulmonary edema. Persistent airway obstruction, bronchiolitis obliterans, bronchiectasis, and hyperreactive airways dysfunction syndrome have been reported after acute, high-dose exposures to ammonia.

Ammonia spray can cause immediate and serious ocular burns. Within a few seconds of injury, it may diffuse through the cornea into the anterior chamber. Permanent impairment of vision and even blindness may follow.

TOXIC DOSAGE/DEATH

Sensitive olfactory properties permit potential victims to detect the pungent odor at 30 ppm, but eye and nasal irritation begins near 50 ppm. Severe symptoms of pulmonary dysfunction appear at ammonia concentrations above 1,000 ppm, and immediate death occurs at concentrations near 1,500 ppm. Levels of ammonia below its threshold limit value (TLV) and short-term exposure limit (STEL) can induce asthma in susceptible persons.

DRUG INTERACTIONS

Chloramine gas (see Bleaches section in Chapter 38, Household Products) may inadvertently be formed when individuals mix ammonia with hypochlorite (i.e., household) bleach. Symptoms such as cough, shortness of breath, and a choking sensation may occur within minutes.

LABORATORY

Analytic Methods

Ammonia may be measured by an enzymatic method.

Blood Levels

While monitoring ammonia levels may be helpful in patients with severe liver dysfunction, there is no evidence that such testing is helpful after ammonia exposures.

TREATMENT

Gut Decontamination

While diluents such as milk or water remain a controversial intervention after ammonia ingestion, there is no evidence that any gut decontamination procedures are at all helpful after ammonia exposures.

Elimination Enhancement

These methods have not been shown to aid in the treatment of ammonia exposures.

SUPPORTIVE MEASURES

- Carefully assess the airway in all individuals, and intubate patients with significant respiratory compromise. Respiratory distress is uncommon but presents occasionally because of soft tissue edema. Unless endotracheal intubation can be accomplished under direct vision, a cricothyroidotomy or tracheostomy may be necessary (blind nasotracheal intubation in this setting is contraindicated). Oxygen is given as indicated.
- The chest x-ray usually is unremarkable. Pulmonary edema may occur in rare instances. Large exposures also can precipitate reactive airways dysfunction.
- Alkali injuries to the eye and skin should be irrigated copiously at least 30 minutes until the eye reaches neutral pH. Topical antibiotics and topical steroids may be required. Alkali injuries to the eye are ophthalmologic emergencies and require ophthalmologic consultation after copious irrigation with saline. Test all patients with conjunctival irritation for corneal abrasions with fluorescein stain and slit-lamp exam.

Questions—Ammonia

1. **All of the following are true concerning ammonia, except**
   A. Ammonia is well-absorbed by the gastrointestinal tract.
   B. Ammonia is water soluble.
   C. Ammonia is metabolized in the liver.
   D. Ammonia is a highly irritating alkaline gas.
   E. Ammonia causes liquefaction necrosis in high concentrations.
2. **Signs and symptoms of ammonia toxicity include all of the following, except**
   A. Laryngospasm
   B. Pulmonary Edema
   C. Seizures
   E. Stridor
   F. Headache
3. **Which is helpful during treatment following ammonia exposure**
   A. Gut decontamination
   B. Supportive respiratory and airway care
   C. Dialysis
   D. Treatment with ammonia antidote kit
   E. Ammonia levels
4. **Chloramine gas, which can cause cough, shortness of breath, and choking, may be formed inadvertently by mixing ammonia with which of the following household products?**
   A. Hydrogen peroxide
   B. Isopropyl alcohol
   C. Household bleach
   D. Lye based soaps
   E. Lauryl sulfate

Sulfur Dioxide

Sulfur dioxide is a primary air pollutant generated by industries that burn fossil fuels. Commercial applications include use in fumigation of fruits and vegetables, bleaching, tanning, brewing, preserving, and refrigeration. Sulfur dioxide also is present as a by-product of smelting, fossil fuel combustion, paper manufacturing, and fabrication of rubber products.

Sulfur dioxide is highly water soluble, so that only a small amount penetrates the lower respiratory tract. Therefore, primarily upper respiratory tract irritation occurs after exposure. Penetration of the lower respiratory tract does occur during increased physical activity, because of mouth breathing. This colorless, irritating gas with a characteristic pungent odor is more than twice as heavy as air.

PATHOPHYSIOLOGY

On contact with moist mucous membranes, sulfur dioxide produces sulfurous acid, which is a direct irritant and inhibits mucociliary transport, as well as bisulfite and sulfite. Most inhaled sulfur dioxide is detoxified by the liver to sulfates. The irritant-induced stimulation of airway sensory end organs causes vagal stimulation and airway smooth muscle contraction. Patients with reactive airways dysfunction syndrome are very sensitive to the bronchospastic properties of sulfur dioxide.

Carbon particles and water droplets carry sulfur dioxide deep into the terminal bronchioles and exacerbate cardiopulmonary disease. Such conditions were blamed for over 4,000 deaths during the 1952 London smog episode. Sulfur oxides and nitrogen oxides are the principal sources of acid rain and snow (defined by a pH under 5.7). Sulfur dioxide mists formed from fossil fuel combustion may float hundreds of miles and are deposited in streams and lakes. Elevated acidity adversely affects fish and tree populations. Concentration, rather than duration of exposure, appears to be the most important determinant of histopathological damage.

CLINICAL PRESENTATIONS

Respiratory tract irritation manifested by cough, burning, lacrimation, conjunctival injection, difficulty in swallowing, and oropharyngeal erythema, occurs after substantial exposures. Vomiting, diarrhea, abdominal pain, fever, headache, vertigo, agitation, tremor, convulsions, and peripheral neuritis also have been noted. Acute high-dose exposures may produce immediate bronchospasm and pulmonary edema with subsequent respiratory failure. Acute high-dose sulfur dioxide exposures have resulted in severe obstructive and restrictive defects 3 months postexposure, which failed to respond to bronchodilators.

Chronic exposure to sulfur dioxide from air pollution has been associated with aggravation of cardiopulmonary conditions such as asthma, COPD, and coronary artery disease. Persistent cough and sputum production has been associated with ambient sulfur dioxide levels in certain communities.

TOXIC DOSAGE/DEATH

Various concentrations of sulfur dioxide are roughly correlated with clinical effects. At 3 ppm, sulfur dioxide has an easily detected odor. Pulmonary effects are unlikely below 5 ppm. Concentrations of 6 to 12 ppm may cause nasal and throat irritation. At 10 ppm, upper respiratory irritation and nosebleeds may occur. Concentrations of 20 ppm are irritating to the eyes and chronic respiratory symptoms may develop at this level. Concentrations of 50 to 100 ppm represent maximum tolerable exposures for 30 to 60 minutes and concentrations of 400 to 500 ppm represent an immediate danger to life.

PREGNANCY/LACTATION

There appears to be no reproductive risk below concentrations of 5 ppm.

TREATMENT

- Remove the patient from the source of contamination and provide immediate support of airway and breathing, as in smoke inhalation.
- Decontaminate eyes and skin with copious irrigation and dilution.

Questions—Sulfur Dioxide

1. **All of the following are true about sulfur dioxide except**
   A. Sulfur dioxide is a primary air pollutant generated by burning of fossil fuels.
   B. Sulfur dioxide is lipid-soluble and penetrates the lower respiratory tract readily
   C. Sulfur dioxide, along with nitrogen oxides, are the principal cause of acid rain.
   D. The most important determinant of histopathologic damage from sulfur dioxide is the concentration rather than the duration of exposure.
   E. Sulfur dioxide produces sulfurous acid on contact with mucous membranes, which causes a direct irritant effect.

2. The clinical manifestations of sulfur dioxide exposure include all of the following except

A. Respiratory tract irritation with cough, burning, and oropharyngeal edema with difficulty swallowing
B. Central nervous system effects including headache, agitation, vertigo, and seizures
C. Coagulopathy resulting in hematuria, epistaxis, gastrointestinal tract bleeding, and intracranial hemorrhage
D. Pulmonary edema and bronchospasm with subsequent respiratory failure
E. Gastrointestinal symptoms including vomiting, diarrhea, and abdominal pain

Nitrogen Oxides

Nitrogen oxides include nitrous oxide, an anesthetic gas (see Chapter 43, Anesthetic Agents), and nitric oxide, a slightly soluble gas that rapidly combines with oxygen to form nitrogen dioxide. Under normal atmospheric conditions, nitrogen dioxide exists in equilibrium with nitrogen tetroxide. These gases are slightly yellow to reddish brown, are heavier than air, and have a faint chlorine bleachlike odor. Nitrogen dioxide produces nitrous and nitric acid on contact with water.

Exposure to nitrogen oxides may occur in industrial, manufacturing, or farm settings. Silos may contain nitrogen dioxide, nitric oxide, and carbon dioxide, because of plant decomposition in the presence of high nitrate levels. Silo filler's disease is a complication of exposure to such irritant gases. Other occupational exposures may result from the manufacture of dyes, fertilizers, celluloid, and lacquers as well as from welding, glass blowing, and food bleaching. Firemen may be exposed to nitrogen oxide during chemical plant fires or from burning mattresses.

The combustion of gas during cooking and the burning of pilot lights releases nitric oxide, nitrogen dioxide, carbon monoxide, carbon dioxide, and water. Nitrogen dioxide, a product of combustion in malfunctioning ice-resurfacing machines, can accumulate in indoor ice-skating arenas that are poorly ventilated.

PATHOPHYSIOLOGY

Because of its poor water solubility, nitrogen dioxide is a mild upper respiratory irritant. This action results from the formation of nitric acid in the presence of water. Nitric acid is destructive to respiratory epithelium and alveolar membranes and may produce metabolic acidosis. Poor initial irritant effects allow widespread dissemination of nitrogen oxides throughout the lungs and diffuse delayed inflammation. Nitrogen dioxide decomposition also may produce nitrates, which are capable of causing vasodilation and mild methemoglobinemia. The fibrotic destruction of terminal bronchioles, termed bronchiolitis obliterans, may occur as a late complication.

Inhalation of nitrogen dioxide causes pulmonary injury that is dose-dependent. The injury is characterized by loss of ciliated cells in the airways and degeneration of alveolar epithelial type I cells leaving the basement membrane denuded. The disappearance of type I cells, which normally cover 97% of the alveolar surface, results in cellular hypertrophy of epithelial type II cells to replace damaged type I cells. Within 72 hours, the denuded basement membrane is repopulated again, but with the rapidly proliferating type II cells.

CLINICAL PRESENTATIONS

The clinical presentation following nitrogen dioxide exposure depends on the duration and intensity of exposure. Initially, mild irritation of the upper respiratory tract, characterized by cough, sore throat, conjunctivitis, dyspnea, headache, vertigo, nausea, rhinitis, somnolence, and chest tightness, occurs. Mild cases become asymptomatic within several hours. The severity of initial symptoms does not correlate well with subsequent pulmonary pathology.

After a latent period of 3 to 30 hours, patients can develop pulmonary edema characterized by fever, tachypnea, tachycardia, hemoptysis, dyspnea, wheezing, cyanosis, and rales, which may result in acute respiratory failure. About half of patients surviving nitrogen dioxide-induced pulmonary edema develop bronchiolitis obliterans within weeks. Occasionally, bronchiolitis obliterans may be the initial presentation with symptoms including progressive dyspnea, cyanosis, cough, and wheezing. Methemoglobinemia and hypotension may complicate nitrogen oxide exposures as well.

Symptoms of silo-filler's disease, a disease following chronic exposures to nitrogen dioxide, resemble influenza and include fever, chills, cough, chest pain, and dyspnea. Most patients completely recover, but others may develop ARDS and/or bronchiolitis obliterans.

TOXIC DOSAGE/DEATH

U.S. ambient air standards allow average nitrogen dioxide levels of 0.05 ppm over 24 hours. Nitrogen dioxide has poor warning properties and frequently is not detectable at concentrations that cause mucosal irritation. At levels of 100 to 150 ppm, toxicity occurs within 30 to 60 minutes, and at levels of 200 to 700 ppm, fatalities result after short exposure.

PREGNANCY/LACTATION

Occupational exposure to nitrous oxide has been associated with decreased fertility.

LABORATORY

Analytic Methods

Pulmonary function tests show obstructive, restrictive, and diffusion defects because of destruction of alveoli, interstitium, and bronchioles.

Blood Levels

Blood levels do not help in the management of nitrogen dioxide and other nitrogen oxides exposures.

TREATMENT

Gut Decontamination

As exposure is airborne, charcoal or any other method of gut decontamination has not proved useful in managing nitrogen oxides exposures.

Elimination Enhancement

These methods would not be expected to be helpful after nitrogen oxides exposures.

Supportive Measures

- Attention to respiratory support similar to smoke inhalation, is necessary. Rescuers should be cautious and wear protective gear if the ambient concentration of nitrogen oxides exceeds 25 ppm or nitrogen dioxide levels exceed 1 ppm.

- Clinical effects are often delayed because of mild irritant properties. The treatment of respiratory and conjunctival irritation is supportive after decontamination.
- Patients who remain asymptomatic several hours after exposure may be treated as outpatients and instructed to return if any symptoms develop.
- Any symptomatic patient should be observed for delayed effects for 24 to 36 hours. Patients who become asymptomatic after 24 to 36 hours of observation may be released, but follow-up should be arranged within several weeks to assess pulmonary status.
- Patients should be screened with chest x-ray, arterial blood gases (including methemoglobin level), and pulmonary function tests. Arterial blood gases may reveal hypoxemia, hypercapnia, and acidosis with early changes in the alveolar-arterial oxygen gradient.
- Early chest x-rays are often normal but serial changes in x-rays parallel changes in the clinical condition. The extent of pulmonary infiltrates does not correlate with prognosis. Watch for development of ARDS manifested by symptoms and signs of increased respiratory distress.
- A nodular pattern predominates in bronchiolitis obliterans, whereas fluffy confluent bilateral infiltrates occur in pulmonary edema. Infiltrates of bronchiolitis obliterans usually clear in 1 to 2 months but may persist.
- The use of corticosteroids has been suggested for the prevention of bronchiolitis obliterans, although the effectiveness of steroids in altering the course of bronchiolitis obliterans has not been confirmed.
- Patients who develop adult respiratory distress should be treated with fluid restriction, oxygen, intubation, and positive end expiratory pressure (PEEP) as necessary. These patients are at high risk of developing bronchiolitis obliterans within several weeks and should be followed closely as outpatients.

Questions—Nitrogen Oxides

1. Which of the following is true?
   A. Decomposition of nitrogen oxide produces nitrates that may lead to methemoglobinemia.
   B. An early complication of nitrogen oxide inhalation is fibrotic destruction of the terminal bronchioles leading to bronchiolitis obliterans.
   C. Nitric acid causes destruction of the respiratory epithelium and respiratory acidosis.
   D. Inhalation of nitrogen dioxide causes injury to the lungs, which is independent of dose.
   E. Nitrogen oxide is a powerful upper respiratory irritant because of its poor water solubility.

2. All are true of the clinical presentation of nitrogen oxide exposure except
   A. Mild throat irritation with cough often is the initial manifestation
   B. The severity of the initial symptoms at the time of exposure correlate well with the subsequent pulmonary pathology
   C. Patients with mild cases of exposure who remain asymptomatic after several hours can safely be discharged home
   D. Patients whose symptoms are mild and resolves within several hours should be admitted to the hospital for 24 to 36 hours of observation.
   E. Central nervous system symptoms include vertigo, somnolence, and coma.

3. Silo filler's disease is an acute illness that is similar to influenza-with fever, chills, and cough that occurs after an acute exposure to nitrogen oxides.
   A. True
   B. False

4. Which of the following is true concerning occupational exposure to nitrogen oxide?
   A. Occupational exposure had been related to increased incidence of birth defects.
   B. The occupational hazard of nitrogen oxide has been minimized because of the ability to detect it in the air at nonhazardous levels.
   C. At levels of 200 to 700 ppm, fatalities can result after only several minutes of exposure.
   D. Occupational exposure has been shown to increase the incidence of coronary artery disease.
   E. In recent years, occupational exposure has been nearly eliminated as a result of diligent testing of worker nitrogen oxide levels.

Phosgene

Phosgene was widely used in World War I as a chemical warfare agent that accounted for 80% of chemical warfare fatalities. It is a colorless gas that is heavier than air. Although phosgene has a musty haylike odor, warning properties are poor and toxic levels are reached before detection. Current uses include the commercial application of phosgene as a chemical intermediate in isocyanate production, and its use in the manufacture of dyestuffs, insecticides, and pharmaceuticals.

The decomposition of heated organochlorine compounds, as in the pyrolysis of polyvinyl chloride or the use of carbon tetrachloride fire extinguishers, produces phosgene. Phosgene also may occur as a decomposition product of arc welding. Phosgene decomposes to carbon monoxide and hydrochloric acid.

PATHOPHYSIOLOGY

Poor water solubility leads to the delayed appearance of clinical signs. Because initial irritating symptoms are mild, direct alveolar damage results in pulmonary edema. The lungs are the principal target organs. Diffuse edema develops in some type II alveolar cells as well as in focal areas of type I cells. Interstitial cells are susceptible to edema and subsequent necrosis. Phosgene also may decrease sympathetic activity, causing vasoconstriction of pulmonary venules and increased alveolar exudates.

CLINICAL PRESENTATIONS

Mild conjunctival and upper respiratory tract irritation occurs initially. Severe mucous membrane irritation in pure phosgene exposures indicates seriously toxic phosgene levels. Delayed pulmonary edema manifested by dyspnea, cough, chest pain, hemoptysis, and cyanosis may occur 2 to 24 hours after exposure. After a moderate phosgene dose, the average clinical latent period lasts 6 to 15 hours.

TOXIC DOSAGE/DEATH

Exposures below 25 ppm/min are harmless. Doses over 150 ppm/min of phosgene will induce pulmonary edema and doses over 300 ppm/min are life threatening.

TREATMENT

Gut Decontamination

As exposure is airborne, charcoal or any other method of gut decontamination has not proved useful in managing phosgene exposures.

Elimination Enhancement

These methods would not be expected to be helpful after phosgene exposures.

Supportive Measures

- The basic approach to phosgene-induced pulmonary edema is supportive, and is similar to that for other respiratory irritants that produce delayed pulmonary edema (e.g., nitrogen oxides, smoke inhalation). Oxygen, ventilator support, and diuretics may be helpful.
- Patients who remain asymptomatic several hours after exposure may be followed as outpatients.
- Patients who develop symptoms after exposure should be observed for the development of delayed pulmonary edema for 24 hours.
- Steroids, both inhaled and systemic, used shortly after exposure may lessen the severity of pulmonary edema.
- The chest x-ray is the most sensitive indicator of early pulmonary edema as manifested by a perihilar haze. Changes in carbon monoxide diffusing capacity may occur within hours of exposure. Blood gases, not blood levels, are important in the management of phosgene toxicity.
- A decrease in the arterial-alveolar oxygen gradient may be an early indicator of pulmonary damage, but values must be correlated with age and preexisting cardiopulmonary disease.

Questions—Phosgene

1. The principal target organs of phosgene toxicity is

A. The kidney
B. The lungs
C. The central nervous system
D. The blood
E. None of the above

2. Delayed pulmonary edema manifested by dyspnea, cough, chest pain, hemoptysis, and cyanosis may occur

A. 5 to 10 hours after exposure
B. 10 to 15 hours after exposure
C. 15 to 20 hours after exposure
D. All of the above
E. None of the above

3. Management of phosgene toxicity includes

A. Blood levels
B. Gut decontamination
C. Blood gases
D. Elimination enhancement
E. None of the above

Chlorine

The deployment of chlorine gas at Ypres in 1915 during World War I initiated modern chemical warfare and led to extensive and controversial studies on the long-term sequelae of chlorine gas exposure. Millions of tons of chlorine are produced for water purification, cloth and paper bleaching, and chemical and plastic processes. Exposures most commonly result from either storage or transportation accidents involving the pressurized liquid form. Other poisonings occur in industrial accidents, school chemistry experiments, accidental release of chlorine from swimming pool operations, and mixing of cleaning agents.

Chlorine is a slightly water-soluble, yellow-green gas. Its pungent odor and irritant action provide good warning properties, although irritation may occur at levels below olfactory detection. Household hypochlorite exposures are less massive than industrial or environmental releases, but can be lethal. When ammonia interacts with hypochlorite-containing products, a combination of monochloramine and dichloramine is produced.

PATHOPHYSIOLOGY

Chlorine is a strong oxidizing agent that forms both hypochlorous and hydrochloric acid on contact with moist mucous membranes. Hypochlorous acid decomposes into hypochloric acid and oxygen free radicals. Tissue damage results from the disruption of cellular proteins. These agents combine with sulfhydryl groups and disulfur bonds and form stable hydrates of organic chlorine. Pulmonary pathological changes include necrosis and sloughing of respiratory epithelium, alveolar exudates, and hyaline membrane formation.

CLINICAL PRESENTATIONS

Mild exposure produces lacrimation, conjunctival irritation, rhinorrhea, cough, headache, sore throat, chest pain, dyspnea, and nausea. Laryngeal edema may produce hoarseness and stridor. As with other halogens (e.g., fluorine, bromine), severe exposures can progress to ulcerative tracheobronchitis, pulmonary edema, and respiratory failure. Corneal abrasions and cutaneous burns also may result from direct exposure. Symptoms usually begin within minutes, and asymptomatic patients may be safely triaged at the exposure site without fear of delayed symptom development.

Restrictive and obstructive defects found on pulmonary function tests may arise acutely because of interstitial edema and bronchospasm. The typical pattern of patients exposed to moderate concentrations of chlorine gas is that of increased airway resistance with normal diffusing capacity. Pulmonary function test abnormalities usually return to normal within several months. Although acute single exposures probably cause minimal, if any, residual pulmonary dysfunction, the issue of permanent pulmonary sequelae has not been settled.

TOXIC DOSAGE/DEATH

The extent of injury following chlorine exposure depends on the concentration and duration of exposure, as well as the water content of tissue involved and the presence of underlying cardiopulmonary disease. Chlorine concentrations roughly correlate with certain clinical parameters. At 0.2 to 3.5 ppm, an odor is detected. Mild mucous membrane irritation that can be tolerated for up to 1 hour occurs at 1 to 3 ppm. 5 to 15 ppm causes moderate irritation of the upper respiratory tract and 30 ppm causes immediate chest pain, vomiting, dyspnea, and cough. At concentrations of 40-60 ppm, toxic pneumonitis and pulmonary edema may occur. A concentration of 430 ppm has been associated with lethality over 30 minutes, and 1,000 ppm has been associated with fatality within minutes.

DRUG INTERACTIONS

Chloramine gas (see Bleaches section in Chapter 38, Household Products) may inadvertently be formed when individuals mix ammonia with hypochlorite bleach. Symptoms such as cough, shortness of breath, and a choking sensation may occur within minutes. Mixing hypochlorite with an acid (such as toilet bowl or tile cleaner) results in the release of chlorine gas.

LABORATORY

Analytic Methods
Ion-selective electrodes and spectrophotometry measure chlorides.

Blood Levels
Following serum chloride levels after chlorine exposures does not help guide management, or reflect clinical pathology.

TREATMENT

Gut Decontamination
As exposure is airborne, charcoal or any other method of gut decontamination has not proved useful in managing airborne chlorine exposures. See Chapter 42, Acids, Bases, and Esophageal Issues chapter for the management of chlorine-containing acids.

Elimination Enhancement
These methods would not be expected to be helpful after chlorine exposures.

Supportive Measures
- The general approach to airborne chlorine exposures is similar to the treatment of smoke inhalation with special attention to initial support of airway and breathing. Humidified oxygen should be given immediately to patients with significant respiratory symptoms.
- Irrigate exposed skin and eyes with copious saline. Be sure to check for corneal abrasions.
- Nausea may be treated with clear liquids and Phenergan.
- Sore throat is treated with humidified air, and throat lozenges as necessary.
- Cutaneous burns are treated as thermal burns after copious irrigation.

Respiratory Failure
- Mild or moderately symptomatic patients may be discharged after several hours of observation if symptoms improve with symptomatic treatment. Patients whose respiratory symptoms persist or deteriorate should be admitted to a direct observation area. These patients are evaluated with arterial blood gases, chest x-ray, and pulmonary function tests. Bronchospasm is treated with inhaled sympathomimetics and humidified oxygen.
- Watch for development of pulmonary edema and laryngeal obstruction. Pulmonary edema may occur up to 24 hours after exposure, sometimes inducing severe hypoxemia in minutes. Patients who are well 24 hours after exposure may be discharged. Intravenous fluids should be given with great caution.
- Corticosteroids are controversial in the patient with pulmonary edema, and clinical studies evaluating their efficacy are lacking.
- Acute hypoxemic respiratory failure generally includes the presence of severe hypoxemia despite oxygen therapy, radiographic evidence of diffuse pulmonary infiltrates, decreased lung compliance and intrapulmonary shunt, and normal cardiac function. The patient with persistent hypoxemia may require positive end-expiratory airway pressure (PEEP), in addition to supplemental oxygen.
- Nebulized sodium bicarbonate may ameliorate respiratory symptoms by neutralizing the acid formed when chlorine gas encounters water in the airways. This may result in an exothermic reaction. Patients should be carefully monitored before and after this procedure. Few clinical studies have confirmed this approach. It is not known if such therapy is safe or effective after severe exposures.

Questions—Chlorine

1. Of the following statements about chlorine which is true
- A. Chlorine is a highly water soluble gas commonly used for water purification and bleaching.
- B. Chlorine is a strong reducing agent that forms hypochloric acid on contact with mucous membranes.
- C. Hypochloric acid causes tissue damage by disruption of cellular proteins.
- D. Household grade chlorine bleach is concentrated to a degree that makes it uniformly toxic.
- E. When household bleach (hypochlorite) is mixed with ammonia, nitrogen oxide gas is produced, which can cause respiratory tract irritation.

2. Which of the following is false concerning the clinical presentation of chlorine gas exposure
- A. Mild exposure produces lacrimation, conjunctival irritation, cough dyspnea and nausea.
- B. Severe exposures can lead to ulcerative tracheobronchitis, pulmonary edema, and respiratory failure.
- C. Symptoms of exposure typically are delayed for several hours and even asymptomatic patients should be admitted to the hospital for observation.
- D. Single acute exposures to moderate levels of chlorine gas may produce increased airway resistance with a normal diffusing capacity.
- E. Pulmonary function abnormalities usually return to normal within several months.

3. Which of the following is false regarding chlorine
- A. The extent of injury depends on the concentration, the duration of exposure, and the water content of the exposed tissue.
- B. Exposure to chlorine gas in concentrations over 1,000 ppm usually is fatal within minutes.
- C. The odor of chlorine gas can be detected at 2 ppm.
- D. At levels of 10 ppm, chlorine gas will commonly cause respiratory tract irritation.
- E. When hypochlorite is mixed with acid cleaning products (toilet or tile cleaner) significant amounts of chlorine gas may be released.

4. All are true regarding the treatment and evaluation of chlorine gas exposure except
- A. Following serum chloride levels has not been proven to be helpful in determining the risk of delayed symptoms or the need for hospitalization.
- B. Humidified oxygen should be given immediately to anyone exposed to significant concentrations of chlorine gas.
- C. Skin decontamination should be started immediately with saline irrigation.
- D. After several hours of observation, patients with improving respiratory symptoms may be safely discharged home with follow-up.
- E. Inhaled sympathomimetics have not been shown useful in treating bronchospasm associated with chlorine gas inhalation.

Metal Fume Fever

Potissier first described metal fume fever in 1822. It results from the inhalation of freshly formed metal oxides, which form when metals are heated above their melting point, as in welding. The most common sites of exposure are brass foundries and zinc smelters. Common synonyms are Monday morning fever, zinc shakes, foundry fever, smelter shakes, copper fever, the smothers, spelter shakes, Braziers' disease, and brass chills. Metals known to cause metal fume fever include antimony, aluminum, arsenic, cadmium, cobalt, copper, iron, lead, magnesium, manganese, mercury, nickel, selenium, silver, tin, and zinc.

PATHOPHYSIOLOGY

The exact mechanism of action is unknown. An immunological connection has been proposed because of the presence of a short-term immunity that correlates to the duration of leukocytosis. The presence of blocking antibodies prevents clinical symptoms while exposure continues, but interruption of exposure allows the buildup of antigen-antibody excess and clinical symptoms. Other proposed mechanisms include a direct toxic effect on the lungs, transient adrenal insufficiency, and direct release of endogenous pyrogens from the leukocytes. Toxicity results only from freshly formed metal oxides, because particles clump upon cooling and do not reach the alveoli.

CLINICAL PRESENTATIONS

Sudden onset of symptoms typically occurs at home 4 to 8 hours after exposure and lasts 12 to 48 hours. Symptoms commonly affect previously unexposed workers or workers who have returned to work after a rest period of several days. Thirst and a metallic taste usually precede the onset of chills, fever, cough, sweating, myalgias, headache, weakness, dyspnea, and nausea. Temperatures up to 39°C may occur 10 to 12 hours after exposure. Expiratory wheezes and metal fume fever are self-limited syndromes, however metals such as mercury and cadmium may produce tracheobronchitis and an ARDS.

LABORATORY

Analytic Methods

There is no analytic method to determine the presence of this entity.

Blood Levels

No blood levels correlate with the diagnosis or prognosis of metal fume fever. Mildly elevated urine levels of heavy metals may occur but are not unequivocally present and do not correlate with clinical effects.

TREATMENT

Gut Decontamination

These methods do not aid in the decontamination of metal fumes.

Elimination Enhancement

These methods do not aid in the elimination of metal fumes or their effects.

Supportive Measures

- The general approach to treatment is recognition of the disease, supportive care, and prevention of exposure. Seriously symptomatic patients should receive chest x-rays, have arterial blood gases determined, and be observed for the development of hemorrhagic tracheobronchitis and pulmonary edema. Chest x-rays usually are normal but may show peribronchiolar cuffing and hazy infiltrates. Rarely, pulmonary edema appears.
- Some metals are directly toxic to lung parenchyma, and differentiation between the initial onset of benign metal fume fever and more serious heavy metal pneumonitis occasionally is difficult.
- A leukocytosis, which may reach 18 to 20,000 WBC / mm^3, can persist for a day after the symptoms subside.
- Pulmonary function tests may indicate reduced lung volumes, small airway obstruction, and decreased CO diffusing capacity but these abnormalities resolve after several months.

Questions—Metal Fume Fever

1. Metals known to cause metal fume fever include all of the following, except

A. Antimony, aluminum, arsenic
B. Barium, boron, beryllium
C. Cadmium, cobalt, copper
D. Magnesium, manganese, mercury
E. Selenium, silver, zinc

2. Metal fume fever

A. Is associated with leukocytosis
B. May be associated with thirst and a metallic taste
C. Commonly occurs in brass foundries and zinc smelters
D. All of the above
E. A and C

Isocyanates

The isocyanates, of which toluene diisocyanate is the most common, are widely used in the production of polyurethane products including plastics, urethane foam, adhesives, and fiber manufacturing. Fires that consume upholstered furniture and thermal insulation often produce isocyanates. Diisocyanates are liquids and include toluene diisocyanate (TDI), methylene bisphenyl isocyanate (MDI), hexamethylene diisocyanate (HDI), and naphthalene diisocyanate (NDI).

The isocyanates are highly reactive chemical compounds. These compounds are strong mucous membrane irritants and pulmonary sensitizers. Methyl isocyanate is a highly reactive chemical intermediate that was used at the Bhopal pesticide manufacturing plant in India, and was responsible for 2,000 deaths. The most common serious side effects of the methyl isocyanate exposure at Bhopal were pulmonary edema and corneal ulceration. Six thousand persons were injured severely with symptoms of respiratory, central nervous system, and circulatory system distress. Approximately 10,000 persons had severe respiratory tract symptoms, but were otherwise unaffected.

PATHOPHYSIOLOGY

These compounds are potent pulmonary sensitizers that cause bronchospasm, even in patients without prior airway hyperreactivity. Diisocyanate compounds act either as inducers of nonspecific bronchial hyperreactivity or as direct pharmacologic agonists. Elevated humoral antibodies have been detected in sensitized workers, but cell-mediated immunity also may produce hypersensitivity reactions. At high doses, toluene diisocyanate may act directly on bronchial mucosa by interfering with cholinergic and adrenergic mechanisms.

CLINICAL PRESENTATIONS

Clinical signs of isocyanate exposure involve mucosal irritation of the respiratory and gastrointestinal tracts. Conjunctival irritation, skin inflammation, nausea, vomiting, and abdominal pain may occur soon after exposure.

Neurologic Effects

Neurologic symptoms include headache, euphoria, ataxia, anxiety, depression, and paranoia that may persist for several weeks. Persistent memory deficits, personality changes, irritability, and depression have been reported after severe exposures to toluene diisocyanate.

Ophthalmologic Effects

Lacrimation, photophobia, profuse lid edema, and superficial corneal abrasions were the most common ophthalmologic effects at Bhopal. No case of blindness or irreversible ocular damage was noted on follow-up examination. Follow-up 3 years after exposure to methyl isocyanate at Bhopal showed an excess of eye irritation, eyelid infection, an apparent increase in cataracts, and a decrease in visual acuity among the exposed.

Pulmonary Effects

Pulmonary symptoms include cough, burning, substernal pain, dyspnea, choking sensation, sputum production, and hoarseness. Bronchospasm manifested by wheezing, rhonchi, dyspnea, and cough may be present. The issue of whether or not diisocyanate exposure in workers causes fixed chronic obstructive pulmonary disease at levels near current federal levels remains controversial. TDI, MDI, and HDI can cause occupational asthma. Hyperreactivity usually resolves after removal from the workplace, but a small subset of sensitized diisocyanate workers may experience persistent asthma symptoms long after removal.

TOXIC DOSAGE/DEATH

TDI may produce bronchospasm in workers at concentrations as low as 1 ppb. Some cross-reactivity occurs between TDI, HDI, and MDI. Odor detection of toluene diisocyanate occurs between 0.02 and 0.05 ppm and symptoms of mucosal irritation begin to appear between 0.05 and 0.1 ppm. All workers develop eye, nose, and throat irritation at 0.5 ppm. Sensitized individuals may manifest symptoms at levels as low as 0.02 ppm. The current US standard is 0.02 ppm as a ceiling value. No changes occurred in pulmonary function tests of workers chronically exposed to levels less than 0.001 ppm.

Exposure experience to methyl isocyanate prior to Bhopal was rare. No effects probably occur below 0.4 ppm, but levels over 21 ppm cause severe irritation. The recognized exposure limit is the same for toluene diisocyanate (0.02 ppm).

DRUG INTERACTIONS

No available data, however other bronchospastic agents such as dusts may conceivably add to the respiratory ailments induced by the isocyanates.

PREGNANCY/LACTATION

Methyl isocyanate is a known fetotoxin.

LABORATORY

Analytic Methods

In the absence of renewed exposure, radioallergosorbent tests (RASTs) may not distinguish sensitive from nonsensitized workers.

Blood Levels

It is possible to monitor exposure to toluene diisocyanate by monitoring plasma concentration of 2,2,4- and 2,6-toluenediamine.

TREATMENT

Gut Decontamination

Few medical data are available to guide gut decontamination. Activated charcoal (1 g/kg) and cathartic may be useful for ingestions, however their efficacy has not been studied formally.

Elimination Enhancement

These methods have not been studied following isocyanate exposures.

Supportive Measures

- Noncardiogenic pulmonary edema and bronchospasm are the most immediate serious clinical consequences of isocyanate exposure. Markedly symptomatic patients should receive oxygen, ventilatory support, and an intravenous line.
- Treatment for asthma includes inhaled sympathomimetics, parenteral sympathomimetics such as epinephrine, and steroids.
- Copiously irrigate contaminated skin and eyes with saline. Mydriatics, systemic analgesics, and topical antibiotics may be used for corneal abrasions.
- There is no effective therapy for sensitized workers except abstinence from exposure to isocyanates.

Questions—Isocyanates

1. Which of the following concerning isocyanates is false?
A. Isocyanates are used widely in the production of polyurethane products.
B. Fires that consume modern upholstered furniture and thermal insulation often produce isocyanates.
C. Isocyanates are highly reactive chemical compounds.
D. These compounds are potent pulmonary sensitizers.
E. Bronchorrhea may occur after significant exposures.

2. ______ is a highly reactive chemical intermediate that was used at the Bhopal pesticide manufacturing plant in India, and was responsible for 2,000 deaths.
A. Methyl isocyanate
B. Toluene diisocyanate
C. Methylene bisphenyl isocyanate
D. Hexamethylene diisocyanate
E. Naphthalene diisocyanate

3. The most common serious side effects after the exposure at Bhopal were
A. Refractory seizures and hemodynamic collapse
B. Coma and dehydration
C. Pulmonary edema and corneal ulceration
D. Desquamative rash and superinfection
E. Burns and dehydration

4. The most immediate serious clinical consequence of isocyanate exposure in the workplace is
A. Rash
B. Gastrointestinal distress
C. Fever
D. Neuropathy
E. Bronchospasm

Lacrimators

Riot control agents are aerosol-dispersed chemicals that produce eye, nose, mouth, skin, and respiratory tract irritation. Most of these symptoms resolve by 30 minutes postexposure, however ocular and mucous membrane symptoms may persist for 24 hours. Three currently used agents include chloroacetophenone (CN), chlorobenzylidenemalononitrile (CS), and dibenzoxazepine (CR). In dilute concentrations, these agents cause profuse lacrimation and blepharospasm as well as cutaneous erythema and pain. Serious systemic toxicity is rare and occurs only when these agents are used in high concentrations within confined spaces.

Tear gases are used by police in crowd-control operations, by the public for personal protection, and by combat forces. Some pulmonary irritants, such as chloropicrin and cyanogen chloride also are lacrimators. Severe traumatic injury from exploding tear gas bombs, as well as lethal toxic injury, has been observed. A tear gas liquid spray made from cayenne peppers may produce serious respiratory problems.

Mace is a 1% solution of CN in a solvent propellant mixture of 4% kerosene, 5% trichloroethane, and Freon 113. A 1-second spray releases 25 mg of CN, but evaporation of the organic solvent may concentrate the mixture in the eyes and intensify damage. Classically, tear gas powder (CN) is combined with a pyrotechnic base that volatilizes and aerosolizes the compound on contact with cool air.

PATHOPHYSIOLOGY

The lacrimators are strong mucous membrane irritants and chemical activators of the lacrimal glands. Both CN and CS are alkylating agents that react with sulfhydryl groups and other nucleophilic sites. Tissue injury and necrosis probably result from the biochemical inhibition of important enzymes. Postmortem findings associated with CN include acute tracheobronchitis with necrosis of the respiratory mucosa and pseudomembrane formation, focal intra-alveolar hemorrhage, early bronchopneumonia, pulmonary edema, cerebral edema, and fatty metamorphosis of the liver.

PHARMACOKINETICS

Absorption

- CS reacts covalently with plasma proteins to form compounds that may be antigenic.

Distribution

- On contact with water, CS hydrolyzes into o-chlorobenzaldehyde and malononitrile.

Elimination

- The kidney excretes o-chlorobenzaldehyde as the metabolites o-chlorohippuric acid (major) and o-chlorobenzoic acid (minor).

CLINICAL PRESENTATIONS

Ophthalmologic Effects

These compounds produce intense blepharospasm, pain, lacrimation, conjunctival erythema, periorbital edema, and a short-duration rise in intraocular pressure. Symptoms diminish generally within 30 minutes postexposure, but the persistence of symptoms depends on the concentration and duration of exposure. Ocular injuries range from conjunctival irritation, ecchymosis, corneal edema, and loss of epithelium to necrotizing keratitis, coagulative necrosis, iridocyclitis, and deformities of the anterior chamber angle.

Pulmonary Effects

Rhinorrhea, nasal irritation and congestion, bronchorrhea, sore throat, cough, sneezing, unpleasant taste, and burning of the mouth occur immediately after exposure and rapidly resolve within minutes postexposure. Prolonged concentrated exposures can produce an acute laryngotracheobronchitis. In doses likely to occur during a riot, pulmonary function tests in human volunteers indicate no adverse effects. RADS may follow a high-level exposure to CS.

Gastrointestinal Effects

Ingestion of CS has led to abdominal cramping and diarrhea.

Dermatologic Effects

Burning and erythema may occur after exposure to lacrimators. Prolonged exposures, particularly those associated with wet clothing or the use of petroleum jelly, can cause second-degree chemical burns. CN is a skin sensitizer and may produce allergic contact dermatitis characterized by pruritus, weeping, and a papulovesicular rash within 72 hours of exposure.

TOXIC DOSAGE/DEATH

Lacrimators are relatively nontoxic except when dispersed in a confined, nonventilated space. CN is the most toxic lacrimator and has accounted for at least five deaths resulting from pulmonary injury and / or asphyxia. Readily apparent irritation occurs at 40 mg/m^3. At higher concentrations, corneal epithelial damage and chemosis develop.

CS is 10 times more potent than CN as a lacrimator, however it is less toxic. CR is the most potent lacrimator with the least systemic toxicity.

LABORATORY

Analytic Methods

Analytic methods for lacrimators include gas chromatographic-mass spectrometric identification procedures. Spectra data and a capillary gas-liquid chromatographic-mass spectrometric method that differentiate and identify CN and CS are available.

Blood Levels

Concentration determinations of these agents do not guide therapy.

TREATMENT

Gut Decontamination

These methods have not been shown useful after airborne exposures.

Elimination Enhancement

There are no data to support the use of these methods after lacrimator exposure.

Supportive Measures

- The immediate priority is removal from exposure and establishment of an airway. The development of laryngeal edema and / or spasm is a theoretical possibility. Patients with respiratory distress should receive oxygen, an evaluation of airway patency and ventilation, an intravenous line, and cardiac monitoring. Severe respiratory injuries can result from gassing in a confined space.
- Obtain arterial blood gases and chest x-rays in these patients. Bronchospasm may contribute to respiratory distress and may be treated with inhaled sympathomimetic drugs. Patients with

respiratory distress should be admitted if symptoms persist several hours. Prophylactic antibiotics and steroids probably are not effective. Humidified oxygen may provide symptomatic relief.

Decontamination

- Remove all contaminated clothing and seal it in a plastic bag.
- Medical personnel should use disposable rubber gloves when handling contaminated clothes.
- If clothing is to be washed, cold water should be used because hot water will cause any residual CS gas to vaporize.

Supportive Care

- The eyes should be examined for corneal abrasions and treated with oral analgesics, topical antibiotics (sulfacetamide), and mydriatics as needed.
- Irrigate ocular injuries with isotonic saline and remove the remaining powder with a cotton wool swab. Any remaining stromal particles should be removed with a needle tip with a slit lamp.
- A significant leukocytosis (i.e., over 20,000 WBC/mm^3) may occur after exposure to chloroacetophenone and can last for several days.
- Vesiculated skin is treated like a second-degree chemical burn.

Questions—Lacrimators

1. Mace contains
A. Chloroacetophenone (CN)
B. Chlorobenzylidenemalononitrile (CS)
C. Dibenzoxazepine (CR)
D. Pepper
E. A product found in nutmegs.

2. Chloroacetophenone is the most toxic lacrimator and has accounted for deaths resulting from pulmonary injury and/or asphyxia.
A. True
B. False

3. Which of the following is false regarding lacrimator exposures?
A. Chlorobenzylidenemalononitrile is 10 times more potent than chloroacetophenone as a lacrimator, however it is less toxic.
B. Dibenzoxazepine is the least potent lacrimator with the least systemic toxicity.
C. Ocular injuries can cause coagulative necrosis, iridocyclitis, and deformities of the anterior chamber angle.
D. Lacrimators are nontoxic except when dispersed in a confined, nonventilated space.
E. In doses likely to occur during a riot, pulmonary function tests in human volunteers indicate no adverse effects.

FLUOROCARBONS

Fluorocarbons are halogenated hydrocarbons. Fluorocarbons that contain chlorine are called chlorofluorocarbons (CFCs). These colorless, noncombustible liquids are used as refrigerants, propellants, degreasers, fire extinguishers, deicers, and agents for cleaning electronic equipment and preparing frozen tissues for histopathology.

Freon is the trade name given to fluoroalkanes widely used as propellants and refrigerants. The two most common fluoroalkanes are dichlorodifluoromethane (Freon 12) and trichloromonofluoromethane (Freon 11). Fluoroalkenes such as tetrafluoroethylene and chlorotrifluoroethylene are polymerized easily by free radical catalysis into nonstick surfaces such as Teflon®. These compounds have relatively low systemic toxicity compared with their chlorinated hydrocarbon counterparts.

Of the more than 36 commercially available fluorocarbons, at least 10 are produced and used in significant quantities. One of these, trichlorotrifluoroethane, is more commonly known as CFC-113 or Freon 113. Freon 113 was used in the industrial setting as a refrigerant, degreaser, and dry-cleaning solvent. CFCs are being phased out to protect the ozone layer. December 31, 1995, was the last day CFCs could be manufactured for use in the Unite States, but export has continued.

Fluorocarbons may be deposited on cigarettes from the air or from a worker's fingers. As the cigarette is smoked, fluorocarbons are burned, or pyrolyzed, and the products of decomposition inhaled with the cigarette smoke. The most common products of such pyrolysis include inorganic fluorides, hydrogen fluoride, carbonyl fluoride, and perfluropropane.

PATHOPHYSIOLOGY

Pyrolysis of fluorocarbon material has been associated with an influenzalike illness (polymer fume fever) and fatal respiratory illnesses in pet birds. Concern over the ability of fluorocarbons to interact with ozone and to deplete the ultraviolet radiation shield of the atmosphere led to restriction of the use of fluorocarbon propellants in the United States. Although fluorocarbons cause cardiac sensitization in certain animal species, rapid elimination prevents the development of cardiotoxic concentrations from aerosol bronchodilator use except at exceedingly high doses.

PHARMACOKINETICS

Absorption

- Absorption of fluorocarbons is much lower after oral ingestion than after inhalation.

Distribution

- The distribution half-life of the common fluorocarbons (e.g., Freon 11 and 12) averages 13 to 14 seconds.
- The lungs generally have the highest fluorocarbon concentrations on autopsy.

Elimination

- The elimination half-life (1.5 hours) is longer than the distribution half-life because of slower release from fat stores.

CLINICAL PRESENTATIONS

Cardiovascular Effects

High concentrations of Freon 11 can cause bradycardia and asystole in dogs. These concentrations are exceeded when plastic bags are filled with Freon propellants in an effort to abuse them. Freon 12, unlike Freon 11, does not appear to suppress spontaneous pacemaker activity. Several cases of sudden death have occurred after the intentional abuse of aerosols containing Freon. Accidental discharge of Freon 113 and Freon 22 has resulted in several deaths, probably from dysrhythmias and asphyxia.

Pulmonary Effects

Perfluoroisobutylene is the most toxic fluoroalkene known, with a toxicity greater than that of phosgene. The lungs are the primary target organs. Fluoroalkanes with mild to moderate pulmonary toxicity include tetrafluoroethylene, hexafluoropropylene, chlorotrifluoroethylene, and dichlorohexafluorobutene. Freons 11 and 12 probably do not cause pulmonary toxicity.

Neurologic Effects

Lightheadedness and altered consciousness may occur at levels above 5% to 15%. A study of refrigerator repairmen intermittently exposed to fluorocarbons revealed an increased incidence of palpitations and lightheadedness compared with a control group. There was no detectable neurologic impairment or electroneurophysiologic abnormality observed.

TOXIC DOSAGE/DEATH

Fatalities attributed to cardiac arrhythmia, asphyxiation, or both have followed occupational exposure to CFC-113 in confined spaces. At least three individuals are known to have suffered from rapid fatal cardiac arrest when they were exposed to a compartment flooded with this gas. Deaths also have been reported following inhalation of Freon 22.

Halon-1301 another fluorocarbon is a commonly used fire extinguisher. Changes in cognitive, psychomotor, and perceptual performance have been reported with exposures between 4% and 7%. At concentrations over 7%, headache, dizziness, disorientation, and coma may occur. At higher levels, cardiac arrhythmias have been observed. Halon-1211 is another widely used extinguishing agent. Several cases of sudden death in teenagers associated with Halon-1211 abuse have been reported.

DRUG INTERACTIONS

Medications that contain ingredients such as epinephrine, norepinephrine, dopamine, isoproterenol, and other sympathomimetic agents may be of concern regarding their ability to induce catecholamine release.

LABORATORY

Analytic Methods

Methods to detect these agents are not routinely available in hospital laboratories.

Blood Levels

A 16-year-old collapsed fatally after exposure to CFC-113. The blood CFC-113 concentration was 2.3 μg/mL.

TREATMENT

Gut Decontamination

These methods have not been shown useful after airborne exposures.

Elimination Enhancement

There are no data to support the use of these methods after fluorocarbon exposures.

Supportive Measures

- Minimize skin contact and absorption. Wear chemical protective clothing such as gloves and aprons. If CFC-113 gets on the skin, promptly wash the contaminated area with soap or a mild detergent and water. Wear splash-proof safety goggles to prevent eye contact. If contact does occur, wash eyes with copious amounts of water.
- Cardiac monitoring is mandatory following significant exposures to these agents as arrhythmias may occur. Avoid epinephrine and sympathomimetics.

Questions—Fluorocarbons

1. Perfluoroisobutylene, the most toxic fluoroalkane known, primarily targets the
A. Liver
B. Upper respiratory tract
C. Lungs
D. Kidney
E. Central nervous system

2. All of the following are true regarding chlorofluorocarbons except
A. They are used as refrigerants and in fire extinguishers
B. They can be polymerized into Teflon®
C. These compounds have relatively low systemic toxicity compared with their chlorinated hydrocarbon counterparts
D. They are being phased out to protect the ozone layer
E. December 31, 1995, was the last day CFCs could be manufactured for use in the United States, but export to foreign countries has continued.

3. Polymer fume fever
A. Has been associated with pyrolysis of fluorocarbon material
B. Is an influenzalike illness
C. Can cause fatalities in pet birds
D. All of the above
E. A and B

4. Which of the following is false?
A. Freon is the trade name given to fluoroalkanes widely used as propellants and refrigerants.
B. The two most common fluoroalkanes are dichlorodifluoromethane (Freon 13) and trichloromonofluoromethane (Freon 14).
C. Fluoroalkenes such as tetrafluoroethylene and chlorotrifluoroethylene are polymerized easily by free radical catalysis into nonstick surfaces
D. A and B
E. B and C

OZONE

Ozone is a naturally occurring, bluish gas that is formed by the action of ultraviolet light on molecular oxygen. The stratosphere contains over 10 ppm and the troposphere, 1 ppm. Ozone provides protection from ultraviolet radiation. It is a potent oxidizing agent that decomposes to oxygen, particularly in the presence of organic material, water vapor, and metals.

Occupational exposures include electric arc welding, mercury vapor lamps, office photocopy machines, water purification, and bleaching. Commercial aircraft flying over 32,000 feet may exceed the recommended occupational ozone exposure limit. Electric storms, high-voltage electrical equipment, and x-ray generators produce ozone. In photochemical smog, ozone represents over 90% of oxidants with high photochemical reactivity, whereas nitrogen dioxide is more common in low-photochemical smog.

Pathophysiology

Ozone has a pungent odor, is poorly water soluble, and is detectable at concentrations below 0.1 ppm. Ozone is more reactive and water soluble than nitrogen dioxide. Ozone primarily causes upper respiratory tract problems, whereas nitrogen dioxide primarily causes lower respiratory tract problems. Ozone is a strong irritant of the eyes, mucous membranes, and upper respiratory tract and exposure to high concentrations of ozone produces damage to type I cells and replacement by metaplastic cuboidal epithelium.

Clinical Presentations

Mild-to-moderate exposure produces primarily upper respiratory tract symptoms and eye irritation (i.e., lacrimation, burning of eyes and throat, nonproductive cough, headache, substernal soreness, bronchial irritation, acrid taste and smell). More severe exposures, such as those seen in industrial settings, may produce significant respiratory distress with dyspnea, cyanosis, and pulmonary edema. Symptoms typically resolve over 1 to 2 weeks, although fatigue, headache, and exertional dyspnea may persist for several months. Chronic low-dose exposure (below 0.5 ppm) probably does not cause pulmonary changes in healthy, nonsmoking adults, although ozone may exacerbate small airway impairment in smokers.

Toxic Dosage/Death

Exposure to high doses (0.6 ppm over several hours) produces airway hyperreactivity unrelated to prior sensitization. Repeated exposure to ozone significantly reduces pulmonary reactivity to a given ozone level.

Laboratory

ANALYTIC METHODS
Methods to detect these agents routinely are not available in hospital laboratories.

BLOOD LEVELS
Following ozone levels does not guide management.

Treatment

GUT DECONTAMINATION
These methods have not been shown useful after airborne exposures.

ELIMINATION ENHANCEMENT
There are no data to support the use of these methods after ozone exposures.

SUPPORTIVE MEASURES
- Treatment is supportive, similar to that for smoke inhalation and chlorine.
- Chest x-rays may show increased bronchovascular markings and bilateral lung densities.

Questions—Ozone

1. **Exposures to ozone include**
   A. Electric arc welding
   B. Office photocopy machines
   C. Bleaching
   D. X-ray generators
   E. All of the above
2. **Ozone causes all of the following, except**
   A. Lower respiratory tract problems
   B. Strong irritation of the eyes
   C. Symptoms that typically resolve over 1 to 2 weeks
   D. Damage to type I cells and replacement by metaplastic cuboidal epithelium
   E. Cyanosis and pulmonary edema in severe cases
3. **Treatment for ozone toxicity is essentially limited to supportive measures.**
   A. True
   B. False

SMOKE INHALATION AND FIRE TOXICOLOGY

More than 2 million Americans sustain burn injuries each year requiring thousands of hospitalizations and many deaths. Most early deaths result from smoke inhalation rather than from direct flame contact. Synthetic materials such as polyurethane and polyvinyl chloride increase smoke toxicity. The most common cause of smoke inhalation-related deaths, by far, is carbon monoxide, a systemic toxin with no irritant properties. Respiratory irritants produce a chemical tracheobronchitis that contributes to thermal injuries of the upper respiratory tract and chemically mediated alveolar injury in the lower respiratory tract. The exact contribution of each irritant in smoke-induced respiratory tract damage is difficult to quantitate in a fire setting.

Combustion

Thermal degradation of organic material in an oxygen-rich environment.

Dusts

Small material, identical to native compound, that is dispersed in air.

Fume

Fumes consist of oxidized solid particles that are derived from a parent material during combustion, which may condense to form large particles ranging from 0.02 to 0.25 μm.

Gas

A formless fluid that completely occupies a given space.

Pyrolysis

Thermal degradation of organic material in an oxygen-poor environment.

Smoke

Smoke is the volatilized product of combustion, which varies significantly depending on the materials involved, the temperature, and the amount of oxygen available.

Vapor

Gaseous phase of volatile liquid.

Pathophysiology

Combustion products depend on the amount of oxygen present in the fire environment. Rarely is a single product produced during a fire, and the products released are difficult to predict. Factors contributing to the production of inhalation injury in the fire setting are varied.

AMOUNTS

Total amount of combustion products absorbed acutely or chronically will affect injury patterns.

GAS TYPES

Specific gases, such as hydrogen cyanide, are more toxic than others. Dilution and pyrolysis are modulated by the relative amounts of oxygen present. The acidity or alkalinity of the gases involved also is a factor.

PARTICLE SIZE

Smoke particles act as vehicles to carry absorbed toxins, such as hydrogen chloride, into the respiratory tract and thus help determine where injury occurs. Particles measuring between 5 and 30 μm affect the nasopharyngeal region, whereas 1 to 5 μm particles affect the large airways of the trachea, bronchi, and bronchioles. Toxin-laden particles smaller than 1 μm reach the alveoli.

PREEXISTING DISEASE

Preexisting diseases, such as cardiopulmonary illnesses, may contribute to inhalational injury.

PROTECTIVE REFLEXES

The effectiveness of protective reflexes, such as coughing, and/or laryngospasm, modulates the potential of inhalational injury. Olfactory fatigue such as that seen in hydrogen sulfide poisoning increases toxic exposure. Obtundation and coma, characterized by loss of cough reflex and laryngospasm, allow deeper penetration of noxious gases.

RESPIRATORY RATE

High-minute volumes, such as those seen in firefighters, increase the volume of inhaled noxious gases.

SOLUBILITY

Ammonia, sulfur dioxide, chlorine gas, nitrogen oxides, and phosgene combine with water to form damaging corrosives. Aldehydes, especially acrolein, produce both mucosal irritation and pulmonary edema. The water solubility of the inhalant and the dose largely determine the anatomic site of injury. Highly soluble gases such as ammonia, formaldehyde, sulfur dioxide, and hydrogen chloride cause immediate upper airway injury. Poorly soluble gases such as nitrogen dioxide and phosgene produce delayed effects on the terminal bronchioles and alveoli. Chlorine gas has intermediate solubility.

TEMPERATURE

Thermal injuries cause primarily upper airway injury above the true vocal cord. Such injuries progress over the first 24 hours. Because of the high heat-absorbing capacity of the upper respiratory tract and the low heat content of hot air, thermal injury below the vocal cords is rare. An exception involves the presence of steam, which has a 4,000-times greater heat capacity than air.

Clinical Presentations

There are no uniform clinical criteria that define the diagnosis of inhalation injury. The absence of pathognomonic signs accounts for the variable incidence of smoke inhalation reported in the literature. Heavy smoke, unconsciousness at the scene, and fire in a poorly ventilated enclosure suggest the presence of smoke inhalation. The vast majority of smoke inhalation victims (90% to 95%) have dyspnea, cough, or hoarseness on arrival at the hospital. Signs include wheezing, carbonaceous sputum, perioral burns, singed nasal hair, cough, rales, rhonchi, cyanosis, tachypnea, confusion, anxiety, stridor, and hemoptysis. Upper respiratory obstruction secondary to edema may increase in the first 24 hours.

There is a poor correlation between the presence of facial burns and respiratory tract damage. Intraoral burns have a better correlation with the presence of pulmonary damage, and the presence of serious cutaneous burns and smoke inhalation indicates a poor prognosis. Carbonaceous sputum, wheezing, and hoarseness appear in less than one-half of smoke inhalation cases. Hemoptysis is rare. On short-term follow-up, single smoke inhalation exposures severe enough to cause transient hypoxemia do not produce chronic respiratory symptoms or functional respiratory impairment.

Airborne toxins involved in smoke inhalation are numerous. The following gases and chemicals may contribute in individual fires. Please see individual toxins elsewhere in this text for specifics regarding their presentations.

SIMPLE ASPHYXIANTS

These chemicals produce hypoxia by displacing oxygen from the environment. A 17% inhaled oxygen content is the safe limit for prolonged exposure. A 5% oxygen content is the minimum compatible with life. Concentrations of 7% produce stupor and memory loss, whereas 10% results in dizziness, dyspnea, and tachypnea. Asphyxiants cause no local irritation or systemic effects but rather displace oxygen. Common asphyxiants include nitrogen in mining and underwater environments, carbon dioxide from grain elevators, silos, dry ice storage and fermentation sites, and methane from organic decomposition sites and mine tunnels. Other combustible fuels such as pentane, hexane, heptane, butane, ethane, and propane can be asphyxiants as well.

SYSTEMIC ASPHYXIANTS

These chemicals produce tissue hypoxia by interfering with oxygen transport or delivery. These include CO, which results from the incomplete combustion of hydrocarbons or the combustion of wood, paper, and cotton. This is the major toxic gas involved in most fires. Cyanide gases are released in fires involving plastics, insecticides, and polyurethanes in industrial settings. Nitriles also result when plastics are burned. Hydrogen sulfide is found in sewers, oil storage tanks, and coal mines. The combustion of nitrite products may produce methemoglobinemia.

RESPIRATORY IRRITANTS

These compounds can produce hypoxia by causing a chemical tracheobronchitis, pulmonary edema, upper airway obstruction, or pneumonia. The anatomic level of injury depends on the ability of the irritant to penetrate the respiratory tract, the duration of exposure, and water solubility. Examples of respiratory irritants include ammonia, acrolein, aldehydes, hydrogen halides, acetic acid, nitrogen oxides, sulfur dioxide, chlorine gas, phosgene, and formaldehyde.

SMOOTH-MUSCLE IRRITANTS

Many organic and chemical substances in the work environment are capable of producing reversible obstructive disease and bronchospasm by immunological and nonimmunological mechanisms. In the fire setting, sulfur dioxide and isocyanates are potent bronchoconstrictors. Sensitized individuals may display marked bronchial hyperreactivity from smoke inhalation.

SYSTEMIC TOXINS

Heavy metals released in fires, such as arsine and stibine gas, lead, mercury, and cadmium, produce toxic effects when inhaled. Metal fume fever, an acute, self-limited, flulike illness resulting from the inhalation of metal oxide fumes, may follow fires as well.

Toxic Dosage/Death

See Carbon Monoxide and Cyanide, above, regarding toxic levels of these common poisons involved in fires.

Laboratory

ANALYTIC METHODS

Xenon 133 radioisotope lung scan is a sensitive early indicator of parenchymal injury and often is positive before the chest x-ray shows abnormalities. The presence of preexisting pulmonary disease, such as COPD, bronchiolectasis, or asthma, reduces sensitivity and specificity. This method defines anatomic rather than physiological abnormality.

Maximum expiratory flow volume (MEFV) and FEV1 are reduced significantly in smoke inhalation patients and in some firefighters immediately after routine firefighting. The prognostic value of FEV1 parameters after smoke inhalation has not been established.

BLOOD LEVELS

See Carbon Monoxide and Cyanide, above, regarding toxic levels of these agents.

Treatment

- Initial attention should focus on safely removing the patient from the hostile environment, establishing an adequate airway, and assisting ventilation as necessary. Early elective nasotracheal intubation (preferably over a bronchoscope) is preferred to crash oral intubation. Tracheostomy should be avoided unless no alternative exists.
- Smoke inhalation victims should receive 100% oxygen unless contraindicated by the presence of severe chronic lung disease.
- Always consider the potential presence of toxins that impair oxygen delivery and utilization such as CO, cyanide, hydrogen sulfide, and methemoglobinemia and give the appropriate antidote when applicable.
- An intravenous line and cardiac monitoring should be established for all moderate or severe inhalation victims. Judicious fluid replacement should follow measurements of blood pressure, urine output, and hemodynamic variables to minimize the development of pulmonary edema.
- Victims exposed to cutaneous toxins (e.g., pesticides) should have clothes removed and washed thoroughly at the accident scene.
- Watch continuously in the first 24 hours for signs of increasing upper airway obstruction. Continuous water bath humidification is preferred to ultrasonic nebulization to better mobilize secretions and reduce deep seeding of bacteria.
- Significantly symptomatic inhalation injuries require arterial blood gases, chest x-ray, ECG, bedside spirometry (FEV1/FVC), and laryngoscopy if upper airway edema is suspected.

FIBEROPTIC BRONCHOSCOPY

- This safe, accurate method allows direct visualization of the airway in patients over 5 years of age. The technique reveals laryngeal, tracheal, and bronchial erythema, edema, necrosis, and soot-laden particles. An additional advantage is the simultaneous placement of a nasotracheal tube and suctioning of the airway.
- This method shows anatomic but not physiological defects, because 25% to 50% of patients with positive findings do not develop clinically significant respiratory complications.

RESPIRATORY ISSUES

- Follow physical signs and arterial blood gases for signs of increasing hypoxemia. A PaO_2 less than 75 mm Hg in well-hydrated, mild, or moderate burn patients suggests inhalation injury. The alveolar-arterial oxygen gradient is an early indication of parenchymal damage, although preexisting pulmonary disease complicates its use.
- Vigorous pulmonary toilet manifested by deep breathing exercises, coughing, and postural drainage is encouraged.
- Watch for pneumonia, which develops as a late complication in up to 15% of smoke inhalation patients. Prophylactic use of antibiotics is unnecessary in this situation and may predispose to the development of antibiotic-resistant strains.
- Most studies indicate that steroids are ineffective. Nonsoluble gases such as phosgene and nitrogen dioxide produce delayed pulmonary edema up to 24 to 36 hours after exposure.
- Bronchospasm and wheezing may respond to β-adrenergic drugs. Do not use epinephrine to treat hydrocarbon inhalation because of enhanced sensitivity to catecholamines. In the setting of most smoke inhalations, epinephrine and terbutaline have been used without complications.
- Progressive hypoxia resulting from pulmonary edema may require continuous positive airway pressure (CPAP), positive-end expiratory pressure (PEEP), and/or mechanical ventilation.

RADIOLOGIC FINDINGS

- Initially, the chest x-ray may be normal, but in serious exposures, changes usually develop within 48 hours. Radiographic abnormalities presenting more than 48 hours after injury are produced by complications of injury (e.g., pneumonia) or treatment.
- The majority of positive radiographs show alveolar and interstitial edema.
- The chest x-ray is not a highly sensitive initial test for smoke inhalation.

Antidotes

See Carbon Monoxide section regarding the use of HBO and Cyanide Poisoning section regarding cyanide antidotes.

Questions—Smoke Inhalation and Fire Toxicology

1. The most common cause of smoke-related deaths is

A. Tracheobronchitis
B. Carbon monoxide
C. Direct alveolar injury by respiratory irritants
D. Direct burn to the oral mucosa
E. None of the above

2. Which of the following is incorrectly defined?

A. Combustion is the thermal degradation of organic material in an oxygen-rich environment.
B. Dusts are the small materials, identical to native compound, that are dispersed in air.

C. Fumes are the formless fluids that completely occupy a given space.
D. Pyrolysis is the thermal degradation of organic material in an oxygen-poor environment.
E. Vapor is the gaseous phase of volatile liquid.

3. There is a poor correlation between the presence of facial burns and respiratory tract damage.
A. True
B. False

4. The minimum percentage oxygen content compatible with life is
A. 1%
B. 5%
C. 10%
D. 15%
E. 21%

Answers

Introduction to Airborne Toxins
1. E 2. C

Indoor Air Pollution
1. E 2. A 3. C 4. A

Outdoor Air Pollution
1. C 2. A 3. D

Carbon Dioxide
1. D

Carbon Disulfide
1. E 2. D 3. D 4. C

Carbon Monoxide
1. B 2. C 3. D 4. C 5. C 6. D
7. D 8. C

Cyanide and Nitriles Poisoning
1. E 2. A 3. E 4. A 5. A 6. B

Hydrogen Sulfide
1. D 2. A

Inhalant Abuse
1. A 2. D 3. B 4. E 5. E 6. B

Introduction to Occupational Lung Disease
1. B 2. C 3. D

Asthma, Bronchitis and Reactive Airways Dysfunction Syndrome
1. D 2. D 3. B 4. A

Hypersensitivity Pneumonitis
1. B 2. B 3. A

Introduction to Pneumoconioses
1. D 2. E

Silicosis
1. B 2. E 3. A

Asbestos-Related Disease
1. B 2. E 3. D

Byssinosis
1. C 2. A

Ammonia
1. A 2. C 3. B 4. C

Sulfur Dioxide
1. B 2. C

Nitrogen Oxides
1. A 2. B 3. B 4. C

Phosgene
1. B 2. D 3. C

Chlorine
1. C 2. C 3. E 4. E

Metal Fume Fever
1. B 2. D

Isocyanates
1. E 2. A 3. C 4. E

Lacrimators
1. A 2. A 3. B

Fluorocarbons
1. C 2. C 3. D 4. B

Ozone
1. E 2. A 3. A

Smoke Inhalation and Fire Toxicology
1. B 2. C 3. A 4. B

SELECTED READINGS

Introduction to Airborne Toxins

1. Sangster B, Meulenbelt J. Acute pulmonary intoxications. Overview and practical guidelines. Netherlands J Med 1988;33:91–100.
2. Smith AG. Toxicology of the lung. Hum Exper Toxicol 1993;12:415–416. Wheeldon EB. Mechanism of lung toxicity. Proc Br Toxicol Soc, September 1992. Hum Exper Toxicol 1993;12:419.

Indoor Air Pollution

1. Angle C. Indoor air pollutants. Adv Pediatr 1988;35:239–280.
2. Brandt-Rauf PW, Andrews LR, Schwarz-Miles J. Sick hospital syndrome. J Occup Med 1991;33:737–739.
3. Samet JM, Marbury MC, Spengler JD. Health effects and sources of indoor air pollution. Part I. Am Rev Respir Dis 1987;136:1486–1508.
4. Samet JM, Marbury MC, Spengler JD. Health effects and sources of indoor air pollution. Part II. Am Rev Respir Dis 1988;137:221–242.
5. Sim MR, Abramson MJ. Indoor air quality and sick buildings. Med J Aust 1991;155:651–52.

Outdoor Air Pollution

1. Abelson PH. Air pollution and acid rain. Science 1985;230:617.
2. De Nevers N. Community air pollution. In: Rom WN, ed. Environmental and occupational medicine. Boston: Little, Brown, 1983, pp. 797–810.
3. Goldstein E, Hackney JD, Rokaw SN. Photochemical air pollution. Part 1. West J Med 1985;142:369–376.
4. Ozone depletion quickens. Lancet 1991;1:1132–1133 (editorial).

Carbon Dioxide

1. Baxter PJ, Kapila M, Mfonfu D. Lake Nyos disaster, Cameroon, 1986: the medical effects of large scale emission of carbon dioxide. Br Med J 1989;298:1437–1441.
2. Johnston RF. The syndrome of carbon dioxide intoxication. Its etiology, diagnosis and treatment. Univ Mich Med Bull 1959;25:280–292.

Carbon Disulfide

1. Corsi A, Maestrelli P, Picotti G et al. Chronic peripheral neuropathy in workers with previous exposure to carbon disulfide. Br J Ind Med 1983;40:209–211.
2. Davidon M, Feinleib M. Carbon disulfide poisoning: A review. Am Heart J 1972;83:100–114.

Carbon Monoxide

1. Chiulli DA, Rivers EP, Kristal S, Smithline HA, Blake H, Reiser E et al. Metabolic abnormalities in patients with severe carbon monoxide poisoning: Insights into pathophysiology. Ann Emerg Med 1992;22:180.
2. Ernst A, Zibrak JD. Carbon monoxide poisoning. NEJM 1998;339(22):1603–1607.
3. Gordon K III. Pulse oximetry in emergency medicine. West J Med 1989;151:67.
4. Grim PS, Gottlieb LJ, Boddie A, Batson E. Hyperbaric oxygen therapy. JAMA 1990;263:2216–2220.
5. Hamilton-Farrell MR, Hanson GC. Hyperbaric oxygen for carbon monoxide poisoning. Lancet 1990;335:550.
6. Krenzelok EP, Full R, Roth R. Carbon monoxide. The silent killer with an audible solution. Clin Toxicol 1995;33:475–486 (abstract 132).
7. Meyers RAM. Carbon monoxide poisoning. J Emerg Med 1984;1:245–248.
8. Tomaszewski CA et al. Use of hyperbaric oxygen in toxicology. Emergency Medicine Clinics of North America 1994;12(2):437–459.

Cyanide And Nitriles Poisoning

1. Graham DL, Laman D, Theodore J et al. Acute cyanide poisoning complicated by lactic acidosis and pulmonary edema. Arch Intern Med 1977;137:1051–1055.
2. Kirk MK, Voorhees SL, Kulig R, Rumack BH. Cyanide leverls after acetonitrile exposure. An in-vitro study. Ann Emerg Med 1990;19:628.
3. Turchen SG, Managuera AS. Severe cyanide poisoning following suicidal ingestion of acetonitrile. Vet Hum Toxicol 1989;31:351.
4. Turchen SG, Manoguerra AS, Whitney C. Severe cyanide poisoning from the ingestion of an acetonitrile-containing cosmetic. Am J Emerg Med 1991;9: 264–267.
5. Vogel SN, Sultan TR. Cyanide poisoning. Clin Toxicol 1981;18:367–83.
6. Way JL. Cyanide intoxication and its mechanism of antagonism. Annu Rev Pharmacol Toxicol 1984;24:451–481.

Hydrogen Sulfide

1. Beauchamp RO Jr, Bus JS, Popp JA et al. A critical review of the literature on hydrogen sulfide toxicity. CRC Crit Rev Toxicol 1984;13:25–97.
2. Burnett WW, King EG, Grace M et al. Hydrogen sulfide poisoning: review of 5 years experience. CMA J 1977;117:1277–1280.
3. Marcus SM. Hydrogen sulfide. Clin Toxicol Rev 1983;5(4):1–2.

Inhalant Abuse

1. Done AK. Sniffing, bagging and huffing. Emerg Med 1979; 9(7):187–195.
2. Flanagan RJ et al. Clinical toxicology of volatile substances. Drug Safety 1990; 5:359–383.
3. Miller NS, Gold MS. Organic solvents and aerosols. An overview of abuse and dependence. Ann Clin Psych 1990;2:85–92.
4. Streicher HZ, Gabow PA, Moss AH, et al: Syndrome of toluene sniffing in adults. Ann Intern Med 1981;94:758–762.
5. Troutman WG. Additional deaths associated with the intentional inhalation of typewriter correction fluid. Vet Hum Toxicol 1987;29:479.
6. Watson JM. Solvent abuse: Presentation and clinical diagnosis. Hum Toxicol 1982;1:249–56.

Occupational Lung Disease

1. Anttila S, Kajalainen A, Taikino-aho O, Kyrronen P, Vainio H. Lung cancer in the lower lobe is associated with pulmonary asbestos fiber count and fiber size. Environ Health Perspect 1993;101:166–170.
2. Brooks SM, Weiss MA, Bernstein IL. Reactive airways dysfunction syndrome (RADS). Persistent asthma syndrome after high level irritant exposures. Chest 1985;88:376–384.
3. Chan-Yeung M, Malo J-C. Occupational asthma. N Engl J Med 1995;333: 107–112.
4. Malmberg P, Rask-Anderson A. Organic dust toxic syndrome. Semin Respir Med 1993;14:38–48.
5. Seaton A. Management of the patient with occupational lung disease. Thorax 1994;49:627–628.
6. Silicosis and Silicate Disease Committee. Diseases associated with exposure to silica and nonfibrous silicate minerals. Arch Pathol Lab Med 1988;112:673–720.

Respiratory Tract Irritants

1. Beswick FW. Chemical agents used in riot control and warfare. Hum Toxicol 1983;2:247–256.
2. Blanc PD. Chlorine gas inhalation. AACT Update 1994;7(4):1–2.
3. Elsayed NM. Toxicity of nitrogen dioxide: an introduction. Toxicology 1994; 89:161–174.
4. Krenzelok E, Mrvos R. Chlorine/chloramine. Clin Toxicol 1995;355–357.
5. Lopez GP, Dean BS, Krenzelok EP. Oral exposure to ammonia inhalants. A report of 8 cases. Vet Hum Toxicol 1988;30:350.
6. Sidell FR. Civil emergencies involving chemical warfare agents: Medical considerations. In: Somani SM, ed. Chemical warfare agents. San Diego: Academic Press, 1992;pp. 341–356.

Fluorocarbons

1. Albrecht WN, Bryant CJ. Polymer-fume fever associated with smoking and use of a mold-release spray containing polytetrafluoroethylene. J Occup Med 1987;29:817–819.
2. Pierce RJ, Seale JP, Ruffin RE. Inhaled respiratory medications and the use of chlorofluorocarbons (CFCs). Med J Aust 1991;154:701–704.
3. Thompson JD, Snodgrass WR. Inflatable toys-an unusual source of Freon toxicity. Vet Hum Toxicol 1991;33:363.

Ozone

1. Lippman M. Health effects of ozone. A critical review. J Am Poll Control Assoc 1989;32:672–695.
2. Rusznak C, Devalia JL, Davies RJ. A hole in our knowledge of ozone toxicity? Allergy 1994;49:21–27.

Smoke Inhalation and Fire Toxicology

1. Becker CE. The role of cyanide in fires. Vet Hum Toxicol 1985;27:487–490.
2. Cahalane M, Demling RH. Early respiratory abnormalities from smoke inhalation. JAMA 1984;251:771–774.
3. Kulig K. Cyanide antidotes in fire toxicology. N Engl J Med 1991;325:1801–1802.
4. McGuigan MA. Smoke inhalation. Clin Toxicol Rev 1985;7(6):1–2.

ACKNOWLEDGMENTS

Thanks to Alison Deutsch, MD, Chris Keyes, MD, MPH, FACMT, and Steven Balser, MD for contributing questions in this chapter.

CHAPTER 46
Hydrocarbons

PETROLEUM DISTILLATES

INTRODUCTION

Petroleum distillates are crude oil by-products that range from petroleum ether to lubricating oils. These products contain varying amounts of saturated and unsaturated aliphatic (straight chain), and aromatic (cyclic) hydrocarbons. The exact content of a petroleum product depends on the particular process used by the manufacturer and is specific for each product.

Hydrocarbon ingestions account for about 5% of all calls reported to poison control centers in the United States. Petroleum distillates represent the most common hydrocarbon exposures. The most common calls about hydrocarbons include gasoline, lacquer thinner, pine oil, furniture polish, kerosene, and charcoal lighter fluid. Petroleum distillates with low surface tension and viscosity are serious aspiration hazards. Viscous by-products are higher-molecular-weight hydrocarbon mixtures, which are usually nontoxic. These include lubricating oil, paraffin wax, asphalt, tar, and petrolatum.

Diesel Oil

Diesel fuel, also called fuel oil, is slightly less volatile but more viscous than kerosene. These products are complex mixtures of C9 and higher hydrocarbons.

Gasoline

Gasoline is almost exclusively a fuel. Additives have included organic lead and cresyl phosphates. The benzene content of American domestic gasoline is lower (0.8–2.0%) than in that of some foreign gasolines (up to 5%). Gasoline is a mixture of C5 to C12 aliphatic hydrocarbons obtained by "cracking" heavy fractions in the boiling range 40–225°C. Appreciable amounts of aromatic hydrocarbons (e.g., xylene) may be found in commercial fuels.

Kerosene

Kerosene consists chiefly of C10 to C16 aliphatic hydrocarbons obtained in the boiling range 175–325°C. Small amounts of unsaturated (e.g., xylene) and saturated (e.g., naphthalene) aromatics appear in these products. Kerosene may be used in lighter fluid, for curing tobacco, in heating, cooling, and jet fuel.

Mineral Seal Oil

Mineral seal oil is a light petroleum fraction obtained between boiling points 200 and 370°C. This product consists mainly of saturated, higher-molecular-weight aliphatic hydrocarbons compared with gasoline and kerosene. Mineral seal oil is used in liquid furniture polish.

Petroleum Ether

Petroleum ether consists primarily of n-pentane and n-hexane, but not benzene or any true ethers.

Petroleum Naptha

Petroleum naphtha represents various mixtures of aliphatic hydrocarbons, C5 to C13, produced at boiling points between 30 and 238°C. This term may refer to any fraction more volatile than kerosene. Occasionally, the term is misused as a synonym for petroleum ether. Petroleum naphtha is used as a lighter fluid.

Rubber Solvent

Rubber solvent consists chiefly of C5 to C9 aliphatic hydrocarbons and is distilled at 38–149°C. This product is less volatile than petroleum ether.

Stoddard Solvent

A higher-boiling fraction of petroleum naphtha, Stoddard solvent (mineral spirits, white spirits) contains straight- and branched-chain hydrocarbons (C9 to C12), naphthalene, and higher aromatic hydrocarbons.

Turpentine

Turpentine is an oleoresin solvent derived from the steam distillation of pine resin. Although technically not a petroleum distillate, most summary articles include turpentine with petroleum distillates because it is an aromatic hydrocarbon with similar properties, toxic effects, and uses. It is used as a solvent for oil-based paints. See Chapter 38, Household Products.

VM and P Naptha

This product, also called varnish maker's and painter's naphtha, or mineral spirits, consists chiefly of C7 to C10 aliphatic hydrocarbons refined at 94–175°C.

Pathophysiology

The primary target organ in serious petroleum distillate ingestion is the lung, where toxicity occurs by aspiration rather than by hematogenous spread. A small amount of intratracheal petroleum distillates can produce severe pulmonary toxicity, whereas only large intragastric quantities produce central nervous system symptoms.

Aspirated hydrocarbons inhibit surfactant, leading to alveolar instability, early distal airway closure, ventilation / perfusion mismatches, and subsequent hypoxemia. Although surfactant loss probably causes the early physiologic abnormalities, direct damage to pulmonary capillaries produces pathologic findings ranging from chemical pneumonitis and hemorrhagic bronchopneumonia to gross pulmonary edema. Initially, cyanosis may result from the replacement of oxygen by vaporized hydrocarbons. Subsequent hypoxemia occurs from surfactant loss and direct alveolar injury. Bronchospasm may contribute to ventilation / perfusion defects.

Aspiration Risks

The physical properties of surface tension, viscosity, and volatility determine the risk for aspiration and therefore have the greatest effect on toxicity. Numerous hydrocarbon products may be abused by inhalation.

SURFACE TENSION

Surface tension is the cohesiveness of molecules on a liquid's surface. Reduced surface tension allows a substance to spread rapidly from the mouth to the trachea.

VISCOSITY

Viscosity, or the tendency to resist flow or change form, provides the best estimate of aspiration potential. Low viscosity allows deep penetration of hydrocarbon into the distal airways.

VOLATILITY

Volatility is the tendency of a liquid to become a gas. Highly volatile hydrocarbons displace alveolar oxygen when aspirated, leading to transient hypoxia. High-viscosity petroleum distillates (e.g., heavy lubricants, mineral oil, and liquid paraffin) produce a lipoid pneumonia that is more localized and less inflammatory than that produced by low-viscosity petroleum distillates such as kerosene or mineral seal oil.

Clinical Groups

Hydrocarbons are classified based on potential clinical effects. Group 1 agents are characterized by high aspiration potential with little central nervous system toxicity (i.e., mineral seal oil, furniture oil polishes). Group 2 agents are characterized by significant central nervous system toxicity with potential aspiration hazard (i.e., methylene chloride, carbon tetrachloride, toluene, xylene, benzene, gasoline, charcoal lighter fluid, mineral spirits, turpentine). Group 3 agents are nontoxic in usual doses ingested, but may lead to lipoid pneumonias on aspiration (i.e., lubricants, motor oil, mineral and baby oils, fuel and diesel oil, suntan lotion, petrolatum).

Clinical Presentations

Moderate fever (38–39°C) may be present after petroleum distillate ingestion, but does not correlate with other clinical symptoms. A majority of admitted patients have fever over 38°C, but three-fourths defervesce in 24 hours.

PULMONARY EFFECTS

Most low-viscosity petroleum distillates produce similar clinical effects, and deaths attributed to petroleum distillates usually result from pulmonary damage. Symptoms of respiratory distress from aspiration usually, but not always, appear within 30 minutes of exposure. Gasping, coughing, and choking are presumptive evidence of aspiration. Signs and symptoms may progress over the first 24 hours, but usually resolve by the third day. Death occurs most commonly within 24 hours.

NEUROLOGIC EFFECTS

Symptoms of central nervous system involvement may result from large intentional ingestions, toxic additives (e.g., aromatic hydrocarbons, insecticides, nitrobenzene, aniline), and aspiration-induced hypoxia. Coma is uncommon and seizures are rare as well. The most serious aspiration pneumonias present with depressed sensorium and lethargy.

GASTROINTESTINAL EFFECTS

Gastrointestinal symptoms are frequent but usually minor, especially after large ingestions. Local irritation of the mouth and pharynx occurs but diarrhea, hematemesis, and melena are rare. Gastrointestinal symptoms are slightly more common in ingestions of furniture polish than in ingestions of other petroleum distillates.

CARDIOVASCULAR EFFECTS

Myocardial involvement is rare after acute ingestions. Sudden deaths secondary to dysrhythmias can occur during solvent abuse, perhaps because of sensitization of the myocardium to endogenous catecholamines.

Toxic Dosage/Death

Although often difficult to assess, ingestion of most petroleum distillates in concentrations below 1–2 mL/kg does not cause systemic toxicity. Substantially larger quantities may be necessary to produce central nervous system depression.

In general, certain hydrocarbons have higher aspiration potential than others. An empirical measure of viscosity is reported in Saybolt Universal Seconds units (SUS). Viscosity is measured by the rate of flow of a liquid through an orifice of standard diameter. Products such as mineral seal oil with 60 SUS are considered to have moderate aspiration potential. Light mineral oil, with 75–86 SUS, is considered to have a low aspiration potential, and gasoline, with 35 SUS, has a very high aspiration potential.

Hydrocarbons may be used as vehicles for more toxic substances (e.g., camphor, pesticides, and heavy metals). These additives may be more toxic than the hydrocarbon; however, most are present at subtoxic levels after acute ingestions.

Treatment

GUT DECONTAMINATION

Gastrointestinal decontamination in accidental petroleum distillate ingestions is not recommended, because of severe aspiration hazard. All contaminated clothing should be removed, and contaminated skin areas washed with green soap and water. Ipecac-induced emesis is not recommended in general. Lavage with cuffed endotracheal protection is indicated in those patients who require decontamination, generally after intentional ingestions. Although activated charcoal does not bind petroleum distillate products and may induce vomiting, *in vitro* studies suggest that large quantities of activated charcoal may bind significant amounts of kerosene and turpentine. Activated charcoal may also be given to adsorb a toxic additive.

ELIMINATION ENHANCEMENT

There are no effective methods to enhance the elimination of these products. Extracorporeal membrane oxygenation is a pulmonary bypass procedure that has been used in adults to provide temporary treatment for reversible pulmonary and cardiac insufficiency. It provides a potentially lifesaving option when a patient fails to respond to conventional therapy for hydrocarbon aspiration.

SUPPORTIVE MEASURES

Respiratory Issues

- The primary threat to life from pure petroleum distillate ingestion is respiratory failure. Patients should be quickly evaluated for signs of respiratory distress (e.g., cyanosis, tachypnea, intercostal retractions, and obtundation) and given oxygen. Patients with inadequate tidal volumes or poor arterial blood gases should be intubated.

- A chest x-ray should be taken immediately after stabilization of breathing and circulation to document aspiration, or lack thereof. Continuous positive airway pressure or positive end-expiratory pressure and intubation may be necessary to maintain adequate oxygenation, but careful observation for the development of pneumothorax must be made during therapy.
- X-ray abnormalities usually appear within 30 minutes, but may develop 12 hours after exposure. Up to 75% of patients hospitalized for suspected hydrocarbon aspiration have chest x-ray abnormalities. Most x-ray changes reach a maximum 72 hours after exposure and clear several days later, although occasionally the changes persist for several months. X-ray changes tend to lag behind clinical improvement.
- The use of steroid therapy in mild to moderate hydrocarbon aspiration pneumonia did not improve outcome in a double blind, controlled human study.
- Present data do not support the use of prophylactic antibiotics. Antibiotics should be reserved for documented bacterial pneumonias, leukocytosis, and fever after the first 24–48 hours.
- Long-term follow-up care with baseline pulmonary function tests should be established to detect the presence of obstructive pulmonary disease, which may be seen in asymptomatic children who previously developed hydrocarbon aspiration pneumonitis.

Cardiovascular Issues

- Since arrhythmias complicate some hydrocarbon ingestions and electrocardiographic evidence of myocardial injury has been reported, intravenous lines and cardiac monitors should be established in symptomatic patients.
- Epinephrine is not recommended for treatment of bronchospasm, because of potential myocardial sensitization to catecholamines. Inhaled bronchodilators are preferred.

Laboratory

- Arterial blood gas abnormalities reflect hypoxemia resulting from ventilation/perfusion mismatching (low PaO_2, low $PaCO_2$), rather than alveolar hypoventilation (high $PaCO_2$).
- Leukocytosis is common during the first 48 hours. Intravascular hemolysis, acute renal failure, elevated hepatic aminotransferases, and coagulopathy develop rarely in gasoline aspiration.
- The urinalysis is usually normal, and renal dysfunction is uncommon.
- Rarely, after aniline or nitrobenzene exposure, methemoglobinemia may be seen.

Admission Criteria

- A number of subgroups are generally admitted. These include symptomatic children who have abnormal initial chest x-rays, patients with suicidal intent or massive ingestion, hypoxic or obtunded patients regardless of x-ray, and patients with a substantially abnormal chest x-ray.
- A number of patients should be admitted after a 6-hour observation period. These include asymptomatic children with mildly abnormal chest x-rays who develop symptoms during the observation period, asymptomatic patients who develop symptoms because of toxic additives (e.g., camphor), mildly symptomatic children who have a normal chest x-ray, but whose symptoms do not improve, and patients for whom follow-up cannot be closely established.
- A number of patients may be safely discharged after 6 hours of observation. These include asymptomatic children with a normal chest x-ray, and asymptomatic children with a mildly abnormal chest x-ray who do not develop symptoms during the observation period.

Questions—Introduction to Petroleum Distillates

1. Hydrocarbon aspiration
A. Is less toxic than ingestion
B. Does not directly damage pulmonary capillaries
C. Inhibits surfactant ultimately leading to hypoxemia
D. Must be in large amounts to produce toxicity
E. Leads to ventilation/perfusion mismatch without bronchospasm

2. The risk for aspiration and thus toxicity from hydrocarbon aspiration is determined by
A. Surface tension
B. Volatility
C. Viscosity
D. All of the above
E. None of the above

3. Respiratory signs of hydrocarbon aspiration
A. Include gasping or coughing
B. Usually do not occur within the first hour after exposure
C. May progress but usually resolve within 24 hours
D. Usually do not include choking
E. Differ from one low-viscosity petroleum distillate to another

4. All of the following systems are commonly vulnerable to a hydrocarbon exposure except
A. Pulmonary
B. Cardiac
C. Central nervous system
D. Renal
E. Gastrointestinal

5. Treatment of hydrocarbon ingestion includes
A. Ipecac-induced emesis
B. Removal of contaminated clothing
C. Dialysis
D. Steroid therapy
E. Prophylactic antibiotics

ALIPHATIC HYDROCARBONS

Aliphatic hydrocarbons are open chain, carbon-containing chemicals derived from petroleum by the cracking, distillation, and fractionation of crude oil. These simple linear carbon chains of variable carbon lengths are subdivided into three groups based on the number of hydrogen atoms. Alkanes (paraffins) are saturated hydrocarbons, alkenes (olefins) are unsaturated hydrocarbons with one or more double bonds, and alkynes (acetylenes) are unsaturated hydrocarbons that contain one or more triple bonds.

Most industrial substances are mixtures of aliphatic hydrocarbons (e.g., gasoline, kerosene, and natural gas), some of which contain substantial aromatic hydrocarbon constituents. Aliphatic hydrocarbons are used in fuels (e.g., natural gas, gasoline, kerosene), propellants, solvents, dyes, inks, plastics and

Answers to questions in shaded boxes appear at the end of the chapter.

coatings, dry cleaning agents, pesticides, and chemical intermediates.

1,3-Butadiene

This olefin compound is a colorless, flammable gas that may reach explosive concentrations without displaying adequate health-warning properties. Synonyms include vinyl ethylene, biethylene, and butadiene. The threshold odor recognition level is 1.3 parts per million (ppm). Little acute toxicity occurs from human industrial exposure, with mild mucous membrane irritation reported between 2,000–18,000 ppm and coughing, drowsiness, and fatigue at higher concentrations. Inhalation exposures between 600–8,000 ppm in animal models have produced lymphomas, reproductive cancers, and thyroid carcinoma as well as teratogenic effects in pregnant rats. Epidemiological studies of workers indicate a definite, but not statistically significant, increase in leukemia and lymphomas. The U.S. National Institute for Occupational Safety and Health (NIOSH) recommends that 1,3-butadiene be considered a potential occupational carcinogen and teratogen.

Butane

Butane is a low-molecular-weight aliphatic hydrocarbon (C4) which is a simple asphyxiant that causes toxicity by displacing oxygen. No systemic carcinogenic or teratogic effects have been directly linked to butane inhalation in the industrial setting. High doses potentially affect the lower respiratory tract. A 19-year-old man developed rapidly progressive bilateral pulmonary infiltrates radiologically consistent with hydrocarbon pneumonitis after inadvertently swallowing butane. A two-year-old girl developed seizures, hypotension, and recurrent ventricular tachycardia after unintentional exposure to a spray can containing butane, isobutane, and propane.

N-Hexane

N-Hexane, a 6-carbon alkane, is usually mixed with other aliphatic hydrocarbons and toluene when used as an industrial solvent and glue. Though it was known as a cause of peripheral neuropathies in Japan by the late 1960s, the first American neurotoxic illness from n-hexane was identified in an Ohio fabrics plant in the early 1970s. N-hexane is used as a solvent and thinner in the rubber, food, pharmaceutical, and perfume industries; as a glue in shoe, tape, and bandage manufacturing; as a cleaning agent in the textile, furniture, and leather industries; and during the chemical production of polypropylene and polyethylene.

2-Nitropropane

This compound is a colorless liquid mononitroparaffin that is commonly used as a solvent for esters, resins, waxes, gums, vinyl polymers, and dyes. Chronic exposure to concentrations above 25 ppm has produced anorexia, nausea, vomiting, headache, and diarrhea in industrial workers. Studies in animals indicate that 2-nitropropane is a central nervous system depressant and pulmonary irritant that may cause methemoglobinemia and Heinz body formation depending on concentration and duration of exposure. High acute industrial exposures in poorly ventilated areas have been associated with acute hepatic failure and death, although these exposures included a variety of solvents. NIOSH has recommended that 2-nitropropane be considered a potential human carcinogen and that its exposures be minimized.

Propane

Like butane, propane is a low-molecular-weight (C3) aliphatic hydrocarbon that is primarily a simple asphyxiant. In high concentrations, propane is a mild narcotic that depresses the sensorium. The U.S. standard is 1,000 ppm (time-weighted average). Propane has been linked to inhalation abuse and death, after it was inhaled by keeping a plastic bag over the face resulting in asphyxia. On autopsy, the highest propane concentrations were found in the brain, followed by the liver, lungs, blood, and kidney. The precise cause of death (dysrhythmia versus hypoxia) was not established.

Pathophysiology

ALIPHATIC HYDROCARBONS

Aliphatic hydrocarbons with less than four carbon atoms are gases (methane, ethane, propane, and butane). Natural gas is a mixture consisting primarily of methane with lesser amounts of ethane, propane, nitrogen, and butane. Gasoline is a complex and variable mixture of higher molecular weight, liquid hydrocarbons. Kerosene contains primarily C10 to C16 hydrocarbons as well as benzene and naphthalene. Certain types of petroleum naphtha consist primarily of aliphatic hydrocarbons, whereas others contain 0–20% aromatic and 40–80% aliphatic hydrocarbons. Coal tar naphtha is principally an aromatic hydrocarbon. Compounds with carbon chains exceeding 16 are solids at room temperature. Paraffin wax is a solid mixture of C16 hydrocarbons used for candles, wax paper, cosmetics, polish, waterproofing, and extracting processes.

N-HEXANE

Chronic neurologic toxicity is probably caused by the oxidation of n-hexane to 2,5-hexanedione. *In vitro* experiments indicate that n-hexane metabolites inhibit glutaraldehyde-3-phosphate dehydrogenase, which supplies energy for the rapid axon protein transport system. The pronounced giant axonal swelling of hexacarbon neuropathy is unique among toxic neuropathies. Orthocresol phosphate, acrylamide, carbon disulfide, and vincristine produce less swelling. Swelling occurs initially in the distal portions of the nerve fiber and then progresses proximally. Nerve fibers may degenerate or demyelinate distal to any swelling. Myelin sheaths are inappropriately thin for their axon diameter. Long, distal nerve sections are the most vulnerable.

About 15% of inhaled n-hexane vapors are absorbed. Deposition of n-hexane within the body depends on tissue lipid content. Studies in animals indicate that n-hexane tissue concentrations are highest in the brain followed by liver, kidneys, and adrenal glands. Large quantities of n-hexane are expired by the lungs after vapor exposures (50–60%). The remaining n-hexane is transformed by the cytochrome P-450 mixed-function oxidase system to 2-hexanol. Further metabolism produces 2,5-hexanedione, which is a common metabolite shared with methyl n-butyl ketone (MBK). 2,5-hexanediol, an intermediate product, is neurotoxic and may be the primary toxic agent in both n-hexane and MBK neurotoxicity.

Clinical Presentations

Low-molecular-weight aliphatic hydrocarbons (e.g., methane) are simple asphyxiants with minimal irritant or systemic effects. These agents may produce myocardial sensitization and dysrhythmias. Higher-molecular-weight aliphatic hydrocarbons are central nervous system depressants at high concentrations. Aspiration of liquid aliphatic hydrocarbons produces a severe chemical pneumonitis. Mild to moderate mucous membrane and respiratory tract irritation may occur depending on vapor concentration. Prolonged skin contact with liquid aliphatic hydrocarbons causes a contact dermatitis secondary to the drying and defatting action of these solvents.

Acute toxicity does not occur with solid aliphatic hydrocarbon compounds. Unsaturated olefins (alkenes) are more potent central nervous system depressants than corresponding saturated linear (alkane) compounds, and are moderate mucous membrane and upper respiratory irritants. Acetylene, the principal alkyne, has low central nervous system depressant effects. Impurities represent the most significant hazard of acetylene exposure. These may include phosphine as well as arsine, hydrogen sulfide, carbon disulfide, and carbon monoxide. Acetone contaminates commercial grades of acetylene, and intentional inhalation of acetylene has resulted in depressed consciousness, metabolic acidosis, hyperglycemia, ketonuria, and elevated creatinine levels.

N-HEXANE

The toxic effects of n-hexane are limited primarily to the peripheral and central nervous systems. Mild skin and mucous membrane irritation may occur at high concentrations. No human experience demonstrates pulmonary damage after inhalation. An exposure level of 100 ppm (time-weighted average) has been recommended.

Chronic exposure to n-hexane vapors produces a motor sensory polyneuropathy in industrial workers. Symptoms include fatigue, muscle weakness, distal paresthesias (upper and lower extremities), pain, and various sensory abnormalities. Usually, sensory disturbances are distal and symmetrical. Signs include muscle atrophy, decreased muscle strength and tone, diminished reflexes with foot drop in severe cases, and distal hypesthesias in the upper and lower extremities with impairment of vibration, temperature, light touch, position, pain, and pressure. Typically, symptoms develop 2–6 months after continuous heavy n-hexane exposure and commonly progress 2–3 months after cessation. Intentional abusers (e.g., glue sniffers) develop a similar symptom pattern, but motor symptoms often are more prominent.

N-Hexane is also a central nervous system depressant that commonly produces headache, nausea, and anorexia at low exposure levels. High concentrations are required to produce confusion, stupor, and coma. Peripheral neuropathies may mask central nervous system abnormalities. Central nervous system abnormalities tend to be permanent, in contrast with the peripheral nervous system in which the nerves regenerate. Spasticity may remain after motor strength and sensation improves. Changes in color vision and retinal pigmentation have been found in chronic industrial exposure.

Drug Interactions

Animal experiments indicate that methyl n-butyl ketone (MBK) enhances the neurotoxicity of n-hexane at low concentrations; therefore, mixed exposures should be avoided. N-Hexane products often are mixtures of aliphatic and aromatic hydrocarbons (e.g., toluene), and it is possible that the combination of chemicals contributes to hexane neuropathies. Methyl ethyl ketone (MEK) probably speeds the development of n-hexane polyneuropathy but does not[1] cause neuropathy by itself.

Treatment

GUT DECONTAMINATION

Ingestion of pure n-hexane is rare. Since n-hexane is a mild to moderate central nervous system depressant, gastric lavage with tracheal protection may be considered for pure hexane ingestions exceeding 2–3 mL/kg.

ELIMINATION ENHANCEMENT

These methods have not been studied in the treatment of n-hexane exposures.

SUPPORTIVE MEASURES

- Severe n-hexane inhalation produces obtundation and coma. Initial attention should be directed toward evaluation and support of respiration after the patient has been removed from the source.
- Cardiac dysrhythmias are a potential complication similar to other hydrocarbon exposures.
- Peripheral and central nervous system symptoms resulting from chronic exposure to N-hexane are treated symptomatically. Mild elevations of hepatic aminotransferase levels have been reported in workers exposed to n-hexane, but no direct link has been established.
- Electrophysiological changes of N-hexane neuropathy include decreased motor and sensory nerve conduction with an increased distal latency period. Electromyography suggests neurogenic disease. Sural nerve biopsies classically show a giant axonopathy with massive accumulation of axon neurofilaments and distal degeneration of myelin sheaths. Severe cases display nerve fiber breakdown (primarily large myelinated fibers) and myelin degeneration more prominently than axonal changes.

Questions—Aliphatic Hydrocarbons

1. Aliphatic hydrocarbons
- A. Are open chain, carbon-containing chemicals
- B. Include alkanes (paraffins), which are saturated hydrocarbons
- C. Include alkenes, which are unsaturated hydrocarbons with one or more double bonds
- D. Include alkynes, which are unsaturated hydrocarbons that contain one or more triple bonds
- E. All of the above

2. Exposure to low-molecular-weight aliphatic hydrocarbons
- A. Often causes significant airway irritation
- B. May produce myocardial sensitization and dysrhythmias
- C. Does not cause asphyxia
- D. Often causes diffuse systemic effects
- E. All of the above

3. Aspiration of liquid aliphatic hydrocarbons
- A. Produces a severe chemical pneumonitis
- B. May produce mucous membrane and respiratory irritation regardless of vapor concentration
- C. Is not associated with skin irritation due to prolonged contact
- D. Has its most significant toxicity related to impurities
- E. All of the above

4. The giant axonal swelling of hexacarbon neuropathy
- A. Is common to all toxic neuropathies

B. Is caused by o-cresol phosphate, acrylamide, carbon disulfide, and vincristine
C. Occurs initially in the distal portions of the nerve fiber and then progresses proximally
D. Causes nerve fibers to degenerate proximal to any swelling which then progresses distally
E. Is most likely to affect long, distal nerve sections

5. **Symptoms of chronic exposure to n-hexane vapors include**
A. Fatigue
B. Muscle weakness
C. Distal paresthesias (upper and lower extremities)
D. Pain
E. All of the above

6. **Symptoms of chronic exposure to N-hexane**
A. Usually develop within one month after continuous heavy exposure to n-hexane
B. Commonly progress for 2–3 months after cessation of exposure
C. Are identical to the pattern of symptoms developed by those who sniff glue
D. Are accompanied by increased reflexes
E. Are not often accompanied by sensory changes

7. **Exposure levels of n-hexane**
A. Have been recommended not to exceed 100 ppm
B. At over 100 ppm over six months have been associated with polyneuropathy
C. Must be long-term and high-dose to cause headache and nausea
D. Are unrelated to the production of confusion and dizziness
E. Have no nationally recommended guidelines

8. **Regarding 1,3-butadiene,**
A. It causes a great deal of acute toxicity from human industrial exposure.
B. Inhalation exposures between 600–8,000 ppm in humans have produced lymphomas, reproductive cancers, and thyroid carcinoma.
C. Studies of exposed workers have shown no increase in leukemia and lymphoma.
D. It is a colorless, flammable gas that may become explosive without warning.
E. It is not considered a potential occupational carcinogen and teratogen.

9. **Butane**
A. Is known to cause systemic effects when inhaled in an industrial setting
B. In high inhaled doses may affect the lower respiratory tract
C. Has never been associated with seizures
D. Is considered a carcinogen and teratogen
E. All of the above

10. **Regarding 2-nitropropane,**
A. Chronic exposure can cause anorexia, nausea, vomiting, headache and diarrhea in humans.
B. It has been shown to cause methemoglobinemia in humans.
C. It has never been implicated in acute hepatic failure.
D. It is considered a teratogen but not a carcinogen.
E. In low inhaled doses, it affects the lower respiratory tract.

11. **Propane**
A. In low concentrations is a mild narcotic
B. Is primarily an asphyxiant
C. Seems to concentrate primarily in the lungs
D. Does not concentrate in the brain
E. In low inhaled doses affects the lower respiratory tract

GASOLINE

Gasoline is a refined petroleum product that is used as a motor fuel. It is highly flammable and potentially explosive and contains more than 250 hydrocarbons and small quantities of additives and blending agents. The composition of gasoline varies depending on geographic region, season, performance requirements, and blending stocks. Benzene, a known hematotoxic agent, is present at an average concentration of approximately 1% in gasoline sold in the U.S., but can be as high as 5% concentration in European formulations.

Exposure to liquid gasoline occurs by unintentional or intentional ingestion, accidental skin contact, or by misuse. Misuse of gasoline, especially to clean and degrease floors, tools and machine parts, represents an important general public risk. Refinery workers and workers involved in removal and maintenance of underground storage tanks are also at risk for exposure to gasoline. Persons who unintentionally ingest gasoline while siphoning, and those who intentionally inhale gasoline vapors to obtain euphoric effects, also risk serious health consequences.

Pathophysiology

Gasoline that contains more than 0.05 g of lead per gram of gasoline is considered leaded gasoline. Organic lead is added to enhance a fuel's octane rating. In 1989, only 10% of the gasoline purchased in the U.S. was leaded gasoline. By 1997, the sale of leaded gasoline in the U.S. was discontinued. Unfortunately, organic lead compounds are still added to gasoline in other countries. Replacements for organic lead (i.e., "antiknock agents") include ethanol, methanol, methyl tertiary butyl ether (MTBE), and tertiary butyl ether (TBE). MTBE has contaminated ground water supplies across the U.S., and its use has become increasingly controversial.

Pharmacokinetics

ABSORPTION

- Inhalation, ingestion, and dermal exposure routes can absorb gasoline.
- The rate of dermal absorption is low compared with gastric absorption, although the aromatic hydrocarbons such as benzene are expected to have higher skin penetration than the alkanes.

DISTRIBUTION

- After unintentional ingestion of gasoline, the highest gasoline concentrations are in the liver, gastric wall, and lungs.
- Service-station attendants, who are exposed to gasoline by dermal contact and inhalation, have elevated blood levels of hydrocarbons such as benzene, toluene, pentane, and hexane.

- Gasoline can be rapidly absorbed through inhalation and skin contact.

ELIMINATION

- Some gasoline hydrocarbons are oxidized by liver microsomal-enzyme systems to products that are readily excreted in the urine.
- Alkanes are stable, saturated compounds that are not metabolized. Most of what is systemically absorbed is excreted unchanged through the lungs.
- After absorption, tetraethyl lead and tetramethyl lead are rapidly dealkylated by the liver to trialkyl metabolites that are toxic. The trialkyl metabolites, which are water soluble, can accumulate in the brain and are slowly metabolized to inorganic lead.
- Ingestion of large amounts of gasoline can result in absorption of methanol in a quantity sufficient to quickly overwhelm the folate-dependent metabolic pathway and produce severe toxicity. See Chapter 17, Alcohols, Glycols and Disulfiram.

Clinical Presentations

Inhalation is the most common route of exposure. The major target organs of gasoline exposure are the central nervous system and the lungs. At high concentrations, gasoline vapor is a respiratory-tract irritant. Pulmonary congestion, edema, acute exudative tracheobronchitis, and intrapulmonary hemorrhage have been observed after gasoline overexposure. High-concentration exposures by any route can cause central nervous system depression. Signs and symptoms may include confusion, tinnitus, disorientation, headache, drowsiness, weakness, seizures, and coma.

Ingestion may cause pain and irritation of the mucous membranes, resulting in nausea, vomiting, abdominal pain, and diarrhea. Severe overexposures may cause degenerative liver and kidney disease. Long-term exposure to gasoline vapor may lead to anemia, hypochromia, thrombocytopenia, and neutropenia. These effects are thought to be due to benzene in gasoline mixtures. Prolonged contact with gasoline can defat skin and cause irritation and dermatitis.

CARCINOGENIC EFFECTS

Epidemiologic studies have not substantiated the carcinogenic effects observed in experimental animals. In 1989, the International Agency for Research on Cancer concluded that gasoline is possibly carcinogenic to humans.

ABUSE

Chronic intentional abuse (e.g., sniffing or "huffing") of gasoline can result in death. Chronic abuse of leaded gasoline may cause a range of neurologic effects, including encephalopathy, ataxia, and tremor. Chronic sniffers of leaded gasoline may show neurologic effects with elevated blood lead levels. Chronic abuse of gasoline through sniffing can cause cardiac dysrhythmias and tachycardia. See the section on Inhalant Abuse in Chapter 45, Airborne Toxins.

Toxic Dosage/Death

Single oral doses of approximately 10 mL/kg may be fatal. Smaller amounts, if aspirated into the lungs, may lead to lipoid pneumonitis. The Occupational Safety and Health Administration (OSHA) short-term exposure limit (STEL) averaged over 15 minutes is 500 ppm for gasoline hydrocarbons and 5 ppm for benzene. The exposure during self-service refueling of automobiles is not likely to be a significant hazard to the public.

Laboratory

ANALYTIC METHODS

Methods to measure gasoline are not generally available in hospital settings.

BLOOD LEVELS

Gasoline levels do not guide therapy.

URINE

Urinary phenol, a biologic indicator of benzene exposure, may be elevated in gasoline-pump workers (average 40 mg/L) compared with persons with no occupational exposure to gasoline (less than 20 mg/L).

Treatment

- Respiratory compromise may require intubation. Persons with suspected ingestion should have a careful pulmonary evaluation, including a baseline chest radiograph to assess possible aspiration. A follow-up chest x-ray should be obtained in about 6 hours if pulmonary symptoms develop. Pulse oximetry or arterial blood-gas analyses may be needed to assess oxygenation.
- If skin or hair has been in contact with liquid gasoline, remove clothing and flush skin and hair with water (preferably under a shower) for 2–3 minutes. Wash with mild soap and rinse thoroughly with water. If eye contact has occurred, the eye should be flushed with water for at least 15 minutes or until pain resolves.
- In most cases, exposure cessation usually leads to complete recovery, even for patients who have evidence of central nervous system toxicity.
- Appropriate laboratory evaluation in the patient with neurologic signs and symptoms includes neurobehavioral testing and electroencephalography.
- See get decontamination and elimination enhancement recommendations in introduction to pretroleum distillations section above.

Questions—Gasoline

1. Gasoline
- A. Is a refined petroleum product generally made of 25 hydrocarbons
- B. Generally has the same composition regardless of season or region
- C. Generally has a concentration of 1–5% benzene
- D. Is not a known public risk
- E. Does not cause risk by skin contact

2. Ingested gasoline
- A. Is less well absorbed than when exposed to the skin
- B. Concentrates in the liver, gastric wall and lungs
- C. Prevents methanol toxicity sustained during inhalation exposure
- D. Is more common than inhaled gasoline
- E. Targets the nervous system and lungs

3. Chronic gasoline inhalation causes
- A. Ataxia
- B. Dysrhythmia

C. Encephalopathy
D. Tremor
E. All of the above

4. Gasoline exposure may lead to
A. Anemia
B. Thrombocytosis
C. Otalgia
D. Dry mucous membranes
E. All of the above

5. Supportive measures for all patients with significant gasoline exposures include
A. Quick delivery of antidote
B. Cleaning the skin with green soap
C. Electroencephalogram
D. Liver function and kidney function testing
E. Head CT

DIMETHYL SULFOXIDE

Dimethyl sulfoxide (DMSO) is widely used as an industrial solvent for both organic and inorganic chemicals. It has been used to treat interstitial cystitis. DMSO has also been used as a vehicle for drugs and has been used to treat certain cutaneous and musculoskeletal disorders with little evidence of beneficial effects. DMSO is a synthetic chemical capable of inducing renal, hepatic, hematopoietic or central nervous system dysfunction when it is administered intravenously. Few controlled clinical studies have been performed in humans.

Pathophysiology

DMSO appears to penetrate cell membranes due to its ability to form hydrogen bonds and to displace water. It has also been reported to exhibit antiinflammatory activity, local analgesia, diuresis, vasodilation, and dissolution of collagen.

Pharmacokinetics

ABSORPTION

- DMSO is well absorbed. Ingestion of 1 g/kg of DMSO results in a peak serum concentration of about 1,000–3,000 μg/mL within 4 hours.

DISTRIBUTION

- Eight hours after the cutaneous application of 2 g of 90% DMSO, 20% remained at the application site. Within 24 hours, 10–15% appears in the urine.

ELIMINATION

- The elimination half-life of oral DMSO is 20 hours, and that of dermal DMSO is about 11–14 hours.
- DMSO is metabolized in humans by oxidation to dimethyl sulfone ($DMSO_2$) or by reduction to dimethylsulfide.
- DMSO is eliminated through the breath and skin and causes a characteristic odor.

Clinical Presentations

A garlic-like taste may remain for 72 hours after its intravesical use. Transient chemical cystitis may follow. Chronic dermal applications of DMSO have resulted in pruritus, urticaria, erythema, eosinophilia, a garlic odor to the breath, fatigue, headache, nausea, dizziness, eye irritation, exfoliation, and pigmentation at the site of application. Mixed sensorimotor peripheral neuropathy and segmental demyelination have been reported.

Dose-dependent intravascular hemolysis with bilirubinemia and hemoglobinuria may follow intravenous use. When used as a penetrating base for other drugs, DMSO may enhance their toxic effects. Abnormalities in renal function tests, hepatic enzymes, and coagulation parameters have been observed. Transient encephalopathy, dysarthria, acute tubular necrosis, disorientation, hypoactive reflexes, and altered consciousness have been described. Symptoms may not clear for 1 week.

Toxic Dosage/Death

Acute tubular necrosis followed two intravenous infusions of 100 g of 20% DMSO.

Drug Interactions

DMSO has been shown to enhance the absorption of heparin, insulin, sodium salicylate, sulfadiazine, and aminophylline in animals.

Pregnancy/Lactation

The U.S. Food and Drug Administration has placed DMSO in pregnancy risk category C. Teratogenic effects have been found in animals. There have been no adequate well-controlled studies in pregnant women. It is not known whether DMSO is excreted in human milk.

Laboratory

ANALYTIC METHODS

DMSO and $DMSO_2$ are measured by flame-ionization or electrocapture gas chromatography after solvent extraction or protein precipitation.

BLOOD LEVELS

Intravenous administration of DMSO led to serum concentrations of DMSO (1,600 μg/mL) and $DMSO_2$ (3,000 mg/mL) which were associated with a severe garlic odor, disorientation, and dysarthric speech.

Treatment

GUT DECONTAMINATION

Ingestion of overdoses of DMSO have not been reported. An attempt should be made to empty the gastric contents with tracheal protection. Emetic agents have not been evaluated.

ELIMINATION ENHANCEMENT

These methods have not been specifically evaluated after DMSO exposure. Renal failure, unresponsive to conservative management, may respond to extracorporeal treatment measures. A paucity of toxicokinetic data does not provide a guide for the clinician.

SUPPORTIVE MEASURES

- Treatment is essentially supportive and symptomatic. Use protective clothing, including gloves and head, foot, and body protection, to minimize skin contact. Use goggles and/or a face shield when a danger of splashing exists. Avoid breathing a spray or mist of DMSO or a high concentration of vapors. Use care in handling solutions of toxic materials in DMSO.

- An overdose of DMSO in the course of intravesical use may result in symptoms of a chemical cystitis. Bladder antispasmodics and analgesic medications may be useful.
- If DMSO is administered by the intravenous route, there may be an increased possibility of central nervous system, renal, hepatic, or hematopoietic dysfunction.
- Excess amounts of DMSO on the skin require vigorous irrigation with water or saline.
- After dermal applications, infrequent elevations of renal function tests and hepatic enzymes may occur. Eosinophilia has been observed and creatine kinase levels may rise. Prothrombin and partial thromboplastin times may shorten.

Questions—Dimethyl Sulfoxide

1. DMSO
  A. Is poorly absorbed
  B. Has the same half-life, whether taken orally or dermally
  C. Is eliminated through breath and skin thus giving an odor
  D. Does not reach peak serum concentration when ingested for 24 hours
  E. Is not metabolized in humans

2. DMSO use is suggested by
  A. A garlic taste
  B. Chemical cystitis
  C. Sensorimotor peripheral neuropathy
  D. Hemolysis with hyperbilirubinemia
  E. All of the above

3. Treatment of DMSO overexposure may include all of the following except
  A. Quick delivery of antidote
  B. Extracorporeal treatment measures, via hemodialysis or hemoperfusion in cases of renal failure
  C. Bladder antispasmodics and analgesics
  D. Irrigation with water or saline if exposure was dermal
  E. Use of protective clothing by caregivers

DIMETHYL SULFATE

Dimethyl sulfate (DMS) is widely used in industry as a methylating agent for the organic synthesis of chemicals, especially in the manufacture of pharmaceuticals, dyestuffs, perfume, and pesticides. It is an industrial chemical that can produce severe ocular reactions and delayed respiratory tract reactions that can terminate fatally. There are no reported natural sources of DMS, but it may be present in the environment because of industrial processes.

Pathophysiology

When DMS encounters a moist mucosal surface, it is hydrolyzed slowly into sulfuric acid, methanol, and methyl hydrogen sulfate. The methanol may be absorbed into the circulation, leading to neurotoxic effects. Sulfuric acid and methyl hydrogen sulfate can induce irritative, anesthetic, and erosive effects on mucosa.

Clinical Presentations

There is usually a latent period of 20 minutes to 12 hours between exposure and onset of symptoms. This delayed effect, and the absence of warning signs (e.g., the absence of color, and a minimal odor), make this compound particularly hazardous. Vital signs may include a rise in body temperature, pulse rate, and respiratory rate. Abnormal breath sounds, wheezing, dry rales, and moist rales may be heard. Congestion and edema of the eyes, pharynx, and uvula may be observed.

Usual clinical manifestations may include skin burns, corneal irritation with photophobia, lacrimation and blurring of vision, oropharyngeal edema with suffocation and hoarseness of the voice, nasal septal necrosis, cough, and dyspnea. Irreversible loss of vision has been reported. Major causes of mortality in DMS intoxication include respiratory failure following mucosal inflammation, edema of major airways, and noncardiogenic pulmonary edema. Other systemic effects can include seizures, delirium, coma, and renal, hepatic, and cardiac failure. DMS is probably carcinogenic in humans. Symptoms may be graded as follows:

IRRITATIVE REACTIONS

Symptoms and signs of mucosal irritation may occur in the eyes, nose, and pharynx, combined with a normal chest x-ray, and no leukocytosis. No systemic signs of intoxication are seen. Patients may be released after symptomatic treatment and medical observation for 24–72 hours.

MILD INTOXICATION

In addition to the above, there are irritative and erosive actions in the respiratory tract manifested by congestion of the pharynx, larynx, and uvula, and abnormal breath sounds. There may be positive findings on chest x-ray and/or leukocytosis. With treatment, patients usually recover in 3–7 days.

MODERATE INTOXICATION

In addition to the manifestations of mild intoxication, necrosis and desquamation of the respiratory mucosa occurs, with more than two of the following: positive chest x-rays showing pneumonia or interstitial pneumonia, leukocytosis, or ECG demonstrating myocardial damage. After treatment and rest, these patients may recover and resume ordinary work.

SEVERE INTOXICATION

In addition to the manifestations of moderate intoxication, patients may exhibit significant laryngeal edema, pulmonary edema, shock, encephalopathy, and/or myocardial damage. Local and systemic supportive treatment is required.

Toxic Dosage/Death

Seemingly minor exposures can prove dangerous. A patient who licked a DMS-covered finger, suffered immediate irritation of the soft palate, laryngeal constriction, and increased salivation that improved on treatment. Unfortunately, 24 hours later there was a sudden onset of glottic edema and death ensued. At autopsy, acute corrosive changes were seen in the upper gastrointestinal tract with edema of the glottis and emphysema of the lungs.

Laboratory

ANALYTIC METHODS

A sensitive gas chromatography-mass spectrometry technique has been developed, and a fully automated gas chromatography method is available for the routine determination of DMS.

BLOOD LEVELS

Following DMS levels in overdose is probably not helpful in guiding treatment, but may demonstrate the presence of this toxin.

Treatment

GUT DECONTAMINATION

Emesis is dangerous because of reexposure of the esophagus to corrosive material and because of the danger of aspiration pneumonia. Gastric lavage can be performed carefully, preferably within one hour of ingestion, with appropriate tracheal protection. Endoscopy will determine the extent of esophageal and gastric injury.

ELIMINATION ENHANCEMENT

There have been no clinical studies on procedures to accelerate the elimination of DMS or its hydrolysis products (e.g., sulfuric acid and methanol) after an exposure. If neurotoxic effects that may be related to methanol poisoning appear, clinical judgment must dictate whether the use of ethanol or hemodialysis is indicated.

SUPPORTIVE MEASURES

- Systemic treatment will depend on the severity of exposure. All patients exposed to DMS should be admitted to a hospital for observation for at least 24 hours.
- All industrial operations using DMS should be carried out in fully enclosed systems with arrangements made for removing spillage. Workers should be supplied with respiratory protective equipment, chemical eye protective wear, protective clothing, and rubber gloves.
- Wash and irrigate all exposed skin thoroughly with water or saline.
- After oral ingestions, treat as a corrosive acid poisoning.
- The ECG may show inversion of T waves and elevation or depression of ST segments, especially in patients with bronchopneumonia, pulmonary edema, and myocardial damage.
- Elevated white blood cell counts may be observed. No abnormalities are usually seen in routine urinalyses, red blood cell counts, or hemoglobin determinations.
- Clinical blood studies for methanol or formate levels are indicated within the first 24 hours if there is evidence of neurotoxicity.

Eye Exposure

- Copious irrigation should be started with water or normal saline for at least 20–30 minutes.
- Most cases of mild corneal and conjunctival injury resolve within 24 hours. Careful ophthalmologic follow-up is indicated for all patients with eye injuries.
- Steroid and antibiotic medication may be instilled for the prevention and treatment of inflammation. Caution must be exercised when using steroids in the presence of corneal injury.

Respiratory Exposure

- Use of antibiotics and humidified oxygen has been recommended.
- Repeated aerosol inhalations composed of dexamethasone 5 mg, aminophylline 0.25 g, and streptomycin 0.5 g or gentamicin 80,000 U in 50 ml normal saline; 10–20 ml/time; 2–8 times/day, have been administered to patients with respiratory tract injury.
- For those who have inhaled high concentrations of DMS, early intravenous administration of hydrocortisone or dexamethasone may prove beneficial.
- Adult respiratory distress syndrome (ARDS) may develop, and continuous, intermittent, positive-pressure oxygen inhalation has been given for 10–16 hours until hypoxia was corrected.
- Lung function tests may show a restrictive pattern when forced expiratory volume in 1 second (FEV1), forced vital capacity (FVC), FEV1/FVC, and carbon monoxide diffusing capacity studies are performed. Periodic chest radiography may indicate peribronchitis, bilateral pulmonary infiltrates, and pulmonary edema.

Questions—Dimethyl Sulfate

1. Dimethyl sulfate (DMS) exposure
A. Usually causes symptoms in 20 minutes to 12 hours
B. Is usually obvious because of its odor and color
C. Does not usually create changes in vital signs
D. Has not been reported to cause irreversible blindness
E. Primarily causes direct cardiac toxicity

2. Intoxication with DMS is categorized as
A. Mild with only mucosal irritation, normal chest x-ray and breath sounds, and no elevation of white blood cells
B. Moderate if there is necrosis of the respiratory mucosa with chest x-ray changes and leucocytosis
C. Moderate if there is necrosis of the respiratory mucosa with chest x-ray changes, normal white blood cell count and normal ECG
D. Severe if ECG changes occur
E. Severe if necrosis of respiratory mucosa occurs

3. Treatment of DMS exposure
A. Depends on the severity of exposure
B. Always includes hospital admission
C. May be managed as a corrosive acid poisoning
D. May include assessment of ethanol or formate levels
E. All of the above

4. If DMS eye exposure occurs,
A. Patients should be informed that blindness is likely.
B. Patients should be informed that no intervention is necessary.
C. Steroid and antibiotic medication may be helpful.
D. Irrigation should not be started until 30 minutes after exposure.
E. Irrigation should continue for 20–30 hours.

STODDARD SOLVENT

"Stoddard Solvent" is the name adopted by the National Association of Dryers and Cleaners to honor W.J. Stoddard for his work with petroleum distillates used in the dry-cleaning industry. It is used in industry as a dry-cleaning solvent, metal degreaser, and extractant. Consumers may be exposed to Stoddard solvent through inhalation or dermal contact with cleaning products, paints, paint thinners, furniture refinishers, pesticides, or residues on dry-cleaned products.

Pathophysiology

Stoddard solvent is a distillation fraction of crude petroleum that contains at least 200 products, predominantly C7 through C12 hydrocarbons. The mixture typically consists of cycloalkanes (naphthenes) and aromatic hydrocarbons (benzene, toluene, and xylene each represent less than 1% of the total mixture.) Although the toxicity of Stoddard solvent is not attributable to any one type of constituent, the aromatic components are considered more toxic than the paraffin or naphthene components.

Clinical Presentations

Acute exposure to Stoddard solvent at air concentrations below the odor threshold produces no adverse health effects. The major effect associated with inhalation of paraffin-like solvents is central nervous system excitation, followed rapidly by central nervous system depression. Reported symptoms of acute exposure to Stoddard solvent include lightheadedness, dizziness, visual disturbances, skin irritation and drowsiness. Although case reports have been published of persons who were exposed to Stoddard solvent and subsequently suffered liver, kidney, or hematologic injury, a causal relationship has not been firmly established. Cardiac dysrhythmias have not been reported in humans after exposure to Stoddard solvent.

RESPIRATORY EFFECTS

Acute exposure to high concentrations of Stoddard solvent can irritate mucous membranes and cause upper respiratory tract irritation. Acute ingestion and aspiration of hydrocarbon mixtures similar to Stoddard solvent have resulted in chemical pneumonitis that mimics adult respiratory distress syndrome (ARDS). Complications of aspiration may also include pulmonary edema, pulmonary emphysema, pneumothorax, pleuritis, pleural effusion, empyema, and pneumatoceles.

NEUROLOGIC EFFECTS

Chronic exposure to Stoddard solvent has been associated with headaches, fatigue, episodes of inebriation, and memory deficits that generally resolve on discontinuation of exposure.

CARCINOGENIC EFFECTS

Data from studies of Stoddard solvent exposure in experimental animals (dermal exposure) and in humans (inhalation exposure) have not conclusively shown that Stoddard solvent is carcinogenic.

Toxic Dosage/Death

The odor threshold for Stoddard solvent is less than 1 ppm. However, after about 6 minutes, the olfactory sense fatigues and Stoddard solvent is no longer detected by smell. Thus odor is not a reliable indicator of exposure and may not provide adequate warning of dangerously high levels.

Pregnancy/Lactation

Stoddard solvent can probably cross the placenta and enter breast milk.

Laboratory

ANALYTIC METHODS

No specific hydrocarbon in the plasma or tissues is a reproducible index of exposure.

BLOOD LEVELS

No specific hydrocarbon in the plasma or tissues is a reproducible index of exposure. Following any particular blood level after exposure does not help guide management.

Treatment

GUT DECONTAMINATION

Gastric decontamination by emesis, lavage, cathartic, and/or activated charcoal is not recommended in most cases.

ELIMINATION ENHANCEMENT

There are no data that hemodialysis or other methods to enhance elimination are helpful in decreasing any ill effects after exposure.

SUPPORTIVE MEASURES

- The person should be removed immediately from the source of exposure. Patients who are asymptomatic after six hours of observation may be discharged from the hospital.
- Remove contaminated clothing and wash exposed areas with mild soap and shampoo, then rinse thoroughly with water. Direct eye splashes should be treated by irrigation with saline or water for 15 minutes or until pain resolves.
- Supplemental oxygen should be administered as needed. Blood gas analysis, chest radiography, ECG monitoring, and baseline liver and kidney function tests should be considered in serious overexposures.
- Corticosteroids and prophylactic antibiotics are not necessary.
- In cases of persistent neurologic symptoms, neuropsychologic testing may be useful for diagnostic purposes and to establish baseline function.

Questions—Stoddard Solvent

1. **Stoddard solvent**
   A. Conclusively causes cancer.
   B. May be associated with headache and ARDS.
   C. Is frequently associated with seizures.
   D. Produces an odor which is always a reliable indicator of exposure.
   E. Represents a single petroleum distillation fraction.
2. **Acute exposure to Stoddard solvent**
   A. Causes incremental central nervous system excitation
   B. Causes cardiac dysrhythmias
   C. Causes immediate progressive central nervous system depression
   D. Produces no adverse health effects below the odor threshold
   E. Has been shown to be carcinogenic
3. **Treatment of Stoddard solvent exposure includes**
   A. Gut decontamination with emesis, lavage, or charcoal
   B. Hemodialysis
   C. Slow removal from source of exposure
   D. Supplemental oxygen
   E. Steroids and antibiotics

AROMATIC HYDROCARBONS

INTRODUCTION

Cyclic or aromatic hydrocarbons are ubiquitous solvents found in gasoline, industrial solvents, glues, cleaners, paint thinners, and degreasers. By definition, they each contain at least one benzene ring. Double fused rings are called naphthalenes and multifused aromatic rings are called polynuclear compounds. Phenol, a benzene ring with an alcohol side group, is described in the Chapter 38, Household Products.

BENZENE

Benzene is the prototype aromatic hydrocarbon, since it is composed of only the benzene ring. It is used widely in the chemical industry as a feedstock for the production of styrene, phenol, and cyclohexane, and less commonly as a solvent. Other industrial applications include the manufacture of detergents, explosives, and pharmaceuticals. This clear, colorless, highly flammable liquid at room temperature is highly volatile and has a pungent aromatic odor.

Benzene is a natural constituent of motor fuels. American gasoline contains an average benzene concentration of 0.8%, and foreign fuels may contain up to 5%. These levels have been reduced due to regulatory standards in recent years. Benzene comprises about 2% of total hydrocarbon emission from a gasoline engine and about 4% of automotive exhaust. Although benzene is a superior solvent for fats, inks, oils, paints, plastics, and rubber, many companies have either reduced the benzene concentration in household products, or reformulated the products to contain the less toxic solvent toluene.

Pathophysiology

Like other aromatic solvents, benzene causes central nervous system depression acutely, but its propensity to produce blood dyscrasias such as myelocytic and monocytic leukemia, and aplastic anemia, apparently is unique.

Pharmacokinetics

ABSORPTION

- Inhalation is the primary route of exposure, with the amount retained varying between 30–80%.
- Initially, both gastrointestinal absorption and pulmonary absorption are rapid.
- Limited absorption does occur through the skin.

DISTRIBUTION

- Studies in animals indicate that maximal concentrations appear in tissues within 3 hours; highest levels occur in fat.
- Maximum benzene metabolite levels appear in the bone marrow and fat.

ELIMINATION

- After cessation of exposure, the lungs excrete unchanged a significant amount of absorbed benzene (10–50%) depending on the quality of body fat and exercise level. Minor amounts are excreted unchanged in the urine and bile.
- Non-expired benzene is biotransformed in the liver by the P450 mixed-function oxidase system, primarily to phenol metabolites.
- The bone marrow possesses a mixed-function oxidase system that may produce the toxic metabolite responsible for benzene-induced hematological abnormalities. Benzene oxide is the most likely toxic metabolite.
- Excretion of phenol metabolites usually is complete in 24–48 hours, with a biological half-life under 12 hours.

Clinical Presentations

Central nervous system depression results from high acute exposures and is characterized by euphoria, headache, nausea, and ataxia followed by staggering gait, stupor, coma, and seizures. Insomnia, agitation, headache, drowsiness, nausea, and anorexia may persist several weeks after exposure. As with other solvents, arrhythmias may develop acutely, perhaps because of myocardial sensitization to endogenous catecholamines. Studies in animals indicate that high concentrations produce mucous membrane and pulmonary irritation, with severe inhalations resulting in noncardiogenic pulmonary edema.

Benzene is hematotoxic after chronic exposures. Bone marrow suppression is well recognized. Benzene-induced leukemia has been less easily accepted, in part because of the difficulty in producing benzene carcinogenicity in animal models.

ANEMIA

Early peripheral depression of blood elements may progress to pancytopenia with bone marrow hyperplasia and then to hypoplasia (aplastic anemia). Reduced blood elements lead to weakness, fatigue, increased infections, and signs of poor blood coagulation such as petechiae, bleeding gums, epistaxis, and gastrointestinal hemorrhage. The hyperplasia stage of aplastic anemia is unique to benzene and may be reversible, although generally aplastic anemia has a poor prognosis. The metabolite responsible for aplastic anemia is believed to be a hydroquinone precursor.

LEUKEMIA

Most, if not all, cases of benzene-induced leukemias are preceded by pancytopenia. Epidemiological studies indicate an increased risk of acute myelocytic and monocytic leukemia in benzene workers with an overall fivefold greater risk for the development of leukemia. For workers exposed more than 5 years, the risk of death from leukemia increased 21 times over that of a control population in one study. Duration of exposure may be less than 1 year but usually exceeds 15 years. Benzene has also been associated with leukemia in several cases of chronic nonindustrial exposure. A metabolite, perhaps an epoxide, is the suspected cause of leukemia. The association between benzene and lymphomas is less clear, although excess lymphoma deaths have been reported in benzene and coal tar workers.

Toxic Dosage/Death

The current U.S. standard for the workplace is designed to prevent chronic hematologic toxicity. Variability of response to benzene-induced hematologic abnormalities does occur, since only a minority of workers exposed to benzene develop hematological changes. Experiments in animals indicate that benzene is a central nervous system depressant with detectable effects around 4,000 ppm and death around 40,000 ppm. Human exposures demonstrate similar effects. The threshold limit for benzene-induced blood dyscrasias has not been firmly established. A lethal dose has been estimated as 100 mL.

In one study, benzene workers exposed to 30–210 ppm benzene over three months to 17 years showed hematological abnormalities, including leukopenia (9.7%), thrombocytopenia (1.84%), leukopenia and thrombocytopenia (2.76%), and mild to moderate hypochromic or normochromic anemia (33% versus 21% in nonexposed controls).

Drug Interactions

Alcohol accelerates urinary phenol excretion, whereas toluene is a competitive inhibitor of benzene biotransformation.

Pregnancy/Lactation

Chromosomal aberrations in workers, human cell cultures, and animals support the role of benzene as a teratogen.

Laboratory

ANALYTIC METHODS

A gas chromatography-mass spectroscopy method has been developed for determination of blood, breath, and urine levels of benzene.

BLOOD LEVELS

Blood benzene levels are useful only for detecting low-level exposures. Exhaled benzene levels may be a more sensitive indicator of the total body burden of benzene than blood levels.

URINE

Urinary phenol collections are the best method for determining occupational benzene exposure. For maximum allowable exposures of 10 ppm for an 8-hour work shift, the urinary phenol level collected postshift should be below 45–50 mg/L. Unexposed persons rarely have urinary phenol levels exceeding 20 mg/L. Dermal application of phenol-containing solutions and ingestion of phenol itself, elevate urinary phenol levels. These non-occupational exposures may complicate interpretations of results.

Treatment

GUT DECONTAMINATION

Gastric decontamination procedures in the setting of hydrocarbon ingestions remain controversial. Emesis has been advocated in alert patients if more than 1 mL of benzene per kilogram has been ingested and less than two hours has passed between exposure and treatment, however lavage with attention to tracheal protection may be safer and equally efficacious. Charcoal may be helpful in cases involving toxic additives. The use of charcoal and cathartics for benzene alone is questionable.

ELIMINATION ENHANCEMENT

These methods are generally not employed in the treatment of hydrocarbon ingestions.

SUPPORTIVE MEASURES

- As with other organic solvents, initial attention after severe acute exposures should be directed toward maintaining ventilation and detecting dysrhythmias. Oxygen, intubation, intravenous lines, and cardiac monitors may be necessary for severe acute exposures.
- Respiratory distress may indicate a hydrocarbon aspiration pneumonitis as well as noncardiogenic pulmonary edema. See the Introduction section for Petroleum Distillates above for treatment guidelines.
- Remove all contaminated clothes and wash exposed skin with green soap and water.
- The treatment of chronic benzene toxicity is supportive and symptomatic, with chemotherapy and bone marrow transplants as therapeutic options for leukemia and aplastic anemia, respectively.

Questions—Benzene

1. Patients are most commonly exposed to benzene
A. Via inhalation
B. Via ingestion
C. Via dermal contact
D. Via accidental ophthalmologic contact
E. There is no single most common route.

2. Hematologic complications of benzene toxicity include all of the following except
A. Depression of all blood elements
B. Weakness, fatigue, infection and poor coagulation
C. Prominent, persistent leukocytosis
D. Bone marrow hyperplasia then hypoplasia
E. Aplastic anemia

3. Benzene-induced leukemias
A. Are usually preceded by leukocytosis
B. Are not more common in benzene workers
C. Are more likely fatal in workers exposed for more than five years
D. Have not been found in chronic nonindustrial exposure
E. Are as closely linked as causal as benzene-induced lymphomas

4. When treating benzene exposed patients,
A. There is no way to detect blood levels.
B. Blood levels may be more sensitive than exhaled levels.
C. Exhaled levels may be more sensitive than blood levels.
D. Urine phenol levels are best to determine non-occupational exposures.
E. Urine phenol levels only reflect inhaled benzene.

5. Benzene exposure treatment includes
A. Avoiding emesis for all patients
B. Inducing emesis in all patients
C. Elimination enhancement
D. Cleansing skin with green soap
E. None of the above

POLYCYCLIC AROMATIC HYDROCARBONS

The field of occupational medicine may have been discovered in 1775, when Percival Pott reported an unusually high incidence of scrotal cancer in chimney sweeps. By the 1930s, this association was attributed to benzopyrene and dibenzanthracene in coal tar. Polycyclic aromatic hydrocarbons (PAHs), found in coal tar and hundreds of other substances, consist of three or more fused benzene rings in varying arrangements that contain only carbon and hydrogen. The carcinogenic form of PAHs results from their oxidation by the mixed-function oxidase system to diol-epoxide derivatives. These compounds contain highly reactive "bay regions" that probably bind covalently to DNA.

Coke oven, coal tar, pitch, asphalt, and carbon black workers are all exposed to PAHs. Naphthalene, which is a coal tar constituent used for mothballs, is not considered a polycyclic aromatic hydrocarbon because it contains only two fused benzene rings. The primary environmental sources of polycyclic aromatic hydrocarbons are forest fires and combustion of fossil fuel, where high temperatures convert organic substances to PAHs. Seafood and agricultural products contain PAHs because of their sedimentation from air and subsequent penetration into water systems. Crude coconut oil, heavily smoked ham, roasted coffee, tea, and charcoal-broiled meat also contain PAHs.

Pathophysiology

The direct covalent binding of carcinogenic agent to DNA, resulting in carcinogenic DNA adducts, may be an essential step in the development of cancer. Polycyclic aromatic hydrocarbon DNA adducts have been detected in lung tissue from patients with lung cancer. Soot, tars, and creosote contain a variety of by-products and contaminants that include PAHs. Epidemiological studies in patients exposed to these agents have demonstrated increased incidences of skin, lung, bladder, and gastrointestinal cancer.

Clinical Presentations

Acute toxicity from PAHs is rarely reported. Exposure to high-risk PAHs via skin and lung absorption results in increased incidences of skin and lung cancer. Certain PAHs are considered carcinogenic, whereas others, such as anthracene and phenanthrene, are not. Coke oven emissions are complex mixtures of coal and coke material that include PAHs, and epidemiological studies of exposed workers has indicated increased incidences of lung and urinary tract cancer. Benzaonthracene, benzopyrene, and dibenzopyrene are suspected carcinogens based on studies in animals that show increased incidences of skin, lung, and liver cancer.

Reported effects associated with chronic exposure to coal tar and its by-products include erythema, burns, warts on sun-exposed areas, and progression to skin cancer. Toxic effects of coal tar are enhanced by exposure to ultraviolet light. Ocular irritation and photosensitivity, cough, bronchitis, and bronchogenic cancer may occur with chronic exposures. Oral effects may include leukoplakia, buccal-pharyngeal cancer, and cancer of the lip. Hematuria, kidney and bladder cancers, and lymphoma have also been associated with chronic exposures.

Toxic Dosage/Death

OSHA permissible exposure limits in air over an 8-hour workday are 0.2 mg/m^3 measured as the benzene-soluble fraction of coal-tar pitch volatiles.

Laboratory

ANALYTIC METHODS

No available data.

BLOOD LEVELS

Benzopyrene (BP) is often measured as an indicator of PAH exposure and may be responsible for an increased risk of lung cancer among smokers, foundry workers, and coke-oven workers. Measurement of BP serum protein adduct concentrations appear to be a useful method by which groups exposed to BP may be biologically monitored.

URINE

Urinary 1-hydroxypyrene (1-OHPY) has promise as a marker of exposures to PAHs.

Treatment

GUT DECONTAMINATION

These methods have not been studied in the treatment of PAH ingestions, however lavage or charcoal use after significant ingestions may be helpful.

ELIMINATION ENHANCEMENT

These methods are generally not employed in the treatment of PAH exposures.

SUPPORTIVE MEASURES

- Ventilatory support should be available in case of an acute inhalation exposure.
- Remove contaminated clothing as soon as possible. Decontaminate the skin by gently scrubbing with soap and water. Ocular exposure should be treated with irrigation and a complete eye examination.
- Periodic evaluation of healthy patients who have been significantly exposed to PAHs, even in the absence of symptoms, is recommended to facilitate early diagnosis and intervention should a malignancy develop.

Questions—Polycyclic Aromatic Hydrocarbons

1. **Polycyclic aromatic hydrocarbon toxicity**
   A. Is most common after acute exposure
   B. Includes skin and lung cancer after skin and lung absorption
   C. Includes cancer regardless of which PAH was the toxin
   D. Commonly includes gynecologic cancers
   E. Is minimized by ultraviolet light
2. **Chronic exposure to PAHs has been associated with**
   A. Cough and pneumonia
   B. Leukoplakia and lip cancer
   C. Hematuria and urine infection
   D. Tinnitus
   E. Vaginitis and vaginal cancer
3. **Useful measurements for acute management of PAH toxicity include**
   A. Benzopyrene as an indicator of PAH exposure
   B. Benzopyrene serum protein adduct concentration to reflect duration of exposure
   C. Urine benzopyrene to reflect quantity of PAH exposure
   D. Serum benzoanthracene
   E. Urine benzoanthracene
4. **Supportive measures in treatment of PAH exposures include**
   A. Ventilatory support of acute inhalation
   B. Skin decontamination with gentle scrubbing
   C. Irrigation if ocular exposure occurred
   D. Periodic follow up despite initial symptoms
   E. All of the above

POLYHALOGENATED BIPHENYLS

Because of their insulating and nonflammable properties, polychlorinated biphenyls (PCBs) have been used as heat exchange and dielectric fluids in transformers and capacitors, hydraulic and lubricating fluids, diffusion pump oils, plasticizers, extenders for pesticides, and as ingredients of caulking compounds, paints, adhesives, and flame retardants. PCBs have also been used in inks and carbonless paper. Polybrominated biphenyls (PBBs) have been used as flame retardants. In 1977, the U.S. Environmental Protection Agency halted the manufacture of PCBs, but did not require the removal of transformers or capacitors containing these agents.

Although PCBs have low acute toxicity, their bioaccumulation in human fat and environmental persistence have resulted in concern over their potential chronic toxicity. The toxicity of polyhalogenated biphenyls received publicity in the U.S. when the consumption of cattle feed inadvertently contaminated with PBBs caused widespread human contamination. Reported symptoms of PBB poisoning include chloracne, arthralgias, fatigue, headache, insomnia, and myalgias.

Syndromes associated with polyhalogenated biphenyls have periodically been described around the world. Contamination of rice bran oil by PCBs produced a disease called *Yusho* ("rice oil disease") in Japan characterized by fatigue, malaise, myalgias, chloracne, jaundice, sensory neuropathies, and serum lipid abnormalities. In 1979, a similar episode called *Ye-cheng* occurred in Taiwan after the consumption of PCB-contaminated rice oil. Symptoms included chloracne, hyperpigmented gums, periorbital edema, and conjunctival irritation. PCB contamination appears more serious than PBB exposure.

Pathophysiology

Polychlorinated biphenyls are halogenated aromatic hydrocarbons that are not naturally present in biological systems. Commercial PCB mixtures contain a variety of the 209 possible chlorobiphenyl isomers. The greater the chlorine content, the more resistant these compounds are to metabolic degradation. PCBs are magnified in the food chain, reaching high concentrations in fish, predators, and humans. All commercial PCB products are contaminated by more toxic polychlorinated dibenzofurans.

Dibenzofuran is an organic compound that contains two benzene rings fused to a central furan ring. Chlorodibenzofurans (CDFs) are a class of organic compounds in which one to eight chlorine atoms are attached to the benzene ring positions of a dibenzofuran structure. Small amounts of CDFs can enter the environment from a number of sources. Accidental fires or breakdowns involving capacitors, transformers, and other electrical equipment that contain PCBs are the main known sources of CDFs in the environment.

Pharmacokinetics

ABSORPTION

- These compounds are absorbed through the lungs, skin, and gastrointestinal tract.
- Chloracne is a marker of systemic as well as cutaneous absorption.

DISTRIBUTION

- Distribution occurs primarily into fat.

ELIMINATION

- Metabolism of these compounds in humans has not been extensively studied.
- PCB biotransformation is slow and depends on chlorine content (i.e., highly chlorinated compounds are metabolized and excreted extremely slowly).
- Half-lives of some of these agents, such as Aroclor 1242, may be 6–7 months. The half-life of Aroclor 1260 may be 33–34 months.

Clinical Presentations

Acute effects after PCB exposures are mild. The most commonly reported symptoms result from eye and skin irritation. Exposures from the release of overheated transformer mist, which contains both PCBs and pyrolysis by-products, results in nausea, eye irritation, sore throat, chest tightness, and headache.

Chloracne is the only overt effect of chronic PCB exposure in humans, but absence of chloracne does not rule out exposure. Chloracne is characterized by straw-colored, cystic lesions, comedos, and pustules. These lesions appear on the head, neck, and trunk, may be refractory to treatment, and can last years. Chloracne typically develops weeks or months after exposure.

A clinical hepatitis and sensory peripheral neuropathy occurred during the *Yusho* epidemic, but elevated hepatic aminotransferase levels were not detected among workers exposed to PCBs. Headache, tremor, insomnia, fatigue, anxiety, and dizziness are reported frequently among PCB-exposed workers. At least one case of neuropsychiatric changes has been associated with chronic PCB exposure and elevated serum PCB levels.

PCB mixtures are definite animal carcinogens causing hepatocellular carcinoma even without gross histological changes. The U.S. Environmental Protection Agency considers PCBs a potential human carcinogen on the basis of animal data. Although epidemiological studies suggest an increased incidence of cancer in occupationally exposed workers, the long-term effect of both acute and chronic exposures remains unknown.

Drug Interactions

PCBs are potent enzyme inducers of both the microsomal monooxygenase or cytochrome P-450 system and the aryl hydrocarbon hydroxylase or cytochrome P-448 system. Patients are encouraged to avoid exposure to other hepatotoxins such as antibiotics or medications with known hepatotoxicity, alcohol, and chlorinated solvents.

Pregnancy/Lactation

Both PCBs and PBBs are excreted in breast milk. Fetuses and neonates are potentially more sensitive to PCBs than adults because of transplacental distribution and physiologic differences. They lack the hepatic microsomal enzyme systems that facilitate metabolism and excretion of PCBs. Furthermore, PCBs accumulate in breast milk. Nursing infants are at additional risk because human milk contains a steroid that inhibits PCB glucuronidation and excretion.

Laboratory

ANALYTIC METHODS

Gas chromatography with electron capture and mass spectrometry quantitate both PCB and PBB levels.

BLOOD LEVELS

Serum PCB levels probably are the best indicator of exposure, but current knowledge of dose-response characteristics is inadequate to correlate acute or chronic effects with a given serum level. Mean serum total PCB levels in the unexposed U.S. population are about 5–7 ppb, with 95% possessing levels below 20 ppb. Follow-up PCB levels in patients poisoned with PCB-contaminated cooking oil demonstrated blood PCB half-lives of more than two years. PCB blood concentrations did not correlate with reported symptoms or signs of headache, dizziness, or sensory neuropathy. This discrepancy may reflect the presence of more toxic contaminants such as dibenzofurans.

Treatment

GUT DECONTAMINATION

There is no specific treatment for PCB toxicity. Activated charcoal has not been proven beneficial, but is not contraindicated.

ELIMINATION ENHANCEMENT

These methods have not been utilized in the treatment of chloracne or chronic PCB or PBB exposures. Since there are no known methods of reducing reserves of PCBs in lipid tissues, attempts to purge the body of PCBs should not be undertaken. Saunas and nutritional therapies have no proven efficacy.

SUPPORTIVE MEASURES

- In cases of ocular PCB splashes, irrigate with tepid water immediately for at least 15 minutes and follow with ophthalmic evaluation. Remove contaminated clothing and discard properly.
- Gently wash affected skin with soap and warm water for at least 15 minutes.
- Initial treatment of chloracne is based on cessation of exposure, good skin hygiene, and use of dermatologic measures commonly employed for acne vulgaris.
- Serum PCB levels, chloracne, and elevated serum hepatic aminotransferase levels help detect high-risk groups.

Questions—Polyhalogenated Biphenyls

1. Polychlorinated biphenyls
- A. Are naturally present in biologic systems
- B. Do not undergo metabolic degradation
- C. Are magnified in the food chain
- D. Are rarely contaminated by substances that are more toxic
- E. All of the above

2. Polyhalogenated biphenyl exposure
- A. Occurs through lung, skin and gastrointestinal tract absorption
- B. Is marked by chloracne
- C. Results in concentration primarily in fat
- D. Results in half-lives which may be longer than two years
- E. All of the above

3. Acute effects of PCB exposures
- A. Are mild
- B. Are more severe than effects over time from chronic exposure
- C. Are usually skin findings
- D. Usually include tinnitus
- E. None of the above

4. PCBs
- A. Induce the cytochrome P-450 system, so hepatotoxin exposure should be avoided
- B. Are not excreted in breast milk
- C. Do not cross the placenta
- D. Are not carcinogenic
- E. All of the above

5. When treating patients with PCB toxicity,
- A. Serum levels correlate with time and dose of exposure
- B. Serum levels correspond with signs and symptoms
- C. Gut decontamination is contraindicated
- D. Elimination enhancement should be undertaken
- E. None of the above

STYRENE

Styrene was discovered in 1827. By the early 1900s, styrene was recognized as an impurity of industrial processes using coal tar and petroleum cracking. Initially, styrene was used primarily in the synthetic rubber industry, but currently most styrene is consumed in plastics, resin, and paints. Styrene production has grown from 30,000 tons in the 1930s to over 7 million tons in the 1970s.

To date, all commercial uses are based on chemical reactions that polymerize or copolymerize styrene. Styrene production consumes 50% of the world's capacity of benzene which, in the form of ethyl benzene, is the base of styrene manufacturing. Styrene is a mild cutaneous and mucous membrane irritant, and a central nervous system depressant. Recent concern over styrene exposure centers on the association of this compound with neurobehavioral abnormalities.

Pathophysiology

Styrene is a colorless to yellowish, opaque oily liquid. The disagreeable, penetrating odor, which is detectable at 0.1–0.5 ppm, provides good warning properties. Mild olfactory fatigue occurs at high concentrations. Synonyms include vinyl benzene, ethylene, styrol, and cinnemenol.

Pharmacokinetics

ABSORPTION

- The primary route of exposure is the lungs, where up to 60% of inhaled vapors are absorbed.
- Gastrointestinal uptake is rapid and substantial. Appreciable absorption may occur through skin.

DISTRIBUTION

- High intravenous styrene doses are distributed rapidly and evenly among organs in animal models, with only minute amounts present after 24 hours.
- Long-term retention of styrene in body fat stores has been reported in workers.

ELIMINATION

- The kidneys excrete small amounts unchanged in the urine.
- Almost all absorbed styrene is metabolized to mandelic acid (70%) and phenylglyoxylic acid (30%), which are excreted unchanged in the urine.
- Styrene oxide is an active metabolite that has a toxicity rating in animal models several times higher than that of styrene.

Clinical Presentations

The most prevalent acute toxic effects in occupational workers are mucosal irritation and mild central nervous system depression. These depend on concentration and duration of exposure. Workers may develop conjunctivitis, nasal irritation, nausea, drowsiness, lightheadedness, ataxia, loss of memory and coordination. Like other aromatic solvents, the defatting action of styrene produces a contact dermatitis. Liver, kidney, and hematological abnormalities have not been linked to styrene toxicity.

Hydrocarbon pneumonitis is a significant risk after styrene ingestions.

"Styrene sickness," characterized by headache, fatigue, weakness, nausea, anorexia, and depression may occur in the occupational setting. One study associated styrene production workers with a peripheral neuropathy characterized by hypoesthesias and decreased peroneal nerve conduction velocities. Chromosomal abnormalities have been reported in some but not all studies of styrene-exposed workers.

Toxic Dosage/Death

The U.S. standard (8-hour time weighted average) is set at 100 ppm to prevent mucous membrane irritation and central nervous system depression. In one study, exposure to concentrations below 26 ppm did not produce central nervous system symptoms or decreased reaction times. Average concentrations of 200 ppm in occupational exposures produce conjunctivitis. Exposure to 376 ppm causes nasal and mucosal irritation within minutes and headache, nausea, and transient impairment of coordination within an hour.

Pregnancy/Lactation

There is no convincing evidence that links occupational styrene exposure to teratogenicity or spontaneous abortions.

Laboratory

ANALYTIC METHODS
Gas chromatography is the preferred detection method.

BLOOD LEVELS
Urine, not blood levels, is generally utilized to confirm exposure.

URINE
Measures of urinary excretion of mandelic and phenylglyoxylic acids provide the best indicators for evaluating the intensity of styrene exposure. Postshift urine samples containing less than 350 mg phenylglyoxylic acid support styrene exposure levels below 100 ppm.

Treatment

GUT DECONTAMINATION
As in benzene and other hydrocarbon ingestions, the utility of gastric emptying procedures remains controversial. The ingested dose of styrene for which emesis has been recommended is 2–3 mL/kg, similar to that for other nonbenzene aromatic hydrocarbons. For patients at risk of aspiration because of obtundation, intubation should precede lavage and emesis should be avoided. The use of activated charcoal and cathartics is questionable.

ELIMINATION ENHANCEMENT
These methods are generally not employed in the treatment of hydrocarbon ingestions.

SUPPORTIVE MEASURES
- The primary toxic effect to be expected in the acute setting is central nervous system depression and, in exceedingly high doses, pulmonary irritation.
- Removal from the source, and evaluation and support of ventilation are the initial priorities.
- The potential for cardiac arrhythmias exists for organic solvents. Significant severe exposures should have cardiac monitoring. Catecholamines (especially epinephrine) should be used cautiously, if at all.
- Inhaled β-2 selective agonists are the drugs of choice for the treatment of bronchospasm.
- Be sure to remove all contaminated clothing and to wash exposed skin with green soap and water.

Questions—Styrene

1. Styrene exposure
- A. Is primarily through the lungs
- B. Is substantially taken up by the gastrointestinal tract
- C. Is appreciable through skin absorption
- D. Results in long-term retention in body fat stores
- E. All of the above

2. Acute toxic effects of styrene exposure
- A. Depend on duration of exposure but not concentration
- B. Have been linked to liver and kidney function abnormalities
- C. Are primarily mucosal irritation and central nervous system depression
- D. All of the above
- E. None of the above

3. Styrene exposed workers
- A. May suffer headache, fatigue, and weakness
- B. Have become schizophrenic after long term exposure
- C. Often suffer loss of peripheral motor control
- D. Have not been shown to have chromosomal abnormalities
- E. All of the above

4. Styrene exposure
- A. Must be below 376 ppm to prevent central nervous system symptoms
- B. Has been shown to produce mucus membrane irritation at 1000 ppm
- C. Has been shown to produce conjunctivitis at 200 ppm
- D. Has been shown to produce coordination impairment at 200 ppm
- E. Is teratogenic

5. Treatment of patients with styrene toxicity
- A. Should have serum levels tested to evaluate the intensity of exposure
- B. Should have emesis induced if 2–3 ml/kg was ingested
- C. Should be offered elimination enhancement
- D. Should not be exposed to β-2 selective bronchodilators
- E. Should be washed gently with vinegar

TOLUENE

Toluene is an excellent solvent for paints, lacquers, thinners, coatings, and glue, and is a popular replacement for the more chronically toxic benzene. Other industrial applications include feedstock for chemical production (e.g., toluene diisocyanate, phenol, benzene, benzoic acid, nitrotoluene, saccharin) and fuel.

Toluene shares the acute central nervous system depressant effects of benzene and generally has more acute toxicity than benzene in animal models. Current controversy centers on the role of toluene in cognitive and psychomotor dysfunction attributed to chronic organic solvent exposures in jobs such as spray painting. Chronic high-dose exposures seen in toluene abuse (i.e., glue sniffers) have been associated with sudden death secondary to dysrhythmias and conduction disturbances, and hepatic, neurologic and renal disorders.

Pathophysiology

Toluene is an aromatic hydrocarbon produced by the addition of a methyl group to the benzene ring. This structural difference makes toluene more lipid soluble and less volatile than benzene. The exact mechanism of action of toluene is not known, although toluene does inhibit bacterial protein synthesis.

Pharmacokinetics

ABSORPTION

- Most exposures involve inhalation. At rest, the lungs retain about 50% of an inhaled dose.
- Toxic effects in humans can occur via ingestion. Absorption is slow through intact skin.

DISTRIBUTION

- Toluene is highly lipid-soluble and poorly water-soluble.
- Highly preferential distribution to fatty tissue occurs after absorption, with high concentrations reached in the lipid-rich structures of nervous tissue.
- The biological half-life varies from several minutes in highly perfused organs to slightly over one hour in fatty tissue.

ELIMINATION

- The lungs excrete about 18% of an absorbed dose unchanged. Minuscule amounts are eliminated unchanged in the urine.
- About 80% of toluene is metabolized via the cytochrome P-450 system to benzylic alcohol. Alcohol and aldehyde dehydrogenase oxidizes benzylic alcohol to benzoic acid. Conjugation of benzoic acid with glycine produces hippuric acid, which is secreted in the urine.

Clinical Presentations

Acutely, toluene causes predominantly depressing effects. Drowsiness, headache, dizziness, and nausea progress to ataxia, confusion, and staggering gait at concentrations near 800 ppm. Early reports of aplastic anemia and leukemia in toluene exposures are now attributed to benzene contamination. Blood dyscrasias resulting from pure toluene exposures have not been reported. Toluene is not a proven carcinogen and is not mutagenic in animal models. Respiratory symptoms are usually minimal.

NEUROLOGIC EFFECTS

Case studies of long-term toluene inhalant abusers (see Chapter 45, Airborne Toxins) describe permanent cerebellar ataxia, encephalopathy manifested by ataxia, tremors, emotional lability, mental status changes, and recurrent headaches with personality changes. Although peripheral neuropathies have been reported in glue sniffers, n-hexane probably accounted for the neurotoxicity. No evidence of impaired nerve conduction and few clinical signs of peripheral neuropathy were apparent in an epidemiological study of workers exposed to toluene and paint solvents.

RENAL EFFECTS

Distal renal tubular acidosis, high anion gap acidosis, hypokalemia, hematuria, proteinuria, and pyuria have been reported in glue sniffers, but the changes usually are reversible. Epidemiological reports have suggested a link between hydrocarbon solvents and proliferative glomerulonephritis (i.e., Goodpasture's syndrome), but toluene has not been directly implicated.

CARDIOVASCULAR EFFECTS

Glue sniffers are subject to sudden death perhaps because of the potential of volatile hydrocarbons to sensitize the myocardium to the arrhythmogenic action of endogenous catecholamines. Animal models show that toluene impairs conduction and myocardial contractility, and one case study documented a profound bradycardia during the initial period of hospitalization after glue sniffing.

DERMATOLOGIC EFFECTS

The highly lipophilic nature of toluene degreases skin, leading to a contact dermatitis with prolonged exposure.

Toxic Dosage/Death

Brief exposure to 100 ppm causes statistical impairment of psychomotor and perceptual performance, suggesting central nervous system dysfunction. Exposure to 500–800 ppm causes headache, drowsiness, nausea, fatigue, weakness, and confusion. Exposure to 800 ppm causes severe fatigue, convulsions, ataxia, and staggering gait that may persist for several days, whereas exposure to 10,000–30,000 ppm has been estimated to produce anesthesia within 1 minute.

Drug Interactions

High doses of n-hexane, methylene chloride, benzene, styrene, and trichloroethylene inhibit toluene biotransformation in animal studies.

Pregnancy/Lactation

No data are available on placental transfer of toluene.

Laboratory

ANALYTIC METHODS

Thin-layer chromatography can separate urinary hippuric, mandelic, and phenylglyoxylic acids after mixed toluene and styrene exposures. High-performance liquid chromatographic methods detect urine hippuric acid and o-cresol levels of 0.05 mg/mL and 0.05 μg/mL, respectively.

BLOOD LEVELS

Blood levels are not routinely helpful in overdose.

URINE

Twenty-four-hour urine collection for toluene metabolites correlates with toluene exposure and toluene blood concentrations. Hippuric acid is a normal constituent of urine therefore amounts of hippuric acid in the urine vary tremendously between patients.

Treatment

GUT DECONTAMINATION

As in benzene and other hydrocarbon ingestions, the utility of gastric emptying procedures remains controversial. The ingested dose of toluene for which emesis has been recommended is 1–2 mL/kg. For patients at risk of aspiration because of obtundation, intubation should precede lavage and emesis should be avoided. The use of activated charcoal and cathartics is questionable.

ELIMINATION ENHANCEMENT

These methods are generally not employed in the treatment of hydrocarbon ingestions.

SUPPORTIVE MEASURES

- Management is supportive, similar to that for inhalation exposures in patients who sniff glue.
- See the Introduction section under Petroleum Distillates above for treatment guidelines of hydrocarbon aspiration.

Questions—Toluene

1. **Toluene exposure**
   A. Through intact skin results in rapid absorption
   B. Is toxic from inhalation but not ingestion
   C. Results in high concentrations in nervous tissue
   D. Is ultimately dealt with via urinary excretion
   E. None of the above
2. **Clinical symptoms to toluene exposure include**
   A. Central nervous system depression
   B. Blood dyscrasias
   C. Cancer
   D. Severe respiratory symptoms
   E. All of the above
3. **All of the following neurologic effects can be due to toluene exposure except**
   A. Cerebellar ataxia
   B. Tremors
   C. Emotional lability
   D. Recurrent headaches
   E. Central nervous system tumors
4. **The following statements about toluene exposure are true except**
   A. Brief exposure to 100 ppm impairs psychomotor and perceptual performance.
   B. Exposure to 500–800 ppm causes headache, drowsiness and confusion.
   C. Exposure to below 500 ppm causes seizures.
   D. Exposure to over 800 ppm causes symptoms that may persist for days.
   E. Exposure to over 10,000 ppm may produce brief anesthesia.
5. **Treatment of toluene-exposed patients**
   A. Depends on serum blood levels
   B. Depends on urine hippuric acid levels
   C. Requires elimination enhancement
   D. Is unlike treatment for other hydrocarbon aspirations
   E. None of the above

XYLENE

Xylene is a widely used aromatic hydrocarbon. Industrial applications include its use as a solvent, cleaning agent and degreaser, and as an aviation fuel. Xylene is a starting material and intermediate for a variety of chemical processes such as the production of phthalic acids used for the manufacture of synthetic fibers, plastics, and enamel.

Pathophysiology

Xylene is an organic solvent produced by the addition of two methyl groups to a benzene nucleus during the distillation of coal tar and petroleum products.

Pharmacokinetics

ABSORPTION

- Pulmonary absorption is rapid, with about 60–65% of a xylene dose retained at rest.
- Absorption through the gastrointestinal tract is also significant. Liquid xylene may be absorbed through intact skin.

DISTRIBUTION

- Studies in animals show that after chronic inhalation, the highest concentrations occur in the adrenal gland, bone marrow, spleen, brain, and blood, respectively.

ELIMINATION

- The lungs excrete only 3–6% of an absorbed xylene dose unchanged. Most of the remainder undergoes oxidative biotransformation to methylbenzoic (toluic) acids.
- Toluic acids are conjugated with glycine and excreted in the urine as methylhippuric acids.
- The half-life of xylene is four hours.

Clinical Presentations

Xylene is a central nervous system depressant that produces lightheadedness, nausea, headache, and ataxia at low doses and confusion, respiratory depression, and coma at high doses. Above 200 ppm, xylene causes conjunctivitis, nasal irritation, and sore throat. It is a potent respiratory irritant at high concentrations. Like other organic solvents, xylene produces a defatting dermatitis with prolonged cutaneous exposure. Transient mildly elevated hepatic aminotransferase levels and reversible renal failure have been reported after large xylene exposures. Hematologic abnormalities reported among organic solvent workers probably occur from benzene contamination.

Toxic Dosage/Death

Studies in animals suggest that xylene is more toxic acutely than benzene and perhaps toluene, but confirmation in humans is limited by mucosal irritant properties present at concentrations over 200 ppm.

Drug Interactions

When consumed before exposure, ethanol decreases the metabolic clearance of xylene by approximately one-half.

Laboratory

ANALYTIC METHODS

Xylene is measured by high-performance liquid chromatography.

BLOOD LEVELS

Rapid xylene clearance from blood (the plasma half-life is four hours) prevents adequate biological monitoring of serum samples.

URINE

Methyl hippuric acid concentrations may be measured in 24-hour urine collections to confirm exposure to xylene.

Treatment

GUT DECONTAMINATION

When seen within two hours of exposure, patients who have ingested large amounts (over 1–2 mL/kg) may benefit from emesis induction if alert. If obtunded, intubation followed by lavage is suggested. Xylene, like other hydrocarbons, may cause severe aspiration pneumonitis. All patients must be directly observed and properly positioned to minimize the risk of aspiration. The use of charcoal and cathartics for xylene ingestion is equivocal.

ELIMINATION ENHANCEMENT

These methods are generally not employed in the treatment of hydrocarbon ingestions.

SUPPORTIVE MEASURES

- Since xylene is a central nervous system depressant, initial attention should be directed toward evaluation and support of ventilation, with oxygen and intubation provided as needed.
- Cardiac monitoring is advisable because of the possibility of cardiac dysrhythmias. Hospitalized patients should receive a complete blood count, liver function tests, and a serum creatinine level.
- Most exposures are either casual contacts in children or mild inhalation exposures in workers. These patients usually respond to removal and supportive care.
- Contaminated clothes should be removed and exposed skin washed with green soap and water.

Questions—Xylene

1. With chronic xylene inhalation, the highest concentration appears to occur in the
   A. Adrenal gland
   B. Bone marrow
   C. Spleen
   D. Brain
   E. Blood

2. Xylene toxicity includes all of the following except
   A. Conjunctivitis
   B. Pharyngitis
   C. Dermatitis
   D. Hepatitis
   E. Cellulitis

3. When treating patients with xylene exposure,
   A. Serum levels are helpful due to xylene's long half-life.
   B. Urine collection of methyl hippuric acid confirms exposure.
   C. Emesis should be induced regardless of the time since ingestion.
   D. Elimination enhancement is standard treatment.
   E. No baseline serum values should be checked.

HALOGENATED HYDROCARBONS

INTRODUCTION

Halogenated hydrocarbons have numerous uses. Paradichlorobenzene is a common ingredient in mothballs, and hexachlorophene is an antiseptic. See Chapter 38, Household Products. Halothane is a commonly used anesthetic gas (see Chapter 43, Anesthetic Agents), and methylene chloride is used as a degreaser and paint remover (see the Carbon Monoxide section in Chapter 45, Airborne Toxins). Numerous other halogenated hydrocarbons are used in the dry cleaning industry, as fumigants, and as solvents.

Pathophysiology

Most halogenated hydrocarbons are clear and colorless liquids that have chloroform-like odors. Most contain impurities such as other chlorinated hydrocarbons. Some, such as carbon tetrachloride, are profound hepatotoxins. All are central nervous system depressants to various degrees. These agents are also capable of myocardial sensitization, perhaps via the release of endogenous catecholamines.

Pharmacokinetics

ABSORPTION

- The pulmonary route is the primary source of toxic exposure to the halogenated hydrocarbons.
- Oral absorption is rapid but less complete than pulmonary absorption.
- Insignificant amounts are absorbed through the skin.

DISTRIBUTION

- Peak blood levels occur soon after inhalation, but peak levels after oral use occur in 1–2 hours.
- Distribution is highest in fat, brain, and blood.

ELIMINATION

- Halogenated hydrocarbons are metabolized in the liver by the cytochrome P-450 system.
- Partial glutathione conjugation may occur.
- Halogenated solvents are also excreted through the lungs.

Clinical Presentations

NEUROLOGIC EFFECTS

Inhalation of halogenated hydrocarbons generally induces central nervous system depression within minutes. Alterations in psychomotor performance occur. Cranial neuropathies have been observed.

GASTROINTESTINAL EFFECTS

Hepatotoxicity and gastrointestinal irritation may occur after significant exposures. Hepatorenal failure beginning a few days after exposure, and deaths have occurred. Centrilobular hepatic necrosis may be observed.

DERMATOLOGIC EFFECTS

"Degreaser's flush" may result from ethanol-induced vasodilation of superficial skin vessels. This typically resolves in about one hour.

RENAL EFFECTS

Halogenated solvents are weakly nephrotoxic. Several anecdotal studies have suggested that a relation may exist between exposure to occupational organic solvents and diseases of the kidney—(particularly malignancy and glomerulonephritis). Definite associations are controversial.

CARDIOVASCULAR EFFECTS

Hypotension and arrhythmias may be seen after halogenated hydrocarbon exposures.

PULMONARY EFFECTS

Upper respiratory tract irritation is common after inhalation. Little alveolar damage is usually observed; however, profound pneumonitis may occur after aspiration.

CARCINOGENIC EFFECTS

Suspected carcinogens include tetrachloromethane, 1-2, dichloroethane, dichloromethane, tetrachloroethylene, and trichloromethane. However, additional studies are required.

PAINTER'S SYNDROME

Headaches, fatigue, difficulties in concentrating, problems with short-term memory, irritability, depression, and alcohol intolerance characterize this syndrome. It has been classified as an occupational disease and has been a cause of premature retirement in Scandinavian countries. Inattention to compounding variables may have led to the erroneous conclusion that chronic solvent exposure causes organic damage to the central nervous system.

Drug Interactions

At least one prospective, case-referred study has suggested that occupational solvent exposure plus alcohol intake may be an important cause of organic brain damage.

Pregnancy/Lactation

Halogenated solvents cross the placenta and may be found in the fetus. No halogenated solvents have been definitively associated with teratogenicity, however.

Laboratory

ANALYTIC METHODS

Gas chromatography with electron capture can be used to determine the concentration of halogenated solvents in biologic samples.

BLOOD LEVELS

While blood levels may confirm exposure to these agents, following concentrations after overdose, misuse, or abuse does not guide therapeutic interventions.

Treatment

GUT DECONTAMINATION

Like other hydrocarbons, the risk of chemical pneumonitis secondary to aspiration is great. Gut decontamination procedures, such as lavage with protected airway, are only recommended in rare cases of large ingestions which have occurred recently. Emesis is contraindicated. Data to support these interventions are controversial and limited. Charcoal use is equivocal, but may be helpful in cases involving additives or polysubstance ingestions.

ELIMINATION ENHANCEMENT

Hemodialysis or hemoperfusion is not likely to remove halogenated hydrocarbons because of the high lipophilic properties of these solvents. Hyperbaric oxygen is experimental.

SUPPORTIVE MEASURES

- Treatment is largely supportive. Watch for cardiac dysrhythmias, aspiration pneumonitis, hepatotoxicity, and hypoxic encephalopathy. Administer oxygen if there is evidence of altered mental status or dyspnea.
- Monitor for arrhythmias for at least 24 hours. Monitor for hepatorenal failure for at least three days after significant exposures. Obtain a chest x-ray, arterial blood gas, electrocardiogram, serum creatinine, and hepatic aminotransferases. Check electrolyte imbalance daily.
- Profound, rare renal failure secondary to these agents may require dialysis.
- Hepatotoxicity, occasionally associated with hepatorenal failure, may be indicated by elevated serum hepatic aminotransferase, bilirubin, alkaline phosphatase, ammonia, creatinine, and lactate levels. In addition, prolonged prothrombin time and hypoglycemia may be seen. Hepatic failure may require fresh frozen plasma, vitamin K, a low-protein diet, neomycin, and lactulose.
- Treat hypotension with volume expansion and pressors as necessary. Avoid epinephrine if possible. Use lidocaine or β-blockers for ventricular arrhythmias.
- Remove all contaminated clothing and wash exposed areas with soap and copious water.
- Ocular exposures require irrigation for 15–20 minutes. Obtain consultation if symptoms persist.

Antidotes

N-acetylcysteine may restore depleted glutathione stores in certain cases, however no adequate clinical studies are available to validate this possible treatment.

Questions—Introduction to Halogenated Hydrocarbons

1. The primary source of toxic exposure to halogenated hydrocarbons is
   A. The oral route
   B. The dermal route
   C. The pulmonary route
   D. The intravenous route
   E. None of the above

2. Painter's syndrome
   A. Is classified as an occupational disease
   B. Has primarily pulmonary symptoms
   C. Is thought to be due to chronic solvent exposure
   D. A and B
   E. A and C

3. "Degreaser's flush," from ethanol-induced vasodilation of superficial skin vessels, typically resolves over six hours.
   A. True
   B. False

CARBON TETRACHLORIDE

Carbon tetrachloride is a well-known hepatotoxin whose use has largely been replaced by less toxic solvents such as methylchloroform, perchloroethylene, and trichloroethylene. The FDA has banned the use of carbon tetrachloride in all products except where it is an unavoidable byproduct. Exposure is now limited to industry where it is used in the production of solvents, aerosol propellants, and refrigerants.

Early applications included its use as a waterless hair shampoo, as an antihelminthic for hookworm, and as an anesthetic. By the 1930s, carbon tetrachloride was widely used as a dry cleaning agent and constituent of fire extinguishers. The recognition of fatalities resulting from the thermal decomposition of carbon tetrachloride to phosgene led to the banning of carbon tetrachloride in fire extinguishers by the early 1960s. Industrial use of carbon tetrachloride as a cleaning agent began declining in the 1950s as toxicity and fatalities became well known.

Pathophysiology

Carbon tetrachloride causes acute fatty degeneration of the liver. The formation and release of low-density lipoproteins are significantly blocked, resulting in the rapid accumulation of fat. A classic yellow fatty liver picture characterizes histologic changes with discrete damage concentrated in the midzonal and centrilobular regions. Although the exact mechanism of hepatic necrosis has not been entirely elucidated, cleavage of the carbon-chlorine bond produces trichloromethyl and monoatomic chlorine-free radicals that lead to lipid peroxidation. Energy processes and protein synthesis in the endoplasmic reticulum subsequently are disrupted.

Pathologically, carbon tetrachloride also produces acute tubular necrosis affecting primarily the proximal tubules and the loop of Henle. Patchy pontine necrosis and demyelination, Purkinje cell damage, cerebellar venous thrombosis, and hemorrhagic infarcts have been identified in several autopsy cases. Such postmortem results suggest that the cerebellum is particularly vulnerable to carbon tetrachloride toxicity.

Pharmacokinetics

ABSORPTION

- Carbon tetrachloride is well absorbed by the lungs and gastrointestinal tract.
- Percutaneous absorption also occurs.

DISTRIBUTION

- Studies in animals indicate that carbon tetrachloride is concentrated in fat.
- Inhalation produces higher levels in liver and kidney than in blood.

ELIMINATION

- The lungs excrete 50–80% of an absorbed dose unchanged. A small part is expired by the lungs or excreted into the urine as carbon dioxide. The remainder is metabolized.
- Formation of free radicals may cause lipid peroxidation and subsequent hepatocellular damage. Chloroform is a recognized metabolite.
- Carbon tetrachloride persists in expired air with an elimination half-life of 9.4 hours after inhalation by rats, and detectable levels remain for 18 days after acute oral exposures.

Clinical Presentations

NEUROLOGIC EFFECTS

Acute exposures present initially with central nervous system depression followed by the development of hepatic and renal dysfunction. Early symptoms include headache, lightheadedness, weakness, blurred vision, ataxia, and depressed levels of consciousness depending on the duration and magnitude of exposure. Immediate fatalities result either from respiratory depression or from dysrhythmias caused by catecholamine sensitization. Visual abnormalities include bilateral visual field constriction, optic atrophy, and amblyopia. Patients may develop tonic-clonic seizures during the initial 24 hours. Toxic effects may resemble encephalitis, with pyramidal tract signs, posterior column deficits (loss of vibration), changes in mentation, and ataxia.

GASTROINTESTINAL EFFECTS

Although hepatic enzymes often rise on the first day, and nonspecific gastrointestinal symptoms may be present, clinical evidence of hepatic disease (i.e., liver tenderness and enlargement, jaundice, dark urine, clay-colored stools) usually does not appear for 2–4 days. Gastrointestinal symptoms may appear with the development of hepatotoxicity. Fever and diarrhea commonly occur after the first day. Liver dysfunction reaches a maximum within three days of exposure, with death from hepatic failure generally occurring within a week. Recovery usually is complete with no long-term sequelae; however, chronic exposure has been associated with cirrhosis. Gastrointestinal or other bleeding may result from the decreased production of clotting factors.

RENAL EFFECTS

Renal disease may appear in the absence of hepatotoxicity. Anuria commonly occurs within three days, with a range of 1–7 days, and may last 15 days. Recovery is usually complete.

DERMATOLOGIC EFFECTS

Like other solvents, carbon tetrachloride can produce a defatting dermatitis characterized by erythema, fissures, and desquamation.

CARCINOGENIC EFFECTS

Relatively small doses of carbon tetrachloride produce hepatocellular carcinoma in hamsters and hepatomas in mice and rats. Data on humans are inadequate to link carbon tetrachloride to liver cancer, but carbon tetrachloride may be a potential carcinogen.

Toxic Dosage/Death

Carbon tetrachloride is a central nervous system depressant that may produce effects at about 150–300 ppm. Headache, dizziness, and drowsiness appear near 2,000 ppm after an exposure of 5–10 minutes. Paresthesias, weakness, slurred speech, and stupor develop within several minutes of exposure to 10,000 ppm. Fatalities occur at concentrations of 20,000 ppm. The estimated fatal adult oral dose is 90–100 mL, but wide variability results from ingestion, and as little as 5–10 mL has been reported to cause death.

Drug Interactions

Aliphatic alcohols including methanol, ethanol, and isopropanol increase carbon tetrachloride hepatorenal toxicity, perhaps by mechanisms that include enzyme induction. Alcoholics appear particularly susceptible to the central nervous system effects of carbon tetrachloride.

Pregnancy/Lactation

Carbon tetrachloride is fetotoxic and teratogenic, and exposure by pregnant individuals should be avoided.

Laboratory

ANALYTIC METHODS

Gas chromatographic analysis accurately and specifically detects carbon tetrachloride.

BLOOD LEVELS

Blood levels are not well correlated with clinical effects.

Treatment

GUT DECONTAMINATION

See the general recommendations in the Introduction section for Halogenated Hydrocarbons above. Since carbon tetrachloride can be absorbed through the skin, all contaminated clothing should be removed and the skin washed with green soap and water.

ELIMINATION ENHANCEMENT

Although hemodialysis has been used in several cases, a lack of pharmacokinetic data restricts our understanding of the usefulness of hemodialysis in eliminating carbon tetrachloride. Carbon tetrachloride apparently is not well removed by hemodialysis. Although case studies have reported the successful use of hyperbaric oxygen (HBO) in treating overdose cases of carbon tetrachloride, the use of HBO in this setting remains experimental.

SUPPORTIVE MEASURES

- Respiratory depression and cardiac dysrhythmias are immediate threats to life. Quick initial evaluation of the adequacy of breathing and circulation should be made.
- Since a major fraction of absorbed carbon tetrachloride is exhaled within the first hour, good tidal volumes should be maintained in severely poisoned patients.
- In serious cases, hepatic aminotransferase levels are usually elevated within the first day. The extent of elevation correlates with severity, and tends to reach a maximum by the third day.
- In cases of renal toxicity, hematuria and proteinuria usually appear before the onset of oliguria.
- Laboratory workup after carbon tetrachloride exposure should include a complete blood count, liver function tests including serum bilirubin and calcium, hepatic aminotransferase levels and prothrombin time, serum creatinine, and urinalysis.
- Patients should be followed daily within the first week for the development of hepatic or renal failure. Patients with abnormal prothrombin times should be followed daily with serial hematocrits and stool guaiacs for the development of gastrointestinal bleeding.

Antidotes

Since reactive metabolites may cause hepatorenal toxicity, intravenous administration of N-acetyl-L-cysteine may reduce complications. Experience with this therapy is limited and investigational but suggests a positive effect. A dosage schedule identical to that for acetaminophen is used, but prolonged therapy may be necessary because of the persistence of carbon tetrachloride.

Questions—Carbon Tetrachloride

1. Carbon tetrachloride is now banned from fire extinguishers.
A. True
B. False

2. Immediate fatalities from carbon tetrachloride exposure result from
A. Respiratory depression
B. Dysrhythmias
C. Liver failure
D. A and B
E. A and C

3. All of the following statements regarding gastrointestinal disease due to carbon tetrachloride exposure are true except
A. Hepatic enzymes often rise on the first day.
B. Clinical evidence of hepatic disease (e.g., liver tenderness) usually develops on the first day.
C. Liver dysfunction reaches a maximum within three days of exposure.
D. Death from hepatic failure generally occurs within a week.
E. Recovery from hepatic dysfunction is usually complete.

CHLOROFORM

Chloroform was first used as a human anesthetic in 1847. It is a potent central nervous system depressant whose use has been limited by its hepatotoxicity and propensity to cause cardiac arrest in high concentrations. Like most chlorinated hydrocarbons, chloroform sensitizes the myocardium to endogenous catecholamines. Chloroform produces a fatty infiltration and necrosis of the liver similarly to carbon tetrachloride, but is a less potent hepatotoxin. Although still used as a solvent, extractant, and chemical intermediary, chloroform has been restricted by the FDA's 1976 ban on chloroform in food, drugs, and cosmetics.

Pathophysiology

This clear, colorless, nonflammable liquid is highly volatile with a sweet odor detectable around 200–300 ppm. Thermal degradation of chloroform produces hydrochloric acid, phosgene, and chlorine, which are potent pulmonary toxins.

Pharmacokinetics

ABSORPTION

- The lungs and gastrointestinal tract rapidly absorb chloroform, with peak blood concentration developing one hour after ingestion.
- Skin absorption occurs but is not extensive enough to produce acute toxicity except after prolonged exposure to damaged skin.

DISTRIBUTION

- Volume of distribution is 2.6 L/Kg.

ELIMINATION

- Considerable species, dose, and individual variation occur. Elimination is mostly expired by the lungs within eight hours. The half-life is 1.5 hours.
- Metabolism of chloroform yields carbon dioxide. Cytochrome P-450 enzymes appear to dechlorinate chloroform to trichloromethanol, which spontaneously dehydrochlorinates to phosgene. Phosgene can react with water to form carbon dioxide or bind to cellular macromolecules.
- Unlike carbon tetrachloride, chloroform does not cause lipid peroxidation, and hepatotoxicity probably results from the covalent binding of toxic intermediates.

Clinical Presentations

NEUROLOGIC EFFECTS

Chloroform is a potent central nervous system depressant that produces symptoms ranging from nausea, lightheadedness, headache, and malaise, to stupor and coma. Central nervous system symptoms appear soon after exposure. Mental status symptoms usually clear by 24 hours, although ingestions complicated by coingestion of ethanol have required mechanical ventilation for three days. Gait instability and slight tremor on finger-to-nose testing have been reported, but signs typically clear in two weeks.

GASTROINTESTINAL EFFECTS

Hepatotoxicity may occur after significant exposures, with elevations of liver function tests typically reaching their peaks in 3–4 days. Permanent sequelae are rare, with levels of hepatic aminotransferase enzymes returning to normal within 6–8 weeks. Prothrombin and hepatic aminotransferase levels usually increase more than serum bilirubin and alkaline phosphatase levels. Chronic industrial exposures may produce gastrointestinal upset and nonspecific symptoms such as dry mouth and malaise, but not hepatotoxicity.

RENAL EFFECTS

Renal damage may develop within 24–48 hours of exposure and is characterized by proteinuria, hematuria, and cellular casts.

PULMONARY EFFECTS

A chemical pneumonitis, resulting from intravenous injection of chloroform, reportedly peaked in three days without requiring intubation. A chemical pneumonitis may follow aspiration of chloroform after ingestion.

CARCINOGENIC EFFECTS

Clinical data have not confirmed the carcinogenic potential of chloroform in humans, although data in animals are sufficient to conclude that chloroform may reasonably be anticipated to be carcinogenic.

Toxic Dosage/Death

Effects such as vertigo and nausea appear at about 1,000–2,000 ppm after ten minutes. Narcosis results from 30–60 minute-exposures to 15,000 ppm. Fatalities typically occur after exposure to 25,000 ppm for 5–10 minutes. Thirty milliliters of ingested chloroform has been suggested as the minimal lethal adult dose, but survival after hepatorenal failure occurred after ingestion of 120 mL.

Drug Interactions

Enzyme inducers such as phenobarbital increase animal hepatotoxicity, and chloroform metabolism appears to deplete hepatic glutathione stores.

Pregnancy/Lactation

Chloroform may be embryotoxic and is known to cross the placenta. There is some evidence that chloroform is mutagenic and carcinogenic.

Treatment

GUT DECONTAMINATION

Emesis is contraindicated as obtundation may occur. The usual measures of decontamination may be helpful; however, data are inadequate to evaluate their efficacy.

ELIMINATION ENHANCEMENT

Hemodialysis has been favorably used in at least one case. However, clinical data on its efficacy are mostly lacking. Renal failure may require dialysis.

SUPPORTIVE MEASURES

- Supportive care is the mainstay of treatment. As with other chlorinated hydrocarbons, cardiac dysrhythmias and respiratory depression are immediate life-threatening complications. Initial attention should be directed toward maintenance of breathing and circulation, with intubation, ventilation, intravenous lines, and cardiac monitoring instituted as indicated.
- Fresh-frozen plasma, vitamin K, a low-protein diet, neomycin, lactulose, and careful fluid and electrolyte balance may be necessary if liver necrosis occurs.
- Significant exposures should be screened for hematopoietic (complete blood count, serum haptoglobin, urinary hemoglobin), renal (urinalysis, serum creatinine), hepatic (hepatic aminotransferases, bilirubin, prothrombin time), and pulmonary (chest x-ray, arterial blood gases) changes as indicated from physical examination.
- It is recommended that renal and hepatic function be followed daily for at least three days.

Antidotes

Although no antidotes have been used effectively, the depletion of glutathione stores suggests that N-acetylcysteine may be effective in overdose. No significant clinical data are available to support its use, however.

Questions—Chloroform

1. **Chloroform is a more potent hepatotoxin than carbon tetrachloride.**
   A. True
   B. False
2. **Chloroform has been banned as a solvent.**
   A. True
   B. False
3. **All of the following may follow chloroform exposure except**
   A. Lightheadedness and headache
   B. Hepatotoxicity

C. Carditis
D. Renal damage
E. Pneumonitis

ETHYLENE DIBROMIDE

Ethylene dibromide (EDB) has been used as a lead scavenger in fuel (similar to ethylene dichloride) and as a soil fumigant. Acute toxicity usually involves cutaneous or mucous membrane irritation and/or gastrointestinal symptoms. At least four fatalities have been attributed to EDB exposure because of intractable metabolic acidosis and hepatorenal failure. Public health concerns centered on the fact that EDB is a potent animal carcinogen. Therefore, the U.S. Environmental Protection Agency banned the use of EDB as a soil fumigant and pesticide and by March 1984, the use of EDB on domestically grown fruits had ceased.

Pathophysiology

EDB is a halogenated hydrocarbon with cardiotoxic and hepatotoxic properties.

Pharmacokinetics

ABSORPTION

- Toxic effects occur after inhalation, skin, and oral exposures.

DISTRIBUTION

- EDB is well adsorbed by wheat products, but during cooking, heat decomposes most EDB to ethylene glycol and inorganic bromide.

ELIMINATION

- Glutathione derivatives are assumed intermediate products of EDB metabolism.
- A carcinogenic metabolite has not been unequivocally identified. However, 2-bromoethanol and bromoacetylaldehyde are suspected carcinogens.

Clinical Presentations

Mild exposure causes headache, nausea, vomiting, abdominal pain, and diarrhea without pulmonary or cardiac problems. EDB is a mucous membrane and cutaneous irritant that produces conjunctival erythema, corneal abrasions, and first- and second-degree chemical burns. Severe exposures produce extensive and generalized necrosis of the heart, skeletal muscle, liver, and kidney which leads to progressive metabolic acidosis, as well as cardiac, renal, and hepatic failure over a course of 12–64 hours. Autopsies reveal extensive putrefaction of the skin and internal organs. Although EDB is considered a central nervous system depressant, exposure to high levels is required to impair consciousness.

EDB is carcinogenic in rats. Epidemiological studies of cancer in humans are inconclusive because of small control groups, inadequate observation periods in relationship to expected latency periods, and incomplete exposure data. A retrospective mortality study of 164 workers exposed to EDB at two plants failed to demonstrate increased mortality.

Toxic Dosage/Death

An intentional ingestion of 140 mg/kg caused the death of a 43-year-old woman. Extensive dermal contact with 0.1% EDB solution for 20–60 minutes produced acute hepatorenal failure and fatal metabolic acidosis.

Laboratory

ANALYTIC METHODS

Serum bromides may be measured via a colorimetric method.

BLOOD LEVELS

Serum bromides are elevated initially and remain elevated for an extended period. Following their concentration does not help guide management of EDB in overdose. In one fatal case, the presenting bromide level was 380 mg/L and the autopsy bromide level 64 hours later was 136 mg/L (normal, 4 mg/L).

Treatment

GUT DECONTAMINATION

Acute ingestions of EDB are rare. The use of lavage and/or activated charcoal may be helpful with the usual dosages and contraindications; however, there are no documented studies to absolutely justify their use.

ELIMINATION ENHANCEMENT

Hemodialysis has been used to correct electrolyte imbalance and renal failure in a severe exposure, but the patient died.

SUPPORTIVE MEASURES

- Victims must be removed from the scene with caution, and an appropriate self-contained breathing apparatus must be used since inappropriately protected rescuers have succumbed to EDB toxicity.
- Exposed attending personnel should be properly gloved and gowned. The exposed individual is rinsed with cold water and washed with mild soap, including nail beds, hair, and skin folds. Washing is then repeated. These measures are critical in severe exposures to reduce the amount of cutaneous EDB absorption.
- Victims may require ventilatory support.
- Elevated levels of serum uric acid, skeletal muscle enzymes (creatine kinase, aldolase), hepatic aminotransferases (lactic dehydrogenase, aspartate aminotransferase), and creatinine have been reported in severely exposed patients who develop hepatorenal failure.
- Intractable metabolic acidosis occurs in fatal cases, but the anion gap calculations must be interpreted with caution because bromides may falsely elevate chloride concentration.

Antidotes

No antidote has been shown effective. Dimercaprol (BAL in Oil) has been suggested as an antidote because of the structural similarity of EDB to methyl bromide, but dimercaprol use is questionable even for methyl bromide.

Questions—Ethylene Dibromide

1. Acute EDB toxicity may include
A. Cutaneous irritation
B. Mucous membrane irritation
C. Gastrointestinal symptoms
D. All of the above
E. None of the above

2. Serum bromide levels
A. Help guide management in overdose
B. Remain elevated over an extended period
C. Are measured via colorimetric methods
D. A and B
E. B and C

3. Dimercaprol (BAL in Oil) is an effective antidote for ethylene dibromide poisoning.
A. True
B. False

ETHYLENE DICHLORIDE

Ethylene dichloride (EDC) is produced primarily for the manufacture of vinyl chloride monomer, a precursor of polyvinyl chloride (PVC) plastic. EDC is a chemical intermediate in the production of solvents (e.g., methylchloroform) and fluorocarbons (i.e., Freon compounds). It has been replaced as a solvent and degreaser by less toxic compounds. EDC is an effective lead scavenger in gasoline, but decreasing consumption of leaded gasoline limits this application.

Pathophysiology

EDC is a colorless, oily liquid with a pleasant, chloroform-like odor and a sweet taste. Although olfactory warning properties are limited by the development of tolerance, this flammable, highly volatile liquid has an odor detectable between 6 and 40 ppm. Like other halogenated hydrocarbons, it acts as a central nervous system depressant, and may sensitize the myocardium.

Clinical Presentations

EDC is a central nervous system depressant that produces symptoms ranging from nausea, vomiting, headache, lightheadedness, and weakness to stupor, dysequilibrium, coma, and respiratory arrest. In severe cases, central nervous system signs appear within several hours of exposure and are followed by a quiescent period. On the second day, oliguria and increased hepatic transaminases may develop. Over the next several days, hepatorenal failure can occur.

Severe ingestions produce widespread organ damage (especially kidney, liver, and adrenal gland) as well as gastrointestinal bleeding. Hepatic and renal effects may accompany massive midzonal hepatic necrosis, acute tubular necrosis, hypoglycemia, hypercalcemia, hypoprothrombinemia, reduced clotting factors, adrenal necrosis, and gastrointestinal hemorrhage. Heavy exposure produces a bluish purple discoloration of the skin, dermatitis, and corneal abrasions. Epidemiological data in humans are inadequate to link EDC in the workplace to cancer.

Toxic Dosage/Death

An ingestion of approximately 15 mL by a 14-year-old boy resulted in fatal hepatorenal failure. EDC should be considered one of the more toxic chlorinated hydrocarbons.

Pregnancy/Lactation

Fetal cardiac defects have been noted after maternal exposure to contaminated water.

Treatment

GUT DECONTAMINATION

Since ethylene dichloride is a potent hepatorenal toxin, all except minor exposures seen within four hours of ingestion should be treated with lavage and/or charcoal, although proof that these methods are helpful is largely lacking in the literature.

ELIMINATION ENHANCEMENT

Hemodialysis is reserved for renal failure.

SUPPORTIVE MEASURES

- As with most chlorinated hydrocarbons, the immediate life-threatening complications are respiratory arrest and cardiac dysrhythmias.
- Initial attention should be directed toward establishing an airway, providing ventilation, and improving circulation as dictated by the clinical situation.
- Contaminated clothes should be removed and exposed skin washed with green soap and water.
- Severe cases require close monitoring of clotting times, serum glucose and calcium levels, as well as hepatic and renal function.

Questions—Ethylene Dichloride

1. Ethylene dichloride causes all of the following symptoms except
A. Central nervous system excitement
B. Hepatorenal failure
C. Gastrointestinal bleeding
D. Skin discoloration
E. Metabolic derangements

METHYL BROMIDE

This simple compound is an inexpensive insect fumigant for soil, grain, fruits, and warehouses. Used commercially, methyl bromide is a chemical intermediate and methylating agent. Less toxic agents have replaced it as a refrigerant and fire extinguisher constituent. Acute, resistant convulsions and severe, permanent mental and neurologic damage characterize methyl bromide intoxication. Supportive treatment is the mainstay of management. See Chapter 48, Pesticides.

Methyl bromide has poor olfactory warning properties which contribute to its toxicity. Fatalities have occurred during the application process, after cleanup operations, and after premature entry into fumigated houses. Methyl bromide is an eye, skin, and mucous membrane irritant that can produce pulmonary edema and coma in high doses. Chronic exposure has been associated with peripheral neuropathies, ataxia, behavioral changes, and mild hepatic and renal dysfunction.

Pathophysiology

Methyl bromide is a delayed pulmonary irritant which, on hydrolysis, produces methanol and hydrobromic acid. Metabolism to methanol may contribute to neurologic and visual changes, although methylation of sulfhydryl groups in vital enzymes is the favored mechanism of action.

Pharmacokinetics

ABSORPTION

- Ready absorption through the lungs provides the usual route of toxicity.

DISTRIBUTION

- Cutaneous absorption occurs but systemic toxicity is usually not significant. Methyl bromide easily penetrates rubber, leather, and cloth, which may lead to direct skin contact and severe chemical burns.

ELIMINATION

- Although the exact mechanism has not been well studied, part of the absorbed methyl bromide is exhaled unchanged and the rest is metabolized to 5-methylcysteine, which is excreted in urine.

Clinical Presentations

Headache, nausea, vomiting, visual changes, confusion, malaise, vertigo, weakness, paresthesias, and dyspnea characterize mild systemic toxicity. Symptoms typically are delayed 4–6 hours or longer. Tremor, ataxia, myoclonus, and behavioral and emotional disturbances may accompany other neurologic changes. Neurologic symptoms may present with or without evidence of pulmonary involvement. Severe exposures produce bronchitis, pneumonitis, pulmonary edema, convulsions, and coma.

Permanent neurologic or psychiatric impairment (e.g., behavioral changes, peripheral neuropathies, and ataxia) can develop after methyl bromide poisoning. Cutaneous exposure can produce erythema and vesicle formation characteristic of a second-degree chemical burn. Chronic methyl bromide toxicity usually is limited to the central nervous system, although a mild elevation of serum hepatic aminotransferase levels has been reported in industrial workers. Optic atrophy may occur. Mild neurologic dysfunction (e.g., decreased finger sensitivity, reduced cognitive performance, and behavioral abnormalities) was detected in a study of soil fumigators.

Toxic Dosage/Death

Contact with skin produces a freezing sensation, so ingestion is rare. At highest risk are workers at fumigation sites where air concentrations range from 30–3,000 ppm (during application) to 4 ppm (five days after application). Tilling the soil nine days after application produces an exposure level of 15 ppm.

Drug Interactions

The use of catecholamines such as epinephrine may synergistically sensitize the myocardium.

Laboratory

ANALYTIC METHODS

Serum bromides may be measured via a colorimetric method.

BLOOD LEVELS

Serum bromide levels usually are elevated and remain above normal for long periods in acute exposures. Blood bromide levels above 5 mg/L may be hazardous in chronic exposures. Bromide blood levels do not, however, accurately predict the clinical course.

Treatment

GUT DECONTAMINATION

These methods are unlikely to be helpful.

ELIMINATION ENHANCEMENT

An anecdotal, uncontrolled report suggests the use of hemodialysis to remove bromide from the blood.

SUPPORTIVE MEASURES

- Management is primarily supportive. The patient should have all contaminated clothing removed and the exposed skin washed with soap and water. Contaminated clothing should not be reworn, since skin lesions may develop, especially from residues present in leather.
- Significant symptomatic exposures should receive an evaluation of pulmonary (arterial blood gases, chest x-ray), hepatic (serum aminotransferase, bilirubin), and renal (creatinine) function.
- See the Introduction section for Hydrocarbons at the beginning of this chapter regarding the treatment of aspiration pneumonitis.

Antidotes

Dimercaprol was found ineffective in a series of seven methyl bromide poisonings. N-acetylcysteine has been suggested, but not proven to be an antidote.

Questions—Methyl Bromide

1. **No fatalities have occurred after premature entry into fumigated houses where methyl bromide was used.**
   A. True
   B. False
2. **Methyl bromide easily penetrates rubber.**
   A. True
   B. False
3. **Symptoms of methyl bromide exposure**
   A. Typically develop immediately after exposure
   B. Always include pulmonary difficulties
   C. May include behavioral and emotional disturbances
   D. Do not progress to permanent neurologic or psychiatric impairment
   E. None of the above

TETRACHLOROETHYLENE

Dry cleaning and textile processing consume two-thirds of the tetrachloroethylene (also called perchloroethylene or PCE) produced. Approximately 15% is used for metal cleaning, and it is the most commonly used degreaser. Other industrial applications include as a chemical intermediary for fluorocarbon production and as an extraction medium.

Although three-fourths of U.S. dry cleaning establishments use PCE (it is an excellent, nonflammable, easily recycled cleaner), exposures exceeding recommended standards are not pervasive. Recent concern about PCE has centered on its potential to produce cancer. NIOSH has recommended that PCE be handled as a potential human carcinogen.

Pathophysiology

Like the structurally related trichloroethylene (TCE), tetrachloroethylene is an excellent solvent that causes pulmonary and mucous membrane irritation, central nervous system depression, contact dermatitis, and hepatic dysfunction in severe exposures.

Pharmacokinetics

ABSORPTION

- PCE is well absorbed through the lungs.
- Although skin absorption occurs, of the five common chlorinated aliphatic hydrocarbon solvents, PCE produced the lowest maximum blood concentration after cutaneous exposure.
- Oral absorption occurs, but toxic effects on humans are not well documented by this route.

DISTRIBUTION

- PCE is highly fat-soluble and is stored in body fat. PCE is distributed to brain, liver and fat.

ELIMINATION

- The lungs excrete most absorbed PCE unchanged. Small amounts (about 3%) are metabolized by the liver to form trichloroacetic acid, which is eliminated by the kidney.
- Elimination is slow (biological half-life is 65 hours for exhaled PCE) because of the continuing release of PCE from fat stores.

Clinical Presentations

NEUROLOGIC EFFECTS

PCE is a central nervous system depressant that causes headache, blurred vision, lightheadedness, nausea, vomiting, confusion, slurred speech, loss of coordination, and memory impairment similar to ethanol intoxication. Heavy inhalations have produced coma and death. Patients recover without permanent neurologic sequelae if respiratory and circulatory support can be provided before hypoxia and shock occurs.

DERMATOLOGIC EFFECTS

Soft tissue contact produces pain and irritation. Defatting properties cause erythema, vesiculation, and fissure formation, which predispose the skin to infection.

GASTROINTESTINAL EFFECTS

Transient hepatic (e.g., elevated aminotransferase levels) and renal (e.g., proteinuria, hematuria) dysfunction have been reported in acute human exposures but no necrosis resulted. The liver is the primary target organ in animals.

CARDIOVASCULAR EFFECTS

Multiple premature ventricular contractions in otherwise healthy workers have been reported in occupational PCE exposures, but no direct link with sudden death has been made. Chronic exposure has not produced cardiovascular toxicity.

CARCINOGENIC EFFECTS

NIOSH has recommended that PCE be considered a potential workplace carcinogen. A small review of 330 deaths in laundry and dry cleaning workers revealed an increased risk for malignant neoplasms, primarily lung and cervical cancers.

Toxic Dosage/Death

Odor threshold is 5–50 ppm. PCE vapor is a mucous membrane and upper respiratory irritant at levels above 75–100 ppm. Exposures between 200–500 ppm produce an intoxicated state that may be confused with ethanol inebriation.

Drug Interactions

The use of catecholamines such as epinephrine may synergistically sensitize the myocardium.

Pregnancy/Lactation

PCE excretion in breast milk has been associated with obstructive jaundice in breast-fed newborn infants.

Treatment

GUT DECONTAMINATION

Although absorption occurs after ingestion, severe intoxications mostly involve inhalation and perhaps some skin absorption. Recommendations for emesis or lavage cannot be based on case studies or other definitive studies. Charcoal is probably unhelpful unless other agents are coingested.

ELIMINATION ENHANCEMENT

There is no data to support the routine use of these methods after PCE exposure or overdose.

SUPPORTIVE MEASURES

- The treatment of acute inhalation exposures is supportive, with initial attention directed towards the evaluation and support of ventilation and circulation.
- Moderate to severe inhalation exposure should receive cardiac monitoring because of the potential of PCE to produce dysrhythmias.
- Hyperventilation may reduce the elimination half-life of PCE from 160 to 30 minutes, but has not altered the terminal elimination half-life. Routine use is not recommended.
- Screen for hepatic and renal dysfunction in severe exposures. Watch for the development of pulmonary edema immediately following exposure. In significant acute exposures, hepatic aminotransferase levels, serum creatinine, and urinalysis should be evaluated.
- In the workplace, PCE concentrations greater than 4 ppm in a worker's breath 16 hours after exposure suggest that a 100-ppm TWA has been exceeded.

Questions—Tetrachloroethylene

1. Trichloroethylene (PCE) is no longer used in the dry cleaning business.
 A. True
 B. False

2. Trichloroethylene exposure
 A. Often produces long-term hepatic effects
 B. Has been linked to sudden cardiac death
 C. Has been associated with increased risk for malignancy in dry cleaning workers
 D. Has been shown to cause renal necrosis
 E. None of the above

TRICHLOROETHANE

Trichloroethane (TCA) is employed in solvents and degreasers, hair sprays and cosmetics. It is used in consumer aerosol products such as oven cleaners, spot removers, furniture polish, automotive lubricants, water repellents, and suede waterproofers. It is also used as a propellant in some decongestant aerosol sprays and as a typewriter correction fluid.

TCA, or methylchloroform, is the most commonly produced chloroethane (i.e., organic compounds with one or more hydrogen atoms replaced by chlorine). Although TCA is not a proven animal or human carcinogen, the U.S. National Cancer Institute has concluded that structurally similar chloroethanes are carcinogenic in mice, and that TCA should be treated with caution in the workplace.

Pathophysiology

Since it is less hepatotoxic than chloroform and carbon tetrachloride, TCA has gained wide acceptance as a substitute for those more toxic compounds. Similar to most other chloroethanes, TCA produces central nervous system depression, mucous membrane and upper respiratory tract irritation, contact dermatitis, and transient hepatic dysfunction.

Pharmacokinetics

ABSORPTION

- TCA is rapidly absorbed through the lungs and gastrointestinal tract.
- Cutaneous absorption is too slow to produce significant toxicity unless trapped against the skin by an impermeable barrier.

DISTRIBUTION

- Wide variations in tissue TCA concentrations occur, with the largest amounts found in lipid-rich brain tissue.

ELIMINATION

- The lungs exhale most of an absorbed dose unchanged. Small amounts (about 10%) are metabolized to trichloroacetic acid and trichloroethanol, which are excreted by the kidneys.
- The half-life of TCA is 53 hours.
- Repeated exposure induces hepatic P-450 mixed-function oxidase enzymes.

Clinical Presentations

NEUROLOGIC EFFECTS

TCA is a central nervous system depressant that can cause headache, lightheadedness, impaired coordination, dysequilibrium, drowsiness, convulsions, gait disturbance, stupor, coma, and death. Peripheral neuropathies or permanent neurologic sequelae have not been directly associated with TCA toxicity.

CARDIOVASCULAR EFFECTS

TCA may produce direct cardiovascular effects. Some animal experiments link TCA to cardiac dysrhythmias. Sudden deaths in glue sniffers have been associated with TCA. The exact role of dysrhythmias in TCA deaths remains to be determined, although premature ventricular contractions and ST depression have been documented in a few patients who underwent TCA anesthesia.

PULMONARY EFFECTS

Prior use of TCA as an anesthetic gas indicated that this compound was not a serious respiratory tract irritant. The use of waterproofing aerosol in a poorly ventilated space has been associated with atelectasis, pleuritic chest pain, hypoxia, tachypnea, and tachycardia which resolved without residual dysfunction in 30 hours.

GASTROINTESTINAL EFFECTS

TCA causes minimal hepatic dysfunction, except in high concentrations.

DERMATOLOGIC EFFECTS

Contact dermatitis with scaling and fissuring may occur with cutaneous exposure.

Toxic Dosage/Death

Minimal impairment of coordination occurs at 1,000 ppm (15 minutes), whereas marked dysequilibrium occurs after 5-minute exposures to 1,700 ppm. The anesthetic concentration range is 10,000–26,000 ppm for 5 minutes. Reversible central nervous system depression has occurred after an accidental ingestion of 600 mg/kg of 95% TCA. Death has occurred in industry, in small, poorly ventilated spaces and with recreational abuse of decongestant aerosols. Autopsy of an 18-year-old seaman revealed a recent myocardial infarction and cerebral edema that were attributed to TCA found in his bunk.

Drug Interactions

The use of catecholamines such as epinephrine may synergistically sensitize the myocardium.

Laboratory

ANALYTIC METHODS

No available data.

BLOOD LEVELS

Exposure to 350 ppm of TCA produces blood levels of approximately 2.67 mg/L, although there is substantial interindividual variation. Following blood levels in overdose has not been shown to be helpful. Fatal serum levels have ranged from 1.7 to 42.0 mg/L.

Treatment

GUT DECONTAMINATION

Emesis is contraindicated. Charcoal is probably unhelpful unless other agents are coingested. See the Introduction section for Hydrocarbons above concerning general guidelines regarding gut decontamination after hydrocarbon ingestions.

ELIMINATION ENHANCEMENT

There is no reported experience with these methods after TCA exposure.

SUPPORTIVE MEASURES

- TCA is less toxic than trichloroethylene at a given concentration, but treatment is similar with initial attention directed toward support of ventilation, correction of hypotension, and cardiac monitoring as indicated.

- Recovery after termination of exposure usually is rapid, with recovery from light anesthesia occurring within five minutes.
- Only severe exposures require laboratory evaluation of liver and kidney function.

Questions—Trichloroethane

1. **TCA is less hepatotoxic than chloroform.**
   A. True
   B. False
2. **TCA exposures can cause**
   A. Seizures and ataxia
   B. Hepatic dysfunction
   C. Sudden death
   D. All of the above
   E. None of the above

TRICHLOROETHYLENE

Trichloroethylene (TCE) was first synthesized in 1864 and introduced into medical practice as a nonflammable narcotic and anesthetic in the early 1900s. Because of its excellent fat solvent properties, TCE has enjoyed widespread industrial use as a degreaser, extraction medium for coffee and spices, as a typewriter correction fluid, and as a household cleaning fluid. It has gradually been replaced by less toxic agents such as trichloroethane (TCA). Approximately 90–95% of TCE is used as a fat solvent for degreasing metal parts. The use of TCE as an anesthetic agent and analgesic has largely been abandoned in medical practice because of its potential cardiotoxicity and hepatotoxicity, but its use in veterinary practice continues.

Most toxicity occurs in industrial cleaning establishments where TCE can produce central nervous system (CNS) depression. High acute doses can cause coma, hepatic and renal failure, and death. TCE can produce euphoria and has consequently been abused for that purpose. Sudden death has occurred both in industrial workers and in TCE vapor abusers, perhaps through the induction of ventricular fibrillation. Current concern has focused on TCE as a potential human carcinogen since it causes hepatocellular carcinoma in mice.

Pathophysiology

Like other halogenated hydrocarbons, TCE may sensitize the myocardium. TCE has been associated with hepatotoxicity and is a known CNS depressant at high doses.

Pharmacokinetics

ABSORPTION

- Inhalation is the usual route of exposure since TCE easily crosses the alveolar membrane. Absorption after ingestion has caused several cases of toxicity, including death.
- TCE can penetrate intact human skin but probably not in quantities sufficient to cause toxicity.

DISTRIBUTION

- Data are limited and tend to indicate that TCE is rapidly cleared from the blood, with the highest concentrations appearing in body fat.

ELIMINATION

- Studies in humans indicate that only small amounts of TCE are excreted unchanged by the lungs.
- TCE is metabolized mostly to trichloroethanol and trichloroacetic acid by hepatic microsomes. Trichloroacetic acid has a longer blood and urine half-life (70–100 hours) than trichloroethanol (10–15 hours) because trichloroacetic acid binds to plasma proteins.
- Metabolic products trichloroethanol and/or chloral hydrate may contribute to the central nervous system depression caused by TCE.
- The metabolite TCE oxide may be involved in mutagenesis and/or carcinogenesis.
- Elimination kinetics indicate that trichloroethanol is the major urinary metabolite and that urinary metabolites can be detected 16 days after exposure.

Clinical Presentations

The most prominent symptom of TCE exposure is CNS depression causing drowsiness, weakness, tremor, dizziness, confusion, and loss of coordination at low levels (200–500 ppm), and coma and respiratory depression at prolonged high levels (5,000 ppm). Sudden death in acute TCE exposures has been attributed to the development of fatal ventricular dysrhythmias.

PULMONARY EFFECTS

TCE is a pulmonary irritant that has produced acute pulmonary edema in an industrial worker who ingested alcohol concomitantly. The exact role of TCE is not clear, since phosgene, chlorine gas, and hydrogen chloride are breakdown products of TCE.

DERMATOLOGIC EFFECTS

TCE can produce a contact dermatitis or act as a sensitizer to cause a generalized exfoliative dermatitis, erythroderma, or papulovesicular dermatitis. TCE exacerbates existing skin lesions and its leaching and drying action reduces resistance to infection. Coingestion with ethanol produces a patchy erythroderma referred to as "degreaser's flush." Vasodilatation involves bilateral and symmetrical areas of the face, neck, back, and occasionally the extremities.

NEUROBEHAVIORAL EFFECTS

Adverse psychological and behavioral abnormalities have been reported in industrial overexposures and include symptoms of headache, fatigue, lightheadedness, depression, insomnia, irritability, and confusion. Cranial and peripheral neuropathies have occurred. Trigeminal neuralgia and facial nerve dysfunction have occurred after exposure to TCE vapor.

GASTROINTESTINAL EFFECTS

Although large TCE exposures produce hepatic and renal dysfunction, studies in animals indicate that TCE is a very weak hepatotoxin compared with chloroform and carbon tetrachloride. Repeat exposures to excessive levels of TCE may result in chemical hepatitis, cirrhosis and hypertension. However, TCE has little if any hepatotoxic effect in the accepted range of occupational TCE exposures. Toxic effects include nausea, vomiting, abdominal cramps, and hepatic dysfunction.

ABUSE

TCE inhalation may be abused in both the workplace and recreational settings. Carbona sniffing (40% TCE) has been associated with renal failure, hepatic necrosis, pulmonary edema, and cardiac hypertrophy consistent with congestive cardiomyopathy. Sudden death has occurred in adolescents recreationally sniffing typewriter correction fluid which contains primarily TCE and trichloroethane.

CARCINOGENIC EFFECTS
Large doses of TCE in mice resulted in a high incidence of hepatocellular carcinoma, leading the National Cancer Institute to suspect that TCE is a potential workplace carcinogen. Adequate studies in humans supporting a cancer link are lacking. One prospective study of 2,646 employees exposed to TCE for periods up to 15 years detected no excess in mortality.

Toxic Dosage/Death
Death secondary to hepatorenal failure occurred in a worker who accidentally drank an unreported amount of TCE. The estimated fatal oral dose in humans is 3–5 mg/kg.

Drug Interactions
Ethanol elevates TCE levels, perhaps by reducing TCE metabolism through competitive inhibition of mixed-function oxidases. Ethanol augments the TCE impairment of visuomotor performance and mental capacity. The well-documented intolerance to ethanol may be explained by the ethanol-induced changes in TCE metabolism.

Pregnancy/Lactation
TCE is fetotoxic in rodents, and there may be an association with congenital heart disease.

Laboratory

ANALYTIC METHODS
Methods to detect TCE are not generally available in hospital settings.

BLOOD LEVELS
The TCE concentration in exhaled air correlates with exposure. An 8-hour exposure to 100 ppm produces TCE levels of 25 ppm immediately and 1 ppm 16 hours after exposure. Trichloroacetic acid accumulates over the course of prolonged exposure.

Treatment

GUT DECONTAMINATION
Activated charcoal and cathartics may be given, although their efficacy has not been studied. Emesis may even be helpful in the alert individual who presents within 30–60 minutes of exposure. Given the hepatorenal toxicity of TCE, gastrointestinal decontamination is recommended for all except casual ingestions when the patient presents within the first 2–4 hours.

ELIMINATION ENHANCEMENT
There is no reported experience with these methods after TCE exposure.

SUPPORTIVE MEASURES
- Most mild exposures respond to removal from the source and supportive care.
- Serious toxicity most often results from hypoxemia or cardiac dysrhythmias so that oxygen, intubation, intravenous lines, and cardiac monitoring should be started initially as the clinical situation dictates. In severely intoxicated patients, arterial blood gases should be obtained. Inhalation victims who show signs of pulmonary toxicity should have a chest x-ray.
- Liver function tests, serum creatinine, coagulation studies (complete blood count, prothrombin time), electrocardiogram and cardiac monitoring may be helpful as well.

Questions—Trichloroethylene

1. Trichloroethylene (TCE) is used mostly
A. As a fat solvent for degreasing metal parts
B. As a dental anesthetic
C. As a postoperative analgesic agent
D. A and B
E. A and C

2. TCE can produce euphoria and has been abused for that purpose.
A. True
B. False

3. The most prominent symptom of TCE exposure is
A. Hypertension
B. Seizures
C. Central nervous system depression
D. Hepatic failure
E. None of the above

VINYL HALIDES

The manufacture of polyvinyl chloride (PVC) from vinyl monomer consumes most of the vinyl chloride produced. Vinyl chloride has many applications, particularly as adhesives, propellants and in plumbing materials. Less common industrial applications include its use as a solvent and chemical intermediate. Vinyl chloride is a flammable gas at room temperature with a pleasant, ethereal odor. Pyrolysis of polyvinyl chloride produces hydrochloric acid fumes as well as smaller quantities of phosgene, chlorine, and aromatic hydrocarbons. These pyrolysis products are potentially toxic to smoke inhalation victims and firefighters.

Vinylidene chloride is used primarily in the plastics industry to form lightweight, pliable products. Direct toxic effects in humans from chronic exposure have not been identified. Concern for the carcinogenic potential of vinylidene chloride results from its structural similarity to vinyl chloride and from animal testing.

Clinical Presentations

NEUROLOGIC EFFECTS
Vinyl chloride is a central nervous system depressant that was once evaluated as a general anesthetic. Acute exposure results in a syndrome similar to that of alcohol intoxication, with lightheadedness, convulsions, ataxia, nausea, and dysequilibrium.

DERMATOLOGIC EFFECTS
Vinyl chloride is a skin irritant, and a pressurized liquid form may produce thermal burns similar to frostbite.

ACRO-OSTEOLYSIS
Acro-osteolysis is a unique occupational disease seen in workers cleaning reaction vessels used in polyvinyl chloride production. Distal phalanges show erosive radiographic changes which consist of loss of the cortex of the tufts and occasional lysis of the

shaft. Changes may be subtle and asymptomatic. Scleroderma-like changes of the dorsal surface of hands and the volar surface of the distal forearm also occur. Raynaud's phenomenon characterizes the disease, with paresthesias, fatigue, arthralgias, pain, and vasoconstriction in response to cold. Immunological abnormalities may occur, suggesting that acro-osteolysis has an immune complex etiology.

HEPATIC EFFECTS

Exposure of workers to vinyl chloride produces an increased incidence of a peculiar form of hepatic fibrosis and angiosarcoma of the liver. Portal fibrosis, a nodular form of capsular fibrosis, and a focal intralobular accumulation of connective tissue characterize the lesion of hepatic fibrosis. The histopathological picture may be confused with cirrhosis. Severe portal hypertension, splenomegaly, and thrombocytopenia may result clinically, but hepatocellular injury is not an early feature of this disease process.

CARCINOGENIC EFFECTS

Vinyl chloride-induced hepatic fibrosis is a precursor to malignant disease. Epidemiological studies of exposed workers show an increased risk of angiosarcoma of the liver as well as of lung, brain, and lymphatic cancer. The use of liver function tests in early cancer detection is questionable, and no clinical sign, symptom, or test is specific for angiosarcoma.

PULMONARY EFFECTS

Case studies have identified pathological lung changes associated with PVC dust exposure (PVC pneumoconiosis) that are characterized by mild lung and chest x-ray abnormalities. Slight exertional dyspnea occurs, although age and smoking are much stronger associated factors. Thermal degradation products of polyvinyl chloride and polyethylene have been associated with bronchospasm in a disease termed "meat wrapper's asthma."

CARDIOVASCULAR EFFECTS

Severe arrhythmias, such as ventricular fibrillation, may be seen.

Toxic Dosage/Death

Vinyl chloride is considered a workplace carcinogen. The U.S. exposure limit is 1 ppm as an 8-hour TWA, with a ceiling of 5 ppm over a maximum of 15 minutes.

Laboratory

ANALYTIC METHODS

Methods to detect vinyl chloride are not generally available in hospital settings.

BLOOD LEVELS

Following vinyl chloride blood levels after exposure does not help guide therapy.

URINE

Urine thiodiglycolic acid detection may indicate recent exposure.

Treatment

GUT DECONTAMINATION

Emesis is contraindicated. Lavage and / or charcoal may be helpful in the alert individual or patient with a protected airway.

ELIMINATION ENHANCEMENT

Studies linking these methods with successful removal of vinyl chloride have not been performed.

SUPPORTIVE MEASURES

- Treatment is symptomatic and supportive. Skin should be thoroughly washed with soap and water and clothes carefully removed. Frostbite injuries are treated with rapid rewarming in saline or water. Eye exposures are irrigated with saline for at least 15 minutes.
- ACLS algorithms are applied to significant arrhythmias.

Questions—Vinyl Halides

1. **Acro-osteolysis**
   A. Is seen in workers cleaning reaction vessels used in polyvinyl chloride production
   B. Consists of loss of cortex and occasional lysis of the shaft of the distal phalanges on radiographs
   C. Causes abnormalities which are always symptomatic
   D. A and B
   E. A and C
2. **Vinyl chloride-induced hepatic fibrosis does not lead to malignant disease.**
   A. True
   B. False

KETONES

INTRODUCTION

Ketones are widely used as solvents for vinyl polymers, resins, lacquers, cotton, pigments, and dyes as well as chemical intermediaries because of their excellent solvent properties, low cost, and mild toxicity. In high concentrations, ketones are central nervous system depressants, but generally they produce only mild cutaneous and mucous membrane irritation. The major exception is methyl n-butyl ketone (MBK), which has been associated with peripheral neuropathies in painters and plastic-coating workers.

METHYL BUTYL KETONE

Methyl n-butyl ketone (MBK) is a clear, colorless solvent with an acetone-like odor.

Pathophysiology

The hexacarbon neuropathies produce a characteristic "dying back" neuropathy with prominent axonal enlargement resulting from neurofilament accumulation that begins distally. Retraction of the myelin sheath occurs, with large myelinated fibers most affected. N-Hexane, acrylamide, and MBK produce similar lesions.

Pharmacokinetics

ABSORPTION

- MBK is well absorbed by the lungs, gastrointestinal tract, and skin.

DISTRIBUTION

- Minimal amounts of absorbed MBK are exhaled unchanged by the lungs.

ELIMINATION

- Most absorbed MBK is metabolized to carbon dioxide and 2,5-hexanedione, which is considered the neurotoxic agent.

Clinical Presentations

MBK produces a distal motor sensory polyneuropathy. Distal paresthesias of the upper and lower extremities occur, with sensory loss involving pinprick, touch, and temperature deficits of the hands and feet. Loss begins symmetrically and distally, with progression proximally. Onset is insidious and may progress after exposure ceases. Recovery is slow and may require several years. Weakness generally is limited to the forearms, head, distal legs, and feet with minimal atrophy. MBK is a mild central nervous system depressant as well as a mild skin and pulmonary irritant.

Toxic Dosage/Death

Epidemiological studies in animals and humans suggest that 1,500 hours of exposure to MBK levels ranging from 200–600 ppm is required to produce peripheral neuropathy.

Laboratory

ANALYTIC METHODS

Peroneal nerve conduction velocities are slowed in MBK neuropathy. Electromyography indicates a neurogenic peripheral neuropathy. Sural nerve biopsies generally show characteristic axonal swelling.

BLOOD LEVELS

Following blood levels after serious exposures does not guide therapy.

Treatment

GUT DECONTAMINATION

Lavage and/or charcoal may be helpful in alert patients with a protected airway.

ELIMINATION ENHANCEMENT

Studies linking these methods with successful removal of MBK have not been performed.

SUPPORTIVE MEASURES

- Skin should be thoroughly washed with soap and water and clothes carefully removed.
- Eye exposures are irrigated with saline for at least 15 minutes.

Questions—Methyl Butyl Ketone

1. Methyl butyl ketone produces
   A. Distal motor sensory mononeuropathy
   B. Proximal motor sensory mononeuropathy
   C. Distal motor sensory polyneuropathy
   D. Proximal motor sensory polyneuropathy
   E. None of the above

2. Which of the following statements regarding methyl butyl ketone toxicity is not true?
   A. Onset of symptoms is acute.
   B. Symptoms occur symmetrically.
   C. Recovery may require several years.
   D. Symptoms may include skin and pulmonary irritation.
   E. None of the above are true.

3. Which of the following is considered the neurotoxic agent after MBK exposure?
   A. Acrylamide
   B. N-Hexane
   C. Carbon disulfide
   D. Methyl ethyl ketone
   E. 2,5-hexanedione

OTHER KETONES

Methyl Ethyl Ketone

Methyl ethyl ketone (MEK) is a widely used solvent. It is a mild central nervous system depressant that can cause contact dermatitis and mucous membrane and eye irritation. MEK probably speeds the development of n-hexane polyneuropathy but does not by itself cause neuropathy. Accidental ingestion of an unreported amount of MEK produced coma, hyperventilation, metabolic acidosis, and tachycardia but no hepatorenal dysfunction or long-term sequelae. Suicidal ingestion of the peroxide of MEK caused a severe metabolic acidosis, hemolysis, esophageal and gastric necrosis, gastric perforation, and death. The current U.S. standard is 200 ppm as an 8-hour TWA.

Methyl Amyl Ketone

Methyl amyl ketone (MAK) is a mucosal and cutaneous irritant with moderate central nervous system depressant properties similar to those of other ketones. It does not cause a peripheral neuropathy in animal models at current exposure standards. The current U.S. standard is 100 ppm as an 8-hour TWA.

Methyl Isobutyl Ketone

Methyl isobutyl ketone (MIK) is another ketone solvent. It is not considered neurotoxic, since the detection of MBK peripheral neuropathy originally occurred after MBK was substituted for MIK as a solvent in a fabric plant. The current U.S. standard is 100 ppm as an 8-hour TWA.

ACETONE

Acetone is the simplest aliphatic ketone. It is a clear liquid with a characteristic aromatic odor and pungent, sweet taste. Commercial applications include its use in nail polish remover, solvents, varnishes, glues, and rubber cement.

Pathophysiology

Acetone is a volatile solvent with narcotic properties. It is a metabolite of isopropyl alcohol. See Chapter 17, Alcohols, Glycols and Disulfiram.

Pharmacokinetics

ABSORPTION

- Acetone is well absorbed by ingestion and inhalation. Dermal absorption is slow.

DISTRIBUTION

- Acetone is distributed through total body water, with a volume of distribution of 0.82 L/kg.

ELIMINATION

- The lungs exhale variable amounts of absorbed acetone unchanged depending on minute volume and alveolar concentration. When normal subjects inhale acetone for two hours, the half-life in alveolar air is about four hours. In overdose however, saturable metabolism and limited clearance prolong the elimination half-life to 25–30 hours.
- The kidneys account for 30% of elimination and are an important route at levels less than 100 mg/dL.
- Acetone is the main product of isopropanol metabolism and contributes to the prolonged effect of isopropanol.

Clinical Presentations

Symptoms of exposure roughly simulate ethanol intoxication, although the anesthetic property of acetone is greater. The characteristic odor of acetone on the breath and ketone in the urine are sensitive indicators of exposure. Lethargy, ataxia, headache, nausea, vomiting, lightheadedness, and incoherent speech occur during mild intoxication. Stupor and coma may appear after serious ingestions. Acetone vapor is an eye and mucous membrane irritant. Large ingestions can produce pharyngeal and soft palate erosions and erythema. Chronic skin contact produces a dry, scaly dermatitis by defatting the epidermis.

Toxic Dosage/Death

Acetone has a relatively low toxicity with no fatalities reported in the industrial setting. Ingestion of 200–400 mL of pure acetone caused CNS depression but no long-term sequelae. A large ingestion did not produce acidosis in a chronic alcoholic with an acetone level of 250 mg/dL.

Pregnancy/Lactation

Acetone exposure has been associated with shortened menstrual cycles, an increased miscarriage rate, and decreased birth weight and length.

Laboratory

ANALYTIC METHODS

Acetone is routinely included in volatile blood screens performed by gas-liquid chromatography.

BLOOD LEVELS

Occurring naturally, acetone is a product of fat metabolism and, in diabetic ketoacidosis, ranges from 10–70 mg/dL. Blood levels greater than 330 mg/L are considered toxic.

Treatment

GUT DECONTAMINATION

Emesis is not advised. Charcoal may adsorb 40% or more acetone and is encouraged if used within a few hours of significant ingestion.

ELIMINATION ENHANCEMENT

No measures to enhance elimination are usually necessary.

SUPPORTIVE MEASURES

- Parents should be warned about potential lethargy, ataxia, and incoherent speech.
- Symptomatic children should be observed for the progression of symptoms as the elimination half-life is over 30 hours.

Questions—Acetone

1. Acetone is now banned from rubber cement and nail polish remover.
A. True
B. False

2. Sensitive indicators of acetone exposure include
A. Malar flushing
B. Characteristic breath odor
C. Urine ketones
D. A and B
E. B and C

3. All of the following have been associated with acetone toxicity except
A. Shortened menstrual cycles
B. Increased miscarriage rate
C. Mucous membrane irritation
D. Lightheadedness
E. Death

CYCLOHEXANONE

Cyclohexanone is a commonly used industrial solvent for cellulose acetate natural resins, vinyl resins, rubber, waxes, and fats. It is also used as a solvent sealer for polyvinyl chloride in many medical devices. It has been found as a contaminant of intravenous dextrose and a parenteral feeding solution used in a newborn special care unit, where it was considered to be leached into infusion fluids from administration sets.

Pathophysiology

Cyclohexanone will dissolve most plastics, resins, and rubber. Cyclohexanone appears to be reduced to cyclohexanol by liver alcohol dehydrogenase. Cyclohexanol is metabolized further by hepatic and microsomal mixed-function oxidase, and the main metabolites are excreted in the urine. Cyclohexanol disappears from the urine after 24 hours. Excretion may continue for at least ten days.

Clinical Presentations

Although cyclohexanone has been associated with central nervous system depression and hepatotoxicity in adults, its toxicity in neonates has not been evaluated. Eye, nose and throat irritation may occur.

Toxic Dosage/Death

Seventy-five ppm has resulted in eye, nose, and throat irritation. The ACGIH threshold limit value (TLV) is 25 ppm as a TWA for a normal 8-hour workday and a 40-hour workweek.

Pregnancy/Lactation

There is little information available on the toxicity of cyclohexanone in neonates.

Laboratory

ANALYTIC METHODS

A sensitive method for determining urinary cyclohexanol involves hydrolysis and gas chromatography with flame ionization detection. Cyclohexanediol is assayed by gas chromatography and mass spectrometry.

BLOOD LEVELS

Urinary cyclohexanol concentrations correlate well with the time-weighted average concentration of cyclohexanone at the workplace.

Treatment

- Management is symptomatic and supportive.

Questions—Cyclohexanone

1. **Cyclohexanone dissolves most plastics, resins and rubber.**
   A. True
   B. False
2. **Neonatal exposure to cyclohexanone**
   A. Has been studied for toxicity evaluation
   B. Has occurred from its leaching into infusion units from administration sets
   C. Should be treated with symptomatic and supportive measures
   D. A and B
   E. B and C

HYDROQUINONE

Hydroquinone is a reducing agent that is used as a photographic developer in black-and-white photography. It is also an antioxidant or stabilizer for certain materials that polymerize, a polymerization inhibitor for vinyl acetate and acrylic monomers, a stabilizer in paints, varnishes, motor fuels, and oils, an intermediate for rubber-processing chemicals, and a source of the production of its mono- and dialkyl ethers. Many of its derivatives are used as bacteriostatic agents.

Hydroquinone exists naturally in pear leaves. "Health teas" prepared from the leaves of blueberry, red whortleberry, cranberry, or bearberry may contain hydroquinone in excess of 1%, capable of causing irritation of the gastrointestinal mucosa and inducing systemic poisoning. A partial list of occupations in which exposure may occur include antioxidant makers, bacteriostatic agent makers, drug makers, fur processors, motor fuel blenders, organic chemical synthesizers, paint makers, photographic developers, plastic stabilizer workers, stone-coating workers, and styrene monomer workers.

Pathophysiology

Hydroquinone is an antioxidant ketone. It is readily absorbed from the gastrointestinal tract and is excreted in the urine as sulfate and glucuronide conjugates.

Clinical Presentations

In July 1977, 544 crew members aboard a U.S. Navy vessel developed an illness characterized by acute nausea, vomiting, abdominal cramps, and diarrhea, all of which resolved within 12–36 hours. Their white blood cell counts were elevated. Drinking water had been contaminated with photographic developer. Fatal cases have been reported after ingestion of 5–12 g of hydroquinone. These doses induced tinnitus, dyspnea, cyanosis, extreme somnolence, a dark color to the urine, icterus of the sclerae, and bile-stained urine.

OPTHALMOLOGIC EFFECTS

Direct acute contamination of the eye with particles of hydroquinone can cause immediate eye irritation. Chronic, low-grade and long-time exposure may result in ulcerations of the cornea with dark brown discoloration and distortion and opacification of the cornea.

DERMATOLOGIC EFFECTS

Skin-lightening preparations containing hydroquinone may produce severe and irreversible cutaneous damage. The effects begin with a darkening and coarsening of the skin, followed by a hyperpigmented papular change.

Toxic Dosage/Death

Hydroquinone ingestion in low doses (300–500 mg daily) may be relatively asymptomatic. In higher doses, it can induce an acute gastroenteritis-like syndrome. When doses of 5–12 g are ingested, death ensues following hemolysis and renal and hepatic failure. Patients who have ingested 5 and 6 g have developed cyanosis and icterus, and died.

Pregnancy/Lactation

No studies have been made to assess the teratogenic potential of hydroquinone.

Laboratory

ANALYTIC METHODS

Liquid chromatographic analysis has been used to quantitate serum hydroquinone levels. High-performance liquid chromatography can also be used for the detection of hydroquinone in water samples.

BLOOD LEVELS

Acutely ill patients with gastrointestinal symptoms following hydroquinone ingestion had serum levels over 0.1 $\mu g/mL$.

URINE

Ingestion of 12 g of hydroquinone led to black-colored urine that tested positive for phenol.

Treatment

GUT DECONTAMINATION

The treatment of oral ingestions is symptomatic and supportive. Gastric lavage has been employed and charcoal may be helpful, but has not been studied.

ELIMINATION ENHANCEMENT

There are no reports of these methods being utilized to treat exposure to hydroquinone.

SUPPORTIVE MEASURES

- Treatment is symptomatic and supportive. On admission, the patient should have access to a source of oxygen, cardiac monitoring, and an intravenous line.
- Dust particles of hydroquinone may remain in the tears for long periods. Treatment of eye contamination consists of immediately flushing with water for 15 minutes and obtaining ophthalmologic consultation.
- Blood should be drawn for a complete blood count, serum aminotransferases, alkaline phosphatase, bilirubin (total and indirect), glucose, creatinine, and blood urea nitrogen. Arterial blood gases and serum electrolytes should be obtained as needed. Hypoglycemia, hypercholesterolemia, leukocytosis, hemoglobinemia, and casts in the urine have been observed after large oral ingestions.
- Since contact with the skin may cause dermatitis, the skin should be thoroughly washed with soap and water.

Questions—Hydroquinone

1. High doses of ingested hydroquinone induce

A. A mild upper respiratory-like illness
B. Bladder irritation mimicking a urinary infection
C. An acute gastroenteritis-like syndrome
D. All of the above
E. None of the above

MISCELLANEOUS HYDROCARBONS

DIBROMOCHLOROPROPANE

1,2-dibromo-3-chloropropane (DBCP) is a soil fumigant and nematocide. A number of pesticide production workers in California exposed to DBCP were found to have a marked reduction in sperm density. These workers had more than 100 hours of estimated exposure in production. The histologic pattern of testicular biopsies showed seminiferous tubules to be the site of damage. The outcome of pregnancies fathered by the exposed men disclosed no evidence of an increase in spontaneous abortion, infant or fetal deaths, or congenital malformations. Permanent destruction of the germinal epithelium occurred in most of the DBCP-sterile persons studied seven years after the termination of exposure.

JET FUEL

Aviation fuel consists primarily of straight-chain and branched-chain alkanes (paraffins), cyclic alkanes (naphthenes), alkenes (olefins), and aromatic hydrocarbons. JP-4 and JP-7 are grades of jet propulsion fuel. Components include benzene, xylene, and toluene. Acute exposure causes central nervous system depression, dizziness, nausea, and vomiting. Chronic exposure is associated with neuropsychiatric disorders and peripheral sensory neuropathy, as well as a dermatitis. Tests of liver function are usually normal. Inhalation may cause respiratory tract irritation. The carcinogenic effects are unknown.

Ingestion may lead to coughing, dyspnea, tachypnea, pulmonary edema, and potentially fatal aspiration pneumonitis. Treatment is symptomatic and supportive. After dermal exposure, remove contaminated clothing and wash skin and hair thoroughly. Eyes should be irrigated with water or saline for at least 15 minutes. After ingestion, gastric emptying is not indicated. Induced emesis or lavage may increase the risk of aspiration. There is no specific treatment for chronic jet fuel toxicity. Recovery occurs within a few days after exposure.

METHANETHIOL

Methanethiol is derived predominantly from the breakdown of methionine or the methylation of hydrogen sulfide. It may be one of the endogenous factors involved in the pathogenesis of hepatic encephalopathy. Methanethiol and dimethyl sulfide (a metabolite) have been found in the urine of patients with fulminant hepatic failure. Methanethiol may be quantified by gas chromatography and mass spectrometry. Occupational exposure to methanethiol may cause headache, nausea, vomiting, eye irritation, chest tightness and wheezing, dizziness, diplopia, and a productive cough.

MONOOCTANOIN

Monooctanoin has been used to dissolve cholesterol gallstones by intrabiliary perfusion. Rapid perfusion may result in respiratory compromise, and cardiac arrest has followed 0.4 mL injected through a central venous catheter. Monooctanoin is a mixture of glycerol esters, principally glyceryl monoactanoate.

Abdominal pain, nausea, vomiting, and diarrhea occur frequently in patients treated with monooctanoin, especially with a rapid rate of perfusion. At least two deaths have been reported from its use. Episodes of dyspnea, hypoxemia, and respiratory compromise have followed intrabiliary monooctanoin use. If symptoms develop, cease use of monooctanoin.

TRIMELLITIC ANHYDRIDE

Trimellitic anhydride is used as a curing agent for epoxy and other resins and as a vinyl plasticizer. It is also found in anticorrosive surface coatings, polymers, paints, dyes, and pharmaceuticals. These products find applications in high-temperature plastics, wire insulation, gaskets, and automobile upholstery.

TMA induces four clinical syndromes in humans, three of which are thought to be immunologically related. The first is an IgE-mediated allergic rhinitis. The second is a late respiratory systemic syndrome characterized by cough, dyspnea, myalgias, fever, and chills that occur 4–12 hours after TMA inhalation. The third is a pulmonary disease and anemia syndrome that is characterized by dyspnea, cough, hemoptysis, and symptoms related to anemia. This syndrome may lead to respiratory failure. A fourth nonimmunologic, irritant syndrome reflects upper airway irritation in response to high concentrations of TMA dust or fumes. Treatment is supportive.

TRIMETHYLAMINE

Trimethylamine is a colorless gas used as an insect attractant, as a warming agent for natural gas, and in organic synthesis. It may be an irritant to the eyes, mucous membranes, and lungs. A "fish odor syndrome," recessively inherited, is probably due to trimethylamine in the sweat. Acid soaps and acid body lotions convert trimethylamine to an odorless oxide.

CREOSOTES

Creosote is a complex mixture of hydrocarbon compounds, including many polycyclic aromatic hydrocarbons. It has been used as a disinfectant and treatment for coughs. Creosote is a potent carcinogen. Skin cancer has been observed in workers exposed to creosote for long periods during timber treatment. The only products now routinely treated with creosotes are commercial wood products such as railroad ties and marine piers.

Creosotes can cause irritation of the skin, mucous membranes, and conjunctiva. The skin may become red, papular, vesicular, or ulcerative. Photosensitization has been observed. Following ingestion of creosote, gastrointestinal irritation (e.g., nausea, vomiting, salivation, and abdominal discomfort) and cardiovascular instability (e.g., tachycardia, hypotension, respiratory distress) may occur. The fatal dose is about 0.1 g/kg body weight. Treatment is symptomatic and supportive.

TETRAHYDROFURAN

Tetrahydrofuran (THF) is an organic solvent liquid belonging to a group of cyclic ethers with an odor similar to acetone. It can dissolve many types of plastics (e.g., polyvinyl chloride, polyurethanes, epoxy compounds, and cellulosics) and a wide range of organic products. Its main applications include the manufacture of glues, paints, varnishes, inks, and wetting and dispersing agents in textile processing. It has recently been used as an iron oxide coating agent employed in the production of audio and video tapes. Tetrahydrofuran forms explosive peroxides when exposed to air.

THF is readily absorbed across the alveolar membrane and from the digestive tract. It can cross the skin in toxic amounts. It is an inhibitor of a number of cytochrome P450-dependent, mixed-function oxidase activities. Metabolic products may possess convulsive properties. Analysis of the breath, blood, and urine is done with gas chromatography.

Tetrahydrofuran is an upper respiratory tract irritant. At high concentrations it is a central nervous system depressant. Symptoms after exposure may include nausea, headache, blurred vision, dizziness, fatigue, tinnitus, chest pain, and cough. Irritation of skin and mucous membranes may occur. An adult ingested tetrahydrofuran and developed abdominal pain, nausea, and vomiting. The patient developed jaundice, oliguria, high fever, and loss of consciousness and died in five days. The two primary signs of intoxication are narcosis and hepatocellular dysfunction.

Treatment is largely symptomatic and supportive. Hepatic aminotransferases may be considerably elevated. The chest x-ray and electrocardiogram are generally normal. Blood counts and renal function tests are usually normal as well. There are no antidotes.

Questions—Miscellaneous Hydrocarbons

1. **Which of the following hydrocarbons is matched to the incorrect use?**
   A. Monooctanoin—Dissolve gallstones
   B. Dibromochloropropane—Nematocide
   C. Creosotes—Jet fuel
   D. Tetrahydrofuran—Iron oxide coating agent
   E. Trimetallic anhydride—Vinyl plasticizer

ANSWERS

Introduction to Petroleum Distillates

1. C 2. D 3. A 4. D 5. B

Aliphatic Hydrocarbons

1. E 2. B 3. A 4. C 5. E 6. B 7. A
8. D 9. B 10. A 11. B

Gasoline

1. C 2. B 3. E 4. A 5. D

Dimethyl Sulfoxide

1. C 2. E 3. A

Dimethyl Sulfate

1. A 2. B 3. E 4. C

Stoddard Solvent

1. B 2. D 3. D

Benzene

1. A 2. C 3. C 4. C 5. D

Polycyclic Aromatic Hydrocarbons

1. B 2. B 3. A 4. E

Polyhalogenated Biphenyls

1. C 2. E 3. A 4. A 5. E

Styrene

1. E 2. C 3. A 4. C 5. B

Toluene

1. C 2. A 3. E 4. C 5. E

Xylene

1. A 2. E 3. B

Introduction to Halogenated Hydrocarbons

1. C 2. E 3. B

Carbon Tetrachloride

1. A 2. D 3. B

Chloroform

1. B 2. B 3. C

Ethylene Dibromide

1. D 2. E 3. B

Ethylene Dichloride

1. A

Methyl Bromide

1. B 2. A 3. C

Tetrachloroethylene

1. B 2. C

Trichloroethane

1. A 2. D

Trichloroethylene

1. A 2. A 3. C

Vinyl Halides

1. D 2. B

Methyl Butyl Ketone

1. C 2. A 3. E

Acetone

1. B 2. E 3. E

Cyclohexanone

1. A 2. E

Hydroquinone

1. C

Miscellaneous Hydrocarbons

1. C

SELECTED READINGS

Introduction to Petroleum Distillates

1. Geehr E. Management of hydrocarbon ingestions. Top Emerg Med 1979;1(3):97–110.
2. Goldfrank L, Kirstein R, Bresnitz E. Gasoline and other hydrocarbons. Hosp Physician 1979;14(9):32–39.
3. McGuigan MA. The management of petroleum distillate hydrocarbon ingestions. Clin Toxicol Rev 1978;1(3):1–2.

Aliphatic Hydrocarbons

1. Gerarde HW. Toxicologic studies on hydrocarbons. Arch Environ Health 1963;6:329–341.
2. Jorgensen NK, Cohr KH. n-Hexane and its toxicologic effects: A review. Scand J Work Environ Health 1981;7:157–168.

Gasoline

1. Edminster SC, Bayer MJ. Recreational gasoline sniffing. Acute gasoline intoxication and latent organolead poisoning. J Emerg Med 1985;3:365–370.
2. Logan D, Dart R. Gasoline Toxicity. Case studies in environmental medicine. 31. Agency for Toxic Substances and Disease Registry, September 1993.

Dimethyl Sulfoxide

1. Greenfield C. Dimethyl sulfoxide toxicity. Lancet 1981;1:276–277.
2. Kligman AM. Topical pharmacology and toxicology of dimethyl sulfoxide-part II. JAMA 1965;193:923–928.
3. Willhite CC, Katz PI. Dimethyl sulfoxide. J Appl Toxicol 1984;4:155–160.

Dimethyl Sulfate

1. Dimethyl sulfate. Environmental Health Criteria 48. Geneva: World Health Organization, 1985, pp. 1–55.
2. Ying W, Jing X, Qin-Wai W. Clinical report on 62 cases of acute dimethyl sulfate intoxication. Am J Ind Med 1988;13:455–462.

Stoddard Solvent

1. Cocchiarella L, Hryhorczuk D, Garrettson LK. Stoddard solvent toxicity. Case studies in environmental medicine. 33. Agency for Toxic Substances and Disease Registry, September 1993.

Benzene

1. Aksoy M, Dincol K, Akgun T, et al. Haematological effects of chronic benzene poisoning in 217 workers. Br J Ind Med 1971;28:296–302.
2. Bond GG, McLaren EA, Baldwin CL, et al. An update of mortality among chemical workers exposed to benzene. Br J Ind Med 1986;43:685–691.
3. Yin S-N, Li G-L, Tain F-D, et al. Leukaemia in benzene workers: A retrospective cohort study. Br J Ind Med 1987;44:124–128.

Polycyclic Aromatic Hydrocarbons

1. Brudzewski J, Shusterman D. Polynuclear aromatic hydrocarbons (PAH) toxicity. Agency for Toxic Substances and Disease Registry. Atlanta. U.S. Department of Health and Human Services, 6/90.
2. Zedeck MS. Polycyclic aromatic hydrocarbons: a review. J Environ Pathol Toxicol 1980;3:537–567.

Polyhalogenated Biphenyls

1. Letz G. The toxicology of PCBs—An overview for clinicians. West J Med 1983;138:534–540.
2. Steele G, Stehr-Green P, Welty E. Estimates of the biological half-life of polychlorinated biphenyls in human serum. N Engl J Med 1986;314:926–927.

Styrene

1. Edling C, Ekberg K. No acute behavioral effects of exposure to styrene: A safe level of exposure? Br J Ind Med 1985;42:301–304.
2. Stewart RD, Dodd HC, Barretta ED, et al. Human exposure to styrene vapor. Arch Environ Health 1968;16:656–662.
3. Tossavainen A. Styrene use and occupational exposure in the plastics industry. Scand J Work Environ Health 1978;4(suppl 2):2–13.

Toluene

1. Carlsson A. Exposure to toluene: Uptake, distribution and elimination in man. Scand J Work Environ Health 1982;8:43–55.
2. Cohr KH, Stokholm J. Toluene. A toxicologic review. Scand J Work Environ Health 1979;5:71–90.
3. Hayden JW, Peterson RG, Bruckner JV: Toxicology of toluene (methyl benzene): Review of current literature. Clin Toxicol 1977;11:549–559.

Xylene

1. Morley R, Eccleston DW, Douglas CP, et al. Xylene poisoning: A report on one fatal case and two cases of recovery after prolonged unconsciousness. Br Med J 1970;3:442–443.

Introduction to Halogenated Hydrocarbons

1. Seaton A, Jellinek EH, Kennedy P. Major neurological disease and occupational exposure to organic solvents. Q J Med 1992;84:707–712.
2. Seedorff L, Olsen E. Exposure to organic solvents. I. A survey on the use of solvents. An Occup Hyg 1990;34:371–378.

Carbon Tetrachloride

1. Koppel C. Carbon tetrachloride poisoning. Lancet 1985;1:1335–1336.
2. Ruprah M, Mant TGK, Flanagan RJ. Acute carbon tetrachloride poisoning in 19 patients. Implications for diagnosis and treatment. Lancet 1985;1:1027–1029.

Chloroform

1. Schroder HG. Acute and delayed chloroform poisoning. Br J Anaesth 1965;37:972–975.
2. Storms WW. Chloroform parties. JAMA 1973;225:160.
3. Waters R: Chloroform—A Study after 100 Years. Madison, Univ. of Wisconsin Press, 1951.

Ethylene Dibromide

1. Jacobs RS. Ethylene dibromide poisoning. JAMA 1985;253:2961.

Ethylene Dichloride

1. National Institute of Occupational Safety and Health: Ethylene Dichloride, Current Intelligence Bulletin 25. Washington, DC, U.S. Government Printing Office, 1978, pp 78–149.

2. Yodiken RE, Babcock JR J.: 1,2-Dichloroethane poisoning. Arch Environ Health 1973;26:281–284.

Methyl Bromide

1. Hine CH. Methyl bromide poisoning: A review of ten cases. J Occup Med 1969;11:1–10.
2. Rathus EM, Landy PJ. Methyl bromide poisoning. Br J Ind Med 1961;18:53–57.

Tetrachloroethylene

1. Centers for Disease Control: Exposure to perchlorethylene in U.S. dry cleaning workers. JAMA 1983;149:3159–3160.
2. Lukaszewski T. Acute tetrachloroethylene fatality. Clin Toxicol 1979;15: 411–415.
3. McMullan JK. Perchloroethylene intoxication. Br Med J 1976;2:1563–1564.

Trichloroethane

1. Bass M. Sudden sniffing death. JAMA 1970;212:2075–2079.
2. Dornette WHL, Jones JP. Clinical experiences with 1,1,1-trichloroethane. A preliminary report of 50 anesthetic administrations. Anesth Analg 1960; 39:249–253.
3. Stewart R. Trichloroethane intoxication: Diagnosis and treatment. JAMA 1971;215:1789–92.

Trichloroethylene

1. Adams RM. Degreaser's flush. West J Med 1976;125:487.
2. Bergman K. Trichloroethylene. Scand J Work Environ Health 1979;5(suppl 1):189–216.
3. Kimbrough RD, Mitchell FL, Hovic VN. Trichloroethylene: An update. J Toxicol Environ Health 1985;15:369–383.

Vinyl Halides

1. Falk H. Vinyl chloride and polyvinyl chloride. In Rom WN (Ed): *Environmental and Occupational Medicine*. Boston, Little, Brown and Co, 1983, pp 579–587.
2. Wilson RH, McCormick WE, Tatum CF, et al.Occupational acro-osteolysis. Report of 31 cases. JAMA 1967;201:577–581.

Ketones

1. Altenkirch H, Mager J, Stoltenburg G, et al. Toxic polyneuropathies after glue sniffing. J Neurol 1977;214:137–152.
2. Mendell JR. Neuropathy and methyl n-butyl ketone. N Engl J Med 1974; 290:1263–1264.
3. Ramu A, Rosenbaum J, Blaschke TF. Disposition of acetone following acute acetone intoxication. West J Med 1978; 129:429–432.

Cyclohexanone

1. Cyclohexanone. Occupational Safety and Health Guidelines for Chemical Hazards. Cincinnati, OH: U.S. Dept Health and Human Services. DHHS (NIOSH) Publication No. 89-104, Supplement II-OHG.

Hydroquinone

1. Carlson AJ, Brewer NR. Toxicity studies on hydroquinone. Proc Soc Exp Biol 1953;84:684.
2. Devillers J, Boule P, Vasseur P, Prevot P, Steinman R, Seigle-Murandi F et al. Environmental and health risks of hydroquinone. Ecotoxicol Environ Safety 1990;19:327–354.

Dibromochloropropane (DBCP)

1. Eaton M, Schenker M, Wharton MD, Samuels S, Perkins C, Overstreet J. Seven-year follow-up of workers exposed to 1,2-dibromo-3-chloropropane. J Occup Med 1986;28:1145–1150.

Jet Fuel

1. Dabney BJ, Brent J. Jet fuel toxicity. Case studies in environmental medicine. 32. Agency for Toxic Substances and Disease Registry, September 1993.
2. Davies NE. Jet fuel intoxication. Aerospase Med 1964;35:481–482.

Methanethiol

1. Garrettson LK, Warren DA. Chronic methanethiol poisoning. Vet Hum Toxicol 1990;32:365.
2. Zreve L, Nagasawa HT. Methanethiol and derivatives in hepatic failure. J Lab Clin Med 1988;111:595–597.

Monooctanoin

1. Minuk GY, Hoofnagle JH, Jones EA. Systemic site effects from the intrabiliary infusion of monooctanoin for the dissolution of gallstones. J Clin Gastroenterol 1982;4:133–135.
2. Monooctanoin for gallstones. Med Lett Drugs Ther 1987; p. 52.

Trimellitic Anhydride

1. Zeiss CR, Wolkonsky P, Pruzansky JJ, Patterson R. Clinical and immunologic evaluation of trimellitic anhydride workers in multiple industrial settings. J Allergy Clin Immunol 1982;70:15–18.

Trimethylamine

1. Ayesh R, Mitchell SC, Zhang A, Smith RL. The fish odour syndrome: biochemical, familial and clinical aspects. Br Med J 1993;307:655–657.

Creosotes

1. Landrigan PJ. Health risks of creosotes. JAMA 1993;209:1309.

Tetrahydrofuran

1. Garnier R, Rosenberg N, Puissant JM, Chauvet JP, Efthymious ML. Tetrahydrofuran poisoning after occupational exposure. Br J Ind Med 1989;46:677–678.
2. Moody DE. The effect of tetrahydrofuran on biological system: does a hepatotoxic potential exist? Drug Chem Toxicol 1991;14:319–342.

ACKNOWLEDGMENT

Thanks to Alison Deutsch, MD for contributing the questions in this chapter.

CHAPTER 47
Metals

INTRODUCTION

Metals are widely found elements and compounds. The inorganic and organic forms of most heavy metals are toxic. The onset of diarrhea, abdominal pain, nausea, vomiting, upper gastrointestinal hemorrhage and a metallic taste in the mouth suggests heavy metal poisoning. Metals are easily detected by various laboratory tests. However, blood, urine, and especially hair levels often do not accurately reflect acute or chronic toxic effects. Patients who have been poisoned by heavy metals may or may not benefit from chelation therapy.

ALUMINUM

Aluminum (chemical symbol Al) is the most abundant element in the earth's crust. Healthy persons on normal diets, including those who cook in aluminum pans, sustain little risk of aluminum toxicity. Poor gastrointestinal absorption of aluminum minimizes the acute oral risk of toxicity.

Pathophysiology

Chronic renal failure patients on long-term dialysis may develop high aluminum serum and tissue concentrations, especially in bone. Aluminum toxicity occurs almost exclusively in patients who are unable to excrete dietary aluminum. Elevated aluminum levels appear to be an important factor in the pathogenesis of dialysis encephalopathy and in one type of dialysis osteomalacia.

Aluminum-containing phosphate binding agents increase gut aluminum absorption and predispose children with renal dysfunction to aluminum toxicity. Children with azotemia, infants receiving aluminum-contaminated intravenous solutions, and uremic neonates drinking powdered milk with a high aluminum content are particularly susceptible to this complication of therapy.

The deposition of aluminum in bone may block the incorporation of calcium into osteoid, leading to osteomalacia. The prevention of calcium deposition in bone leads to return of the calcium to the circulation with a rise in the serum calcium level. The elevated levels in turn inhibit the release of parathyroid hormone by the parathyroid glands. In addition, aluminum may be a factor in the etiology of anemia in chronic renal failure.

Pharmacokinetics

ABSORPTION

- The normal ingestion of aluminum in the diet is about 3–5 mg/day.
- The total body burden is maintained at about 30 mg.
- Patients on antacid or phosphate binding therapy may yield a positive balance to the extent of 200–300 mg/day.

DISTRIBUTION

- Most of the tissue aluminum stores (about 30–50 mg) reside in bone.
- At least 50% of serum aluminum is bound to proteins, which include both albumin and transferrin.

ELIMINATION

- The kidney can excrete up to 0.5 mg/24 hours.
- Insoluble aluminum compounds such as aluminum hydroxide mixture, which contain varying amounts of the hydroxide, oxide, carbonate, or bicarbonate, are slowly but incompletely converted to aluminum chloride in the stomach.
- Current data indicate that biliary excretion is the major route of excretion, but renal elimination appears more important after large aluminum loads.

Clinical Presentations

Encephalopathy, osteomalacia, and microcytic anemia secondary to aluminum toxicity are more likely to occur in individuals who take aluminum-containing phosphate binders or who are exposed to high levels of parenteral aluminum.

Hypercalcemia, a reversible microcytic anemia, vitamin D refractory osteodystrophy, and progressive encephalopathy may characterize aluminum toxicity. In one study, hemodialysis patients with higher serum aluminum levels appeared to exhibit a decline in visual memory, vocabulary scores, and a decrease in concentration and frontal lobe functions. Symptoms usually develop insidiously over months to years in chronic renal failure patients unless dietary aluminum loads are excessive. Even in the absence of severe anemia or microcytosis, aluminum contributes to anemia in dialysis patients, in part by impairing iron utilization.

DIALYSIS ENCEPHALOPATHY

Classical dialysis encephalopathy initially presents with a mild speech disturbance characterized by stuttering or stammering that most frequently occurs immediately following dialysis. This is associated with subtle mental changes such as directional disorientation and personality changes. As the disease progresses, the speech disorder is intensified and is accompanied by twitching, myoclonus, motor apraxia, seizures, visual and auditory hallucinations, and paranoid and suicidal behavior. Ultimately, patients may become immobile, mute, and obtunded. Death may follow 6–9 months after the onset of symptoms. If begun early enough, chelation therapy with deferoxamine appears to be effective in treating dialysis encephalopathy.

OCCUPATIONAL EXPOSURE

Pulmonary fibrosis and asthma have been reported in some workers heavily exposed to fine aluminum dust. A severe encephalopathy with incoordination, intention tremor, and cognitive deficits has been reported in aluminum workers with pulmonary fibrosis. Symptomatic workers may demonstrate a frequent loss of balance and memory loss. A neurologic syndrome observed among workers in the pot room of aluminum smelting plants, previously termed "pot room palsy" is characterized by incoordination, poor memory, impairment in abstract reasoning, and depression.

ALUM IRRIGATIONS

Continuous bladder irrigation with potassium aluminum sulfate (alum) can induce an increase in serum aluminum levels that can lead to fatal encephalopathy. The development of lethargy, confusion, seizures, or metabolic acidosis in a patient receiving intravesical alum mandates cessation of treatment, supportive measures, and the selection of an alternative modality to control hematuria.

PEDIATRIC EFFECTS

Plasma aluminum levels may become elevated in infants with normal renal function who are consuming high doses of aluminum-containing antacids. Infants at particular risk of aluminum intoxication are those born prematurely and those with impaired renal function.

BONE EFFECTS

Transiliac bone biopsy remains the "gold standard" for the diagnosis of aluminum-related bone disease in patients on regular hemodialysis, but it is an invasive and painful procedure. There is some suggestion that patients who have had a parathyroidectomy may be particularly prone to aluminum-related bone disease.

Toxic Dosage/Death

A study of 10,646 patients undergoing long-term hemodialysis suggests that mortality was 18% higher in patients with serum aluminum levels between 1,520 and 2,220 mmol/L and increased to 60% higher for patients with aluminum levels above 7,410 mmol/L. These data suggest that patients undergoing long-term hemodialysis should have periodic surveillance of the serum aluminum level, and that in those with plasma levels of 1,570–2,220 mmol/L or higher, use of aluminum salts to control serum phosphorous levels should be reconsidered.

Drug Interactions

Aluminum hydroxide may decrease fluoride and tetracycline absorption.

Pregnancy/Lactation

Pregnancy risk factor C.

Laboratory

ANALYTIC METHODS

Aluminum may be detected by flameless atomic absorption spectrometry.

BLOOD LEVELS

Serum levels of aluminum are helpful but do not accurately reflect total body burden since aluminum is highly protein bound. Normal individuals possess serum aluminum levels below 10 μg/mL, whereas chronic dialysis patients without toxicity develop levels up to 50 μg/mL. Serum aluminum levels above 60 μg/mL indicate increased absorption.

Potential toxicity occurs with levels above 100 μg/mL, and clinical symptoms usually are present when serum aluminum levels exceed 200 μg/mL. There are few data to correlate plasma and bone aluminum levels. This suggests that plasma aluminum levels do not necessarily reflect the status of total body aluminum.

Treatment

GUT DECONTAMINATION

Presumably, lavage and/or charcoal may be helpful after large ingestions of aluminum-containing products, but there is little clinical experience with these entities.

ELIMINATION ENHANCEMENT

Hemodialysis and charcoal hemoperfusion may remove serious aluminum burdens; however, their role in acute intoxications is limited.

SUPPORTIVE MEASURES

- The co-administration of an H2-receptor antagonist such as ranitidine can reduce absorption from aluminum-containing phosphate binders, resulting in lower plasma aluminum concentrations after one month, together with a decrease in urinary aluminum excretion and a decrease in desferrioxamine-induced plasma aluminum.
- The U.S. Food and Drug Administration (FDA) has recommended that dialysis facilities routinely evaluate dialysate delivery systems, including dialysate concentrate transfer and storage devices. When elevated serum aluminum levels are found, corrective actions such as avoiding aluminum-based phosphate binders and initiating chelation therapy are undertaken.
- Aluminum neurotoxicity may be managed with discontinuation and deferoxamine therapy.
- Aluminum is radiopaque. Foreign bodies as small as 0.5 mm x 0.5 mm x 1 mm can be clearly visualized when projected away from underlying bone. Aluminum foreign bodies that are embedded in larger body parts or that have been swallowed or aspirated may not be detected radiographically. Swallowed aluminum pull tabs are difficult to detect radiographically.

Antidotes

DEFEROXAMINE

Deferoxamine (DFO) has been used to treat dialysis encephalopathy and osteomalacia. The use of deferoxamine for aluminum-toxic dialysis patients has been suggested for serum levels of aluminum between 100 and 200 μg/mL. Deferoxamine also has been used to diagnose aluminum-related osteodystrophy. After a deferoxamine infusion of 40 mg/kg over 2 hours, an increment in plasma aluminum concentration of 200 μg/L identified 35 of 37 patients with biopsy-proven aluminum-related osteodystrophy. Calcium disodium EDTA does not appear as effective as deferoxamine in chelating aluminum.

Hemoglobin levels, mean cell volume, and mean cell hemoglobin concentrations may respond to a 3-month course of deferoxamine. Therapy with DFO significantly improved anemia in patients when sufficient levels of erythropoietin were present to stimulate erythropoiesis. Care must be taken to replete iron stores during therapy to avoid iron deficiency

Questions—Aluminum

1. Which of the following statements is false?

A. Aluminum (chemical symbol A) is the most abundant element in the earth's crust.
B. Poor gastrointestinal absorption of aluminum minimizes the acute oral risk of toxicity.
C. Chronic renal failure patients on long-term dialysis may develop high aluminum serum and tissue concentrations, especially in bone.
D. Aluminum toxicity occurs almost exclusively in patients who are unable to excrete dietary aluminum.
E. Elevated aluminum levels appear to be an important factor in the pathogenesis of dialysis encephalopathy and in one type of dialysis osteomalacia.

2. Which of the following statements is false?

A. Aluminum-containing phosphate binding agents increase gut aluminum absorption and predispose children with renal dysfunction to aluminum toxicity.
B. Children with azotemia, infants receiving aluminum-contaminated intravenous solutions and uremic neonates drinking powdered milk with a high aluminum content are particularly susceptible to renal toxicity.
C. The deposition of aluminum in bone may block the incorporation of calcium into osteoid, leading to osteomalacia.
D. Aluminum may be a factor in the etiology of polycythemia.
E. Hypercalcemia, a reversible microcytic anemia, vitamin D refractory osteodystrophy, and progressive encephalopathy may characterize aluminum toxicity.

ANTIMONY

Antimony (chemical symbol Sb) is widely used in the production of alloys and is commonly found in ores associated with arsenic. Patients at risk from the adverse effects of antimony compounds include those treated with anti-leishmaniasis agents and workers occupationally exposed to dusts and fumes containing antimony.

Trivalent antimony compounds were used for the treatment of trypanosomiasis and leishmaniasis between 1908 and the 1920s. Because of their toxicity the trivalent antimony compounds were superseded by the less toxic pentavalent compounds in the 1920s. For the past 50 years, pentavalent antimonials have been the main drugs used for the management of visceral, cutaneous, and mucocutaneous leishmaniasis.

Pathophysiology

Antimony is similar to arsenic in its generalized effect and its affinity for sulfhydryl groups on many enzymes. It is primarily an irritant.

Pharmacokinetics

ABSORPTION

- Antimony compounds are poorly absorbed from the gastrointestinal tract.

DISTRIBUTION

- Trivalent antimony compounds rapidly leave the plasma, but remain in the circulation bound to erythrocytes. They react with the red cell membrane and interfere with hemoglobin function.
- Pentavalent antimony is largely recovered from the plasma.

ELIMINATION

- The kidney excretes about 10% of the trivalent form in 24 hours.
- Fifty to sixty percent of the pentavalent form is found in the urine within 24 hours.

Clinical Presentations

Stibine gas (SbH_3) exposure produces a clinical picture similar to that of arsine gas (AsH_3). Stibine gas appears when antimony alloys are treated with acids. Clinical features include hemolytic anemia, myoglobinuria, renal failure, weakness, profuse vomiting, nausea, headache, abdominal and low back pain, and hematuria. Vomiting is usually prominent.

Reversible side effects that are commonly associated with pentavalent antimonial therapy but seldom require discontinuing therapy include arthralgias, myalgias, increases in hepatocellular enzymes, and flattening or inversion of T-waves on electrocardiogram. Prolongation of the corrected QT interval and concave ST segments are considered ominous signs. A prospective study has shown an excess of lung cancer in exposed workers with a carcinogenic latency of 20 years.

Toxic Dosage/Death

Occasional deaths that may have been due to cardiotoxicity have been reported, but they occurred in association with either high daily doses or with underlying cardiac disease. The OSHA permissible exposure limit in air as a time-weighted average (TWA) is 0.5 mg antimony/m_3.

Pregnancy/Lactation

An increased incidence of spontaneous abortion may be associated with antimony exposure.

Laboratory

ANALYTIC METHODS

Antimony levels may be determined by atomic absorption spectrophotometry.

BLOOD LEVELS

Mean normal serum values for antimony are 0.05–0.5 μg per 100 mL.

Treatment

GUT DECONTAMINATION

Treatment of an acute oral antimony intoxication includes gastric lavage, which, due to the slow absorption rate of antimony, can be used even several hours after ingestion. Repeated charcoal installations (1 g/kg body weight) may be useful.

ELIMINATION ENHANCEMENT

Dialysis may theoretically be useful in removing pentavalent antimony; however, this method has not been clinically tested in humans. The role of exchange transfusion is not clear.

SUPPORTIVE MEASURES

- Fluid, electrolyte, and blood losses must be replaced. Be sure to monitor for dysrhythmias.

Antidotes

Chelation with British Anti-Lewisite (BAL) for serious antimony exposures should be employed, as in arsenic intoxication. Dimercaptosuccinic acid (DMSA) and dimercaptopropane sulfonic acid (DMPS) have been proposed for the treatment of antimony intoxicants. There is no evidence that BAL is useful for stibine gas exposure.

Questions—Antimony

1. Which of the following statements is false?

A. Antimony (chemical symbol Sb) is widely used in the production of alloys and is commonly found in ores associated with arsenic.
B. Patients at risk from the adverse effects of antimony compounds include those treated with anti-leishmaniasis agents and workers exposed to dusts and fumes containing antimony.
C. Because of their toxicity, the pentavalent antimony compounds were superseded by the less toxic trivalent compounds in the 1920s.
D. For the past 50 years, antimonials have been the main drugs used for the management of visceral, cutaneous, and mucocutaneous leishmaniasis.
E. Antimony is similar to arsenic in its generalized effect and its affinity for sulfhydryl groups on many enzymes.

2. Which of the following statements is false?

A. Stibine gas (SbH_3) exposure produces a clinical picture similar to that of arsine gas (AsH_3).
B. Stibine gas appears when antimony alloys are treated with bases.
C. Clinical features of stibine gas exposure include hemolytic anemia, myoglobinuria, renal failure, weakness, profuse vomiting, nausea, headache, abdominal and low back pain, and hematuria.
D. Reversible side effects that are commonly associated with antimonial therapy but seldom require discontinuing therapy include arthralgias, myalgias, increases

in hepatocellular enzymes, and flattening or inversion of T-waves on electrocardiogram.

E. Chelation with British Anti-Lewisite (BAL) for serious antimony exposures may be helpful.

ARSENIC

Arsenic (chemical symbol As) is the fiftieth most abundant element in the earth's crust. It is widely known as a homicidal agent. However, not all poisonings are intentional. The nonspecific, multiorgan effect of this odorless, tasteless compound has made it a favorite agent of detective stories. Accidental contamination of food and drink has caused several epidemics of polyneuropathy. Clare Booth Luce developed arsenic intoxication while she was the American ambassador to Italy in the 1950s. Apparently, arsenic-laden paint chips fell from the ceiling of the U.S. embassy in Rome and contaminated her food.

Arsenic has been used to treat protozoa, helminths, amoeba, spirochetes, and trypanosoma, but has been superseded by therapy that is more effective. Currently, commercial applications include its use as a wood preservative, pesticide, rodenticide, veterinary antihelminthic, and ant paste. The burning of arsenic-treated wood in home stoves can produce toxicity. Commercial applications of arsenic compounds include herbicides, glassware, marine paints, alloy makers, pigment production, and the use of arsine gas in the semiconductor industry to produce microchips.

Arsenic compounds are by-products of lead, copper, and gold extraction, and arsenic has been an occasional contaminant of well water and food. Homeopathic medications may also contain arsenic. The two most commonly found organic, nontoxic variants of arsenic found in food regularly consumed by humans are arsenobetaine and arsenocholine.

Pathophysiology

Arsenic disrupts metabolic pathways by inhibiting oxidative phosphorylation and consequently producing widespread effects. Arsenic binds to the sulfhydryl cofactor, dihydrolipoate, which inhibits the pyruvate and succinate oxidative pathways. The body also substitutes arsenic for phosphorus, which inhibits oxidative phosphorylation, but that mechanism appears less important than sulfhydryl inhibition.

Pharmacokinetics

ABSORPTION

- Pentavalent arsenic is well absorbed through the gut, but the trivalent form is more lipid-soluble.
- Toxicity results from the arsenite form, especially by dermal absorption.
- Inhalation can result in symptomatic chronic exposure, particularly with arsine gas.
- Arsenic compounds are well absorbed parenterally within 24 hours.

DISTRIBUTION

- Arsenic initially localizes in the blood bound to globulin. Redistribution occurs within 24 hours to the liver, lungs, intestinal wall, and spleen, where arsenic binds to the sulfhydryl groups of tissue proteins. Only small amounts of arsenic penetrate the blood-brain barrier.
- Arsenic replaces phosphorus in the bone, where it may remain for years. Within 30 hours postingestion, arsenic deposits in the hair.
- Arsenic levels in hair sections may provide an indication of the time of exposure based on length from growth site. The hair of an individual who died 6 to 8 hours after ingestion of an arsenic overdose generally does not contain arsenic.

ELIMINATION

- The half-life of inorganic arsenic in blood is about 2 hours, and the half-life of methylated metabolites ranges from 5 to 20 hours. The half-life of organic arsenic is 4–6 hours.
- After arsenobetaine and arsenocholine are ingested, they are rapidly cleared in the urine, where they are completely excreted within 1–2 days.

Clinical Presentations

Abdominal pain, bloody diarrhea, albuminuria, and a garlic odor suggest acute arsenic toxicity. Signs of chronic arsenic poisoning may follow acute arsine gas exposure and include coryza, paresthesias, garlic perspiration, keratosis, hair loss, hyperpigmentation, Mees lines (horizontal white lines on nails), and anemia. Late sequelae of chronic arsenic poisoning may include a Wernicke-like encephalopathy, gangrene of the extremities (endarteritis obliterans), esophageal varices secondary to portal hypertension, anemia, leukopenia, squamous cell carcinoma of the skin, lung cancer, nasal septal perforations, and possibly visceral tumors including hepatic angiosarcoma.

ACUTE EFFECTS

Prominent gastrointestinal symptoms develop within 30 minutes to 2 hours after ingestion and include vomiting, bloody diarrhea, severe abdominal pain, and burning esophageal pain. Garlic odor on the breath and salivation may be present. Severely poisoned patients develop symptoms of shock secondary to vasodilation and myocardial depression. The development of cerebral edema leads to headache, delirium, coma, and convulsions. Death usually results from circulatory failure within 1–4 days. Later sequelae of toxicity include jaundice, renal failure, and peripheral neuropathy.

CHRONIC EFFECTS

The diagnosis of chronic arsenic poisoning may be difficult because of its insidious presentation and its nonspecific symptoms. Early features typically involve the gastrointestinal tract (diarrhea, abdominal pain) and the skin (hyperpigmentation and hyperkeratosis, especially on the palms and the soles, in 50% of cases). A symmetrical sensory neuropathy with paresthesias and loss of vibratory or position sense also develops after chronic exposure. Other signs and symptoms of chronic exposure include localized edema (face, ankles), sore throat, stomatitis, pruritus, coryza, lacrimation, salivation, perspiration, garlic odor, vitiligo, and alopecia.

ARSINE GAS EFFECTS

The classic presentation of arsine exposure involves a latent period up to 24 hours, followed by the onset of abdominal pain, hemolysis, and renal failure. Constitutional signs such as headache, lightheadedness, malaise, and weakness may occur initially. Gastrointestinal signs may include nausea, vomiting, and abdominal pain. Hyperkalemia, anemia and dark red urine (hemoglobinuria) indicate severe hemolysis. Bronze-colored skin also may appear, but jaundice and hepatotoxicity occur rarely. Renal failure is associated with hemolysis and probably results from myoglobinuria.

Toxic Dosage/Death

The pentavalent form (arsenate or the organic form) is less toxic than the trivalent form (arsenite or the inorganic form) because it is less soluble. Insoluble arsenic salts (e.g., arsenic trioxide, and lead arsenate) and organic alkane arsenates possess substantially fewer toxic properties than soluble inorganic arsenic compounds (e.g., sodium arsenite, arsenic acid, and arsenious acid). The most toxic form is arsine gas (AsH_3).

Toxicity occurs depending on the compound and form involved. Less than 1 mg/kg of arsenic can cause serious illness in children, and 2 mg/kg can cause death. The lethal range is 120–200 mg, although survival may occur at higher levels in adults. An ingestion of 9–14 mg of arsenic trioxide by a 16-month-old produced significant signs of poisoning which required chelation therapy. Single, low-dose pentavalent arsenate ingestions (e.g., less than 5 mL of 3% sodium arsenate-containing ant killers) is associated with little toxicity and can be managed at home. The need for chelation following exposure to pentavalent compounds requires further study.

Arsine gas, a hazard from leaking cylinders and semiconductor factories, is a colorless, nonirritating gas that has poor olfactory warning properties and evolves when arsenic compounds are exposed to acid. Immediate death occurs at 150 ppm. Fatalities with extensive hemolysis result in 30 minutes from exposure to 25–50 ppm, and in less than 30 minutes at 100 ppm.

Pregnancy/Lactation

Inorganic arsenic crosses the placenta. A 22-year-old female at 20 weeks gestation ingested 340 mg of sodium arsenate and delivered a healthy infant at 36 weeks. At birth, 24-hour urinary arsenic levels were 50 μg/L in the infant and 100 μg/L in the mother. Dimercaprol appears to be safe in these unusual cases. D-penicillamine has been associated with teratogenicity.

Laboratory

ANALYTIC METHODS

The current standard for arsenic analysis is atomic absorption spectroscopy, which measures total arsenic and does not distinguish between pentavalent arsenic, trivalent arsenic, or organic arsine.

BLOOD LEVELS

The short half-life of arsenic in the blood means that blood arsenic levels are less useful than urine levels unless exposure occurs on the same day. Serum arsenic levels are detectable only during the first 2–4 hours after ingestion.

URINE

Most persons have urine levels below 50 μg/L. If the levels are between 100 and 200 μg/L, arsenic intoxication should be suspected unless there is heavy consumption of seafood or work exposure. Urine arsenic levels above 200 μg/L usually indicate significant acute exposure and suggest the need for hospitalization and chelation. Levels may remain elevated for 1–2 months after systemic arsenic absorption.

HAIR

Hair analysis for arsenic is a semireliable method for confirming chronic toxicity. It does not discriminate between externally deposited arsenic and arsenic found within the hair shaft.

Treatment

GUT DECONTAMINATION

Activated charcoal, lavage and/or cathartics may be used but their efficacy is unclear.

ELIMINATION ENHANCEMENT

Hemodialysis may be considered in arsenic poisoning when the ingested dose is massive and signs of systemic involvement are present. These include hypotension, mental confusion, coma, oliguria, and/or lactic acidosis. Dimercaprol should be administered in combination with hemodialysis to avoid the possible deleterious effects of arsenic redistribution.

SUPPORTIVE MEASURES

- Follow fluid/electrolyte balance carefully since arsenic causes vasodilation. Treat hypotension with fluids before using vasopressors.
- Obtain an electrocardiogram and monitor the patient's cardiac rhythm.
- Follow renal and hepatic function with serum creatinine and hepatic enzymes.
- Obtain a baseline chest x-ray. Pulmonary edema is a rare complication, and respiratory failure secondary to neuromuscular weakness may develop several weeks after severe poisoning.

Arsine Gas

- A self-contained breathing apparatus, full-face mask, protective clothing, and boots should be worn in areas where arsine gas has been lurking.
- Victims should be washed thoroughly. An intravenous line should be established and fluids administered during transport and management in the hospital.
- Evaluate and support ABCs (airway, breathing and circulation) and provide oxygen by mask. Monitor cardiac rhythm and obtain a 12-lead electrocardiogram.
- Laboratory tests should include a urine dipstick for occult blood and hemoglobin. Obtain a complete blood count, electrolytes, blood urea nitrogen, creatinine, bilirubin, lactate dehydrogenase, blood type and screen as hemolysis may be quite severe.
- If there is evidence of acute hemolysis, alkalinize the urine with sodium bicarbonate (50–100 mEq in 1 liter of 5% dextrose) and administer intravenously to maintain a urine output at 2–3 cc/kg/hr. Consider furosemide or mannitol. Follow blood urea nitrogen, creatinine, and fluid status closely because renal failure may result in acute fluid overload.
- If there is a significant rapid drop in hematocrit and/or physical signs of intravascular hemolysis (e.g., severe abdominal pain, jaundice and shock), consider exchange transfusion after consultation with a medical toxicologist. Prepare for dialysis in case of renal failure. Shock may occur and should be treated appropriately.
- Dimercaprol and other chelating agents are not effective for arsine exposure. Arsine does not produce the classical symptoms of arsenic poisoning.

Antidotes

BRITISH ANTI-LEWISITE

British Anti-Lewisite (BAL) in Oil (dimercaprol) is indicated in all serious acute arsenic exposures except for arsine gas. The actual dosage range depends on the severity of exposure. A typical dosage schedule for arsenic toxicity is 3–5 mg/kg intramuscularly every 4 hours for 2 days, 3 mg/kg intramuscularly every 6 hours for 1 day, and then 3 mg/kg intramuscularly every 12 hours for 7 days until symptoms clear or the urine arsenic level drops below 50 μg/24 hours.

BAL therapy is effective for hematologic manifestations of chronic arsenic poisoning but not for neurologic symptoms. Side effects of BAL therapy may include urticaria, a burning sensation in the lips, mouth, and throat, fever, conjunctivitis, headache, transient leukopenia and/or hypotension.

PENICILLAMINE

This compound provides adjunctive therapy in serious ingestions and produces fewer adverse reactions than BAL. Serious side effects from d-penicillamine usually occur from long-term use (e.g., optic neuritis and nephrotoxicity). Sensitivity reactions to penicillamine include fever, rashes, leukopenia, eosinophilia, and thrombocytopenia. The dose for adjunctive chelation in children is 100 mg/kg/day for 5 days in four oral doses up to 1 g/d and up to 500 mg four times a day in adults. Reconsider its use after a 5-day rest period if symptoms reappear and the urine arsenic levels remain elevated. The use of penicillamine is contraindicated in penicillin-sensitive patients.

OTHERS

Dimercaptosuccinic acid (DMSA) is used orally and may be useful in the prolonged or late treatment of human arsenic poisoning and in the chelation of organoarsenates. Dimercaptopropane sulfonate (DMPS) produces a water-soluble complex with arsenic that appears less likely than the lipophilic BAL-arsenic complex to penetrate the central nervous system.

Questions—Arsenic

1. Which of the following statements concerning arsenic is true?

A. Arsenic (chemical symbol Ar) is the fiftieth most abundant element in the earth's crust.
B. The nonspecific, multiorgan effect of this smelly, tasteless compound has made it a favorite agent of detective stories.
C. Accidental contamination of food and drink has caused several epidemics of polyneuropathy.
D. Arsenic has been used to treat protozoa, helminths, amoeba, spirochetes, trypanosoma, and HIV but has been superseded by therapy that is more effective.
E. The body substitutes arsenic for ferric ions, which inhibit oxidative phosphorylation, but this mechanism appears less important than sulfhydryl inhibition.

2. Commercial applications of arsenic include its use as a

A. Degreaser
B. Wood preservative
C. Pesticide
D. All of the above
E. B and C

3. Arsenic compounds are by-products of lead, copper, and gold extraction, and arsenic has been an occasional contaminant of well water and food.

A. True
B. False

4. Which of the following statements is false?

A. The two most commonly found organic, nontoxic variants of arsenic found in food regularly consumed by humans are arsenobetaine and arsenocholine.
B. Arsenic disrupts metabolic pathways by inhibiting oxidative phosphorylation and consequently producing widespread effects.
C. Arsenic binds to the sulfhydryl cofactor, dihydrolipoate, which inhibits the pyruvate and succinate oxidative pathways.
D. Trivalent arsenic is well absorbed through the gut, but the pentavalent form is more lipid-soluble.
E. Arsenic levels in hair sections may provide an indication of the time of exposure based on length from growth site.

5. Which of the following is not typical of arsenic exposure?

A. Abdominal pain
B. Bloody diarrhea
C. Albuminuria
D. Garlic odor
E. Hyperpyrexia

6. The classic presentation of arsine exposure involves a latent period up to 24 hours, followed by the onset of abdominal pain, hemolysis, and renal failure.

A. True
B. False

7. Which of the following statements is false?

A. BAL in Oil is indicated in all serious acute arsenic exposures except for arsine gas.
B. BAL therapy is effective for neurologic manifestations of chronic arsenic poisoning but not for hematologic symptoms.
C. Side effects of BAL therapy may include urticaria, fever, conjunctivitis, headache, transient leukopenia and/or hypotension.
D. Penicillamine provides adjunctive therapy in serious arsenic ingestions and produces fewer adverse reactions than BAL.
E. Reactions to penicillamine may include rashes, eosinophilia, and thrombocytopenia.

BARIUM

Barium sulfate used for contrast radiography is extremely insoluble and is practically nontoxic. Acid-soluble barium salts (acetate, carbonate, chloride, hydroxide, nitrate, and sulfide) are highly toxic after ingestion. Barium (chemical symbol Ba) poisoning can result in a rapid onset of gastrointestinal symptoms, paralysis, cardiac dysrhythmias, hypertension, and death. Hypokalemia after overdose may be severe (i.e., below 2.0 mEq/L). Magnesium levels usually remain normal. The benign pneumoconiosis, baritosis, results from inhalation of sulfate and oxide salts as fine dusts.

A remarkable example of mass barium poisoning was experienced in 1943 in the Szechuan province of China where an endemic form of periodic paralysis known as Pa Ping was traced to massive contamination of table salt by barium chloride.

Pathophysiology

Barium initially stimulates striated, cardiac and smooth muscle and depresses serum potassium, which is forced intracellularly. Subsequent muscle weakness may result from a direct depolarizing effect and neuromuscular blockade. Peak serum barium levels appear within two hours in overdose. Normal barium levels do not exceed 0.4 μg/mL. After overdose, barium levels fall quickly with an elimination half-life of three hours.

Clinical Presentations

Within 1–2 hours of barium salt ingestion, patients may experience tingling around the mouth, diarrhea, vomiting, and colicky abdominal pain. Hypertension may be observed. In 2–3 hours, the tingling moves from the face to the hands, pupillary reactions are impaired, muscle stretch reflexes become depressed, muscle twitching is noticeable, and flaccid weakness begins to spread through the muscles of the upper and lower extremities. In some cases, complete flaccid quadriplegia develops within a few hours. In other cases, paralysis becomes severe on the second day of illness. Sensation is always preserved despite subjective paresthesias.

In most cases, symptoms abate by 24 hours and patients are ambulatory within 48 hours. Long-term prognosis is favorable, but the acute syndrome, which can also include cardiac dysrhythmias, can be fatal and must be treated promptly. Death may ensue in a few hours from cardiac arrest or respiratory paralysis unless potassium is vigorously administered.

Toxic Dosage/Death

Oral ingestion of 0.8–1.5 g of absorbable barium chloride or barium carbonate (used for glazing pottery) may lead to hypokalemic paralysis and death.

Treatment

GUT DECONTAMINATION

Gastric lavage with saline may be helpful. The addition of 5–10 g of sodium sulfate or 30 g of magnesium sulfate to the lavage solution may prevent severe barium poisoning by precipitating insoluble barium sulfate.

ELIMINATION ENHANCEMENT

Barium sulfate is excreted in the feces, and it is unlikely that diuresis, dialysis, or hemoperfusion will be effective.

SUPPORTIVE MEASURES

- The cardiac rhythm and serum potassium concentration must be monitored closely.
- In reported cases of barium poisoning, the serum potassium level has remained low until large amounts of potassium are administered. Barium and potassium appear to compete in their interaction with potassium conductance channels. Administered potassium continues to enter muscle until serum potassium rises high enough to displace barium from potassium channels.
- Administer generous amounts of fluid, but monitor the urine and serum for evidence of renal failure. Administration of a large volume of fluid allows barium to be "flushed out" by the resulting diuresis.
- X-rays of the abdomen may indicate the presence of radiopaque concentrations in the small intestine and colon.

Questions—Barium

1. Which of the following statements is true?

A. Barium sulfate used for contrast radiography is insoluble and can be extremely toxic.

B. Acid-soluble barium salts (acetate, carbonate, chloride, hydroxide, nitrate, and sulfide) are rarely toxic after ingestion.

C. Barium (chemical symbol Ba) poisoning can result in a rapid onset of gastrointestinal symptoms, paralysis, cardiac dysrhythmias, hypertension, and death.

D. Hyperkalemia after overdose may be severe.

E. The rapidly malignant pneumoconiosis, baritosis, results from inhalation of sulfate and oxide salts as fine dusts.

2. Which of the following statements is false?

A. Barium initially stimulates striated, cardiac and smooth muscle and depresses serum potassium, which is forced intracellularly.

B. Within 1–2 hours of barium salt ingestion, patients may experience tingling around the mouth, diarrhea, vomiting, and colicky abdominal pain.

C. Barium sulfate toxicity may be associated with paralysis.

D. Oral ingestion of absorbable barium chloride or barium carbonate (used for glazing pottery) may lead to hypokalemic paralysis and death.

E. Barium sulfate is excreted in the feces and it is unlikely that diuresis, dialysis, or hemoperfusion will be effective.

BERYLLIUM

Beryllium (chemical symbol Be) is the fourth lightest element. It is used in alloys for space exploration, military equipment, and nuclear reactors. Exposure to beryllium can cause chronic granulomatous disease similar to sarcoidosis and miliary tuberculosis. In contrast to sarcoid involvement, ocular involvement is absent. Multisystem involvement may include the lymph nodes, spleen, liver, myocardium, kidney, and bone.

Pathophysiology

Acute beryllium exposures produce chemical pneumonitis and pulmonary edema. This metal is a cutaneous sensitizer and primary skin irritant that produces contact dermatitis, skin granulomas, and ulcers.

Clinical Presentations

The lung is the primary target organ, with a defect occurring in carbon monoxide diffusing capacity. Multisystem involvement may include the lymph nodes, spleen, liver, myocardium, kidney, and bone. Hypercalcemia may occasionally develop. This metal is a cutaneous sensitizer and primary skin irritant that produces contact dermatitis, skin granulomas, and ulcers. Exposure to beryllium can cause an acute pneumonitis and chronic granulomatous disease similar to sarcoidosis and miliary tuberculosis. Initially, nonspecific symptoms appear and are followed by dyspnea and cough. Symptoms are progressive and steroids may help blunt the course of the disease.

The diagnosis of chronic beryllium disease requires at least four of the following six features and must include at least one of the first two: epidemiologic evidence of significant beryllium exposure, presence of beryllium in lung tissue, lymph nodes, or urine, evidence of lower respiratory tract disease and a clinical course consistent with beryllium disease, radiologic evidence of interstitial disease consistent with a fibronodular process, evidence of a restrictive or obstructive ventilatory defect or diminished carbon monoxide diffusing capacity, and pathologic changes consistent with beryllium disease.

Chronic beryllium disease may develop decades after exposure and is a progressive granulomatous disease that may lead to reduced lung volume, dyspnea, and diffuse irregular opacities on radiography. Chronic beryllium disease involves a cell-mediated immune response.

Toxic Dosage/Death

Chronic occupational exposure studies have shown an excess of lung cancer 15 years after initial exposure among patients with chronic berylliosis, and among some who had experienced acute berylliosis. Specific doses have not been identified.

Laboratory

ANALYTIC METHODS

Persons with chronic beryllium disease have cell-mediated immune responses to beryllium that can be detected by beryllium-specific blast transformation of lung lymphocytes obtained through bronchoalveolar lavage. A beryllium-specific lymphocyte transformation blood test appears to be a sensitive screening test that may be useful in preventing chronic beryllium disease by early diagnosis in a subclinical phase. Not all individuals with a positive test may have beryllium disease at the time of their initial evaluation.

In patients with chronic beryllium disease, beryllium acts as a class II-restricted antigen, stimulating local proliferation and accumulation in the lung of beryllium-specific CD4 (helper/inducer) T cells. The Kveim test is reported to be consistently negative in beryllium disease, but also has a high false-negative rate (20%) in sarcoidosis. Thus, a negative result cannot be taken as compelling evidence of beryllium disease when signs are consistent with either diagnosis.

BLOOD LEVELS

No definitive blood level helps guide the identification or management of beryllium exposure.

Treatment

GUT DECONTAMINATION

These methods have not been utilized in the treatment of beryllium exposures.

ELIMINATION ENHANCEMENT

These methods have not been utilized in the treatment of beryllium exposures.

SUPPORTIVE MEASURES

- Treatment of acute beryllium disease includes removal from exposure, bed rest, oxygen, mechanical ventilation as required, and corticosteroids.

Antidotes

Aurin tricarboxylic acid effectively protected monkeys exposed to lethal quantities of beryllium, but no data on humans are available to substantiate its safety or effectiveness.

Questions—Beryllium

1. Which of the following statements is false?
- A. Beryllium (chemical symbol Be) is the fourth lightest element.
- B. Beryllium is used in alloys for space exploration, military equipment, and nuclear reactors.
- C. Exposure to beryllium can cause chronic granulomatous disease similar to sarcoidosis and miliary tuberculosis.
- D. Acute beryllium exposures cause profound cardiotoxicity.
- E. Beryllium is a cutaneous sensitizer and primary skin irritant that produces contact dermatitis, skin granulomas, and ulcers.

2. Criteria for the diagnosis of chronic beryllium disease may include
- A. Epidemiologic evidence of significant beryllium exposure
- B. Presence of beryllium in lung tissue, lymph nodes, or urine
- C. Evidence of apical respiratory tract disease
- D. Radiologic evidence of interstitial disease consistent with a fibronodular process
- E. A, B and D

BISMUTH

Bismuth is a brittle metal (chemical symbol Bi) used in alloys. In the United States bismuth subsalicylate, the active ingredient in Pepto-Bismol®, is considered safe in doses up to 4.8 g daily, but there is insufficient evidence to establish its effectiveness as an antinauseant or antiemetic. Bismuth subsalicylate (BSS) is a highly insoluble salt of trivalent bismuth and salicylic acid. Each molecule contains 58% bismuth and 42% salicylate by weight. See Chapter 11, Salicylates.

Between 1973 and 1980 approximately 1,000 cases of bismuth-related neurotoxicity were reported in France, Australia, Belgium, Switzerland, and Spain. In France, the neurotoxicity was associated with the use of a bismuth substrate. All patients recovered within two to 12 weeks after ceasing bismuth administration. Bismuth salts were placed under prescription control, and other restrictions were initiated.

Pathophysiology

Bismuth strongly associates with the mucosal surface of the stomach and may be responsible for the cytoprotective properties of Pepto-Bismol. See the section on Bismuth Subsalicylate (Pepto-Bismol®) in Chapter 30, Gastrointestinal Toxicology. Pharmacologically active bismuth compounds have been subdivided into four groups.

Group 1 compounds are simple inorganic salts and subsalts of bismuth such as bismuth subcarbonate, and bismuth subnitrate. These compounds are insoluble in water in the absence of complexing agents, with minimal bismuth absorption and virtually no toxicity. Group 2 substances are predominantly lipid-soluble organic compounds and complexes of bismuth such as bismuth subgallate. They are easily absorbed, lead to high bismuth blood levels, and are neurotoxic and possibly hepatotoxic.

Group 3 agents are predominantly water-soluble organic compounds and complexes of bismuth that are stable enough to be absorbed and also lead to high bismuth blood levels. Renal damage is a prominent feature of the toxicity syndrome in many of these compounds. An example is bismuth triglycollamate. Group 4 compounds are water-soluble organic complexes of bismuth that decompose in the gastrointestinal system with the ultimate production of simple insoluble bismuth compounds such as bismuth subchloride and bismuth sulfide. Minimal absorption and practically no toxicity are characteristic features.

Pharmacokinetics

ABSORPTION

- Absorption of the salicylate in bismuth subsalicylate (BSS) occurs in the small intestine.

DISTRIBUTION

- BSS is mostly hydrolyzed in the stomach to form bismuth oxychloride and salicylic acid.
- In the small intestine, nondissociated BSS reacts with other anions (bicarbonate and phosphate) to form bismuth subcarbonate and bismuth phosphate salts, which are highly insoluble.

ELIMINATION

- In the colon, nondissociated BSS and other bismuth salts react with hydrogen sulfide produced by anaerobic bacteria to produce bismuth sulfide, a highly insoluble black salt responsible for darkening of the stool.
- Unchewed and undissolved Pepto-Bismol® tablets are radiopaque.

Clinical Presentations

Symptoms of systemic intoxication are similar to those of lead and mercury. Increased salivation, a bismuth line (bluish discoloration of the gums), pyorrhea, and loss of teeth have been observed. Permanent discoloration of the skin and ulcerative stomatitis with or without colitis is rarely seen. Methemoglobin may follow the reduction of bismuth substrate to nitrate. Diminished renal function with severe nephrosis and renal failure has been observed, in addition to hepatic degeneration and peripheral neuritis.

NEUROLOGIC EFFECTS

Despite the relative safety of oral bismuth preparations, encephalopathy has been reported after large or repetitive ingestions of water- or lipid-soluble salts. Altered mental status, ataxia, myoclonus, and a specific electroencephalographic abnormality characterize the encephalopathy. Death has followed bismuth encephalopathy. Osteoarthropathy may complicate bismuth encephalopathy. Osteoporosis and osteomalacia may follow increased bismuth levels in bone.

CHRONIC EFFECTS

Chronic ingestion results in stomatitis, black spots on the mucosa and gums (bismuth lines), salivation, and pathologic fractures. Chronic toxicity results in encephalopathy and acute nephrotoxicity following the use of bismuth salts.

Toxic Dosage/Death

Daily doses of 5.2–9.4 g of Pepto-Bismol® daily led to a fatal encephalopathy in seven days. Blood bismuth levels were 200 μg/L (normal is 5 μg/L) and urine levels were 2,960 μg/L.

Laboratory

ANALYTIC METHODS

Bismuth may be quantified in urine, blood, or serum by electrothermal atomic absorption spectrophotometry or a reverse-phase high-performance liquid chromatography (HPLC) method.

BLOOD LEVELS

Blood concentrations are not a reliable marker for neurotoxicity. However, blood levels from 1,500–2,000 μg/L (normal is less than 20 μg/L) have been associated with bismuth encephalopathy. No relationship is apparent between blood and urine bismuth concentrations, and blood and cerebrospinal fluid bismuth concentrations. Hyperdensities in the basal ganglia, cerebellum, and cerebral cortex in one series were most marked when bismuth blood levels exceeded 2,000 μg/L.

Treatment

GUT DECONTAMINATION

These methods have not been evaluated after bismuth overdose.

ELIMINATION ENHANCEMENT

The role of hemodialysis has not been evaluated.

SUPPORTIVE MEASURES

- Treatment of overdose is largely symptomatic and supportive. Even after large overdoses, the prognosis is good. The main therapeutic measure in bismuth encephalopathy is to withdraw bismuth from the patient. Benzodiazepines or other anticonvulsants may be useful for myoclonic seizures, but few studies have been performed to support this or any other intervention.
- A radiopaque substance may be seen on a plain film of the abdomen in the large intestine of patients with bismuth encephalopathy.
- A characteristic EEG in bismuth toxicity displays low voltage and diffuse beta-frequencies bilaterally, maximal in the frontal and central areas and accentuated by hyperventilation.
- On CT scan, an increase in density may be seen in the cortex of the cerebral hemisphere and in the basal ganglia. This increased density may be caused directly by the presence of bismuth, which is radiopaque.

Antidotes

Chelating agents may be effective before tissue binding has occurred. D-penicillamine does not appear to facilitate excretion of bismuth. Dimercaprol (BAL in Oil) has enhanced bismuth clearance in at least two patients with myoclonic encephalopathy due to bismuth salt intoxication. Dimercapto-1-propane sulfonic acid (DMPS) has led to a tenfold increase in urinary clearance of bismuth with clinical improvement of encephalopathy.

Questions—Bismuth

1. Which of the following statements is false?

A. Bismuth is a brittle metal (chemical symbol Bi) used in alloys.

B. Bismuth subsalicylate is the active ingredient in Pepto-Bismol®.

C. Bismuth subsalicylate (BSS) is a highly insoluble salt of trivalent bismuth and salicylic acid.
D. Numerous cases of bismuth-related neurotoxicity have been reported in Europe.
E. The salicylate in bismuth subsalicylate is benign and not a factor in BSS poisoning.

2. **Which of the following statements about bismuth toxicity is false?**
A. Symptoms of systemic intoxication are similar to those of iron and antimony.
B. Increased salivation, a bismuth line (bluish discoloration of the gums), pyorrhea, and loss of teeth have been observed.
C. Methemoglobin may follow the reduction of bismuth substrate to nitrate.
D. Diminished renal function with severe nephrosis and renal failure has been observed, in addition to hepatic degeneration and peripheral neuritis.
E. Despite the relative safety of oral bismuth preparations, encephalopathy has been reported after large or repetitive ingestions of water- or lipid-soluble salts.

CADMIUM

Cadmium (chemical symbol Cd) is a nonessential trace metal that progressively accumulates in the body, particularly in the kidney. Cadmium poisoning is a rare type of heavy-metal poisoning associated with industrial exposures, ingestion of contaminated shellfish, or drinking of acidic beverages from contaminated vessels. It causes leg cramps, nausea, vomiting, and diarrhea. Acute exposures usually occur in the workplace via inhalation and initially affect the lungs. Chronic exposures produce renal dysfunction, emphysema, and osteomalacia.

Environmental exposures involve zinc and lead smelters (i.e., cadmium is a common contaminant of metal ores), electroplated ice trays, as well as contaminated foodstuffs (e.g., rice, cigarettes, and soil). Environmental contamination in Japan caused a disease called *Itai-Itai* ("ouch-ouch"), which was characterized by severe arthralgias and osteomalacia in middle-aged postmenopausal women with low calcium and vitamin D intake.

Cadmium also appears in the workplace in solder, as a neutron absorbent in the nuclear industry, in alkaline storage batteries, as an amalgam in dentistry, and as a stabilizer for polyvinyl chloride, engravings, and pigments. Some occupations at risk include alloy makers, battery makers, engravers, textile workers, welders, solder workers, and zinc and lead refiners.

Pathophysiology

The kidney is the main target organ for chronic exposure. Proximal tubular dysfunction characterized by proteinuria, aminoaciduria, and glycosuria occurs. Renal failure is rare. High acute exposure produces delayed pulmonary edema progressing to interstitial fibrosis. Chronic effects include emphysema and chronic bronchitis. A weak epidemiological association exists between lung carcinoma and chronic cadmium exposure.

Clinical Presentations

The initial presentation after acute inhalation simulates metal fume fever with symptoms (e.g., fever, headache, dyspnea, pleuritic chest pain, conjunctivitis, rhinitis, sore throat, cough) developing 4–12 hours after exposure. Depending on the exposure level, noncardiogenic pulmonary edema may appear which can progress to death. Respiratory failure may ensue in 3–10 days. Acute gastroenteritis results from ingestion and is characterized by the sudden onset of vomiting, diarrhea, and abdominal pain.

Other cadmium-related signs and symptoms include "yellow teeth lines," tubular or glomerular insufficiency (characterized by microhematuria, proteinuria, and hypertension), vertigo, fatigue, urinary calculi, osteopenia, osteomalacia, rhinitis, anosmia, anorexia, and dyspnea. *Itai-Itai* disease is associated with impaired urine concentration. The overall IARC classification of cadmium is 'probably carcinogenic to humans.'

Toxic Dosage/Death

A suicidal ingestion of 150 g of cadmium chloride produced facial edema, vomiting, hypotension, respiratory arrest, metabolic acidosis, pulmonary edema, oliguria, and finally death 30 hours postingestion.

Pregnancy/Lactation

There appears to be a maternal-fetal gradient of blood cadmium. The birth weight of offspring of mothers who smoke cigarettes is decreased, but this has not been definitely attributed to cadmium exposure without smoking.

Laboratory

ANALYTIC METHODS

Quantitation of urine cadmium is accomplished with electrothermal atomic absorption spectrometry. The detection limit of urinary cadmium is 0.08 $\mu g/L$.

BLOOD LEVELS

The concentration of cadmium in the blood in normal populations is about 0.4–1.0 $\mu g/L$ for nonsmokers and 1.4–4.0 $\mu g/L$ for smokers. Values in occupationally exposed populations range from 10 to 100 $\mu g/L$. Levels above 0.7 $\mu g/dL$ indicate significant exposure. Blood cadmium levels in workers involved in an outbreak of cadmium intoxication in a jewelry factory were higher than those in unexposed workers. A dose-response relationship was observed between blood cadmium levels and symptoms of dyspnea, chest pain, dyscrasia, and dizziness.

URINE

When the urinary excretion of cadmium is less than 2 $\mu g/24$ hours, the risk of occurrence of renal effects remains low. The urine level best reflects total body burden, although some authors believe that an increased cadmium level requires the concomitant presence of renal damage.

Treatment

GUT DECONTAMINATION

Charcoal is not useful.

ELIMINATION ENHANCEMENT

These methods have not been used in the treatment of cadmium exposures.

SUPPORTIVE MEASURES

- Watch carefully for delayed pulmonary edema after acute inhalation.
- Symptomatic patients should be hospitalized.
- Hospitalize all patients in whom chelation is indicated.

Antidotes

Calcium disodium EDTA is the chelator of choice for acute cadmium exposures. Dimercaptosuccinic acid (DMSA) may have a role in enhancing cadmium excretion and may be of clinical use in acute oral intoxication by cadmium compounds. Clinical studies confirming these observations remain to be done. BAL in Oil (dimercaprol) increases nephrotoxicity and is therefore not indicated. Chronic exposures require no chelation, and treatment involves removal from contamination.

Questions—Cadmium

1. **Which of the following statements about cadmium poisoning is false?**
   A. Cadmium (chemical symbol Cm) is an essential trace metal that progressively accumulates in the body, particularly in the kidney.
   B. Cadmium poisoning is a rare type of heavy-metal poisoning associated with industrial exposures and ingestion of contaminated shellfish.
   C. Chronic exposures produce renal dysfunction, emphysema, and osteomalacia.
   D. Environmental contamination in Japan caused a disease called *Itai-Itai* ("ouch-ouch").
   E. Cadmium also appears in the workplace in solder and may appear as an amalgam in dentistry.
2. **The initial presentation after acute cadmium inhalation simulates metal fume fever with symptoms (fever, headache, dyspnea, pleuritic chest pain, conjunctivitis, rhinitis, sore throat, cough) developing 4–12 hours after exposure.**
   A. True
   B. False
3. **Signs of cadmium exposure include all of the following except**
   A. Vomiting, diarrhea, and abdominal pain
   B. "Yellow teeth lines"
   C. Seizures
   D. Tubular or glomerular insufficiency
   E. Urinary calculi
4. **The chelator of choice for acute cadmium exposures is**
   A. Calcium disodium EDTA
   B. Dimercaprol (BAL in Oil)
   C. Deferoxamine
   D. D-Penicillamine
   E. Sodium Diethyldithiocarbamate

CHROMIUM

Chromium (chemical symbol Cr) compounds are both skin and pulmonary sensitizers. They can produce irritation of the conjunctiva and mucous membranes, nasal perforation, and contact dermatitis (e.g., "blackjack disease" in card players and dealers exposed to chromium in green felt). Exposure to chromium compounds is primarily industrial. Epidemiologic studies have detected an increased incidence of lung cancer in workers exposed to hexavalent chromium compounds. Trivalent chromium compounds are relatively harmless.

Pathophysiology

The toxicity of chromium is due to the oxidizing properties of the hexavalent compounds and to pH. Chromic acid has a pH of 5 and ammonia dichromate has a pH of 13. Hexavalent chromium in dichromate compounds binds nonspecifically to proteins and nucleoproteins and is specifically taken up into red cells and platelets. It is reduced to trivalent chromium. This conversion, and perhaps the intermediate pentavalent chromium, produces free-radical damage to mitochondria, particularly in kidney tubules and hepatocytes.

Pharmacokinetics

ABSORPTION

- The lungs and gastrointestinal tract readily absorb toxic hexavalent chromium compounds (e.g., sodium, potassium, ammonium, and chromium trioxide, and chromic acid).
- Bivalent and trivalent forms (e.g., chromic oxide, chromic sulfate, and other salts) are relatively insoluble, poorly absorbed, and usually not of any clinical importance.

DISTRIBUTION

- Once absorbed, chromium is rapidly excreted mainly via the urinary tract.
- It is widely distributed to the kidneys and liver.

ELIMINATION

- The elimination half-life of hexavalent chromium is 15–41 hours.

Clinical Presentations

Ingestion of hexavalent compounds usually leads to abdominal pain, vomiting, diarrhea, and intestinal bleeding. Death may ensue due to circulatory collapse. If the patient survives the initial phase, renal tubular damage may occur. Hepatic failure, severe coagulopathy, and/or intravascular hemolysis have been observed. An adult who suffered full-thickness burns of the left calf (1% of body surface) from a concentrated chromic acid solution developed nausea and vomiting within one hour and complete anuria within 24 hours.

Dichromate dust can cause conjunctivitis, chronic penetrating lesions of the skin, lacrimation, and ulceration of the nasal septum. Vertigo, thirst, abdominal pain, vomiting, oliguria, anuria, shock, seizures, severe coagulopathy, intravascular hemolysis, and a hepatorenal syndrome can follow large doses of dichromate. There is an increased incidence of bronchogenic carcinoma in workers exposed to chromate dust. The risk of dying from respiratory cancer among chromate workers is more than 20 times that of a control population and the latent period appears relatively short.

Toxic Dosage/Death

As little as 500 mg of ingested hexavalent chromium (such as chromic acid or chromium trioxide) may cause life-threatening toxicity in adults. Lethal doses of 1–2 g have been reported. Potassium dichromate at doses of 0.5–0.8 g may be lethal. Death has occurred after a 10% skin surface burn. A 15-year-old who ingested a few grains of potassium dichromate vomited, became unconscious, and died in 12 hours. Her blood level was 3.5 μg/dL. High chromate concentrations were found in the liver, kidney, and stomach.

Pregnancy/Lactation

The hexavalent form crosses the placenta and may be found in breast milk.

Laboratory

ANALYTIC METHODS

Chromium is measured by flameless atomic absorption spectrometry.

BLOOD LEVELS

Toxic levels include blood concentrations greater than 2.65 μg/100 mL and urine levels exceeding 3.7 μg/L.

HAIR

Hair chromium concentrations may be used as indices of industrial exposure to trivalent chromium.

Treatment

GUT DECONTAMINATION

Nasogastric lavage with an ascorbic acid solution and intravenous doses of ascorbic acid may theoretically reduce hexavalent chromium to the less toxic trivalent state. Studies to prove the clinical efficacy of this regimen are lacking however.

ELIMINATION ENHANCEMENT

Survival in at least two cases of chromic acid ingestion and one case of potassium dichromate has been achieved with vigorous hemodialysis. Treatment of chromic acid burns by peritoneal dialysis has been less successful. The efficacy of exchange transfusion has not been established.

SUPPORTIVE MEASURES

- Treatment is symptomatic. Administer oxygen as required for respiratory compromise.
- Esophagoscopy may be required to evaluate gastrointestinal burns.
- Large-dose intravenous therapy with ascorbic acid has been recommended in uncontrolled *in vitro* studies. Theoretically, ascorbic acid may reduce hexavalent chromium to the less toxic trivalent form. Chromium dermatitis has also been treated with topical ascorbic acid. Further studies are necessary to confirm or deny the efficacy of these interventions.
- Monitor renal and hepatic function.

Antidotes

The efficacy of BAL has not been established. Dimercapto-propane-sulfonic acid (DMPS) was given to a man who fell into a pool of chromic acid. His urine chromium level rose to 13,614 μg/mL and he survived. Treatment using intravenous N-acetylcysteine and hemodialysis was associated with hepatic and renal improvement in an adult who ingested sodium dichromate. Further studies are required.

Questions—Chromium

1. Which of the following statements about chromium poisoning is false?

A. Chromium (chemical symbol Cr) compounds are both skin and pulmonary sensitizers.
B. They can produce irritation of the conjunctiva and mucous membranes, nasal perforation, and contact dermatitis (e.g., "blackjack disease" in card players and dealers exposed to green felt).
C. Exposure to chromium compounds is primarily household and extremely rare.
D. Epidemiologic studies have detected an increased incidence of lung cancer in workers exposed to hexavalent chromium compounds.
E. Trivalent chromium compounds are relatively harmless.

2. True statements about chromium exposure include all of the following except

A. Ingestion of hexavalent compounds usually leads to abdominal pain, vomiting, diarrhea, and intestinal bleeding.
B. Death may ensue due to circulatory collapse.
C. Hepatic failure, severe coagulopathy, and/or intravascular hemolysis have been observed.
D. Dichromate dust can cause conjunctivitis, chronic penetrating lesions of the skin, lacrimation, and ulceration of the nasal septum.
E. Respiratory cancer from chromate has only been recognized in animals.

COBALT

Chronic exposure to cobalt (chemical symbol Co) produces "hard-metal pneumoconiosis" in industrial workers. This term derives from the use of cobalt in the manufacture of heat-resistant hard-metal alloys. The acute form of the disease resembles a hypersensitivity reaction with malaise, cough, and wheezing. The chronic form progresses to cor pulmonale. Epidemics of "beer drinker's cardiomyopathy" resulted from the use of cobalt as a defoaming agent, and similar cardiac dysfunction may appear in those who work with hard metals. Chronic administration of this essential trace element (cobalt is a component of vitamin B12) may cause goiter and reduced thyroid activity.

Hard metal interstitial lung disease was first described in 1940, and hard metal occupational asthma in 1967. Both disorders are considered idiopathic reactions to the cobalt component of hard metal, although nickel may play a part as well. "Hard metal" is an alloy consisting of tungsten carbide (usually 75–95%) and cobalt (5–25%) as a matrix. Others metals that may be added include titanium, nickel, chromium, niobium, vanadium, and tantalum. Hard metal is 90–95% as hard as diamond. Tungsten carbide is inert and cobalt is considered the cause of associated lung damage.

Pathophysiology

Both the obstructive and the interstitial syndromes in hard metal disease are responses to the inhalation of cobalt. Histologic abnormalities in subjects chronically exposed to cobalt dust include an interstitial pneumonitis (fibrosing alveolitis) with infiltrates of lymphocytes, macrophages, plasma cells, and eosinophils. A more characteristic feature is the presence of multinucleated giant cells of macrophage and monocyte origin within the alveoli and bronchoalveolar lavage fluid.

Pharmacokinetics

ABSORPTION

- Absorption depends on numerous factors including the solubility of the specific cobalt compound, coingested material and individual variation.
- Absorption may occur via the lungs.

DISTRIBUTION

- Cobalt is found in highest concentration in the liver followed by the kidney.

ELIMINATION

- Most elimination of cobalt occurs via the kidney.
- The half-life of an absorbed dose is several days.

Clinical Presentations

Hard metal lung disease is an occupational pulmonary disease generally found in patients who work as grinders of material made from tungsten carbide. It can occur as an interstitial lung disease with all the classical signs of pulmonary fibrosis and as an obstructive airway syndrome. Hard metal lung disease often starts as an allergic alveolitis that can progress to severe fibrosis if the exposure is not stopped. Hard metal asthma may be an IgE-antibody-mediated syndrome due to cobalt reactivity. Nickel, as well as cobalt, sensitivity may play a role in hard metal asthma.

COBALT LUNG

Interstitial lung disease attributed to cobalt not alloyed to carbides of hard metals may induce cough, chest tightness, dyspnea, weight loss, a severe restrictive defect, and a markedly decreased diffusing capacity. It may be accompanied by the presence of multiple multinucleated giant cells in the bronchoalveolar lavage. This condition may show a rapidly fatal progression.

COBALT CARDIOMYOPATHY

Industrial cobalt exposure may cause fatal cardiomyopathy in adults employed in the hard metal industry. In the 1960s, after a large number of beer drinkers in three countries consumed beer to which cobalt chloride or cobalt sulfate had been added, an abrupt onset of left and right heart failure was reported. Overall mortality approached 50%.

CANCER

Some data suggest that metallic cobalt and certain cobalt compounds (e.g., cobalt oxide, sulfide, chloride, acetate and naphthenate) are probable chemical carcinogens and that such exposure has been associated with lung cancer.

Toxic Dosage/Death

An 11-year-old who swallowed two magnets consisting of 40% cobalt developed vomiting, weight loss, polycythemia, thyromegaly, metabolic acidosis, and cardiomyopathy. An abdominal radiograph showed an opaque mass in the stomach. His serum cobalt level was 4.1 $\mu g/dL$ (normal 0.35–1.7 $\mu g/dL$) and his urine cobalt value was 1,700 $\mu g/L$ (normal 1–7 $\mu g/L$). Clinical improvement followed chelation with calcium disodium EDTA.

Pregnancy/Lactation

Occupational reports suggest that a woman can have a successful pregnancy despite severe pulmonary dysfunction secondary to hard metal lung disease.

Laboratory

ANALYTIC METHODS

Respiratory function tests may show evidence of restrictive lung disease and a decrease in the diffusion capacity of carbon monoxide. Flame or flameless atomic absorption and / or inductively coupled plasma analysis may measure cobalt.

BLOOD LEVELS

Following cobalt levels will not assist in the clinical management of cobalt exposure.

Treatment

GUT DECONTAMINATION

There are no clinical reports documenting positive interventions with these methods.

ELIMINATION ENHANCEMENT

There are no clinical reports documenting positive interventions with these methods.

SUPPORTIVE MEASURES

- Chest x-ray may reveal bilateral linear shadows, a reticulonodular pattern, or a nodular pattern.
- Interruption of exposure usually leads to a rapid regression of complaints and a partial improvement of lung function.
- Steroids and / or cyclophosphamide may be helpful in the treatment of hard metal lung disease.

Antidotes

Animal experiments suggest that N-acetylcysteine (NAC) may be helpful, but there are no human studies to corroborate these findings. Calcium disodium EDTA may be helpful as well.

Questions—Cobalt

1. **Which of the following statements about cobalt poisoning is false?**
   A. Chronic exposure to cobalt (chemical symbol Co) produces "hard-metal pneumoconiosis" in industrial workers.
   B. Acute cobalt poisoning resembles a hypersensitivity reaction with cough and wheezing.
   C. Epidemics of "beer drinker's cardiomyopathy" resulted from the use of cobalt as a defoaming agent, and similar cardiac dysfunction may appear in those who work with hard metals.
   D. Chronic administration of this essential trace element (cobalt is a component of vitamin B12) may cause hyperthyroidism.
   E. "Hard metal" is an alloy consisting of tungsten carbide (usually 75–95%) and cobalt (5–25%) as a matrix.
2. **Which of the following pulmonary diseases may follow occupational exposure to cobalt?**
   A. Hard metal lung disease

B. Pulmonary fibrosis
C. Obstructive airway syndrome
D. All of the above
E. A and B

3. Nickel, as well as cobalt, sensitivity may play a role in hard metal asthma.
A. True
B. False

COPPER

Copper (chemical symbol Cu) contamination of food and beverages can produce an acute gastrointestinal illness. Sources include beverages from vending machines, copper or brass vessels, and rarely drinking water. In India, copper has been used as a suicidal agent. The medicinal use of copper as an emetic was discontinued because of its toxicity. Reports of chronic liver disease, diffuse pulmonary fibrosis, and angiosarcoma in workers and children following copper exposure require further confirmation by controlled studies.

Wilson's disease is an autosomal recessive metabolic disease that results from a gene alteration. Low concentrations of ceruloplasmin allow accumulation of large quantities of copper in the liver, brain and other organs. Accumulation results from the inability to excrete copper in bile.

Pathophysiology

Copper is an essential trace element that catalyzes processes in heme synthesis and iron absorption.

Pharmacokinetics

ABSORPTION

- Systemic bioavailability of edible copper (5 mg/day) is 30%.
- The usual intake of copper in the U.S. population averages 1 mg/d.
- A controlled study of copper balance suggests that 0.8 mg of copper/day may be close to the copper requirement for young adults.
- Copper (metallic and/or its azide salt) may be absorbed from the skin.

DISTRIBUTION

- Copper is present in serum in two different forms. The first form reacts directly with the copper colorimetric reagent, sodium diethyldithiocarbamate and is loosely bound to serum albumin. This function is cytotoxic. This small fraction is concerned with the transportation of copper from the gastrointestinal tract to tissues, and from one tissue to another.
- The larger fraction of serum copper is tightly bound to the serum copper enzyme ceruloplasmin.
- About 7% of copper is loosely bound to albumin, and 93% is bound to ceruloplasmin.
- The apparent volume of distribution of copper is 1.95 L/kg.

ELIMINATION

- The half-life of copper in healthy individuals is about 26 days.
- About 0.1–1.3 ng of copper is excreted through the bile daily and lost in the feces.
- If a large amount of copper is suddenly released from the liver, it is taken up by erythrocytes and a hemolytic crisis may occur.

Clinical Presentations

RENAL EFFECTS

Copper causes a focal necrosis of the proximal tubules. The Fanconi syndrome, characterized by tubular proteinuria, generalized aminoaciduria, phosphaturia, uricosuria and hypercalciuria, may result from a direct toxic effect of copper or from associated hemolysis. A syndrome of intravenous copper intoxication due to copper released from tubing during hemodialysis includes nausea, vomiting, abdominal pain, diarrhea, anxiety, and depression.

SYSTEMIC EFFECTS

Myalgias, abdominal pain, diarrhea, acidosis, pancreatitis, methemoglobin formation, and hemolysis are indicative of copper intoxication. Copper may be a factor in the development of childhood cirrhosis.

CHRONIC EFFECTS

Airborne dusts of inorganic copper salts have low toxicity. "Vineyard sprayer's lung disease" has been associated with airborne copper sulfate. This is a histiocytic granulomatous lung and liver disease occurring in individuals exposed to copper sulfate spray for 2–15 years.

DERMATOLOGIC EFFECTS

Chronic copper poisoning has occurred after repeated application of a copper-containing topical cream to eczematous skin. The application of copper crystals to granulomatous tissue with burns has resulted in chronic poisoning with skin darkening. The most common form of skin contamination by copper is the production of green hair discoloration. The green hue is produced by an increased absorption of copper into the hair from copper algicides used in swimming pools.

WILSON'S DISEASE

Clinical manifestations of Wilson's disease include liver failure, dysarthria, dysphagia, ataxia, hemolytic anemia, renal tubular dysfunction and renal stones. Kayser-Fleischer rings are corneal deposits of copper.

SPIRITUAL WATER

Overdosage of copper salts is common in developing countries because of its wide use in various traditional preparations. Poisoning is due to the ingestion of "spiritual green water" following distribution to members of spiritual churches. Within a few hours of ingestion, greenish vomiting and abdominal pain are seen. Anuria may supervene within 24 hours. Flapping tremor, toxic psychosis, hemolytic anemia, and jaundice may follow within a few days. Patients may die within a few days of hemodialysis.

Toxic Dosage/Death

Renal failure and death may follow ingestion of as little as 1 g of copper sulfate. Ingestion of 10–20 g of copper sulfate is usually lethal. Hemodialysis has not prevented death in such cases. Fortunately, fatal poisoning is rare.

Laboratory

ANALYTIC METHODS

Copper is measured by inductively coupled plasma emission spectroscopy.

BLOOD LEVELS

The normal serum concentration of copper ranges from 70 to 155 μg/dL. Patients with metal fume fever following exposure to metallic copper demonstrate copper levels over 160 μg/dL. The mean value of normal ceruloplasmin is 30 mg/100 mL. Ingestion of 20–30 mL of copper sulfate led to a blood copper level of 1.25 μg/mL in a patient who died. The plasma copper concentration in a series of fatal cases involving copper ranged from 9.8 to 46 mg/L.

Treatment

GUT DECONTAMINATION

Vomiting usually makes lavage unnecessary. Charcoal may be used but its role is unproved.

ELIMINATION ENHANCEMENT

Removal of copper by dialysis may be useful in the early stages of poisoning when the metal is still present in the circulation as free copper.

SUPPORTIVE MEASURES

- Treatment is primarily symptomatic and supportive.

Antidotes

Chelating agents are recommended in severe poisoning, but few pharmacokinetic data on humans exist to guide their use. Either intravenous calcium disodium EDTA or intramuscular dimercaprol is the agent of choice in severe ingestions. D-penicillamine may be administered orally, if tolerated, to patients who are not allergic to penicillin. D-penicillamine is preferred for the treatment of Wilson's disease. The copper-chelating drug tetrathiomolybdate, used in Wilson's disease, has been associated with pancytopenia and has not been reported in acute copper poisoning.

Questions—Copper

1. Wilson's disease
   A. Is associated with high ceruloplasmin levels
   B. Is associated with too much copper and zinc
   C. Is an idiosyncratic disease
   D. Is an autosomal recessive, inherited metabolic disease that results from a gene alteration
   E. Is associated with "bronze diabetes"

2. Which of the following is not associated with copper exposure?
   A. The Fanconi syndrome, characterized by tubular proteinuria, generalized aminoaciduria, phosphaturia, uricosuria and hypercalciuria
   B. Myalgias, abdominal pain, diarrhea, acidosis and pancreatitis
   C. Kayser-Fleischer rings
   D. Green hair discoloration
   E. Neonatal jaundice

3. Overdosage of copper salts is common in developing countries because of its wide use in various traditional preparations.
   A. True
   B. False

GERMANIUM

Germanium (Ge) is a trace metal used industrially because of its semiconductive properties. It is an element with chemical properties similar to those of silicon, tin, arsenic, and antimony. The daily intake by humans is about 1 mg, in foods such as oats and barley. It is rapidly absorbed in the gastrointestinal tract and excreted mainly through the kidneys. Germanium-containing organic molecules are under investigation for their ability to modulate immune responses.

The role of germanium in human biology is unknown. In Japan, the United Kingdom, the U.S. and the Netherlands it has been used as a health food supplement. When used in doses of 50–250 mg/d for several months or longer, germanium dioxide has been associated with severe renal dysfunction. At least one case of fatal lactic acidosis has been reported in a 43-year-old female who abused germanium.

Questions—Germanium

1. Which of the following statements about germanium is false?
   A. Germanium is a trace metal used industrially because of its semiconductive properties.
   B. It is an element with chemical properties similar to those of silicon, tin, arsenic, and antimony.
   C. The role of germanium in human biology is well described in vitamin metabolism.
   D. Germanium has been used as a health food supplement.
   E. Germanium dioxide has been associated with severe renal dysfunction.

GOLD

Gold (chemical symbol Au) compounds are used in dentistry, as food coloring agents, in the treatment of pemphigus and in certain psoriatic patients who do not respond to non-steroidal anti-inflammatory agents. In the form of gold sodium thiomalate, gold therapy is an acceptable treatment for rheumatoid arthritis.

Pathophysiology

All anti-rheumatic gold compounds contain gold in the gold I oxidation state. The adverse effect of gold-containing antirheumatics appear to be caused by gold III, an oxidation product of gold I.

Clinical Presentations

Adverse reactions which occur during therapy include interstitial pneumonitis, dermatitis, stomatitis, bone marrow suppression, nephrotic syndrome, nephritis, and hepatitis. An encephalopathy also has been associated with gold therapy.

GOLD LUNG

Gold lung is a rare toxic side effect of gold therapy that may begin after a 300–1,000 mg total gold dose has been administered. Dyspnea suddenly appears over a period of 2–10 days. The chest x-ray shows diffuse bilateral pulmonary shading. The prognosis is good after simple withdrawal of the gold. Lung function tests show a restrictive defect. Impairment of lung function may be permanent.

NITRITOID REACTION

The nitritoid reaction, a rare side effect of treatment with sodium aurothiomalate, consists of a brief episode of facial flushing, nausea, dizziness, and occasionally hypotension. It occurs several minutes after an intramuscular injection and appears unpredictably during the first week after gold treatments are begun.

GASTROINTESTINAL EFFECTS

Gold-induced enterocolitis may follow treatment with either injected or orally administered gold and may involve any segment of the gastrointestinal tract. Presenting symptoms may include fever, nausea, vomiting, and abdominal cramps with diarrhea. This condition may end fatally. Self-limited intrahepatic cholestasis with eosinophilia may be observed after gold injections.

HEMATOLOGIC EFFECTS

Idiosyncratic agranulocytosis and aplastic anemia have been reported following gold therapy. Spontaneous neutrophil recovery may take 15–30 days after drug withdrawal. Enlarged regional lymph nodes following prolonged gold therapy may contain deposits of elemental gold.

RENAL EFFECTS

Proteinuria occurs in 2–20% of patients treated with injected gold and may be sufficiently severe to cause the nephrotic syndrome in 10–30% of those affected. Membranous glomerulonephritis may occur. Proteinuria usually resolves when the drug is stopped. Renal function does not deteriorate.

Toxic Dosage/Death

A 53-year-old was accidentally injected with an intramuscular dose of 450 mg of sodium aurothiomalate. Palpebral edema and a rash were observed in 30 minutes. His gold blood level reached 2,970 μg/dL without significant toxicity. The patient was treated with BAL and recovered.

Drug Interactions

The nitritoid reaction may be more common if an angiotensin-converting-enzyme inhibitor is added to the regimen of gold therapy.

Laboratory

ANALYTIC METHODS

Gold is measured by atomic absorption spectrometry.

BLOOD LEVELS

Following gold levels does not guide therapy or management in overdose. In one case, the peak serum gold level was 5 mg/dL after an injection of 500-mg gold aurothiomalate.

Treatment

GUT DECONTAMINATION

Limited experience with gold-containing products makes recommendations regarding methods of gut decontamination unhelpful.

ELIMINATION ENHANCEMENT

These methods have not been utilized in managing gold overdose.

SUPPORTIVE MEASURES

- Steroids may be helpful for pneumonitis, but more studies are needed.

Antidotes

BAL in Oil (dimercaprol) has been utilized as a chelator after large gold exposures.

Questions—Gold

1. **Which of the following is not associated with gold exposure?**
   A. All anti-rheumatic gold compounds contain gold in the gold I oxidation state.
   B. Epistaxis frequently follows intense exposure to gold vapor.
   C. Encephalopathy
   D. Nephrotic syndrome
   E. Interstitial pneumonitis
2. **The nitritoid reaction, a rare side effect of treatment with sodium aurothiomalate, consists of a brief episode of facial flushing, nausea, dizziness, and occasionally hypertension. It occurs hours after an intravenous injection and appears predictably in 10 minutes after gold treatments are begun.**
   A. True
   B. False

IRON

Iron (chemical symbol Fe) remains a significant and potentially deadly cause of metal poisoning in the United States. Thousands of reported exposures are made to poison centers each year. An overdose of chewable vitamins with iron remains one of the most commonly encountered potential poisonings in children. Most exposures involve children less than 6 years of age. Most of these patients remain asymptomatic or develop minimal toxicity. Concentrated iron supplement overdoses more often result in serious sequelae and may be fatal.

Chewable vitamins may enhance iron absorption so that "low" doses can cause systemic effects. Patients may die and present to the emergency room at any stage of iron poisoning. If a patient does not develop symptoms within 6 hours after ingestion, it is unlikely that iron toxicity will develop. The introduction of the antidote deferoxamine has reduced the mortality in hospitalized patients from 50% to less than 2%.

Pathophysiology

Iron is an essential element of hemoglobin and red blood cell homeostasis. It is also found in myoglobin and numerous enzymes. Toxic doses of iron overwhelm normal gastrointestinal regulatory mechanisms and can lead to massive iron absorption. Major toxicity occurs when serum iron levels exceed the iron-binding capacity of transferrin. Free circulating iron damages systemic blood vessels.

The release of the potent vasodilator ferritin and, possibly, the release of serotonin and histamine potentiate the vascular damage caused by free serum iron. Iron can produce cerebral edema by an unknown mechanism. In severe iron overdose, coagulative necrosis with platelet aggregation appears similar to the damage caused by corrosive agents.

Pharmacokinetics

ABSORPTION

- The kinetics of iron absorption after ingestion of chewable vitamins are not fully understood; however, it appears that iron is very well absorbed from this form.
- Iron is absorbed through the mucosal barrier in the ferrous ($^{2+}$) state where it oxidizes to the ferric ($^{3+}$) state and attaches to the storage protein, ferritin. The control of iron stores depends on variation in absorption rather than excretion.
- Absorption has occurred through aspiration, ingestion, and burned skin.

DISTRIBUTION

- Iron is released from ferritin to the globulin transferrin in the plasma and then transported to blood-forming sites.

ELIMINATION

- The natural elimination of iron by the body is extremely limited and occurs by blood loss or desquamation of gastrointestinal mucosa.
- Adults lose up to 2 mg of iron daily.

Clinical Presentations

Classically, severe iron toxicity presents in four phases. Some variation may exist depending on form, individual variation, and quantity.

INITIAL PERIOD

A severe hemorrhagic gastritis characterizes the initial period 1/2–2 hours after ingestion. Vomiting is probably the most sensitive indicator of serious iron ingestion. Diarrhea is a less sensitive but more specific indicator of serious iron ingestions. Central nervous system signs such as lethargy and coma and cardiovascular symptoms (e.g., pallor, tachycardia, and hypotension) may be seen early in severe ingestions.

QUIESCENT PERIOD

During this period (variable, up to 12 hours), a deceptive improvement and stabilization occur, which may result in premature discharge from health care facilities. Alternating periods of lethargy may appear during this stage. In severe overdoses, this quiescent period may be brief.

RECURRENT PERIOD

Systemic symptoms that are life-threatening predominate during this phase (12–48 hours). Gastrointestinal tract signs include hematemesis, melena, and gastrointestinal perforation. Increasing lethargy, metabolic acidosis, coma, convulsions, vasomotor collapse, cyanosis, and pulmonary edema may occur. Hepatorenal failure with coagulation defects and hypoglycemia may develop toward the end of this phase.

LATE PERIOD

Gastric scarring and pyloric obstruction may appear during late recovery (4–6 weeks).

GASTROINTESTINAL EFFECTS

The corrosive effect of iron can result in stomach and intestinal erosions and ulcerations. There is a lack of correlation between the severity of intestinal damage and death. Pyloric obstruction and intestinal scarring are rare, late complications. Circulating free iron initially accumulates in Kupffer cells and later the hepatocytes. The effects on the liver are highly variable and range from no abnormalities to massive periportal necrosis. Hepatic damage may progress to hepatic failure with hypoprothrombinemia and hypoglycemia. Hepatorenal syndrome may occur. Free iron inhibits the thrombin-induced conversion of fibrinogen to fibrin and, therefore, directly affects coagulation.

CARDIOVASCULAR EFFECTS

Fatty degeneration of the myocardium can occur in iron poisoning. Iron acts on the vascular system to increase venous pooling (increased capillary permeability) and decrease cardiac output (reduced postarteriolar and venous tone). Hypotension may result. Proposed etiologies for postarteriolar dilation include a direct iron effect, ferritin release, and serotonin/histamine release.

RENAL EFFECTS

Masses of iron-containing granules accumulate in the capsular space and tubule lumen. However, tubular degeneration is rare. Interference with oxidative enzymes, the release of hydrogen with formation of ferric hydroxides, and the accumulation of lactic acid from anaerobic metabolism may all result in severe metabolic acidosis. Ferrous ions catalyze lipid peroxidation that can disrupt mitochondrial membranes and the Krebs cycle. Iron also shunts electrons from the electron transport system by acting as an electron sink.

HEMATOLOGIC EFFECTS

Depression of activities of factors V, VII, IX, and X and fibrinogen are typical abnormalities. The prothrombin time and partial thromboplastin time are increased. The coagulopathy may be biphasic with the initial phase occurring within hours of the overdose. It is reversible and serum iron-dependent. The second, later phase is characterized by hepatotoxicity with resultant coagulopathy and usually occurs at least 24 hours after ingestion. Coagulopathy is reversible and is dependent on the serum iron concentration.

Toxic Dosage/Death

Less than 20 mg of elemental iron ingested per kilogram is generally nontoxic. Clinical toxicity is expected following an ingestion of at least 20 mg/kg of elemental iron, and decontamination is generally recommended at this level. Ingestions greater than 60 mg/kg are considered serious.

The amount of elemental iron in ferrous fumarate is 33%, in ferrous chloride 28%, ferrous sulfate (the most common source) 20%, ferrous chloride 20%, and ferrous gluconate 12%. Ingestion of as few as 5–6 tablets of a high-potency preparation can be fatal in a 10-kg child. Death has been reported after the ingestion of 542 mg of elemental iron, and survival has followed the ingestion of 3.9 g of elemental iron.

Pregnancy/Lactation

Iron is classified as pregnancy risk category A, and the antidote chelator deferoxamine is classified as pregnancy risk category C. A study of iron overdose and deferoxamine treatment in pregnancy concluded that iron overdose does not appear to be markedly fetotoxic. First-trimester overdose is so rarely reported that even a large poison center is unlikely to estimate its consequences reliably. There is no evidence that deferoxamine adversely affects the outcome of pregnancy, so it should not be withheld if needed. More vigorous teratologic studies of deferoxamine are required.

Laboratory

ANALYTIC METHODS

Iron may be measured by inductively coupled plasma emission spectroscopy. The administration of deferoxamine interferes with chromogenic methods of iron determination but not with atomic absorption spectrophotometry.

BLOOD LEVELS

Normal serum iron levels are 0–100 μg/dL. Although serum iron levels cannot always be correlated with the severity of intoxication, patients are at risk if free iron exists in the plasma (i.e., the serum iron level exceeds the total iron-binding capacity or TIBC). Serum iron levels may be interpreted as follows:

100–350 μg/dL	Definite poisoning, questionable toxicity
350–500 μg/dL	Potentially serious toxicity
500–1,000 μg/dL	Definite serious toxicity
Over 1,000 μg/dL	Potentially fatal

Peak serum iron levels occur 2–4 hours after ingestion and correlate best with potential toxicity. Serum iron levels drawn more than 4–6 hours after ingestion may underestimate toxicity because of the binding of iron to ferritin and the distribution of iron into the tissues.

A serum iron level less than the TIBC does not rule out acute iron poisoning. The presence of a serum iron level greater than the TIBC is not always associated with clinical symptoms or the occurrence of vin-rose urine after deferoxamine challenge. Glucose levels over 150 mg/dL and white blood cell counts over 15,000/mm^3 do not indicate iron levels over 300 μg/dL. Deferoxamine, by providing iron-binding sites, may cause falsely elevated measurements of TIBC. The unreliability of the TIBC as a decision-making factor in the initiation of deferoxamine therapy may be due to a laboratory aberration in cases of iron poisoning.

Fewer than 10% of patients with serum iron levels below 500 μg/dL will develop cardiovascular collapse or coma. For chewable vitamins, 2-hour serum iron levels are too early to predict peak levels and to identify the potential for systemic toxicity. The value of serum iron levels after chewable multivitamin ingestion remains to be established.

Vomiting, diarrhea, leukocytosis (i.e., over 15,000/mm^3), hyperglycemia (i.e., over 150 μg/dL), and radiopacities have been associated with serum iron concentrations greater than 300 μg/dL, but not always. At concentrations greater than 500 μg/dL, coma and/or the combination of leukocytosis, radiopacities, and an increased anion gap are commonly observed. The wide range of serum iron values from groups with and without cardiovascular symptoms make the interpretation of individual values difficult.

Treatment

GUT DECONTAMINATION

Activated charcoal is ineffective. The iron-deferoxamine complex does adsorb onto charcoal with an affinity similar to that of salicylates. Gastric emptying techniques such as emesis or lavage may be helpful in the alert patient shortly after ingestion; however, the efficacy of these interventions after spontaneous emesis is probably small. Lavage may not be helpful if a significant period of time (i.e., greater than 2 hours) has passed or pill fragments are large. If abdominal x-ray reveals a significant amount of iron tablets in the stomach, these methods may be more relevant.

Lavage solutions other than saline, including deferoxamine, sodium bicarbonate, magnesium hydroxide and Phospho-Soda have been suggested. The theory that these agents might decrease the solubility of iron by chemical transformation has not been proven.

Iron tablets may form concretions or adherent masses that are resistant to decontamination measures and endoscopic removal. Continuing release of iron from large bezoars may produce delayed elevation of iron levels, gastrointestinal inflammation, hemorrhage, and scarring. In situations in which serum iron levels rose and the concretions failed to progress down the gastrointestinal tract, gastrotomy has reduced toxic effects and prevented perforations.

ELIMINATION ENHANCEMENT

Whole-bowel irrigation may be preferred if x-ray reveals progression of a significant number of pills beyond the stomach. Whole-bowel irrigation in the treatment of acute iron poisoning appears to be a safe, effective means of gastrointestinal decontamination in severe iron poisoning. Because iron has a well-known corrosive effect on gastrointestinal mucosa, late presentation after acute iron ingestion may lead to significant gastrointestinal damage. Ileus, bowel obstruction, perforation, or significant gastrointestinal hemorrhage are contraindications to whole-bowel irrigation.

There is a suggestion based on an animal study that continuous arteriovenous hemofiltration may be useful to remove iron in severe iron intoxication, especially in the presence of renal failure. Exchange transfusion represents another potential method for iron removal and in experimental animals has removed more iron than intravenous deferoxamine. The clinical efficacy of such removal remains uncertain, since deferoxamine chelates only free iron, whereas exchange transfusion removes both free and bound iron. Hemodialysis removes the iron-deferoxamine complex but not the iron itself. Its use is limited to those patients with impaired renal function.

SUPPORTIVE MEASURES

- The first priority in iron overdose is attention to airway, breathing and circulation. An intravenous line should be established, saline infused and a cardiac monitor applied.
- Abdominal x-rays can confirm the diagnosis of iron poisoning when positive, but cannot exclude it if negative. Although chewable vitamins with iron are radiopaque, visualization of these tablets clinically is unlikely.
- Observation alone is usually sufficient when a child has ingested less than 20 mg/kg of elemental iron and the abdominal x-ray is negative.
- In patients who are symptomatic, a bolus of 20 mL/kg of normal saline should be quickly administered. Shock is treated with saline, Trendelenburg position, and vasopressors if necessary.
- Arrhythmias may respond to conventional ACLS protocols.
- Laboratory investigations should include serum iron levels, total iron binding capacity (TIBC), creatinine, electrolytes, glucose, complete blood count, prothrombin time, baseline liver function tests, and arterial blood gases in seriously poisoned patients.
- Waiting for a TIBC to return, or for the appearance of vin rose urine after deferoxamine (see below), should not delay gut decontamination and stabilization measures in significant overdoses. The treatment of a seriously ill patient with suspected iron toxicity should be prompt (e.g., deferoxamine) and not await the return of a serum iron level.

Antidotes

DEFEROXAMINE

Chelation therapy with deferoxamine mesylate (DFO or Desferal®) is indicated in all symptomatic patients who exhibit more than transient minor symptoms. It is also indicated in patients with evidence of lethargy, significant abdominal pain, hypovolemia, or acidosis and in patients with abdominal radiographs demonstrating multiple radiopacities. The great majority of these patients will go on to develop symptomatic iron poisoning.

Vin-rose urine is an insensitive marker for significantly elevated serum iron levels or serious iron poisoning. The absence of vin-rose urine after DFO use does not rule out acute iron toxicity or the need for DFO therapy. A DFO challenge test is therefore not useful. Any symptomatic patient with a serum iron level greater than 300–350 $\mu g/dL$, regardless of the TIBC, should be treated with deferoxamine. A conservative approach without deferoxamine therapy may be considered when serum iron levels are below 500 $\mu g/dL$ in asymptomatic patients, as well as in those with self-limited, non-bloody emesis or diarrhea without other symptoms.

Intravenous DFO is the preferred route for acute iron poisoning. The recommended dose level of deferoxamine mesylate is 15 mg/kg/hour by continuous intravenous infusion, although there are few controlled clinical studies to support this dose. Infusions of 25 mg/kg/hour for 12 hours/day for 3 days in an infant with iron levels over 15,000 $\mu g/dL$ have been used. The iron-deferoxamine complex, ferrioxamine, is poorly absorbed from the gastrointestinal tract. It is not degraded to any appreciable extent and is rapidly excreted unchanged in the urine. Deferoxamine is rapidly metabolized mainly in the plasma, probably by an enzyme belonging to the alpha globulins.

IgE-mediated anaphylaxis following deferoxamine seldom occurs. Rapid infusion over 15 mg/kg/hr can cause histamine release and hypotension, especially in the presence of hypovolemia. Yersinia enterocolitica septicemia, after iron overdose treated with deferoxamine, may be due to iron enteritis or to iron/deferoxamine-induced growth promotion. There appears to be a relationship between iron-overload states and yersinia with or without deferoxamine. Mucormycosis and pneumocystic infection may occur in iron-overdose patients treated with deferoxamine.

Questions—Iron

1. Which of the following statements is false?
- A. Iron (chemical symbol Fe) remains a potentially deadly cause of metal poisoning in the U.S.
- B. Overdose of chewable vitamins with iron remains one of the most commonly encountered potential poisonings in children.
- C. Most toxic exposures involve adventurous adolescents and ironworkers.
- D. Patients may die or present to the emergency room at any stage of iron poisoning.
- E. The antidote deferoxamine has reduced mortality in hospitalized patients from 50% to less than 2%.

2. Which of the following statements is false?
- A. Iron is an essential element of hemoglobin and red blood cell homeostasis.
- B. Toxic doses of iron overwhelm normal gastrointestinal regulatory mechanisms and can lead to massive iron absorption.
- C. Ferritin-bound iron damages systemic blood vessels.
- D. Iron can produce cerebral edema.
- E. In severe iron overdose, coagulative necrosis with platelet aggregation appears similar to the damage caused by corrosive agents.

3. Vomiting is probably the most sensitive indicator of serious iron ingestion.
- A. True
- B. False

4. Which association with the clinical stages of iron poisoning is false?
- A. Quiescent period—During this period (variable, up to 12 hours) a deceptive improvement and stabilization occur.
- B. Recurrent period—Systemic symptoms that are life-threatening predominate during this phase (12–48 hours).
- C. Initial period—Hemorrhagic gastritis characterizes the initial period (less than 2 hours after ingestion).
- D. Late period—Gastric scarring and pyloric obstruction may appear during the late recovery phase (2–3 days).
- E. None of the above.

5. Definite poisoning and questionable toxicity occurs at what iron levels?
- A. 10–20 $\mu g/dL$
- B. 100–350 $\mu g/dL$
- C. 350–500 $\mu g/dL$
- D. 500–1000 $\mu g/dL$
- E. Over 1,000 $\mu g/dL$

6. A serum iron level less than the TIBC does not rule out acute iron poisoning.
- A. True
- B. False

7. Vomiting, diarrhea, leukocytosis (i.e., over 15,000 mm^3), hyperglycemia (i.e., over 150 mg/dL), and radiopacities are always associated with serum iron concentrations greater than 300 $\mu g/dL$.
- A. True
- B. False

8. Reasonable, proven treatment option(s) after serious iron ingestions in otherwise normal individuals include
- A. Activated charcoal
- B. Deferoxamine
- C. Sodium bicarbonate lavage
- D. Hemodialysis
- E. B and C

9. Vin-rose urine is a sensitive marker for elevated serum iron levels or serious iron poisoning.
- A. True
- B. False

LEAD

Lead has been used for multiple purposes for centuries. It has been smelted, ingested as a homeopathic medicine, applied as a cosmetic, painted on buildings, and glazed on ceramic pots since earliest recorded times. By the time of the fall of the Roman Empire, an estimated 40 million tons of lead were produced, primarily as a by-product of silver mining. Lead may be the oldest recognized chemical toxin. A Greek poet-physician first described lead poisoning in the second century BC.

Lead serves no known useful biologic purpose. Humans accumulate lead in their bodies based on environmental exposure. Lead toxicity in adults results primarily from workplace exposure via inhalation. Lead exposure can occur by ingestion because of the lack of proper hygiene in lead-contaminated environments and, in countries that still use it, from leaded gasoline exposure. In the United States, an important reason for the nationwide decline of blood lead is the reduction of lead from many sources, and, most of all, the near-complete elimination of lead from gasoline.

Non-occupational sources of exposure include hobbies, lead-lined containers, absorption of lead from bullets lodged near orthopedic joints, and home-distilled whiskey. Acidic foods such as fruit and vegetable juice can release lead from improperly fired ceramic glazes leading to increased lead consumption. Gunshot wounds in adults and children may lead to anorexia, abdominal pain, vomiting, anemia, encephalopathy, and seizures. Many factors may lead to gunshot-induced lead poisoning. These include the surface area and location of retained lead particles, the length of time that one is exposed to lead, and whether the lead is coated or not.

Although current legislation limits the paint content of lead to less than 0.06%, some paints in old homes built before 1940 contain lead in concentrations exceeding 50%. Renovation of these homes can result in significant lead contamination. Lead toxicity in children usually results from oral exploration of a contaminated environment. Sources include old lead-based house or bridge paints, drinking water, lead-glazed pottery, lead in dust or top soil (e.g., near smelter dumps, burning battery casings, freeways), and traditional folk remedies. Lead sulfide is a component of black eye makeup found in Nigeria, India, and the Arab world. Gasoline sniffing in adolescents has caused elevated lead levels. Lead may contaminate heroin and has caused toxicity in drug abusers.

Pathophysiology

Chronic lead exposure may cause subtle neuropsychiatric, reproductive, and renal effects. Blood lead levels once thought to be safe have been associated with IQ deficits, behavior disorders, slowed growth, and impaired hearing. Children are particularly susceptible to lead-induced impairment of neuropsychological development because of their reduced ability to excrete lead and their enhanced absorption of lead compared with adults. The effect of low-level lead exposure on adults is less clear.

HEMATOLOGIC EFFECTS

Impaired heme biosynthesis occurs with increasing lead levels. Sensitive inhibition occurs when lead blocks the conversion of δ-aminolevulinic acid to porphobilinogen. Lead inhibits the enzyme (ferrochelatase) which helps insert ferric ion (3+) into protoporphyrin during the formation of heme in bone marrow normoblasts. This inhibition results in elevated free erythrocyte protoporphyrin (FEP) levels, which are a sensitive screening measure of the effect of lead. FEP levels begin to increase at lead levels of 15 μg/dL, before evidence of anemia begins.

NEUROLOGIC EFFECTS

Segmental demyelination of peripheral nerves leads to decreased motor nerve conduction velocity. In adults, peripheral neuropathy is the most common neurologic manifestation of lead toxicity, whereas encephalopathy appears more frequently in children. Lead apparently passes the blood-brain barrier more easily in children and disrupts mitochondrial function, leading to coma and convulsions. Cerebral edema is a late complication of lead encephalopathy, and coma appears in the absence of cerebral edema. Subtle neuropsychiatric changes (e.g., hyperactivity, learning disorders, and fine motor dysfunction) may represent "subclinical" neuropathy.

RENAL EFFECTS

Lead toxicity produces lesions of the proximal tubule and loops of Henle characterized by round acidophilic intranuclear inclusion bodies. A Fanconi syndrome develops which includes aminoaciduria, phosphaturia, glycosuria, and renal tubular acidosis. Kidney lesions usually are reversible. End-stage lead nephropathy is characterized more by chronic interstitial disease than by glomerular disease. Lead decreases the tubular secretion of uric acid, causing a higher incidence of gout, but factors other than lead exposure account for most cases of renal failure in patients with gout.

Pharmacokinetics

ABSORPTION

- An adult absorbs about 5–10% of an ingested lead dose and the remainder appears in the feces.
- In small children, gastrointestinal absorption of lead is higher and approaches 40%.
- Decreased iron, calcium, and zinc levels increase lead absorption.
- Gastric acid solubilizes lead salts, and lead absorption occurs in the small bowel by both active and passive transport.
- From 50 to 70% of an inhaled dose is absorbed if the particle size allows the material to reach the alveoli.
- Although inorganic lead does not pass through skin, organic lead alkyls (e.g., tetraethyl lead) do in sufficient quantities to produce toxicity after heavy exposure.

DISTRIBUTION

- In the circulation, 95% of lead exists in the red blood cells (RBC). The lead in erythrocytes has a half-life of 35 days and distributes into soft tissue or bone stores. Hence, blood lead levels may not reflect the total body burden.
- About 10% of the total body lead burden equilibrates in soft tissue (e.g., kidney, liver and nervous tissue) where the half-life is 40 days.
- Bones are the major depositories for lead in the body, with about 90% of the total body lead burden existing in the skeleton.
- The half-life of lead in bone is 20–30 years.
- Some equilibration between bone and blood lead does occur. Up to 70% of blood lead may derive from the bones, and during pregnancy more lead is mobilized from bone stores.

ELIMINATION

- The kidney filters lead unchanged, although at high levels some active tubular transport occurs. The excretion rate is dependent on the glomerular filtration rate and renal plasma flow.
- The kidney accounts for 75% of daily lead loss.

Clinical Presentations

Neurasthenic symptoms are most common in adults. Acute lead exposures may cause colicky abdominal pain, constipation, arthralgias, headache, and weakness. There is some evidence to suggest that lead may play a primary role in hypertension through direct effects on arterioles and through metabolic processes related to calcium metabolism.

NEUROLOGIC EFFECTS

Lead toxicity produces a classic motor neuropathy. Extensor weakness (wrist drop) occurs at high levels and paresthesias are uncommon. Motor conduction velocities and distal latency may be significantly prolonged or delayed without evidence of clinical lead toxicity, but sensory conduction velocities are usually normal. Acute encephalopathy occurs infrequently in adults. Seizures, obtundation, and confusion are the most common signs of lead encephalopathy, with headache and optical neuritis occurring less frequently. Subtle effects on personality, memory, learning, reaction time, psychomotor function, and motor coordination have been reported in lead workers with lead levels greater than 40 $\mu g/dL$.

HEMATOLOGIC EFFECTS

Anemia is the most common hematological manifestation and increases in frequency and severity with increasing lead levels. Basophilic stippling is uncommon but is highly suggestive of lead intoxication. Neither anemia nor basophilic stippling is a sensitive indicator of lead intoxication since concurrent congenital defects in heme synthesis may be required to express the anemia. Eosinophilia appears more often in lead-intoxicated patients but does not demonstrate a clear dose-response effect.

PEDIATRIC EFFECTS

Anorexia, lethargy, vomiting, and colicky abdominal pain are the most common symptoms in children. Irritability, lethargy, and ataxia may be early signs of acute encephalopathy. Convulsions and coma are a hallmark of acute encephalopathy. Other symptoms include bizarre behavior, ataxia, apathy, and memory loss. Chronic low-level lead exposure may cause decreased intelligence, behavioral and learning disorders, and deficits in visuomotor function, perceptual integration, and verbal abstraction.

Toxic Dosage/Death

There is substantial epidemiologic evidence of adverse effects of lead at blood levels as low as 20 $\mu g/dL$. Data indicate that moderate lead poisoning (25–55 $\mu g/dL$) can cause neurobehavioral and intelligence deficits. Obvious clinical symptoms may not occur until 60 $\mu g/dL$ in children and 80 $\mu g/dL$ in adults. Patients in whom occupational exposure resulted in blood lead levels of 40–60 $\mu g/dL$ have shown evidence of impaired performance on verbal concept formation, visuomotor performance, memory, and mood in the absence of peripheral nervous system derangement.

Pregnancy/Lactation

Workplace exposures have raised questions about stillbirths, spontaneous abortions, and decreased sperm counts. There appears to be an association between high blood lead concentrations (i.e., 40–70 $\mu g/dL$) and adverse reproductive effects on sperm counts and hormonal parameters. Whether lead exposure *in utero* results in an increased incidence of congenital malformation is unclear. Major malformations have rarely been reported. Lead is readily transferred from the mother to the developing infant during pregnancy. The cord blood lead concentration is approximately 85–90% as high as the mother's blood lead concentration.

Laboratory

ANALYTIC METHODS

Serum lead is measured by flameless atomic absorption spectrometry. Free and zinc protoporphyrin tests are measured by high-pressure liquid chromatography with fluorometric endpoint.

BLOOD LEVELS

Whole Blood Lead Concentration

The whole-blood lead level is the best measure of recent exposure. Nonspecific subjective symptoms (e.g., fatigue, headache, sleep disturbances, constipation, and abdominal pain) do not correlate well with elevated lead levels in workers. Lead-free Vacutainer tubes should be used unless a batch of Vacutainers has been specifically tested for lead contamination.

Free Erythrocyte Protoporphyrin Test

The free erythrocyte protoporphyrin (FEP) test is the best screening test for chronic but not acute lead intoxication. All children between 9 months and 6 years of age should receive an FEP test. Although the FEP is a better measure of body lead burden (i.e., soft tissue levels) than blood lead, both tests should be used to estimate body lead burden since iron deficiency anemia causes an elevation of the FEP. Elevation of FEP persists long after the cessation of lead exposure.

An FEP level higher than 35 $\mu g/dL$ and a blood lead level higher than 10 $\mu g/dL$ indicate excess lead exposure and require further medical evaluation and environmental investigation. An elevated FEP level indicates impairment of the heme biosynthetic pathway. FEP levels are sensitive screening tests for iron deficiency, and iron status should be assessed in any child with an elevated FEP level (i.e., greater than 35 $\mu g/dL$).

RBC Zinc Protoporphyrin Test

The RBC zinc protoporphyrin test measures the effects of lead on bone marrow that has occurred in the preceding 120 days. Zinc protoporphyrin levels begin to increase at blood lead concentrations of 15–25 $\mu g/dL$ in children, 20–25 $\mu g/dL$ in female adults, and 30–40 $\mu g/dL$ in adult males. The zinc protoporphyrin level is more sensitive to an elevated body lead burden than blood lead and may correlate well with anorexia, weight loss, joint pain, and anemia. The zinc protoporphyrin concentration may not be a sensitive indicator of lead levels in the absence of iron deficiency.

δ-Aminolevulinic Acid Dehydratase Inhibition

The inhibition of δ-aminolevulinic acid dehydratase is the most sensitive indicator of the effect of lead, with changes initially detected at blood lead levels as low as 10 $\mu g/dL$. The FEP is a more practical screening method.

Treatment

GUT DECONTAMINATION

Recent, witnessed episodes of significant lead paint chip ingestion may benefit from ipecac. Abdominal x-ray may help confirm ingestion. In an acute lead ceramic glaze ingestion, the potential for ongoing absorption of large amounts of lead from the gut makes gastrointestinal contamination reasonable. No unanimity exists regarding optimal evacuation techniques.

ELIMINATION ENHANCEMENT

Hemodialysis appeared to enhance the excretion of calcium disodium EDTA chelated lead in one adult who ingested 40 g of lead oxide. Little confirmatory evidence of the usefulness of hemodialysis is available. Whole-bowel irrigation has shown some usefulness in the prevention of lead toxicity by removing a lead glaze preparation from the gastrointestinal tract.

SUPPORTIVE MEASURES

Screening

- Screening for lead poisoning requires (a) determining the child's risk for high-dose lead exposure by asking a few questions; (b) measuring blood lead levels in children who are at the greatest risk for high-dose lead poisoning when they are 6 months old; (c) measuring blood lead levels in children who are at lower risk for high-dose lead exposure at 12–15 months of age; and (d) conducting necessary follow-up blood lead testing of children.
- Screening should be done using a blood lead test, since erythrocyte protoporphyrin levels are not sensitive enough to identify more than a small percentage of children with blood lead levels between 10–25 μg/dL and miss many with blood lead levels 25 μg/dL or more.
- The free erythrocyte protoporphyrin test is a good test for chronic but not acute lead intoxication. All children between 9 months and 6 years of age should receive an FEP test.
- Because almost all children in the U.S. are at risk for lead poisoning (although some children are at higher risk than others), all children should be screened. In areas of high risk, screening should begin at 6 months of age and continue at least through the age of 4 years and, in some cases, until 6 years of age or older.

Radiology

- The flat plate (plain film) of the abdomen is significant only if positive and indicates a recent ingestion (24–36 hours) of lead.
- The width and density of lead lines on long-bone radiographs (wrist, knee) can reflect a chronic exposure. These opacities represent dense zones of calcium rather than actual lead deposition and appear in children of 9 months to 5 years during the age of rapid bone growth. The development of long-bone opacities requires 4–8 weeks of heavy exposure.
- Radiographs may demonstrate lead lines in chronic plumbism at blood lead levels considerably less than 50 μg/dL.

Blood Lead Levels 20–24 μg/dL.

- Only very minimal data exist about chelating children with blood lead levels below 25 μg/dL, and such children should not be chelated except in the context of approved clinical trials.
- A child with a confirmed blood lead level of 20–24 μg/dL will require individual case management by a pediatric health-care provider. The child should have an evaluation with special attention to nutritional and iron status.
- The parents should be taught about (a) the causes and effects of lead poisoning, (b) the need for more routine blood lead testing, (c) possible sources of lead intake and how to reduce them, (d) the importance of adequate nutrition and of food high in iron and calcium, and (e) resources for further information.
- Sequential measurements of blood lead levels along with review of the child's clinical status should be done at least every 3 months. Iron deficiency should be treated promptly. Children with blood lead levels in this range should be referred for environmental investigation.
- Identifying and eradicating all sources of excessive lead exposure is the most important intervention for decreasing blood lead levels.

Blood Lead Levels 25–44 μg/dL

- For this blood lead range, the effectiveness of chelation therapy in decreasing the adverse effect of lead on children's intelligence has not been shown.
- Patients with blood lead levels of 25–45 μg/dL need aggressive environmental intervention. The minimum medical management for children with these blood lead levels is to decrease exposure to all sources of lead to ensure that the child's blood lead levels decrease.
- If blood lead levels persist in this range despite repeated environmental study and abatement, some patients may benefit from (oral) chelation therapy.
- Treatment regimens vary from clinic to clinic. Some practitioners treat children with lead levels in this range with D-penicillamine.
- Some practitioners use DMSA in children with blood lead levels of 20–35 μg/dL if (a) blood levels remain refractory despite attempted chelation with D-penicillamine or calcium disodium EDTA, or (b) for children with complications from D-penicillamine.
- Many experienced practitioners decide whether to use chelation therapy on the basis of the results of carefully performed calcium disodium EDTA mobilization tests.

Blood Lead Levels 45–69 μg/dL

- Chelation therapy is indicated in patients with blood lead levels between 45 and 70 μg/dL.
- DMSA may be potentially useful in asymptomatic children with no clinical signs of lead encephalopathy and with a blood lead level of 35–70 μg/dL. Children with these blood levels may receive outpatient DMSA therapy if (a) their environment is assessed to be safe; (b) an abdominal radiograph does not contain radiopaque densities, and (c) the family is likely to comply with medication administration and appropriate medical follow-up.
- In the absence of clinical symptoms suggesting encephalopathy (e.g., obtundation, headache, and persistent vomiting), patients may be treated with succimer (DMSA) at 30 mg/kg per day for 5 days, followed by 20 mg/kg per day for 14 days.
- Children may need to be hospitalized for the initiation of therapy to monitor for adverse effects and institute environmental abatement. Discharge should be considered only if the safety of the environment after hospitalization can be guaranteed.
- An alternate regimen involves calcium disodium EDTA as inpatient therapy at 25 mg/kg per day for 5 days.
- A second course of chelation therapy with calcium disodium EDTA may be required if the blood lead level rebounds to 45 μg/dL within 7–14 days. Allow 5–7 days before beginning a second course of calcium disodium EDTA. If blood lead in hospitalized children remains 35 μg/dL after chelation with calcium disodium EDTA, DMSA may also be considered.
- Before chelation with either agent is begun, if an abdominal radiograph shows that enteral lead is present, bowel decontamination may be considered as an adjunct to treatment.

Blood Lead Levels greater than 70 μg/dL

- Patients with blood levels greater than 70 μg/dL or with clinical symptoms suggesting encephalopathy require inpatient chelation therapy using the most efficacious parenteral agents available.
- Lead encephalopathy is a life-threatening emergency that should be treated using contemporary standards for intensive care treatment of increased intracranial pressure, including appropriate pressure monitoring, osmotic therapy, and drug therapy in addition to chelation therapy.

- Therapy is initiated with intramuscular dimercaprol at 25 mg/kg per day divided into six doses. The second dose of dimercaprol is given four hours later, followed immediately by intravenous calcium disodium EDTA at 50 mg/kg/d as a single dose infused during several hours or as a continuous infusion.
- Current labeling of calcium disodium EDTA does not support the intravenous route of administration, but clinical experience suggests that it is safe and more appropriate in the pediatric population.

Antidotes

CALCIUM DISODIUM EDTA

A calcium disodium EDTA mobilization test is used to determine whether a child with an initial confirmatory blood lead level of 25–41 μg/dL will respond to chelation therapy with a brisk lead diuresis. Because of the cost and staff time needed for quantitative urine collection, this test is used only in selected medical centers where large numbers of lead-poisoned children are treated. Children whose blood lead levels are 45 μg/dL or over do not require a provocative chelation test but should be referred for appropriate chelation therapy immediately.

The outcome of the provocative chelation test is determined not by a decrease in the blood lead level but by the amount of lead excreted per dose of calcium disodium EDTA given. This ratio correlates well with blood lead levels. In one study almost all children with blood lead levels of 45 μg/dL had positive provocative tests, 76% of the children with blood lead levels of 35–44 μg/dL had positive test results, and 35% of the children with blood lead levels of 25–34 μg/dL had positive test results. This test should not be done until the child is iron-repleted, since iron status may affect the outcome of the test.

DIMERCAPROL

Like most chelating agents, dimercaprol (British Anti-Lewisite or BAL in Oil) contains ligands that bind heavy metals in preference to the body's sulfhydryl groups. The resulting chelated mercaptide product is less toxic and more easily excreted from the body than the heavy metals. The dimercaprol-metal complex can disassociate and release the bound metal, particularly at low pH or low dimercaprol concentrations.

Hypertension and tachycardia may occur frequently, and dose-related adverse effects may last several hours postingestion. Blood pressure should be monitored, and dimercaprol must be given cautiously in hypertensive patients. Dimercaprol must be administered by deep intramuscular injection because of its propensity to produce pain and sterile abscesses at the injection site. It must never be given intravenously. Fever occurs commonly in children following the second or third dose and frequently persists until dimercaprol is withdrawn.

Dimercaprol is potentially nephrotoxic. The drug must be used with caution in patients with renal dysfunction and oliguria. Alkalinization of the urine may produce disassociation of the dimercaprol-metal complex and may prevent renal toxicity. Dimercaprol elimination requires hepatic metabolism and must be used cautiously, if at all, in patients with hepatic dysfunction.

DMPS

Although 2,3 dimercapto-1-propane-sulfonic acid (DMPS) has shown promise in the treatment of lead poisoning, patients have developed Stevens-Johnson syndrome following its administration. There is a need for further study.

DMSA

The FDA approved succimer (DMSA) in 1991 for treating children with blood lead levels greater than 45 μg/dL. Regardless of the blood lead concentration, chelation therapy should never be used as a substitute for environmental assessment and abatement of lead hazards for lead-poisoned children. Succimer appears to be an effective oral chelating agent. Its selectivity for lead is high, whereas its ability to chelate essential trace metals is low. Although its use to date has been limited, succimer appears to have promising potential, and a broader range of clinical research studies in children is being undertaken.

Succimer is chemically similar to BAL, but is more water-soluble, has a high therapeutic index, and is absorbed from the gastrointestinal tract. It is effective when given orally and produces a lead diuresis comparable to that produced by calcium disodium EDTA. Diuresis lowers blood lead levels and reverses the biochemical toxicity of lead, as indicated by normalization of circulating aminolevulinic acid dehydrase levels. Children with blood lead levels of 45 μg/dL who are being treated with succimer should, if possible, be hospitalized until their blood lead levels fall below 45 μg/dL and the lead hazards in their homes are abated or alternative lead hazard-free housing has been identified.

Experience using DMSA in children with a blood lead value of 70 μg/dL or more is extremely limited, and at this time it is not recommended for use in high-level lead poisoning. Accordingly, at present BAL and calcium disodium EDTA are recommended to treat children with blood lead levels equal to or greater than 70 μg/dL. Multiple courses of DMSA may be required because of the rebound in blood lead levels after cessation of a course of treatment. A post-rebound blood lead level of 15 μg/dL has been used as an endpoint of therapy.

Toxicity due to succimer appears to be minimal. The most common adverse effects reported in clinical trials in children and adults were primarily gastrointestinal and included nausea, vomiting, diarrhea, and appetite loss. Rashes, some necessitating discontinuance of therapy, have been reported in about 4% of patients. Though succimer holds considerable promise for the outpatient management of lead poisoning, clinical experience with succimer is limited. DMSA has been placed in pregnancy category C. Transmission via breast milk is unknown.

D-PENICILLAMINE

D-penicillamine enhances the urinary excretion of lead, although not as effectively as calcium disodium EDTA. Its specific mechanism and site of action are not well understood. The FDA has approved D-penicillamine for the treatment of Wilson's disease, cystinuria, and severe, active rheumatoid arthritis. Until the approval of succimer, it was the only commercially available oral chelating agent. It can be given over a long period (weeks to months). D-penicillamine has been used mainly for children with blood lead levels greater than 45 μg/dL.

Toxic side effects (albeit minor in most cases) occur in as many as 33% of patients given the drug. The main side effects of D-penicillamine are reactions resembling those of penicillin sensitivity, including rashes, leukopenia, thrombocytopenia, hematuria, proteinuria, hepatocellular enzyme elevations, and eosinophilia. Anorexia, nausea, and bloating are commonly seen. Of most concern, however, are isolated reports of nephrotoxicity, possibly from hypersensitivity reactions. For these reasons, patients should be carefully and frequently monitored for clinically obvious side effects, and frequent blood counts, urinalyses, and renal function tests should be performed.

D-penicillamine should not be given on an outpatient basis if exposure to lead is continuing or the physician has doubts about compliance with the therapeutic regimen. D-penicillamine should not be administered to patients with known penicillin allergy. The drug should be continued until lead levels are less than 15 $\mu g/dL$. Rebound following cessation of therapy may raise the lead level an additional 25% from its nadir.

Questions—Lead

1. Which of the following statements is false?
A. Lead toxicity in adults results primarily from workplace exposure via accidental ingestion.
B. In the U.S., an important reason for the nationwide decline of blood lead is the reduction of lead from many sources, and, most of all, the near-complete elimination of lead from gasoline.
C. Non-occupational sources of exposure include hobbies, lead-lined containers, and home-distilled whiskey.
D. Acidic foods such as fruit and vegetable juice can release lead from improperly fired ceramic glazes, leading to increased lead consumption.
E. Gunshot wounds in adults and children may lead to anorexia, abdominal pain, vomiting, anemia, encephalopathy, and seizures from lead absorption.

2. Which of the following statements is false?
A. Impaired heme biosynthesis occurs with increasing lead levels.
B. Sensitive inhibition occurs when lead blocks the conversion of δ-aminolevulinic acid to porphobilinogen.
C. Lead inhibits the enzyme (ferrochelatase) which helps insert ferric ion ($^{3+}$) into protoporphyrin during the formation of heme in bone marrow normoblasts.
D. Inhibition of ferrochelatase results in decreased free erythrocyte protoporphyrin (FEP) levels, which are a sensitive screening measure of the effect of lead.
E. FEP levels begin to increase at lead levels of 15 $\mu g/dL$, before evidence of anemia begins.

3. Wrist drop may occur at slightly elevated lead levels and paresthesias are uncommon.
A. True
B. False

4. Which of the following observations about neurologic signs of lead poisoning is false?
A. Segmental demyelination of peripheral nerves and decreased motor nerve conduction velocity.
B. In adults, peripheral neuropathy is the most common neurologic manifestation of lead toxicity, whereas encephalopathy appears more frequently in children.
C. Cerebral edema is an early complication of lead encephalopathy
D. Subtle neuropsychiatric changes may represent "subclinical" neuropathy.
E. Coma may occur after significant exposures.

5. ________ is/are the major depository for lead in the body
A. The spleen
B. The bones
C. The liver
D. The kidneys
E. The muscles

6. The free erythrocyte protoporphyrin (FEP) test is the best screening test for acute but not chronic lead intoxication.
A. True
B. False

7. Basophilic stippling is uncommon but is highly suggestive of lead intoxication.
A. True
B. False

8. In the circulation, what percentage of lead exists in the red blood cells?
A. 5%
B. 10%
C. 50%
D. 95%
E. 100%

9. Lead serves no known useful biologic purpose.
A. True
B. False

10. The RBC zinc protoporphyrin test measures the effects of lead on bone marrow that has occurred in the preceding year.
A. True
B. False

11. The width and density of lead lines on long-bone radiographs (wrist, knee) can reflect a chronic exposure. These opacities represent dense zones of calcium rather than actual lead deposition and appear in children of 9 months to 5 years during the age of rapid bone growth.
A. True
B. False

12. Which of the following about antidotal therapy in lead poisoning is false?
A. A calcium disodium EDTA mobilization test is used to determine whether a child with an initial confirmatory blood lead level of 25–41 $\mu g/dL$ will respond to chelation therapy with a brisk lead diuresis.
B. Dimercaprol is potentially nephrotoxic.
C. Although 2,3 dimercapto-1-propane-sulfonic acid (DMPS) has shown promise in the treatment of lead poisoning, patients have developed Stevens-Johnson syndrome following its administration.
D. Experience of using DMSA in children with a blood lead value of 70 $\mu g/dL$ is recommended for use in high-level lead poisoning.
E. D-penicillamine enhances the urinary excretion of lead, although not as effectively as calcium disodium EDTA.

LITHIUM

Lithium (chemical symbol Li) is used for manic-depressive affective disorders, as an adjunctive therapy of depressive disorders, and for mania control in children and adolescents. It has been used for the treatment of alcoholism, to control schizoaffective disorders, as prophylaxis of cluster headaches, and to ameliorate chemotherapy-induced neutropenia. Lithium is also used industrially in nuclear reactor coolant, alkaline storage batteries, and alloys. Fortunately, occupational lithium toxicity is rare.

Lithium has a narrow toxic therapeutic index, with most common poisonings resulting from altered drug kinetics during chronic therapeutic use. Side effects include thirst, polyuria, resting tremor, acne, and hypothyroidism. Rare effects include dysarthria, ataxia, impaired cognition, pseudotumor cerebri, alopecia, keratoderma, psoriasis of the fingernails, restless legs syndrome, rhabdomyolysis and reduced renal tubular concentrating ability.

Pathophysiology

The exact mechanism of lithium is unclear. Lithium effects result from its substitution for body cations, resulting in multisystemic actions. A partial substitution for normal cations causes changes in ion exchange and transfer in cellular processes. Incorporation of lithium into membrane structures may alter responses to hormones and the coupling of energy processes.

NERVOUS SYSTEM

The major target organs of lithium toxicity are the central nervous system and kidneys. Persistent high brain concentrations in chronic overdose patients may account for slow neurologic improvement despite low serum lithium levels. Equilibrium between the cerebrospinal fluid and serum is rapid, but cerebrospinal fluid levels do not accurately reflect brain lithium levels.

RENAL SYSTEM

Up to 5% of patients treated with lithium for a long period develop renal insufficiency. Both glomerular and tubular functions are affected. Lithium is capable of causing a major disturbance in water balance manifested as polyuria and secondary polydipsia. A decreased urinary concentrating ability (i.e., nephrogenic diabetes insipidus) with a disturbed responsiveness of the distal nephron to the action of ADH (vasopressin) is demonstrable. The symptoms are largely reversible on cessation of lithium or reduction of the dose.

CARDIOVASCULAR SYSTEM

Cardiac complications are common but rarely serious in chronic overdose. Sinus node dysfunction is the most common lithium-related conduction defect. Both the sinus node dysfunction and cardiac repolarization delays may be treated by oral potassium chloride. Dysrhythmias are rare and hypotension is usually secondary to coma. Cardiac arrest may be observed during chronic lithium therapy. Sinus arrest and asystole due to serum lithium intoxication may be seen in patients with preexisting conduction tissue disease. Lithium may depress serum potassium concentrations.

RESPIRATORY SYSTEM

Severe lithium intoxication may rarely yield adult respiratory distress syndrome (ARDS). Echocardiogram and a normal pulmonary capillary wedge pressure may confirm the diagnosis of noncardiogenic pulmonary edema with normal ventricular function.

ENDOCRINE SYSTEM

Lithium is concentrated in the thyroid gland and can reach levels 2.5–5 times those of its concentration in the serum. Lithium inhibits thyroid hormone synthesis and metabolites at five different stages. Lithium intoxication may exacerbate preexisting hypothyroidism to the point of respiratory arrest and myxedema coma. Thyrotoxicosis has developed in the course of lithium therapy despite the suppressive effect of lithium on thyroid hormone synthesis and release. Long-term lithium therapy may lead to laboratory evidence of hyperparathyroidism manifested by elevated serum calcium, ionized calcium, and parathormone levels.

Pharmacokinetics

ABSORPTION

- Nearly complete lithium absorption occurs from the gastrointestinal tract, with peak therapeutic levels appearing 30 minutes to 2 or 3 hours postingestion. Clinically significant delayed absorption may develop in an overdose situation up to 72 hours postingestion.
- The bioavailability of lithium is over 95%.

DISTRIBUTION

- Peak plasma levels of lithium are generally 0.8–1.5 mmol/L.
- The volume of distribution is 0.6 L/kg.
- Plasma protein binding is 10%.

ELIMINATION

- No hepatic metabolism of lithium occurs, and glomerular filtration eliminates the entire dose.
- The proximal renal tubules resorb 60–70% of the filtered lithium load, whereas no absorption occurs in the distal tubules.
- Hyponatremia reduces lithium clearance, and alkaline urine increases lithium clearance.
- The elimination half-life of lithium is 24 hours.

Clinical Presentations

Three types of lithium poisoning are generally recognized. These include acute, acute on chronic, and chronic poisoning. Acute poisoning may be voluntary or accidental. Acute poisoning carries less risk and patients usually show only mild symptoms independent of their serum lithium concentration. Nausea, vomiting, and diarrhea may occur in chronic ingestions and acute ingestions. More severe symptoms may appear if lithium elimination is impaired.

Acute on chronic poisoning, (i.e., an acute overdose in patients who are under lithium treatment) may be associated with severe symptoms. In this type of poisoning, serum concentrations above 3–4 mmol/L are usually associated with profound toxicity.

Chronic or therapeutic poisoning occurs in patients who are under lithium treatment. These patients can develop progressive lithium toxicity following an increase in dosage, a decrease of lithium renal elimination, or during an intercurrent disease. Severity of symptoms usually correlates well with serum concentrations, although features of toxicity may also be present at concentrations below 1.5 mmol/L.

NEUROLOGIC EFFECTS

Mental status changes are the most common manifestation of toxicity and may develop in 90% or more of patients affected. Encephalopathy characterized by disorientation, incoherence, and poor memory may appear several hours to several days after an acute overdose or during maintenance therapy and can progress to paralysis, stupor, seizures, and coma. Additional neurologic effects may include a Parkinsonian syndrome, myoclonus, choreoathetosis, proximal muscle weakness, fasciculations, gait disturbances, incontinence, and corticospinal tract signs.

Lithium administered to patients with preexisting neurologic disease (e.g., stroke) may, at low to therapeutic plasma levels, enhance disabling neurologic symptoms. Lithium may affect the peripheral nervous system at both therapeutic and toxic levels. Permanent cerebellar degeneration manifested by truncal ataxia, hyperreflexia, and an intention tremor have occurred after lithium overdose. Seizures can develop in patients with serum levels in both the therapeutic and toxic ranges. Photophobia is rare but has been reported.

CARDIOVASCULAR EFFECTS

Serious cardiac complications usually appear in comatose patients. ST-T wave changes similar to those in hypokalemia often occur. Impaired conduction is an uncommon complication and includes sinoatrial block, sinus and junctional bradycardia, first-degree atrioventricular block, intraventricular conduction delay and QT prolongation. Hypotension is a secondary event usually resulting from volume depletion. Hypertension occurs rarely but may be severe.

RENAL EFFECTS

Lithium produces transient natriuresis, nephrogenic diabetes insipidus, and partial distal renal tubule acidosis in therapeutic doses. Lithium intoxication causes mild renal dysfunction and is rarely associated with acute renal failure.

CHRONIC INTOXICATION

Patients with chronic lithium intoxication experience a period of days to a few weeks with slight "nervous" symptoms. This may be accompanied by moderately elevated serum lithium, serum creatinine concentrations, and serum urea concentration. Cerebrovascular deterioration, cerebellar dysfunction, and abnormal T waves are observed in patients with chronic lithium intoxication. T-wave abnormalities may distinguish patients with acute from chronic intoxication.

Patients with chronic lithium intoxication appear to be at greater risk of life-threatening events. Patients who have become chronically intoxicated from lithium have a delayed resolution of toxicity following the return of lithium concentrations to therapeutic levels when compared with those with acute overdoses.

Toxic Dosage/Death

A single ingestion of 40 mg of lithium salt per kilogram by a patient with a history of prior lithium use is capable of producing toxic lithium blood levels (>2 mEq/L).

Drug Interactions

Acute ethanol consumption has little effect on lithium except for a mild increase in peak lithium levels. If lithium and chlorpromazine are used in combination, the withdrawal of lithium may be associated with a prolonged QTc interval, low serum potassium, and ventricular fibrillation. Cisplatin effects on the glomeruli and tubules may either increase or decrease the serum lithium concentration. Lisinopril may induce elevations of lithium serum concentrations with toxic central nervous system effects.

Agents that may reduce lithium clearance include the thiazides, non-steroidal anti-inflammatory drugs such as ibuprofen, phenytoin, and tetracycline. Agents that can increase lithium clearance include theophylline, verapamil, acetazolamide and sodium bicarbonate.

Pregnancy/Lactation

Lithium crosses the placenta readily. Fetal serum concentrations approximately equal maternal serum levels. Toxicity has been noted in newborns of mothers taking lithium and is manifested by hypotonicity, lethargy, and cyanosis. Lithium may be one of the causes of the "floppy baby" syndrome.

The best estimate of the risk of major congenital anomalies among the children of women treated during early pregnancy is about 4–12% in cohort studies. The prevalence of congenital anomalies in untreated comparison groups was 2–4%. Patients who decide to conceive while taking lithium and who subsequently continue to take it should be counseled regarding the slightly increased risks of cardiovascular and other malformations in the fetus. Lithium has been classified as pregnancy risk category D.

Lithium is excreted into breast milk. Infant serum and milk levels are approximately equal. Although no toxic effects in infants have been reported, The American Academy of Pediatrics considers lithium to be contraindicated during breast feeding.

Laboratory

ANALYTIC METHODS

Lithium is measured in serum via an ion-selective electrode.

BLOOD LEVELS

Serum levels do not always correlate with symptoms, in part because of drug interactions and coexisting disease processes. Clinical effects appear related to the duration of increased levels as well as to the serum lithium level. Single acute overdoses may produce less severe toxicity than chronic intoxication at the same serum lithium level because of rapid absorption and slow distribution. Erythrocytes may alter serum lithium levels by concentrating lithium, thereby causing toxicity with "normal" serum (but not whole blood) levels. Seizures may occur in susceptible patients at therapeutic doses documented by normal serum lithium levels.

In acute overdose, lithium levels may be quite elevated without the patient exhibiting significant toxicity. Peak serum concentrations may occur much later after a large overdose than after a therapeutic dose. Severe toxicity may not occur after levels have peaked. This may present a confusing picture of a patient who is deteriorating while lithium levels are falling. Thus, the eventual severity of toxicity cannot accurately be predicted by either the presenting clinical status or buy lithium levels. Patients can deteriorate late after presentation.

Treatment

GUT DECONTAMINATION

Charcoal is not useful. Lavage may be helpful if the patient has ingested a large amount of lithium and presents shortly after ingestion. No clinical data on humans are available to guide the administration of cathartics.

ELIMINATION ENHANCEMENT

Hemodialysis

Hemodialysis significantly increases lithium clearance, with lithium extraction higher from serum than from whole blood or red blood cells. In a chronic intoxication case, hemodialysis decreased the lithium serum half-life from 54 to 25 hours. On average, four hours of hemodialysis will reduce the plasma lithium concentration by 1.0 mEq/L, since rebound of lithium concentration may occur after dialysis. A dialysis time of 10–12 hours is suggested.

Indications for hemodialysis include unstable patients (i.e., those with coma, convulsions, or respiratory failure and/or progressive clinical deterioration). Hemodialysis may also be considered in patients who chronically take lithium with serum levels over 4 mEq/L, and in acute poisoning in patients with serum lithium levels over 6–8 mEq/L. Repeat dialysis may be needed to compensate for a rebound of serum levels.

Concentration alone, particularly in stable individuals, should not dictate the use of hemodialysis. Dialysis usually is unnecessary in patients with levels below 2.5 mEq/L. Hemodialysis is not an emergency treatment in lithium poisoning. Single acute ingestions resulting in serum lithium levels over 4.0 mEq/L have been managed successfully without dialysis in patients without prior lithium exposure. Forced diuresis/saline diuresis has resulted in serious problems with electrolyte balance and is inferior to dialysis.

Whole-Bowel Irrigation

Whole-bowel irrigation with polyethylene glycol electrolyte lavage solution at a rate of 2 L/hr for five hours, if begun within one hour after ingestion, has been shown in at least one study to be effective for acute ingestions of sustained-release lithium.

Hemodiafiltration

Continuous arteriovenous hemodiafiltration (CAVH) can rapidly eliminate toxic quantities of lithium, does not require a hemodialysis-trained staff, and is now available in an increasing number of intensive care units. The rebound increase in lithium concentrate after cessation of CAVH suggests that optimal therapy with this technique will require about 24 hours of treatment.

Sodium Polystyrene Sulfonate

Hemodialysis is the treatment of choice for severe lithium intoxication. However, this may present a problem for facilities without dialysis equipment or in which there is a long delay before dialysis can be accomplished. Sodium polystyrene sulfonate administered to healthy volunteers after ingesting 0.5 mEq/kg (18.5 mg/kg) of lithium significantly decreased lithium absorption. This study suggested that sodium polystyrene sulfonate may be given to patients immediately or soon after the ingestion of a significant acute overdose of lithium when hemodialysis cannot be instituted promptly.

SUPPORTIVE MEASURES

- In the obtunded patient, cumulative control of the airway, breathing, and circulation is the first priority. The patient should have access to a cardiac monitor and an i.v. line.
- Patients with serum lithium levels less than 2.5 mEq/L can usually be treated with saline infusion unless they exhibit moderate or severe neurotoxicity or have significant underlying cardiac or renal disease. In the absence of these factors, a rapid i.v. infusion of normal saline, 1–2 liters over 6 hours, may be sufficient.
- Frequent monitoring of sodium levels is mandatory. Lithium may impair renal-concentrating ability and can cause hypernatremia, as well as hypercalcemia and hypoparathyroidism.
- If the admitting serum level is 2.5–4.0 mEq/L and there is no significant toxicity, a trial of saline infusion may be begun unless contraindicated by severe neurologic dysfunction, renal insufficiency, or congestive heart failure.
- Admit all symptomatic patients and asymptomatic patients with a lithium serum level exceeding 2.0 mEq/L. After serial serum levels at least four hours apart confirm a declining level, the asymptomatic patient may be discharged if the lithium level is below 2.0 mEq/L. Psychiatric counseling may be appropriate before discharge. Factors contributing to toxicity (e.g., dehydration and loop diuretics) should be addressed.
- Periodic serum calcium measurements would appear to be indicated in chronic lithium use. If hypercalcemia is mild (less than 2.8 mmol/L), no further action is indicated. If levels are higher, consider stopping lithium, if possible.
- Hyperbilirubinemia has been observed after therapeutic use.

Questions—Lithium

1. Which of the following statements concerning lithium is false?

A. Lithium (chemical symbol Li) is used for manic-depressive affective disorders, as an adjunctive therapy of depressive disorders, and for mania control in children and adolescents.
B. Lithium is used industrially in nuclear reactor coolant, alkaline storage batteries, and alloys. Fortunately, occupational lithium toxicity is rare.
C. Lithium has a narrow toxic therapeutic index, with most common poisonings resulting from altered drug kinetics during chronic therapeutic use.
D. Side effects include thirst and polyuria.
E. The exact mechanism of lithium is well established.

2. Which of the following statements concerning lithium is false?

A. Lithium effects result from its substitution for body anions, resulting in multisystemic actions.
B. Incorporation of lithium into membrane structures may alter responses to hormones and the coupling of energy processes.
C. The major target organs of lithium toxicity are the central nervous system and kidneys.
D. Persistent high brain concentrations in chronic overdose patients may account for slow neurologic improvement despite low serum lithium levels.
E. Equilibrium between the cerebrospinal fluid and serum is rapid, but cerebrospinal fluid levels do not accurately reflect brain lithium levels.

3. Most patients treated with lithium for a long period develop renal insufficiency.

A. True
B. False

4. Which of the following observations about the endocrine effects of lithium is false?

A. Lithium is concentrated in the thyroid gland and can reach levels 2.5–5 times those of its concentration in the serum.
B. Lithium inhibits thyroid hormone synthesis and metabolites at five different stages.
C. Lithium intoxication may exacerbate preexisting hypothyroidism to the point of respiratory arrest and myxedema coma.
D. Long-term lithium therapy may lead to laboratory evidence of hypoparathyroidism manifested by decreased serum calcium, ionized calcium, and parathormone levels.
E. Thyrotoxicosis has developed in the course of lithium therapy.

5. Mental status changes are the most common manifestation of toxicity and may develop in ________ or more of patients affected.

A. 10%
B. 25%
C. 50%
D. 90%
E. 100%

6. **Although no toxic effects in infants have been reported, the American Academy of Pediatrics considers lithium to be contraindicated during breast feeding.**
   A. True
   B. False
7. **Serum levels of lithium do not always correlate with symptoms, in part because of drug interactions and coexisting disease processes.**
   A. True
   B. False
8. **On average, four hours of hemodialysis will reduce the plasma lithium concentration by 1.0 mEq/L since a rebound of the lithium concentration may occur after dialysis.**
   A. True
   B. False

MAGNESIUM

Magnesium (chemical symbol Mg) is the second most abundant intracellular cation and is an essential component of all enzyme processes that involve the transfer of phosphate in nucleotide triphosphate reactions (e.g., ATP). Magnesium is commonly used to control hypertension, to prevent seizures in preeclampsia, to stop premature labor, to treat Torsade de Pointes cardiac arrhythmias after surgery and myocardial infarction, and to maintain normal circulating concentrations of calcium and magnesium. Poisoning from magnesium can result from ingestion (e.g., Epsom Salts, magnesium citrate cathartics), and from occasional excess intravenous administration.

Magnesium hydroxide laxatives administered to infants and neonates may induce symptoms of severe magnesium intoxication with elevated serum magnesium levels. In adults, toxicity is rare in the absence of renal failure since the kidney excretes moderate excesses of magnesium effectively. In the infant or neonate, renal immaturity may be a factor. An additional cause of hypermagnesemia may be the erroneous ordering of "one amp" of magnesium sulfate intravenously. A 50-mL vial of 50% magnesium sulfate may be erroneously given instead of a standard ampule containing 2 mL of 50% solution. Such incidents may lead to severe magnesium intoxication and death.

Pathophysiology

Magnesium, with sodium, potassium, and calcium, represents a vital inorganic cation whose actions are vital to cell homeostasis. In normal humans, magnesium appears to increase cardiac output and heart rate and produce a decrease in systolic arterial pressure and systemic vascular resistance. This is accompanied by a vasodilation of the coronary arteriolar bed. Parenteral magnesium prolongs conduction through the sinoatrial and atrioventricular nodes. Magnesium also increases AV nodal refractoriness in normal humans and may be useful in the treatment of paroxysmal atrial fibrillation with a rapid ventricular response.

Hypermagnesemia impairs neuromuscular junction transmission by decreasing acetylcholine release from the presynaptic membrane, by diminishing the depolarizing action of acetylcholine at the postsynaptic junction, and by impairing postsynaptic junction sensitivity to acetylcholine.

Pharmacokinetics

ABSORPTION

- Magnesium is rapidly and completely absorbed.
- The gut absorbs about 30% of an orally administered dose.
- The glomerulus filters and the proximal tubule resorbs 95% of the filtered load. Glomerular filtration rates below 30 mL/min predispose patients to hypermagnesemia.
- Both magnesium resorption and calcium resorption in the kidney are closely related. A common carrier exists for both calcium and magnesium, in addition to separate active processes.

DISTRIBUTION

- Magnesium is primarily an intracellular (46%) and skeletal (53%) ion.
- Less than 1% of total body magnesium is found in the extracellular compartments.
- Total serum magnesium concentrations reflect free or ionized (55%), chelated (12%), and protein-bound (33%) fractions. The free form is the active form of magnesium.
- A decrease in albumin lowers total serum levels without affecting the ionized level. Alkalosis increases and acidosis decreases protein binding.
- Low serum magnesium levels may not indicate cellular magnesium deficiency. Tissue magnesium deficiency may exist with normal serum magnesium levels.

ELIMINATION

- Magnesium is excreted via the kidneys.

Clinical Presentations

Magnesium is a calcium antagonist. Magnesium causes clinical changes similar to those seen with administration of calcium blocking agents. These changes include peripheral vasodilation, flushing, decrease in blood pressure, and decrease in the strength of cardiac conduction. Excess magnesium decreases impulse transmission across the neuromuscular junction. This may lead to impairment of respiratory function and apnea, an effect that is antagonized by calcium. When deep tendon reflexes are absent, respiration must be closely monitored.

Bradycardia and hypotension due to the direct vasodilator and ganglionic blocker effects of magnesium on peripheral arteries and arterioles may be observed at plasma levels of 4–5 mEq/liter. At plasma magnesium concentrations of 5–10 mEq/liter the PR, QRS, and QT intervals may increase. Cardiopulmonary arrest with coma, nonreactive pupils, flaccid extremities, loss of deep tendon reflexes, and no response to painful stimulus may be observed early after magnesium overdose.

Magnesium serum levels of 9–12 mEq/L may cause respiratory arrest and cardiovascular collapse. Coma has been reported with serum levels of 9.5 mmol/L (23 mg/dL). Extensive hypermagnesemia can cause parasympathetic blockade and fixed dilated pupils, in addition to neuromuscular blockade, mimicking a midbrain syndrome, and resulting in a pseudocomatose state.

Toxic Dosage/Death

Iatrogenic hypermagnesemia with respiratory depression has been reported in patients with mild renal dysfunction who received doses of hemiacidrin and magnesium citrate. A patient with normal kidney function developed symptomatic hypermagnesemia (respiratory arrest, bradycardia) after receiving 90 g of magnesium sulfate over 18 hours. As a tocolytic agent, magnesium sulfate is administered as a 4.0 g intravenous loading dose, followed by 1.0–2.0 g/hour. An accidental infusion at 1.5 g/hour into the epidural space of a 40-week pregnant patient in early labor was well tolerated.

Drug Interactions

Aminoglycosides should not be used concurrently since they may potentiate the neuromuscular blockade of magnesium.

Pregnancy/Lactation

Magnesium sulfate is classified as pregnancy risk category B.

Laboratory

ANALYTIC METHODS

Magnesium is measured via a spectrophotometric method.

BLOOD LEVELS

Serum levels may not reflect tissue levels. The plasma magnesium concentration usually exceeds 4 mEq/liter before any signs or symptoms of magnesium excess appear. At blood levels of 4 mEq/liter, a decrease or disappearance of deep tendon reflexes appears. Somnolence is observed at levels of 4–7 mEq/liter and flaccid paralysis of voluntary muscles at 10 mEq/liter or greater. Complete heart block and cardiac arrest in asystole may occur at levels of 15 mEq/liter or greater.

Treatment

GUT DECONTAMINATION

Magnesium may be eliminated by enema if it is in the bowel. Activated charcoal does not absorb magnesium salts.

ELIMINATION ENHANCEMENT

Hemodialysis effectively removes magnesium and often is necessary to correct the associated renal dysfunction. Serum magnesium levels over 8 mEq/L suggest the need for dialysis. Exchange transfusion has been instituted in a neonate with severe magnesium intoxication. If renal function is normal, intravenous furosemide (40 mg, adults, 1 mg/kg infants and children) may be administered with replacement of urine volume by 0.90% saline. Forced diuresis with mannitol (25 g by rapid i.v. infusion) may also be useful.

SUPPORTIVE MEASURES

- Discontinue administration of magnesium by all routes.
- Monitor serum electrolytes, calcium, phosphorus, renal function, fluid intake, urinary output, and electrocardiogram. Intravenous lines, oxygen, and cardiac monitor must be available.
- If patient is symptomatic (e.g., central nervous system depression) and has electrocardiographic changes and/or a serum magnesium level over 2.9 mEg/L, begin calcium therapy.
- Pacemaker therapy may be useful in refractory hypotension.
- Parenteral administration of magnesium lowers plasma calcium concentrations in both normal and hypoparathyroid patients. Electrolytes must be followed closely. The anion gap may be unchanged and the osmolal gap may be increased.

Antidotes

CALCIUM

Calcium is an antagonist of magnesium action. The exact mechanism of action is unknown, but calcium may displace magnesium from cell membranes. Treat with calcium when serum magnesium levels exceed 5 mEq/L and the patient exhibits symptoms. The adult dose of calcium gluconate is 10 mL of a 10% solution over several minutes. The dose may be repeated once and the calcium level should be rechecked. Intravenous calcium gluconate is less irritating than calcium chloride.

Questions—Magnesium

1. **Magnesium is a calcium agonist.**
   A. True
   B. False

2. **Clinical changes seen with the administration of magnesium include all of the following, except**
   A. Peripheral vasodilation
   B. Increase in blood pressure
   C. Impairment of respiratory function
   D. Loss of deep tendon reflexes
   E. Bradycardia

3. **Regarding magnesium,**
   A. It does not have cardiovascular effects.
   B. It is a calcium antagonist thereby producing peripheral vasodilation, flushing, decrease in blood pressure and slowing of cardiac conduction.
   C. Serum levels correlate well with cellular magnesium levels.
   D. It is used to treat Torsade de Pointes.
   E. B and D

4. **Magnesium toxicity**
   A. Never occurs because it is an inert substance
   B. Only occurs when serum levels reach greater than 7 mEq/liter
   C. May be treated with calcium gluconate
   D. Is less likely to occur in patients with renal failure
   E. May cause hyperreflexia by increasing transmission across the neuromuscular junction

5. **Magnesium excess can cause**
   A. Increased cardiac output
   B. Hyperreflexia
   C. Vasoconstriction
   D. Hypersensitivity to painful stimuli
   E. All of the above

6. **Symptoms of hypermagnesemia usually do not appear until the plasma concentration exceeds**
   A. .04 mEq/L
   B. .4 mEq/L
   C. 4 mEq/L
   D. 40 mEq/L
   E. 400 mEq/L

7. **Treatment of hypermagnesemia may include**
   A. Enema
   B. Activated charcoal
   C. Forced diuresis
   D. A and B
   E. A and C

MANGANESE

Manganese (chemical symbol Mn) comprises 0.1% of the earth's crust. It is used to increase the strength of steel alloys and is an essential co-factor for certain enzymes. Manganese toxicity can be manifested by a rare central nervous system disease generally resulting from chronic occupational exposure to the dust from manganese ore or fumes in steel processes. The lungs may also be effected adversely after chronic exposures. The progressive psychiatric disturbance known as "manganese madness" includes apathy, somnolence, confusion, and bizarre behavior. A Parkinsonian syndrome may dominate the clinical picture as well.

Pathophysiology

The two main target organs affected by chronic exposure to manganese dust are the lungs and the central nervous system. Neurologic lesions seen after excessive manganese exposure are found in the globus pallidus and striatum sections of the basal ganglia rather than in the substantia nigra as seen in Parkinson's disease. Neurologic symptoms improve after withdrawal from exposure but many symptoms persist.

Pharmacokinetics

ABSORPTION

- Absorption from the gastrointestinal tract occurs in the divalent and tetravalent forms.
- The solubility of manganese dioxide and other inhaled manganese compounds is poor.

DISTRIBUTION

- The highest levels of manganese appear in liver, muscle, erythrocytes, pancreas and pituitary.

ELIMINATION

- Elimination occurs primarily by excretion in bile.
- Renal excretion is small.

Clinical Presentations

Dermal and oral toxicity is low because of the low solubility of manganese.

NEUROLOGIC EFFECTS

"*Locura manganica*" or "manganese madness" is the insidious onset of psychiatric symptoms, including apathy, insomnia, confusion, bizarre behavior, visual hallucinations, emotional lability, decreased libido, impotence, and anxiety. Neurologic manifestations may include nystagmus, disequilibrium, paresthesias, memory impairment, a vocal pattern described as "whispering speech," problems with fine motor movement, lumbosacral pain, urgency, and incontinence. The neurologic syndrome is similar to Parkinson's disease with tremor, ataxia, loss of memory, flat affect, muscle rigidity, and gait disturbances.

RESPIRATORY EFFECTS

A metal fume fever syndrome may occur after exposure to high concentrations of manganese oxide. No known permanent pulmonary sequelae develop after acute manganese exposure. The most common respiratory symptom is dyspnea. Because of its low solubility in water, airborne manganese does not cause oral or dermal problems. Instead, it may penetrate the lower respiratory tract leading to the development of pneumonitis, pneumonia, and bronchitis.

HEPATIC EFFECTS

Patients with manganism toxicity may develop pathologic hepatic changes such as increased Golgi bodies and dilated biliary canaliculi, but rarely develop clinical hepatitis.

Toxic Dosage/Death

Studies in workers exposed to manganese suggest that exposure to airborne dust above current recommendations for one year or more may lead to clinical signs of intoxication, especially respiratory symptoms, changes in lung ventilatory parameters, alteration of neurofunctional performances, and hypercalcemia.

Pregnancy/Lactation

Manganese passes the placental barrier and is found in breast milk. Very high exposures to manganese have been associated with impotence.

Laboratory

ANALYTIC METHODS

Manganese may be measured by flameless atomic absorption spectrophotometry.

BLOOD LEVELS

Normal manganese levels for blood are 2.0–8.0 $\mu g/dL$, and for urine, 0.1–0.8 $\mu g/dL$. Neurologic symptoms may be associated with blood manganese levels of 3.0–5.6 $\mu g/dL$.

Treatment

GUT DECONTAMINATION

There is limited clinical data to confirm or deny the efficacy of these methods. Charcoal is probably not helpful.

ELIMINATION ENHANCEMENT

Dialysis has not been utilized to treat the effects of manganese poisoning.

SUPPORTIVE MEASURES

- One study suggests that symptoms of chronic manganese poisoning may be ameliorated by treatment with sodium para-aminosalicylic acid (6 g/day in 500 mL of 10% glucose solution by intravenous drip). Confirmatory studies will be required to evaluate this proposal.
- Other treatments which have been used with limited success include L-dopa, 5-hydroxytryptophan, scopolamine, procyclidine, and trihexyphenidyl.
- Diagnostic tests suggestive of excessive manganese exposure include elevated urine and serum manganese levels, a positive response to calcium disodium EDTA chelation, and reversal or improvement after L-dopa treatment. None of these tests is highly specific or sensitive for manganese toxicity.
- Standard heavy-metal screens only detect mercury, arsenic, bismuth, and antimony. If another heavy metal is suspected, a screen for it must be specifically requested.
- Preliminary studies indicate that magnetic resonance imaging (MRI) appears to be effective in visualizing manganese in the basal ganglia. Serial MRI changes clearing in 5–7 months are characteristic of manganese encephalopathy.

Antidotes

Chelation therapy with calcium disodium EDTA may improve an acute manganese-induced psychosis but probably will not alter chronic neurologic symptoms.

Questions—Manganese

1. Which of the following statements about manganese is false?
   A. Manganese (chemical symbol Mn) comprises 0.1% of the earth's crust.
   B. Manganese toxicity can be manifested by a rare central nervous system disease generally resulting from chronic occupational exposure to the dust from manganese ore or fumes in steel processes.
   C. The progressive psychiatric disturbance known as "manganese madness" includes apathy, somnolence, confusion, and bizarre behavior.
   D. A seizure disorder resembling Huntington's chorea may dominate the clinical picture as well.
   E. Neurologic lesions seen after manganese exposure are found in the globus pallidus and striatum sections of the basal ganglia rather than the substantia nigra as seen in Parkinson's disease.

2. A metal fume fever syndrome may occur after exposure to high concentrations of manganese oxide. No known permanent pulmonary sequelae develop after acute manganese exposure.
   A. True
   B. False

MERCURY

The National Institute of Occupational Safety and Health (NIOSH) indicates that about 150,000 people in the United States are exposed to mercury (chemical symbol Hg) at work every year. Industries that routinely use mercury or mercury-based compounds include chlor-alkali facilities, manufacturers of mercury-filled instruments (e.g., barometers, thermometers, manometers), manufacturers of lighting (e.g., including neon, fluorescent lamps, and high-temperature mercury vapor lamps), and producers of batteries and electrical switches when mercury is used for thermostats and silent contacts. Mercury is also used to refine gold and other ores.

Dentists in the U.S. use over 100 tons of mercury annually. Individual dentists in private practice use an average of 2–3 pounds of mercury per year. About 100 million fillings per year in the U.S. involve the use of amalgam. About 14% of dental operating rooms exhibit levels of total mercury concentration (vapor and particulates) that exceed recommended threshold limits. Many dentists still knead the amalgam mass in the palms of their hands. Mercury droplets sometimes fall to the floor where they are allowed to remain and vaporize.

Mercury was introduced during carrotting, the process of rubbing fur with mercuric nitrate to produce felt. Subsequent heating released mercury vapor that was inhaled during the later phases of felt-hat manufacturing. In 1860, J.A. Freeman of Orange, New Jersey described "hatter's shakes." These characteristic tremors were sometimes called "the Danbury tremor" in reference to Danbury, Connecticut, a former center for the hat-making industry. Common wisdom deemed hatters "mad" because of the curious jerking gait, extreme shyness, and stammering speech the hatters exhibited. The notion that mercury accounted for the name of the "Mad Hatter" gained credibility after the publication of Alice's Adventures in Wonderland in 1865.

In 1948, Warkany and Hubbard made the connection between mercury and acrodynia ("pink disease"). As late as 1952, before the removal of calomel (mercuric oxide) from teething powders, acrodynia accounted for 3.6% of all admissions to a children's hospital in England. Various forms of mercury can cause acrodynia, among them mercury vapor, phenylmercuric compounds, mercurous and mercuric salts, and ammoniated mercury ointment. Cases have involved school children who brought metallic mercury home and inhaled mercury vapor for long periods. Liquid mercury certainly remains an attractive hazard.

ORGANIC MERCURY

In the 1950s, an epidemic of methyl mercury poisoning developed in Minamata, Japan, affecting over 2,500 individuals. MRIs showed brain damage in areas of the brain concerned with coordination, balance, and sensation. Prominent choreoathetosis, ataxia, spasticity and seizures developed. These symptoms generally improved; however, cortical blindness and constricted visual fields persisted. Methyl mercury easily crosses the blood-brain barrier, while inorganic mercury crosses the blood-brain barrier poorly.

ELEMENTAL MERCURY

Potential sources of elemental mercury in the home include mercury switches and mercury-containing devices such as thermometers, thermostats, and barometers. Family members may also bring into the home elemental mercury obtained from laboratories, dental offices, or other industrial sources. A small vial (e.g., 5 mL) of elemental mercury spilled on a rug can lead to the development of symptoms in a child (e.g., anorexia, irritability, insomnia, stomatitis, and red, painful hands).

INORGANIC MERCURY

Inorganic mercury poisoning may be associated with the ingestion of pesticides, antiseptics, and germicides. Ingestion of a stool fixative containing 4.5% mercuric chloride resulted in immediate oropharyngeal burns, salivation, vomiting, abdominal pain and guaiac-positive stool.

Pathophysiology

Mercury exists in elemental (liquid or "quicksilver"), organic and inorganic forms. Mercury blocks catechol methyl transferase, the enzyme that converts catecholamines to metanephrine. Elevated levels of epinephrine and norepinephrine can be found in the urine. Vanillylmandelic acid and homovanillic acid in the urine are increased. Sweating, tachycardia, hypertension, and occasional glucosuria may be related to sympathetic overactivity.

Pharmacokinetics

ABSORPTION

- In humans, mercury distributes to all parts of the body on absorption, reaching a peak over 1–2 days.
- About 10 minutes is required for a tablet of mercuric bichloride to be absorbed from the stomach. It is then widely distributed to the liver, kidney, blood, and muscle.
- After inhalation, elemental mercury is readily absorbed through the alveolar membrane and is transported by blood to the brain and other tissues of the nervous system.

DISTRIBUTION

- Elemental mercury easily penetrates the blood-brain barrier and accumulates in brain tissue. The same areas of the brain are affected by both inorganic and organic mercury.
- In humans, brain mercury concentrations are highly correlated with total mercury concentrations in abdominal muscles.
- High levels accumulate in the cerebellum, brainstem (inferior olive nucleus, subthalamic nucleus), and choroid plexus.

ELIMINATION

- Excretion of mercury from mercuric bichloride takes place through the large bowel, kidney, liver, gastric mucosa, salivary glands, and skin.
- Mercury is converted in blood to mercuric ions, which are then excreted in the urine and feces.
- Elimination of elemental mercury occurs primarily in the urine, with a half-life of about 60 days.
- After oxidation, elemental mercury may act as mercuric or divalent mercury and is therefore identical to the chemical form that occurs after dissociation of mercuric salts. The dissociated mercuric ion may then lead to renal tubular danger similar to that seen after an ingestion of mercuric chloride or the mercurial diuretics.
- The loss of mercury from the lungs has a half-life of 1.7 days, from the kidney 64 days, and from the head 21 days.
- After the first week, about 19% of a retained dose is eliminated through fecal excretion (50%), expired breath (37%), and urinary excretion (13%).

Clinical Presentations

Three signs characterize the diagnosis of industrial mercurialism: gingivitis, tremor of the extremities, and emotional instability. The clinical course reflects an insidious onset and a slow and progressive evolution. Mercurialism, although a chronic intoxication most of the time, occasionally assumes the features of an acute overdose. Gingivitis, salivation, and a metallic taste are often present.

ACRODYNIA

The onset of acrodynia (also known as 'pink disease') in children is often insidious, with anorexia, insomnia, and irritability. This is often attributed to teething. Sweating may be profuse, often leading to miliaria-type rashes. Photophobia may occur and children may bury their heads in pillows or blankets to avoid light. The hands and feet become puffy, pink, painful, paresthetic, perspiring, and peeling. Children frequently rub their hands together resulting in shedding of skin, denudation, and secondary infection. In severe cases, teeth are shed with ulceration of the gums. The muscles are weak and the limbs can be hyperextended. Hypertension is usually present.

Clinical findings are less severe in older children. The extremities are not as pink since the palms and soles are thicker. Asocial outbursts, fatigue, and insomnia may be observed. Alopecia is often present. Hypertension and hypotension may be observed as well. In adults, the presenting symptoms are insomnia, thirst, abdominal pain, aching extremities, and psychologic disturbance. A study of mercury levels in dentists suggested that dentists with high tissue mercury levels may develop polyneuropathies, mild visuographic dysfunction, and evidence of mild neuropsychopathy. Cases of acrodynia are currently rare.

INORGANIC MERCURY

Following an ingestion of inorganic mercury such as mercuric chloride, some patients may remain asymptomatic, but the majority develop gastrointestinal symptoms. Of this latter group, some may develop renal lesions that terminate fatally. Burning mouth, sore throat, nausea, and vomiting with severe gingivitis, stomatitis, and esophageal erosions may develop after inorganic mercury ingestion. Abdominal pain, weakness, fatigue, pallor, hematemesis, hematochezia, shock, and vascular collapse may follow. Patients who develop renal involvement almost invariably have severe gastrointestinal symptoms.

In most types of inorganic mercury poisoning, toxicity results from absorption of the mercuric ion. Mercurous chloride laxative ingested over a long period may produce toxic effects of mercury on the kidneys, gastrointestinal tract, and central nervous system. Chronic mercury poisoning due to mercurous chloride-containing laxative preparations should be suspected in patients with a history of laxative abuse who present with renal failure, colitis, dementia, or tremor.

ELEMENTAL MERCURY

Elemental mercury vapor is absorbed rapidly through the lungs, reaching the blood and entering the brain. A clinical picture evolves that may be divided into three phases. The initial phase (first few days after exposure) is manifested as metal fume fever or a flulike illness characterized by chills, fever, aching muscles, dryness in the mouth and throat, and headache. The intermediate phase (symptoms present two weeks after exposure) can be defined as the period during which severe multiorgan symptoms (central nervous system, respiratory tract, and gastrointestinal and urologic systems) may be involved. Severe cases may progress to noncardiogenic pulmonary edema with dyspnea, cyanosis, and a chest x-ray exhibiting extensive bilateral infiltrates. Complications include subcutaneous emphysema, pneumomediastinum, pneumothorax, and death.

The classic symptoms of metallic mercury vapor poisoning may include (a) intention tremor; (b) erethism (loss of memory, lack of self control, irritability, excitability, loss of self confidence, drowsiness, and depression); and (c) gingivitis. In severe cases, delirium with hallucinations, suicidal melancholia, or manic-depressive psychosis may occur. Shyness and loss of appetite may occur. Rarely, acute renal failure, hepatocellular dysfunction, and seizures occur. Subcutaneous injections cause local abscesses and pulmonary embolization, but systemic symptoms are unusual. A late, third phase involves a period when central nervous symptoms persist and other organ complaints resolve. Thus, acute exposure to elemental mercury and its vapor can induce acute inorganic mercury toxicity and cause long-term, probably irreversible, neurologic sequelae.

INTRAVENOUS MERCURY INJECTIONS

Injected mercury can pass through the pulmonary capillary bed and can be observed in systemic sites such as the liver, lungs, kidneys, brain, or heart where it can oxidize to mercuric ion and produce toxic effects. Pulmonary embolism from metallic mercury is rare. It may occur after a deliberate intravenous injection of mercury as a suicide gesture, in the presence of drug abuse or severe psychiatric disturbance, with the hope of increasing athletic and sexual performance, and accidentally during right heart catheterization while sampling blood with mercury-containing syringes. The term "quicksilver" may be the origin of the misconception that mercury quickens a boxer's punches. Injection of mercuric chloride has led to nausea, vomiting, darkened gums, abdominal pain, and anemia.

The patient who has injected mercury intravenously may experience pleuritic pain, exertional dyspnea, and fatigue. There may be a low-grade fever and a posterior pleural rub. Repeated hemoptysis has been observed. Respiratory symptoms are relatively uncommon. The patient may have mild dyspnea or transient chest pain. Mercury emboli have little or no effect on pulmonary function. Spirometry may be normal or show a reversible restrictive pattern. Metallic mercury causes a local chronic inflammation with progressive fibrosis with globules of metal still evident several years later.

NEUROLOGIC EFFECTS

Tremor, rigidity, and truncal unsteadiness impairing gait may produce a Parkinsonian syndrome suggesting involvement of the basal ganglia and cerebellum. Involvement of the corpus callosum may be involved as indicated by performance on tests showing no improvement on switching to the preferred from the non-preferred hand. Defects in memory suggest involvement of the temporal lobe.

DERMATOLOGIC EFFECTS

The skin is affected by mercury used in skin lightening creams, mercury used in soap, topical ammoniated mercury, mercuric oxide used in the treatment of eczema, topical metallic mercury, and by contact allergy. Mercury intoxication following the cutaneous application of inorganic mercury has been reported in the treatment of infected eczema or impetigo by application of different mercury salts.

OPHTHALMOLOGIC EFFECTS

The brown reflex is evidence of protracted mercury exposure and persists unchanged for years after removal from mercury exposure. The brown reflex of the anterior lens capsule is bilateral and symmetrical and varies in intensity from light brown to coffee brown (mercurialentis). Fine punctate opacities are present bilaterally and are most evident in the anterior cortex of the lens. Well-marked vascularity is observed at the corneoscleral junction. Visual fields are usually normal.

CARCINOGENIC EFFECTS

Mercury compounds are genotoxic mainly by inhibiting the mitotic spindle, but the direct mutagenic effect of the inorganic forms seems to be low. The effect on the spindle mechanism is probably the high affinity of mercury for sulfhydryl groups in the spindle apparatus. Cytogenetic studies in subjects exposed to mercury vapor have in most cases shown no effect on chromosomes.

RENAL EFFECTS

The kidney has a remarkable capacity to concentrate mercury and is a target organ following exposure to mercury. The potential of mercuric salts (e.g., mercuric chloride) to produce overt renal tubular damage is well documented. The evidence that human exposure to metallic mercury vapor produces renal damage is less convincing. The nephrotoxicity associated with mercury may be manifested as either an acute tubular necrosis or as an immune complex glomerulonephritis. The nephrotic syndrome may develop secondary to a membranous glomerulonephritis. Complement tests are normal. Antinuclear antigen titers, renal venograms and intravenous pyelograms are normal.

There are two types of proteinuria associated with mercury toxicity: a glomerular proteinuria and a tubular proteinuria. Glomerular proteinuria is characterized by the leakage of serum proteins (predominantly high-molecular-weight) through damaged glomeruli and is thought to represent an idiosyncratic immune-complex glomerulonephritis. Tubular proteinuria consists of a variety of proteins and enzymes. Many of these markers are low-molecular-weight proteins normally filtered through the glomerulus and then reabsorbed in the proximal tubules. Tubular proteinuria may be a more sensitive marker for mercury toxicity.

Toxic Dosage/Death

Normal blood mercury levels are 60 nmol / L and normal urine mercury levels are 60 nmol / L. Signs of mercury poisoning are seldom observed in individuals with less than 750–1,000 nmol (150–200 μg) per liter of urine. This may correspond to an air exposure of about 30 μg / m^3, a urine mercury excretion of about 195 nmol / L, and a blood level of mercury of about 100 nmol / L.

Pregnancy/Lactation

Women of childbearing age should not be exposed to mercury vapor if at all possible. Children born of mothers with a history of inorganic mercury exposure must be regularly evaluated by a neurologist who is aware of the occupational history. The rate of spontaneous abortion was higher than controls among the wives of 152 workers occupationally exposed to mercury vapor in one study. In Sweden, a study of infants born to dentists, dental assistants, or dental technicians indicated no increase in stillborns, spontaneous abortions, or malformations.

The highest concentration of mercury is found in the placenta, suggesting a barrier role. *In vitro* studies of the human placenta suggest that the mercuric ion may interfere with placental amino acid transfer and with placental oxygen consumption rate. This may indicate a role for the mercuric ion in impaired organogenesis in early pregnancy or deranged fetal growth during the last trimester.

Laboratory

ANALYTIC METHODS

Flameless atomic absorption spectrometry will detect as little as 1 ppb (1 ng / mL) of mercury. High-performance liquid chromatography can also be used to detect mercuric compounds. An atomic absorption method has been described to determine total mercury and selectively inorganic mercury. Organic mercury is measured as the difference between total and inorganic mercury.

BLOOD LEVELS

Blood mercury levels up to 50–70 nmol / L may be considered "normal." If the blood mercury levels exceed 150 nmol / L, control measures to reduce mercury exposure (blood, urine mercury levels) should be initiated. If the ratio of blood to urine mercury concentration is over 1, repeat the investigations in 2–4 weeks. If the mercury level in the blood still exceeds 150 nmol / L and the ratio still exceeds 1, special attention is recommended. At blood levels over 300 nmol / L, all exposure to mercury should cease. The blood level of mercury from amalgam is estimated as 1.12 ng Hg / mL, whereas toxic signs of mercury intoxication begin at blood levels of about 30 ng / mL.

URINE

The normal level of urine mercury is considered less than 1 mg / mL. Basal urinary excretion of mercury can be normal even in overt acrodynia. One hundred μg / L of mercury in urine usually requires treatment, and levels of 50 μg / L and lower are considered safe. However, urinalysis often yields unreliable results, and normal levels are not yet clearly established. Nonetheless, careful behavioral and neurologic monitoring is recommended when urine levels are 100 μg / dL or greater.

Urine mercury levels are correlated with the number of hours of practice / week and with the number of amalgam restorations per week. In one study of dentists, the mean urinary mercury levels were 14.2 μg / liter urine and about 1.3% had levels greater than 100 μg / L, a level at which physiologic effects from mercury may first appear. Group average urine levels over 50 μg / L should arouse suspicion and levels above 100 μg / L call for correction of a faulty work situation. An individual with urine levels over 200 μg / L on two successive tests should be removed from exposure until the level has fallen below 50 μg / L. Clinical poisoning does not normally occur with levels below 300 μg / L unless kidney function is impaired.

HAIR

Hair analysis may indicate past exposure resulting from a concentration of mercury in sulfhydryl groups at a particular place on the hair. External contamination is a potential source of inaccurate analysis, particularly with methyl mercury compounds, which are more readily absorbed on the hair shaft than inorganic mercury. Hair analysis continues to require controlled clinical confirmatory studies.

Treatment

GUT DECONTAMINATION

These methods are generally not applicable. Emesis and / or lavage with a protected airway may theoretically be useful after a large elemental mercury ingestion.

ELIMINATION ENHANCEMENT

Charcoal hemoperfusion and hemodialysis are ineffective in removing mercury even after the patient has been treated with dimercaprol (BAL in Oil). N-acetylcysteine may be clinically useful in the removal of mercury from the body during hemodialysis for acute mercury poisoning, but additional study is needed. Charcoal hemoperfusion does not offer a useful alternative to accelerate the elimination of mercury. Hemodialysis, peritoneal dialysis, hemofiltration, and hemodialysis with N-acetylcysteine infusions have all been tried in patients with acute renal failure, but have had limited success in reducing the body load of mercury. Plasma exchange may be useful in association with chelation therapy during the early phase of intoxication.

Extracorporeal regional coupling hemodialysis (ERCH) induces a more than tenfold greater removal of mercury into dialysate compared with hemodialysis. This procedure may prove to be useful to enhance the removal of mercury in mercuric chloride-induced renal failure. If treatment is begun soon after exposure to methyl mercury and before the appearance of signs and symptoms, the incidence and severity of methyl mercury poisoning may potentially decrease.

SUPPORTIVE MEASURES

- The FDA advises consumers that it is not necessary to have amalgam fillings removed. There is no valid data to demonstrate that the fillings are harmful in clinical use or that removing them would prevent adverse health effects or reverse the course of existing illness.
- Attempts to remove spilled elemental mercury often fail and may disperse the mercury over a larger surface area. The problem may require removal of contaminated carpeting or vacuuming with a specialized industrial mercury vacuum.
- Despite elevated blood and urine mercury levels, routine clinical testing such as physical examination, blood chemistries, and urinalysis are generally normal after mercury exposures. More sensitive indicators of toxicity may include evaluation of neuropsychologic symptoms, elevated urinary N-acetyl-β-d-glucosaminidase (NAG) levels, decreased motor nerve conduction velocities, and the presence of lenticular opacities on slit-lamp examination.
- After intravenous injection of mercury, there may be a moderate increase in the white blood cell count. The electrocardiogram will usually be normal. Pelvic and abdominal x-rays may indicate mercury in the paraspinal and pelvic areas in addition to the injection site.
- Radionuclide images may indicate pleural effusions and multiple bilateral pulmonary emboli. The chest radiograph may exhibit multiple fine, radiodense, spherical particles in the lungs and a pooled metallic density in the right ventricle by echocardiography. Despite its striking radiographic appearance, mercury that has embolized to the lung does not cause significant vascular obstruction as judged by angiography.
- Following an intravenous injection of mercury, neurologic examination may be within normal limits. The cerebrospinal fluid results may also be noncontributory. Neuropsychologic testing may reveal severely impaired performance in memory, new problem solving, learning efficiency, and sustained attention / concentration. Psychologic symptoms may include depression, emotional lability, and anxiety.
- Chest x-rays, pulmonary function tests, and electrocardiograms are usually not significantly abnormal in mercury-exposed workers.
- Treatment of acrodynia requires careful monitoring of fluids and electrolyte balance. Patients with acrodynia should avoid high ambient temperatures as this may exacerbate profuse sweating.
- Studies of evoked somatosensory potential have a potential use as an efficient early warning system for the prevention of mercury-induced clinical symptoms. Visually evoked responses may indicate an effect on the nervous system many years after exposure to inorganic mercury has ceased.

Antidotes

DIMERCAPROL

Dimercaprol (British Anti-Lewisite or BAL in Oil) is an option in the treatment of self-administered intravenous mercury poisoning even months after the original exposure. Patients may continue to respond clinically and exhibit positive effects in both the urine and blood mercury levels.

DMPS

2,3-Dimercaptopropane-1-sulfonic acid (DMPS) is an investigational drug used under U.S. Food and Drug Administration (FDA) guidelines. DMPS is less toxic than DMSA (succimer, meso 2,3-dimercaptosuccinic acid). In oral doses of 100 mg twice daily, DMPS has significantly increased the urinary excretion of mercury. Maculopapular rashes, erythema multiforme, and mucous membrane reactions (mouth ulcers) can develop after a course of DMPS treatment.

DMSA

DMSA (succimer, meso 2,3-dimercaptosuccinic acid) has been approved by the FDA for the treatment of lead poisoning in children with blood levels above 45 μg / dL. It has been shown to be of possible use as an antidote in poisoning from mercury, arsenic, cadmium, antimony, tellurium, gold, zinc, nickel, platinum, silver, cobalt, and tin. Doses of 30 mg / kg / day for 5 days followed by 20 mg / day for 14 days led to a threefold increase in urinary mercury excretion with a decrease in the blood mercury concentration. Longer courses of therapy or sustained therapy may have a larger impact on total body mercury elimination following elemental mercury exposure.

D-PENICILLAMINE

Penicillamine therapy may be helpful in mild cases, but may not be worth its adverse effects. Even with the use of chelating agents, mercurialism may take months or years to recover and mental deterioration may be permanent. Therapy with chelating agents may or may not be warranted.

N-ACETYLCYSTEINE

The principal target organs for mercuric chloride-induced toxicity are the kidneys. Nonprotein sulfhydryl groups may be directly involved in mercury entry into the tubular cells. Glutathione plays a role in this process. Its high concentration in renal tissue may explain the accumulation of mercury in the kidney. Animal studies suggest that the nephrotoxic effects of mercuric chloride are either enhanced by glutathione depletion or prevented by glutathione augmentation. N-acetylcysteine promotes a significant increase in renal nonprotein sulfhydryl content and may be helpful after mercury exposures.

Questions—Mercury

1. **Which of the following statements concerning acrodynia is false?**
   A. The onset of acrodynia in children is often insidious, with anorexia, insomnia, and irritability.
   B. Sweating may be profuse in acrodynia.
   C. The hands and feet in patients with acrodynia are puffy, pink, painful, paresthetic, perspiring, and peeling.
   D. In adults, the presenting symptoms are insomnia, thirst, abdominal pain, aching extremities, and psychologic disturbance.
   E. Acrodynia, or "pink disease," is still common among dentists.
2. **Which of the following statements concerning mercury is true?**
   A. Following an ingestion of inorganic mercury such as mercuric chloride, patients may remain asymptomatic, but the majority develop gastrointestinal symptoms.
   B. Patients who develop renal involvement almost invariably have gastrointestinal symptoms.
   C. Mercurous chloride laxative ingested over a long period may produce toxic effects of mercury on the kidneys, gastrointestinal tract, and central nervous system.
   D. All of the above
   E. A and C
3. **Injected mercury can pass through the pulmonary capillary bed and can be observed in systemic sites such as the liver, lungs, kidneys, brain, or heart where it can oxidize to mercuric ion and produce toxic effects.**
   A. True
   B. False
4. **Which of the following symptoms are associated with erethism?**
   A. Lack of self control
   B. Irritability
   C. Shyness
   D. All of the above
   E. A and B
5. **Organic mercury**
   A. Was associated with an epidemic in Minamata, Japan, affecting over 2,500 people.
   B. Can cause brain damage in areas of the brain concerned with color recognition and speech. Prominent choreoathetosis, ataxia, spasticity and seizures develop.
   C. Easily crosses the blood-brain barrier.
   D. All of the above
   E. A and C
6. **Elemental liquid mercury**
   A. Is totally benign
   B. Can volatilize into inhalable toxin
   C. Is no longer used in light switches and barometers
   D. All of the above
   E. B and C
7. **Inorganic mercury may be associated with the ingestion of pesticides or germicides.**
   A. True
   B. False
8. **In humans, mercury distributes to all parts of the body, reaching a peak over 1–2 days.**
   A. True
   B. False
9. **Mercury intoxication following the cutaneous application of inorganic mercury has been reported in the treatment of infected eczema or impetigo by the application of different mercury salts.**
   A. True
   B. False
10. **Charcoal hemoperfusion and hemodialysis are effective in removing mercury.**
    A. True
    B. False
11. **Chelators which may be helpful in mercury poisoning include each of the following except**
    A. Dimercaprol
    B. DMPS
    C. DMSA
    D. Deferoxamine
    E. D-Penicillamine

MOLYBDENUM

Molybdenum (chemical symbol Mo) is used in stainless steel and cast iron alloy production. It is an essential element in humans, as enzymes involved in carbon, sulfur and nitrogen metabolism require it. Molybdenum increases the production of xanthine oxidase and is a cofactor required for transferases to bind iron.

Symptoms of molybdenum exposure may include decreased appetite, listlessness, weakness, fatigue, anorexia, headache, arthralgias, myalgias, chest pain, nonproductive cough, and diarrhea. Patients with high molybdenum levels can develop gout-like attacks and a hypochromic microcytic anemia. A pneumoconiosis has been associated with chronic molybdenum exposure. Chronic molybdenism causes testicular atrophy.

Questions—Molybdenum

1. Which of the following has not been associated with molybdenum?
A. Myalgias
B. Gout-like attacks
C. Macrocytic anemia
D. Testicular atrophy
E. Pneumoconiosis

NICKEL

Nickel (chemical symbol Ni) is a silver-white metal widely used in industry. The largest nickel source found in the atmosphere is from fuel oil combustion. Other sources of atmospheric emissions include mining and refining operations, municipal waste incinerators, and windblown dust. Nickel sources in water soil include stormwater runoff and wastewater from municipal sewage treatment plants. Consumer products contribute little to exposure. Nickel occurs in most food items. The highest level of exposure to nickel comes from dietary intake.

Acute nickel toxicity generally occurs from exposure to nickel carbonyl. This product is considered one of the most toxic chemicals used in industry. Severe pulmonary and gastrointestinal effects may follow exposure to this agent. Nickel sulfate exposure may be fatal and may produce evidence of respiratory, circulatory, and neurologic distress. Nickel is a common sensitizing agent, and allergic contact dermatitis from nickel in industry and jewelry is quite prevalent.

Pathophysiology

Nickel readily crosses the cell membrane via calcium channels and competes with calcium for specific receptors. Although a nickel deficiency disease has not been identified in humans, circumstantial evidence and the fact that nickel is an essential element in several animal species suggest an essential status of nickel.

Pharmacokinetics

ABSORPTION

- The absorption of soluble nickel compounds is rapid. Insoluble compounds are only partially absorbed by the gastrointestinal route.
- Some absorption may occur via the lungs.

DISTRIBUTION

- Albumin is the main transport protein in blood.
- After absorption, concentrations are highest in the kidneys, lungs, liver, and pituitary gland.

ELIMINATION

- Absorbed nickel is excreted predominantly in the urine. It is also excreted in perspiration and is deposited in the hair.
- The half-life of nickel in the serum is 11 hours.

Clinical Presentations

NICKEL CARBONYL

Nickel carbonyl is the most toxic form of nickel. Immediate symptoms following exposure include nausea, vertigo, headache, dyspnea, and chest pain. Severe pulmonary symptoms and death may occur in the following days.

NICKEL HYPERSENSITIVITY

Asthma, urticaria, erythema multiforme, contact dermatitis, and hand eczema may follow the use of objects made with nickel. Stainless steel sutures may induce a hypersensitivity reaction in a patient allergic to nickel. Patch tests may be useful. Nickel disposable surgical skin clips may be contraindicated in patients with nickel allergy.

CARCINOGENICITY

Occupational exposure to nickel refinery dust, which contains nickel subsulfide, has been associated with an increased risk of lung and nasal cancers, and possibly cancer of the larynx. Nickel subsulfide is considered a known human carcinogen. Nickel carbonyl is a probable human carcinogen. Metallic nickel, nickel oxide, and soluble nickel salts may be associated with lung and nasal sinus cancer.

Toxic Dosage/Death

Following an exposure to an air concentration of nickel carbonyl over 50 mg/m^3, symptoms referable to the respiratory and nervous system may appear within 30 minutes to one hour followed within 24 hours by serious life-threatening events. Fatalities usually occur after 4–11 days and are attributed to neurologic and respiratory toxicity.

A fatal case of nickel poisoning by the oral route occurred in a 2-year-old who ingested 15 g of nickel sulfate crystals. Ingestion of 0.5–2.5 g of nickel sulfate led to transient symptoms and full recovery in 32 workers who drank water contaminated with both nickel sulfate and chloride.

Pregnancy/Lactation

No human studies are available relative to effects of nickel on pregnancy or lactation. Nickel crosses the placental barrier in animals and may do so in humans.

Laboratory

ANALYTIC METHODS

Electrothermal atomic absorption spectrometry is useful for determinations of nickel concentration in the urine.

BLOOD LEVELS

Normal levels of nickel have been reported to be less than 0.1 mg/kg in tissues, 3–7 $\mu g/L$ in whole blood, 1–5 $\mu g/L$ in blood serum, and 2–4 $\mu g/L$ in urine.

Treatment

GUT DECONTAMINATION

Little data are available to guide management with these modalities.

ELIMINATION ENHANCEMENT

Hemodialysis may be an option in cases involving renal failure; however, the effectiveness of this intervention has not been documented.

SUPPORTIVE MEASURES

- Mild cases of nickel carbonyl inhalation can be treated with bed rest after removal from exposure. Bronchodilators and oxygen may be useful.
- No evidence exists to support the efficacy of topical Dithiocarb or disulfiram in the treatment of nickel dermatitis.

- Exposure to nickel carbonyl fumes may induce a leukocytosis that may parallel the severity of intoxication. Eosinophilia is usually not found. Transient elevations of blood reticulocytes, urine albumin, and serum bilirubin may follow nickel sulfate ingestion.
- The electrocardiogram may show sinus tachycardia, bradycardia, heart block and toxic myocarditis manifested by changes in ST and T-waves, and QT interval prolongation.

Antidotes

DITHIOCARB AND DISULFIRAM

Sodium diethyldithiocarbamate (DDC or Dithiocarb) is an investigational antidote in the U.S. Animal studies indicate that it may be effective when it is administered parenterally shortly after exposure. Disulfiram may be effective because it is metabolized to two molecules of Dithiocarb; however, there are currently insufficient data to support its use. Data on Dithiocarb and disulfiram have not been subjected to controlled clinical studies.

Questions—Nickel

1. **Which of the following statements is false?**
   A. Nickel (chemical symbol Ni) is a silver-white metal widely used in industry.
   B. The largest nickel source found in the atmosphere is from coal mining operations.
   C. Acute nickel toxicity generally occurs from exposure to nickel carbonyl.
   D. Nickel sulfate exposure may be fatal and may produce evidence of respiratory, circulatory, and neurologic distress.
   E. Nickel is a common sensitizing agent, and allergic contact dermatitis from nickel in industry and jewelry is quite prevalent.
2. **An investigational antidote in the U.S. which may be effective against nickel is**
   A. Sodium diethyldithiocarbamate
   B. Succimer
   C. Ascorbic acid
   D. DMPS
   E. Dimercaprol

PALLADIUM

Palladium (chemical symbol Pd) occurs in nature with platinum or gold. It is found in nickel sulfide ores. Palladium compounds include palladium chloride, palladium iodide, palladium oxide, palladium nitrate and palladium trifluoride. Allergy to palladium may be manifested by urticaria, rash, bronchospasm and eosinophilia. No cases of occupational poisoning from palladium or its compounds have been reported. In Austria, palladium has been used to replace amalgam in dental fillings because of concerns about mercury toxicity. Contact dermatitis has been reported.

Questions—Palladium

1. **Palladium (chemical symbol Pm) occurs in nature with platinum or gold. It is found in nickel sulfide ores.**
   A. True
   B. False

PHOSPHORUS

Phosphorous (chemical symbol P) occurs in numerous forms. Originally, the match industry used phosphorus extensively but the occurrence of "phossy jaw" (i.e., painful, suppurative mandible enlargement) from chronic industrial phosphorus poisoning led to a prohibitive tax. Exposures may occur from suicidal ingestion of fire crackers called "totes," or accidental ingestion of yellow phosphorus rodenticides. Less toxic red phosphorus and phosphorus sesquisulfide have replaced toxic yellow phosphorus in matches. Red phosphorous is nonvolatile, insoluble, and unabsorbable.

Occupational exposure involves acetyl cellulose makers, bronze alloy makers, munitions workers, smoke bomb and incendiary makers, pesticide rat poison workers, fertilizer makers, electroluminescent-coating makers, and semiconductor workers. Elemental yellow phosphorus causes second- and third-degree burns on skin contact and may cause systemic symptoms from absorption. The compound is highly toxic.

Phosphine is used in the semiconductor industry, grain fumigation and rodenticides. Phosphine gas exposures can cause gastrointestinal tract symptoms, as well as respiratory, cardiovascular, and central nervous system changes resulting from metabolic changes. See Chapter 48, Pesticides.

Pathophysiology

Yellow phosphorus is a general protoplasmic poison that uncouples oxidative phosphorylation. Pathological changes can include severe ulcerative gastritis, rarely with luminescent stools, acute yellow liver atrophy, and proximal renal tubular and cortical necrosis. Chronic degenerative bone changes and osteoporosis, especially of the mandible ("phossy jaw"), occur after chronic phosphorus exposure. There is a subsequent predisposition to fracture and infection. Fatty degeneration of the myocardium with necrosis can also occur with yellow phosphorus.

Pharmacokinetics

ABSORPTION

- Elemental yellow phosphorus is well absorbed from the skin and gastrointestinal tract.
- Phosphine toxicity results from inhalation.
- Red phosphorus is practically unabsorbable.

DISTRIBUTION

- Targets of yellow phosphorous poisoning include the GI tract, liver, kidney, and bone.

ELIMINATION

- The lungs and gut excrete yellow phosphorus, but little elimination occurs via the kidneys.

Clinical Presentations

YELLOW PHOSPHORUS

The classical presentation of acute yellow phosphorus toxicity appears in three stages. Severe gastrointestinal irritation manifested by nausea, vomiting, hematemesis, and abdominal pain occurs early. Diarrhea, mucosal burns, garlic breath and luminescent stools / vomitus appear infrequently. Phosphorus is corrosive to skin and can cause dermatitis. In severe cases, coma and cardiovascular collapse may follow the gastrointestinal phase.

An asymptomatic phase appears hours to 2–3 days postingestion. Later, systemic toxicity occurs and is characterized by lethargy, stupor, coma, restlessness, hypotension, shock, hepatorenal dysfunction, bleeding, vomiting, and diarrhea. Central nervous system involvement portends a critical prognosis. Indicators of poor prognosis include generalized muscle tenderness and a clouded sensorium. Little prognostic value results from the degree of liver enlargement, severity of abdominal pain, intensity of jaundice, or extent of elevation of hepatic aminotransferase levels.

PHOSPHINE GAS

Prominent clinical manifestations of acute phosphine gas exposure include headache, fatigue, nausea, vomiting, cough, dyspnea, paresthesias, jaundice, ataxia, intention tremor, weakness, and diplopia. On autopsy, fatal cases have revealed centrilobular necrosis of the liver, congestive heart failure with pulmonary edema, and focal myocardial necrosis.

Toxic Dosage/Death

A low-birth-weight infant of 28 weeks was inadvertently administered 460 mg of phosphorus daily instead of 46 mg as a preventive measure for metabolic bone disease. The infant developed apneic attacks with cyanosis, a distended abdomen, generalized muscle spasms, extreme hypocalcemia, and hyperphosphatemia. The acute fatal dose of elemental yellow phosphorus is 15–100 mg.

Laboratory

ANALYTIC METHODS

Phosphorous is measured by spectrophotometry.

BLOOD LEVELS

Following blood levels after overdose has not been helpful in managing ill effects.

Treatment

GUT DECONTAMINATION

Lavage with 1:5,000 potassium permanganate solution (using 500 mL in a child and 1–2 L in an adult) has been advocated, but has yet to be conclusively proven to be efficacious and safe. Saline lavage may be performed as well.

ELIMINATION ENHANCEMENT

Exchange transfusions are questionably effective. Hemodialysis is recommended only if renal failure develops.

SUPPORTIVE MEASURES

- Monitor all ill patients in an intensive care setting. Watch for dysrhythmias and replace fluids/electrolytes as needed. Follow calcium, magnesium, phosphorus, glucose, prothrombin time, renal and liver function and complete blood count daily.
- For phosphorus burns, copious irrigation with 2% copper sulfate may be helpful.
- Since yellow phosphorus ignites at 34°C, cover any particles present in the skin with mineral oil. Be sure to protect patients' and health care workers' skin from the corrosive action of phosphorus with gloves and careful washing of all vomitus and stools.

Questions—Phosphorus

1. Which of the following statements is false?
A. "Phossy jaw" is a painful, suppurative mandible enlargement from chronic industrial phosphorus exposure.
B. Red phosphorous has been used in rodenticides.
C. Yellow phosphorous may cause burns and is highly toxic.
D. Phosphine gas can cause gastrointestinal tract symptoms, as well as respiratory, cardiovascular, and central nervous system changes resulting from metabolic changes.
E. Yellow phosphorus is a protoplasmic poison that uncouples oxidative phosphorylation.

2. Phosphorous exposure rarely yields luminescent stools.
A. True
B. False

PLATINUM

Platinum (chemical symbol Pt) is well known for its use in the chemotherapeutic agent cis-platinum. See Chapter 44, Chemotherapeutic Drugs. Platinum and its alloys appear in jewelry, the chemical and electrical industries, dentistry, and fiberglass production. Complex platinum salts are catalysts in the preparation of sulfuric acid in the petroleum and pharmaceutical industries. Because of the extensive use of platinum in catalytic converters, the automobile industry consumes the majority of platinum.

Pathophysiology

Workplace toxicity results from the potent sensitizing properties of platinum salt complexes but not from platinum itself. These low-molecular-weight compounds (in particular, the compounds containing halogen ligands such as chloride) induce immediate hypersensitivity (type I) reactions. Other group VIII metal salts (e.g., palladium and rhodium) appear to be poor skin sensitizers. Cisplatin (Platinol®) inhibits DNA synthesis by forming cross-links and denaturing the double helix.

Clinical Presentations

Wheezing, tightness of the chest, dyspnea, and cough characterize platinum-induced asthma. Symptoms usually abate soon after terminating exposure. Nasal and conjunctival irritation, sore throat, and rhinitis also may occur. Signs of platinum dermatitis include erythema, urticaria, vesiculation, and fissures.

CISPLATIN TOXICITY

Nausea and vomiting occur in almost all patients, but diarrhea is uncommon. Nephrotoxicity develops in two-thirds of patients, manifested by acute tubular necrosis of the distal convoluted tubules. Large single doses with vigorous prehydration and the use of osmotic diuretics help reduce but do not eliminate toxicity. Hypomagnesemia, leukopenia, and thrombocytopenia (onset at 6–26 days) may occur. Normocytic anemia appears in 9–40% of patients. Ototoxicity is often non-reversible and is characterized by tinnitus and hearing loss. Peripheral neuropathies, memory loss, and intention tremor may develop. Allergic reactions involve skin rash and rarely anaphylaxis.

POTASSIUM CHLOROPALATINITE

Potassium chloropalatinite is a soluble, nonorganic salt of platinum used in photography, in the chemical and electrical industries, in electroplating, and in the manufacture of catalysts. Oliguric renal failure, metabolic acidosis, fever, muscle cramps, gastroenteritis, and rhabdomyolysis have been associated with overdose.

Toxic Dosage/Death

A 31-year-old who ingested 10 mL of a photographic tonic solution containing 600 mg of potassium chloropalatinite developed acute oliguric renal failure, metabolic acidosis, fever, muscle cramps, gastroenteritis, and rhabdomyolysis.

Laboratory

ANALYTIC METHODS

Blood and urine platinum levels may be obtained by atomic absorption spectrophotometry.

BLOOD LEVELS

Following blood levels of platinum in overdose has not been shown to be helpful in management.

Treatment

GUT DECONTAMINATION

Charcoal has not been shown to be helpful after platinum exposures.

ELIMINATION ENHANCEMENT

These methods have not been reported to be helpful after platinum exposure.

SUPPORTIVE MEASURES

- Control dust exposures by providing adequate ventilation. Bronchospasm may respond to β-agonist inhalational therapy.
- Decontaminate affected areas by washing thoroughly and treat symptoms supportively.

Questions—Platinum

1. Which of the following statements concerning platinum is false?

A. Platinum and its alloys appear in jewelry, the chemical and electrical industries, dentistry, and fiberglass production.
B. Workplace toxicity results from the potent sensitizing properties of platinum but not from platinum salts.
C. Other group VIII metal salts (e.g., palladium and rhodium) appear to be poor skin sensitizers.
D. Cisplatin inhibits DNA synthesis by forming cross-links and denaturing the double helix.
E. Ototoxicity from cis-platinum is often non-reversible and is characterized by tinnitus and hearing loss.

POTASSIUM

Potassium (chemical symbol K) is an essential intracellular ion involved in all phases of cellular homeostasis. Potassium is fundamentally involved in cellular electrical conduction. It is found in numerous chemical agents, is used to replace potassium loss due to diuretics, is used to treat cardiac glycoside toxicity, and is used to treat hypokalemia from any cause. Potassium is also found in salt substitutes. Like magnesium toxicity, hyperkalemia often results from reduced renal excretion in association with potassium loads. Patients with normal renal function rarely develop hyperkalemia.

Electrocardiographic changes and arrhythmias characterize overdose with potassium. Certain potassium compounds have been associated with individual profiles in overdose. These include ingestion of potassium bichromate match heads which can lead to acute renal failure, and potassium permanganate poisoning which may be associated with acute hemorrhagic pancreatitis that can terminate fatally. Potassium perchlorate has been associated with aplastic anemia.

Pathophysiology

Potassium is an intracellular ion involved in cellular homeostasis and electrical conduction.

Pharmacokinetics

ABSORPTION

- Potassium is well absorbed in the small intestine.

DISTRIBUTION

- Potassium is found in all body tissues and fluids.
- The intracellular fluid compartment contains 98% of the body's potassium.

ELIMINATION

- The half-life of potassium chloride is 16 seconds.
- Potassium is primarily eliminated via the kidney; however, some is excreted in feces and sweat.
- Renal potassium excretion depends on chloride ion concentration, acid-base status, and adrenal hormone secretion.

Clinical Presentations

The clinical picture of hyperkalemia depends on the serum potassium level, the chronicity of elevated levels, underlying cardiovascular disease, and the concomitant enhancement of hyperkalemia by hyponatremia, hypomagnesemia, or acidosis. Neuromuscular signs may include weakness, paresthesias, hyporeflexia, and paralysis.

Cardiovascular signs may include bradycardia, slowed conduction, hypotension, ventricular fibrillation, and asystole. The patient may develop serious cardiac problems without prominent early symptoms of systemic toxicity. The sequential electrocardiographic manifestations of hyperkalemia include tall, peaked T-waves, depressed S-T segments, decreased amplitude of R-waves, P-R interval prolongation, decreased P waves, widened QRS complexes, Q-T prolongation, sine wave appearance, and asystole.

Small-bowel ulcerations may follow the use of enteric-coated potassium chloride tablets, and local pain and inflammation may result from intravenous administration of potassium chloride. Slow-release potassium tablets in overdose may lead to serious arrhythmias and death.

Toxic Dosage/Death

Cardiac manifestations of toxicity are frequent at potassium levels above 8 mEq/L and rare below 6.5 mEq/L. A patient who ingested 100 slow-release potassium tablets developed ventricular tachycardia and survived. A 27-year-old who ingested 60 tablets of sustained-release potassium chloride (Slow-K®) developed first-degree heart block, wide QRS complexes, and tall T-waves. The plasma potassium concentration was 91 mmol/L and the patient survived.

Drug Interactions

Hyperkalemia may be exacerbated by potassium-sparing diuretics and many agents capable of inducing renal failure.

Pregnancy/Lactation

Pregnancy risk factor A.

Laboratory

ANALYTIC METHODS

Potassium is measured by atomic absorption spectrometry or ion-selective electrode.

BLOOD LEVELS

A normal potassium concentration is 3.5–5.3 mEq/L. Factitious hyperkalemia may result from the release of intracellular potassium stores (e.g., hemolyzed blood samples, prolonged tourniquet time, and thrombocytosis).

Treatment

GUT DECONTAMINATION

Approximately 1 mEq of potassium is removed per gram of cation-exchange resin (e.g., sodium polystyrene sulfonate or Kayexalate®) administered. The resin compounds exchange sodium for potassium and therefore should be used cautiously in patients with cardiac and renal dysfunction. The oral dose is 20–50 g of Kayexalate® dissolved in 100–200 mL of 20% sorbitol. The dose is repeated every four hours up to four or five daily doses until the potassium level returns to normal. Alternative rectal administration involves the suspension of 8 g of Kayexalate® and 50 g of sorbitol in 200 mL of water, given as a retention enema.

ELIMINATION ENHANCEMENT

Dialysis effectively removes potassium. Patients who cannot tolerate fluid loads or those with severe renal dysfunction benefit from early hemodialysis.

SUPPORTIVE MEASURES

- Every patient with suspected hyperkalemia should receive an electrocardiogram as well as measurement of serum electrolytes, creatinine, BUN and calcium levels.
- The presence of electrocardiographic evidence of hyperkalemia or serum potassium levels exceeding 7.5 mEq/L indicates a medical emergency requiring an intravenous line and constant cardiac monitoring. Serious dysrhythmias may occur suddenly despite moderate elevations of serum potassium.
- Symptomatic hyperkalemia and hyperkalemia with evidence of EKG changes should be treated with Kayexalate® and the following antidotes depending on the degree of abnormality.

Antidotes

CALCIUM

The intravenous injection of 5–10 mL of 10% calcium gluconate in adults over a 2-minute period antagonizes the cardiac and neuromuscular effects of hyperkalemia. The dose may be repeated in ten minutes if needed. Calcium must be used cautiously in patients who also receive digitalis preparations. The duration of action is approximately one hour.

SODIUM BICARBONATE

The intravenous injection of 50 mEq of bicarbonate in adults over a 5-minute period causes the rapid movement of potassium into the cells. The dose may be repeated in 10–15 minutes if needed. The onset of action is within 15 minutes, and the duration is 1–2 hours. Cardiac and renal dysfunction may limit the use of bicarbonate because of high sodium and fluid loads.

GLUCOSE AND INSULIN

The administration of glucose (one ampule of 50 mL of D50W) and 5–10 units of regular insulin over a 5-minute period in adults causes an intracellular shift of potassium. The effects appear in 30–60 minutes and last several hours.

Questions—Potassium

1. **Symptomatic hyperkalemia may be treated with all of the following, except**
   A. Calcium
   B. Insulin and dextrose
   C. Kayexalate®
   D. Sodium bicarbonate
   E. Fluid restriction

SELENIUM

Selenium (chemical symbol Se) is widely used in industry in electronics, glass, explosives, ceramics, steel, and pigment manufacturing. Chronic elemental selenium exposure can cause dental caries, but adverse effects are unusual. Selenious acid is the most toxic form of selenium and usually causes fatalities. It is a component of gun-bluing solution. Medicinal uses of selenium include antidandruff shampoos, dietary supplements, and the treatment of cystic fibrosis. While human toxicity is rare, it can be deadly.

Pathophysiology

Selenium is an essential trace metal that inactivates sulfhydryl groups in certain enzymes, and is a component of glutathione peroxidase.

Pharmacokinetics

ABSORPTION

- Selenious acid is well absorbed from the lungs and gastrointestinal tract.
- Selenious acid, selenium dioxide and selenium oxychloride may be absorbed through the skin.

DISTRIBUTION

- Selenium is distributed to all soft tissues, especially liver and kidney.
- Protein binding is 95%.
- Fifty percent of selenious acid is excreted renally.

ELIMINATION

- The half-life of selenium is 116 days, and the half-life of selenious acid is 1.2 days.

Clinical Presentations

SELENIOUS ACID

Selenious acid ingestions are almost invariably fatal. Stupor, respiratory depression, hypotension, and death result several hours after ingestion. Severe hypotension develops from decreased contractility (from a toxic cardiomyopathy) and from low peripheral vascular resistance. Postmortem examination has demonstrated myocardial and pulmonary infarction, ascites, obstructive bronchial plugs, interstitial pulmonary emphysema, bronchopulmonary dysplasia, and barotrauma.

CHRONIC EFFECTS

Chronic exposure to selenium compounds resembles arsenic toxicity. Hair loss, white horizontal streaking on fingernails, paronychia, fatigue, irritability, hyperreflexia, nausea, vomiting, garlic odor on breath, and metallic taste characterize chronic toxicity. Muscle tenderness, tremor, lightheadedness, and facial flushing may be seen in selenite poisoning.

INHALATIONAL EFFECTS

Selenium dusts produce respiratory tract irritation manifested by nasal discharge, loss of smell, epistaxis, and cough. Accidental inhalation of hydrogen selenide gas produced upper respiratory tract irritation and wheezing followed in 18 hours by progressive dyspnea, pneumomediastinum, and markedly reduced expiratory flow rates. Improvement occurred over five days, but some restrictive and obstructive changes remained three years later.

Toxic Dosage/Death

Elemental selenium is generally nontoxic in therapeutic doses (50–200 μg/d). The estimated ingested dose of superpotent selenium in a series of toxic cases ranged from 27 to 2,310 μg, with nausea, vomiting, nail changes, fatigue, and irritability as the most common manifestations.

The ingestion of 22 mg of sodium selenate per kilogram produced minimal toxicity despite a substantial rise in blood level. Consumption of 1–5 mg/kg of sodium selenite by five adults caused nausea, vomiting, abdominal pain, and tremor that resolved in 24 hours. Selenate is the least toxic inorganic selenium form; selenite is more toxic.

Selenious acid is the most toxic inorganic selenium compound. A 15-mL ingestion of gun bluing solution (2% selenious acid) by a 2-year-old and a 30–60 mL ingestion by an adult have resulted in death. Selenium dioxide is a white crystalline solid that decomposes in water to selenious acid. An estimated 10-g oral dose produced apnea and asystole within 8 hours of ingestion.

Pregnancy/Lactation

Selenium readily crosses the placenta. There have been no reports of abortion following selenium use.

Laboratory

ANALYTIC METHODS

A fluorometric assay of total selenium in plasma and urine has a limit of detection of 10 μg/L. Stable isotope dilution gas chromatography-mass spectrometry can be used for the determination of Selenium in urine samples.

BLOOD LEVELS

Serum selenium levels may be elevated after chronic exposures but do not correlate well with symptoms. In a fatal case, the plasma selenium level reached 285 μg/mL on the first hospital day and returned to normal by day 4.

Treatment

GUT DECONTAMINATION

Emesis after selenious acid ingestion is contraindicated. Since this acid may cause profound systemic poisoning and death, decontamination with (gentle) gastric lavage and charcoal may be indicated. Factors to consider in the decision to use these measures include the time since exposure, the amount of spontaneous emesis, the clinical condition of the patient, and the amount ingested.

ELIMINATION ENHANCEMENT

These methods have not been reported following acute selenium ingestions.

SUPPORTIVE MEASURES

- Management of chronic intoxication is supportive with elimination of the selenium source.
- The treatment of ingestions of compounds containing selenious acid (i.e., gun bluing solutions) is not well studied. Even small amounts of this chemical are potentially lethal. All patients who ingest selenious acid should be hospitalized for observation.
- Gun bluing compound containing selenious acid is corrosive and will produce esophageal burns.
- Treatment includes cardiopulmonary monitoring in an intensive care setting, intravenous saline infusion, supplemental oxygen, and ventilation as needed.
- Skin exposures are treated with aggressive irrigation. Ten-percent sodium thiosulfate solution may decrease pain and necrosis following dermal exposure.
- Laboratory abnormalities may include thrombocytopenia, moderate hepatorenal dysfunction, and elevated serum creatine kinase levels. The electrocardiogram may demonstrate ST elevations and T-wave changes characteristic of myocardial infarction.

Antidotes

There are no antidotes to selenious acid toxicity. British Anti-Lewisite (BAL) and calcium disodium EDTA may enhance renal toxicity and are contraindicated.

Questions—Selenium

1. Which of the following statements about selenium is false?

A. Selenium is widely used in industry in electronics, glass, explosives, ceramics, steel and pigment manufacturing.
B. Chronic elemental selenium exposure can cause dental caries, and adverse effects from selenium are common.
C. Selenious acid is the most toxic form of selenium and usually causes fatalities.
D. Medicinal uses of selenium include antidandruff shampoos, dietary supplements, and the treatment of cystic fibrosis.

E. Selenium is an essential trace metal that inactivates sulfhydryl groups in certain enzymes.

2. **Selenious acid (gun-bluing solution) ingestions are almost invariably fatal. Severe hypotension develops from a toxic cardiomyopathy and from low peripheral vascular resistance.**
   A. True
   B. False

SILVER

Silver (chemical symbol Ag) is available in sulfadiazine cream (Silvadene®) used for burns, colloidal silver iodide, and certain eye drops. Silver nitrate ointment and solution have well-established roles in the prophylaxis of perinatal gonococcal conjunctivitis. Silver nitrate may be locally corrosive.

Silver is also used in the photographic and electronics industries. Advertising materials in health food stores have promoted colloidal silver protein for numerous diseases. Colloidal silver proteins have been touted as powerful antimicrobials against viruses, bacteria, parasites, fungi, herpes, Candida, and tuberculosis.

Argyria is an irreversible blue-gray pigmentation of the skin found in patients who have ingested silver compounds for prolonged periods. It is commonly caused by mechanical impregnation of the skin by small silver particles in workers involved in silver mining, and in the manufacture of silverware, metal alloys, metallic films, electroplating solutions, and photographic processing.

Pathophysiology

Silver is not an essential mineral supplement and has no known physiologic function. It has a strong affinity for sulfhydryl groups and proteins.

Clinical Presentations

Neurologic deficits and diffuse silver deposition in visceral organs have been reported with long-term use of oral silver products. Renal damage and metal fume fever have been reported with high silver exposures. Argyria is manifested by blue-gray skin changes. Bronchitis, cough, bronchospasm, hypertension, black nail and feces pigmentation, and proteinuria have been reported after exposures.

Treatment

GUT DECONTAMINATION

Charcoal and / or lavage may be helpful after significant ingestions.

ELIMINATION ENHANCEMENT

These methods have not been utilized after silver ingestions.

SUPPORTIVE MEASURES

- Bronchospasm may respond to nebulized β-agonists.
- Skin contamination by silver nitrate is treated with aggressive cleansing with soap and water.

Questions—Silver

1. **Argyria**
   A. Like acrodynia, is associated with too much mercury
   B. Is a reversible blue-gray pigmentation of the skin found in patients who have ingested silver compounds for prolonged periods
   C. Is commonly caused by mechanical impregnation of the skin by small silver particles in workers involved in silver mining
   D. All of the above
   E. B and C

2. **Bronchitis, cough, bronchospasm, hypertension, black nail and feces pigmentation, and proteinuria have been reported after exposures to silver.**
   A. True
   B. False

TELLURIUM

Tellurium (chemical symbol Te) is a white elemental metal whose chemical behavior is similar to that of selenium. Tellurium is used as a component of many alloys. It is a powerful carbide stabilizer and is used in the synthetic rubber, glass, and steel production industries. Tellurium is absorbed by ingestion, by inhalation, and through the skin. Tellurium compounds are reduced to the relatively harmless elemental tellurium and methyl telluride. Ninety percent of the body stores of tellurium is in bone.

Clinical Presentations

About 15 mg of tellurium in humans can cause a garlic odor lasting over 200 days. Workers exposed to tellurium fumes may experience a garlic odor of the breath and sweat, dryness of the mouth, metallic taste, nausea, anorexia, weight loss, decreased sweating, dry itchy skin, gastrointestinal disturbances, and somnolence. Loss of consciousness and death following inadvertent ingestion of sodium tellurium has been reported.

Treatment

SUPPORTIVE MEASURES

- There has been no effective treatment reported for tellurium poisoning.

Questions—Tellurium

1. **Which of the following statements about tellurium is false?**
   A. Tellurium (chemical symbol Te) is a white elemental metal whose chemical behavior is similar to that of selenium.
   B. Tellurium is absorbed by ingestion, by inhalation, and through the skin.
   C. Ninety percent of the body stores of tellurium is in bone.
   D. Tellurium can cause a bitter almond odor.
   E. Symptoms of tellurium exposure may include dryness of the mouth, metallic taste, nausea, anorexia, and weight loss.

THALLIUM

Thallium (chemical symbol Tl) is a toxic metal found in granite, shale and volcanic rock. It is found in smelters and has been used in alloys for its anticorrosive properties. It is used in nuclear medicine to image cardiac muscle. Most recent uses include the manufacture of imitation jewelry pigments, low-temperature thermometers, semiconductors, scintillation counters, and optical lenses. It is odorless and tasteless and was used as a rodenticide until it was banned in 1975. It has also been used as a depilatory and to treat syphilis.

Pathophysiology

Thallium behaves biologically like potassium. It accumulates in the nervous system, liver and muscle. Thallium inhibits certain enzyme systems, interferes with disulfide bond formation, and damages ribosomes, adversely affecting protein synthesis.

Clinical Presentations

The clinical picture of thallium intoxication is variable. However, the diagnosis should be suspected in the presence of (a) alopecia and skin rash, (b) painful peripheral neuropathy, and (c) confusion and lethargy. The first symptoms of poisoning occur within hours and include nausea, vomiting, abdominal pain, diarrhea, tachycardia, and headache. Within hours to days, the next stage of poisoning typically involves alopecia. A characteristic dark, pigmented band may appear in scalp hair within four days. Neurologic symptoms may appear in 2–5 days and include confusion, hallucinations, and convulsions.

Cardiovascular signs may include tachycardia and hypertension. In severe cases coma, respiratory paralysis, and death can occur within one week. When smaller doses are taken, a painful peripheral sensorimotor neuropathy and ataxia are the outstanding symptoms. Other neurologic features include cranial nerve palsies, optic neuropathy, choreoathetosis, tremor, and encephalopathy.

CHRONIC EFFECTS

Scalp alopecia is the best known symptom of chronic thallium poisoning, which begins days after ingestion and is typically completed within one month. Skin may be involved by acneiform eruptions, a papulomacular rash, and dystrophy of the nails (Mees lines). Autonomic dysfunction, hypertension, cardiomyopathy, electrocardiographic changes, testicular toxicity, hypokalemia, renal failure, abnormal liver function, leukocytosis, and thrombocytopenia have been reported.

Ophthalmologic manifestations include eyelid lesions, ophthalmoplegia, nystagmus, optic neuritis, keratitis and lens opacities. Optic atrophy as a sequel to thallium-induced toxic optic neuropathy is well reported. Functional changes include impairment of contrast sensitivity, abnormal color vision, impaired visual acuity, and scotomas. Optic neuropathy and cranial nerve palsies are the most marked features.

Toxic Dosage/Death

The average lethal adult dose is 1 g of soluble thallium salt. Survival has been reported after 1.3-g ingestions by adults and death has resulted from a 3.2-g ingestion.

Pregnancy/Lactation

Thallium does cross the placental barrier, and has produced alopecia and nail abnormalities in a fetus exposed in the last trimester.

Laboratory

ANALYTIC METHODS

Thallium is detected by flameless atomic absorption spectrometry.

BLOOD LEVELS

Normal reference values are less than 10 ng/mL.

Treatment

GUT DECONTAMINATION

Gastric lavage and multiple-dose activated charcoal have been suggested as treatment modalities. Unlike other heavy metals, thallium is adsorbed to charcoal.

ELIMINATION ENHANCEMENT

Whole-bowel irrigation may be helpful in individuals who ingest large quantities of thallium. In cases of renal insufficiency, charcoal hemoperfusion and/or hemodialysis may be helpful. Forced diuresis may be equally as efficacious.

SUPPORTIVE MEASURES

- Initial support focuses on airway, breathing and circulatory issues.
- Potassium administration, while probably associated with increased elimination, may be dangerous and is not generally advised. Thallium is not easily chelated.
- Thallium is radiopaque and may be detected by x-ray.
- Tests of contrast sensitivity and color vision are useful in the early detection of optic neuropathy in thallium intoxication.

Antidotes

PRUSSIAN BLUE

Prussian blue (potassium ferric hexacyanoferrate) is possibly effective in thallium toxicity. Thallium is exchanged for potassium in a molecular lattice and subsequently the complex is excreted in the feces. Prussian blue is not commercially available or approved for use. The dose is 250 mg/kg/d in four divided doses orally or through a nasogastric tube.

Questions—Thallium

1. Which of the following statements about thallium is false?

A. Thallium is used in nuclear medicine to image cardiac muscle.
B. Thallium is odorless and tasteless and was used as a rodenticide until it was banned in 1975.
C. Thallium behaves biologically like calcium.
D. Thallium inhibits certain enzyme systems, interferes with disulfide bond formation, and damages ribosomes, adversely affecting protein synthesis.
E. Thallium may cause alopecia.

2. Prussian blue (potassium ferric hexacyanoferrate) is possibly effective in thallium toxicity. Prussian blue is not commercially available or approved for use in the U.S.

A. True
B. False

TIN

Tin (chemical symbol Sn) is used in the manufacture of aerosol cans, paints, to coat copper wire, and in solder. Inhalation of dust or fumes of tin and tin oxide can result in a benign pneumoconiosis known as stannosis. Inorganic tin is relatively nontoxic. Although the corrosive properties of metallic tin salts produce gastrointestinal disturbances in high dose, poor oral absorption limits systemic toxicity.

Tributyltin oxide may induce occupational asthma. Its addition to indoor paint can induce eye and throat irritation, loss of appetite, nausea and vomiting, and a burning sensation in the nose. Inorganic tin may cause metal fume fever. Organic tins, such as triethyltin, have been used as fungicides, stabilizers and catalysts.

Pathophysiology

Tin may involve the uncoupling of oxidative phosphorylation. Morphologic changes after trimethyltin intoxication are confined to the nervous system.

Clinical Presentations

An acute limbic-cerebellar syndrome has followed inhalation of trimethyl tin. Hearing loss, confabulation, hyperphagia, disturbed sexual behavior, nystagmus, partial and tonic-clonic seizures, and a sensory neuropathy characterize this syndrome. Increased intracranial pressure, paralysis, tonic-clonic seizures, and death have characterized oral triethyltin (a contaminant in the production of the bactericidal drug Stalinon®) exposure.

Toxic Dosage/Death

A toxic oral dose of triethyltin has been estimated as 70 mg.

Treatment

GUT DECONTAMINATION

Lavage may be helpful after large ingestions but has not been studied.

ELIMINATION ENHANCEMENT

There are no published reports regarding these methods after tin exposures.

SUPPORTIVE MEASURES

- Decontamination of skin involves thorough cleansing with soap and water.
- Ocular exposures require irrigation with normal saline.

Questions—Tin

1. **Organic tin is relatively nontoxic.**
   A. True
   B. False
2. **Tributyltin oxide may induce occupational asthma.**
   A. True
   B. False
3. **Tin may involve the uncoupling of oxidative phosphorylation.**
   A. True
   B. False
4. **An acute limbic-cerebellar syndrome has followed inhalation of trimethyl tin characterized by hearing loss, confabulation, hyperphagia, disturbed sexual behavior, nystagmus, seizures, and a sensory neuropathy.**
   A. True
   B. False

TITANIUM

Titanium (chemical symbol Ti) is found in titanium dioxide, a white pigment used in paints, linoleum lacquers, leather, inks, rubber, soaps, textiles, ceramics, and plastics. It is approved by the U.S. Food and Drug Administration for use in adhesives, cellophane, cosmetics, paper products, poultry products, and to whiten salads and spreads.

Pathophysiology

Titanium is a respiratory irritant.

Clinical Presentations

Titanium dioxide exposure has been associated with alveolar cell hyperplasia and fibrosis. Chemical pneumonitis, pharyngeal edema, and upper airway irritation may occur. In one study of workers exposed to titanium dioxide there was no association with an increased risk of lung cancer, chronic respiratory disease, or chest x-ray abnormalities. In some subjects there may be evidence of hypersensitivity to titanium. Cataracts, conjunctivitis and keratitis have been described.

Treatment

GUT DECONTAMINATION

Dilution may be helpful after oral exposures. The use of charcoal has not been studied.

ELIMINATION ENHANCEMENT

These methods have not been utilized after titanium exposures.

SUPPORTIVE MEASURES

- Decontamination is initiated with dry wiping of the skin or eyes followed by irrigation with saline or water. Treatment is primarily symptomatic and supportive.

Questions—Titanium

1. **The titanium used in paints is non-toxic.**
   A. True
   B. False

URANIUM

Uranium (chemical symbol U) is well known for its nuclear applications. It is also used in large incandescent lamps, in gyro compasses and as mordant in the silk and wood industries. Adverse effects from uranium mining result from the inhalation of radon daughters. The decay of uranium and ultimately radium produces radon, which in turn forms short-life radon daughters (e.g., isotopes of lead, bismuth, and polonium). These products attach to dust particles that may be inhaled by workers.

Pathophysiology

Uranyl ion complexes with bicarbonate and produces acute renal proximal tubular damage.

Clinical Presentations

Renal tubular damage has been described. Cancer, both dermatologic and pulmonary, may be associated with prolonged exposures. alpha radiation delivers 95% of the radiation dose to the tracheobronchial epithelium. Mortality of uranium miners from lung cancer and chronic lung disease strongly depends on radon exposure, cigarette smoking, and height. Although both squamous and oat cell tumor types display a dose-response effect, there is some difference in the strength of the association.

Toxic Dosage/Death

Although gamma radiation is present in all uranium mines, levels rarely exceed the acceptable standard of 5 rads per year. Renal tubular damage occurs with doses exceeding 0.1 mg/kg.

Treatment

- A forced alkaline diuresis with sodium bicarbonate after large uranium exposures may be nephroprotective. All exposed surfaces should be irrigated thoroughly.
- A Geiger counter may help monitor decontamination procedures.

Questions—Uranium

1. The decay of radium produces plutonium, which in turn forms short-life radon daughters.
A. True
B. False

VANADIUM

Vanadium (chemical symbol V) is a corrosion-resistant metal used in hard steel alloys. It is used in jet engines and in the production of pesticides, inks, dyes and pigments. Vanadyl sulfate has been used by athletes to enhance weight training.

Pathophysiology

Clinical effects probably result from the oxidizing ability of vanadium. Vanadium decreases alveolar macrophage viability and is a respiratory irritant. It causes a redistribution of iron, chromium and other metals.

Pharmacokinetics

ABSORPTION

- Inhalation of dusts is the major route of absorption in workers.
- Vanadium salts are poorly absorbed from the gastrointestinal tract.

DISTRIBUTION

- Vanadium is quickly distributed to the kidneys, liver and lungs.
- The bones and teeth ultimately retain the highest concentrations of vanadium.

ELIMINATION

- Most ingested vanadium is eliminated via the feces and most absorbed vanadium is excreted via the kidneys.
- Excretion is relatively rapid and occurs within days.

Clinical Presentations

Upper respiratory tract irritation characterized by wheezing, cough, pneumonitis and rhinitis has followed exposure to vandium dust in the workplace. Nonspecific symptoms such as headache, weakness, tinnitus and palpitations have also been reported. There are no studies describing the carcinogenicity of vanadium.

Treatment

GUT DECONTAMINATION

There is little clinical evidence to support the use of these methods.

ELIMINATION ENHANCEMENT

Hemodialysis or other methods to enhance elimination are not described in the literature.

SUPPORTIVE MEASURES

- Treatment is symptomatic and supportive.

Questions—Vanadium

1. Which of the following statements about vanadium is false?
A. Vanadium (chemical symbol V) is a corrosion-resistant metal used in hard steel alloys.
B. Vanadium is used in jet engines and in the production of pesticides, inks, dyes and pigments.
C. Vanadyl sulfate has been used by athletes to enhance weight training.
D. Clinical effects probably result from the reducing ability of vanadium.
E. Vanadium decreases alveolar macrophage viability and is a respiratory irritant.

ZINC

Zinc (chemical symbol Zn) is an essential metal used in metal alloys, for the manufacture of brass, and for the galvanizing of iron. Inhalation of zinc oxide is the most common cause of metal fume fever. Uses of zinc oxide include pharmaceutical manufacturing, rubber formulation, as a vulcanizing agent, and as a white pigment. Occupational exposures involve galvanizers, electroplaters, and welders where zinc-containing alloys are heated.

Zinc chloride is used in soldering flux, dry battery cells, oil refining, dentists' cement, and taxidermy. Exposed workers include military personnel, rubber workers, textile finishers, embalmers, and dental cement makers. Metallic zinc provides a protective coating for other metals. Zinc gluconate has been touted as a cure for the common cold. Zinc phosphide has been used as a rodenticide. Zinc deficiency has been associated with growth retardation, anorexia, delayed sexual maturation, iron-deficiency anemia, and alterations of taste.

Pathophysiology

Zinc is an essential co-factor in DNA synthesis, reproduction, bone formation, growth, behavioral responses and wound healing. Zinc interferes with copper absorption by inducing the formation of metallothionein. Metallothionein has a higher affinity for copper than for zinc; therefore more copper is bound and excreted in the feces.

Pharmacokinetics

ABSORPTION

- Absorption occurs in the small intestine, and zinc oxide is probably absorbed via the lungs as well.

DISTRIBUTION

- Zinc is 99% protein bound.
- Zinc is present in all body tissues, mostly in the bone and muscle.

ELIMINATION

- Zinc is mostly eliminated through fecal excretion.

Clinical Presentations

METAL FUME FEVER

Metal fume fever (see Chapter 45, Airborne Toxins) resembles a flulike illness. Onset occurs in 4 to 6 hours, generally on the evening after exposure to fumes. Signs and symptoms include fatigue, chills, fever, myalgias, cough, dyspnea, leukocytosis, thirst, metallic taste, and salivation. Illness is generally self-limited with resolution of symptoms appearing in 36 hours. The chest x-ray is usually clear. Tolerance develops in workers, but may be lost over the weekend ("Monday morning fever").

Physical findings may vary from person to person. Fever, sweating, tachycardia, chills, pleural friction rub, and pulmonary rales have been described. Pulmonary function study results may be normal or may show acute changes consistent with reduced lung volumes and decreased carbon monoxide diffusing capacity. Over time, pulmonary function abnormalities revert to normal.

RESPIRATORY EFFECTS

Autopsies after zinc chloride exposures have revealed severe inflammation of the upper respiratory tract mucosa and pulmonary edema. Severe adult respiratory distress syndrome (ARDS) and death have followed exposure to hexite smoke.

GASTROINTESTINAL EFFECTS

Zinc concentrates in the pancreas. Hyperamylasemia has been reported in human beings with oral or parenteral zinc toxicity. Later development of chronic pancreatic exocrine deficiency may occur. After ingestion of zinc compounds, nausea, vomiting and abdominal pain may occur. Zinc chloride is a corrosive in high concentrations.

CHRONIC EFFECTS

Patients who receive zinc supplementation may develop copper deficiency and hyperceruloplasminemia. Sideroblastic anemia has been associated with copper deficiency, and copper excretion is enhanced by the ingestion of zinc.

Toxic Dosage/Death

Death has followed exposure to a zinc chloride-containing smoke bomb. Hypotension, diarrhea, vomiting, pulmonary edema, jaundice, hyperamylasemia, oliguria, anemia, and thrombocytopenia occurred after a suicidal zinc sulfate injection.

Pregnancy/Lactation

Pregnancy risk factor C. Zinc is an essential element for normal fetal growth. Reproductive abnormalities have not been demonstrated in mothers taking zinc during their pregnancies.

Laboratory

ANALYTIC METHODS

Zinc is detected by inductively coupled plasma emission spectroscopy.

BLOOD LEVELS

Normal values for plasma zinc are less than 1.5 $\mu g/mL$. Following zinc levels after overdose has not been shown to be useful.

Treatment

GUT DECONTAMINATION

The usual measures for decontamination such as lavage and charcoal may be administered, although patients usually have sufficient vomiting to not require them.

ELIMINATION ENHANCEMENT

Whole-bowel irrigation was useful in improving rectal elimination in one patient who had ingested 50 zinc sulfate tablets.

SUPPORTIVE MEASURES

- As zinc chloride and zinc acetate may be corrosive, immediate irrigation with saline is required after eye or skin involvement.
- Laboratory studies may reveal leukocytosis after zinc exposures. Lactate dehydrogenase may be elevated. Abdominal flat plate may demonstrate radiopaque tablets after large ingestions.

Antidotes

Plasma zinc may decrease after chelation with calcium disodium EDTA with improvement of lethargy and hypertension. D-penicillamine has increased mortality in animal models, and N-acetylcysteine has been found to increase urinary zinc excretion in rats.

Questions—Zinc

1. **Zinc is an essential co-factor in DNA synthesis, reproduction, bone formation, growth, behavioral responses and wound healing.**
   A. True
   B. False
2. **Patients who receive zinc supplementation may develop copper deficiency and hypoceruloplasminemia.**
   A. True
   B. False

ZIRCONIUM

Zirconium (chemical symbol Zr) is used in certain deodorant sticks and poison ivy lotions. Subcutaneous granulomas can develop from these dermal applications, probably because of hypersensitivity reactions. Minimal industrial toxicity apparently occurs, and at least one study of occupational zirconium inhalation failed to detect pulmonary abnormalities. Nonetheless, a sarcoid/granulomatous type of chronic pulmonary hypersensitivity reaction has been reported following long-term exposure to zirconium. Zirconium can also cause an acute and fulminant allergic alveolitis-like hypersensitivity reaction. Treatment is symptomatic and supportive.

Questions—Zirconium

1. **Dermal applications of zirconium may be associated with subcutaneous granulomas.**
   A. True
   B. False

ANSWERS

Aluminum
1. A 2. D

Antimony
1. C 2. B

Arsenic
1. C 2. E 3. A 4. D 5. E 6. A 7. B

Barium
1. C 2. C

Beryllium
1. D 2. E

Bismuth
1. E 2. A

Cadmium
1. A 2. A 3. C 4. A

Chromium
1. C 2. E

Cobalt
1. D 2. D 3. A

Copper
1. D 2. E 3. A

Germanium
1. C

Gold
1. B 2. B

Iron
1. C 2. C 3. A 4. D 5. B 6. A 7. B
8. B 9. B

Lead
1. A 2. D 3. B 4. C 5. B 6. B 7. A
8. D 9. A 10. B 11. A 12. D

Lithium
1. E 2. A 3. B 4. D 5. D 6. A 7. A
8. A

Magnesium
1. B 2. B 3. E 4. C 5. A 6. C 7. E

Manganese
1. D 2. A

Mercury
1. E 2. D 3. A 4. D 5. E 6. B 7. A
8. A 9. A 10. B 11. D

Molybdenum
1. C

Nickel
1. B 2. A

Palladium
1. B

Phosphorus
1. B 2. A

Platinum
1. B

Potassium
1. E

Selenium
1. B 2. B

Silver
1. C 2. A

Tellurium
1. D

Thallium
1. C 2. A

Tin
1. B 2. A 3. A 4. A

Titanium
1. B

Uranium
1. B

Vanadium
1. D

Zinc

1. A   2. B

Zirconium

1. A

SELECTED READINGS

Aluminum

1. Garrett RJ, Mulcahy D, Carmody M, et al. Aluminum encephalopathy: clinical and immunological features. Q J Med 1988;69:775–783.
2. Lione A. Aluminum toxicology and the aluminum-containing medications. Pharmacol Ther 1986;29:255–285.
3. Winship KA. Toxicity of aluminum: a historical review. I. Adverse Drug React Toxicol Rev 1992;11:123–141.

Antimony

1. Aaseth J. Recent advances in therapy of metal poisoning with chelating agents. Hum Toxicol 1983;2:257–272.
2. Winship KA. Toxicity of antimony and its compounds. Adverse Drug React Acute Pois Rev 1987;2:67–90.

Arsenic

1. Gorby MS. Arsenic poisoning. West J Med 1988;149:308–315.
2. Kleinfeld MJ. Arsine poisoning. J Occup Med 1980;22:820–821.

Barium

1. Boehmert M. Soluble barium salts. Clin Toxicol Rev 1988;10(5):1–2.
2. Scharn TF, Olbricht CH, Schuler A, et al. Barium carbonate intoxication. Intensive Care Med 1991;17:60–62.
3. Stedwell RE, Allen KM, Binder LS. Hypokalemic paralyses: a review of the etiologies, pathophysiology, presentation and therapy. Am J Emerg Med 1992;10:143–148.

Beryllium

1. Aronchik JM. Chronic beryllium disease. Radiol Clin N Amer 1992;30:1209–1217.
2. Hooper WF. Acute beryllium lung disease. NC Med J 1981;42:551–553.
3. Kriebel D, Brain JD, Sprince NL, et al. The pulmonary toxicity of beryllium. Am Rev Respir Dis 1988;137:464—473.
4. Williams WJ. Beryllium disease. Postgrad Med J 1988;64:511–516.

Bismuth

1. Basinger MA, Jones MM, McCroskey SA. Antidotes for acute bismuth intoxication. J Toxicol Clin Toxicol 1983;20:159–165.
2. Bierer DW. Bismuth subsalicylate: history, chemistry and safety. Rev Infect Dis 1990;12(Suppl 1):S3–S8.
3. Slikkerveer A, Helminth RB, Jong HB, et al. Development of a therapeutic procedure for bismuth intoxication using chelating agents. Hum Exp Toxicol 1993;12:77–78.
4. Winship KA. Toxicity of bismuth salts. Adverse Drug React Acute Pois Rev 1982;2:103–121.

Cadmium

1. Agency for Toxic Substances and Disease Registry: Toxicological Profile for Cadmium. March, 1989;TSDR / TP-88 / 08.
2. Kressel J. Cadmium. Clin Toxicol Rev 1983;5:1–2.

Chromium

1. Barceloux, DG. Chromium. Clin Tox 1999;37(2):173–194.
2. Bradberry, SM, Vale, JA. Therapeutic review: Is ascorbic acid of value in chromium poisoning and chromium dermatitis? Clin Tox. 1999;37(2):195–200.
3. Schonwald S. Chromium. Clin Toxicol Rev 1989;11(5):1–2.

Cobalt

1. Barceloux, DG. Cobalt. Clin Tox 1999;37(2):201–216.
2. Jarius JQ, Mammond E, Meier R, et al. Cobalt cardiomyopathy. A report of two cases from mineral assay laboratories and a review of the literature. J Occup Med 1992;34:620–6.

Copper

1. Barceloux, DG. Copper. Clin Tox 1999;37(2):217–230.

Germanium

1. Germanium danger. Lancet 1989;2:755 (editorial).
2. Van der Spoel JI, Stricker BHC, Esseveld MR, et al. Dangers of dietary germanium supplements. Lancet 1990;336:117.

Gold

1. Barelli A, Calimici A, Pala F. Gold salts acute poisoning: a case report. Vet Hum Toxicol 1987;29(Suppl 2):108–110.
2. Cohen MAH. Adverse reactions to gold compounds. Adverse Drug React Acute Poison Rev 1988;4:163–178.

Iron

1. Bosse GM. Conservative management of patients with moderately elevated serum iron levels. Clin Toxicol 1995;33:235–240.
2. Cheney K, Gumbiner C, Benson B, et al. Survival after a severe iron poisoning treated with intermittent infusions of deferoxamine. Clin Toxicol 1995;33:61–66.
3. Chyka PA, Butler AY. Assessment of acute iron poisoning by laboratory and clinical observations. Am J Emerg Med 1993;11:99–103.
4. Durbin DR, Wood BP. Acute iron poisoning and gastrointestinal decontamination procedures. Am J Dis Child 1992;146:765–766.
5. Mills KC, Curry SC. Acute iron poisoning. Emerg Med Clin North Am 1994;12:397.
6. Yatscoff RW, Wayne EA, Tenenbein M. An objective criterion for the cessation of deferoxamine therapy in the acutely iron poisoned patient. Clin Toxicol 1991;29:1–10.

Lead

1. Graef J. Lead poisoning management. II. Clin Toxicol Rev 1992;14(9):1–2.
2. Graef J. Lead poisoning. I. Clin Toxicol Rev 1992;14(8):1–2.
3. Graef J. Lead poisoning. III. Therapeutic protocols. Clin Toxicol Rev 1992;14(12):1–2.
4. Lovejoy FH, Shannon M, Woolf AD. Recent advances in clinical toxicology. Curr Probl Pediatr 1992 (March), pp. 119–129.

Lithium

1. Arden A. Clinical features and management of lithium poisoning. Med Toxicol 1988;3:18–32.
2. Schonwald S. Lithium. Clin Toxicol Rev 1990;12(7):1–2.
3. Shannon MW, Eisen T, Linakus J, et al. Clinical features of acute versus chronic lithium intoxication. Ann Emerg Med 1990;19:630.

Magnesium

1. Mordes JP, Wacker WEC. Excess magnesium. Pharmacolog Rev 1978;29:274–286.2. Graber TW, Yee AS, Baker FJ. Magnesium: Physiology, clinical disorders and therapy. Ann Emerg Med 1981;10:49–57.
3. Hoffman RS, Smilkstein MJ, Rubenstein F. An "amp" by any other name: the hazards of intravenous design. JAMA 1989;261:557.
4. Jones J, Heiselman D, Dougherty J, et al. Cathartic-induced magnesium toxicity during overdose management. Ann Emerg Med 1986;15:1214–1218.

Manganese

1. Barceloux, DG. Manganese. Clin Tox, 1999;37(2):293–307.

Mercury

1. Baratz R. Dental amalgam. Heavy metal. Harvard Health Letter. 1991; 16(11):4–5.
2. Davis LE, Kornfeld M, Mooney HS, et al. Methylmercury poisoning: long-term clinical, radiological, toxicological and pathological studies of an affected family. Ann Neurol 1994;35:680–688.

3. Elemental mercury vapor poisoning-North Carolina 1988. MMWR 38:770–777.
4. Hancocks S. Is dental amalgam bad for you? Br Med J 1991;302:488.
5. McLauchlan GA. Acute mercury poisoning. Anesthesia 1991;46:110–112.
6. Swineheart LT. Elemental mercury exposure. Pediatrics 1988;81:743–744.

Molybdenum

1. Barceloux, DG. Molybdenum. Clin Tox 1999;37(2):231–237.

Nickel

1. Barceloux, DG. Nickel. Clin Tox 1999;37(2):239–258.
2. Bradberry, SM, Vale, JA. Therapeutic review: Do diethyldithiocarbamate and disulfiram have a role in acute nickel carbonyl poisoning? Clin Tox 1999;37(2):259–264.
3. Zhicheng S. Acute nickel carbonyl poisoning: a report of 179 cases. Br J Ind Med 1986;43:422–424.

Palladium

1. Mastromatteo E. Palladium alloys and compounds. In: Parmeggiani L, ed. *Encyclopaedia of occupational health and safety*. 3rd ed. Geneva: International Labour Office 1991; pp. 1587–1588.

Phosphorus

1. Augenstein WL, Sokol R, Kulig K, et al. Phosphine poisoning: a report of six cases. Vet Hum Toxicol 1988;30:344.
2. Casteel SW, Bailey EM Jr. A review of zinc phosphide poisoning. Vet Hum Toxicol 1986;28:151–154.
3. Gupta S, Ahlawat S. Aluminum phosphide poisoning—a review. Clin Toxicol 1995;33:19–24.

Platinum

1. Vaisrub S. Humble therapeutic beginnings for a noble metal. JAMA 1979;241:2738.
2. Woolf AD, Ebert TH. Toxicity after self-poisoning by ingestion of potassium chloropalatinite. Clin Toxicol 1991;29:467–472.

Potassium

1. Restuccio A. Fatal hyperkalemia from a salt substitute. Am J Emerg Med 1992;10:171–173.
2. Saxena K. Clinical features and management of poisoning due to potassium chloride. Med Toxicol Adverse Drug Exp 1989;4:429–443.
3. Steedman DJ. Poisoning with sustained release potassium. Arch Emerg Med 1988;5:206–211.

Selenium

1. Barceloux, DG. Selenium. Clin Tox 1999;37(2):145–172.
2. Sioris LJ, Guthrie K, Pentel PR. Acute selenium poisoning. Vet Hum Toxicol 1980;22:364.

Silver

1. Karakashian GV, Burnett JW. Argyria. Cutis 1989;43:209.
2. Raiber A, Bruner B. Ingestion of concentrated silver nitrate. A report of two cases. Vet Hum Toxicol 1987;29:321–322.

Tellurium

1. Finkel AJ, Hamilton A, Hardy HL. Tellurium. In: Finkel AJ, ed. *Hamilton and Hardy's industrial toxicology*. 4th ed. Bristol, UK: John Wright, 1983; pp. 128–130.
2. Shie MD, Deeds FE. The importance of tellurium as a health hazard in industry. Public Health Perspect 1970;35:939–954.

Thallium

1. Stack AM. Thallium. Clin Toxicol Rev 1992;14(4):1–2.
2. Wax PM. Tortilla the votoxicosis. Clin Toxicol 1995;33:265.

Tin

1. Leikin, JB, Paloucek, FP. *Poisoning and Toxicology Handbook*, 2nd Edition, 1996-97.Lexi-Comp, Inc. Cleveland, OH. 1995; pp.1028–29.
2. Wax PM, Dockstader L. Tributyl tin use in interior paints: a continuing health hazard. Clin Toxicol 1995;33:239–241.

Titanium

1. Chen JL, Fayerweather WE. Epidemiologic study of workers exposed to titanium dioxide. J Occup Med 1988;30:937–942.

Uranium

1. Archer VE. Health concerns in uranium mining and milling. J Occup Med 1981;23:502–05.
2. Leikin, JB, Paloucek, FP. *Poisoning and Toxicology Handbook*, 2nd Edition, 1996-97.Lexi-Comp, Inc. Cleveland, OH. 1995; p.1036.

Vanadium

1. Barceloux, DG. Vanadium. Clin Tox 1999;37(2):265–278.
2. Leikin, JB, Paloucek, FP. *Poisoning and Toxicology Handbook*, 2nd Edition, 1996-97.Lexi-Comp, Inc. Cleveland, OH. 1995; p.1037.

Zinc

1. Barceloux, DG. Zinc. Clin Tox 1999;37(2):279–292.
2. McKinney PE, Brent J, Kulig K. Zinc chloride ingestion in a child: Exocrine pancreatic insufficiency. Ann Emerg Med 1995;25:562.

Zirconium

1. Bartter T, Irwin RS, Abraham JL, et al. Zirconium compound-induced pulmonary fibrosis. Arch Intern Med 1991;151:1197–1201.

CHAPTER 48
Pesticides

INTRODUCTION

Pesticide poisoning is an important cause of worldwide morbidity and mortality. It has been estimated that there are 3 million severe cases of acute pesticide poisoning each year with some 220,000 deaths. 95% of fatal pesticide poisonings occur in developing countries. Serious cases of pesticide poisoning are more likely to occur in adults than in children. More than 1,000 biocides and 25,000 formulations currently are in use. California leads the United States in both volume of pesticides used and pesticide-related illnesses. Both severe accidental and intentional illness results from the misapplication of these potent compounds.

Well-publicized epidemics in Iraq, Morocco [tri-o-cresyl phosphate (TOCP)], and in the United States (TOCP in alcoholic beverages) have resulted from ingestion of contaminated food and beverage products. When pesticide ranks for all age groups were combined, the east south central and west south central states of the United States were the highest ranked regions. A general trend of increasing pesticide concentrations with increasing age appears to exist, indicating that continued exposure results in higher levels of toxins in human adipose tissue because of bioaccumulation. The ultimate correlation of this data with scientific proof that toxic chemicals in the environment pose significant threats to humans has not yet been defined.

INSECTICIDES

ORGANOPHOSPHATES

Although phosphates and phosphonates were synthesized over 75 years ago, commercial interest in organophosphate compounds did not develop until late in World War II when German scientists developed tetraethyl pyrophosphate (TEPP) as a nicotine insecticide substitute. Soon thereafter, the German group developed dimefox, sarin, tabun, and parathion. In the United States, organophosphates cause numerous poisonings each year. In California, four out of five systemic poisonings from agricultural chemicals result from exposure to organophosphate compounds. Organophosphates have relatively high acute toxicity but low chronic toxicity.

Farmhands can acquire a chronic low-level exposure known as "orange-picker's flu" characterized by nausea, weakness, and headache. Several well-recorded epidemics of severe extremity motor weakness and mild sensory impairment resulted from TOCP contamination, and cooking oil containing TOCP (Morocco, 1959). Mass intoxication occurred in the southern United States during the 1930s when TOCP was employed as an adulterant of Jamaica Ginger ("Jake"), a popular alcohol-containing drink of the Prohibition Era. The resulting neurologic syndrome was known as Ginger "Jake" Paralysis or "Jack-Leg" because of its predilection for paralysis of the lower extremity. Gastrointentinal (GI) complaints were followed by the resolution of symptoms, and then by delayed neuropathic change often with permanent sequelae.

Diagnosis of acute organophosphate toxicity includes a reliable history, evidence of exposure to organophosphate (garlic odor), signs or symptoms of cholinergic excess, improvement with atropine or pralidoxime, and inhibition of cholinesterase in blood. A diagnosis of mild-to-moderate acute organophosphate poisoning rarely is justified unless a number of conditions are present. These include a reliable history of exposure to an organophosphate pesticide, a latent interval of not more than a few hours between the last exposure and the onset of illness, a clinical picture in which typical signs and symptoms are present, reduction of plasma and red blood cell (RBC) cholinesterase activity to a level substantially below 50% of baseline values, and an acute illness that is not substantially longer than 48 hours.

Pathophysiology

Organophosphates complex with acetylcholinesterase enzymes, leading to their deactivation. The resultant accumulation of large amounts of acetylcholine causes initial stimulation, then exhaustion of cholinergic synapses. Gamma-aminobutyric acid (GABA) and dopamine pathways provide compensatory inhibition to counteract the excessive cholinergic activity produced by these agents.

Pharmacokinetics

ABSORPTION

- Most organophosphate compounds are rapidly and well absorbed from the skin, conjunctiva, GI tract, and lungs.

DISTRIBUTION

- Most organophosphates are polar, water-soluble chemicals, but a few compounds possess high-partition coefficients (e.g., dichlofenthion), which may lead to delayed, prolonged symptoms.

ELIMINATION

- These chemicals are detoxified by cytochrome P450-mediated monooxygenases in the liver, but some metabolites are more toxic than parent compounds (i.e., conversion of the thiono groups on parathion, diazinon, and malathion to oxons).
- Metabolites usually are detected from 12 to 48 hours postexposure.

Clinical Presentations

Neurologic effects of organophosphate poisoning primarily depend on the balance between muscarinic and nicotinic receptors, and contributions of the central nervous system. Miosis is the most constant sign, but its absence does not exclude organophosphate poisoning. Muscle fasciculations are a highly reliable sign of organophosphate poisoning. The presence of excessive secretions (e.g., lacrimation and bronchorrhea) is also helpful in confirming the diagnosis.

Symptoms develop several hours postexposure, but symptoms can occur 5 minutes after massive ingestions. Another etiology should be considered if symptoms appear more than 12 hours postexposure, and the diagnosis of acute organophosphate poisoning is equivocal if symptoms begin after more than 24 hours. The exceptions are highly lipid-soluble compounds, which can cause mild initial symptoms followed by cholinergic crisis in 40 to 48 hours.

The duration of illness depends on the severity of poisoning, because several months may be required for cholinesterase activity to return to normal levels. Symptoms of mild to moderate organophosphate poisoning usually resolve within a month. Episodes of headache, visual disturbances, nausea, and vomiting may persist 10 weeks after an acute exposure.

NEUROLOGIC EFFECTS

Numerous central nervous system symptoms have been associated with organophosphate poisoning. These include giddiness, tension, anxiety, restlessness, emotional lability, excessive dreaming, insomnia, nightmares, headache, tremor, apathy, depression, drowsiness, difficulty in concentrating, confusion, slurred speech, ataxia, weakness, coma with absence of reflexes, Cheyne-Stokes respirations, convulsions, and depression of respiratory and circulatory centers with dyspnea, cyanosis, and hypotension.

MUSCARINIC EFFECTS

Muscarinic effects result from potentiation of post-ganglionic parasympathetic activity on smooth muscle. Physiological effects include intestinal, bronchial, and bladder smooth-muscle contraction, pupillary constriction and decreased reactivity, secretory gland stimulation, slowing of the sinus node and atrioventricular conduction, and ventricular dysrhythmias.

NICOTINIC EFFECTS

Nicotinic effects result from accumulation of acetylcholine at the motor end plate and autonomic ganglia, leading to persistent depolarization of skeletal muscles.

CHOLINERGIC EFFECTS

The mnemonic DUMBELS describes signs of cholinergic excess: **D**iarrhea, **U**rination, **M**iosis, **B**ronchospasm, **E**mesis, **L**acrimation, and **S**alivation.

ODOR

A garliclike odor emanating from the patient or involved container may aid in the diagnosis. The organic solvent in which the organophosphate is dissolved may mask the odor.

DERMATOLOGIC EFFECTS

Organophosphate compounds can produce dermal irritation, but most are weak sensitizers. Malathion in a 10% concentration induces contact sensitization in almost one-half of those exposed.

PULMONARY EFFECTS

Bronchorrhea may be a predominant and life-threatening sign of cholinergic excess. Organophosphates may cause noncardiogenic pulmonary edema or adult respiratory distress syndrome (ARDS). The differential diagnosis of toxin-induced ARDS includes phosgene, nitrogen dioxide, narcotics, phenothiazines, salicylates, and paraquat exposure.

RENAL EFFECTS

Immune complex nephropathy with renal dysfunction and massive proteinuria may occur several weeks after malathion exposure.

PANCREATIC EFFECTS

Pancreatitis after ingestion of organophosphates may terminate fatally. Pancreatic enzyme estimation in serum or urine, as well as imaging procedures such as ultrasound or computed tomography, should be performed in cases of parathion ingestions.

MUSCULOSKELETAL EFFECTS

Organophosphate compounds produce muscle weakness by cholinergic excess initially. Fasciculations progress to paralysis resulting from depolarization and desensitization blocks at the neuromuscular junction. See Intermediate Syndrome section.

CARDIOVASCULAR EFFECTS

Depending on the agent, absorption, and amount employed, patients may have elevated blood pressure and tachycardia (e.g., nicotinic) rather than bradycardia or hypotension (e.g., muscarinic effects). Torsade de pointes and atrial dysrhythmias (e.g., atrial fibrillation) have been associated with organophosphate poisoning. QT prolongation, ST-T wave abnormalities, and premature ventricular contractions occur commonly in seriously poisoned patients. Fatal dysrhythmias may develop 24 to 48 hours after ingestion.

INTERMEDIATE SYNDROME

An intermediate paralytic syndrome has been described that follows exposure to certain organophosphate insecticides. The syndrome begins 24 to 96 hours after poisoning. Patients develop muscle weakness primarily involving the proximal limb muscles, cranial nerves, and muscles of respiration. Cholinergic symptoms resolve before the onset of muscle weakness. Patients may die from respiratory depression. Unfortunately, none of the symptoms respond to conventional antidotes such as atropine or pralidoxime. Symptoms typically resolve within 4 to 18 days. The intermediate syndrome probably is a result of long-lasting cholinesterase inhibition. Finally, muscle weakness may be a result of demyelination of nerves. This begins 2 to 3 weeks after intoxication and spares the muscle of respiration. Recovery may not be complete.

DELAYED NEUROTOXICITY

Wallerian degeneration or "dying-back" of axons may occur, rather than demyelination. The process begins as a focal lesion, primarily in large myelinated fibers, and leads to axon death distal to the lesion. Polyneuropathy has been described in those exposed to organophosphates. Suggested diagnostic criteria for an organophosphate delayed syndrome include a history of severe acute organophosphate poisoning about 1 to 6 weeks prior to the onset, symptoms and signs of polyneuropathy, denervation changes shown by electromyography, slow recovery, and reasonable exclusion of other nervous disease. The cerebrospinal fluid is usually normal with the exception of a slight rise in protein.

PSYCHIATRIC EFFECTS

Persistent neurobehavioral symptoms may develop. Persistent neurological and behavioral abnormalities attributed to organophosphate exposure include drowsiness, mental confusion, anxiety, emotional lability, depression, fatigue, and irritability. Most of the persistent symptoms that develop after acute organophosphate exposure resolve within 1 year.

Toxic Dosage/Death

Full recovery from most organophosphate exposures generally occurs within 10 days when optimum treatment has been quickly instituted. Fatality usually occurs in untreated, severely intoxicated patients within 24 hours.

Drug Interactions

Patients who develop low plasma cholinesterase activity after organophosphates exposure may develop apnea after administration of succinylcholine. Phenothiazines and antihistamines have anticholinesterase activity and may potentiate organophosphate toxicity. Central nervous system depressants, such as opiates, may increase the likelihood of respiratory arrest.

Pregnancy/Lactation

Patients who ingest organophosphorous insecticides during the second or third trimesters of pregnancy have been treated successfully with atropine and pralidoxime and later delivered healthy newborns with no significant abnormalities. During early pregnancy, plasma cholinesterase levels fall but they return to normal levels by the third trimester.

Laboratory

ANALYTIC METHODS

Gas chromatographic techniques are available to identify organic phosphate metabolites of malathion, diazinon, and parathion in both blood and urine. Urine screens are qualitative tests that indicate exposure but do not correlate with symptoms or cholinesterase activity.

BLOOD LEVELS

While blood levels are available, proof of significant exposure relies more on the inhibition of cholinesterases.

RED BLOOD CELL CHOLINESTERASE

Inhibition of acetylcholinesterase is a confirmatory test for organophosphate poisoning but is not diagnostic when used alone. The RBC cholinesterase level is the preferred index of toxic exposure, because it measures the same enzyme active in nervous tissue and is less labile than the plasma cholinesterase level. RBC cholinesterase regenerates slowly (0.5% to 1% per day) and, in severe poisoning, may be depressed up to 3 months after acute exposure. In mild-to-moderate toxicity, these levels typically return to baseline values within several weeks. Preexposure baseline levels should be established for any worker frequently exposed to organophosphates.

PLASMA (PSEUDO) CHOLINESTERASE

The liver produces most of the plasma (pseudo) cholinesterase, but this enzyme also is found in nervous tissue, pancreas, heart, and white matter. Greater daily variations in plasma cholinesterase occur compared with RBC cholinesterase. Plasma cholinesterase levels both decline and regenerate more quickly than RBC cholinesterase levels, with an initial rapid increase followed by slower recovery. Typically, plasma cholinesterase levels are depressed for a maximum of 1 to 3 weeks after organophosphate poisoning. The rate of decline may be more important in mild-to-moderate poisoning than the amount of depression. Acute symptoms develop after a 50% decrease in baseline cholinesterase levels.

Because of the wide range of normal values for RBC and plasma cholinesterase, these levels may be normal in symptomatic patients exposed to organophosphates. Both plasma and RBC cholinesterase levels should be drawn in all patients with suspected organophosphate toxicity. A 15% to 20% or greater increase in the plasma cholinesterase level drawn 3 to 5 days later indicates a high likelihood of organophosphate poisoning. In equivocal cases, a baseline RBC cholinesterase level should be established by serial measurements and compared with immediate postexposure values. RBC cholinesterase levels rather than plasma levels are recommended as an endpoint, because the RBC levels more closely reflect physiological effects in the nervous tissue. Generally, acute exposures are classified as mild (20% to 50% of baseline), moderate (10% to 20% of baseline), and severe (10% or less of baseline).

Treatment

GUT DECONTAMINATION

Most organophosphate insecticides contain hydrocarbon solvents, which are severe aspiration hazards. The usual measures of gastric decontamination such as activated charcoal and cathartics may be used when the patient presents within 4 hours after exposure, however extreme caution must be exercised to avoid aspiration.

ELIMINATION ENHANCEMENT

Because effective antidotes are available, methods to enhance removal are seldom necessary. Charcoal hemoperfusion may be helpful in malathion poisoning, however its effectiveness is limited by a short duration of effective removal afforded by the hemoperfusion column, and by the wide distribution of malathion in the body. Over a prolonged time in severe, acute malathion poisoning, the column must be changed as it becomes saturated.

SUPPORTIVE MEASURES

- Immediate life-threatening symptoms usually are respiratory problems resulting from weakness of respiratory muscles, central depression of respiration, bronchospasm, bronchial secretions, and pulmonary edema, which all result in hypoxemia. Frequent suctioning, endotracheal intubation, and / or assisted ventilation may be necessary to maintain adequate oxygenation. Monitor PaO_2 carefully with arterial blood gases in an intensive care setting.
- Although cardiovascular function generally is maintained, the use of atropine and the presence of hypoxemia require continuous cardiac monitoring and an intravenous (IV) line for at least 48 hours in serious poisonings. Patients with QT prolongation should be monitored until the QT interval returns to normal.
- Because organophosphates may be absorbed through intact skin, be sure to remove all contaminated clothing. Wash contaminated skin with water and then mild soap. Tincture of green soap, which contains alcohol, is an effective means of removing fat-soluble compounds. The entire area, including the nails, intertriginous areas, and groin area, should be rewashed with soap and water.
- Diazepam is the drug of choice for convulsions. Avoid parasympathomimetic agents such as physostigmine or succinylcholine, as these may potentiate anticholinesterase activity.
- Persistent central nervous system effects such as irritability, nervousness, fatigue, lethargy, impaired memory, depression, psychosis, and peripheral neuropathies have been reported. Serial examinations and exclusion of other possible etiologies must be entertained.
- The patient must avoid reexposure until cholinesterase activity is over 75% of normal.
- Reported laboratory abnormalities include leukocytosis with a left shift, reduced eosinophil, lymphocyte, and monocyte counts, hyperglycemia, glycosuria, albuminuria, acetonuria, ketoacidosis, and hyperamylasemia. No prolonged effect on liver function, coagulation, skin, or respiratory tract has been documented.

Antidotes

ATROPINE

Atropine antagonizes both muscarinic and central nervous system effects of organophosphate poisoning by alleviating excessive bronchial secretions, salivation, sweating, anorexia, nausea, chest tightness, abdominal cramps, vomiting, and bradycardia. Atropine has no effect on muscle weakness or respiratory failure seen in severe poisoning, because this drug does not reactivate cholinesterase enzymes. For symptomatic patients, 2 to 4 mg is used intravenously in adults or 0.015 to 0.05 mg / kg in children every 15 minutes as needed.

Atropinization may be needed for up to 48 hours in cases of moderate toxicity. Atropine is metabolized rapidly, and large doses often are needed within the first 24 hours. Seriously poisoned patients develop marked resistance to the usual doses of atropine and may even require grams of antidote for many days. The drying of secretions, rather than dilated pupils, is the effective endpoint of atropine titration.

Do not wait for the return of cholinesterase levels before treating significantly symptomatic patients with atropine. Alternate routes for atropine administration (when rapid IV access cannot be achieved) include the intraosseous route in children and nebulized atropine by inhalation in adults. During antidote administration, the patient should be followed closely for signs of respiratory failure and atropinization in an intensive care setting. The patient should be observed at least 48 hours after the last dose of atropine.

PRALIDOXIME

Pralidoxime (2-PAM) is a specific antidote that effectively reverses phosphorylation of the cholinesterase when given within 24 hours and perhaps up to 36 to 48 hours postexposure. 2-PAM ameliorates muscle weakness, fasciculations, and alterations of consciousness (e.g., coma in parathion poisoning). It does not relieve bronchospasm or bronchorrhea and must be given concurrently with atropine. The indication for 2-PAM use in organophosphate poisonings is respiratory depression or muscle weakness.

The dosage is 1 to 2 g in adults or 25 to 50 mg / kg in children, given over 3 to 5 minutes. Rapid injection may cause tachycardia, laryngeal spasm, muscle rigidity, or transient neuromuscular blockade. If symptoms recur, a constant 2.5% pralidoxime IV infusion may be started in adults at 500 mg/hour, or repeat bolus doses (0.5 to 1 g or 10 to 25 mg/kg every 8 hours) may be given. It may take days until residual insecticide is cleared from body stores. Adverse reactions to 2-PAM may mimic both atropine and organophosphate poisoning. The kidney rapidly excretes 2-PAM in the urine and toxic levels of 2-PAM may accumulate in the presence of renal dysfunction.

Questions—Organophosphates

1. **Which of the following concerning organophosphates is false?**
   A. Organophosphates have relatively high acute toxicity but low chronic toxicity.
   B. Farmhands can acquire a chronic low-level exposure known as orange-picker's flu characterized by nausea, weakness, and headache.
   C. Epidemics of severe extremity motor weakness and mild sensory impairment have resulted from tri-o-cresyl phosphate (TOCP) contamination.
   D. Mass intoxication has occurred when TOCP was employed as an adulterant of Jamaica Ginger ("Jake"), a popular alcohol-containing drink of the Prohibition Era.
   E. Acute organophosphate poisoning has not been reported in the United States for years.
2. **Organophosphates may be absorbed through intact skin.**
   A. True
   B. False
3. **Which of the following concerning organophosphates is true?**
   A. Organophosphates are detoxified by cytochrome P450-mediated monooxygenases in the liver, but some metabolites are more toxic than parent compounds.
   B. Miosis is present in all patients exposed.
   C. A garliclike odor emanating from the patient or involved container may aid in the diagnosis.
   D. All of the above
   E. A and C
4. **An intermediate paralytic syndrome has been described that follows exposure to certain organophosphate insecticides. The syndrome begins 24 to 96 hours after poisoning. Patients develop muscle weakness primarily involving the distal limb extensors and urinary control.**
   A. True
   B. False
5. **Which of the following are true?**
   A. Atropine antagonizes both muscarinic and central nervous system effects of organophosphate poisoning.
   B. Atropine has no effect on muscle weakness or respiratory failure seen in severe poisoning.
   C. After 3 mg of atropine is used, its effect in organophosphate poisoning is minimal.
   D. All of the above
   E. A and B
6. **Pralidoxime**
   A. Effectively reverses phosphorylation of cholinesterase
   B. Relieves bronchospasm and bronchorrhea
   C. Is used if respiratory depression or muscle weakness accompany organophosphate use
   D. All of the above
   E. A and C
7. **Wallerian degeneration involves demyelination of nerve fibers.**
   A. True
   B. False
8. **Inhibition of acetylcholinesterase is diagnostic of organophosphate poisoning.**
   A. True
   B. False

CARBAMATES

Carbamate pesticides, like organophosphates, cause a decrease in cholinesterase activity. These poisonings are less severe than organophosphates however, because they bind reversibly to the active site on the cholinesterase enzyme, in contrast to the organophosphate pesticides which, over time, bind irreversibly. Carbamates cause the same excess in muscarinic stimulation and nicotinic stimulation, followed by weakness, as seen in organophosphate poisonings, but for a relatively shorter duration. Examples include methomyl, carbaryl, and aldicarb. Methomyl is a broad-spectrum carbamate insecticide used on various vegetable crops (e.g., cabbage and broccoli).

Hexapropymate is a carbamate sedative-hypnotic drug that, in overdose, resembles meprobamate or barbiturate intoxication and may lead to fatalities. Hypothermia, severe respiratory depression, and prolonged coma may require a long period of assisted ventilation.

Pathophysiology

Carbamylation of acetylcholinesterase produces accumulation of acetylcholine and the picture of muscarinic and nicotinic poisoning. Spontaneous hydrolysis of the carbamate-cholinesterase complex occurs *in vivo*, leading to disappearance of clinical effects within 24 hours.

Pharmacokinetics

ABSORPTION

- Carbamates are absorbed readily through the lungs, gastrointestinal tract, and skin.
- Absorption by the respiratory tract depends on the vapor pressure of individual insecticides. Carbaryl and aldicarb display low inhalation toxicity because of their high vapor pressures.

DISTRIBUTION

- Carbamates poorly penetrate the blood-brain barrier, producing minimal effects on brain cholinesterase activity and few central nervous system symptoms.
- The volume of distribution of carbaryl is 32.9 L/kg.

ELIMINATION

- Most of these insecticides undergo hydroxylation, hydrolysis, and conjugation by the liver and are then excreted in the urine within several days.
- Following first-order kinetics, the half-life of carbaryl is 1.30 hours and the half-life of α-naphthol is 1.13 hours.

Answers to questions in shaded boxes appear at the end of the chapter.

Clinical Presentations

Clinical symptoms after exposure to methomyl and other carbamates are similar to those produced by organophosphates, although of lesser intensity and duration. Symptoms usually develop within 15 minutes to 2 hours and last several hours unless continued absorption occurs from clothing. Typical manifestations of cholinesterase inhibition include nausea, miosis, headache, lacrimation, salivation, vomiting, and abdominal pain. Dyspnea, tremors, muscle twitching, ataxia, and headache also may appear. Symptoms beyond 24 hours probably do not result from carbamate intoxication. The electrocardiogram (ECG) after methomyl exposure may exhibit sinus tachycardia or T-wave changes. Such changes may revert to preexposure status within 1 week.

Toxic Dosage/Death

Fatalities have followed ingestions of methomyl. Patients ingesting large doses, from 2 to 16 g of methomyl have developed symptoms of cholinesterase inhibition and survived. However, a lethal dose may be as low as 12 to 15 mg/kg.

Laboratory

ANALYTIC METHODS

High-pressure liquid chromatography, gas chromatography, and gas chromatography/mass spectrometry methods are available.

BLOOD LEVELS

Measuring RBC and plasma cholinesterase are often not helpful as carbamates have only a transient effect (1 to 2 hours) on these levels.

Treatment

GUT DECONTAMINATION

Methods for elimination are not recommended in view of the short action of the carbamates and the effectiveness of atropine. Container identification is important to determine appropriate therapeutic measures, as the vehicle (e.g., hydrocarbon) may be as toxic as the insecticide.

ELIMINATION ENHANCEMENT

Again, no methods are recommended, because of the short clinical effect of carbamates and the presence of an effective antidote (i.e., atropine).

SUPPORTIVE MEASURES

- Immediate life-threatening symptoms usually result from weakness of the respiratory muscles, central respiratory depression, bronchospasm, bronchial secretions, and pulmonary edema, all of which may result in hypoxemia. Frequent suctioning, endotracheal intubation, and ventilatory assistance may be required.
- Patients should be admitted to an intensive care facility where access to a central line, oxygen, and cardiac monitoring is available. Administer fluids to replace losses.
- Be sure to remove contaminated clothing and wash the contaminated skin, as in organophosphate treatment. Exposure after spraying will require careful washing of the entire (e.g., nails, intertriginous areas) body with tincture of green soap. Health personnel should use rubber gloves and avoid direct contact with contaminated material.
- Avoid central nervous system depressants (e.g., opiates); they may increase the possibility of respiratory arrest. Monitor the PaO_2 with repeat arterial blood gases.
- There may be a decrease in plasma cholinesterase concentrations but no decrease in RBC cholinesterase levels. Cholinesterase determination should be done within 4 hours of exposure. Such determinations generally are not important as carbamates only have a transient effect on cholinesterase levels.
- Lactate dehydrogenase (LDH) levels may be elevated after methomyl exposure. Leukocytosis may occur.

Antidotes

ATROPINE

Atropine is the antidote of choice in carbamate poisoning. Although the total amount of required atropine usually is less than in organophosphate exposures, the same initial doses are recommended. Patients generally require approximately 6 to 12 hours of atropine treatment, but all significantly poisoned patients should be observed at least 24 hours after the last atropine dose. Atropine (0.6 mg IV in adults and 0.05 mg/kg in children) may be useful without reaching complete atropinization (e.g., dilated pupils, dry or red skin, confusion, tachycardia, fever ileus). It can be administered every 15 minutes as needed. Significant poisoning may require at least 24 hours of observation after the last atropine dose.

PRALIDOXIME

The use of 2-PAM is indicated as an adjunct to atropine in serious, potentially fatal poisonings with unknown cholinesterase inhibitors. 2-PAM is indicated in poisoning involving both organophosphates and carbamate compounds together, and if a patient with known carbamate poisoning does not respond to atropinization. 2-PAM may reduce the effectiveness of atropine (especially when used to treat carbaryl poisoning).

Questions—Carbamates

1. Which of the following concerning carbamates is false?

A. Carbamates only yield muscarinic poisoning, in contrast to organophosphates, which produce muscarinic and nicotinic poisoning.
B. Carbamates are absorbed readily through the lungs, gastrointestinal tract, and skin.
C. Clinical symptoms after exposure to methomyl and other carbamates are similar to those produced by organophosphates, although of lesser intensity and duration.
D. Fatalities have resulted from carbamate exposures.
E. Methods for elimination are not recommended in view of the short action of the carbamates and the effectiveness of atropine.

2. Carbamate pesticides are less severe than organophosphates because they bind reversibly to the active site on the cholinesterase enzyme, in contrast to the organophosphate pesticides which, over time, bind irreversibly.

A. True
B. False

3. Which of the following concerning carbamates is true?
A. Atropine is the antidote of choice in carbamate poisoning.
B. The total amount of required atropine usually is less than in organophosphate exposures.
C. The use of pralidoxime is not indicated as an adjunct to atropine in carbamate poisoning.
D. A and C
E. A and B

4. An intermediate paralytic syndrome has been described that follows exposure to certain carbamate as well as organophosphate insecticides.
A. True
B. False

ORGANOCHLORINES

Most organochlorine pesticide compounds have been replaced by organophosphates. The US Environmental Protection Agency (EPA) banned many organochlorine compounds (e.g., DDT, and endrin) because these products are stored indefinitely in human tissue. DDT is dichlorodiphenoxyltricholoroethane. Lindane is the most common organochlorine currently available as a garden spray and as a scabicide (Kwell®). Human exposures occur through the ingestion of contaminated foodstuffs or water, inhalation of vapor, or absorption through skin. Outbreaks of poisoning from contaminated food sources characteristically involve headaches, vomiting, restlessness, irritability, vertigo, twitching, confusion, stupor, coma, and convulsions.

Pathophysiology

Lindane is directly absorbed by parasites and subsequently causes their demise by overstimulating their nervous system. These drugs also interfere with synaptic GABA receptors.

Pharmacokinetics

ABSORPTION

- Organochlorines are well absorbed from the lungs, gastrointestinal tract, and skin.
- Topically, approximately 10% of an applied dose of lindane is absorbed, but lipid solvents increase dermal penetration.

DISTRIBUTION

- Although serious toxicity occurs after ingestion of lindane, less than 0.1% of an ingested dose of lindane pellets appeared in the blood in one study.
- Lindane accumulates in organs to a lesser extent than other organochlorines.

ELIMINATION

- Most organochlorines are metabolized slowly and are excreted primarily in the feces.
- Excretion occurs in a few days (lindane, methoxychlor, chlordane, and toxaphene), weeks to months (dieldrin, aldrin, endrin, and heptachlor), or months to years (DDT, chlordecone, mirex, and the β isomer of hexachlorocyclohexane).
- Hepatic enzyme induction can result from exposure to certain organochlorine insecticides.

Clinical Presentations

Intoxication from acute oral exposures generally begins within 45 minutes to several hours. Subacute toxicity has been reported after the extensive and careless use of chlordane over several weeks. Symptoms included paresthesias, anorexia, nausea, fatigue, and malaise. Organochlorines may enhance myocardial irritability, leading to cardiac dysrhythmias after heavy exposures. Endosulfan may cause vomiting within an hour, in addition to hypotension, seizures, fever, metabolic acidosis, and elevation in liver function enzymes.

NEUROLOGIC EFFECTS

Organochlorines are central nervous system stimulators that produce apprehension, excitability, paresthesias, dizziness, headache, disorientation, and tremor progressing to stupor, coma, and convulsions in severe cases. Serious complications involve seizures with resultant hypoxemia, severe metabolic acidosis, and death

PULMONARY EFFECTS

The solvent vehicle of organochlorine insecticides is capable of producing a hydrocarbon pneumonitis after aspiration. Pulmonary edema has been reported after intentional lindane ingestion, but the exact role of aspiration in producing these changes is not clear.

HEMATOLOGIC EFFECTS

Several anecdotal reports have implicated lindane as a cause of aplastic anemia, agranulocytosis, and bone marrow hypoplasia. No cases of blood abnormalities have been reported after the therapeutic use of lindane (Kwell®) despite documented dermal absorption.

MISCELLANEOUS EFFECTS

Persistent symptoms may include headache, chest pain, fatigue, irritability, difficulty concentrating, and decreased libido. The International Agency for Research on Cancer lists DDT as "probably carcinogenic to humans," although data are not sufficient for adequate assessment. Myoglobinuria, acute renal failure, and a proximal myopathy have been reported after lindane ingestion. Almost 50% of dichlorobromopropane (DCBP) workers have low sperm counts, compared with only 10% of nonexposed workers.

Toxic Dosage/Death

The oral lethal adult dose of aldrin ranges from approximately 3 to 7 g. Ingestion of 6 g of chlordane by adults has resulted in death and less than 2 g has produced stupor and seizures. The acute adult lethal dose of Dieldrin is approximately 1.5 to 5 g. Endrin, a stereoisomer of dieldrin, has a similar toxicity, producing death after a 6-g ingestion.

The fatal dose of lindane in adults is approximately 10 to 30 g. Doses of 1.6 and 45 g are capable of producing seizures in young children and adults, respectively. A single application of lindane to adults may lead to seizures. Ingestion of as little as 250 mg of lindane may lead to seizures within 30 minutes.

Pregnancy/Lactation

Organochlorine insecticides (e.g., DDT) appear in breast milk. Breast milk may be considered a main route for the elimination of heptachlor (now outlawed) from the mother's body. Lindane crosses the placenta. Intrauterine death has been attributed to lindane. Lindane levels in human blood and placental and fetal tissues are higher in cases of spontaneous abortion and prematurity than in normal-term pregnancies. Lindane is categorized as pregnancy risk category B.

Laboratory

ANALYTIC METHODS

Electron-capture gas chromatographic procedures can detect organochlorine insecticides, but these levels are not useful for clinical management. Gas-liquid chromatography of blood or urine within 72 hours is required to detect high levels of lindane.

BLOOD LEVELS

The presence of organochlorines in blood or tissue is not necessarily an indication of poisoning, because most US citizens have residual organochlorine residues, especially in fat depots.

Treatment

GUT DECONTAMINATION

Syrup of ipecac and lavage are not recommended as a high potential for seizure activity and aspiration exists. Furthermore, most organochlorine insecticides contain organic solvents, which are severe aspiration hazards. As certain organochlorines may have substantial enterohepatic recirculation, activated charcoal may reduce the half-life in certain cases and should be considered in serial doses for significant poisonings.

ELIMINATION ENHANCEMENT

The use of cholestyramine, 3 to 8 g four times a day, has increased fecal excretion and reduced the mean half-life of chlordecone. Dialysis, diuresis, and hemoperfusion are ineffective because of extensive tissue binding and large volumes of distribution.

SUPPORTIVE MEASURES

- Seizures are treated with diazepam. Seizures, hypoxemia, and resultant acidosis are immediate life-threatening emergencies. Moderately to severely poisoned patients should have intravenous lines and a cardiac monitor.
- Skin decontamination (removal of contaminated clothes, washing of area with water and green or mild soap) is necessary to prevent continued dermal absorption. Be careful not to cross-contaminate health personnel.

Antidotes

Cholestyramine resin has been touted anecdotally as being helpful in lindane ingestions.

Questions—Organochlorines

1. **Which of the following concerning organochlorines is false?**
   A. Organochlorines are central nervous system stimulators that may produce seizures.
   B. Organochlorines may enhance myocardial irritability, leading to cardiac dysrhythmias after heavy exposures.
   C. Numerous blood abnormalities have been reported after dermal absorption of lindane.
   D. The solvent vehicle of organochlorine insecticides is capable of producing a hydrocarbon pneumonitis after aspiration.
   E. Several anecdotal reports have implicated lindane as a cause of aplastic anemia, agranulocytosis, and bone marrow hypoplasia.
2. **Almost 50% of dichlorobromopropane (DCBP) workers have low sperm counts.**
   A. True
   B. False
3. **Which of the following concerning DDT is true?**
   A. DDT has been banned in the United States.
   B. DDT takes months to be eliminated.
   C. It has been classified as "probably carcinogenic to humans."
   D. All of the above
   E. B and C
4. **Most organochlorine pesticide compounds have been replaced by organophosphates.**
   A. True
   B. False
5. **Atropine is an effective antidote against organochlorine exposures.**
   A. True
   B. False

DIETHYLTOLUAMIDE

Diethyltoluamide (DEET) is a commonly used insecticide available in numerous preparations to repel mosquitos and other insects. The American military finds 75% DEET useful to protect its forces in jungles infested with disease-carrying mosquitos. Yet preparations containing 100% DEET are available in the United States, some of which may be used in children.

The optimal concentration of DEET for prevention of tick bites is unknown. Repeated cutaneous application of varying concentrations of DEET in children can lead to behavioral abnormalities, ataxia, encephalopathy, seizures, coma, and even death. Ingestion of DEET has resulted in hypotension, seizures, coma, and death, as well.

Pathophysiology

DEET is highly lipophilic. Adverse effects are secondary to hypersensitivity reactions, direct central nervous system toxicity, and interference with ammonia metabolism.

Pharmacokinetics

ABSORPTION

- Oral and dermal routes absorb DEET. 9% to 56% of a topical dose is absorbed within 6 hours.
- Peak plasma concentration for GI and dermal absorption sites usually is reached within 1 hour.

DISTRIBUTION

- The volume of distribution of DEET is 2.1 L/kg.
- DEET and its metabolites can be detected in the urine for 2 weeks and from the skin and adipose tissues for 1 to 3 months after dermal application.

ELIMINATION

- About 10% to 15% of each dose can be recovered unchanged from the urine.
- Plasma half-life is 2.5 hours. The urinary half-life of DEET is 4 hours.
- DEET is eliminated by hepatic oxidative metabolism through the P450 enzyme system. It exhibits some enterohepatic recirculation.

Clinical Presentations

Ingestion of DEET may cause coma, seizures, and hypotension within 1 hour of ingestion. Seizures may begin 8 to 48 hours after last using DEET. Toxic psychosis has been described after daily application of a 70% solution of DEET. Immediate-contact urticaria and a general pruritus that led to a generalized angioedema have been described. A Reyelike syndrome and increased ammonia have been described in a child with carbomoyl transferase deficiency.

Toxic Dosage/Death

Frequent applications of DEET in infants have caused encephalopathy and death. A 14-year-old who ingested 50 cc of 95% DEET became hypotensive and seized. The same ingestion caused death in a 26-year-old. A DEET level of 24 mg/dL was reported after one fatal case.

Laboratory

ANALYTIC METHODS

A procedure for monitoring DEET in urine and serum by high-performance liquid chromatography has been described.

BLOOD LEVELS

Blood levels do not guide management in overdose.

Treatment

GUT DECONTAMINATION

Syrup of ipecac is contraindicated. Decontaminate with gastric lavage after ingestion if gag reflex is intact and airway is protected. Repetitive doses of activated charcoal may be useful because of possible enterohepatic recirculation. Do not use emetics because of the rapid onset of seizures.

ELIMINATION ENHANCEMENT

Dialysis rarely has been used to enhance the elimination of DEET.

SUPPORTIVE MEASURES

- Seizures are treated with diazepam and phenytoin.
- For dermal exposure, remove clothing and wash skin thoroughly with tepid water and soap.
- Apply repellent sparingly only to exposed skin or clothing. Avoid applying high-concentration products to eyes. Avoid applying repellents to portions of children's hands that are likely to have contact with eyes or mouth.
- Wear long sleeves and long pants, when possible, and apply repellent to clothing to reduce exposure to DEET. Wash repellent-treated skin after coming indoors.
- Never use repellents on wounds or irritated skin. Use repellent sparingly as one application generally will last 4 to 8 hours. Saturation does not increase efficacy.

Questions—Diethyltoluamide

1. Which of the following concerning DEET is false?

A. DEET is highly lipophilic.
B. The optimal concentration of DEET for prevention of tick bites is unknown.
C. The American military has not found DEET effective against disease-carrying mosquitos.
D. Frequent applications of DEET in infants have caused encephalopathy.
E. Repeated cutaneous application of varying concentrations of DEET in children can lead to behavioral abnormalities, ataxia, seizures, coma, and even death.

PYRETHRUM AND PYRETHROIDS

Pyrethrum is a natural derivative of the chrysanthemum plant. Because synthetic derivatives are effective "knock-down" agents for flying insects, the pyrethrins are common components of household insecticide sprays. Cost, high biodegradability, and low photostability limit the use of pyrethrins to synergistic action in combination pesticides. The production of synthetic pyrethroids began in 1950 in order to alleviate the disadvantages of the natural pyrethrins. Examples of these products include allethrin, bioresmethrin, permethrin, decamethrin, and fenvalerate.

Pathophysiology

The synthetic pyrethroids delay closure of the sodium channel. Apparently, the pyrethroid molecule holds the activation gate in the open position yielding insect death.

Pharmacokinetics

ABSORPTION

- These agents are absorbed rapidly after oral ingestion, but poorly absorbed through the skin.
- There is a large first-pass effect in the liver.

DISTRIBUTION

- Pyrethrins are distributed widely through tissues, including brain.

ELIMINATION

- Elimination is primarily hepatic. These products are slowly eliminated in bile and urine.

Clinical Presentations

Mammalian toxicity to pyrethrums is extremely low, in part because of poor bioavailability and a large first-pass extraction by the liver. The clinical manifestations of inhalation exposure include rhinitis, sneezing, scratchy throat, oral and laryngeal mucosal edema. Lower respiratory tract signs may include cough, shortness of breath, wheezing, and chest pain.

An asthmalike reaction may occur with acute exposures in sensitized patients. Hypersensitivity pneumonitis has been reported. About 50% of persons sensitive to ragweed exhibit cross-sensitivity to pyrethrum. Synthetic pyrethroids, in contrast, are neither cutaneous sensitizers nor irritants. Although these compounds do not cause signs of inflammation such as edema, erythema, or vesiculation, they may produce paresthesias after contact.

Toxic Dosage/Death

The estimated lethal dose of pyrethrum in humans is over 1 g/kg. Death has been reported after ingestion of a pyrethrin shampoo.

Pregnancy/Lactation

Pregnancy risk category C. As skin absorption is poor, these agents are preferred over lindane during pregnancy for the treatment of lice.

Treatment

GUT DECONTAMINATION

Emesis should not be induced when petroleum distillate additives are present unless the product ingested is estimated to contain a near lethal dose (1 g/kg) of pyrethrum or pyrethrins. The alert person with an intact gag reflex and sublethal pyrethrum ingestion may be given a slurry of activated charcoal. Oils and fats, including milk, promote the intestinal absorption of pyrethrums and should be avoided.

ELIMINATION ENHANCEMENT

Dialysis has not been utilized in the treatment of pyrethrin overdose.

SUPPORTIVE MEASURES

- Treatment is supportive, and most casual exposures require only decontamination. Additives such as petroleum distillates may represent a greater toxic threat to the patient than the active ingredient itself. Pulmonary and allergic sequelae are treated symptomatically with airway maintenance, oxygen, and ventilatory assistance as required.
- Standard drugs and management protocols may be used for treatment of bronchospasm and anaphylaxis. Rare instances of seizures are treated with diazepam.
- Topical vitamin E may ameliorate the paresthesias that accompany contact with certain synthetic pyrethroids.
- The ECG may indicate ST-T changes, sinus tachycardia, and ventricular premature beats.

Questions—Pyrethrum and Pyrethroids

1. Which of the following concerning pyrethrums is false?

A. Pyrethrins are common components of household insecticide sprays.
B. The synthetic pyrethroids delay closure of the calcium channel in insects.
C. Mammalian toxicity to pyrethrums is extremely low, in part because of poor bioavailability and a large first-pass extraction by the liver.
D. About 50% of persons sensitive to ragweed exhibit cross-sensitivity to pyrethrum.
E. Pyrethrum is a natural derivative of the chrysanthemum plant.

2. Pyrethrum toxicity is limited to the skin.

A. True
B. False

RODENTICIDES

INTRODUCTION

Rodenticides have long been present in our environment. As early as the 16th century, strychnine was used in Germany to combat the growing presence of rodents. Through the years, science has produced various strategies to eliminate these pests. Highly toxic agents have included metals such as arsenic, thallium, and yellow phosphorous (see Chapter 47, Metals).

Strychnine produced many deaths in the 1920s as rat pellets appeared with tempting sugar coatings and children inadvertently ate them. Sodium monoflouroacetate (Compound 1080®) interferes with the Krebs cycle in rodents. Others include the highly toxic vacor, long acting coumarin anticoagulants, and the cardiac glycoside, red squill.

SODIUM MONOFLUOROACETATE

Sodium Monofluoroacetate (Compound 1080®) is a rodenticide, which is metabolized to toxic fluorocitrate. Fluoroacetic acid is the major isolate of the poisonous South African gifblaar plant. Monofluoroacetic acid produces toxicity when livestock consume plants from the South American genus *Palicourea* and the Australian genera *Gastrolobium*, *Oxylobium*, and *Acacia*.

Pathophysiology

The parent compound is metabolized to fluorocitrate, which blocks the Krebs cycle in rodents.

Pharmacokinetics

ABSORPTION

- Sodium monofluoroacetate is absorbed from the gastrointestinal tract, lungs, and mucous membranes but probably not from intact skin.

DISTRIBUTION

- Sodium monofluoroacetate appears to have wide distribution to rodent tissues including brain.

ELIMINATION

- Sodium monoflouroacetate is metabolized to fluorocitrate.

Clinical Presentations

A latent period of 30 to 150 minutes precedes the onset of GI symptoms. Initially, nausea, vomiting, and abdominal pain may occur, followed by anxiety, agitation, muscle spasm, stupor, seizures, and coma. Sinus tachycardia and hypotension are common cardiovascular signs. The cardiac rhythm may deteriorate into ventricular tachycardia or fibrillation. Renal failure may occur within 3 to 4 days. Late cerebellar degeneration, cerebral atrophy, and polyneuropathy have been associated with suicidal ingestions.

Toxic Dosage/Death

Estimates of the mean lethal human dose range from 2 to 10 mg/kg with a mean of 5 mg/kg, similar to values for strychnine. Survival, despite renal failure, was reported after a 400-mg adult suicide attempt.

Laboratory

ANALYTIC METHODS

Normal human body fluids and tissues contain fluoride and citrate but no fluoroacetate. Both gas-liquid and high-performance liquid chromatographic techniques are available to detect fluoroacetate in biologic specimens.

BLOOD LEVELS

Following blood levels in overdose is not helpful.

Treatment

GUT DECONTAMINATION

Avoid syrup of ipecac as seizures may occur. Gastric lavage, possibly with magnesium sulfate, and charcoal use with a protected airway may be helpful (albeit unstudied) interventions.

ELIMINATION ENHANCEMENT

There have been no documented cases of hemodialysis being helpful in overdose.

SUPPORTIVE MEASURES

- The approach to sodium monofluoroacetate-poisoned patients primarily is supportive.
- Pay careful attention to respiratory status, pH, and cardiac rhythm in moderate to severe poisonings. Metabolic acidosis may occur.
- Hyperglycemia, hyperuricemia, elevated serum hepatic aminotransferases, and elevated creatinine levels have been observed. Hypocalcemia is treated with IV calcium gluconate.
- Seizures are treated with diazepam and procainamide may help treating arrhythmias.

Antidotes

Animal studies suggest that calcium gluconate in combination with sodium succinate may offer a promising therapy modality in sodium fluoroacetate intoxication. Clinical studies with these chemicals have not been performed.

Questions—Sodium Monofluoroacetate

1. **Sodium monofluoroacetate is a rodenticide, which is metabolized to toxic fluorocitrate, which blocks the Krebs cycle in rodents.**
   A. True
   B. False

STRYCHNINE

Strychnine poisoning, while common earlier this century, is now a relatively rare occurrence. It first was used medically in 1540 and was introduced in Germany in the sixteenth century as a rodenticide. It was used as recently as the 1960s in cathartics, stimulants, and tonics. Many tablets had brightly colored sugar or sweet chocolate coatings and were attractive to children.

Strychnine-containing medications are no longer found in American pharmacies, but strychnine still is found in some veterinary preparations, rodenticides, avicides, and occasionally in adulterated street drugs such as cocaine. Strychnine, a basic alkaloid, is an odorless, bitter-tasting crystalline material derived from the ripe seeds of the Strychnos plant, *S. nux vomica*, a tree native to India.

Pathophysiology

Strychnine prevents the uptake of glycine at inhibitory synapses, especially in the ventral horns of the spinal cord. This results in a net excitatory effect, with minimal sensory stimulation, and diffuse muscle contractions. A clinical picture of convulsive activity in an awake patient with no postictal phase has been associated with strychnine use.

Pharmacokinetics

ABSORPTION

- Strychnine is absorbed rapidly from the gastrointestinal tract or nasal mucosa.
- The half-life of absorption is about 15 minutes.

DISTRIBUTION

- There is little protein binding. The volume of distribution in one patient was 13 L/kg.

ELIMINATION

- Metabolism is by first-order kinetics primarily by enzymatic degradation involving the liver microsomal system. The half-life is about 10 hours.
- Less than 1% of the product is excreted unchanged in the urine.

Clinical Presentations

Onset of symptoms usually begins 15 to 30 minutes following ingestion and as soon as 5 minutes after inhalation. Initial symptoms include apprehension, a heightened sense of awareness, and muscle spasms. Generalized hyperreflexia and hypersensitivity to stimuli usually are present. This is followed by overwhelming convulsions, typically lasting 30 seconds to 2 minutes, often precipitated by minimal external stimuli. Opisthotonic posturing develops with the back arched, extremities hyperextended, and the jaw tightly clamped. Facial muscle spasm may be so violent as to produce a sardonic smile (*risus sardonicus*). Muscle relaxation occurs between convulsions.

The patient generally maintains a clear sensorium during and after the convulsions which is of major diagnostic importance. Most patients do not tolerate more than five convulsive episodes, and death commonly occurs within several hours of ingestion. Respiratory arrest secondary to spasm of the respiratory muscles is the usual fatal event. Prognosis for survival is good if the patient survives beyond 5 hours.

Complications from strychnine-induced muscle spasms include hypoxia, hyperthermia, cardiac arrest, rhabdomyolysis, and acute renal failure. Chest muscle and diaphragmatic spasm may result in hypoxia and hypercarbia. Excessive muscle activity, if not controlled, may result in hyperthermia and rhabdomyolysis. Acute renal failure has resulted from rhabdomyolysis. Severe metabolic acidosis may be present. The differential diagnosis includes tetanus, rabies, meningitis, hysteria, and ingestions of phenothiazines, cocaine, phenycyclidine (PCP), chlorinated hydrocarbons, isoniazid, or other substances that may cause myoclonus or seizures.

Toxic Dosage/Death

Fatal doses of strychnine are reported to be as low as 5 to 10 mg but more significantly, survival can follow ingestion of very high doses (over 3.5 g). Strychnine ingestion should be considered in all cases of seizures of obscure etiology, especially if the person is an agricultural worker or is known to have access to the poison.

Pregnancy/Lactation

Risk to the fetus correlates with oxygen status and metabolic abnormalities of the mother.

Laboratory

ANALYTIC METHODS

Strychnine may be detected in the gastric aspirate, urine, blood, and tissues through a variety of methods. Thin-layer chromatography (TLC) gives reliable qualitative information, while high-performance liquid chromatography (HPLC) provides quantitative data. For most purposes, it is adequate to confirm strychnine poisoning with a qualitative test such as TLC.

BLOOD LEVELS

Following blood levels is generally not helpful in overdose, as treatment is generally required long before these levels can be obtained. Blood levels are not reliable.

Treatment

GUT DECONTAMINATION

Syrup of ipecac is absolutely contraindicated as the onset of convulsions may be rapid and vomiting may elicit muscle spasms or at least complicate their management. Gastric lavage should always follow protection of the airway because pharyngeal stimulation may result in uncontrolled convulsions. Activated charcoal may be administered with a protected airway as well.

ELIMINATION ENHANCEMENT

IV fluid sufficient to maintain a brisk urine output is indicated pending assessment of myoglobinuria. Measures to enhance elimination, such as forced diuresis and peritoneal dialysis, have not been studied adequately enough to be recommended.

SUPPORTIVE MEASURES

- Treatment is directed at preventing absorption, reversing hypoxia and acidosis, minimizing muscle spasm, and maintaining an adequate urine output. Early aggressive airway management is the priority.
- Serial physical examinations and appropriate surgical consultation should be done to assess for compartment syndromes.
- Aggressive control of seizures is the key to successful management. Diazepam is considered the first-line drug for this purpose and large total doses may be required (e.g., more than 1 mg/kg). Lorazepam and barbiturates also may be effective.
- If control of convulsions is unsuccessful following IV benzodiazepines and barbiturates, neuromuscular blockade with an agent such as pancuronium (0.04 to 0.1 mg/kg) may be necessary.
- Follow creatine phosphokinase as it relates to muscular breakdown, potassium, bicarbonate, arterial blood gases, and renal function. ECG may reflect hyperkalemia or acidosis.

Questions—Strychnine

1. Which of the following concerning strychnine is false?
A. Strychnine, a very effective poison, is still used frequently in deadly suicide attempts.
B. Strychnine prevents the uptake of glycine at inhibitory synapses, especially in the ventral horns of the spinal cord.
C. Spasms and seizures are classic signs of strychnine poisoning.
D. The patient generally maintains a clear sensorium during and after the convulsions of strychnine poisoning which is of major diagnostic importance.
E. Syrup of ipecac is absolutely contraindicated as the onset of convulsions may be rapid and vomiting may elicit muscle spasms or at least complicate their management.

2. If control of seizures as a result of strychnine is unsuccessful following IV benzodiazepines and barbiturates, neuromuscular blockade with an agent such as pancuronium may be necessary.
A. True
B. False

3. Strychnine, a basic alkaloid, is an odorless, bitter-tasting, white crystalline material derived from the ripe seeds of the Strychnos plant, *S. nux vomica*, a tree native to India.
A. True
B. False

VACOR

Vacor (N-3-pyridylmethyl-N-p-nitrophenylurea or PNU) is related to alloxan and streptozotocin, both of which are potent β cell pancreatic toxins. It was used widely as a rat killer until commercial distribution was voluntarily suspended in 1979. Nonetheless, stores of PNU may still be found under sinks and in closets.

Pathophysiology

PNU probably produces toxic effects by reducing intracellular synthesis of NAD and NADH (oxidized and reduced nicotinamide adenine dinucleotide). Extensive destruction of pancreatic β cells occurs and the marked insulinopenia in the presence of normal glucagon levels suggests a specific β cell cytotoxic effect. New-onset, insulin-dependent diabetes with orthostatic hypotension and autonomic dysfunction characterizes PNU toxicity.

Clinical Presentations

Clinical features of PNU poisoning usually simulate diabetic ketoacidosis. Serum glucose levels display a triphasic response: transient hyperglycemia, hypoglycemia lasting up to 48 hours, and permanent glucose intolerance with the development of ketoacidosis. Symptoms may include nausea, vomiting, abdominal pain, diffuse myalgias, polyuria, polydipsia, malaise, weakness, and dyspnea. Seizures may occur. A dysautonomic state with orthostatic hypotension and postural lightheadedness also may be prominent. Other manifestations of the autonomic neuropathy include dysphagia, impotence, urinary retention, and constipation or diarrhea. A peanut odor may aid the diagnosis of PNU poisoning.

Toxic Dosage/Death

Between 1976 and 1980, the use of PNU in attempted suicides caused 30 cases of severe diabetes mellitus in the United States. The estimated lethal human dose is 5 mg/kg.

Treatment

GUT DECONTAMINATION

Gastrointestinal decontamination with lavage and/or activated charcoal may be effective within the first several hours of exposure, but patients usually present after that time period.

ELIMINATION ENHANCEMENT

These methods have not been reported in the treatment of PNU poisoning.

SUPPORTIVE MEASURES

- As autonomic instability may ensue, monitor blood pressure and vital signs closely. Orthostatic hypotension unresponsive to fluid challenge has been treated with 0.3 mg of fludrocortisone per day, but clinical response was limited.
- Treatment of the PNU-poisoned patient is similar to the treatment of diabetic ketoacidosis (e.g., intravenous fluids, low-dose continuous insulin therapy, potassium replacement, and acid-base monitoring). Altered mental status and seizures are treated with IV dextrose because hypoglycemia occurs early in the course of PNU poisoning.

Antidotes

NICOTINAMIDE

Nicotinamide (not niacin or nicotinic acid) has effectively protected experimental animals from streptozotocin and alloxan-induced pancreatic cytotoxicity when administered within 3 hours of exposure. Recommended adult doses are 500 mg either intravenously or intramuscularly, followed immediately by 300 mg every 4 hours for 48 hours and then 100 mg 4 times a day for 2 weeks. A maximum human nicotinamide dose has not been determined.

Questions—Vacor

1. Which of the following concerning Vacor is false?
   A. Vacor is related to alloxan and streptozotocin, both of which are pancreatic β cell toxins.
   B. Vacor was used widely as a rat killer until commercial distribution was voluntarily suspended in 1979. Nonetheless, stores of PNU may still be found under sinks and in closets.
   C. Extensive destruction of pancreatic beta cells causes profound hyperglycemia.
   D. A peanut odor may aid the diagnosis of vacor poisoning.
   E. Nicotinamide has protected experimental animals from streptozotocin and alloxan-induced pancreatic cytotoxicity when administered within 3 hours of exposure.

RED SQUILL

This rodenticide is a natural plant product that contains cardiac glycosides. Its potential toxicity to humans is low, because it is poorly absorbed from the gut, contains low glycoside concentrations, and possesses a strong emetic action that substantially limits absorption. Consequently, the compound is practically nontoxic. Treatment involves gut decontamination and a search for signs/symptoms of digitalis poisoning. See Chapter 26, Cardiovascular Toxicology.

Questions—Red Squill

1. Red squill, a potent cardiac glycoside botanical, causes bradycardia in susceptible hosts.
   A. True
   B. False

HERBICIDES

INTRODUCTION

Herbicides are used chiefly to kill weeds. Examples include paraquat, diquat, chlorophenoxy compounds, chlorates, ioxynil, bromoxynil, and glyphosate. Certain chlorophenoxy herbicides, 2,4-D and 2,4,5-T, were used extensively in the Vietnam War in Agent Orange. Toxic dioxins contaminated Agent Orange and have been responsible for periodic toxic outbreaks around the world.

PARAQUAT

Paraquat (1,1′-dimethyl-4, 4′-dipyridylium), a toxic herbicide capable of producing multisystem organ failure and pulmonary fibrosis in fatal ingestions, was introduced in 1962. By 1971, at least 124 deaths were reported from suicidal and accidental ingestions. Mortality from accidental ingestion has ranged from 33% to 50% and correlates roughly with blood levels.

Paraquat is used as a desiccant, contact herbicide, defoliant, and plant growth regulator. Paraquat has been sprayed on marijuana plants to discourage illicit smoking. Paraquat is classified for restricted use and is limited to use by or under the supervision of certified pesticides applicators. It is the most important bipyridyl herbicide. Although deaths are reported from accidental paraquat exposure by inhalation and transdermal absorption, the method for suicide is nearly always oral ingestion.

Pathophysiology

Paraquat is reduced to an unstable free radical that then is reoxidized to produce a superoxide radical. Superoxide radicals destroy lipid membranes, damage alveolar integrity, and induce fibrotic changes. The earliest observed pulmonary changes occur in type I alveolar epithelial cells. Alveolar type II cells represent another cell type that shows overt damage during paraquat toxicity. The onset of a proliferative phase occurs several days after paraquat ingestion and is characterized by a rapidly forming, extensive fibrosis.

Pharmacokinetics

ABSORPTION

- Following inhalation, paraquat is poorly absorbed because most aerosolized particles have a diameter greater than 5 mm and cannot reach the alveolar barrier. Only a few cases of systemic paraquat poisoning by the inhalational route have been described.

- Paraquat cannot be absorbed significantly through intact human skin. However, damage to the skin, either by paraquat itself or by other means, allows greater systemic absorption.
- Systemic absorption of paraquat following subcutaneous administration is about 10% of the administered dose. Absorption after ingestion is small, ranging from 1% to 5% of the quantity ingested. Absorption is rapid, with the peak plasma level occurring 2 to 4 hours after ingestion.

DISTRIBUTION

- The lungs are the principal target organs for paraquat toxicity. The uptake of paraquat by lung tissue in the human is an early process that is essentially complete at the time of presentation to medical facilities.
- The kinetics of paraquat in the lungs show a rapid decline with an elimination half-life of 20 minutes, followed by a slower decline with a half-life of about 50 hours.
- Peak paraquat concentrations in the lungs is reached 4 to 5 hours after IV administration and 5 to 7 hours after ingestion, if renal function is normal.
- The apparent volume of distribution ranges from 1.2 to 1.6 L/kg.
- Muscle may represent an important reservoir, explaining the long persistence of paraquat in plasma and urine for several weeks or months after poisoning.

ELIMINATION

- Plasma paraquat concentration exhibits a mean distribution half-life of 5 hours and a mean elimination half-life of 8 hours. Renal elimination is rapid, with 80% to 90% being excreted in the first 6 hours and urinary recovery being almost 100% complete by 24 hours.
- Paraquat is not metabolized, but is reduced to an unstable free radical that is then reoxidized to produce a superoxide radical.

Clinical Presentations

A typical form of acute poisoning follows ingestion of the liquid form. Ingestion of 30 to 50 mg/kg of paraquat is equivalent to a single swallow of 12% to 20% concentrated commercial products. Buccopharyngeal, esophageal, epigastric, and gastric pain resulting from the herbicide's causticity immediately follow ingestion. Vomiting usually ensues, even in the absence of emetic additives in the commercial preparation. Abdominal pain and diarrhea are noted occasionally. Caustic lesions of the lips, oral cavity, and gastrointestinal tract are established over the first few hours. Fiberoptic esophagogastroscopy frequently shows mucosal lesions. These usually are superficial, although several cases of gastric perforation and massive gastrointestinal hemorrhage have been reported.

Two to 5 days after ingestion, renal failure and hepatocellular necrosis may develop. Hypovolemia secondary to gastrointestinal fluid losses and decreased oral fluid intake is common. Paraquat itself has direct renal toxicity. It generally causes a pure tubulopathy with proximal predominance, which evolves to full recovery without sequelae. The liver lesion caused by paraquat is centrilobular hepatocellular necrosis and is most often moderate.

Delayed development of pulmonary fibrosis generally is responsible for the poor prognosis in acute paraquat poisoning. Clinically and radiographically, this appears several days after ingestion, however alveolar-capillary abnormalities are present much earlier. A decrease in the carbon monoxide diffusing capacity may be noted from the first day. Pulmonary fibrosis leads rapidly to the development of refractory hypoxemia, resulting in death over a period of 5 days to several weeks. Neither spontaneous nor assisted artificial ventilation can delay the fatal outcome.

OPHTHALMOLOGIC EFFECTS

Several cases of ocular damage have been reported in workers who accidentally splash paraquat into their eyes. Anterior uveitis, corneal lesions, severe ocular surface destruction and/or variable degrees of conjunctivitis have followed initial irritation. Healing of ocular lesions may take 2 to 10 weeks but recovery generally is complete.

MARIJUANA

No cases of paraquat pulmonary toxicity have ever been documented among smokers of paraquat-treated marijuana. It has been shown that the temperatures generated by smoking inactivate the paraquat.

CARCINOGENIC EFFECTS

No direct evidence associating paraquat with cancer in humans has been found. Based on an increased incidence of squamous cell carcinoma in the head region of rats, the EPA has classified paraquat as a possible human carcinogen.

Toxic Dosage/Death

Any oral exposure to the commercial 20% concentrate should be considered potentially fatal. Adult ingestions exceeding 50 mL of concentrated paraquat solution are universally fatal, whereas 10 to 50 mL of concentrate can be fatal. The lethal adult dose ranges from 3 to 6 g. Although it is absorbed poorly through the skin, several cases of dermal exposure to concentrate have been reported, including the death of one worker with chronic skin abrasions. One patient died of paraquat poisoning following insertion into the vagina of a tampon inadvertently soaked in paraquat. Inhalation of paraquat spray is unlikely to produce toxic effects, because of the size of spray droplets.

Mild poisoning follows the ingestion or injection of 20 mg of paraquat ion per kilogram. Patients are asymptomatic or develop vomiting and diarrhea. Full recovery occurs, but there may be a transient fall in the carbon monoxide diffusing capacity and vital capacity. Moderate to severe poisoning follows the ingestion or injection of 20 to 40 mg of paraquat ion per kilogram. Patients suffer vomiting and diarrhea and develop generalized symptoms indicative of systemic toxicity. Pulmonary fibrosis develops in all cases, but recovery may occur. In addition, renal failure and sometimes hepatic dysfunction may supervene. Death occurs in the majority of cases, but can be delayed for weeks.

Acute fulminant poisoning follows the ingestion of more than 40 mg of paraquat ion/kg. In addition to nausea and vomiting, there is marked ulceration of the oropharynx with multiple organ (cardiac, respiratory, hepatic, renal, adrenal, pancreatic, and neurologic) failure. In this group, the mortality is 100%. Death may occur within 24 hours of the overdose, but is never delayed for more than 1 week. In cases of massive ingestion (greater than 55 mg/kg of paraquat), patients usually survive for less than 4 days and die in a setting of cardiogenic shock.

Drug Interactions

Three chronic rum drinkers who drank 80 g of ethanol per day survived after each had drunk more than 20 mL of "Gramoxone" (20% paraquat). The exact mechanism of interaction remains to be elucidated.

Pregnancy/Lactation

No epidemiologic studies have been performed on the possible reproductive effects of paraquat in humans. Exposures that have been fatal to mothers also have been fatal to term fetuses. Paraquat crosses the placenta and may be concentrated in the fetus. In one study, levels in amniotic fluid and fetal and cord blood exceeded those in maternal blood. The value of cesarean operations in these patients is unclear. No fetus has survived after significant exposures.

Laboratory

ANALYTIC METHODS

Paraquat and diquat may be assayed in serum and urine simultaneously using second-derivative spectroscopy. The method is less sensitive than high-pressure liquid chromatography, however serum analyses are complete within 10 minutes and urine samples within 5 minutes. A radioimmunoassay also has been proposed.

BLOOD LEVELS

There appears to be prognostic value of paraquat plasma levels. Patients whose plasma levels are less than those on a plot joining 2 mg/L at 4 hours after ingestion and 0.1 mg/L at 24 hours after ingestion tend to survive. Those with plasma levels above this line at comparable times, tend to die. Serum levels greater than 0.2 μg/mL at 24 hours and 0.1 μg/mL at 48 hours are usually associated with a fatal outcome.

Paraquat plasma levels also may predict the circumstances of death. Plasma paraquat concentrations greater than 10 mg/L suggest that death will occur from cardiogenic shock during the first 2 days after ingestion, while plasma concentrations less than 10 mg/L suggest a late death from pulmonary fibrosis. Patients whose initial plasma paraquat concentrations exceed 3 mg/L do not survive, regardless of the time after ingestion and therapeutic modalities.

URINE

All patients who die in less than 24 hours appear to show urine paraquat levels up to 10 μg/mL. When paraquat concentrations are less than 1 μg/mL, all patients survive. In one study of 30 patients, those who died from pulmonary fibrosis had urine levels between 1 and 1,000 μg/mL.

Treatment

GUT DECONTAMINATION

There is no definite evidence that gastric lavage is of any value in the treatment of paraquat poisoning in humans. If this procedure is used, any possible benefit is likely to be confined to the first hour following ingestion. No clinical or experimental studies involving the use of syrup of ipecac in paraquat poisoning have been reported. Whole-gut lavage has not improved outcome to date and may produce pulmonary edema in compromised patients.

There is no evidence to demonstrate an improved prognosis associated with the administration of Fuller's Earth and activated charcoal has not been shown to reduce systemic absorption significantly enough to affect either the morbidity or mortality in cases of paraquat poisoning. The cation resin Kayexalate® ultimately may be used to adsorb paraquat, however further studies are needed.

ELIMINATION ENHANCEMENT

As plasma paraquat levels peak early in the course of poisoning, intervention with hemodialysis or hemoperfusion should be attempted early, probably within 10 to 12 hours, before absorbed paraquat is distributed extensively to tissues. No patient whose initial plasma paraquat concentration was greater than 3 mg/L has survived, regardless of the time after ingestion when plasma levels were measured and despite treatment with hemoperfusion.

Because of the relative ease with which continuous arteriovenous hemofiltration (CAVH) can be performed, its low cost compared with hemoperfusion or hemodialysis, and the continuous nature of the procedure, CAVH still may be worth considering in paraquat poisoning. It may be used in those patients who have developed renal failure or while patients are being prepared for hemoperfusion. Additional studies still are needed.

SUPPORTIVE MEASURES

- Patients who ingest paraquat should be treated as medical emergencies even if asymptomatic. All patients exposed to paraquat should be washed thoroughly with soap and water.
- In the first 2 hours following ingestion, upper gastrointestinal endoscopy is recommended to identify the extent and severity of any mucosal lesions in the esophagus or stomach.
- Meticulous attention to supportive care has improved the prognosis of poisoned patients and remains the mainstay of treatment for paraquat poisoning. Management includes protection of the airway, maintenance of the circulation, frequent monitoring of vital signs and blood gases, treatment of secondary infection, adequate pain relief, prevention or treatment of renal failure, replacement of blood losses, treatment of complications such as arrhythmias and seizures, and counseling of the patient and family.
- Perform rapid qualitative analysis for paraquat on urine and gastric fluid. If the qualitative test for urinary paraquat remains negative over the first 24 hours, serious toxicity is unlikely.
- Hypokalemia is reported to be induced by paraquat itself and/or an additive and may be a good prognostic indicator. The interval of time from ingestion to admission, serum creatinine concentration, serum potassium concentration, and arterial blood HCO_3 may bear a significant relationship to the prognosis of acute paraquat poisoning.
- Radiologic changes do not always parallel the severity of clinical symptoms. The chest x-ray may be normal, particularly in those patients who die soon after ingestion from multiorgan failure. More often, patchy infiltration develops, which may progress to opacification of one or both lung fields.
- Long-term use of paraquat has been found safe under appropriate conditions of hygiene, with protective equipment, and avoidance of aerosol inhalation.

ANALGESIA

- Pain and distress should be reduced to a minimum. It is difficult to abolish the severe pain produced by local ulceration. Mouthwashes, ice-cold fluids, local anesthetic sprays, and lozenges all have been employed with varying degrees of success.
- Opiates may be required eventually in most patients to relieve pain and distress.

LUNG TRANSPLANTATION

- Lung transplantation would appear to be useful in a patient with extensive irreversible pulmonary fibrosis from paraquat toxicity, but with reversible damage to all other organs.

- Unfortunately, in the few situations where this has been attempted, there was new uptake by the transplanted lung of paraquat sequestered in other organs and the subsequent development of paraquat toxicity. Lung transplantations have not reduced mortality because either the transplanted lung developed toxicity or technical complications have led to death.
- High-dose cyclophosphamide and dexamethasone appear unlikely to improve the prognosis of paraquat poisoning.

Antidotes

Paraquat-specific antibodies have reduced the uptake of a toxic concentration of paraquat by type II cells *in vitro*, but no clinical studies have validated the usefulness of this procedure. No antidote can be recommended currently on the basis of convincing evidence obtained in patients.

Questions—Paraquat

1. **Which of the following concerning paraquat is false?**
   A. Paraquat is a toxic herbicide capable of producing multisystem organ failure and pulmonary fibrosis in fatal ingestions.
   B. Mortality from accidental ingestion has ranged from 33% to 50% and correlates roughly with blood levels.
   C. Paraquat has been sprayed on marijuana plants to discourage illicit smoking.
   D. Paraquat has caused numerous fatalities in marijuana smokers.
   E. The method for suicide nearly always is oral ingestion.
2. **Following inhalation, paraquat is absorbed poorly because most aerosolized particles have a diameter greater than 5 mm and cannot reach the alveolar barrier.**
   A. True
   B. False
3. **Delayed development of pulmonary fibrosis generally is responsible for the poor prognosis in acute paraquat poisoning. Clinically and radiographically, this appears several days after ingestion, however alveolar-capillary abnormalities are present much earlier.**
   A. True
   B. False
4. **Which of the following concerning paraquat is false?**
   A. Oral exposure to the commercial 20% concentrate should be considered potentially fatal.
   B. Adult ingestions greater than 50 mL of concentrated paraquat solution may be well tolerated.
   C. Death can be delayed for 2 to 3 weeks.
   D. In cases of massive ingestion, patients usually survive for less than 4 days and die in a setting of cardiogenic shock.
   E. There appears to be some prognostic value from paraquat plasma levels.
5. **Fuller's earth may be an effective antidote if given early.**
   A. True
   B. False

DIQUAT

Diquat is a dipyridyl herbicide used less frequently than paraquat. Although diquat is less toxic in animal models than paraquat, seven deaths were reported by 1983 in the English-language medical literature.

Pathophysiology

The mechanism of toxicity is similar to that of paraquat, in which superoxide radicals destroy lipid membranes, however diquat does not cause pulmonary lesions, because of its lower affinity for lung tissue. The activity of diquat, as well as paraquat, may be based on the liberation of hydrogen peroxide, leading to tissue destruction.

Pharmacokinetics

ABSORPTION

- Humans are poisoned by oral and, rarely, pulmonary routes.

DISTRIBUTION

- In rats, 90% of an oral dose remains in the feces.

ELIMINATION

- The majority (90%) of an absorbed dose is excreted unchanged by the kidneys within 24 hours. No metabolites are known.

Clinical Presentations

Gastrointestinal complications include vomiting, mucosal ulcers, diarrhea, and ileus. Sequestration of fluids in the gastrointestinal tract may cause hypovolemia. Myocardial necrosis and ventricular dysrhythmias occur in severe poisoning. Central nervous system effects may include coma, seizures, and pontine hemorrhage. Hepatic and renal damage are usually mild. Progressive pulmonary fibrosis is not seen in diquat survivors.

Acute and persistent parkinsonism has followed exposure of the hand to an aqueous solution of 10% diquat dibromide. This may relate to the chemical similarity between diquat and MPTP (methyl-g-phenyl-tetrahydropyridine) known to elicit chronic parkinsonism in humans.

Toxic Dosage/Death

Deaths have occurred after an ingestion of 20 to 50 mL of Reglone® (diquat 20 g/100 mL). Mortality in reported cases approaches 50% despite a lower LD50 (400 mg/kg) than for paraquat (25 to 50 mg/kg). Survival has been reported after ingestion of 300 mL of 20% diquat.

Laboratory

ANALYTIC METHODS

An enzyme-linked immunosorbent assay is available to determine the diquat level in human tissues. A pyrolysis gas chromatography method is available for determination of diquat levels.

BLOOD LEVELS

Diquat serum levels of 0.45 μg/mL and 4.5 μg/mL have been associated with fatalities.

Treatment

GUT DECONTAMINATION

Gastric lavage should be considered early in treatment, but care must be exercised because of the expected occurrence of extensive tissue necrosis in the esophagus and stomach.

ELIMINATION ENHANCEMENT

In one case of a 24-year-old who developed systemic symptoms and mild nonoliguric renal failure, hemoperfusion over 12 hours did not remove significant amounts of diquat.

SUPPORTIVE MEASURES

- The general approach to diquat intoxication is similar to that for paraquat poisoning.
- Prompt aggressive therapy remains the hallmark of effective therapy, even in those who have a relatively symptom-free initial interval.

Questions—Diquat

1. Which of the following concerning diquat is false?
 A. Diquat is a herbicide used less frequently than paraquat.
 B. Mortality has not been reported from diquat.
 C. Diquat does not cause pulmonary lesions.
 D. Acute and persistent parkinsonism has followed exposure to diquat dibromide.
 E. There are antidotes for diquat poisoning.

CHLOROPHENOXY COMPOUNDS AND DIOXIN

Chlorinated phenoxy acid compounds represent a significant class of herbicides. Acute toxic reactions to chlorophenoxy compounds are rare. 2,4-dichlorophenoxy acetic acid (2,4-D) is the most popular herbicide among the chlorinated phenoxy acid compounds. This chemical group has received extensive publicity because the dioxin 2,3,7,8-tetrachlorodibenzo-p-dioxin (TCDD) that causes mutagenic, teratogenic, and carcinogenic changes in animal models is a by-product of production of the herbicides 2,4-D and 2,4,5-trichlorophenoxy acetic acid (2,4,5-T).

Large-scale exposure to dioxins occurred after the use of the herbicide mixture Agent Orange (50% 2,4 D and 50% 2,4,5-T) in Vietnam. The EPA has since removed 2,4,5-T from the commercial market. Toxic effects of TCDD result from occupational exposures during the production of trichlorophenol and hexachlorophene, from manufacturing accidents and from environmental contaminations. Burning of coal and incineration of municipal waste produce dioxins, but usually in minute amounts. Delineation of the exact clinical effects from dioxins is difficult, because pure exposures are rare. Suspected subacute features are hepatic enlargement, chloracne, neuromuscular symptoms, and deranged porphyrin metabolism.

The largest known contamination from dioxin occurred between 1962 and 1970, when 12 million gallons of Agent Orange, a defoliant mixture contaminated with a form of the most toxic dioxin (TCDD), were sprayed over southern and central Vietnam. Several areas of the United States have been contaminated because of industrial discharges or spraying of dirt roads with dioxin-contaminated waste oils. Three areas that have received notoriety are the Love Canal in Niagara Falls, New York, Times Beach, Missouri, and Newark, New Jersey. The most highly publicized accident affecting a residential population was an explosion at a chemical plant that resulted in an airborne discharge of dioxins over Seveso, Italy, in 1976. More than 37,000 people lived in an area that may have been contaminated by dioxins. There were no deaths from acute poisoning.

Pathophysiology

Dioxins and furans are terms applied to polychlorinated dibenzo-p-dioxins and polychlorinated dibenzofurans. Because TCDD is the most thoroughly studied and most toxic of the 75 dioxin isomers, the term TCDD is used interchangeably with dioxins throughout.

Pharmacokinetics

ABSORPTION

- Dioxins enter the body by ingestion, inhalation, and dermal absorption.

DISTRIBUTION

- Dioxins distribute to organs according to lipid content and readily accumulate in body fat.

ELIMINATION

- Metabolism of TCDD primarily is by hepatic detoxification, with the major metabolites consisting of hydroxylated or methoxylated TCDD derivatives. These are excreted as glucuronide and sulfate conjugates.
- The half-life of TCDD ranges from several hours (on the surface of plants) to 7.1 years (in human serum and adipose tissue).

Clinical Presentations

The onset of symptoms after an acute exposure to TCDD-containing substances can take days to weeks and may include skin, eye, and respiratory tract irritation, headache, dizziness, and nausea. Many signs and symptoms are nonspecific. No deaths from systemic dioxin toxicity in humans have been reported. Only two clinical effects have been observed repeatedly in exposed populations: chloracne and transient hepatic effects. Soft-tissue sarcomas, lymphomas, peripheral neuropathy, birth defects, and reproductive effects have been studied but remain unconfirmed.

DERMATOLOGIC EFFECTS

Acneform lesions may appear as early as 1 to 3 weeks after dioxin exposure. The lesions are small, pale yellow cysts that arise from altered differentiation of acinar sebaceous basal cells in keratinocytes. The acne primarily involves the face and upper body. Most cases of chloracne resolve in 1 to 3 years. Chloracne also can be caused by chloro- and bromonaphthalenes, polychlorinated and polybrominated biphenyls (PCBs, PBBs), pentachlorophenol, and tetrachlorobenzene. See Chapter 46, Hydrocarbons. The absence of chloracne does not rule out dioxin exposure. Other reported dermal effects include hyperpigmentation, hirsutism, increased skin fragility, and vesicular eruptions on exposed areas of the skin.

HEPATIC EFFECTS

There is no evidence that TCDD causes long-term hepatotoxicity in humans. Some studies have shown a transient increase in liver enzymes without clinical disease. Epidemiologic studies of TCDD-exposed workers have shown no difference in serum levels of hepatic enzymes compared with those of matched controls. Intentional ingestion of 2,4-D produces rhabdomyolysis, hepatitis, and metabolic acidosis.

CARCINOGENIC EFFECTS

The EPA and the National Institute of Occupational Safety and Health (NIOSH) consider TCDD to be a "cancer promoter" in conjunction with certain other chemicals. NIOSH classifies TCDD as a "potential occupational carcinogen." The EPA considers TCDD to be a probable human carcinogen. Several Swedish occupational studies and American case studies suggest an increased incidence of soft tissue sarcomas and lymphomas among workers exposed to phenoxy acid herbicides, but other studies have failed to substantiate the increased risk.

Toxic Dosage/Death

Death has followed ingestion of 80 mg/kg of 2,4-D in a 75 kg student. Toxic or lethal doses of the chlorophenoxy compounds or dioxin have generally not been identified.

Pregnancy/Lactation

Studies of Vietnam servicemen possibly exposed to Agent Orange revealed no overall increase of debilitating birth defects in their progeny. Studies of the Seveso area have failed to demonstrate an increased risk of birth defects resulting from dioxin exposure. Spontaneous abortion rates in exposed mothers did increase after the 1976 Seveso dioxin accident, but no difference was observed between women from areas of low, moderate, and high contamination. Data collected after the Seveso incident failed to demonstrate any increased risk of birth defects associated with TCDD. Because of the lipophilic nature of milk, nursing females decrease their body burden of TCDD through lactation.

Laboratory Tests

ANALYTIC METHODS

A high-performance liquid chromatographic assay useful as an aid in the diagnosis of acute poisoning by 2,4-D and related components has a limit of detection of 20 μg/mL. Analyses of serum or fat TCDD levels by gas chromatography-mass spectroscopy are expensive and time-consuming and are not recommended.

BLOOD LEVELS

Some researchers believe that serum levels correlate with adipose tissue levels in persons with long-term exposure. Vietnam veterans who were heavily exposed to Agent Orange exhibited an increase in both blood and adipose tissue levels of TCDD. Many people in the Seveso, Italy, accident had TCDD levels 1,000 times greater than the average found in the general unexposed population and did not experience illness. All who developed severe chloracne had TCDD levels over 12,000 ppt. The results were 3,000 to 4,000 times higher than background human levels. These data suggest that chloracne is not the most sensitive marker of overt exposure to TCDD but that the actual measurement of TCDD in human samples may be helpful.

Treatment

GUT DECONTAMINATION

The usual measures of gut and skin decontamination (lavage, and/or charcoal) are recommended within the first several hours.

ELIMINATION ENHANCEMENT

Four patients who had ingested from 40 to 160 g of 2,4-D were treated with hemodialysis. Three were admitted in coma within 2 to 3 hours of ingestion. Recovery followed hemodialysis in three patients and hemodialysis and resin hemoperfusion in the fourth. One study of 38 patients with herbicide poisoning suggested that alkaline diuresis should be used to treat acute poisoning with chlorophenoxy herbicides in the presence of coma or other poor prognostic indicators, such as acidemia or if plasma total chlorophenoxy concentrations are 0.5 g/L or more.

SUPPORTIVE MEASURES

- Treatment of chronic exposure to dioxin-containing agents is primarily supportive. It is most important to remove the patient from the source of exposure.
- Chloracne often is refractory and unresponsive to common acne treatments. Long-term topical treatment with dilute retinoic acid and administration of tetracycline to treat secondary pustular follicles has been used. In severe cases, acne surgery or dermabrasion may be effective.
- Moderately to severely 2,4-D-poisoned patients should receive the following tests: serum aldolase, creatinine, electrolytes, hepatic aminotransferase, and urinalysis.

Questions—Chlorophenoxy Compounds and Dioxin

1. **Which of the following is the most popular chlorinated phenoxy acid herbicide?**
   A. 2,4,5-trichlorophenoxy acetic acid (2,4,5-T)
   B. 2,4-dichlorophenoxy acetic acid (2,4-D)
   C. 2,3,7,8-tetrachlorodibenzo-p-dioxin (TCDD)
   D. 2-chloronaphthalene
   E. 2,4,5,7-tetrachlorobenzene
2. **Which of the following is a by-product of production of the herbicides 2,4-D and 2,4,5-trichlorophenoxy acetic acid (2,4,5-T)?**
   A. 2,3,7,8-tetrachlorodibenzo-p-dioxin (TCDD)
   B. Agent Orange
   C. 2,4-DDT
   D. PCBs
   E. PBBs
3. **Which of the following has not been associated with chloracne?**
   A. Bromonaphthalene
   B. Chloronaphthalene
   C. Polybrominated biphenyls
   D. Dioxins
   E. Ethylene dioxide
4. **The two clinical effects repeatedly observed in dioxin-exposed populations include**
   A. Chloracne and transient hepatic effects
   B. Chloracne and bronchospasm
   C. Hepatoma and pruritus
   D. Hirsutism and loss of libido
   E. Cancer and hyponatremia
5. **Dioxins definitely have been associated with cancer.**
   A. True
   B. False
6. **Studies of Vietnam servicemen possibly exposed to Agent Orange revealed no overall increase of debilitating birth defects in their progeny.**
   A. True
   B. False

CHLORATES

Sodium chlorate is a strong oxidizing agent used commercially in the manufacture of explosives and dyestuffs, and in tanning. This compound also is a nonselective herbicide. Its toxicity is relatively low and reports of accidental, suicidal, and homicidal poisoning are rare. This white crystalline powder may be mistaken for sugar with fatal results. Toxicity has been reported after ingestion of match heads and inhalation of atomized spray.

Pathophysiology

Sodium chlorate is a powerful oxidizing agent that causes methemoglobinemia, hemolytic anemia, and direct nephrotoxic effects. Coma and death within hours can result from tissue hypoxia from methemoglobinemia, hyperkalemia from massive hemolysis, or acute renal failure compounded by hemoglobinuria.

Clinical Presentations

Within 2 to 24 hours, gastrointestinal symptoms develop including nausea, vomiting, diarrhea, and abdominal pain. After absorption, hemoglobin rapidly oxidizes to methemoglobin, leading to cyanosis, dyspnea, and coma in severe cases. Intravascular hemolysis also can occur. Seven of 14 patients in the largest published chlorate poisoning series developed acute renal failure within 48 hours of hospital admission. Disseminated intravascular coagulation also may occur.

Toxic Dosage/Death

The acute lethal dose in adults is approximately 20 to 35 g. Survival after ingestion of 45 and 100 g resulted after the use of sodium thiosulfate and prompt management of renal failure by peritoneal dialysis. Potassium chlorate is more lethal (12 g in an adult, 5 g in a child, and 1 g in an infant) than the sodium salt.

Treatment

GUT DECONTAMINATION

The usual measures of gut decontamination (i.e., lavage, and/or activated charcoal) may be useful within the first several hours after exposure, however the effectiveness of charcoal has not been established.

ELIMINATION ENHANCEMENT

Sodium chlorate is freely dialyzable, and hemodialysis or early exchange transfusion is recommended, particularly when renal failure is present. Such procedures may prevent hemolysis, which may be fatal.

SUPPORTIVE MEASURES

- Obviously ill patients should be evaluated for the adequacy of airway, ventilation, and circulation. Methemoglobin levels, complete blood count, serum electrolytes, and creatinine should be drawn immediately after the establishment of adequate ventilation and an IV line. The patient should receive cardiac monitoring and supplemental oxygen. Signs of hyperkalemia may include widening of the QRS and PR prolongation.
- Blood abnormalities may include normocytic normochromic anemia, thrombocytopenia, free plasma haptoglobin, polymorphonuclear leukocytosis, Heinz bodies, ghost cells, dark brown "chocolate" serum, methemoglobin levels exceeding 10%, mildly elevated hepatic aminotransferases, hyperkalemia, and elevated serum creatinine.
- Proteinuria and hemoglobinuria may also be present.

Antidotes

SODIUM THIOSULFATE

Sodium thiosulfate either orally or intravenously (2 to 5 g in 200 mL of 5% sodium bicarbonate) inactivates chlorate ion and is a potentially useful antidote based on anecdotal reports.

METHYLENE BLUE

Methemoglobin can be reduced to hemoglobin by the IV use of methylene blue, however methylene blue may have minimal effect in the treatment of chlorate intoxication. The clinical course of chlorate poisoning appears to be determined by hemolysis, disseminated intravascular coagulation, and renal failure.

Questions—Chlorates

1. Chlorates have been used for all of the following, except
A. Jet fuel
B. Explosives
C. Dyestuffs
D. Tanning
E. Match heads

2. Potential treatments after chlorate exposure include
A. Hemodialysis
B. Methylene blue
C. Sodium thiosulfate
D. All of the above
E. B and C

GLYPHOSATE

Glyphosate is a broad-spectrum herbicide used in crop, noncrop, and aquatic weed control. Glyphosate has been combined with a surfactant, polyoxethyleneamine. Glyphosate-surfactant herbicide concentrate (Roundup®) has been ingested in suicide attempts. The toxic syndrome consists of mucosal and gastrointestinal irritation, hypotension, metabolic acidosis, pulmonary insufficiency, and oliguria. Most deaths have followed suicide attempts and a few deaths have followed accidental ingestions, usually in children.

Pathophysiology

Glyphosate is a useful herbicide because it effectively inhibits plant aromatic amino acid biosynthesis. Some data indicate that glyphosate may interfere with mitochondrial oxidative phosphorylation, but tachypnea, tachycardia, and significant hyperpyrexia usually are not observed clinically. The profound hypotensive shock observed in many of the nonsurvivors combined with a relative absence of hypovolemia suggests a direct cardiotoxic effect.

Clinical Presentations

A toxic syndrome may follow the ingestion of a large volume of glyphosate consisting of oral-pharyngeal, mucosal, and GI irritation, hypotension, pulmonary insufficiency, metabolic acidosis, and oliguria. Effects on organs other than the gastrointestinal tract tend to occur with increasing amounts ingested. There may be a low-grade fever after 6 to 24 hours. In severe poisoning, mental status alteration may develop after up to 6 hours, often attributable to hypoxia or hypotension. A sore throat, burning sensation in the mouth and throat, salivation, erythema, and oral ulcerations have been observed.

GASTROINTESTINAL EFFECTS

Spontaneous vomiting, nausea, epigastric and abdominal pain, diarrhea, and dysphagia are seen. Hematemesis, bloody stool, and acute pancreatitis have been observed. Erosions of the pharynx and larynx were described in one series. The esophagus was involved in 39% of cases with development of esophageal ulcers, superficial or corrosive esophagitis with mucosal edema, erosions, and hemorrhage. Transmural injury or perforation has not been observed. The stomach usually is involved with gastritis and ulceration and the duodenum is involved in about 26% of patients with duodenitis or duodenal ulcer. Colitis has been observed rarely. Aminotransferases (AST, ALT) may be mildly elevated and jaundice is not seen.

PULMONARY EFFECTS

Asymptomatic mild hypoxemia may be detected by arterial blood gas analysis. More serious involvement ranges from alveolar or interstitial infiltrates seen on a chest x-ray, tachypnea, dyspnea, cough, and bronchospasm, to cyanosis, aspiration pneumonia, frank pulmonary edema, and respiratory failure. Lung injury may be a result of toxic effects of both glyphosate and surfactant.

CARDIOVASCULAR EFFECTS

Hypotensive shock is often observed within hours of glyphosate ingestion. In survivors, this may be transient. In one series, hypotensive shock occurred in all nonsurvivors. The hypotension may respond initially to position change, hydration, and pressor amines, but later may become refractory to these measures. Hypovolemia does not appear to be the cause.

RENAL EFFECTS

Renal abnormalities may include oliguria, anuria, and infrequent gross or microscopic hematuria. Blood urea nitrogen and serum creatinine tend to be normal or slightly elevated initially. A metabolic acidosis has been observed in those with serious poisoning, hypoxemia, or anuria. Lactate production may be a factor. In some fatal cases, the metabolic acidosis has not responded to bicarbonate therapy.

MISCELLANEOUS EFFECTS

Confusion and coma may appear. Glyphosate does not appear to exert a primary toxic effect on bone marrow and hemolysis has not been documented. No platelet or coagulation abnormalities have been reported. Temporary conjunctival irritation can occur from ocular exposure. No significant absorption occurs through the skin. Prolonged contact can lead to a "detergent dermatitis." Glyphosate does not appear to induce skin irritations, photo irritation, skin sensitizations, or photosensitization.

Toxic Dosage/Death

Asymptomatic patients in one series appeared to ingest about 5 to 50 mL and mild symptoms were observed with ingestions of 5 to 150 mL. Moderate symptoms followed 20 to 500 mL, and severe symptoms with 85 to 200 mL. Gastric and esophageal abnormalities may follow ingestion of as little as 25 mL of glyphosphate. Ingestions of 30 to 60 mL of the concentrate may lead to emesis, pharyngeal pain, and nausea within 15 minutes. Survivors usually have ingested no more than 100 to 120 mL of the concentrate. A minimal lethal dose of 150 mL has been suggested.

Adults over 40 years of age who have ingested over 100 to 150 mL of glyphosate appear to be at the highest risk of a fatal outcome. Patients may appear to do well for hours and then slowly lapse into a hypotensive, nonhypovolemic shock that can be refractory to fluids and pressor amines and often ends fatally. Individuals have survived ingestion of up to 500 mL of the Roundup® concentrate with mild-to-moderate symptomatology but fatalities have followed ingestions of only 100 mL of the concentrate. Death may be associated with severe hypotension, shock, renal failure, or respiratory distress syndrome.

Laboratory

ANALYTIC METHODS

Gas chromatography, high-performance liquid chromatography, gas chromatography-mass spectrometry, and nuclear magnetic resonance spectroscopy can quantitate glyphosate. There is no clinical assay available to measure the surfactant.

BLOOD LEVELS

Blood levels are not good prognostic indicators of severity of poisoning. In one study, survivors had glyphosate plasma levels of 725 μg/mL. Two nonsurvivors had plasma glyphosate levels of 918 μg/mL and 1,515 μg/mL, respectively.

Treatment

GUT DECONTAMINATION

If emesis has not occurred, the patient presents within 4 hours of ingestion, and about 0.5 mL/kg body weight of concentrate has been ingested, gastric lavage may be indicated. Protect against aspiration by frequent oral suctioning, placing the patient in the left lateral decubitus position, and inserting a cuffed endotracheal tube during lavage, as required. Activated charcoal may adsorb the surfactant. There is no clinical evidence to support the use of multiple doses of activated charcoal or cathartic.

ELIMINATION ENHANCEMENT

There is no evidence to support the use of forced diuresis. Care must be taken to monitor fluid balance and prevent either fluid depletion or fluid overload. Hemodialysis or hemoperfusion have not been studied systematically, but may be useful in view of the low molecular weight and the low volume of distribution seen in dogs. Hemodialysis is indicated for renal failure and intractable metabolic acidosis.

SUPPORTIVE MEASURES

- Patients who have ingested more than 0.5 mL/kg of Roundup® should be admitted to an intensive-care facility for evaluation and monitoring. Patency of the airway, respirations, and circulation are the first priorities. Intravenous lines should be established immediately. Careful monitoring of the status of pulmonary, cardiovascular, and renal functions is essential. Administer 100% oxygen initially. Respiratory distress may require cricothyroidotomy if excessive swelling contraindicates endotracheal intubation.
- Do not administer buffering agents (e.g., antacids) because they may induce an exothermic reaction without altering the pH. Attempt to avoid further emesis by limiting the oral fluid intake.

- Glyphosate surfactant herbicide is not an organophosphate compound. Do not give atropine or 2-pralidoxime (2-PAM).
- Wash contaminated skin with mild soap and water. Irrigate exposed eyes with normal saline or water for at least 15 to 20 minutes. Artificial tears may relieve residual irritation. If irritation persists, call an ophthalmologist.

GASTROINTESTINAL CONSIDERATIONS

- Rinsing the mouth with water may soothe mucosal lesions and remove residual toxin. Topical anesthetics such as viscous lidocaine may be useful for oral pain in a conscious, alert patient.
- Patients should not be fed orally until endoscopy has confirmed the extent of injury.
- H2-blockers such as cimetidine, ranitidine, and other similar drugs may be considered.
- Serial abdominal examinations, and, if indicated, radiography and water-soluble contrast studies may aid in the management of gastric or duodenal ulcers.
- Steroids have not been systematically evaluated in this ingestion. Antibiotics should be reserved for documented infections.

CARDIOVASCULAR CONSIDERATIONS

- Hypotension may develop hours after ingestion. Cardiac monitoring should be available.
- If hypotension develops, treat initially with IV fluids and place the patient in the Trendelenburg position. If the patient is unresponsive to fluid challenges, use pressor amines.
- A central venous pressure line or Swan-Ganz catheter may be necessary to guide fluid therapy when clinically indicated. An arterial line for constant blood pressure monitoring is advisable.
- Fluid overload may lead to pulmonary edema.

PULMONARY CONSIDERATIONS

- Respiratory function should be evaluated by serial chest x-rays, arterial blood gas determination, and clinical evidence of signs of respiratory distress. Adequate oxygenation may require intubation, assisted ventilation, high inspiratory oxygen flow rates, and positive end-expiratory pressure (PEEP).
- Use antibiotics for documented infection.
- When fluid overload or left ventricular failure is evident, furosemide may be useful.
- Morphine may compromise blood pressure, depress cardiac output, and/or impair central respiratory drive.

RENAL EFFECTS

- Urine output should be monitored hourly. Adequate circulating volume and systolic blood pressure should be ensured. Do not use diuretics for volume depletion or hypotension. Mannitol may precipitate pulmonary edema and should not be used in an anuric patient.
- Dialysis is indicated for renal failure. Treat significant acidosis with bicarbonate infusion. Failure to reverse acidosis may be an indication for hemodialysis to correct acid-base balance.

OCCUPATIONAL PRECAUTIONS

- Wear chemical-resistant gloves, head covering, long-sleeved shirt, long pants, and shoes with socks. Avoid getting glyphosate surfactant herbicide concentrate on the skin or eyes.
- Launder clothing worn during application of the herbicide separately from the family laundry.
- Children and pets should be kept from close contact with an area sprayed for 24 hours after use. Store in its original container, in a secure place, away from children and pets.
- Do not pour unused product down sinks or into showers.

ANCILLARY TESTS

- Monitor white cell count, hematocrit, hemoglobin, electrolytes, blood urea nitrogen, creatinine, bilirubin, amylase, hepatic aminotransferases, acid-base status, arterial blood gas, chest x-ray, central venous pressure, pulmonary capillary wedge pressure, and cardiac output as clinically indicated.
- About one-half of patients exhibit a leukocytosis especially in severe cases. Hyperglycemia has been observed in 30% of patients in one series. Serum amylase frequently is elevated from salivary gland irritation. Elevations in serum aminotransferases and bilirubin may be seen.
- The ECG may exhibit sinus tachycardia or sinus bradycardia. Atrioventricular block and ventricular ectopy also have been observed.

Questions—Glyphosate

1. Which of the following about glyphosate poisoning is true?

A. Glyphosate is a broad-spectrum herbicide used in crop, noncrop, and aquatic weed control.
B. Glyphosate-surfactant herbicide (Roundup®) has been ingested in suicide attempts.
C. A toxic syndrome may follow the ingestion of a large volume of glyphosate consisting of oral-pharyngeal, mucosal, and gastrointestinal irritation, hypotension, pulmonary insufficiency, metabolic acidosis, and oliguria.
D. All of the above
E. A and B

2. There is no evidence to support the use of forced diuresis in glyphosate poisoning.

A. True
B. False

FUNGICIDES AND MOLLUSCICIDES

INTRODUCTION

Fungicides are compounds used to kill fungi and molds. Examples include the dithiocarbamates and pentachlorophenol. Molluscicides such as metaldehyde kill molluscs, marine invertebrates such as snails.

PENTACHLOROPHENOL AND DINITROPHENOL

Pentachlorophenol is used as a wood preservative, fungicide, and bactericidal agent. In contrast to creosote-treated lumber, pentachlorophenol-impregnated wood retains its natural appearance, emanates little odor, and accepts paint easily. Tetrachlorophenols also have insecticidal and fungicidal properties, but these uses are much more limited.

Nitrophenolic and nitrocresolic compounds are aromatic nitro chemicals used as dyestuffs, chemical intermediaries, explosive agents (dinitrophenol), and herbicides. Pentachlorophenol produces a hypermetabolic state similar to that produced by dinitrophenol, leading to hyperpyrexia, cerebral edema, convulsions, and coma. Most toxic effects result from the occupational use of pentachlorophenol in poorly ventilated areas.

In a St. Louis newborn nursery epidemic, laundry products were mistakenly washed in 23% sodium pentachlorophenate. Affected infants developed respiratory distress, tachycardia, diaphoresis, tachypnea, hepatic enlargement, and metabolic acidosis after the percutaneous absorption of pentachlorophenol. Chronic exposures result from inhabitation of pentachlorophenol-heated log homes and cause elevated serum and urine pentachlorophenol levels as well as skin lesions, respiratory tract irritation, and headaches. Dioxin-contaminated pentachlorophenol has led to several cases of chloracne in workers exposed to these solutions.

Pathophysiology

Pentachlorophenol and dinitrophenol inhibit oxidative phosphorylation, leading to a heat-exhaustion or heat-stroke picture. Pentachlorophenol is a selective inhibitor of P450 hepatic microsomal enzymes. The presence of methemoglobinemia also may contribute to toxicity. Postmortem examination after pentachlorophenol poisoning has revealed severe centrilobular congestion, fat droplets in the liver, proximal renal tubules, and myocardium, cerebral edema, pulmonary edema, and alveolar hemorrhage.

Pharmacokinetics

ABSORPTION

- Toxicity occurs via the pulmonary, gastrointestinal, and dermal routes.
- In the animal model, pentachlorophenol is 20 times more toxic by inhalation than ingestion and 10 times better absorbed by the lungs than the skin.
- The presence of organic solvents as vehicles or open skin lesions increases absorption.

DISTRIBUTION

- Significant amounts of pentachlorophenol have been reported in serum, adipose, and urine.
- The liver and kidney accumulate between 65% to 83% of total body stores of pentachlorophenol.

ELIMINATION

- The kidney excretes 75% of an orally administered dose of pentachlorophenol unchanged and 12% as the conjugated form.
- After oral exposure, peak plasma levels occur in about 4 hours and decline with a plasma half-life of 27 to 35 hours.
- After continued exposure to high levels, elimination pathways become saturated and toxic levels build rapidly.

Clinical Presentations

Within several hours of exposure to pentachlorophenol and/or dinitrophenol, fever, perspiration, headache, malaise, abdominal pain, anorexia, nausea, vomiting, weakness, myalgias, and thirst may develop. In severe cases, these symptoms progress to coma, convulsions, cerebral edema, and vascular collapse. Chronic poisoning is often difficult to detect because symptoms can be vague and include anorexia, weight loss, weakness, dizziness, headache, personality changes, anxiety, urticaria, pemphigus vulgaris, and chloracne. Fever is seen in chronic, as well as acute, intoxication. Upper respiratory complaints, conjunctivitis, and sinusitis also have been seen.

Prolonged exposure to pentachlorophenol may be a factor in hirsutism and alopecia. Workers with documented skin contact with pentachlorophenol that has been contaminated with dioxins, and dibenzofurans have an increased risk of chloracne. Yellow staining of the skin suggests a diagnosis of nitrophenol poisoning but does not correlate with blood level, route of intoxication, or severity. Pentachlorophenol is considered a potential carcinogen because of the carcinogenicity of structurally similar compounds. Although it has not proven to be mutagenic or teratogenic, the chlorinated phenols may act as promoters or cocarcinogens.

Toxic Dosage/Death

Pentachlorophenol is a highly toxic substance that produces severe toxic effects in adults after ingestion of 2 g.

Pregnancy/Lactation

Prolonged exposure to pentachlorophenol may be a factor in unexplained infertility, repeated abortions, and other endocrine and immunologic disorders in women.

Laboratory

ANALYTIC METHODS

Electron-capture gas chromatography of a methyl or ethyl derivative is the preferred method of analysis of pentachlorophenol.

BLOOD LEVELS

In nonoccupationally exposed individuals, blood pentachlorophenol concentrations range up to 1 mg/L. Occupational exposure of workers exposed to pentachlorophenol in a wood factory indicated that plasma PCP concentrations varied from 50 to 200 μg/L in workers without direct exposure and from 500 to 600 μg/L in workers handling and applying PCP on the wood. Obvious intoxication occurs with blood pentachlorophenol levels exceeding 40 mg/L. One postmortem blood study of an occupational exposure revealed a level of 162 ppm.

Treatment

GUT DECONTAMINATION

The usual measures of gastrointestinal decontamination (i.e., lavage and activated charcoal) may be used within the first several hours of exposure.

ELIMINATION ENHANCEMENT

Exchange transfusions were used successfully in ill infants exposed to pentachlorophenol, but the exact role of this procedure in altering outcome was not well documented. Although forced diuresis reduced the total body stores of pentachlorophenol, the clinical efficacy of this procedure in acute poisoning is unproved.

SUPPORTIVE MEASURES

- Solutions spilled on the skin should be removed promptly by thorough washing with soap and water. Eyes should be flushed thoroughly to remove residual chemicals.
- The use of aspirin is not recommended to control fever because salicylates also uncouple oxidative phosphorylation.
- Pentachlorophenol reduces both glomerular filtration rates and tubular function. An increased anion gap and a metabolic acidosis have been observed in acute pentachlorophenol poisoning.

- A typical odor of pentachlorophenol can be noted in the urine after a massive acute poisoning in addition to proteinuria, acetone, and an aminoacidosis.

Questions—Pentachlorophenol and Dinitrophenol

1. Which of the following is false?
A. Pentachlorophenol is used as a wood preservative, fungicide, and bactericidal agent.
B. Nitrophenolic and nitrocresolic compounds are aromatic nitro chemicals used as dyestuffs, chemical intermediaries, explosive agents and herbicides.
C. Pentachlorophenol produces a hypermetabolic state similar to that produced by dinitrophenol, leading to hyperpyrexia, cerebral edema, convulsions, and coma.
D. Dioxin-contaminated pentachlorophenol has led to several cases of chloracne in workers exposed to these solutions.
E. The hyperpyrexia induced by pentachlorophenol is effectively treated with salicylates.

DAMINOZIDE

Daminozide (Alar) has been widely used as a chemical plant growth regulator to retard growth and enhance color, particularly in apples. Studies in the 1970s suggested that daminozide was carcinogenic in animals. This effect appears largely due to its hydrolysis product 1,1-demethylhydrazine. In February 1989, the EPA stated that daminozide posed a significant risk of cancer in humans however a month later the EPA reversed its advice. Nonetheless, the manufacturer voluntarily withdrew the chemical from the United States market but is still selling it to the United Kingdom.

By 1990, the Food and Drug Administration and Consumers Union found little detectable daminozide on apples in the United States. There have been no confirmed cases of acute poisoning from ingesting legally applied pesticides on food. There have been no epidemiologic studies indicating an actual human cancer incidence following the use of daminozide on apples.

Questions—Daminozide

1. Daminozide (Alar) retards growth by enhancing color in apples.
A. True
B. False

2. Daminozide (Alar) has been definitively linked with cancer.
A. True
B. False

DITHIOCARBAMATES AND THIOCARBAMATES

In addition to their fungicidal applications, dithiocarbamates and thiocarbamates are used as rubber accelerators, vulcanizers, seed disinfectants, and insecticides. Compounds of this class usually have low acute toxicity. Critically ill patients probably suffer from the effects of the vehicle or another pesticide. Some members of this group (e.g., thiram) are structurally similar to disulfiram (Antabuse®) and patients rarely manifest the alcohol-disulfiram reaction to the above chemicals. The medical literature on human exposure to these compounds is scant, but studies in animals suggest that contact dermatitis and thyroid hyperplasia may occur after exposure.

Previously, dithiocarb was recommended as a chelator for thallium poisoning. Dithiocarb has been used to treat nickel dermatitis and nickel carbonyl poisoning. It is an investigational drug in the United States and is classified as an orphan drug. These compounds do not have the cholinergic properties of structurally related carbamate insecticides. The usual measures for gut and skin decontamination are recommended for large doses. Disulfiram-alcohol reactions usually last several hours and respond to fluids, oxygen, and analgesics. Dysrhythmias may develop, and patients with serious reactions should be monitored.

Questions—Dithiocarbamates and Thiocarbamates

1. Possible applications of dithiocarbamates include all of the following, except
A. Alcohol withdrawal
B. Nickel toxicity
C. Thallium toxicity
D. Rubber acceleration
E. Fungicide

METALDEHYDE

Metaldehyde is a molluscicide. European uses for metaldehyde include Meta-fuel tablets, which are portable energy products and equally common sources of poisoning. European metaldehyde concentrations in commercial molluscicides may reach 50%. During 1997 there were 402 exposures of metaldehyde reported to the American Association of Poison Control Centers National Data Collection System. Most reports concerned children less than 6 years and almost all were accidental. A small number exhibited life-threatening symptomatology. There were no deaths.

In the United States, metaldehyde formulations are limited to concentrations less than 4% by weight and occasionally contain other toxins such as carbaryl, arsenate, and organophosphates. Although serious metaldehyde poisonings are rare in the United States, several accidental and suicidal deaths resulting from ingestion of Meta-fuel tablets have been reported in Europe.

Pathophysiology

Metaldehyde is a tetramer composed of an eight-member ring containing aldehyde molecules. Metaldehyde rapidly hydrolyzes to acetaldehyde in the stomach, and has been postulated to cause seizures by affecting the concentration of the inhibitory central neurotransmitter GABA in the brain. As metaldehyde also increases monoamine oxidase activity and decreases central serotonin levels, formation of acetaldehyde may not be the sole mechanism of toxicity.

Clinical Presentations

Metaldehyde produces predominantly gastrointestinal and central nervous system effects such as nausea, vomiting, muscle spasms, salivation, seizures, and coma. Reported signs and symptoms include erythema and edema of the extremities, dermatitis, confusion, agitation, dilated pupils, fever, cyanosis, and respiratory distress. Mild symptoms resolve within 24 to 48 hours.

Laboratory

ANALYTIC METHODS

A gas chromatographic assay for use with plasma or urine has a sensitivity of 1 μg/mL for urine and 2 μg/mL for plasma.

BLOOD LEVELS

Ingestion of about 100 to 150 mg/kg of metaldehyde leads to peak serum levels 35 hours after ingestion and urine levels of 53 μg/mL in 14 hours. Acetaldehyde levels in the serum were less than 1.0 μg/mL.

Treatment

GUT DECONTAMINATION

Within the first several hours, gastric lavage and activated charcoal may be helpful. Syrup of ipecac is contraindicated. Casual contact with 4% metaldehyde products in asymptomatic children (i.e., a taste) probably requires no decontamination measures.

ELIMINATION ENHANCEMENT

Hemodialysis is probably not effective.

SUPPORTIVE MEASURES

- Maintenance of adequate oxygenation, control of seizures, and prevention of pulmonary aspiration are the major treatment goals in serious metaldehyde ingestions.
- Arterial blood gases should be followed closely and intubation performed as indicated.
- Seizures may persist despite the use of diazepam, phenobarbital and/or phenytoin. Paraldehyde should not be used as an anticonvulsant.

Questions—Metaldehyde

1. Which of the following is false?

A. Metaldehyde is a molluscicide.
B. Europeans have used a nontoxic form of metaldehyde called Meta-fuel as a portable energy product.
C. Most reports of metaldehyde exposure concern young children and accidental ingestions.
D. Although serious metaldehyde poisonings are rare, several accidental and suicidal deaths have been reported.
D. Metaldehyde rapidly hydrolyzes to acetaldehyde in the stomach, and has been postulated to cause seizures by affecting the concentration of GABA in the brain.

FUMIGANTS

INTRODUCTION

Fumigants are agents used to sterilize products. Agents used as fumigants include many chemical families. Examples include the hydrocarbons naphthalene and paradichlorobenzene. Halogenated hydrocarbons used as fumigants include methylene chloride, methyl bromide, chloroform, carbon tetrachloride, ethylene dichloride, ethylene dibromide, dichloropropene, dichloropropene plus dichloropropane, and dibromochloropropane. Many of these agents are described in Chapter 46, Hydrocarbons.

Other agents include oxides and aldehydes such as ethylene oxide, formaldehyde, propylene oxide, paraformaldehyde, and acrolein. Sulfur compounds used as fumigants include sulfur dioxide, sulfuryl fluoride, and carbon disulfide. Phosphorus compounds such as phosphine gas, and nitrogen compounds such as hydrogen cyanide and acrylonitrile also are used as fumigants. See Chapter 45, Airborne Toxins.

Naphthalene, methylene chloride, methylbromide, chloroform, carbon tetrachloride, ethylene dichloride, ethylene dibromide, dibromochloropropane, dichloropropane, paradichlorobenzene, ethylene oxide, formaldehyde, acrolein, sulfur dioxide, carbon disulfide, hydrogen cyanide, and acrylonitrile are discussed in other chapters.

PHOSPHOROUS COMPOUNDS

Aluminum Phosphide

Aluminum phosphide is used as a grain preservative. Fumigation depends on the release of phosphine gas from the aluminum phosphide when it encounters the moisture in grain. Oral aluminum phosphide is a commonly used agent for self-poisoning in India. In the presence of moisture in humans, aluminum phosphide releases phosphine, which can cause severe pulmonary edema. Taken orally, phosphine is liberated in the stomach causing gastrointestinal irritation and intractable peripheral circulatory failure. Occupational phosphine exposure also has occurred.

Phosphine Gas

Industrial exposures occur in the production of acetylene gas or when it is used as a doping agent for the manufacture of silicon crystals. Aluminum phosphide grain fumigants and zinc phosphide rodenticides release phosphine gas on contact with moisture, leading to fatalities. This gas has a garlic odor and causes severe GI symptoms. In severe cases coma, convulsions, hypotension, and pulmonary edema develop. Unlike arsine gas, phosphine gas does not produce hemolytic anemia.

Zinc Phosphide

Zinc phosphide produces immediate toxicity by the production of phosphine gas. Zinc phosphide has been used as a rodenticide. Signs and symptoms of toxicity include nausea, vomiting, dyspnea, and changes in mental status. Immediate death results from pulmonary edema. Delayed effects follow the absorption of phosphide and affect primarily the liver, heart, and kidneys. Delayed death may be a result of direct cardiotoxicity. Aggressive airway management and circulatory support are critical.

Pathophysiology

The exact mechanism of action of aluminum phosphide is not known. In animals, it induces a noncompetitive inhibition of mitochondrial cytochrome oxidase. Cytochrome C oxidase activity is likely inhibited primarily in the myocardium.

Clinical Presentations

ALUMINUM PHOSPHIDE

Following an ingestion of aluminum phosphide, patients will present with profuse vomiting and upper abdominal pain. Tachycardia, an altered sensorium, anemia, and pulmonary edema also may characterize clinical presentations. Intractable multisystem failure and shock is usually present. Death may occur within hours to days.

PHOSPHINE GAS

Symptoms from acute phosphine gas exposure generally are transient and findings are often absent on physical examination and laboratory tests. Patients with mild toxicity recover. Significant exposures can cause GI tract symptoms as well as respiratory, cardiovascular, and central nervous system changes resulting from metabolic changes. Prominent clinical manifestations of acute phosphine gas exposure include headache, fatigue, vomiting, cough, dyspnea, paresthesias, jaundice, ataxia, intention tremor, weakness, and diplopia.

On autopsy, fatal cases revealed centrilobular necrosis of the liver, congestive heart failure with pulmonary edema, and focal myocardial necrosis. If patients survive the initial 6 to 24 hours, the ARDS may supervene. If the patient reaches the hospital with significant hypotension, death is a probable outcome.

Workers engaged in fumigation of stored grains may report minor symptoms such as cough, dyspnea, chest tightness, headache, giddiness, numbness, lethargy, anorexia, and epigastric pain.

Toxic Dosage/Death

Phosphine concentrations in the work environment ranged from 0.17 to 2.11 ppm when workers involved in fumigation became ill. Clinical effects from phosphine may occur at levels below the olfactory threshold of 1.5 to 3 ppm. Less than 500 mg is a usual lethal dose of aluminum phosphide in India.

Laboratory

ANALYTIC METHODS

Phosphorous is measured by spectrophotometry.

BLOOD LEVELS

A normal phosphorous level in an adult man or woman is 2.5 to 5.0 mg/dL. Following blood levels after overdose has not been helpful in managing ill effects.

Treatment

GUT DECONTAMINATION

If fumigant liquid or solid has been ingested less than several hours prior to treatment, quantities remaining in the stomach should be removed as effectively as possible by gastric intubation, aspiration, and lavage after all possible precautions have been taken to protect the respiratory tract from aspirated gastric contents.

ELIMINATION ENHANCEMENT

Exchange transfusions are questionably effective. Hemodialysis is recommended only if renal failure develops.

SUPPORTIVE MEASURES

- Quickly evaluate the ABCs (**a**irway, **b**reathing, and **c**irculation). Rescuers should wear fully self-contained breathing apparatus and agent-specific protective clothing and gloves. Flush the victim with water. If gas is likely to be trapped in clothing (i.e., significant exposure in an enclosed area), remove and double-bag clothing.
- Treatment with fluids, bicarbonate, oxygen, and vasopressors has been unsuccessful in many patients with severe poisoning. Steroids appear to be ineffective. Vitamin E may prevent liver damage from phosphorus-induced lipoperoxidation, but this needs to be additionally studied.
- Pulmonary edema and shock are treated symptomatically. The ECG has revealed a subendocardial infarction in a few patients and occasional transient atrial fibrillation. ST elevation or depression, a wandering pacemaker, and heart block also have been observed.
- Laboratory tests generally include a complete blood count, electrolytes, BUN, creatinine, liver enzymes, calcium, magnesium, and blood gases.
- Clinical diagnosis can be confirmed by analysis of gastric aspirate or breath, both of which blacken a paper impregnated with silver nitrate.

Questions—Phosphorous Compounds

1. Which of the following is false?

A. Aluminum phosphide is used as a grain preservative.
B. In the presence of moisture, aluminum phosphide releases phosphine, which can cause pulmonary edema.
C. Phosphine gas has a pearlike odor and causes severe gastrointestinal symptoms.
D. Zinc phosphide produces immediate toxicity by the production of phosphine gas.
E. Zinc phosphide has been used as a rodenticide.

2. If patients survive the initial 6 to 24 hours, the adult respiratory distress syndrome may supervene after phosphine gas exposure.

A. True
B. False

CHLOROPICRIN

Chloropicrin was initially synthesized in 1848. It was used as a tear gas during World War I because of its irritant properties. Since 1917, it has been used as an insecticide and fumigant. Chloropicrin is used as a fumigant for cereals and grains and as a soil insecticide. A small amount of chloropicrin is added to other toxic, odorless fumigants or utilized as a prewarning gas in ship fumigation before introducing cyanogen gas. The water solubility of chloropicrin is very low and its toxicity appears to be intermediate between chlorine and phosgene. Less water-soluble agents such as chloropicrin tend to damage the lower respiratory tract.

Clinical Presentations

Human exposure results in lacrimation, cough, nausea, vomiting, and skin irritation. Aspirations can causes vomiting and choking. Pulmonary edema has caused death within hours.

Toxic Dosage/Death

A concentration of 15 ppm cannot be tolerated longer than 1 minute and exposure to 4 ppm for a few seconds is temporarily disabling because of its irritant effects. Concentrations of 0.3 to

0.37 ppm can lead to painful eye irritation in 3 to 30 seconds. Exposure to air containing 4 mg/L chloropicrin for a few seconds renders a soldier unfit for fighting and 15 mg/L results in respiratory tract injury. A lethal exposure in humans is approximately 119 ppm for 30 minutes, or 0.8 mL/L. Death usually results from pulmonary edema.

Laboratory

ANALYTIC METHODS

Gas chromatography-mass spectrometry has been used to identify chloropicrin.

BLOOD LEVELS

Following blood levels has not been reported as being helpful in guiding management.

Treatment

SUPPORTIVE MEASURES

- Treatment includes flushing contaminating fumigants from the skin and eyes with copious amounts of water for at least 15 minutes, removal to fresh air immediately, intravenous fluids, pressors, position change, and controlling seizures.
- Pulmonary edema is treated with diuretics, following blood gases and intubation, as required.

Questions—Chloropicrin

1. **Death from chloropicrin usually results from refractory seizure activity.**
   A. True
   B. False

ANSWERS

Organophosphates

1. E 2. A 3. E 4. B 5. E 6. E 7. B 8. B

Carbamates

1. A 2. A 3. E 4. B

Organochlorines

1. C 2. A 3. D 4. A 5. B

Diethyltoluamide

1. C

Pyrethrum and Pyrethroids

1. B 2. B

Sodium Monofluoroacetate

1. A

Strychnine

1. A 2. A 3. A

Vacor

1. C

Red Squill

1. B

Paraquat

1. D 2. A 3. A 4. B 5. B

Diquat

1. B

Chlorophenoxy Compounds and Dioxin

1. B 2. A 3. E 4. A 5. B 6. A

Chlorates

1. A 2. D

Glyphosate

1. D 2. A

Pentachlorophenol and Dinitrophenol

1. E

Daminozide

1. B 2. B

Dithiocarbamates and Thiocarbamates

1. A

Metaldehyde

1. B

Phosphorous Compounds

1. C 2. A

Chloropicrin

1. B

SELECTED READINGS

Introduction to Pesticides

1. Hayes WJ Jr. Toxicology of Pesticides. Baltimore: Williams and Wilkins, 1975, 317.
2. Murphy SD. Toxic effects of pesticides. In Klaassen CD, Amdur MO, Doull J (eds): Casarett and Doull's toxicology: The basic science of poisons, 3rd ed. NY: Macmillan, 1986.

Organophosphates

1. Coye MJ, Barnett PG, Midtling JE, et al. Clinical confirmation of organophosphate poisoning by serial cholinesterase analysis. Arch Intern Med 1987; 147:438–442.

2. Le Blanc FN, Benson BE, Gilg AD. A severe organophosphate poisoning requiring the use of an atropine drip. Clin Toxicol 1986;24:69–76.
3. Senanayake N, Karalliedde L. Neurotoxic effects of organophosphorus insecticides. N Engl J Med 1987;316:761–763.
4. Worrell C. The management of organophosphate intoxication. South Med J 1975;68:335–339.

Carbamates

1. Jackson RJ, Stratton JW, Goldman LR, et al. Aldicarb food poisoning from contaminated melons. California MMWR 1986;35:254–257.

Organochlorines

1. Coble Y, Hildebrant P, Davis J, et al. Acute endrin poisoning. JAMA 1967;202:489–493.
2. Davies JE, Dedhia HV, Morgade C, et al. Lindane poisonings. Arch Dermatol 1983;119:142–144.
3. Jaeger V, Podczeck A, Haubenstock A, et al. Acute oral poisoning with lindane solvent mixtures. Vet Hum Toxicol 1984;26:11–14.

Diethyltoluamide

1. De Garbino JP, Labrode A. Toxicity of an insect repellent: N-N-diethyltoluamide. Vet Hum Toxicol 1983;25:422–423.
2. Reuveni H, Yagupsky P. Diethyltoluamide-containing insect repellent; Adverse effects on worldwide use. Arch Dermatol 1982;118:582–583.

Pyrethrum and Pyrethroids

1. Flannigan SA, Tucker SB, Key MM, et al. Synthetic pyrethroid insecticides: A dermatological evaluation. Br J Ind Med 1985;42:363–372.
2. Wouters W, Van den Berken J. Review: Action of pyrethroids. Gen Pharmacol 1978;9:387–398.

Sodium Monofluoroacetate

1. Egekeze JO, Oehme FW. Sodium monofluoroacetate (SMFA, Compound 1080): A literature review. Vet Hum Toxicol 1979;21:411–416.

Strychnine

1. Gordon AM Jr, Richards DW. Strychnine intoxication. JACEP 1979;8:520–522.
2. McGuigan MA. Strychnine. Clin Toxicol Rev 1983;6(2):1–2.

Vacor

1. Johnson D, Kubie P, Levitt C. Accidental ingestion of Vacor rodenticide. Am J Dis Child 1980;134:161–164.
2. Prosser PR, Karam JH. Diabetes mellitus following rodenticide ingestion in man. JAMA 1978;239:1148–1150.

Paraquat

1. Bismuth C, Garnier R, Dally S, et al. Prognosis and treatment of paraquat poisoning: A review of 28 cases. J Toxicol Clin Toxicol 1982;19:461–474.
2. Crome P. Paraquat poisoning 1986. Lancet 1986;1:333–334.

Diquat

1. Mahieu P, Bonduelle Y, Bernard A, et al. Acute diquat intoxication: Interest of its repeated determination in urine and the evaluation of renal proximal tubule integrity. Clin Toxicol 1984;22:363–369.

Chlorophenoxy Compounds and Dioxin

1. Berwick P. 2,4-Dichlorophenoxyacetic acid poisoning in man. Some interesting clinical and laboratory findings. JAMA 1970;214:1114–1117.
2. Hoffman RE, Stehr-Green P, Webb KB, et al. Health effects of long term exposure to 2,3,7,8-tetrachlorodibenzo-p-dioxin. JAMA 1986;255:2031–2038.
3. Safe SH. Comparative toxicology and mechanism of action of polychlorinated dibenzo-p-dioxins and dibenzofurans. Am Rev Pharmacol Toxicol 1986; 26:371–399.
4. Stevens KM. Agent Orange toxicity: A quantitative perspective. Hum Toxicol 1981;1:31–39.
5. Wells WDE, Wright N, Yeoman WB. Clinical features and management of poisoning with 2,4-D and mecoprop. Clin Toxicol 1981;18:273–276.

Chlorates

1. Helliwell M, Nunn J. Mortality in sodium chlorate poisoning. Br Med J 1979;1:1119.
2. Steffen C, Wetzel E. Pathologic aspects of chlorate poisoning. (Abstr) Hum Toxicol 1985;4:541–542.

Glyphosate

1. Hoogheem TJ. The safety of Roundup pesticide. JAMA 1989;262:2679.
2. Jackson JR. Toxicity of herbicide containing glyphosate. Lancet 1988;1:414.
3. Tominack RL, Yang GY, Tsai WJ, Chung HM, Deng JF. Taiwan National Poison Center Survey of glyphosate-surfactant herbicide ingestions. Clin Toxicol 1991;29:91–109.

Pentachlorophenol and Dinitrophenol

1. Wood S, Rom WN, White GL, et al. Pentachlorophenol poisoning. J Occup Med 1983;25:527–530.

Daminozide

1. Alar withdrawn in US. Lancet 1989;1:145 (editorial).
2. Ames BN, Gold LS. Pesticides, risk and applesauce. Science 1989;224:755—756.

Dithiocarbamates and Thiocarbamates

1. Fishbein L. Environmental health aspects of fungicides. Dithiocarbamates. J Toxicol Environ Health 1976;1:713–735.

Metaldehyde

1. Booze TF, Oehme FW. Metaldehyde toxicity: A review. Vet Hum Toxicol 1985;27:11–19.

Phosphorous Compounds

1. Augenstein WL, Sokol R, Kulig K, Rumack BH. Phosphine poisoning: a report of six cases. Vet Hum Toxicol 1988;30:344.
2. Casteel SW, Bailey EM Jr. A review of zinc phosphide poisoning. Vet Hum Toxicol 1986;28:151–154.
3. Gupta S, Ahlawat S. Aluminum phosphide poisoning-a review. Clin Toxicol 1995;33:19–24.

Chloropicrin

1. Gonmonri K, Muto H, Yamamoto T, Takahashi K. A case of homicidal intoxication by chloropicrin. Am J Forensic Med Pathol 1987;8:135–138.

CHAPTER 49
Chemical Warfare

INTRODUCTION

Forms of chemical warfare include nerve gases, vesicants such as mustard gas, lacrimators, incapacitating agents, lung-damaging agents (e.g., choking agents such as phosgene and chlorine), and blood agents (e.g., cyanogens). Nerve agents (organophosphates) may be taken up by inhalation (e.g., during manufacturing and processing, during application of insecticides in agriculture, or during exposure as nerve agents on the battlefield), orally (e.g., in suicide attempts with insecticides), and percutaneously. See Chapter 48, Pesticides. Mustard gas is a vesicant that was first employed offensively by the German Army at Ypres, Belgium, on the evening of July 12, 1917. Vesicant agents act on mucous membranes, lungs, skin, and blood-forming organs. They incapacitate far more than they kill.

Lacrimators, or tear gases, are used routinely to control riots and may be utilized on the battlefield. Although generally incapacitating, death has only been reported from these agents in rare, isolated cases. See Chapter 45, Airborne Toxins. Incapacitating agents act on the central nervous system to produce incapacitation. Few are potent or safe, or possess the necessary physical and chemical properties to make them useful as potential chemical agents. Of these few, an atropinelike drug, quinuclidinyl benzilate (BZ), and lysergic acid diethylamide (LSD) have been identified as potential adjuncts to chemical warfare. BZ appears to block the action of acetylcholine both peripherally and centrally, but unlike atropine, it produces predominantly central rather than peripheral effects. High doses produce a delirium that renders one unable to perform tasks.

Lung-damaging agents were introduced in World War I. These heavier-than-air agents may be inhaled on the battlefield and cause incapacitating pulmonary edema and irritation. Although not widely used in war for many years, these agents may accompany the pyrolysis of plastics, and may be present in numerous industrial settings. Blood agents (e.g., cyanogens) produce their effects by interfering with oxygen utilization at the cellular level. Inhalation is the usual route of entry. The French initiated the use of cyanide agents in 1916 with the employment of shells filled with hydrogen cyanide. As cyanide is extremely volatile, its vapor was lighter than air and it was almost impossible to establish a lethal concentration in the field by this means of delivery. To overcome this problem, cyanogen chloride and cyanogen bromide were produced, whose vapors were heavier than air. See Chapter 45, Airborne Toxins.

Questions—Introduction to Chemical Warfare

1. **Mustard**
   A. Is primarily a lung-damaging agent
   B. Is primarily a blood agent
   C. Kills more people than it incapacitates
   D. Has only been used since the 1950s
   E. None of the above
2. **Blood agents**
   A. Have always been delivered in lethal concentrations
   B. Are delivered intravenously
   C. Are delivered via inhalation
   D. All of the above
   E. None of the above

NERVE AGENTS

Nerve agents, prepared for use in chemical warfare, are organophosphate compounds similar to the organophosphates used as pesticides (see Chapter 48, Pesticides). Exposure to very small amounts of certain nerve agents can induce severe muscarinic, nicotinic, and central nervous system effects that can lead to death.

The principal nerve agents are Tabun (GA), Sarin (GB), Soman (GD), and VX. The G agents are fluorine- or cyanide-containing organophosphates. In field concentrations, they are odorless. Clothing releases G agents for about 30 minutes after contact with vapor. The V agents are sulfur-containing organophosphorous compounds. They affect the body in essentially the same manner as G agents. The nerve agents are all viscous liquids, not nerve gas *per se*. The vapor pressure of the G-series nerve agents is sufficiently high for the vapors to be lethal rapidly. GB is largely a vapor hazard. VX is of such low volatility that it is mainly a liquid contact hazard. G agents spread rapidly on surfaces such as skin. VX spreads less rapidly.

Pathophysiology

Toxic manifestations and lethality following nerve agent exposure follow the irreversible phosphorylation of the serine-containing active site of the enzyme acetylcholinesterase. A variety of proteolytic enzymes also may be inhibited by organophosphates (e.g., chymotrypsin and trypsin). Minor changes in coagulation parameters (PT, APTT, and fibrinogen) are observed following soman poisoning in rabbits and significant changes are seen in alkaline phosphatase, calcium, and creatine phosphokinase activity.

Sarin can cause myonecrosis. Acetylcholine accumulation is involved in the calcium flux into skeletal muscle fibers during anticholinesterase poisoning. This phenomenon with organophosphate anticholinesterases may be linked to organophosphate-induced myopathy.

Clinical Presentations

MUSCARINIC EFFECTS

Muscarinic effects after moderate exposure include miosis, blurring of vision, eye pain on focusing, frontal headache, rhinorrhea, tightness in the chest, bronchoconstriction, increased secretions, cough, occasional nausea, and vomiting. Following systemic absorption, muscarinic effects become increasingly pronounced. Symptoms include prolonged wheezing, dyspnea, chest pain, bronchorrhea, cough, cyanosis, pulmonary edema, anorexia, vomiting, abdominal cramps, heartburn, diarrhea, tenesmus, and involuntary defecation. Other cholinergic signs such as sweating, increased salivation, increased lacrimation, bradycardia, and involuntary micturition may occur.

NICOTINIC EFFECTS

The appearance of moderate-to-severe muscarinic effects is followed by the increased appearance of nicotinic effects. These include involuntary muscular twitching, scattered muscular fasciculations, muscle cramps, fatigue, weakness, and ultimate paralysis. The skin may be pale, and blood pressure may rise from transitory vasoconstriction resulting from cholinergic stimulation of sympathetic ganglia and possibly from the release of epinephrine.

Fascicular twitching, which usually appears first on the eyelids and in the facial and calf muscles, may become generalized. Rippling movements are seen under the skin, and twitching movements appear in all parts of the body. This is followed by severe generalized muscular weakness, including the muscles of respiration. Respiratory movements become more labored, shallow, and rapid then slow and intermittent. Later respiratory muscle weakness may become profound and contribute to respiratory depression.

CENTRAL NERVOUS SYSTEM EFFECTS

Central respiratory depression may be a major cause of respiratory arrest. Other signs of central nervous system compromise include generalized weakness, seizures, loss of consciousness, coma, and hypotension. Delayed or chronic effects include giddiness, anxiety, restlessness, emotional lability, insomnia, headaches, tremor, depression, concentration difficulties, confusion, slowness of recall, slurred speech, and ataxia.

Answers to questions in shaded boxes appear at the end of the chapter.

CHRONIC EFFECTS

Nerve agents do not appear to cause mutations or cancer and probably do not damage fetuses or induce reproduction dysfunction. Agents GA and GB have caused delayed neuropathy in susceptible animals. Agent VX is not known to cause delayed neuropathy. Acute lethality is of more immediate concern than delayed neuropathy in the evaluation of exposed persons.

Specific Nerve Agent Exposures

SARIN

In March 1995, six people were killed and about 600 injured when poison fumes believed to be sarin overwhelmed rush-hour subway commuters in Tokyo. Passengers began coughing and complaining of headaches, diminished vision, and nausea. Several collapsed onto the floor. As trains pulled into stations, passengers staggered out onto the platforms and collapsed with bubbles coming from their mouths. In some cases, blood poured from their noses. In June 1994, seven people died in a mysterious case of gas poisoning in Matsumoto, Japan. Sarin also was blamed for that outbreak and the method of gassing was unclear.

SOMAN

Soman 25%, 1 mL, splashed into and around the mouth of a 33-year-old man. Signs and symptoms included coma, labored respirations, miosis, injected conjunctivae, oral and nasal secretions, trismus, nuchal rigidity, muscular fasciculations, hyperactive deep-tendon reflexes, and tachycardia. He was treated with atropine (20 mg over a 2-day period), pralidoxime chloride (2-PAM) 2 mg over 30 minutes in an intravenous (IV) infusion, oxygen, nasopharyngeal suction, and prochlorperazine for nausea. No detectable RBC-ChE was observed for 10 days. The patient recovered in about 1 week after a period of psychologic instability.

VX

Diarrhea and transient nausea can occur within 3 to 4 hours after VX 4.0 mg/kg is administered orally. RBC cholinesterase is depressed to 70% below normal values. Spontaneous recovery has occurred in some subjects within 24 to 48 hours. Pralidoxime chloride, 5 to 30 mg/kg, was administered 5 to 48 hours after VX and all subjects exhibited reactivation of 70% of the inhibited enzyme.

Subjects given 1.5 mg/kg intravenously experience lightheadedness, dizziness, nausea, and vomiting within 1 hour. An increase in heart rate and blood pressure is observed at 3 hours. RBC-ChE is depressed to 20% of normal in subjects with symptoms and to 28% of normal in subjects without symptoms. Spontaneous recovery is observed at 1% per hour over 70 hours.

Laboratory

ANALYTIC METHODS

A capillary column gas chromatography-mass spectrometry method is available for tabun determinations. Gas chromatography retention indices have been determined for 22 chemical warfare agents.

BLOOD LEVELS

Following blood levels of serious nerve agents is generally not time-effective. Following RBC cholinesterase levels is ultimately more meaningful in determining patient progress and the severity of initial poisoning.

Treatment

GUT DECONTAMINATION

Charcoal may be helpful in minor, oral ingestions. Perform gastric lavage as required. If water or food contaminated with a large amount of nerve agent has been ingested, colicky abdominal pain, substernal tightness, increased salivation, and possibly vomiting may occur within 30 minutes.

ELIMINATION ENHANCEMENT

Extracorporeal detoxification is not likely to be useful, as the Vd of these agents is high.

SUPPORTIVE MEASURES

- Move victim from the contaminated site. In cases of respiratory distress, treat with oxygen, endotracheal intubation, assisted ventilation, frequent airway suctioning, and positive end-expiratory pressure for severely hypoxic patients.
- Improve tissue oxygenation before atropine is begun to lessen risk of ventricular fibrillation.

COMMUNITY EMERGENCY RESPONSE

- Full-scale emergency response requires localization of the source of an agent, identification of a chemical warfare agent (e.g., tank truck, burning warehouse, and unidentified shell fragments), isolation of the agent by a trained response team that prevents access to the area and limits spread of the agent, neutralization, and evacuation.
- A "hot line," or clearly demarcated line dividing those considered "dirty" (contaminated) and those considered "clean," must be established. The line must be upwind from the accident and the medical first-aid facility is further upwind.
- Anyone crossing the "hot line" into the "dirty" area must wear protective clothing and must undergo decontamination before returning to the "clean" area. Anyone in the "dirty" area at the time of an accident should be decontaminated before passing to the "clean" area.
- Decontamination should be performed ideally by trained and protected emergency personnel, taking the utmost care to avoid self-contamination.

REMOVAL OF THE TOXIC COMPOUND

- Responders should protect themselves from contamination (protective mask, wearing rubber gloves, heavy rubber apron, or encapsulation). After percutaneous exposure, carefully remove clothes with appropriate protective clothing and shield.
- Any item removed from the patient should be maintained in the "dirty" area until it can be properly handled. Expendable materials should be burned or buried with a quantity of bleach slurry to ensure destruction of the agent. Burning will cause toxic vapors and protection of individuals in the vicinity and downwind must be borne in mind.
- Wash skin with soap and water. Alkalis and hypochlorite solutions inactivate nerve agents, including household bleach. At field medical units, a 0.5% solution of calcium hypochlorite has been used for removing nerve agent from the skin of some casualties.

OCULAR CONSIDERATIONS

- Do not use your fingers or gloved hand for holding the eyelids apart. Open the eyes as wide as possible, and pour water or saline solution slowly while tilting the head to one side.
- Keep the mouth closed to prevent absorption through the mucous membranes.

- If skin contamination occurs while flushing the eyes, then decontaminate the face with hypochlorite solution or another suitable solution.
- Ocular pain relief is obtained with local instillation of atropine ophthalmic ointment (1%) repeated every several hours as required for 1 to 3 days.

GAS MASKS

- The Gulf War in the Middle East provided Israel with a national experience on the effects of preparation for a chemical warfare attack. Seven people were reported to have died of asphyxia because of their failure to remove the protective plastic seal on gas mask filters.
- Transient hypoxia and syncope may be observed in those with cardiopulmonary disorders.
- A purpuric rash, "suction purpura," facial contact urticaria, and dermatographism was transiently experienced. Other effects included heightened anxiety, panic attacks, claustrophobia, hyperventilation, exacerbations of asthma, and angina.

PROPHYLAXIS

- Pyridostigmine pretreatment appears to protect guinea pigs from the lethal actions of soman and sarin, however pretreatment with pyridostigmine alone provides little or no protection against incapacitation or lethality induced by soman or sarin. See Pyridostigmine section below.
- Clonidine appears to protect animals against soman-induced acute and chronic toxicity, including the toxic behavioral, autonomic, and cardiovascular symptoms.
- Diazepam, when used with atropine-oxime mixture, affords considerable anticonvulsant protection against anticholinesterases.
- Neostigmine and pyridostigmine should be used only cautiously during the cholinergic phase or during any intermediate syndromes as they may produce definite and prolonged inhibition of plasma cholinesterase.

Antidotes

Over the past 50 years, a series of chemical countermeasures have been developed, including atropine, the oximes, and pyridostigmine. Atropine effectively ameliorates most muscarinic effects by itself, but has little effect on nicotinic effects such as muscle twitching and flaccidity. Oximes are useful in countering nicotinic effects, but do not function well without atropine. Pyridostigmine appears to assist in protecting the body against soman toxicity when given prophylactically, but is not effective as treatment by itself. Pyridostigmine is relatively ineffective for the treatment of poisoning with other nerve agents (e.g., tabun, sarin, and VX).

ATROPINE

United States soldiers carry three atropine autoinjectors, each containing 2 mg of atropine citrate. These autoinjectors permit rapid intramuscular (IM) injection of antidote through protective clothing and underlying garments. Medical personnel carry additional atropine autoinjectors and are trained to inject more atropine as required. Heart rate and pupil sizes are not reliable indicators of adequate atropinization. Atropine can be given as often as every 5 minutes until secretions are minimal and respirations are adequate. Some patients require 15 to 20 mg in the first 3 minutes after exposure. Atropine effects without nerve agent challenge last about 3 to 5 hours after 1 or 2 injections, and 12 to 24 hours after marked atropinization.

Labored breathing, including coughing, noisy breathing, wheezing, and gasping for air, indicates the need for administration of additional atropine. When adequate atropine has been given, labored breathing efforts will be relieved. Used alone, atropine has little influence on the mortality rates in potentially fatal apneic cases. Assisted ventilation in these cases is much more effective. The combination of adequate atropinization plus assisted ventilation is more effective in saving life than assisted ventilation alone.

OXIMES

2-PAM is used as an adjunct to atropine. 2-PAM may reduce the time required for assisted ventilations. It is administered to all symptomatic patients after a nerve gas exposure. Pralidoxime mesylate (P2S) is effective against the neuromuscular block in animals produced by sarin, but much less effective against the block produced by tabun. Pralidoxime as the chloride (2-PAM) or mesylate (P2S), is best administered in a dose of 30 mg/kg body weight over a 30-minute period every 4 to 6 hours, preferably by IV injection, but it also can be given by IM injection. Oxime concentrations over 4 μg/mL can be maintained for 3 to 6 hours after IM injections of 30 mg/kg of either oxime (chloride or mesylate). A suggested initial dose for children is 15 to 25 mg/kg and 15 mg/kg for infants.

Obidoxime is claimed on the basis of *in vitro* studies to be about 20 times more effective than pralidoxime in reactivating phosphorylated cholinesterase and to be capable of penetrating the blood-brain barrier. In cases of organophosphate poisoning in man, it appears to be about as effective as 2-PAM. See Oximes below, as well as Chapter 5, Antidotes and Chapter 48, Pesticides.

Questions—Nerve Agents

1. Nerve agents cause all of the following except
   A. Cancer
   B. Fascicular twitching
   C. Respiratory arrest
   D. Seizures
   E. Hypotension

2. Nerve agents
   A. Generally are odorless
   B. Are viscous liquids, not gases
   C. Spread rapidly on skin
   D. All of the above
   E. None of the above

3. Sarin is a nerve agent that
   A. Is not believed to have been used since the 1950s
   B. Is thought to have been used in the Japan subway exposure of 1995
   C. Has no published reports of presumed exposures
   D. Has been studied closely in search of a dose response curve
   E. None of the above

4. Soman exposure
   A. Has been associated with transient diarrhea and nausea
   B. Has been found to cause significant depression of RBC-cholinesterase
   C. Has never been survived by humans
   D. Has never been described in humans
   E. None of the above

5. **Following RBC cholinesterase levels in patients with nerve agent exposure**
   A. Helps determine patient progress
   B. Does not reflect severity of initial poisoning
   C. Is less timely than following blood levels of nerve agents
   D. A and B
   E. A and C

6. **Antidotes for nerve agent exposure include**
   A. Atropine and 2-PAM for all symptomatic patients
   B. Obidoxime
   C. Diazepam for seizure activity
   D. A and B
   E. All of the above

7. **Emergency response to nerve agent exposure should include**
   A. Skin washing with acid
   B. Mouth breathing to protect sensitive intranasal membranes
   C. Inactivation of the agent with alkalis and hypochlorite solutions
   D. Setting up a "clean area" where contaminated clothing can be cleaned
   E. All of the above

8. **Ocular pain from nerve agent exposure**
   A. Should be treated with dilute bleach
   B. Should be treated with water or saline
   C. Should be treated with atropine sulfate ointment
   D. Is not common so would suggest an alternate exposure
   E. None of the above

9. **Antidotes for nerve agent exposures**
   A. Include atropine for amelioration of nicotinic effects
   B. Include oximes for countering muscarinic effects
   C. Include pyridostigmine for treating acute symptoms
   D. All of the above
   E. None of the above

10. **Atropine autoinjection**
   A. May be performed through protective clothing
   B. Causes significant impairment when given without nerve agent challenge
   C. Should not be monitored by heart rate and pupil size
   D. All of the above
   E. None of the above

OXIMES

Pralidoxime chloride (2-PAM) is currently is the only oxime antidote approved by the Food and Drug Administration (FDA) for clinical use in organophosphate poisoning. 2-PAM appears to be useful in all types of organophosphate insecticide poisoning irrespective of the route of exposure.

Obidoxime (Toxogonin®) is claimed on the basis of *in vitro* studies to be about 20 times more effective than pralidoxime in reactivating phosphorylated cholinesterase and to be capable of penetrating the blood-brain barrier. In cases of organophosphate poisoning in man, it appears to be about as effective as 2-PAM. Obidoxime, although recommended by some governments (e.g., Israel) as a preferred oxime, may be hepatotoxic, may be less effective alone against soman, and is associated with some minor side effects that could render it a problem in military use.

Pathophysiology

Pralidoxime contains an oxime group that dissociates a nerve agent moiety from an acetylcholinesterase molecule, reactivating the enzyme and gradually restoring normal skeletal muscle function. Pralidoxime itself has little or no apparent central nervous system effects because it does not appear to cross the blood-brain barrier easily. Most oximes act largely at nicotinic receptor sites to normalize skeletal muscle activity and have little activity at muscarinic sites. They may greatly enhance the effects of atropine at muscarinic sites, however.

Pralidoxime counters inhibited acetylcholinesterase (AChE), exhibits hydrolytic power against the active inhibitor, and has a weak, direct, anticholinesterase effect. Its main effect remains the reversal of cholinergic effects at peripheral nicotinic sites. No oxime appears able to prevent the development of organophosphate-induced delayed neuropathy. 2-PAM alone, or with atropine, appears to reduce mortality following poisoning with organophosphate insecticides.

Pharmacokinetics

PRALIDOXIME

Absorption

- Oral doses of the oximes are relatively slow for use in emergencies, either military or civilian.

Distribution

- Titration of the IV dose of 2-PAM may be effective in patients who have breakthrough nicotinic symptoms (fasciculations) secondary to organophosphate poisoning while on IV bolus therapy.
- Pralidoxime is distributed widely in most body fluids and is not highly bound to plasma proteins.
- The volume of distribution of 2-PAM (central compartment) is 0.27 L/kg. The volume of distribution of pralidoxime mesylate or P2S (central compartment) is 0.20 L/kg.

Elimination

- Pralidoxime is excreted rapidly in the urine.
- The oral elimination half-life of P2S is about 94 minutes and the oral elimination half-life of 2-PAM is about 160 minutes after doses of 2 to 9 grams.
- The half-life of 2-PAM after 2.5 to 10 mg/kg IM is about 77 minutes. The IV half-life of P2S is about 84 minutes and that of 2-PAM is 78 minutes.

OBIDOXIME

Absorption

- After oral ingestion of 1 gram of obidoxime, plasma concentrations of about 1 μg/mL are obtained in 1 to 2 hours.
- Plasma levels of 4 μg/mL or more are reached with doses of 7 grams and above, levels at which subjects often note tightness in the cheeks, faces that feel numb, and coolness in the throat.

Distribution

- The apparent volume of distribution of obidoxime is 0.173 L/kg.

Elimination

- About 2.2% of an oral dose are excreted in the urine over 24 hours.

- The elimination half-life of obidoxime after oral use is 2.64 hours.
- After IV use, 68% of a dose is recovered in the urine.
- The elimination half-life of obidoxime after IV use is 1.20 hours.

Clinical Presentations

PRALIDOXIME

Following rapid parenteral infusions of higher doses (over 10 mg/kg) of the oximes (2-PAM, and P2S), pain at the site of injection, nausea, vomiting, diarrhea, headaches, dizziness, tachycardia, hypertension, nervousness, malaise, and blurred vision may be experienced. An increase in the amplitude of T-waves and an increase in the PR interval may accompany this on electrocardiographic tracings. At higher-than-therapeutic doses, pralidoxime may inhibit acetylcholinesterase and block neuromuscular transmission.

OBIDOXIME

Obidoxime intramuscular injections are often followed by pain at the site and a symptom complex consisting of a generalized "hot feeling" over the upper part of the body within several minutes of injection. At 5 to 15 minutes, this becomes localized to the face, with a feeling of tightness or numbness of the circumoral area. A hot feeling around the throat with a menthol taste is observed within 1 to 3 minutes of injection. All symptoms appear to subside within 1 to 2 hours.

Toxic Dosage/Death

Oral use of 8 to 9 grams of 2-PAM may induce diarrhea, anorexia, and malaise. At doses of 30 to 45 mg/kg, IV P2S causes a marked increase in both systolic and diastolic pressure.

Drug Interactions

Total clearance is depressed when 2-PAM is given with thiamine. Alkalinization with sodium bicarbonate appears to augment the protective efficacy of 2-PAM. Pralidoxime is more likely to be excreted in acid urine.

Pregnancy/Lactation

2-PAM is classified as pregnancy risk category C.

Treatment

- Treatment is primarily symptomatic and supportive.

Questions—Oximes

1. **Which of the following is/are approved by the FDA for clinical use in organophosphate poisoning?**
   A. Pralidoxime chloride (2-PAM)
   B. Obidoxime (Toxogonin®)
   C. Pralidoxime mesylate (P2S)
   D. All of the above
   E. A and C
2. **Obidoxime**
   A. Can penetrate the blood-brain barrier
   B. Is probably more effective than 2-PAM
   C. May be hepatotoxic
   D. All of the above
   E. A and C
3. **Pralidoxime**
   A. Contains an oxime that dissociates a nerve agent moiety from acetylcholinesterase molecules
   B. Counteracts central nervous system effects by crossing the blood-brain barrier
   C. Acts at muscarinic receptors to normalize skeletal muscle activity
   D. Enhances the effects of atropine at nicotinic sites
   E. A, C and D
4. **Only pralidoxime is able to prevent the development of organophosphate-induced delayed neuropathy.**
   A. True
   B. False

PYRIDOSTIGMINE

Pyridostigmine has been utilized as a pretreatment against possible nerve gas exposure. The use of atropine and the oximes may be insufficient for protection against the toxic effects of GD (soman), even if they are administered immediately after exposure. Even with good training and the ability to don a mask rapidly, some soldiers on a chemical battlefield may be at risk for absorbing up to five times the lethal dose of GD during an intense chemical attack.

Therefore, a preexposure treatment agent has been sought. Pretreatment is not effective against sarin and VX challenge. When used for soman challenge, it should be followed by atropine and an oxime. Pyridostigmine by itself does not provide protection without the use of these antidotes. It is an antidote "enhancer" rather than a "true" antidote. It appears to enhance the efficacy of the other antidotes within 1 to 3 hours of taking the first tablet. Maximal benefit appears to develop with time and may be reached when a tablet is taken every 8 hours.

Pathophysiology

The possible protective action of carbamates such as pyridostigmine appears to depend on the ability of the carbamate to reversibly inhibit about 20% to 40% of red blood cell acetylcholinesterase, forming a semistable carbamylated enzyme that then can spontaneously break down to liberate the enzyme. The fraction of the enzyme in the tissues that is carbamylated will be protected against phosphorylation by subsequent organophosphate poisoning.

The gradual decarbamylation of the enzyme, in parallel with the relatively rapid removal or destruction of the organophosphate, releases sufficient acetylcholinesterase to maintain life. Protection against soman-induced lethality is related to the degree of carbamylation of red blood cell AChE just before the challenge.

Pharmacokinetics

ABSORPTION

- The bioavailability of oral pyridostigmine is 7.6%.
- Peak plasma concentrations of 35-65 ng/ml after oral intake are reached in about 1.7 hours.

DISTRIBUTION

- After IV injection of pyridostigmine 2.5 mg, the plasma elimination half-life is 1.52 hours, the apparent volume of distribution is 1.43 L / kg, and the plasma clearance is 0.65 L / kg / hour.
- After oral administration of 120 mg, the elimination half-life is 1.78 hours, apparent volume of distribution 1.64 L / kg and plasma clearance 0.66 L / kg / hour.

ELIMINATION

- From 75% to 90% of the dose is excreted in the urine unchanged.

Clinical Presentations

Pyridostigmine poisoning is diagnosed by medical history, presence of cholinergic signs, response to atropine administration, and determination of serum cholinesterase activity. Patients with preexposure cholinesterase values in the upper normal range may exhibit a 60% inhibition of their cholinesterase activity and still have values above the lower limits of normal. Plasma cholinesterase levels may be reduced 30% to 50% before signs or symptoms are evident.

CHOLINERGIC CRISIS

Pyridostigmine overdosage may lead to a cholinergic crisis characterized by nausea, vomiting, diarrhea, excessive salivation and sweating, increased bronchial secretions, miosis, lacrimation, bradycardia or tachycardia, cardiospasm, bronchospasm, hypotension, incoordination, blurred vision, muscle cramps, weakness, fasciculation, and paralysis. At very high doses, agitation, restlessness, confusion, visual hallucinations, and paranoid delusions may be observed. Death may result from cardiac arrest or respiratory paralysis and pulmonary edema. Weakness in myasthenia gravis patients that begins approximately 1 hour after drug administration suggests overdosage. Edrophonium can be used to distinguish cholinergic crises from myasthenic crises.

BROMIDE INTOXICATION

Pyridostigmine bromide in sufficient doses can produce bromide intoxication characterized by a low or negative anion gap, falsely elevated serum chloride level, neurologic changes, headache, agitation, weakness, slurred speech, confusion, delusions, hallucinations, stupor, and coma. Dermatologic changes may include acnelike lesions on the face and trunk, and pyoderma gangrenosum-like lesions (bromoderma).

Toxic Dosage/Death

Pyridostigmine bromide, 30 mg orally, was self-administered every 8 hours by 41,650 soldiers in Israel while under threat of nerve agent attack for 1 to 7 days in January 1991. About half of those who ingested pyridostigmine noted physiologic changes that were not incapacitating such as increased flatus, abdominal cramps, soft stools, and urinary urgency. Headaches, rhinorrhea, diaphoresis, and tingling of the extremities occasionally were observed. Less than 0.1% had effects sufficient to discontinue the drug. A few noted acute elevations in blood pressure.

Drug Interactions

Antimuscarinics such as atropine, glycopyrrolate, and scopolamine are antagonizers of pyridostigmine action. Thiopental may enhance the ability of pyridostigmine to precipitate bronchospasm. It also may potentiate the bradycardia and drop in cardiac output and blood pressure occasionally observed with pyridostigmine. Diazepam used as an anesthetic induction agent may enhance the cardiovascular depressant effects of pyridostigmine shock. Pyridostigmine reverses the neuromuscular blocking effect of neuromuscular blockers. Isoflurane use in a pyridostigmine-treated patient may decrease the requirement for succinylcholine. Pyridostigmine inhibits the enzyme (i.e., plasma cholinesterase) that hydrolyzes ester-type local anesthetics, prolonging their action.

Pregnancy/Lactation

Pregnancy risk category C. Pyridostigmine is excreted into breast milk however is felt to be compatible with breast-feeding by the American Academy of Pediatrics.

Laboratory

ANALYTIC METHODS

Pyridostigmine is identified and quantitated by high-performance liquid chromatography.

BLOOD LEVELS

Studies in patients with pyridostigmine overdose suggest that no clear correlation exists between the extent of cholinesterase inhibition and the incidence and severity of cholinergic signs. Clinical recovery appears to precede the spontaneous recovery of the enzyme.

Treatment

GUT DECONTAMINATION

Charcoal may be helpful in overdose. As patients may develop increased secretions and breathing difficulties, a protected airway is a vital consideration.

ELIMINATION ENHANCEMENT

There is no data supporting the use of hemodialysis in pyridostigmine overdose.

SUPPORTIVE MEASURES

- The treatment of patients with carbamate poisoning consists of general supportive care, including establishment of an airway, stabilization of vital signs, and use of atropine as indicated.

Antidotes

An antimuscarinic (e.g., atropine) is the drug of choice for pyridostigmine overdose. In adults, an initial intravenous dose of 2 mg of atropine given every 5 to 30 minutes may be required to reach atropinization. If poisoning is moderate, 1 to 4 doses may be sufficient.

Questions—Pyridostigmine

1. Pyridostigmine

A. Has been used as a pretreatment against possible nerve gas exposure
B. Does not provide protection without the use of other antidotes
C. Is not effective against sarin and VX
D. All of the above
E. A and C

2. **The possible protective action of carbamates such as pyridostigmine appears to depend on its ability to reversibly inhibit about 20% to 40% of red blood cell acetylcholinesterase, forming a semistable carbamylated enzyme that can spontaneously break down to liberate the enzyme.**
   A. True
   B. False
3. **Pyridostigmine overdose may lead to a cholinergic crisis characterized by**
   A. Nausea, vomiting, diarrhea
   B. Excessive salivation and sweating
   C. Blurred vision
   D. Paralysis
   E. All of the above
4. **Pyridostigmine bromide can produce bromide intoxication characterized by a low or negative anion gap, acnelike lesions, headache, agitation, weakness, slurred speech, confusion, delusions, hallucinations, stupor, and coma.**
   A. True
   B. False

VESICANT AGENTS

The German Army at Ypres, Belgium, first employed mustard gas, on July 12, 1917. From 1917 until the end of World War I, British casualties from mustard gas amounted to at least 125,000 with about 1,859 deaths. In World War II, no chemical agents were used, but from 1945 to 1948, large stockpiles of chemical weapons, including mustard gas, were dumped into the Baltic Sea. Corrosion ultimately weakened these containers and some shells broke when they were hauled onto fishing trawlers in 1984, leading to mustard-gas poisoning of 23 fishermen. Mustard gas also appears to have been used by Iraqi forces during the Iran-Iraq conflict.

Vesicant, or blister, agents act on the eyes, mucous membranes, lungs, skin, and blood-forming organs. They incapacitate far more people than they kill. Sulfur and nitrogen mustards are insidious in action, with little or no pain at the time of exposure. Signs of injury may not appear for hours.

Pathophysiology

Mustards are powerful alkylating agents and react with amino, thiol, carboxyl, hydroxyl, and primary phosphate groups. Because of its alkylating and electrophilic properties, mustard gas is able to change the structure of nucleic acids, cellular membranes, and proteins. Mustard gas causes a cross-linking of the two complementary strands in the DNA molecule. This cross-linking prevents the separation of the strands required for normal replications of the DNA molecule and so interferes with DNA syntheses and cellular division. Mustard gas may induce long-term mutagenic and carcinogenic changes.

Clinical Presentations

SULFUR MUSTARDS

Mustard gas (either vapor or liquid) causes damage to the skin, eyes, respiratory system, and gastrointestinal tract, as well as having a general effect on the body similar to that of radiation.

Dermatologic Effects

Different skin effects appear at different points following significant exposure. Erythema may appear at 1 hour. Raised erythema (edema) may appear at 2 to 3 hours. Pinhead vesication appears in 13 to 22 hours, vesicles coalescing into blisters at 16 to 48 hours, and maximum blisters or necrosis appear at 42 to 72 hours. The skin denudes in 6 to 9 days, and healing may take up to a month.

Ocular Effects

Initial gas exposure causes no symptoms, but after a delay of 4 to 6 hours, conjunctival irritation, lacrimation, photophobia, dryness, pain, blepharospasm, and corneal ulceration may develop. The periocular area may become red and edematous. In severe cases, blindness may occur. Recovery from a mild conjunctivitis may take 1 to 2 weeks, from a severe conjunctivitis, 2 to 5 weeks, and from mild corneal involvement, 2 to 3 months. A delayed keratopathy may develop decades later.

Respiratory Effects

After a delay of 24 hours, inhalation of the gas initially produces hoarseness, which may progress to loss of voice. Cough, fever, dyspnea, rhonchi, and rales may develop. Pneumonia frequently intervenes and symptoms may persist for years.

Gastrointestinal Effects

Ingestion of food or water contaminated by liquid mustard can produce nausea, vomiting, pain, bloody diarrhea, and prostration resulting from dehydration.

Systemic Effects

Dizziness, anorexia, lethargy, and general malaise may follow exposure. Fatalities may follow severe exposure and are largely a result of respiratory complications.

Long-Term Effects

Eye problems and recurrent bronchopneumonia may persist for many months. Exposure of human research subjects to mustard gases during World War II led to asthma, chronic bronchitis, emphysema, chronic laryngitis, corneal opacities, chronic conjunctivitis, and ocular keratitis. Other long-term effects may include respiratory cancer (especially nasopharyngeal, laryngeal and lung), skin cancer, pigmentation abnormalities of the skin, chronic skin ulceration and scar formation, recurrent ulcerative disease of the eye (including opacities), bone marrow depression, psychologic disorders, and sexual dysfunction.

Studies of workers in British mustard-gas manufacturers suggest an increased death rate from respiratory tract malignancies. An increased death rate from respiratory tract malignancies also has been observed in Japanese and German mustard gas factories. Only a marginal increase in lung cancer was found in exposed servicemen from the United States 46 years later.

NITROGEN MUSTARDS

In single exposures, nitrogen mustards irritate the eyes in doses that do not significantly damage the skin or respiratory tract. Ingestion of 2 to 6 mg of nitrogen mustard may result in nausea and vomiting.

Respiratory Effects

Symptoms and signs may be similar to those following exposure to mustard gas. Residual effects may include a persistent cough and low-grade fever for a few weeks. Severe exposures may terminate in a fatal pneumonia.

Systemic Effects

Nitrogen mustard exposure following absorption from the skin, respiratory tract, or gastrointestinal tract may exert profound effects on hematopoietic and lymphoid tissue. Degenerative bone marrow changes may be detected within 12 hours and may progress to severe aplasia. There may be leukocytosis for a few hours, followed by severe lymphopenia, granulocytopenia, thrombocytopenia, and a moderate anemia.

ARSENICAL VESICANTS

Arsenical vesicants are more dangerous as liquids than as vapors. As liquids, they cause severe burns of the eyes and skin. These agents are chlorinated arsine compounds. Dichloroarsine is also known as lewisite. Pulmonary edema, diarrhea, restlessness, weakness, hypothermia, and hypotension have been observed in animals.

Dermatologic Effects

Stinging pain usually is felt in 10 to 20 seconds after contact with liquid arsenical vesicants. In a few minutes, it becomes a deep, aching pain. In about 5 minutes, a gray area of dead epithelium appears, resembling that seen in corrosive burns. The pain lessens in 48 to 72 hours. Erythema and blisters are similar to the other vesicants. If the arsenical vesicant burn is large and deep, there may be considerable necrosis of tissue, gangrene, and slough.

Ocular Effects

Liquid arsenical vesicants cause severe damage to the eye, including the cornea, iris, and conjunctivae, which may terminate in permanent damage or blindness.

Respiratory Effects

Respiratory lesions are similar to those following mustard gas. Pulmonary edema and pleural effusion may be observed.

PHOSGENE OXIME

Phosgene oxime (CX or dichloroformoxime) has a disagreeable penetrating odor. CX is very irritating to the mucous membranes of the eyes and nose. Within 30 seconds, exposure to liquid or vapor can produce pain and skin necrosis at the site of contact. The original blanched area becomes brown in 24 hours, followed by eschar formation in 1 week. The eschar sloughs in about 3 weeks. Healing may be delayed for several months.

Laboratory

ANALYTIC METHODS

A method for quantitation of exposure to mustard gas was used to test urine samples of Iranian patients, victims of an alleged mustard-gas attack in March 1984. The method analyzes thiodiglycol in the urine. The method is sensitive to 1 ng/mL. Thiodiglycol values also may be obtained from skin analysis. Unmetabolized mustard gas has been analyzed by a gas chromatography-mass spectrometry method.

BLOOD LEVELS

Urine thiodiglycol levels found in Iranians ranged from 5 to 336 ng/mL in one study and from 1 to 30 ng/mL in another.

Treatment

SULFUR MUSTARD

Skin Considerations

- If erythema has not appeared, areas of skin contamination may be decontaminated with immediate use of wipes containing hydroxyethane 72%, phenol 10%, sodium hydroxide 5%, ammonia 0.2%, and water and a pad impregnated with chloramine B.
- Cut away and discard hair contaminated with liquid mustard. If the above substances are not available, use 0.5% aqueous sodium hypochlorite solution for decontamination of the skin and hair. Wash off the decontaminating solutions within 3 to 4 minutes, if possible.
- If erythema of the skin has appeared, soap and water is the best decontaminant. If mild, no treatment is required. If pruritus exists, use topical steroid creams or calamine lotion containing 1% each of phenol and menthol.
- Contaminated clothing should be removed promptly outside the treatment facility to prevent more severe burns and to lessen the vapor hazard to patients and attendants.
- If blisters have been broken after mustard exposure, remove the ragged roof and if not broken, drain under aseptic conditions. Clean the area with tap water or saline with application of petrolatum gauze when the areas are small. For large blisters, apply a thick layer of 10% mafenide acetate or silver sulfadiazine burn cream. Appropriate antibiotic drugs may be given locally or systemically as indicated.
- Antihistamines or opioids may not control intense burning pain during skin healing. Considerable relief has been observed with the use of carbamazepine 200 mg three times daily.

Ocular Considerations

- Self-aid should be performed within 2 minutes of exposure. Sterile petroleum jelly may be used to prevent the lid margins from sticking together.
- Mild mustard conjunctivitis lesions may require little treatment. A steroid antibiotic eye ointment can be applied. Ophthalmic ointment such as 5% boric acid ointment will provide lubrication and minimal antibacterial effects.
- If injuries are more severe, edema of the lids, photophobia, and blepharospasm may obstruct and alarm the patient. The lids may be gently forced open to provide assurance that the patient is not blinded. Pain is controlled by systemic narcotic analgesics.
- Severe photophobia and blepharospasm are treated with one drop of atropine sulfate solution (1%) instilled in the eye three times daily. To prevent infection, a few drops of 15% solution of sodium sulfacetamide should be instilled every 4 hours. Other antibacterial ointments may be substituted.
- Do not bandage the eye. The lids should not be allowed to stick together. Dark glasses or an eyeshade may be worn for photophobia.

Respiratory Tract Considerations

- Mild respiratory tract injury with hoarseness and sore throat only, usually requires no treatment. Cough may be relieved by codeine-containing cough syrups. Laryngitis and tracheitis may be treated symptomatically with steam or sterile cool mist inhalations. For more severe respiratory tract injury, hospitalize.
- Treat chemical pneumonitis initially with broad-spectrum antibiotics. Perform culture and sensitivity studies on sputum. Use appropriate specific antibiotics.

- Severely affected patients may need assisted ventilation and oxygen enriched air.

Systemic Mustard Poisoning

- Atropine subcutaneously (0.4 to 0.8 mg) may be useful in reducing gastrointestinal activity.
- Discomfort and restlessness may be treated with sedatives, but also may be a manifestation of hypovolemic shock from severe systemic injury.
- If severe systemic poisoning is present (i.e., manifested by vomiting, diarrhea, leukopenia, hemoconcentration, and/or shock), maintain adequate nutritional status and replace loss of fluid and electrolytes. Monitor leukocytes and hemoglobin.
- IV sodium thiosulfate, 35 grams or 500 mg/kg, if given within 20 to 30 minutes of exposure, may prevent or reduce damage from mustard gas. However, mustard gas is an alkylating agent that binds strongly to proteins, and it is unlikely that sodium thiosulfate will be very effective after a severe exposure.
- Most patients exposed to mustard gas recover completely. Only a small proportion will have long-term eye or lung damage.

NITROGEN MUSTARD

Skin Considerations

- Liquid nitrogen mustards are absorbed through the skin slower than mustard gas.
- Decontamination should be performed within 2 to 3 hours of exposure even if erythema is already present and no liquid nitrogen mustard is visible on the skin.

Ocular Considerations

- Treat as with mustard gas. Lesions and symptoms may be more severe than with mustard and frequent instillations of atropine may be required for pain from ciliary spasm.

Respiratory Tract Considerations

- Treat as for sulfur mustard gas exposure.

Systemic Nitrogen Mustard Poisoning

- Frequent hematologic evaluations (i.e., hematocrit, peripheral blood counts, and platelets) will be required. Vomiting and diarrhea will require IV fluids with electrolyte or volume expanders.
- Isolate against infection. Use antibiotics vigorously as indicated.
- Use sedatives, opiates, and atropine as indicated.

ARSENICAL VESICANTS

Skin Considerations

- If seen before actual vesication has occurred, dimercaprol (BAL) ointment should be tried. BAL is rubbed in with the fingers, allowed to remain at least 5 minutes, and then washed off with water.
- BAL may cause temporary stinging, itching, or urticarial wheals. Treatment of erythema, blisters, and denuded areas is similar to that for mustard lesions.
- For larger skin area exposure (over 20% of body surface area or less than 20% if deep lesions) hospitalization is required. Debride wound, treat with 10% mafenide acetate burn cream or silver sulfadiazine burn cream.

Ocular Considerations

- Treatment is largely symptomatic. Occlusive dressings or pressure should be avoided.
- Atropine ointment, sulfacetamide solution, and sterile petrolatum may be applied as indicated.

Systemic Arsenical Vesicant Poisoning

- Systemic treatment with BAL is indicated in patients with cough, dyspnea, frothy sputum, and signs of pulmonary edema. It also is indicated for patients with significant skin burn.
- Treatment includes local dimercaprol ointment and intramuscular injection of BAL in oil (10%).
- Further trials are required with newer analogues of BAL, meso-dimercaptosuccinic acid, and the sodium salt of 2,3 dimercapto-1-propanesulfonic acid.

PHOSGENE OXIME

- If possible, flood the contaminated area as soon as possible with copious amounts of water. See sulfur mustard gas decontamination.

Antidotes

There are no specific antidotes for mustard agent poisoning. Exposure to lewisite can effectively be countered by treatment with British anti-lewisite after time lapses of as much as 1 hour.

Questions—Vesicant Agents

1. Vesicant or blister agents
- A. Act on the eyes, mucous membranes, lungs, skin, and blood-forming organs
- B. Kill more than they incapacitate
- C. Generally cause extreme pain at the time of exposure
- D. All of the above
- E. B and C

2. Mustards
- A. Are powerful alkylating agents
- B. Change the structure of nucleic acids, cellular membranes, and proteins
- C. May induce long-term mutagenic and carcinogenic changes
- D. All of the above
- E. B and C

3. Sulfur mustard exposure
- A. Causes profound conjunctival irritation, initially
- B. Causes pinhead vesication within an hour
- C. Causes fever and dyspnea within minutes
- D. Causes refractory seizures in high doses
- E. None of the above

4. Which of the following is false?
- A. Nitrogen mustard exposure following absorption from the skin, respiratory or gastrointestinal tracts may exert profound effects on hematopoietic and lymphoid tissue.
- B. Arsenical vesicants are more dangerous as vapors than as liquids.
- C. Dichloroarsine also is known as lewisite.

D. Liquid arsenical vesicants cause severe damage to the eye, including the cornea, iris, and conjunctivae, which may terminate in permanent damage or blindness.
E. Phosgene Oxime liquid or vapor can produce pain and skin necrosis at the site of contact within 30 seconds.

ANSWERS

Introduction To Chemical Warfare

1. E 2. C

Nerve Agents

1. A 2. D 3. B 4. B 5. A 6. E 7. C
8. C 9. E 10. D

Oximes

1. A 2. E 3. A 4. B

Pyridostigmine

1. D 2. A 3. E 4. A

Vesicant Agents

1. A 2. D 3. E 4. B

SELECTED READINGS

Introduction to Chemical Warfare

1. Corupton JAF. Military chemical and biological agents. Clinical and toxicology properties. Caldwell, NJ: Telford Press; pp. 253–335.
2. Diller WF. Therapeutic strategy in phosgene poisoning. Toxicol Ind Health 1985;1:93–99.
3. Vick JA, Froehlich H. Treatment of cyanide poisoning. Milit Med 1991; 156:330–339.

Nerve Agents

1. Minton N, Murray SG. A review of organophosphate poisoning. Med Toxicology 1988;3:350–375.
2. Sidell FR. Clinical considerations in nerve agent intoxication. In: Somani SM, ed. Clinical warfare agents. San Diego: Academic Press, 1992; pp. 155–194.

Oximes

1. Barr SJ. Chemical warfare agents. Top Emerg Med 1985;7(1):62–70.
2. Marrs TC. Toxicology of oximes used in treatment of organophosphate poisoning. Adverse Drug React Toxicol Rev 1991;10:61–72.

Pyridostigmine

1. Almog S, Winkler E, Amitai Y, Dani S, Shefi M, Tirosh M, Sherner J. Acute pyridostigmine overdose: A report of nine cases. Isr J Med Sci 1991;27: 659–663.
2. Barr SJ. Chemical warfare agents. Top Emerg Med 1985;7(1):62–70.
3. Gunderson CH, Lehmann Cr, Sidell FR, Jabbai B. Nerve agents. A review. Neurology 1992;42:946–950.

Vesicant Agents

1. Newman-Taylor AJ, Marris AJR. Experience with mustard gas casualties. Lancet 1991;337:242.
2. Schonwald S. Mustard gas. The PSR Quarterly 1992;2(2):92–97.
3. Wormser U. Toxicology of mustard gas. Trends Pharmaceut Sci 1991; 12:164–167.

ACKNOWLEDGMENT

Thanks to Alison Deutsch, MD for contributing many of the questions in this chapter.

CHAPTER 50
Radiation Toxicology

RADIATION POISONING

INTRODUCTION

Radiation is characterized as either ionizing or nonionizing. Ionizing radiation disrupts neutral atoms by dislodging orbital electrons. Ion pairs, consisting of a dislodged electron and the residual atom, are formed when this occurs. Ion pairs are chemically reactive and may produce toxic agents, such as free radicals, which can interfere with cell processes. Nonionizing radiation does not dislodge orbital electrons and does not destroy the physical integrity of an impacted atom.

IONIZING RADIATION

Ionizing radiation is part of the natural environment. Since the discovery of x-rays and radioactivity, it has become part of the work environment as well. Background radiation varies between 100 and 1,000 mrad per year. Maximum annual permissible total body dose by radiation standard for the general public is 500 mrad. Radiation workers are permitted to receive a dose ten times higher (e.g., 5,000 mrad). Radiation exposure from television sets, watch and clock dials, and reactors are several orders of magnitude below background.

Ionizing radiation is used in (a) diagnostic radiology, including diagnostic x-ray, fluoroscopy, angiography, dental radiography, and computerized axial tomography (CAT) scanners; (b) therapeutic radiology; (c) dermatology; (d) nuclear medicine in diagnostic and therapeutic procedures; and (e) radiopharmaceutical laboratories.

Absorbed Dose

The amount of radiation that the body absorbs.

α Particles

An ionized helium nucleus (2 protons and 2 neutrons). α particles usually have energies of 4 to 8 million electron volts (MeV). They travel a few centimeters in air and up to 60 μm into tissue. The high energy and short path result in a dense track of ionization along the tissues with which the particles interact. They can be stopped by a thin sheet of cardboard because of their relatively large mass. α particles will not penetrate the skin, and thus are not an external hazard. However, if α-emitting elements are inhaled, ingested, or absorbed through open wounds, serious problems such as cancer may develop. Radium implants are examples of α particle emitters.

β Particles

β particles interact much less readily with matter than do α particles and will travel up to a few centimeters into tissue or many meters through air. Exposure to external sources of beta particles is potentially hazardous, but internal exposure is more hazardous.

Curie

A measure of a substance's radioactivity. 1 curie (Ci) = 3.7 × 1,010 disintegrations per second.

Exposure

The amount of radiation to which the body is exposed.

γ Rays

Are electromagnetic energy emitted from an atom's nucleus. They have a range of many meters in air and many centimeters in tissue and, like β particles, constitute a biologic hazard both internally and externally.

Millirem (MREM)

Is equivalent to 10^{-3} rem. 1 mrem = 0.01 mSV (millisievert).

Protons

Protons are produced by high-energy accelerators and are quite effective in producing tissue ionization. The path length of a proton is somewhat longer than that of an α particle of equivalent energy.

Rad

Acronym for radiation absorbed dose. A unit that measures the absorbed dose of ionizing radiation. 1 Rad = 100 ergs/gm = 0.01 Gray (Gy).

Radioactive Half-Life

The time required for the radioactivity of an isotope to decrease by 50%.

Rem

Acronym for roentgen equivalent man. The dosage of any ionizing radiation that will cause biologic injury to human tissue equal to the injury caused by 1 roentgen of x-ray or gamma-ray dosage. 1 rem = 0.01 sievert (SV).

Roentgen

Unit of measure for quantity of ionization produced by x-radiation or γ radiation. 1 Roentgen = 2.58×10^{-4} coulomb/kg.

X-Rays

Electromagnetic energy emitted from displaced electrons. X-rays generally have longer wavelengths, lower frequencies, and lower energies than gamma rays. The biologic effects of x-rays and gamma rays are better known than those of any of the other forms of ionizing radiation. X-rays may be encountered during the use of electronic tubes and electron microscopes.

Questions—Ionizing Radiation

1. **Radiation is measured by**
   A. Measuring the charge that it emits
   B. Measuring the light that it emits
   C. Measuring the mutations that it causes (long term)
   D. Measuring the toxic effects that it produces (short term)
2. **Which of the following does not employ ionizing radiation?**
   A. CT scanners
   B. Diagnostic nuclear medicine
   C. Angiography
   D. Ultrasound

RADON

Radon is an odorless, colorless, inert, gaseous element produced during the decay of uranium and ultimately radium, a ubiquitous element found in rock and soil. The US Environmental Protection Agency (EPA) suggests that homes should be tested for radon. Radon passes into the home through cracks in solid floors, construction joints, cracks in walls, gaps in suspended floors, gaps around service pipes, cavities inside walls, and the water supply. Radon's half-life, 3.8 days, provides sufficient time for it to diffuse through soil and into homes, where further disintegration produces more chemically and radiologically active radon progeny, so-called "radon daughters."

These radon progeny include four isotopes with half-lives less than 30 minutes, and are the major source of human exposure to α radiation. α radiation can cause cellular transformation in the respiratory tract, which may result in lung cancer. The EPA estimates that approximately 14,000 deaths annually in the United States are the result of lung cancer caused by indoor radon exposure. It also has been estimated that approximately 14% of all current cases of lung cancer are attributable to radon.

Underground uranium mines found throughout the world pose the greatest risk because of their high concentration of radon. Iron ore, potash, tin, gold, zinc, and lead mines also have been found to have significant levels of radon. Radon exposure causes no acute or subacute health effects, no irritating effects, and has no warning signs at levels normally encountered in the environment.

The only established human health effect currently associated with residential radon exposure is lung cancer. Factors that may intensify human exposure risks from radon include cigarette smoking, job-related radiation exposures, high ambient radon levels, a long duration of exposure, and a high average minute ventilation (e.g., children). Even conservative estimates suggest that radon is one of the most important environmental causes of death.

Questions—Radon

1. **Radon's primary effect on humans is**
   A. It causes gastrointestinal cancers.
   B. It causes lung cancer by direct γ radiation when it is inhaled.

Answers to questions in shaded boxes appear at the end of the chapter.

C. It causes lung cancer primarily by diffusing from uranium mines.
D. It causes lung cancer by disintegrating into daughter products, which are inhaled.

2. **Which is true?**
   A. Radon causes no short-term health effects.
   B. Radon causes a negligible amount of lung cancers.
   C. Radon is difficult to detect in the environment at any level.
   D. Radon is a form of radium.

RADIATION ACCIDENTS

A radiation accident is defined as an uncontrolled exposure to radiation or radioactive materials causing injury or contamination. Radiation accidents have been rare in the past, but with the increasing use of ionizing radiation in industry, research, power production, defense, and in the diagnosis and treatment of disease, the possibility of an increased number of injuries associated with radiation exists. Selected examples of radiation accidents include the mishandling and/or misadministration of therapeutic or diagnostic radionuclides; careless use or loss of radiography sources; failure of safety-systems in x-ray or γ-ray producing devices; and, in very rare instances, release of radioactive materials in transportation accidents. There are four general types of radiation accidents involving humans.

Irradiation

A type of radiation accident in which the victim has been irradiated by penetrating radiation to the whole body or some part of the body. The irradiated patient may have been exposed to electromagnetic radiation from an x-ray machine, an accelerator, or from a sealed source containing a γ emitter. Sources of high-energy electrons (betatrons) also can produce this type of injury. Exposure may be to a part of the body or to the whole body.

External Contamination

A type of radiation accident in which the victim has received surface contamination with radionuclides. The victim who has been contaminated by radionuclides in an accident may, depending on the degree of contamination, be cared for with strict isolation precautions to prevent the transfer of radionuclides to other personnel or other areas of the hospital. The contaminant can be in the form of liquids or particulate matter. The latter may range from powdery, invisible substances to large particles. The contaminant can consist of radionuclides that emit particulate radiation (α or β radiation), or electromagnetic radiation (x-rays, γ rays), or combinations of these.

Internal Contamination

Radiation accidents in which victims have been contaminated internally with radionuclides such as by inhalation, ingestion, injection, or absorption through skin or wounds. Accident victims with internal contamination usually present no special hazard to medical laboratory personnel. An example includes Thorotrast (25% thorium dioxide), a radiologic contrast agent used between 1928 and 1955, which was abandoned following a report of hepatic angiosarcoma and the development of a wide range of malignancies, mainly of hepatic origin.

Combination Contamination

Radiation accidents with combinations of these problems. These patients may also have complicating medical and surgical problems.

Pathophysiology

The different types of ionizing radiation vary in their penetrative powers, as well as in the number of ions they produce while traversing matter. Ionizing radiation is produced naturally by the decay of radioactive elements or artificially by such devices as x-ray machines. A radioactive element is one that spontaneously changes to a lower-energy state, emitting particles and gamma rays from the nucleus in the process. The particles commonly emitted are α or β particles. X-rays are produced when high-energy electrons strike atoms of a suitable target such as tungsten. When these fast-moving electrons approach the electrical field around the nuclei of the target material, the electrons are deflected from their path and release energy in the form of high-energy electromagnetic radiation (x-rays).

Clinical Presentations

ACUTE EFFECTS

Tissues typically involved in acute radiation poisoning include the bone marrow, gut, skin, and epithelium of the upper digestive tract and bladder. Bone marrow depression, mucositis, epithelitis, epilation, and gastrointestinal (GI) upset represent failure of the integrity of proliferative compartments of local cell-renewal systems.

INTERMEDIATE EFFECTS

Intermediate effects result from injury to cells of a slowly proliferating cell-renewal system, possibly endothelium or connective tissue. Radiation pneumonitis and pericarditis are particularly important intermediate effects. They occur shortly after irradiation and usually are transient, mild in severity, and not associated with permanent sequelae. Radiation pneumonitis is characterized by the insidious onset of cough, dyspnea, and fever, usually occurring 6 to 12 weeks after radiotherapy.

The chest roentgenogram and computed tomographic (CT) scan of the thorax show changes that vary from an ill-defined, nonhomogeneous opacification to a dense alveolar infiltrate associated with air bronchograms. A characteristic feature of the roentgenographic infiltrate is that is has a sharply defined border that corresponds to the edge of the radiation field. Radiation pneumonitis probably represents a form of immunologically mediated hypersensitivity pneumonitis.

LATE EFFECTS

Late radiation sequelae are directly related to the total effective dose received by the limiting normal tissue within a treatment portal. Although it is assumed endothelium or connective tissue, the nature of this critical target tissue is by no means certain. The development of tissue necrosis, fistulas, and fibrosis is related to total effective radiation dose. Late complications may occur as early as a few months to as long as several years after irradiation. Unlike acute and intermediate radiation reactions, however, these complications are chronic and not always amenable to surgical correction. Moreover, they do not necessarily bear any relation to prior acute or intermediate reactions. It is the development of these late effects that limit the total effective dose delivered to a tumor.

CANCER

The induction of cancer is a particularly important late side effect of cancer treatment and of significant radiation accidents. Several epidemiologic studies demonstrate increased risks of leukemia and solid tumors in patients exposed to radiotherapy. Large increases in leukemia risk also have been observed after chemotherapy with alkylating agents. While almost all types of cancer can be caused by exposure to ionizing radiation, certain organs such as the thyroid gland and the female breast appear to be more radiosensitive than others. The full incidence of thyroid cancers may not be expressed for 30 years. The incidence of thyroid cancer in children in parts of the former Soviet Union affected by fallout from the Chernobyl reaction continues to rise.

Toxic Dosage/Death

NUCLEAR ACCIDENTS

There is no convincing evidence of a cause-effect relationship between nuclear facilities and cancer occurrence in nearby populations (e.g., Three Mile Island). However, between 1944 and 1988, 3,005 recorded nuclear misadventures occurred worldwide. The explosion and fire at the Chernobyl nuclear power plant on April 16, 1986, was the most significant nuclear event in terms of acute injuries, deaths, the amount of radioactivity released into the environment, the size of the affected area, and the magnitude of long-term consequences since the bombings of Hiroshima and Nagasaki. It was the worst commercial nuclear power plant disaster in history and the second to involve a meltdown of nuclear fuel, 7 years after the first at Three Mile Island in 1979.

The 31 deaths resulting from the Chernobyl reactor accident approximated the total number of accidental radiation deaths occurring in the world during the previous 42 years. It is now estimated that approximately 50 individuals were irradiated with doses greater than 500 rad (5 Gy), approximately 100 received doses of between 300 rad (3 Gy) and 500 rad, and perhaps another 100 received doses of between 100 rad (1 Gy) and 300 rad. In general, measurable whole body doses of ionizing radiation, as witnessed at Chernobyl and other nuclear accidents, yield predictable physiologic signs and symptoms.

Clinical effects may be correlated with whole-body doses of ionizing radiation. 0 to 25 rad generally produce no acute clinical effects, but may be associated with a small increase in risk of delayed cancer and genetic effects. 25 to 100 rad produce a temporary reduction in lymphocytes and neutrophils. Minimal symptoms, such as nausea, vomiting, diarrhea, and fatigue typically are seen with 100 to 200 rad exposures. 200 to 300 rad exposures yield nausea and vomiting on the first day, followed by a 2-week latent period characterized by anorexia, malaise, and hematopoietic subsyndrome. Recovery occurs within 3 months.

Higher exposures produce more devastating effects. 300 to 600 rad exposures are characterized by nausea, vomiting, and diarrhea within a few hours, followed by anorexia and malaise in one week. By the third week, hemorrhage, purpura, and GI inflammation are typical, and death may occur. Indeed, eventual death may be associated with 50% of individuals exposed at this level. At 600 to 1,000 rad, vomiting occurs quickly in all individuals. Diarrhea, hemorrhage, and fever follow within one week, and death generally follows. Higher exposures are characterized by certain death, preceded by severe vomiting and hemodynamic collapse within minutes to hours.

Pregnancy/Lactation

The possibility of pregnancy should be considered in deciding whether to examine a woman of reproductive age with x-rays. In the first 10 days after menstruation, it is unlikely that there is a conceptus and x-radiation is unlikely to be an additional risk. During the rest of the first month, any risk is likely to be so small that no special limitation on diagnostic exposures is required. During the second month of gestation, malformation of specific organs has occurred in experimental animals exposed to radiation. Between 8 and 15 weeks after conception, irradiation of the forebrain may result in mental retardation, but no evidence of this has been shown in the first 8 weeks.

Practical guidelines for the use of x-rays assume that a woman in her reproductive years is pregnant unless proved otherwise. Generally acceptable proofs that she is not pregnant include onset of menses in the last 10 days, oral contraceptive use, intrauterine device use, surgical sterilization, or a negative pregnancy test. If a woman may be in the first trimester of pregnancy, avoid inclusion of the pelvis in the primary x-ray beam if possible. Where feasible, always shield the pelvis and abdomen of women when performing diagnostic roentgenographic studies.

If there is a valid medical indication to perform a diagnostic study using radiation on a pregnant woman, this generally will outweigh the remote possibility of harm to the patient or her fetus. If a woman receives a relatively large amount of radiation (5 to 15 rads) to the pelvis in the first trimester of pregnancy, the increased risk of a congenital anomaly of the fetus is estimated at 1% to 3%.

Treatment

INTERNAL CONTAMINATION

- Following internal contamination, there usually is a period before the radionuclide has been absorbed, transported, and taken up by tissue cells. The absorption from the lung, gut, or wound sometimes can be reduced by chemical manipulation in the GI tract, or by hastening the passage of the material through the body.
- Alkalizing the stomach may, in some instances, cause the formation of relatively insoluble hydroxides or keep the pH high enough to reduce solubility of some metal salts.
- The administration of a cathartic such as magnesium sulfate will shorten the intestinal transit time, thereby reducing absorption and radiation exposure to the gut wall and nearby tissues.
- Once absorbed, uptake can be reduced by the use of blocking agents, isotopic dilution, or chelating agents. A blocking agent is a chemical that saturates a tissue with a nonradioactive element, thereby reducing the uptake of the radionuclide. Chelating agents bind metals into complexes, prevent tissue uptake and enhance urinary excretion.
- Chelating agents such as EDTA, DTPA, BAL, penicillamine, or deferoxamine sometimes are useful after uptake has occurred, but their effectiveness is greatly reduced.

TREATMENT AT CHERNOBYL

- In general, treatment consisted of burn therapy, platelet and red blood cell transfusions, prophylactic antibiotics, specific antibiotic therapy when infections developed, fluid maintenance, and parenteral hyperalimentation. Patients were placed in single rooms with sterile precautions and laminar air flow facilities.
- Those with estimated exposures of 500 rad or more were candidates for bone marrow transplantation.

- All of the fatalities had received doses of more than 600 rad (6 Gy) to bone marrow plus severe β-radiation burns of the skin, and in many cases also thermal burns. Potassium iodide was administered to much of the population near the accident site.
- Of the potential radionuclides that may be released in a nuclear reactor accident, radioiodines, particularly iodine 131, are the most significant. This was confirmed in the Chernobyl accident. Huge, volatile quantities typically are found in the reactor core. Iodine is absorbed rapidly and completely by the GI tract within 30 to 60 minutes of ingestion and subsequently is concentrated by the thyroid gland. Major nonthyroidal effects are dose-dependent, and include sialadenitis and certain skin reactions.

Questions—Radiation Accidents

1. The acute effects of radiation typically involve
   A. Skin
   B. Mucous membranes
   C. Bone marrow
   D. All of the above

2. Which of the following is not an example of a radiation accident?
   A. Misadministration of a nuclear medicine dose
   B. Radiation therapy administered to an incorrect patient
   C. Radiation spill in the nuclear medicine lab
   D. Performing an ultrasound exam with a vaginal probe when the exam was ordered transabdominally

3. Which of the following cancer rates increases in people who have been exposed to large doses of ionizing radiation?
   A. Leukemia
   B. Thyroid cancer
   C. Breast cancer
   D. All of the above

4. The most significant nuclear accident to have occurred is
   A. Three Mile Island
   B. Chernobyl
   C. Hiroshima
   D. Nagasaki

5. Regarding x-rays of women who might be pregnant,
   A. The pelvis and lower abdomen should not be shielded unless they are included in the exam.
   B. The greatest risk to the fetus is during the first 10 days after menses.
   C. An x-ray should be performed if there is a valid medical indication for it.
   D. The risk of an anomaly is as high as 50% during first trimester x-rays.

NON-IONIZING RADIATION

Electromagnetic Spectrum

The term "radiation" simply means energy transmitted by waves. Ionizing radiation, such as that associated with x-rays and γ rays at the higher end of the electromagnetic spectrum, has enough energy to strip electrons from atoms. The lower end of the electromagnetic spectrum includes nonionizing electric, magnetic, and microwave fields produced by everyday electrical appliances. Electric fields from most appliances primarily create charges of current on or near the surface of the body and not in the internal organs. Magnetic fields, however, pass through the body and actually induce electric currents within the body.

The strength of a magnetic field is measured in units of gauss (G) or milligauss (mG = 1/1000th of a gauss). (The international standard unit is microtesla, which is the same as 10 milligauss.) The typical American home has a background magnetic field level (away from any appliances) ranging from 0.5 to 4.0 mG. Higher frequency nonionizing radiation, such as microwaves, can heat up biologic tissue by vibrating molecules.

Electromagnetic Waves

The term "electromagnetic field" applies to a type of energy that exists in the air. These fields have two components, as the name implies: an electric charge and a magnetic attraction. Light, radio waves, radar, x-rays, and γ rays are all forms of electromagnetic radiation. Physically, they differ from one another only in frequency. The higher the frequency, the more energy contained in the field. The strongest 60-Hz field produced by high-voltage power lines and generators does not damage DNA, even in someone standing very close.

Electric charges create electric fields. Electric charges that move (i.e., electric current) create magnetic fields. An appliance that is plugged in, and therefore connected to a source of electricity, has an electric field even when the appliance is turned off. To produce a magnetic field, the appliance must not only be plugged in, but also operating, so that current is flowing. The electric component influences primarily those particles at the surface of a nearby object, whereas the magnetic field penetrates to the interior. Ambient levels of the two components vary from place to place. Someone walking underneath a high-voltage power line has relatively high exposure to both.

Infrared Radiation

Infrared radiation (IR) falls between microwaves and visible light in the electromagnetic spectrum. The biologic effects associated with IR exposure revolve around its ability to heat tissue. The eye is particularly sensitive to IR. Corneal, iritic, and lenticular lesions have been observed in experimental studies. The prevalence rates of subcapsular, cuneiform, and nuclear cataracts were found to be elevated among glassworkers exposed to IR when compared with an unexposed group.

Lasers

"Laser" is an acronym for Light Amplification by Stimulated Emission of Radiation. Thus, the laser is a device that produces and amplifies light. Lasers vary greatly in their output power, from a few milliwatts in a helium-neon gas laser, to thousands of watts in a carbon dioxide gas laser. Lasers are capable of operating continuously or in pulses, with millions of watts of power in each pulse. When light emerges from a laser, it does not diverge (spread) significantly. Thus, energy is not greatly dissipated as the beam travels. Laser light is very close to being monochromatic or one color or wavelength of light.

Laser light can be very intense and can be used to destroy microscopic amounts of tissue—quantities too small for a surgical blade. The type of tissue that is affected by a laser can be adjusted through the choice of wavelength because different tissues may absorb light of different colors. Common lasers used in medicine include four types introduced 15 to 20 years ago: the carbon dioxide, argon, neodymium/YAG, and ruby varieties. Devices to deliver light virtually anywhere have been developed. Fiberoptic bundles now can be passed into areas heretofore thought unreachable, such as small blood vessels. Kidney stones also have been disintegrated with lasers. Laser beams can treat an abnormal growth of blood vessels in the retina, a common complication of diabetes. Recently, lasers have been used to target arterial plaques of atherosclerosis.

Unfortunately, lasers are associated with numerous hazards. These include radiation, because most lasers have high voltage power supplies, fire, and explosions. Electric shocks also are a potential danger. Most accidents occur during setup or alignment procedures when goggles are not worn. Laser radiation may be absorbed, scattered, or reflected from biologic tissues. In most cases, a combination of all of these effects occurs. Carbon monoxide, chloride, and fluorine toxic vapors may be produced from cutting, welding, and heat-treating. Some lasers also are quite loud and may be a nuisance. Theoretically, cancer cells may spread during vaporization processes.

Magnetic Resonance Imaging (MRI)

Felix Block and Edward Purcell first demonstrated nuclear magnetic resonance principles in 1946, and jointly received the Nobel Prize for Physics in 1952 for their discoveries. Electromagnetic signals are acquired from the body using nuclear magnetic resonance phenomena with a static magnetic field, gradient magnetic fields, and radiofrequency magnetic fields. The static magnetic field produced by the main magnet determines the resonant radiofrequency of the nuclei of interest. Time-varying magnetic fields occur during switching of the magnetic gradients used for spatial localization of the acquired nuclear magnetic resonance signal. Computers process this information and present an image, a spectrum, or localized nuclear magnetic resonance parameter data. Various imaging techniques and spectroscopy acquisition protocols are used.

Risks to health from MRI theoretically include adverse effects of whole or partial body exposure to the static magnetic field and adverse effects of exposure to time-varying magnetic fields. Other theoretical risks include adverse effects of absorption of energy from magnetic fields, hazards from high acoustic noise levels, hazards from laser beams used in patient positioning, electrical and mechanical hazards, and/or insufficient image or spectral quality resulting in reduced clinical utility. Due to the configuration of the system and the length of the examination, some patients become claustrophobic. Radiofrequency magnetic fields occur at the resonant frequency of the nuclei of interest. Radiofrequency absorption in a patient may cause systemic and local thermal injury.

The field near the magnet, that is, the fringe field, may be strong enough to attract ferromagnetic objects such as tools with great force, causing a collision. The field in or near the magnet may fatally interfere with the operation of devices such as cardiac pacemakers. The static magnetic field may move or dislodge ferromagnetic materials within the patient's body such as intracranial aneurysm clips, shrapnel fragments, and mobile prostheses constructed of ferromagnetic material, each of which may cause life-threatening situations.

Static hardware, including most of that used for orthopedic and spinal work (with the exception of halo fixation devices) does not contraindicate MRI; the procedure should, however, be stopped if patients experience pain in the region of large implants. Ventricular shunts used to treat hydrocephalus and most hemostatic clips do not pose problems. Nonmagnetic dental implants are harmless as are intrauterine and diaphragm contraceptive devices. Some penile and inflatable breast implants may, however, be hazardous. Prosthetic heart valves are compatible with magnetic resonance imaging.

Microwaves

Microwave field intensity is described by both electric field strengths (volts per minute) and power density (milliwatts per square centimeter). Microwaves encompass a range of electromagnetic nonionizing radiation whose energy levels and tissue penetration depend on wavelength. All radar systems, microwave ovens, diathermy machines, and a variety of industrial heat sources produce specific wavelengths of microwave energy to achieve their effects. Microwave interference with cardiac pacemakers has resulted in shielding of current devices. Lenticular opacities have been associated with short- and long-term exposures to microwaves.

Ultrasound

Ultrasound is the mechanical vibration of an elastic medium that is produced in the form of alternating compressions and expansions. The vibration may be produced by continuous or impulse sound in the form of a sequel of interrupted vibrations. The medical uses of ultrasound include therapeutic, surgical, and diagnostic procedures. Ultrasound does not produce tissue ionization. No epidemiologic studies have indicated that diagnostic ultrasound results in any measurable or significant biologic effects.

Although exposure to ultrasound does not appear to pose a human health risk, exposure to audible high frequency radiation above 10 kHz can result in a syndrome involving nausea, headaches, tinnitus, pain, dizziness, and fatigue. Temporary hearing loss and threshold shifts also are possible from high-frequency ultrasound radiation. Low-frequency ultrasound radiation may produce local effects when a person touches parts of materials being processed by ultrasound. Exposure to powerful sources of ultrasound may result in damage to peripheral nervous and vascular structures at the points of contact.

Ultraviolet Radiation

Ultraviolet-A (UVA) light is closest to the visible spectrum. Ultraviolet-B (UVB) has a shorter wavelength, is more energetic, and has a greater potential to cause injury. Protection from sun damage depends mainly on the absorption of UVB. Compared with natural UVB radiation, fluorescent lighting is unlikely to be a significant factor in the induction of skin cancer by UVB radiation.

Two different types of tanning occur in response to ultraviolet radiation (UVR) exposure—immediate tanning, which is more correctly termed "immediate pigment darkening," and delayed tanning. Immediate pigment darkening begins during exposure and is maximal at the end of the radiation period. It is a transient grayish-brown discoloration of the skin induced by UVA and exposure to certain visible light wavelengths. Persistence of the effect depends on the duration of exposure. The darker the natural skin and previously acquired tan, the more pronounced the response.

Delayed tanning occurs 48 to 72 hours following UVR exposure, peaks in 7 to 10 days, and persists for several weeks to months. It can be maintained by repeated exposure to UVR. Considerably larger doses of UVA than UVB are required for delayed tanning. UVA radiation is not uniformly effective in producing a tan. UVB radiation, particularly the shorter wavelengths, is most efficient in causing erythema and sunburn. UVA also can cause erythema, but levels 800 to 1,000 times higher than those of UVB are required.

Visual Display Terminals

It was originally feared that working with visual display terminals (VDTs) potentially caused three types of adverse health effects: cataracts, adverse pregnancy outcomes, and skin rashes. Initial concerns focused on radiation such as x-rays, microwaves, or UVR. Despite the fact that computer monitors do not emit microwaves or other significant radiation, some companies have done brisk business selling lead-lined aprons to worried computer operators.

Epidemiologic studies have failed to demonstrate an increased occurrence of spontaneous abortion or malformed children in relation to VDT use. VDTs do not cause permanent ocular damage, but the use of these terminals, often combined with a change in work routine, may be associated with ocular and general musculoskeletal discomfort. Representative equipment has been monitored for all forms of electromagnetic and other emissions, and the levels have been below presently accepted standards of exposure.

Clinical Presentations

LASER OPHTHALMOLOGIC EFFECTS

For visible and infrared radiation, the eye is generally the most critical organ in terms of vulnerability to laser radiation. Infrared radiation can cause thermal injury to the cornea and conjunctiva. The biologic response to ultraviolet laser radiation is similar to that produced by noncoherent UVR sources. Photophobia, tearing, conjunctival discharge, surface exfoliation, and stromal haze are the expected consequences of exposure to these lasers.

LASER DERMATOLOGIC EFFECTS

The biologic consequences of irradiating the skin with laser radiation are considered less than those to the eye, because skin damage is often repairable or reversible. On the other hand, exposure of the skin to high levels of optical radiation can cause depigmentation, severe burns, and possible damage to underlying organs. The effects of UVR laser radiation on the skin are the same as for UVR from conventional sources: erythema from acute exposure and accelerated skin aging and skin cancer from chronic exposure.

CANCER AND NONIONIZING RADIATION

During the past 20 years, a number of poorly designed studies have suggested an increased risk of cancer induced by electromagnetic fields. However, numerous potential confounders of these studies have been identified, making interpretation of their results complicated and controversial. In general, reviews of cancer studies and electromagnetic fields (i.e., generally from overhead power lines) indicate that there is no evidence of carcinogenic hazard from exposure of paternal gonads, the fetus, children, or adults to extremely low frequency electromagnetic fields. Such fields may be associated with residences near major sources of electricity, the use of electrical appliances, and/or work in the electronic and telecommunication industries.

PHOTOSENSITIVITY AND PHOTODAMAGE

People take drugs or apply cosmetics with photosensitizing potential to enhance their tans. Individuals using medications or using topical agents known to be sensitizing should avoid sun exposure altogether, if possible, and absolutely shun any form of UVA from artificial sources. Those who then use UVA "sunbeds" may develop a severe photosensitivity reaction. Sunbeds also can cause photodermatosis or polymorphous light eruption. Symptoms include a transient, irritating, papular reaction. Immunologic changes, both cutaneous and systemic, have been seen after exposure to UVR from a sunbed. Excessive use of UVA sunbeds produces skin fragility and blistering. It also may cause melanocytic lesions with malignant potential.

Although UVB is responsible for much of the dermal connective-tissue destruction in the photoaging process, high-intensity UVA also can enhance loss of elasticity. Other effects related to photoaging include the development of actinic or "solar" keratoses. Actinic keratoses are most common in older people, but may be seen in younger individuals exposed to sunlight over a prolonged period (e.g., beach lifeguards, outdoor laborers, farmers, and sailors). Other solar-induced skin changes include a severe form of skin wrinkling that occurs on the posterior portion of the neck, facial telangiectasias, especially on the cheeks, nose, and ears, and increased vascular fragility.

PHOTOCARCINOGENESIS

UVR acts at all three of the recognized stages of carcinogenesis—initiation, promotion, and progression. The most common skin cancer in the United States is basal-cell carcinoma. It occurs with greatest frequency in men who spend much time outdoors and who may posses other high-risk characteristics such as fair skin. Another common skin cancer in whites is squamous-cell carcinoma, which also may be related to UVR skin exposure.

The incidence of cutaneous malignant melanoma (CMM) has markedly increased in the last 10 years. In 1990, it was predicted that 27,600 people in the United States would develop melanoma and 6,300 die from it. A history of sunburn is significantly more common in individuals with CMM. There is a markedly lower incidence of CMM and actinic keratoses in races with deeply pigmented skin than in whites. People with fair skin, blond or red hair, or marked freckling on the upper back are more likely to get melanoma. In addition, at increased risk are people who have actinic keratoses, usually developing after age 40. Merely living closer to the equator, which increases exposure to ultraviolet light, may be a predisposing factor.

Treatment

SKIN PROTECTION

- Treatment of photodamaging radiation is fundamentally protective and preventative. In addition to wearing protective clothing or staying out of the sun and not using tanning devices, the primary method of mitigating most harmful effects of UVR is the use of sunscreens.
- There are two types of topical sunscreens, (1) chemical sunscreens that provide protection by absorbing UVR, and (2) physical sunscreens that block UVR from reaching the skin.
- Ultraviolet-absorbing preparations may contain one or more chemical entities in a carrier base and are intended to be applied as a thin film to exposed skin.
- Sunscreens should be used on sun-exposed skin by individuals habitually exposed to the sun, by people with fair skin types, and by those who are hypersensitive to sunlight.
- Frequent use of sunscreens should become a standard procedure for children.
- Bald-headed men should apply sunscreens to the exposed area regularly. Additional applications should be made following swimming, after exercise that has caused profuse sweating, or when clothing or beach towels have rubbed off part of the original application.

- Physical sunscreens contain materials such as zinc oxide, talc, or titanium dioxide in an ointment base. These preparations scatter ultraviolet and visible radiation and are opaque to all wavelengths of light. They are effective and useful in protecting selected areas of the body (e.g., the nose) if applied thickly, but may be cosmetically unappealing.

OCULAR PROTECTION

- The cornea filters most UVR, however the lens absorbs nearly all ultraviolet from 295 to 400 nm. UVR from sunlight is an important risk factor in forming cataracts.
- Ocular exposure to UVB can be reduced by wearing a wide-brimmed hat and by wearing UVR-absorbing sunglasses at times of maximal exposure to sunlight.
- The Sunglass Association of America, in cooperation with the Food and Drug Administration (FDA), adopted a voluntary program in 1990 to provide information about light absorption of sunglass lenses. The tag on any pair of nonprescription sunglasses distributed under the program states that it meets or exceeds requirements for one of three categories: cosmetic, general purpose, or special purpose.

Questions—Nonionizing Radiation

1. **Regarding nonionizing radiation, which of the following is false?**
   A. Infrared is a type of nonionizing radiation.
   B. The difference between ionizing radiation and nonionizing radiation is that nonionizing radiation does not remove electrons from atoms.
   C. Nonionizing radiation is not harmful to humans.
   D. Magnetic fields are a type of ionizing radiation.
2. **Which of the following are hazards of lasers?**
   A. Fire
   B. Electric shocks
   C. Eye injury
   D. All of the above
3. **Hazards of MRI machines include all of the following except**
   A. Interference with cardiac pacemakers
   B. Dislodgement of shrapnel that may be within a patient
   C. Induction of cardiac irregularities
   D. Attraction of ferromagnetic objects into the magnet at high velocities
4. **Which of the following is true?**
   A. At diagnostic levels, ultrasound does not cause clinically significant biologic effects.
   B. Ultrasound can causes tissue ionization when used at high frequencies.
   C. Fluorescent lighting is a significant contributing factor in the development of skin cancers.
   D. Both UVA and UVB contribute to suntans.
5. **Which of the following is true?**
   A. Long-term use of television monitors (video display terminals) increases the risk of spontaneous abortion by at least 50%.
   B. The most sensitive organ to the effects of laser radiation is the eye.
   C. Increased cancer risk has been linked conclusively to electromagnetic fields.
   D. Laser radiation has significantly different effects on skin than light from conventional sources.
6. **People who are taking photosensitizing medications are safe from UVA radiation.**
   A. True
   B. False
7. **The nonionizing radiation that is most important in development of skin cancer is ultraviolet.**
   A. True
   B. False
8. **Currently, the primary method of protecting the skin from the damaging effects of the sun is by use of sunscreens.**
   A. True
   B. False
9. **Ultraviolet absorbing sunglasses do not help in protecting the eye from UVR.**
   A. True
   B. False
10. **In the eye, most of the UVR is absorbed by the**
   A. Cornea
   B. Lens
   C. Retina
   D. Macula

CONTRAST MEDIA

INTRODUCTION

Ten to 15 million intravascular contrast media-assisted radiologic examinations are conducted each year in North America. Although adverse side effects are infrequent, a detailed knowledge of the variety of side effects, their likelihood in relationship to preexisting conditions, and their treatment is required to assure optimal patient care.

The exact incidence of adverse side effects after the administration of intravascular contrast media is not known. Underreporting or variation in categorization of reactions affects statistics regarding incidence. Most mild side effects are reported to occur in 5% to 12% of all patients who receive ionic, high-osmolar contrast media. Many patients will experience warmth or heat, which is often not recorded. Use of low-osmolar ionic and nonionic contrast media is associated with a lower overall incidence of adverse side effects, particularly serious life-threatening ones.

Serious contrast reactions are rare and are estimated to occur in 1 or 2 per 1,000 examinations using high-osmolar contrast media. The precise incidence of fatalities related to contrast material also is unknown. Deaths from high-osmolar contrast media have been reported between 1/40,000 and 1/170,000 intravenous (IV) administrations. The incidence of fatal outcomes after a contrast-medium reaction has decreased for high-osmolar contrast media to 0.9/100,000, essentially a rate equivalent to that observed with nonionic agents.

Higher-Osmolality Contrast Agents

HOCA have been utilized in radiologic examinations for approximately 60 years. There has been profound improvement in the quality of these agents in terms of their usefulness and safety. They generally are regarded as safe and effective, however pretreatment with steroids may decrease patient risk.

Lower-Osmolality Contrast Agents

Because of occasional discomfort associated with the use of HOCA, and associated uncommon, severe adverse reactions, the search for improved contrast agents continues. Lower-osmolality contrast agents (LOCA), most of which are nonionic compounds, have been developed. Such nonionic agents are associated with less discomfort and have a low incidence of adverse effects.

LOCA generally are used/preferred in patients with a history of adverse reaction to contrast material, with the exception of a sensation of heat, flushing, or a single episode of nausea or vomiting. They also are used in patients with a history of asthma or allergy, and patients with known cardiac dysfunction (e.g., recent or potentially imminent cardiac decompensation, severe arrhythmias, unstable angina pectoris, recent myocardial infarction, and pulmonary hypertension).

Other situations in which LOCA may be preferred include patients with sickle cell disease, patients at increased risk for aspiration, patients who are anxious about the contrast procedure, patients in whom communication cannot be established regarding risk factors, patients who request or demand the use of LOCA, patients undergoing painful angiographic procedures, and in patients at high risk (e.g., infants, the elderly, diabetics, and those with renal impairment, and/or hemoglobinopathies).

Questions—Introduction To Contrast Media

1. **Regarding high-osmolar contrast media**
   A. They generally are considered safe and effective for diagnostic use.
   B. The fatality rate is between 1 per 4,000 and 1 per 8,000 examinations.
   C. They are as safe as low-osmolar contrast media.
   D. All of the above
2. **Regarding lower-osmolality contrast agents**
   A. There have been no reported deaths when using them.
   B. They should be used in patients who have experienced a warm or hot sensation when receiving high-osmolar contrast previously.
   C. They tend to cause more discomfort than higher-osmolality contrast agents.
   D. They should be used in high-risk patients instead of higher-osmolaltiy contrast agents.

SPECIFIC CONTRAST MEDIA

Angiography

Contrast agents include water-soluble molecules that are easily distributed through blood vessels. They have low viscosity and high radiodensity.

Cholecystography

Oral cholecystographic media represent small monomeric molecules to facilitate absorption. They require conjugation with glucuronic acid to reach sufficient molecular weight for biliary excretion. Examples include ipodates, iocetamic acid, iopanoic acid, and sodium tyropanoate. Iopanoic acid (Telepaque®) is an ionic monomeric contrast agent frequently used as a cholecystographic contrast medium. Doses up to 75 grams have been associated with nausea, vomiting, diarrhea, hypotension, coronary insufficiency, hepatic necrosis, renal failure, and death.

Treatment is essentially symptomatic and supportive. IV fluids, alkalinization of urine, and cholestyramine as a chelator of iopanoic acid have been suggested, but not proven, in overdose. Cardiac and respiratory monitoring should be instituted in an intensive care facility. IV agents represent larger dimeric molecules that do not require conjugation. Examples include salts of iodipamide, iodoxamic acid, ioglycamic acid, and iotroxic acid.

Computerized Tomography

Contrast media may be used in conjunction with computerized tomography (CT) to study the GI tract and other organs. Agents are absorbed or nonabsorbed, iodinated, water-soluble agents. They are high in osmolality (i.e., are associated with less water absorption and rapid transfer through the gut). Examples include ionic media such as Renografin®.

Gastrointestinal Studies

Contrast agents represent nonabsorbable media that homogeneously coat GI mucosa. They do not interact with GI secretions, or leave radiographic artifacts. Barium sulfate is the fundamental example. Low-density suspensions of barium sulfate used for bronchography have been considered relatively harmless in the bronchial tract, but aspiration of a low-density suspension in the elderly can be associated with pneumonia.

Lymphangiography

Contrast agents have high radiodensity and are water-insoluble media that persist in lymph nodes. Iodized oil is an example, as is Iotasul, a nonionic dimer.

Magnetic Resonance Imaging

Contrast agents are complexes that enhance MRI. Examples include gadolinium, manganese, iron, and gadopentetic acid. IV gadopentetate, used as a contrast agent for MRI, has been associated with anaphylactoid reactions, seizures, headache, nausea, hypotension, and a transient increase in serum iron values. There have been few vital sign or electrocardiogram (ECG) abnormalities. Similar experience has followed the use of gadoteridol.

Myelography

Contrast agents are nonionic, water-soluble, and have good tolerance. They are well visualized and miscible with cerebrospinal fluid. They are removed from the subarachnoid space by normal pharmacokinetic mechanisms. Examples include metrizamide and iohexol. In myelography, nonionic contrast material is used exclusively because of reductions in arachnoiditis and because removal is unnecessary.

Inadvertent administration, by the intrathecal route, of ionic contrast media (e.g., diatrizoate, iodamide, and ioxithalamate) instead of iopamidol has led to fatalities. When accidental intrathecal accidents occur with ionic contrast agents, appropriate circulatory support, intrathecal lavage, and anticonvulsant therapy are necessary elements in patient management. Despite the low but still present risk of seizures after myelography, patients are instructed not to drive or be alone for 24 hours after the procedure.

Urography

Contrast agents are small molecules and highly water-soluble substances with low protein-binding, and high plasma concentrations. They are given intravenously. Examples include ionic monomers such as diatrizoates, iothalamates, metrizoates, iodamide, and ioxithalamate. Use of a high-dose, high-osmolarity contrast agent (meglumine iothalamate) during excretory urography has led to cardiopulmonary failure. Urography in infants with diatrizoate sodium has led to fatalities.

Clinical Presentations

Contrast-media reactions vary in severity. The majority of adverse side effects are mild or moderate non-life–threatening events that require only observation, reassurance, and support. The dose, route, and rate of delivery of contrast media affect the frequency and severity of contrast reactions. All adverse side effects, regardless of their degree or mode of presentation, may portend or progress to a worse event. Contrast-media reactions are usually evident within the first 5 to 20 minutes after administration. They may uncommonly be delayed up to 24 to 48 hours. They may appear after single or multiple intravascular injections. Types of contrast media reactions include, (1) anaphylactoid, allergic or idiosyncratic reactions, (2) chemotoxic or vasomotor, nonidiosyncratic reactions, (3) combinations of these or, (4) organ-specific, local reactions.

ANAPHYLACTOID REACTIONS

Anaphylactoid reactions are observed in less than 5% of examinations using radiopaque agents, ranging from skin reactions to irreversible shock. A history of allergy increases the likelihood of reactions at least two- to threefold. Patients who have had anaphylactoid reactions to contrast material have a 35% to 60% chance of having a second reaction on rechallenge.

CARDIOPULMONARY EFFECTS

Cardiovascular and/or pulmonary changes include cardiac ischemia resulting in pain and arrhythmia. Premature ventricular contractions with ectopy may be seen after contrast medium administration. ECG changes occur in up to 33% of patients with atherosclerotic disease or coronary artery disease and in about 5% of normal patients. Cardiac signs and symptoms may be accompanied by shortness of breath. Hypoxia may predispose to arrhythmias, especially in patients with preexisting coronary artery disease or pulmonary disease. Rapid progression to ventricular tachycardia, fibrillation, and shock with cardiac arrest may occur. Increased airway resistance and bronchoconstriction may occur in asthmatic patients.

Noncardiogenic pulmonary edema has been reported following the intravascular administration of contrast materials. Patients with a history of contrast-related pulmonary edema probably should be given prophylactic corticosteroids, but recurrence of pulmonary edema has been described despite pretreatment with prednisone and diphenhydramine. Both ionic and nonionic contrast media may impair unloading of oxygen from hemoglobin in the capillary blood. Large volumes of such contrast media may lead to serious adverse effects in patients with leftward shifts of the oxyhemoglobin dissociation curve, such as in neonates with intracardiac shunts or adult smokers with severe coronary artery disease.

CHEMOTOXIC EFFECTS

Chemotoxic side effects include neurotoxicity, cardiac depression, arrhythmias, ECG changes, and renal injury. Chemotoxic side effects appear to relate to the cation content and the ionic nature of contrast materials that dissociate in solution. Nonionic contrast media are associated with fewer such chemotoxic side effects.

GASTROINTESTINAL EFFECTS

Oral iohexol has been associated with nausea, vomiting, abdominal pain, hypotension, and difficulty breathing.

NEUROLOGIC EFFECTS

Neurologic signs such as headache, visual blurring, global amnesia, blindness, encephalopathy, dizziness, sensory changes, transient paresis, or seizures are observed infrequently after intravascular administration of contrast media. Patients undergoing cerebral angiography or direct opacification of the aortic arch are most at risk of irreversible neurologic damage resulting from air or plaque emboli. Nonionic compounds appear to have low rates of neurotoxic reactions. With higher doses, above 4.5 grams iodine, the rate of neurotoxic adverse reactions increases.

OSMOTIC EFFECTS

Osmotic effects include changes in plasma volume, changes in vascular permeability, vasodilatation, local discomfort or pain, hypotension, and vasomotor instability.

RENAL EFFECTS

Acute renal failure following injection of water-soluble contrast media has been reported with many agents currently in use. Clinically, patients develop acute tubular necrosis, presenting with oliguria within 24 hours after exposure to the agent. Renal function usually is restored within 2 to 3 weeks. It is not well established whether low osmolar contrast causes renal failure less frequently than high osmolar contrast.

Dehydration compromises renal function. Hence, all patients undergoing examination involving contrast media should be adequately hydrated. Patients with multiple myeloma are particularly prone to renal failure after the use of intravenous contrast agents.

THROMBOEMBOLIC EFFECTS

Thromboembolic events causing myocardial infarction and stroke have been reported during angiographic procedures with both ionic and nonionic contrast media. Meticulous intravascular administration technique is necessary to minimize clotting and thromboembolic events. The difference between ionic and nonionic contrast media and their relation to thromboembolic complications appears to be small, although the incidence of thrombus formation at the site of coronary intervention is somewhat increased with both low- and high-osmolality media. Caution should be exercised when using nonionic contrast media in high-risk patients such as the elderly and in those with defects in the coagulation system that may lead to thrombosis.

THYROID EFFECTS

Radiocontrast agents contain iodide atoms that are covalently bound to a phenolic ring, and these compounds cannot be metabolized *in vivo* by deiodinating enzymes. Contaminating free iodide is present in these preparations, and the free iodide is probably responsible for effects on the thyroid gland. Following ingestion of iodine or the use radiologic iodinated contrast media, diverse changes in thyroid status may occur.

VASOVAGAL EFFECTS

Apprehension, confusion, sweating, unresponsiveness, and loss of bowel or bladder function often accompany the combination of hypotension and bradycardia, a so-called vasovagal reaction. The etiology is unknown, but it can be aggravated by fear and anxiety and, if untreated, may progress to cardiopulmonary arrest. The cardiac effects of increased vagal tone include depressed sinoatrial (SA) and atrioventricular (AV) nodal activity, inhibition of AV conduction, and peripheral vasodilatation. Hypotension is out of proportion to the bradycardia and persists after the bradycardia has been corrected by treatment with atropine.

Drug Interactions

Verapamil and contrast media may exhibit a synergistic effect on the sodium/calcium ratio, which can result in cardiac side effects. The epileptogenic properties of chlorpromazine can be potentiated by intrathecal injection of contrast media. Radiographic contrast agents may impede the fibrinolytic effect of thrombolytic drugs. Patients who have received interleukin-2 therapy may develop fever, chills, rash, nausea, vomiting, urticaria, diarrhea, hypotension, and dyspnea following administration of ionic and nonionic contrast media.

Treatment

- In patients with normal renal function, few precautions are necessary, and HOCAs can be used, unless they are contraindicated because of an increased risk of allergic or hemodynamic side effects.
- Patients with preexisting renal impairment may benefit from 0.45% saline intravenously for 12 hours before and 12 hours after the administration of contrast agents.
- Pretreatment protocols including steroids and antihistamines may be used to prevent reactions to contrast material.
- Nausea and vomiting generally resolves spontaneously and does not require specific treatment.

CONTRAST MEDIA REACTIONS

- The American College of Radiology recommends treatment protocols for those who develop acute reactions to iodinated contrast media. Urticaria is treated with antihistamines such as diphenhydramine, and rarely requires epinephrine in disseminated cases. Facial edema and/or bronchospasm are treated with epinephrine. β-Agonist inhalers are used to treat bronchospasm as well. Anaphylaxis may require fluids and/or pressors for hypotension, liberal use of epinephrine intravenously, as well as Trendelenburg positioning.

Questions—Specific Contrast Media

1. Which of the following is an incorrect match?
A. Contrast for the gastrointestinal tract—nonabsorbable
B. Contrast for angiography—water soluble
C. Contrast for lymphangiography—water soluble
D. Contrast for myelography—water soluble

2. Which of the following is true?
A. Most contrast reactions require medical treatment.
B. Most contrast reactions occur within 20 minutes of administration of contrast.
C. If a patient has received contrast previously without an adverse reaction, it is exceedingly unlikely that a reaction will occur with a second dose.
D. All contrast reactions are capable of causing diarrhea.

3. Which is true regarding anaphylactoid reactions?
A. Skin reactions, including hives, is a type of anaphylactoid reaction that can be caused by contrast administration
B. Cardiopulmonary collapse can be caused by contrast administration
C. A previous anaphylactoid reaction is a risk factor for developing another anaphylactoid reaction when giving a second dose of contrast
D. All of the above

4. Regarding neurologic effects from contrast agents
A. Neurologic effects are not associated with myelography.
B. Neurologic effects occur in slightly over 5% of contrast administrations.
C. The risk of a neurologic event is higher when undergoing cerebral angiography.
D. All of the above

5. Regarding renal toxicity from contrast agents.
A. Overhydration predisposes a patient to renal failure.
B. It is rare for renal function to recover.
C. It is usually part of an anaphylactoid reaction.
D. Renal failure can occur with higher- or lower-osmolality contrast agents.

Additional Questions—Radiation Toxicology

1. The primary risk of x-irradiation to a fetus is
A. 10 days after menses
B. Approximately 2 weeks after conception
C. Between 8 and 15 weeks after conception
D. Between 24 and 36 weeks after conception
E. 36 weeks after conception until birth

2. Treatment of acute radiation exposure may include
A. Antibiotics
B. Bone marrow transplantation
C. Potassium iodide
D. Electrolyte repletion
E. All of the above

3. Approximately what percentage of lung cancer is a result of radon?
A. less than 1%
B. 1% to 2%
C. 5% to 10%
D. 10% to 20%
E. 40%

4. Which of the following forms of radiation have the weakest statistical association with health effects on humans?
A. Infrared radiation
B. Magnetic fields
C. Lasers
D. Microwaves
E. Ultraviolet radiation

5. **Which is not an early symptom of acute radiation poisoning?**
   A. Mucositis
   B. Diarrhea
   C. Epilation
   D. Renal failure
   E. Bone marrow depression
6. **Which is false?**
   A. Ultraviolet-A radiation is more responsible for photoaging of skin than ultraviolet-B radiation.
   B. Actinic keratosis can be seen in young people.
   C. Vascular fragility can occur as a result of ultraviolet exposure.
   D. Basal-cell carcinomas, squamous-cell carcinomas, and melanomas are all associated with increased exposure to the sun.
   E. Sunblocks cannot totally eliminate the possibility of damage from radiation.
7. **Which contrast medium has the lowest incidence of side effects?**
   A. Barium sulfate in the gastrointestinal tract.
   B. Low-osmolar contrast injected intravenously
   C. High-osmolar contrast injected intravenously
   D. Low osmolar contrast injected intra-arterially
   E. High osmolar contrast injected intra-arterially
8. **Which contrast reaction does not require treatment?**
   A. Shortness of breath
   B. Hypotension
   C. Vomiting
   D. Seizures
   E. Urticaria
9. **Which of the following has been responsible for the most risk from radiation exposure?**
   A. Airplane travel
   B. Nuclear reactors
   C. Appliances (e.g., television sets, microwave ovens)
   D. Radon
   E. Electric outlets
10. **Late effects of radiation include all of the following except**
   A. Gastrointestinal hemorrhage
   B. Lung fibrosis
   C. Fistulas
   D. Anemia
   E. Malignant tumors

Case Study (Question 11)

A 29-year-old female undergoes an uneventful barium enema. Two days later, she reports that she has a positive pregnancy test and is concerned about the possible effects on her fetus.

11. **Which of the following should be done first?**
   A. Review the barium enema to determine an approximate dose to the fetus.
   B. An ultrasound examination to determine the age of the fetus.
   C. A review of the barium enema to determine if the patient was adequately shielded.
   D. Determination of the date of the patient's last menstrual period.
   E. Review her history for other possible radiation exposures.

Case Study (Question 12)

A 35-year-old male patient is undergoing an IVP examination with low osmolar contrast. Immediately after the contrast is injected, he experiences nausea and vomiting that continues unabated for 3 to 4 minutes.

12. **At this point, which of the following should be given?**
   A. Cimetidine
   B. Vistaril
   C. Compazine
   D. Benadryl
   E. No treatment

ANSWERS

Ionizing Radiation

1. A 2. D

Radon

1. D 2. A

Radiation Accidents

1. D 2. D 3. D 4. B 5. C

Nonionizing Radiation

1. C 2. D 3. C 4. D 5. B 6. B 7. A
8. A 9. B 10. B

Introduction To Contrast Media

1. A 2. D

Specific Contrast Media

1. C 2. B 3. D 4. C 5. D

Radiation Toxicology

1. C 2. E 3. D 4. B 5. D 6. A 7. A
8. C 9. D 10. A 11. D 12. E

SELECTED READINGS

Radiation Toxicology

1. American College of Radiology. Manual of Iodinated Contrast Media 1991; 20–21.
2. Becker DV. Reactor accidents. Public health strategies and their medical implications. JAMA 1987;258;649–654.
3. Bentur Y. Ionizing and nonionization radiation in pregnancy. In: Koren G, ed. Maternal-fetal toxicology. New York: Marcel Dekker, 1990; pp. 205–251.
4. Brent RL. X-ray, microwave and ultrasound: the real and the unreal hazards. Pediatr Ann 1989;9:43–47.

5. Connor S. No risk of cancer from electromagnetic fields. Br Med J 1992;304:938–939.
6. Council on Scientific Affairs. Harmful effects of ultraviolet radiation. JAMA 1989;262:380–384.
7. Council on Scientific Affairs. Lasers in medicine and surgery. JAMA 1986;256:900–907.
8. Finch SC. Acute radiation syndrome. JAMA 1987;258:164–167.
9. Hendricks WM. How much sun is enough? NCMJ 1989;50:272–273, 435–440.
10. Leonard RB, Ricks RC. Emergency department radiation accident protocol.Ann Emerg Med 1980;9:462–470.
11. Marwick C. More studies pending of low-dose radiation. JAMA 1990;264:944.
12. Woolf AD. Radon. Clin Toxicol Rev 1991;43:1–2.
13. Yalow RS. Concerns with low(c)level ionizing radiation. Mayo Clin Proc 1994;69:436–440.

ACKNOWLEDGMENT

Thanks to Michael Leviton, MD for contributing the questions in this chapter.

CHAPTER 51
Plastics, Resins, and Plasticizers

INTRODUCTION

Plastics have become an ubiquitous and increasingly important part of our society. Numerous applications, from packaging to medicine, from building materials to film, pervade our environment. Acrylates, commonly used in orthopedics and dentistry, may induce a wide variety of symptoms including contact dermatitis, peripheral neuropathy, occupational asthma, hypotension, atrioventricular block, and cardiac arrest.

Cyanoacrylates are used as adhesives and may lead to an allergic type of asthma. Accidental ocular exposure may cause corneal damage. These compounds may lead to skin bonding that can often be treated conservatively by simple manipulation. Chronic dermatitis may follow their use on fingernails. Other plastics, such as multifunctional acrylates (MFAs) and methacrylates are used in photocurable coatings such as ultraviolet (UV) curing inks, paints, dental sealants, resins, and varnishes. Fluoropolymers such as polytetrafluoroethylene are used in the treatment of vocal cord disorders and urinary incontinence. Toxic respiratory tract effects have been observed during manufacture.

The Food and Drug Administration (FDA) has approved plastic for use on food. Many tests have been performed at temperatures up to 250 to 300°F. The use of polymer materials in microwaves that are capable of heating foods to 500°F ultimately may lead to an increased rate of polymer (and monomer) transfer to food, in addition to other thermal degradation products. Additives, including antioxidants, brighteners, colorants, and lubricants may be used in plastics used for food use.

An increasing number of plastics are being used in the food packaging industry. These include polyethylene, polypropylene, ethylene-vinyl acetate copolymer, vinyl plastics, and vinyl copolymers. Polyvinyl chloride (PVC) is used in trays, inserts, and shrink-wrap. Vinyl chloride is used to wrap cheese and as an over-wrap for paper-wrapped products. Polystyrene is used for yogurt and cottage cheese containers. Styrene-acrylonitrile is commonly used for measuring cups and juice squeezers. Acrylonitrile-butadiene-styrene (ABS) is used for margarine tubs. Nylons are used to vacuum-seal bacon and cheese. Polyethylene terephthalate is used for boil-in-the-bag foods and polycarbonates are used for nondisposable plates and cups.

Questions—Introduction to Plastics, Resins and Plasticizers

1. Acrylates have been associated with the following
A. Contact dermatitis
B. Peripheral neuropathy
C. Hypotension
D. Occupational asthma
E. All of the above

2. The transfer of plastics to food during heating occurs at temperatures of
A. 200°F
B. 300°F
C. 500°F
D. 700°F
E. Never occurs

PLASTICS

Polymethacrylates are used in the manufacture of dentures, denture bases, and filling materials. In the orthodontics market, methacrylates have found acceptance as sealants painted over teeth, which act as barriers to tooth decay. Polymethacrylates also are used in the manufacture of artificial nails, as bone cement, and for preparation of soft and hard contact lenses.

Primary uses for cyanoacrylates include skin closure, immobilization of grafts for hair transplants, local hemostasis, closure of gingival flaps in periodontal surgery, and restorative procedures on teeth or on fixed dental prostheses. Cosmetic applications, such as gluing of nail overlays, synthetic eyelashes, eyebrows, small hairpieces, and facial prostheses, also seem to be common. Industrial and consumer grades of these adhesives include Crazy Glue® and Durabond®.

Commercial preparations are often modified by the addition of fillers such as talc, powdered glass, alumina, and fumed silica, most of which are not resorbable and can act as embedded foreign bodies in tissue. In addition, these preparations incorporate strong desiccating agents and stabilizers to prevent premature curing in the reopenable container.

Cyanoacrylate nail glue (Superglue®) may be mistaken for prescribed eye drops. Many bottles used for nail glue appear identical to those used for ophthalmic solutions. Poorly sighted individuals, careless persons, and children are at risk for this error. Treatment of the resultant upper to lower lid adhesion and transient keratoconjunctivitis may require use of scissors or eye pads saturated with tap water.

Pathophysiology

The basic structure of acrylic monomers is the ester of acrylic acid. A side or "R" group determines the properties of each ester and the polymer it forms. Cyanoacrylate monomers usually are synthesized by condensation of formaldehyde and a cyanoacetate. This produces a polycyanoacrylate that then is depolymerized to yield the monomer, decomposing to formaldehyde and a cyanoacetate. This degradation mechanism probably is the major cause of tissue toxicity of cyanoacrylate adhesives.

Pharmacokinetics

ABSORPTION

- A peak venous blood level of methacrylate in patients receiving cement insertion into the femur and acetabulum is noted 3 minutes after insertion.

DISTRIBUTION

- Methylmethacrylate is present in blood cells in concentrations twice as large as plasma.
- It disappears from plasma at a rate at least 10 times faster than from the cells.
- Methylmethacrylate appears to be broken down exclusively in the plasma phase. The cells act as a storage place from which the monomer is released into the plasma.

ELIMINATION

- The half-life of methylmethacrylate (MMA) in whole blood at 20°C is 3 hours.
- MMA is not found in the urine of healthy controls.

Clinical Presentations

Systemic reactions to the odor of orthopedic cement, characterized by hypertension, dyspnea, and generalized erythroderma, have been reported. Increased complaints of respiratory, cutaneous, and genitourinary problems have been observed in workers exposed to MMA. Dental students have experienced nausea and anorexia while working with MMA.

DERMATOLOGIC EFFECTS

The acrylic bone cement used in orthopedic surgery leaves some residual monomer unpolymerized. These monomers penetrate most rubber and polyvinyl gloves but thick butyl rubber gloves may prevent the development of contact dermatitis. Many orthopedic surgeons have acquired allergic contact dermatitis from the acrylic monomers and have shown strongly positive patch-test reactions to MMA. Loss of fingernails may be the result of an allergic reaction to an acrylic nail preparation. A history of skin disease during childhood or allergic rhinitis may predispose an individual to the dermatologic effects caused by MMA.

CARDIOVASCULAR EFFECTS

Several cases of intraoperative cardiac arrest have been reported in patients undergoing hip replacements, although the occurrence is rare. Hypotension occurs during 50% to 80% of total hip replacements. The drop in blood pressure rarely exceeds 15 mm Hg, reaches its maximum 30 to 60 seconds following insertion of the prosthesis, and usually returns to normal in 90 seconds. A second-degree atrioventricular block and bradycardia that progressed to a fatal third-degree heart block has been reported during hip arthroplasty using MMA cement.

NEUROLOGIC EFFECTS

A generalized sensorimotor peripheral neuropathy of the axonal degeneration type may follow inhalational exposure to MMA monomer. Between 3% and 5% of MMA is unreacted monomer, posing an occupational hazard to dental technicians who may experience feelings of numbness, coldness, and pain. Irritability, rapid fatigue, and headache have been observed in workers engaged in pouring MMA into forms. Drowsiness, headache, and nausea have followed exposure to ethyl and butyl acrylate. Repeated dermal application of MFAs may lead to seizures, tremors, or ataxia.

RESPIRATORY EFFECTS

At high concentrations, MMA causes irritation to the respiratory tract. A transient decrease in PaO_2 occurs within seconds after application of MMA and is reversed within minutes. Inhalation of thermal degradation products of plastic fumes from heated PVC or polyethylene meat-wrapping film may cause bronchospasm or "meat wrappers" asthma. Patients may have a history of preexisting bronchospastic disease. Alkyl cyanoacrylates (ethyl cyanoacrylate, methyl cyanoacrylate) appear to act as allergens, including an immunologic reaction (type I) leading to the development of asthma with sneezing, nasal discharge, coughing, stridor, and dyspnea.

POLYMER FUME FEVER

Polymer fume fever is an influenzalike syndrome starting 2 to 3 hours after exposure to polymers, which clears up spontaneously within 36 to 48 hours. It has been observed in the home after utensils have been overly heated. In comparison to metal fume fever, exposures producing polymer fume fever are more likely to result in pulmonary consolidation associated with radiologic abnormalities. Unlike metal fume fever, polymer fume fever episodes appear to have little or no tendency to diminish in intensity after serial daily exposure.

CARCINOGENIC EFFECTS

The International Agency for Research on Cancer has labeled three plastic compounds as carcinogenic with varying degrees of certainty. These include vinyl chloride (definite), acrylonitrile (probable), and chloroprene (under suspicion). One study concluded that there was no evidence to support the hypothesis that MMA is a human carcinogen. Elevated colorectal cancer incidence has been observed in workers employed in the production of polypropylene. Polyp prevalence rates also appear elevated in such workers.

OCULAR EFFECTS

Cyanoacrylate applied superficially to the cornea of animals produces a mild corneal haze and mild inflammatory reaction that clears in 1 week. MFAs are severe eye and skin irritants.

Pregnancy/Lactation

There is one report of an increase in spontaneous abortion in women employed in polystyrene manufacture. MFAs do not appear to be potent fetotoxins or teratogens.

Laboratory

ANALYTIC METHODS

Gas chromatography with a flame ionization detector is used to detect monomer in blood and can detect concentrations as low as 1 ppm.

BLOOD LEVELS

Blood levels do not impact the clinical management of individuals with potential exposures.

Treatment

GUT DECONTAMINATION

Charcoal may be useful in isolated cases of oral plastic ingestion, however formal studies have not been done.

ELIMINATION ENHANCEMENT

No experience with elimination enhancement of plastic materials has been documented in the literature.

SUPPORTIVE MEASURES

- Treatment of adverse reactions to MMA monomer or polymer is largely symptomatic and supportive. The prophylactic administration of blood and fluids, such as 500 mL of blood and 2,000 mL of balanced salt solution, before cement insertion may be helpful in limiting the intraoperative hypotensive response to these agents.
- To prevent dermatitis, orthopedic cement can be mixed mechanically and applied with a spatula.
- Skin contamination with acrylates can be cleaned with alcohol or methylethylketone and the hands washed with ample soap and water.
- Asthma from cyanoacrylates is treated symptomatically.
- Adherence of cyanoacrylates to the corneal conjunctiva, skin, or eyelid may require (a) copious irrigation of the exposed surface with tepid tap water for at least 15 minutes, (b) application of mineral oil to the external eyelid surface after irrigation, and (c) referral to an appropriate health care facility for ophthalmologic evaluation.
- Acetone has been used to remove adhesive from fingernails.

Questions—Plastics

1. Contact dermatitis to methylacrylate has been seen in all of the following except

A. Orthopedists performing hip and bone replacements
B. Ophthalmologists performing cataract surgery
C. Adults and children with a history of asthma exposed to Crazy Glue® or Dermabond®
D. Patients who use fake nails, synthetic eyelashes, or small hairpieces

2. A 23-year-old male presents to your emergency department (ED) complaining of shortness of breath after his first day in a meat-packing plant. On physical exam, what finding would you be most unlikely to find?

A. Sneezing, nasal discharge
B. Cough, stridor
C. Irregular heart beat
D. Wheezing

3. The International Agency for Research on Cancer (IARC) has labeled the following chemical as a definite carcinogenic agent:

A. Vinyl chloride
B. Methylacrylate
C. Acrylonitrile
D. Chlorophene

4. An elderly female presents to the ED with c/o her eyes being glued shut by her grandson while she was napping. What is your first action?

A. Apply mineral oil.
B. Refer directly to ophthalmology.
C. Apply tepid water for at least 15 minutes.
D. Contact social worker regarding elder abuse.

5. Evidence based medicine supports the use of the following in treatment of acrylate exposure

A. Charcoal will increase the elimination time.
B. Urinary excretion will be enhanced by alkalinization.
C. Monitoring of blood levels should be done to guide treatment.
D. None of the above

ETHERS AND EPOXY RESINS

Acrylamide is a colorless solid also known as propanamide, acrylamide monomer, and acrylic amide. Most toxic exposures occur during its use as a soil waterproofing agent in mining and tunneling operations. Other industrial applications include its use in the production of grouts and dyes and as a sizing agent in the paper and permanent press fabric industries.

Dimethylformamide (DMF) is a versatile and widely used laboratory and industrial solvent. It is used primarily in the manufacture of polyurethane products and acrylic fibers, as well as in the production of pharmaceuticals, pesticides, and other products. It also is present in textile dyes, pigments, paint strippers, and coating, printing, and adhesive formulations. In veterinary medicine it is used as a vehicle for drug administration. Clinical studies suggest an association between DMF and liver damage, and that DMF may have a role as a possible carcinogen in view of an association it has with testicular cancer.

Dimethylacetamide (DMAC), like DMF, can induce liver damage in man. A relationship exists between the amount of DMAC absorbed and the amount of its metabolite monomethylacetamide excreted in the urine. High doses induce mental changes that are reversible. Dimethylacetamide is a colorless liquid that exhibits wide organic and inorganic solubility and water miscibility. Dimethylacetamide has solvent properties and is widely used in the production of plastics, resins, synthetic fibers, gums, and as a booster solvent in coatings and adhesive formulations.

Pathophysiology

Acrylamide neurotoxicity resembles the ''dying back'' peripheral neuropathy of tri-o-cresyl phosphate (TOCP) in which the distal regions of the longest and largest axons are affected. Acrylamide may inhibit energy production of distal nerves through progressive inhibition of glycolytic enzymes involved with rapid axonal transport.

Pharmacokinetics

ABSORPTION

- DMAC is readily absorbed in man after oral, dermal, or inhalation exposure.
- After absorption, DMAC undergoes sequential demethylation to the monomethyl derivative (N-methylacetamide, MMAC) and the demethylated product, acetamide.
- DMF is absorbed readily through the skin, respiratory system, and gastrointestinal tract.

DISTRIBUTION

- The urinary concentration of N-methylformamide probably is the best index of worker exposure to DMF. Concentrations of N-methylformamide in the urine that do not exceed 40 to 50 mg/gram of creatinine, suggests an exposure that is possibly safe with regard to acute and long-term effects of DMF on liver function.

ELIMINATION

- About 2% of a dose of DMAC are recovered in the urine as MMAC after inhalation and 10% is recovered after inhalation plus skin exposure.
- In workers continuously exposed to DMAC vapor (inhalation plus skin) about 13.5% of an estimated dose is excreted as MMAC in the urine.
- Urinary MMAC may reflect the amount of DMAC in occupational air.

- For each part per million of DMAC in air, approximately 10 ppm MMAC appear in the end of shift urine sample. A buildup of urine MMAC during the week may be due to dermal contact.
- DMF is metabolized by N-demethylation to methylformamide and formamide, which are largely excreted in the urine.
- The amount of N-methylformamide recovered in the urine represents only 2% to 6% of the dose of DMF inhaled. A substantial portion of an absorbed dose of DMF is excreted unchanged in the expired breath.

Clinical Presentations

ACRYLAMIDE

Severe exposure to acrylamide may produce central nervous system symptoms including confusion and hallucinations. Subacute intoxication may cause drowsiness, loss of concentration, and ataxia. Hypotension, seizures, gastrointestinal bleeding, and adult respiratory distress syndrome may be seen with large acrylamide ingestions. Symptoms of peripheral neuropathy and hepatotoxicity may appear within 3 days.

Long-term acrylamide exposure produces a motor and sensory polyneuropathy that is insidious and distal in onset. The presence of ataxia and, occasionally, dysarthria and tremor suggests midbrain involvement. Signs and symptoms include weakness, paresthesias, fatigue, lethargy, decreased pinprick sensation, vibratory loss, decreased reflexes, and positive Romberg sign. Severity is worse distally. Desquamation of the palms and soles, sweating, and peripheral vasoconstriction is more prominent in acrylamide peripheral neuropathy compared with other industrial neuropathies. Recovery typically occurs within several months to a year of cessation of exposure, although severe exposures may result in permanent sequelae.

DIMETHYLFORMAMIDE

Complaints of abdominal pain, nausea, vomiting, dizziness, headaches, loss of appetite, and alcohol intolerance have been reported in workers exposed to DMF. DMF has been associated with liver damage, skin problems, weakness and constipation. Long-term studies of workers exposed to DMF indicate a possible role for this chemical in the development of testicular cancer, however animal studies have not demonstrated that DMF is mutagenic or carcinogenic. The International Agency for Research on Cancer has classified DMF as a possible carcinogen. DMF hepatotoxicity is believed to be dose-dependent. Hepatic necrosis and steatosis have been observed on liver biopsy specimens from exposed workers. The long-term hepatic effects of DMF exposure are not known.

DIMETHYLACETAMIDE

Jaundice has been observed in workers exposed to high levels of DMAC with skin penetration contributing to this effect. Hepatomegaly secondary to DMAC exposure is well recognized. Doses of DMAC given to patients with advanced malignancies may induce depression, lethargy, confusion, and disorientation. Hallucinations (primarily visual), perceptual distortions, and delusions are common. Workers chronically exposed to DMAC may exhibit varying evidence of hepatotoxicity. DMAC appears to be noncarcinogenic.

Toxic Dosage/Death

Acrylamide polymer is nontoxic. Toxicity from acrylamide can result from handling of the crystalline powder, primarily through cumulative skin absorption. DMF exposure to air concentrations of 3,500 ppm is considered immediately dangerous to life or health. The concentration of DMAC considered an immediate danger to life and health is 400 ppm.

Drug Interactions

Ingestion of alcohol during or after an exposure to DMF can produce a disulfiramlike reaction, with facial flushing, dizziness, sweating, nausea, palpitations, breathlessness, and loss of consciousness. This probably is due to the inhibition of acetaldehyde dehydrogenase by methylformamide.

Pregnancy/Lactation

No studies in human pregnancy or lactation are available.

Laboratory

ANALYTIC METHODS

DMAC in air is measured by gas chromatography with a flame ionization detector. Urine levels of MMAC are measured by gas chromatography. DMF and methylformamide in blood may be measured after extraction into ethanol by nitrogen-selective gas chromatography. Methylformamide in the urine is quantified by flame-ionization gas chromatography.

BLOOD LEVELS

A relationship exists between the amount of DMAC absorbed and the amount of MMAC excreted in the urine so that biomonitoring of urinary metabolites may indicate situations in which total exposure, both dermal and inhalation, are excessive.

Treatment

GUT DECONTAMINATION

Charcoal may be useful in isolated cases of oral epoxy or resin ingestion, however formal study has not been done.

ELIMINATION ENHANCEMENT

No experience with elimination enhancement of epoxy or resin materials has been documented in the literature.

SUPPORTIVE MEASURES

- Workers exposed to DMAC and DMF should be informed about potential adverse health effects. Workers must be trained to avoid skin contact and to use appropriate protective equipment and work practices.
- Employees should institute engineering controls to ensure that DMF exposure does not exceed the National Institute for Occupational Safety and Health (NIOSH) recommended and permissible exposure limits.
- Saline irrigation and slit lamp investigation should follow eye exposure to any of these agents.
- Skin exposure is followed by prompt and extensive irrigation with water.
- Oral ingestion of epoxy and resin materials is treated supportively.
- Elevation of serum aminotransferase has been observed following occupational exposure to DMAC and DMF. Liver function tests should be obtained in patients with significant DMAC and DMF exposures within 24 hours and followed weekly. Resolution of the abnormal liver enzymes may take up to 1 to 7 months. Elevations of creatine phosphokinase (CPK) may follow exposure to DMF.

Questions—Ethers And Epoxy Resins

1. **Dimethylformamide**
   A. May be associated with testicular cancer
   B. Can induce liver damage
   C. Induces reversible mental status changes
   D. A and B
2. **DMAC is widely absorbed through**
   A. Dermal exposure
   B. Oral exposure
   C. Inhalation
   D. All of the above
3. **Exposure to DMAC**
   A. Is best indicated by measuring urinary concentration of n-methylformide
   B. Is safe at levels up to 100 mg/kg of creatinine
   C. Is not measured in urine after skin exposure
   D. Is directly related to urinary DMF levels after respiratory exposure
4. **Subacute intoxication of acrylamide may cause**
   1. Hypotension
   2. Seizures
   3. Gastrointestinal bleeding
   4. Peripheral neuropathy and hepatotoxicity
   A. 1 and 2
   B. 1 and 3
   C. 1, 2, and 3
   D. All of the above
5. **Ingestion of alcohol during or after exposure to DMF can produce all except**
   A. Facial flushing
   B. Paralysis
   C. Nausea, palpitations
   D. Loss of consciousness

PLASTICIZERS

Chemicals referred to as a plasticizers are added to vinyl plastics to make them more pliable. Vinyl plastic is used in the manufacture of blood bags and associated medical devices used in the collection, processing, storing, and dispensing of blood components. It is also used in numerous consumer products such as imitation leather, rainwear, footwear, upholstery, flooring, tablecloths, shower curtains, food packaging materials, and children's toys. Cling films, the thin, clear, flexible plastic films used for packaging foods, are made from PVC or vinylidene chloride (VDC) copolymers. Plasticizers provide flexibility to these substances.

The most widely used plasticizer worldwide, particularly for medical devices, is a phthalic acid ester known as di (2-ethyl hexyl) phthalate or DEHP. DEHP is not bound chemically to the vinyl plastic, but is dissolved physically into it. DEHP may be leached from PVC containers by numerous drugs. The possibility therefore exists for migration of the plasticizer from the plastic film. It is insoluble in water but soluble in fat and can therefore migrate into food containing fats and oils. Because plasticizers are fat soluble, cling films should not be used to wrap food with a high fat content. Plasticizers also used in PVC cling films are di-2-ethyl hexyl adipate (DEHA) and polymeric species.

Limited data exist on exposure to di-n-butylphthalate, a liquid used to make soft plastics, paints, glue, insect repellents, hair spray, nail polish, and rocket fuel. Glo sticks and other glow products are very popular with children, especially in the summer months. They provide a heatless chemical luminescence in an array of vivid colors. Contact of any body parts with the liquid contents induces a burning sensation. Little or no morbidity is observed, however workers may develop hypertension, pain, numbness, spasm, reflex disturbances, depression of vestibular function, and hyperbilirubinemia after extended exposure. Eye irrigation, gut dilution, and washing with soap is adequate treatment in most cases.

Pharmacokinetics

ABSORPTION

- DEHP may enter the body through the lungs, skin, or gastrointestinal tract, as well as through direct injection. It readily forms aerosols.
- It is absorbed rapidly and extensively following oral administration.
- DEHP is absorbed primarily as its nondeesterified metabolite, MEHP. Hydrolysis occurs in intestinal cells, mucosa cells, blood, and tissues. Little DEHP is detected in the body after oral exposure.
- MEHP undergoes oxidative metabolism to yield 13 or more metabolites excreted in the urine.

DISTRIBUTION

- In one case, the elimination half-life of DEHP was approximately 10 hours.
- The apparent volume of distribution of DEHP is 0.06 L/kg.

ELIMINATION

- Approximately 4.5% to 15% of a single oral dose of 10 to 30 grams of DEHP is excreted as urine metabolites. These oxidized metabolites are excreted in humans as glucuronides.

Clinical Presentations

Based on animal data, DEHP may have potential toxicity in the heart, lungs, liver, and reproductive organs in man. There have been no specific defined lesions in humans associated with its use. Limited data in man seem to suggest that humans exposed to "normal" amounts of phthalates are not susceptible to cytogenic effects. Patients repeatedly exposed to phthalate esters in infusion fluids have not been adequately studied to prove a causal relationship between exposure and possible renal pathology. The inhalation of DEHP has been associated with pulmonary dysfunction and bronchial asthma. Exposure of workers to high levels of mixed phthalates in the workplace area may produce transient irritation of the nose and throat.

Laboratory

ANALYTIC METHODS

Liquid-liquid extraction followed by capillary gas chromatography has been developed to screen solutions leached from packaging material. This procedure screens for metabolites of DEHP.

BLOOD LEVELS

Plasma concentrations of DEHP- and MEHP-derived metabolites may be determined by gas chromatography-chemical ionization spectrometry. DEHP metabolites in urine samples may be of use in monitoring occupational exposure to DEHP.

Treatment

GUT DECONTAMINATION

Charcoal may be useful in plasticizer ingestion, however formal studies have not been done.

ELIMINATION ENHANCEMENT

No experience with elimination enhancement of plasticizer materials has been documented in the literature. It is known, however, that significant amounts of these materials may be leached from tubing involved in exchange transfusions.

SUPPORTIVE MEASURES

- Saline irrigation and slit lamp investigation should follow eye exposure to any of these agents.
- Skin exposure is followed by prompt and extensive irrigation with water.
- Oral ingestion of plasticizer materials is treated supportively.

Questions—Plasticizers

1. All of the following are true about DEHP except
 A. Is physically dissolved into vinyl
 B. Is rarely used
 C. Has the potential to migrate from plastic film
 D. Is used in blood bags, intravenous bags, and medical components

2. Plasticizers
 A. Are soluble in water
 B. Are soluble in oil
 C. Are added to vinyl to make it stiffer
 D. Will not leach from cling wrap into food with high fat content

3. All of the following are true about DEHP except
 A. Is absorbed into the lungs, skin, gastrointestinal tract
 B. Is directly measurable in the body after oral exposure
 C. Is eliminated as urine metabolites
 D. Readily forms aerosols

4. Exposure to phthalates is associated with
 A. Bronchial asthma
 B. Is directly measurable in the body after oral exposure
 C. Pulmonary dysfunction
 D. A and C

5. Treatment of a patient exposed to DEHP includes
 1. Immediate irrigation of the eyes
 2. IV fluids, supportive measures
 3. Alkalinize urine
  A. 1 and 2
  B. 1 and 3
  C. 2 and 3
  D. All of the above

ANSWERS

Introduction To Plastics, Resins And Plasticizers

1. E 2. C

Plastics

1. B 2. C 3. A 4. C 5. E

Ethers And Epoxy Resins

1. D 2. D 3. A 4. D 5. B

Plasticizers

1. B 2. B 3. B 4. D 5. A

SELECTED READINGS

Plastics

1. Blais P, Campbell RW. Cyanoacrylates in medicine. Can Med Assoc J 1982;126:227–228.
2. De Fonsek ACP. Danger of instant adhesives. Br Med J 1976;2:234.
3. Rajanieni R. Clinical evaluation of occupational toxicity of methylmethacrylate monomer in dental technicians.J Soc Occup Med 1986;36:56–59.

Acrylamide

1. Donovan JW, Pearson T. Ingestion of acrylamide with severe encephalopathy, neurotoxicity, and hepatotoxicity. Vet Hum Toxicol 1987;29:462.
2. Garland TO, Patterson MWH. Six cases of acrylamide poisoning. Br Med J 1967;4:134–138.
3. Le Quesne PM. Clinical and morphological findings in acrylamide toxicity. Neurotoxicology 1985;6:17–24.

Dimethylacetamide

1. Kennedy GL Jr. Biological effects of acetamide, formamide and their monomethyl and dimethyl derivatives. CRC Crit Rev Toxicol 1986;17:129–182.
2. Proctor NH, Hughes JP, Fischman ML, Hathaway GW. The chemical hazards. In: Proctor NH, Hughes JP, Fischman ML, eds. Chemical hazards of the work place, 2nd ed. New York: Van Nostrand Reinhold, 1989; pp. 206–207.

Dimethylformamide

1. Baselt RC, Cravey RH. Disposition of toxic drugs and chemicals in man. 3rd ed. Chicago: Year Book, 1989; pp. 280–282.
2. NIOSH alert on DMF. [DHHS (NIOSH) 90–105].
3. Scailteur V, Lauwerys RR. Dimethylformamide (DMF) hepatotoxicity. Toxicology 1987;43:231–238.

Plasticizers

1. Milkov LE, Aldryeva MV, Poporia TB et al. Health status of workers exposed to phthalate plasticizers in the manufacture of artificial leather and films based on PVC resins. Environ Health Perspect 1973;3:175–178.
2. Rubin RJ, Ness PM. What price progress? An update on vinyl plastic blood bags. Transfusion 1989;29:358–361.

ACKNOWLEDGMENT

Thanks to Ann Marie Testarmata, MD for contributing the questions in this chapter.

PART

V

Natural Toxins

CHAPTER 52

Snakes, Reptiles, and Amphibians

INTRODUCTION TO SNAKES

All snakes belong to the order Squamata, suborder Serpentes, characterized by scaly skin, absence of movable eyes, and elongated bodies without appendages. About 120 species of snakes reside in the United States, 26 of which are considered poisonous. Members of the Crotalidae (pit viper) family inflict the vast majority (95%) of poisonous snakebites. The three main genera in this family are Crotalus (rattlesnake), Agkistrodon (copperhead and cottonmouth), and Sistrurus (pygmy rattler and Massasauga). Rarely, envenomation results from foreign snakes imported to private or public collections (about 2% of poisonous snakebites).

More than 5,000 snakebites were reported to the American Association of Poison Control Centers (AAPCC) Toxic Exposure Surveillance System (TESS) by 66 poison centers in 1997. Only two deaths were reported. Within the last 40 years, improved supportive care and the aggressive use of antivenin have significantly reduced mortality and morbidity.

Not all bites by poisonous snakes result in envenomation, or deposition of venom into a victim. Rattlesnakes fail to inject venom in up to 20% of bites. Coral snake bites are often superficial, leading to an even lower rate of envenomation. The highest rates of venomous snakebites occur in the southern United States. Enzyme-refined equine antivenoms are clinically effective against hemostasis disorders, hypotension, and postsynaptic neurotoxicity, but much less effective against presynaptic neurotoxicity, nephrotoxicity, and local necrosis.

Nonvenomous Snakes

Of the thousands of people bitten by snakes in the United States each year, more than 80% are not envenomated. Patients bitten by a nonvenomous snake usually can be discharged after tetanus toxoid inoculation and local wound care. If the snake cannot be identified, the patient should be observed closely for 4 to 6 hours for symptoms and signs of envenomation. Prophylactic antibiotic therapy usually is unnecessary. Persistently tender snakebite wounds may contain an embedded tooth fragment that can be detected radiographically.

Venomous Snakes

There are five families of venomous snakes. The Viperidae include vipers, adders, pit vipers, and rattlesnakes. The Elapidae include cobras, kraits, mambas, coral snakes, and terrestrial Australasian venomous snakes. American venomous snakes include certain Crotalidae, or pit vipers, and certain Elapidae, or coral snakes. The Colubridae are black-fanged, arboreal snakes such as the African boomslang and twig snakes. The Hydrophiidae include sea snakes. See Chapter 53, Marine Toxicology and Mammals. The Atractaspididae include burrowing asps or stiletto snakes (formerly known as burrowing or mole vipers) and adders.

Crotalidae (Pit Vipers)

Four characteristics generally separate poisonous pit vipers (Crotalidae family) from most nonpoisonous snake species. These include a triangular or arrow-shaped head (compared with a smooth tapered body and narrow head of nonpoisonous snakes), facial pits located between the nostril and eye (this organ functions as a heat and vibration sensor), vertical, elliptical pupils (in contrast to the round pupil of nonpoisonous varieties; however, poisonous coral snakes do have round pupils), and a single row of subcaudal scales (compared with a double row in nonpoisonous snakes). Coloration and diamondback patterns do not exclusively identify rattlesnakes because nonpoisonous snakes mimic these markings as defensive mechanisms. All pit vipers have movable fangs that inject a controlled amount of venom (compared with the fixed fangs of the Elapidae).

The typical victim of a pit viper is a young male (11 to 35 years of age, with highest incidence between 11 and 19 years) who is bitten on the hand while trying to handle the snake. The male/female ratio of victims is 4:1. Women more commonly sustain a bite on the leg during an inadvertent encounter. Overall, about two-thirds of bites involve the upper extremity, one-third involve the lower extremity, and less than 1% occur on other body parts. Because snakes either hibernate or are inactive during winter, the peak snakebite season is April through October.

COTTONMOUTHS (*AGKISTRODON PISCIVORUS*)

The prominent white buccal mucosa gives this genus its common name. Mature members have a dark olive color, a heavy body, and a broad head. Commonly, they inhabit a semiaquatic environment, which leads to their other common name, water moccasin. No rattles are present.

COPPERHEADS (*AGKISTRODON CONTORTRIX*)

The head of these snakes is solid copper to red-brown. The rest of the body is marked with dark cross bands that resemble dumbbells. The highland moccasin is another common name. These snakes possess no rattles.

MASSASAUGA (*SISTRURUS CATENATUS*)

These shy and gentle snakes of the rattlesnake species are classified as *S. catenatus*. The Massasauga is distinguished from true rattlesnakes (Crotalus) by nine large shields arranged in rows across the crown of its head. In contrast, *Crotalus* species have small crown scales. Generally, the Massasauga inhabits bogs or swamps but moves to drier places in summer. The desert Massasauga lives in the Sonoran desert region of the southwestern United States. It has a slender tail or small rattles and averages 18 to 28 inches in length.

PYGMY RATTLER (*SISTRURUS MILIARIUS*)

The other member of the *Sistrurus* genus has a small, slender body that seldom exceeds 30 inches in length. Like the Massasauga, the pygmy rattler displays characteristic dorsal head scales. The *Sistrurus* genus is considered more primitive than true rattlesnakes (*Crotalus*) and may represent an evolutionary "side path" in the development of the true rattlesnake.

TRUE RATTLESNAKES (*CROTALUS*)

Although all pit vipers share the aforementioned four characteristics, variations in color and body features separate genera. Most, but not all, rattlesnakes (genus *Crotalus*) have a set of interlocking, terminal horny segments known as rattles. A characteristic buzzing sound, similar to the sound of escaping steam, may occur before a strike. Each molting (average of three to four times per year) adds a rattle, but trauma or congenital abnormalities may lead to their absence.

Elapidae (Coral Snakes)

Two genera of poisonous coral snakes, *Micrurus* and *Micruroides*, represent this family in the United States. Coral snakes are slender snakes ranging from 2 to 4 feet with brightly colored rings circling the body, but not the head or tail. In North America, the coral snake's red and yellow rings are contiguous, whereas nonvenomous snakes that mimic coral snakes have a black ring separating the red and yellow rings. The famed mnemonic "Red on yellow, kill a fellow. Red on black, good for Jack" helps differentiate the coral snake from nonpoisonous snakes.

In contrast to pit vipers, coral snakes have round pupils, fixed fangs, small heads, and no facial pits. Generally, coral snakes are docile, preferring to chew rather than bite, because their fangs are fixed. The Eastern coral snake (*Micrurus fulvius fulvius*) inhabits the southern United States from Arkansas to Florida and the Texas coral snake (*Micrurus fulvius tenere*) extends to west Texas. The Arizona or Sonoran coral snake (*Micruroides euryoxanthus*) is found in the Southwestern United States.

Questions—Introduction to Snakes

1. **Most snakes in the United States are considered poisonous.**
   A. True
   B. False
2. **Which of the following is/are true?**
   A. Coral snakes have round pupils, fixed fangs, small heads, and no facial pits.
   B. Cottonmouths (*Agkistrodon piscivorus*) get their name from their white buccal mucosa.
   C. There are ten families of venomous snakes.
   D. All of the above
   E. A and B
3. **Four characteristics generally separate poisonous pit vipers (Crotalidae family) from most nonpoisonous snake species. These include all of the following except**
   A. A triangular or arrow-shaped head
   B. Facial pits located between the nostril and eye
   C. Diamondback patterns
   D. Vertical, elliptical pupils
   E. A single row of subcaudal scales
4. **Copperheads**
   A. Have copper-colored heads
   B. Possess rattles
   C. Are also called highland moccasins
   D. All of the above
   E. A and C
5. **The typical victim of a pit viper is**
   A. A young female
   B. Bitten on the arm
   C. Bitten in January in the United States
   D. All of the above
   E. None of the above

CROTALIDAE

True Rattlesnakes

There are 32 species of rattlesnakes comprising 65 to 70 subspecies. 15 species are limited to the United States. Rattlesnakes can be found in every state on the U.S. mainland except Maine and Delaware.

EASTERN DIAMONDBACK

The eastern diamondback rattlesnake (*Crotalus adamanteus*) is the largest rattlesnake, with some reported as long as 7 feet. The highly specialized sidewinder species uses a peculiar type of lateral motion for rapid movement over the smooth hot desert terrain, as little contact with the hot ground is required.

MOJAVE RATTLESNAKE

The Mojave rattlesnake (*Crotalus scutulatus scutulatus*) is a clinically important species because its venom causes delayed neurotoxic effects that are not accompanied by the usual tissue damage used to estimate toxicity. Recognition of this species is necessary to treat the neurologic sequelae of envenomation properly. This snake is easily confused with the western diamondback species (*Crotalus atrox*). The Mojave rattlesnake favors flat grassland or brushy desert and rarely is found in more rocky, hilly terrain. Rhomboid markings are found on a brownish yellow to green background, with a tail characterized by white rings twice the size of the black rings. The basal rattle is yellow or white.

WESTERN DIAMONDBACK

Eastern and western diamondback rattlesnakes are the most dangerous species, accounting for many fatalities but only 10% of bites. One western diamondback (*C. atrox*) specimen lived more than 24 years. Variations occur in size, coloring, and distribution as well as venom potency. The western diamondback has white and black tail rings of equal width and a black basal rattle. It is the largest rattlesnake in the Western United States.

PATHOPHYSIOLOGY

Snakes are carnivores that use their venom primarily as an offensive weapon to obtain food. The potency of the venom allows the prey only several minutes to withdraw from the scene before its death. Crotalus venoms are rich in enzymes such as hyaluronidase, which causes rapid spread of venom through tissue by hydrolyzing connective tissue. Proteases digest tissue proteins and peptides, resulting in severe tissue damage. Phospholipases hydrolyze lipids and enhance disruption of neurotransmission, at both the presynaptic and postsynaptic levels. Other enzymes present include transaminase, ribonuclease, deoxyribonuclease, phosphomonoesterase, phosphodiesterase, DNase, ATPase, alkaline phosphatase, acid phosphatase, and endonuclease. Crotalus species do not contain acetylcholinesterase enzymes.

The snake cannot accurately follow prey more than 20 feet and usually stays within that distance after a strike. The best sensory modalities of the pit vipers are vibration and smell. Vision is poor with probably no color discrimination, and pit vipers are deaf. Most rattlesnakes crawl at speeds of about 3 miles per hour. Rattlesnakes usually, but not always, strike from a coiled position. The strike averages 8 ft/second and generally occurs in a slightly downward position. Accurate bites are limited to half the body length of the snake, which indicates that 10 to 15 feet is a safe distance to avoid bites. Reflex actions may cause bites up to 1 hour after a snake has died, even after decapitation.

Facial Pit

The facial pit contains thermal receptors that can detect changes of as little as 2°C one foot in front of the nose. This unique thermal sensory organ is approximately 5 mm in depth and is located below the eyes and nostrils in a depression of the maxil-

Answers to questions in shaded boxes appear at the end of the chapter.

lary bone. Because it is highly sensitive to temperature change, the facial pit allows the snake to recognize warm-blooded foes. The presence of humans probably overwhelms the sensory mechanism because of our relatively large size.

Fangs

Pit vipers have movable fangs that rest on the roof of their mouth and rotate forward during a strike. They are hollow modified upper maxillary teeth and length varies between 8 and 19 mm. This potentially allows intramuscular penetration, although even subfascial injections are uncommon. Most envenomations result from subcutaneous deposition of venom, but venom may penetrate superficial abrasions.

The pattern of fang marks depends on the strike. The most common pattern is two marks, 2 to 4 mm apart, depending on the size of the snake. Because reserve fangs gradually move into place, three fangs may be present and victims may display one, two, three, or more (multiple strikes) marks. Teeth patterns alone do not discriminate between venomous and nonvenomous snakes. A bite of nonvenomous snakes, rats, bees, or plant thorns may be confused with fang marks. Commonly, nonvenomous snakes leave a horseshoe-shaped row of multiple teeth marks.

Venom Glands

Venom glands are modified parotid glands. Contraction of voluntary muscles causes venom discharge, so that the snake controls the amount of venom injected. The venom sac contains a lethal adult dose of venom. Fortunately, the snake usually does not discharge the whole sac. Venom is a complex mixture consisting of enzymes, metal ions, biogenic amines, lipids, free amino acids, large and small proteins, and polypeptides that have only partially been identified. Snake venom composition and toxic properties vary between *Crotalus* species, perhaps because of local evolutionary pressure. Venom may vary seasonally because of changes in feeding patterns or physiological responses such as hibernation. Individual variation occurs within the same species because of such factors as age and time from last feeding. Rattlesnakes are venomous from birth.

CLINICAL PRESENTATIONS

Severity varies greatly between bites. The seriousness of an envenomation is determined by presenting signs, symptoms, and laboratory abnormalities. About 20% of *Crotalus* bites do not result in envenomation and produce no toxic effects. Severity depends on numerous factors including age (children have more severe reactions), amount of venom injected, toxicity of specific venom involved (species, individual, and seasonal variation), size of the snake, protective clothing, health of the victim, condition of the snake, type of treatment rendered, pathogens in the mouth of the snake, and individual patient susceptibility.

Crotalus envenomation classically presents with visible fang marks (one or more), immediate burning without severe pain, and localized edema that develops within 5 minutes of the bite. Swelling usually progresses to involve the whole extremity within 1 hour, but remains subcutaneous. Elevations of intracompartment pressures are small provided there is no muscle necrosis from a subfascial envenomation. The intensity of the pain is correlated with the amount of edema, rather than a direct action of the venom. Species variation does occur. The eastern diamondback produces the most severe swelling, for example, and the Mojave rattlesnake the least. Tender regional lymph nodes may be palpable.

Venom affects almost every organ system with the exception of the brain, which appears resistant to direct toxic effects. The primary target organs are the hematologic, cardiovascular, respiratory, and central nervous systems. Renal dysfunction may result from hypoperfusion, hemoglobinuria, and perhaps a direct effect on the kidney.

Dermatologic Effects

Serious local dermatologic changes characterize *Crotalus* envenomation because of the presence of proteases and hyaluronidase. Cutaneous manifestations of envenomation are fang marks, edema, ecchymosis, vesiculation, and necrosis. Generalized petechiae and purpura appear rarely and are associated with thrombocytopenia, especially in previously damaged skin. Ecchymoses resulting from extravasation of blood from damaged vessels occurs within several hours. Clear or hemorrhagic vesicles and petechiae may appear distant to the fang marks on the same extremity.

Necrosis results from untreated bites and was common before development of an effective antivenin. If burning pain or edema more than 2 cm from a fang mark has not developed within an hour, envenomation probably has not occurred. Despite significant discoloration and swelling of extremities, arterial pulses generally increase after envenomation. Decreased skin temperature in the extremity suggests ischemia.

Neurologic Effects

Most rattlesnake envenomations cause relatively minor changes in neuromuscular transmission as compared with coral snake envenomations. The major exception is Mojave rattlesnake envenomation, which produces respiratory paralysis that may result in death. The neurotoxin appears to act on presynaptic acetylcholine release. Mojave rattlesnake envenomation can produce respiratory paralysis after an 8 to 12 hour delay, with little or no preceding local pain or systemic symptoms.

Hematologic Effects

A wide spectrum of coagulation and platelet disorders as well as microangiopathic hemolytic anemia can develop after envenomation. Both hypofibrinogenemia and thrombocytopenia without significant coagulopathy may result from envenomation. A consumptive coagulopathy (DIC) can occur after *Crotalus* envenomation and is characterized by elevated levels of fibrin-split products, thrombocytopenia, and hypofibrinogenemia. Clinically, the syndrome is manifested by petechiae, bleeding from gums and puncture sites, hematomas, melena, epistaxis, and hematuria. Rarely, intracerebral, intracardiac, and retinal hemorrhage results.

Cardiovascular Effects

Although some venoms (e.g., those of Mojave and Southern Pacific rattlesnakes) contain a direct cardiotoxin, hypotension usually results from extravasation caused by intimal injury and changes in vascular resistance. Released serotonin and bradykinin also may contribute to hypotension. Large volumes of fluid may diffuse across injured capillaries. Hypotension usually results from third spacing of fluid. Pulmonary edema may result from extravasation of proteins through damaged alveolar membranes.

Systemic Symptoms

The development of systemic symptoms (e.g., perioral paresthesias and facial fasciculations) indicates a moderate to severe envenomation. Weakness, diaphoresis, lightheadedness, and nausea commonly occur. Muscle fasciculations may involve the head and neck in addition to the extremities. Paralysis is more common with the eastern diamondback and Mojave rattlesnakes, but otherwise is rare. Seizures are not a usual part of the clinical picture.

PREGNANCY/LACTATION

Antivenin may be used in pregnancy where it can prevent envenomation-induced abortions.

LABORATORY

Analytic Methods

Enzyme-linked immunoassay techniques have been developed in experimental laboratories to detect North American pit viper venom in samples taken from the bite area. Plasma and urine venom levels frequently are too low to be detected. Potentially, such assays can differentiate snakebites from other injuries and envenomations, determine the genus and occasionally the species involved, and detect the presence of specific antibodies in human populations. Unfortunately, the materials are available only in specialized laboratories.

Blood Levels

No specific blood level can diagnose or predict the severity of a crotalid bite.

TREATMENT

Gut Decontamination

These methods play no role in the treatment of crotalid bites.

Elimination Enhancement

Although the kidney excretes venom, no such measures have been seriously considered, especially since an antidote is available.

Supportive Measures

- All asymptomatic patients suspected of being envenomated should be observed for at least 4 to 8 hours. All envenomated patients require observation in an intensive care setting.
- Suspected Mojave rattlesnake envenomations should be observed for 24 hours.
- Hypotension is treated by starting two intravenous (IV) lines for the administration of saline. Large volumes may be required. Whole blood may be needed if hemolysis or bleeding reduces the hemoglobin level. Vasopressors may be required.
- Allergic reactions to snake bites are uncommon, except in those patients such as snake handlers who sustain multiple bites. Anaphylaxis or allergic reactions to antivenin may require fluids, diphenhydramine, and epinephrine with cardiac monitoring, and / or steroids.
- Pulmonary edema may complicate severe envenomations and should be treated like the adult respiratory distress syndrome. Respiratory depression is uncommon except as a complication of shock and Mojave rattlesnake envenomations.
- Mild sedatives and analgesics (e.g., acetaminophen, codeine) may be required. More potent analgesics must be used cautiously to avoid respiratory depression. Aspirin is contraindicated because of its enhancement of platelet dysfunction.
- Surgical incisions and fasciotomies should be avoided unless there is objective evidence of vascular compromise (e.g., elevated compartment pressures and distal sensory / motor dysfunction). Most envenomations result in superficial rather than subfascial swelling.
- Steroids should be reserved for those patients who develop serum sickness. There is no convincing evidence that steroids favorably affect the outcome of human or animal envenomation. Malaise, fever, headache, gastrointestinal upset, arthralgias, myalgias, lymphadenopathy, skin lesions, peripheral neuritis, meningismus, and renal dysfunction can characterize serum sickness.

Gradation Of Envenomation

- Numerical grading (0 to 5) has been replaced by a minimal / moderate / severe classification system. This system is more accurate and predictive of the required amount of antivenin.
- Minimal manifestations are confined to the bite area. Systemic symptoms and laboratory abnormalities are absent or insignificant.
- Moderate tissue damage extends beyond the immediate bite area. Significant systemic symptoms and signs appear along with moderate laboratory changes (i.e., thrombocytopenia, decreased fibrinogen and hemoconcentration).
- Severe tissue destruction extends to the entire extremity. Serious systemic symptoms or signs are present. Very significant laboratory abnormalities appear.

First-Aid

- Proper first-aid measures after envenomation constitute an area of controversy in which many recommendations have not been adequately researched. Above all else, move the victim to a medical facility as soon as possible, because antivenin administration is the most important treatment measure.
- Remove all constricting items, such as rings, immediately. Put the victim at rest, give reassurance, and keep warm, since activity may increase the spread of venom. Lightly immobilize the injured part below the heart.
- If possible, obtain the snake for identification, taking extreme care to avoid additional bites (envenomation is possible an hour after snake death). The snake must not be directly handled.
- Application of a lightly constricting band above the swelling (that admits a finger beneath it) is commonly recommended to prevent lymphatic spread of the venom. While a constrictive band may limit systemic spread of venom, increased local morbidity may occur and increased venom concentration at the bite site may cause increased necrosis.
- Incision and drainage are recommended only in the unusual circumstance where medical help is over 30 to 40 minutes away, and the incision / suction procedure is started within 5 minutes of the bite. Surgical drainage has no value in a medical facility where antivenin is available.
- A constriction band is placed just proximal to the wound, and the incision is made through the fang marks. This procedure is probably not effective after 10 to 15 minutes, because venom spreads rapidly from the site of envenomation. Proper technique involves parallel incisions through the fang marks, about 1 cm in length, just through the skin (no deeper than 3 mm). Avoid cross-incision (cruciate incisions), because of poor wound healing. Use of a commercial suction device is preferable to suction by mouth, which may contaminate the wound much like a human bite.
- Although cryotherapy has some strong proponents, most authorities advise against the use of ice packs, cold packs, or ice water soaks.
- Do not give alcohol or drugs in the field, and do not wait to evaluate the seriousness of the envenomation, since early administration of antivenin is most effective.
- Tourniquets should not be removed in the emergency department until intravenous lines are established and antivenin therapy is ready.

Wound Care

- The affected area is cleansed with medium-pressure irrigation (e.g., 18-gauge needle and syringe) using very dilute povidone-iodine (Betadine®) solution. The wound may be left open

or gently covered with nonadherent hydrophilic dressings (e.g., Xeroform®).
- For the first 3 days, the extremity should be immobilized below the heart in a position that facilitates rehabilitation.
- Give tetanus booster if the person has not been adequately immunized within 5 years.
- Prophylactic antibiotics are appropriate for high-risk wounds (e.g., severe envenomations, those patients who received incision and drainage by the human mouth, and bites on the hand or foot in which puncture wounds tend to produce infection).
- Gram-negative organisms in the mouth of the North American pit viper require broad-spectrum coverage.
- Debridement of hemorrhagic blebs and necrotic tissue should be delayed for 3 days until hemostasis is normal.

Ancillary Tests

- Labs (e.g., fibrinogen, fibrin-split products, platelets, PT, PTT, and complete blood count) are followed for the development of defibrination syndrome. Often the coagulopathy is a benign process that does not result in bleeding. Heparin is not indicated. Treatment, when needed, involves the use of fresh-frozen plasma, cryoprecipitates, and platelet packs.
- Early hematologic changes may include hemoconcentration, hypofibrinogenemia, and thrombocytopenia. A rebound thrombocytosis may occur 36 hours after envenomation. Anemia may result from hemolysis or bleeding. Clotting times typically are prolonged and fibrinogen may be depleted for several days, but complications usually develop only in severe cases. The PTT is prolonged earlier and more often than the PT.
- Urinalysis may indicate hematuria, glycosuria, proteinuria, or myoglobinuria. Serum electrolytes, creatinine, and blood urea nitrogen also are followed. A chest x-ray, arterial blood gases, and electrocardiogram (ECG) may be indicated in severe envenomations, particularly in patients older than 40 years.

ANTIDOTES

Polyvalent Crotalidae Antivenin

Antivenin is a lyophilized powder of refined horse serum produced by immunization of horses with the venoms of *Crotalus atrox* (western diamondback), *Crotalus adamanteus* (eastern diamondback), *Crotalus durissus terrificus* (South American rattlesnake), and *Bothrops atrox* (fer-de-lance). Because pit viper venoms have basic antigenic characteristics, the antivenin is effective against poisonous American pit vipers, including rattlesnakes, pygmy rattlesnakes, cottonmouths, and copperheads as well as the fer-de-lance, Cantil, and Central and South American bushmaster.

Antivenin is necessary for all significant *Crotalus* envenomations unless the risks significantly outweigh the benefits. The only absolute contraindication to antivenin use is the lack of signs of envenomation. A relative contraindication is horse serum sensitivity. Dosing depends on gradation of envenomation. The most serious adverse reaction to polyvalent crotalidae antivenin is a type I anaphylactic reaction to the horse serum, especially in patients with horse serum sensitivity. Up to 80% of patients who receive antivenin may develop serum sickness within 3 weeks (average, 3 to 14 days). Fever, headache, myalgias, arthralgias, and urticaria characterize this. Patients who receive more than seven vials invariably develop serum sickness.

Sensitivity Testing

Sensitivity testing is the best way to measure human sensitivity to horse serum, although 1% of patients with a negative skin test can develop immediate, though not usually severe, hypersensitivity reactions. Sensitivity testing should not be done in patients for whom antivenin is not needed, because such testing itself may sensitize patients and complicate future antivenin administration. Before testing, a history should be obtained about horse serum sensitivity because these patients are at higher risk of anaphylactic reactions. The physician must be prepared to treat an anaphylactic reaction before administering the test. An IV line should be in place, and oxygen, epinephrine, and diphenhydramine immediately available.

For patients without horse serum sensitivity, sensitivity testing is performed by intradermally injecting 0.02 mL of horse serum diluted 1:10 into one location and injecting 0.02 mL of normal saline in the opposite extremity as a control. A wheal and erythema indicate a positive reaction. Occasionally, patients may develop generalized urticaria, pruritus, or bronchospasm. No reaction by 20 to 30 minutes indicates a negative reaction. For patients suspected of horse serum sensitivity, the horse serum should be diluted 1:100 (10 times weaker) and administered in the same acute care setting under direct observation. Not all patients with positive skin tests will have immediate hypersensitivity reactions when antivenin is given slowly.

The use of antivenin in a patient with a positive skin test requires careful clinical judgment, since withholding antivenin in severe envenomations may result in loss of life or limb. Pretreatment with diphenhydramine and careful, slow antivenin titration, as well as the use of subcutaneous epinephrine for reactions, may be helpful. Be prepared for severe reactions in an acute care setting. Difficult patients may respond to antivenin infusions and simultaneous epinephrine infusion in a separate line, but this method requires considerable judgment.

PATHOPHYSIOLOGY

Antivenin neutralizes pit viper venom but does not reverse local injury. Early administration (ideally within 4 hours) is necessary to prevent local and systemic injury before vascular destruction restricts antivenin delivery to tissues.

DOSAGE

The amount used depends on the clinical grading of severity. Typical dosages are 5 to 8 vials for minimal, 8 to 12 vials for moderate, and 12 to 30 or more vials for severe rattlesnake bites. Additional 5-vial incremental doses may be added to the 500-mL saline bottle if local or systemic signs progress. The circumference of the bitten extremity should be measured at points 10 and 20 cm above the bite every 15 minutes during antivenin administration as one guide to the dosage required (systemic signs and symptoms are the other).

Children typically have more severe reactions to a given envenomation because of the greater amount of venom per body weight and, therefore, tend to require more antivenin than adults. Giving antivenin by clinical grading accounts for this difference. The exact dose depends on the patient's response as determined by progression of extremity swelling and systemic symptoms. In geographic areas in which the Mojave rattlesnake is found, the administration of 10 vials of antivenin may be considered despite the lack of symptoms whenever envenomation by this species is strongly suspected. All patients with suspected Mojave rattlesnake bites should be observed in an intensive care unit and given antivenin when any symptoms develop.

Because IV administration of antivenin is the most effective route, antivenin should not be given intramuscularly, not in a digit, and not at the site of the bite. For adults, the appropriate number of antivenin vials is added to 500 mL of normal saline and then piggybacked to the main IV line. For children, the volume is decreased proportionally so that the reconstituted vials may be diluted 1:1 in normal saline and added to a microdrop set.

The diluted antivenin is started slowly with careful observation for signs of an allergic reaction (e.g., pruritus, urticaria and flushing). If such symptoms develop, the infusion is stopped and fluids and diphenhydramine are given. If no reaction occurs within the first 5 to 10 minutes, the infusion rate should be increased to administer the entire dose of antivenin within the first 2 to 4 hours after envenomation. Antivenin is less effective 8 hours after envenomation and of questionable value after 24 hours, except in reversing coagulation defects.

Questions—True Rattlesnakes

1. **Rattlesnake envenomation capable of significant neuromuscular toxicity is associated with the**
   A. Cottonmouth
   B. Mojave rattlesnake
   C. Copperhead
   D. Western diamondback
   E. Eastern diamondback
2. **Rattlesnakes can be found in every state on the U.S. mainland except**
   A. Arizona and Utah
   B. Alaska and Hawaii
   C. North Carolina and South Carolina
   D. Maine and Delaware
   E. Arizona and New Mexico
3. **The number of crotalidae antivenin vials needed to combat the effects of a bite is based on**
   A. The patient's weight
   B. Time since the patient was bitten
   C. The clinical grading of severity
   D. All of the above
   E. A and C
4. **Which of the following is false?**
   A. The eastern diamondback rattlesnake is the largest rattlesnake.
   B. The Mojave rattlesnake is easily confused with the western diamondback.
   C. Eastern and western diamondback rattlesnakes are the most dangerous species, accounting for many fatalities but only 10% of bites.
   D. All of the above
   E. None of the above
5. **Snakes are herbivores that use their venom primarily as a defensive weapon when attacked.**
   A. True
   B. False
6. **Crotalid venom contains numerous enzymes including**
   A. Hyaluronidase, which causes hemolysis
   B. Proteases, which digest tissue proteins
   C. Phospholipases, which hydrolyze lipids
   D. Acetylcholinesterase enzymes, which degrade cholinergic transmission
   E. B and C
7. **Reflex actions may cause bites up to 1 hour after a snake has died, even after decapitation.**
   A. True
   B. False
8. **The facial pit contains thermal receptors that can detect changes of as little as 2°C one foot in front of the nose. Because it is highly sensitive to temperature change, the facial pit allows the snake to recognize warm-blooded prey and foes.**
   A. True
   B. False
9. **Teeth patterns alone do not discriminate between venomous and nonvenomous snakes; however, nonvenomous snakes commonly leave a horseshoe-shaped row of multiple teeth marks.**
   A. True
   B. False
10. **Antivenin is a lyophilized powder of refined horse serum produced by immunization of horses with various crotalid and other snake venoms.**
    A. True
    B. False
11. **Hematologic disorders that can develop after rattlesnake envenomation include**
    A. Hyperfibrinogenemia
    B. Thrombocytopenia without significant coagulopathy
    C. A consumptive coagulopathy
    D. All of the above
    E. B and C

Pigmy Rattlesnakes and Massasaugas

Sistrurus snakes include the pigmy rattlesnake (*Sistrurus Miliarius*) and Massasaugas (*Sistrurus catenatus*). Both comprise three subspecies each, and are distributed throughout the United States. Generally, *Sistrurus* snakes are gentler than *Crotalus* rattlesnakes and are highly secretive.

CLINICAL PRESENTATIONS

Envenomations involve the same organ systems as *Crotalus* bites, but the clinical picture usually is much less severe. Often bites occur without envenomation. The clinical picture of *Sistrurus* envenomation more closely resembles copperhead than *Crotalus* bites. Edema is much less severe, but hemorrhagic blebs frequently occur after Massasauga envenomation. Some nausea develops, but vomiting, paresthesias, and fasciculations are uncommon. Laboratory abnormalities and fatalities are rare.

TREATMENT

- Management of *Sistrurus* envenomation is similar to *Crotalus* protocols, with gradation of clinical symptoms and administration of Antivenin (Crotalidae) Polyvalent as needed.
- Often, antivenin is not necessary.

Questions—Pygmy Rattlesnakes and Massasaugas

1. **Which of the following is false?**
   A. *Sistrurus* snakes include the pygmy rattlesnake and Massasaugas (*Sistrurus catenatus*).
   B. *Sistrurus* envenomations involve the same organ systems as *Crotalus* bites, but the clinical picture usually is much less severe.
   C. The clinical picture of *Sistrurus* envenomation more closely resembles copperhead than *Crotalus bites.*

D. Management of *Sistrurus* envenomation, unlike *Crotalus* bites, does not require the administration of antivenin
E. Hemorrhagic blebs frequently occur after Massasauga envenomation

Copperheads

Five species of copperheads (*Agkistrodon contortrix*) range from the eastern United States to southern Texas. The average adult copperhead is 60 to 90 cm and has a large coppery head, a thick body with reddish brown hourglass designs, and a rattleless tail. This species is found in mountains, wooded hillsides, and in the south near streams and lowlands. Their bite is the least venomous among North American pit vipers.

CLINICAL PRESENTATIONS

Copperhead bites produce less swelling and ecchymosis than do bites of other North American pit vipers, but pain may be out of proportion to local tissue injury. Systematic symptoms, especially fasciculations, are unusual. Thrombinlike enzymes that produce coagulation defects *in vitro* have been isolated from copperhead venom. The resultant incomplete splitting of fibrin fails to activate clot-stabilizing factors.

TREATMENT

- Most of the medical literature does not deal specifically with copperhead bites but considers them together with *Crotalus* envenomations.
- General wound care, first aid, and antivenin administration are the same as for *Crotalus* envenomations.

ANTIDOTES

Polyvalent crotalidae antivenin is effective as with the *Crotalus* group, but usually only children or the elderly require its use.

Questions—Copperheads

1. **The copperhead's bite is the least venomous among North American pit vipers.**
   A. True
   B. False

Cottonmouth

Three cottonmouth (*Agkistrodon piscivorus*) species are distributed across the semiaquatic environments of the southeastern United States. A unique white buccal mucosa on a dark head, a broad heavy body, and a rattleless tail characterize this species. The cottonmouth shares pit viper characteristics with rattlesnakes.

CLINICAL PRESENTATIONS

Cottonmouth bites produce an envenomation intermediate in severity between those of rattlesnakes and copperheads. The clinical manifestations should be graded similarly to rattlesnake envenomation.

TREATMENT

- See general guidelines under True Rattlesnakes, above.

ANTIDOTES

Polyvalent crotalidae antivenin is effective and should be used in the same manner as after rattlesnake envenomation.

Questions—Cottonmouth

1. **Cottonmouths are shy snakes whose bite may be treated with polyvalent crotalidae antivenin. Their prominent rattles generally hint at their whereabouts.**
   A. True
   B. False

ELAPIDAE

The Sonoran or Arizona coral snake (*Micruroides euryoxanthus*) appears primarily in Arizona. The Texas coral snake (*Micrurus fulvius tenere*) is found in Texas, Louisiana, and Arkansas and the Eastern coral snake (*Micrurus fulvius fulvius*) ranges across the southeastern United States. These snakes belong to the Elapidae family and differ anatomically and clinically from *Crotalus* species. Coral snakes account for only 1% to 2% of annual poisonous snakebites in the United States.

A small, round head and a tricolored, slender body consisting of wide black and red bands separated by yellow or white stripes characterize this genus. Their eyes are round, and their fangs are fixed. Bites leave a row of teeth marks rather than fang marks, because the coral snake needs prolonged contact (about 30 seconds) to work venom into the skin. This secretive snake avoids human contact and most bites result from molestation of the snake.

Pathophysiology

Coral snake venom is primarily a neurotoxin and causes little local tissue reaction. Systemic neurologic reactions are common. The rate of fatalities from bites of the eastern coral snake (i.e., not the Arizona coral snake) is about 9% compared with 0.2% for pit viper bites.

Clinical Presentations

Some pain may be present at the bite site, but usually edema, erythema, and pain are minimal. Typically, several hours after envenomation, neurologic signs and symptoms develop. Euphoria, lightheadedness, or drowsiness appears first. Fasciculations, tremor, weakness, increased salivation, and nausea and vomiting then occur. Symptoms may progress to bulbar palsy, paralysis, and respiratory depression after 5 to 10 hours manifested by diplopia, slurred speech, ptosis, dysphagia, and dyspnea. Convulsions can develop in small children.

Symptoms may be delayed 7 to 10 hours after coral snake bites and no local reaction may be present to confirm envenomation. Death may occur within 24 hours because of respiratory depression, although hypotension and cardiovascular collapse may contribute to mortality. The Arizona coral snake causes headache, blurred vision, abdominal pain, and gait disturbances, but usually not the serious central nervous system symptoms associated with Texas and eastern coral snakes.

Treatment

SUPPORTIVE MEASURES

- First-aid recommendations are similar to those involving crotalidae (see above). Capture of the snake is an important measure to help identify the species if it can be done promptly, safely, and with minimal hazard to both victim and rescuer.
- Transport the patient to an emergency medical facility as soon as possible.

- All victims of coral snake envenomations should be carefully observed for at least 24 to 48 hours.
- Narcotics such as morphine that depress respirations should be avoided. Do not give alcohol to the victim.
- Tourniquets are controversial and may not be effective, although isolated studies have suggested that pressure wrapping and immobilization may decrease the spread of venom.

Antidotes

CORAL SNAKE ANTIVENIN

North American coral snake (*M. fulvius*) antivenin is an effective antidote and is recommended for all Texas and eastern coral snake envenomations. The same precautions, including skin testing and the quick availability of epinephrine and other measures, should be used as for the administration of polyvalent crotalidae antivenin. Serum sickness may develop similar to that following administration of polyvalent crotalidae antivenin and is treated in a similar fashion.

Approximately 3 to 5 vials of antivenin should be given in 250 to 500 mL of normal saline after a negative skin test. The antivenin should be administered as soon as possible without waiting for symptoms to develop. An additional 3 to 5 vials should be given if neurotoxic signs develop. There is no antivenin available for the Arizona or Sonoran coral snake (*Micruroides euryoxanthus*).

Questions—Elapidae

1. Which of the following concerning *Elapidae* is/are true?
   A. A small round head and a tricolored, slender body consisting of wide black and red bands separated by yellow or white stripes characterizes this genus.
   B. *Elapidae* fangs are retractable and are often left in bite wounds.
   C. Coral snake venom is primarily a cardiotoxin.
   D. All of the above
   E. B and C

2. Signs of coral snake envenomation may include
   A. Minimal edema, erythema, and pain at the bite site.
   B. Complete heart block
   C. Arrhythmias
   D. Torsade de pointes
   E. None of the above

3. North American coral snake (*M. fulvius*) antivenin is an effective antidote and is recommended for all Texas and eastern coral snake envenomations.
   A. True
   B. False

COLUBRIDAE

This snake family comprises 1,400 species or about two-thirds of the world's snakes. 38 genera have been identified in the United States. Generally, snakes from this family are not considered poisonous because they lack the specialized venom-injecting apparatus seen in the *Crotalidae* and *Elapidae*. Their small size and difficulty in injecting venom contribute to their designation as nonpoisonous. Both rear-fanged (opisthoglyphous) and nonfanged (aglyphous) colubrids possess a Duverney's (parotid) gland, which is located above the rear maxillary teeth and contains toxic saliva.

Clinical Presentations

Most colubrid bites result only in minor abrasions and anxiety, because envenomation apparently requires continued contact. Certain colubrid species, some of which are imported into the United States, appear to cause envenomation with prolonged (e.g., 30 second) bites. An imported red-neck keelbuck bite (*Rhabdophis subminatus*) has produced prolonged defibrination, headache, nausea and vomiting within 4 hours. A severe consumptive coagulopathy subsequently developed with thrombocytopenia, absent fibrinogen, depressed factors V and VIII, and elevated fibrin degradation products.

Bites by the Japanese colubrid snake known as yamakagashi (*Rhabdophis trigrinus*), a close relative of the American garter snake, have produced nausea, vomiting, headache, and coagulation disorders that have resulted in massive ecchymosis and hematuria. Two nonindigenous African colubrid species, the twig snake and boomslang, are considered venomous and have caused fatalities.

Treatment

- Experience with treatment procedures is limited. First aid primarily involves dislodging the snake.
- Hemorrhage can be a serious threat to life. Hematemesis and hematuria may require cryoprecipitate, packed red blood cells, and fresh-frozen plasma transfusions. Heparin and epsilon-aminocaproic acid are not recommended.

Antidotes

The effectiveness of colubrid antivenins is not known, and their use should probably be avoided except in severe envenomations.

Questions—Colubridae

1. Most U.S. colubrid bites result only in minor abrasions and anxiety, because envenomation apparently requires continued contact.
   A. True
   B. False

2. Some colubrid bites around the world have been deadly.
   A. True
   B. False

EXOTIC SPECIES

Both legally and illegally imported snakes for private collections and zoos can represent a significant health hazard. Almost 10% of the 75,000 snakes imported annually are venomous and account for 1% to 2% of reported venomous bites. Local or regional consultants should be contacted concerning special care or the use of antivenin. An antivenin index is kept by the Arizona Poison Information Center. Injuries and death because of snakes occur in most parts of the world especially in the tropics where they may represent a major health problem. While by no means exhaustive, the regional list below describes some of the better known venomous snakes.

Africa

In the savanna regions of West Africa, the carpet viper (*Echis carinatus*) is the most important cause of snakebite morbidity and mortality. The carpet viper is probably responsible for more deaths and injuries caused by snakebite than any other species. It may cause thousands of deaths a year in the savannah region of Nigeria alone. The Gabon viper (*Bitis Gabonica*) can cause neurologic, respiratory, cardiac, and hematologic symptoms. In North Africa scorpion stings are medically more important than snakebites.

Australia

There are over 120 species of snake in Australia or 6% of the world's snakes. About 60% of these are from the *Elapidae* family. It has been estimated that Australia possesses 40% of the world's elapid snakes, and about 23% of all venomous snakes in the world. Nevertheless, the reported mortality as a result of snakebite is only two or three per year. Up to 500 cases of envenomation occur requiring antivenom per year, and about 3,000 bites remain asymptomatic and require no treatment.

The Australian small-scaled snake (*Oxyuranus microlepidotus*) or inland taipan, is an elapid that is potentially the most poisonous snake in the world. Signs of Australasian elapid envenomation include vomiting, headaches, localized pain of the lymph nodes, abdominal pain, loss of consciousness, shortness of breath, cyanosis of the lips and gums, and a heavy sensation of the limbs. Australian elapids induce a coagulopathy characterized by defibrination and normal platelet counts. Factors V and VIII, protein C, and plasminogen are significantly depleted. Monovalent antivenoms may be employed to neutralize the five major groups of Australian snake venom.

Burma

Each year 10,000 snakebites, from 144 species, occur in Burma with an estimated 1,000 lives lost. Russell's viper is perhaps the most venomous snake in Burma and is responsible for 85% of poisonous snakebites and 95% of the fatalities due to venomous snakebites. Cobra bites are responsible for 5% of deaths resulting from venomous snakebites in Burma.

In minimal envenomations from Russell's viper, there are mild symptoms and slight local swelling. If severe, hemorrhagic effects such as bleeding gums, epistaxis, hemoptysis, hematemesis, hematuria, orbital edema, and subconjunctival hemorrhages may be observed in a few hours. Shock may be seen. The prothrombin time is much prolonged and the plasma fibrinogen extremely low. Polyvalent cobra venom is available. After antivenom therapy, the coagulation time can return to normal within 2 to 3 hours.

Central America

Bothrops asper is responsible for the majority of snakebites in Central America. Venoms from the adult snake induce myonecrosis, hemorrhage, edema, defibrination, systemic hemorrhage, cardiovascular shock, and acute renal failure. The newborn snake exhibits higher lethal, hemorrhagic, edema-forming, and proteolytic activities than the adult does. In Costa Rica, hospital admissions for snakebites have been estimated as high as 22.4 per 100,000 population per year, with five deaths per 100,000 mostly from bites by *Bothrops asper*.

China

In China, there are 200 species, 62 genera, and 8 families of snakes. 57 species are considered venomous. Many snakes are captured, sold and used for their venoms, skin (arts and crafts), bile (traditional medicine), and meat (food). The Shanghai Institute of Biological Products for the whole country produces antivenoms. No statistical data on snakebites are readily available. Antivenom against *Agkistrodon blomhoffi brevicaudus* can be used for snakebite of all species of *Agkistrodons*. The antivenoms of *Elapidae* and *Viperidae* are very specific. The banded krait (*Bungarus multicinctus*) often induces respiratory arrest and multisystem organ failure. Antivenom and respiratory support are essential for survival.

Europe

The common European adder (*Vipera berus*), *Vipera aspis*, *Vipera ammodytes*, and *Vipera ursini* are found in Europe. Snakebites are relatively rare. Only 14 deaths from *Vipera berus* have been reported in Britain during the last 100 years. In England and Wales, only one death from adder bite was recorded from 1950 to 1972, but there were 61 deaths from bee or wasp stings. The last adder bite death in Germany was in 1959. In France, about 1,000 to 2,000 bites, mostly from *Vipera aspis* and *Vipera berus* are reported each year.

Vipera venoms contain hyaluronidase and proteolytic enzymes, which cause local damage to subcutaneous structures and capillary endothelium. Direct neurotoxic activity has been associated with *V. ammodytes*, and cardiotoxicity has followed bites from *V. berus* and *V. aspis*. Histamine, bradykinin, prostaglandins, and serotonin may be released during reaction to a *Vipera* bite. *Vipera* envenomation is characterized by edema, relatively little local pain, vomiting, abdominal pain, diarrhea, leukocytosis, shock, confusion, somnolence, and occasional loss of consciousness. Bronchospasm, renal dysfunction, fever, exanthem, coagulopathy, and hemolysis may be observed.

Supportive care has been the mainstay of treatment in symptomatic cases. An antivenom from Zagreb may be helpful. Reassurance, immobilization of the bitten limb, tetanus protection, volume substitution, and correction of acid-base balance and electrolyte abnormalities will suffice in most cases. Severe reactions may require high-dose steroids and inotropic drugs. Anaphylactic reactions may require epinephrine, antihistamines, and corticosteroids.

Hong Kong

Snakebites in Hong Kong are most commonly from *Trimeresurus albolabris* (the white-lipped pit viper or bamboo snake). Most induce a coagulopathy, probably resulting from the presence of a thrombinlike substance that induces defibrination and secondary fibrinolysis. Increased blood concentration of fibrin degradation products is the most sensitive test for detecting the abnormality, although a decrease in fibrinogen concentration and thrombocytopenia also are seen. Problems remain with the purification of the antivenom and its use probably should be restricted to high-risk patients. Fatalities rarely have occurred.

India

There are four medically important venomous land snakes in India. These include the Indian krait (*Bungarus caeruleus*), the common cobra (*Naja naja*), the saw-scaled viper (*Echis carinatus*), and Russell's viper (*Vipera russelli*). Only Russell's viper has been locally reported as a cause of renal failure. Peritoneal dialysis has been shown to be an adequate form of treatment for many of these patients. Nevertheless, thousands of deaths from snakebite are reported annually.

The frequency of snakebites peaks in the rainy season, which coincides with increased agricultural operations. Farmers and their families are the main victims. Vasculotoxic and neuroparalytic signs predominate. In addition to general supportive care, polyvalent antivenom is the mainstay of treatment. Neostigmine with atropine may be used to reverse paralysis. Ventilatory support is essential. Whole blood transfusions and transfusions of fibrinogen with heparin may be used to correct bleeding diatheses.

Israel

Of the 35 or more snake species of Israel, eight are venomous and belong to three families. These include six species of *Viperidae*, one *Elapidae* species (*Walterinnesia aegyptia*) and one *Atractaspididae* species (*Atractaspis engaddensis*). *Vipera palestinae* is the most clinically important snake of Israel, accounting for 100 to 300 bites/year and rare fatalities. Symptoms include weakness, restlessness, vomiting, profuse perspiration, and abdominal pain. Diarrhea, hypotension, tachycardia, angioneurotic edema, and swelling of the bitten extremity may follow. Monospecific antivenom is available and effective for *Vipera palestinae* bites.

Japan

Rhabdophis tigrinus (family Natricidae) and *Agkistrodon blomhoffi blomhoffi* (family Crotalidae) are the most common venomous snakes in Japan. Others are found in the Ryuku archipelago and include *Callophis* species (family Elapidae) and *Trimeresurus* species (family Crotalidae) or habu. Antivenom against habu is commercially produced.

Malaysia

In Malaysia, 17 of 105 strictly land snakes are venomous and dangerous to man. All 14 species of fresh-water snakes are harmless, but all of the 22 species of sea snakes are venomous. The family Viperidae is represented by two genera, the *Agkistrodon* with a single species, and *Trimeresurus* with seven species. All the dangerous land snakes found in Malaysia belong to the Elapidae family and include cobras, kraits, and coral snakes. Most snake species are forest dwellers. The genus *Agkistrodon* (family Viperidae) is represented by one species, *Calloselasma rhodostoma*, which probably is the most common cause of snakebite in Malaysia. It produces local swelling and/or systemic poisoning with blood clotting abnormalities or shock. Antivenom treatment may not prevent hemorrhage.

Middle East

Echis coloratus (family Viperidae) inhabits the arid zones of the Middle East, including the Jordan valley, Judean desert, and northern Negev. *Echis carinatus* is the other major snake causing envenomation in this area. The venom of all species of Echis causes hemostatic failure, with disseminated intravascular coagulation and occasional thrombocytopenia. Unlike *E. coloratus*, untreated envenomation by *E. carinatus* is associated with overt bleeding and 10% to 20% mortality mostly because of cerebral hemorrhage. Antivenom for Echis snakes is available.

New Guinea

The Papuan black snake, *Pseudechis papuanus*, is a main cause of serious snakebites in Southern Papua. The New Guinea death adder (*Acanthophis antarcticus*) produces venom that appears to act postsynaptically by blocking cholinergic receptors causing a severe flaccid paralysis and death from respiratory failure. Polyvalent Papuan antivenom is available. Nonspecific death adder, taipan, black snake, or brown snake antivenoms are available. Anticholinesterases administered together with atropine may be useful during the initial stage of envenomation from death adders.

Persian Gulf

The Arabian Peninsula and the waters that surround it harbor at least 51 species of snake, of which 18 are poisonous. Of the land snakes, at least nine must be considered dangerous. These include Innes' cobra (*Walterinnesia aegypti*), the Arabian cobra (*Naja naja arabicus*), the sand viper (*Ceristes Cerastes gasperittii*), the Levant viper (*Vipera lebitina*), *Pseudocerastes persica fieldi*, the puff adder (*Bitis lactesis*), the burrowing adder (*Atractaspis microlepidota andersoni*), the carpet viper (*Echis carinatus*), and *Echis coloratus*. All nine types of sea snakes in the area are dangerous.

Philippines

The snake fauna of the Philippines is related to those in Malaysia and Western Indonesia, but it lacks the genera *Bungarus* and *Agkistrodon*. Out of more than 60 species, seven are venomous. Three are *Trimeresurus* (family Crotalidae) and four are elapids (family Elapidae). Probably the most important snake in the Philippines is the Philippine cobra (*Naja naja philippinensis*). Cobras are the leading cause of snakebite death in the Philippines.

The Philippine cobra produces a clinical syndrome significantly different from other Asian cobras in which local swelling and necrosis but not paralysis are the most distinctive features. Neurotoxicity dominates the clinical picture and can be severe in the absence of any swelling or necrosis at the bite site. Neurotoxic signs may not occur until 24 hours after a bite, however ptosis may occur as early as 5 minutes. Respiratory dysfunction and apnea may begin in 10 minutes, but usually take longer. Arrhythmias and hypotension may occur in some patients with severe respiratory paralysis and may be related to hypoxemia.

South America

In Brazil, snakes of genus *Bothrops* (lance-headed vipers) are responsible for more than 80% of bites in which the snake is identified. These pit vipers also are the most common cause of envenomation in other parts of Latin America. Since the introduction of antivenom, case fatality has decreased dramatically. Acute renal failure is the major cause of death. Shock, intracranial hemorrhage, and blood incoagulability also have been reported with *Bothrops* envenomation.

The jararaca (*Bothrops jararaca*) is responsible for 90% of all snakebite cases in southeastern Brazil. Swelling, ecchymosis, necrosis, coagulopathy, and spontaneous systemic bleeding may follow envenomation. The bleeding often is correlated with the presence of thrombocytopenia. Systemic envenomation with *B. jararaca* may result in incoagulable blood. These phenomena also have been seen with *Bothrops atrox*.

Sri Lanka

Sri Lanka has one of the highest incidences of death from snakebite in the world. The snakes of Sri Lanka include all the known families of venomous or medically important snakes such as the kraits and cobra (family Elapidae), sea snakes (family Hydrophiidae), Russell's viper, saw-scaled viper, hump-nosed viper, and green pit viper (family Viperidae). The common krait (*Bungarus caeruleus*), cobra (*Naja naja naja*), and Russell's viper (*Vipera russelli pulchella*) account for 97% of deaths due to snakebite envenomation in Sri Lanka.

The victims of the common krait (*Bungarus caeruleus*) run a greater risk of death than from any other snake in Sri Lanka. Most of these deaths occur without receiving antivenom. The Elapidae family is the most important group of snakes in Sri Lanka. Their venom is mainly neurotoxic. Lyophilized polyvalent antivenoms effective against the venoms of Indian, *Naja naja, Bungarus caeruleus, Vipera russelli,* and *Echis carinatus* are available.

Thailand

There are 160 species and 9 families of snakes in Thailand. 46 species in 2 families are deadly. Each year thousands of individuals are bitten and hundreds die. The Siamese cobra (*Naja kaouthia*) induces the highest mortality rate. The spitting cobra (*Naja sputatrix*) can spit venom several feet toward the head or face of an enemy. Permanent blindness may result. The king cobra (*Ophiophagus hannah*) is perhaps the longest venomous snake in the world. Bites may be fatal in 3 minutes. The banded krait (*Bungarus fasciatus*) is the least aggressive venomous snake in Thailand, but produces a potent neurotoxin. Russell's viper (*Vipera russelli siamensis*) makes a hissing sound when disturbed, feeds at night on rodents, birds, and frogs and induces varying degrees of acute renal failure in man.

Viper bite treatment aims at prevention of the venom from reaching the systemic circulation, neutralization of circulating venom, correction of venom-induced abnormalities, and general supportive care. Specific antivenom is used when the nonclotted blood or venous clotting time lasts longer than 30 minutes. Monovalent antivenom, 4 to 6 vials, is administered in normal saline, 250 mL IV over 30 minutes and repeated in 6 hours if indicated. Heparin infusion may be helpful after a Russell's viper bite.

Questions—Exotic Species

1. **Which of the following country/snake associations is wrong?**
   A. Thailand—Cobras
   B. Brazil—Bothrops
   C. Sri Lanka—Kraits
   D. Europe—Adders
   E. Hong Kong—Crotalidae
2. **Both legally and illegally imported snakes for private collections and zoos can represent a significant health hazard. Almost 50% of the 750,000 snakes imported annually are venomous and account for 5% of reported venomous bites.**
   A. True
   B. False

COLORADO RIVER TOAD

The Colorado River Toad (*Bufo alvarius*) is the most toxic toad in North America. Salivation, cyanosis, cardiac dysrhythmias, dyspnea, and seizures are common complications of the ingestion of *Bufo alvarius* by domestic animals. The dried venom of the *B. alvarius* or Colorado River toad contains 5-methoxy-N, N-dimethyltryptamine (Meo-DMT), a hallucinogen related to N, N-dimethyltryptamine. "Smoking toad" induces hallucinations lasting about 5 minutes. A clinical picture of profound drooling, seizure activity, arrhythmias, and cyanosis may follow the oral application of a toad to an individual's tongue. Such activity is called "toad kissing." See Chapter 20, Hallucinogenic Drugs.

In general, toad venoms contain biogenic amines (e.g., epinephrine and norepinephrine), indolalkylamines (bufotenins), cardioactive steroids similar to digitalis compounds (bufotalin or bufogenins), and conjugates of bufogenins (bufotoxins). A 5-year-old boy who placed a toad in his mouth developed drooling and generalized tonic-clonic seizures within 15 minutes. Seizures lasted 1 hour until controlled by diazepam and phenobarbital in the emergency department. Physical examination revealed a total left-sided hemiparesis, Babinski sign, slurred speech, tachypnea, tachycardia, and systolic hypertension. The serum potassium level was 2.5 mEq/L. The neurologic deficit resolved over 1 week on high-dose hydrocortisone sodium succinate.

Questions—Colorado River Toad

1. **"Kissing" or "smoking" toad may cause**
   A. Hallucinations
   B. Seizures
   C. Salivation
   D. All of the above
   E. A and C
2. **The dried venom of the *Bufo alvarius* or Colorado River toad contains**
   A. LSD
   B. Tryptamine
   C. A hallucinogen related to N, N-dimethyltryptamine
   D. Cannabinoids
   E. Phencyclidine

COLOMBIAN POISON-DART FROG

The Colombian poison-dart frog group contains some of the most toxic substances known to man. The skin secretions of Colombian poison-dart frogs contain the steroidal alkaloid, batrachotoxin, pumiliotoxins B and C, isodihydrohistrionicotoxin, and gephyrotoxin. Dysrhythmias and atrial arrest develop after the application of batrachotoxin to isolated cardiac muscle preparations in animal models. At least three species of frogs (*Phyllobates terribilis, Phyllobates bicolor, Phyllobates aurotaenia*) from lower Central America and northwestern South America possess the powerful poison batrachotoxin. Birds of the *Pitohui* species from New Guinea recently have been identified as containing homobrachotoxin, a toxin that resembles batrachotoxin.

One freshly caught *Phyllobates terribilis* frog (the most dangerous species) contains up to 1.9 mg of batrachotoxin. The lethal dose in humans ranges from 0.02 to 0.2 mg. This toxin depolarizes electrical membranes by increasing the permeability to sodium ions. Fast axonal transport also is blocked at high concentrations. In contrast with the sodium-channel blockers, tetrodotoxin and saxitoxin, batrachotoxin activates the sodium channel by binding to a separate and distinct site. This results in stabilization of the sodium channel in an open conformation. This toxin produces swelling of the axon at the node of Ranvier and extracellular fluid accumulation along the axon.

Questions—Colombian Poison-Dart Frogs

1. **The Colombian poison-dart frog group contains some of the most toxic substances known to man. The skin secretions of Colombian poison-dart frogs contain the steroidal alkaloid**
   A. Tetrodotoxin
   B. Batrachotoxin
   C. Cicutoxin
   D. Botulinum toxin
   E. Saxitoxin
2. **Birds of the *Pitohui* species from New Guinea have recently been identified as containing homobrachotoxin, a toxin that resembles batrachotoxin.**
   A. True
   B. False
3. **Colombian poison-dart frog toxin depolarizes electrical membranes by increasing the permeability to sodium ions. It activates the sodium channel by binding to a separate and distinct site. This results in stabilization of the sodium channel in a closed conformation.**
   A. True
   B. False

GILA MONSTER

Only two lizards of the family Helodermatidae are considered venomous, containing rudimentary grooved teeth and venom glands located in the lower jaw. These two species are the Gila monster (*Heloderma suspectum*) and the beaded lizard, escorpion (*Heloderma horridum*). The Gila monster appears primarily in the Great Sonoran Desert. Two subspecies are the banded Gila monster and the reticulated Gila monster. These creatures are large (30 to 40 cm), slow-moving, nocturnal lizards that live 10 to 25 years. They possess sharp claws on short, stout legs, and flat, relatively large heads with blunt snouts.

Pathophysiology

A primitive injection apparatus consists of grooved teeth that connect by a duct to the lower mandibular venom glands. Envenomation requires prolonged contact and a grinding motion. Bites may be tenacious, requiring minutes to several hours to disengage. Because the venom is used primarily for defense, bites in humans are rare and usually result from careless handling of captured lizards. Lizard venom has much lower enzymatic activity than rattlesnake venom and consists primarily of phospholipase A, hyaluronidase, serotonin, protease, and kallikrein. The toxin helothermine has been isolated from *Heloderma horridum horridum* (Mexican beaded lizard) venom.

Clinical Presentations

Most bites cause local tissue injury, pain, and minor systemic complaints such as weakness, lightheadedness, paresthesias, muscle fasciculations, diaphoresis, nausea, and chills. Edema is usually minimal but, beginning about 15 minutes after envenomation, may extend slowly over a 4- to 8-hour period. The delayed appearance and slow progression of edema help differentiate the bite of the lizard from that of the rattlesnake.

Pain, a consistent symptom, may be severe for several hours and last for 8 hours. The wound may remain tender for several weeks. Hypotension is a potential complication and should respond to fluid challenges. Clotting abnormalities in humans have not been reported, but patients who are discharged should be warned about such possibilities and instructed to return if increased bruising or bleeding occurs. Deaths from Gila monster envenomation have not been well documented.

Treatment

- The most important measure is detachment of the tenacious creature from the victim with whatever means are available. Pulling the reptile by the tail has been suggested, but increased tissue destruction may result.
- Irrigate and debride the wound, taking care to remove embedded teeth. Teeth do not appear on x-rays.
- Peripheral nerve blocks may help relieve pain. Check the distal neurovascular system carefully and make serial assessments.
- Prophylactic antibiotics are unnecessary. Give tetanus prophylaxis as needed.
- Analgesics should be given as needed to provide relief while observing the usual precautions.
- Treat hypotension with fluids.
- Laboratory abnormalities are usually minimal. Coagulation studies have been normal in envenomated victims despite very early experimental work that suggested bleeding abnormalities in experimental animals.
- Intraventricular conduction defects and T-wave inversions have been reported.

Questions—Gila Monster

1. **Which of the following about Gila monsters is/are true?**
   A. Only two lizards of the family Helodermatidae are considered venomous, containing rudimentary grooved teeth and venom glands located in the lower jaw.
   B. The Gila monster appears primarily in the Great Sonoran and Sahara Deserts.
   C. Envenomation requires prolonged contact and a grinding motion. Bites may be tenacious, requiring minutes to several hours to disengage.
   D. All of the above
   E. A and C
2. **Clotting abnormalities are frequent after Gila monster envenomations.**
   A. True
   B. False

NEWT

The skin and internal organs of several species of newts possess tetrodotoxin, the same neurotoxin that causes hypotension and respiratory paralysis following puffer fish ingestion. Ingestion of a newt (*Taricha granulosa*) has produced paresthesias and a fatal cardiopulmonary arrest within 2 hours, however patients have survived the consumption of five newts. Variations in the presence of the neurotoxin probably account for differences in clinical presentation. The East Coast species found in the Carolinas (*Notophthalmus*) is much less potent in animal studies than the West Coast variety (*Taricha*). Treatment is supportive, with early gut decontamination recommended. Patients should be observed for 24 hours for signs of respiratory depression and hypotension.

Questions—Newt

1. **Several species of newts contain**
   A. Tetrodotoxin
   B. Cicutoxin
   C. Grayanotoxin
   D. Saxitoxin
   E. Batrachotoxin

ANSWERS

Introduction To Snakes

1. B 2. E 3. C 4. E 5. E

True Rattlesnakes

1. B 2. D 3. C 4. E 5. B 6. E 7. A
8. A 9. A 10. A 11. E

Pigmy Rattlesnakes and Massasaugas

1. D

Copperheads

1. A

Cottonmouth

1. B

Elapidae

1. A 2. A 3. A

Colubridae

1. A 2. A

Exotic Species

1. E 2. B

Colorado River Toad

1. D 2. C

Colombian Poison-Dart Frogs

1. B 2. A 3. B

Gila Monster

1. E 2. B

Newt

1. A

SELECTED READINGS

Snakes, Reptiles, and Amphibians

1. Blackman JR, Dollon S. Venomous snakebite: Past, present, and future treatment options. J Am Board Fam Pract 1992;53:399–405.
2. Clement JE, Pietrusko RG. Pit viper snakebite envenomation in the United States. Clin Toxicol 1979;14:515–538.
3. Dart RC, Horowitz R, Gomez H. Management of poisonous snakebite in the United States. Rocky Mountain Poison and Drug Center and University of Colorado, Denver, CO. Revised September 18, 1994.
4. Davidson T, Schafer S, Jones J. North American pit vipers. J Wilderness Med 1992;3:397–421.
5. Harris JB. Toxic constituents of animal venoms and poisons: 1. Incidence of poisoning, clinical and experimental studies and reptile venoms. Adverse Drug React Acute Poisoning Rev 1982;1:65–92.
6. Hitt M, Ettinger DD. Toad toxicity. N Engl J Med 1986;314:1517.
7. Hooker KR, Caravati EM. Gila monster envenomation. Ann Emerg Med 1994;24:731.
8. Kunkel DB, Curry SC, Vance M, et al. Reptile envenomations. J Toxicol Clin Toxicol 1983-1984;21:503–526.
9. Minton SA. Beware: Nonpoisonous snakes. Clin Toxicol 1978;15:259–265.
10. Russell FE, Carlson RW, Wainschel J et al. Snake venom poisoning in the United States: experience with 550 cases. JAMA 1975;233:341–344.
11. Russell FE, Picchioni AL. Snake venom poisoning. Clin Toxicol Consult 1983;5:73–87.
12. Sutherland SK. Treatment of snakebite. Aust Fam Physician 1990;19:1–13,21–41.
13. Warrell DA, Fenner PJ. Venomous bites and stings. Br Med Bull 1993;49:423–439.
14. Watt CH. Poisonous snake bite treatment in the United States. JAMA 1978;240:654–656.
15. Wingert WA, Sullivan JB. Snakebite management: Which approach to use. Emerg Med Rep 1984;5:37–44.
16. Wingert WA. Poisoning by animal venoms. Top Emerg Med 1980;2(3):89–118.

CHAPTER 53
Marine Toxicology and Mammals

INTRODUCTION

Marine animals may be classified as invertebrates or vertebrates. Invertebrates include the Coelenterata, which are represented by over 9,000 species. Three major groups of Coelenterata characterized by a large gastric cavity surrounded by tentacles that possess venomous nematocysts include the Hydrozoa (e.g., hydroids, fire coral, and Portuguese Man-of-War), Scyphozoa (e.g., sea wasp, sea nettles, and true jellyfish) and the Anthozoa (e.g., sea anemones, true coral, and soft coral).

Other invertebrates include the Porifera (sponges). This group contains over 4,000 species, at least 13 of which can cause a contact dermatitis. Of the 45,000 species of Mollusca, oysters, clams, and scallops are responsible for most toxic effects in humans. At least 18 of 400 Conus species produce envenomation. Another invertebrate, the blue-ringed octopus of Australia, produces allergic reactions and neuromuscular depression. At least 80 of the 600 species of Echinodermata are venomous. This group contains sea urchins, starfish, and sea cucumbers.

Vertebrate marine animals include the Scorpionida. Three groups of Scorpionida of interest to the toxicologist include the Pterois (e.g., lionfish, also known as the zebra fish, and turkey fish), the Scorpoena (e.g., sculpin, bullrout, and California scorpion fish), and the Synaceja (e.g., stonefish). Other toxic marine vertebrates include the weever fish, ratfish, dogfish, toadfish, catfish, stingray, and sea snakes (Hydrophiidae). All 52 species of sea snakes are venomous, being marine relatives of cobras and kraits.

Ingestion of marine creatures may be associated with a broad range of toxicities. Please see Chapter 41, Food Poisoning for an elucidation of ciguatera poisoning, scromboid, paralytic shellfish poisoning, tetrodotoxin, neurotoxic shellfish poisoning, and other toxins.

INVERTEBRATES

Coelenterata

Contact with coelenterates accounts for most marine envenomations. Coelenterates, a group of invertebrates, comprise more than 9,000 species, of which approximately 100 belonging to the phylum Cnidaria are recognized as venomous. As noted above, the Cnidaria are subdivided into Hydrozoa (e.g., Portuguese Man-of-War), Scyphozoa (e.g., jellyfish and sea nettle) and Anthozoa (e.g., sea anemone and corals). Cnidaria inflict their stings with organelles called nematocysts located in their epithelial tissues.

A single enclosed cavity characterizes each species and functions as both a gastrointestinal tract and a circulatory system. Long tentacles surround the only entrance. Two morphological forms of coelenterates (polyp, medusa) appear alternately during their life cycle. The polyp is a sedentary form that attaches to objects with its caudal end. Feeding occurs through its oral end, which is surrounded by tentacles. The medusa form is a free-floating, domelike cavity that on its concave undersurface has a mouth surrounded by tentacles. Within these tentacles are numerous stinging cells called nematocysts, which range in size from 5 μm to over 1 mm. The highest concentrations of nematocysts appear near the mouth and outer surfaces of the tentacles.

Although there are at least 17 types of nematocysts, most resemble a tightly coiled tube surrounded by a venom capsule or cnidoblast. On top of this capsule is a trap door called the operculum. The harpoonlike hollow tube is discharged through the operculum by a trigger (the cnidoblast) that is sensitive to both osmolar changes and mechanical stimulation. The coiled tube is capable of penetrating the human epidermis as well as some soft-shelled marine animals and thus transfers small amounts of venom to the victim. Large coelenterates may discharge hundreds of thousands of nematocysts.

Atlantic Portuguese Man-of-War

Also called *Physalia Physalia*, its habitat includes the Atlantic Ocean and Caribbean Sea. The gastric cavity is 5 to 10 cm in diameter, similar to the Pacific variety, but the tentacles are longer and more numerous. These free-swimming coelenterates (cnidarians) are composed of a carbon monoxide/nitrogen-filled float with a crest (pneumatophore) that functions as a sail. The similarity of the body and long tentacles to a Portuguese admiral's hat prompted the name Portuguese man-of-war. These organisms are predators that use several markedly elongated tentacles called fishing tentacles to trap prey.

Box Jellyfish

This coelenterate is also known as *Chironex Fleckeri*, "box jelly," "cubomedusan," "cubo," "fire medusa," "indringa," and "seastinger." It is reportedly the most venomous of all sea creatures. There are two species indigenous to the Southern Pacific Ocean (*Chironex fleckeri*–Australia, and *Chiropsalmus quadrigatus*–Philippines). It can be very difficult to see a box jellyfish in the water under natural conditions. Their relative transparency makes them almost invisible, except to trained spotters, even in clear sunlit seawater.

Corals

This group constitutes the major portion of coral reefs, where their calcified exoskeletons surround small anemonelike polyps. Mechanical trauma is the major clinical problem, since they do not envenomate.

Hydroids

These marine animals, also called fire coral, appear as upright, branching, calcareous growths and inhabit tropical and subtropical waters including the Florida Keys and the Caribbean Sea. Although they are not true corals, they live in coral reefs. Fire coral contains a yellow exoskeleton composed of numerous pores through which polyps protrude to cause envenomation.

Pacific Portuguese Man-of-War

Also called *Physalia Utriculus* or bluebottle, this smaller version of the Atlantic variety is distributed across the Pacific and Indian oceans. The body rarely grows larger than 8 to 10 cm in diameter, and the tentacles seldom reach 30 m.

Scyphozoa

These jellyfish species are ubiquitous throughout United States coastal waters. The sea nettle (*Chrysaora quinquecirrha*) found near Chesapeake Bay and North Carolina sounds, especially in late summer, is one of the most common and best-studied species. An estimated 500,000 annual jellyfish envenomations occur in the Chesapeake Bay and an estimated 200,000 occur in Florida.

Sea Anemones

These marine organisms (Anthozoa) develop stationary polyps with tentacles surrounding the mouth on an oral pole. The caudal pole stabilizes the body by forming attachments to an object. The polyps possess modified nematocysts, which are infrequent causes of envenomation and produce lesions similar to those produced by jellyfish.

PATHOPHYSIOLOGY

Clinical responses after coelenterate envenomation result from direct toxic effects, since repeat envenomations display similar symptoms. No cases of immunity to coelenterate stings have been reported; however, allergic reactions may play a significant role in some human envenomations. The major component of Portuguese Man-of-War venom produces vasoconstriction, pain, and histamine release. It appears to be 5-hydroxytryptamine (serotonin), but most venom is not well characterized.

Other constituents isolated from various coelenterate species include ATPase, hyaluronidases, fibrinolysin, a peripheral calcium antagonist, a neurotoxic agent (tetramine), and other low-weight-molecular fractions that cause hemolysis, local necrosis, and myocardial depression.

CLINICAL PRESENTATIONS

Portuguese Man-of-War

Portuguese Man-of-War envenomation causes painful, linear, erythematous, vesicular lesions on the skin. Pain usually resolves within 24 hours. However, cutaneous signs such as hemorrhagic vesicles, and urticaria may persist up to a month. Systemic symptoms include headache, lightheadedness, malaise, muscle cramps, diaphoresis, and syncope. Recurrent eruptions at the site of envenomation, persistent granulomatous lesions, and activation of herpes labialis after the envenomation are unusual sequelae. Subcutaneous fat atrophy, granuloma annulare, and keloid formation may occur at the site of injury.

Documented fatalities have occurred from the Atlantic Portuguese Man-of-War, but death after a Pacific *Physalia* sting has not been reported. A scuba diver was a victim in one of the fatalities when stung by the multi-tentacled Atlantic *Physalia*. By contrast, a single-tentacled *Physalia*, typified by the Australian bluebottle, inflicts a common, nonserious jellyfish sting characterized by a painful, "beaded" urticarial eruption.

Scyphozoa and Anthozoa

Scyphozoa and Anthozoa envenomation produces primarily local effects of erythematous papular lesions around which vesicles may develop within 24 hours. Pustules and necrosis are uncommon. Lymphadenopathy may appear, but usually there are no systemic complaints. These envenomations are less severe than Portuguese man-of-war envenomations.

Sea Bather's Eruption

Sea bather's eruption ("sea lice") has been reported predominantly in the Florida Keys. It is an intensely pruritic, vesicular or maculopapular eruption primarily affecting skin surfaces covered by swimwear. Symptoms begin within 24 hours of ocean exposure, last 3–5 days, and usually resolve spontaneously. The larvae of *Linuche Unguiculata* ("thimble jellyfish") likely cause the eruption.

Hydroids

Most hydroids produce mechanical injury to unprotected extremities on contact, resulting in erythema, edema, and pruritus that can progress to an indolent ulcer. Members of the Leptomedusae order cause a more severe contact dermatitis characterized by vesicular lesions, including erythema multiforme. Systemic reactions manifested by abdominal pain, diarrhea, fever, and muscle spasm, occasionally occur. *Milleporae* (fire coral) produces a painful, erythematous wound that occasionally develops irregular, necrotic borders and indolent ulcers, which may require months to heal.

TREATMENT

Scyphozoa and Anthozoa

- Analgesics and / or antihistamines may be required after simple stings.
- Current first-aid advice is to douse the sting area with vinegar. When vinegar is not available, rescuers should pick off adherent tentacles with their fingers (there is little danger of significant stinging through the rescuers' fingers) or a knife before the application of compressive, immobilizing bandages.
- Vinegar saturation of the bandage-covered sting area should be carried out when able.
- A slurry of baking soda may also inactivate unexploded nematocysts by topical application for at least 30 minutes. Aluminum subacetate 10 to 20% solution (Burow's solution) may also be used.
- Wash the area with sea (salt) water and apply a steroid cream or lotion (e.g., triamcinolone 0.1%).
- If ulcerating lesions develop, clean the area with Burow's solution and cover with dry dressings.
- Administer appropriate tetanus prophylaxis.

Portuguese Man-of-War

- Systemic symptoms may require circulatory and, for children swallowing tentacles, respiratory support. First aid is similar to that for coelenterate venom.
- Vinegar appears to be effective in fixing the nematocysts and may be used in place of alcohol.
- Steroids have not been proven to be beneficial, and no antivenin is available.
- Intravenous 10% calcium gluconate (5–10 mL for an adult) may provide temporary relief from muscle spasms.

Box Jellyfish

- Treatment measures for the Portuguese Man-of-War and box jellyfish are similar.
- Solutions of 3–10% acetic acid (in vinegar) have been shown to rapidly inactivate the penetrating nematocysts of *Chironex fleckeri*.
- A sheep antivenom is available against *Chironex* in Australia and should be given intravenously as one vial (20,000 units) in all serous envenomations. Fluids, vasopressors, and antidysrhythmic agents may be required in severe envenomations. Beneficial effects appear maximal when the antivenom is given within 4 to 6 hours after a serious *Chironex* envenomation.
- Treatment for pulmonary edema and pain following jellyfish envenomation may require large doses of meperidine or morphine, and / or phentolamine (5 mg slowly i.v. followed by 10 mg i.v. repeated when necessary) for treatment of hypertension, shaking, and sweating.
- Symptomatic management of pulmonary edema may require i.v. diuretics, opiates, or nitrites. Swan-Ganz catheterization may be required to monitor pressure so that i.v. nitroprusside, dopamine, or dobutamine can be administered. Endotracheal intubation and intermittent positive-pressure ventilation may also be necessary.
- Anaphylaxis from jellyfish envenomations is treated by first addressing the "ABC's." Epinephrine, antihistamines, aggressive hydration and / or steroids may be required.
- Verapamil may be useful for arrhythmias. Use of verapamil in mice after intravenous challenge with box jellyfish venom suggests that calcium antagonists may be useful in the acute treatment of box jellyfish stings.

Sea-Bather's Eruption

- Treatment of sea bather's eruption has included antihistamines and antipruritic agents. Topical steroids may also be used.
- All treatments may be disappointing in severe cases.
- Topical agents (e.g., isopropyl alcohol, vinegar, papain, baking soda, and / or aluminum sulfate) are unlikely to be effective in neutralizing venoms after a sting has occurred.
- Changing swimwear and showering are probably effective in preventing stings.

Hydroids/Fire Coral/Corals

- Wounds require thorough exploration and irrigation after local anesthesia. The wound must be inspected and, if necessary, probed carefully to detect any remaining skeletal fragments.
- Copious irrigation with saline should follow exploration. For grossly contaminated wounds, the povidone-iodine solution Betadine® may be added in very dilute form to the irrigating solution.
- After thorough cleansing, facial wounds can be closed. Old wounds (i.e., extremity wounds presenting 6–8 hours after injury) may benefit from delayed primary closure.
- Prophylactic antibiotics have not been effective in this setting.

Questions—Coelentera

1. Stinging cells within coelenterate tentacles are called

A. Scyphozoa
B. Medusae
C. Nematocysts
D. Pedicellaria
E. Cnidariae

Answers to questions in shaded boxes appear at the end of the chapter.

2. **Which of the following associations is incorrect?**
   A. Atlantic portuguese man-of-war—Carbon monoxide and nitrogen filled pneumatophore
   B. Box Jellyfish—Venomous South Pacific creatures
   C. Corals—Venom released with physical trauma
   D. Sea Nettle–Thousands of annual U.S. envenomations
   E. Sea Anemone—Stationery polyps and rare envenomation

3. **Signs of Portuguese Man-of-War envenomation may include**
   A. Painful, linear, erythematous, vesicular lesions on the skin
   B. Hemorrhagic vesicles
   C. Headache, lightheadedness and muscle cramps, diaphoresis
   D. All of the above
   E. A and B

4. **Sea bather's eruption ("sea lice") is probably caused by**
   A. The larvae of *Linuche Unguiculata* ("thimble jellyfish")
   B. *Milleporae* (fire coral) spines
   C. Leptomedusae slime
   D. Sea nettle stings
   E. Anthozoa envenomation

5. **Treatment options include all of the following, except**
   A. Scyphozoa and Anthozoa—vinegar
   B. Portuguese Man-of-War—vinegar, i.v. calcium gluconate
   C. Box Jellyfish—antivenin, vinegar, antiarrhythmics
   D. Sea-Bather's Eruption—isopropyl alcohol, papain
   E. Corals—wound exploration and irrigation

Porifera

At least 13 Porifera (sponge) species are considered toxic. Case studies of sponge toxicity have included the Caribbean and Hawaiian fire sponge (*Tedania ignis*), the Western Tropical Atlantic poison burn sponge (*Fibula nolitangere*), the Northeastern American red sponge (*Microiona prolifera*), and the Southern Australian stinging sponges (*Neofibularia mordens*, and *Lissodendoryx* sp).

PATHOPHYSIOLOGY

The constituents of Porifera are not well defined, but envenomation can occur after the sponge is removed from seawater if the specimen remains wet. A dry sponge is not toxic, but wetting may reactivate the toxin. Secondary inhabitants of sedentary sponges (e.g., coelenterates) are responsible for a contact dermatitis that produces local necrosis in divers and is referred to as "sponge diver's disease." Calcareous spicules may contaminate the wound and contribute to mechanical trauma, but chemical toxins clearly are involved. Vibrio species may produce secondary wound infections.

CLINICAL PRESENTATIONS

Symptoms present as a contact dermatitis similar to Rhus dermatitis (poison oak or ivy). Typically, the victim develops a transient burning pruritus and erythema on direct contact, which has been described as "putting your hand in a hornet's nest." Several hours later, mild edema, pain, and stiffness occur, followed by the appearance of vesicles that drain a seropurulent fluid. Lesions may last several weeks, with desquamation resulting after 2–3 weeks. Anaphylactoid reactions after sponge stings remain a potential complication.

TREATMENT

- The wounds are cleansed thoroughly with saline and very dilute povidone-iodine (Betadine®), taking care to remove all spicules.
- Adhesive or cellophane tape may speed spicule removal.
- Acute symptoms respond to dilute vinegar soaks (30-mL vinegar per liter of water) or 5% acetic acid soaks several times per day for 5–30 minutes.
- The patient must be followed for signs of infection. Lymphadenopathy may result from the envenomation alone.
- Desquamation occurs despite vinegar soaks.
- Steroids, antihistamines, and antibiotics do not appear to alter the course of the acute lesions. Delayed reactions, however, may result from hypersensitivity and may respond to steroids or antihistamines.

Questions—Porifera

1. **Which of the following statements regarding Porifera is false?**
   A. May cause a contact dermatitis similar to Rhus dermatitis (poison oak or ivy)
   B. Are toxic when wet or dry
   C. Envenomation may respond to vinegar soaks.
   D. Can cause anaphylaxis
   E. May cause lesions which last for weeks

Mollusca

Marine Snails

The tropical marine snail (*Conidae* species) is most abundant in shallow waters, where it lives among coral reefs. Many species may be present on the same reef. An attractive shell covers this cone-shaped univalve. The largest species, *Conus geographicus*, can attain a length up to 15 cm. These creatures are nocturnal predators that feed on worms by paralyzing them with a detachable radula tooth. During the day, the snail burrows under sand or stones.

Of approximately 400 species, at least 18 have been reported to be venomous, with most envenomations involving careless handling of shells or inadvertent contact while digging in sand or coral debris. The universal presence of a venom apparatus, however, makes all Conus species potentially toxic to humans. Thin-shelled species with wide openings have a more developed venom apparatus and are therefore potentially more harmful.

Blue-Ringed Octopus

The blue-ringed octopus (*Hapalochlaena maculosa*) is the only member of Cephalopoda (octopus, squid, cuttlefish) believed to be a toxic danger to humans. The blue-ringed octopus is a small creature found in the warm shallow waters of Australia. Rarely does this octopus exceed 20 cm in length. Dark brown bands cover both the body and the arms and contain blue rings, which become an iridescent blue when the octopus is disturbed. The small size and brilliant variable colors allow easy identification. Envenomations commonly occur when this small, colorful octopus is placed on the unsuspecting victim's hand for display.

PATHOPHYSIOLOGY

Snails

The extensible snail proboscis contains a small (6–8 mm) hollow tooth (radula tooth) at its base that forcefully injects venom into the victim. The rest of the venom apparatus lies within the body cavity of the snail and consists of a muscular venom bulb, a long, highly convoluted venom duct, and a radula sheath where the radula teeth are produced. The venom is not well characterized, but the main component is a neurotoxin that varies significantly in potency among species.

Blue-Ringed Octopus
A sharp beak is located in the center of the origin of the arms, behind which is an area connected to posterior salivary glands. At least two low-molecular-weight neurotoxins, as well as hyaluronidase, are present. The initial bite leaves two small puncture wounds and may not be painful despite serious envenomation.

CLINICAL PRESENTATIONS

Snails
Symptoms vary considerably among both patients and species. Local effects may include immediate pain (like a wasp sting) followed by local edema and erythema, which usually resolve within an hour. Hypoesthesia, hyperesthesias, local cyanosis, and ischemia may occur in more serious envenomations, and the swelling and sensitivity may last several weeks.

More serious cases involve generalized muscle weakness and paralysis characterized by hoarseness, dysphagia, diplopia, perioral paresthesias, slurred speech, weakness, and dyspnea. Nausea may be present, but other gastrointestinal symptoms are usually absent. Symptoms generally resolve within 6–8 hours, but ventilatory support has been required in some cases to maintain adequate oxygenation. At least one death has been reported after a *C. geographicus* sting.

Blue-Ringed Octopus
Lightheadedness, weakness, nausea, and vomiting may begin within 10 minutes of envenomation and may be followed by slurred speech, dysphagia, paresthesias, muscle weakness, blurred vision, diplopia, and, in severe cases, respiratory paralysis. Myoclonic jerks and muscle spasms may complicate the clinical picture.

Symptoms usually resolve within 24 hours. Fatalities have resulted from respiratory depression. Pruritus and generalized urticaria have developed 12 hours after envenomation, followed by joint effusions which required several weeks to resolve. Such reactions suggest the possibility of anaphylactoid, and perhaps anaphylactic, reactions after blue-ringed octopus bites.

TREATMENT

Conus Envenomation
- Hot water immersion (110–115°F) for 30 minutes may provide some relief. After immersion, analgesics may be given to provide pain relief although symptoms usually abate by one hour.
- Patients with systemic symptoms should be observed for signs of respiratory depression for at least six hours. Rarely is ventilatory support necessary.
- No antivenin is available.

Blue-Ringed Octopus
- Local suction and pressure immobilization have been suggested. Wound excision is not recommended. Hot water immersion appears to have no benefit.
- Patients displaying neurotoxic effects should be observed for 4–6 hours and admitted to an intensive care facility if symptoms progress.

Questions—Mollusca

1. Which of the following statements is true?
A. All tropical marine snails are venomous.
B. Marine snails can grow up to one foot in length.
C. The blue-ringed octopus is the only member of Cephalopoda (octopus, squid, cuttlefish) believed to be a toxic danger to humans.
D. Snail venom primarily contains hemolysin.
E. Blue-ringed octopus envenomation has not been associated with fatalities

Echinodermata

This phylum includes sea urchins, starfish, and sea cucumbers. Approximately 80 of 6,000 species are considered venomous to humans. The toxins vary in chemistry and modes of action. Actions in experimental animals include erythrocyte hemolysis, heart block, hypotension, neuromuscular blockage, and release of histamine.

Sea Urchins
Sea urchins (*Echinoidea*) are part of the 1% of echinoderm species that are venomous. They are ubiquitous creatures that resemble pincushions and are covered by calcareous skeletons surrounded by numerous movable calcium carbonate spines. The sharp spines are brittle and easily detach when touched by the victim. Most injuries result from either stepping on or carelessly handling the spines. Certain species (e.g., *Areosoma*) have well-developed venom spines, and others (e.g., *Tripneustes* and *Toxopneustes*) have developed specialized venom organs called pedicellaria.

Starfish
Starfish (*Asteroidea*) are widely distributed in tropical waters. A few species (*Acanthaster*) produce a slimy venomous substance that may cause a contact dermatitis. Crown-of-thorns (*Acanthaster planci*) is an attractive starfish that possesses dorsal spines covered with a sheath that secretes venom. This organism is plentiful in the Great Barrier Reef off the coast of Australia.

Sea Cucumbers
Sea cucumbers are sausage-shaped, wormlike echinoderms found in both shallow and deep water. They are bottom dwelling scavengers.

PATHOPHYSIOLOGY

Sea Urchins
The globular body of sea urchins is covered with calcareous spines of many sizes and shapes, some of which contain poison glands. Between the spines are small pincerlike organs called pedicellaria, which also serve as venom organs. Traumatic injury by penetration of the spines may occur without envenomation. All species are capable of inflicting mechanical trauma, and local tissue reaction may result from retained debris and calcareous material.

Sea urchin venom contains primarily serotonin, steroid glycosides, acetylcholinelike substances, quaternary ammonium bases, and phosphagens. The *Tripneustes* genus produces histamine and bradykininlike products within the pedicellaria that can cause severe pain and cranial nerve paralysis.

Starfish
Needle-sharp dorsal spines may pierce the victim's skin on contact.

Sea Cucumbers
Sea cucumbers produce a chemical toxin known as holothurin in glands along the side and ventral surface. Structurally, holothurin is a cardiac glycoside that causes intense inflammation.

CLINICAL PRESENTATIONS

Sea Urchins
Contact with sea urchin spines produces intense pain, with some localized erythema and edema. Colored sea urchins may leave multiple punctate discolorations within human skin when the spines fracture. Inflammation develops in response to retained fragments and may require weeks to months for complete resolution. Painless granulomas, 1–5 mm in diameter, may develop 2–12 months after envenomation.

Spines embedded near nerves and joint spaces, particularly in the hand, occasionally produce complications. Such irritation may cause hyperesthesias, sensory deficits, and painful joints. Infrequently reported systemic symptoms include weakness, nausea, syncope, lightheadedness, paresthesias, muscle spasm, dyspnea, and, rarely, respiratory depression.

Stepping on a sea urchin may result in a puncture wound, and the brittle spine may break and remain embedded in the wound. A foreign-body reaction, pain, and secondary infection may follow. If the spine is left *in situ*, a granuloma forms or the spine may be absorbed within 48 hours. Surgical removal may be required.

Starfish
Usually, the victim develops a painful erythematous lesion that resolves in several hours. Muscle paralysis, nausea, vomiting, and paresthesias have been reported in severe cases. As in sea urchin stings, granulomas may develop.

Sea Cucumbers
Contact with the venom results in a macular-papular eruption. Eye irritation may be severe, with permanent corneal opacities leading to blindness. Furthermore, the sea cucumber may secrete undigested nematocysts in its own defense. Contact with these nematocysts produces signs of coelenterate envenomation.

TREATMENT

Sea Urchins
- Hot water immersion in nonscalding water for 30–90 minutes and thorough wound cleansing are advisable, as in sea coral treatment. Analgesics may be necessary after hot water immersion.
- Detached pedicellaria may secrete venom for several hours, so a careful search should be made to remove these structures.
- Surgical excision of embedded spines may be helpful but is not indicated as a routine matter since fragmentation of the spines may lead to further injury or infection. Attempts to remove these spines may require radiological direction.
- Chronic granulomas usually require complete excision, since spontaneous intradermal or steroid-induced resolution is rare.
- Ammonia, systemic steroids, and prophylactic antibiotics have not been shown to be efficacious. Applying steroid ointment may treat mild echinoderm stings.
- Severe poisoning may require cardiopulmonary support as indicated until the venom is metabolized.

Starfish
- Hot water immersion may be helpful. Embedded spines should be removed.
- Steroid creams, antibiotics, and ammonia soaks have unproven efficacy.

Sea Cucumbers
- Follow the coelenterate treatment plan if the skin eruption simulates coelenterate envenomation.

Questions—Echinodermata

1. Which of the following associations is incorrect?
A. Sea urchins (Echinoidea)–venomous
B. *Acanthaster* starfish–contact dermatitis
C. Sea cucumbers–holothurin
D. Sea urchins–foreign body reactions
E. Sea cucumbers–edible, essentially harmless

VERTEBRATES

Scorpaenidae

This group is the most dangerous bony fish family and consists of 30 genera. Approximately 80 of the 350 species are venomous. Widely distributed, these tropical fish generally inhabit sandy, rocky, or coral coastlines in shallow water. Classification is based on the morphology of the venom apparatus.

Pterois
This group contains beautiful, graceful fish that are aquarium favorites. Examples include lionfish, turkey fish, zebra fish, butterfly cod, tiger fish, featherfish, and firefish. The most commonly encountered species is the lionfish (*Pterois volitans*), which is also known as feather fish, firefish, scorpion fish, tiger fish, zebra fish, or even turkey fish. This beautiful Asian tropical fish responds aggressively to perceived threats by erecting venomous spines.

Scorpaena
Examples include the scorpion fish and sculpin. Most envenomations occur when a fisherman removes the fish from either a hook or net and accidentally touches a retractable venomous spine. Scorpion fish are bottom-dwelling fish that inhabit shallow waters off the coasts of California and Hawaii. The annual number of scorpion fish stings there may approach 250 to 300.

Synaceja
The stonefish (*Synaceja trachynis*) is a well-camouflaged bottom-dweller. It is quite dangerous and has caused numerous fatalities, generally when accidentally touched. The bony plate that covers the facial region from the eyes to the gill helps identify this diverse family. Generally, they conceal themselves in the shallow waters of coral reefs, kelp beds, and rocky coastline, where inadvertent contacts may occur with humans. Its distribution is limited to the tropical Pacific, and it may be encountered in Hawaii. Fatalities have been reported in Australia.

PATHOPHYSIOLOGY
The venoms of most species of the Scorpaenidae are antigenically and pharmacologically similar. A nondialyzable, high-molecular-weight, heat-labile protein component produces vasodilation, hypotension, muscular weakness, and respiratory paralysis. The venom remains potent up to 24–48 hours after

the fish has died. Although the venom's potency is similar among the species, differences in amount and delivery mechanisms cause a wide variation in symptoms.

Pterois
Long thin spines are associated with small venom glands covered by a thin integumentary sheath but no venom ducts. The venom is released into the wound when the force of the puncture tears away the spine's sheath. Symptoms usually are localized to the area of trauma.

Scorpaena
A thick integumentary sheath capable of producing significant systemic symptoms covers long heavy spines with moderate-sized venom glands.

Synaceja
This group possesses the most sophisticated venom apparatus, with short, thick spines, well-developed venom glands, and very thick sheaths.

CLINICAL PRESENTATIONS
Although species vary widely in their clinical effects, all produce an extremely painful sting. Substantial local swelling, hyperesthesias, paresthesias, erythema, and pain extending up the involved extremity may occur. Pain typically reaches a maximum in 60–80 minutes and usually resolves within 24 hours. Complications may include sloughing of tissue at the envenomation site which may require weeks to heal, secondary infection, cutaneous granulomas, and persistent paresthesias and hypesthesias. Regional lymphadenopathy with local tenderness has been reported as a direct toxic effect without evidence of infection.

Systemic symptoms present less commonly. Rarely, mild hypotension, tachycardia, dyspnea, pallor, diaphoresis, vomiting, headache, muscle cramps, tremor, and generalized weakness appear. Stonefish produce the most severe envenomations, and fatalities may occur within six hours from respiratory paralysis. Serious manifestations may include bradycardia, syncope, dysrhythmias, hypotension, convulsions, paralysis, and pulmonary edema.

TREATMENT
- Since Scorpaenidae venom is heat-labile, rapid hot water immersion for 30–60 minutes at 45°C (110–115°F) is the most effective first-aid measure. Intradermal emetine, procaine, epinephrine, and potassium permanganate have been recommended to neutralize the venom, but there is little clinical or experimental support for these therapies.
- Relief generally occurs soon after immersion, and the soaks may be stopped after complete relief.
- Narcotic analgesics should be withheld until hot water immersion is complete to prevent scalding.
- Local wound care includes irrigation, debridement, and tetanus prophylaxis as needed.
- Prophylactic antibiotics are not recommended, but the patient should be warned about signs and symptoms of infection. Antihistamines, epinephrine, corticosteroids, and local excision are generally not effective for these envenomations.
- Magnesium sulfate (Epsom salts) soaks twice a day for several days may provide symptomatic relief for persistent symptoms.
- Systemic symptoms may require fluids to correct hypotension.

ANTIDOTES

Antivenin
Most serious stonefish envenomations require antivenin, a horse serum product. One vial is given intravenously after skin testing is adequate. Bites of other members of the Scorpionida usually do not require antivenin.

Questions—Scorpaenidae

1. **Examples of venomous fish include all of the following, except**
   A. Lionfish
   B. Turkey fish
   C. Scorpion fish
   D. Cod fish
   E. Scorpion fish
2. **Rapid hot water immersion for 30–60 minutes at 45°C (110–115°F) is the most effective first-aid measure for treating Scorpaenidae envenomations.**
   A. True
   B. False
3. **The stonefish (*Synaceja trachynis*) is a well-camouflaged bottom-dweller. It is quite dangerous and has caused numerous fatalities, generally when accidentally touched.**
   A. True
   B. False

Weever Fish

The weever fish (*Echiichthys Vipera*) is the most venomous fish present in the temperate zone. It is found in European costal waters, the eastern Atlantic Ocean, and the Mediterranean Sea. This short, stout fish ranges from 14 cm to 46 cm. This sedentary fish prefers shallow water where it partially buries itself in the mud or sand awaiting prey such as crab or shrimp. Bathers may tread on the partially submerged dorsal spines and receive envenomation. Fishermen may sustain stings while handling fish caught in nets. In France, the weever fish is considered a delicacy and is widely sold.

PATHOPHYSIOLOGY
The dorsal spines of the weever fish contain two grooves composed of holocrine glandular tissue. Like those of the lionfish, the spines are covered with a thin integument of stratified columnar epithelium that ruptures during contact with the victim and thus releases the venom. The venom contains several heat-labile proteins, including a high-molecular-weight protein, a kinin or kininlike substance, and possibly serotonin as well as adrenaline, noradrenaline, histamine, and several enzymes. Albumins and mucopolysaccharides in the venom cause wheal-and-flare reactions in subcutaneous injections and are lethal to animals.

CLINICAL PRESENTATIONS
Immediately after envenomation, intense pain develops which may be excruciating and difficult to control with analgesics. Erythema and edema occur within several hours. Local trauma may be significant, since the spines are strong enough to penetrate shoe leather. Systemic symptoms are unusual but may include headache, delirium, nausea, vomiting, diaphoresis, syncope, and hypotension. Death is extremely rare and thought to be secondary to respiratory failure.

TREATMENT

- The best first-aid measure is immediate hot water immersion (110–115°F) for 30–60 minutes.
- Local wound care requires irrigation, cleansing, and debridement. Tetanus immunizations should be updated. Otherwise, treatment is supportive and infection is rare.

Questions—Weever Fish

1. Weever fish
   A. Are considered a delicacy by the French
   B. Produce a heat-stabile venom
   C. Can cause local or systemic symptoms
   D. All of the above
   E. A and C

Catfish

Although most of the 1,000 catfish species are freshwater, bottom-dwelling scavengers, a few species are found in salt water. Freshwater fishes of North America include the brown bullhead (*Ictaluri nebulosus*), white catfish (*Ictaluri catus*), blue catfish (*Ictaluri furcatus*), channel catfish (*Ictaluri punctatus*), and Carolina mudtom (*Noturus furiosus*). The marine catfish (*Plotosus pineatus*) frequents kelp beds and is capable of inflicting serious envenomations. The majority of envenomations occur when fishermen handle the catfish during extrication from nets or hooks.

Several interesting characteristics of different catfish species have been observed. Members of one South American species have suctorial lips that allow them to scale cliffs; male sea catfish incubate and hatch eggs in their mouths; small Amazon catfish are able to penetrate the human urethra, requiring endoscopic removal; and electric catfish possess electric plates capable of stunning and killing prey.

Toxicity results from venom, delivered when a spine punctures the victim, and from a skin toxin found over the entire surface of the catfish. Death has been reported, but symptoms are usually limited to the involved extremity and respond within hours to supportive therapy.

The major groups of persons at risk for catfish envenomation are fishermen and water-sports participants. Worldwide, saltwater fishermen have sustained many serious envenomations from the Arabian Gulf catfish (*Aurius thalasinus*) and the potentially lethal Oriental catfish (*Plotosus lineatus*), which possesses one of the most potent known marine toxins. In North America, the Carolina mudtom (*Noturus furiosus*) and the Ictalurids (genus *Ictaluri*) are most commonly responsible for dangerous catfish envenomations. This group includes the brown bullhead (sp. *nebulosus*), channel catfish (sp. *punctatus*), blue catfish (sp. *furcatus*), and white catfish (sp. *catus*).

PATHOPHYSIOLOGY

Like the weever fish, the catfish possesses dorsal and pectoral spines able to penetrate human skin and envenomate the victim when the integumentary sheath is torn and the venom gland is exposed. The venom contains several toxic low-molecular-weight protein fractions. Although mudtoms (*Noturus*) appear most toxic to humans, studies in animals suggest that species differences do not entirely account for the wide variation in venom potency.

The stinging apparatuses of the catfish are the bony dorsal and pectoral fins, each of which contains a spine attached to venom glands in its leading edge. The spines have a series of razor-sharp teeth that act as barbs, and extraction of these brittle structures is difficult. The spines normally lie flat against the side of the fish, but they extend when the fish is frightened or excited.

A second mechanism of catfish toxicity, crinotoxicity, has been found in some catfish species (*A. thalasinus* and *P. lineatus*). Crinotoxins are proteinaceous toxins found in catfish epidermal secretions that coat the entire body, including the fins. Agitation of the catfish causes locked extension of fins and secretion of the crinotoxins.

CLINICAL PRESENTATIONS

Envenomation produces painful puncture wounds and paresthesias, which may extend along the whole extremity. Symptoms often resolve in several hours. Edema and erythema may appear. Localized hypesthesias, regional lymphadenopathy, mild fever, and necrosis result from more severe envenomations. Local spasm and muscle fasciculations have been reported.

Other localized symptoms commonly found with catfish envenomation are erythema, cyanosis, edema, sweating, lymphangitis, and muscle fibrillation. Any of these may progress to involve the entire extremity. Wounds inflicted by catfish spines often bleed more freely than expected for their size. Systemic findings occur less frequently in catfish envenomation and may include fever, convulsive muscular contractions, coagulopathy, palpitations, nausea, hypotension, weakness, and altered level of consciousness.

TREATMENT

- Management is supportive and similar to that for Scorpaenidae envenomations, although the venom may not be as heat-labile.
- The affected body part should be immersed in hot water (110°F) for at least 30 minutes. Hot water immersion, originally thought to provide relief through toxin inactivation, may result in at least partial symptomatic improvement through reversal of painful vascular and muscular spasm.
- Opiate analgesics may be required to control pain, but local anesthesia with bupivacaine may reduce the need for systemic analgesics.
- Good wound care is important, since secondary infection is a common complication. Optimal wound outcome depends on removal of foreign material and consideration of secondary bacterial infection. Deep wounds should be cultured.
- Bacteremia resulting from wound infection with *Aeromonas* or *Vibrio* is more likely in patients with diabetes, cirrhosis, or the immunocompromised. Tetracycline, β-lactamase-stable β-lactams, and aminoglycosides may be necessary to eradicate *Aeromonas* or *Vibrio* infections.
- Radiograph or ultrasound may localize embedded material, since catfish barbs are often radiopaque.
- Tetanus prophylaxis is given when indicated.
- Inpatient therapy may be required in patients with deep wounds, long delays in wound care, wounds with retained foreign material, wounds with spine penetration of sterile body cavities, and wounds with persistent inflammatory changes.

Questions—Catfish

1. Which of the following statements regarding catfish is false?
   A. Members of one South American species have suctorial lips that allow them to scale cliffs.
   B. Certain male sea catfish incubate and hatch eggs in their mouths.

C. Small Amazon catfish are able to penetrate the human urethra
D. Electric catfish possess electric plates capable of stunning and killing prey.
E. Catfish venom contains antibiotic proteins.

2. Which of the following statements regarding catfish is true?
A. All catfish are fresh water scavengers.
B. The majority of envenomations occur when fishermen handle the catfish during extrication from nets or hooks.
C. The Oriental catfish (*Plotosus lineatus*) possesses one of the most potent known marine toxins and is potentially lethal.
D. All of the above
E. B and C

Stingrays

Stingrays constitute one of the largest and most important groups of venomous marine animals. Almost 1,500 attacks on humans occur annually in the United States. Stingrays (elasmobranchs) range in size from several inches in diameter to over 14 feet. Stingrays inhabit temperate, subtropical, and tropical waters, and 11 species are present in U.S. coastal waters. The favorite habitats of these passive, reclusive creatures are sandy or muddy bottoms of sheltered lagoons and estuaries, where they feed on crustaceans and mollusks.

Their excellent camouflage and habit of submerging in the bottom allow accidental contact with exposed human extremities. Rarely, envenomation occurs on the chest or abdomen while a human is swimming. Typically, an individual's foot stimulates the stingray to thrust its tail forward, driving its spine deep into the victim's foot or lower leg.

PATHOPHYSIOLOGY

All stingrays possess one or several bony, serrated spines located on the dorsal surface of their powerful tail. A thin layer of skin called the integumentary sheath surrounds the elongated spine and covers two ventrolateral grooves that contain venom glands. As in other venomous vertebrates (e.g., scorpion fish), this sheath breaks upon contact with the victim, allowing the venom to enter the wound. The powerful tail and serrated spines may inflect severe trauma and are capable of penetrating the abdomen or throat. At least two deaths have occurred in children who received eviscerating abdominal wounds.

Significant family variation exists in the development of the venom apparatus. The Gymnuridae possess the weakest system, and the Urolophidae the strongest. The Dasyatidae, commonly found off U.S. coastal waters, possess a partially developed venom apparatus. Many stingrays lose or tear their integumentary sheaths. Stings often result in trauma without envenomation. Experimental studies reveal that the venom contains cardiotoxins, respiratory depressants, and perhaps convulsants. Other fractions include phosphodiesterase, 5′-nucleotidase, and serotonin.

CLINICAL PRESENTATIONS

Symptoms of envenomation typically begin within 10 minutes and are characterized by intense pain out of proportion to the degree of trauma. Edema around the wound is a constant finding but is variable in extent. Cyanosis or erythema may surround the wound edges. Stings may cause severe lacerations from 5–20 cm long, usually on a lower extremity. The edges of the wound tend to become necrotic. Debris, including portions of the integumentary sheath, may contaminate the wound, and bleeding often is profuse. The pain peaks within 90 minutes if untreated and may last 12–48 hours.

Systemic symptoms vary considerably and may include abdominal pain, nausea and vomiting, muscle cramps, diaphoresis, tachycardia, syncope, headache, and muscle fasciculations. Cardiac dysrhythmias, hypotension, convulsions, and death rarely occur.

TREATMENT

- Primary treatment is hot water immersion at (110–115°F) for 30–60 minutes. After it is soaked, the wound is debrided and copiously irrigated with dilute povidone-iodine (Betadine®) solution since secondary infection is common.
- Local anesthesia may be used to search for remnants of the integumentary sheath and to excise devitalized tissue. Grossly contaminated wounds or wounds older than six hours may be managed by delayed primary closure.
- Prophylactic antibiotics are not necessary, but updating tetanus immunization is imperative, since a case of tetanus after stingray envenomation has been reported.
- There are no adequate clinical data to support the use of steroids, cryotherapy, potassium permanganate, ammonia, or antihistamines.

Questions—Stingrays

1. Which of the following statements regarding stingrays is false?
A. Stingrays constitute one of the largest groups of venomous marine animals.
B. Stingrays range in size from several inches in diameter to over 14 feet.
C. Typically, an individual's foot stimulates the stingray to thrust its tail forward, driving its spine deep into the victim's foot or lower leg.
D. Stingrays possess serrated spines on the dorsal surface of their powerful tail.
E. Stings are always associated with envenomation.

2. Regarding stingray stings,
A. Symptoms of envenomation typically begin within 10 minutes and are characterized by intense pain out of proportion to the degree of trauma.
B. Edema around the wound is a constant finding.
C. Stings may cause severe lacerations.
D. Systemic symptoms vary considerably and may include abdominal pain, and muscle cramps.
E. All of the above

Sea Snakes

This group comprises the true sea snakes (*Hydrophiidae*) and the sea kraits (*Laticaudinae*). These close relatives of the cobra (Elapidae) family are the most biologically successful reptiles and probably the most abundant in the world. See Chapter 52, Snakes, Reptiles and Amphibians. There are 52 species, all of which are venomous. Generally, these snakes are docile creatures. They capture small fish around rocky bottoms and coral reefs. Most bites occur in fishermen who inadvertently handle the snakes in their fishing nets. Less often, bites result when victims walk in shallow water, particularly near river estuaries.

Sea snakes may be 3–9 feet long and swim in an undulating fashion, powered by a flat, paddle-shaped tail. True sea snakes have nostril valves. Their habitats include the Indian and Pacific oceans but not the Atlantic Ocean or Caribbean Sea. *Pelamis platurus* is the most common species, extending from the west coast of the Americas to the east coast of Africa. Sea kraits are less aquatic than true sea snakes, seeking rock crevices or land debris during inactive periods. Most sea snake species, except for the *Pelamis* species, are bottom feeders that spend little time at the surface.

PATHOPHYSIOLOGY

Sea snakes possess two to four hollow maxillary fangs with associated venom glands. Most bites do not result in envenomations because the fangs are short (2–3 mm) and easily dislodged. Fang marks are characterized by several (usually up to four) small puncture wounds that may be hard to detect because of the absence of erythema and edema. Multiple bite marks and serrated lacerations suggest serious envenomation when accompanied by symptoms.

The venom contains at least three neurotoxic compounds which inhibit postsynaptic neuromuscular transmission. In addition, the venom appears to be myotoxic but not hemotoxic, producing skeletal muscle necrosis, myoglobinuria, and hyperkalemia. Because of the high potency of the venom (greater than that of terrestrial snakes), mortality reported in published studies of sea snake bites before antivenin was available approximated 10%.

CLINICAL PRESENTATIONS

Characteristically, sea snake envenomations do not produce initial pain and swelling. This fact distinguishes sea snake bites from stings of other marine animals. Neurologic symptoms typically begin within 30–60 minutes (range, 15 minutes to 8 hours) of envenomation and may include myalgias, malaise, anxiety, euphoria, diaphoresis, and vomiting. Serious signs include bulbar palsy (characterized by dysphagia, ptosis, extraocular muscle weakness, pupillary dilation, and dysphonia), progressive muscle weakness, respiratory depression, cyanosis, and coma.

Most sea snake bites do not result in envenomation. Bites that do not produce symptoms by 6–8 hours can safely be categorized as bites without envenomation. In general, serious envenomations are obvious within two hours unless tourniquets have been used. Envenomated patients may benefit from antivenin.

TREATMENT

- Sea snake venom is rapidly absorbed (within 5 minutes in experimental animals) and probably spreads through lymphatic drainage and capillaries. A lymph-restrictive tourniquet may be useful only if applied within the first 5–10 minutes of envenomation. Previously applied tourniquets should not be removed until intravenous lines can be established and respiratory equipment is available to support the patient, since clinical deterioration has been reported after such removal.
- Tourniquets have no place in hospital management. Reassurance, immobilization of the affected limb in a dependent position, and immediate medical attention at a facility that possesses antivenin are key first-aid measures.
- The effectiveness of incision and drainage even within the first 10 minutes is controversial and probably questionable.
- Follow the patient closely for signs of respiratory failure.
- Monitor urinary myoglobin. Maintain an alkaline urine and adequate diuresis (2–3 mL/kg/h) if significant myoglobinuria exists.
- As hyperkalemia and renal failure may complicate rhabdomyolysis, daily serum potassium and creatinine levels should be obtained.

ANTIDOTES

Antivenin

Polyvalent equine sea snake antivenin is indicated in all significantly symptomatic patients (e.g., moderate or severe myalgias or any neurologic signs) after skin testing for horse serum sensitivity. Antivenin should be administered soon, since it is most effective when given within 8 hours of envenomation. The initial dose is one vial, with further vials titrated to the patient's condition.

Questions—Sea Snakes

1. **All sea snakes are venomous.**
   A. True
   B. False
2. **Characteristically, sea snake envenomations do not produce initial pain and swelling, and this distinguishes sea snake bites from stings of other marine animals.**
   A. True
   B. False
3. **Polyvalent equine sea snake is indicated in all significantly symptomatic patients after skin testing for horse serum sensitivity.**
   A. True
   B. False

Miscellaneous Venomous Vertebrates

DOGFISH

The dogfish (*Squalus*) is a member of the shark order and is present throughout the ocean temperate zones (tropics to sub-Antarctic seas). They prefer cool waters and protected bays, where they feed on a variety of vertebrate and invertebrate marine animals. Thick venomous spines protrude from the front of each dorsal fin and can produce painful, erythematous, and edematous puncture wounds. Systemic symptoms are rare but may be serious.

PUFFERFISH

Pufferfish, a delicacy in Japan and Asia, contain the deadly neurotoxin tetrodotoxin. The skin and internal organs of several species of newts possess the same toxin. Tetrodotoxin causes hypotension and respiratory paralysis following pufferfish ingestion and has been associated with numerous, well-documented fatalities.

RATFISH

Ratfish (Chimaeridae) are relatives of stingrays and sharks and prefer the cool waters of the Pacific Ocean from Alaska to Baja California. They have large heads and a tapered body. A large venomous spine is located in front of the first dorsal fin which can produce a painful sting.

TOADFISH

The toadfish (Batrachoididae) is found on the Atlantic Coast from Massachusetts to Central America, particularly in shallow areas near river mouths and estuaries. They are bottom-dwelling fish with large mouths and flat heads that often hide in sand, rocks, or kelp beds. Two venomous spines project from the dorsal fin to cause local pain and swelling.

OTHERS

Other types of fish which produce local, painful puncture wounds include dragon fish, sea robins, flying gurnards, goose fish, rabbit fish, surgeon fish, scats, moray eels, and stargazers. Thorough irrigation and removal of debris along with hot water immersion at 45°C (110–115°F) for 30–60 minutes remain the cornerstones of treatment.

Questions—Miscellaneous Venomous Vertebrates

1. Which of the following associations is incorrect?
- A. Dogfish (*Squalus*)—Thick venomous dorsal spines
- B. Pufferfish—Batrachotoxin
- C. Ratfish (Chimaeridae)—Relatives of stingrays, large venomous spine
- D. Toadfish (Batrachoididae)—Venomous dorsal spines
- E. Dragon fish, sea robins, flying gurnards, goose fish—Hot water immersion

MAMMALS

The male Australian duckbilled platypus (*Ornithorhynchus anatinus*) has venomous spurs on its hind legs that produce pain and edema, but no serious envenomations have been reported. Shrews possess submaxillary venom glands that potentially could cause poisoning, but human envenomation is not well described. The Australian echidna has venomous spines on its hind legs. The Haitian insectivore (*Solenodon paradoxes*) has also been recognized as being venomous.

Birds of the *Pitohui* species from New Guinea have recently been identified as containing homobrachotoxin. This toxin resembles one found in South American poison dart frogs. See Chapter 52, Snakes, Reptiles and Amphibians regarding poisonous frogs, toads, newts and salamanders.

TREATMENT

- There are few venomous mammalian species, and envenomations are not well described.
- Mammalian bites may produce a variety of infectious complications as well as transient serious diseases such as rabies.

Questions—Mammals

1. Toxic birds from New Guinea have been found that contain which type of toxin?
- A. Homobrachotoxin
- B. Tetrodotoxin
- C. Botulinum toxin
- D. Grayanotoxin
- E. Cyanogenic glycosides

2. The following mammals may be considered venomous except
- A. The Australian *Echidna*
- B. Siberian snow leopard
- C. Certain shrews
- D. The Australian duck-billed platypus
- E. The Haitian insectivore *Solenodon paradoxes*

Answers

Coelenterata

1. C 2. C 3. D 4. A 5. D

Porifera

1. B

Mollusca

1. C

Echinodermata

1. E

Scorpaenidae

1. D 2. A 3. A

Weever Fish

1. E

Catfish

1. E 2. E

Stingrays

1. E 2. E

Sea Snakes

1. A 2. A 3. A

Miscellaneous Venomous Vertebrates

1. B

Mammals

1. A 2. B

SELECTED READINGS

Marine Toxicology

1. Auerbach PS, Halstead BW. Hazardous marine life, in Auerbach PS, Geehr EC (eds): *Management of Wilderness and Environmental Emergencies*. New York, MacMillan, 1983.
2. Auerbach PS. Marine envenomations. N Engl J Med 1991;325:486–493.
3. Halstead BN: *Poisonous and Venomous Marine Animals of the World*. Princeton, NJ, Darwin Press, 1978.
4. Kizer KW: Marine envenomations. J Toxicol Clin Toxicol 1983–1984;21:527–555.
5. McGoldrick J, Marx JA. Marine envenomations. I. Vertebrates. J Emerg Med 1991;9:497–502.
6. McGoldrick J, Marx JA. Marine envenomations. II. Invertebrates. J Emerg Med 1992;10:71–77.

Mammals

1. Dumbacher JP, Beehler BM, Spande TF, et al. Homobrachotoxin in the genus Pitohui: Chemical defense in birds? Science 1992;258:799–801.
2. Holloway M. The Pitohui: The colorful bird that looks better than it tastes. Sci Am 1993;258:20–22.

CHAPTER 54
Arthropods

INTRODUCTION

The phylum Arthropoda is the largest division in the animal kingdom representing about 80% of known animals. It contains six major groups that comprise approximately 900,000 species. Insecta is the largest group of arthropods. Orders include the Hymenoptera (bees, wasps, hornets and ants), Lepidoptera (butterflies, moths and caterpillars), Siphonaptera (fleas), Anoplura (body lice), Diptera (mosquitoes, sandflies, midges, black flies, gnats, and tsetse flies), Hemiptera (bed bugs, kissing bugs and wheel bugs), Cleoptera (beetles), Thysanoptera (thrips), Myriapoda (millipedes or Diplopoda and centipedes or Chilopoda), and Arachnida (mites, ticks, chiggers, spiders including tarantulas and scorpions).

Pathophysiology

Clinical effects result from numerous mechanisms including physical trauma, injection of venom (e.g., black widow spider and scorpion), introduction of sensitizing material that produces reactions varying from local edema (e.g., mosquito) to anaphylaxis (e.g., Hymenoptera), tissue invasion (e.g., scabies), and bacterial infection. A foreign-body reaction (e.g., secondary to retained insect parts such as tick mouthparts or Hymenoptera ovipositor), and contact skin reactions (e.g., the blister beetle's body fluid contains a vesicant called cantharidin) may also occur. Diseases carried by arthropods include trypanosomiasis, Rocky Mountain spotted fever, malaria, and encephalitis.

Questions—Introduction to Arthropods

1. Which of the following mechanisms does not contribute to morbidity from arthropod bites?
A. Venom
B. Foreign-body reaction
C. Bacterial superinfection
D. Insect pH
E. Allergic reactions

HYMENOPTERA

Characteristics of this group include two pairs of wings, one pair of antennae, three body segments (head, abdomen, and thorax) and, in females, a tubular ovipositor that has become a stinging apparatus. Apoidea include bumblebees, honeybees and solitary bees. Vespoidea include wasps, hornets and yellow jackets. Formicoidea include ants.

AFRICAN BEES

The African bee (*Apis mellifera scutellata*) was introduced to Brazil in 1957 and colonies reached the United States in the late 1980s. These bees can survive in areas with mean high temperatures of at least 60°F. When disturbed, these African bees can inflict hundreds of stings within several minutes. They attack in large numbers and have led to the development of hypersensitivity with the risk of fatal anaphylaxis. Multiple stings are necessary to cause death by direct toxicity, but as few as 30–50 stings have proved fatal in children.

ANTS

Members of all but one of the ant families bite and sting. The fire ant (*Solenopsis richteri* and *invicta*) is the most vicious species. It was introduced to the U.S. around 1920. Colonies are now present in 13 southern states from North Carolina to Texas. Only the presence of low temperatures (below 12°C) limits the distribution of fire ants. The fire ant is bright red and inhabits a loose dirt mound about 30 cm around and 5–10 cm high.

Most ants (e.g., harvester or agricultural ants) grasp skin with their jaws and then sting or spray locally irritating venom, which causes burning and itching. Fire ants are extremely prolific and possess volatile tempers, as displayed by the ferocity of their attack when their nest is disturbed. Trespassers can receive 3,000–5,000 stings within seconds by the ant swarm. Fire ant workers have well-developed abdominal stinging organs. They attach themselves to their victim with powerful jaws and then pivot, inflicting multiple stings in a circular fashion.

BUMBLEBEES

Bumblebees are the most primitive social bees. They are found throughout the Temperate Zone and are unfairly feared because of their large size and loud noise.

HONEYBEES

This social bee forms a sophisticated colony or hive and produces honey commercially. Generally, bees are not aggressive and sting only when disturbed or when their hive is threatened. The barbed stinger contains two lancets that serve as plungers, which force about 50 μg of venom down a poison canal. When piercing, these lancets become firmly attached to human skin, resulting in disengagement of the whole apparatus from the abdomen. The eviscerated bee soon dies, but the reflex action of attached muscles may continue to inject more venom. See the section on African Bees.

HORNETS

Hornets possess a truncated abdomen and a shorter waist than wasps. Hornets are aerial or ground nesters and are mild mannered unless their hive is threatened.

SOLITARY BEES

This group comprises thousands of species (e.g., miner, carpenter, mason, cuckoo, etc.), that live alone and usually are named for their particular habitat.

WASPS

An egg-shaped abdomen supported on the thorax by a slender stalk characterizes this group. Wasps consume only liquid food. Polistes wasps may seek indoor shelter during winter but usually are not aggressive. Yellow jackets (see below) are scavengers with ill tempers and may attack without provocation. As one of the most aggressive and vicious stinging insects, the yellow jacket produces envenomations that are the most common cause of insect-induced anaphylactic reactions.

The stinging apparatus of the wasp family differs from that of bees by the absence of barbs. This feature allows the wasp to withdraw and, if desired, to reinsert the stinger. Retained stingers are uncommon, but multiple stings from the same wasp are possible.

YELLOW JACKETS

Characteristic yellow and black stripes distinguish the nonstinging male from the stinging, black-faced female. See the section on Wasps above.

Answers to questions in shaded boxes appear at the end of the chapter.

Pathophysiology

Limited local reactions result from biological amines within venom. Most insect sting allergies are either local or systemic type I immediate hypersensitivity reactions mediated by IgE antibodies. Almost all persons manifesting allergies to an insect sting have elevated serum IgE antibodies directed against the specific venom. Although IgE is thought to be the primary immunoglobulin responsible for anaphylaxis, homocytotropic IgG or activated complement contributes to the degranulation of mast cells and basophils.

Sensitized individuals synthesize excessive IgE antibodies when reexposed to Hymenoptera venoms. Such antibodies cause the release of substances that result in vasoconstriction and smooth muscle contraction. Although venom composition among the Hymenoptera varies, cross-reactivity definitely occurs, as evidenced by the fact that death has resulted from a wasp sting in a bee-sensitized individual. Generally, yellow jacket venom is the most potent sensitizer.

Bees

Bee venom contains dopamine, histamine, phospholipase A2, hyaluronidase, and toxic peptides including a hemolysin called mellitin, the neurotoxin apamin, and a mast cell degranulator. Mellitin enhances phospholipase A2 activity and may be the main toxin as well as the primary constituent of bee venom (50% dry weight). In studies in animals, this toxin releases histamine from mast cells and serotonin from platelets. It contracts smooth muscle of the ileum, blocks synaptic transmission in the isolated diaphragm, and produces inflammation.

Mellitin increases guanylate cyclase activity in animal models, but is an important allergen only in a few patients. Phospholipase A2 and hyaluronidase probably are the main immunogens. Apamin is a unique toxin isolated from *Apis mellifera* which crosses the blood-brain barrier and exhibits biological activity in small animals. Its role in human toxicity, however, is unclear. The venom of African honeybees is similar to the venom of European honeybees.

Fire Ants

Formicoidea (fire ant) venom contains mainly alkaloids. Some bactericidal activity is believed to account for the low incidence of secondary bacterial infection. Local tissue reactions most often result from the direct effect of the venom on mast cell membranes, resulting in the release of histamine. The presence of low-molecular-weight proteins provides a pathophysiological basis for hypersensitivity reactions.

Wasps and Hornets

Vespoidea venom is similar but not identical to bee (Apoidea) venom. Both wasp and hornet venoms contain serotonin. Hornet venom has the most concentrated source of acetylcholine. Vespoidea venom contains various vasoactive kinins that have not been purified.

Clinical Presentations

Hymenoptera envenomations produce sharp stabbing pain followed for several minutes by burning pain, which is at times severe. A wheal and flare forms with central erythema surrounded by a whitish ring and subsequent edema, which usually resolves in several hours. Pruritus and a feeling of warmth may persist for several hours.

Fire ants produce a wheal-and-flare reaction, followed in 24 hours by the formation of a sterile pustule, which is painful and lasts 3–10 days. Characteristically, multiple bites occur in a circular pattern. However, the absence of pustules does not rule out fire ant bites. Sensitized individuals may develop erythema and edema up to 10 cm surrounding the bite, whereas unsensitized patients show only mild circumferential erythema. Fire ant bites may be confused with blister beetle bites, which produce bullous rather than pustular lesions.

EXCESSIVE LOCAL REACTIONS

An exaggerated response may cause extended swelling that involves the whole extremity without producing systemic effects. These large local reactions seldom cause serious sequelae unless important structures are involved. For example, a pharyngeal sting obtained during a motorcycle ride may require nasotracheal intubation.

Severe local symptoms and signs peak between 48–72 hours after envenomation and last up to one week. Within the first 2–3 days, local reaction must be differentiated from infection. Generally, pain and tenderness are greater when infection complicates the bite. Red streaks radiating up the extremity are indications of lymphangiitis and occur more often after yellow jacket stings than after bee envenomations.

SYSTEMIC EFFECTS

Target organs may include those of the cardiovascular, respiratory, hematologic, gastrointestinal, genitourinary, and dermatologic systems. Systemic symptoms range from urticaria, pruritus, anxiety and flushing to anaphylaxis. Visual abnormalities (e.g., amblyopia) and gastrointestinal symptoms such as diarrhea and abdominal pain are characteristic of insect sting allergies.

Moderate effects may include generalized angioedema, tightness of the chest or constriction of the throat, lightheadedness, gastrointestinal symptoms such as nausea, vomiting, or abdominal pain, and/or facial edema. Severe signs may include dyspnea, hoarseness, confusion, weakness, wheezing, and a feeling of impending disaster. Signs of shock including hypotension, loss of consciousness, incontinence, and/or cyanosis may also be seen. Reversible myocardial ischemia and pulmonary edema may occur in susceptible older patients.

ANAPHYLACTIC REACTIONS

Hymenoptera envenomations are responsible for approximately half of the 50–100 reported annual deaths following anaphylactic reactions. The actual incidence may be higher. Although most fatalities occur in adults over 40, most severe reactions occur in males younger than 20. Outcome may depend on the ability to withstand cardiovascular stress.

Adults with positive venom skin tests and previous severe reactions (e.g., manifested by laryngeal edema, severe bronchospasm, and/or hypotension) have a 60% chance of having the same severe symptoms if bitten by the same insect. The use of venom immunotherapy reduces the chance of severe reactions in adults to 5%. There are no reliable criteria to predict the occurrence of anaphylaxis, since a previous reaction is not a reliable indicator of future reactions unless the prior reaction was severe. Fatal cases often have no prior reaction.

SERUM SICKNESS

Delayed symptoms of serum sickness may occur up to 10–14 days after envenomation and include fever, malaise, lymphadenopathy, headache, arthralgias, myalgias, and urticaria. Local tissue necrosis may also result from delayed hypersensitivity.

RENAL EFFECTS

Renal dysfunction secondary to rhabdomyolysis from a hornet sting and nephrotic syndrome has been reported. Acute renal failure may develop from hypotension and rhabdomyolysis caused by multiple African bee envenomations.

NEUROLOGIC EFFECTS
Severe neurologic effects have been temporally related to Hymenoptera envenomation, although the role of hypotension or anatomic abnormalities in these patients has not been clarified. Most neurologic reactions are delayed in onset. Multiple sclerosis, cerebral infarct, myasthenia gravis, optic neuritis, and Guillain-Barré syndrome have been reported after Hymenoptera stings. Extrapyramidal disorders have occurred after Hymenoptera stings as well.

HEMATOLOGIC EFFECTS
Acute hemolytic anemia occurred 12–18 hours after a wasp bite in a child and one week after a wasp bite in an adult. Hemolysis as well as self-limited thrombotic thrombocytopenic purpura (TTP) resulted from a Hymenoptera sting in a 44-year-old adult.

Toxic Dosage/Death

The more rapid the onset of symptoms, the greater the risk of death. The majority of fatalities occur within the first hour. Respiratory obstruction accounts for most deaths. The remaining causes of death are divided between acute anaphylactic shock and thrombotic or hemorrhagic complications.

Headache, fever, muscle spasm, convulsions, and death have resulted from multiple stings. Five hundred simultaneous bee stings may be lethal, but survival after more than 2,000 bee stings has been reported. Diarrhea, vomiting, lightheadedness, and transient loss of consciousness are the most common symptoms. Toxic reactions in an adult are unlikely with fewer than 100 honeybee stings, but may be quite serious in children.

Drug Interactions

Several case studies suggest that the concomitant ingestion of nonsteroidal anti-inflammatory medications can worsen the clinical effect of Hymenoptera envenomation.

Treatment

GUT DECONTAMINATION
These methods are not applicable to the treatment of Hymenoptera envenomation.

ELIMINATION ENHANCEMENT
In severe cases, hemodialysis should be considered not only for the treatment of renal failure, but also for removal of circulating low-molecular-weight venom components such as mellitin.

SUPPORTIVE MEASURES

Bee Venom
- Supportive therapy must be started immediately. Airway management and assurance of adequate ventilation and oxygenation are the first priorities.
- Aggressive fluid resuscitation may be necessary if shock is present, and increased fluid requirement will be obvious in patients who exhibit vomiting and diarrhea. Maintenance of adequate cardiac output and blood pressure is vital.
- Both H1 (e.g., diphenhydramine) and H2 (e.g., ranitidine) blockers should be given intravenously to treat the vascular effects of histamine in bee venom.
- Epinephrine (0.3–0.5 mL of 1:1,000 epinephrine, subcutaneously) should be administered with any sign(s) of systemic involvement. It may be difficult to distinguish systemic toxic effects from anaphylaxis when relatively small numbers of stings are sustained.
- Over the ensuing two days, acute renal failure may occur due to rhabdomyolysis with myoglobinuria, hemoglobinuria, renal ischemia, or immune mechanisms. Monitoring urine output, hemoglobinuria, electrolytes, creatinine, BUN and urinalysis is indicated. The patient should also be monitored for intravascular hemolysis.
- Continuous electrocardiographic monitoring should be done routinely because of the possibility of rare myocardial damage, arrhythmia, and hyperkalemia.
- If only a few stings are sustained, the stingers should be removed within one minute of the attack. Studies have shown that the entire contents of domestic bee venom sacs are empty within two minutes of the time when the stinger is embedded in the skin.
- When large numbers of stings are sustained, transportation to an emergency department and treatment for the toxic effects of venom must be started immediately, even if the initial presentation is suggestive of an allergic reaction.

Treatment of Anaphylactic Reactions
- Anaphylactic reactions are medical emergencies that require the prompt use of epinephrine. Most deaths occur within the first hour and result from respiratory obstruction secondary to edema in patients who have not received parenteral epinephrine.
- Immediately provide oxygen and assisted ventilation if necessary, and establish an intravenous line and cardiac monitoring. Most patients will require intravenous fluids beginning with a 10–20 mL/kg bolus of normal saline. Bronchodilator aerosol therapy and/or endotracheal intubation may be necessary as well.
- All patients who display signs of a systemic reaction (generalized urticaria, angioedema, respiratory distress, or shock) should receive epinephrine immediately. For patients not in shock, 0.01 mL/kg up to 0.3–0.5 mL of 1:1,000 epinephrine should be given subcutaneously. The dose may be repeated every 15 minutes because of its short half-life.
- The presence of shock may limit the effectiveness of subcutaneously administered epinephrine because of poor absorption, but definitive studies have not established safe and therapeutic dosages for intravenous epinephrine in anaphylaxis.
- The same dose of 1:10,000 epinephrine may be carefully administered intravenously over 10–15 minutes. Patients with cardiovascular disease and those over 40 years of age will require careful cardiac monitoring for evidence of ischemia or dysrhythmias.
- Patients who are on long-term β-agonist therapy (e.g., asthmatics) may require larger doses of epinephrine for therapeutic effect. Patients receiving β-blocker drugs may not respond well to epinephrine, since cyclic AMP release may actually decrease in the presence of unopposed α-adrenergic stimulation. Patients with β-blockade may be refractory to epinephrine and require an intravenous isoproterenol drip.
- Vasopressors with strong α-adrenergic agonist properties (e.g., norepinephrine) may be necessary to support blood pressure unresponsive to fluids and epinephrine.
- Other intravenous medications should include an H1 blocker (e.g., diphenhydramine, 1.5 mg/kg), an H2 blocker (e.g., cimetidine, 7.5 mg/kg), and corticosteroids (e.g., methylprednisolone, 50 mg, or hydrocortisone, 200 mg).

Prevention of Anaphylaxis

- All individuals with a history of systemic reactions to bee stings should carry an anaphylaxis emergency treatment kit that allows for two doses of epinephrine (e.g., two EpiPen® injectors) whenever engaged in outdoor activities.
- These individuals should consult an allergist for venom skin testing and possible venom immunotherapy, although it is unclear as to whether current bee venom immunotherapy schedules are effective in preventing toxic reactions to multiple bee stings.
- For 4–6 weeks after an episode of multiple stings, allergic skin-test reactivity to bee venom may be found because of sensitization by the episode or from preexisting sensitivity.
- A warning bracelet or tag should be worn.

Antidotes

ANTIVENOM

No antivenom product is available to immediately counteract systemic or anaphylactic effects of Hymenoptera venom. Although controversy remains over how effectively venom immunotherapy reduces mortality, most authorities now recommend desensitization for those patients with prior immediate serious systemic symptoms (respiratory distress, generalized urticaria, hypotension, and collapse). Commercial preparations of venom from honeybee, yellow jacket, white-faced hornet, yellow hornet, fire ant, and wasp are now available in the U.S. for diagnosis and immunotherapy.

Questions—Hymenoptera

1. Which of the following statements is false?
A. African bees can inflict hundreds of stings within several minutes.
B. All ants are capable of biting and stinging.
C. The fire ant is the most vicious ant species.
D. Fire ant workers have well-developed abdominal stinging organs.
E. Generally, bees are not aggressive and sting when disturbed or when their hive is threatened.

2. The most common cause of insect-induced anaphylactic reactions is
A. Bumble bees
B. Hornets
C. Yellow jackets
D. Fire ants
E. Honey bees

3. The primary immunoglobulin responsible for anaphylaxis is
A. IgA
B. IgD
C. IgG
D. IgE
E. IgC

4. Although venom composition among the Hymenoptera varies, cross-reactivity definitely occurs. A wasp sting, for example, can cause anaphylaxis in a bee-sensitized individual.
A. True
B. False

5. The main component of bee venom is
A. Dopamine
B. Histamine
C. Apamin
D. Epinephrine
E. Mellitin

6. Which of the following statements is false?
A. Hymenoptera envenomations are responsible for approximately half of the annual deaths following anaphylactic reactions in the U.S.
B. Adults with previous severe reactions to Hymenoptera bites have a 100% chance of having severe symptoms if bitten by the same insect.
C. Fatal cases often have no prior reaction to Hymenoptera bites.
D. Delayed symptoms of serum sickness may occur up to 10–14 days after Hymenoptera envenomation and include fever, lymphadenopathy, headache, arthralgias, myalgias, and urticaria.
E. A and C

7. Which of the following has/have been reported after Hymenoptera stings?
A. Multiple sclerosis
B. Myasthenia gravis
C. Optic neuritis
D. Guillain-Barré syndrome
E. All of the above

8. Which of the following may be helpful in treating anaphylaxis?
A. H1 blockers
B. H2 blockers
C. Steroids
D. All of the above
E. A and C

9. No antivenom product is available to immediately counteract systemic or anaphylactic effects of Hymenoptera venom.
A. True
B. False

LEPIDOPTERA

Lepidopterism is a common problem in the southern U.S., where stinging moths cause symptoms similar to those induced by venomous caterpillars. There are about ten families of venomous caterpillars and moths. The most common stinging caterpillar is the puss caterpillar (*Megalopyge opercularis*), which is also known as the woolly slug. This flat, ovoid creature reaches 35 mm in length and feeds on common shade tree leaves.

Other irritating species include the range caterpillar (*Hemileuca olivae*), flannel moth caterpillar (*Lagoa crispata*), spiny caterpillar (*Automeris io*), saddleback caterpillar (*Sibine stimula*), oak slug (*Euclea delphinii*), and tussock moth caterpillar (*Hemerocampa* spp). The gypsy moth caterpillar (*Lymantria dispas*) can cause papulovesicular dermatitis of the delayed hypersensitivity type in certain individuals.

Pathophysiology

Hairs act as irritants and produce characteristic pruritic erythematous lesions at contact sites.

Clinical Presentations

Specialized hollow spines with venom glands at their base act as the venom apparatus. The chitinous spines are capable of penetrating the human epidermis and causing contact urticaria. Secondary infection may produce residual scarring. Systemic reactions to North American species do not occur; however, muscle spasms, paresthesias, dizziness, diaphoresis, nausea, abdominal pain, joint stiffness, and lymphadenopathy have been described elsewhere.

Treatment

- Adhesive tape may aid spine removal. Tetanus status should be addressed.
- Steroids and antihistamines may be necessary if a hypersensitivity reaction is suspected (e.g., gypsy moth dermatitis).
- Calamine lotion and soothing soaks with Epsom salts or Domeboro solution may suffice.

Questions—Lepidoptera

1. **The primary skin irritant from caterpillar exposures is/are**
   A. A slimy skin secretion
   B. Tiny teeth
   C. Tiny hairs
   D. Venom secreted from their feet
   E. Pollen
2. **Systemic reactions from North American moth and caterpillar exposures may include muscle spasms, paresthesias, abdominal pain and joint stiffness.**
   A. True
   B. False

SIPHONAPTERA

Fleas are dark, shiny, wingless, blood-sucking insects that can live for several months in rugs and furniture without a meal and can jump several feet (100 times their own length). They are intermittent feeders that choose covered areas of skin to avoid light.

Pathophysiology

Although fleas are important disease vectors (e.g., murine typhus and plague), their primary clinical manifestation is the appearance of bite sensitivity. Fleas usually prefer specific hosts (e.g., dogs, cats, birds, and even humans) but attack humans in the absence of their normal host (e.g., when the pet dog leaves home temporarily).

Clinical Presentations

Flea bites are characteristically arranged in groups of urticarial lesions, often in lines limited by tight clothing. A central punctum occurs, which may be hemorrhagic. Flea bites are common in children and may account for the majority of papular urticarial lesions. In Africa and Latin America, the jigger flea or chigoe (*Tunga penetrana*) burrows underneath the stratum corneum of the toes and fingernails, producing paronychia.

Treatment

- Removal of fleas is the most important preventive measure.
- Calamine lotion and oral antihistamines are effective antipruritic agents. Cool wet compresses may provide symptomatic relief.
- Application of a menthol or benzocaine-containing ointment three to four times a day can provide relief from the burning and pain associated with flea bites.

Questions—Siphonaptera

1. **Fleas**
   A. Can fly
   B. Must eat every 2–3 days
   C. Produce deadly venom
   D. Prefer specific hosts, but are capable of biting additional ones if necessary
   E. A and B

ANOPLURA

Lice infestations (pediculosis) result from three types of lice and produce three clinical syndromes.

BODY LICE

Involvement by the body louse (*Pediculus humanus corporis*) most frequently occurs in lower socioeconomic groups. Most lice live on clothing and bedding, and a few attach to body hairs.

HEAD LICE

Infestations of hair by the head louse (*Pediculus humanus capitis*) cause scalp itching, seen most frequently on the back of the neck in school children.

PUBIC LICE

Pubic, axillary, and rarely eyelash involvement by the crab or pubic louse (*Phthirus pubis*) causes intense pruritus. This entity typically occurs in adults who contract it through infested sexual partners or clothing.

Pathophysiology

These blood-sucking insects require human contact to complete their life cycle. Bites precipitate excoriations and occasionally urticaria. Fertilized females deposit oval egg sacs called nits on hair shafts, readily visible to the human eye. The scurrying crablike insect often is felt but not seen. Body lice are found in clothing seams of infested patients, who are commonly inactive individuals with poor hygiene. Lice can transmit diseases such as epidemic typhus (Rickettsia prowazekii), trench fever (Rickettsia quintana), and epidemic relapsing fever (Borrelia recurrentis).

Clinical Presentations

Pruritus and excoriation are the most common manifestations of infestation, with crusted secondary lesions, regional lymphadenopathy, and a morbilliform rash developing in chronic cases. Occasionally, blue macules (maculae caeruleae) about 5 mm in diameter are seen on the lower abdomen after pubic lice infestations and probably represent altered blood pigment.

Treatment

- Management is similar to that for scabies infestations. See section on Arachnida.
- Hair is initially washed and nits are combed out.
- Pediculicides include 1% lindane (Kwell® shampoo) and Rid® (0.3% pyrethrin synergized with 3% piperonyl butoxide). Rid® is an over-the-counter product that is equally efficacious and less toxic than lindane; however, more mucous membrane irritation and allergic reactions occur.
- Temperatures above 52°C destroy lice and eggs. Washing clothes and sheets in hot water, drying for 20 minutes, ironing, dry cleaning, and even storage for 2 weeks in plastic bags (life cycle is 30 days) eliminate infestations. Fumigation is not necessary.
- Body lice are treated symptomatically with calamine lotion and laundering of clothing and linens.

Questions—Anoplura

1. Which of the following is not transmitted by lice?
A. Plague
B. Typhus
C. Trench fever
D. Relapsing fever
E. None of the above

2. Lice require human contact to complete their life cycle.
A. True
B. False

DIPTERA

Blood-sucking insects (biting flies and mosquitoes) of this order are characterized by a single pair of wings. The second pair of wings has been replaced by small knobbed structures that function as stabilizers.

CULICIDAE
Mosquitoes are aquatic breeders found worldwide, even beyond the Arctic Circle. They cause lesions that may become bullous and excoriated. Transmitted diseases include filariasis, dengue fever, and malaria.

PHLEBOTOMUS
Sand flies are tiny, 1–3 mm hairy gnats that breed in dark, damp crevices during the day. The female feeds exclusively on blood at night.

SIMULIIDAE
Black flies, midges, and buffalo flies are 1–5 mm flies that have a hump-backed appearance and breed in fast-flowing streams. Black flies swarm in late spring and early summer. Biting midges swarm at sunset and form dense clouds. This distinguishes them from night-biting sand flies and day-biting black flies.

STOMOXYS CALCITRANS
The stable fly is physically similar to the common housefly and breeds around farm animals. A blood-sucking fly may either feed at one spot for several minutes or move to a different location.

TABANIDAE
The horse fly is a large (20 mm), slow-moving, blood-sucking insect that usually is easily repelled.

Pathophysiology

Bites from these insects consist of a stabbing or piercing motion with a bayonet-like proboscis, which inflicts minimal physical trauma. Injected fluids produce local tissue damage as well as local hypersensitivity reactions.

Clinical Presentations

Black flies produce an extremely painful, pruritic, erythematous lesion that usually begins one hour after they bite. The lesion may develop into a nodular, eczema-like patch or a hard pigmented nodule. Black flies may also cause an anaphylactic reaction characterized by fever, edema, malaise, and leukocytosis. Anaphylactoid reactions may result from antigen-antibody complex deposition.

Treatment

- The area is washed with an antiseptic solution such as povidone-iodine (Betadine®).
- Antibiotic ointment applied to horse and stable fly bites may prevent infection.
- Calamine lotion and oral antihistamines are effective antipruritic agents. Cool wet compresses may provide symptomatic relief.

Questions—Diptera

1. Blood-sucking insects include each of the following, except
A. Mosquitoes
B. Gypsy moths
C. Sand flies
D. Midges
E. Horse flies

2. Black flies can cause an anaphylactic reaction characterized by fever, edema, malaise, and leukocytosis.
A. True
B. False

HEMIPTERA

Reduviid Bug

Reduviid "kissing" bugs (*Triatoma protracta*) are black or brown, 2.5–4 cm in length, and have a long triply segmented proboscis or beak that they use to suck blood painlessly. Their usual habitat is the den of wild rodents or opossums, but this insect can readily adapt to human habitats. Fifteen species are found in the U.S. in a crescent-shaped distribution from Florida to northern California.

PATHOPHYSIOLOGY
Triatoma spend daylight hours in dark protected areas and feed at night. They inflict multiple, painless bites in areas not covered by tight-fitting clothes. These bugs are vectors for trypanosomiasis.

CLINICAL PRESENTATIONS

Clinical features of bites are distinctive but not pathognomonic. Commonly, this bug inflicts multiple erythematous, pruritic nodules clustered in a single area. A protein in the saliva causes allergic reactions ranging from pruritus, urticaria, lightheadedness, and gastrointestinal upset to anaphylaxis.

TREATMENT

- Medications containing menthol, phenol, or camphor may relieve itching.
- The presence of systemic reactions necessitates a search for the offending insects and their eradication from the home.
- Lesions should be observed for secondary infections.

Bedbugs

Bedbugs (*Cimex lectularius*) are large, flat brown bugs that hide in protected crevices during the day and feed at night on exposed skin. Cosmopolitan and well adapted to human habitats, the female bugs lay eggs in cracks of floors and furniture.

PATHOPHYSIOLOGY

Mature bugs emerge after 1 or 2 months to feed on humans at night. They produce several linear, often hemorrhagic lesions.

CLINICAL PRESENTATIONS

Bedbugs typically inflict linear bites, do not produce sensitization, and leave a characteristic track of black or brown excrement, in contrast to kissing bugs. Sensitivity reactions generally do not occur, but anaphylaxis from bedbug bites has been reported.

TREATMENT

- Treatment is supportive, with cool, wet compresses and mild analgesics.

Wheel Bug

The wheel bug (*Arilus cristatus*) is a 4-cm-long bug with a characteristic coglike wheel on its prothorax and a narrow head with a stout proboscis. This mild-mannered bug uses its snout to produce a temporarily painful laceration that usually heals without complications.

Questions—Hemiptera

1. **Which of the following associations is incorrect?**
   A. Reduviid bugs—Multiple erythematous, pruritic nodules clustered in a single area
   B. Bedbugs—Linear bites
   C. Bedbugs—Tracks of black or brown excrement
   D. Wheel bug—Rubber feeders
   E. Wheel bug—Painful laceration

CLEOPTERA

Blister beetles (*Meloidae*) contain a powerful vesicant, such as the cantharidin of the Spanish fly (*Lytta vesicatoria*). The hemolymph of the beetle causes 5–50 mm vesicles or bullae several hours after the beetle is crushed on the skin. Apparently, the beetle does not bite or sting. It lives in brush, and exposure is accidental. Commonly, contact occurs painlessly during handling of garden plants (*Epicanta* species) in the eastern U.S. Blebs erupt 2–5 hours after contact and may be painful and hemorrhagic. A severe conjunctivitis can develop if contaminated hands rub the eyes.

Treatment

- Treatment is supportive. Application of steroid cream to skin blebs may be helpful.
- Lesions usually subside in 2–3 days.

Questions—Cleoptera

1. **Blister beetles**
   A. Contain the vesicant cantharidin
   B. Bite and inject toxin
   C. Are dangerous to handle
   D. All of the above
   E. A and C

MYRIAPODA

Chilopoda

The western U.S. centipede (*Scolopendra*) is responsible for most domestic Myriapoda bites, since the smaller eastern centipede seldom bites. Centipedes are nocturnal, predatory animals that feed on small vertebrates. The blue-to-chestnut-brown giant desert centipede (14–16 cm long), (*Scolopendra heros*), is found in Arizona, Southern California, Texas, Georgia, Kansas, Louisiana, and parts of Mexico.

PATHOPHYSIOLOGY

Centipedes have powerful claws on their front segment beneath the mouth, which are connected by ducts to poisonous glands. Their bite releases venom containing enzymes, small peptides, and possibly serotonin and produces a hemorrhagic punctum with surrounding erythema and edema, similar to a hornet sting.

CLINICAL PRESENTATIONS

Pruritus, pain, rare lymphangiitis, lymphadenopathy, and local necrosis may follow envenomation. Myonecrosis, compartment syndrome of the lower extremity, and subsequent dysfunction of the peroneal nerve have resulted from its bite. Rhabdomyolysis has caused renal failure, metabolic acidosis, hyperphosphatemia, hypocalcemia, and hyperuricemia. An ingestion of a centipede (*Scutigera morpha*) by a 6-month-old resulted in lethargy and marked hypotonia. He vomited a few times and slowly improved over 48 hours with no specific treatment.

TREATMENT

- Management is supportive. Anesthetic infiltration may be transiently helpful.
- Steroids may be useful in severe cases, but experience is too limited to be conclusive.
- Patients bitten by *Scolopendra heros* should be warned about the possibility of a muscle compartment syndrome.

Diplopoda

Millipedes have two pairs of legs per body segment, compared with one pair for centipedes, and lack poisonous glands. They have a specialized gland that projects irritant fluid several centimeters. This agent produces skin and mucous membrane irritation. The defensive fluid contains organic acids, phenol, cresols, and quinones. Skin lesions begin as a brown-stained area, and may progress from erythema and edema to vesiculation and exfoliation. Eye involvement by South Seas species has resulted in chemosis, periorbital edema, corneal ulceration, and blindness.

Questions—Myriapoda

1. Which of the following statements is false?
A. The western U.S. centipede is responsible for most domestic Myriapoda bites.
B. Centipedes are strict herbivores.
C. Centipedes can grow to be 16 cm long.
D. Centipedes have powerful claws on their front segment beneath the mouth, which are connected by ducts to poisonous glands.
E. Rhabdomyolysis has followed centipede bites.

2. Millipedes have two pairs of legs per body segment, compared with one pair for centipedes, and lack poisonous glands.
A. True
B. False

ARACHNIDA

Mites

These ubiquitous creatures are barely visible to the naked eye but can cause significant pruritic dermatoses. A variety of nonburrowing mites produce multiple, often excoriated lesions without central puncta. They should be considered when a patient has unexplained pruritus, closely associated persons have similar lesions, and other insects have been excluded. Sources and species are widely varied.

Scabies
Scabies (*Sarcoptes scabiei*) are mites that attack humans most frequently and appear to affect humans in epidemics based on 30-year cycles. These mites complete their life cycle in humans unless interrupted by an effective miticide.

Trombiculidae
This group includes chiggers in the U.S. and harvest mites in Europe. The larval stages produce chicken pox-like lesions.

PATHOPHYSIOLOGY

Scabies
Female scabies burrow into epidermis at a rate of 2 mm/day for 1–2 months before laying 10–20 eggs and dying. In about three weeks, larvae emerge from tunnels. Females then burrow again, repeating the cycle. Infestation requires close personal contact, since the mite lives only several days away from humans and can neither jump nor fly.

Chiggers
After hatching, the larvae crawl along the ground onto grass, where humans acquire them from walking or lying on the grass, generally in late summer.

CLINICAL PRESENTATIONS

Scabies
Scabies lesions produce an intense pruritus, especially at night, on areas excluding the head and neck. Their burrows resemble black threads 5–20 mm long that end in vesicles, and classically appear in skin folds such as the webs between fingers, wrists, elbows, umbilicus, lower abdomen, genitalia, gluteus, and breast. Secondary changes may result from hypersensitivity (i.e., urticaria, excoriation, and eczema) or bacterial infection. Scraping of burrows from unexcoriated areas with a sterile scalpel may reveal mites, mite parts, or black fecal material.

Chiggers
Chigger lesions are usually seen on belt lines, ankles, or moist intertriginous areas where larvae pierce the skin and release a digestant that liquefies epidermal cells. First, a small macule with a red, pinpoint mite at its center appears. Within 24 hours, an intensely pruritic papule surrounded by a clear vesicle develops. The lesion may become ecchymotic. The engorged mite falls off after 3–4 days. A 0.5–2.0-cm lesion persists for several weeks and eventually crusts, similar to chicken pox.

TREATMENT

Scabies
- Lindane (Kwell®) effectively eliminates most infestations of this mite, although its use is somewhat controversial.
- An alternative medication for use in pregnant women and children is crotamiton (Eurax®), but this drug is less effective and requires a second application 24 hours later.
- The patient takes a warm shower or bath using soap, and then applies miticide over the entire body from the neck down, specifically including spaces between fingers and toes. The lotion is left on for 8–12 hours and then washed off thoroughly. The process may be repeated in one week, but usually is not necessary.
- The patient, sexual contacts and family members must clean all clothes, bed linen, and towels.

Chiggers
- Treatment is supportive. Watch for secondary infection.
- Application of an ointment containing 5–10% sulfur and 1% phenol may relieve pruritus and remove the mites.

Questions—Mites

1. Which of the following statements is false?
A. Scabies are mites.
B. Chiggers are mites.
C. Scabies jump from one host to another.
D. Female scabies burrow into epidermis at a rate of 2 mm/day.
E. Scabies lesions produce an intense pruritus, especially at night, on areas excluding the head and neck.

2. Chigger lesions are usually seen on belt lines, ankles, or moist intertriginous areas where larvae pierce the skin and release a digestant that liquefies epidermal cells.
A. True
B. False

Ticks

Hard body (*Ixodidae*) and soft body (*Argasidae*) ticks are strongly clinging blood-sucking insects. They are found worldwide, and usually are acquired in rural areas. They possess an ovoid body (fused thorax and abdomen) with prominent legs and may reach 1.5 cm when engorged.

PATHOPHYSIOLOGY

Ticks in all stages (larva, nymph, adult) attack humans by painlessly attaching to the host with strong teeth reinforced by cementlike secretions.

CLINICAL PRESENTATIONS

Granulomas as large as 2 cm may develop, but usually resolve spontaneously in several months. Hard ticks are disease vectors for typhus, viral encephalitis, tularemia, Colorado tick fever, Lyme disease, Rocky Mountain spotted fever, and a symmetrical ascending paralysis known as tick paralysis. The latter disease results from the secretion of a neurotoxin in certain species.

TREATMENT

- Thirty-percent N-butyl acetanilide solution is a good tick repellent.
- Organic solvents and chloroform encourage ticks to dislodge.
- Mechanical force increases the secretion of toxins and may leave mouth parts engaged in the host. Care must be taken to sterilely dislodge these parts.

Questions—Ticks

1. Hard ticks are vectors for each of the following diseases except

A. Lyme disease
B. Trypanosomiasis
C. Rocky Mountain spotted fever
D. Tick paralysis
E. Typhus

2. Which of the following statements is false?

A. Ticks may possess hard or soft bodies.
B. Certain ticks may possess a neurotoxin.
C. Ticks are found only in North and South America.
D. Ticks are blood-sucking insects.
E. Ticks can attack humans in all stages of development.

Spiders

INTRODUCTION

All but two of 20,000 American spider species are venomous, but only about 50 species have fangs capable of penetrating human skin. Spiders are ubiquitous and are found in concentrations up to two million per acre of grassland. They generally live for 1–2 years. Anatomically, the spider consists of cephalothorax (fused head and chest) and an abdomen, with four pairs of legs protruding from the thorax, as opposed to Hymenoptera (i.e., ants, bees, wasps), which have six legs. Spiders depend primarily on a sense of touch, since they are extremely shortsighted. Two clawlike fangs, the celicerea, protrude from their head and are connected to venomous glands believed to be under voluntary control.

Spiders molt 5–10 times before maturity. During this period they shed their hard shells and may change coloration or markings. Although their venom is more potent than pit viper venom, small quantities and weak injection mechanisms limit seriously venomous spiders to the *Latrodectus* and *Loxosceles* genera. Some examples include:

Garden Spiders

Argiope spiders (black or yellow) can inflict noticeable skin lesions on humans.

Golden Orb Weaver

Chiracanthium or running spider envenomation produces urticarial and necrotic lesions. Envenomation may cause pain without inflammation.

Latrodectus

These include the nefarious black widow spider. The venom is primarily neurotoxic, producing little local tissue reaction.

Liocranoides

The North American running spider is capable of producing a necrotic lesion.

Loxosceles

These include brown recluse spiders. Clinical problems range from mild local necrosis to rare hemolysis, coagulopathy, and death. At least four species, excluding Loxosceles species, indigenous to the U.S. are capable of producing necrotic lesions.

Phidippus

This jumping spider is probably the most common cause of necrotic arachnidism and is characterized by short legs, white stripes, and fluorescent green mouth parts. A bite produces a sharp, painful site that may develop into urticarial swelling and pruritus lasting several days.

Wolf Spider

Lycosa spiders can inflict noticeable skin lesions on humans.

Questions—Introduction to Spiders

1. Very few of the 20,000 American spider species are venomous.

A. True
B. False

2. Which of the following associations is incorrect?

A. Spiders–four pairs of legs
B. Hymenoptera–six legs
C. Spiders–two clawlike fangs
D. Jumping spider–necrotic arachnidism
E. Latrodectus–brown recluse

LOXOSCELES

Loxosceles spiders are also called brown recluse spiders, fiddlebacks, violin, or brown spiders. This rapidly expanding group includes at least 54 species and is found throughout the world. Thirteen species are indigenous to the U.S. These spiders are medium-sized and nondescript. Their short-haired body is 9–12 mm long and their color varies from fawn to dark brown depending on molting. The dorsal cephalothorax has a violin-shaped dark brown to yellow marking, with the larger end cephalad. The presence of three rather than four pairs of eyes is a distinctive but not unique feature.

This shy creature, which is well adapted to indoor living, prefers quiet areas such as clothes and storage closets. Their reclusive habits make them difficult to eradicate in human dwellings. Upon confrontation, these spiders usually retreat rapidly on long legs. They bite when threatened and when no escape route exists. Bites probably are much more prevalent than originally suspected. Fortunately, most bites are painless and people usually respond with mild reactions. The *Loxosceles reclusa* spider is the most widely reported species and is found from the east coast to California, with highest concentrations in the southeast. The term "brown recluse" technically applies only to this species.

PATHOPHYSIOLOGY

Loxosceles venom is primarily cytotoxic. Almost all of the venom consists of spreading factors and enzymes such as hyaluronidase, collagenase, esterase, protease, phospholipase, deoxyribonuclease, ribonuclease, and dipeptides. Hyaluronidase is apparently not responsible for the dermonecrosis associated with these spiders.

Purified venom produces direct cellular injury in human tissue cultures. Experimental laboratory data indicate that rapid coagulation and occlusion of small vessels lead to dermonecrosis. The exact component responsible for this has not been delineated, but once coagulation begins, a cascade of coagulation mediators causes a progression to necrosis.

Necrosis is greater in fatty areas of the buttocks, thighs, and abdomen and the venom may act directly on fatty tissue. *In vitro* experiments indicate that *Loxosceles reclusa* venom attaches directly to red blood cell membranes and causes structural changes. Venom attachment to erythrocyte membranes apparently is a prerequisite for hemolysis in human cells.

CLINICAL PRESENTATIONS

Dermatologic Effects

The progression of necrotic lesions varies widely depending on host immunity. Necrosis may occur rapidly within several hours or slowly over several days. Accurate descriptions of Loxosceles bites are complicated by the fact that the biting spider is usually not identified and the offending spider is only implicated by circumstantial evidence. Typical lesions produce pain and erythema within 1–2 hours of envenomation after little initial pain. This is followed by the formation of a bleb surrounded by a whitish ring of ischemia.

Ecchymosis may surround the evolving bleb, the center of which turns blue as necrosis ensues. After several days the bleb bursts, the blue necrotizing lesion widens, the edges become uneven, and the center sinks. In about seven days, a black eschar forms which sloughs within several weeks and may require 6–8 weeks to fill.

Large areas of necrosis have been reported at areas distant from the primary bite site, and lesions that are more serious definitely occur in fatty areas. A rapidly expanding lesion may spontaneously regress before necrosis occurs. Color and configuration differentiate Loxosceles bites from nonnecrotic ones, since the latter bites remain raised and erythematous. Loxosceles lesions are often confused with other necrotic spider bites, other arthropod bites, and systemic disease.

Systemic Effects

Systemic reactions occur uncommonly and do not correlate with the severity of cutaneous lesions. Typically, systemic symptoms develop within 24–48 hours of envenomation and are characterized by fever, chills, malaise, nausea, vomiting, myalgias, hemolysis, and/or consumptive coagulopathy (DIC). Coma, convulsions, and renal dysfunction are probably secondary effects. Hemolytic anemia may be insidious, often requiring 2–3 days to develop.

LABORATORY

Analytic Methods

A passive hemagglutinated inhibition test to diagnose brown recluse spider bite envenomation has been proposed but further studies are necessary.

Blood Levels

No routine laboratory tests are available to diagnose necrotic arachnidism.

TREATMENT

Wound Care

- Local treatment has been controversial. Some advocate early excision and others suggest that such therapy is ineffective, expensive, and disfiguring. Surgical intervention may be necessary for cosmetic purposes, especially when the lesion exceeds 4 cm at 12 hours after envenomation. Successful surgical management may result from allowing necrosis to delineate and then excising it with wide margins.
- Inadequately controlled and documented human cases, as well as the difficulty in predicting the course of cutaneous lesions, make incisional therapy controversial.
- Cleansing with bactericidal agents, tetanus prophylaxis as indicated, immobilization, elevation, serial observation, and antipruritic agents are the mainstays of treatment.
- Infections are uncommon but do occur.

Medical Management

- Systemic steroids are of unproven benefit.
- The use of polymorphonuclear leukocyte inhibitors such as dapsone has been suggested for large violaceous lesions on the basis of laboratory data. However, methemoglobinemia has complicated dapsone use.
- Serious adverse effects, the small scale of studies in humans, and the fact that leukocyte migration may only be a secondary phenomenon limit the human use of dapsone for Loxosceles envenomations at this time. The use of dapsone in the management of the local lesion has not been validated in a controlled clinical study and cannot be recommended.

Systemic Considerations

- All patients with systemic reactions should be followed in the hospital for evidence of hemolysis, coagulopathy, and renal failure.
- Systemic corticosteroids have not been proven effective in controlled studies.
- Rarely, a consumptive coagulopathy appears with depressed levels of fibrinogen, clotting factors, and platelets, as well as increased fibrin degradation products. Treatment for hemolysis and coagulopathy is supportive (i.e., RBC transfusions, platelets, cryoprecipitate, and fresh-frozen plasma).
- The white blood cell count may rise to 20,000–30,000 cells per cubic millimeter in the absence of secondary infection.
- Patients with systemic symptoms should receive a complete blood count including platelets, coagulation profile, urinalysis, electrolytes, liver function tests, and serum creatinine.

ANTIDOTES

Effective Loxosceles antivenin is currently not available in the U.S.

Questions—Loxosceles

1. **Which of the following statements about Loxosceles spiders is false?**
   A. They are called fiddlebacks, violin, or brown spiders.
   B. Their ventral cephalothorax has a violin-shaped red marking, with the larger end caudad.
   C. They have three, rather than four pairs of eyes.
   D. Upon confrontation, these spiders usually lunge at their prey.
   E. B and D
2. **Most brown recluse spider bites are painless and people usually respond with mild reactions.**
   A. True
   B. False
3. **Loxosceles venom is primarily**
   A. Nephrotoxic
   B. Cardiotoxic
   C. Cytotoxic
   D. Neurotoxic
   E. Hepatotoxic
4. **Which of the following statements concerning Loxosceles bites is true?**
   A. Necrosis may occur rapidly within several hours or slowly over several days.
   B. Systemic reactions occur uncommonly and do not correlate with the severity of cutaneous lesions.
   C. Large areas of necrosis can occur in areas distant from the primary bite site.
   D. All of the above
   E. A and B
5. **Early excision of necrotic sites is the accepted standard for treatment of Loxosceles bites.**
   A. True
   B. False

LATRODECTUS

These widow spiders are found in all parts of the world except at ecological extremes. The female is one of the larger female spiders, with a leg span of 5 cm and a body length of 1.5 cm. *Latrodectus mactans* females have a characteristic red hourglass spot on the dorsal surface of their black, shiny bodies, but the *tredecimguttatus* subspecies has two red marks that do not meet. Female widows are venomous from birth, but their venom toxicity is seasonal and greatest in warmer months.

Only three species are predominantly black (*mactans*, *hesperus*, and *variolus*). The other two species are more commonly brown (*geometricus*) or orange-red (*bishopi*). Marked intraspecies variation may occur as a result of molting. The black spiders become darker with less prominent red spots on each of nine moltings. In fact, black widow spiders can turn brown and then revert to the original color. The male has more colorful white markings and is smaller than the female at maturity. Its smaller venom apparatus and less aggressive nature make it clinically insignificant.

These shy trapping spiders use their venom to paralyze entrapped prey and then suck the hemolymph. They form irregular, untidy three-dimensional webs in dark, hidden protected places such as crevices, ground cover, stone walls, woodpiles, barns, stables, and outdoor toilets. A period of postcopulation lassitude allows the male spider to escape unless the female has a voracious appetite. Contrary to popular belief, both females and males may be found living together. Although earlier encounters involved bites to the buttocks and genitalia during outdoor toilet use, the body part most commonly bitten now is the hand. At least one of the five known U.S. Latrodectus species is present in every state.

PATHOPHYSIOLOGY

Latrodectus species contain one of the more potent neurotoxins known. Although at least seven protein fractions have been isolated from Latrodectus venom (e.g., hyaluronidase, phosphodiesterase, GABA, and 5-hydroxytryptamine), only a high-molecular-weight neurotoxin appears to affect mammals. Variation occurs among species. Animal susceptibility is also variable. Camels and horses are quite sensitive, whereas rats are not.

The venom produces a nonspecific spontaneous release of neurotransmitters, including GABA, norepinephrine, and acetylcholine, by facilitating exocytosis of synaptic vesicles. The postsynaptic membrane probably is morphologically unaffected. The venom binds specifically to nerve membrane and forms ion channels that allow the influx of calcium ions. High concentrations of calcium apparently facilitate the release of neurotransmitters by endogenous electrical stimulation while inhibiting venom-induced release.

CLINICAL PRESENTATIONS

Latrodectus bites usually cause a mild needleprick sensation that often goes unnoticed. Typically, two erythematous fang marks appear about 1 mm apart with slight swelling. The site may later develop into urticaria and pruritus but not necrosis. Frequently, local symptoms subside within a few minutes. Initially, pain may begin in regional lymph nodes, usually in the axilla or inguinal area. Generalized symptoms may start 15 minutes to six hours after envenomation. These are characterized by muscle spasms of the upper body in upper extremity bites or abdominal cramps in lower extremity bites.

In one series of patients envenomated by *L. mactans*, the most frequent symptoms were bite site pain, abdominal cramping, pain and weakness in the lower extremities, and chest tightness or pain. The most frequent signs were erythema at the bite site, abdominal tenderness or rigidity, lower leg cramps, tachypnea, restlessness, and hypertension. Chest or abdominal pains may become severe. Nausea, vomiting, headache, tremulousness, anxiety, sweating, lacrimation, salivation, and increased bronchorrhea may develop. Hyperesthesias (especially in the feet), paresthesias, ptosis, increased deep tendon reflexes, and convulsions may occur. Most envenomations by the Latrodectus species produce symptoms that peak in 3–4 hours.

The misdiagnosis of latrodectism as an acute abdomen is well reported, but the absence of true abdominal tenderness to palpation or rebound in spider bite victims should easily differentiate the two. Symptoms subside in several hours to several days but subjective symptoms of weakness, headache, insomnia, myalgias, and malaise may last for weeks. Envenomation from Latrodectus is rarely fatal. Persons at the extremes of life, those with preexisting cardiovascular disease and pregnant women are most vulnerable. Blood pressure elevation occurs commonly and is a significant risk to susceptible patients.

TREATMENT

- Treatment is generally self-limited and requires only supportive care and occasional pain relief. Warm moist compresses may be soothing. There are no effective first-aid measures.
- Wounds should be cleaned and tetanus prophylaxis given as indicated.
- Generalized spasms may respond to the judicious use of intra-

venous morphine under careful direct observation to prevent respiratory depression.

- Intravenous methocarbamol (Robaxin®) has been used to combat serious muscle spasms; however, methocarbamol is probably inferior to calcium (see below) for pain relief.
- Diazepam (Valium®) has also been used for sedation and spasm relief but has not been shown to be superior to either calcium gluconate or methocarbamol.
- Uncontrolled clinical case studies suggest that intravenous dantrolene sodium (0.5–0.9 mg/kg) followed by a maximum of 25 mg orally every four hours for six doses produced good muscle relaxation in five of six patients with mild side effects.

ANTIDOTES

Calcium Gluconate

Although widely touted as the first-line treatment of severe envenomation by black widow spiders, a review of 163 cases found calcium gluconate largely ineffective for pain relief compared with a combination of intravenous opioids and benzodiazepines. The usual dose of 10% intravenous calcium gluconate for Latrodectus spider bites is 0.2 mL/kg up to 10 mL given slowly with continuous cardiac monitoring. The period of analgesia lasts between 30 minutes and four hours, but the failure to provide relief within one hour of injection suggests that further doses will not be effective. Calcium chloride is more irritating to tissues, and therefore the gluconate solution is preferred.

Antivenin

Muscle spasms, pain, and elevated blood pressure may be refractory to treatment with calcium gluconate, diazepam, and methocarbamol and only temporarily decreased with meperidine. Latrodectus antivenin may shorten the duration of symptoms in severe envenomations. All symptoms can resolve following the use of this specific equine-derived antivenom. The antivenin blocks the ability of venom to bind to presynaptic membrane and has been useful as late as 46 hours postenvenomation.

Latrodectus antivenin is available and is effective for all U.S. species. Since the antivenin is derived from horse serum, sensitivity testing must be performed before administration. Prior or current evidence of horse serum sensitivity is a contraindication, especially since most patients can be managed with supportive care. Anaphylactic reactions are rare but serum sickness may occur. Antivenin is generally reserved for either pediatric or geriatric populations and those with cardiovascular disease. The usual dosage is one or two vials diluted in 50–100 mL of saline and infused over one hour. Symptoms usually resolve within an hour. The antivenin has been used successfully in pregnant women. Death has followed its use in a patient with bronchial asthma.

Questions—Latrodectus

1. **Which of the following statements concerning Latrodectus spiders is false?**
   A. These widow spiders are found in all parts of the world except at ecological extremes.
   B. *L. mactans* females have a characteristic red hourglass spot on the dorsal surface of their black, shiny bodies.
   C. Female widows are venomous when mature, and their venom toxicity is constant throughout the year.
   D. Not all Latrodectus spiders are black.
   E. They form irregular, untidy three-dimensional webs in dark, hidden protected places.
2. **Black widow females typically eat their mates and cannot live together.**
   A. True
   B. False
3. **The human body part most commonly bitten by black widows is**
   A. The hand
   B. The buttocks
   C. The genitalia
   D. The foot
   E. The face
4. **The most frequent symptoms associated with black widow spider bites are**
   A. Bite site pain, abdominal cramping, lower extremity pain and chest tightness
   B. Pruritus at the bite site, profound weakness, and incontinence
   C. Severe gastroenteritis followed by seizures and coma
   D. Skin and myonecrosis, rash
   E. Cardiovascular collapse and death
5. **The following may be helpful in treating symptoms from black widow spider bites:**
   A. Narcotic analgesics
   B. Latrodectus antivenin
   C. Diazepam
   D. Calcium gluconate
   E. All of the above

Tarantulas

Beginning in the 17th century, panic spread from the southern Italian city of Taranto throughout Europe concerning spider bites that caused muscle contractions and pain. The spider involved was believed to be the largest European spider, the wolf spider (*Lycosa tarantula*). The name tarantula has limited zoologic meaning, since the term has been used to refer to any big spider. Such hysteria led to the development of a special dance called the tarantella designed to protect the envenomated victim.

Concern over the tarantula persists today despite the fact that the widow spider (Latrodectus), not the wolf spider, was probably responsible for the envenomations. The mild-mannered North American tarantula species can produce a bite similar to a Hymenoptera sting; however, systemic toxicity does not occur. Urticarial hairs on the abdomen of the tarantula may cause dermatitis and conjunctivitis on contact.

TREATMENT

Local therapy (i.e., ice packs, cleansing) is usually all the treatment necessary.

Questions—Tarantulas

1. **Which of the following statements about tarantulas is false?**
   A. The tarantella, a dance, developed in response to tarantula hysteria.
   B. Hairs on the tarantula may cause contact dermatitis in humans.
   C. Strictly speaking, the tarantula is not a spider.

D. The tarantula is also called the wolf spider.
E. Systemic toxicity has not been associated with tarantula bites.

Scorpions

Scorpions are among the oldest land animals, dating back almost 400 million years. They have been known to inflict pain since at least the 3rd century BC. Although all of the known 650 species cause painful stings, only a few are very dangerous (e.g., Mexican *Centruroides suffusus*, Brazilian *Tityus serrulatus*, North African *Leiurus quinquestriatus*).

The only dangerous scorpion species in the U.S. is *Centruroides sculpturatus*. Numerous deaths from this scorpion have been reported. Most envenomations in healthy patients over ten years of age result in only local pain, but significant respiratory distress can occur in children under six years of age. The most serious envenomations occur in children under age ten. Examples of scorpion species include:

Buthus tamualus

Toxic myocardial effects (i.e., acute pulmonary edema secondary to congestive heart failure) are more common than neurotoxic effects in red scorpion (*Buthus tamulus*) envenomations seen in India. Signs of autonomic stimulation following *B. tamulus* envenomation include pain at the sting site, local edema, cool extremities, urticaria, vomiting, profuse sweating, priapism, salivation, hypertension, brady- and tachyarrhythmias, and ventricular premature contractions. Numerous electrocardiographic changes may be seen as well.

Centruroides sculpturatus

Centruroides sculpturatus is found in Arizona, parts of Texas, New Mexico, Northern Mexico, small desert sections of eastern California, and Lake Mead in Nevada. The body of the scorpion consists of a cephalothorax, an abdomen, and a six-segmented tail that terminates in a bulbous enlargement called the telson. Within this structure lie the stinger and venom apparatus. Two venom glands are located within the telson, with independent ducts leading to an opening near the stinger. This small (13–75 mm), hairless creature passes through four color phases ranging from the characteristic yellow-brown, to striped.

This scorpion is a climbing rather than a burrowing species that prefers areas around trees. Climbing characteristics cause it to sting unsuspecting humans who fail to look beneath objects to which the scorpion is attached. It tends to rest its tail on the ground rather than carry it arched overhead like most scorpions. The scorpion is a nocturnal feeder that eats small insects and spiders by clasping them in its claws and stinging them to death by thrusting its stinger from the arched tail. Scorpions hibernate during winter and seek shelter during the day.

Leiurus quinquestriatus

Leiurus quinquestriatus stings in tropical and subtropical areas have been reported to induce bradycardia, tachycardia, and hypertension in children. Heart failure, pulmonary edema, abdominal pain, nausea, vomiting and pancreatitis may be seen in older children and adults. Perioral paresthesias have been described after envenomation by *L. quinquestriatus*.

PATHOPHYSIOLOGY

Scorpion venom contains a complex mixture of constituents, but five neurotoxins appear to constitute the clinically important component. One class of neurotoxins induces a slow inward sodium current that prolongs the action potential so that a given stimulus causes greater sodium channel activation. Other neurotoxins are stabilizers that reduce sodium channel flow during depolarization. These effects on sodium gating occur at preterminal sites, resulting in the release of neurotransmitters at the neuromuscular junction and repetitive enhanced axonal discharges. The North African species *L. quinquestriatus* possesses a cardiotoxic toxin, producing peripheral vascular collapse, hypotension, and pulmonary edema.

CLINICAL PRESENTATIONS

Most *C. sculpturatus* envenomations are minor. In one patient series, 92% were treated successfully at home with conservative therapy of cold compresses and mild analgesics. Most bites in adults result in local pain, similar in severity to Hymenoptera envenomation. Swelling, erythema, and ecchymosis, however, are usually not present in scorpion envenomations. Mild palpation usually produces moderately severe pain. Symptoms usually resolve within ten hours and are inversely related to age. Some symptoms in severely envenomated infants have lasted for 30 hours.

Neurologic Effects

Cranial nerve dysfunction may include blurred vision, disconjugate gaze, hypersalivation, dysphagia, slurred speech, tongue fasciculations, or upper airway obstruction. Somatic and skeletal dysfunction may manifest as increased involuntary activity (e.g., myoclonic jerks), restlessness, and hemiballismus.

Pediatric Effects

Children are more severely affected with pain, restlessness, and roving eye movements. Hyperexcitability is very common in infants. Typically, initial intense pain is followed within minutes to several hours by hyperexcitability, increased salivation, tachypnea, muscle fasciculations, muscle spasms, paralysis, and respiratory failure. Symptoms generally reflect sympathetic, parasympathomimetic, and neuromuscular excitation followed by exhaustion.

Sympathetic effects may include tachycardia, hypotension, diaphoresis, mydriasis, piloerection, hyperthermia, and hyperactivity. Parasympathomimetic signs are salivation, lacrimation, urination, defecation, and gastric distension. Hyperesthesias, muscle fasciculations, opisthotonus, disconjugate gaze, nystagmus, and convulsions may occur. Respiratory effects include stridor, cyanosis, and dyspnea.

LABORATORY

Analytic Methods

Specific laboratory tests are usually not helpful in the management of scorpion envenomations.

Blood Levels

Blood levels do not help identify or aid in the management of scorpion envenomations.

TREATMENT

- Most envenomations produce no serious side effects and may be treated with local ice application, local anesthetic injection, and analgesics such as codeine.
- Management of severe human scorpion envenomation should be directed toward neutralizing the overstimulated autonomic nervous system. All patients with systemic manifestations such as severe hypertension, hypovolemia, and pulmonary edema or patients in shock should be admitted to a critical care unit under close electrocardiographic and, if necessary, invasive hemodynamic monitoring.

- Management should include sedation, fluid replacement, and afterload reduction in severe cases. Patients with respiratory failure or with central nervous system disturbances should be mechanically ventilated. Acid-base imbalance should be corrected.
- Children under three years of age are at the greatest risk of developing respiratory failure and frequently require hospital admission. All patients below one year of age and older children with neurologic signs require monitoring in an intensive care unit.
- Routine laboratory tests in severe envenomations should include a complete blood count, electrolytes, creatinine, and urinalysis. Arterial blood gases may be helpful in cases involving respiratory distress.
- Fluid loss due to vomiting, perspiration, and increased salivation may complicate the clinical course. Every effort should be directed toward correcting fluid balance.
- Phenobarbital (5–10 mg / kg intravenously) may improve neurologic symptoms such as agitation or hyperactivity but probably does not decrease the duration of symptoms. Large phenobarbital doses may depress respirations and may have contributed to the mortality and morbidity seen in earlier studies.
- No rational basis exists for the use of antihistamines, corticosteroids, or calcium in the treatment of scorpion stings.
- Rhythm disturbances and conduction abnormalities may be observed after *B. tamulus* and other scorpion stings, sometimes in the presence of pulmonary edema. These abnormalities are of short duration, are rarely sustained, and usually do not need a specific treatment except on the rare occasions that tachyarrhythmias contribute to the hemodynamic failure.
- Propranolol has effectively and rapidly reversed tachydysrhythmias but has not improved other hemodynamic or neurologic parameters.

ANTIDOTES

Antivenin

Goat antivenin is available in Arizona but government regulations restrict its use to Arizona. One to two vials of antivenin have been used safely in over 30 patients, with only one case of urticaria reported and no cases of serum sickness. Most patients who benefit from the use of scorpion antivenom may develop rash, urticaria, or serum sickness within two weeks of administration.

Symptoms improve within an hour and resolve within several hours. To date, no multicenter prospective clinical trials have demonstrated the efficacy and safety of scorpion antivenin, but the antivenin appears effective in severe envenomations. Antivenin appears to shorten the duration of respiratory failure and may prevent rhabdomyolysis. Its use carries a potential for anaphylaxis and an increased risk for a delayed reaction.

Questions—Scorpions

1. The only dangerous scorpion species in the U.S. is
A. *Centruroides sculpturatus*
B. *Leiurus quinquestriatus*
C. *Buthus tamulus*
D. *Lycosa tarantula*
E. *Apis mellifera scutellata*

2. Which of the following statements is false?
A. *C. sculpturatus* is found in the U.S. southwest.
B. The six-segmented tail of a scorpion is called the telson.
C. *C. sculpturatus* is a climbing rather than a burrowing species that prefers areas around trees.
D. *L. quinquestriatus* stings in tropical and subtropical areas have been reported to induce bradycardia, tachycardia, and hypertension in children.
E. *C. sculpturatus* venom contains primarily neurotoxins.

3. Most *C. sculpturatus* envenomations are minor and are successfully treated at home.
A. True
B. False

4. *Buthus tamulus*
A. Can cause toxic myocardial effects
B. Is called the red scorpion
C. Can cause electrocardiographic changes
D. All of the above
E. A and C

Answers

Introduction to Arthropods

1. D

Hymenoptera

1. B 2. C 3. D 4. A 5. E 6. B 7. E
8. D 9. A

Lepidoptera

1. C 2. B

Siphonaptera

1. D

Anoplura

1. A 2. A

Diptera

1. B 2. A

Hemiptera

1. D

Cleoptera

1. E

Myriapoda

1. B 2. A

Mites

1. C 2. A

Ticks

1. B 2. C

Introduction to Spiders

1. B 2. E

Loxosceles

1. E 2. A 3. C 4. D 5. B

Latrodectus

1. C 2. B 3. A 4. A 5. E

Tarantulas

1. C

Scorpions

1. A 2. B 3. A 4. D

SELECTING READINGS

Arthropods

1 Anderson PC, Necrotizing spider bites. Am J Fam Pract 1982;26:198–203.
2. Barnard JH. Studies of 400 Hymenoptera sting deaths in the United States. J Allergy Clin Immunol 1973;52:259–264.
3. Bawaskar HS, Bawaskar PH. Scorpion sting: a review of 121 cases. J Wilderness Med 1991;2:164–174.
4. Berger RS. Management of brown recluse spider bite. JAMA 1984;251:889.
5. Binder LS. Acute arthropod envenomation. Incidence, clinical features and management. Med Toxicol Adverse Drug Exp 1989;4:163–173.
6. Clark RF, Wethern-Kestner S, Vance MV, et al. Clinical presentation and treatment of black widow spider envenomation: a review of 163 cases. Ann Emerg Med 1992;21:782–787.
7. Frankland AW, Lessott MH. Allergy to bee stings: A review. J R Soc Med 1980;73:807–809.
8. Gueron M, Margulic G, Ilia R, et al. The management of scorpion envenomation. Toxicon 1993;31:1071–1083.
9. Maretic Z: Latrodectism: Variation in clinical manifestations provoked by Latrodectus species of spiders. Toxicon 1983;21:457–466.
10. McCormick MA: Black widow spiders. Clin Toxicol Rev 1983;5(10):1–2.
11. Reisman RE. Insect stings. N Engl J Med 1994;331:523–527.

CHAPTER 55
Herbal Medicines, Volatile Oils and Plant Dermatitis

HERBAL TEAS

Interest in herbal medicine has recently increased, possibly as a by-product of the vast publicity accorded the toxins and carcinogens in our environment. Toxicity from herbs may result from causes other than an exaggerated pharmacological response to excessive ingestion. Chamomile, for example, is a popular tea that may cause allergic rhinitis or even anaphylactic shock in patients with ragweed sensitivity. Herbal intoxication can cause a wide range of symptoms because of multiorgan involvement.

Misidentification represents another serious hazard. The inadvertent brewing of tea from foxglove (*Digitalis purpurea*), instead of the similar, nontoxic comfrey plant has caused several fatalities. In addition, certain herbs may be contaminated with toxic substances. For example, atropine poisoning has occurred after the consumption of burdock (*Arctium minus*) root tea, which normally does not contain atropine-like alkaloids.

A number of common teas, volatile oils, and herbal remedies are described below. The field of botanical toxicology is huge, and these examples represent a mere sampling of interesting and commonly encountered toxins. The list is by no means exhaustive. Some (e.g., foxglove and mate) are reviewed in other chapters. While some toxins are extremely well-documented, an element of folklore and "less than rigorous" methods have characterized certain elements of this literature.

Chaparral

The chaparrals are a group of closely related wild shrubs found in the deserts of the American Southwest and Mexico. Chaparral is derived from the ground leaves of the creosote bush. It is found in health food stores as leaflets and twigs. Chaparral has been used by Native Americans in teas, capsules, and tablet form for a variety of disorders. Nordihydroguaiaretic acid and related lignins appear to be antioxidants at the cellular level. Chronic ingestion of chaparral may be associated with acute or chronic hepatotoxicity. In 1992, the U.S. FDA issued a warning following four cases of chaparral hepatitis.

TREATMENT

- Cessation of use may lead to improvement in liver function.

Germander

The blossoms of wall germander have been used in preparations of herbal teas to form medicinal liquor in which germander is mixed with various other herbs. Germander may induce hepatitis. These preparations may contain a variety of herbs and plants including valerian, asafetida, skullcap, gentian, senna, Chinese herbs, mistletoe, and chaparral leaf.

TREATMENT

- Treatment is supportive.

Ginseng

Ginseng has been used in traditional Chinese medicine for several thousand years for cardiovascular collapse, fatigue, cardiac disease, Addison's disease, dyspepsia, neurosis, cancer, anemia, and leukopenia. Ginseng has been known in the U.S. since colonial times. George Washington mentioned the gathering of this plant in his diary, and Daniel Boone was known to be active in the ginseng trade.

Ginseng is a native plant of the Eastern United States and Canada that grows in shady hardwood forests between Quebec and Georgia. The vast majority of American ginseng is shipped to the Orient, where this root is preferred to oriental ginseng (*Panax pseudoginseng*). Recently, American consumption of the oriental root has increased, but the U.S. still exports most American ginseng root to the Orient.

PATHOPHYSIOLOGY

The most characteristic compounds in ginseng roots are ginsenosides, and most biologic effects have been ascribed to these compounds. Ginsenosides, being glycosylated steroids, are very difficult to analyze and quantify in small amounts. No estrogens are present, but ginseng produces an estrogen-like effect on human vaginal epithelium and may influence corticosteroid secretion through the adrenal-pituitary axis. Two ginseng saponins have anti-inflammatory properties.

CLINICAL PRESENTATIONS

The average therapeutic dose is 2–3 grams, although doses up to 50 grams have been prescribed, resulting in insomnia, depression, and nervous disorders. Ingestion of ginseng root can result in general arousal and excitation. In one well-controlled study of night-shift nurses, the use of 1–2 grams of Korean ginseng failed to improve the mood or sense of well-being more than a placebo. Cerebral arteritis has been reported after ingestion of a large quantity of ginseng extract (about 25 grams drug weight).

Chronic excessive consumption has resulted in hypertension, insomnia, skin eruptions, and morning diarrhea. About 10% of chronic users develop hypertension. The estrogen-like effects of ginseng have produced diffuse breast nodules and mastalgia, and may cause postmenopausal bleeding. Hypertension and depression may result from withdrawal after chronic use.

TREATMENT

- Treatment is supportive.

Pyrrolizidine Alkaloids

The pyrrolizidine alkaloids compose 180 compounds that occur in at least eight plant families, but four genera—*Heliotropium*, *Crotalaria*, *Senecio*, and *Symphytum*—have accounted for most toxic ingestions. The last genus includes common comfrey (*Symphytum officinale*), prickly comfrey (*Symphytum asperus*), and Russian comfrey (*Symphytum uplandicen*). They produce hepatic veno-occlusive disease in sporadic cases after consumption of teas, or in epidemics when these herbs contaminate cereal.

Over 150 pyrrolizidine alkaloids have been isolated. Herbalists have employed comfrey as a demulcent, an antihemorrhagic, an antirheumatic, and an anti-inflammatory agent. The dried roots and the dried or fresh leaves are used, orally or topically. Comfrey may be the most widely recognized source of dietary pyrrolizidine alkaloids in developed countries.

Other examples include *Senecio longilobus* (Sunflower) tea, which has produced fatal hepatic necrosis simulating Reye's syndrome in a 2-month-old, *Gynura segetum*, a native Chinese herb, and comfrey-pepsin preparations. Consumption of bread contaminated by *Heliotropium* seeds caused an outbreak of hepatic veno-occlusive disease in Afghanistan. Ingestion of bread contaminated by *Crotalaria* seeds, and bush teas produced from *Crostalacia* leaves, have also caused veno-occlusive liver disease.

PATHOPHYSIOLOGY

An essential structural requirement for toxicity is the presence of an unsaturated pyrrolizidine ring structure. The pyrrolizidine alkaloids themselves are not toxic and are largely cleared from the body in 24 hours. They are activated in the liver, where they are metabolized by mixed-function oxidase to pyrrolic dihydroalkaloids, which are reactive alkylating agents. These metabolites induce liver cell necrosis and vascular lesions characterized by primary pulmonary hypertension. Characteristic hepatic veno-occlusive lesions, endothelial proliferation, arterial hypertrophy, pulmonary hypertension, right ventricular hypertrophy, and cor pulmonale are probably due to the release of pyrrole metabolites by the liver.

CLINICAL PRESENTATIONS

Large doses over a number of days produce occlusion of hepatic venules and the clinical picture of Reye's syndrome characterized by vomiting, progressive hyperpnea, and encephalopathy. In pyrrolizidine poisoning jaundice, ascites, hepatomegaly, hypoglycemia, and massive elevations of serum hepatic aminotransferase levels are prominent. In epidemic settings, the symptoms are more insidious and begin with anorexia, lassitude, and weight loss. Subsequently, ascites, edema, emaciation, hepatomegaly, and splenomegaly develop. Prolonged pyrrolizidine alkaloid consumption can cause pulmonary artery hypertension, leading to cor pulmonale and right ventricular hypertrophy.

TOXIC DOSAGE/DEATH

Liver toxicity follows consumption of herbal teas for up to several years. A high level of comfrey consumption as salad is about 5–6 leaves daily. Intake from comfrey tea is at the same level. A dose of 70–147 mg of *Senecio* alkaloids has been associated with liver cirrhosis in a 6-month-old girl. Children appear to be more susceptible than adults. Herbal preparations of comfrey-pepsin from leaves and roots may contain total pyrrolizidine levels of 270 mg and 2,900 mg per kilogram, respectively.

TREATMENT

- Management is entirely supportive. Hepatic necrosis represents the greatest threat to life.
- Laboratory studies demonstrate hepatic necrosis with coagulopathies, hypoglycemia, leukocytosis, hyperbilirubinemia, and grossly elevated hepatic aminotransferase levels.
- Profound hypoglycemia is a definite risk. Any obtunded patient should receive intravenous glucose immediately after blood samples are drawn.
- The diagnosis of pyrrolizidine alkaloid poisoning can only be made by excluding other causes of hepatic failure, by recognizing pathognomonic histopathologic changes in hepatic biopsy specimens, and by analyzing for pyrrolizidine alkaloids in herbal preparations to which the patient has been exposed.

Questions—Herbal Teas

1. All of the following herbal teas are associated with liver disease except
A. Russian comfrey
B. Ginseng
C. Chaparral
D. Germander
E. Prickly comfrey

2. Large doses of pyrrolizidine alkaloids such as *Heliotropium* can cause
A. A clinical picture of Reye's syndrome
B. Insidious symptoms of anorexia, lassitude, and weight loss
C. Significant elevation of aminotransferases
D. A and B
E. All of the above

3. Which of the following statements about herbal teas is true?
A. Liver toxicity is from acute ingestion of large doses, not chronic ingestions.
B. Hyperglycemia is a common metabolic derangement in acute overdose.
C. Children appear to be more susceptible to herbal tea toxicity than adults.
D. All of the above
E. None of the above

4. Chronic excessive consumption of ginseng typically causes
A. Insomnia
B. Hypotension
C. Constipation
D. All of the above
E. None of the above

Answers to questions in shaded boxes appear at the end of the chapter.

VOLATILE OILS

Volatile or essential oils are widely used as rubefacients, in teas, as flavoring agents in numerous foods and candies, in anesthetics and in fragrances. "Essential" refers to "essence." While small doses are generally well tolerated, well-known patterns of morbidity have been associated with certain volatile oils.

Oil of wintergreen, for example, contains methyl salicylate and may be associated with typical signs of salicylate poisoning. See Chapter 11, Salicylates. Camphor, an agent found in numerous topical preparations, may cause refractory seizures. See Chapter 39, Over-The-Counter Products. Nutmeg oil can be abused as a hallucinogen (see Chapter 20, Hallucinogenic Drugs), and turpentine oil, a solvent and cleaning agent, can cause a toxic pneumonitis (see Chapter 46, Hydrocarbons). Absinthe, a flavoring agent in alcoholic drinks consisting of a mixture of volatile oils, can cause ataxia, vertigo and gastrointestinal distress. See Chapter 56, Beans, Houseplants and Food Plants.

Cinnamon Oil

Cinnamon oil is easily obtained from pharmacies in 5–10-mL amounts for use as a flavoring agent and in craft items. Cinnamon oil abuse in young adolescents follows sucking on toothpicks or fingers dipped in cinnamon oil. A rush or sensation of warmth, facial flushing, and oral burning may be experienced. No residual symptoms have been observed. Cinnamon oil contains local mucous membrane irritants such as cinnamaldehyde. Prolonged skin contact (over 48 hours) from a cinnamon oil spill has produced superficial partial-thickness burns.

TREATMENT

- Treatment is symptomatic and supportive.

Citronella Oil

Oil of citronella is a fragrant, volatile oil obtained by distillation from fresh grass of *Cymbopogon nardus Rendle* or *Cymbopogon winterianus Jowitt* (family Gramineae). The main constituents are geraniol and citronellol. Countries producing this oil include Sri Lanka, Indonesia, and Taiwan. Citronella oil is used in perfumery, in insect repellents, and other veterinary products. A 21-month-old child drank three teaspoons of a preparation containing oil of citronella. The child developed cyanosis, seizures, and vomiting and died in five hours. The child had been given an emetic of salt and water that may have contributed to the clinical course.

TREATMENT

- Treatment is symptomatic.

Clove Oil

Clove oil contains 84–88% eugenol used as an anesthetic for dental procedures, a flavoring agent in foods and pharmaceuticals, in the manufacture of textiles, and in herbal medicines. Ingestion can lead to central nervous system depression, seizures, a coagulopathy, lactic acidosis and hepatic dysfunction. Like acetaminophen it is metabolized by glucuronide and sulfate conjugates in the liver. Animal studies suggest that the hepatic damage is reversed by N-acetylcysteine. Evidence for this in humans is not available.

Clove oil is obtained from the dried flower buds or leaves of the *Syzygium aromaticum* (*Eugenia caryophyllus*) tree of the myrtle family (Myrtaceae). Consumption of 5–15 mL of clove oil may induce a high anion gap acidosis, seizures, coagulopathy, acute liver damage, behavioral changes, and coma. A clove oil spill may lead to a stinging erythematous reaction with diminished sweating and reduced sensation in affected areas.

TREATMENT

- Treatment is symptomatic and supportive.
- Gastric lavage was used safely in one patient.

Eucalyptus Oil

Eucalyptus oil contains 70% eucalyptol, which is absorbed rapidly from the gastrointestinal tract. Cineol, a skin irritant, is a major component of eucalyptus oil. Transient coma has followed ingestion of as little as 1 mL, and fatalities have resulted from the consumption of 3.5 mL. Seizures are common and rapid in onset, similar to camphor.

Symptoms may include headache, ataxia, delirium, obtundation, coma, convulsions, hypotension, hyperpnea, and gastrointestinal distress. Premature ventricular contractions and apnea in one child have been reported. Ingestion of "taste" amounts seems to be relatively harmless. Survival has been reported with ingestion of 21–30 mL in an 8-year-old, 23 mL in an adult, and 120–240 mL in a treated adult.

TREATMENT

- Activated charcoal should be administered with tracheal protection instead of syrup of ipecac because of the rapid onset of seizures and coma.
- Treatment is supportive and all ingestions should be considered serious.

Margosa Oil

Margosa oil is a yellowish extract of neem tree seeds (*Azadirachta indica*) and is an infant folk remedy in India and Southeast Asia. Vomiting usually starts within 15 minutes–4 hours of ingestion and is followed by lethargy, tachypnea, seizures, and coma. Liver dysfunction is unusual.

TREATMENT

- Treatment requires control of seizures, correction of cerebral edema, hydration, respiratory support, and a search for associated infection.

Pennyroyal Oil

Pennyroyal oil is a volatile oil derived from *Mentha pulegium* and *Hedeoma Pulegeoides*, indigenous plants present from Canada to Florida and west to Nebraska. Herbalists use pennyroyal oil as an abortifacient and to induce menses. Toxic effects usually result from the misuse of the herb in folk medicine. The toxin pulegone is the ketone, cyclohexanone, which constitutes 85% of pennyroyal oil and produces direct hepatic damage.

Pennyroyal oil consumption produces direct toxic effects on the gastrointestinal tract and the liver. Depending on the dose, the clinical presentation may include nausea, vomiting, abdominal pain, burning of the throat, seizures and dizziness followed by liver dysfunction. Ten milliliters of this compound has produced gastrointestinal distress, and 30 mL has resulted in fatal hepatic necrosis.

In fatal cases, hepatomegaly, coagulation abnormalities, renal failure, shock, consumptive coagulopathy and hepatorenal failure have developed.

TREATMENT

- The usual measures of decontamination (e.g., charcoal and lavage) may be helpful in patients who have ingested significant amounts of pennyroyal oil (i.e., more than a taste) and who present within several hours.

- Asymptomatic patients or those whose symptoms subside within four hours postingestion may be discharged. Symptomatic patients should be admitted.
- No methods to enhance elimination are available and there are no antidotes.
- Patients who are admitted should have a complete blood count, electrolytes, creatinine, liver function tests, urinalysis, and coagulation profiles.
- Hepatic necrosis usually occurs within 24 hours. Such patients should be observed for development of bleeding secondary to coagulation abnormalities and treated with platelet packs, fresh-frozen plasma, and blood transfusions as necessary.
- Seizures are self-limited and should respond to diazepam.

Sassafras Oil

Teas from the root bark of the sassafras tree (*Sasafras albidum*) contain safrole. The aromatic oil has 80% safrole, which is hepatotoxic and hepatocarcinogenic in animal models. Safrole is a potent inhibitor of some liver microsomal enzymes, and major root extracts cause ataxia, ptosis, hypersensitivity to touch, hypothermia, and central nervous system depression in mice. Although a single sassafras tea bag may exceed the calculated human toxic dose, no clinical data on humans are available to assess or confirm toxicity to humans. An adult who ingested 5 mL of sassafras oil developed vomiting, "shakiness," flushing, and tachycardia. A 72-year-old who drank ten cups of sassafras tea developed diaphoresis and hot flashes that resolved on cessation of drinking the tea.

TREATMENT

- Treatment is symptomatic and supportive.

Tea Tree Oil

Oil of Melaleuca has been promoted as a remedy for certain skin conditions. Melaleuca oil is extracted from the leaves of the Australian *Melaleuca alternifolia* tree (where it is also known as tea tree oil) and contains 50–60% terpenes and related alcohols. It has been used as an antiseptic and antifungal agent. Ingestion of 100% Melaleuca oil has led to confusion, inability to walk, disorientation, ataxia, and a eucalyptus-like odor on the breath.

TREATMENT

- Recovery follows treatment with activated charcoal.
- Treatment is symptomatic and supportive.

Questions—Volatile Oils

1. Which of the following oils is commonly used to repel insects?
A. Cinnamon oil
B. Citronella oil
C. Clove oil
D. Eucalyptus oil
E. None of the above

2. Which of the following may be used by herbalists as an abortifacient and to induce menses?
A. Clove oil
B. Eucalyptus oil
C. Pennyroyal oil
D. Sassafras oil
E. None of the above

3. Pennyroyal oil produces direct toxic effects on the gastrointestinal tract and the liver.
A. True
B. False

MISCELLANEOUS HERBAL REMEDIES

There are literally thousands of herbal remedies used in folk medicine in the U.S. and around the world. Many have been used for centuries. It is not unusual for patients who use traditional medicines to seek advice and treatment with traditional ethnic practitioners before resorting to more conventional medical advice. While by no means exhaustive, a few observations about some popular herbal remedies follow.

Absinthe

Absinthe or wormwood (*Artemisia absinthe*) is a toxic liquor. Absinthe was a flavoring and coloring agent in alcoholic drinks. See Chapter 56, Beans, Houseplants and Food Plants. It contains a volatile oil, thujone, and is now banned in the U.S. It caused "absinthism," which includes psychosis, hallucinations, and intellectual deterioration. It is rumored to have produced effects in the artist Van Gogh. Its central nervous system effects are similar to camphor. It produces ataxia, vertigo, headache, vomiting, diarrhea, and diaphoresis.

Aconitum

Aconite (*Aconitum napellus*) is known as monkshood or wolfsbane. See Chapter 57, Wild Plants, Mushrooms and Mycotoxins. Fatal doses include 5 mL of aconite tincture, 2 mg of pure aconite, and 1 gram of the plant.

Aloe

Aloe (*Aloe vera, barbadensis, officinalis*) soothes skin burns and rashes. Aloe may cause hypersensitivity, skin irritation, diarrhea, vomiting, and red urine.

Ayurvedic Medicines

In India, a widely practiced type of traditional medicine is known as Ayurveda, which employs preparations such as vegetable products, animal products, metals (often lead and mercury) and minerals. Modern pharmaceuticals, such as penicillin, are even prescribed by traditional healers. Other indigenous drugs are analgesics, antipyretics, and corticosteroids.

Ayurvedic traditional medicine preparations, commonly known as bhasmas, are administered orally for systemic use or are applied locally. In Ayurvedic medicine, lead is regarded as an aphrodisiac and its reputed role may have been to counter the impotence associated with autonomic neuropathy in the diabetic male. Bhasmas are fine ashes of metals and metallic salts (iron, copper, etc.) and a variety of natural products (oyster shells, conches). The ingredients are subjected to several cycles of heating, cooling, and grinding until the preparation turns to a fine ash. All contain polycyclic aromatic hydrocarbons. They may be significantly contaminated with benzo(a)pyrene, a chemical carcinogen.

Gymnema (*Gymnema sylvestre*) has been used by Ayurvedic practitioners in India for centuries either alone or as a compound of Tribang shia, a mixture of tin, lead, zinc, Gymnema Sylvestre leaves, neom (*Melia azadirachta*) leaves, *Enicostenna littorale*, and janbul (*Eugena jambolana*) seeds. It has also been used in traditional African medicines. It appears to have hypoglycemic properties.

Birch Bark

Birch bark (bark leaves, *Betula* species) contains methylsalicylate. See Chapter 11, Salicylates.

Black Balls

Black balls are also called *Tung Shueh* pills. They contain diazepam, heavy metals and steroids.

Black Cohosh

Black cohosh (*Cimicifuga racemosa*) has estrogenic effects and has been used for "female complaints" and other disorders. Adverse effects of this plant include nausea, vomiting, dizziness, and weakness. Tannin is also present and has the potential for liver damage.

Black Snake Root

Black snake root (Zygandenus species), similar to veratrine, can produce hypotension and bradycardia.

Boui-Ougi-Tou

Boui-ougi-tou is a mixture of Chinese crude drugs containing glycyrrhizin, which has been associated with a Fanconi syndrome in an anecdotal report of a patient who survived.

Buckthorn

Buckthorn (*Hipothae momnoides*) is suspected to contain anthraquinones, which can produce severe watery diarrhea. Buckthorn (Rhamnus species) bark yields a toxin that causes spinal cord demyelination and paralysis. It has been used as a cathartic. See Chapter 57, Wild Plants, Mushrooms and Mycotoxins.

Burdock Root

Burdock root (*Articum minus*) has anticholinergic activity.

Bush Tea

Bush tea (Crotalaria species) contains pyrrolizidine alkaloids, which are hepatotoxic. See the section on Pyrrolizidine Alkaloids.

Cantharidin

One of the best known traditional medicines responsible for acute poisoning is the cantharidin beetle. There are over 300 species producing cantharidin belonging to the Meloidae family in South Africa. It is ground to a powder and has been used as an aphrodisiac, abortifacient, and for purifying the blood. Seletsa poisoning produces severe gastrointestinal irritation and ulceration. Nephrotoxicity occurs with hematuria and dysuria, and fatalities are relatively common.

Cantharidin is a toxic terpenoid produced by beetles. The dried and powdered blister beetle is termed cantharides. Cantharidin was for many years wrongly believed to be an aphrodisiac ("Spanish Fly") and an abortifacient based on its tendency to cause marked irritation to the genitourinary system leading to priapism in men and pelvic congestion in women. In overdose, it may lead to death.

Capsicum

Capsicum (Capsicum peppers) contains capsaicin, an alkaloid contained in various capsaicin red peppers (used as a herbal remedy for pain for centuries) and exhibits widespread pharmacologic properties, notably on type C nociceptive afferent nerve fibers. It is believed to deplete substance P, a neurotransmitter of pain. The application of capsaicin produces desensitization to thermal, chemical, and mechanical stimuli in a dose-dependent manner. See Chapter 56, Beans, Houseplants and Food Plants.

Cassia Species

Cassia species (*Senna*), cascara sagrada (*Rhamnus purshiana*) contain strong botanical laxatives and diuretics. Frequent use has been associated with a laxative abuse syndrome including severe electrolyte disturbances leading to cardiac dysrhythmias. See Senna below.

Catnip

Catnip (*Nepeta cataria*) is a mild central nervous system stimulant and hallucinogen. It is used by insufflation.

Chamomile

Chamomile teas are members of the Composita family. *Anthemis cotula* is found in the western U.S. It has been recommended for its antispasmodic and carminative actions. It is made from the fragrant pollen-laden flowering heads that have a cross-allergic reaction with other members of the Composita family, including ragweed, asters, and chrysanthemums. A single cup can cause allergic reactions such as anaphylactoid reactions, hives, and respiratory distress. In Mexico, it is called Manzanilla.

Ch' an Su

Ch' an Su, a traditional Chinese medication, is used as a topical anesthetic and cardiac medication and contains bufadienolides. It has been used as an aphrodisiac ("rock hard") and caused deaths. Cardioactive steroids, including bufadienolides, have a narrow therapeutic index, and unintentional therapeutic intoxication is well documented. These steroids can adversely affect the myocardium, and the most life-threatening manifestations of toxicity include arrhythmias, ventricular ectopy, sinus bradycardia, atrial arrhythmias, and hyperkalemia. Cardiac steroids are also found in nontraditional therapies such as oleander (*Nerium oleander*) and foxglove (*Digitalis purpurea*) teas.

Chaparral

Chaparral, from the leaves of the creosote bush (*Lares tridentas*), is recommended as an antioxidant or free-radical scavenger to retard aging and treat a variety of skin disorders. It has been used as a traditional Indian medicine. It contains nordihydroguaiaretic acid, a potent antioxidant that can act as a cyclooxygenase and lipoxygenase pathway inhibitor. See the section on Herbal Teas.

Chromium

Trivalent chromium is not truly an herbal product, but a heavy metal. It has been used by body builders to enhance glucose utilization and increase lean body mass. Toxicity is unlikely with a single acute dose. The minimum daily dose of chromium has not been established; however, 50–200 mg appears to be safe. Long-term exposure to other chromium salts is a possible carcinogen. See Chapter 47, Metals.

Chu an wu

Chu an wu may be made from toad venom (*Bufo melanosticus*), which contains bufotoxins structurally and pharmacologically similar to digoxin. Patients may present with symptoms of digoxin poisoning.

Chuifong Tokuman

Chuifong tokuman, a pharmaceutical product manufactured in Hong Kong, is a combination product containing diazepam, hydrochlorothiazide, mefenamic acid, dexamethasone, lead, and cadmium. It is not approved by the U.S. Food and Drug Administration (FDA) and is not legal for sale or importation into the U.S. *Chuifong tokuman* may increase the body burden of cadmium. Renal tubular cell damage has been reported after cadmium exposures. See Chapter 47, Metals.

Chuen Lin

Chuen Lin (*Coptis chinensis/japonicum*) is a tonic used in infants and may displace bilirubin from serum protein binding sites, causing hyperbilirubinemia.

Clove Oil

Clove cigarettes contain an essential oil, eugenol 60%, and tobacco 40%. Smoking has been known to cause epistaxis, respiratory problems, hemoptysis, and death, in addition to the hazards of tobacco. See the section on Volatile Oils.

Cocoa Beans

The cocoa bean contains theobromine, which is dangerous to dogs if ingested. Sixty milliliters has caused death in a 30-pound dog.

Comfrey

Comfrey and Russian comfrey are used as herbal teas and digestive aids, which have been linked to pyrrolizidine poisoning and liver damage (veno-occlusive disease, hepatic failure and hepatic carcinogenicity). Epidemics have occurred in India, Afghanistan, and Jamaica due to contamination of grain and bush tea. See the section on Pyrrolizidine Alkaloids.

Daidzin

The root of the kudzu vine has been used by traditional Chinese healers to treat alcohol abuse. An extract of the herb *Radix puerariae* contains daidzin and may reduce the craving for alcohol. Controlled clinical studies have not yet been performed.

Ephedra

At least six different ephedrine alkaloids have been isolated from Chinese ephedra medications. Of these, ephedrine, pseudoephedrine, and norephedrine (phenylpropanolamine) are commonly used in the U.S. as decongestants or bronchodilators. The other three—methylephedrine, methylpseudoephedrine, and norpseudoephedrine—are not available in the U.S. in pharmaceutical dosage form. Erythroderma has followed ingestion. In the U.S., ephedrine is legal and can be obtained in over-the-counter diet and pep pills. Activated charcoal may be useful in the overdose patient. Nifedipine and phentolamine or nitroprusside may be required to control hypertension in overdose.

Eucalyptus Oil

Eucalyptus oil contains 38–68% eucalyptol. The toxic dose of a 100% solution is 3.5–5 mL. As little as 1 mL may be fatal in a child. Eucalyptus oil can cause gastrointestinal upset, seizures, and coma. The toxin is eucalyptol. The onset of symptoms may occur within 10–20 minutes. Ingestion can cause rapid onset of convulsions and apnea, aspiration pneumonia, bronchospasm, and permanent neurologic sequelae. See the section on Volatile Oils.

European Mistletoe

European mistletoe (*Viscum album*) is cardiotoxic and produces vasoconstriction. The American mistletoe (*Phoradendron flavescens*) is also cardiotoxic and has potential vasopressor effects. See Chapter 56, Beans, Houseplants and Food Plants.

Fang-Ji

Fang-ji is derived from *Aristolochia fangchi* and contains aristolochic acid, which is nephrotoxic. Chinese herb nephropathy may be associated with an increased risk for developing urothelial tumors.

Feverfew

Feverfew or *Tanacetum parthenium* (*Chrysanthemum parthenium*) has been used for the treatment of disorders often controlled by aspirin such as fever, rheumatic inflammations, and migraine. Feverfew is taken orally either as fresh leaves or in tablets. *T. parthenium* is a short bushy perennial. The plant is rich in sesquiterpene lactones, principally parthenolide. It appears to inhibit platelet aggregation, histamine release from mast cells, and the production of prostaglandins, thromboxanes, and leukotrienes. Symptoms such as mouth ulcers, swollen lips, and abdominal pain have been reported. It does not appear to be mutagenic. Management is supportive.

Garlic

Garlic (*Allium sativum*) and onions (*Allium cepa*) are members of the Liliaceae or lily family. They have been used as traditional culinary adjuncts since ancient times. In 1944, allicin (diallyl disulfide), the antibacterial agent in garlic, was isolated. Fresh garlic may be effective against various Gram-positive and Gram-negative organisms, including strains that are resistant to other antimicrobials. Recently garlic's fibrinolytic activities, prophylactic activities against hypercholesterolemia, hyperlipidemia, and atherosclerotic plaque formation have been recognized. It is claimed to retard aging. See Chapter 56, Beans, Houseplants and Food Plants.

Gan Mao Tong Pian

Gan mao tong pian contains phenylbutazone and may induce aplastic anemia.

Ginseng

Ginseng (*Panax quinquefolium* native to North America or *Panax ginseng* native to Korea) is recommended for many ailments. It has been used in China for the treatment of impotence, fatigue, ulcers, and stress. It is a composite of many active compounds. There are two types of ginseng, and both contain saponin glycosides that are reported to produce direct central nervous system stimulation and arousal. It increases gastrointestinal motility.

Ginseng metabolically affects glucose metabolism and lowers blood glucose. It increases erythropoiesis, increases iron absorption, lowers cholesterol, and increases blood pressure. Some varieties produce paradoxical hypotension due to the presence of damarenetriol glycosides. Chronic or excessive use can produce a ginseng-abuse syndrome characterized by diarrhea, nervousness, insomnia, hypertension, tachycardia, and increased motor and cognitive activity. Treatment is to discontinue use and monitor blood pressure and blood glucose. See the section on Herbal Teas.

Germander

Germander, wild germander, wall germander, or ortealine in the United Kingdom (*Teucrium chamaedrys*) comes in the form of a tea or capsule used for weight loss and anal pruritus. It has produced hepatitis and hepatotoxic death. In April 1992, it was prohibited from sale in France after it was believed to have produced 26 cases of hepatitis. See the section Herbal Teas.

Golden Seal

Golden seal (*Hydrastis canadensis* and other Hydrastis species) is a natural laxative. Golden seal in overdose has produced nausea, vomiting, diarrhea, and paresthesias. In very large amounts, hypotension, respiratory depression, and seizures can occur. See Chapter 57, Wild Plants, Mushrooms and Mycotoxins.

Gordolobo Yerba

Some Jamaicans and Mexicans consume a product called *gordolobo yerba* (*Senecio longilobus*), which contains pyrrolizidine alkaloids and can produce fulminant liver disease. See the Pyrrolizidine Alkaloids section.

Groundsel

Groundsel (*Senecio vulgaris, Senecio spartoides*) contains pyrrolizidine, which is hepatotoxic and has produced cirrhosis in children fed a tea containing this product. See the Pyrrolizidine Alkaloids section.

Hai Ge Fen

Hai Ge Fen (clamshell powder) may be contaminated with copper, chromium, arsenic, or lead. See Chapter 47, Metals.

Heliotropium

Heliotropium, used as an anticonvulsant, has produced two deaths in American Indians because of intrinsic pyrrolizidine alkaloids. See the Pyrrolizidine Alkaloids section.

Herbal Balls

Herbal balls are aromatic, malleable, earth-toned, roughly spherical, hand-rolled mixtures of primarily herbs and honey. They are 1.5–2.5 cm in diameter and weigh 2.5–9.0 grams. These balls are factory-produced, patented medicinal agents manufactured in mainland China. The recommended adult dose of the preparation is two herbal balls daily, which can provide up to 73 mg of arsenic and over 1,200 mg of mercury. Such doses can induce chronic arsenic sulfide poisoning or chronic mercury sulfide poisoning. See Chapter 47, Metals.

Hops

Hops (*Humulus lupulus*) may contain lupulin, which can produce intravascular hemolysis and paroxysmal nocturnal hemoglobinuria.

Jin Bu Huan

Jin Bu Huan is a Chinese herbal medication derived from plants of the genera *Stephania* and *Corydalis* and is used for relieving pain. Rapid-onset, life-threatening bradycardia, central nervous system and respiratory depression have been associated with its use. Hepatotoxicity (hepatitis) has been observed. Botanical ingredients may be incorrectly identified on the labeling. Clinical studies suggest that its biochemical action is similar to that of reserpine-like drugs.

Kava-Kava

Kava-kava (*Piper methysticum*) or kava contains methysticine, which causes ataxia, blurred vision, central nervous system intoxication, deafness, skin yellowing, and dermatosis. See Chapter 56, Beans, Houseplants and Food Plants.

Kelp

Kelp has high sodium and potassium content.

Khat

Khat (*Catha edulis*) is a hallucinogen and stimulant from a plant grown in East Africa and the Arabian Peninsula. See Chapter 20, Hallucinogenic Drugs. The active ingredient is norpseudoephedrine. Methcathinone, a designer stimulant from Russia, is a derivative of cathinone, a potent amphetamine-like constituent occurring naturally in the fresh evergreen leaves of khat. It belongs to the class of phenylalkylamine alkaloids.

A medieval Arabic medical treatise recommends chewing khat leaves to avoid hunger and fatigue. Khat use has mainly occurred in North Yemen, Ethiopia, Kenya, adjacent Djibouti, and Somalia. In the U.S., Switzerland, and several other countries its use is prohibited. It may produce hypertension, cerebral hemorrhage, myocardial infarction, and pulmonary edema. The l-isomer of methcathinone parallels the physiologic parameters of d-amphetamine.

Kola Nut

Kola nut (*Cola nitida*) contains caffeine and theobromine, which act as stimulants.

Ibogaine

Ibogaine (*Tabernanthe ibogafrom*) is a hallucinogen classified since 1967 as a drug similar to LSD. It is an extract obtained from the roots of a flowering shrub native to the West African nation of Gabon. Ibogaine is classified by the U.S. government as a Schedule I drug, which indicates no medical value and a high potential for abuse.

Juniper

Juniper (*Juniperus macropodia*) is a hallucinogen, but renal toxicity and gastrointestinal irritation may also occur.

Kampo

Traditional Chinese herbal medicines imported from China into Japan are referred to as *Kampo* medicines containing magnolol, an inhibitor of 11-beta-hydroxysteroid dehydrogenase. Magnolol can be isolated from the urine.

Kohl

Kohl is a cosmetic predominantly used as an eye makeup in Morocco, Mauritania, Great Britain, and the U.S. When tested, samples have contained more than 50% lead, often as galena, or lead sulfide, in addition to ground antimony.

Kombucha

Kombucha "mushroom" tea is a popular health beverage made by incubating the *Kombucha* mushroom in sweet black tea. Although advocates of *Kombucha* tea have attributed many therapeutic effects to the drink, its beneficial and adverse effects have not been determined scientifically. Beneficial effects attributed to consumption of *Kombucha* tea have included prevention of cancer, relief of arthritis, treatment of insomnia, and stimulation of regrowth of hair. Because the tea is believed to stimulate the immune system, it has become popular among persons with human immunodeficiency virus (HIV) infection. In addition, the tea has become popular among the elderly (who are less likely to try alternative therapies).

The *Kombucha* "mushroom" is a symbiotic colony of several species of yeast and bacteria that are bound together by a surrounding thin membrane. Although the composition of the *Kombucha* colony varies, some of the species reportedly found in the mushroom include *S. ludwigii*, *S. pombe*, *Bacterium xylinum*, *B. gluconicum*, *B. xylinoides*, *B. katogenium*, *Pichia fermentans*, and *Torula* species. There are at least two commercial producers of *Kombucha* mushrooms in the U.S.

Kudzu

Kudzu is a fast-growing vine native to the tropics, China, and Japan. It is used as fodder, as a ground cover crop, and to control soil erosion. It has taken hold in the moist southern regions of the U.S. Several isoflavones have been identified in an extract of kudzu root (*radix puerariae*). The isoflavones may be reversible inhibitors of alcohol dehydrogenase and may enhance the management of alcoholism. Management is supportive.

Kushtay

Preparations called *"kushtay"*, used especially as tonics and aphrodisiacs, contain oxidized heavy metals such as arsenic, mercury, tin, zinc, and lead. A typical *kushtay* may contain 10–12% of each of several of these metals. See Chapter 47, Metals.

Kyushin

Kyushin, a popular Chinese medicine used in Japan, exhibits immunoreactive digoxin-like activity. The major component is *Chan-su*, the dried venom of the Chinese toad (*Bufo bufo gargarizans Cantor*), which contains several cardiotoxic steroids such as cinobufagin, bufotalin, and bufalin. The chemical structures of these chemicals are similar to that of digoxin.

Lead

Lead poisoning due to traditional ethnic remedies has been reported in a number of countries. Asian preparations are often "tonics" and aphrodisiacs, which appear to be a particular hazard. Analysis of such remedies may disclose the presence of lead oxide, lead sulfate, and lead nitrate. See Chapter 47, Metals.

Licorice

Licorice (*Glycyrrhiza glabra*) can produce mineralocorticoid effects, sodium retention, edema, hypertension, and hypokalemia. Licorice root has been used as a laxative, to treat gastritis, and to treat peptic ulcer disease. The principal toxic component of licorice root is 10–20% glycyrrhizic acid. Glycyrrhetic acid inhibits both hepatic and renal 11-β hydroxysteroid dehydrogenases. This enzyme converts active cortisol to inactive cortisone and is present in the kidneys, gonads, placenta, lungs, and intestinal mucosa.

A mineralocorticoid effect may be seen with chronic ingestion. Chronic excess consumption leads to weakness, edema, weight loss, hypertension, hypokalemia, and confusion. Licorice candy, licorice-flavored soft drinks, medicinals, chewing tobacco, and chewing gum may be toxic when excessive amounts are consumed chronically.

Lobelia

Lobelia (*Lobelia inflata*) contains lobeline, atropine, scopolamine and pyridine alkaloids, which can produce anticholinergic actions and may be a potential hepatotoxin.

Ma Huang

Ma Huang (Ephedra sinica) or Chinese ephedra is an ephedra herb that has been widely banned. It contains ephedrine and pseudoephedrine in the Asiatic species. North American varieties are high in tannins, and ten species native to North America contain no useful alkaloids. Symptoms are palpitations, vomiting, tingling, and numbness of the extremities.

Mandrake

Mandrake (*Mandragon officinarum*) or "Satan's apple" contains scopolamine and hyoscyamine and can produce anticholinergic effects. Mandrake (*Podophyllum peltatum*) resins also produce keratolytic effects, hypotension, and seizures after ingestion. The ripe fruit is nontoxic.

Manzanilla

See Chamomile tea in the section on Chamomile above.

Mate

Mate (*Ileus paraguayensis*) may contain caffeine and pyrrolizidine alkaloids, which may be hepatotoxic and hallucinogenic. See Chapter 56, Beans, Houseplants and Food Plants.

Miracle Herb

See the section on *Chuifong Tokuman*.

Melaleuca Oil

Melaleuca oil from leaves of *Melaleuca alternifolia* contains 50–60% terpenes and related alcohols and produces central nervous system depression. It is used for skin conditions.

Mercury

Certain Chinese patent medicines contain cinnabar (mercuric sulfide) and calomel (mercurous chloride). The influx of new immigrants to North America has resulted in an increase in the availability and use of mercury. See Chapter 47, Metals.

Mescal Bean

Mescal bean derives from *Sophora secundiflora* that grows on an evergreen shrub in the southwestern U.S. and northern Mexico. It has been used as a hallucinogen; half of a seed has produced toxicity. A suicide attempt using this shrub resulted in myoclonic jerking, seizures, hypertension, and hypotension. See Chapter 56, Beans, Houseplants and Food Plants.

Mistletoe

Mistletoe berry tea (*Phoradendron flavescens*) is a cardiotoxin with vasopressor effects. See Chapter 56, Beans, Houseplants and Food Plants.

Moonseed

Moonseed (*Menispermaceae*) contains a toxin with convulsant properties.

Mormon Tea

Mormon tea (*Ephedra nevadensis*) contains ephedrine and can result in symptoms of sympathomimetic overdose.

Morning Glory Seeds

Morning glory seeds (*Ipomea purpora orviolacea* or *Rivea corymbosa*) are used as a hallucinogen. One seed can contain up to 25 mg of lysergic acid. It may produce nausea, vomiting, confusion, and coma. See Chapter 20, Hallucinogenic Drugs.

Naoyanghua

This Chinese herbal medicine contains atropine. Ingestion may lead to symptoms of anticholinergic poisoning.

Nutmeg

Nutmeg is the dried ripe fruit of *Myristica fragrans*, a tree native to the South Pacific islands. Ground nutmeg is a cooking spice. Nutmeg contains volatile terpenes and aromatic ethers. The perceptible dose is 5–15 grams (1–3 ground nutmeg seeds) of myristica oil or nutmeg oil. It is a carminative in a dose of 0.03 mL. It is used as a hallucinogen in doses of 2–4 teaspoonfuls. It can cause gastrointestinal upset, agitation, coma, miosis, hypertension, and dry mouth. See Chapter 20, Hallucinogenic Drugs.

Oleander

Oleander tea (*Nerium oleander*) contains cardiac glycosides, which can produce malignant dysrhythmias and cardiac arrest. See Chapter 57, Wild Plants, Mushrooms and Mycotoxins.

Panagamate

See the section on Vitamin B-15 below.

Paraguay Tea

Paraguay tea (*Ilex paraguayensis*) contains caffeine, theophylline, and essential oils. It is used medicinally as a bowel antispasmodic. It also contains belladonna alkaloids (atropine, scopolamine, and hyoscyamine) that can produce toxic anticholinergic symptoms. See the section above on Mate.

Paraphenylenediamine

Paraphenylenediamine (PPD), an aromatic diamine, is a hair dye used as a cosmetic in Africa, the Middle East, and countries of the Indian subcontinent. It is commonly mixed with henna (leaves of *Lausonia alba*) and applied to color the palms of the hands and soles of the feet and to dye hair a dark red shade. Ingestion may be fatal. In the Sudan, it is a frequent cause of suicidal poisoning.

Passionflower

Passionflower may produce convulsions and hypotension.

Paylooah

Paylooah is used in Southeast Asia for rash or fever. It is an orange-red powder and may contain lead.

Pennyroyal Oil

Pennyroyal oil (*Mentha pulegium* and *Hedeoma pulegeoides*) has oxytocic properties and has been used as an abortifacient. It has also been used for the regulation of menstruation. It contains pulegone, an aromatic ketone, as its main toxin, which is bioactivated to a hepatotoxin by cytochrome P-450. The mechanism of toxicity may also be due to an epoxide metabolite. Pennyroyal oil has produced gastrointestinal bleeding, seizures, hematuria, shock, hepatotoxicity, and death. See the Volatile Oils section.

Periwinkle

Periwinkle yields vinca alkaloids used for cancer treatment. Periwinkle rose (*Cathararhus rosus*) is a hallucinogen, but may cause seizures, gastrointestinal upset, hepatotoxicity, and alopecia.

Pokeweed

Pokeweed (*Phytolacca americana, Phytolacca decandra*) is called inkberry and Jerusalem artichoke. It contains saponins, triterpenes, and glycoproteins. Pokeweed may produce decreased vision, respiratory depression, seizures, and cardiac dysrhythmias. It has a mitogen action and may produce fulminant bloody diarrhea. It may be tolerated when rinsed twice in boiling water. See Chapter 57, Wild Plants, Mushrooms and Mycotoxins.

Quinghaosu

Quinghaosu (artemisinine) is a sesquiterpene lactone peroxide derived from the leaves of the Chinese medicinal herb *quinghao*, a traditional Chinese medication used for the treatment of febrile illnesses. Artemisinine and its derivatives (e.g., dihydroartemisinine) appear to have antimalarial activity. Reported toxic effects include first-degree heart block, a dose-related decrease in reticulocyte and neutrophil counts, an increase in serum aspartate aminotransferase, abdominal pain, and diarrhea. Significant toxicity has been infrequent.

Rattlesnake Capsules

Rattlesnake capsule ingestion is a common practice among Mexican-Americans in the Los Angeles area. It is a Mexican folk remedy used to treat cancer, diabetes, arthritis, and skin disorders. The reptile is decapitated, skinned, dried in the sun, pulverized, placed in capsules, and sold under various names—*vibora de cascabel*, *polvo de vibora*, and *carne de vibora*—without prescription. *Salmonella arizonae* infections may follow its use.

Royal Jelly

Royal jelly (queen bee jelly) is a milky white viscid secretion from the salivary glands of the worker hive bee *Apis mellifera* (Apidae). It is essential for the development of queen bees. Royal jelly has been used as a "general tonic" and has been incorporated in some cosmetic preparations for its supposed beneficial effect on skin tissue. Consumption of royal jelly (about 2 capsules) has produced severe respiratory distress, asthma, anaphylaxis, and death.

Sapo

Sapo is obtained from the skin of the frog *Phyllomedusa bicolor* and is used by the Peruvian Matses Indians in shamanic limiting practices. Active peptides induce severe gastrointestinal and cardiovascular toxicity in humans.

Sassafras

Sassafras (*Sassafras albidum*) contains safrole and derivatives that are carcinogenic in animals. It may be associated with hepatic tumors. The FDA has banned safrole-containing products. Safrole inhibits microsomal enzymes. In animals, ataxia, hypothermia, central nervous system depression, hepatotoxicity and hepatic tumors have occurred. See the section on Herbal Teas.

Senna

Senna (*Cassia acutifolia* or *Cassia angustifolia*) is a natural laxative. However, a large dose can cause diarrhea. Senna contains three classes of anthranoids with laxative activity. Tetany associated with hypokalemia and hypocalcemia has been associated with chronic ingestion of excessive amounts of senna. Osteomalacia and arthropathy have also followed senna abuse. Hepatitis has been reported as well as pericentral hepatic vein necrosis. Anthraquinones such as rhein anthron in rhubarb have been associated with liver disease.

Sho-Saiko-To

This herbal medicine has been used in the treatment of cirrhosis of the liver and is associated with an increase in cytokine production. Controlled clinical studies have yet to be performed.

Silver

In the 19th century, colloidal silver proteins (CSPs) were promoted as cure-alls to prevent and treat diseases such as tetanus and rheumatism. Up until World War II, CSPs were widely used to treat colds and gonorrhea. However, in recent decades, the medicinal use of silver has largely been replaced by safer and more effective therapies.

Since 1990, interest has resurged in promoting CSP products as "essential" mineral supplements with multiple health claims. For example, advertising materials in health food stores promote CSP use in more than 650 different diseases. Colloidal silver proteins are being touted as powerful antimicrobials against viruses, bacteria, parasites, and fungi, including human immunodeficiency virus (HIV), herpes, Candida, and tuberculosis. CSPs have also been advertised as "an immune system stimulant and antiinflammatory agent" for use in diabetes, chronic fatigue syndrome, allergies, and cancer.

Silver is not without toxicity. Silver accumulates in the body and may result in bluish skin discoloration (argyria). Argyria is irreversible and has no effective treatment. In addition, neurologic deficits and silver deposition in visceral organs have been reported with long-term use of oral silver products. Renal damage and metal fume fever have been reported with silver exposures.

Simplex Plus

Simplex plus is mainly a bitter alkaloid of the plant *Menispermum condense* and has been promoted as a muscle-building and testosterone-increasing agent. Plant steroids are used in the manufacture of steroidal drugs, but there is no scientific evidence that natural steroids are converted into testosterone in the human body.

Skullcap

See the section on Germander.

Slang Nut

Slang nut in Thailand and Southeast Asia is called *Salang chai nut*, which contains strychnine from *Strychnos nux vomica*.

Snakeroot

Snakeroot (*Rauwolfia serpentina*) contains reserpine, which can produce hypotension, bradycardia, and central nervous system intoxication.

Sulfur

Elemental sulfur is widely used as a folk remedy. It is usually combined with a sweet syrup or molasses. Its internal uses include intestinal "spring-cleaning," treatment for dyspnea, and as a "tonic." Its usefulness for these indications is subject to doubt, but it is generally considered harmless. Sulfur is used widely in the treatment of dermatologic disease. The lethal oral dose in humans is estimated to be between 0.5–5.0 mg/kg. There is no evidence that sulfur ingestion by humans leads to hydrogen sulfide toxicity.

Tansy Ragwort

Tansy ragwort (*Senecio jacobea*) contains hepatotoxic pyrrolizidine alkaloids.

Thiazolidine Carboxylic Acid

In Mexico, Europe, and Central and South America, thiazolidine carboxylic acid is available as a "hepatoprotector" under a variety of trade names. It has been claimed that the drug "reactivates the enzymatic processes of the liver, normalizes the transaminases and shortens the icteric and recuperation periods." Ingestions have resulted in coma, seizures, acidosis, and hypoglycemia. Many patients have also exhibited fever, tachycardia, respiratory distress, and miosis.

Tonka Bean

Tonka bean (*Dipteryx odoratum* and *Doumarouna oppositofilia*) contains coumarin and produces prolonged prothrombin time and bleeding.

Tung Shueh

Tung Shueh pills (see section entitled Black Balls) contain mefenamic acid and diazepam, neither of which is listed on the label. Acute renal failure has followed the use of mefenamic acid, phenylbutazone, and aristolochic acid in these preparations.

Tu-San-Chi

Tu-san-chi (*Gynura segetum*) contains hepatotoxic pyrrolizidine alkaloids.

Urginea Maritima

The most important plant sources of cardiac glycosides are digitalis (foxglove), strophanthus, and squill. Squill is *Urginea maritima*, the sea onion that grows near the Mediterranean shore and in the southwest region of Turkey. The bulb, and possibly the whole plant, contains several related steroidal cardioactive glycosides that exert digitalis-like toxicity. Ingestion of squill as a folk remedy may result in fatal toxicity. Red squill has been used as a rodenticide. In patients presenting with gastrointestinal symptoms and bradyarrhythmias due to presumed poisoning by herbal medicines, cardiac glycoside poisoning should be suspected.

Valerian

Valerian (*Valeriana officinalis*) has been used since the Middle Ages as a sedative and antispasmodic. It is a herbaceous perennial widely distributed in the temperate regions of North America, Europe, and Asia. Valerian is widely used in traditional Chinese and Indian medicines. In the U.S., valerian is sold in natural food stores as a sleep-promoting herbal preparation, or combined with other herbal products. In Europe, valerian is used as a homeopathic remedy.

Dried valerian root has a characteristic malodorous aroma. The plant consists of essential oils (valerianic acid and valenol), valepotriates (nonglycoside iridoid esters), and a small number of alkaloids. The valepotriates appear to be the most active of these chemicals.

Valerian increases the quality of sleep and decreases sleep latency. Valerian has relaxant effects on gastrointestinal smooth muscle, as well as coronary dilating and antiarrhythmic properties. An intravenous injection of raw valerian root with tap water has caused drowsiness, dilated pupils, chest pain, hypotension, hypocalcemia, hypophosphatemia, and hyperkalemia. Adverse reactions associated with chronic use include headaches, excitability, cardiac disturbances, and hepatotoxicity.

Vitamin B-15

Vitamin B-15 or panagamate is not a B vitamin and is obtained from apricot seeds. It is similar to laetrile. It has the potential to cause cyanide poisoning if ingested. Chapter 56, Beans, Houseplants and Food Plants.

Woodruff

Woodruff (*Galium segetum*) contains coumarin, which can cause prolonged prothrombin time and bleeding.

Wormwood

See the section on Absinthe.

Yangjinhua

Yangjinhua, the dried flowers of *Datura metel L*, are used in southern Asia and southern China for treating bronchial asthma and chronic bronchitis. This preparation contains scopolamine, hyoscyamine, and atropine, which can account for anticholinergic poisoning. Symptoms may include dry mouth, dilated pupils, agitation, tachycardia, tachypnea, unsteady gait, hallucinations, coma, and death.

Yellow Root

See the section on Golden Seal.

Yixin Wan

Yixin Wan is a nonprescription Chinese medication that contains toad venom (*Ch'an Su*), ginseng, pearl (*Chem Chu*), and musk (*She Hsiang*). The product is sold in the U.S. in ethnic grocery stores and pharmacies. Toad venom contains a digitalis-like immunoreactive cardiotrophic substance (bufotoxin). Bufotalin, a major bufotoxin in toad venom, has a chemical structure similar to digitalis. Anecdotal reports indicate that therapeutic levels of serum digoxin and atrioventricular node conduction dysfunction have followed ingestion of *Yixin Wan*.

Yohimbe

Yohimbe, or *YoYo* (*Corynanthe yohimbine*) is used as an aphrodisiac and hallucinogen. In overdose, it may cause hypertension, weakness, and paralysis.

Questions—Miscellaneous Herbal Remedies

1. Which of the following associations is correctly matched?
   A. Absinthe—Severe watery diarrhea
   B. Birch bark—Psychosis, hallucinations
   C. Black cohosh—Estrogenic effects
   D. *Boui-ougi-tou*—Methylsalicylate
   E. Buckthorn—Fanconi syndrome

2. Which of the following associations is incorrectly matched?
   A. Bush tea—Hepatotoxicity
   B. Cantharidin—Beetle toxin aphrodisiac
   C. Cassia—Senna laxative
   D. Catnip—Free radical scavenger
   E. *Chuen Lin*—Neonatal hyperbilirubinemia

3. Which of the following associations is correctly matched?
A. Ephedra—Pseudoephedrine
B. *Hai ge fen—Ephedra sinica*
C. *Ma huang*—Scopolamine
D. Mormon Tea—Clamshell powder
E. Mandrake—*Ephedra nevadensis*

4. Which of the following is cardiotoxic?
A. Germander
B. Goldenseal
C. Juniper
D. *Kyushin*
E. None of the above

5. Licorice can produce
A. Mineralocorticoid effects
B. Sodium retention
C. Edema
D. Hypertension
E. All of the above

PLANT DERMATITIS

Introduction

Plant dermatitis represents a significant medical problem, especially during the warmer months when both pollen levels and plant exposures are high. Skin eruptions also may appear during winter months as certain species store their allergenic chemicals in their roots and stems. Weeds, garden flowers, native vegetation, vegetables, sawdust, and plant products probably contain thousands of chemicals that can produce a contact dermatitis caused by either direct irritation or an allergic reaction.

Clinically, plant dermatitis can be subdivided into four categories: airborne allergic dermatitis, direct contact allergic dermatitis, primary skin irritation, and phytophotodermatitis. Not all of these categories are mutually exclusive, since some plants that cause primary skin irritation may sensitize the patient to further exposures. Treatment remains similar and depends on the severity rather than the type of dermatitis. Fluctuation in chemical content caused by genetic factors, plant composition, environmental conditions, and seasonal changes combines with host susceptibility to cause a significant variation in clinical response to dermatitis-inducing plant chemicals.

Airborne Allergic Plants

Ragweed (*Ambrosia*) is the most common causative agent of airborne contact dermatitis, but a variety of plants produce similar symptoms depending on locality. These plants produce dermatitis when airborne allergens settle on exposed skin. Seasonal variation of plant dermatitis parallels that of respiratory allergies, which provides a diagnostic clue to the presence of airborne dermatitis. However, the same person may develop skin eruptions from exposure to several different pollens present in different seasons. Furthermore, plants that produce direct contact dermatitis (e.g., poison ivy / oak) may produce a clinical picture of airborne dermatitis when plant substances are burned and the allergens are absorbed into the airborne ash.

PATHOPHYSIOLOGY

Certain plant pollens contain oleoresins that penetrate exposed skin and act as a hapten to produce a delayed hypersensitivity reaction. The protein portion of the pollen causes allergic rhinitis and asthma. Failure to develop hypersensitivity symptoms does not guarantee a lack of response to the oleoresins, which reside in the nonprotein portions of the pollen.

CLINICAL PRESENTATIONS

Airborne contact dermatitis presents as generalized eczematous lesions on exposed areas that may be confused with neurodermatitis or phytophotodermatitis. Pruritic macules or papules may form on exposed areas, but vesicular or bullous lesions are rare. In contrast to the linear, vesicular lesions of direct contact dermatitis, airborne pollens produce almost uniform involvement of the hands, face, and other exposed areas.

TREATMENT

- Treatment is based on severity of symptoms, similar to contact dermatitis.
- Steroid creams, anti-pruritics, cool compresses and / or systemic steroids may be helpful in individual cases.

Direct Contact Allergic Dermatitis

Classic delayed hypersensitivity reactions develop to direct contact with a variety of plants of which members of the Anacardiaceae family are the most common sensitizers. Up to two million cases of Toxicodendron (poison oak, ivy, and sumac) dermatitis occur annually in the U.S. Primrose dermatitis (*Primula obconica*) is more common in the United Kingdom.

The presence of oleoresin antigens on pets or clothing may spread the inflamed lesions to unexposed areas. The severity of the dermatitis depends on the degree of exposure to the sensitizing agent as well as individual sensitivity. Hence, lesions may develop after numerous previously asymptomatic exposures. Cross-reactivity to antigens within the same plant family (e.g., Toxicodendron) often occurs, but usually no correlation is found between contact dermatitis and allergic rhinitis.

It has been estimated that 50–65% of the U.S. population is sensitive to Toxicodendron oleoresins. This indicates that this genus contains the most common potent dermatitis-inducing plants. Of all members of the animal kingdom, only humans and a few primates are sensitive to these plant species. All ages, races, and sexes are susceptible, but infants are not easily sensitized.

Eastern Poison Oak

This erect, deciduous, woody shrub has triple leaflets similar to those of poison ivy but the leaf edges are sinuate like oak leaves. Eastern poison oak is less commonly present than poison ivy in an area bounded by Texas, northern Florida, and New Jersey.

Poison Ivy

Poison ivy is found in North and South America as well as eastern Asia. This species is found in every state except California and Nevada. Poison ivy is most abundant along the rocky coasts of New England, sandbars off New Jersey and Long Island, and throughout the Carolinas. It usually grows as a woody vine but occasionally is an erect shrub that may reach 15–20 feet in height. Leaves are pointed and hairless and grow in three leaflet clusters on a short stalk. Their bright green color turns shades of red, yellow, and brown in the fall. Poison ivy is unrelated to cultivated garden ivies.

Poison Sumac

Poison sumac grows predominantly in swamps and bogs east of the Mississippi River. It grows as a wood shrub (5–8 feet) or as a small tree (up to 25 feet) with light gray bark. Leaves appear as 7–13 leaflet clusters arranged in pairs, with a terminal leaflet at the end of the stem. Leaflet margins are smooth and pointed.

Western Poison Oak

Western poison oak grows only on the Pacific Coast from Canada to Mexico. It is a woody, deciduous shrub that sends many stems from its underground roots. Leaves appear in clusters of three and resemble oak leaves.

PATHOPHYSIOLOGY

Urushiol is the antigenic oleoresin component responsible for the delayed hypersensitivity dermatitis. It can retain its sensitizing potency indefinitely in the dry state. Clothing, domestic animals, shoes, and even oleoresin underneath fingernails may reexpose the patient. Urushiol is nonvolatile. Airborne exposures occur only when smoke carries the urushiol on dust particles.

Urushiol has been fractionated into four constituent catechols. Similar catechols appear in all poisonous members of the Anacardiaceae family but individual concentrations vary because of genetic and environmental factors. The antigenic structure is an orthocatechol. As catechols are soluble in rubber, rubber gloves will not prevent dermatitis. Soap and water degrade urushiol. Thorough machine washing will remove dried urushiol from clothes.

Catechols are haptens that almost immediately penetrate the skin and conjugate with skin proteins to form complete antigens. No amount of washing will remove the catechol-protein complex formed. Immunocompetent lymphocytes carry these complexes to the reticuloendothelial system where humoral factors produce a generalized state of cutaneous sensitivity. Subsequently, a delayed hypersensitivity reaction occurs.

CLINICAL PRESENTATIONS

Typically, burning pruritic erythema in the configuration of linear scratch marks appears about 24–48 hours after exposure. Depending on sensitivity, the onset may be as soon as 6–12 hours or as late as 5–6 days. Raised lesions (i.e., papules) follow, and finally vesiculation develops. Lesions usually appear first on exposed areas. Secondary lesions may appear on the genitals or other areas to which the catechols have spread.

By three days, the skin's moisture inactivates the oleoresin on the skin. Hence, spread after three days results from reexposure to dried urushiol on domesticated animals or inanimate objects. The lesions may leak fluid (which is nonantigenic) until a crust forms. In the majority of cases, the dermatitis is self-limited and disappears within 2–3 weeks. Hyperpigmentation is common in black-skinned races.

The most common complications are secondary infections. Rarely, scarlatiniform eruptions or erythema multiforme results from the systemic absorption of catechols. Membranous nephropathy, proliferative glomerulonephritis, and arteritis have been associated with Toxicodendron exposures, particularly when commercial poison oak extract has been administered. Proteinuria, edema, lethargy, and, in severe cases, fever, anuria, congestive heart failure, and death have been reported.

Ingestion of leaves may produce a severe gastroenteritis and pruritus ani. The idea that American Indians developed immunity to Toxicodendron by chewing its leaves has not been documented. Rarely, Toxicodendron species may produce urticaria, allergic rhinitis, and asthma. The differential diagnosis includes phytophotodermatitis, Portuguese Man-of-War envenomation, and caterpillar dermatitis.

TREATMENT

- Fluorinated steroid gels and creams may be applied 2–3 times daily for mild cases, but are probably not effective for more severe lesions.
- Cold water compresses or soaks three to four times daily are recommended for weeping or pruritic lesions during the acute phase. The addition of Domeboro's solution may provide additional relief. Tepid showers are preferred to hot showers since heat may cause vasodilation, erythema, and edema.
- Calamine lotion is useful to help dry lesions between soaks, but topical antihistamines are not recommended because of potential sensitization. Zirconium-containing products produce granulomas and therefore are contraindicated.
- Adequate doses of systemic corticosteroids given early in severe, edematous cases provide quick relief and may blunt the usual course. At least 40 mg of prednisone daily is necessary initially. The dose is subsequently tapered. At times, prolonged therapy (5–6 weeks) is needed.
- Oral antihistamines are given for their sedative and antipruritic effects, but do not alter the course of the lesions.

Supportive Measures

- All contaminated clothing and domestic animals should be washed with soap and water.
- Since the catechols are quickly fixed to skin proteins, washing more than one hour after exposure does not alter the course of the dermatitis.
- Bullous lesions should be protected with bulky dressings (e.g., Kerlix®) and not iatrogenically ruptured. The dressing may be soaked off with cool water to prevent disruption of the bullae.
- The skin lesions should be observed for signs of secondary infection (e.g., increasing redness, warmth, pain).
- At the present time, current commercial extracts are not recommended for desensitization.

Questions—Plant Dermatitis

1. **Airborne contact dermatitis generally produces uniform involvement of the hands, face and other exposed areas.**
   A. True
   B. False
2. **Steroid creams are generally unhelpful in the treatment of ragweed-caused dermatitis.**
   A. True
   B. False
3. **The severity of dermatitis caused by poison ivy is related to**
   A. The degree of exposure
   B. The race of the patient
   C. Individual sensitivity
   D. A and B
   E. A and C
4. **Which of the following statements about direct contact allergic dermatitis from plant exposure is true?**
   A. Onset of scratch marks may occur between six hours and six days after exposure.

B. Spread after three days is usually due to reexposure to dried urushiol.
C. The most common complication is erythema multiforme.
D. A and B
E. A and C

Answers

Herbal Teas

1. B 2. E 3. C 4. A

Volatile Oils

1. B 2. C 3. A

Miscellaneous Herbal Remedies

1. C 2. D 3. A 4. D 5. E

Plant Dermatitis

1. A 2. B 3. E 4. D

SELECTED READINGS

Miscellaneous Herbal Remedies and Volatile Oils

1. Atherton DJ, Rustin MN, Brostoff J. Need for correct identification of herbs in herbal poisoning. Lancet 1993;341:637–638.
2. Chan TYP, Chan JCN, Tomlinson B, et al. Chinese herbal medicines revisited: a Hong Kong perspective. Lancet 1993;342:1532–1534.
3. D'Arcy PF. Adverse reactions and interactions with herbal medicines. I. Adverse reactions. Adverse Drug React Toxicol Rev 1991;10:189–208.
4. D'Arcy PF. Adverse reactions and interactions with herbal medicine. II. Drug interactions. Adverse Drug React Toxicol Rev 1993;12:147–162.
5. De Smet PAGM. Health risks of herbal remedies. Drug Safety 1995;13: 81–93.
6. Guang-Sheng D. Important Chinese herbal remedies. Clin Ther 1987; 9:345–357.
7. Huxtable RJ. The harmful potential of herbal and other plant products. Drug Safety 1990;5(Suppl 1):126–136.
8. Huxtable RJ: The myth of beneficent nature. The risks of herbal preparations. Ann Intern Med 1992;117:165–166.
9. Mofenson HC, Caraccio TR, Brody G, et al. Herbal products. Poison Perspective for Health Professionals 1994;13:54–62.
10. Perharic L, Shaw D, Murray V. Toxic effects of herbal medicines and food supplements. Lancet 1993;342:180–181.
11. Savage A, Hutchings A. Poisoned by herbs. Br Med J 1987;295:1650–1651.
12. Tai Y-T, But PP, Young K, et al. Adverse effects from traditional Chinese medicine. Lancet 1993;341:892–893.

Plant Dermatitis

1. Fisher AA: The notorious poison ivy family of Anacardiaceae plants. Cutis 1977;20:570–595.
2. Logan PC, Parker GF: Poison ivy (Rhus) dermatitis. Am Fam Phys 1972;6: 62–66.
3. Mitchell JC, Rosk AJ: Diagnosis of contact dermatitis from plants. Int J Dermatol 1977;16:257–266.

ACKNOWLEDGMENT

Thanks to Alison Deutsch, MD for contributing the questions in this chapter.

CHAPTER 56
Beans, Houseplants, and Food Plants

INTRODUCTION

Exposure to potentially poisonous plants is a common occurrence in homes, gardens, and natural environments as reflected by calls to poison control centers. Generally, between 5% and 10% of calls to these centers concern plant exposures. In 1997, plant exposures represented 5.6% (123,139) of the calls reported to the American Association of Poison Control Centers (AAPCC) National Data Collection System. Exposures to houseplants are consistently common because of the easy accessibility of houseplants to inquisitive toddlers.

A few plant species may produce serious toxicity. These include oleander (*Nerium oleander*), foxglove (*Digitalis purpurea*), jequirity pea (*Abrus precatorius*), castor beans (*Ricinus communis*), water hemlock (*Cicuta maculata*), Jerusalem cherry (*Solanum pseudocapsicum*), tree tobacco (*Nicotiana glauca*), jimsonweed (*Datura stramonium*), false hellebore (*Veratrum* species), plants containing pyrrolizidine alkaloids (e.g., *Senecio longilobus* teas), autumn crocus (*Colchicum autumnale*), and hepatotoxic mushrooms (*Amanita phalloides, Amanita virosa*). Each year a few deaths from plant poisonings occur in the United States.

A number of beans, seeds, houseplants, and food plants are described below. The field of botanical toxicology is huge, and these examples represent a mere sampling of interesting and commonly encountered toxins. The list is by no means exhaustive. While some toxins are extremely well-documented and described, an element of folklore and less-than-rigorous methods have characterized certain elements of this literature.

GENERAL APPROACH TO PLANTS

Once a toxic ingestion is recognized, a portion of the offending plant, tree, or mushroom should be collected if possible. A working relationship with a botanist or the local poison control center represents a valuable resource to identify these substances.

Pathophysiology

Toxic plant substances belong to a relatively few broad categories of compounds. Major groupings of these compounds include alkaloids, glycosides, proteinaceous compounds, organic acids, alcohols, resins, resinoids (including phenolics), mineral toxins, and nonorganic compounds. Botanicals may affect any organ system.

Clinical Presentations

GASTROINTESTINAL EFFECTS

Pokeweed (*Phytolacca americana*) and holly bush (*Ilex* species) are common causes of gastroenteritis. The toxalbumin-containing plants, castor bean (*R. communis*) and jequirity bean (*A. precatorius*), produce a severe gastroenteritis and, rarely, multiorgan failure.

CARDIOVASCULAR EFFECTS

Common oleander (*N. oleander*), lily of the valley (*Convallaria majalis*), foxglove (*D. purpurea*), and yellow oleander (*Thevetia peruviana*) contain cardiac glycosides resembling digitalis.

SEIZURES

Water hemlock (*Cicuta* species) ingestions can produce convulsions within 30 to 60 minutes of exposure. Chinaberry (*Melia azedarach*), moonseed (*Menispermum canadense*), and *Coriaria myrtifolia* contain potential convulsants. Occasionally, convulsions have resulted from serious ingestions of *Aconitum* (monkshood), *Taxus* (yew), and *Veratrum* plant species.

NICOTINE TOXICITY

Several plant species contain nicotinelike toxins, including the golden chain tree (*Laburnum anagyroides*), tree tobacco (*N. glauca*), Indian tobacco (*Lobelia inflata*), and poison hemlock (*Conium maculatum*). Nausea, vomiting, salivation, and abdominal cramps begin soon after exposure and are followed by headache, confusion, tachycardia, mydriasis, fever, and ataxia.

ANTICHOLINERGIC TOXICITY

Atropine, scopolamine, and hyoscyamine appear in a variety of plants, the most common of which are jimsonweed (*D. stramonium*), deadly nightshade (*Atropa belladonna*), henbane (*Hyoscyamus niger*), angel's trumpet (*Brugmansia* species, formerly *Datura sauveolens*), and matrimony vine (*Lycium halimifolium*). Clinical manifestations of toxicity are similar to those of classic atropine poisoning with headache, nausea, dry skin and mouth, tachycardia, mydriasis, and urinary retention.

HALLUCINATIONS

Nutmeg (*Myristica frangans*), the ergot fungus (*Claviceps purpurea*), morning glory seeds (*Ipomoea violacea*), peyote (*Lophophora williamsii*), *Mimosa species*, psilocybin-containing mushrooms (e.g., *Psilocybe* or *Panaeolus*), ibotenic acid-containing mushrooms (e.g., *Amanita muscaria*), and marijuana (*Cannabis* species) possess mind-altering properties.

RENAL EFFECTS

Rhubarb plants contain soluble oxalate crystals, which can produce renal failure after chronic consumption. Decreased renal function may be associated with *A. phalloides* poisoning. Autumn crocus (*C. autumnale*), podophyllum resin, and *Cortinarius* mushrooms can produce primary renal dysfunction.

HEPATIC EFFECTS

Hepatotoxic mushrooms are well described. Less well known are the pyrrolizidine alkaloids, which produce hepatic failure both sporadically (e.g., when ingested as teas from *Senecio longilobus*) and epidemically (e.g., consumption of cereals contaminated by *Crotalaria* or *Heliotropium* seeds). Akee fruit, a South African tuber (*Callilepis laureola*), and sassafras root also cause hepatic dysfunction in severe cases.

Treatment

GUT DECONTAMINATION

The majority of casual ingestions require no specific therapy. Emesis is still preferred to lavage in many pediatric household cases because plant particles are difficult to remove by gastric tube. Activated charcoal absorbs most alkaloids well and should be administered in almost all symptomatic cases.

ELIMINATION ENHANCEMENT

Most plant poisonings respond to supportive care. Hemoperfusion has been used after *A. phalloides* and *Podophyllum* poisoning, but its precise role remains controversial.

SUPPORTIVE MEASURES

- If the patient is symptomatic after botanical poisoning, basic blood tests such as electrolytes, complete blood count, and renal and hepatic function tests should be obtained.
- Toxic screens and urinalysis may be helpful in specific cases.
- Electrocardiographic monitoring is indicated in cardiac glycoside poisonings (*D. purpurea, N. oleander*) and anticholinergic or cholinergic ingestions.

Antidotes

Few antidotes to plant poisonings are available. Laetrile toxicity has been treated successfully with use of the Lilly Cyanide Kit. Digoxin-specific Fab fragments have been administered to symptomatic patients who ingest digitalis-containing plants.

Questions—General Approach to Plants

1. **Plants known for their cardiotoxicity include all of the following except**
   A. Common oleander (*Nerium oleander*)
   B. Chinaberry (*Melia azedarach*)
   C. Lily of the valley (*Convallaria majalis*)
   D. Foxglove (*Digitalis purpurea*)
   E. Yellow oleander (*Thevetia peruviana*)
2. **Plants known for their anticholinergic toxicity include all of the following except**
   A. Jimsonweed (*Datura stramonium*)
   B. Deadly nightshade (*Atropa belladonna*)
   C. Henbane (*Hyoscyamus niger*)
   D. Angel's trumpet (*Brugmansia* species)
   E. Lily of the valley (*Convallaria majalis*)
3. **Plants known for hallucinations include all of the following except**
   A. *Aconitum* (monkshood)
   B. Nutmeg (*Myristica frangans*)
   C. Ergot fungus (*Claviceps purpurea*)
   D. Morning glory seeds (*Ipomoea violacea*)
   E. Peyote (*Lophophora williamsii*)
4. **Plants known to cause seizures include all of the following except**
   A. *Abrus precatorius*
   B. Water hemlock (*Cicuta* species)
   C. Moonseed (*Menispermum canadense*)
   D. *Coriaria myrtifolia*
   E. Serious *Veratrum* plant ingestions

BEANS AND SEEDS

Ornamental beans are used widely in jewelry, crafts, rituals, and herbal medicines. While many are harmless, some are quite dangerous. Examples are two of the most potent parenteral toxins in the animal kingdom, abrin and ricin. *Abrus precatorius*

Answers to questions in shaded boxes appear at the end of the chapter.

is an ornamental vine that grows profusely throughout southern Florida. Its seeds contain the toxalbumin abrin and commonly decorate necklaces and rosaries. The castor bean plant (*Ricinus communis*) is grown commercially as the source of castor oil and has naturalized in southern California.

Castor Beans

Castor beans grow on a large shrub that grows on woody stalks, 4 to 12 feet high, with wide palmate green-red leaves. Three of the mottled gray-white seeds are found in each soft-spined brown capsule. These are clustered together on a central stalk. Documentation of the use of castor bean extracts dates back to Egypt where it was used as a salve. Over the years, this plant has enjoyed widespread use ranging from the treatment of rhinitis in China to the eradication of gonorrhea in the Dominican Republic. Currently, the plant is grown commercially for the lubricating quality of its oil and the purgative effect of its extract.

PATHOPHYSIOLOGY

The toxicity of this plant results from the effects of ricin, which is one of the most toxic parenteral substances in the plant kingdom. Ricin contains two polypeptide chains held together by a single disulfide bond. Chain B is a lectin that binds to the surface of the cell to facilitate toxin entry into the cell. Chain A disrupts protein synthesis by activating the 60S ribosomal subunit. The pulp of the seed contains allergenic glycoproteins, which cause allergic dermatitis, rhinitis, and asthma in sensitized industrial workers.

CLINICAL PRESENTATIONS

A study of 424 cases of castor bean intoxication revealed symptoms including acute gastroenteritis, fluid and electrolyte depletion, gastrointestinal bleeding, hemolysis, and hypoglycemia. Fourteen patients died of hypovolemic shock. The clinical severity of the intoxication cannot be predicted on the basis of the number of beans ingested. The most common initial symptoms result from gastrointestinal irritation and include burning in the alimentary tract, nausea, vomiting, diarrhea, and colicky abdominal pain. In severe poisoning, these symptoms progress to hemorrhagic gastritis and dehydration.

There is a latent period for nonallergenic reactions, which has been reported to vary between 2 and 24 hours. Serious oral ingestions appear early with severe gastrointestinal symptoms. The primary target organs are the kidney, liver, and pancreas, although the inhibition of protein synthesis by ricin may affect any organ. The significance of hemolysis after oral ingestions is unclear because most series do not report evidence of hemolysis. Although toxic effects from ricin usually require several hours to develop, allergic reactions in sensitized individuals may occur immediately after exposure. Severe orbital edema and urticaria have been reported from casual contact with a castor-bean necklace.

TOXIC DOSAGE/DEATH

Although ricin is present throughout the plant, the seeds contain the highest concentration. Toxic cases involve ingestion of well-masticated seeds. Whole seeds are nontoxic. In animal models, ricin ranks among the three most toxic parenteral substances by weight in the world. At least several well-masticated seeds are required to produce significant toxicity. An Indian series of 57 children revealed that 22 displayed evidence of shock. The average ingestion was four to five seeds, with a maximum of 15. No deaths were reported.

An infamous case of ricin poisoning involved a 49-year-old Romanian exile who died 3 days after the injection of a 1.52-mm platinum sphere into his thigh at a London bus stop. The sphere contained a 0.28-mm^3 hole. Fever, leukocytosis, and progressive hypotension similar to septic shock characterized his illness. The West London coroner ruled that his death was a homicide, most likely the result of ricin poisoning. Ricin is several hundred times more toxic when administered parenterally than by ingestion.

The lethal dose of ricin in man has been estimated to be 1 mg/kg body weight (about eight seeds). Predicting severity on the basis of seed ingestion is difficult both because of incomplete intestinal absorption of ricin and because of its variable release from the hard seed coat. Any ingestion should be considered dangerous, especially in children. Because of the potential of anaphylaxis, one seed may be fatal.

TREATMENT

Gut Decontamination

Every patient should receive the usual measures to prevent absorption (i.e., lavage, charcoal, and cathartics) after the usual precautions and contraindications are observed.

Elimination Enhancement

Ricin (water-soluble) is not dialyzable, and little is excreted in the urine. Therefore, hemodialysis or forced diuresis is not indicated.

Supportive Measures

- Attempt to identify the plant and seed. Radioimmunoassays of ricin are available but levels do not aid management.
- The maintenance of fluid and electrolyte balance is the most important aspect of supportive care.
- Screening for liver, renal, pancreatic, and red blood cell dysfunction is important. Useful laboratory tests include a complete blood count, electrolytes, blood urea nitrogen, creatinine, glucose, prothrombin time, liver enzymes, amylase, and urinalysis.
- Symptomatic patients should be hospitalized. Asymptomatic patients may be discharged with instructions to return immediately should symptoms develop. Asymptomatic pediatric patients who have ingested several beans should be observed for at least 4 to 6 hours postingestion.
- Initial daily outpatient follow-up for several days is important to identify target organ toxicity for those patients released.

Questions—Castor Beans

1. The toxic substance in castor beans is
A. Tetrodotoxin
B. *Digitalis alkaloids*
C. *Veratrum*
D. Ricin
E. Abrin

2. Although castor bean toxin is present throughout the plant, seeds contain the highest levels.
A. True
B. False

Fava Beans

Vicia faba is cultivated widely in Canada and often grown as an ornamental vine in the United States. It is of European origin and often cultivated there. Fava beans grow on a coarse erect annual vine without tendrils. Fruit are up to 14 inches long and are a thick many-seeded legume. The large seeds are compressed or globular, and variously colored from green to purple or blue.

PATHOPHYSIOLOGY

A hemolytic syndrome associated with favism has been recognized since antiquity. Glucose-6-phosphate dehydrogenase (G6PD) deficiency is the most common disease-producing enzyme disorder of humans with an estimated 7% of the world's population carrying the gene. The G6PD gene is located on the X chromosome. It is inherited in a sex-linked manner and is fully expressed in hemizygote males and homozygous females. A high incidence of low activity G6PD variants is typical of the Mediterranean area and the Middle East in addition to Taiwan and South China. About 12% of black American men are reported to have the deficiency.

G6PD catalyzes the first step in the hexose-monophosphate pathway. This results in reduction of the cofactor nicotinamide adenine dinucleotide phosphate (NADP) to NADPH. NADPH is necessary to protect the sulfhydryl groups of enzymes and the β-chain of hemoglobin from oxidation. This protection is mediated by glutathione. In the absence of adequate G6PD activity, hemolysis is the primary effect of an oxidative stress. Sensitivity to favism is a poorly understood phenomenon.

CLINICAL PRESENTATIONS

About 10% to 20% of G6PD-deficient individuals who consume fava beans experience fava crises. The first symptoms of favism are malaise, generalized weakness to severe lethargy, nausea and vomiting, headache, and lumbar or abdominal pain. Chills, tremors, and fever are often present. After a delay of up to 48 hours, jaundice may appear accompanied by enlargement of the spleen and liver. A few hours after fava bean intake, hemoglobinuria begins and may continue for several days. Anemia and reticulocytosis follow. In most cases, the hemolysis is self-limited.

TREATMENT

Gut Decontamination

Unintentional large fava bean ingestions may benefit from gut decontamination with emesis and/or lavage and charcoal.

Elimination Enhancement

Renal failure from hemolysis may benefit from dialysis.

Supportive Measures

- The disorder induces a self-limited to low-grade hemolytic anemia, light or no hemoglobinuria, and slight jaundice.
- It may require no treatment or only supportive therapy (i.e., intravenous hydration to maintain urine output and diuresis to prevent precipitation of hemoglobin in the kidneys).
- If anemia is life-threatening, transfusion is required.

Questions—Fava Beans

1. Which of the following is false?

A. Glucose-6-phosphate dehydrogenase (G6PD) deficiency is the most common disease-producing enzyme disorder of humans affecting an estimated 7% of the world's population.
B. All G6PD-deficient individuals who consume fava beans experience fava crises.
C. The G6PD gene is located on the x chromosome. It is inherited in a sex-linked manner and is fully expressed in hemizygote males and homozygous females.
D. In the absence of adequate G6PD activity, hemolysis is the primary effect of oxidative stress.
E. A high incidence of low activity G6PD variants is typical of the Mediterranean area and the Middle East in addition to Taiwan and South China.

Jequirity Beans

This native Indian plant is a perennial vine used as a natural ornamental cover in tropical regions such as southern Florida and the Florida Keys. 3- to 8-mm ovoid seeds are distinctive features of this plant. Most of the seed is a bright scarlet, with the hilum end of the seed appearing jet-black. Three varieties of seeds are found. The toxic properties of abrin have been long recognized. In India, where the plant is native, abrin has been administered as both an animal and a human poison. In addition, certain African and Madagascar tribes used the toxin as an ordeal poison. The seeds appear sporadically in beadwork and jewelry, and tourists may unintentionally expose their children to inherent toxic.

PATHOPHYSIOLOGY

The jequirity bean contains N-methyltryptophan, abric acid, glycyrrhizin (the active principle of licorice), a lipolytic enzyme, and abrin. Structurally, abrin has the same two-subunit configuration as ricin. The β chain (haptomere) on each abrin molecule binds to nonreducing β-galactosyl residues of cell surface glycoproteins. The internalization of the abrin molecule mediated by the β chain conceivably occurs by endocytosis. Once inside, the α chain (effectomere) possesses enzymatic activity that inhibits protein synthesis by binding to the 60S ribosomal subunit after a 30-minute delay. The roots contain glycyrrhizin, the active ingredient in licorice. A clinical syndrome of hyperaldosteronism characterized by sodium retention and hypertension may develop.

CLINICAL PRESENTATIONS

Serious abrin ingestion produces a severe gastroenteritis several hours after consumption and is followed by the development of diarrhea that may become bloody. Symptoms may last as long as 10 days. Anecdotal cases report the delay of symptoms up to 2 days, but no case histories document such a long onset of action in serious poisonings. Most ingestions involve children who do not develop symptoms. Jequirity beans are highly antigenic and may produce anaphylactic reactions.

TOXIC DOSAGE/DEATH

Reported fatalities associated with abrin consumption occur after a 3- to 4-day course and are characterized by persistent gastroenteritis. The exact mechanism of death is not known.

TREATMENT

Gut Decontamination

Because of the potent toxicity of abrin, all patients who ingest the seeds and are seen within 4 hours of ingestion should receive lavage and/or charcoal.

Elimination Enhancement
There is no effective method to enhance elimination.

Supportive Measures
- Careful fluid and electrolyte replacement is the most important aspect of management. In general, supportive care is similar to that for castor bean poisoning.
- Asymptomatic children may be observed at home and symptomatic patients should be hospitalized.

Questions—Jequirity Beans

1. **Which of the following concerning jequirity beans is false?**
   A. 3- to 8-mm ovoid seeds are distinctive features of this plant. Most of the seed is a bright scarlet, with the hilum end of the seed appearing jet-black.
   B. The toxic properties of abrin have only recently been recognized.
   C. The seeds appear sporadically in beadwork and jewelry, and tourists may unintentionally expose their children to the toxic substances.
   D. Structurally, abrin has the same two-subunit configuration as ricin.
   E. The roots of the jequirity bean plant contain glycyrrhizin, the active ingredient in licorice. Clinical hyperaldosteronism characterized by sodium retention and hypertension may develop.
2. **Which of the following concerning jequirity beans is false?**
   A. Serious abrin ingestion produces a severe gastroenteritis within minutes of consumption and is followed by the development of diarrhea that may become bloody.
   B. Symptoms may last as long as 10 days.
   C. Most ingestions involve children who do not develop symptoms.
   D. Jequirity beans may produce anaphylactic reactions.
   E. Abrin inhibits protein synthesis

Mescal Beans

The Texas mountain laurel plant is a woody, evergreen shrub with alternate, pinnate leaves that is native to the southwestern United States and adjacent Mexico. Hard, colorful seeds are yellow to scarlet in color and about 1 cm long. American and Mexican Indians have used the bean in religious ceremonies for many years. Today, the seeds are more commonly used as a good luck charm. No evidence supports the association of mescal bean ingestion with hallucinations.

PATHOPHYSIOLOGY
Of the seven quinolizidine alkaloids found in mescal beans, the major toxic constituent appears to be cytisine (0.25%). By contrast, the more toxic golden chain seeds (*Laburnum anagyroides*) have a cytisine concentration four times greater. Pharmacologically, cytisine resembles nicotine.

CLINICAL PRESENTATIONS
In those children who are symptomatic, the most common presentation is vomiting and abdominal pain with delirium, drowsiness, diarrhea, and sore mouth occurring occasionally. The only reported human intoxication resulted from the self-administration of the powder from one quarter of a *Sophora speciosa* seed. The experimenter developed headache, paresthesias, lightheadedness, and difficulty in walking within 2 hours, followed by diarrhea. A "peculiar numbness in the spinal column" lasted over 24 hours.

TOXIC DOSAGE/DEATH
The lethal human dose is not known.

TREATMENT

Gut Decontamination
All patients who ingest the seeds and are seen within 4 hours of ingestion should receive syrup of ipecac and/or lavage, and charcoal.

Elimination Enhancement
There is no effective method to enhance elimination.

Supportive Measures
- Management is primarily supportive.
- Poisoning is unlikely unless teas or large quantities (probably over 20 beans) are ingested.

Questions—Mescal Beans

1. **Which of the following about mescal beans is false?**
   A. Hard, colorful seeds are yellow to scarlet in color and about 1 cm long.
   B. American and Mexican Indians have used the bean in religious ceremonies for many years.
   C. Evidence supports the association of mescal bean ingestion with hallucinations.
   D. Of the seven quinolizidine alkaloids found in mescal beans, the major toxic constituent appears to be cytisine.
   E. Golden chain seeds (*Laburnum anagyroides*) also contain cytisine.

Other Beans and Seeds

GOLDEN CHAIN SEEDS
L. anagyroides or golden chain is a beautiful flowering tree native to southern Europe and grown in the northern United States and southern Canada as an ornamental tree. Flowers mature into green pods containing two to seven kidney-shaped seeds. Most poisonings occur in children between July and September when they ingest the attractive pods and seeds. Laburnum contains the toxic alkaloid cytisine, which is pharmacologically similar to nicotine and lobeline.

The estimated lethal dose is 0.5 mg/kg. Most children who ingest seeds develop no symptoms and the remainder develop mild to moderate symptoms when one to ten seedpods are consumed. Symptoms usually start 1/2 to 4 hours after ingestion, most commonly with nausea, vomiting, abdominal pain, pallor, lightheadedness, drowsiness, and ataxia. Dilated pupils, tachycardia, paralysis, and delirium may occur in cases that are more serious. Symptoms usually resolve within 12 hours and rarely require more than 12 to 24 hours for resolution. Management is supportive. Decontamination measures are indicated for ingestion of more than one to two seeds after the usual precautions have been observed.

INDIAN CLUSTER BEANS
Native to tropical Asia, Indian cluster bean plants or guar plants grow throughout India and Pakistan and have been growing

in the United States since the early 1900s. The guar plant is a nitrogen-fixing annual that bears pods, each containing a number of seeds. Guar has been used in the management of hypercholesterolemia and as an over-the-counter diet pill. Guar gum contains about 80% guaran. The guar gum is isolated from the endosperm of the Indian cluster bean. Esophageal and small bowel obstruction have been reported following use of guar gum "diet pills" in tablet and capsule formulations. Management has included endoscopic removal from the esophagus or stomach. This is difficult because of its tenacious sticky consistency. Surgery has been required for small bowel obstruction.

JATROPHA SEEDS

The black seeds of unripe Jatropha fruit are known in the Philippines as "tuba-tuba." Children commonly ingest them. A prospective study describes vomiting, abdominal pain, nausea, muscle twitching, weakness, salivation, and sweating following their ingestion. Most patients only require supportive therapy. The toxicity may be caused by ricin and tannic acid.

LUPIN BEANS

Lupins are legumes cultivated extensively in Australia, South America, Eastern Europe, and the Mediterranean as supplemental feed for livestock. Humans ingest lupins as bean dishes, appetizers, or in high-fiber breads, pastas, and biscuits containing lupin flour. There are two forms of lupin toxicity: an alkaloid-induced syndrome and mycotoxin (phomopsin)-induced hepatotoxicity (*Lupinosis*). Quinolizidine alkaloids are present in lupin plants, and the beans are responsible for acute lupin toxicity. Fatalities among children and moderately severe acute anticholinergic reactions have been reported. A motor neuron disease associated with chronic and excessive consumption of lupin beans has been observed.

MUCUNA PRURIENS

An outbreak of acute toxic psychosis in Mozambique followed ingestion of the seeds of *Mucuna pruriens*, also known as *feijao nacaca* in Mozambique and as cowhage, kaunch, and pica-pica in other countries. The seeds contain levodopa, N,N-dimethyltryptamine (DMT), bufotenine, 5-methoxy-N,N-dimethyltryptamine (5-Meo-DMT), and other alkaloids.

QUINOLIZIDINE ALKALOIDS

Various *Thermopsis* species are found in the foothills and plains of the Rocky Mountains. Common names include golden banner, false lupine, buckbean, buffalo pea, yellow bean, and mountain *Thermopsis*. The seeds contain the highest plant concentration of quinolizidine alkaloids. Symptoms may follow ingestion of the flowers or blossoms. *T. rhombifolia* contains numerous alkaloids. The two principal alkaloids of the group are anagyrine and thermopsine. The most studied of the group are cytisine, the primary toxin of *L. anagyroides*, which exerts a nicotinelike effect and anagyrine, a teratogen in cattle. No specific toxic dose is known for humans, but a handful of seeds produce symptoms.

Symptoms seen in quinolizidine alkaloid poisoning include abdominal pain, cramping, vomiting, convulsions, and death via respiratory paralysis. Serious cytisine ingestion may exhibit nausea, abdominal pain, vomiting, stupor, giddiness, muscular weakness, incoordination, and ataxia followed by respiratory paralysis. If emesis has occurred, induction of emesis may not be necessary. If emesis has not occurred or the patient is seen during the first few hours, vomiting may be helpful followed by charcoal. Children should be observed for 4 to 6 hours for unusual lethargy, ataxia, delirium, or convulsions.

SUNFLOWER SEEDS

Eating excessive sunflower seeds can cause pain on defecation. Clinical features include obstipation, rectal pain with defecation, and a "crunchy" sensation on rectal examination after ingestion of unhusked sunflower seeds. Rectal pain is from undigested shards impinging on the delicate anoderm. Attempts to defecate enhance the symptoms. Treatment involves disimpaction under general anesthesia or enemas requiring nitrous oxide anesthesia.

Questions—Other Beans and Seeds

1. Which of the following is not associated?
- A. Golden chain seeds—Cytisine, which is pharmacologically similar to nicotine and lobeline
- B. Golden chain seeds—Dilated pupils, tachycardia, paralysis, and delirium in serious cases
- C. Guar gum diet pills—Esophageal and small bowel obstruction
- D. Lupins—Pyrrolidine alkaloids
- E. Quinolizidine alkaloids—Abdominal pain, cramping, vomiting, convulsions, and death via respiratory paralysis

HOUSEPLANTS

As the popularity of indoor plants spreads, exposure of curious toddlers to toxic plants also increases. In 1997, plant exposures represented 5.6% of the calls reported to the AAPCC National Data Collection System. The five most common plant exposures in decreasing order were pepper, philodendron, poinsettia, peace lily, and holly. Most toxic effects resulted from the irritant properties of *Araceae* species, poinsettias, and holly berries on the buccal mucosa and the gastrointestinal tract. Deaths caused by this group of plants are not well documented in the medical literature. In most cases of houseplant ingestion, only symptomatic care and parental observation are required.

Dieffenbachia

Dieffenbachia is a popular ornamental plant that has broad, shiny leaves and grows to 6 feet. This tropical American native has leaves that may be spotted or variegated. The toxic effects of *Dieffenbachia* are limited to its mucosal irritant properties. *Dieffenbachia* contains calcium oxalate crystals, which are believed to cause the irritation. *Dieffenbachia* leaves contain raphide crystals (needle-shaped crystals arranged in compact bundles) that have the potential to penetrate buccal mucosa when cut. These raphides are contained within special cells known as idioblasts that forcibly extrude the raphides in response to mechanical or chemical forces.

The stalk of the *Dieffenbachia* produces the most severe reaction. The leaves and stems are less stringent. The oral toxicity is well described in plant toxicology textbooks. *Dieffenbachia* species cause salivation and severe swelling of the lips, mouth, and tongue, which may lead to interference with swallowing and breathing. In addition, contact with the eye can produce conjunctivitis and perhaps corneal abrasions. Although rare, an occupational contact dermatitis in gardeners has been confirmed.

TREATMENT

- Most encounters involve casual contact.
- Usually demulcents (milk, water) and cold packs are all that is required.

- The most severe sequela appears to be the potential for respiratory obstruction, which progresses over the first 6 hours. Only those patients with significant edema require medical observation.
- Otherwise, only symptomatic care with topical agents (e.g., Cepacol®, Orabase Plain®) is necessary. Severe cases require analgesics.
- Antihistamines are of questionable value because the role of histamine-induced edema is unclear.

Holly

The genus *Ilex* contains 300 to 350 species found throughout regions with temperate and tropical climates, where they grow as deciduous and evergreen shrubs and trees. They have bright green leaves, often with hard teeth on the leaf margins, which discourage leaf consumption. The red or black berries (Christmas holly) are attractive ornaments, especially to curious children.

PATHOPHYSIOLOGY

Polyphenols, saponins, triterpenes, steroids, and alkaloids have been extracted from *Ilex opaca*. Although saponins are present in both fruit and leaf extracts, the limited oral bioavailability of saponins makes systemic toxicity by the oral route unlikely.

CLINICAL PRESENTATIONS

Ilex species produce gastrointestinal distress in some but not all ingestions. Case studies of toxic effects in humans are rare. A set of identical twins ingested a "handful of holly berries" after which 15 mL of syrup of ipecac was given. Over the next 6 hours, the twins vomited 40 to 50 times. The following day, several loose stools were passed and mild vomiting continued, but symptoms resolved completely by 30 hours postingestion.

TREATMENT

- Treatment is supportive. Casual ingestions (e.g., a few berries) require no decontamination measures.
- Patients with large ingestions may benefit from administration of syrup of ipecac and activated charcoal.

Mistletoe

Mistletoe is a semiparasitic perennial that grows chiefly on oak trees. It grows as a 1- to 4-ft bush in the oak branches and is distinguished from the oak by light green leaves and hairy stems. Small white berries grow in grapelike clusters. Several species are present in the United States, including the familiar Christmas mistletoe (*Phoradendron flavescens*). The dominant European mistletoe species is *Viscum album*, which has been studied extensively for its cardiotoxin. Mistletoe has a long medicinal history. Mistletoe is a favorite extract of herbalists who have advocated its use in infertility, epilepsy, asthma, and nervous tension. The berries and leaves are used commonly as Christmas ornaments.

PATHOPHYSIOLOGY

Mistletoe contains gastric irritating alkaloids, cardiac toxins, and lectins. Extracts from European mistletoe are known as viscotoxins and are physiologically similar to cobra venom. Viscotoxin causes vasoconstriction, bradycardia, and negative inotropic effects when administered intravenously to cats. Viscotoxin apparently alters cell membrane permeability by displacing calcium. In high doses, viscotoxin arrests papillary muscle preparations in systole. Extract of the American mistletoe, *Phoradendron serotinum*, has effects quantitatively different from those of the European viscotoxin. A parenteral dose of phoratoxin 10 times greater is required to produce the same bradycardia, hypotension, and decreased inotropy seen after viscotoxin administration.

CLINICAL PRESENTATIONS

All parts of the plants are poisonous. The berries have been a common source of gastrointestinal poisoning. One fatality was associated with the use of a tea brewed from mistletoe berries as an abortifacient. Ingestion of large quantities of berries causes gastroenteritis. Mistletoe contains a number of potential toxins (e.g., phenylethylamine, tyramine), but the ability of a parenteral cardiotoxin (e.g., viscotoxin, phoratoxin) to be absorbed from the gastrointestinal tract has not been documented. Although anecdotal reports support the cardiac toxicity of these agents, the severity of their human cardiotoxicity remains to be documented.

TREATMENT

- The ingestion of 1 to 3 berries or 1 to 2 leaves probably does not cause toxic effects in a child.
- Because mistletoe causes gastrointestinal symptoms in large doses, syrup of ipecac should be administered for significant ingestions (i.e., more than one to three berries) in children unless contraindicated.
- The potential for adverse cardiac effects theoretically exists. Patients who manifest dysrhythmias or electrolyte imbalance should be hospitalized for observation overnight.
- Asymptomatic patients may be discharged after several hours of observation. "Mistletoe hepatitis" remains a curiosity and should be considered in serious or chronic ingestions.

Poinsettia

Poinsettia is a popular indoor Christmas ornamental plant with large (3- to 6-in) alternating leaves and prominent red, pink, yellow, or cream bracts clustered at the tops of the stems. Poinsettia toxicity is limited to its ability to produce local irritation, contact dermatitis, mucosal burns, and keratoconjunctivitis.

TREATMENT

- Treatment is supportive.

Questions—Houseplants

1. Which of the following is not associated?
A. Poinsettia—Mucosal burns and keratoconjunctivitis.
B. *Dieffenbachia*—Calcium oxalate crystals
C. Mistletoe—Viscotoxin
D. Mistletoe berries—Gastrointestinal poisoning
E. Holly—Uniform systemic toxicity by the oral route

FOOD PLANTS

Absinthe

In the first century AD, a wine fortified with extract of wormwood (*Artemisia absinthium*) was described as "absinthites" by Pliny the Elder. A stronger drink, with 70% to 80% alcohol by volume, was developed by a Frenchman who sold the recipe to M. Pernod in 1797. Absinthe was widely enjoyed in 19th century Europe. Vincent van Gogh was known to repeatedly drink absinthe and painted a still life with absinthe. Edouard Manet painted the Absinthe Drinker (1859), and Edgar Degas painted "L'Absinthe" in 1876. Some countries have banned absinthe.

PATHOPHYSIOLOGY

Wormwood is a perennial shrub native to Europe, but is also grown in the northeast and north central United States. A deleterious compound in absinthe that appears to produce hallucinations and psychosis is a terpene, thujone. Thujone occurs in a variety of plants, including tansy (*Tanacetum vulgare*), sage (*Salvia officinalis*), and white cedar (*Thuja occidentalis*). Wormwood is bitter because of a compound called absinthin.

CLINICAL PRESENTATIONS

Ingestion of absinthe may lead to a group of symptoms described as "absinthism" characterized by digestive disorders, thirst, restlessness, vertigo, tremor, numbness of extremities, diminished intellect, delirium, paralysis, and death. Fifteen grams of the volatile oil can cause convulsions and coma in humans.

TREATMENT

- Treatment is symptomatic and supportive.

Question—Absinthe

1. Which of the following is false?
   A. Absinthe was widely enjoyed in 19th century Europe.
   B. Vincent Van Gogh was known to repeatedly drink absinthe and painted a still life with absinthe.
   C. Some countries have banned absinthe.
   D. A deleterious compound in absinthe that appears to produce hallucinations and psychosis is a terpene, thujone.
   E. Ingestion of absinthe may lead to a group of symptoms described as "absinthism" characterized by delirium, paralysis, and obsessive-compulsive disorder.

Ackee Fruit

Sapida is a native of West Africa and was introduced to Jamaica in 1778 by Thomas Clark. It was named after the infamous Captain Bligh who took the breadfruit tree to the West Indies. Ingestion of unripe akee fruit causes Jamaican vomiting sickness and occurs among poor children who use the akee as a food staple. The tree grows in Florida, but the fruit commonly is not eaten outside of Jamaica. Typically, each fruit contains three glassy black seeds surrounded by a thick oily white aril. This aril can be eaten when mature, but at other stages of development is poisonous.

PATHOPHYSIOLOGY

A water-soluble toxin called hypoglycin has been isolated from unripe fruit. This compound produces hypoglycemia by inhibition of hepatic gluconeogenesis. A metabolite of hypoglycin reduces the cofactors coenzyme A and carnitine essential to the oxidation of long-chain fatty acids. Sequestration of these factors alone may not be the primary factor causing hypoglycemia. Limited fatty acid oxidation and the sustained formation of isovaleric acid also require coenzyme A. Thus, the inhibition of fatty acid oxidation has a role in the impaired gluconeogenesis.

CLINICAL PRESENTATIONS

The syndrome of Jamaican vomiting sickness is similar to Reye's syndrome and is characterized by gastrointestinal distress and central nervous system depression. Severe cases display hypoglycemia and fatty infiltration of the liver and kidney. Nausea, vomiting, and abdominal pain are usually, but not always, the first symptoms and appear several hours after ingestion of unripe acee fruit. After a brief quiescent period, vomiting, lethargy, convulsions, coma, and death may occur 2 to 12 hours postexposure. Metabolic acidosis is present in most severe cases. Hypoglycemia does not explain the entire clinical picture, because vomiting and central nervous system depression can occur in the absence of hypoglycemia.

TREATMENT

- The usual measures of decontamination may be beneficial within the first several hours of poisoning, although vomiting usually is a prominent part of the clinical syndrome.
- All patients should receive measurements of serum glucose and arterial pH. The presence of any degree of obtundation mandates immediate administration of glucose.
- Treatment is primarily supportive with restoration of fluid, electrolyte, glucose, and pH balance.
- Liver function tests and serum creatinine and glucose levels should be followed closely.

Question—Ackee Fruit

1. The active toxin in ackee fruit is called
   A. Hyperglycin
   B. Hypoglycin
   C. Ackrin
   D. Jamatoxin
   E. Abrin

Betel Nut

The Ministry of Health and Family Welfare for India has included betel nut or supari as a food item "injurious to health" because of its causal association with oral cancer. Supari is chewed alone or as pan, a mixture of supari, lime, and other ingredients with or without tobacco wrapped in a betel leaf (*Piper betel*). Pan masala is a concentrated powdered form of the preparation used in pan.

About six reduced pyridine alkaloids are present in betel nuts. Arecaidine may have carcinogenic effects and may be a factor in the associated increased incidence of oral cancer. Arecoline, a major component of the Areca (betel nut), is a cholinergic agent of similar structure to methacholine. Asthmatics challenged with inhaled arecoline respond with bronchoconstriction.

TREATMENT

- Treatment is symptomatic and supportive.

Question—Betel Nut

1. Betel nut has been associated with
   A. Esophageal cancer
   B. Gastric cancer
   C. Retroperitoneal fibrosis
   D. Thyroid cancer
   E. Oral cancer

Cyanogenic Plants

About 150 plant species contain cyanogenetic glycosides, which yield hydrocyanic acid upon hydrolysis. See Chapter 45, Airborne Toxins, for more about cyanide poisoning. Cyanogenic plants include apricot (*Prunus armeniaca*), bitter almond (*Prunus dulcis*), peach (*Prunus persica*), apple (*Malus domestica*), black or wild cherry (*Prunus serotina*), hydrangea (Saxifragaceae family), jetbead or jetberry bush (*Rhodotypos scandens*), Puerto Rican lima bean (*Phaseolus lunatus*), cassava (*Manihot esculenta*), choke cherry (*Prunus virginiana*), and elderberry (*Sambucus mexicana*).

AMYGDALIN

Amygdalin, which is the diglycoside of mandelonitrile, probably was the first complex glycoside described. In 1830, French chemists isolated amygdalin from bitter almonds. The ancient Egyptians probably used amygdalin as a means of capital punishment known as "penalty of the peach." Apricot, peach, cherry, and apple kernels as well as the stems, leaves, and roots of many rose family species contain amygdalin. The presence of amygdalin alone in these kernels is not dangerous, however; the crushed, moistened seed releases an enzyme, emulsin, that catalyzes the hydrolysis of amygdalin to glucose, benzaldehyde, and cyanide. Amygdalin is much more toxic (perhaps 40 times) when ingested than when administered intravenously.

LAETRILE

Laetrile is a purported cancer chemotherapeutic agent that is composed primarily of d-amygdalin. Laetrile itself is relatively free of hydrolytic enzymes therefore intravenous administration usually does not produce cyanide poisoning. Proponents suggest that laetrile releases hydrocyanic acid in the presence of β-glucuronidase, which allegedly occurs in higher, lethal concentrations in malignant compared with normal cells. Clinical trials have failed to support the efficacy of laetrile in cancer treatment, and several cyanide fatalities have been associated with accidental and intentional ingestion of laetrile.

Clinical Presentations

The clinical picture of amygdalin poisoning mimics cyanide poisoning. The rapid onset of dyspnea, cyanosis, vomiting, diaphoresis, weakness, lightheadedness, and excitement followed by convulsions, stupor, disorientation, paralysis, weakness, coma, and cardiovascular collapse characterizes cyanide toxicity. Symptoms typically start within one half hour of consumption and progress quickly. Ingestion of 45 mL of laetrile has caused severe headache, dizziness, coma, and convulsions within minutes. Consumption of 48 apricot kernels as a milkshake caused vomiting, headache, flushing, diaphoresis, and lightheadedness after 1 hour, which rapidly subsided after syrup of ipecac-induced emesis at an emergency department. Ingestion of 12 bitter almonds has produced vomiting, abdominal pain, coma, lactic acidosis, and pulmonary edema starting within 15 minutes.

Treatment

- Treatment is identical to that for cyanide poisoning. When nitrates are administered to children, appropriate adjustments for weight and hemoglobin content must be made to avoid fatal methemoglobinemia.
- Mild-to-moderate ingestions may require only decontamination and supportive care.
- Alteration in mental status, severe acidosis, continuous seizures, or refractory hypotension indicates the need for antidotal therapy.
- Clinical features that suggest response to antidotes include normalization of blood pressure, pulse, mentation, cessation of seizure activity, and return of spontaneous respirations.

Question—Cyanogenic Plants

1. Cyanogenic plants include all of the following except
   A. Apricot (*Prunus armeniaca*)
   B. Bitter almond (*Prunus dulcis*)
   C. Peach (*Prunus persica*)
   D. Apple (*Malus domestica*)
   E. Rhubarb (*Polygoniaceae*)

Garlic

Garlic has been used as a medicine in many cultures as reported in folk medicine literature. It has been utilized as an antipyretic, antibiotic, antifungal, and antiviral agent. Preliminary data indicate that it may affect antifibrinolytic activity in humans, decrease atherosclerotic plaque formation, and decrease lipid and cholesterol levels in man. Most of these claims have not been subjected to controlled clinical studies.

PATHOPHYSIOLOGY

Garlic contains about 0.5% of a volatile oil composed of sulfur-containing compounds (diallyl disulfide, diallyl trisulfide, and methylallyl trisulfide). The enzyme allicinase converts alliin (5-allyl-L-cysteine sulfoxide) to 2-propenesulfene acid, which dimerizes to form allicin. Allicin gives the pungent characteristic odor to crushed garlic and probably is the cause of skin reactions.

CLINICAL PRESENTATIONS

Adverse effects have included arrhythmias, asthma, contact dermatitis, and partial-thickness, second-degree burns.

TREATMENT

- Management is supportive and symptomatic.
- Topical burns will respond to sterile dressings.

Questions—Garlic

1. Allicin gives the pungent characteristic odor to crushed garlic and probably is the cause of skin reactions.
   A. True
   B. False

Ginkgo

The ginkgo is the world's oldest living tree species. The extract of its fruit has been used for peripheral arterial disease and organic brain syndromes in the elderly. There is little controlled clinical evidence to support its use.

PATHOPHYSIOLOGY

The ginkgo contains a number of terpenes, proarthocyanidines, heterosides, and bioflavones. Its terpenoids include ginkgolides and bilobalides.

CLINICAL PRESENTATIONS

Ingestion of ginkgo extract has been associated with mild gastrointestinal disturbance and headache. The whole ginkgo plant has been associated with severe allergic reactions. Ginkgolides and bilobalides are structurally similar to the allergens of poison ivy, mango rind, and cashew nut shell oil. Contact with the fruit pulp can cause erythema, edema, vesicles, and itching.

TREATMENT

- Treatment is symptomatic and supportive.
- There are no desensitization preparations in clinical use.

Questions—Ginkgo

1. Which of the following concerning ginkgo is false?
   A. The ginkgo is the world's oldest living tree species.
   B. The extract of its fruit has been used for peripheral arterial disease and organic brain syndromes in the elderly.
   C. There is little controlled clinical evidence to support its use.
   D. Only its leaves have been associated with severe allergic reactions.
   E. Ingestion of ginkgo has been associated with mild gastrointestinal disturbance and headache.

Kava

Kava is an intoxicating drink prepared from the rhizome of *Piper methysticum*. The pulverized roots are steeped in water. The plant is indigenous to the islands of the South Pacific.

PATHOPHYSIOLOGY

Lactones (kavaine, dihydrokavaine, methysticine, dihydromethysticine, desmethoxyyanogonin, and yanogonin) are major constituents of kava resin. This extract reportedly produces sedation, protection from electric shock, local anesthetic action, smooth muscle relaxation, and potentiation of barbiturate narcosis. The plasma elimination half-life of kavaine is 2.8 to 6.7 hours.

CLINICAL PRESENTATIONS

Kava drinkers may develop shortness of breath, malnutrition, and loss of body fat. Albumin and plasma proteins are decreased. A scaly ichthyotoxic skin rash may be present. Its main effect appears to be on the liver, kidneys, blood, and lungs where it induces biochemical and functional evidence of damage. Signs suggestive of central dopaminergic antagonism, including dystonic reactions and dyskinesias, have been observed.

TREATMENT

- Reduction of consumption of kava and improvement of nutrition appear to be reasonable approaches to lessening the problems induced by this drink.

Questions—Kava

1. Kava drinkers may develop shortness of breath, malnutrition, and loss of body fat.
   A. True
   B. False

Mate

Mate (i.e., Paraguay Tea) is a beverage, not a plant, and is prepared from the leathery leaves of *Ilex paraguayensis*, a species of holly that is found in South America. In areas where mate is drunk, it largely replaces coffee and tea. The leaves are plunged into hot water.

PATHOPHYSIOLOGY

Yerba mate contains phenylpropanoids, including caffetannin, yielding caffeic acid when hydrolyzed, chlorogenic acid, neochlorogenic acid, and isochlorogenic acid. The beverage contains caffeine (about 2%), theobromine, and theophylline.

CLINICAL PRESENTATIONS

Heavy use of yerba mate has been associated with a high risk of esophageal cancer. This may be from the hot drinks, rather than the alkaloids. Clinical effects associated with xanthines, such as palpitations, arrhythmias, and/or seizures, are possible theoretically.

TREATMENT

- Treatment is symptomatic and supportive.

Questions—Mate

1. Which of the following about mate is false?
   A. Mate is also called Paraguay Tea
   B. Mate is a plant, not a beverage
   C. In areas where mate tea is drunk, it largely replaces coffee and tea.
   D. The beverage contains caffeine (about 2%), theobromine, and theophylline.
   E. Heavy use of yerba mate has been associated with a high risk of esophageal cancer.

Pepper

Pepper is a ubiquitous spice on American tables and is found around the world in numerous cuisines. Topical capsaicin has been used for the treatment of neuralgia associated with herpes zoster infection, psoriasis, diabetic neuropathy, pruritus related to hemodialysis, and posttraumatic amputation stump pain. Workers exposed to hot chili cayenne peppers (*Capsicum annum*) may experience an increase in cough ("chili workers' cough"). Capsaicin, the active principle of hot peppers (genus *capsicum*), has been a subject of child abuse. Chili peppers are edible and nontoxic in usual doses. Certain dog and human repellent products contain up to 10% oleum capsicum.

PATHOPHYSIOLOGY

Capsaicin is the alkaloid responsible for the mucosal irritant properties of the fruit. Capsaicin reduces vasodilation and heat pain thresholds and directly excites nociceptors, leading to increased pain sensitivity. Repeat exposure to capsaicin causes desensitization to the effect of the chemical.

CLINICAL PRESENTATIONS

Contact with products containing capsaicin produces local irritation and lacrimation. The use of dried red chili peppers (*Capsicum annuum cultivar*) caused severe burning of the fingertips of a man who earlier had sustained abrasions of the fingers. The name "Hunan hand" was given to this syndrome, which is caused by the volatile oils activating dermal pain fibers. Ingestion of large quantities of jalapeno peppers has led to lacrimation, rhinorrhea, dysuria, and burning discomfort on defecation within 24 hours. Black pepper (*Piper nigrum*) has caused asphyxia when deliberately poured down children's throats.

TREATMENT

- Management is entirely supportive and involves cleansing of the affected area with water.
- Cases of aspiration may require bronchoscopy and pulmonary lavage.
- Immersion of irritated skin areas in vinegar (5% acetic acid) may provide relief even if initiated 30 minutes or longer after

exposure. Several hours of bathing may be required in severe cases.

Questions—Pepper

1. Capsaicin has been used for all of the following except
   A. Neuralgia associated with herpes zoster infection
   B. Psoriasis
   C. Diabetic neuropathy
   D. Sciatica
   E. Posttraumatic amputation stump pain

2. Ingestion of large quantities of jalapeno peppers has led to lacrimation, rhinorrhea, dysuria and burning discomfort on defecation within 24 hours.
   A. True
   B. False

Rhubarb

Rhubarb is a garden vegetable plant with large, leathery, heart-shaped leaves and a reddish color. The stalks are used as a vegetable and for making pies. Consumption of rhubarb leaves as a food substitute for spinach was encouraged in England during World War I until several deaths were attributed to the ingestion of cooked leaves. The dried roots have been used medicinally as a cathartic and as a tonic.

PATHOPHYSIOLOGY

The leaf blade is the toxic part of the plant, containing less than 1% soluble oxalates. The stalks have much lower oxalate levels and therefore are edible. Cooking does not make rhubarb leaves edible. The soluble oxalates are absorbed readily from the gastrointestinal tract. Systemic formation of calcium oxalate may produce hypocalcemia. Precipitation of insoluble salts in the renal system may lead to kidney dysfunction and electrolyte imbalance.

CLINICAL PRESENTATIONS

Symptoms may result from the mucosal irritant effect of oxalate on the gastrointestinal tract and include sore throat, nausea, vomiting, anorexia, diarrhea, and abdominal pain. Hematochezia or hematemesis may be present. Symptoms typically begin within 6 to 12 hours but may be delayed 24 hours. Kidney dysfunction and electrolyte imbalance are the major causes of death and appear after signs of gastrointestinal distress develop. One month may be required for renal function to return to normal. Anuria, oliguria, proteinuria, hematuria, and oxaluria are present in severe cases. Paresthesias, tetany, hyperreflexia, muscle twitches, and muscle cramps reflect hypocalcemia. Seizures may complicate the clinical course and usually result from hypocalcemia.

TREATMENT

- Patients who ingest rhubarb leaves and are seen early in their clinical course (4 to 6 hours after ingestion) should receive syrup of ipecac and/or charcoal after the usual precautions have been observed.
- Gastric lavage with 0.15% calcium hydroxide (lime water) to precipitate insoluble calcium oxalate in the gastrointestinal tract has been suggested for serious ingestions, but no clinical substantiation of this intervention exists.
- Generous fluid replacement should be given to promote the excretion of calcium oxalate crystals from the kidney tubules.
- Symptomatic patients should receive a complete blood count, and serum electrolytes, including calcium and kidney function tests (creatinine, urinalysis). Kidney function may deteriorate over the first week and careful management of fluid and electrolyte balance may be necessary.
- Intravenous calcium may be necessary to reverse oxalate-induced hypocalcemia.

Questions—Rhubarb

1. The most toxic part of the rhubarb plant is
   A. The leaf blade
   B. The roots
   C. The stems
   D. The flower
   E. All parts of the plant are equally toxic.

2. Which of the following regarding the clinical effects of rhubarb is false?
   A. Symptoms may result from the mucosal irritant effect of oxalate on the gastrointestinal tract and include sore throat, nausea, vomiting, anorexia, diarrhea, and abdominal pain.
   B. Hematochezia or hematemesis may be present.
   C. Symptoms typically begin immediately.
   D. Kidney dysfunction and electrolyte imbalance are the major causes of death and appear after signs of gastrointestinal distress develop.
   E. Paresthesias, tetany, hyperreflexia, muscle twitches, and muscle cramps reflect hypocalcemia.

Solanine Plants

Potatoes belong to the nightshade family (Solanaceae), which contains a number of poisonous species because of the presence of alkaloids such as solanine. These glycoalkaloids usually appear in nontoxic amounts. Human poisoning occurs after consumption of green or stressed potatoes. The toxic alkaloids are produced by the periderm, the cortex, and areas of high metabolic activity such as the eyes and sprouts. Trauma, sunlight, and adverse storage conditions favor solanine production. Because of the bitter taste of the alkaloids, solanine poisoning is rare except in times of food shortages. Peeling and boiling remove most solanine. Sweet potatoes (*Ipomoea batatas*) belong to a different plant family.

The tomato (*Lycopersicin esculentum*) is closely related to *Solanum* and at one time was considered a *Solanum* species. Glycoalkaloids of the solanine type are present in tomato leaves and vines but not in the fruit. These alkaloids produce a poisoning syndrome similar to that of solanine when the stems or vines are consumed; however, reported cases of human toxicity are rare. The toxicity of the "nightshade" family has been known since ancient times.

PATHOPHYSIOLOGY

Solanum species contain the toxic glycoalkaloid solanine. Solanine actually is a mixture of two classes of glycosides, solanines and chaconines. Six of these glycosides have been isolated from the potato plant. These compounds all contain solanidine, but differ with respect to the composition of the sugar chain. Because solanidine is structurally similar to steroids, its proposed biosynthetic pathway is from acetate through cholesterol. Solanine is poorly absorbed from the gastrointestinal tract. Although solanine exists throughout the plant, its concentration varies over a wide range because of a host of environmental and genetic factors. Ripe fruit contains the least solanine.

CLINICAL PRESENTATIONS

Gastrointestinal and neurologic symptoms predominate in cases of solanine poisoning depending on the amount ingested. Vomiting, headache, and flushing were the most common symptoms reported in children ingesting plant parts. Symptoms began 7 to 19 hours after ingestion, with vomiting, diarrhea, anorexia, and malaise as the most common symptoms. Nongastrointestinal symptoms included fever, altered mental status, restlessness, headache, and hallucinations. Hypotension, tachycardia, and stupor out of proportion to fluid and electrolyte imbalance may occur. Deaths have been associated with consumption of toxic potatoes, but those reports involved malnourished patients who may not have received adequate care.

TREATMENT

- Gut decontamination may be useful for those patients who are seen early (i.e., within 4 hours) and who do not have spontaneous vomiting and diarrhea. General supportive care is the key to treatment.
- Fluid status should be evaluated in every patient by means of orthostatic pulse and blood pressures. Electrolytes should be checked on those patients who exhibit profound changes or who take medications that alter fluid or electrolyte balance. An intravenous line should be established in those patients who exhibit orthostatic hypotension or neurologic signs.
- For seriously ill patients who do not respond to fluid replacement, cardiac monitoring and vasopressors may be needed.
- Seizures are treated with diazepam.

Questions—Solanine Plants

1. Which of the following does not contain solanine?
A. Wild tomato
B. Potato
C. Eggplant
D. Nightshade
E. Sweet potato

2. Which of the following about solanine is false?
A. Human poisoning may occur after consumption of green or stressed potatoes.
B. Trauma, sunlight, and adverse storage conditions favor solanine production in potatoes.
C. Peeling and boiling remove most solanine.
D. Glycoalkaloids of the solanine type are present in tomato leaves and vines but not in the fruit.
E. Solanine is well absorbed from the gastrointestinal tract.

Answers

General Approach to Plants
1. B 2. E 3. A 4. A

Castor Beans
1. D 2. A

Fava Beans
1. B

Jequirity Beans
1. B 2. A

Mescal Beans
1. C

Other Beans and Seeds
1. D

Houseplants
1. E

Absinthe
1. E

Ackee Fruit
1. B

Betel Nut
1. E

Cyanogenic Plants
1. E

Garlic
1. A

Ginkgo
1. D

Kava
1. A

Mate
1. B

Pepper
1. D 2. A

Rhubarb
1. A 2. C

Solanine Plants
1. E 2. E

SELECTED READINGS

General Approach to Plants

1. Blackwell WH. *Poisonous and medicinal plants.* Englewood Cliffs, NJ: Prentice-Hall, 1990.
2. D'Arcy PF. Adverse reactions and interactions with herbal medicines. I. Adverse reactions. Adverse Drug React Toxicol Rev 1992;10:189–208.
3. Frohne D, Pfander HJ. *A colour atlas of poisonous plants.* London: Wolfe Publishing, 1984.

4. Huxtable RJ. The harmful potential of herbal and other plant products. Drug Safety 1990;5(Suppl 1):126–136.
5. Larkin T. Unsafe herbs. FDA Consumer 1993;14:5–10.
6. Ogzewalla CD, Bonfiglio JF, Sigell LT. Common plants and their toxicity. Pediatr Clin North Am 1987;34:1557–1598.

Beans and Seeds

1. Challoner KR, McCarron MM. Castor bean intoxication. Ann Emerg Med 1990;19:1177–1183.
2. Lowen RJ, Alam FKA, Edgar JA. Lupin bean toxicity. Med J Aust 1995; 162:256–257.
3. Makalinao IP. A descriptive study on the clinical profile of Jatropha seed poisoning. Vet Hum Toxicol 1993;35:330.
4. Phillips RW, Moses FR. Sunflower seed syndrome: A prickly proctological problem. Ann Emerg Med 1991;20:1049–1050.

Houseplants

1. Spiller HA, Willias DB, Gorman SE, Sanftleban J. Retrospective study of mistletoe ingestion. Clin Toxicol 1995;33:475–486 (abstract 156).

Food Plants

1. Arnold WN. Absinthe. Sci Am 1989;260(6):112–117.
2. Blanc P, Liu D, Juarez C, Boushey HA. Cough in hot pepper workers. Chest 1991;99:27–32.
3. CDC. Toxic hypoglycemic syndrome-Jamaica 1989-1991. MMWR 1992;41:53–55.
4. Editor. India: Betel nut warning. Lancet 1993;341:819.
5. Editor. Kava. Lancet 1988;1:258–259.
6. Mate. Lawrence review of natural products. St. Louis: Facts and Comparisons, April 1988.
7. Olin BR, ed. The Lawrence review of natural products. St. Louis: Facts and Comparisons. Ginkgo. February 1988.
8. Roser D. Garlic. Lancet 1990;335:114–115.
9. Shragg TA, Albertson TE, Fisher CJ. Cyanide poisoning after bitter almond ingestion. West J Med 1982;136:65–69.

CHAPTER 57

Wild Plants, Mushrooms, and Mycotoxins

TREES, SHRUBS AND FLOWERS

A number of common trees, shrubs, and flowers are described below. The field of botanical toxicology is huge, and these examples represent a mere sampling of interesting and commonly encountered toxins. The list is by no means exhaustive. While some toxins are extremely well-documented and described, an element of folklore and less-than-rigorous methods have characterized certain elements of this literature.

ACONITUM

The aconite root has been used for 2,000 years in Eurasia as a homicidal agent, arrow poison, and medicinal drug. The crude drug "bushi," obtained from Aconitum roots, has been administered to improve metabolism and to cure dysuria, cardiac weakness, gout, neuralgias, and rheumatism. Rat studies suggest that ignavine, an Aconitum root alkaloid, has antiinflammatory properties.

Pathophysiology

Aconitum contains the potent poisons aconitine, mesaconitine, and jesaconitine, which are C19 diterpenoid ester alkaloids. Experimentally, aconite induces atrial and ventricular dysrhythmias after direct application to the myocardium. In addition to the cardioactive alkaloid, Aconitum roots contain physiologically active catecholamine analogs.

Clinical Presentations

Aconite poisoning produces intoxication similar to that of veratrum alkaloids except that paresthesias are more prominent and persistent. See Veratrum section. Soon after ingestion, numbness and tingling of the tongue, throat, and mouth begins, followed within 2 to 6 hours by nausea, salivation, and generalized weakness. Convulsions have occurred 5 hours postingestion. Mild symptoms usually resolve within 24 hours, but weakness, paresthesias, pruritus, and numbness may persist for several weeks.

Cardiotoxicity commonly complicates serious aconitine poisoning and is characterized by hypotension, shock, conduction delays, and dysrhythmias beginning within 6 hours of ingestion. Sinus bradycardia with first-degree atrioventricular block, supraventricular tachycardia and hypotension, multiple premature ventricular contractions, bundle branch block, junctional escape rhythms, ventricular tachycardia, and Torsade de Pointes have been reported. Serious ventricular dysrhythmias occur within 24 hours of ingestion, but ST-T wave abnormalities and conduction delays may persist for several days.

Toxic Dosage/Death

Most of the toxic effects of aconite result from the accidental, suicidal, or homicidal ingestion of aconitine powder, especially in India where the paste is used to relieve neuralgias and dental pain. The Aconitum root rarely is confused with horseradish. All parts of the plant contain toxic alkaloids, but the alkaloid content and composition varies throughout the year. Ingestion of 3 to 10 mg has produced paresthesias, nausea, vomiting, weakness, and cardiac dysrhythmias.

Treatment

GUT DECONTAMINATION

Because all parts of the Aconitum plant contain aconitine, decontamination with syrup of ipecac, gastric lavage, charcoal and/or cathartics is reasonable in those patients who ingest more than a taste of the plant.

ELIMINATION ENHANCEMENT

These methods generally are not utilized in the treatment of aconitum exposures.

SUPPORTIVE MEASURES

- Toxicity is difficult to predict because of alkaloid variability, however a 2- to 4-hour observation period generally is appropriate. Symptomatic patients should be hospitalized for 24 hours with cardiac monitoring.
- Symptomatic patients (e.g., those with protracted vomiting and weakness) should receive an intravenous (IV) line, oxygen, and cardiac monitoring, and should be monitored for at least 24 hours. Cardiovascular collapse and ventricular dysrhythmias represent the greatest risk to life.
- Lidocaine has not been tested in the clinical setting of aconitine poisoning, but is an effective antiarrhythmic agent for ventricular dysrhythmias. Procainamide and diphenylhydantoin have been successful clinically and experimentally in suppression of ventricular dysrhythmias resulting from aconite poisoning.

- Respiratory and central nervous system depression is not a common feature of aconitine toxicity and usually results from poor perfusion or coingestion of another drug.

Questions—Aconitum

1. Aconite poisoning produces intoxication similar to
A. Abrin
B. Cytisine
C. Veratrum
D. Ricin
E. Solanine

2. Signs of aconite poisoning include all of the following except
A. Numbness and tingling of the tongue, throat, and mouth
B. Convulsions
C. Hypotension, shock, conduction delays, and dysrhythmias
D. Nausea and vomiting
E. Exfoliative rash

BANEBERRY

The baneberry plant is a tall perennial herb with thick roots and large, compound leaves composed of toothed edges. The white flower produces attractive red berries. The western baneberry (red fruit) occurs in Alaska to central California, and Arizona to Montana. The eastern baneberry (*Actaea pachypoda*) produces white fruit in rich woodlands from Canada to Georgia and west to the Rocky Mountains. The European variety may be more toxic.

The rootstock, sap, and berries contain glycosides or essential oils that produce gastroenteritis.

Ingestion of six berries produces gastroenteritis within 30 minutes. Confusion, headache, and distorted visual perception have been reported, followed by tachycardia, abdominal pain, lethargy, dry mouth, and eructation.

Treatment

- Decontamination measures are reasonable if given within the first several hours.

Questions—Baneberry

1. Baneberry ingestion is associated with gastroenteritis.
A. True
B. False

BRACKEN

Bracken is found in mountainous areas. Occasionally, the fronds are put into floral displays and are used in table decorations. Bracken contains thiaminase, which destroys thiamine and results in a vitamin B deficiency poisoning in horses and cattle. It has not been reported to be toxic to children when ingested. Bracken is carcinogenic in animal species perhaps due to shimic. Further data are required to establish a firm carcinogenic association with bracken.

Treatment

- Decontamination measures generally are not necessary.

Questions—Bracken

1. Bracken causes vitamin B deficiency in horses and cattle, however human toxicity has not been well established.
A. True
B. False

BUCKEYE

These deciduous trees and shrubs contain palmately divided leaflets on a long stalk. Yellow, red, and white flowers produce a characteristic three-compartment fruit surrounded by a leathery husk that encloses brown, glossy seeds. Seven native species appear throughout the United States.

This genus contains the alkaloid aesculin, which is capable of causing weakness, ataxia, dilated pupils, nausea, vomiting and obtundation. Most ingestions of horse chestnut by children result in no symptoms. GI distress is the most common symptom complex.

Treatment

- Only ingestion of several horse chestnuts or more requires decontamination.

Questions—Buckeye

1. Buckeye toxin is called
A. Aesculin
B. Buckrin
C. Alkaline
D. Abrin
E. Tetrodotoxin

BUCKTHORN

This poisonous shrub grows along canyons and gullies of the southwestern United States and northern and central Mexico. The common buckthorn is an ornamental plant used as a hedge and is now naturalized in the eastern United States. A brownish black berry matures from clusters of greenish flowers.

Pathophysiology

The seeds of *Karwinskia humboldtiana* contain an unidentified neurotoxin that produces an ascending paralysis similar to Guillain-Barré syndrome. Injection of the toxin into experimental animals produces a segmental demyelination of peripheral nerves, probably because of disruption of Schwann cell metabolism. Common buckthorn contains glycosides that are strong cathartics.

Clinical Presentations

Chronic consumption of *Karwinskia humboldtiana* has caused a progressive, symmetrical polyneuropathy that resulted in flaccid quadriplegia and respiratory insufficiency complicated by pneumonia. Sural nerve biopsy revealed segmental demyelination. Exposure to common buckthorn causes primarily diarrhea but no serious symptoms.

Answers to questions in shaded boxes appear at the end of the chapter.

Treatment

- Decontamination is not necessary.

Questions—Buckthorn

1. **Buckthorn has been associated with a neurotoxin that can cause an ascending paralysis similar to Guillain-Barré syndrome.**
   A. True
   B. False

BULBS

Daffodil bulbs contain a high concentration of the GI irritant alkaloid lycoramine. Lesser amounts of lycoramine are present in the stems, leaves, and flowers. A second, more powerful alkaloid is galanthamine. This compound appears in the bulb, but its contribution to toxicity has not been delineated. In animal models, both alkaloids are powerful GI irritants and central nervous system stimulants and can cause death.

Poisoning most often occurs when daffodil bulbs are mistaken for edible bulbs such as onions. Vomiting, abdominal pain, lightheadedness and occasionally diarrhea appear soon after ingestion and symptoms usually resolve within 3 hours. Similar GI symptoms may occur after consumption of jonquil (*Narcissus jonquilla*) leaves, except that symptoms may last over 24 hours. Plant and flower parts may cause a dermatitis ("lily rash") commonly seen in horticulturists. Other members of the family Amaryllidaceae, such as amaryllis, produce self-limited GI symptoms.

Zygandenus Species

Zygandenus species are perennial herbs with narrow, grasslike leaves (appearing mostly at the base) and thick, horizontal rootstock. Yellow or whitish-green flowers form along the top of a central stalk. Most poisonings involve mistaken ingestion of the onionlike bulbs. *Zygandenus* bulbs lack the characteristic onion odor. About 15 species are found throughout the United States. They apparently vary in their toxicity. Animal and human poisonings are reported more commonly from the western United States.

Zygandenus species contain veratrumlike alkaloids (see Veratrum section) that decrease blood pressure and heart rate as well as suppress respiration in experimental animals. The primary effects of these alkaloids are hypotension, bradycardia, GI distress and neurologic depression. Cardiovascular changes are thought to result from changes in autonomic function. Hypotension develops secondary to peripheral venodilation rather than bradycardia. Toxicity has resulted from consumption of both bulbs and blossoms.

Other Gastroenteritis-Producing Bulbs

Other bulbs may produce GI symptoms, although their toxicity in humans is not well documented in the medical literature. Fluid and electrolyte imbalance represents the major concern in those patients demonstrating protracted vomiting or diarrhea. Decontamination measures are appropriate after ingestions that are more than a casual contact.

Hyacinth (*Hyacinthus orientalis*), a member of the lily family, contains a toxic alkaloid. Iris plants may cause mucosal irritation as well as GI symptoms, but the course usually is mild and self-limited. Illness resulted from the prolonged use of bulbs as food sources during World War II in Holland. Buttercup (*Ranunculus spp*), a native California species, contains an irritant oil called protoanemonin, which is mildly toxic to the GI tract.

Treatment

- The usual measures of decontamination are recommended within the first several hours if copious vomiting has not occurred. Because of the rapid onset of action, such measures are probably not beneficial after 3 to 4 hours.
- Atropine usually reverses bradycardia but may not improve perfusion. Because of vasodilation, hypotension is treated with fluids and vasopressors if necessary. Patients with vital sign abnormalities or central nervous system depression should be observed for 12 to 24 hours.

Questions—Bulbs

1. **Which of the following is false?**
   A. Daffodil bulbs contain a high concentration of a hallucinogen.
   B. Amaryllis produces self-limited gastrointestinal symptoms.
   C. *Zygandenus* species are perennial herbs that are often mistaken for onionlike bulbs.
   D. *Zygandenus* species contain veratrumlike alkaloids that decrease blood pressure and heart rate as well as suppress respiration in experimental animals.
   E. Illness resulted from the use of bulbs as food sources during World War II in Holland.

COLCHICINE

Colchicine is approved for the treatment of acute gouty arthritis, for which it was first used in 1763. Colchicine is an alkaloid that can be obtained from the autumn crocus and glory lily. The bulb of the autumn crocus contains colchicine (0.8% by weight) and tubers of the glory lily contain about 0.3% by weight. Most serious ingestions result from the suicidal ingestion of colchicine tablets, which also are used to treat familial Mediterranean fever. Occasionally, the tubers of the glory lily have been mistakenly consumed because of their similarity to sweet potatoes.

Colchicine is a potent GI toxin and causes intractable multiorgan failure when ingested in large doses (over 0.8 mg/kg). Fatalities from suicidal ingestion of colchicine tablets are well reported in the medical literature. Toxic effects result from consumption of parts of these plants, but the severe reactions seen in colchicine tablet overdoses are less common because of the large volume of plant material needed to cause a toxic reaction.

Pathophysiology

Colchicine binds to tubulin and prevents its polymerization into microtubules. This antimitotic property disrupts the spindle apparatus that separates chromosomes during metaphase. Cells with high metabolic rates (e.g., intestinal epithelium, hair follicles, and bone marrow) are the most suppressed. Such inhibition of cellular division does not account for the multiorgan failure seen in severe colchicine overdoses. The variable effects of colchicine may depend on its binding to the protein subunit of microtubules with subsequent disruption of microtubule function.

Pharmacokinetics

ABSORPTION

- Colchicine is rapidly absorbed from the GI tract (30 to 120 minutes for peak plasma levels).

DISTRIBUTION

- The apparent volume of distribution exceeds total body water (about 2.2 L/kg) with an extremely short plasma half-life (20 minutes).

ELIMINATION

- Colchicine is primarily deacetylated by the liver, although as much as 20% may be excreted unchanged by the kidney.
- Large amounts of both parent drug and metabolites are excreted in the bile and intestinal secretions, so that enterohepatic circulation probably is significant.

Clinical Presentations

GASTROINTESTINAL EFFECTS

All seriously poisoned patients develop signs of GI distress manifested by nausea, vomiting, diarrhea, and abdominal pain within 1 to 6 hours of ingestion. A neurogenic rather than direct irritant action is the suspected cause. In experimental studies, atropine and anesthesia abolish the diarrhea of colchicine excess and colchicine has no direct stimulant action on isolated segments of the small bowel. Volume depletion and hypotension may occur during this period. An ileus commonly develops within the first several days and persists for a week.

MULTISYSTEM FAILURE

Life-threatening complications often develop 24 to 72 hours postingestion. Increasing hypoxemia results from diffuse interstitial and alveolar edema presumably caused by capillary leakage, because pulmonary capillary wedge pressures usually are normal. Confusion and delirium may develop secondary to poor cerebral perfusion or because of direct cerebral toxicity. Papilledema, coma, seizures, and cerebral edema have complicated a few fatal colchicine overdose cases. *Gloriosa* tuber ingestion has resulted in an ascending polyneuropathy characterized by stocking-glove anesthesia, weakness, and loss of deep tendon reflexes that required 4 weeks to resolve.

RENAL EFFECTS

Dysuria, hematuria, and proteinuria are common, however renal dysfunction probably is secondary to hypoxia, hypotension, and myoglobinuria. The contribution of direct colchicine toxicity to renal failure is unclear, but severe renal dysfunction is not a prominent part of most fatal overdose cases. Rhabdomyolysis may occur in acute poisoning, with dramatic increases in muscle enzymes and myoglobinuria.

HEMATOLOGIC EFFECTS

In the initial stage, a peripheral leukocytosis occurs frequently, with numerous immature myeloid cells. Bone marrow suppression follows and reaches a nadir between the fourth and seventh day after ingestion. A consumptive coagulopathy also may be seen during this period. A lack of bone marrow suppression suggests mild toxicity.

CARDIOVASCULAR EFFECTS

Sudden cardiac arrest has occurred between 36 and 54 hours after ingestion despite adequate oxygenation and fluid and electrolyte replacement. Most deaths result from shock within the first 72 hours. Patients with hemodynamic features of cardiogenic shock or patients in whom plasma infusion fails to improve the cardiac index have a poor prognosis. Direct myocardial toxic effects have not been documented.

RECOVERY PHASE

By the 10th day, most organ systems show definite signs of improvement. A rebound leukocytosis often occurs. Alopecia begins by the 12th day and is complete by 3 weeks after ingestion. Hair regrowth begins after the first month. Complete recovery from acute complications characterizes the convalescent period. Fever may be a persistent part of the clinical picture for the first several weeks but rarely exceeds 39°C. Sepsis is a well-recognized complication of colchicine overdose and should be considered whenever clinical deterioration occurs.

Toxic Dosage/Death

In one series, patients who ingested less than 0.5 mg of colchicine per kilogram survived with supportive care, whereas those who consumed more than 0.8 mg/kg invariably died. However, adults have died from ingestions reported to be in the range of 8 to 12 mg, in part because of individual sensitivity. Most fatalities occur within the first 24 to 72 hours. Because colchicine is a potent poison, children who ingest more than one tablet (0.5 mg) should receive decontamination measures. Plant toxicity is more difficult to predict, but decontamination measures also should be used in all patients except those who ingest small amounts during exploratory activity. All symptomatic patients should be medically evaluated.

Laboratory

ANALYTIC METHODS

Although colchicine can be measured in body fluids by high-performance liquid chromatography, these determinations are not clinically useful in case management.

BLOOD LEVELS

Postmortem colchicine blood concentrations definitely do not correlate with the severity of ingestion. A 2-hour postingestion colchicine level was 250 μ/L in a 39-year-old woman who consumed 18 to 21 g of colchicine, but no drug was detected at death 40 hours postingestion.

Treatment

GUT DECONTAMINATION

The usual measures of decontamination may be useful even 24 hours after ingestion in colchicine plant ingestions. A postmortem examination 30 hours after glory lily ingestion in one case revealed 196 mg of colchicine in the victim's stomach. The enterohepatic circulation of colchicine suggests that serial activated charcoal may be useful, although human cases are too rare to support clinical trials. Paralytic ileus may complicate serial-activated charcoal therapy and necessitate its discontinuance.

ELIMINATION ENHANCEMENT

Serial-activated charcoal is a theoretical method of enhancing elimination. There is no evidence that hemoperfusion or hemodialysis increases elimination of colchicine, especially in view of its large volume of distribution and limited renal excretion.

SUPPORTIVE MEASURES

- Initially, hypotension represents the most serious risk. An IV line with fluid replacement (normal saline or Ringer's lactate)

should be established first and then vasopressors given if the hypotension does not respond to fluid challenges.
- Symptomatic patients (e.g., those with nausea, vomiting, diarrhea, dyspnea) should be hospitalized for fluid replacement and medical observation in a monitored setting. Respiratory dysfunction usually is secondary to the adult respiratory distress syndrome, which commonly presents 24 to 36 hours postingestion. Follow respiratory status closely, because increasing hypoxemia suggests the onset of this syndrome.
- Fluid administration often requires hemodynamic monitoring to replace losses accurately. The hemodynamic response to fluid administration has prognostic value as those patients who show continuing cardiogenic shock have a poor prognosis.
- Frequent monitoring of electrolytes is necessary in the first several days. Electrolyte abnormalities may persist for a week. Hypoglycemia, myoglobinuria, and creatine kinase levels also should be checked. Urinary alkalinization may be necessary if myoglobinuria persists.
- A consumptive coagulopathy may appear within the first several days and usually responds to vitamin K and fresh-frozen plasma. The prothrombin time, partial thromboplastin time, and platelet count should be monitored daily for the first several days and then as indicated. Fibrinogen and fibrin split product levels also should be obtained if a coagulopathy is suspected.
- Daily complete blood count levels are important to detect either hemolytic anemias or upper GI hemorrhages. Transfusions of both platelet packs and packed red blood cells may be needed.
- Sepsis may complicate the clinical course, especially during the nadir of bone marrow suppression between the fourth and seventh days. Patients who have fever and/or hemodynamic instability should have blood cultures and perhaps broad-spectrum antibiotic coverage. Fever is not a specific sign of infection, because it often accompanies overdose.
- Hypothermia is a poor prognostic sign and should be treated with the usual passive rewarming measures.
- Hepatic aminotransferase levels may be elevated moderately, but fulminant hepatic failure is not a common occurrence. Hyperamylasemia has been reported. Hypocalcemia, hypophosphatemia, and hypokalemia may persist for days.
- Metabolic acidosis may be present initially but usually responds to supportive care. Rhabdomyolysis and myoglobinuria may occur as a result of direct muscle damage.
- The electrocardiogram (ECG) may show signs of myocardial injury, with both creatine kinase and initial MB isoenzyme fractions increased.

Questions—Colchicine

1. Which of the following about colchicine is false?
  A. Colchicine is used for the treatment of gouty arthritis.
  B. Colchicine is an alkaloid that can be obtained from the autumn crocus and glory lily.
  C. Colchicine is a potent gastrointestinal toxin and causes intractable multiorgan failure when ingested in large doses.
  D. Colchicine binds to tubulin and prevents its polymerization into microtubules.
  E. Colchicine does not affect the central nervous system, as transfer across the blood-brain barrier is quite limited.

2. All seriously colchicine-poisoned patients develop signs of gastrointestinal distress manifested by nausea, vomiting, diarrhea, and abdominal pain within 1 to 6 hours of ingestion.
  A. True
  B. False

CYCADS

Cycads are tropical plants with palmlike leaves that grow outward encircling a central trunk. The seeds of the false sago palm have been used as a dietary staple for the Chamorro indigenous population of the Mariana Islands in the Western Pacific. The leaves and seeds of the false sago palm contain a glycoside, cycasin, and an unusual nonprotein amino acid found in the pea, *Lathyrus sativus* (see Sweet Pea and Lathyrism) called BMAA. Much evidence links motor neuron disease parkinsonism in Guam to BMAA.

Treatment

- Treatment of this syndrome is symptomatic and supportive. If children ingest the seeds, syrup of ipecac or gastric emptying reduces exposure.

Questions—Cycads

1. Cycads, tropical plants found in Guam, have been associated with Parkinsonism.
  A. True
  B. False

DAPHNE

Daphne is a small, deciduous shrub that grows 1 to 4 feet high and has simple alternate leaves. Small lilac-purple, fragrant flowers appear before the leaves. It is cultivated throughout the United States as an ornamental shrub and has naturalized in the eastern United States. All plant parts contain a glycoside in which the aglycone is dihydroxycoumarin. The toxin has been called daphnin, but is not well characterized. An extract of the seed known as mezerein has been identified and has been shown to possess activity against lymphocytic leukemia in mice. Reports of Daphne toxicity are rare. Frequently mentioned symptoms in textbooks include local irritation, nausea, vomiting, abdominal pain, weakness, and diarrhea, which may become bloody.

Treatment

- Treatment consists of decontamination and supportive care.

Questions—Daphne

1. Daphne has been associated with multisystem failure and irreversible pulmonary fibrosis.
  A. True
  B. False

DOG'S MERCURY

Dog's mercury is a common woodland plant found in Britain with serrate, opposite leaves and clusters of flowers on a central stalk. The American species is a common weed found in uncultivated areas. The active principle is thought to be the volatile basic oil mercurialine. Ingestion of a tea made from *Mercurialis perennis* produced severe gastroenteritis and trace hemoglobinuria without liver or renal dysfunction. Pronounced anisocytosis was present in blood smears, but no changes in hemoglobin concentration occurred. Hemolysis, hepatic centrilobar necrosis, and GI distress occur in animal poisoning but have not been reported in human poisoning.

Treatment

- Treatment is supportive.

Questions—Dog's Mercury

1. **Hemolysis, hepatic centrilobar necrosis, and gastrointestinal distress have been reported in human poisoning from dog's mercury.**
   A. True
   B. False

FOXGLOVE

Foxglove is a beautiful biennial herb with simple toothed leaves and a central stalk of purple, pink, yellow, or white tubular flowers. It is a popular ornamental flower found in the western United States. Digitalis leaf is obtained for medicinal use by the grinding and milling of *Digitalis purpurea* leaves. Foxglove contains a number of cardiac glycosides, the most prominent of which is digitoxin. The cardiac glycosides of *Digitalis purpurea* are hydrolyzed to digitoxin, gitoxin, and gitalin with only small amounts of digoxin formed from liver metabolism. *Digitalis purpurea* toxicity may be prolonged because of the long serum half-life of digitoxin (4 to 5 days).

Clinical Presentations

Foxglove toxicity resembles oleander and digitoxin poisoning. GI symptoms develop within several hours and may be followed by confusion, cardiac conduction defects, hyperkalemia, and dysrhythmias. Visual disturbances such as yellow haloes are classic symptoms of Digitalis leaf poisoning but usually are not seen with commercial digoxin poisoning. Ventricular tachycardia, junctional rhythms, and atrial fibrillation with high-grade atrioventricular block have been reported in foxglove tea poisoning.

Treatment

- Management is similar to that for oleander and digoxin poisoning.
- Elevated digitoxin levels confirm toxicity (in the absence of simultaneous consumption of Digitalis preparations) but do not guide management, because of cross-reactivity.

Antidotes

There is little published clinical experience with botanical cardiac glycoside poisoning and the use of digoxin Fab fragments.

Questions—Foxglove

1. **Which of the following is false?**
   A. Digitalis is derived from foxglove.
   B. The most common cardiac glycoside in digitalis is digitoxin.
   C. Foxglove toxicity resembles oleander and digitoxin poisoning.
   D. Fab fragments routinely have been used to counteract the toxicity of Foxglove tea poisoning.
   E. Ventricular tachycardia, junctional rhythms, and atrial fibrillation with high-grade atrioventricular block have been reported in foxglove tea poisoning.

GOLDENSEAL

Goldenseal is a stout perennial found deep in rich woods from Vermont to Arkansas in the United States. It produces dark red berries in April and May and green-white flowers. The rhizomes are golden yellow and knotted in appearance. Goldenseal has been used as a uterine hemostatic. Goldenseal had gained the reputation of being able to prevent the detection of morphine, marijuana, or cocaine in urine samples. Studies have found no basis for this belief.

Goldenseal contains the alkaloids hydrastine (about 4%) and berberine (up to 6%) with smaller amounts of hydrastinine, canadine, and related alkaloids. Berberine has weak antibiotic activity and some antineoplastic activity. Hydrastine can cause exaggerated reflexes, hypertension, convulsions, and death from respiratory failure. Large doses of the plant irritate the mouth and throat, and can cause nausea, vomiting, diarrhea and paresthesias. Central nervous system stimulation and respiratory failure induced by the plant can be fatal.

Treatment

- Treatment is supportive.

Questions—Goldenseal

1. **Goldenseal has gained a reputation**
   A. As an easily acquired, "legal" hallucinogen
   B. For its purported ability to prevent the detection of marijuana or cocaine in urine samples.
   C. As a "natural" antiinflammatory agent
   D. As a "natural" abortifacient
   E. None of the above

JIMSONWEED AND ANTICHOLINERGIC PLANTS

Datura grows as a weed throughout the United States, particularly in rich, disturbed soils such as barnyards. There are more than a dozen species of this naturalized Asian plant, with *Datura stramonium* being most common in the eastern United States. Its toxic, mind-altering properties have been known since ancient times. Selected References to Datura may be found in Homer's *Odyssey* and in Shakespeare's *Romeo and Juliet* and *Antony and Cleopatra*. Historical accounts in the United States date back to 1676 when British soldiers sent to Jamestown to put down the Bacon rebellion mistakenly ate Datura, "the effect of which was a very pleasant comedy, for they turned natural fools upon it for several days."

Datura is a common annual weed that grows 3 to 6 feet high and emits a rank odor. It has a simple, large, white taproot and a strong, dichotomous stem. The leaves are large, waxy, and dark green with pointed margins and scalloped borders. Attractive, white tubular flowers bloom in late spring and grow 3 to 4 inches long. Later, a green burrlike fruit appears that ripens in early fall. The dried pod may contain up to 500 2 to 3 mm kidney-shaped seeds.

All parts of the Datura plant are poisonous. Toxic effects have been reported after ingestion of teas brewed from plant parts, ingestion of leaves and flowers, and smoking of stramonium cigarettes. Seed ingestion now is the most common route of toxicity. Over-the-counter asthma preparations containing Datura products have been marketed for years and abused by the teenage population. The most common intoxication now involves teenagers seeking the mind-altering properties of the seeds, which appear in the autumn.

Pathophysiology

The toxins in *Datura* species are tropane belladonna alkaloids (e.g., atropine, hyoscyamine, and scopolamine), which possess strong anticholinergic properties. See Chapter 34, Anticholinergic Drugs. The exact concentration of specific alkaloids varies between species as well as with cultivation, environmental, and storage factors. Because there are structural similarities between these alkaloids, they are absorbed easily from mucous membranes, skin, and intestinal tract. Other anticholinergic plants include:

ATROPA BELLADONNA

A. belladonna (Deadly Nightshade) contains the alkaloid 1-hyoscyamine which represents about 75% of total alkaloid content, with most of the remainder being scopolamine. The roots and leaves have the highest total alkaloid content followed by seeds and berries.

HYOSCYAMUS NIGER

H. niger (Henbane) contains tropane alkaloids, with the leaves containing from 0.05% to 0.15% of the total alkaloid content. Like *A. belladonna*, most of the alkaloids are 1-hyoscyamine and the rest are primarily scopolamine (1-hyoscine).

MANDRAGORA OFFICINARUM

M. officinarum (Mandrake) contains 1-hyoscyamine and scopolamine, as well as small amounts of the unidentified alkaloid mandragorine.

Clinical Presentations

The classical presentation for Datura toxicity is the anticholinergic poisoning syndrome described by the phrase "blind as a bat, hot as a hare, dry as a bone, red as a beet, and mad as a wet hen." Symptoms begin within 2 to 6 hours after ingestion. See Chapter 34, Anticholinergic Drugs. Consumption of Datura tea may result in symptoms within 5 to 10 minutes. Dryness of the mouth frequently is the earliest sign of intoxication followed by pupillary dilation.

The classical presentation of a severe intoxication is fever, erythema, dilated pupils, blurred vision, delirium, and hallucinations. Hallucinations usually involve simple images in natural colors, in contrast with the brilliant displays seen with lysergic acid diethylamide (LSD). The presence of bowel sounds and diaphoresis suggests an adrenergic (e.g., cocaine, amphetamine) poisoning rather than an anticholinergic (e.g., jimsonweed) one. Seizures may occur but are uncommon. Symptoms usually resolve in 24 to 48 hours, although pupillary dilation may continue up to 1 week.

Toxic Dosage/Death

In case studies the amounts ingested have not been determined well enough to predict symptoms from the history of ingestion. Based on calculations of hyoscyamine content, 50 to 100 Datura seeds contain the equivalent of 3 to 6 mg of atropine, which would cause severe intoxication upon ingestion. Fatalities usually result from trauma or drowning rather than direct toxic effects.

Treatment

GUT DECONTAMINATION

Patients seen early in their course (4 to 6 hours) may benefit from the usual measures of gut decontamination. Generally, tropane alkaloids are well absorbed in solution although their anticholinergic properties may delay absorption of vegetable matter and seeds. Hence, symptomatic patients with an intact gag reflex may benefit from emetics or lavage 12 to 24 hours after ingestion.

ELIMINATION ENHANCEMENT

Enhancement of elimination of atropine by extracorporeal means (e.g., peritoneal dialysis, hemoperfusion) has not been evaluated but is not likely to be effective in view of the large volume of distribution. In overdoses reported to date, recovery has been achieved without these procedures.

SUPPORTIVE MEASURES

- Patients with mild symptoms may be discharged from the emergency department after 4 to 6 hours of observation if symptoms are improving.
- Most patients respond well to supportive and protective measures. The patient should be placed in a calm, reassuring environment with a familiar person. Pharmacological intervention should be limited to patients who fail to respond to a calm environment and present a danger to themselves.
- Laboratory elevations of aspartate aminotransferase, lactate dehydrogenase (LDH), and bilirubin levels and prothrombin time have been reported.
- Valium and hydroxyzine have been used for agitation, but care must be exercised not to heavily sedate these patients. Because of their anticholinergic properties, phenobarbital, phenothiazines, and haloperidol should not be used.
- Vital signs should be monitored every 15 to 20 minutes until improvement is noted. Hypertension usually is transient and requires no therapy. Hyperthermia may be treated with a cooling blanket or a sponge bath. Catheterization may be necessary for urinary retention.
- Patients requiring physostigmine should be admitted for at least 24 hours of observation.
- Patients who exhibit central nervous system symptoms (e.g., disorientation, hallucinations, and delusions) should be observed until those symptoms resolve.

Antidotes

PHYSOSTIGMINE

Physostigmine is an antagonist to serious atropine poisoning (e.g., severe central nervous system or peripheral anticholinergic symptoms, dysrhythmias, seizures, hypertension and/or hallucinations). The initial adult dose is 1 to 2 mg (0.01 to 0.03 mg/

kg) intramuscularly or intravenously over 2 to 5 minutes. Improvement usually is seen within 15 minutes and a second dose may be repeated in 20 to 30 minutes.

Cholinergic excess manifested by bradycardia, heart block, and excessive secretions may accompany physostigmine use, and must be carefully monitored. Repeated doses should be given only if symptoms reappear. Relative contraindications to the administration of physostigmine include a history of cardiovascular disease, gangrene, asthma, glaucoma, and GI or genitourinary obstruction.

Questions—Jimsonweed and Anticholinergic Plants

1. Which of the following is anticholinergic?
A. Hyoscyamine
B. Atropine
C. Scopolamine
D. All of the above
E. B and C

2. Which of the following is not an anticholinergic plant?
A. *Datura stramonium*
B. *Atropa belladonna*
C. *Hyoscyamus niger*
D. *Mandragora officinarum*
E. *Lantana camara*

LABURNUM

Laburnum or golden chain is a beautiful flowering tree native to southern Europe and grown in the northern United States and southern Canada as an ornamental tree. Flowers bloom in May and June and mature into green pods containing two to seven kidney-shaped seeds. Most poisonings occur in children between July and September when they ingest the attractive pods and seeds. Laburnum ingestion is a common occurrence in England however serious toxicity is rare.

Pathophysiology

Laburnum contains the toxic alkaloid cytisine, which is structurally and pharmacologically similar to nicotine and lobeline. Laburnum seeds are said to contain 1% cytisine by weight. The estimated lethal dose is 0.5 mg/kg. Prediction of symptoms remains difficult, especially because cytisine content varies throughout the season.

Clinical Presentations

Most children who ingest seeds develop no symptoms. Some develop mild to moderate symptoms when 1 to 10 seedpods are consumed. Symptoms start 1/2 to 4 hours after ingestion and include nausea, vomiting, abdominal pain, pallor, lightheadedness, drowsiness, and ataxia. Dilated pupils, tachycardia, paralysis, and delirium may occur in serious cases. Death is believed to be the result of respiratory depression. Symptoms typically resolve within 12 hours and rarely require more than 12 to 24 hours for resolution.

Treatment

- Decontamination measures are indicated for ingestion of more than one to two seeds after the usual precautions have been observed. Management is supportive.
- Most children can be safely discharged after 4 to 6 hours of observation, providing vital signs and physical examination have returned to normal.

Questions—Laburnum

1. Cytisine, the toxin found in laburnum, is structurally related to
A. Ricin
B. Grayanotoxin
C. Nicotine
D. Sea anemone toxin
E. Atropine

LANTANA

Lantana is a perennial shrub with simple, serrated leaves and heads of multicolored flowers. It is used as an ornamental shrub in California and the southern United States, where it has become established in the wilds, along fences, and ditchbanks. Poisonings in grazing animals are frequent. Lantana consumption by grazing animals has caused widespread livestock loss in South Africa, Australia, India, Mexico, and the United States. A variety of Lantana species occur throughout the world, but *Lantana camara* appears to be the most widespread and toxic to animals.

Pathophysiology

The major toxin in *L. camara* appears to be lantadene A, a triterpenoid that is structurally identical to rehmannic acid. Lantadene B is a structurally similar substance extracted from *L. camara* but appears to be pharmacologically inactive. Lantadene A content varies between plant parts and season. In children, ripe berries appear nontoxic, whereas green berries ingested in the spring and fall have produced serious toxic effects and death. The exact mechanism of toxicity is not known. Lantana poisoning in animals causes widespread changes in mitochondrial, microsomal, and membrane enzymes.

Clinical Presentations

In animals grazing on Lantana, an acute cholestatic jaundice develops and is characterized by weakness, vomiting, anorexia, jaundice, conjunctivitis, blindness, mucosal ulcerations, and photosensitization. Death can occur within 7 to 10 days. The chronic form is similar, but dehydration and renal failure are more prominent.

In children, ingestion of green berries may cause nausea, vomiting, lethargy, depressed respiration and tendon reflexes, dilated pupils, and death. Symptoms begin within 2 to 3 hours and at least one reported death from acute pulmonary edema and cardiovascular collapse has occurred 2 hours after ingestion.

Treatment

- The mainstay of management is decontamination followed by supportive care.
- Children should be observed closely for 4 to 6 hours postingestion, and a physician should evaluate symptomatic children.

Questions—Lantana

1. **In children, green Lantana berries appear nontoxic, whereas ripe berries ingested in the spring and fall have produced serious toxic effects and death.**
   A. True
   B. False

LILY OF THE VALLEY

Lily of the valley is a native European plant that is grown as a garden flower in the United States. A related species, *Convallaria Montana*, grows in the Appalachian Mountains. It is a perennial plant with slender rootstock and fragrant white bell-shaped flowers originating from a central stalk. The leaves are long and broad, typical of the lily family. The plant contains cardiac glycosides, called convallatoxins, but apparently these glycosides are less potent than digoxin or digitalis.

Clinical Presentations

Human toxic reactions are poorly reported in the medical literature. GI distress is the most common side effect, although the potential for a digitalislike poisoning (i.e., like oleander poisoning) exists when large quantities or teas have been ingested.

Treatment

- Because of the low potency of *Convallaria*, small ingestions probably do not require decontamination. Large ingestions may benefit from decontamination and supportive care.

Questions—Lily Of The Valley

1. **Lily of the valley contains a well documented, deadly cardiac glycoside.**
   A. True
   B. False

NICOTINE AND LOBELINE

Nicotine products for cigars, cigarettes, and pipes occur in nature. See Nicotine section, Chapter 38, Household Products.

Pathophysiology

Initially, nicotine stimulates sympathetic and parasympathetic ganglia via a direct acetylcholinergiclike action on the ganglion. This stimulatory phase may be brief and is followed by prolonged ganglionic blockade resulting from persistent depolarization. Similar excitatory-inhibitory phases occur in the cardiovascular and central nervous systems and at the neuromuscular junction.

NICOTIANA TABACUM

Nicotine is the major toxic alkaloid of commercial tobacco with a concentration in tobacco leaves ranging from 1.5% to 4% by dry weight. The blending of tobacco in cigarettes and cigars results in an average nicotine content of 1% to 2%. Hence, an average cigarette contains between 10 to 20 mg of nicotine.

NICOTIANA GLAUCA

This plant contains the alkaloid anabasine, which is pharmacologically similar to nicotine. Anabasine is a minor alkaloid in the common tobacco plant, but is present in the *N. glauca* leaf at a concentration of 1.3% by weight.

LOBELIA INFLATA

L. inflata contains at least 14 different piperidine alkaloids of which lobeline is the principal one with a concentration of approximately 0.3%. Structurally and pharmacologically, lobeline is similar to nicotine. The dried herb was used by eastern North American Indians as a purgative and emetic. Interestingly, the North American Indians also incorporated the herb into tobacco leaves for smoking. Lobeline sulfate has been advocated in tablets as a tobacco substitute to aid people in breaking the smoking habit, but its efficacy is questionable.

Pharmacokinetics

ABSORPTION

- Nicotine is well absorbed from the skin, lungs, and GI tract, and poisonings have been documented from all three routes of exposure.
- Peak nicotine levels in smokers appear about 10 minutes after inhalation.
- Nicotine appears to be poorly absorbed in the acid pH of the stomach, and in fact some nicotine excretion occurs into the stomach. Clinical ingestion of liquid nicotine pesticides (40% nicotine concentrations) however, has resulted in death within 5 to 10 minutes.

DISTRIBUTION

- Nicotine toxicity is characterized by a rapid onset of action (30 to 60 minutes).
- Dermal absorption of a 95% nicotine solution has resulted in coma and respiratory failure.
- Intravenously administered nicotine in doses commonly found in cigarettes has a volume of distribution of 1.7 times body weight.

ELIMINATION

- About 80% to 90% of administered nicotine is metabolized rapidly by the liver into inactive compounds such as cotinine and nicotine-1′-N-oxide, which then are excreted by the kidney.
- The amount of nicotine excreted unchanged by the kidney varies with urinary pH.

Clinical Presentations

The onset of symptoms after nicotine exposures usually is rapid (15 to 30 minutes) beginning with GI distress manifested by vomiting, nausea, salivation, abdominal pain, and diarrhea. Neurologic symptoms of headache, diaphoresis, ataxia, lightheadedness, weakness, confusion, and, in severe poisonings, convulsions and coma follow. Miosis, lacrimation, bronchorrhea, loss of deep tendon reflexes, fasciculations, and paralysis may be seen. Paralysis of respiratory muscles may occur and necessitates intubation.

Transiently, hypertension and tachycardia may develop followed by hypotension, bradycardia, and cardiovascular collapse. Symptoms in mild poisonings resolve in several hours. In severe poisoning, 24 hours may be required for restoration of homeostasis. Leukocytosis and glycosuria may be seen, but most laboratory values are normal. Deaths have been associated with the mistaken consumption of tobacco leaves.

TREE TOBACCO

The ingestion of tree tobacco leaves (*N. glauca*) has resulted in a nicotinelike poisoning, with initial hypertension and coma followed by neuromuscular blockade and respiratory failure requiring intubation for 24 hours. Symptoms, however, were delayed (1 hour to onset of symptoms), perhaps because of slower absorption of anabasine. Anabasine, not nicotine, is likely teratogenic.

GREEN TOBACCO SICKNESS

Picking green tobacco in a moist environment has been associated with an occupational disease called green tobacco sickness. Characteristic symptoms include headache, pallor, nausea, vomiting, weakness, lightheadedness, and abdominal pain. The disease is self-limited and resolves by the following day. Cigarette smokers rarely display symptoms of green tobacco sickness, suggesting that a tolerance to nicotine may be developed through chronic smoking.

Toxic Dosage/Death

The estimated lethal adult dose of nicotine is 60 mg. This amounts to the nicotine content of three to six cigarettes. The extraction of the nicotine from five to 10 cigarettes in hot water and the subsequent administration of the fluid as an enema have resulted in moderately severe poisoning. Although most cases of cigarette consumption by children result in no or mild symptoms, severe poisonings characterized by depressed respirations, dysrhythmias, and convulsions have been reported after the ingestion of two cigarettes by 9- and 10-month-old infants. Flaccidity, bradycardia, and sinoatrial block developed in an infant who reportedly ingested one-half of a cigarette.

Treatment

GUT DECONTAMINATION

Most children only taste tobacco and develop no symptoms. Ingestion of more than one half to one cigarette may lead to symptoms and consumption of more than two cigarettes may cause serious effects. Decontamination measures are indicated in children who ingest more than one cigarette. Charcoal and lavage are preferable to ipecac because of rapid onset of nicotine effects.

ELIMINATION ENHANCEMENT

Continuous nasogastric suction and serial activated charcoal are theoretically advantageous, but have not been tested in the clinical setting. Acidification of urine also has theoretical advantages, but its complicated effects and nicotine's short duration of action limits the use of acid diuresis.

SUPPORTIVE MEASURES

- Serious poisonings are followed in an intensive care setting for the development of respiratory failure within the first 12 hours. Seizures are treated with diazepam.
- As respiratory failure represents the greatest risk to life, an initial evaluation must be done to ensure adequate ventilation. Patients with altered sensorium should receive intravenous lines, cardiac monitoring, oxygen, and arterial blood gases in addition to the usual doses of glucose and naloxone.
- The initial hypertension and tachycardia should not be treated aggressively unless they represent a definite risk, because a depressive phase of bradycardia and hypotension often follows.
- All skin contaminated with nicotine solutions must be thoroughly washed with a nonalkaline soap and cool water.

Antidotes

Atropine may improve bradycardia and hypotension but does not reverse muscular weakness.

Questions—Nicotine and Lobeline

1. Initially, nicotine stimulates sympathetic and parasympathetic ganglia via a direct acetylcholinergic-like action on the ganglion. This stimulatory phase may be brief and is followed by prolonged ganglionic blockade resulting from persistent depolarization.

A. True
B. False

2. Severe poisonings characterized by depressed respirations, dysrhythmias, and convulsions have been reported after the ingestion of how many cigarettes by 9- and 10-month-old infants?

A. 1
B. 2
C. 5
D. 10
E. 20

OLEANDER

The Greeks, Romans, and Hindus all considered the oleander seriously toxic. Although the root and the bark have been used in India for skin diseases and leprosy, the whole plant is considered poisonous. Preparations of oleander have been used as rodenticides and insecticides as well as remedies for indigestion, malaria, and venereal disease. The most commonly mentioned folk use is as an abortifacient. The Chinese used oleander extract for the treatment of mental disorders. The highest percentages of cardiac glycosides are found in seed, stems, and roots, followed by the fruit and leaves, but the leaves contain the greatest oleandrin concentrations.

In the United States, oleander is present throughout the temperate regions from California to Florida, and is used extensively in dry climates as a flowering shrub along roadsides and in gardens. The plant appears throughout the world in Mediterranean climates, including India and China. Australia, Hawaii, and southern Florida have a similar plant, the yellow oleander (*Thevetia peruviana* and *Thevetia thevetioides*).

Pathophysiology

Serious toxic effects result from the presence of numerous cardiac glycosides. Over 400 cardiac glycosides have been isolated in the plant kingdom, with most concentrated in the milkweed (*Asclepiadaceae*), figwort (*Serophulariaceae*), lily (*Liliaceae*), and dogbane (*Apocynaceae*) families. The venom of the cane toad (*Bufo marinus*) also contains substantial amounts of cardiac glycosides. In addition to common oleander (*Nerium*) and yellow oleander (*Thevetia*), numerous plants are known to contain cardiac toxins.

Common oleander contains at least five cardiac glycosides (oleandrin, digitoxigenin, neriin, folinerin, and rosagenin) that apparently exert a digitoxinlike effect by inhibiting the sodium-potassium adenosine triphosphatase enzyme system. The resulting toxic syndrome resembles digitalis poisoning with marked hyperkalemia, conduction abnormalities, and ventricular arrhythmias in serious ingestions.

Clinical Presentations

Oleander poisoning may resemble digitoxin poisoning with predominantly GI and cardiac symptoms. Signs of digitalis poisoning include hyperkalemia, conduction abnormalities, and ventricular arrhythmias. Nausea and vomiting usually occur within several hours. Serious toxic effects and potential mortality may result from cardiotoxicity, but well documented cases of serious toxicity are lacking.

Toxic Dosage/Death

Ingestion of large amounts of oleander probably is required to cause toxic effects. A reported ingestion of three leaves by a 7-year-old resulted in a right bundle branch block but no symptoms.

Treatment

GUT DECONTAMINATION

Any symptomatic patient, any patient who ingests more than one leaf, or any patient suspected of ingesting more than one leaf should be given the usual measures to prevent absorption and should be referred to an emergency department or private physician. Serial charcoal has theoretical value since the pharmacokinetics of oleander are similar to those of digitoxin which has significant enterohepatic circulation.

ELIMINATION ENHANCEMENT

These methods generally are not utilized in the treatment of oleander exposures.

SUPPORTIVE MEASURES

- Casual contact by children usually does not result in serious morbidity.
- If the child is alert and the parents are absolutely convinced that the child ingested less than a leaf or flower, then such a child may be observed at home after emesis is induced.
- Serious mortality results from ventricular dysrhythmias. Prolonged EKG monitoring is required in serious cases.
- Hyperkalemia, elevated digoxin levels, conduction block, and ventricular ectopy are markers of serious toxicity. Serial potassium and creatinine levels should be monitored until a trend is established. Monitoring may be discontinued after normal sinus rhythm returns.
- Careful attention should be given to maintaining fluid and electrolyte balance.

Antidotes

Hemodynamic decompensation may require the temporary use of a cardiac pacemaker and digoxin-specific Fab antidote fragments. Doses of 200 mg and 480 mg intravenously have reportedly improved oleander intoxication; however, experience is limited.

Questions—Oleander

1. Oleander has been used for all of the following, except
A. As a rodenticide
B. As an antipruritic
C. As an insecticide
D. As an abortifacient
E. To treat mental disorders

2. All of the following contain cardiac glycosides, except
A. Milkweed (*Asclepiadaceae*)
B. Henbane (*Hyoscyamus niger*)
C. Figwort (*Serophulariaceae*)
D. Lily (*Liliaceae*)
E. Dogbane (*Apocynaceae*)

3. Which of the following is false?
A. The one cardiac glycoside in common oleander exerts a digitoxinlike effect by inhibiting the sodium-potassium adenosine triphosphatase enzyme system.
B. Signs of digitalis poisoning may include hyperkalemia, conduction abnormalities, and ventricular arrhythmias in serious ingestions.
C. Fab antidote fragments have been used to treat oleander poisoning.
D. A large amount of oleander is potentially lethal.
E. Oleander is common in the United States.

PODOPHYLLUM

American Indians used Mayapple roots medicinally as a cathartic. Since 1942, podophyllum resin, which is an extract of dried mandrake rhizomes and roots, has been used to cure warts, especially *condyloma acuminatum*. Two semisynthetic derivatives of podophyllotoxin have been tested for the treatment of acute leukemias and lymphomas.

Pathophysiology

Podophyllum resin extract, which often but incorrectly has been named "podophyllin," contains at least 16 active physiological compounds including podophyllotoxin, picropodophyllin (i.e., the cis isomer of podophyllotoxin), α- and β-pellatins, and quercetin. Podophyllum resin is a potent spindle poison that blocks mitosis in metaphase, similar to colchicine. Most human poisonings result from either topical application or ingestion of the commercial extract. Podophyllum resin solutions contain from 5% to 25% podophyllum resin concentrations as well as vehicles such as tincture of benzoin, salicylic acid, cantharidin, penederm, castor oil, ethanol, and acetone.

Clinical Presentations

Features of systemic toxicity include nausea, vomiting, peripheral neuropathy, fever, obtundation, coma, hypotension, oliguria, hyperpnea, adynamic ileus, and death. Symptoms may be delayed more than 10 hours. Overexposure causes neurologic, GI, and hematological toxicity that occasionally result in fatalities. Hematological suppression reaches a peak within 4 to 5 days. Bone marrow aspiration in several poisoning cases has revealed sudden maturational arrest of both erythroid and myeloid precursors. Rarely, poisoning results from consumption of unripe fruit or plant parts and causes primarily diarrhea.

NEUROLOGIC EFFECTS

Patients may develop changes in sensorium and peripheral neuropathies. In serious cases, lethargy and obtundation develop after 12 hours and may progress to convulsions, confusion, delirium, and prolonged coma. Over the course of several days, a symmetrical motor / sensory peripheral neuropathy develops distally and is characterized by profound bilateral weakness in the upper and lower extremities. Loss of deep tendon reflexes, vibration, position sense, and distal light touch occur. Changes in sensorium may require 10 to 15 days to clear.

RENAL EFFECTS

Renal failure has developed despite normal renal perfusion. This may represent a direct toxic effect to the kidney. Glycosuria and pyuria have been reported, but renal failure is uncommon.

PULMONARY EFFECTS

Direct pulmonary toxicity has not been reported, although tachypnea likely occurs as a result of respiratory compensation for a metabolic acidosis. The generalized weakness seen in severe poisonings may contribute to respiratory depression and the need for intubation in comatose patients. Previously, hyperventilation was thought to result from direct central neurogenic stimulation.

Toxic Dosage/Death

Death has resulted from ingestion of as little as 350 mg, whereas survival has occurred after 2.8 g and 10 g. Bone marrow suppression and a severe motor/sensory neuropathy developed in a 20-year-old woman when 3 mL of a 20% podophyllum resin solution was applied to *condyloma acuminatum*. The calculated dose was 150 mg. A child who received syrup of ipecac for the ingestion of 10 mL of an 8% podophyllum resin solution was discharged from the emergency department 6 hours after ingestion. Upon returning to the emergency department 9 hours postingestion, she was comatose, hypotensive, and hyperpyrexic.

Treatment

GUT DECONTAMINATION

Because of its oral toxicity, all patients who ingest podophyllum resin should be decontaminated. The usual measures of decontamination including syrup of ipecac, gastric lavage, and charcoal should be used for patients seen within 4 hours of exposure after standard precautions are observed.

ELIMINATION ENHANCEMENT

Hemodialysis probably is not effective because of the high lipid solubility of podophyllum resin. Hemoperfusion rapidly decreases plasma podophyllotoxin concentrations as assayed by thin-layer liquid chromatography however, the pharmacokinetics and plasma podophyllotoxin levels are not well enough understood to indicate whether or not hemoperfusion alters clinical outcome.

SUPPORTIVE MEASURES

- Any topical podophyllum resin solution should be removed with soap and water. Symptomatic patients should be hospitalized and observed for at least 24 hours. Children who ingest potentially toxic quantities (i.e., one swallow or 5 mL of the 20% podophyllum resin solution) should be directly observed for at least 8 hours.
- Serum electrolytes, fluids, and serum calcium levels should be followed closely.
- Metabolic acidosis may occur, especially in patients who are hyperventilating.
- Although fever may be seen with overdose, its presence also may indicate infection in patients whose susceptibility to infection peaks around 4 to 5 days postexposure. All patients who deteriorate during this period should have blood drawn for culture. Clinical judgment dictates the necessity of broad-spectrum antibiotics.
- In severe poisonings, complete blood counts, platelet counts, and coagulation profiles should be determined daily and replacement therapy with platelets, and red blood cell transfusions may be necessary. Initially, a profound leukocytosis may be present along with metamyelocytes and immature band forms.
- Severe poisonings have resulted in mild to moderately elevated levels of creatine kinase and hepatic aminotransferases, as well as hypocalcemia.

Questions—Podophyllum

1. Which of the following is false?
   A. Podophyllum is found in Mayapple roots
   B. Podophyllum resin, which is an extract of dried mandrake rhizomes and roots, has been used to cure warts, especially *condyloma acuminatum*
   C. Podophyllum also is called podophyllin.
   D. Podophyllum resin is a potent spindle poison that blocks mitosis similar to colchicines.
   E. Most human poisonings result from either topical application or ingestion of podophyllum commercial extract.

2. Which of the following is not associated with podophyllum poisoning?
   A. Urinary incontinence
   B. Nausea and vomiting
   C. Peripheral neuropathy
   D. Coma and death
   E. Renal failure

POISON HEMLOCK

Conium maculatum was used by the early Greeks as a means of suicide. Socrates probably died from *Conium* poisoning, as was the custom in Greek executions, although the characteristic ascending paralysis and terminal asphyxia of *Conium* poisoning are not well described in historical accounts.

Poison hemlock is a biennial weed that has a large taproot and lacy, fernlike leaves that reach 8 to 10 feet in height. The leaves are multiple pinnate and deeply divided into minute leaflets. The flowers are white and clustered into multiple umbrella-shaped groups. Conium grows as a luxuriant weed along roadsides, ditches, and open areas throughout the United States, especially in the north. Poisonings usually result from mistaken identification by people foraging for natural food. The plant may be mistaken for wild carrots, the leaves for parsley, and the seeds for anise; however, the bitter taste of the plant usually discourages consumption.

Pathophysiology

Conium toxicity results from piperidine alkaloids, such as coniine, which are structurally related to the pyridine nicotine. These propylpiperidine alkaloids are among the simplest alkaloids and appear in other plant families (e.g., *Crassulaceae* and *Punicaceae*). Symptoms appear similar to those of nicotine poisoning. Alkaloid content varies significantly between species, plant parts, and geographic locations. As the plant matures, alkaloid concentration increases respectively in the stems, leaves, and fruit, but the roots consistently contain the largest alkaloid concentrations.

Clinical Presentation

Toxicity to animals has been reported widely in the veterinary literature and includes ataxia, salivation, convulsions, and coma.

Based on their structural similarity to nicotine and on data in animals, these alkaloids produce initial stimulation (tremor, ataxia, mydriasis), nausea, vomiting, and sore throat followed by cardiorespiratory depression (bradycardia, paralysis, coma) and ascending paralysis. Death results from respiratory failure. The usual absence of convulsions distinguishes coniine toxicity from the more deadly *Cicuta* (water hemlock) poisoning in which seizures are common.

Treatment

- There is scant information to guide treatment, however, usual decontamination measures and supportive care probably are warranted.

Questions-Poison Hemlock

1. **Which of the following concerning poison hemlock is false?**
   A. *Conium maculatum* was used by the early Greeks as a means of suicide and Socrates probably died from *Conium* poisoning.
   B. The plant may be mistaken for wild carrots, the leaves for parsley, and the seeds for anise however, the bitter taste of the plant usually discourages consumption.
   C. *Conium* toxicity results from piperidine alkaloids, such as coniine, which are related structurally to ricin.
   D. As the plant matures, alkaloid concentration increases respectively in the stems, leaves, and fruit, but the roots consistently contain the largest alkaloid concentrations.
   E. These alkaloids produce initial stimulation (tremor, ataxia, mydriasis), vomiting, and sore throat followed by cardiorespiratory depression (bradycardia, coma) and ascending paralysis.
2. **The usual absence of convulsions distinguishes coniine toxicity from the more deadly *Cicuta* (water hemlock) poisoning in which seizures are common.**
   A. True
   B. False

POKEWEED

Pokeweed is a native weed of the eastern United States and grows abundantly in rich, moist areas in open fields and roadsides. Occasionally, it grows on the West Coast. The Indians used it medically for a purgative and for relief from rheumatism. Folk remedies include its use as a salve and bronchodilator. Poke salad is a regional delicacy of the rural southern United States. Pokeweed is a large, shrublike, perennial herb that regrows from a long fleshy taproot each spring.

Pathophysiology

The plant contains a powerful GI irritant, phytolaccine, which causes symptoms ranging from a burning sensation of the alimentary tract to severe hemorrhagic gastritis. As the plant matures, this toxin increases in concentration. Five nonspecific mitogens have been isolated, which have hemagglutinating as well as mitotic activity. Noncardioactive steroids and triterpenoid glycosides (saponins) also are present in significant quantities. Saponins may potentiate GI toxicity and, when administered parenterally, produce vasodilation.

Controversy continues over the question of whether or not any part of the plant is edible. There is no question that toxicity varies between susceptible individuals, parts of the plant, and time of year. The root is the most toxic part. In order of decreasing toxicity are the leaves, the stems, and the berries. Green berries are more toxic than mature ones, whereas young leaves may be less toxic than older ones.

Clinical Presentations

Early GI symptoms predominate in pokeweed poisoning, and severity depends on the type of ingestion. Symptoms in an outbreak of poke salad poisoning included nausea, stomach cramps, vomiting, headache, dizziness, burning of mouth or stomach, and diarrhea. The mean onset of illness was 3 hours and the duration was 1 to 48 hours.

Poisoning from poke salad tea and poke root tea is more severe and immediate (15 to 30 minutes to onset of illness). Symptoms may include lethargy, weakness, respiratory depression, convulsions, paresthesias, syncope, blurred vision, vertigo, sweating, salivation, and urgency. Peripheral and central cholinergic symptoms have been suggested as a prominent part of severe intoxication. Death has been reported in the literature from a large ingestion of poke berries.

Treatment

GUT DECONTAMINATION

Because pokeweed contains a powerful GI toxin, the usual measures should be undertaken to prevent absorption if vomiting hasn't occurred already. Patients who present hours after ingestion or who display profuse diarrhea and vomiting probably will not benefit from emetics and cathartics.

ELIMINATION ENHANCEMENT

These methods are usually not utilized in the treatment of pokeweed exposures.

SUPPORTIVE MEASURES

- Therapy should be directed toward maintaining fluid and electrolyte balance. Serious intoxications involve ingestion of pokeweed teas and usually result in significant GI symptoms within 1 hour. These patients should be hospitalized and monitored for secondary hypotension and electrolyte imbalance.
- Symptoms rarely last more than 36 hours and there have been no reports of long-term sequelae.

Antidotes

Because of the prominence of cholinergic symptoms, atropine has been considered beneficial by some, but there has been no documentation of its usefulness in the literature.

Questions—Pokeweed

1. **Which part of the pokeweed plant is the most toxic?**
   A. The leaves
   B. The stems
   C. The berries
   D. The flowers
   E. The root

2. **Poisoning from poke salad tea can be severe and immediate and include lethargy, weakness, respiratory depression, convulsions, paresthesias, syncope, vertigo, sweating, salivation, and urgency.**
   A. True
   B. False

RHODODENDRON

The toxicity of honey collected from bees frequenting rhododendron leaves has been recognized since ancient times. Xenophon in the Anabasis reported the poisoning of his troops by the honey of *Rhododendron ponticum* flowers, and Pompey's army was massacred by King Pontus' army while they were disabled after honey ingestion in a similar area in northern Asia Minor.

Azaleas and rhododendrons belong to the same genus, *Rhododendron*, which contains over 800 species. Because of the presence of many hybrid forms, some commercial species are difficult to identify. These beautiful flowering evergreen or rarely deciduous shrubs belong to the family Ericaceae (heath), which contains a number of well-known toxic substances.

Pathophysiology

Some confusion exists over the terminology of the poisonous principles of the *Ericaceae* because of the numerous toxins present. Andromedotoxin was the name given to the toxic substance isolated from *Rhododendron chrysanthum* by Archangelsky in 1899. Now the toxins have been identified as diterpene polyalcohols possessing the andromedane skeleton and are termed grayanotoxins, asebotoxins, rhodojaponins, and lyoniatoxins. The pharmacology of andromedotoxin most closely resembles that of grayanotoxin I, which is a potent hypotensive agent. Grayanotoxin, batrachotoxin, veratridine, and aconitine possess similar structural groups that modulate the sodium gate and maintain the sodium channel in the open position.

Clinical Presentations

The toxicity of honey collected from bees frequenting rhododendron leaves is characterized by nausea, vomiting, lethargy, weakness, and paresthesias, which may last several days. The ingestion of 75 mL of Turkish honey containing grayanotoxin produced coma, convulsions, bradycardia, and atrioventricular block in a 27-year-old woman. A series of 152 azalea exposures revealed only one significantly symptomatic patient who developed protracted vomiting and mild hypertension.

Not all *Rhododendron* species produce toxic nectar, and predicting which hybrids will secrete toxic nectar is difficult. Consumption of rhododendron leaves and flowers by a 4-year-old child resulted in vomiting and abdominal pain within 2 hours, followed by an apneic spell and cyanosis for 30 seconds. Subsequent cardiac monitoring revealed a sinus bradycardia of 60 beats / minute, which responded to subcutaneous atropine. No neuromuscular weakness, ventricular dysrhythmias, or hypotension was noted.

Thirty patients with food poisoning resulting from honey were seen in Turkey from 1983 to 1986. Symptoms included hypotension, bradycardia, nausea, vomiting, sweating, dizziness, impaired consciousness, exhaustion, fainting, blurred vision or diplopia, cyanosis, and chills. The amount of toxic honey ingested ranged between 2 teaspoonfuls to 5 tablespoonfuls. Symptoms began within 30 minutes to 2 hours. Bradycardia, junctional rhythm, complete atrioventricular block, and Wolff-Parkinson-White syndrome with sinus bradycardia were often observed.

Treatment

- Most children who sample rhododendron plants will be asymptomatic. For those patients who ingest more than a whole leaf or flower, the usual decontamination measures are reasonable after the necessary precautions are observed.
- A physician should observe symptomatic patients for 4 to 6 hours with monitoring of vital signs.
- Atropine may be useful if bradycardia is reducing cardiac output.

Questions—Rhododendron

1. **Which of the following is false?**
   A. The toxicity of honey collected from bees frequenting rhododendron leaves has been recognized since ancient times.
   B. Azaleas and rhododendrons belong to the same genus, *Rhododendron*, which contains over 800 species.
   C. Toxins derived from rhododendron are called grayanotoxins, asebotoxins, rhodojaponins, and lyoniatoxins.
   D. Grayanotoxin can cause refractory hypertension from α stimulation and may be responsible for intracerebral bleeds.
   E. The toxicity of honey collected from bees frequenting rhododendron leaves is characterized by nausea, vomiting, lethargy, weakness, and paresthesias, which may last several days.
2. **Toxins known to modulate the sodium gate and maintain the sodium channel in the open position include all of the following except**
   A. Grayanotoxin
   B. Batrachotoxin
   C. Nicotine
   D. Veratridine
   E. Aconitine
3. **All *Rhododendron* species produce toxic nectar.**
   A. True
   B. False

SNAKEROOT

Snakeroot is a common weed found along roadsides in the East and Midwest. It is a perennial herb with large ovate toothed leaves on long stalks. Clusters of white flowers produce small fruit.

Pathophysiology

The entire plant contains the higher alcohol tremetol and certain glycosides, which accumulate in the milk of cows grazing on this plant. The afebrile epidemic illness known as "milk sickness" results from ingestion of contaminated milk. In colonial times and particularly during the first half of the 19th century, milk sickness caused numerous deaths. The rayless goldenrod

(*Haplopappus heterophyllus*) in the Southwest also contains tremetol and causes milk sickness.

CLINICAL PRESENTATIONS

Milk sickness is an insidious disease causing weakness, nausea, vomiting, tremors, headache, constipation, dizziness, delirium, and, in serious cases, coma, convulsions, and death. Recovery often is prolonged. Autopsy reveals fatty degeneration of the liver and kidney. Modern milk-processing procedures have eliminated milk sickness, but consumption of unprocessed milk represents a potential danger.

Treatment

- Decontamination measures generally are not necessary and treatment is supportive.

Questions—Snakeroot

1. Which of the following about snakeroot is false?
A. It is a common weed.
B. The entire plant contains the higher alcohol tremetol and certain glycosides that accumulate in the milk of cows grazing on this plant.
C. The afebrile epidemic illness known as "milk sickness" occurs in cows that ingest snakeroot.
D. Death has occurred from milk sickness.
E. Milk sickness causes weakness, nausea, vomiting, tremors, headache, constipation, dizziness, coma, and convulsions.

SNOWBERRY

The snowberry is a low-growing deciduous shrub that grows in woodlands and open areas of the northern United States and Canada. In Europe, the species is cultivated as an ornamental hedge. The white, waxy berries mature in summer and fall and may remain on the shrub after leaves drop.

Pathophysiology

The alkaloid chelidonine has been isolated from *Symphoricarpos albus* but does not account for its toxicity. Additional compounds reported to be present include aesculin, sitosterol saponins, tannins, terpenes, triglycerides, sugars, coumarins, flavonoids, and secologanin. It is unknown which, if any, of these compounds cause adverse effects.

Clinical Presentations

Most children who ingest snowberries remain asymptomatic. Vomiting, to date, has been the only complication. Heavy consumption of snowberries before 1900 was reported to cause GI distress, delirium, and obtundation, but no fatalities.

Treatment

- Decontamination probably is not necessary unless more than several berries have been ingested.

Questions—Snowberry

1. Heavy consumption of snowberries before 1900 was reported to cause gastrointestinal distress, delirium, and obtundation, but no fatalities.
A. True
B. False

SWEET PEA AND LATHYRISM

Lathyrism is a chronic disease resulting from excessive ingestion of certain *Lathyrus* (e.g., *Lathyrus sativus*) peas. Human lathyrism is a spastic lower-extremity paraplegia that has been recognized since the time of Hippocrates. The disease occurred in concentration and prisoner-of-war camps in World War II and still is a public health problem in parts of India.

An animal disease affects primarily collagen tissue and is called osteolathyrism and a human variety is a neurologic disease called neurolathyrism. There are more than 100 *Lathyrus* species in the United States and Europe, and several of these species (e.g., *hirsutus*, *latifolius*, *odoratus*, *pusillus*, *sphaericus*, *splendens*, *lactiflorus* species *alefeldii*, *sylvestris*, and *tingitamus*) have been associated with toxic effects in animals.

Pathophysiology

NEUROLATHYRISM

Neurolathyrism and bone changes seen in humans probably result from the neurotoxin β-N-oxalylamino-1-alanine, which is structurally similar to the putative neurotransmitter glutamate. Experimentally, this neurotoxin is a potent excitatory 1-amino acid and may disrupt the central nervous system neurotransmitter activity of glutamate.

OSTEOLATHYRISM

The toxin in experimental osteolathyrism is β-aminopropionitrile, which is not present in the *Lathyrus* species causing toxic effects in humans. This toxin in animals appears to cause the formation of abnormal collagen with poor tensile strength. Animals fed peas from species containing β-aminopropionitrile develop skeletal deformities and aortic aneurysms when these nitriles are incorporated into collagen in place of amino acids.

Clinical Presentations

Consumption of 300 g of *L. sativus* daily for 3 months is required to produce a spastic, ataxic paraplegia, which preferentially affects young males. Of concentration camp victims who developed this syndrome, about 80% had upper motor neuron lesions, 15% had both upper and lower lesions, and 5% had peripheral neuropathies. Symptoms include motor and sensory complaints (the lower extremities), GI distress, bladder and sexual dysfunction, and neurasthenic (i.e., insomnia, thirst, and short-term memory loss) problems. Acute toxic effects from single *Lathyrus* ingestions have not been reported.

Treatment

- Management involves primarily supportive care. Decontamination is not necessary for the usual childhood ingestion.

Questions—Sweet Pea and Lathyrism

1. Which of the following is false?
A. Lathyrism is a chronic disease resulting from excessive ingestion of certain *Lathyrus* (e.g., *L. sativus*) peas.
B. Human lathyrism is a spastic gastrointestinal disease that has been recognized since the time of Hippocrates.
C. Lathyrism occurred in concentration and prisoner-of-war camps in World War II and is still a public health problem in parts of India.
D. An animal disease affects primarily collagen tissue and is called osteolathyrism.
E. Decontamination is not necessary for the usual childhood ingestion.

VERATRUM

Veratrum species are tall, perennial herbs with alternate, pleated leaves. Small flowers emerge from a large terminal panicle. A native of moist woodlands in the Southeast, *Veratrum viride* (also called False Hellebore or Hellebore) is found from Canada and northern United States to North Carolina, Georgia, and Tennessee. *Veratrum album* is a European species that has been associated with severe poisoning when the pulverized root has been marketed as a sneezing powder. *Veratrum* alkaloids contained within all plant parts have been used medicinally for the treatment of hypertension and agriculturally as a pesticide.

Pathophysiology

Toxin production varies between species. *V. viride* produces substantial amounts of hypotensive alkaloids whereas *Veratrum californicum* contains little. Veratridine, a *V. album* alkaloid, is an experimental agent used to study neurotransmitter release. The afferent vagal fibers of the coronary sinus and left ventricle appear to be most sensitive to the depolarizing effects of *Veratrum* alkaloids. Reflex cardiac parasympathetic stimulation then results in bradycardia and hypotension.

Clinical Presentations

GI distress and sneezing develop within 30 to 60 minutes of inhalation or ingestion because of direct stimulation of peripheral receptors. An initial burning sensation is followed by pain in the upper abdomen, nausea, vomiting, diaphoresis, blurred vision, lightheadedness, and confusion. Dilated pupils and syncope may occur. Subsequently, hypotension and bradycardia may develop.

Massive *Veratrum* overdoses can produce digitalislike cardiotoxicity characterized by sinoatrial and atrioventricular blocks and ventricular dysrhythmias. Myalgias and paresthesias may be seen but myoclonus and seizures occur only when large doses have been ingested. Eye contact may result in severe conjunctival irritation, lacrimation, and erythema.

Treatment

- The usual measures of decontamination may be used but the rapid onset of symptoms and profuse vomiting often make such measures superfluous.
- Cardiac monitoring and ECGs should be instituted in severely poisoned patients because of the potential of digitalislike dysrhythmias. Symptoms and signs (with the exception of eye irritation) usually resolve within 12 to 15 hours.

Antidotes

Atropine usually reverses the bradycardia but only partially improves hypotension. Fluids and vasopressors may be required.

Questions—Veratrum

1. Massive *Veratrum* overdoses can produce digitalislike cardiotoxicity characterized by sinoatrial and atrioventricular blocks and ventricular dysrhythmias.
A. True
B. False

2. Veratrum toxicity is associated with hellebore plants.
A. True
B. False

WATER HEMLOCK

At least nine distinct species occur throughout the United States and all these species grow along moist areas such as marshes or streams. Common species include *Cicuta maculata*, *Cicuta bulbifera*, *Cicuta occidentalis*, *Cicuta douglasi*, and *Cicuta vagans*. Most human toxic reactions result when adults mistake *Cicuta* for wild edible species such as wild carrot and Jerusalem artichoke or when children eat wild vegetation. There are no medicinal uses. The first recorded case of *Cicuta* toxicity appeared in 1679 and Stockbridge reported three cases in the United States in 1814.

Water hemlock is a perennial weed that has multiple, thick, tuberous roots and a hollow stalk reaching 8 feet high. The leaves are large and divided into narrow leaflets several inches long with saw-toothed borders. Small white clustered flowers appear in an umbrella shape by June or July.

Pathophysiology

Boehm isolated a toxic substance in 1876 from a European species, which he named oenanthotoxin. Later, this compound was identified as a highly unsaturated higher alcohol. Thin-layer chromatographic, high-performance liquid chromatographic and mass spectrometric techniques are available to identify oenanthotoxin. Cicutoxin, isolated from the species *Cicuta virosa*, is an isomer of oenanthotoxin. Cicutoxin is the most violent indigenous poison in North America and is next only to *Amanita* species in reported lethality. Although most cases involve ingestion, the toxin may be absorbed through the skin.

All parts of the plant are considered poisonous; however, case studies clearly demonstrate that the root is the most toxic portion. Most poisonings occur in the spring when roots are exposed easily and *Cicuta* species are confused with edible plants. The ingestion of a piece of one *Cicuta* root has resulted in the death of an 8-year-old boy.

Clinical Presentations

Cicuta toxicity is one of the best described serious plant poisonings in the American literature. Between 1900 and 1975, one case series identified 83 cases of *Cicuta* poisoning with an overall mortality rate of 30%. In the typical case, severe GI symptoms such as nausea, vomiting, and abdominal pain begin within 15 to 90 minutes of ingestion and are rapidly followed by convulsions and coma.

Major toxicity results from the central nervous system stimulant properties of cicutoxin, and this property distinguishes it from coniine (poison hemlock), which causes central nervous system depression. Death results from status epilepticus, perhaps caused by excessive stimulation of cholinergic receptors in the basal ganglia and brain stem. Hypotension results from fluid depletion secondary to GI distress. Salivation, diaphoresis, flushing, and dizziness also are common symptoms. Several case studies have documented the presence of opisthotonus and hemiballismus.

Treatment

GUT DECONTAMINATION

Decontamination with lavage may be helpful, but tracheal protection is vital given the propensity for seizures associated with this plant. Syrup of ipecac is contraindicated. Charcoal may be helpful.

ELIMINATION ENHANCEMENT

Hemodialysis and hemoperfusion have been used in a case of *Cicuta* poisoning that resulted in status epilepticus.

SUPPORTIVE MEASURES

- Immediate attention should be directed toward airway, breathing, and circulation. As patients may suddenly seize, an IV line must be established immediately.
- Muscle spasticity usually responds to diazepam. Exceedingly high creatine kinase levels suggest direct muscle toxicity. Grossly elevated muscle enzyme levels suggest the need for alkalinization of the urine and good urine volumes.
- Several authors have reported transient hematuria, glycosuria, and proteinuria. Hypotension, hypertension, bradycardia, and tachycardia have been reported. Significant dysrhythmias or conduction disturbances have not been reported.
- In the emergency department, adult patients who convulse should receive diazepam first and then at least 1 g of phenytoin (maximum of 40 mg/minute with vital signs and rhythm constantly monitored). Ventilation, acid-base status, electrolytes, and volume status are followed carefully. Appropriate laboratory studies include a complete blood count, electrolytes, muscle enzymes, creatinine, arterial blood gases, and urinalysis.
- All patients with central nervous system symptoms (including spasticity) or cardiac instability should be admitted. All other patients should be observed at least 4 to 6 hours before discharge.

Antidotes

No specific antidotes are available. In animal studies, anticholinergic agents do not alleviate seizures or the cholinergic effects of *Cicuta* toxicity.

Questions—Water Hemlock

1. **Water hemlock is so named because**
   A. Water is an effective antidote if taken early.
   B. Ingestion of water with the plant liberates toxin.
   C. The toxin is quite clear and resembles water.
   D. The plants usually grow near water.
   E. Toxic symptoms produce profound salivation, urination and diaphoresis.
2. **Which of the following is false?**
   A. Numerous water hemlock species occur throughout the United States.
   B. Most human toxic reactions result when adults mistake *Cicuta* for wild edible species such as wild carrot and Jerusalem artichoke or when children experiment with wild vegetation.
   C. Cicutoxin, derived from water hemlock, is the most violent indigenous poison in North America and is next only to *Amanita* species in reported lethality.
   D. Although most cases involve ingestion, cicutoxin may be absorbed through the skin.
   E. Cicuta toxicity is extremely rare and poorly described.
3. **Toxicity results from the stimulant properties of cicutoxin, and this property distinguishes it from coniine (poison hemlock), which causes central nervous system depression.**
   A. True
   B. False

WISTERIA

12.5 to 15 cm wisteria pods contain 3 to 5 seeds, which are flat, nearly circular, and brown. The known toxins are wistarin, alectin, and a glycoside. About 3 hours following ingestion of 2 to 10 seeds, headache, nausea, vomiting, diarrhea, dizziness, abdominal pain, and drowsiness may ensue. There have been no fatalities reported.

Treatment

- A leukocytosis may be present. Treatment is largely symptomatic and supportive.

Questions—Wisteria

1. **Wisteria seeds may be associated with seizures and fatalities.**
   A. True
   B. False

YEW

The yew is a tall tree native to mountain gorges in mixed evergreen forests from northern California to Alaska and Montana. The tree has drooping branches and alternate branchlets with needlelike leaves about 2 cm long. A fleshy red cup called an aril encloses hard seeds. *Taxus cuspidate* (Japanese yew) and *Taxus baccata* (European variety) are cultivated as ornamental shrubs. *Taxus canadensis* is a native eastern United States species. Aqueous extracts have been used for years in Indian folk medicine (e.g., crude drug called Zarnab) for the cardiotonic, expectorant, antispasmodic, diuretic, and antiseptic properties.

Pathophysiology

The main toxins are the alkaloids taxine A and taxine B, which are found in all parts of the tree except the fleshy red part of the berry. These compounds are capable of causing hypotension, bradycardia, and depressed myocardial contractility similar to digitalis poisoning. The diterpene Taxol® appears to be a major cytotoxic and antileukemic constituent of *Taxus brevifolia*.

Clinical Presentations

Most casual ingestions result either in no symptoms or in mild GI distress. Symptomatic patients have toxic reactions within 1 to 3 hours and usually display only GI distress. Before 1900, deaths were reported in children who masticated the seeds and developed convulsions. Ingestion of four to five handfuls of yew leaves by a mental patient has also resulted in death. Within 1 hour, lightheadedness, nausea, and abdominal pain developed and were followed by coma, tachycardia, bundle branch block resembling hyperkalemia, ventricular flutter, QRS prolongation, respiratory arrest, and cardiac standstill. Chewing yew needles has resulted in anaphylactic shock. Cutting yew wood also has been associated with contact dermatitis.

Treatment

- Alert children who ingest more than several seeds should receive the usual decontamination measures after the standard precautions have been observed.
- Those patients who remain asymptomatic or have only mild GI distress may be released after 4 hours. Serious ingestions require oxygen, an intravenous line, and cardiac monitoring in an intensive care setting.

Questions—Yew

1. **The fleshy red yew berry is the most toxic part of the plant.**
   A. True
   B. False
2. **The alkaloids taxine A and taxine B found in yew plants are capable of causing hypotension, bradycardia, depressed myocardial contractility and conduction delay, similar to digitalis poisoning.**
   A. True
   B. False
3. **The diterpene Taxol® appears to be a major antileukemic constituent of *Taxus brevifolia*.**
   A. True
   B. False

MUSHROOMS

INTRODUCTION

Although only about 2% of the 5,000 U.S. mushroom species are poisonous, serious poisonings continue to result from the inability of patients to distinguish toxic from nontoxic mushrooms. The actual incidence of mushroom toxicity is difficult to estimate because poisoning often occurs in clusters and the law does not require the reporting of adverse reactions from mushroom ingestion. California consistently leads the nation in annual mushroom fatalities. In the United States, adult fatalities generally are limited to the consumption of several amatoxin-containing species of *Amanita* (e.g., *phalloides*, *verna*, *virosa*, and *ocreata*) and *Galerina*.

Pathophysiology

Two higher fungus divisions (Basidiomycetes and Ascomycetes) contain the poisonous mushroom species. Since fungi contain no chlorophyll, they must obtain their nutrients from decaying organic matter (as a saprophyte) or from living organisms (as a parasite).

Mycelia

Mycelia are an extensive network of minute underground tubules (i.e., hyphae) that extend several hundred feet and live for years in the pursuit of nutrients. At times, a specific mycelium develops a mutually beneficial relationship with higher plant roots and together they are known as a mycorrhiza.

Mushroom

The mushroom portion of the fungus is the reproductive structure that grows from an underground mycelium as a densely packed cap and stipe (stalk) of interwoven hyphal strands. This structure contains the spores that upon germination form new mycelia. Variation in size, shape, color, and spore and other microscopic structures aids in the identification of mushroom species.

Classification

Mushroom toxicity has been divided into seven categories based on target organ and the onset of symptoms. Because adequate mushroom specimens often are unavailable for identification, a clinical classification provides an excellent mechanism to guide medical treatment. Individual variations in susceptibility and the co-ingestion of other mushroom species may limit the usefulness of this classification. The best aid to treatment remains the accurate identification of the species involved. This often requires an experienced mycologist and a microscope.

Identification

There are no visible signs present on all mushrooms to indicate toxicity. The distinguishing characteristics of each mushroom must be learned species by species. The annulus is a ring of tissue (skirt) left on the stalk when the veil covering the gill breaks. The pileus is the mushroom cap. Spores are minute, uniquely shaped reproductive units that are analogous to seeds in higher plants. The application of Meltzer's reagent aids in the differentiation of spore species. Spores that turn blue after contact with Meltzer's reagent are referred to as amyloid and those that do not turn blue are called nonamyloid.

A partial veil is a membrane that covers the gills of some immature mushrooms. The remnant is the annulus when left on the stipe. Occasionally, the partial veil adheres to the cap margin (i.e., appendiculate margin). A universal veil is a membrane that covers the entire immature mushroom. After maturation, the mushroom expands, breaking through the universal veil. Some species leave a remnant at the base of the stipe known as the volva. Gills or lamellae are vertical plates on the undersurface of the cap on which spores form and are released.

Estimating Toxicity

Because of limited knowledge, species variation, and individual susceptibility, a priori determination of clinical effects is difficult. The seriousness of toxicity depends on a number of variables. Some mushrooms require cooking (e.g., *Clitocybe nuda*) to remove toxins; however, deadly amatoxins are not altered by any method of preparation. The toxicity of the *Coprinus atramentarius* species requires the ingestion of alcohol within several days of consumption. Concurrent ingestion does not cause adverse symptoms.

Only large ingestions, or consumption on consecutive days of certain species (e.g., early morel or *Verpa bohemica*) produces toxic effects. Some species (e.g., *Paxillus involutus*) are poisonous in one geographical area but edible in another. Some mushrooms are edible when they are young or fresh but toxic when old, decayed, or traumatized, similar to some fruits and vegetables (e.g., potatoes). Some mushroom toxins (e.g., phallotoxin) are severely toxic when injected but nontoxic when given orally because of poor absorption. Amatoxin concentrations vary both between species (some edible species have minute amounts) and within the same species.

Treatment

GUT DECONTAMINATION

Activated charcoal and a cathartic, orally or by nasogastric tube, should be administered instead of syrup of ipecac. If feasible, and when indicated, send gastric aspirate or emesis, along with any remaining mushrooms, to a mycologist for identification.

ELIMINATION ENHANCEMENT

Dialysis may be required to support nephrotoxicity from certain mushrooms.

SUPPORTIVE MEASURES

- The often repeated dictum "There are old mushroom hunters and bold mushroom hunters, but there are no old, bold mushroom hunters" is an appropriate admonition. Mushroom ingestions can be deadly and each ingestion must be taken seriously. Maintain supportive measures, including airway support, intravenous fluids, and vasopressors (if needed).
- Points of history to obtain should include a history of ingestion, how many types of mushrooms were ingested, the time of ingestion, if anyone else ate them, and what the current symptoms are.
- Obtain a history of symptom presentation with emphasis on chronology. Usually, potentially lethal mushrooms produce symptoms 6 hours or longer after ingestion, whereas nonlethal mushrooms produce symptoms within 6 hours. However, keep in mind a variety of mushrooms could have been eaten, and early symptoms do not rule out a potentially serious poisoning.
- Try to perform a preliminary identification of mushroom and spores. Many mycologists can assist with mushroom identification by telephone. Prepare a spore print if possible.
- If the ingested mushroom is suspected to be in the cyclopeptide group, (i.e., *Amanita phalloides* and *Galerina autumnalis*), admit the patient and follow hepatic and renal functions until recovery.
- Consider the use of specific antidotes when indicated (see specific mushroom groups below).

PITFALLS IN MUSHROOM TREATMENT

- Mushroom poisoning actually may represent an allergic reaction or food poisoning.
- Symptoms actually may be secondary to pesticides sprayed on the mushroom, secondary to edible mushrooms being laced with drugs (i.e., phencyclidine) or from a concomitant medical or surgical disease.
- Never assume that all persons ingesting the same mushroom must become ill. Never assume that if symptoms occur before 6 hours postingestion, deadly *Amanitas* could not have been eaten.
- Patients should not be discharged without follow-up after recovering from GI symptoms when those symptoms developed more than 6 hours postingestion.
- In most cases of mushroom poisoning, supportive care and close follow-up can lead to a favorable outcome. It is always recommended to contact your regional Poison Center for assistance with any mushroom ingestion.

Questions—Introduction to Mushrooms

1. Most U.S. mushroom species are poisonous.
A. True
B. False

2. Which of the following aid in identification of mushroom species?
A. Color
B. Smell
C. Solubility in water
D. Solubility in alcohol
E. All of the above

3. Mushrooms are toxicologically grouped based on
A. Size
B. Solubility in water
C. Seasonal growth patterns
D. Geographic locale
E. Target organ and the onset of symptoms

CYCLOPEPTIDES (GROUP I)

The cyclopeptide amatoxins contained within certain *Amanita* and *Galerina* species cause severe hepatorenal dysfunction and gastritis. *A. phalloides* causes more than 50% of all mushroom poisonings. The *Amanita* genus accounts for 95% of mushroom related fatalities. Appropriately, *A. phalloides* has been named the "death cap," while several *Amanita* species (i.e., *virosa*, *verna*, *bisporigera*, and *ocreata*) are known as the "destroying angel." *A. phalloides* is the predominant European poisonous mushroom. Frequently, this mushroom is ingested when it is mistakenly identified as *Tricholoma equestre*. Several other *Amanita* species (e.g., *virosa*, *verna*, *brunescens*, *ocreata*, and *bisporigera*) are more prevalent than *A. phalloides* in the United States. Many victims consider themselves experts who have consumed wild mushrooms on previous occasions without adverse effects. Rarely, fatalities have resulted from other North American mushroom species belonging to the *Galerina* genus (i.e., *autumnalis*, *marginata*).

Amanita phalloides

A. phalloides appears to be spreading rapidly along the east and west coasts of the United States. Although the mature *A. phalloides* mushroom often has a distinctive olive green cap, white gills, and veil at the base of the stem, even experts, especially in its immature stages can misidentify it. Other toxic *Amanita* species have white gills and caps and are difficult to distinguish from each other with the unaided eye.

Although trauma may alter distinguishing characteristics, certain physical mushroom structures of the toxic *Amanita* species are reviewed here as an aid to emergency department management and not as a guide for mushroom hunters. These include a ring around the stalk ("ring of death"), a cup or volva at the bottom of the stalk ("cup of death"), white spores and usually white gills, gills that physically do not attach to the stalk (twisting off the stalk should leave the gills intact) and thin-walled, spores that have a positive (blue) amyloid reaction to Meltzer's reagent.

Galerina

Galerina compounds include at least seven cyclic heptapeptides (phalloidins), eight cyclic octapeptides (amatoxins), and five virotoxins (e.g., alaviroidin, viroisin, deoxoviroisin, and viroidin). Although phalloidin is a potent parenteral animal hepatotoxin, it has poor oral bioavailability and probably is not involved in human poisoning. Phallotoxins are bicyclic peptides containing cysteine, whereas virotoxins are monocyclic peptides containing d-serine.

Pathophysiology

Of the amatoxins, α-amanitin is the chief component and, together with β-amanitin, probably produces the hepatorenal syndrome seen with mushroom ingestions. Amatoxins probably are present in all mushroom species and occur in minute amounts in several edible mushroom species. *A. phalloides* is the most toxic species and contains 2 to 3 mg of amatoxin per gram of dry tissue. One to three fresh mushrooms (50 g) probably contain sufficient quantities of amatoxin to be lethal.

Amatoxins are potent inhibitors of cellular protein synthesis. They inhibit RNA polymerase II within the nucleoplasm at very low concentrations and thus interfere with both RNA and DNA transcription. Those cells with the highest replication rates and most direct contact with the amatoxins (e.g., liver, kidney, and intestinal cells) develop necrosis. In fact, much of the GI damage in dogs is confined to the duodenum, where biliary secretion (i.e., enterohepatic circulation) occurs. Deadly amatoxins are not altered by any method of food preparation.

Amatoxin concentrations vary significantly between species, with some American samples of *Amanita virosa* containing small amounts of amatoxin. *Amanita bisporigera* appears to be the most toxic American species and *Amanita verna* contains variable amounts of amatoxins. Generally, other toxic *Amanita* species contain less amatoxin. Interestingly, the *Galerina* species, similar to the toxic *Amanita* species, can produce a fatal hepatorenal dysfunction and yet they contain no phallotoxins. This observation further supports the concept that amatoxins are the primary toxic constituents.

Pharmacokinetics

ABSORPTION

- Amatoxins are rapidly absorbed from the GI tract and subsequently can be detected by radioimmunoassay in the serum and urine of poisoned patients.

DISTRIBUTION

- Amatoxins may remain in the gastric aspirate more than 48 hours, probably because of their biliary excretion, but they disappear from serum within 24 hours.
- Both enterohepatic circulation and resorption of glomerular filtrate potentially augment toxicity.

ELIMINATION

- Amatoxins are excreted rapidly in the urine. Urine concentrations reflect serum concentrations several hours previously.
- In dogs, 85% of α-amanitin is excreted within 6 hours, with a calculated elimination half-life of 22 hours.
- Blood and amniotic fluid samples taken from a woman in the eighth month of pregnancy suggested that amatoxins do not cross the placental barrier.

Clinical Presentations

Typically, 6 to 24 hours (average, 10 to 12 hours) pass between the ingestion of amatoxin and the onset of symptoms. This delayed onset is an important but not sensitive sign of cyclopeptide ingestion. Most nonlethal mushrooms produce toxic effects soon after ingestion. Presumably, the latent period represents the time required for the amatoxins to bind to intranuclear RNA polymerase II and disrupt protein synthesis. Characteristically, cyclopeptide poisoning has three stages.

GASTROENTERITIS PHASE

A profuse, choleralike diarrhea characterized by the abrupt onset of severe abdominal pain, nausea, vomiting, and bloody diarrhea marks the onset of toxicity. Usually this phase lasts about 24 hours. Fever, tachycardia, hyperglycemia, dehydration, and electrolyte imbalance may complicate this phase.

LATENT PHASE

With adequate fluid and electrolyte replacement, a remission of symptoms occurs with a subclinical elevation of serum hepatic aminotransferase enzymes. If mushroom-related toxicity is not suspected during this 12 to 24 hour latent phase, the patient may be misdiagnosed as having gastroenteritis and discharged.

HEPATORENAL PHASE

Within 3 to 4 days of ingestion, hepatic dysfunction becomes clinically obvious, and jaundice, delirium, confusion, hypoglycemia, and coma develop despite adequate fluid replacement. Coagulopathies, metabolic acidosis, conduction abnormalities, hemorrhage, and sepsis frequently complicate severe cases. Renal failure is present in most fatal cases but occasionally may be the dominant feature. Renal toxicity results from direct nephrotoxicity, hypovolemia, or both.

SYSTEMIC EFFECTS

Cardiovascular and central nervous system effects are believed to be secondary to hepatorenal failure. Autopsies have demonstrated cerebral edema and cerebellar tonsillar herniation with fatty infiltration and mild hemorrhage of the subendocardial region. Neuropathological changes as well as cardiovascular changes are variable and nonspecific, especially in view of the hyperpyrexia, sepsis, and cardiovascular collapse seen in terminal cases.

Toxic Dosage/Death

Mortality rates vary between 10% and 40% because of the wide variation in the amount of toxin ingested, individual susceptibility, and the patient's condition on admission. Previous estimates of a 90% mortality rate vastly overrated *Amanita* toxicity. In a European *Amanita* toxicity series, children under 10 years of age displayed a higher mortality rate that approached 50%. Death usually results from hepatorenal failure 3 to 7 days postingestion. In most fatalities, encephalopathy, coma, and renal insufficiency have developed.

Laboratory

ANALYTIC METHODS

The Meixner test is a field test for the presence of amatoxins that is highly sensitive, but negative results do not guarantee edibility. The test is based on the acid-catalyzed reaction of amatoxin with lignin. Cheap pulp paper, which contains high lignin concentrations, is required. Thin-layer chromatography assays have been developed with documented standards to detect α-amanitin levels around 50 μg/mL. Radioimmunoassay techniques have been developed to detect amatoxin levels as low as 0.5 ng/mL in gastric, serum and urine samples.

BLOOD LEVELS

Blood levels may identify *Amanita*, however concentrations may not correlate with significance of exposure. Amatoxins are found in the serum as late as 30 hours after ingestion in concentrations of 0.5 to 24 ng/mL.

Treatment

GUT DECONTAMINATION

Induction of emesis is not beneficial more than 4 hours after ingestion. The delay in presentation beyond 4 hours after ingestion is a common occurrence because of the delayed toxicity of *Amanita*. Activated charcoal and cathartics have been recommended, but their exact role has not been defined. Potentially, such therapy is efficacious because of enterohepatic circulation of the amatoxin within the first 36 hours. Serial activated charcoal need not be continued more than 48 hours postingestion.

ELIMINATION ENHANCEMENT

Amatoxins are dialyzable and eliminated by glomerular filtration. Conceivably, forced diuresis may enhance elimination. Clinical trials to assess the efficacy of forced diuresis have not been done. Charcoal hemoperfusion within 24 hours of ingestion was administered to eight victims of *A. phalloides* poisoning in one series. No fatalities occurred; however, the severity of poisoning has been questioned and no pharmacokinetic data were supplied to document extraction ratios. The use of hemodialysis has been limited to reversing the effects of renal dysfunction.

SUPPORTIVE MEASURES

- Initial treatment requires the restoration of fluid and electrolyte balance. Obtunded patients should receive IV glucose immediately because of the common complication of hypoglycemia.
- Patients have presented to an emergency department in cardiac arrest resulting from fluid loss and massive GI hemorrhage. Fresh-frozen plasma and vitamin K may be needed in addition to packed red blood cell transfusions and balanced electrolyte infusions.
- Routine laboratory tests for symptomatic cases include a complete blood count, electrolytes, blood urea nitrogen, creatinine, prothrombin time, bilirubin urinalysis, and blood glucose. Determinations should be repeated daily until clinical improvement occurs.
- Serum hepatic aminotransferases generally are lower in survivors than nonsurvivors, but they are not accurate predictors of survival. Elevated serum amylase levels have been reported in up to 50% of *A. phalloides* poisonings. Blood ammonia levels are not elevated until the advanced stages of hepatic failure.
- Orthotopic liver transplantation was performed in a 3-year-old girl who survived fulminant hepatic failure with neurologic deficits. Technically, such a procedure is difficult and must be performed within a brief period of 2 to 4 days postingestion to be effective.
- Cardiovascular and central nervous system changes probably reflect either underlying disease or secondary changes resulting from poor perfusion. Elevated creatine kinase levels and bradycardia have been reported.
- A severe dynamic ileus may complicate the hepatorenal phase of mushroom poisoning and has been reported in both *A. phalloides* and *Galerina* poisoning.

Antidotes

A variety of drugs including the silymarin group, penicillin G, rifampicin, thioctic acid, insulin, human growth hormone, cytochrome c, aucubin (iridoid glucoside of *Aucuba japonica*), and vitamin C have been suggested for the treatment of *Amanita* poisoning. None of these drugs have been tested in controlled clinical trials.

THIOCTIC ACID

Thioctic acid is a coenzyme of the Krebs cycle and has few adverse effects except for hypoglycemia. It has been used extensively in Eastern Europe since 1968 and has been credited with lowering mortality. The dose is 50 to 150 mg every 6 hours titrated to clinical response. Studies in animals have not documented the beneficial effect of thioctic acid, and its efficacy remains unproved.

SILIBININ

Silibinin is a constituent of the extract silymarin derived from the milk thistle *Silybum marianum*. Studies in animals suggest that this derivative reduces hepatic damage even when given 24 hours after *A. phalloides* administration, perhaps through inhibition of amatoxin uptake by hepatocytes. In a retrospective, uncontrolled Austrian study, the administration of IV silibinin (20 to 50 mg/kg/day in four doses) and penicillin was associated with a favorable outcome in all but one of 18 *A. phalloides* cases.

PENICILLIN

Penicillin appears to displace amatoxin from plasma protein-binding sites, allowing for increased renal excretion. It also may inhibit the penetration of amatoxin into hepatocytes. In one retrospective clinical study of 205 patients, doses of 300,000 to 1,000,000 units of benzyl penicillin daily tended to be more often associated with survival than below 300,000 U/day. Despite experimental data, the overall survival of patients treated with penicillin is not impressively higher than that of the total population.

Questions—Cyclopeptides (Group I)

1. Which of the following is false?

A. The *Amanita* genus accounts for 95% of mushroom related fatalities.
B. Cyclopeptide amatoxins can cause severe hepatorenal dysfunction and gastritis.
C. *Amanita phalloides* has been named the "death cap" and several *Galerina* species are known as the "destroying angel."

D. Many victims of amanita poisoning consider themselves experts who have consumed wild mushrooms on previous occasions without adverse effects.
E. *Amanita phalloides* mushrooms are found in the United States.

2. Physical mushroom structures of the toxic *Amanita* species include
A. A ring around the stalk ("ring of death")
B. A cup or volva at the bottom of the stalk ("cup of death")
C. A bright red cap ("cap of death")
D. All of the above
E. A and B

3. Mortality rates approach 90% after *Amanita* ingestions.
A. True
B. False

4. Deadly hepatic consequences of *Amanita phalloides* ingestion generally become apparent.
A. Within 1 hour
B. Within 1 day
C. Within 3 to 4 days
D. Within 1 week
E. Within 1 month

5. Which of the following concerning antidotes to cyclopeptide mushrooms is/are false?
A. Thioctic acid is a coenzyme of the hexose-monophosphate shunt that has been used extensively in Eastern Europe and has been credited with lowering mortality.
B. Silibinin is a constituent of the extract silymarin derived from the milk thistle *Silybum marianum*. Studies in animals suggest that this derivative reduces hepatic damage when given 24 hours after *Amanita phalloides* administration.
C. Penicillin appears to improve survival from sepsis associated with end-stage *Amanita phalloides* ingestions.
D. All of the above
E. A and C

6. Boiling *Amanita* mushrooms effectively removes all inherent toxins.
A. True
B. False

GYROMITRIN (GROUP II)

The genus *Gyromitra* contains some of the most prized edible mushrooms of all, the morels. Gyromitrin is one of nine different hydrazones found in variable amounts in *Gyromitra* species. Its hydrolysis to monomethylhydrazine (a compound used for rocket fuel) causes gastritis. Less often, hemolysis, hepatorenal dysfunction, coma, convulsions, and death occur after ingestion. Not all species of *Gyromitra* contain the relatively unstable gyromitrin, and concentration varies dramatically even within the same species. Several fatalities have been reported.

Gyromitra esculenta is a serious health hazard in Poland where improper consumption accounts for nearly one-quarter of mushroom-related fatalities. There are at least eight species of Gyromitra (including *esculenta*) in the United States, which contain variable amounts of gyromitrin. All are nongilled fungi. Caps are yellow-brown to dark-red and have irregularly wrinkled deep convoluted tops. The cap size varies between 1 and 5 inches.

Pathophysiology

Gyromitrin is the most toxicologically important of the nine hydrazones isolated from *G. esculenta*. Structurally, gyromitrin is an aldehyde that hydrolyzes in the body to N-monomethylhydrazine. Gyromitrin is heat labile, although simple parboiling does not guarantee edibility. Toxic concentrations vary with climatic conditions as well as other undetermined variables, so that people who previously have consumed them without difficulty may develop adverse reactions.

Clinical Presentations

Humans who ingest gyromitrin develop gastroenteritis 6 to 8 hours later, similar to those who eat amatoxin-containing mushroom species. Symptoms may include dizziness, fatigue, nausea, vomiting, severe headache, and abdominal pain. In mild cases, vomiting may persist for several hours but nonspecific symptoms may persist for several days. In severe cases, hepatic failure may develop over the next several days complicated by hypoglycemia and hypovolemia. Most gyromitrin ingestions result in mild symptoms; however, seizures, coma and death have been reported in severe cases.

Laboratory

ANALYTIC METHODS

Ultraviolet spectrophotometric methods have been developed to detect gyromitrin after extraction by thin-layer chromatography.

BLOOD LEVELS

Following blood levels after exposure does not always correlate with clinical presentation.

Treatment

GUT DECONTAMINATION

Most patients present after methods of decontamination would be expected to be beneficial. The use of activated charcoal and a cathartic is a reasonable treatment modality, although no human or animal data are available to guide the therapy of gyromitrin toxicity. Syrup of ipecac or lavage may be used if the patient presents within 4 hours of ingestion when the usual precautions are observed.

ELIMINATION ENHANCEMENT

No methods have been studied in human gyromitrin toxicity.

SUPPORTIVE MEASURES

- Depletion of fluids, electrolytes, and glucose is the most common complication of severe gyromitrin poisoning. Rarely, coma and convulsions may compromise the airway, requiring ventilatory support.
- In severe cases, baseline laboratory analysis should include a complete blood count, electrolytes, creatinine, liver function tests (including prothrombin time), glucose, and urinalysis (including a screen for hemoglobinuria).
- Gyromitrin-induced hepatic encephalopathy requires the same supportive treatment used in *A. phalloides* poisoning.
- Drugs that require cytochrome P-450 metabolism (e.g., phenobarbital) may have exaggerated effects because of gyromitrin-induced disruption of the cytochrome P-450 pathway and should be used with caution.

Antidotes

PYRIDOXINE

Pyridoxine (25 mg/kg up to a daily adult dose of 15 to 20 g) has been recommended for the neurological symptoms of gyromitrin poisoning based on the similarity between gyromitrin and hydrazine toxicity. Pyridoxine increases the formation of GABA in the presence of toxic levels of isoniazid and its hydrazine, but the activation of GABA transamination by pyridoxine may actually lead to decreased brain GABA. Which actual effect predominates in humans remains to be documented.

Although sensory neuropathies have been reported in chronic megavitamin overdose, large pyridoxine doses have few reported side effects. Doses administered for central nervous system symptoms of gyromitrin toxicity are similar to those used for isoniazid toxicity.

Questions—Gyromitrin (Group II)

1. **The genus *Gyromitra* contains some of the most prized edible mushrooms of all, the morels.**
   A. True
   B. False
2. **Gyromitrin, a hydrazone found in variable amounts in *Gyromitra* species, is hydrolyzed to monomethylhydrazine, a compound used in rocket fuel.**
   A. True
   B. False
3. **Large gyromitrin ingestions**
   A. Have caused death
   B. Have caused seizures
   C. Have caused gastritis
   D. All of the above
   E. A and B
4. **Pyridoxine has been recommended for the neurological symptoms of gyromitrin poisoning based on the similarity between gyromitrin and hydrazine toxicity.**
   A. True
   B. False

MUSCARINE (GROUP III)

Only three genera of mushrooms (*Amanita*, *Inocybe*, and *Clitocybe*) are reported to contain muscarine while several other genera (*Boletus*, *Hebeloma*, *Mycena*, and *Omphalotus*) are suspected of containing muscarine. Muscarine was first isolated from *A. muscaria* in 1868; however, this mushroom contains such toxicologically insignificant amounts that other physiologically dissimilar compounds are responsible for *A. muscaria* toxicity.

Clitocybe are widely distributed species that occasionally inhabit lawns and parks. They often are found in close association with other genera of fungi. This makes identification difficult. They have white-tan to gray caps, fleshy central stalks, and adnate to decurrent gills. Inocybe mushrooms are usually found in oak and pine woods. They are small, brown mushrooms with conical, fibrillose caps and adnate whitish to tobacco brown gills.

Ingestion of *Clitocybe* or *Inocybe* mushrooms usually produces a mild cholinergic excess syndrome within 30 minutes. Serious toxicity is relatively unusual, perhaps because of the inaccessible habitat of some toxic species, poor oral bioavailability of muscarine, and general unattractiveness as a forage food. This type of mushroom poisoning is the only one for which atropine is a specific antidote.

Pathophysiology

Muscarine is responsible for the parasympathomimetic effects of *Inocybe* and *Clitocybe*. *Inocybe napipes* contains the highest concentration of muscarine by dry weight of the 30 North American *Inocybe* and eight North American *Clitocybe* species known to contain this toxin. Physiologically, muscarine stimulates postganglionic cholinergic fibers, producing increased muscle tone and gastro-urinary mobility, bradycardia, miosis, diaphoresis, and salivation. Muscarine is heat stable so that cooking does not produce edible species.

Clinical Presentations

Typically, symptoms begin within 15 minutes to 1 hour with headache, nausea, vomiting, and abdominal pain followed by salivation, lacrimation, diarrhea, diaphoresis, miosis, and blurred vision. Bronchoconstriction may lead to dyspnea and wheezing. The presence of diaphoresis is an important diagnostic sign and strongly suggests muscarinic poisoning unless hypovolemic shock is present. Elevated liver function tests have been reported in *Clitocybe* ingestions. Cardiovascular effects include bradycardia, hypotension, and shock. Symptoms usually are mild, however, and generally abate within 2 to 6 hours. Death is uncommon.

Ingestions of jack o'lantern mushrooms (*Omphalotus illucens*) has led to vomiting, diarrhea, weakness, tiredness and the feeling of being cold. Recovery is complete within 18 hours. Abdominal cramping, dizziness, and diaphoresis also may occur.

Treatment

GUT DECONTAMINATION

Syrup of ipecac may be given to alert patients if they present within several hours of ingestion, although spontaneous vomiting may preclude its use. Activated charcoal may be useful, but cathartics are rarely necessary because of cholinergic stimulation. Patients who remain asymptomatic need not be decontaminated unless a toxic co-ingestion is suspected.

ELIMINATION ENHANCEMENT

No methods have been shown to enhance the elimination of muscarine mushrooms.

Supportive Measures

- Although rare, death may result from inability to control respiratory secretions, bronchospasm, and cardiovascular collapse. Such patients require oxygen, suctioning intravenous lines, cardiac monitoring, and, if indicated, intubation.
- Symptoms resolve within 24 hours so that observation beyond that time is rarely necessary. Be sure to watch for fluid depletion and treat accordingly.
- Elevated levels of liver function tests and hypokalemia have been observed after jack o'lantern mushroom poisoning (*Omphalotus illucens*).

Antidotes

ATROPINE

Atropine is a specific antidote that should be used to dry secretions. Atropine specifically antagonizes the effect of muscarine. A useful IV starting dose is 0.2 mg for children under 2 years of age, 0.3 mg for children 2 to 4 years, 0.4 mg for children 4 to 10 years, 0.6 mg for children 10 to 14 years, and 0.8 to 1 mg for adults. Additional smaller doses may be given, adjusted to the clinical response. Drying of secretions should be used as an endpoint along with rhythm monitoring to prevent excessive atropinization.

Questions—Muscarine (Group III)

1. **Muscarine**
   A. Is the major toxin in *Amanita muscaria*
   B. Causes a cholinergic toxidrome
   C. Is heat labile
   D. All of the above
   E. A and B
2. **Which of the following is/are true?**
   A. Atropine may be helpful in treating signs and symptoms of muscarine poisoning.
   B. Death from *Clitocybe* ingestions is common.
   C. *Inocybe* ingestion demonstrates parasympathomimetic effects.
   D. All of the above
   E. A and C

COPRINE (GROUP IV)

The North American species *Coprinus atramentarius* (inky cap) produces coprine, a toxin that interacts with ethanol to cause a disulfiramlike reaction. Although hyperacetaldehydemia is present in coprine toxicity, similar to the disulfiram-ethanol reaction, disulfiram has not been isolated consistently from *C. atramentarius*. The exact toxic mechanism remains unclear because elevated aldehyde levels alone do not reproduce either coprine or disulfiram-ethanol toxicity in experimental animals. Instead, the toxic component probably is a derivative of glutamine.

Coprinus species are gilled fungi with convex to parabolic caps that often fold over the stalk like an umbrella. The common name "inky cap" derives from the propensity of the gills to dissolve into an inky, black fluid upon maturity.

Pathophysiology

The *Coprinus* species do not contain disulfiram. Chemical and data suggest another active compound. Aldehyde dehydrogenase inhibition is not the mechanism of action of coprine because coprine is a poor inhibitor of this enzyme. Although unproved, the toxic effects of coprine more likely result from altered neurotransmitter concentrations.

Clinical Presentations

Sensitivity to ethanol occurs as soon as 2 hours (average, 3 to 6 hours) after the consumption of *Coprinus* mushrooms and may last up to 72 hours. Typically, symptoms begin soon after ethanol ingestion (15 to 20 minutes) and spontaneously resolve in 3 to 6 hours. The intensity of symptoms is related to the quantities of *Coprinus* mushrooms and ethanol ingested, as well as the time elapsed between mushroom and ethanol consumption.

Common symptoms include severe headache, facial flushing, paresthesias, lightheadedness, orthostatic hypotension, vomiting, palpitations, tachycardia, diaphoresis, and chest pain. Shock, metabolic acidosis, cardiac dysrhythmias, and myocardial infarction have complicated disulfiram-ethanol reactions. Such adverse symptoms represent a theoretical danger in coprine-ethanol interactions, especially in patients with underlying cardiovascular disease.

Treatment

GUT DECONTAMINATION

These measures usually are unnecessary, especially because spontaneous vomiting frequently occurs and the reaction rarely lasts more than several hours.

ELIMINATION ENHANCEMENT

No methods to enhance elimination have been used clinically. The use of hemodialysis to remove alcohol has theoretical benefit only in the critically ill patient.

SUPPORTIVE MEASURES

- Adequate fluid and electrolyte management is the most important aspect of supportive care. Reactions are usually mild and self-limited.
- Patients should be warned to avoid all alcohol-containing products (including cold remedies and medical elixirs) for 72 hours. Phenothiazine antiemetics should be avoided because their α-adrenergic-blocking properties may exacerbate hypotension.
- Coprine toxicity should be treated similarly to the disulfiram-ethanol reaction. Hypotension and cardiac dysrhythmias present the most immediate threat to life.
- Patients with vital sign abnormalities or those with cardiovascular disease should receive cardiac monitoring, oxygen, and an IV line. Initially, hypotension should be treated with fluids.
- For those patients remaining hypotensive, a direct-acting vasopressor (e.g., Levophed®) should be used because norepinephrine stores may be depleted in the coprine-ethanol syndrome.

Antidotes

Propranolol has been recommended for the treatment of supraventricular tachycardia and anxiety (10 to 15 mg orally) but is not well tested. Antihistamines, ascorbic acid, and iron salts have not been effective in human trials, at least in the disulfiram-ethanol reaction.

Questions—Coprine (Group IV)

1. **Which of the following is true?**
   A. The North American species *Coprinus atramentarius* (inky cap) produces coprine, a toxin that interacts with ethanol to cause a disulfiramlike reaction.
   B. Disulfiram is consistently isolated from *Coprinus atramentarius*.

C. Sensitivity to ethanol occurs as soon as 2 hours after the consumption of *Coprinus* mushrooms and may last up to 72 hours.
D. All of the above
E. A and C

2. Shock, metabolic acidosis, cardiac dysrhythmias, and myocardial infarction have complicated disulfiram-ethanol reactions.
A. True
B. False

IBOTENIC ACID AND MUSCIMOL (GROUP V)

A. muscaria and *A. pantherina* are the two major North American species that contain psychoactive isoxazole derivatives. As with hallucinogenic psilocybin mushrooms (group VI), the onset of central nervous system symptoms occurs in 30 to 60 minutes. Isoxazole compounds produce alterations in visual perception rather than formed hallucinations seen with the indole derivatives (psilocybin and psilocin). *A. muscaria* contains only minute amounts of muscarine, and the syndrome caused by its ingestion cannot be characterized as cholinergic or anticholinergic. Occasionally, both these species are intentionally ingested for their psychoactive properties.

A. muscaria (Fly Agaric) is white, has gills free from the stalk, and a 3 to 4 inch orange-red cap with distinctive white to pale yellow warts on top. An annulus and a distinguishing volva of concentric rings are present, slightly differing from those of other *Amanita* species. *A. pantherina* is most abundant during the rainy seasons of spring, summer, and fall. It has the distinctive pileal warts, white gills, annulus, and bulbous volva at the stalk's base of *A. muscaria*, but possesses more sheathing. The pileus (cap) is tan to yellow-brown to dark brown.

Pathophysiology

The isoxazole compounds, ibotenic acid, and its decarboxylated derivative muscimol account for most (e.g., muscle spasm, confusion, intoxication, drowsiness, and sleep) but not all the symptoms of poisoning. Muscimol appears to be several times more active than ibotenic acid. Determination of clinical toxicity by ingestion history is complicated by the fact that considerable variation occurs both in individual isoxazole compounds and in total isoxazole content within the same species. *A. muscaria* appears to contain a greater concentration of isoxazole compounds (0.17% to 1.0% dry weight) than *A. pantherina* (0.02% to 0.53%).

Experimental studies suggest that muscimol acts on GABA receptors, whereas ibotenic acid affects glutamic acid receptors by changing membrane permeability and resting potential. The psychoactive properties of muscimol may result from its action on GABA receptors in the brain where, at least in the rat model, muscimol is a weak, noncompetitive inhibitor of central GABA uptake. Both isoxazole derivatives can be detected in the urine within 1 hour of ingestion.

Clinical Presentations

Depending on the amounts of isoxazole compounds consumed, symptoms may appear within 30 minutes to several hours and include dizziness, ataxia, euphoria, muscle twitches, and initial psychic stimulation followed by a dream-filled sleep. More severe ingestions produce visual disturbances, fever, confusion, myoclonus, mydriasis, seizures, and coma. Symptoms are transient, last about 6 hours and rarely simulate either a cholinergic or anticholinergic syndrome. Vomiting is not a prominent part of the clinical picture. Some patients may have residual headaches for days.

Treatment

GUT DECONTAMINATION

Measures of decontamination (syrup of ipecac / lavage, charcoal, cathartics) may be useful within the first several hours of ingestion, although agitation may make these procedures technically difficult. For this reason, activated charcoal is preferred to lavage in the alert patient.

ELIMINATION ENHANCEMENT

No methods to enhance elimination have been used clinically.

SUPPORTIVE MEASURES

- General supportive care is the mainstay of treatment because most ingestions require observation and no medications. Short-acting hypnotic agents should be used with caution since studies suggest that isoxazole compounds potentiate their effect by inhibiting the formation of microsomal enzymes. Nonpharmacologic intervention is preferred unless seizures or airway compromise necessitates treatment.
- *A. pantherina* often contains compounds, in addition to ibotenic acid and muscimol, that can produce anticholinergic effects.

Antidotes

Atropine most likely will exacerbate symptoms and should not be given. Experimentally, muscimol symptoms are not ameliorated by physostigmine.

Questions—Ibotenic Acid and Muscimol (Group V)

1. Which of the following concerning group V mushrooms is/are false?
A. *Amanita muscaria* and *Amanita Psilocybe* are the two major North American species that contain psychoactive isoxazole derivatives.
B. Isoxazole compounds produce alterations in visual perception rather than formed hallucinations seen with mushrooms containing indoles.
C. *Amanita muscaria* contains only minute amounts of muscarine, and the syndrome caused by its ingestion cannot be characterized as cholinergic or anticholinergic.
D. Ibotenic acid and its decarboxylated derivative muscimol account for most (e.g., muscle spasm, confusion, intoxication, drowsiness, and sleep) but not all the symptoms of poisoning in this group.
E. A and C

2. Muscimol ingestions may produce visual disturbances, fever, confusion, myoclonus, mydriasis, seizures, and coma.
A. True
B. False

HALLUCINOGENIC MUSHROOMS (GROUP VI)

The use of hallucinogenic mushrooms predates the arrival of the Spaniards in the New World because the Aztecs consumed a substance called teonanacatl (God's flesh) in religious ceremonies. Later, *Psilocybe mexicana* was discovered to be the active component of teonanacatl. The use of mushrooms by native Americans to produce mystical revelations during religious ceremonies continued into the 20th century. Psilocybin and the less stable psilocin were isolated in 1958 from mushrooms used in Mazatec Indian ceremonies in the state of Oaxaca, Mexico. These compounds have LSD-like properties and produce alterations of autonomic function, motor reflexes, behavior, and perception. During the 1960s, Aldous Huxley and Carlos Castaneda popularized recreational ingestion of psilocybin-containing mushrooms in the western United States.

Patients typically present to emergency departments with dysphoric and sympathomimetic symptoms that are transient, lasting less than 12 hours. The potential for self-inflicted or accidental trauma during periods of altered behavior represents the greatest health hazard, although persistent psychiatric symptoms have been rarely reported.

The principal hallucinogenic mushrooms in North America are found primarily in the Pacific Northwest, Hawaii, Texas, and Florida and are grouped into three genera. *Panaeolus* mushrooms have a thin stalk, dark purple to black spores, and a convex to parabolic pileus. The North American *Psilocybe* species has long thin stalks with a conical or bell-shaped pileus and dark brown to purple-brown spores. Characteristically the stalk turns blue upon handling and common names include liberty cap, blue legs, and magic mushrooms. *Gymnophilus* mushrooms have a broad yellow to orange cap, a thick stalk, and rusty orange spores, and usually grow in the woods on buried logs.

Pathophysiology

The active constituents of these mushrooms probably are indole compounds derived from tryptamine. Psilocybin and its less stable metabolite psilocin are the best known active compounds, but their effects may not entirely explain the range of symptoms caused by hallucinogenic mushrooms. Wide variation occurs in clinical response. Agitation and hallucination were reported after ingestion of 10 mushrooms in one case; however, another patient complained of only abdominal pain after consuming 200 mushrooms. The concentration of active ingredients in these species is so low that consumption of one or two mushroom caps does not result in symptoms. Most patients have eaten large quantities to experience the psychotomimetic effects.

Clinical Presentations

Patients usually present to an emergency department within 4 hours of ingestion with symptoms of lightheadedness, weakness, and anxiety that began 30 to 60 minutes after ingestion. Most symptoms resolve within 4 hours and persistence of dysphoric symptoms past 12 hours is rare. Persistent neurologic symptoms composed primarily of flashback phenomena are well recognized but are uncommon complications of psilocybin ingestion.

Mydriasis and blurred vision are common, but other sympathomimetic signs such as tachycardia, hypertension, and hyperreflexia are seen in fewer than one half of emergency department patients. Dysphoria, disorientation, ataxia, agitation, and aggressive behavior may appear after ingestions. Antisocial behavior represents the greatest danger to life. Hallucinations occur in less than half of patients who ingest these mushrooms. Visual hallucinations are more common than auditory hallucinations; however, alterations in perception occur in almost all patients and involve primarily distortion of shapes and colors.

Coma, convulsions, hyperthermia, and death have been reported after large ingestions in small children. Adult seizures also have been reported in psilocybin intoxication. Several cases of IV administration of psilocybin extract have been associated with vomiting, myalgias, hyperpyrexia, hypoxemia, and mild methemoglobinemia.

Treatment

GUT DECONTAMINATION

Although recommended by some authorities, decontamination measures may be technically difficult and most patients can be managed by supportive care alone. Within 2 hours of ingestion, syrup of ipecac may be used in the alert patient, but in patients in which decontamination measures have not been used, no complications have been reported. The one exception would be the rare case of a large ingestion in a small child seen within 4 hours of consumption.

ELIMINATION ENHANCEMENT

No methods to enhance elimination have been used clinically.

SUPPORTIVE MEASURES

- Most patients who ingest psilocybin-containing mushrooms do not present to a hospital and usually suffer no ill effects.
- For those who do go to a hospital, dysphoria is the major complaint and a quiet, supportive environment (darkened room with familiar faces) and calm reassurance are all that is usually necessary. Diazepam (oral or IV) may be needed for sedation and chlorpromazine should be reserved for frank hallucinations.
- Mild elevations of LDH, serum aspartate aminotransferase, and alkaline phosphatase have been reported but probably are not clinically important.

Questions—Hallucinogenic Mushrooms (Group VI)

1. Hallucinogenic mushrooms include
A. *Panaeolus* mushrooms
B. *Psilocybe* species
C. *Gymnophilus* mushrooms
D. All of the above
E. B and C

2. Death has been reported in small children after *Psilocybe* ingestion.
A. True
B. False

3. The active constituents of hallucinogenic mushrooms are
A. Nicotinic compounds
B. Isoxazole compounds
C. Muscarinic compounds
D. Hydrazone compounds
E. Indole compounds

GASTROENTERITIS-PRODUCING MUSHROOMS (GROUP VII)

The rapid onset of GI distress is the most common adverse reaction to mushroom ingestion. A large group of mushrooms is capable of producing these unpleasant, but seldom dangerous, reactions. In general, symptoms appear within 2 hours of ingestion and include malaise, weakness, nausea, vomiting, and diarrhea that may turn bloody. Fluid and electrolyte imbalance and the co-ingestion of hepatotoxic mushrooms (e.g., group I or II) represent the greatest danger. The clinical course of isolated ingestion of group VII mushrooms is usually mild, with resolution occurring within 24 hours.

Pathophysiology

Since most GI irritants remain unidentified, most mechanisms of action are also unknown. Because many reactions are idiosyncratic, the role of allergic reactions has been suggested as a possible mechanism. No cases of anaphylactic reactions to mushroom ingestions have been reported despite the fact that the diversity of higher fungi suggests that haptens may be present.

The structures of the toxins within this group have not been elucidated, except for those of *Chlorophyllum molybdites*, *Gomphus floccosus*, and *Lactarius* species. Cooking appears to inactivate many gastritis-inducing mushroom toxins but does not guarantee the absence of side effects.

Clinical Presentations

AGARICUS HONDENSUS

Consumption of this mushroom results in fever, a mildly elevated serum alkaline phosphatase, and a gastroenteritis that resolves within 48 hours with supportive care.

CHLOROPHYLLUM MOLYBDITES

Ingestion of this mushroom produces a self-limited gastroenteritis characterized by nausea, vomiting, and diarrhea within 1 to 3 hours of consumption. Initially, the stool is watery, but subsequently bloody diarrhea develops along with fecal leukocytes. Shaking chills, diffuse abdominal pain, and myalgias occasionally are present, and symptoms resolve within 24 to 48 hours. GI hemorrhage with disseminated intravascular coagulation has followed ingestion of *C. molybdites*. Mature *C. molybdites* specimens ("green parasol") are recognized easily by their gills, which are green because of mature spore deposits.

CLITOCYBE NEBULARIS AND TRICHOLOMOPSIS PLATYPHYLLA

These mushrooms usually are considered edible but may cause gastroenteritis in a limited number of susceptible people. Typically, the symptoms of nausea, vomiting, lightheadedness, headache, and diarrhea begin 2 to 6 hours after ingestion and resolve in 24 to 48 hours.

ENTOLOMA LIVIDUM

This mushroom has been associated with the rapid onset of gastroenteritis (chills, nausea, vomiting, crampy abdominal pain) and mild elevation of hepatic aminotransferase levels. Acute symptoms resolve within 12 hours and loose stools improve within 48 hours.

Treatment

GUT DECONTAMINATION

These methods are generally unnecessary as vomiting occurs spontaneously.

ELIMINATION ENHANCEMENT

No methods to enhance elimination have been used clinically.

SUPPORTIVE MEASURES

- Treatment is entirely supportive. Fluid and electrolyte imbalance is the most common serious adverse effect. Most symptoms resolve within 24 to 48 hours with supportive care.
- The most important diagnostic point is to exclude group I (cyclopeptide) and group II (gyromitrin) poisonings through history and either specimen identification or spore analysis. GI irritants and hepatotoxic mushrooms may be co-ingested.
- Antiemetics may be helpful.

Questions—Gastroenteritis-Producing Mushrooms (Group VII)

1. **Gastroenteritis-producing mushrooms (group VII) seldom are dangerous.**
   A. True
   B. False
2. **Among mushrooms, only group VII mushrooms produce gastroenteritis.**
   A. True
   B. False

CORTINARIUS (GROUP VIII)

Several species of the genus *Cortinarius* (*speciosissimus*, *orellanus*, *splendena*, *venenosus*) have produced irreversible renal failure in European and Japanese patients. Some patients later required renal transplantation to restore normal kidney function. Poisoning by this mushroom group first was reported in Poland and subsequently has been seen in Scotland, France, Switzerland, Finland, and Sweden. Although *Cortinarius* toxicity has not been reported in the United States, many representatives of this genus do appear in North America. *Cortinarius* species have robust, colored (purple, orange, greenish yellow) fruit bodies with characteristic rusty orange gills, a partial veil hanging over the gills, a thick stalk with striae, and a bulbous base.

Pathophysiology

Two bipyridyl toxins, orelline and orellanine, have been isolated from *Cortinarius orellanus*, but the mechanism of action and its pharmacokinetics are not well understood. These 2,2-bipyridine compounds are structurally related to paraquat and diquat. Cooking or drying does not reduce toxicity.

Clinical Presentations

Typically, gastritis appears about 36 hours postingestion and is followed by anorexia, headache, chills, thirst, myalgias, and oliguria over the next week. Patients may present with renal failure between 3 and 17 days after *Cortinarius* ingestion. Consumption of *Cortinarius* mushrooms produces a severe interstitial nephritis, pronounced focal tubular damage, and early fibrosis between damaged tubules. Glomeruli are minimally involved. A few cases of poisoning involving hepatocellular damage have been reported after *C. orellanus* ingestion, but no liver damage has been demonstrated in *Cortinarius speciosissimus* poisoning cases.

Treatment

GUT DECONTAMINATION

Measures of decontamination (syrup of ipecac / lavage, charcoal, cathartics) may be useful within the first several hours of ingestion.

ELIMINATION ENHANCEMENT

The use of hemodialysis for supportive care markedly reduces fatalities. Clinical evidence supporting hemoperfusion remains anecdotal.

SUPPORTIVE MEASURES

- The mainstay of treatment is supportive care with careful management of fluid and electrolyte balance. Hospitalization may be prolonged because of slow return of kidney function.
- In more severe cases, irreversible renal disease occurs, requiring kidney transplantation.

Questions—Cortinarius (Group VIII)

1. ***Cortinarius* mushrooms are well known for producing**
   A. Hepatotoxicity
   B. Renal failure
   C. Pulmonary toxicity
   D. Hematologic toxicity
   E. Cardiotoxicity
2. **Although *Cortinarius* toxicity has not been reported in the United States, many representatives of this genus do appear in North America.**
   A. True
   B. False
3. **Major toxicity from *Cortinarius* mushrooms may occur within minutes in severe cases.**
   A. True
   B. False

MYCOTOXINS

INTRODUCTION

Mycotoxins are a by-product of mold (microscopic fungi) metabolism and produce toxic reactions known as mycotoxicoses upon inhalation or consumption by humans or animals. The toxic metabolites appear in mold after maximum growth is reached. Hence, the mycotoxicoses differ from the infectious fungal diseases called mycoses (e.g., blastomycosis, histoplasmosis, and coccidioidomycosis), that require fungal replication within a host to produce disease. Typically, disease occurs after consumption of contaminated food that no longer contains live mold.

Historically the first documented mycotoxicoses occurred in the Middle Ages during the epidemics of hallucinations, delirium, convulsions, and gangrene known as St. Anthony's Fire. By the 1850s, the ergot alkaloids of the fungus *Claviceps purpurea* were recognized as the causative toxin, and the disease was called ergotism.

Renewed interest in mycotoxicoses resulted from the isolation and identification of a mycotoxin called aflatoxin (*Aspergillus flavus* toxin) derived from the mold *Aspergillus flavus* in Ugandan peanuts. Consumption of these contaminated peanuts by turkeys and ducks caused hundreds of thousands of animal deaths in the early 1960s. Subsequently, aflatoxin B1 was described as the most potent naturally occurring carcinogen and considerable research interest in the role of mycotoxins in human health ensued.

Fungi are ubiquitous and can grow on almost any substrate. Five major mycotoxin groups occur in North America. Aflatoxin is common under warm humid conditions. Zearalenone is most commonly reported in the north central cornbelt. Trichothecene mycotoxins, especially deoxnivalenol, are common in cool damp regions. Ochratoxin is reported in the Carolinas and Canada, and ergot infects small grains such as barley, rye, and wheat in the northern Great Plains.

Pathophysiology

Fungi species that produce mycotoxins are mostly pathogens and plant decomposers. Cultivation and storage practices usually minimize unfavorable conditions but climatic stress (e.g., drought) may strain normal safety standards. Factors affecting mycotoxin production include species variation, presence of mycoviruses that induce toxin production, mechanical damage, geographic distribution of mycotoxin-producing fungi, and climatic conditions at both harvest and storage time.

HEPATIC EFFECTS

Aflatoxins are the best studied mycotoxins and are suspected of causing both acute hepatocellular disease and hepatocarcinoma. Other animal hepatotoxins include sporidesmin, ochratoxin, and rubratoxin.

RENAL EFFECTS

Both citrinin and ochratoxin A are nephrotoxic in pigs. High dietary ochratoxin A has been associated with areas where Balkan nephropathy is endemic. Acute renal failure after excessive beer consumption may result from a barley mycotoxin, perhaps on an antigenic basis.

CARDIOVASCULAR EFFECTS

A mycotoxin (citreoviridin) isolated from penicillin mold growing on yellow rice (*Penicillium citreo-viride*) has caused paralysis, convulsions, and cardiac failure in experimental animals. A similar disease known as cardiac beriberi was once common in the Orient. Available data are not sufficient to strongly support a definite link between this disease and citreoviridin.

DERMATOLOGIC EFFECTS

The trichothecene mycotoxins produce photosensitivity dermatitis along with hemorrhage and desquamation when applied to the skin of experimental animals. Similarly, butenolide and other photosensitizing furocoumarins occur in the pink rot fungus, *Sclerotinia sclerotinorium,* which appears in celery.

REPRODUCTIVE EFFECTS

Zearalenone is a naturally occurring, nonsteroidal, estrogenic product of the cereal fungus *Fusaria* that causes vulvar and uterine enlargement in animals. This toxin has not produced documented adverse effects in man.

RESPIRATORY EFFECTS

Aflatoxins appear to separate into particles smaller than 7 μm, so average dust samples may underestimate their presence. Both alveolar cell carcinoma and colon cancer have been reported in workers exposed to aflatoxin by inhalation.

Questions—Introduction to Mycotoxins

1. Mycotoxins are
A. Molds
B. Muscular poisons
C. A by-product of mold metabolism
D. Fungi
E. Poisons that destroy grain

ERGOTS AND DERIVATIVES

Ergots are molds with vasoconstrictive properties that have a fascinating and long history. Overdose produces two characteristic mycotoxic syndromes with well known constellations of symptoms. The mold *Claviceps purpurea* and related fungi mold invade rye ovaries and produce a purplish black mass called a sclerotium, which replaces kernels. Sclerotia are composed of densely packed mycelia and represent the mold's body. Sclerotia contain powerful ergot alkaloids that are ingested when the contaminated rye is consumed as bread. The term ergot applies both to the sclerotia produced by the *C. purpurea* mold and to the ergotamine alkaloids within it.

From the 9th to the 19th century, recurrent epidemics of ergotism highlighted European history. A "gangrenous" and a "convulsive" syndrome were recognized. The more widely recognized syndrome was the "gangrenous type" characterized by hypesthesia, paresthesias, and hemorrhagic bullae that progressed to dry gangrene and black mummification of involved body parts. The term "holy fire" or St. Anthony's Fire was given to this malady as numerous victims claimed that a pilgrimage to St. Anthony's Shrine relieved their symptoms. As the mold did not infect rye in the area of the shrine, spontaneous cures may actually have occurred.

Vertigo, headache, tinnitus, sensual disturbances, hallucinations, muscle spasms, GI upset, and convulsions characterized the "convulsive type" of ergotism. One ergot alkaloid, isoergine (lysergic acid amide) has one-tenth of the mind-altering potency of the structurally related compound LSD. Morning glory seeds contain the same alkaloid and were used by the Aztec Indians as a ceremonial hallucinogen. Geographical differences in alkaloid production and host susceptibility probably accounted for the variation in expression of these two syndromes.

Ergot was used as an herb by midwives long before its discovery as a uterine stimulant by Lonicer in 1582. Ergot was first mentioned in 1677 in the English literature as a cause of epidemics, but not until the middle 19th century was ergot recognized as a parasitic fungus. It has been theorized that ergotism may explain the physical afflictions and vivid imagery presented at the Salem Witchcraft Trials from 1691 to 1692.

In 1918, the active principle ergotamine was isolated from ergot. Medical uses have included the treatment of pruritus, diabetes, hyperthyroidism, and psychosis, but by the 1950s, administration was restricted to the treatment of migraine headaches and postpartum hemorrhage. Improved agricultural and storage practices have virtually eliminated epidemic ergotism, although sporadic episodes have occasionally occurred.

Current therapeutic uses of ergot alkaloids include vascular headache prophylaxis and treatment, uterine atonia, senile dementia, orthostatic circulatory disturbances, hyperprolactinemic infertility, and adjunctive treatment of Parkinsonism. Ergotamine tartrate is administered for the relief of migraine and related headaches. Combination tablets include ergotamine plus phenobarbital and belladonna alkaloids, and ergotamine plus caffeine (Cafergot®). Hydrogenated ergot alkaloids are used for symptoms of idiopathic decline in mental activity of the elderly. Hydergine is a mixture of dihydrogenated ergot alkaloids.

Ergonovine is used to treat postpartum hemorrhage and to assess coronary artery disease. Methysergide has been used for migraine treatment but the development of retroperitoneal fibrosis has limited its use. Methylergonovine (Methergine®) is used in the management of postpartum hemorrhage. Bromocriptine is used to manage amenorrhea, to suppress postpartum lactation, and as an adjunct in the treatment of Parkinson's disease. Bromocriptine has also been used to treat the neuroleptic malignant syndrome.

Pathophysiology

All ergot alkaloids are derivatives of the tetracyclic compound 6-methylergoline, which is a lysergic acid base structurally similar to biogenic amines such as dopamine, serotonin, and norepinephrine. The majority of the alkaloids can be divided into three groups based on side-chain substitution. Several pharmacologically active substances (e.g., tyrosine, tryptophan, tyramine, histamine, histidine, choline, and acetylcholine) have been isolated from sclerotia, but their clinical significance is questionable.

Ergot compounds act on several different receptors (e.g., noradrenaline, dopamine, serotonin) as both agonists and antagonists. Ergotamine is the prototype of the ergot alkaloid compounds producing peripheral vasoconstriction. Vasospasm results from both its central sympatholytic and its peripheral α-adrenergic effects mediated by α-adrenergic and serotonin agonism. Although both veins and arteries are affected, distal arteries most commonly are involved symmetrically. Focal neuropathies may result from constriction of nutrient vessels to peripheral nerves or from local arterial vasoconstriction.

Bromocriptine is a long-acting dopamine agonist that has central stimulating effects, which may exacerbate bipolar affective disorders. Bromocriptine is a synthetic brominated ergopeptide derivative with powerful dopaminergic agonist properties used to suppress postpartum lactation. Bromocriptine has moderate emetic activity and mild α-adrenergic-blocking properties in the animal model. See Chapter 37, Dopaminergic Drugs.

Pharmacokinetics

ABSORPTION

- Most ergot alkaloids, with the exception of bromocriptine, are incompletely absorbed.
- Oral therapeutic doses of ergotamine and dihydrogenated ergot alkaloids possess a highly variable bioavailability because of large, first-pass hepatic extractions.
- Caffeine increases the rate and completeness of intestinal absorption, perhaps by increasing the dissolution rate in the alkaline pH of the small intestine.
- Rectal administration produces higher but more delayed peak plasma levels reflecting a substantial first-pass effect. Intramuscular bioavailability also is incomplete and variable.

DISTRIBUTION

- Ergotamine is rapidly distributed in tissues and displays a 3-minute distribution half-life after parenteral administration. Ergotamine has an approximate volume of distribution of 2 L/kg.

ELIMINATION

- Ergot alkaloids are metabolized primarily by the liver. A significant first-pass extraction occurs and accounts for higher ergotamine plasma levels after rectal administration.
- Mean initial elimination half-lives range from 1.4 to 6.2 hours, with bromocriptine exhibiting the longest elimination phase.
- About 80% to 90% of an intravenous ergot alkaloid dose is excreted in the feces through the bile.
- Urinary excretion is small.

Clinical Presentations

The sporadic cases of ergotism seen today result from either an acute excessive ingestion, chronic consumption of therapeutic doses, or recent ingestion of small amounts of ergot drugs in hypersensitive individuals. Ergot alkaloid overdose is rare. Accidental parenteral administration of ergonovine to newborn infants produced cutaneous erythema and hemorrhagic buds on the extremities, groin, and genitalia. A neonate who received ergometrine developed respiratory depression and convulsions, which required endotracheal intubation. Cerebral edema, hemorrhagic gastritis, and peripheral cyanosis have occurred in a fatal case of Cafergot® ingestion.

Typically, symptoms including restlessness, agitation, lethargy, coma, nausea, vomiting, tachycardia, or hypotension present within 4 hours of ingestion. Manifestations of ischemia may be delayed and include cyanosis, cold extremities, paresthesias, and pain. Bromocriptine overdoses usually are mild, presenting with vomiting, mild hypotension, and diaphoresis.

Chronic ergotism may present with symmetrical, bilateral, peripheral vascular insufficiency affecting the lower more than the upper extremities. Ischemia may develop in a variety of vascular beds, leading to diffuse and variable symptoms. After discontinuation of ergotamine, the course of peripheral ischemia is variable. Improvement may begin within 24 hours but may be delayed for several days. Although peripheral pulses may reappear early, several weeks may be required for normalization of the distal circulation as seen on angiography.

Ergotamine has been associated with vascular insufficiency in the cerebral, mesenteric, renal, ophthalmic, and coronary arteries. Toxicity of chronic ergot alkaloid poisoning is highly individual and dependent on a number of variables. The presence of vascular disease and the sensitivity of individual vascular beds may affect susceptibility. Symptoms and signs of chronic toxicity may include intermittent claudication, cold extremities, pain, numbness, cyanosis, paresthesias, pallor, malaise, nausea, vomiting, abdominal pain, and edema. Seizures, coma, confusion, diarrhea, syncope, diplopia, blurred vision, psychosis, and bradycardia are uncommon but have been reported.

Untoward side effects of pharmacological doses of ergotamine are common. Nausea and vomiting are the most common complaints and appear to be dose related. Ergotamine directly stimulates the chemoreceptor trigger zone in the medulla oblongata. Other problems include headache, lightheadedness, peripheral vasoconstriction, malaise, spasms, and paresthesias.

Toxic Dosage/Death

The acute toxic dosage of ergots is not well established, in part because of marked individual susceptibility to the vasoconstrictive properties of ergotamine. A single ergotamine rectal suppository may produce paresthesias, weakness, difficulty in walking and painful muscle spasms. A 0.5-mg intramuscular ergotamine dose was associated with atrial fibrillation and precordial pain lasting 3 to 4 hours in a 36-year-old woman.

A reported 12-mg ergotamine ingestion in a 14-month-old child was fatal, whereas an approximately 15-mg ingestion in a 13-month-old child resulted in reversible hypotension and coma. Given such variability, all children who accidentally ingest ergotamine should be observed closely at least 24 hours. Ingestion of more than 1 mg/kg should be considered serious and direct medical observation is advised.

Drug Interactions

Propranolol may exacerbate the peripheral vasoconstricting properties of ergot alkaloids. Oral contraceptives and smoking may contribute to vasospasm. As bromocriptine is a potent dopamine agonist, its use represents a theoretical risk for adverse interactions with antipsychotics.

Pregnancy/Lactation

Bromocriptine is pregnancy risk category C. Ergotamine is pregnancy risk category D, as it possesses oxytocic properties.

Laboratory

ANALYTIC METHODS

Methods to detect or quantify ergots are not generally available in hospital settings.

BLOOD LEVELS

Adverse reactions are more likely to occur when ergotamine levels exceed 1.8 ng/mL, but generally ergotamine levels are not useful in managing toxic effects. Objective signs of a toxic reaction (e.g., peripheral ischemia) may be found despite the absence of detectable ergotamine levels. Clinical assessment is more reliable than measurement of ergotamine levels.

Treatment

GUT DECONTAMINATION

Activated charcoal should be administered within several hours of ingestion to those patients who do not spontaneously vomit and who ingest more than 0.5 mg of ergotamine per kilogram. Methysergide and bromocriptine are less toxic and decontamination measures are only necessary for ingestions exceeding 1.0 to 1.5 mg/kg.

ELIMINATION ENHANCEMENT

The large apparent volume of distribution and small blood levels of ergotamine suggest that hemodialysis, peritoneal dialysis, diuresis, and hemoperfusion probably would not be effective.

SUPPORTIVE MEASURES

- Signs of peripheral ischemia determine the need for angiography, which often helps exclude thrombosis and other causes of poor perfusion in questionable cases. Withdrawal of ergot alkaloids is mandatory. Reduction of precipitating factors such as hepatic and renal insufficiency, smoking, febrile illness, thyrotoxicosis, drugs such as oral contraceptives and beta-blocking agents, is potentially helpful.
- IV and intraarterial nitroprusside therapy has been used successfully to reverse severe vasospasm. The successful use of sympathetic blockade, surgical sympathectomy, low-molecular-weight dextrans, and anticoagulants has been highly variable.
- Low-dose heparin has been recommended in all cases of ergotamine vasospasm, even if arterial thrombosis is not suspected

on arteriogram. In less severe cases, oral vasodilators may be effective and provide the advantage of not requiring intravenous lines and constant blood pressure monitoring.

- Ergonovine-induced coronary vasospasm during assessment of angina pectoris has responded to sublingual or intravenous nitroglycerin. Intravenous nitroglycerin may also reverse peripheral ischemia without untoward effects.
- An ECG and cardiac monitoring are important adjuncts in managing ergot overdoses. Cardiac arrest secondary to ventricular dysrhythmias has been reported both in acute massive ergotamine / caffeine overdose and during therapeutic assessment of coronary artery disease. Advanced Cardiac Life Support (ACLS) criteria are used as management guidelines.
- Lab abnormalities in bromocriptine overdose may include mildly elevated creatine kinase and alkaline phosphatase levels, but their clinical significance is unclear.

Questions—Ergots and Derivatives

1. **Which of the following is false?**
   A. Ergots are molds with vasoconstrictive properties.
   B. The mold *Claviceps purpurea* and related fungi mold invade rye ovaries and produce a purplish black mass called a sclerotium, which replaces kernels.
   C. Sclerotia contain powerful ergot alkaloids that are ingested when the contaminated rye is consumed as bread.
   D. The term ergot applies both to the sclerotia produced by the *Claviceps purpurea* mold and to the ergotamine alkaloids within it.
   E. The term "holy fire" or St. Anthony's Fire was applied to patients during the Middle Ages because of the hyperpyrexia associated with its toxicity.
2. **The "convulsive type" of ergotism is associated with each of the following except**
   A. Vertigo
   B. Resolution of headache
   C. Tinnitus
   D. Hallucinations
   E. Seizures
3. **Improved agricultural and storage practices have eliminated ergotism around the world.**
   A. True
   B. False
4. **Current therapeutic uses of ergot alkaloids include each of the following except**
   A. Vascular headache prophylaxis
   B. Vascular headache treatment
   C. Hyperprolactinemic infertility
   D. Parkinsonism
   E. Uterine fibroids
5. **Which of the following is false?**
   A. Ergonovine is used to treat postpartum hemorrhage and to assess coronary artery disease.
   B. Methysergide has been used for migraine treatment but the development of fibrosis has limited its use.
   C. Methylergonovine (Methergine®) is used in the management of postpartum hemorrhage.
   D. Bromocriptine is used to manage amenorrhea, to enhance postpartum lactation, and as an adjunct in the treatment of Parkinson's disease.
   E. Bromocriptine has been used to treat the neuroleptic malignant syndrome.
6. **Symptoms of ergotism may include**
   A. Restlessness and agitation
   B. Coma
   C. Hypotension
   D. All of the above
   E. A and B
7. **Manifestations of ischemia as a result of ergotism may be delayed and may include**
   A. Purpura
   B. Hot extremities
   C. Paresthesias
   D. Exfoliative dermatitis
   E. None of the above
8. **Ergotamine has been associated with vascular insufficiency in the cerebral, mesenteric, renal, ophthalmic and coronary arteries.**
   A. True
   B. False
9. **Methysergide has been used for migraine treatment but the development of retroperitoneal fibrosis has limited its use.**
   A. True
   B. False

AFLATOXINS

Aflatoxins are metabolites of the ubiquitous *Aspergillus flavus* and *Aspergillus parasiticus* fungi. Between 20% and 98% of *A. flavus* strains produce aflatoxin. Foodstuffs most commonly contaminated by aflatoxins include peanuts, cottonseed, maize, Brazil nuts, and pistachios. Of the major grains used for human consumption in the United States (i.e., wheat, rye, oats, and corn), significant aflatoxin contamination appears only in corn. During 1977, as much as two thirds of the corn crops of some states were contaminated at harvest.

Aflatoxin has oncogenic and immunosuppressive effects that may influence the pattern of infection with the human immunodeficiency virus (HIV). Heroin may be contaminated with aflatoxin. Intravenous heroin users may inject aflatoxin B1 into their systemic circulation and suppress cell-mediated immunity.

Pathophysiology

Aflatoxins are unique among naturally occurring substances, as they are composed of highly substituted coumarin compounds that contain an unusual fused dihydrofurofuran configuration. The aflatoxins are divided into two major groups. Of the four major aflatoxins (B1, G1, B2, G2), B1 is the most potent and most common. Whenever they occur as food contaminants, aflatoxin B1 is always present. Aflatoxins are densely fluorescent. The B refers to blue, while the G signifies green fluorescence.

The acute hepatocellular necrosis seen in experimental animals probably results from a number of intracellular interactions, whereas the carcinogenic potential of aflatoxin probably depends on its metabolic activation to a DNA alkylating agent such as 2,3-epoxide. Aflatoxin B1 reduces hepatic glycogen stores and causes the accumulation of hepatic lipids in experimental animals. Changes in DNA equilibrium may cause permanent transcriptional changes.

Rather than act as a primary carcinogen, aflatoxin may suppress cell-mediated immunity and increase the number of hepatitis B virus carriers. This increased incidence of chronic infection may contribute to higher incidences of hepatocellular carcinomas in aflatoxin-exposed human populations, in contrast to animals in which active metabolites may play a more important role.

Pharmacokinetics

ABSORPTION

- Although few quantitative data on aflatoxin absorption exist, animal and human cases associated with aflatoxin to date involve ingestion.
- Chronic low-dose occupational exposure presumably by the pulmonary route has been associated with carcinoma of the lungs and colon, but the link is unsubstantiated.

DISTRIBUTION

- The half-life of aflatoxin B1 is 36 minutes and its volume of distribution is 14% of body weight.

ELIMINATION

- Almost all primary biotransformations of aflatoxin B1 occur in the liver via hydroxylation.
- The route of activation is to the reactive hydrophilic aflatoxin B1 2-3-epoxide. This may be the most important product from the carcinogenic point of view. This highly reactive substance can combine with DNA bases such as guanine to produce alterations in DNA.
- The metabolite aflatoxin M1 retains acute oral toxicity in contrast to other metabolites.

Clinical Presentations

A positive correlation between aflatoxin ingestion and human liver cancer has been observed in population studies in which the incidence of hepatocellular carcinoma has been correlated with aflatoxin intake. However, primary hepatocellular carcinoma is one of the most common cancers of developing countries where mycotoxins, hepatitis B virus, malnutrition, and parasitic infections frequently coexist, confounding epidemiological studies. Hepatic aflatoxin levels were detected in a majority of Indonesian patients with hepatocellular carcinoma in one series and were detected in an American hepatitis B virus carrier who developed hepatocellular cancer.

Kwashiorkor, a widespread and serious disorder of children in the tropics, may be associated with ingestion of aflatoxins by infants. Exposure to aflatoxins may begin prenatally, persist during breast-feeding, and continue into adult life. Aflatoxins may increase neonatal susceptibility to infection and jaundice, increase childhood susceptibility to infections and malignant disease, compromise normal response in prophylactic envenomations, and play a role in the pathogenesis of diseases in heroin addicts. Acute fatal aflatoxin poisoning may appear as "hepatitis"; however, the subject demands additional exploration.

Some have suggested that Reye's syndrome (acute encephalopathy with fatty degeneration of the viscera and particularly the liver) is associated with exposure to aflatoxin. Except for a few sporadic cases in which aflatoxins were identified in necropsy tissue or blood, most cases of aflatoxin-associated Reye's disease appear in Thailand and not in countries where aflatoxins commonly contaminate food. Acute hepatitis manifested by jaundice, ascites, portal hypertension and death secondary to massive GI bleeding was reported after heavy aflatoxin consumption in India and in Kenya.

Toxic Dosage/Death

Aflatoxin levels are regulated by the Food and Drug Administration (FDA), which recognizes that aflatoxins can develop both in the field and in storage. Aflatoxin cannot be totally eliminated from foodstuffs. Current guidelines limit aflatoxin levels to 20 ppb in all animal feed crops except cottonseed meal for which the limit was recently raised to 300 ppb.

Consumption of aflatoxin in many parts of the world varies from 0 to 30,000 ng/kg/day. In most areas, consumption varies from 10 to 200 ng/kg/day. Maize grain samples from two Kenyan homes where eight people died of hepatic failure revealed aflatoxin B1 levels of 12 and 3.2 ppm, while samples from unaffected homes had maximum levels of 0.5 ppm.

An outbreak of food poisoning, which resulted in 13 pediatric deaths, occurred in Malaysia during the Chinese festival of the Nine Emperor Gods in 1988. The food poisoning was attributable to aflatoxins and boric acid. Clinical features included an initial Reye-like syndrome with vomiting, fever, diarrhea, abdominal pain, seizures, and coma. Patients died in acute hepatic and renal failure.

Pregnancy/Lactation

Transplacental transfer of aflatoxin B1 may play a biologic role in the initiation of primary hepatocellular carcinoma in progeny. Aflatoxin may be secreted in breast milk.

Laboratory

ANALYTIC METHODS

Radioimmunoassays and the Enzyme Linked Immunosorbent Assay (ELISA) method are the most sensitive indices of exposure. High-performance liquid chromatography is also accurate.

BLOOD LEVELS

Levels of serum aflatoxin do not correlate with toxicity.

URINE

Aflatoxin-guanine adduct concentration may provide a marker for liver cancer risk.

Treatment

- Management is supportive together with reduction of exposure levels. Good cultivation and storage techniques represent the best method of reducing aflatoxin levels in food.
- Currently, the FDA samples suspected interstate food shipments (e.g., peanuts, corn, pecans, and walnuts) for aflatoxin levels.
- Aflatoxins are avidly adsorbed by activated charcoal under experimental conditions. Alkaline conditions also destroy mycotoxins.

Questions—Aflatoxins

1. Which of the following is false?

A. Aflatoxins are metabolites of ubiquitous *Aspergillus* fungi.
B. Heroin may be contaminated with aflatoxin.
C. Aflatoxins are divided into two major groups based on their fluorescence.
D. Aflatoxins are proven direct hepatic carcinogens.
E. Levels of serum aflatoxin do not correlate with toxicity.

2. **Foodstuffs commonly contaminated by aflatoxins include all of the following, except**
   A. Peas
   B. Peanuts
   C. Cottonseed
   D. Brazil nuts
   E. Pistachios
3. **Of the major grains used for human consumption in the United States, significant aflatoxin contamination appears in**
   A. Wheat
   B. Barley
   C. Oats
   D. Corn
   E. Rice
4. **Aflatoxin has been implicated as a causative factor in**
   A. Hepatocellular carcinoma
   B. Kwashiorkor
   C. Hepatitis
   D. Reye's syndrome
   E. All of the above

TRICHOTHECENES

The trichothecene mycotoxins constitute a group of more than 40 sesquiterpene compounds produced by a variety of widely distributed fungi. The name trichothecene derives from the mold *Trichothecium roseum* from which the mycotoxin trichothecene was isolated in 1948. The fungus genus *Fusarium* is the most important source of trichothecenes because of its prolific mycotoxin production and diverse worldwide habitat. Other genera involved in trichothecene mycotoxin production include *Cephalosporium, Gibberella, Myrothecium, Trichothecium,* and *Trichoderma.*

Four naturally occurring trichothecenes have been identified in agricultural products, including T-2 toxin, 4-deoxnivalenol (DON, vomitoxin), diacetoxyscirpenol (DAS, anguidine), and nivalenol. The mycotoxin T-2 toxin has been isolated from samples of a suspected outbreak of human alimentary toxic aleukia (ATA) and speculation persists that a trichothecene mycotoxin was responsible for numerous ATA fatalities that occurred in Russia during World War II.

The first well-described veterinary mycotoxicosis was the Russian horse disease called stachybotryotoxicosis, which was characterized by pancytopenia and mucosal ulcerations. The recognition by Nikita Khruschev of the need for clean, uncontaminated straw to prevent disease in transport horses was a key factor in his early rise to power, in part because of the importance of these horses to the pre-World War II Russian economy.

Pathophysiology

Trichothecenes are potent inhibitors of protein synthesis and are particularly active at the 80 S ribosomal subunit. Trichothecene mycotoxins are potent inhibitors of protein synthesis in eukaryotic cells and appear to block synthesis at the initiation, elongation, and termination phases.

Pharmacokinetics

ABSORPTION

- T-2 toxin is well absorbed orally.

DISTRIBUTION

- Rapid distribution to the liver is completed within 3 hours.
- Peak tissue levels occur by 1 to 4 hours, with the highest concentrations in the liver.

ELIMINATION

- About 50% of T-2 toxin are excreted presumably as metabolites in the feces within 24 hours.
- The elimination half-life is approximately 22 hours.

Clinical Presentations

There are no well-documented cases of clinical exposure of humans to trichothecenes. When administered chronically to animals, trichothecenes produce a variety of pathological responses including cutaneous inflammation and necrosis, mucous membrane lesions, GI inflammation and hemorrhage, petechiae, ecchymosis, granulocytopenia, and anemia. Carcinogenesis has not been linked to trichothecenes.

Although these mycotoxins have not been conclusively implicated in human disease, strong circumstantial evidence has associated trichothecenes with the fatal epidemics of alimentary toxic aleukia seen in Russia between 1931 and 1947. Clinically, signs and symptoms of trichothecene mycotoxicosis are similar to those of radiation toxicity. The most prominent manifestations include fever, nausea, vomiting, diarrhea, leukopenia, bleeding, and sepsis.

Recent concern about trichothecenes has centered on the alleged use of these mycotoxins in chemical warfare. The American government described the release of small yellow particles (termed yellow rain) from low-flying planes on rural civilian populations in Cambodia, Laos, and Afghanistan. Victims reported painful skin lesions, lightheadedness, dyspnea, and a rapid onset of hemorrhaging, incapacitation, and death in susceptible individuals.

Survivors allegedly developed a radiation-type sickness that was consistent with trichothecene toxicity. Data were consistent with mycotoxicosis, but an exact cause-effect relationship could not be established despite the fact that trichothecene toxins were found in the kidney, liver, and intestine of victims. Such findings are controversial, since the presence of mycotoxin may represent contamination from naturally occurring phenomena such as honeybee excretions.

Toxic Dosage/Death

Because toxicity has not been firmly established, toxic levels cannot be accurately determined.

Laboratory

ANALYTIC METHODS

Gas-liquid chromatography sensitivity for T-2 toxin is 0.03 to 0.05 ng/L (ppb) and gas chromatography-mass spectrometry is slightly more sensitive (0.02 ng/L).

BLOOD LEVELS

Blood levels of T-2 toxin have not been shown to correlate with clinical effects.

Treatment

- Because little is known about trichothecenes, treatment is entirely supportive.
- Sodium hypochlorite, common bleach, decomposes trichothecenes, but the toxicity of the breakdown products is unknown.

- Activated charcoal appears to be an effective antidote for treatment of T-2 toxicosis in mice.

Questions—Trichothecenes

1. The first well-described veterinary mycotoxicosis was the Russian horse disease called stachybotryotoxicosis, which was characterized by pancytopenia and mucosal ulcerations.
A. True
B. False

2. There are no well-documented cases of clinical exposure of humans to trichothecenes.
A. True
B. False

3. "Yellow Rain"
A. Is another name for acid rain
B. Refers to the release of small yellow particles from low-flying planes on rural civilian populations in Cambodia, Laos, and Afghanistan
C. May represent a form of chemical warfare using trichothecenes
D. Is a term used to describe a skin condition associated with trichothecenes
E. B and C

OTHER MYCOTOXINS

Butenolide

This compound is a photosensitizing furocoumarin that is produced in celery by the pink rot fungus *Sclerotinia sclerotinorium*. Celery harvesters frequently develop bullous photosensitivity dermatitis when this organism invades the celery crop.

Citrinin

This toxin was first isolated from *Penicillium citrinum* in 1931 and since that time has been identified in several species of *Penicillium* and *Aspergillus*. Renal damage in experimental rats is the most common pathological lesion caused by citrinin. Despite more than 30 years of clinical research, the role of citrinin as a human toxin or food contaminant remains unclear. Potentially, humans risk exposure through milk, eggs, and meat.

Mildewed Sugar Cane Poisoning

Mildewed sugar cane poisoning is an acute intoxication resulting from ingestion of mildewed sugar cane. It is characterized by toxic encephalopathy following initial GI symptoms and by a delayed dystonia in severe cases. There have been 217 outbreaks of acute mildewed sugar cane poisoning between 1972 and 1989 in China resulting in 884 patients and 88 deaths. Epidemiologic and experimental studies have found that 3-nitropropionic acid, a mycotoxin produced by *Arthrinium*-contaminated sugar canes, is the probable etiologic factor of the disease.

Initial symptoms are nausea, vomiting, abdominal pain without diarrhea, and anorexia that follows headache and dizziness. Coma and convulsions develop within 3 to 18 hours. Coma lasted 20 days in one case. Motor aphasia, inability of voluntary movement, and urinary and fecal incontinence have been reported. The focal cerebral impairments were reversible. Computerized tomography scans indicate bilateral lenticular lesions in the putamen and pallidum. Treatment is symptomatic and supportive.

Ochratoxins

Ochratoxin A was the first toxin isolated from *A. ochraceus*. Subsequently, a dozen other *Aspergillus* and *Penicillium* species were identified as ochratoxin producers. Ochratoxin contamination has been reported in Canada, Denmark, Poland, Sweden, Yugoslavia, and the United States. Ochratoxin A is the most abundant and toxic of the five metabolites in the ochratoxin group.

Experimentally, ochratoxins produce kidney damage when fed to ducklings, dogs, chickens, rats, mice, and trout. They have been implicated as a probable cause of porcine nephropathy in Denmark. Balkan endemic nephropathy in man is a chronic kidney disease of rural Bulgaria, Romania, and Yugoslavia. Striking pathological similarities between porcine nephropathy and Balkan endemic nephropathy suggest a common origin. Supportive circumstantial evidence for this link includes the frequent isolation of *Penicillium* species from food samples in endemic areas. However, no definite proof of such a relationship currently exists.

Rubratoxins

Penicillium rubrum and *Penicillium purpurogenum* produce rubratoxins. Rubratoxins cause liver, renal, and central nervous system damage in experimental animals. Their role in human disease is unclear since their actual existence in toxin-contaminated foodstuffs is unknown. Some authors believe that rubratoxins may act synergistically with other mycotoxins such as aflatoxins to produce animal diseases including moldy corn toxicosis.

Zearalenone

Zearalenone is a phenolic lactone derived from several *Fusarium* species. Low temperatures enhance production. Zearalenone is a natural contaminant of corn and occasionally appears in cereals and feeds depending on climatic conditions. This compound has been found at levels of 13 $\mu g/kg$ in cornflake samples. High levels (8 to 53 mg/kg) were reported to contaminate South African beer derived from corn and sorghum.

In several *Fusarium* species, zearalenone appears to control sexual development. Mammals and, in particular, swine are particularly sensitive to its estrogenic activity, displaying vulval, uterine, and breast enlargement as well as ovarian atrophy, vaginal prolapse, and infertility at feed levels of 1 mg/kg. There have been no reports of adverse effects in man.

Questions—Other Mycotoxins

1. Which association is not correct?
A. Butenolide—Bullous photosensitivity dermatitis in celery handlers
B. Mildewed sugar cane poisoning—3-nitropropionic acid
C. Ochratoxins—Thrombocytopenic purpura seen in Africa
D. Rubratoxins—Penicillium products
E. Zearalenone—Uterine and breast enlargement in swine

Answers

Aconitum

1. C 2. E

Baneberry

1. A

Bracken

1. A

Buckeye

1. A

Buckthorn

1. A

Bulbs

1. A

Colchicine

1. E 2. A

Cycads

1. A

Daphne

1. B

Dog's Mercury

1. A

Foxglove

1. D

Goldenseal

1. B

Jimsonweed and Anticholinergic Plants

1. D 2. E

Laburnum

1. C

Lantana

1. B

Lily of the Valley

1. B

Nicotine and Lobeline

1. A 2. B

Oleander

1. B 2. B 3. A

Podophyllum

1. C 2. A

Poison Hemlock

1. C 2. A

Pokeweed

1. E 2. A

Rhododendron

1. D 2. C 3. B

Snakeroot

1. C

Snowberry

1. A

Sweet Pea and Lathyrism

1. B

Veratrum

1. A 2. A

Water Hemlock

1. D 2. E 3. A

Wisteria

1. B

Yew

1. B 2. A 3. A

Introduction to Mushrooms

1. B 2. A 3. E

Cyclopeptides (Group I)

1. C 2. E 3. B 4. C 5. E 6. B

Gyromitrin (Group II)

1. A 2. A 3. D 4. A

Muscarine (Group III)

1. B 2. E

Coprine (Group IV)

1. E 2. A

Ibotenic Acid and Muscimol (Group V)

1. A 2. A

Hallucinogenic Mushrooms (Group VI)

1. D 2. A 3. E

Gastroenteritis-Producing Mushrooms (Group VII)

1. A 2. B

Cortinarius (Group VIII)

1. B 2. A 3. B

Introduction to Mycotoxins

1. C

Ergots and Derivatives

1. E 2. B 3. B 4. E 5. D 6. D 7. C
8. A 9. A

Aflatoxins

1. D 2. A 3. D 4. E

Trichothecenes

1. A 2. A 3. E

Other Mycotoxins

1. C

SELECTED READINGS

Aconitum

1. Bissett NG. Arrow poisons in China: Part II. Aconitum—botany, chemistry and pharmacology. J Ethnopharmacol 1981;4:247–336.
2. Saito H, Veyama T, Naka N, et al: Pharmacological studies of ignavine, an Aconitum alkaloid. Chem Pharm Bull 1982;30:1844–1850.

Baneberry

1. Bacon AE. An experiment with the fruit of red baneberry. Rhodora 1903;5:77–79.

Bracken

1. Spoerke D, Evans B, Linaburg B. The hidden hazards in house and garden plants. Missoula, MT: Pictorial Histories, 1991, p. 142.
2. Trotter WR. Is bracken a health hazard? Lancet 1990;336:1563–1564.

Buckthorn

1. Calderon-Gonzalez R, Rizzi-Hernandez H. Buckthorn polyneuropathy. N Engl J Med 1967;277:69–71.

Bulbs

1. Litovitz TL, Fahey BA. Please don't eat the daffodils. N Engl J Med 1982;306:547.
2. O'Leary SB. Poisoning in man from eating poisonous plants. Arch Environ Health 1964;9:216–242.
3. Spoerke DG, Spoerke SE. Three cases of Zygandenus (death camas) poisoning. Vet Hum Toxicol 1979;21:346–347.

Colchicine

1. Boehnort M, McGuigan MA. Colchicine. Clin Toxicol Rev 1983;5(12):1.
2. Murray SS, Kramlinger KG, McMichan JC, et al. Acute toxicity after excessive ingestion of colchicine. Mayo Clin Proc 1983;58:528–532.
3. Stapczynski JS, Rothstein RJ, Gaye WA, et al. Colchicine overdose: Report of two cases and review of the literature. Ann Emerg Med 1981;10:364–368.

Cycads

1. Editorial. A poison tree. Lancet 1987;2:947–948.

Daphne

1. Kupchan SM, Baxter RL. Mezerein: Antileukemic principles isolated from Daphne mezereum. Science 1975;187:652–653.

Dog's Mercury

1. Rugman F, Melchan J, Edmondson J. Mercurialis perennis (dog's mercury) poisoning. A case of mistaken identity. Br Med J 1983;287:1924.

Foxglove

1. McGuigan MA. Plants—Cardiac glycosides. Clin Toxicol Rev 1984;6(8):1–2.

Goldenseal

1. Dombek C, ed. Lawrence review of natural products. St. Louis: Facts and Comparisons, May 1994.

Jimsonweed and Anticholinergic Plants

1. Brown JK, Malone MH. "Legal highs"—Constituents, activity, toxicology, and herbal folk lore. Clin Toxicol 1978;12:1–31.
2. CDC. Jimson weed poisoning Texas, New York and California, 1994. MMWR 1995;44:41–44.
3. Gowdy JM. Stramonium intoxication: A review of symptomatology in 212 cases. JAMA 1972;221:585–587.

Laburnum

1. Bramley A, Goulding R. Laburnum "poisoning". Br Med J 1981;283:1220–1221.
2. Dale HH, Laidlow PP. The physiological action of cytisine, the active alkaloid of laburnum (Cytisus laburnum). J Pharmacol Exp Ther 1912;3:205–221.
3. Mitchell RG. Laburnum poisoning in children. Report of 10 cases. Lancet 1951;2:57–58.

Lantana

1. Sharma OP. Review of the biochemical effects of Lantana camara toxicity. Vet Hum Toxicol 1984;26:488–493.

Nicotine and Lobeline

1. Lavoie FW, Harris TM. Fatal nicotine ingestion. J Emerg Med 1991;9:133–136.
2. Lockhart LP. Nicotine poisoning. Br Med J 1933;1:246–247.
3. McGee D, Brabson T, McCarthy J, Picciotti M. Four-year review of cigarette ingestions in children. Pediatr Emerg Care 1995;11:13–16.
4. McGuigan MA. Nicotine. Clin Toxicol Rev 1982;4(6):1–2.

Oleander

1. Krenzelok, EP. Plantlore Debunked. Clin Tox 1999;37(4):53–24.
2. Radford DJ, Gilles AD, Hinds JA, et al. Naturally occurring cardiac glycosides. Med J Aust 1986;144:540–544.
3. Safadi R, Ley I, Amitai Y, Caraco Y. Beneficial effect of digoxin-specific Fab antibody fragments in oleander intoxication. Arch Intern Med 1995;155:2121–2125.

Podophyllum

1. Balucani M, Zellers PD. Podophyllum resin poisoning with complete recovery. JAMA 1964;189:639.
2. Cassidy DE, Drewry J, Fanning JP. Podophyllum toxicity: A report of a fatal case and a review of the literature. J Toxicol Clin Toxicol 1982;19:35–44.
3. Rate RG, Leche J, Chervenak C. Podophyllin toxicity. Ann Intern Med 1979;90:723.

Poison Hemlock

1. Keeler RF, Balls LD. Teratogenic effects in cattle of Conium maculatum and Conium alkaloids and analogs. Clin Toxicol 1978;12:49–64.
2. Ober WB. Did Socrates die of hemlock poisoning? NY State J Med 1977; 77:254–258.

Pokeweed

1. Jaeckle KA, Freeman FR. Pokeweed poisoning. South Med J 1981;5:639–640.
2. Lewis WH, Smith PR. Pokeroot herbal tea poisoning. JAMA 1979;242:2759–2760.

Rhododendron

1. Gossinger H, Hruby K, Haubenstock A. Cardiac arrhythmias in a patient with grayanotoxin-honey poisoning. Vet Hum Toxicol 1983;25:328–329.
2. Klein-Schwartz W, Litovitz T. Azalea toxicity. An overrated problem. Clin Toxicol 1985;23:91–101.
3. Leach DG. The history of rhododendron poisoning. Garden J 1967;17:15–18.
4. Yavuz H, Ozel A, Akkus I, Erkul I. Honey poisoning in Turkey. Lancet 1991;337:789–790.

Snakeroot

1. Jordan EO, Harris MN. Milk sickness. J Infect Dis 1909;6:401–505.

Snowberry

1. Lewis WH. Snowberry (Symphoricarpos) poisoning in children. JAMA 1979; 242:2663.

Sweet Pea and Lathyrism

1. Paissios CS, Demopoulos T. Human lathyrism: A clinical and skeletal study. Clin Orthop 1982;23:236–249.
2. Weaver AL, Spittell JA. Lathyrism. Mayo Clin Proc 1964;39:485–489.

Veratrum

1. Carlier P, Efthymiou ML, Garnier R, et al. Poisoning with Veratrum containing sneezing powder. Hum Toxicol 1983;2:321–325.
2. Nelson DA. Accidental poisoning by Veratrum japonicum. JAMA 1954; 156:33–35.

Water Hemlock

1. Costanza DJ, Hoversten VW. Accidental ingestion of water hemlock. Report of two patients with acute and chronic effects. Calif Med (West J Med) 1973;119(2):78–82.
2. Knutsen OH, Paszkowski P. New aspects in the treatment of water hemlock poisoning. Clin Toxicol 1984;22:157–166.
3. Miller MM. Water hemlock poisoning. JAMA 1933;101:852–853.

Wisteria

1. Rondeau ES. Wisteria toxicity. Clin Toxicol 1993;31:107–112.

Yew

1. Burke MJ, Siegel D, Davidow B. Anaphylaxis. Consequence of yew (Taxus) needle ingestion. NY J Med 1979;79:1576–1577.
2. Porter KAM, Kroll S. Yewberry ingestion. Br Med J 1982;284:116.
3. Thompson J. Poisoning by yew berry. Lancet 1868;95:530.

Mushrooms

1. Lincoff G, Mitchel DH. Toxic and hallucinogenic mushroom poisoning. A handbook for physicians and mushroom hunters. New York: Van Nostrand Reinhold, 1977; pp. 156–157.
2. Trestrail JH. Mushroom poisoning in the United States. An analysis of 1989 United States Poison Center data. Clin Toxicol 1991;29:459–465.

Ergots and Derivatives

1. Caporael LR. Ergotism: The satan loosed in Salem? Science 1976;192:21–26.
2. Fuller JG. *The Day of St. Anthony's Fire.* New York, MacMillan Co, 1968.
3. Glazer G, Myers KA, Davids ER. Ergot poisoning. Postgrad Med J 1966; 42:562–568.
4. Merhoff GC, Porter JM. Ergot intoxication: Historical review and description of unusual clinical manifestations. Ann Surg 1974;180:773–779.
5. Warren DE, Nakfoor E. Acute overdose of bromocriptine. Drug Intell Clin Pharm 1983;17:394.

Mycotoxins

1. Arstwick PKC. Mycotoxins. Br Med Bull 1975;31:222–229.
2. Denning D. Aflatoxin and human disease. Adverse Drug React Acute Pois Rev 1987;4:175–209.
3. Forgacs J. Mycotoxicoses: The neglected diseases. Feedstuffs 1962;34:124–134.

ACKNOWLEDGMENT

Thanks to Alison Deutsch, MD for contributing questions in this chapter.

Index